Contemporary Medical Imaging

Series Editor
U. Joseph Schoepf

More information about this series at:
http://www.springer.com/series/7687

U. Joseph Schoepf
Editor

CT of the Heart

Second Edition

Humana Press

Editor
U. Joseph Schoepf
Department of Radiology
Center for Advanced Imaging Research (CAIR)
Medical University of South Carolina
Charleston, SC
USA

Originally published in the series: Contemporary Cardiology
Contemporary Medical Imaging
ISBN 978-1-60327-236-0 ISBN 978-1-60327-237-7 (eBook)
https://doi.org/10.1007/978-1-60327-237-7

Library of Congress Control Number: 2018966541

This Humana Press imprint is published by the registered company Springer Science+Business Media, LLC part of Springer Nature
The registered company address is: 233 Spring Street, New York, NY 10013, U.S.A.

This book is dedicated to my mother Ursula Schoepf and my late father, Josef Schoepf.

Foreword to the First Edition

Radiologic technology has made dramatic advances in the last 25 years, and none have been more impressive than those in computed tomography (CT). The progress in the speed of obtaining images, computing, postprocessing, and spatial resolution has been incredible. The result is that CT has moved from displaying purely morphologic information to providing valuable physiologic data as well. Whether with electron beam or multidetector-row CT, advances are impressive and nowhere have the applications been more useful and dramatic than in the heart.

This multiauthored book, *CT of the Heart*, edited by U. Joseph Schoepf, MD, is a splendid rendition of the state-of-the-art in CT imaging of the heart; however, where appropriate, it also features comparisons with other technical approaches, such as magnetic resonance and ultrasound. The contributors are leading radiologists, cardiologists, physicists, engineers, and basic and clinical scientists from Europe, the United States, Israel, and Japan.

The entire contents are meticulous and comprehensive, from the introduction about the past, present, and future of CT of the heart, through the technical underpinning of the method and the various clinical, physiologic, and pathologic applications of CT in studying the heart.

This book fills an immense need, particularly at a time when cardiac screening with CT, whether one agrees with this practice or not, is a reality. Furthermore, with the rapid increase of aging populations in the industrialized world, noninvasive diagnostic approaches are increasingly needed. As technology continues to advance and applications of CT to heart studies expand, it is my hope that the editor will bring this book up to date with a new edition.

Alexander R. Margulis, MD, DSc (HON)
Clinical Professor of Radiology
Weill Medical College of Cornell University,
New York, NY, USA

Foreword

CT imaging of the heart and coronary vessels has emerged over the past two decades as one of the most important and dynamic advances in medicine. Heart disease is the leading cause of death in the United States and worldwide, challenging health systems and health providers on how best to diagnose and manage their patients. CT imaging helps address these questions through the remarkable and important information it provides about both cardiovascular anatomy and function.

The first edition of *CT of the Heart: Principles and Applications* edited by U. Joseph Schoepf was excellent. The book was very well received and widely used. Dr. Schoepf chose a multiauthor format that allowed him to invite key leaders in each aspect of the subject to contribute their special knowledge—physicists, engineers, radiologists, cardiologists, and others. Their presentations were outstanding—richly illustrated and put in appropriate context with other methods.

The second edition of *CT of the Heart* promises to build on the excellence of the first edition by maintaining the strategy of selecting the most expert people as authors. To this end, Dr. Schoepf has maintained the multiauthor format in the second edition, now inviting over 170 people from around the globe as contributors. The authorship list is a true "Who's Who" of people working in the field.

Two things happen over time that make new editions of even the most classic medical texts vital and important. These are implicit in the subtitle of the first edition of *CT of the Heart* and are advancements in the science and technology underlying the subject and advancements in the accumulated knowledge about the role and efficacy of clinical applications. In the decade between editions, it is fair to say that the pace of technology development has steadily increased and that new applications have been added to clinical practice. Dr. Schoepf and his coauthors address these important advances in the second edition. The discussion of each topic is designed to bring it up to date, and several new chapters have been added to cover new areas of technology development and clinical application. As in the first edition, the discussions are meticulous and comprehensive.

Another feature of *CT of the Heart* that will be useful to readers is the separation of chapters into categories of "Where We Were," "Where We Are," and "Where We Are Going." Too often in textbooks, there is not a clear separation of material covering topics recognized as well established versus emerging topics that are important in comprehensive understanding of a subject but not yet in routine clinical use. The 14 chapters in the section on "Where We Are Going" bespeak the dynamic advances being made in CT imaging. Topics in this section include new approaches to anatomic and functional applications such as new approaches to myocardial perfusion imaging but also the potential roles of radiomics, big data, and machine learning.

CT of the Heart will be invaluable for students and trainees seeking to learn the subject as well as established physicians looking for definitive reference information or for ideas about how to continue to advance their practices. Since the second edition has the same attributes that made the first edition a trusted resource, it will soon be regarded in the same way. Dr. Schoepf and his coauthors are to be congratulated for producing such a high-quality and timely text.

James H. Thrall, MD
Chairman Emeritus, Department of Radiology
Massachusetts General Hospital
Boston, MA, USA

Distinguished Taveras Professor of Radiology
Harvard Medical School
Boston, MA, USA

Preface

Ποταμοῖσι τοῖσιν αὐτοῖσιν ἐμβαίνουσιν, ἕτερα καὶ ἕτερα ὕδατα ἐπιρρεῖ... – Herakleitos

More than a decade has passed since the publication of the first edition of *CT of the Heart*. And what a ride it's been since then! From the perch of today's technology, with lightning-fast acquisition speeds and temporal resolution, massive tube power, yet gentle techniques, the evolution could not have been more dramatic. Back then we were mostly still living in the dark ages of 16-slice multidetector-row CT technology, with 64-slice CT faintly on the horizon.

While we have been experiencing the evolution of cardiac CT as a continuum, for many the introduction of 64-slice CT technology constitutes the pivotal breaking point in history, whence the clinical use of cardiac CT became more broadly established for the first time. In the subsequent years, we all expected a revolution, a wildfire to happen, with cardiac CT ensconcing itself rapidly, profoundly, and irrevocably in all arenas of cardiovascular medicine. It did not happen quite as fast as many had betted on, causing a degree of disillusionment in some quarters. After all, it may not be a bad thing that not every latest flash in the pan gets embraced by mainstream medicine overnight.

But then something quite rare and precious happened; the field of believers in this technology came together and, in a manner unprecedented in medical imaging, piece by piece built the evidence that incrementally drove this test to new heights and today forms the foundation for the ever-growing importance of cardiac CT. In fact, we submit that cardiac CT may be considered a beacon, a blueprint, and prime example of how the value of a medical test can be unequivocally proven and supported via the generation of high-level evidence, a formidable challenge that the field of medical imaging has mostly unsuccessfully grappled with to date. This is what this book is about; while in the first edition we mainly investigated a fascinating new instrument looking for an application, we now have a vast realm of guideline-driven, robust, and beneficial clinical applications that are enabled by an enormous and ever-growing field of technology. Accordingly, the focus has shifted from a technology-centric to a more patient-centric appraisal. While the specifications and capabilities of the CT system itself remain front and center as the basis for diagnostic success, much of the benefit derived from cardiac CT today comes from avant-garde technologies enabling enhanced visualization, quantitative imaging, and functional assessment, along with exciting deep learning, and artificial intelligence applications. Long have we passed the stage of a mere tool for noninvasive coronary artery stenosis detection in the chest pain diagnostic algorithms; cardiac CT has proven its value for uses as diverse as personalized cardiovascular risk stratification, prediction, and management, diagnosing lesion-specific ischemia, guiding minimally invasive structural heart disease therapy, and planning cardiovascular surgery, among many others.

In the Preface to the first edition of *CT of the Heart*, we stated that we do not claim to have all the answers. That is still the case; but we have vastly more answers and enough to know that cardiac CT is here to stay and bound to occupy the space that we originally envisioned. In some more regulated and resource-conscious economies, we already see cardiac CT positioned as the entrance test and gatekeeper to any type of chest pain work-up, invasive or not. However, also in less progressive, more entrenched, and conflicted healthcare systems around the globe, this test is now quickly gaining ground and will even more so with newer generations of healthcare providers who are less enamored with outdated testing strategies of the past.

Like the first edition, the second edition of *CT of the Heart* is again a snapshot of the *status quo*, of the current state-of-the-art, and of a success story in the care for our patients which still keeps rapidly evolving. Yet, we have a much clearer view now of what we have accomplished, where we are, and where we are going.

While the first edition was the work of many, the second edition is the result of the work of even more. An astounding array of the great houses in cardiac imaging, giants in the field, came together to present our readers with the most comprehensive, coherent, up-to-date, and in-depth review of cardiac CT principles and applications. We are grateful beyond limits to this exalted, respected group of experts who poured their genius into this tome. Finally, this work would not have come to fruition without the invaluable help of Taylor M. Duguay and Dante Giovagnoli in our lab and Margaret Burns of Springer, who so skillfully and deftly steered the production of this second edition. We hope that this work will inspire and guide current and future leaders in healthcare in their quest to optimally harness the powers of a disruptive, amazing technology, to the benefit of our patients worldwide.

Charleston, SC, USA U. Joseph Schoepf

Contents

Contributors

Suhny Abbara, MD, FACR, FSCCT Department of Radiology, Cardiothoracic Imaging Division, UT Southwestern Medical Center, Dallas, TX, USA

Moritz H. Albrecht, MD Department of Diagnostic and Interventional Radiology, University Hospital Frankfurt, Frankfurt am Main, Germany

Hatem Alkadhi, MD, MPH, EBCR Institute of Diagnostic and Interventional Radiology, University Hospital Zurich, Zurich, Switzerland

Thomas Allmendinger, PhD Department of Computed Tomography, Siemens Healthcare GmbH, Forchheim, Germany

Amadeus Altenburger, Dr. med Department of Diagnostic and Interventional Radiology and Neuroradiology, Klinikum Augsburg, Augsburg, Germany

Kweku Appau, MD Department of Cardiology, Emory University School of Medicine, Atlanta, GA, USA

Christoph Artzner, MD Department of Radiology, Duke University Medical Center, Durham, NC, USA

Department of Diagnostic and Interventional Radiology, University of Tuebingen, Tubingen, Germany

Anil Attili, MD Department of Radiology, Division of Cardiothoracic Radiology, University of Michigan, Ann Arbor, MI, USA

Adefolakemi Babatunde, MD Cardiovascular Division, Department of Medicine, Washington University School of Medicine, St. Louis, MO, USA

Fabian Bamberg, MD, MPH Department of Diagnostic and Interventional Radiology, University of Tuebingen, Tubingen, Germany

Gorka Bastarrika, MD, PhD, EBCR Cardiothoracic Imaging Division, Department of Radiology, Clínica Universidad de Navarra, Pamplona, Spain

Richard R. Bayer II, MD Division of Cardiovascular Imaging, Department of Radiology and Radiological Science, Medical University of South Carolina, Charleston, SC, USA

Division of Cardiology, Department of Medicine, Medical University of South Carolina, Charleston, SC, USA

Raveen Bazaaz, MD Heart and Vascular Institute, University of Pittsburgh Medical Center, Pittsburgh, PA, USA

Hans-Christoph R. F. Becker, MD Department of Radiology, Stanford University, Stanford, CA, USA

Daniel Berman, MD Department of Imaging and Medicine and the Burns Allen Research Institute, Cedars-Sinai Medical Center, Los Angeles, CA, USA

Philipp Blanke, MD Department of Radiology, University of British Columbia, Vancouver, BC, Canada

Daniel T. Boll, MD Department of Radiology, University of Basel, Basel, Switzerland

Marques L. Bradshaw, MD Department of Radiology and Radiological Sciences, Vanderbilt University School of Medicine, Nashville, TN, USA

Herbert Bruder, PhD Department of Computed Tomography, Siemens Healthcare GmbH, Forchheim, Germany

Patricia Carrascosa, MD, PhD Department of Cardiovascular Imaging, Diagnóstico Maipú, Buenos Aires, Argentina

Damiano Caruso, MD Department of Radiological Sciences, Oncological and Pathological Sciences, University of Rome "Sapienza", Latina, Italy

Csilla Celeng, MD Department of Radiology, Heart and Vascular Center, Semmelweis University, Budapest, Hungary

Siyu Chen, BS Department of Radiologic Imaging, Fuwai Hospital, Chinese Academy of Medical Sciences and Peking Union Medical College, National Center of Cardiovascular Diseases, Beijing, China

Yundai Chen, MD, PhD Division of Cardiovascular Imaging, Department of Radiology and Radiological Science, Medical University of South Carolina, Charleston, SC, USA

Department of Cardiology, People's Liberation Army General Hospital, Beijing, China

Leonid Chepelev, MD, PhD Department of Radiology, University of Ottawa Faculty of Medicine, Ottawa, ON, Canada

Ottawa Hospital Research Institute, Ottawa, ON, Canada

Salvatore A. Chiaramida, MD Division of Cardiology, Department of Medicine, Medical University of South Carolina, Charleston, SC, USA

Yeon Hyeon Choe, MD, PhD Department of Radiology, HVSI Imaging Center, Heart Vascular Stroke Institute, Samsung Medical Center, Sungkyunkwan University School of Medicine, Seoul, South Korea

Byoung Wook Choi, MD, PhD Department of Radiology, Yonsei University School of Medicine, Severance Hospital, Seoul, South Korea

Jin-Ho Choi, MD Division of Cardiology, Department of Medicine (J-H C), Samsung Medical Center, Sungkyunkwan University School of Medicine, Seoul, South Korea

Shahryar M. Chowdhury, MD, MSCR Division of Pediatric Cardiology, Department of Pediatrics, Medical University of South Carolina, Charleston, SC, USA

Adriaan Coenen, MD Departments of Radiology and Cardiology, Erasmus University Medical Center, Rotterdam, The Netherlands

Andrew Crean, BSc, BM, MRCP, MSc, FRCR, MPhil Department of Cardiology, Ottawa Heart Institute, University of Ottawa, Ottawa, ON, Canada

Marco Das, MD, PhD Department of Radiology and Nuclear Medicine, Maastricht University Medical Center, Maastricht, The Netherlands

CARIM School for Cardiovascular Diseases, Maastricht University Medical Center, Maastricht, The Netherlands

Carlo N. De Cecco, MD, PhD Department of Radiology and Radiological Science, Medical University of South Carolina, Charleston, SC, USA

Domenico De Santis, MD Department of Radiological Sciences, Oncological and Pathological Sciences, University of Rome "Sapienza", Latina, Italy

Division of Cardiovascular Imaging, Department of Radiology and Radiological Science, Medical University of South Carolina, Charleston, SC, USA

Annemarie M. den Harder, MD, PhD Department of Radiology, University Medical Center Utrecht, Utrecht, The Netherlands

Karin E. Dill, MD Department of Radiology, UMass Medical Center, Worcester, MA, USA

Ian R. Drexler, MD, MBA Department of Radiology, Weill Cornell Medicine, New York, NY, USA

Taylor M. Duguay, BS Division of Cardiovascular Imaging, Department of Radiology and Radiological Science, Medical University of South Carolina, Charleston, SC, USA

Ullrich Ebersberger, MD Department of Cardiology and Intensive Care Medicine, Heart Center Munich-Bogenhausen, Munich, Germany

Division of Cardiovascular Imaging, Department of Radiology and Radiological Science, Medical University of South Carolina, Charleston, SC, USA

Heidi A. Edmonson, PhD Department of Radiology, Mayo Clinic, Rochester, MN, USA

Marwen Eid, MD Division of Cardiovascular Imaging, Department of Radiology and Radiological Science, Medical University of South Carolina, Charleston, SC, USA

Ahmed Hamdy, MD Department of Radiology, Mie University Hospital, Tsu, Japan

Christian D. Eusemann, PhD Department of Collaborations, Siemens Medical Solutions USA, Inc., Malvern, PA, USA

Lloyd M. Felmly, MD Department of Surgery, Division of Cardiothoracic Surgery, Medical University of South Carolina, Charleston, SC, USA

Gudrun M. Feuchtner, MD Department of Radiology, Innsbruck Medical University, Innsbruck, Austria

Aloke V. Finn, MD CVPath Institute, University of Maryland, Gaithersburg, MD, USA

Thomas G. Flohr, PhD Department of Computed Tomography, Siemens Healthcare GmbH, Forchheim, Germany

Kunihiko Fukuda, MD Department of Radiology, The Jikei University School of Medicine, Tokyo, Japan

Michael Gebhard, MD Department of Diagnostic and Interventional Radiology and Neuroradiology, Klinikum Augsburg, Augsburg, Germany

Lucas L. Geyer, MD Division of Cardiovascular Imaging, Department of Radiology and Radiological Science, Medical University of South Carolina, Charleston, SC, USA

Institute for Clinical Radiology, Ludwig-Maximilians-University Hospital Munich, Munich, Germany

Brian B. Ghoshhajra, MD, MBA Division of Cardiovascular Imaging, Department of Radiology, Massachusetts General Hospital/Harvard Medical School, Boston, MA, USA

Cardiac MR PET CT Program, Massachusetts General Hospital, Boston, MA, USA

Frank Gijsen, PhD Department of Biomedical Engineering, Erasmus University Medical Center, Rotterdam, The Netherlands

Harold Goerne, MD Department of Radiology, Cardiothoracic Imaging, UT Southwestern Medical Center, Dallas, TX, USA

Orly Goitein, MD Department of Diagnostic Imaging, Chaim Sheba Medical Center, Ramat Gan, Israel

Katharine Grant, PhD Siemens Medical Solutions USA, Inc., Malvern, PA, USA

Daniel B. Green, MD Department of Radiology, Weill Cornell Medicine, New York, NY, USA

David Gregg, MD Division of Cardiology, Department of Medicine, Medical University of South Carolina, Charleston, SC, USA

B. Kelly Han, MD Department of Advanced Congenital Cardiac Imaging, Minneapolis Heart Institute and the Children's Hospitals and Clinics of Minnesota, Minneapolis, MN, USA

Thomas Henzler, MD Institute of Clinical Radiology and Nuclear Medicine, University Medical Center Mannheim, Medical Faculty Mannheim, Heidelberg University, Heidelberg, Germany

Anthony M. Hlavacek, MD Department of Pediatrics, Division of Pediatric Cardiology, Medical University of South Carolina, Charleston, SC, USA

Udo Hoffmann, MD Department of Cardiovascular Imaging, Massachusetts General Hospital, Boston, MA, USA

Jin Hur, MD, PhD Department of Radiology, Yonsei University School of Medicine, Severance Hospital, Seoul, South Korea

Lynne M. Hurwitz, MD Department of Radiology, Duke University Medical Center, Durham, NC, USA

Gregory Jackson, MD Department of Cardiology, Medical University of South Carolina, Charleston, SC, USA

Brian Jacobs, BS Department of Radiology and Radiological Science, Medical University of South Carolina, Charleston, SC, USA

Michael A. Kadoch, MD Department of Radiology, University of California, Davis, CA, USA

Steffen Kappler, Dr. rer. Nat Department of Computed Tomography, Siemens Healthcare GmbH, Forchheim, Germany

Ella A. Kazerooni, MD, MS, FACR Department of Radiology, Division of Cardiothoracic Radiology, University of Michigan, Ann Arbor, MI, USA

Sung Mok Kim, MD Department of Radiology, HVSI Imaging Center, Heart Vascular Stroke Institute, Seoul, South Korea

Kakuya Kitagawa, MD, PhD Department of Radiology, Mie University Hospital, Tsu, Japan

Friedrich Knollmann, MD, PhD Department of Radiology, UCDavis Health, Sacramento, CA, USA

Brian S. Ko, MBBS (Hons), PhD Department of Medicine Monash Medical Centre (MMC), Monash Cardiovascular Research Centre, MonashHEART, Monash Health and Monash University, Melbourne, Australia

James M. Kofler, PhD Department of Radiology, Mayo Clinic, Jacksonville, FL, USA

Madeleine Kok, MD, PhD Department of Radiology and Nuclear Medicine, Maastricht University Medical Center, Maastricht, The Netherlands

CARIM School for Cardiovascular Diseases, Maastricht University Medical Center, Maastricht, The Netherlands

Frank D. Kolodgie, PhD CVPath Institute, Gaithersburg, MD, USA

Márton Kolossváry, MD Cardiovascular Imaging Research Group, Heart and Vascular Center, Semmelweis University, Budapest, Hungary

Eli Konen, MD Department of Diagnostic Imaging, Chaim Sheba Medical Center, Ramat Gan, Israel

B. Krauss, PhD Siemens Healthcare GmbH, Forchheim, Germany

Shaw Hua Kueh, MBChB Department of Radiology, University of British Columbia, Vancouver, BC, Canada

Joan M. Lacomis, MD Department of Radiology, Thoracic Imaging Division, University of Pittsburgh Medical Center, University of Pittsburgh School of Medicine, Pittsburgh, PA, USA

Scott P. Landreth Department of Radiology and Radiological Science, Medical University of South Carolina, Charleston, SC, USA

Hwa Yeon Lee, MD, PhD Smile Radiologic Clinic, Seoul, South Korea

Jongmin Lee, MD, PhD Department of Radiology, Kyungpook National University, School of Medicine, Daegu, South Korea

Nam Ju Lee, MD Department of Radiology, Mayo Clinic, Rochester, MN, USA

Alan C. Legasto, MD Department of Radiology, Weill Cornell Medicine, New York, NY, USA

Jonathon A. Leipsic, MD Department of Radiology, St. Paul's Hospital, Providence Healthcare, Vancouver, BC, Canada

Shuai Leng, PhD Department of Radiology, Mayo Clinic, Rochester, MN, USA

John R. Lesser, MD, FACC, FAHA Minneapolis Heart Institute Foundation, Minneapolis, MN, USA

Virginia W. Lesslie, BS Division of Cardiovascular Imaging, Department of Radiology and Radiological Science, Medical University of South Carolina, Charleston, SC, USA

David C. Levin, MD Department of Radiology, Thomas Jefferson University Hospital, Philadelphia, PA, USA

Ana Paula S. Lima, MD Department of Radiology and Biomedical Imaging, University of California San Francisco, San Francisco, CA, USA

Fay Y. Lin, MD Department of Radiology, NewYork-Presbyterian Hospital and the Weill Cornell Medical College, New York, NY, USA

Harold Litt, MD, PhD Department of Radiology, Perelman School of Medicine of the University of Pennsylvania, Philadelphia, PA, USA

Sheldon E. Litwin, MD Division of Cardiology, Department of Medicine, Medical University of South Carolina, Charleston, SC, USA

Bin Lu, MD Department of Radiologic Imaging, Fuwai Hospital, Chinese Academy of Medical Sciences and Peking Union Medical College, National Center of Cardiovascular Diseases, Beijing, China

Guang Ming Lu, MD Department of Medical Imaging, Jinling Hospital, Medical School of Nanjing University, Nanjing, Jiangsu, China

Manoj Mannil, MD, MSc Institute of Diagnostic and Interventional Radiology, University Hospital Zurich, Zurich, Switzerland

Mohamed Marwan, MD Department of Medicine, Cardiology and Angiology, Universitätsklinikum Erlangen, Erlangen, Germany

Pál Maurovich-Horvat, MD, PhD, MPH Cardiovascular Imaging Research Group, Heart and Vascular Center, Semmelweis University, Budapest, Hungary

C. H. McCollough, PhD Department of Radiology, Mayo Clinic, Rochester, MN, USA

Felix G. Meinel, MD Department of Diagnostic and Interventional Radiology, Rostock University Medical Center, Rostock, Germany

Nandini (Nina) M. Meyersohn, MD Division of Cardiovascular Imaging, Department of Radiology, Massachusetts General Hospital/Harvard Medical School, Boston, MA, USA

Casper Mihl, MD, PhD Department of Radiology and Nuclear Medicine, Maastricht University Medical Center, Maastricht, The Netherlands

CARIM School for Cardiovascular Diseases, Maastricht University Medical Center, Maastricht, The Netherlands

James K. Min, MD Department of Radiology, NewYork-Presbyterian Hospital and the Weill Cornell Medical College, New York, NY, USA

John F. Mooney, MBB Department of Radiology, University of British Columbia, Vancouver, BC, Canada

Hiroyoshi Mori, MD CVPath Institute, Gaithersburg, MD, USA

Pamela B. Morris, MD Seinsheimer Cardiovascular Health Program, Department of Medicine and Cardiology, Medical University of South Carolina, Charleston, SC, USA

Giuseppe Muscogiuri, MD Centro Cardiologico Monzino, IRCCS, Milan, Italy

John W. Nance, MD Department of Radiology, Medical University of South Carolina, Charleston, SC, USA

Koen Nieman, MD, PhD Stanford University, School of Medicine, Cardiovascular Institute, Stanford, CA, USA

Iclal Ocak, MD Department of Radiology, Thoracic Imaging Division, University of Pittsburgh Medical Center, University of Pittsburgh School of Medicine, Pittsburgh, PA, USA

Maksymilian P. Opolski, MD, PhD Department of Interventional Cardiology and Angiology, Institute of Cardiology, Warsaw, Poland

Karen G. Ordovas, MD, MAS Department of Radiology, University of California San Francisco, San Francisco, CA, USA

Kotaro Ouchi, MD, PhD Department of Radiology, The Jikei University School of Medicine, Tokyo, Japan

Gert Jan Pelgrim, PhD Department of Radiology, University of Groningen, University Medical Center Groningen, Groningen, The Netherlands

Laura J. Pierce, MPA, RT (CT) Department of Radiology, Duke University School of Medicine, Durham, NC, USA

Todd Pietila Materialise USA Biomedical Engineering, Plymouth, MI, USA

Gianluca Pontone, MD, PhD, FESC, FSCCT Centro Cardiologico Monzino, IRCCS, Milan, Italy

Andrew N. Primak, PhD Department of Diagnostic Imaging, Siemens Healthineers, Malvern, PA, USA

Gregorio Rábago, MD Department of Cardiac Surgery, Clínica Universidad de Navarra, Pamplona, Spain

Mark Rabbat, MD, FSCCT Department of Medicine, Division of Cardiology, Loyola University Chicago, Chicago, IL, USA

Department of Medicine, Division of Cardiology, Edward Hines Jr. VA Hospital, Hines, IL, USA

Prabhakar Rajiah, MBBS, MD, FRCR Department of Radiology, Cardiothoracic Imaging Division, UT Southwestern Medical Center, Dallas, TX, USA

Matthias Renker, MD Department of Cardiology, Kerckhoff Heart and Thorax Center, Bad Nauheim, Germany

Xinshuang Ren, MD Department of Radiologic Imaging, Fuwai Hospital, Chinese Academy of Medical Sciences and Peking Union Medical College, National Center of Cardiovascular Diseases, Beijing, China

Asim Rizvi, MD Department of Radiology, Dalio Institute of Cardiovascular Imaging, NewYork-Presbyterian Hospital and the Weill Cornell Medical College, New York, NY, USA

Department of Radiology, Mayo Clinic, Rochester, MN, USA

Sebastian Rogowski, MD Department of Cardiology and Intensive Care Medicine, Heart Center Munich-Bogenhausen, Munich, Germany

Hadi Mirhedayati Roudsari, MD Department of Radiology, NewYork-Presbyterian Hospital and the Weill Cornell Medical College, New York, NY, USA

Alan Rozanski, MD Department of Cardiovascular Medicine, Gagnon Cardiovascular Institute, Morristown Medical Center, Morristown, NJ, USA

The Division of Cardiology, Mount Sinai St. Luke's Hospital, Mount Sinai Heart, New York, NY, USA

Geoffrey D. Rubin, MD, MBA Department of Radiology, Duke University School of Medicine, Durham, NC, USA

Ronen Rubinshtein, MD Department of Cardiovascular Medicine, Lady Davis Carmel Medical Center, The Ruth and Bruce Rappaport School of Medicine, Technion-Israel Institute of Technology, Haifa, Israel

John A. Rumberger, PhD, MD Department of Cardiac Imaging, The Princeton Longevity Center, Princeton, NJ, USA

Frank J. Rybicki, MD, PhD Department of Radiology, University of Ottawa Faculty of Medicine, Ottawa, ON, Canada

Ottawa Hospital Research Institute, Ottawa, ON, Canada

Pooyan Sahbaee, PhD Siemens Medical Solutions USA, Inc., Malvern, PA, USA

Toru Sakuma, MD, PhD Department of Radiology, The Jikei University School of Medicine, Tokyo, Japan

Arnold M. R. Schilham, PhD Department of Radiology, University Medical Center Utrecht, Utrecht, The Netherlands

Christopher L. Schlett, MD, MPH Department of Diagnostic and Interventional Radiology, University Medical Center Freiburg, Freiburg, Germany

Bernhard Schmidt, PhD Department of Computed Tomography, Siemens Healthcare GmbH, Forchheim, Germany

Paul Schoenhagen, MD Imaging Institute, Cleveland Clinic, Lerner College of Medicine, Cleveland, OH, USA

Jan-Erik Scholtz, MD Cardiac MR PET CT Program, Massachusetts General Hospital, Boston, MA, USA

Florian Schwarz, PD Dr. med Department of Diagnostic and Interventional Radiology and Neuroradiology, Klinikum Augsburg, Augsburg, Germany

Chris Schwemmer, MSc Department of Computed Tomography, Siemens Healthcare GmbH, Forchheim, Germany

Stephanie Sellers, MSc Department of Radiology, University of British Columbia, Vancouver, BC, Canada

Michael D. Shapiro, DO Department of Medicine, Division of Cardiovascular Medicine, Oregon Health & Science University, Portland, OR, USA

James V. Spearman, MD Department of Radiology and Radiological Science, Medical University of South Carolina, Charleston, SC, USA

David Steflik, MD Department of Pediatrics, Division of Pediatric Cardiology, Medical University of South Carolina, Charleston, SC, USA

Arthur E. Stillman, MD, PhD Department of Radiology and Imaging Science, Emory University School of Medicine, Atlanta, GA, USA

Pal Spruill Suranyi, MD, PhD Division of Cardiovascular Imaging, Department of Radiology and Radiological Science, Medical University of South Carolina, Charleston, SC, USA

Division of Cardiology, Department of Medicine, Medical University of South Carolina, Charleston, SC, USA

Richard A. P. Takx, MD, MSc, PhD Department of Radiology, University Medical Center Utrecht, Utrecht, The Netherlands

Christian Tesche, MD Division of Cardiovascular Imaging, Department of Radiology and Radiological Science, Medical University of South Carolina, Charleston, SC, USA

Department of Cardiology and Intensive Care Medicine, Heart Center Munich-Bogenhausen, Munich, Germany

Christian Thilo, MD Department of Cardiology, Klinikum Augsburg, Herzzentrum Augsburg-Schwaben, Augsburg, Germany

Quynh A. Truong, MD, MPH, FACC Department of Radiology, Weill Cornell Medicine, New York, NY, USA

Seth Uretsky, MD Department of Cardiovascular Medicine, Gagnon Cardiovascular Institute, Morristown Medical Center, Morristown, NJ, USA

Marly van Assen, MSc Department of Radiology, University of Groningen, University Medical Center Groningen, Groningen, The Netherlands

Department of Radiology and Radiological Science, Division of Cardiovascular Imaging, Medical University of South Carolina Charleston, SC, USA

Edwin J. R. van Beek, MD, PhD Edinburgh Imaging Facility QMRI, University of Edinburgh, Edinburgh, UK

Akos Varga-Szemes, MD, PhD Division of Cardiovascular Imaging, Department of Radiology and Radiological Science, Medical University of South Carolina, Charleston, SC, USA

Renu Virmani, MD CVPath Institute, Gaithersburg, MD, USA

Rozemarijn Vliegenthart, MD, PhD Department of Radiology, University of Groningen, University Medical Center Groningen, Groningen, The Netherlands

Department of Radiology and Radiological Science, Division of Cardiovascular Imaging, Medical University of South Carolina Charleston, SC, USA

Andrew Voigt, MD Heart and Vascular Institute, University of Pittsburgh Medical Center, Pittsburgh, PA, USA

Charles S. White, MD Department of Diagnostic Radiology, University of Maryland Medical Center, Baltimore, MD, USA

Joachim E. Wildberger, MD, PhD Department of Radiology and Nuclear Medicine, Maastricht University Medical Center, Maastricht, The Netherlands

CARIM School for Cardiovascular Diseases, Maastricht University Medical Center, Maastricht, The Netherlands

Martin J. Willemink, MD, PhD Department of Radiology, University Medical Center Utrecht, Utrecht, The Netherlands

Michelle C. Williams, MBChB, PhD Edinburgh Imaging Facility QMRI, University of Edinburgh, Edinburgh, UK

Eric E. Williamson, MD Department of Radiology, Mayo Clinic, Rochester, MN, USA

Arik Wolak, MD Department of Cardiology, Shaare Zedek Medical Center, Jerusalem, Israel

Pamela K. Woodard, MD Mallinckrodt Institute of Radiology, Washington University School of Medicine, St. Louis, MO, USA

Junjie Yang, MD Division of Cardiovascular Imaging, Department of Radiology and Radiological Science, Medical University of South Carolina, Charleston, SC, USA

Department of Cardiology, People's Liberation Army General Hospital, Beijing, China

Weihua Yin, MD Department of Radiologic Imaging, Fuwai Hospital, Chinese Academy of Medical Sciences and Peking Union Medical College, National Center of Cardiovascular Diseases, Beijing, China

Seung Min Yoo, MD, PhD Department of Radiology, CHA University Bundang Medical Center, Bundang, South Korea

Long Jiang Zhang, MD, PhD Department of Medical Imaging, Jinling Hospital, Medical School of Nanjing University, Nanjing, Jiangsu, China

Mathis Zimmermann, Dipl Ing, MBA Digital Health Services, Siemens Healthineers, Malvern, PA, USA

Peter L. Zwerner, MD Division of Cardiology, Department of Medicine, Medical University of South Carolina, Charleston, SC, USA

The original version of the book was revised. The correction to the book is available at https://doi.org/10.1007/978-1-60327-237-7_69

Part I

Where We Were

History of Cardiac CT: A Personal Story

1

John A. Rumberger

As the story goes, Wilhelm Conrad Röentgen, a physicist, was working late in his laboratory in Wurzburg, Germany, experimenting with a vacuum tube made of glass. He was using this to generate beams of electrons and wrapped the tube with black paper to avoid viewing the electric discharge occurring in the gas inside the vacuum tube. When he started his experiment, he noted that a piece of coated paper lying near the tube began to glow. He was astonished and did another experiment where he held a thick book between the tube and the paper – however, the "rays" simply passed through the book, as if totally unobstructed. When Röentgen looked at the coated paper it showed a shadowy outline of the bones in his hand. This was November 8, 1895, and the world of the "X-ray" has never looked back.

The "X-ray" has been intimately linked to the ability to see "inside" the body since the late nineteenth century; but it remained a projection image with superposition of all the densities of the tissue placed between the anode and the cathode. To separate these various tissue densities, a thin cross-sectional image would be of significant benefit as the various organs can be separated from their surrounding tissues of fat, muscle, and bone.

The birth of clinical X-ray computed tomography (CT) was not realized until about 80 years after Röentgen's discovery. At the time of this writing, an estimated 90,000 peer reviewed scientific articles have been published on or about CT. A dominant majority of these articles deal with body organs and processes that either do not move during the image acquisition or, in the case of lung imaging, when motion can be suspended long enough to get "static images." In the case of cardiac CT imaging, however it is a different story and has been a difficult challenge to image an object that is constantly moving in four dimensions and cannot be, safely, stopped. Cardiac CT and my personal involvement with cardiac CT interestingly started nearly at the same time as the development of commercial CT in general.

J. A. Rumberger (✉)
Department of Cardiac Imaging, The Princeton Longevity Center, Princeton, NJ, USA
e-mail: jrumberger@theplc.net

In the Beginning, There Was Mathematics

The story of cardiac CT, and all CT for that matter, begins with mathematics that allow us to "reconstruct" the density/tissue characteristics of an "unknown" object placed in a black box as light [or later X-ray] of known intensity is shown through. Pierre Bouguer, credited in about 1729, noted that the absorption of light through an object is directly proportional to its thickness [or path length]. Lambert later popularized this observation in a paper from 1760. August Beer discovered another light attenuation factor in 1852 noting that light absorbance was proportional to the concentrations of the attenuating "unknown object." The modern Lambert-Beer law combines these two observations and correlates the changes in light energy to both the concentration of the attenuating "unknown" object and the thickness of the unknown object. Since visible light is part of the electromagnetic energy spectrum, this can apply to the application of X-rays as well. The general application of the Lambert-Beer law to X-ray imaging is shown in Fig. 1.1.

Referring to Fig. 1.1, the unknown object of density μ represents a "pixel" [i.e., picture element] size of 1×1. If we know the incident radiation and the output radiation after passing through the unknown object, as well as the distance between these measurements, the Lambert-Beer law then provides an equation with only one unknown, i.e., μ. What if I wanted to determine the density of four unknown μ objects? I can use the Lambert-Beer law to set up four equations in four unknowns or a field of view of 2×2 pixels as shown in Fig. 1.2. However, the ability to solve pixel density resolutions of 80×80 pixels [as was used on the first-generation clinical CT scanner] was simply too daunting a task until the modern development of the computer. The "exact solutions" for the individual μ, to speed up the mathematical solutions,

U. J. Schoepf (ed.), *CT of the Heart*, Contemporary Medical Imaging, https://doi.org/10.1007/978-1-60327-237-7_1

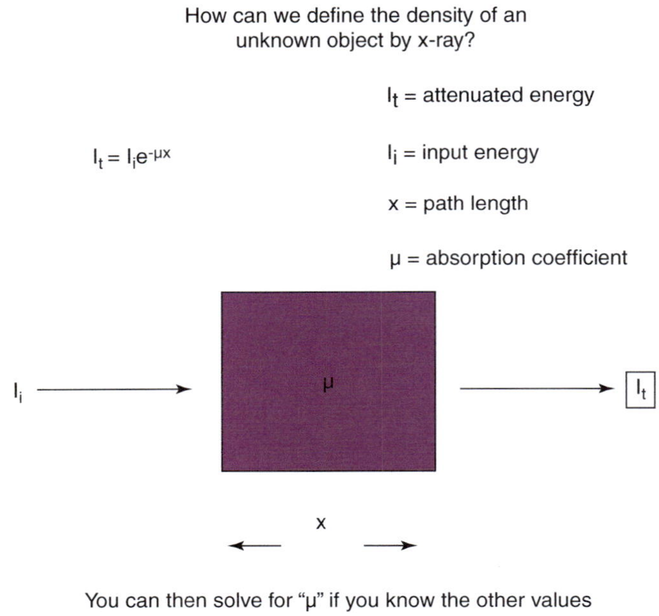

Fig. 1.1 The Lambert-Beer law applied to X-ray

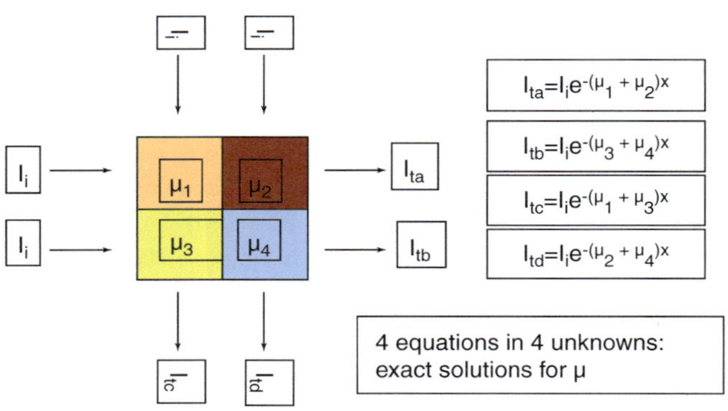

Fig. 1.2 The exact solution of the Lambert-Beer law for four unknown objects of density μ

initially involved various "iterative" methods. The final solutions reached in a series of best guesses and comparisons with the actual data. The original mathematics was part of the ART [algebraic reconstruction theory] algorithm [1].

In 1963 another physicist in South Africa, Allan Cormack, was working on improving the dose calculations used in radiation therapy planning, but knowledge of cross-sectional density distributions was required. He developed the first concept of image reconstruction from projections [2]. This became the basis for another image reconstruction called "back projection" [later improved to reduce noise at the edges of objects and called "filtered back projection"] [3].

Attainment of Reality in Clinical Medicine: The EMI Scanner

Modern X-ray CT was developed by Sir Godfrey Hounsfield while working for Electronic and Musical Industries Ltd. [EMI] in England. A prototype scanner using an X-ray tube was developed in 1969/1970 and a clinically applicable scanner installed at the Atkinson Morley Hospital in a London suburb in 1971; the first clinical results were presented in 1973 [4]. At first only the brain could be imaged due to very long acquisition times in which the patient was required to be very still [and surrounded by a water phantom]. The first clinical CT scanner in the USA was installed at the Mayo Clinic in Rochester, Minnesota, in 1973.

As an interesting personal anecdote, the engineer installing the scanner at the Mayo Clinic was named David King and had worked closely with Hounsfield in England. David King, later the founder of "calcium club" [see further discussion below] and acknowledged as the "father" of coronary artery calcium scanning, told me a story. When Hounsfield and colleagues at EMI contemplated the "world's" eventual needs for such a unique brain imaging device, they estimated that probably less than a hundred scanners would be eventually made and sold. After 1 week at the Mayo Clinic, and after performing more head/brain CT scans than had been done in the past 2 years in England, David told Godfrey – "Maybe you might want to increase your estimation of the world's need for the EMI scanner".

By 1975 a second-generation EMI scanner, the first prototype "body scanner" was introduced. Acquisition times per slice were about 20 s, and it used iterative reconstruction techniques although the much faster filtered back projection method was now established. Because of the success of the EMI scanner, many other commercially available scanners were quickly introduced by other manufacturers that, like EMI itself, eventually went under, while others such as the Picker, Siemens, and GE survived. But the die was cast. In 1979 both Hounsfield and Cormack received the Nobel Prize in Physiology and Medicine for the development of the CT scanner.

The Dynamic Spatial Reconstructor

There were several attempts to using "conventional" CT scanning in the early 1980s to study the cardiovascular system, mainly viewing patency of coronary artery bypass grafts and looking for aortic dissections [5]. Already there was a clear advantage noted in cardiac CT over the conventional M-mode/sector echocardiographic examinations and plane chest X-rays that were "state of the art" at the time for imaging of the chest and heart.

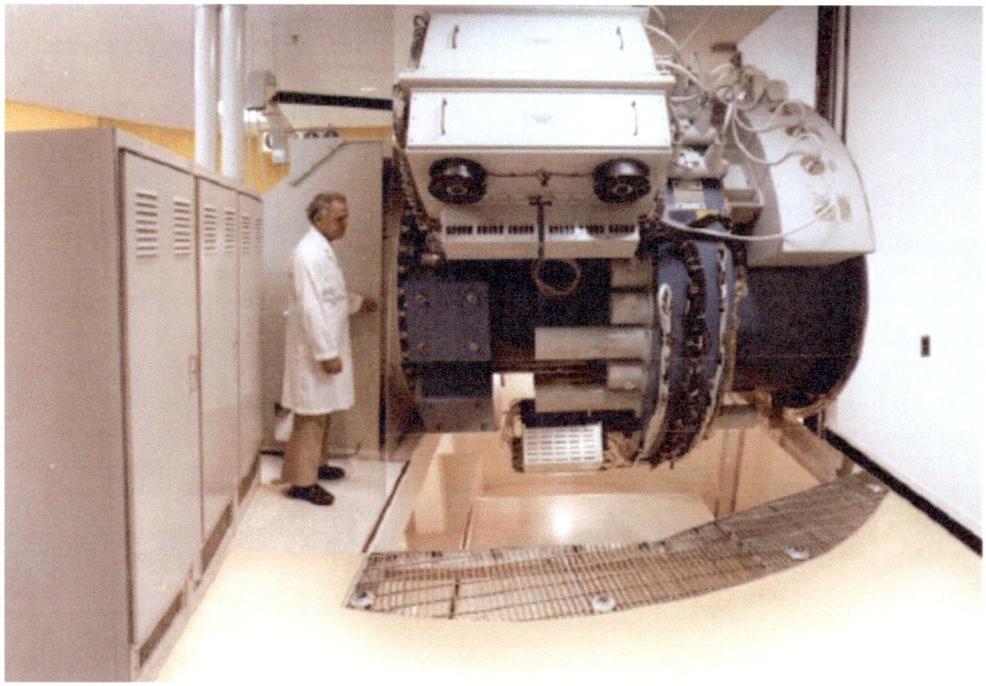

Fig. 1.3 The dynamic spatial reconstructor. (With permission of the Mayo Foundation for Medical Education and Research. All rights reserved)

The Biodynamics Research Laboratory at the Mayo Clinic had a long and storied history with aviation medicine in World War II and under the directorship of Dr. Earl H. Wood did the first human centrifuge experiments studying "G" force [i.e., gravity] effects on pilots during flight and combat. Along with the US government, they developed the first "G-suits," and after the war Dr. Wood was awarded a special commendation by President Harry S. Truman.

The idea of using X-ray CT to study the moving heart dated to the first body images produced using the EMI body scanner; but despite some success as noted by Brundage et al. [5], the spatial resolution and most importantly the temporal resolution were not sufficient for most clinical cardiac work. The idea of developing a CT scanner fast enough to make "stop action" images of the beating heart was first realized in the Biodynamics Research Laboratory where, under NIH funding, they introduced the Dynamic Spatial Reconstructor (DSR) in 1975.

The DSR was imagined as a specialized cardiac CT scanner using conventional X-rays with photomultiplier tubes and fluoroscopic projection imaging applied in a unique manner (Fig. 1.3). The original design was to use 28 pairs of X-ray sources and 28 direct line visualization fluoroscopic units. This vast array [requiring literally two floors with gantry and imaging chain] was then rotated at high speed as images of the beating heart were acquired using intra-arterial injection of iodinated contrast over a period of about 20 s. Using ART reconstruction methods, a temporal resolution of 16 msec/image could be realized as well as spatial resolution approaching 1 mm. However, only 14 sets of X-ray/fluoroscopic units were installed due to technical difficulties and funding. Later the fluoroscopic units were replaced by CCDI cameras. Image reconstruction however was arduous and could take as long as several weeks to be completed. Specialized software was developed to review and analyze the data. Countless contributions to the world of cardiac CT were introduced by the investigators working on multiple aspects of the DSR project [6–8]. I can recall at one of my earliest American Heart Association conventions as a cardiology fellow seeing the astounding video presented by Dr. Eric Ritman, the then head of the biodynamics research unit, showing detailed anatomy of adult patients in 3-D and, with time added, in 4-D. Unfortunately, the DSR was not a commercially viable enterprise and was decommissioned in 2002. By that time cardiac imaging using MDCT was developing rapidly.

Electron Beam CT

In the early 1970s, the initial applications to develop a specialized cardiac CT scanner given to the NIH were of two distinctly different designs. The X-ray tube/fluoroscopic unit design as noted above was eventually used for the DSR. However, another design using scanning electron beams was discussed.

The scanning electron beam approach eventually proved to be the superior design for practical clinical applications and for commercial product success. However, this required many years in development. Two early designs, one by Iinuma et al. [9] at JEOL, a Japanese manufacturer of electron microscopes, and by Haimson [10] resulted in prototype machines but were abandoned. Published in the same issue as Reference [8], citing the initial DSR results, was a third design, originating with Dr. Douglas Boyd [11, 12]. This eventually resulted in the development of what is now called EBCT [electron beam computed tomography].

In 1984 Dr. Boyd and colleagues, working initially under the aspics of the University of San Francisco Physics Laboratory, developed a commercially viable electron beam scanner. A for-profit company, Imatron Inc., was developed, and then it was time to sell the scanners to academic institutions for cardiac research. It was initially called "ultrafast CT."

The design was radically different from conventional CT at the time. The idea behind ultrafast CT was a large bell-shaped X-ray tube. An electron beam [think back to the initial experiments of Röentgen] emitted from the cathode is focused into a narrow beam and then, by means of powerful electromagnets, deflected to impinge on a small focal spot on an annular tungsten target anode. The electron beam [and of course the focal spot] was electronically swept along at semicircular array along 210° of arc (Fig. 1.4). In order to perform a true cross-sectional image, the beam sweep must be at least 180° plus the width of the "fan beam," which for the Imatron scanner was 30°. To acquire rapid heart scans without table movement, ultrafast CT included four anodes and two detector arrays, each offset along the z-axis to acquire eight interleaved slices covering 8 cm of the heart. Although very fast speeds were possible, since there were no moving parts, as with then and current CT scanners, the limited tube current (650 mA) required slower speeds for acceptable mAs values and associated image quality. However, with ultrafast CT temporal resolution speeds of 50 msec and 100 msec, this was 10–20 times faster than possible at that time from conventional CT [and frankly would not be possible with mechanical CT until 20+ years later].

I started my cardiology fellowship in 1981 at the University of Iowa under the mentorship of the late Dr. Melvin Marcus. Dr. Marcus had already distinguished himself as a leader in the world of coronary physiology. The initial experiments were done in laboratory animals, but he longed to be able to study in detail human cardiac and coronary physiology. Recall this was a time early in the developments of nuclear perfusion imaging and the 30° and 60° "sector" two-dimensional echocardiograms. The only way to evaluate for the severity of coronary artery disease was direct invasive angiography.

Mel had published a paper showing that patients with severe aortic stenosis and severe left ventricular hypertrophy, but no evidence for obstructive coronary disease, evaluated in the operating room using a Doppler coronary flow meter placed directly on the coronary arteries, could result in decreased coronary artery flow reserve and angina related to the left ventricular hypertrophy [13]. If only he could study such phenomenon in adult patients outside of the operating room.

Dr. Marcus had heard of the potential for ultrafast CT to do noninvasive human "experiments" of cardiac structure, function, and flow. The University of Iowa agreed to purchase Imatron scanner #3, and I was sent to the UCSF Physics Laboratory, along with the late Dr. Andrew

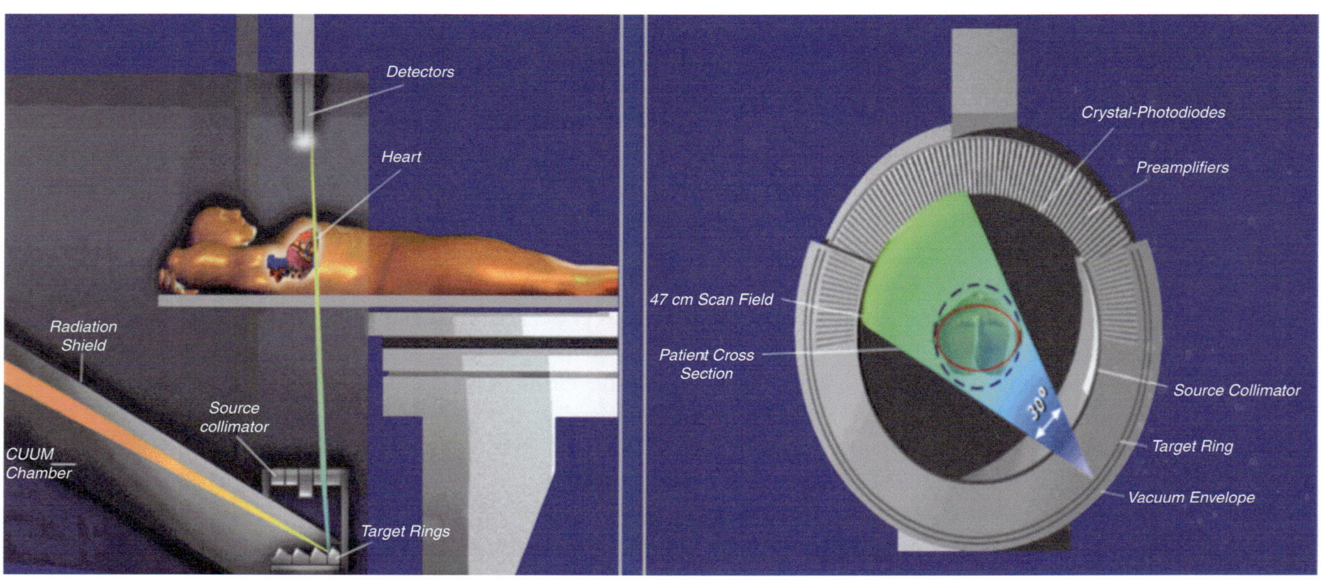

Fig. 1.4 Schematic of electron beam tomography. (Personal archives, John A. Rumberger, MD)

J. Feiring, to begin validation studies using ultrafast CT for two important parameters: accurate definition of global left ventricular muscle mass and regional myocardial perfusion.

During our time in South San Francisco, I got to know, learn from, admire, and befriend the "greats" in early cardiac CT including Dr. Bruce Brundage [cardiology], Dr. Charles Higgins [radiology], and Dr. Martin Lipton [radiology]. After many errors, trials, false endings, and misunderstandings of the physics of CT and image reconstructions, we were successful with our two primary objectives [14, 15].

Over the next 15 years, our laboratory at the University of Iowa and later at the Mayo Clinic, along with scores of other investigators all over the world, used ultrafast CT [later called simply electron beam CT (EBT/EBCT)] to validate a number of potential human clinical cardiac situations including quantitation of left ventricular regurgitant volumes [16], visualization of coronary artery bypass graft patency [17], segmental left ventricular systolic function [18], regional left ventricular diastolic function [19, 20], regional radius to wall thickness rations in normal volume overloaded left ventricle [21], right ventricular assessment in patients under consideration for lung transplantation [22], post-infarct left ventricular and right ventricular remodeling during the first year after myocardial infarction [23, 24], and revalidation of measurements of myocardial perfusion in animal models [25] and in humans [26].

Imatron, as a stand-alone provider of ultrafast CT, had many "suiters" during the years beginning with Picker International and later with Siemens. These associations later proved to be economically fatal.

Despite these and many other publications, imaging of the heart using CT was considered at the time as a "niche" and likely not to be applied widely in clinical medicine as magnetic resonance imaging and two-dimensional [and eventually three] echocardiography, both not involving exposure to ionizing radiation, gained more and more applications and notoriety. Ultrafast CT/EBT needed a "unique" application to clinical cardiology.

There had been reports as early as the 1960s using the presence of coronary artery calcification, detected at fluoroscopy, as a noninvasive definition of coronary atherosclerotic plaque. Early investigations at the University of Chicago showed a correlation with coronary obstructive disease and non-quantitation of coronary artery calcification using ultrafast CT [27]. However, it was the publication of a study from Mt. Sinai hospital by Agatston and Janowitz that set the course for the use of quantitated coronary artery calcium score [Agatston score] as a surrogate for clinical coronary artery atherosclerosis [28].

David King [as identified previously] was then the "scientific director" of Imatron and visited all US and foreign ultrafast CT installed sites to interest researchers in CAC [coronary artery calcification]. At the time, we had two installations of EBT at the Mayo Clinic, and we were imaging cardiac physiology [as noted above] and exploring applications of fast imaging of the respiratory system [cine angiographic imaging of patients with sleep apnea and exploring the application of ultrafast CT in detecting pulmonary emboli].

David tried to interest me in CAC in the early 1990s. I had four comments: (1) We know that CAC is associated with atherosclerosis, but it does not tell us the severity of coronary stenosis, (2) I am happy studying cardiac/coronary physiology that I know can be done with EBT, (3) I am not interested, and (4) find somebody else at Mayo that might find CAC valuable… *Should such comments strike me down as I stand.*

Dr. William Stanford and I edited the first book on *Ultrafast Cardiac CT* in 1992 [29]. At that time, we discussed the physics of CT imaging and had many of our colleagues submit chapters on their ultrafast CT research. One such chapter was from Drs. Agatston and Janowitz on the clinical applications of CAC scanning. I edited the chapter and felt that the "suggestions" for applications were a bit "imaginative," and I asked them to "tone it down" for the eventual publication.

I was aware peripherally of the research my colleagues Dr. Robert Schwartz in collaboration with a well-known cardiac pathologist, Dr. William Edwards, in looking at CAC in autopsy hearts using EBT. At the same time, epidemiologists from the University of Michigan, Drs. Pat Peyser and Lawrence Bielak, were conducting studies in the "Rochester Family Heart Study" looking at CAC in residents of Olmsted County, MN., in relationship to coronary angiography [30].

At the Mayo Clinic, we required all our internal medicine residents to participate in at least one research project during their residency. Dr. Brent Simons, who had been involved with Drs. Schwartz and Edwards in the pathologic studies of CAC versus coronary plaque studies, came to me to discuss his data and how to best analyze the information. He basically had a listing of CAC area measurements using EBT made at 3 mm intervals from the ostium of the autopsy coronary arteries and representative coronary histologic atherosclerotic plaque areas from the same coronary segments. I was not his academic advisor but suggested we start with a simple linear correlation of CAC areas versus histologic plaque areas. At the time the best program was called "Lotus 123." I took the data and displayed the information. What I saw was astounding and provocative: there was a clear, albeit scattered, linear correlation between CAC area and comparable atherosclerotic plaque area. I turned to Brent and said, quite literally: "Where the hell did you get these data?"

From that point on, I had a mission, and we published several papers from this dataset and a subsequent dataset using non-decalcified autopsy coronary segments as compared with CAC images using EBT [31, 32]. My initial "bias" that CAC could not define percent stenosis was subsequently shown to be a consequence of coronary artery remodeling during atherosclerotic plaque development [33].

As interest, all around the world, began to develop regarding the use of CAC as a "screening" method to define coronary atherosclerosis, David King formed the "calcium club." We would have meetings in the AM prior to the American College of Cardiology and American Heart Association annual meetings discussing the latest CAC research from around the world. Many of the well-known cardiologists of the time would attend these meetings only to dismiss such information during the true scientific presentations. The "calcium club" however was a popular forum to openly discuss research and advance ideas among like-minded colleagues. In fact, the original members of the calcium club founded the Society of Atherosclerosis Imaging [SAI] and later incorporated the Society of Cardiovascular Tomography [SCCT]. Some of the "issues" between the calcium club and established conventional cardiology, interested in obstructive disease and development of angioplasty and stents, somewhat congruous with detecting nonclinical atherosclerosis by CAC, are featured in the documentary "The Widowmaker" [34].

Although there are likely thousands of publications from all parts of the world regarding cardiac CT using EBT, the "holy grail" was the potential to image the coronary arteries in vivo. EBT had superior temporal resolution and, for a long time, superior spatial resolution over conventional CT. Dr. Stephan Achenbach and colleagues in 1995 first published the use of EBT in quantitative imaging of the coronary arteries [35]. Following that publication, the labeling of cardiac CT as a "niche" changed dramatically.

Despite the potential advantages of EBT over, at the time, conventional CT in terms of cardiac imaging, no more than 110 Imatron scanners were manufactured/installed. Many are still installed and operational across the world using cannibalized parts from other scanners or via post-market jerry rigging. They were temperamental, difficult to maintain, and very expensive. In 1999 EBT, a niche scanner might cost $1.5 million, while conventional CT used for thoracic and body imaging might cost <$0.7 million. The final curtain was the incorporation of Imatron in 2001 by General Electric. The swan song of EBT was the GE "e-Speed," a "stripped down" scanner with improved spatial resolution to 1.5 mm versus 3 mm, but was not sufficient to compete in the world striving to be able to image the coronary arteries, which are on the order of 3–4 mm or less in diameter. The e-speed was abandoned by GE within a few years of its introduction.

MDCT

Conventional CT in the 1980s, as opposed to using a scanning electron beam as noted above, had a disadvantage for imaging the heart due to the physical time required to move a heavy X-ray tube, resulting in temporal resolution on the order of 1000 msec, a spatial resolution of 5–6 mm, and the physical attachment to the scanning gantry of the electrical connection receiving the electronic data. This tethering required that a 230-degree arc for the rotation of the X-ray tube about the patient had to be "returned" or wound back to its original position and the scanning table advanced a predetermined distance before another tomographic image could be taken.

"Slip-ring" technology introduced in 1989 gave way to the "uncoupling" of the data acquisition system [DAS] from the X-ray gantry allowing continuous scanning along with synchronized and graduated scanner table motion. Thus, contiguous X-ray tomograms could be acquired during graduated increments of the imaging table covering more of the body in less time than had been previously possible with prior generations of CT scanners. The CT scanner, untethered, can produce a spiral or helical imaging path through the body. Helical CT provides no obvious slice Z-positions, and any arbitrarily selected slice plane is equivalent to any other. Thus, once helical data are acquired, slices may be reconstructed at any Z-position.

The speed of imaging a body part was improved significantly by the introduction of slip-ring technology, but only one slice could be imaged at a single time. Multislice imaging, looking at multiple slices acquired at the same time, would afford a better temporal and spatial imaging of the heart.

In 1998 Elscint, an Israeli based operation, introduced the "dual-slice" CT scanning able to acquire two contiguous scans at one sweep of the X-ray source/detector pair – thus halving the time required for a chest or body scan. Elscint was absorbed by Picker International eventually but then Picker folded. Siemens and GE followed suit with their introductions – later four-slice CT and eight-slice CT. With the introduction of multislice CT scans came the implication that these would replace EBT in terms of cardiac imaging. However, these "wannabees" simply could not duplicate the spatial and temporal resolution of EBT in terms of cardiac imaging.

In 2002 I reviewed an article detailing the use of Siemens 16-slice MDCT [multi-detector CT] and its application to noninvasive coronary angiography [36]. The spatial resolution of MDCT was superior to EBT, and with the use of beta-blockade to lower the heart rate, spectacular images as compared with conventional angiography were finally available. For the first time, I realized that multislice conventional

CT could, indeed, duplicate and improve on the prior studies using EBT. We were ready to "take it up a notch."

Quickly the numbers of simultaneous "slices" were increased to 32-, 42-, and finally to the current state-of-the-art 64-slice MDCT. The industry has not stopped at 64 slices, moving to 256 and even 320 slices acquired at a single sweep of the scanner gantry. Faster rotational speeds, along with mathematical algorithms, have reduced spatial resolution to 0.4 mm or better as well as duplicating EBT temporal resolution to <100 msec.

Scores of publications using 16+ MDCT have duplicated the original cardiac research initially done using EBT, and 64+-slice MDCT is now used routinely in the outpatient and inpatient facilities to define CAC and coronary artery atherosclerotic plaque severity and type in the outpatient and inpatient situations.

Conclusions

> "Those that do not remember the past are bound to repeat it." *[George Santayana, 1863–1952 in George Santayana (1905) Reason in Common Sense, p. 284, volume 1 of The Life of Reason]*

I have lived the history of cardiac CT and am still doing and teaching it – the awe has not left me wondering. The pages to follow in this book will define far better than I can the wonder of the physics, mathematics, and computer science that has, along with the manufacturing of MDCT, come together to establish cardiac CT as a mainstream and in many instances a primary or initial imaging tool for studying the heart and coronary arteries, going full circle with the initial efforts to define cardiac size, function, and flow which begun now nearly 40 years ago.

References

1. Budinger TF, Gullberg GT. Three dimensional reconstruction in nuclear medicine emission imaging. IEEE Trans Nucl Sci. 1974;NS-12:2–21.
2. Cormack A. Representation of function by its line integrals with some radiological applications. Part I. J Appl Phys. 1964;35:2722.
3. Ramachandran GN, Lakshminarayanan AV. Three-dimensional reconstruction from radiographs and electron micrographs: application of convolutions instead of Fourier transforms. Proc Natl Acad Sci USA. 1971;68:2236–40.
4. Hounsfield GN. Computerized transverse axial scanning (tomography). 1. Description of system. Br J Radiol. 1973;46:1023–47.
5. Brundage BH, Lipton MJ. The emergence of computed tomography as a cardiovascular technique. Am Heart J. 1982;103:313–6.
6. Sinak LJ, Hoffman EA, Schwartz RS, Smith HG, Holmes DR, Bove AA, Robb RA, Holmes DJ, Ritman EL. Three dimensional cardiac anatomy and function in heart disease in adults: initial results with the Dynamic Spatial Reconstructor. Mayo Clin Proc. 1985;60:383–92.
7. Ritman EL, Kinsey JH, Robb RA, Gilbert BK, Harris LD, Wood EH. Three-dimensional imaging of heart, lungs, and circulation. Science. 1980;210(4467):273–80.
8. Robb RA, Sinak LJ, Hoffman EA, Kinsey JH, Harris LD, Ritman EL. Dynamic volume imaging of moving organs. J Med Syst. 1982;6(6):539–54. PubMed PMID 7183727.
9. Iinuma TA, Tateno Y, Umegake Y, et al. Proposed system for ultrafast computed tomography. J Comput Assist Tomogr. 1977;1:494–9.
10. Haimson J. X-ray source without moving parts for ultra-high speed tomography. IEEE Trans Nucl Sci. 1979;26:2857–61.
11. Boyd DP, Gould RG, Quinn JR, et al. A proposed dynamic cardiac 3-D densitometer for early detection and evaluation of heart disease. IEEE Trans Nucl Sci. 1979;26:2724–7.
12. Boyd DP. Computerized transmission tomography of the heart using scanning electron beams. In: Higgins CB, editor. CT of the heart and the great vessels: experimental evaluation and clinical application. Mount Kisco: Futura Publishing Company; 1983.
13. Marcus ML, Doty DB, Hiratzka LF, Wright CB, Eastham CL. Decreased coronary reserve – a mechanism for angina pectoris in patients with aortic stenosis and normal coronary arteries. N Engl J Med. 1982;307:1362–6.
14. Feiring AJ, Rumberger JA, Skorton DJ, Collins SM, Higgins CB, Lipton MJ, Ell S, Marcus ML. Determination of left ventricular mass in the dog with rapid acquisition cardiac CT scanning. Circulation. 1985;72:1355.
15. Rumberger JA, Feiring AJ, Lipton MJ, Higgins CB, Ell S, Marcus ML. Use of ultrafast CT to quantitate myocardial perfusion: a preliminary report. J Am Coll Cardiol. 1987;9:59–69.
16. Reiter SJ, Rumberger JA, Stanford W, Marcus ML. Quantitative determination of aortic regurgitant volumes by cine computed tomography. Circulation. 1987;76:728–35.
17. Stanford W, Rooholamini M, Rumberger JA, Marcus ML. Evaluation of coronary bypass graft patency by ultrafast CT. J Thorac Imaging. 1988;3:52–5.
18. Feiring AJ, Rumberger JA, Reiter SJ, Collins SM, Skorton DJ, Rees M, Marcus ML. Sectional and segmental variability of left ventricular function: experimental and clinical studies using ultrafast computed tomography. J Am Coll Cardiol. 1988;12:415–25.
19. Rumberger JA, Weiss R, Feiring AJ, Stanford W, Hajduczok Z, Rezai K, Marcus ML. Patterns of regional diastolic function in the normal human left ventricle: an ultrafast computed tomographic study. J Am Coll Cardiol. 1989;14:119–26.
20. Rumberger JA, Bell MR, Stanson AF, Sheedy PF, Behrenbeck T. Assessment of left ventricular diastolic function in man using ultrafast computed tomography. Am J Cardiac Imaging. 1990;4:130–7.
21. Feiring AJ, Rumberger JA. Ultrafast computed tomography analysis of regional radius-to-wall thickness ratios in normal and volume-overloaded human left ventricle. Circulation. 1992;85:1423–32.
22. Vigneswaran WT, McDougall JC, Olson LJ, Breen JF, McGregor CGA, Rumberger JA. Right ventricular assessment in patients presenting for lung transplantation. Transplantation. 1993;55:1051–5.
23. Rumberger JA, Behrenbeck T, Breen JR, Reed JE, Gersh BJ. Nonparallel changes in global chamber volume and muscle mass during the first year following transmural myocardial infarction in man. J Am Coll Cardiol. 1993;21:673–82.
24. Hirose K, Shu NH, Reed JE, Rumberger JA. Right ventricular dilatation and remodeling the first year after an initial transmural wall myocardial infarction. Am J Cardiol. 1993;72:1126–30.
25. Wolfkiel CJ, Ferguson JL, Chomka EV, Law WR, Labin IN, Tenzer ML, Booker M, Brundage BH. Measurement of myocardial blood flow by ultrafast computed tomography. Circulation. 1987;76:1262–73.
26. Bell RM, Lerman L, Rumberger JA. Validation of minimally invasive measurement of myocardial perfusion using electron beam

computed tomography and application in human volunteers. Heart. 1999;81:628–35.
27. Tannenbaum SR, Kondos GT, Veselik KE, Prendergast MR, Brundage BH, Chomka EV. Detection of calcific deposits in coronary arteries by ultrafast computed tomography and correlation with angiography. Am J Cardiol. 1989;63:870–2.
28. Agatston AS, Janowitz WR, Hilder FJ, Zusmer NR, Viamonte M, Detrano R. Quantification of coronary artery calcium using ultrafast computed tomography. J Am Coll Cardiol. 1990;15:827–32.
29. Stanford W, Rumberger JA. In: Stanford W, Rumberger JA, editors. Ultrafast computed tomographic cardiac imaging: principles and practice. Mt Kisco, NY: Futura Publishing Company; 1992.
30. Kaufmann RB, Sheedy PF 2nd, Maher JE, Bielak LF, Breen JF, Schwartz RS, Peyser PA. Quantity of coronary artery calcium detected by electron beam computed tomography in asymptomatic subjects and angiographically studied patients. Mayo Clin Proc. 1995;70:223–32.
31. Simons DB, Schwartz RS, Edwards WD, Sheedy PF, Breen JF, Rumberger JA. Non-invasive definition of anatomic coronary artery disease by ultrafast CT: a quantitative pathologic study. J Am Coll Cardiol. 1992;20:1118–26.
32. Rumberger JA, Simons DB, Fitzpatrick LA, Sheedy PF, Schwartz RS. Coronary artery calcium areas by electron beam computed tomography and coronary atherosclerotic plaque area: a histopathologic correlative study. Circulation. 1995;92:2157–62.
33. Sangiorgi G, Rumberger JA, Severson A, Edwards WD, Gregoire J, Fitzpatrick LA, Schwartz RS. Arterial calcification and not lumen stenosis is highly correlated with atherosclerotic plaque burden in humans: a histologic study of 723 coronary artery segments using non-decalcifying methodology. J Am Coll Cardiol. 1998;31:126–33.
34. http://www.nytimes.com/2015/02/27/movies/review-the-widow-maker-a-heart-care-documentary.html?_r=0.
35. Moshage W, Achenbach S, Seese B, Bachmann K, Kirchgeorg M. Coronary artery stenoses: three-dimensional imaging with electrocardiographically triggered, contrast-agent enhanced, electron beam CT. Radiology. 1995;196:707–14.
36. Rumberger JA. Non-invasive coronary angiography using CT – ready to kick it up another notch? Circulation. 2002;106:2036–8.

Evolution of Radiation Dose from Cardiac CT

2

Manoj Mannil and Hatem Alkadhi

Cardiac imaging with computed tomography (CT) remains a challenging task requiring both a high spatial resolution for imaging of the relatively small coronary arteries and a high temporal resolution for providing motion-free images of the heart. In parallel to technological advances, tireless efforts to simultaneously reduce radiation dosages were implemented. As in any given body region, these measures are based on the following two principles: restricting the total number of cardiac CT examinations by close adherence to guidelines and recommendations and reducing the radiation of each individual CT study according to the "as low as reasonably achievable" (ALARA) principle while maintaining a diagnostic image quality [1]. This chapter focuses on the latter.

Introduction of various CT protocol developments and software modifications such as tube current modulation, automatic tube potential selection, electrocardiography (ECG) pulsing, and iterative reconstruction enabled the decrease of ionizing radiation dose in one order of magnitude over the last two decades [2] (Table 2.1).

ECG Gating

Cardiac CT imaging must be performed with ECG gating, in order to freeze all images in defined time points of the cardiac cycle. At normal heart rates, least cardiac motion occurs during diastole, when the ventricles are filling. Three

Table 2.1 Abbreviations and terms for cardiac CT imaging

Abbreviations and terms	Description
AEC	Automatic exposure control mechanism for dose optimization in CT, which adapts tube current according to the part of the body being scanned to obtain the desired image quality
CTDI	Computed tomography dose index: Radiation dose of a single slice from the primary beam and scatter from surrounding slices, in milligrays [mGy]
CTDIvol	Computed tomography dose index volume: A measure describing the radiation dose factoring in pitch, which represents the average radiation dose in three dimensions and is typically reported in milligrays [mGy]
DLP	Dose length product reflects the total energy absorbed attributable to a complete CT scan acquisition and is determined by multiplying the CTDIvol by the scan length [mGy*cm]
ECG pulsing	Modulation of the tube current according to the electrocardiogram (ECG). Peak tube output during a selected pulsing window and reduction of the tube output to approximately 25% during remaining parts of the cardiac cycle
IR	Iterative reconstruction: Image reconstruction algorithm that localizes and selectively removes image noise. Repetitive comparison of reconstructed images with a computed expected data set
Pitch	Defined as table distance traveled in one 360° gantry rotation divided by beam collimation in single-slice CT or total thickness of all simultaneously acquired slices in multislice CT
Reconstructed slice thickness	Width of a single slice in the reconstructed image [mm]. The greater the slice thickness, the more X-ray photons are present in the raw data for reconstructing the image, with an effect on image noise similar to that of increasing the tube current
TCM	Tube current modulation automatically adapts the mAs delivered during the CT scan based on patient thickness determined from the topogram

M. Mannil (✉) · H. Alkadhi
Institute of Diagnostic and Interventional Radiology, University Hospital Zurich, Zurich, Switzerland
e-mail: manoj.mannil@usz.ch

U. J. Schoepf (ed.), *CT of the Heart*, Contemporary Medical Imaging, https://doi.org/10.1007/978-1-60327-237-7_2

approaches for ECG gating are currently used: (1) retrospective ECG gating with spiral data acquisition, (2) prospective ECG gating with a sequential (or "step-and-shoot") data acquisition, and (3) prospective ECG gating with spiral data acquisition and high pitch.

Retrospective ECG Gating

In retrospective ECG-gating techniques, partially overlapping multi-detector CT projections are continuously acquired in the spiral mode, and the ECG signal is simultaneously recorded. Software algorithms are then used to sort the data from different phases of the cardiac cycle by progressively shifting the temporal window of acquired helical projection data relative to the R wave (Fig. 2.1). Every position of the heart is covered by a detector row at every point of the cardiac cycle. Therefore, the scanner table continuously moves but advances not more than the total width of the active detectors for each heartbeat [3]. For a gapless volume coverage of the heart in each cardiac phase, a low table feed (pitch <1) is required, which has to be adapted to the heart rate of the patient: the higher the heart rate, the faster the table can move. Using a 4-cm detector enables covering the entire heart volume in 3–4 heartbeats [4]. Due to the low pitch of this imaging technique, the same anatomic area is repeatedly exposed to ionizing radiation during consecutive rotations of the gantry, which results in a relatively higher radiation dose as compared to the other ECG-gating techniques described below. Radiation dose values of up to 21 mSv have been initially reported for this technique with 64-slice CT.

The use of ECG pulsing allows for modulation of the tube current according to the ECG. The peak tube output is generated during a selected pulsing window, usually during diastole. During the remaining parts of the cardiac cycle, the tube output is reduced to approximately 25%. Most scanners allow to adjust the ECG-pulsing window width according to the heart rate, in order to be as narrow as possible for maximal radiation exposure reduction while being as wide as reasonable to obtain diagnostic image quality at the same time [5]. Modern ECG-pulsing algorithms are able to automatically detect arrhythmia and switch off ECG pulsing during ectopic heartbeats.

When combining retrospective ECG gating with optimized tube voltage and tube current in combination with modern iterative reconstruction algorithms, radiation doses can be as low as 4–6 mSv per cardiac CT examination with this technique.

Prospective ECG Gating in the Sequential Mode

Prospective ECG triggering uses the ECG signal to limit scanning to time points defined prior to the data acquisition, usually during diastole. Projection data are acquired during more than half a gantry rotation. The total number of slices produced per heartbeat during this half rotation of the gantry is proportional to the number of rows of active detectors. As

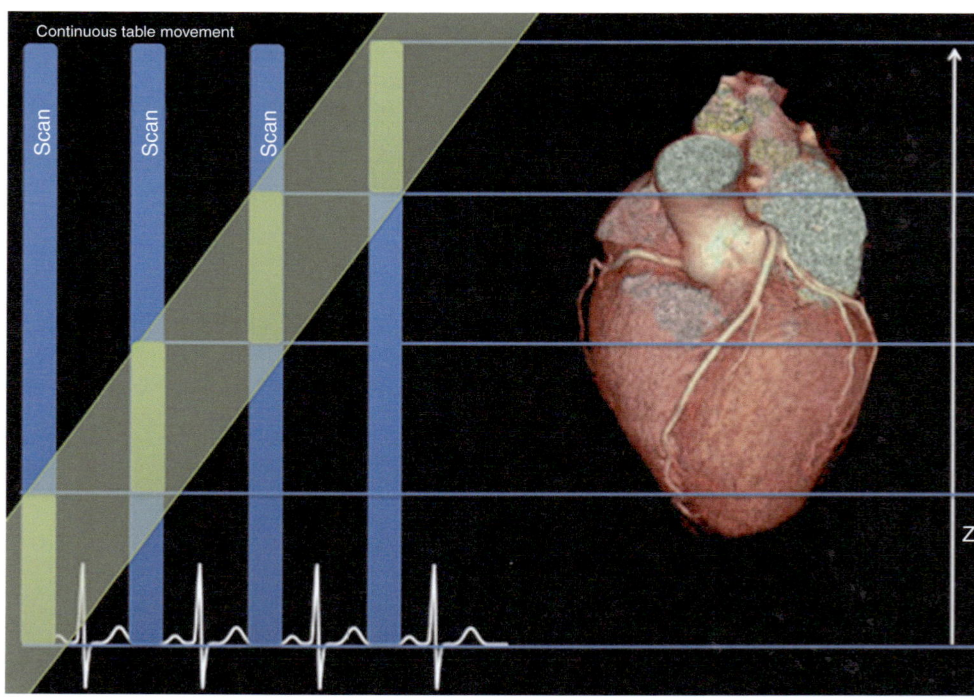

Fig. 2.1 Retrospective ECG-gated cardiac CT in the spiral mode with continuous table movement. The ECG of the patient is schematically shown at the bottom. Data can be retrospectively reconstructed at each after data acquisition at each time point of the cardiac cycle. (Modified from Flohr et al. [4], with permission)

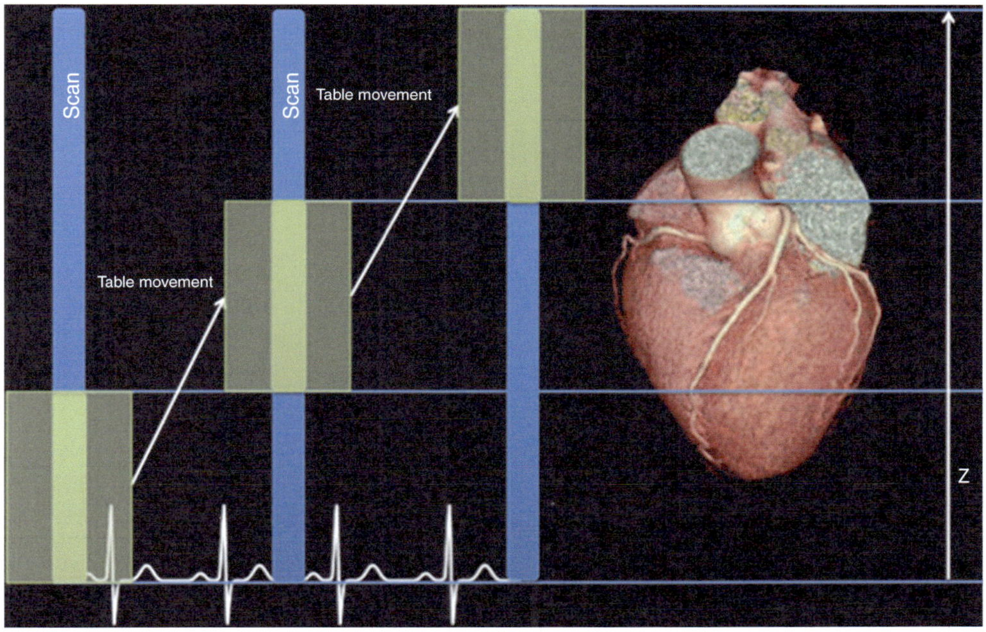

Fig. 2.2 Principle of prospective ECG-gated sequential (or "step-and-shoot") scanning. The ECG of the patient is schematically shown at the bottom. The blue lines indicate the z-positions of the individual detector rows of a multirow detector relative to the patient. Axial (sequential) scan data are acquired with a user-selectable temporal distance to the preceding R wave. After each axial scan, the table moves to the next z-position. Scan data are typically acquired at every second heartbeat. (Modified from Flohr et al. [4], with permission)

axial (rather than helical) scanning is used, the table is not moving during but only in-between data acquisition. The table has to move by the total collimation width after each acquisition (sequential or "step-and-shoot" mode) (Fig. 2.2). About 12 cm of scanning in the z-axis is required to cover most adult hearts; the total number of heartbeats and number of image stacks for a cardiac CT study depend on the width of the detector. However, as the scan is sequentially obtained, there is minimal flexibility in retrospectively choosing different phases of the cardiac cycle for image reconstruction. This minimal flexibility can be circumvented by using the technique of "padding." Padding allows for acquisition of images in additional cardiac phases by extending the mandatory minimum acquisition time. There is a trade-off between acquisition flexibility and radiation dose. Extensive use of padding is associated with a greater radiation dose. For instance, a 100 millisecond increase in padding results in a 45% increase in radiation dose [6]. A recent meta-analysis showed that prospective ECG gating is associated with an average radiation dose of 2.7 mSv [7]. Currently, prospective ECG gating is the most widely used technique for data acquisition in cardiac CT [2, 8].

Prospective ECG Gating with Spiral Acquisition and High Pitch

Since the commercial launch of dual-source CT technology in 2005, further reduction of ionizing radiation was achieved through use of prospective ECG gating with high pitch. In this mode, data is acquired in a spiral fashion, while the table runs with a high pitch (e.g., 3.2 with third-generation dual-source CT, equivalent to a table feed of 737 cm/s).

Using this technique yields a "snapshot" scan of the entire heart within one cardiac cycle, usually during diastole. While pitch in a single-source CT is limited to values of approximately 1.5 to ensure gapless volume coverage along the z-axis, a dual-source CT system contains a second X-ray tube at 90° offset, which acquires scan data at the same angular position at a quarter rotation later. This facilitates a maximum pitch of 3.2–3.4, depending on the scanner generation, within a limited scan field of view (FOV) covered by both detectors (Fig. 2.3). A quarter rotation of data per measurement system is used for image reconstruction, and each individual axial image has a temporal resolution of a quarter of the gantry rotation time. The ECG is used to prospectively trigger the start of table motion and the start of the high-pitch spiral. A requirement for usage of this technique is generally a stable sinus rhythm with heart rates ≤60 bpm with second-generation dual-source CT and ≤70 bpm with third-generation dual-source CT (Fig. 2.4).

The effective radiation dose of a prospectively ECG-gated high-pitch cardiac CT can be well below 1 mSv [9, 10]. In contrast to prospective ECG gating, where additional X-ray exposure along the entire width of the detector is generated at every slice, the high-pitch mode generates superfluous X-rays exposing the entire width of the detector only at the beginning and at the end of the spiral path. This explains the further reduction of radiation exposure when using this mode [1].

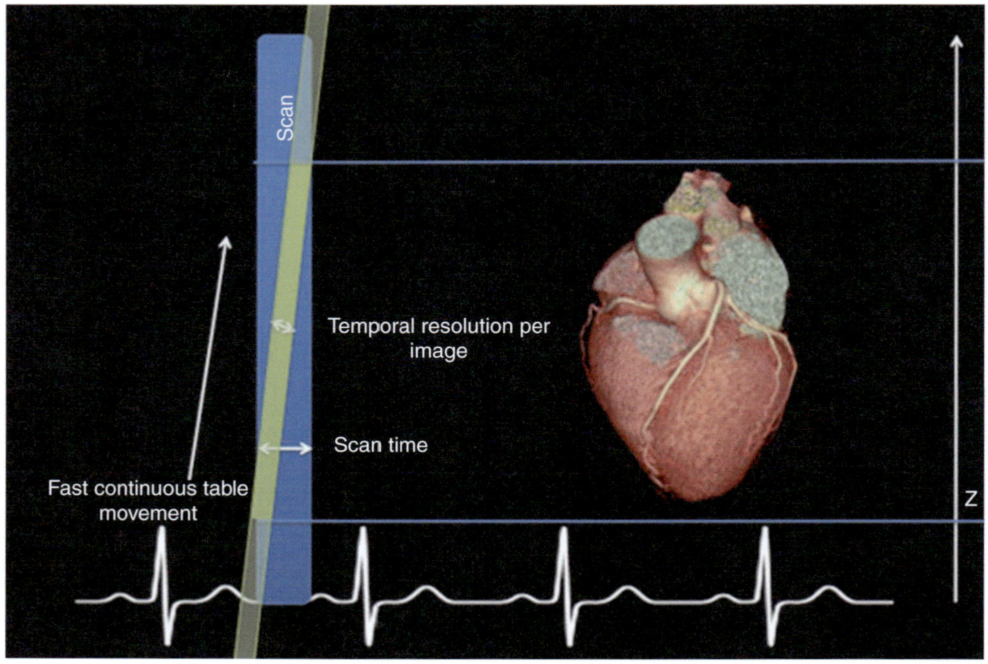

Fig. 2.3 ECG-gated high-pitch mode. The ECG of the patient is schematically shown at the bottom. The table is moved at very high speed, sufficient to cover the entire heart volume within a single diastole. At each z-position, only the minimum amount of scan data necessary for image reconstruction is acquired. The temporal resolution per image is therefore close to a quarter of the gantry rotation time; and there is a slight phase shift of the reconstructed images along the z-axis. (Modified from Flohr et al. [4], with permission)

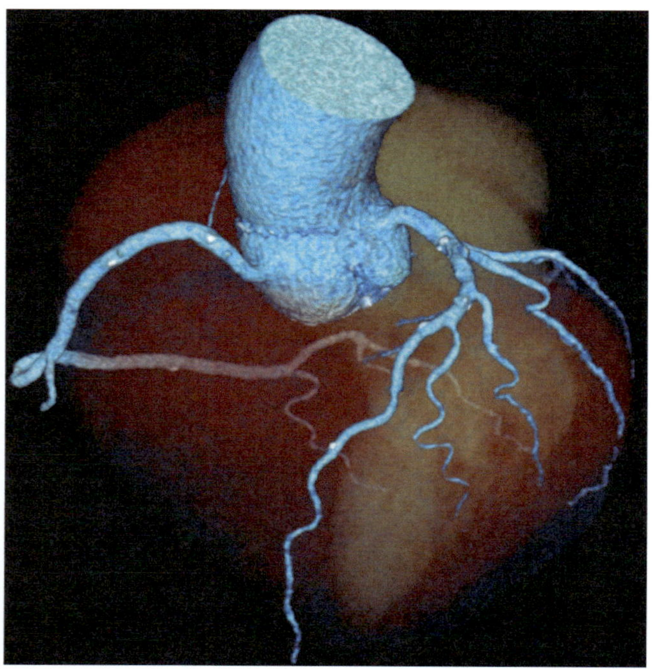

Fig. 2.4 3D image of the coronary artery tree with volume rendering of image data acquired with the high-pitch mode on a third-generation dual-source CT scanner. Estimated effective radiation dose was 0.4 mSv

Tube Current Modulation and Tube Voltage Adaptation

Both tube current modulation and tube voltage adaptation can be used for all scan protocols described above. Tube current modulation is defined as automatic adjustment of the tube current to account for differences in body shape and attenuation depending on the body region scanned. Lowering and optimizing the tube voltage represent another important approach for dose reduction, as radiation dose varies with the square of the tube voltage. Initial investigations with 16-/64-slice CT systems comparing 120- and 100-kV tube voltage CT protocols have shown that decreased tube voltages reduce overall radiation dose at the expense of increased image noise. The signal-to-noise (SNR) and contrast-to-noise ratios (CNR), however, remain unaffected, as decreased tube voltages approach the k-edge of iodine (33.2 keV), which results in higher attenuation of iodinated contrast. With an increase in both parameters, signal/contrast and noise, the overall ratios for SNR and CNR remain unaffected [11–13]. Recently, automatic tube potential selection algorithms became available which automatically lower the tube potential according to patient size, diagnostic task, and scanner tube current limits. This measurement is reported to yield a dose reduction between 20% and 50% in nonobese patient populations. For larger patients, however, image quality may deteriorate beyond diagnostic quality [14].

Iterative Reconstruction (IR)

Iterative reconstruction (IR) is a technique that incorporates statistical modeling in image reconstruction with the main aim to reduce image noise. This technique can be also used for reducing the radiation dose (usually through reduced tube current) while maintaining the image quality of the examination [1, 10]. Similar to the options tube current modulation and tube voltage adaptation, IR can be applied for all scan protocols described above.

Filtered Back Projection (FBP)

Until recently, CT images were almost exclusively reconstructed with filtered back projection (FBP), largely due to the fact that FBP generates diagnostic images at a low level of computational complexity. In FBP the X-ray beam assumes a pencil shape, and the X-ray source is aligned in a parallel fashion to a linear X-ray detector array. For image generation, the X-ray source is rotated over a certain angle, allowing for intensities to be measured at the detector. These intensities are described as an integral function for a specific angle and the shift in the position of the X-ray tube. After this, the reconstruction process involves solving an integral equation by inversion or so-called back projection. Despite its ability to rapidly reconstruct images, FBP has various limitations, in particular increased image noise, which is most prominent in low tube current imaging, poor contrast resolution, and streak artifacts. This is primarily due to the inherent failure of the FBP algorithm to account for image noise that results from Poisson statistical variations in the number of photons across the imaging plane, leading to an inverse relationship between radiation dose and image noise. Until the recent introduction of IR, lowering image noise could only be achieved at the expense of increased radiation dose. Attempts at so-called image-based denoising through smoothing algorithms and filters (convolution kernels) allow for noise reduction but result in compromised spatial resolution and image fidelity [15].

Iterative Reconstruction (IR)

In principle, IR techniques attempt to localize and selectively remove image noise by frequent comparison with a canvas. This is achieved through a process of modeling the imaging acquisition process, including fluctuations in photon statistics, the optics system, and various aspects of X-ray interactions to generate an expected data set, which is then compared to the actually acquired data set. The differences between these two are used to identify and remove noise, and the process is repeated multiple times until the updated data converges with or approximates the expected data to maximize image optimization.

Initially, *statistical* IR was introduced in CT imaging. It deals with noise due to fluctuations in photon statistics by assigning a relatively higher weighting to data with low statistical uncertainty (low noise) and lesser weighting to data with high statistical uncertainty (high noise). It operates in either the "raw data domain" with subsequent reconstruction using the "noise-reduced" data or in the "image domain" after IR. More recently, IR algorithms that model for the physical three-dimensional nature of the system optics (geometric modeling of the focal point of the X-ray tube and pixel detector) and the interaction of photons in the transmission between the X-ray tube, isocenter, and detector (physical modeling) have been developed and are collectively referred to as model-based IR [15]. Current IR algorithms typically combine statistical modeling with model-based IR. In hybrid IR algorithms, the imaging data can be blended with traditional FBP at certain thresholds. The iteratively reconstructed CT images are generally less noisy and possess an improved image resolution and edge detection compared to images acquired with FBP (Fig. 2.5).

Due to this circumstance, diagnostic images can be achieved even at lower tube currents when using IR instead of FBP, and radiation exposure can be significantly decreased. Many studies have evaluated noise and dose reduction with IR algorithms across multiple vendors (Table 2.2). In summary they demonstrate either (1) improved noise properties with IR compared to FBP when images from the same patients are reconstructed using both algorithms (intraindividual analysis) or (2) preserved subjective image quality and quantitative noise properties among patients undergoing IR image reconstruction with low-radiation dose techniques (reduced tube current and/or potential) compared to FBP algorithms with standard dose techniques (interindividual analysis). For instance, performing prospectively ECG-gated high-pitch coronary angiography with third-generation dual-source CT and using advanced modeled IT at a 70 kVp tube voltage result in a reduced image noise and improved overall image quality compared to standard FBP reconstructions at an average effective dose of only 0.3 mSv [15, 16].

Limiting the Scan Length

Limiting the scan length, or z-axis coverage, to exactly encompass the heart and coronary arteries represents another important factor for reducing the radiation dose cardiac CT. Traditionally, each cardiac CT examination starts with acquisition of a scout view for planning the scan length of the examination. It is a common practice to obtain an unenhanced low-dose calcium scoring scan, whose scan length is usually planned on the scout view. Then, contrast-enhanced CT coronary angiography is performed for diagnosing or excluding coronary artery stenoses. Due to the limited anatomic information provided by the scout view, the exact cranio-caudal extent of the coronary arteries cannot be discerned on a scout view. Therefore, the region of the carina is frequently used as the upper border and the cardiac apex as the lower border of the scan length of CT coronary angiography.

Alternatively, scan length can be determined by using the axial images from calcium scoring for identifying the table position at the origin of the left main artery and that

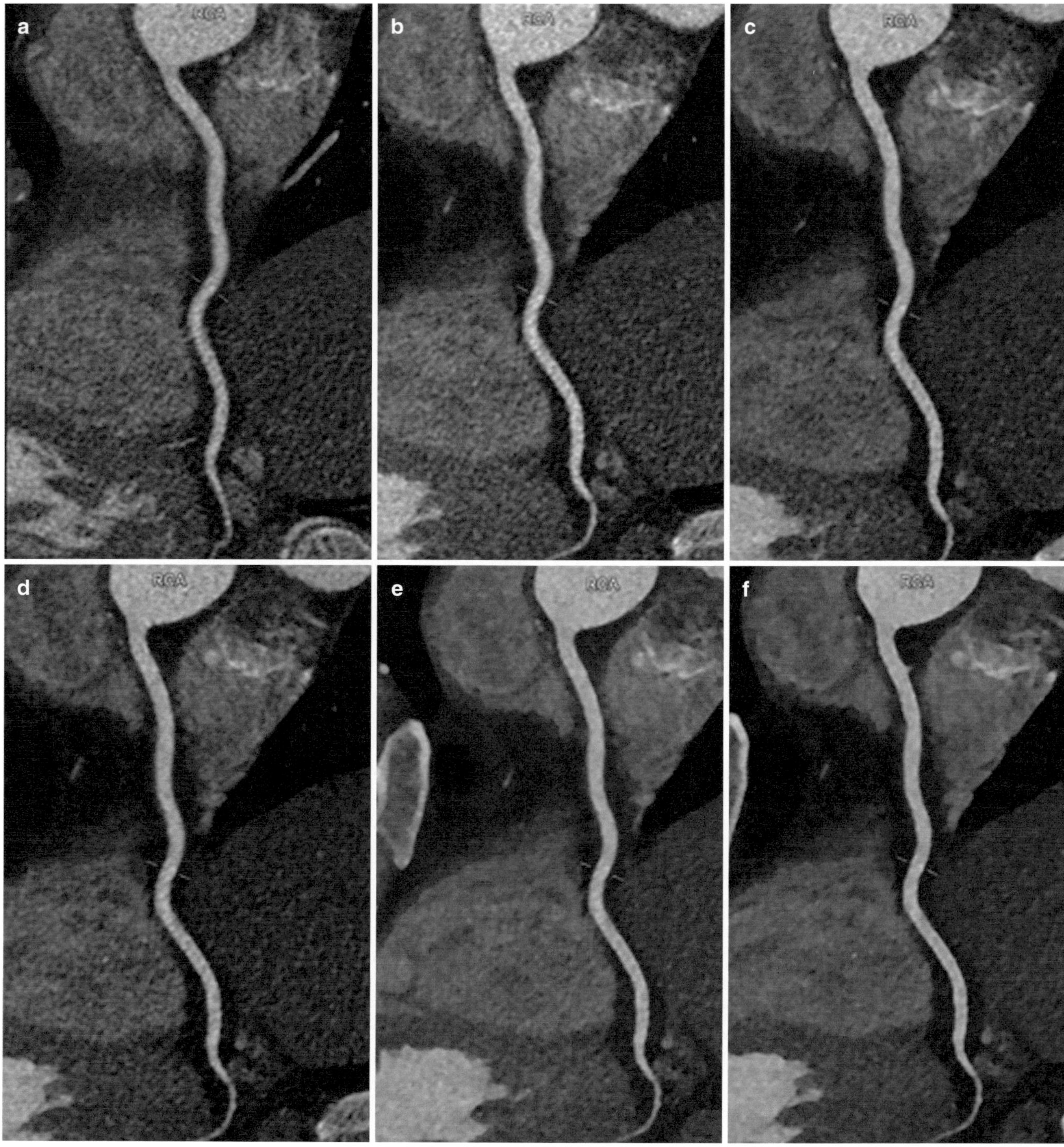

Fig. 2.5 Multiplanar reformations of the right coronary artery using (**a**) filtered back projection (FBP), (**b**) advanced modeled iterative reconstruction (ADMIRE) strength level 1, (**c**) ADMIRE strength level 2, (**d**) ADMIRE strength level 3, (**e**) ADMIRE strength level 4, (**f**) ADMIRE strength level 5. Note the continuous decrease of image noise and the improved vessel sharpness from FBP to ADMIRE images

Table 2.2 Iterative reconstruction algorithms by vendor

Iterative reconstruction technique	Vendor	Type
Adaptive statistical iterative reconstruction (ASIR)	General Electric (GE) Healthcare	Hybrid
Model-based iterative reconstruction (MBIR-Veo)	General Electric (GE) Healthcare	Model-based
Adaptive statistical iterative reconstruction (ASIR-V)	General Electric (GE) Healthcare	Hybrid
iDose	Philips Healthcare	Hybrid
Iterative model reconstruction (IMR)	Philips Healthcare	Model-based
Iterative reconstruction in image space (IRIS)	Siemens Healthcare	Hybrid
Sinogram-affirmed iterative reconstruction (SAFIRE)	Siemens Healthcare	Hybrid
Advanced modeled iterative reconstruction (ADMIRE)	Siemens Healthcare	Hybrid
Adaptive iterative dose reduction (AIDR)	Toshiba	Hybrid
Adaptive iterative dose reduction 3D (AIDR 3D)	Toshiba	Hybrid

of the cardiac apex. The scan length for CT coronary angiography can be then planned by adding around 1 cm to the cranial and around 1 cm to the lower border to account for possible changes in inspiration depth between calcium scoring and CT coronary angiography. Using this approach might lead to another reduction of radiation exposure of around 16% [17].

Clinical Relevance of Dose Reduction and Cancer Risk

Raised awareness of medical practitioners and stringent application of the aforementioned dose reduction techniques have been proven to be effective. Cardiac CT is well established for certain indications, e.g., for ruling out obstructive coronary artery disease at a low-to-intermediate pretest probability [18]. For determining whether all efforts in minimizing ionizing radiation are relevant requires comparison of the clinical benefit of the CT examination with the potential and theoretical cancerogenic risk of the procedure.

Reports on cancer risk in medical imaging are mainly derived from extrapolations of risk estimates to low levels of radiation and multiplications with a large number of exposed individuals. However, the data extrapolation is not reliable below an exposure of 100 mSv. Therefore, various different hypotheses about extrapolation of radiation risk to lower radiation doses were formulated, including a linear no-threshold model which indicates that each level of radiation is associated with a risk to the patient and that there is no lower threshold for this risk. Still, the American Association of Physicists in Medicine considers risks of medical imaging at effective doses <50 mSv for single procedures or <100 mSv for multiple procedures over short-time periods as too low to be epidemiologically detectable. While there is no evidence between radiation from medical imaging and cancer induction in a general adult population, it is in the best interests of the patients to keep the ionizing radiation exposure ALARA, without loss of diagnostic information.

Summary

Recent technological advances in cardiac CT imaging, ranging from automated exposure control, tube voltage optimization, scan length adjustments, evolution of ECG-gating techniques, and iterative reconstruction post-processing, have reduced radiation doses in one order of magnitude over the last decade. Continuous efforts in the optimal selection of each of the techniques help in keeping the radiation exposure to each individual adult patient so low that the assumed theoretical radiation risk from cardiac CT can be neglected.

References

1. Alkadhi H, Leschka S. Radiation dose of cardiac computed tomography - what has been achieved and what needs to be done. Eur Radiol. 2011;21(3):505–9.
2. den Harder AM, Willemink MJ, de Jong PA, Schilham AM, Rajiah P, Takx RA, et al. New horizons in cardiac CT. Clin Radiol. 2016;71(8):758–67.
3. Desjardins B, Kazerooni EA. ECG-gated cardiac CT. AJR Am J Roentgenol. 2004;182(4):993–1010.
4. Flohr TG, De Cecco CN, Schmidt B, Wang R, Schoepf UJ, Meinel FG. Computed tomographic assessment of coronary artery disease: state-of-the-art imaging techniques. Radiol Clin North Am. 2015;53(2):271–85.
5. Leschka S, Scheffel H, Desbiolles L, Plass A, Gaemperli O, Valenta I, et al. Image quality and reconstruction intervals of dual-source CT coronary angiography: recommendations for ECG-pulsing windowing. Investig Radiol. 2007;42(8):543–9.
6. Labounty TM, Leipsic J, Min JK, Heilbron B, Mancini GB, Lin FY, et al. Effect of padding duration on radiation dose and image interpretation in prospectively ECG-triggered coronary CT angiography. AJR Am J Roentgenol. 2010;194(4):933–7.
7. von Ballmoos MW, Haring B, Juillerat P, Alkadhi H. Meta-analysis: diagnostic performance of low-radiation-dose coronary computed tomography angiography. Ann Intern Med. 2011;154(6):413–20.
8. Menke J, Unterberg-Buchwald C, Staab W, Sohns JM, Seif Amir Hosseini A, Schwarz A. Head-to-head comparison of prospectively

triggered vs retrospectively gated coronary computed tomography angiography: meta-analysis of diagnostic accuracy, image quality, and radiation dose. Am Heart J. 2013;165(2):154–63. e3.
9. Meyer M, Haubenreisser H, Schoepf UJ, Vliegenthart R, Leidecker C, Allmendinger T, et al. Closing in on the K edge: coronary CT angiography at 100, 80, and 70 kV-initial comparison of a second- versus a third-generation dual-source CT system. Radiology. 2014;273(2):373–82.
10. Gordic S, Desbiolles L, Sedlmair M, Manka R, Plass A, Schmidt B, et al. Optimizing radiation dose by using advanced modelled iterative reconstruction in high-pitch coronary CT angiography. Eur Radiol. 2016;26(2):459–68.
11. Leschka S, Stolzmann P, Schmid FT, Scheffel H, Stinn B, Marincek B, et al. Low kilovoltage cardiac dual-source CT: attenuation, noise, and radiation dose. Eur Radiol. 2008;18(9):1809–17.
12. Hausleiter J, Martinoff S, Hadamitzky M, Martuscelli E, Pschierer I, Feuchtner GM, et al. Image quality and radiation exposure with a low tube voltage protocol for coronary CT angiography results of the PROTECTION II Trial. JACC Cardiovasc Imaging. 2010;3(11):1113–23.
13. Hausleiter J, Meyer T, Hadamitzky M, Huber E, Zankl M, Martinoff S, et al. Radiation dose estimates from cardiac multislice computed tomography in daily practice: impact of different scanning protocols on effective dose estimates. Circulation. 2006;113(10):1305–10.
14. Park YJ, Kim YJ, Lee JW, Kim HY, Hong YJ, Lee HJ, et al. Automatic Tube Potential Selection with Tube Current Modulation (APSCM) in coronary CT angiography: comparison of image quality and radiation dose with conventional body mass index-based protocol. J Cardiovasc Comput Tomogr. 2012;6(3):184–90.
15. Naoum C, Blanke P, Leipsic J. Iterative reconstruction in cardiac CT. J Cardiovasc Comput Tomogr. 2015;9(4):255–63.
16. Hell MM, Bittner D, Schuhbaeck A, Muschiol G, Brand M, Lell M, et al. Prospectively ECG-triggered high-pitch coronary angiography with third-generation dual-source CT at 70 kVp tube voltage: feasibility, image quality, radiation dose, and effect of iterative reconstruction. J Cardiovasc Comput Tomogr. 2014;8(6):418–25.
17. Leschka S, Kim CH, Baumueller S, Stolzmann P, Scheffel H, Marincek B, et al. Scan length adjustment of CT coronary angiography using the calcium scoring scan: effect on radiation dose. AJR Am J Roentgenol. 2010;194(3):W272–7.
18. Hausleiter J, Meyer T, Hermann F, Hadamitzky M, Krebs M, Gerber TC, et al. Estimated radiation dose associated with cardiac CT angiography. JAMA. 2009;301(5):500–7.

The Long March into Clinical Practice: Cardiac CT and Its Competitors

3

Seth Uretsky, Alan Rozanski, and Daniel Berman

In the early twentieth century, control of infectious diseases, increasing longevity, and poor lifestyles resulted in chronic diseases becoming the major cause of disability and death [1]. By the 1920s, coronary artery disease (CAD) became the leading cause of death in the United States. As treatments emerged to treat CAD, it became important to develop means for identifying those patients at risk for developing the disease and its complications. Initial diagnostic work in this regard was initiated even prior to the advent of exercise electrocardiography. In the 1920s, Master developed his famous "two-step" stress test [2], which allowed physicians to assess patients' functional capacity in a semiquantitative manner and to provoke angina symptoms through physical activity. In the 1950s, treadmill testing was implemented, and in 1963, Robert Bruce published his protocol for performing graded multistage treadmill exercise with electrocardiographic monitoring [3], a protocol that is still used today. This development of the Bruce protocol treadmill exercise was timely since the 1960s saw the introduction of cardiac catheterization and coronary bypass surgery. With this dramatic new treatment option, a need emerged to accurately identify those patients who were at risk for cardiac events and thus potential beneficiaries of coronary artery bypass surgery.

Epidemiological study in the 1960s and 1970s refined the use of exercise electrocardiography for diagnostic and prognostic testing [4]. Various aspects of the exercise electrocardiographic response were identified as predictors of adverse outcomes, including the magnitude, time to onset, and postexercise duration of exercise ST segment depression. In addition, patients' overall exercise capacity, as assessed by exercise duration during Bruce protocol exercise ECG, was found to be a potent predictor of patient risk [5].

In the mid-1970s, the field of cardiac imaging emerged due to the introduction of radionuclide imaging techniques. Since then, the field of noninvasive cardiac imaging has grown markedly. Today, many different forms of noninvasive tests can be used for the work-up and management of patients in clinical practice, as listed in Table 3.1. While these tests vary markedly in their capabilities, they remain focused on three principal needs in cardiology: (1) to screen for latent CAD in asymptomatic subjects, (2) to establish the presence or absence of CAD in patients presenting with chest pain symptoms (diagnostic testing), and/or (3) to evaluate patients' clinical risk for developing future cardiac events (prognostic testing). Herein, we review the development of these imaging modalities and the future competition that will shape how these modalities will be used in clinical practice.

The Advent of Nuclear Cardiology

The first cardiac imaging approach to be applied for diagnostic and prognostic testing was exercise-rest myocardial perfusion imaging (MPI). This new imaging technology became possible due to the application of gamma-emitting monovalent cations which could be actively extracted by the myocardium, such as potassium-43 [6], and its analogues, rubidium-81 [7] and thallium-201 [8]. The initial uptake of these analogues was found to correlate with the distribution of myocardial blood flow over a wide range of flow rates, making these agents well suited for cardiac imaging at stress as well as during rest imaging. Redistribution thallium-201 imaging became a useful method for assessing myocardial viability. Exercise MPI, initially employed using a planar technique, was soon shown to have both higher sensitivity

S. Uretsky (✉)
Department of Cardiovascular Medicine, Gagnon Cardiovascular Institute, Morristown Medical Center, Morristown, NJ, USA
e-mail: seth.uretsky@atlantichealth.org

A. Rozanski
Department of Cardiovascular Medicine, Gagnon Cardiovascular Institute, Morristown Medical Center, Morristown, NJ, USA

The Division of Cardiology, Mount Sinai St. Luke's Hospital, Mount Sinai Heart, New York, NY, USA

D. Berman
Department of Imaging and Medicine and the Burns Allen Research Institute, Cedars-Sinai Medical Center, Los Angeles, CA, USA

U. J. Schoepf (ed.), *CT of the Heart*, Contemporary Medical Imaging, https://doi.org/10.1007/978-1-60327-237-7_3

Table 3.1 Noninvasive techniques for the work-up of patients

Exercise electrocardiography
Stress-rest myocardial SPECT perfusion imaging
Stress-rest position emission tomography
Exercise radionuclide ventriculography
Stress echocardiography
Stress magnetic resonance imaging (MRI)
Coronary artery calcium scanning
Coronary computed tomography angiography
Carotid ultrasound
Femoral ultrasound

and specificity than its then only competitor for the detection of CAD – exercise ECG. In the early days of nuclear cardiology imaging, another radionuclide technique, exercise radionuclide ventriculography (RNV), performed by using either the first pass or multiple-gated equilibrium technique, was also found to have higher sensitivity and specificity than exercise ECG. Then, after the advent of single-photon emission computed tomography (SPECT) MPI in the early 1980s, exercise SPECT-MPI became favored over both exercise planar MPI and exercise RNV, due to this technique's enhanced ability to size the magnitude of stress-induced myocardial ischemia. Alongside these developments was the creation of semiquantitative and quantitative scoring systems to determine the severity of perfusion defects on SPECT-MPI as well as software that allowed for easy processing, display, and analysis of the images. A universal scoring system helped decrease inter- and intra-observer variability and effective communication of results.

Other important developments in the 1980s included the introduction of PET imaging for assessing myocardial perfusion and myocardial viability, the initiation of pharmacologic testing with dipyridamole for those patients who could not exercise, and the development of Tc-99m sestamibi and tetrofosmin, which considerably improved image quality due to the shorter half-life of Tc-99m versus thallium-201 which allowed for higher injected doses which led to improved image quality. Subsequently, the development of ECG-gated SPECT imaging in the mid-1990s introduced the assessment of left ventricular ejection fraction and regional wall motion analysis, which could be assessed in myocardial segments containing myocardial perfusion defects [9].

A further key component of the growth of nuclear cardiology studies was the inclusion of scientists and clinicians in the field, with the scientists helping emphasize the importance of standardization of acquisition and processing methods and providing development of objective quantitative analysis methods which provided a "second expert opinion" in interpretation. These methods were first developed for planar imaging methods [10] and then subsequently were applied in SPECT-MPI [11]. For the latter, the advent of the polar map, with comparison of a patient's studies to normal limits, allowed easy appreciation of the presence and location of perfusion defects. The quantitation became a standard part of the imaging methods.

As investigators and clinicians became seasoned in the application of nuclear cardiology, they established many principles regarding the correct validation of testing. Three principles that are particularly applicable to the tests which have since followed are reviewed below.

Characterizing the Full Extent of Test Abnormality

Investigators in nuclear cardiology sought from the onset to evaluate all potential information that could be derived from the scintigraphic images. Early work established that the extent of perfusion defects (i.e., the area of ischemic myocardium) and the severity of perfusion defects (ranging from very mild abnormality to the complete absence of uptake) provided complementary and independent information. For example, in a follow-up of 1689 diagnostic patients who underwent exercise thallium-201 MPI, Ladenheim et al. [12] found that both the number and severity of perfusion defects within six myocardial regions were related to adverse cardiac outcomes; when both extensive and severe ischemia were present, adverse events increased in exponential fashion (Fig. 3.1). Other examples of ischemic parameters that could be used to characterize the presence of either extensive or severe ischemia for thallium-201 MPI, sestamibi MPI, or stress echo are shown in Table 3.2. For example, the identification of transient ischemic dilation was identified as a variable that predicted both extensive and severe CAD [13], with extensive ischemia needed to induce left ventricular dilation postexercise and severe ischemia needed to maintain dilation during the postexercise phase.

To convey the information regarding ischemic extent and severity to physicians, investigators developed routine semiquantitative analysis of MPI studies based on the visual scoring of the degree of radiotracer reduction in each segment of the myocardium. This led to the further development of summed segmental scores at stress, rest, and their difference [14]. A later development was the conversion of these scores into a percent of the myocardium involved for ischemia and total defect severity [15], first based on a 0–4 scoring of 20 myocardial segments and later, of 17 segments.

Combining Clinical and Physiological Data

The combined assessment of clinical and imaging data can also improve risk assessment. This point was also well illustrated by the abovementioned study by Ladenheim et al. (see Fig. 3.1) [12]. For any given level of ischemia, the cardiac event rate was increased approximately threefold among

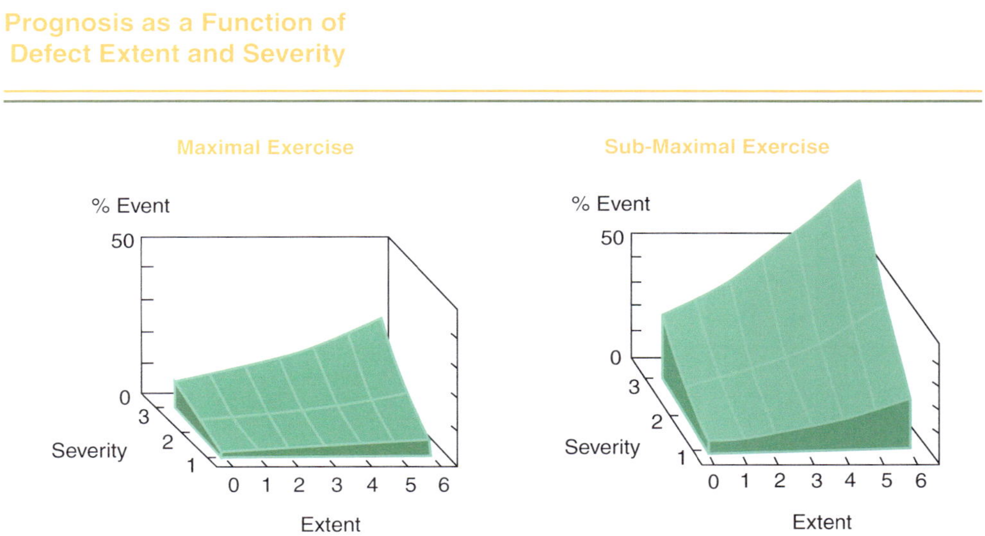

Fig. 3.1 Frequency of cardiac events on the orthogonal z axis according to the extent of myocardial ischemia, ranging from 0 to 6 myocardial zones (x axis); the severity of defects, ranging from none (score of 0) to severe (score of 3) on the y axis; and the patients are divided according to those who showed both for patients achieving >85% of maximal predicted heart rate (left graph) and those achieving <85% of maximal predicted heart rate (right graph). The extent and severity of ischemia were both independently correlated to cardiac event rates. (From Ladenheim et al. [12], with permission)

Table 3.2 Extent and severity of ischemia parameters

Study	Ischemic	
	Extent	Severity
Number of perfusion defects	++++	
Severity of perfusion defects		++++
Lung thallium-20 uptake	+++	+
Delayed thallium redistribution		++++
Stunned myocardium on gated SPECT		++++
Transient ischemic dilation of the LV	++++	++++
Number of stress-induced WMA	++++	
Severity of WMA		++++
Decrease in LVEF	+++	++

those patients who could not exercise to at least 85% of their maximal predicted heart rate on treadmill exercise. Today, many patients are studied by pharmacologic stress due to an inability to exercise. The mere inability to perform treadmill exercise also increases mortality risk by at least twofold compared to patients who can exercise (Fig. 3.2) [16]. The further consideration of CAD risk factors does not generally influence short-term risk assessment, but it plays an important role in complementing the results of stress testing for predicting long-term risk (Fig. 3.3) [17, 18].

The Assessment of Incremental Information

The early investigators in nuclear cardiology recognized that it was insufficient to merely demonstrate that radionuclide imaging had superior test sensitivity and specificity compared to exercise ECG. Rather, they also addressed whether nuclear stress testing added to risk prediction when all of the more readily available clinical information and results of exercise electrocardiography were first factored into their risk analysis. Analyses of multiple patient populations consistently demonstrated that radionuclide imaging provided substantial additional risk prediction [19, 20]. Since then, the demonstration of incremental information is on the basis by which any new imaging modality is evaluated.

Finally, a key component of the growth of nuclear cardiology was the formation in 1993 of the American Society of Nuclear Cardiology (ASNC). The organization, formed predominantly by cardiologists, became an advocate for the method and laid the ground work for cardiologists employing the novel methods as part of their own clinical armamentarium—as occurred with echocardiography. The ASNC had a profound effect on the success of the field.

Summarizing key components of the success of nuclear cardiology might be the following: (1) recognition of the need for comprehensive databases containing clinical ECG, and comprehensive nuclear variables regarding the extent and severity of ischemia and scarring and follow-up for cardiac events, resulting in a large body of published evidence regarding diagnosis and prognosis and the incremental information in large patient populations could be reported; (2) recognition of the need for standardization of methodology for acquisition and processing and interpretation, along with automated quantitative analytic tools; (3) the development of vasodilator stress so that the method could be utilized in patients who could not exercise; (4) prominent role played

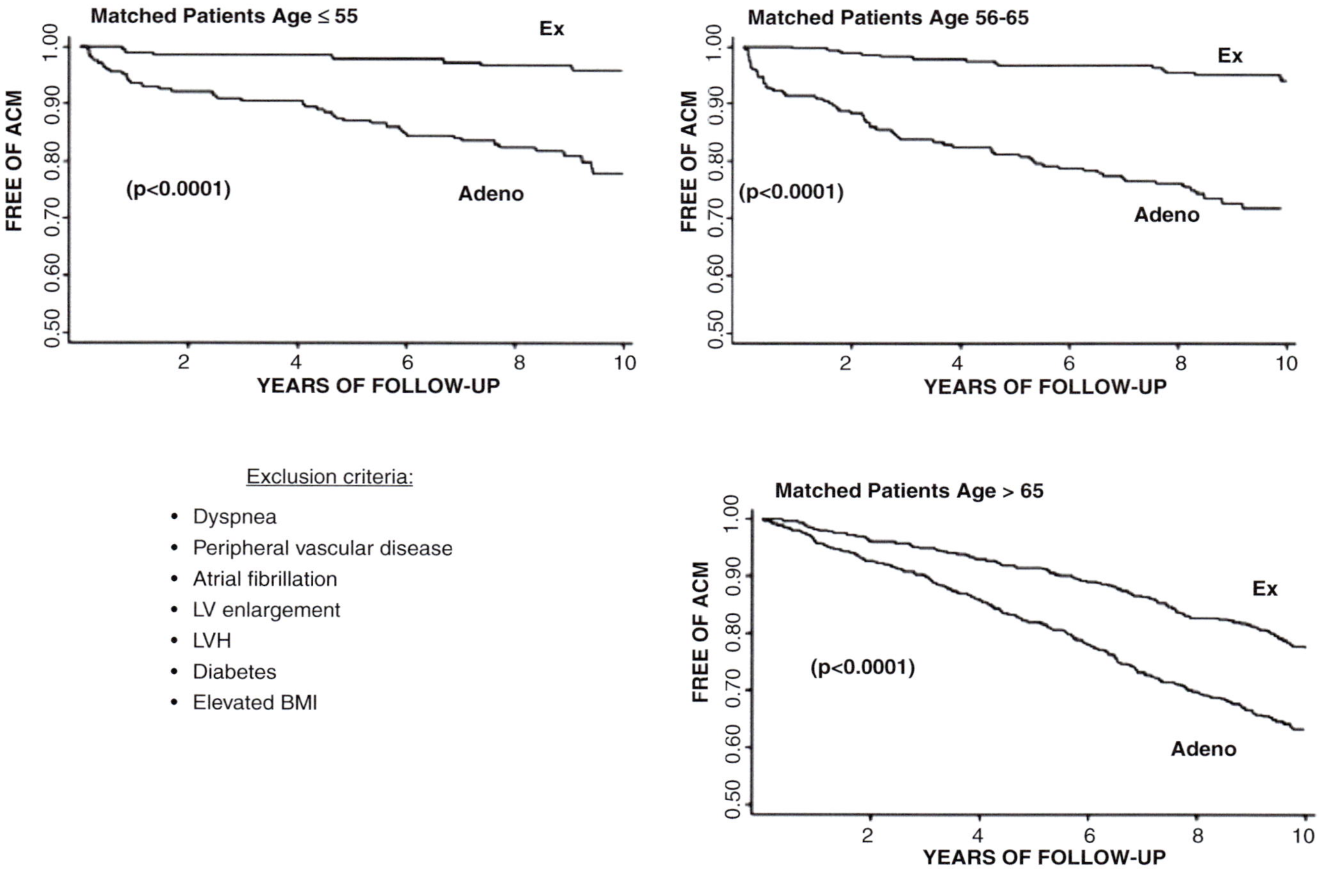

Fig. 3.2 Comparison of cumulative survival among exercise and adenosine patients with normal SPECT-MPI studies who were risk factor-matched using propensity analysis. The patients were subdivided by age. (From Rozanski et al. [16], with permission)

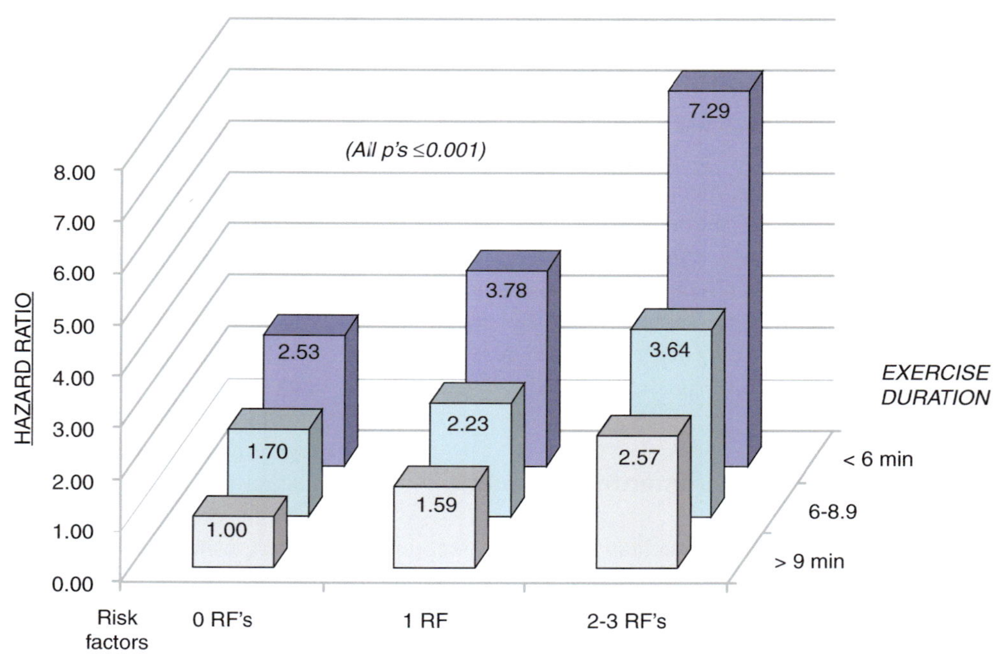

Fig. 3.3 Age- and gender-adjusted hazard ratios for all-cause mortality according to a number of CAD risk factors among patients with normal SPECT-MPI study, divided according to exercise duration. (From Rozanski et al. [17], with permission)

by clinical cardiologists who control the patient referrals; and (5) the development of a professional society that could be an advocate for all aspects of the field.

The Advent of Stress Echocardiography

Resting echocardiography has long been a mainstay for the evaluation of cardiac structure and function, valvular heart disease, congenital heart disease, cardiac masses, and pericardial disease. In the 1980s, postexercise stress echocardiography was introduced as a new method for evaluating patients, followed later by the application of echocardiography during dobutamine infusion. Because stress echocardiography lagged approximately 5–10 years behind the introduction of nuclear cardiology, the application of this technology was able to rely heavily on the principles established by nuclear cardiology for its own validation. For example, just like with the extent and severity perfusion defects, the extent and severity of stress-induced echocardiographic wall motion abnormalities proved to be potent predictors of patient risk [21]. Generally, stress echocardiography has become employed for similar clinical indications and in the same general populations as stress radionuclide imaging. Among differences between the methods are the commercial availability of validated quantitative analytic methods for nuclear cardiology methods, perceived less dependence on the operator expertise, and ease with which the method can be applied to patients who cannot exercise using vasodilator stress.

The Advent of Magnetic Resonance Imaging (MRI)

MRI applications for cardiovascular disease were first developed in the 1980s and began to be applied clinically in the 1990s. MRI has a number of clinical utilities. First, MRI has the ability to differentiate different types of soft tissue from each other and assess and quantify myocardial fibrosis/scar and edema. Second, because of its ability to image the entire chest in any imaging plane, MRI has become a gold standard for assessing left and right ventricular structure and function. Third, MRI can be used for assessment of cardiovascular masses, valvular heart disease, and cardiac masses. Fourth, the development of myocardial delayed enhancement techniques allowed MRI to become a mainstay in assessing myocardial viability and the assessment of cardiomyopathies.

In addition, MRI had also been used as an alternative method to assess patients during pharmacologic stress. Stress MRI techniques can be applied in either of two ways: (1) use of perfusion techniques such as those developed in nuclear cardiology and (2) use of wall motion techniques as developed for stress echocardiography. Either stress technique, combined with the functional and viability images, gives the clinician the ability to assess wall motion, myocardial viability/scar, and myocardial ischemia in one test.

Despite the broad capabilities of cardiac MRI and its introduction only a decade after nuclear cardiology methods, it remains used in only a small number of centers in the United States. In stress testing as an example, while it is estimated that at most a few hundred thousand cardiac MRI procedures are performed in the United States per year, the number of stress echocardiography procedures is an order of magnitude greater than this and of nuclear cardiology procedures approximately two orders of magnitude greater than this. Understanding this lack of growth of cardiac MRI may provide insight into the development of cardiac CT. MRI utilizes expensive equipment, costing approximately ten times that of a nuclear cardiology scanner and much more than that compared to echocardiography equipment. Given this, it is not suitable for office practice. The method has required a great deal of expertise from technologists, to a greater extent than with nuclear or echocardiographic methods. The interpretation of cardiac MRI is more complex than that of nuclear cardiology or echocardiography studies, requiring greater training of the physician interpreters. Standardized, validated automated quantitative analytic software has not become available. While echocardiography and nuclear cardiology became part of the standard curriculum of cardiology fellows over the last two decades, this training in cardiac MRI was far more limited, being available in a limited number of programs. Finally, while echocardiography and nuclear methods were almost always contained within cardiology divisions, in only a small number of centers in the United States is cardiac MRI within cardiology. Strong collaboration between cardiology and radiology in cardiac MRI has not been common.

The Advent of Coronary Artery Calcium Scanning

The advent of coronary artery calcium (CAC) scanning with electron beam CT in the later part of the 1980s and 1990s ushered in the beginning of a new era in the use of cardiac imaging in asymptomatic patients, which is beginning to profoundly affect the future course of noninvasive cardiac testing. The test is easily performed, not requiring a great deal of technical expertise. An objective, quantitative analytic method has been available since soon after its introduction, providing what became described as a single number—the Agatston score—which has become the standard approach since its introduction for expressing the results of the scan and improved our ability to screen for CAD since the presence of CAC serves as a highly sensitive and specific marker for the presence of underlying atherosclerosis.

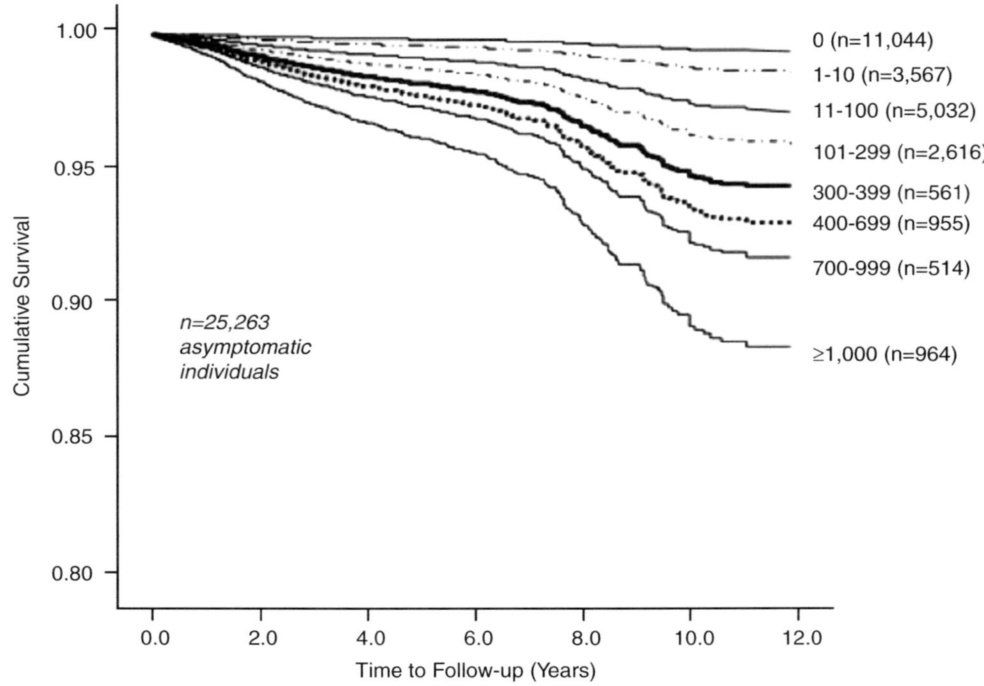

Fig. 3.4 Risk-adjusted cumulative survival among asymptomatic patients undergoing CAC scanning. For each increment in the CAC score, there was a significant increase in all-cause mortality. (From Budoff et al. [23], with permission)

Importantly, patho-anatomic correlations in the 1990s by Rumberger et al. established a proportional relationship between the CAC score and the overall burden of coronary atherosclerosis [22]. Consistent study has demonstrated that cardiac risk increases in direct proportion to increasing degrees of CAC abnormality [23–25]. For example, in a long-term follow-up of 25,263 asymptomatic subjects who underwent CAC scanning, Budoff et al. demonstrated an increase in risk in association with each increment of CAC score increase (Fig. 3.4) [23]. Even a very low CAC score, in the range of 1–9, establishes the presence of atherosclerosis. Such low scores suffice to increase the risk for cardiac events by twofold compared to a CAC score of zero.

As with cardiac stress testing, investigators recognized the need to assess whether CAC scanning added incremental information to the assessment of cardiac risk by global algorithms, such as the Framingham Risk Score, which incorporate age, gender, and consideration of CAD risk factors. A potential limitation of such scores is their reliance on only current risk factor status, without consideration of the chronicity of the risk factors. Moreover, these algorithms only provide a *probabilistic* assessment of the likelihood of CAD based on populations, whereas CAC scanning provides a marker of disease in an individual patient, representing the lifetime effect of all risk factors on the coronary vasculature. Numerous studies have demonstrated that CAC scanning provides incremental prognostic information compared to CAD risk factors and global algorithms [26, 27]. For instance, within the MESA study, the CAC score potently stratifies risk among all FRS subgroups including those with low and high FRS scores (Fig. 3.5) [27].

In addition, the CAC score has been shown to provide superior risk stratification compared to other methods used to screen for CAD. An important analysis in this regard was provided by Yeboah et al. within the MESA population, who assessed 1330 subjects with an intermediate FRS by 6 separate measurements: the ankle-brachial index, brachial flow-mediated dilation, carotid intima-media thickness, consideration of one's family history of premature CVD, high-sensitivity C-reactive protein, and assessment of one's CAC score [28]. Over a mean follow-up of 7.5 years, subjects were assessed for the occurrence of incident CVD. Other than CAC scanning, the other five screening measurements failed to provide a significant discrimination for predicting incident CVD. By contrast, CAC scanning was highly predictive. In addition, the net reclassification improvement provided by CAC scanning in the intermediate risk MESA subjects was substantially greater than that provided by the other scanning techniques evaluated by Yeboah et al. (Table 3.3) [28].

Several aspects of CAC scanning, however, led to a lag in its becoming a routine part of clinical cardiology until recent years. These include the manner in which it was introduced as a commercial screening test, its initial perception as being a diagnostic test (shown to have low specificity for obstructive coronary artery disease), the backlash from expert consensus panels and guidelines committees from its endorsement, and the persistent lack of coverage of the method, making it available only to patients who can afford to pay for their own scans.

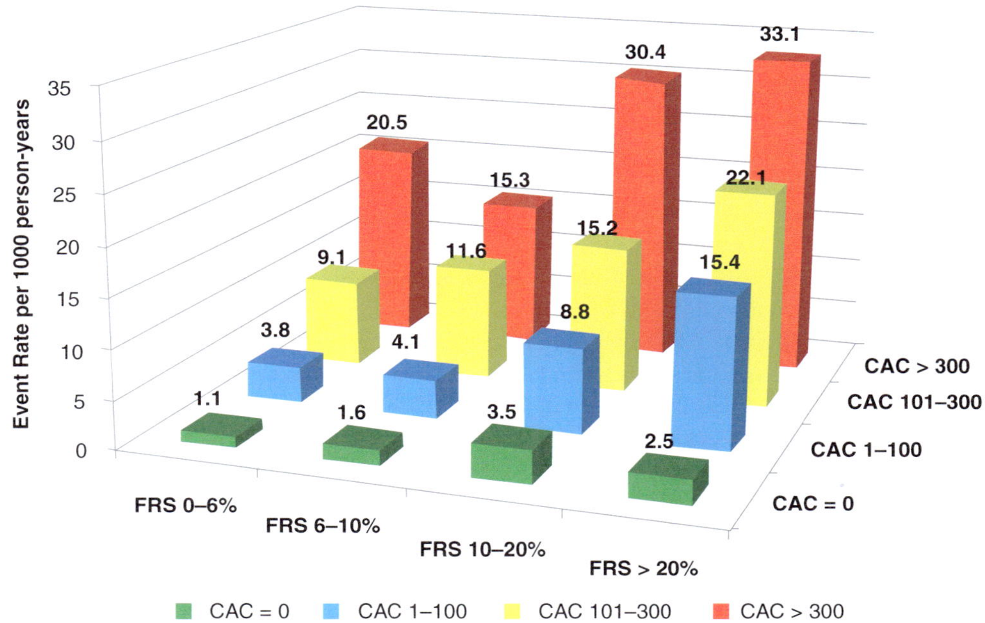

Fig. 3.5 Total cardiac event rates (per 1000 person-years) according to the combined consideration of coronary artery calcium scores and calculated Framingham Risk Score (FRS) category within the MESA study. (From Silverman et al. [27], with permission)

Table 3.3 Comparison of net reclassification improvement among 1330 intermediate Framingham risk subjects in the MESA study

Variables	% NRI
Brachial FMD	2.4%
Ankle-brachial index	3.6%
Hs-CRP	7.9%
Carotid IMT	10.2%
Family history	16.0%
Coronary artery calcium	65.9%

The Advent of Coronary CT Angiography (CCTA)

Coronary CT angiography became possible only after multislice scanners with rotation speeds became commercially available in the early 2000s—with the general availability of 64 slice scanners beginning around 1995. It was thus introduced at a time in which its developers could learn from the history of the other methods. Continual hardware and software improvements have led to faster and higher quality scans (improved spatial and temporal resolution) and the ability to perform these scans with very low radiation exposure.

Lessons learned from the experience with the earlier methods were applied to coronary CTA. These included the following:

1. The need for systematic development of databases within multiple centers that contained comprehensive clinical and coronary CTA data as well as follow-up information for cardiac events, which then could result in rapid published evidence for the field in diagnosis and prognosis. Importantly, this need was recognized in centers around the world, such that multicenter registries became possible.
2. The need for cardiologists and radiologists and imaging scientists to be involved in order to have the source of patient referrals and the physicians who generally control the expensive scanners both being advocates of the methods.
3. The need for standardization of acquisition, processing, and interpretation methods.
4. The need for a professional organization to be an advocate for all aspects of the development of the field.

Thus, in 2007, only a few years after the introduction of the 64-slice scanners, the Society of Cardiovascular CT (SCCT) was formed, to support research and education in cardiac CT and, from its beginning, dedicated to having the organization be a collaborative effort between cardiologists and radiologists.

Using the databases that had become part of imaging practice, early studies focused on the accuracy of CCTA in detecting stenosis compared to invasive coronary angiography, in which it far surpassed the accuracy of the other noninvasive imaging techniques—not surprisingly, since they were both anatomic imaging methods. The prospectively defined databases provided the tool for rapid reporting of multiple studies showing the prognostic value of CCTA above baseline CAD risk factors and commonly used risk stratification schemes. Further, since centers around the world had learned the need for prospective databases, it was possible to have multicenter registries that quickly amassed large numbers of patients with comprehensive clinical and coronary CTA data. The desire of many leaders in the field to provide evidence that would lead to broad dissemination of the method and importantly to payor coverage and inclusion in guidelines led multiple investigators to pool their data in such a fashion that individual centers might not be recognized for their contribution, but the overall field could have the opportunity to rapidly gain strength. Exemplifying this, in a very large registry of 23,854 patients without known CAD in the Coronary CT Angiography Evaluation for Clinical Outcomes: An International Multicenter (CONFIRM) registry, there was a significant association between mortality and CCTA findings, according to analysis of obstructive CAD by either a per-patient, per-vessel, or per-segment basis [29]. Outcome studies have consistently demonstrated that the absence of CAD by CCTA is associated with an excellent prognosis and a very long "warranty period."

The excellent diagnostic and prognostic accuracy of CCTA makes it an attractive test in diagnostic populations. The high negative predictive accuracy of CCTA among patients with a low to intermediate risk of CAD—with the ability to define absent or minimal CAD in a large proportion of patients undergoing testing—makes it superior to stress testing for the diagnostic work-up of patients in this patient cohort.

The Advent of Comparative Effectiveness Research

While each of the imaging modalities reviewed above have diagnostic and prognostic effectiveness, the newer imaging modalities, such as the CAC scan and coronary CTA, have to date been limited in terms of third-party insurance coverage. This limited coverage has its roots in two important developments over the prior decade. First, the development of a marked increase in the use of stress imaging modalities between 2000 and 2006 [30] caught the attention of Congress in the United States and has led to demands to curb the growth of cardiac testing in general. Thus one aspect of the success of nuclear cardiology served to slow the growth of coronary CTA, as coverage was not as easily gained. This demand has led to important methods for restraining medical costs, such as the advent of appropriateness criteria, precertification, and reduced medical reimbursement. Moreover, concerns for the rising costs of testing have led to the development of a new standard for evaluating the efficacy of cardiac tests. For decades, cardiac tests were evaluated solely according to their diagnostic and prognostic efficacy. Demonstration of such efficacy was sufficient to gain third-party insurance coverage. Instead, cardiac tests are now evaluated according to a standard of "therapeutic efficacy," as illustrated in Fig. 3.6 [31]. Whereas in the past, it was sufficient to demonstrate that a test merely *predicts* clinical outcomes, third-party carriers now demand evidence that a new test will also *improve* clinical outcomes or reduce costs, thereby providing value (Fig. 3.7). The optimal outcome is to demonstrate that a test leads to reduction in hard cardiac events, including cardiac death and myocardial infarction. However, demonstration of improvement in intermediate outcomes such as reduction in the number of invasive coronary angiograms that reveal nonobstructive CAD, reduction in time in the emergency department, and fewer admissions for chest pain in patients who prove not to have acute coronary syndromes. These might also include evidence that a

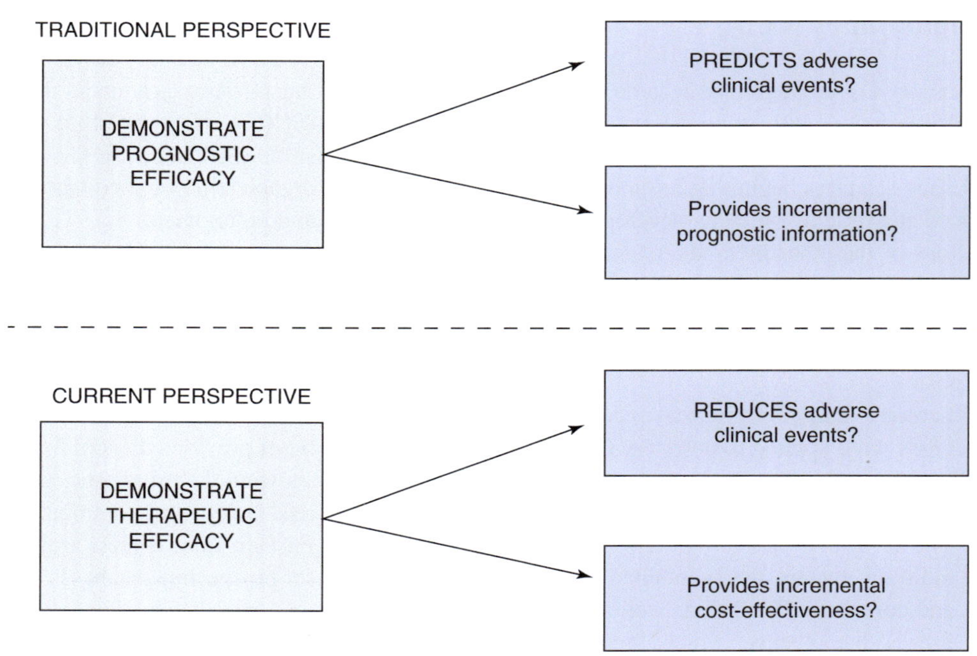

Fig. 3.6 Traditional versus new standard for assessing the efficacy of cardiac tests. Traditionally, the efficacy of cardiac tests was assessed according to their ability to predict adverse clinical events (prognostic efficacy). Now, tests are also evaluated according to their ability to reduce adverse clinical events (therapeutic efficacy). (From Rozanski et al. [31], with permission)

new test leads to a reduction in CAD risk factors. On the side of costs a new test would show, reduced downstream medical testing, and interventions, such as percutaneous coronary interventions and coronary bypass surgery, and unnecessary hospital admissions.

Because of today's multiplicity of cardiac tests, third-party carriers also require demonstration of how new tests compare to existing tests or clinical management strategies with respect to their ability to improve clinical outcomes and reduce downstream medical costs and medical resource utilization. This has led to a new era of comparative effectiveness research. A basic algorithm for performing such research is schematized in Fig. 3.8. This research takes the form of prospective randomized trials in which a cohort of patients is either randomized to usual medical care/conventional testing or a new proposed imaging modality. Patients are then followed for a specified period of time and then assessed for the relative frequency of clinical events or other specified outcomes.

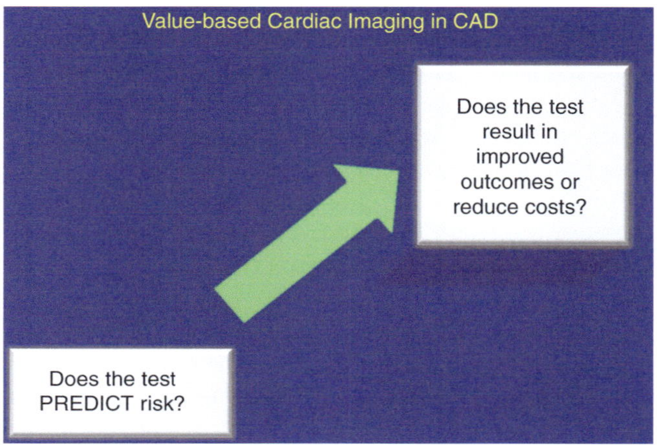

Fig. 3.7 Concepts of value-based cardiac imaging in CAD

The last decade has seen a proliferation of cardiac imaging trials designed to compare new imaging modalities versus usual care or prior imaging modalities. Most of this research has centered upon the use of coronary CTA as the experimental imaging modality. To date, coronary CTA has been evaluated in three clinical settings: its use for the work-up of patients presenting to emergency departments (ED), patients admitted to the hospital for clinical work-up, and patients being evaluated for chest pain in outpatient settings. Comparative effectiveness trials involving coronary CTA that have been done in the ED setting are listed in Table 3.4 [32–40].

In a meta-analysis of imaging trials, Hulten et al. found that randomization to coronary CTA [41] resulted in decreased length of stay and decreased costs in the emergency department rather than usual care in the ED. However coronary CTA was associated with an increase in referral for invasive coronary angiography.

Two small trials have assessed the use of CTA in the inpatient setting. The cardiac CT in the treatment of acute chest pain (CATCH) study randomized 600 patients to CCTA or standard of care. The results showed a similarly low frequency of events in both randomized arms, but the duration of follow-up was short [39]. In the Prospective First Evaluation in Chest Pain Trial (PERFECT), 411 patients admitted to the hospital for the work-up of chest pain were randomized to either CCTA or stress testing, using either stress echo or stress MPI [38]. The study showed no differ-

Fig. 3.8 Paradigm for conducting comparative effective research for cardiac imaging tests

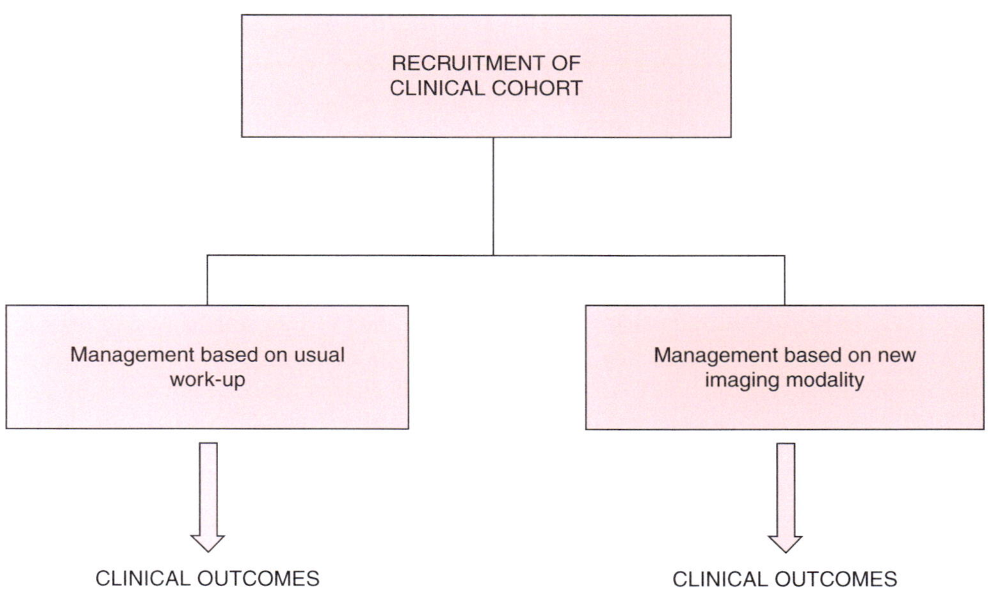

Table 3.4 Randomized prospective comparative effectiveness studies for CCTA

Study	*n*	Setting	Comparison	
			CCTA	SOC
Goldstein et al. [32]	197	ED	CCTA	SN
CT-STAT [33]	699	ED	CCTA	SN
ACRIN-PA [34]	1370	ED	CCTA	ET, SI
ROMICAT II [35]	1000	ED	CCTA	SOC
PROMISE [36]	10,003	Outpatient	CCTA	ET, SE, SN
Levsky et al. [37]	400	Inpatient	CCTA	SN
PERFECT [38]	411	Inpatient	CCTA	SE, SN
CATCH [39]	600	Inpatient	CCTA	ET, SN
SCOT-HEART [40]	9849	Outpatient	ET + CCTA	ET

CCTA coronary CT angiography, *ED* emergency department, *ET* exercise testing, *SE* stress echocardiography, *SI* stress imaging, *SN* stress nuclear, *SOC* standard of care

ence in downstream testing, hospitalization, or morbidity/mortality within the two arms of the study. As with some of the ED studies, there was a higher frequency of invasive coronary angiography and revascularization procedures within the coronary CTA arm.

Two large randomized trials have compared coronary CTA vs. either usual care or stress testing in the outpatient setting. The Scottish Computed Tomography of the HEART Trial (SCOT-HEART) trial randomized patients with chest pain syndromes to coronary CTA or usual care [40]. The coronary CTA arm demonstrated increased accuracy and certainty in the diagnosis of angina—the primary aim of the trial. There was a trend toward a decrease in hard cardiac events. When a delay in implementation of changes in therapeutic decision-making in the Scottish system was taken into account, a 50% reduction in myocardial infarction and cardiac death was observed [42]. Those who underwent coronary CTA also had a higher frequency of initiation of medical therapies and cancelation of therapies based on the results of the coronary CTA.

The largest imaging trial to date has been the Prospective Multicenter Imaging Study for Evaluation of Chest Pain (PROMISE) [35]. In the PROMISE study, 10,003 symptomatic patients were randomized to CCTA or stress testing. At a median follow-up of 2 years, there was no difference in clinical outcomes, but there was a higher frequency of invasive angiography in the CCTA arm. However, among those referred for ICA, 72% of patients in the coronary CTA arm had obstructive CAD, compared to only 48% of patients in the stress testing arm. Of note, however, the prevalence of obstructive CAD was far lower in the PROMISE trial than anticipated (10.7% observed versus 53.3% predicted), and the overall event rate was very low. These crucial factors seriously limited the overall utility of this study. Nevertheless, the study demonstrated that coronary CTA had comparable efficacy compared to stress testing in the PROMISE cohort.

In part based on the SCOT-HEART findings, the NICE criteria in Great Britain now have coronary CTA as the first-line test of choice in patients with acute or stable chest pain syndromes. While the growth of coronary CTA in the United States has been slowed by lack of commercial coverage, its growth worldwide has been dramatic.

Coronary CTA and Its Competitors

There has increasingly been a recognition in each field that both anatomic and physiologic measures are needed for comprehensive use of noninvasive imaging in guiding patient management. For coronary CTA, this recognition has led to the development of stress CT perfusion (CTP) and, more recently, attempts to assess coronary physiology through CT fractional flow reserve ($FFR_{CT)}$. Both approaches have been supported by a series of recent prospective multicenter trials [43–46]. Further, the ability of coronary CTA to evaluate coronary plaque, with its potential to provide automated quantitative assessments of the global coronary plaque burden of lipid-containing plaque, non-calcified plaque, and calcified plaque, as well as adverse plaque characteristics, is being developed. Quantitative plaque assessment may provide important key to prediction of cardiac events and to monitoring the effects of medical therapy. It is likely that the profound ability of coronary CTA to detect CAD, evaluate its extent and severity, assess its physiologic significance, and provide quantitative measures of plaque and plaque vulnerability will revolutionize cardiac imaging. Furthermore, the previous high radiation doses initially associate with coronary CTA have been dramatically reduced with new instrumentation and new modes of acquisition.

These and other newer advances of CCTA are covered within the chapters of this book. Of note, however, many of the "competitors" of CCTA are also "on the march," benefiting from important improvements in their technology.

Advances in Nuclear Cardiology

Nuclear cardiology has enjoyed substantial technological improvements in recent years. The recent development of solid-state detectors (e.g., cadmium zinc telluride) and improved collimation has resulted in improved energy resolution and reduction in undesirable scatter events. Application of attenuation correction is used to improve the accuracy of SPECT-MPI by eliminating artificial defects, thus permitting a higher frequency of stress-only imaging studies. The combination of new SPECT camera instrumentation with current improvements in reconstruction software is not only improved image quality but also markedly reduced radiation exposure to patients during the MPI scan. With new systems, stress-only SPECT-MPI can be performed with radiation doses as low as 1 mSv. The improvements in software have also improved the automation of quantitative analysis of MPI images and now permit the incorporation of all observed variables for decision-making through the application of machine learning.

PET MPI is performed with very low radiation doses—in the range of 1 mSv. Importantly, PET MPI provides a measurement of absolute stress myocardial blood flow and coronary flow reserve. These features provide information that adds to the prognostic value of perfusion defect assessment and provides a better understanding of the cause of patients' symptoms [47] (Fig. 3.9). A new PET scanning agent with ideal perfusion tracer characteristics—F-18 flurpiridaz— is undergoing phase III clinical trials [48] (Fig. 3.10). This agent will allow use of PET MPI without the need for an expensive on-site generator or cyclotron and can also be used with exercise. Further, PET is routinely performed with cardiac CT, allowing the routine measurement of CAC—thus adding competition to coronary CTA. SPECT CT systems are also becoming more common. These developments could allow for the improved effect of MPI testing on outcomes, by assessment of coronary atherosclerosis as well as myocardial perfusion.

Advances in Stress Echocardiography

As with the other imaging modalities, there have been important advances in the technical capabilities of stress echocardiography. Manufacturing improvements have improved the post-processing of ultrasound studies and increased the temporal resolution of the acquired images. Contrast echo has improved endocardial definition, further improved resolution, and decreased the number of nondiagnostic studies. In addition, newer ultrasound approaches for assessing peripheral arterial beds allow application of echocardiography for the detection of subclinical atherosclerosis. This includes the potential use of three-dimensional carotid ultrasound to characterize carotid plaque burden. In the BioImage Study, carotid plaque burden was comparable to CAC scanning for predicting adverse cardiac events [49]. Femoral ultrasound can also be used for identifying atherosclerotic plaques in this vascular bed. In the Aragon Workers' Health Study,

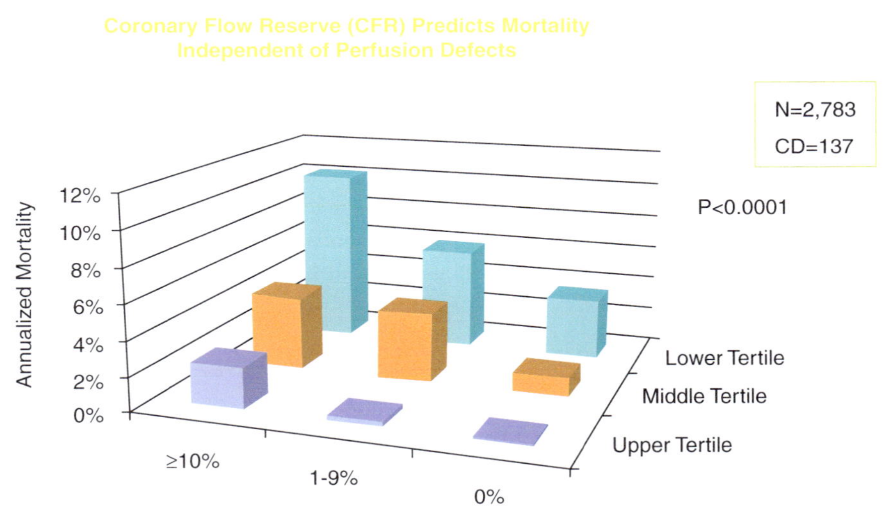

	≥10%	(n)	1-9%	(n)	0%	(n)
Upper Tertile	2.4%	(119)	0.3%	(195)	0.1%	(614)
Middle Tertile	4.4%	(217)	4.0%	(202)	1.1%	(509)
Lower Tertile	10.2%	(416)	6.0%	(190)	3.6%	(321)

Murthy VL, *et al. Circulation 2011*

Fig. 3.9 Unadjusted annualized cardiac mortality by tertiles of CFR and categories of stress SPECT-MPI perfusion defect (PD). CD = cardiac mortality. For each category of perfusion finding, there is increasing mortality associated with decreasing tertiles of CFR. (From Murthy et al. [47], with permission)

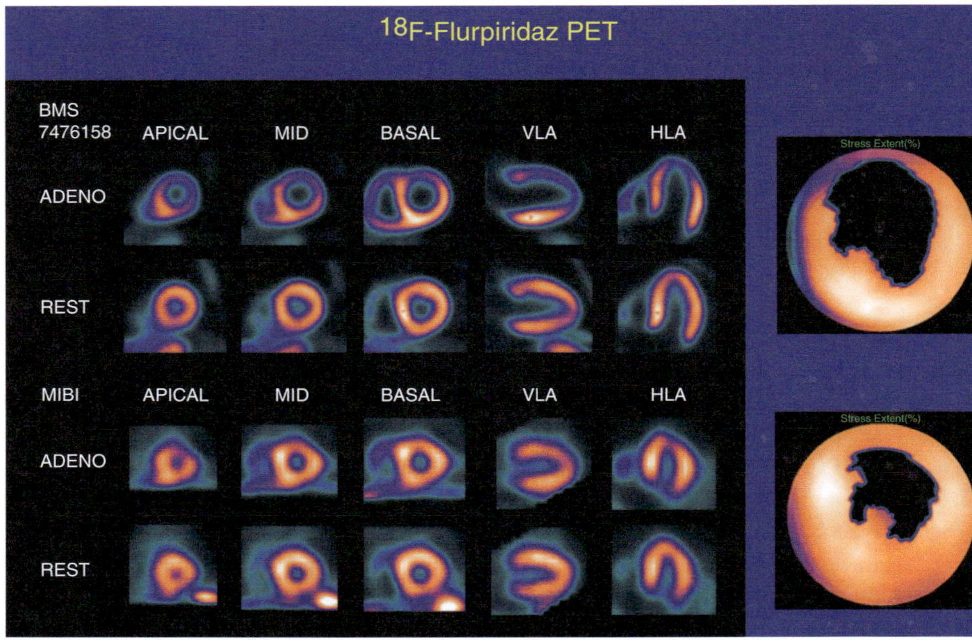

Fig. 3.10 Adenosine stress (adeno) and rest apical, mid-ventricular, and basal short-axis and vertical and horizontal mid-ventricular long-axis views acquired with flurpiridaz F-18 PET (top) and Tc-99m sestamibi (MIBI) SPECT bottom. Quantitative polar maps reconstructed from the same PET and SPECT studies are shown on the right. The extent and severity of induced perfusion defect are more apparent in the PET images. The quantitative TPD with the 99mTc-sestamibi SPECT study was 17% and was 32% with flurpiridaz F-18 PET. (From Berman et al. [56], with permission)

assessment of the femoral arteries revealed greater plaque detection than assessment of atherosclerosis by carotid ultrasound or CAC scanning [50]. A high sensitivity for detecting atherosclerotic plaque by femoral ultrasound was also demonstrated in the Progression of Early Atherosclerosis Study [51]. Ultrasound approaches could thus be used to assess stress-induced ischemia as well as subclinical atherosclerosis, if routine combination of plaque imaging and cardiac imaging were performed.

Advances in Cardiac MRI

Technological advances also continue to improve the capabilities of cardiac MRI. Recent advances include the advent of 3-Tesla scanners and the refinement of MRI sequences to allow shorter breath holds. In addition, emerging modalities such as T1 mapping and 4D flow sequences are refining the diagnostic capabilities of MRI. Importantly, major strides are being made in the standardization of cardiac MRI acquisition and processing methods, reducing the reliance on technical expertise. In the United States, it is anticipated that approval of a gadolinium contrast agent for myocardial perfusion may allow for a broader dissemination of information regarding the method.

Advances in CAC Scanning

The technological advances with CT have also benefited CAC scanning by permitting studies that can now be obtained with less than 1 mSv of radiation exposure. Until recently, emphasis with CAC scanning has been placed almost exclusively on the total Agatston CAC score. However, recent studies suggest that additional useful information may be obtained from the CAC scan, including assessment of the number of CAC plaques, the density of the plaques, and pericardial fat [52, 53].

Future Directions

As the technical capabilities of CCTA and its competitors improve, the new field of cardiac comparative effectiveness research will need to develop accordingly. As today's imaging technologies reach a relative technical maturation, there will be impetus to compare these imaging modalities with new prospective randomized imaging trials which will seek to determine the relative effectiveness of these imaging competitors for improving medical outcomes. These imaging trials will seek to determine which techniques provide the most effective reduction in adverse clinical events in the most economical way. These trials may also consider combinations of technologies that can be used in a cost-effective manner. For example, whereas exercise electrocardiography, a technique that has not changed since the 1960s, provides only limited diagnostic and prognostic information, its utility can be enhanced by combining it with a CAC scan into a hybrid test that has been termed the "treadmill calcium test" [54]. Similarly, MPI scans can now be combined with atherosclerosis imaging using combined SPECT/CT and PET/CT camera systems. These test combinations will deserve strong consideration as trials are developed to determine the optimal method for the work- up patients for diagnostic and prognostic assessment.

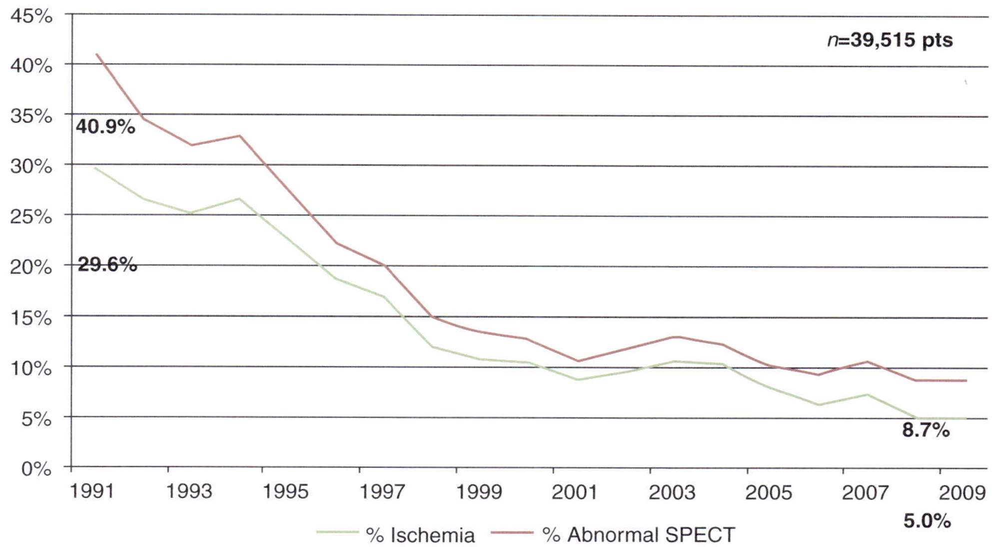

Fig. 3.11 The temporal prevalence of abnormal SPECT-MPI studies and ischemic SPECT-MPI studies between 1991 and 2009. (From Rozanski et al. [55], with permission)

An experience that has been garnered over four decades has taught us that there is no one ideal imaging test for all clinical scenarios. Rather, the value of a test is always dependent upon the goal of testing and upon disease and/or ischemic prevalence. Notably, the frequency of inducible ischemia is itself a now changing variable, as the frequency of inducible myocardial ischemia recedes due to enhanced prevention and the earlier detection of CAD in modern clinical practice (Fig. 3.11) [55]. In various settings, such as the ED, imaging technologies will also compete against more effective serum markers of disease, such as high-sensitivity troponin assays. Thus, the future assessment of what constitutes optimal imaging technologies is likely to be a dynamic process. What is certain, however, is that as our imaging capabilities improve, they are likely to retain and even grow in the central role that they have assumed for screening, diagnostic assessment, and/or risk stratification among patients with suspected and known CAD.

The rapid evolution of new medical devices and therapies and the increasing numbers of patients being studied or treated based on these developments are leading to an unsustainable increase in health-care costs. In the United States, there will be a transition from a volume-based health-care reimbursement to a value-based reimbursement. Inherently, as with any commodity, value is a function of quality and cost. In cardiology, quality ultimately implies not just risk stratification but an improvement in outcomes or reduction in costs. In the patient with CAD, these outcomes might be reduced cardiac events such as death or myocardial infarction or improvement in quality of life and other measures. In the future, whether the payer is the government, insurance companies, or the patients themselves, it is likely that only those approaches that provide value will be purchased. In imaging, this implies an increasing penetrance of value-based imaging, with growth in testing in areas of proven value and reduction of testing in areas in which value is not provided or has not been shown. Provision of value will be the metric upon which imaging tests will be judged. The long march into clinical practice of cardiac CT will be inherently linked to the evidence of the value of this powerful modality.

References

1. Dalen JE, et al. The epidemic of the 20(th) century: coronary heart disease. Am J Med. 2014;127(9):807–12.
2. Master AM. The two-step exercise electrocardiogram: a test for coronary insufficiency. Ann Intern Med. 1950;32(5):842–63.
3. Bruce RA, et al. Exercising testing in adult normal subjects and cardiac patients. Pediatrics. 1963;**32**:SUPPL 742–56.
4. Coplan NL. Evaluation of patients for coronary artery bypass surgery: the role of exercise testing. Am Heart J. 1991;122(6):1800–2.
5. Mark DB, et al. Exercise treadmill score for predicting prognosis in coronary artery disease. Ann Intern Med. 1987;106(6):793–800.
6. Zaret BL, et al. Noninvasive regional myocardial perfusion with radioactive potassium. Study of patients at rest, with exercise and during angina pectoris. N Engl J Med. 1973;288(16):809–12.
7. Berman DS, et al. Noninvasive detection of regional myocardial ischemia using rubidium-81 and the scintillation camera: comparison with stress electrocardiography in patients with arteriographically documented coronary stenosis. Circulation. 1975;52(4):619–26.
8. Wackers FJ, et al. Prognostic significance of normal quantitative planar thallium-201 stress scintigraphy in patients with chest pain. J Am Coll Cardiol. 1985;6(1):27–30.
9. Germano G, et al. Quantitative LVEF and qualitative regional function from gated thallium-201 perfusion SPECT. J Nucl Med. 1997;38(5):749–54.
10. Garcia EV, Maddahi J, Berman DS, Waxman A. Space-time quantitation of thallium-201 myocardial scintigraphy. J Nucl Med. 1981;22(4):309–17.
11. Garcia EV, Van Train K, Maddahi J, Prigent F, Friedman J, Areeda J, Waxman A, Berman DS. Quantification of rotational thallium-201 myocardial tomography. J Nucl Med. 1985;26(1):17–26.

12. Ladenheim ML, et al. Extent and severity of myocardial hypoperfusion as predictors of prognosis in patients with suspected coronary artery disease. J Am Coll Cardiol. 1986;7(3):464–71.
13. Weiss AT, et al. Transient ischemic dilation of the left ventricle on stress thallium-201 scintigraphy: a marker of severe and extensive coronary artery disease. J Am Coll Cardiol. 1987;9(4):752–9.
14. Berman DS, et al. Separate acquisition rest thallium-201/stress technetium-99m sestamibi dual-isotope myocardial perfusion single-photon emission computed tomography: a clinical validation study. J Am Coll Cardiol. 1993;22(5):1455–64.
15. Hachamovitch R, et al. Comparison of the short-term survival benefit associated with revascularization compared with medical therapy in patients with no prior coronary artery disease undergoing stress myocardial perfusion single photon emission computed tomography. Circulation. 2003;107(23):2900–7.
16. Rozanski A, et al. Comparison of long-term mortality risk following normal exercise vs adenosine myocardial perfusion SPECT. J Nucl Cardiol. 2010;17(6):999–1008.
17. Rozanski A, et al. Long-term mortality following normal exercise myocardial perfusion SPECT according to coronary disease risk factors. J Nucl Cardiol. 2014;21(2):341–50.
18. Supariwala A, et al. Influence of mode of stress and coronary risk factor burden upon long-term mortality following normal stress myocardial perfusion single-photon emission computed tomographic imaging. Am J Cardiol. 2013;111(6):846–50.
19. Hachamovitch R, et al. Incremental prognostic value of myocardial perfusion single photon emission computed tomography for the prediction of cardiac death: differential stratification for risk of cardiac death and myocardial infarction. Circulation. 1998;97(6):535–43.
20. Kang X, et al. Incremental prognostic value of myocardial perfusion single photon emission computed tomography in patients with diabetes mellitus. Am Heart J. 1999;138(6 Pt 1):1025–32.
21. Yao SS, et al. Practical applications in stress echocardiography: risk stratification and prognosis in patients with known or suspected ischemic heart disease. J Am Coll Cardiol. 2003;42(6):1084–90.
22. Rumberger JA, et al. Coronary artery calcium area by electron-beam computed tomography and coronary atherosclerotic plaque area. A histopathologic correlative study. Circulation. 1995;92(8):2157–62.
23. Budoff MJ, et al. Long-term prognosis associated with coronary calcification: observations from a registry of 25,253 patients. J Am Coll Cardiol. 2007;49(18):1860–70.
24. Detrano R, et al. Coronary calcium as a predictor of coronary events in four racial or ethnic groups. N Engl J Med. 2008;358(13):1336–45.
25. Polonsky TS, et al. Coronary artery calcium score and risk classification for coronary heart disease prediction. JAMA. 2010;303(16):1610–6.
26. Nasir K, et al. Interplay of coronary artery calcification and traditional risk factors for the prediction of all-cause mortality in asymptomatic individuals. Circ Cardiovasc Imaging. 2012;5(4):467–73.
27. Silverman MG, et al. Impact of coronary artery calcium on coronary heart disease events in individuals at the extremes of traditional risk factor burden: the Multi-Ethnic Study of Atherosclerosis. Eur Heart J. 2014;35(33):2232–41.
28. Yeboah J, et al. Comparison of novel risk markers for improvement in cardiovascular risk assessment in intermediate-risk individuals. JAMA. 2012;308(8):788–95.
29. Min JK, et al. Age- and sex-related differences in all-cause mortality risk based on coronary computed tomography angiography findings results from the International Multicenter CONFIRM (Coronary CT Angiography Evaluation for Clinical Outcomes: An International Multicenter Registry) of 23,854 patients without known coronary artery disease. J Am Coll Cardiol. 2011;58(8):849–60.
30. Shaw LJ, et al. Why all the focus on cardiac imaging? JACC Cardiovasc Imaging. 2010;3(7):789–94.
31. Rozanski A, Muhlestein JB, Berman DS. Primary prevention of CVD: the role of imaging trials. JACC Cardiovasc Imaging. 2017;10(3):304–17.
32. Goldstein JA, et al. The CT-STAT (coronary computed tomographic angiography for systematic triage of acute chest pain patients to treatment) trial. J Am Coll Cardiol. 2011;58(14):1414–22.
33. Goldstein JA, et al. A randomized controlled trial of multi-slice coronary computed tomography for evaluation of acute chest pain. J Am Coll Cardiol. 2007;49(8):863–71.
34. Litt HI, et al. CT angiography for safe discharge of patients with possible acute coronary syndromes. N Engl J Med. 2012;366(15):1393–403.
35. Douglas PS, et al. Outcomes of anatomical versus functional testing for coronary artery disease. N Engl J Med. 2015;372:1291–300.
36. Hoffmann U, et al. Coronary CT angiography versus standard evaluation in acute chest pain. N Engl J Med. 2012;367(4):299–308.
37. Levsky JM, Travin MI, Haramati LB. Coronary computed tomography angiography versus radionuclide myocardial perfusion imaging in patients with chest pain admitted to telemetry: a randomized, controlled trial. Ann Intern Med. 2016;164(2):133–4.
38. Uretsky S, et al. Comparative effectiveness of coronary CT angiography vs stress cardiac imaging in patients following hospital admission for chest pain work-up: the Prospective First Evaluation in Chest Pain (PERFECT) Trial. J Nucl Cardiol. 2017;24(4):1267–78.
39. Linde JJ, et al. Long-term clinical impact of coronary CT angiography in patients with recent acute-onset chest pain: the randomized controlled CATCH trial. JACC Cardiovasc Imaging. 2015;8(12):1404–13.
40. Investigators, S.-H. CT coronary angiography in patients with suspected angina due to coronary heart disease (SCOT-HEART): an open-label, parallel-group, multicentre trial. Lancet. 2015;385(9985):2383–91.
41. Hulten E, et al. Outcomes after coronary computed tomography angiography in the emergency department: a systematic review and meta-analysis of randomized, controlled trials. J Am Coll Cardiol. 2013;61(8):880–92.
42. Williams MC, et al. Use of coronary computed tomographic angiography to guide management of patients with coronary disease. J Am Coll Cardiol. 2016;67(15):1759–68.
43. Cury RC, et al. Dipyridamole stress and rest myocardial perfusion by 64-detector row computed tomography in patients with suspected coronary artery disease. Am J Cardiol. 2010;106(3):310–5.
44. Min JK, et al. Diagnostic accuracy of fractional flow reserve from anatomic CT angiography. JAMA. 2012;308(12):1237–45.
45. Norgaard BL, et al. Diagnostic performance of noninvasive fractional flow reserve derived from coronary computed tomography angiography in suspected coronary artery disease: the NXT trial (analysis of coronary blood flow using CT angiography: next steps). J Am Coll Cardiol. 2014;63(12):1145–55.
46. Rocha-Filho JA, et al. Incremental value of adenosine-induced stress myocardial perfusion imaging with dual-source CT at cardiac CT angiography. Radiology. 2010;254(2):410–9.
47. Murthy VL, et al. Improved cardiac risk assessment with noninvasive measures of coronary flow reserve. Circulation. 2011;124(20):2215–24.
48. Berman DS, et al. Phase II safety and clinical comparison with single-photon emission computed tomography myocardial perfusion imaging for detection of coronary artery disease: flurpiridaz F 18 positron emission tomography. J Am Coll Cardiol. 2013;61(4):469–77.
49. Baber U, et al. Prevalence, impact, and predictive value of detecting subclinical coronary and carotid atherosclerosis in

asymptomatic adults: the BioImage study. J Am Coll Cardiol. 2015;65(11):1065–74.
50. Laclaustra M, et al. Femoral and carotid subclinical atherosclerosis association with risk factors and coronary calcium: the AWHS study. J Am Coll Cardiol. 2016;67(11):1263–74.
51. Fernandez-Friera L, et al. Prevalence, vascular distribution, and multiterritorial extent of subclinical atherosclerosis in a middle-aged cohort: the PESA (progression of early subclinical atherosclerosis) study. Circulation. 2015;131(24):2104–13.
52. Berman DS, Arnson Y, Rozanski A. Coronary artery calcium scanning: the Agatston score and beyond. JACC Cardiovasc Imaging. 2016;9(12):1417–9.
53. Rozanski A, Slomka P, Berman SD. Extending the use of coronary calcium scanning to clinical rather than just screening populations: ready for prime time. Circ Cardiovasc Imaging. 2016;9(5):e004876.
54. Rozanski A, Cohen R, Uretsky S. The coronary calcium treadmill test: a new approach to the initial workup of patients with suspected coronary artery disease. J Nucl Cardiol. 2013;20(5):719–30.
55. Rozanski A, et al. Temporal trends in the frequency of inducible myocardial ischemia during cardiac stress testing: 1991 to 2009. J Am Coll Cardiol. 2013;61(10):1054–65.
56. Berman DS, Germano G, Slomka PJ. Improvement in PET myocardial perfusion image quality and quantification with flurpiridaz F 18. J Nucl Cardiol. 2012;19(Suppl 1):S38–45.

Part II

Where We Are: Human Requisites

4 Cardiac Computed Tomography: A Team Sport

Sheldon E. Litwin

Nature abhors a vacuum. – Attributed to Aristotle
All politics are local. – Attributed to Tip O'Neill

Historical Perspective

The concepts underlying computed tomography (CT) were first developed by Godfrey Hounsfield and Allan Cormack in the early 1970s [1]. Although Hounsfield attempted to use gated CT for cardiac imaging in the mid-1970s [2], nearly 30 years elapsed before this became a reality in clinical medicine. In the mid-2000s, a number of hardware and software advances including the use of multiple rows of detectors and helical imaging allowed us to overcome the technical limitation imposed by cardiac and respiratory motion. The long slow road to the advent of modern cardiac CT was followed by a decade of accelerated development and refinement of the hardware, imaging approaches, processing techniques, and interpretation skills. This rapid expansion led to somewhat of a vacuum in the proprietorship of this field.

Nature Abhors a Vacuum

As one would expect, the initially empty space surrounding the rapidly expanding use of cardiac CT strongly attracted enterprising individuals with a variety of backgrounds and training. The sudden realization that we could noninvasively image coronary arteries at high spatial resolution was a powerful draw for cardiologists who have always been fascinated by coronary anatomy. The striking views of the heart and vasculature that could be created using newer approaches such as curved multiplanar reconstructions and three-dimensional volume rendering also proved irresistible to radiologists. Given a history of struggles over ownership of other cardiac imaging modalities such as invasive or catheter-based coronary angiography and nuclear cardiology, it is not altogether surprising that tensions also developed in this new landscape. The term "tribalism" refers to a strong cultural or ethnic identity that separates one group from another. In medicine, tribes are most often defined by specialty or departmental affiliations. The conflicts that exist regarding the modern practice of cardiac CT generally relate to debates over which medical specialty is best suited to oversee the equipment and technologists, the interpretation of the images, communications with referring providers, and the financial aspects of the service being rendered. An underlying premise in the dispute is that cardiologists have traditionally "owned" the body part being studied (the heart) while radiologists have been the keepers of the CT scanner. Before discussing the arguments put forth over these issues more specifically, it is worth recalling that the pioneers in this field were an engineer and a physicist, not cardiologist or radiologist. Arguably, neither medical specialty owns exclusive rights to the use of this imaging modality for evaluation of the heart.

Imaging Turf Wars

The term "turf war" has been used to describe a dispute between criminals and gangs over the right to operate within a particular area. More recently this term has been aptly applied to conceptually similar struggles in the medical field. A recent Internet search of the terms "medical turf wars" yielded >240,000 hits. Obviously, this is a topic that has commanded quite a bit of attention. Cardiac CT is not the only battleground, but it is one of the arenas where the tug-of-war has been relatively public. The degree of conflict over cardiac CT and the various solutions to the struggle have varied rather widely in different parts of the country or the world. From the "30,000 foot view," it is relatively easy to see the benefits of a cooperative approach to running a cardiac CT program with the opportunity for input and active participation from all interested and qualified parties.

S. E. Litwin (✉)
Division of Cardiology, Department of Medicine, Medical University of South Carolina, Charleston, SC, USA
e-mail: litwins@musc.edu

U. J. Schoepf (ed.), *CT of the Heart*, Contemporary Medical Imaging, https://doi.org/10.1007/978-1-60327-237-7_4

However, many complexities such as institutional tracking of individual physician or departmental productivity can easily derail the ideal vision of how to optimally deliver a clinical service. It is typically easier to endorse the broad concept of truly integrated cardiac imaging services, than it is to bring that concept to fruition at one's own institution. At a national or international level, organizations like the Society for Cardiac Computed Tomography bring together many individuals with a variety of backgrounds. The shared enthusiasm for cardiac CT allows such a group to have communal goals such as increasing availability, standardizing reporting, improving insurance coverage, and other factors relevant to this imaging modality. The big picture notwithstanding the primacy of local politics often wins out to the detriment of many.

Competition Versus Collaboration

The issue at hand is how to effectively bring together the competing groups in a fashion that is mutually beneficial and results in the best and most efficient patient care. Most would agree that cardiologists and radiologists bring unique and complementary skill sets and knowledge bases to the discipline of cardiac CT. Cardiologists have substantial familiarity with cardiac and coronary anatomy and physiology and are accustomed to looking at moving (cine) images of the heart. Assessment of global function, regional wall motion, and heart valves is second nature to most cardiologists. However, they are less likely to be comfortable with CT technology, injection protocols, recognition of artifacts, use of conventional CT imaging planes, image post processing, and evaluation of extra-cardiac anatomy. In contrast, radiologists tend to be more adept at performing mental three-dimensional reconstructions of anatomy while viewing axial images and are highly familiar with most of the anatomy in the chest outside of the heart. They are usually very comfortable performing post processing of images and manipulating volumetric data sets. However, many radiologists are less at ease with viewing and interpreting dynamic images, such as those of the beating heart. Radiologists may also have less familiarity with the clinical implications of using certain descriptive terms such as "coronary artery disease," which can be used with reference to nonobstructive coronary atherosclerosis, although this terminology is frequently assumed to mean that obstructive plaques are present.

The advantages of a collaborative approach to the development and management of a cardiac CT program are abundantly clear. Unfortunately, major barriers to cooperation still exist. Some of the more important obstacles include tradition, departmental silos, turf, time, billing, volume of studies, maintenance of interpretive competency, management of equipment, supervision of technical staff, and location of services. Workflow for cardiologists and radiologists has traditionally been different, and this impacts the ability to work together in a seamless fashion. Radiology reading rooms are often physically located near the CT scanners where cardiac imaging is performed, and hence, radiologists are more immediately available to troubleshoot issues at the time of scans and to do immediate wet reads. Cardiologists on the other hand have conventionally spent much of their time seeing patients in an office or hospital setting and doing invasive or noninvasive procedures in areas that are distant from the CT scanner. Thus, they are generally less available for immediate issues related to the scan procedures. Use of cardiac CT in the emergency department for evaluation of chest pain is one of the most rapidly growing indications for the technique. To make the test most valuable to patients and to the system, rapid interpretation is necessary. A shortened time to diagnosis is one of the major advantages of cardiac CT compared to other approaches. Again, this favors the use of interpreting physicians who have proximate access to computer workstations with post processing capability and the hardware and software solutions for immediate reporting. In most institutions, the volume of cardiac CT scans is still relatively low, and it is challenging for individual practitioners to maintain competency if this volume is spread among multiple different readers. All of these issues are potentially solvable in an era where increasing numbers of CT technologists are trained in performing ECG-gated acquisitions without the need for physician supervision and thin client or cloud-based image interpretation can be done anywhere.

Perhaps the most vexing challenge to shared ownership and management of cardiac CT programs relates to the economic issues resulting from the ever-increasing pressure to raise productivity and lower costs for health systems. As a means to achieve this goal, many systems closely track individual physician revenues or relative value units (aka, RVUs). In general, only one physician can be the official interpreter of a test. That person is also the one who bills for the interpretation. This focus on individual productivity, rather than team work, has an obvious chilling effect on any arrangement that results in splitting of reimbursement or on any process that may slow down the pace of interpreting studies (i.e., joint reading sessions). The technical charges associated with a procedure generally only go to one department – again, a strong disincentive to cross-departmental collaboration. Coming up with equitable ways to share revenues, or to assign credit for communal work or program building, does not fit very with most current accounting systems.

Creativity and thinking outside the customary departmental structures are needed to make a program work. A commitment from hospital, departmental, and division leaders is a necessity in order to overcome the many obstacles. The creation of service lines is one approach to breaking down departmental barriers. However, in most cases, the service line is not the fiscal accounting unit, and the solid and dotted lines on the new organizational charts become blurred. Frequently radiology is considered to be a service unit, like anesthesiology and pathology, and is not included as part of a cardiovascular service line. To be successful, there is a need for real equality among the participants, with each member of the team playing an important role. Transparency about financial issues and clear delineation of responsibilities and roles must exist. Excellent communication, shared values, and mutual respect are cornerstones of a successful program, but these are not things that are taught in medical school nor nurtured in subsequent training. It is often easier to retreat to the tribal mentality, than to expend the effort to bridge political divides.

When cardiac CT is practiced as a team sport, it creates many rich opportunities. As in any team sport, individuals play different positions, and the depth of talent on any team, not the skill of one or a few individuals, typically determines its success. The analogy to the varying contributions of cardiologists and radiologists to the sport of cardiac CT is apt. Jointly managed programs have clear symbiosis when it comes to education of medial trainees who can greatly benefit from the collective wisdom of diverse teachers. Research programs, as well, are much more likely to thrive when the ideas of many are allowed to come together. Intriguingly, the progressive push toward value-based health care, which emphasizes the importance of population health and cost effectiveness, rather than volume of procedures or tests, may be the thing that ultimately eliminates departmental silos and reduces economic competition within institutions. If and when this enlightened approach to health care becomes engrained, other benefits such as improved radiation stewardship [3], more flexible night and weekend coverage, and reduction of layered or redundant testing may become easier to realize. As in any group practice, veneration among the involved individuals is the foundation upon which teamwork is built.

The field of cardiac CT is still relatively young and the optimal organization of a program represents a moving target. A number of forces will affect how CT programs are actualized as the field matures. It is likely that CT will progressively assume portions of the diagnostic imaging volume previously performed in nuclear laboratories or in the invasive angiography suite. If this comes to pass, there will be a need for many more physicians who are competent to interpret cardiac CT and perhaps competition will wane. "Miniaturization" and reduced cost of CT hardware may allow decentralization of cardiac CT imaging locations into smaller hospitals and clinics. Recently an imaging think tank was convened to discuss the future of cardiac imaging [4]. The group made many recommendations including redefining a cardiac imager as someone with a high level of expertise in at least one imaging modality, but not necessarily more than one modality. In an accompanying editorial, the authors made the case that such an approach may work well in academic institutions or large hospitals, but is not well suited to regional hospitals or smaller systems where most clinical care actually occurs. They opined that we should instead direct our efforts toward developing imagers with a broader skill and knowledge base [5]. Using this approach, they believe that clinicians will be more likely to choose an optimal test for an individual patient based on their specific characteristics, rather than choosing on the basis of existing practice patterns or local islands of expertise. How we train the next generation of cardiac imagers is likely to affect what the imaging teams of the future will look like and how they will function. Hopefully that future health-care system will be focused more on health and less on politics. In the meantime, efforts to forge a permanent partnership between the radiology and cardiology communities can yield benefits for all.

References

1. Hounsfield GN. Historical notes on computerized axial tomography. J Can Assoc Radiol. 1976;27(3):135–42.
2. Sagel SS, et al. Gated computed tomography of the human heart. Investig Radiol. 1977;12(6):563–6.
3. Douglas PS, et al. Developing an action plan for patient radiation safety in adult cardiovascular medicine. Proceedings from the Duke University Clinical Research Institute/American College of Cardiology Foundation/American Heart Association Think Tank Held on February 28, 2011. J Nucl Cardiol. 2012;19(3):534–50.
4. Douglas PS, et al. The future of cardiac imaging: report of a think tank convened by the American College of Cardiology. JACC Cardiovasc Imaging. 2016;9(10):1211–23.
5. Marwick TH, Chandrashekhar Y, Narula J. Training in multimodality CV imaging: is there an inclusive model? JACC Cardiovasc Imaging. 2016;9(10):1235–7.

Cardiac CT: Credentialing and Accreditation

5

James M. Kofler, Heidi A. Edmonson, Shuai Leng, and Eric E. Williamson

Accreditation of Cardiac CT Scanners: Scanner and Technologist Requirements

There are currently four different organizations recognized by the Centers for Medicare and Medicaid Services (CMS) as accreditors for CT imaging, including the American College of Radiology (ACR), the Joint Commission (TJC), the Intersocietal Accreditation Commission (IAC, formerly Intersocietal Commission for the Accreditation of Vascular Laboratories (ICAVL)), and RadSite [1]. In addition to general CT imaging accreditation, the ACR has a specific cardiac module, and the IAC has accreditation programs for coronary calcium scoring CT and coronary CTA exams. TJC and RadSite have no specific cardiac requirements for CT scanners, although RadSite requires submission of a sample cardiac case if cardiac CT is part of the clinical practice. The commonality of all four accreditors is that the CT equipment specifications and performance meet all state and federal requirements. Beyond this requirement, the criterion for equipment accreditation and the technologist credentials differs among the accreditors.

The ACR CT Accreditation Program

Scanner Requirements

The ACR requires submission of clinical examples, which are assumed to represent the best work of the site, not just typical cases. The type and number of clinical cases depend on the number and type of modules that are being submitted for accreditation. The module choices are adult abdomen, adult head, pediatric abdomen, pediatric head, and adult and/or pediatric cardiac CT (http://www.acraccreditation.org/~/media/ACRAccreditation/Documents/CT/Requirements.pdf?la=en). For the application of the cardiac module, if one or more other modules are included in the same application, at least one clinical adult coronary CTA case must be submitted, unless the unit is used solely for patients of 18 years of age or younger, in which case a pediatric cardiac examination is required. If the unit is used for both adult and pediatric patients, then at least one pediatric cardiac CT exam is required to be submitted. The non-cardiac modules require submission of additional cases specific to the module. For accreditation applications specific to a cardiac module, the requirements are as follows: adult-only cardiac CT requires two coronary CT clinical cases; pediatric-only cardiac CT requires two pediatric cases; and for both adult and pediatric cardiac CT, at least one (of three) clinical case must be a pediatric patient (http://www.acraccreditation.org/~/media/ACRAccreditation/Documents/CT/Requirements.pdf?la=en). Complete case sets must be submitted for each CT unit application, including a copy of the clinic protocol for each. Full details on the required cases for submission are available from the ACR [2]. Minimum criteria for scan parameters for various exams, including cardiac exams, are listed in the ACR accreditation program Testing Instructions [3]. The clinical images are reviewed by multiple radiologist reviewers who use a range of criteria, such as image quality, appropriateness of scan parameters, scan range, etc., to determine if the submission meets the requirements for ACR accreditation.

The ACR also requires phantom testing and radiation dosimetry measurements for accreditation. This testing must be completed by a "qualified medical physicist" (QMP), which is defined in the personnel requirements [4]. The imaging phantom required for the physics testing was developed specifically for the ACR accreditation program and is available through a separate vendor (Gammex 464, Sun Nuclear, Middleton, WI). Sections of the phantom are designed to measure CT number accuracy, low-contrast resolution, and image uniformity. Phantom measurements are acquired using the site's clinical scan parameters for the relevant protocols, depending on the modules included for the submission, but none include cardiac-specific protocol

J. M. Kofler (✉)
Department of Radiology, Mayo Clinic, Jacksonville, FL, USA
e-mail: jkofler@mayo.edu

H. A. Edmonson · S. Leng · E. E. Williamson
Department of Radiology, Mayo Clinic, Rochester, MN, USA

U. J. Schoepf (ed.), *CT of the Heart*, Contemporary Medical Imaging, https://doi.org/10.1007/978-1-60327-237-7_5

testing. Radiation dosimetry measurements and images must also be submitted. These are also acquired using the site's clinical scan parameters, but, again, none are specific to cardiac CT imaging. Tolerances are provided for measured values, most of which, if exceeded, count as "minor" demerit points for the submission. A unit may have up to six minors before failing the application. More severe issues can result in a "major," which is automatic failure. Some examples of major issues are excessive dose, gross misuse of certain technical parameters, and excessive image artifacts. Sites may also fail if the submitted images were acquired using parameters that are substantially different from those listed in the scan protocol. The detailed instructions for the physics tests for accreditation submission are available from the ACR [3].

The ACR also requires an ongoing CT quality assurance program, which includes involvement from the technologist, radiologist, and medical physicist. The program requires acceptance testing at scanner installation and routine physics testing done at least annually, completed by a QMP, and including reports and documentation. The technologist must perform daily measurements on the scanner prior to scanning patients. The measurements include recording of the CT number of water and image noise values, as well as a visual inspection for artifacts. The technologist must also perform monthly visual checks of basic system operating and safety features. All measurements must be recorded and available for review by the medical physicist or an ACR inspector. All required and suggested tests, including tolerances, are described in the ACR CT QC Manual [5]. The ACR also has requirements for CT protocol maintenance, in which a team consisting of at least a technologist, medical physicist, and radiologist review protocol items such as appropriateness, clarity of the instructions, and dose optimization opportunities. Although the ongoing quality assurance (QA) component of the ACR accreditation program involves many individuals, it is ultimately the responsibility of the radiologist to ensure that all aspects of the program are being met.

Technologist Requirements

Technologists must meet all three of the following criteria for ACR accreditation: (1) ARRT registered (RT) and radiography (R) and/or computed tomography (CT) certified and/or NMTCB registered (CNMT) and/or unrestricted state license; (2) documented training and experience in CT; and (3) documented training and experience in operating CT equipment, radiation physics, and protection. Passing an advanced examination for CT certification is recommended. For registered technologists, the continuing education requirements of the certifying organization, including credits pertinent to CT, must be met. Maintaining good standing status within the certifying organization is sufficient proof of meeting the continuing education credits. For state-licensed and other technologists, 24 h of continuing education, relevant to CT imaging, radiological sciences, and patient care, is required. In these cases, a documentation of the continuing education credits must be provided to the ACR.

The IAC Accreditation Program

Scanner Requirements

The IAC has several exam-specific accreditation programs, including coronary calcium scoring CT, coronary CTA, vascular CTA, neurological CT, sinus and temporal bone CT, and body CT. The general program includes basic guidelines and requirements for such items as image archive, timely reporting, policies and procedures for patient safety, and a pathway to report incidents and adverse events, among others. Details can be found in the IAC CT Standards [6]. The roles of the personnel and supervisory staff, as well as facility requirements, are also listed in this document.

For coronary calcium scoring, a multi-detector system of four slices or greater must be used, with a recommended rotation time of ≤0.5 s. The software and reconstruction systems must have the following capabilities: provide visual representation of coronary calcium exceeding protocol thresholds; quantify coronary calcification using Agatston and mass and/or volume scoring methodologies; and provide user interaction with quantitative program to allow selecting or deselecting coronary calcification based on visual inspection.

For coronary CTAs (used for coronary arteries and coronary bypass grafts), the CT scanner must have ≥64 slices, a rotation time of ≤0.5 s, and a dual auto-injector. The associated software must meet the following requirements: (1) are capable of displaying data as maximum intensity projection (MIP), thick or thin slices, multi-planar reformats, and data in a curve plane reformat; (2) create 3D images and rotate about all three axes; (3) provide measurements as described in a facility-specific protocol; (4) simultaneously load multiple phases; and (5) perform quantification of coronary calcium.

General CT requirements are that all data be reviewed digitally on a monitor which is sufficient to prevent any loss of resolution and with standard window/level settings and which can also be adjusted manually. The datasets must be DICOM compatible, and the systems must have the capability to optimize the field of view based on patient size and protocol.

The IAC also requires a quality improvement (QI) program, which includes quality control testing, acceptance testing after installation or major repair or upgrade, and room shielding verification. QI program oversight should be done by a QI committee which consists of the technical director, medical director, service engineer, and/or site-appointed medical physicist. The facility must have at least one QI meeting per year to review the results of the QI program.

Acceptance testing includes measurements of image quality, system performance characterization, and radiation dose. The system parameters must be compared to the manufacturer's specifications. Daily and periodic QC tests are to be performed as suggested by the manufacturer. The daily tests, which would be completed by a technologist, include the measurement of the CT number of water and another reference material, measurement of image noise, and visual artifact assessment. Additionally, the proper functioning of the audible and visual patient safety equipment must be verified. Annual performance checks are also required to be completed by a qualified medical physicist. The tests include basic image quality and system checks and are listed in the standards manual [6]. A QI committee and/or the medical director must evaluate the physicist's recommendations for the type of testing, frequency, and designated personnel to perform the test(s). Preventive maintenance service is also required at least annually for each scanner at the site. All QC testing, including preventative maintenance records, must be documented and maintained at the facility.

As part of the QI program, facilities must have a process to assess the exam appropriateness and to evaluate aspects of the technical quality, including review of clinical images for suboptimal image quality or artifacts, completeness of the study, adherence to protocol, and any patient or facility safety concerns. The interpretive quality should be evaluated, such as through peer review, including the final report completeness and timeliness. Radiation safety items must also be recorded, including documentation of the expected dose ranges based on patient-specific characteristics, comparison of doses for each protocol, and tracking of repeated CT exams. Proper usage of dose reduction must be documented, and staff occupational exposures must be monitored.

The IAC accreditation program also has criteria and guidelines for minimum procedure volumes, indication verification, and ensuring that the CT test is appropriately ordered and scheduled. A list of elements for examination performance is also included, as well as parameters that should be included in the scan protocol.

Technologist Requirements

All technologists performing CT scans must meet at least one of the following criteria: (1) the American Registry of Radiologic Technologists (ARRT) or the Canadian Association of Medical Radiation Technologists (CAMRT) certification in CT imaging (i.e., ARRT(R) ARRT(CT)), (2) an appropriate nationally recognized credential in another medical imaging field (i.e., CNMT, ARRT(R), ARRT(R)(MR)), or (3) a 12-month full-time clinical CT experience under direct supervision of a credentialed technologist plus one of the following – completion of a formal 2-year program (or equivalent) in another medical imaging profession (with focus on radiation physics) or completion of a bachelor's degree in another medical imaging profession (with focus on radiation physics).

The technologists must have at least 15 h of Category 1 AMA or RCEEN-approved CT-related continuing education credits over a period of 3 years. Three of the 15 h must be related to radiation safety.

The Joint Commission Accreditation Program

Scanner Requirements

The Joint Commission diagnostic imaging accreditation program includes CT but with no specific requirements for cardiac imaging. TJC has requirements for annual testing of the CT scanners, including measuring standard image quality metrics and radiation dose, as well as display device monitoring tests, although measurement methods and tolerances are not provided. A complete list of the required tests can be found in the Joint Commission Diagnostic Imaging Requirements [7]. The requirements also include shielding design for new installations or remodels, including verification afterward.

TJC accreditation program mandates that patient age and recent imaging be considered when deciding the most appropriate type of imaging. The CT protocols must be based on current standards of practice, which includes clinical indication, contrast administration, etc. The protocols must be reviewed and kept current with input from an interpreting radiologist, medical physicist, and lead technologist.

Patient radiation doses must be documented in the patient record, in a retrievable format (if the scanner is capable of producing dose metrics). Some tracking or recording of patient doses is also necessary to meet the requirement that any incidents where the dose exceeds a pre-defined dose range must be reviewed and analyzed. These doses then need to be compared to external benchmarks.

Technologist Requirements

The site must have documentation that the technologists who perform CT participate in ongoing education in radiation dose optimization techniques and tools for pediatric and adult patients, as well as training in safe scanner operation. Specific hours of required training are not provided.

The RadSite Accreditation Program

Scanner Requirements

The requirements for accreditation are detailed in the RadSite Accreditation Standards [8]. Clinical patient images must be submitted for each CT unit. A selection of choices is listed for each type of exam, including neuroimaging, musculoskeletal, and body [9]. A minimum of three adult cases and protocols, as well as one pediatric case, if applicable, must be included in the submission. For scanners that perform cardiac imaging, at least one cardiac exam must be submitted, as listed in the requirements for body scanners. Clinical exam submissions must also include the clinical indication and any post-processed images, as well as the clinical report. A list of scan parameters for various exams, as well as pass/fail examples, is included in the Standards document. Some examples for failing the submission include incomplete coverage, excessive dose, or inappropriate scan parameters. The Standards document also includes samples of the image quality scoring sheet, which contains all of the elements that are part of the review process. An on-site audit checklist is also provided, such that sites can be prepared for an on-site inspection.

The RadSite accreditation program requires annual QA testing that includes basic image quality and dose metrics and is completed by a qualified medical physicist. There are several phantom options available for testing, and tolerances are listed for each for the various required tests. Phantom images must be supplied for adult and pediatric head and abdomen exams that have been acquired using the site's clinical protocol, and the dose for each of these must be within the listed limits. The physicist's report for each unit applying for accreditation must be included in the submission materials. Preventative maintenance, including documentation, is also required.

Technologist Requirements

For CT accreditation, the technologists must meet the following requirements: have registration or certification from the American Registry of Radiologic Technologists (ARRT); trained and/or hold current, unrestricted registration(s) or be licensed in each of the modalities performed; have an associate's or bachelor's degree in radiologic science whenever required, with requisite job experience; and complete ongoing education as required by the license, certification, and medical director's directives. Validated credentials by the technologist's internal credentialing program are sufficient evidence of meeting these requirements.

Credentialing of Physicians Interpreting Cardiac CT

Unlike accreditation, which focuses on the technical aspects of cardiac CT and the equipment used to perform it, credentialing refers to the process used to ensure that the practitioners who interpret these studies are competent to do so. In the United States, credentialing is the responsibility of the hospital or imaging center where these studies are performed or interpreted.

US hospitals employ credentialing committees to review physician qualifications. It is the responsibility of the committee to ensure individual physicians have the medical knowledge, technical skills, and clinical judgment to perform their assigned duties. Once a physician has been credentialed at an individual hospital, he or she must apply to be recredentialed every 3 years to maintain hospital privileges [10].

The credentialing committee is also responsible for determining hospital privileges for each practitioner. Determination of criteria for individual staff privileges is at the discretion of the committee. Examples of criteria for the practice of cardiac CT could include specifying residency and/or fellowship subspecialty training, minimum numbers of cases read and reported, or completion of a certifying examination.

Recommendations for Physician Training in Cardiac CT

Several different organizations have published training guidelines and recommendations for certification of specialists who are to interpret cardiac CT studies. Although none of these recommendations has been universally adopted, each represents an effort to improve patient safety through standardization of training for physicians. Several of these consensus documents are detailed below.

Conjoint Committee of Australian and New Zealand Practitioners: Training Requirements for CTCA Specialists

In 2009, a conjoint committee comprised of members of the Australasian Association of Nuclear Medicine Specialists (AANMS), the Cardiac Society of Australia and New Zealand (CSANZ), and the Royal Australian and New Zealand College of Radiologists (RANZCR) published a summary statement detailing their recommendations for training in coronary CT angiography. This document has been revised several times, most recently in 2014 [11].

The conjoint committee describes two distinct levels of specialist training. Level A training allows the practicing physician to interpret coronary CT angiography independently and without supervision. Level B training allows the practitioner to operate independently and to supervise the training and recertification of other physicians. The training consists of didactic work as well as a mix of live and "library" cases, each of which needs to have been supervised by a Level B specialist.

Level A Training

A. 40 hours of didactic coursework, including 20 h of "hands-on" training
B. 150 coronary CTA cases, including:
   (a) 50 live cases
   (b) 50 cases with correlation of findings to other modalities
   (c) 25 cases with non-coronary cardiac findings
   (d) 25 cases with non-cardiac findings

Level B Training

A. Level A training requirements
B. 150 coronary CTA cases beyond those provided for Level A (total of 300 cases), including:
   (a) 50 live cases (total of 100 live cases)
   (b) 30 cases with correlation of findings (total of 80 correlated cases)

Upon completion of their training, physicians can apply for recognition of training, which functions as certification by the conjoint committee. Recertification is available for practitioners who document a minimum of 300 cases (for Level A) or 600 cases (for Level B) within a 3-year recertification period.

American College of Cardiology Recommendations for Training in Cardiovascular CT: COCATS 4 Task Force 7

In 2015, the American College of Cardiology (ACC) published its recommendations for fellows-in-training to become proficient in cardiac CT. This document was endorsed by the American Society of Nuclear Cardiology (ASNC), the Society for Cardiovascular Angiography and Interventions (SCAI), the Society of Atherosclerosis Imaging and Prevention (SAIP), and the Society of Cardiovascular Computed Tomography (SCCT). The recommendations are designed to meet the competency-based parameters endorsed by the American College of Graduate Medical Education (ACGME) and are intended to address the six ACGME core competencies for medical education [12].

As with the Australia and New Zealand guidelines, these recommendations delineate distinct levels of proficiency that can be attained with different amounts of training. Unlike the conjoint committee's document, these recommendations only cover fellows during their initial training. Recommendations for established practitioners are not included. Details of these training recommendations can be found in Table 5.1.

Level 1 Training

Level 1 training is the minimum basic level of training needed to gain basic familiarity with the principles of cardiac CT. Practitioners who have Level 1 training can be considered to be educated consumers but are not expected to be able to interpret CT scans independently. This training consists of approximately 1 month of intensive exposure to cardiac CT and should include mentored interpretation of at least 50 scans with correlation to other cardiac imaging. For at least 15 of these studies, it is expected that the trainee will be present during the performance of the examination.

Level 2 Training

Level 2 training is the minimum level of training needed for independent interpretation of cardiac CT studies. Trainees should complete at least 1 additional month of training in addition to the requirements for Level 1 and interpret at least 200 additional cardiac CT studies, of which 65 require the trainee be present during performance of the examination. Additionally, the trainee is expected to review all CT cases for non-cardiac findings.

Level 3 Training

Level 3 training allows the practitioner to supervise an independent cardiac CT facility or direct an academic cardiac CT practice. The ACC recommendations specify that this level of training requires additional time beyond the standard 3-year cardiovascular fellowship and is expected to include training in at least one other cardiac imaging modality. Additionally, Level 3 training should involve participation in research, teaching, and the administrative aspects of running a cardiac CT service.

Certification in Cardiac CT

Although credentialing standards for individual physicians are determined by the hospitals where they work and do not necessarily include completion of a certification examination, two different organizations in the United States provide certification for specialists in cardiac CT. Each of these certificates is designed to allow qualified practitioners from varying medical specialties to demonstrate proficiency in the performance and interpretation of cardiac CT.

CBCCT Certification in Cardiac CT

In 2008, the Certification Board of Cardiovascular Computed Tomography (CBCCT) began offering a certification examination in cardiac CT. The examination is a computer-based test offered every 2 years and consists of up to 175 multiple choice questions on a variety of topics relating to cardiac CT (http://www.cccvi.org/cbcct) [13].

Qualified physicians who pass the examination are granted certification, which is valid for a period of 8 years. Recertification is accomplished through maintenance of a valid medical license and appropriate medical board certification, supplemented by continued medical education and

Table 5.1 Core competency components and curricular milestones for training in cardiovascular computed tomography

		Milestones (months)			
	Competency component	12	24	36	Add
Medical knowledge					
1	Know the principles of cardiovascular computed tomographic scanning and the scanning modes		I		
2	Know the risks and safety measures for cardiovascular computed tomographic scanning, including radiation reduction strategies			I	
3	Know the appropriate indications for cardiovascular computed tomography for screening or evaluating symptoms in patients with suspected cardiac disease		I		
4	Know the indications, potential adverse effects, prevention, and treatment of complications of iodinated contrast agent use in cardiovascular computed tomographic studies		I		
5	Know the indications and protocols for beta-adrenergic blocking drugs and nitroglycerin during cardiovascular computed tomographic studies			II	
6	Know the principles of cardiovascular computed tomographic scan collimation, temporal resolution, table speed, field of view, and window and level view settings			II	
7	Know the principles of post-processing methods for cardiovascular computed tomographic scanning			II	
8	Know the algorithms used for reconstruction, and recognize and isolate causes of artifacts			II	
9	Know the principles of quantitative coronary artery calcium scoring			II	
10	Know normal chest anatomy and common incidental extra cardiac findings			II	
11	Know the characteristic cardiovascular computed tomographic images of normal cardiac chambers and great vessels, normal coronary arteries and veins, and normal variants			I	
12	Know the characteristic cardiovascular computed tomographic findings of coronary atherosclerosis including plaque morphology and assessment of stenosis severity			II	
13	Know the characteristic cardiovascular computed tomographic findings of anomalous coronary arteries and other common congenital anomalies			II	
14	Know the characteristic cardiovascular computed tomographic findings in postoperative cardiac surgical patients including internal mammary artery and saphenous vein bypass grafts			II	
15	Know the characteristic cardiovascular computed tomographic findings of acquired and congenital valvular disease			II	
16	Know the characteristic cardiovascular computed tomographic findings of left atrial and pulmonary and coronary venous abnormalities			II	
17	Know the characteristic cardiovascular computed tomographic findings of pericardial disease			II	
18	Know the characteristic cardiovascular computed tomographic findings of cardiomyopathies and infiltrative myocardial diseases			II	
19	Know the differential diagnosis of cardiac masses identified by cardiovascular computed tomography			II	
20	Know the characteristic cardiovascular computed tomographic findings of common diseases of the aorta and great vessels			II	
21	Know the characteristic cardiovascular computed tomographic findings of pulmonary embolism and primary and acquired pulmonary vascular diseases			II	
22	Know when to request help with the interpretation of difficult studies, such as patients with complex congenital heart disease			I	
	Evaluation tools: conference presentation, direct observation, and in-training examination				
Patient care and procedural skills					
1	Skill to appropriately utilize cardiovascular computed tomography in the evaluation and management of patients with known or suspected cardiovascular disease			I	
2	Skill to integrate cardiovascular computed tomographic findings with other clinical information in patient evaluation and management			I	
3	Skill to recognize and treat contrast-related adverse reactions	I			
4	Skill to independently perform and interpret cardiovascular computed tomography			II	
5	Skill to perform and interpret hybrid CT/SPECT and CT/PET imaging				III
	Evaluation tools: conference presentation, direct observation, and logbook				
Systems-based practice					
1	Incorporate appropriate use criteria, risk/benefit, and cost considerations in the use of cardiovascular computed tomography and alternative imaging modalities		I		
	Evaluation tools: conference presentation, direct observation, and multisource evaluation				
Practice-based learning and improvement					
1	Identify knowledge and performance gaps and engage in opportunities to achieve focused education and performance improvement			I	

Table 5.1 (continued)

Competency component		Milestones (months) 12	24	36	Add
2	Utilize point-of-care educational resources (e.g., guidelines, appropriate use criteria, and clinical trial results)			I	
	Evaluation tools: conference presentation, direct observation, and reflection and self-assessment				
Professionalism					
1	Work effectively in an interdisciplinary cardiovascular computed tomographic imaging environment		I		
2	Reliably obtain patient-informed consent, ensuring that patients understand the risks and benefits of, and alternatives to, cardiovascular computed tomographic testing		I		
3	Know and promote adherence to clinical practice guidelines		I		
	Evaluation tools: conference presentation, direct observation, and multisource evaluation				
Interpersonal and communication skills					
1	Communicate testing results to physicians and patients in an effective and timely manner		I		
	Evaluation tools: direct observation and multisource evaluation				

From Garcia et al. [12], with permission
Add additional months beyond the 3-year cardiovascular fellowship, *CT* computed tomography, *PET* positron emission tomography, *SPECT* single-photon emission computed tomography

ongoing interpretation of a minimum of 150 cardiac CT studies over a 36-month period. Details regarding eligibility requirements for initial certification are available on the CVCCT website [cccvi.org].

ACR Certificate of Advanced Proficiency in Cardiac CT

In 2008, the American College of Radiology developed a certification examination for practitioners to demonstrate advanced competency in cardiac CT. Initially, this examination included a live workstation case review. The current examination is computer-based and consists of 100 multiple-choice questions administered over a 2-h period at more than 850 testing centers around the world.

The ACR Certificate of Advanced Proficiency (CoAP) examination covers a wide variety of topics related to cardiovascular CT (http://www.acr.org/Education/Exams-Certifications/CoAP). Successful completion of the examination conveys a certificate which is valid for a period of 10 years. Eligibility requirements to sit for the examination and a list of designated testing centers are available on the ACR website [acr.org] [14].

Conclusion

Although accreditation of equipment and credentialing of practitioners are not the first topics that come to mind when discussing cardiac CT, each is important for establishing and maintaining a successful cardiovascular imaging program. As cardiovascular CT continues to develop as an imaging subspecialty, maintenance of certification and employment of appropriate technology will become increasingly important as means of demonstrating expertise in this rapidly changing field.

References

1. https://www.cms.gov/Medicare/Provider-Enrollment-and-Certification/SurveyCertificationGenInfo/Accreditation-of-Advanced-Diagnostic-Imaging-Suppliers.html. Accessed 27 Oct 2016.
2. CT Accreditation Program Requirements. http://www.acraccreditation.org/~/media/ACRAccreditation/Documents/CT/Requirements.pdf?la=en. Accessed 27 Oct 2016.
3. American College of Radiology CT Accreditation Program Testing Instructions. http://www.acraccreditation.org/~/media/ACRAccreditation/Documents/CT/CT-Accreditation-Testing-Instructions.pdf?la=en. Accessed 27 Oct 2016.
4. Personnel Requirements for Medical Physicists and MR Scientists. http://www.acraccreditation.org/Revised-Program-Requirements. Accessed 27 Oct 2016.
5. 2012 Computed Tomography Quality Control Manual, available from the American College of Radiology (http://www.acr.org/Education/Education-Catalog/Products/8336734).
6. The IAC Standards and Guidelines for CT Accreditation. http://www.intersocietal.org/ct/standards/IACCTStandards2015.pdf. Accessed 27 Oct 2016.
7. Diagnostic Imaging Requirements. https://www.jointcommission.org/assets/1/18/AHC_DiagImagingRpt_MK_20150806.pdf. Accessed 27 Oct 2016.
8. RadSite MAP Accreditation Standards, version 2 (MAP v 2.2), available on request from http://www.radsitequality.com/cms-accreditation-requirments. Accessed 27 Oct 2016.
9. http://www.radsitequality.com/cms-accreditation-requirments with permission.
10. National Association Medical Staff Services. www.namss.org/portals/0/education. Accessed 15 Jan 2017.
11. Training Requirements for CTCA Specialists, Version 4 (Rep.). 2014 Conjoint Committee for Recognition of Training in Computed Tomography Coronary Angiography.
12. Garcia MJ, Blankstein R, Budoff MJ, Dent JM, Drachman DE, Lesser JR, et al. COCATS 4 task force 7: training in cardiovascular computed tomographic imaging. J Am Coll Cardiol. 2015;65(17):1810.
13. Latest News-Certification Board of Cardiovascular Computed Tomography. http://www.cccvi.org/cbcct. Accessed 28 Oct 2016.
14. Cardiac CT Certificate of Advanced Proficiency (CoAP Exam). http://www.acr.org/Education/Exams-Certifications/CoAP. Accessed 28 Oct 2016.

Part III

Where We Are: Technical and Operational Requisites

Cardiac CT Platforms: State of the Art

6

Bernhard Schmidt, Katharine Grant, Thomas G. Flohr, and Thomas Allmendinger

Shorter scan times and the desire for higher resolution were the driving forces behind the development of spiral scanning in 1990 and the first multi-detector row computed tomography (CT) systems in 1998 [1–6]. With the introduction of ECG-gated scanning on four-slice CT scanners in 1999, the first step toward cardiac imaging with multi-detector row computed tomography (MDCT) had been made.

Available since 2004, 64-slice CT systems are currently considered prerequisite for routine cardiac imaging in clinical scenarios [7–10], and with its introduction, the task of imaging coronary arteries and calcium scoring replaced EBCT (electron beam CT) completely. 64-slice CT scanners allowed for comprehensive diagnosis of morphology and cardiac function within one integrated CT examination, including high-resolution imaging of the coronary arteries [11–14]. Improved temporal resolution (< 200 ms) was enabled by faster gantry rotation times down to 0.33 s and leading to an increased clinical robustness of ECG-gated scanning techniques at higher heart rates [9, 10]. ECG-gated 64-slice CT also started being used for rapid triage of patients with acute chest pain in the emergency room and for diagnosis of pulmonary embolism, aortic dissection or aneurysm, or significant coronary artery disease in one scan.

Despite the new clinical opportunities and the increasing use of CT for routine cardiac imaging, several challenges still remained: For high heart rates, multi-segment reconstructions allowing for temporal resolutions beyond half the rotation time were still desired for robust imaging of coronary arteries. Multi-segment reconstructions unfortunately do not guarantee images with a well-defined improved temporal resolution in combination with the need for redundant data and thus due to acquisitions with reduced pitch resulting in substantially increased patient dose values [15]. Irregular or arrhythmic heart rates posed a challenge for artifact-free combination of images that were reconstructed from multiple cardiac cycles into a single volume, often yielding "stack artifacts" in these cases. Moreover, calcium blooming was still an issue – mainly due to operation in an X-ray tube limited, and therefore noise-dominated regime, resulting in the routine application of medium-sharp reconstructions in cardiac images exhibiting the undesired blooming of high-contrast calcium. Adaption of X-ray tube voltages (kVs) to lower kVs to reduce patient dose was used in particular for regular contrast-enhanced scans, to improve image quality in pediatric patients. These adaptations occurred manually, often on weight-based selection criteria, and application was limited to a select group of the general population due to the demand of high X-ray tube current capacities required for cardiac imaging [16]. Finally, scan times for coronary CTAs were still in the range of 10–15 s given the limited detector coverage and the lack of alternative scan technology.

In 2004, all major CT vendors offered 64-slice CT scanners. The remaining challenges of cardiac CT imaging, the pursuit for even more clinical applications, the risk that MR imaging could further improve on and replace CT for not just functional but for morphological imaging, the tenacious competition of the vendors, and the relentless improvements in engineering and scientific innovations, made cardiac imaging the main driving force for further CT innovations, technical developments, and new CT platforms. In contrary to previous innovations, technical solutions and directions of development differed substantially between different vendors, ranging from wide detector systems with single-source systems over two X-ray source systems with a single detector to systems with two X-ray tubes and two detectors.

In 2005, a dual-source CT (DSCT) system, i.e., a CT system with two X-ray tubes and two corresponding detectors offset by 90°, was introduced [17]. It provided improved

B. Schmidt (✉) · T. Allmendinger · T. G. Flohr
Department of Computed Tomography, Siemens Healthcare GmbH, Forchheim, Germany
e-mail: bernhard.schmidt@siemens.com

K. Grant
Siemens Medical Solutions USA, Inc., Malvern, PA, USA

U. J. Schoepf (ed.), *CT of the Heart*, Contemporary Medical Imaging, https://doi.org/10.1007/978-1-60327-237-7_6

temporal resolution of 83 ms independent of the patient's heart rate as compared to 165–190 ms with MDCT systems at that time. DSCT scanners proved to be well suited for integrated cardiothoracic examinations even in acutely ill patients and for the triage of patients with acute chest pain [18]. The introduction of dual-energy scanning with DSCT enabled tissue characterization and provided combined functional and morphological information, i.e., to depict local perfusion deficits in the lung parenchyma in patients with pulmonary embolism [19, 20].

The second and third generations (introduced in 2009 and 2013, respectively) of DSCT systems offer high-pitch scan modes which enabled coverage of the heart in a single cardiac cycle [21, 22]. In addition, high-resolution CT scans of the entire thorax in less than 1 s scan time with an acquisition time per image better than 100 ms were now possible [23, 24]. These scan modes are potentially advantageous for evaluating the lung parenchyma and vascular structures in patients who have difficulty complying with breath-holding instructions [25]. High-pitch scan modes have also been used for fast CTA scans of the aorta [26]. Combined with ECG triggering, they provide adequate visualization of the coronary arteries, the aortic valve, the aorta, and the iliac arteries in one scan at low radiation dose, which is beneficial in the planning of transcatheter aortic valve replacement (TAVR) procedures [27, 28].

Another challenge for CT is the visualization of dynamic processes in extended anatomical ranges, i.e., to characterize the inflow and outflow of contrast agent in the arterial and venous system in dynamic CT angiographies or to determine the enhancement characteristics of the contrast agent in volume perfusion studies. One way to address this problem is by utilizing wide-area detectors large enough to cover organs such as the heart, the kidneys, or the brain in one axial scan. Besides temporal resolution, registration or mismatch artifacts from the combination of multiple cardiac cycles or slabs in *z*-direction are another challenge, naturally leading to the idea of increasing the detector coverage to such a level that the entire heart is covered in a single prospectively gated sequential acquisition. Meanwhile, two vendors have introduced CT scanners with 16 cm detector coverage at isocenter, providing 320 × 0.5 mm collimation at 0.28 s rotation time or 256 × 0.625 mm collimation at 0.28 s rotation time [29]. Additionally these scanners have the potential to acquire dynamic volume data by repeatedly scanning the same anatomical range without table movement (e.g., [30–32]).

In the following sections, after a short historic review of EBCT, general technical demands of MDCT for cardiac image quality are discussed. Then a technical overview of the main currently available platforms and CT systems is provided, and details about advantages and technical challenges of the different approaches are discussed.

From EBCT to Multi-detector CT for Cardiac Imaging

EBCT

Generation of X-rays for medical imaging is typically accomplished by using X-ray tubes. Electrons emitted from a cathode are accelerated by a high-voltage power source and collide with the anode, at which X-rays are generated by the interaction of electrons within the anode material. For CT imaging, X-ray attenuation data from multiple angles around the patient are required. Thus, first CT systems were equipped with X-ray tubes set up opposite a detector, which in conjunction rotated around the patients at rotation times of about 5 s or longer. Mechanical constraints and challenges with rotating components, mainly data and power transmission, prevented continuous rotation at faster rotation times back then. Unfortunately, for cardiac imaging in particular, faster rotation times were desired to minimize motion artifacts and provide better temporal resolution. Already in the late 1970s, electron beam scanners were proposed with the goal of providing a substantially higher temporal resolution for cardiac imaging by avoiding rotating parts. In the early 1980s, D.P. Boyd – a Stanford researcher and partner in the radiology department at the University of California, San Francisco (USA) – invented the first clinically used EBCT system: "Electron beam control assembly and method for a scanning electron beam computed tomography scanner." It related to "… a high speed multiple section computed-tomographic (CT) x-ray transmission scanner and more particularly to a multiple target scanning-electron beam x-ray source providing rapid scan …" (see also Figs. 6.1 and 6.2) [33]. Instead of rotating tube and detector around the patient, a stationary detector ring is used for data acquisition. To generate X-rays, an electron beam originating from an electron gun is deflected and steered over an anode that was ringlike enclosing the patient. Temporal resolutions of 100 ms and shorter were possible. The main application – in particular in the early days of EBCT – was the detection and quantification of coronary calcium at dose levels of about 0.6 mSv [34]. Later on, studies reported the use of EBCT for coronary CTA imaging [35], assessment of ventricular anatomy and function [36], as well as myocardial perfusion [37].

Despite the unquestionable benefit of high temporal resolution of EBCT, only a few systems were installed worldwide, by the end of 1987 about 14 units. The high price, low production volume, system design issues (e.g., the inability to use scatter collimators), and limited clinical benefit beside the heart were preventing cardiologists and radiologists to invest into an EBCT system. Finally, the limited spatial resolution was yet another factor making the already niche scanner even less attractive. Although with the latest generation of EBCTs (GE's e-Speed), slice thicknesses of 1.5 mm were

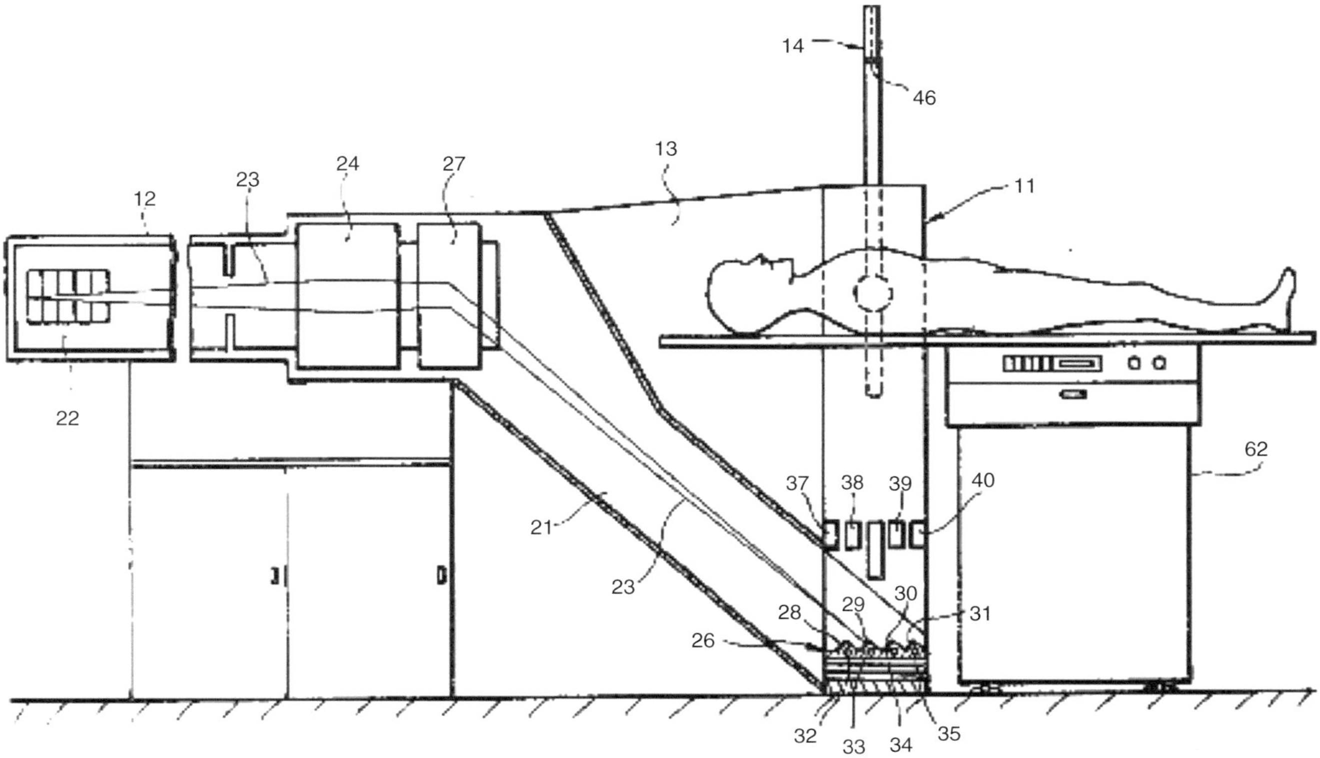

Fig. 6.1 Illustration of an EBCT (electron beam computerized tomography) system – taken from Boyd's patent in 1982; US 4352021: Electrons emitted from the electron gun [22] are accelerated and steered around the patient. The electron beam hitting the target rings [28–31] created X-rays at the respective position on the ring. From there the X-rays passed through the patient to the detector [14] on the opposite end of the scan tube tomography system. (From US patent US4352021 https://www.google.com/patents/US4352021?dq=us+patent+4352021&hl=en&sa=X&ved=0ahUKEwitp6_N38vYAhXDY98KHT01DXwQ6AEIJzAA)

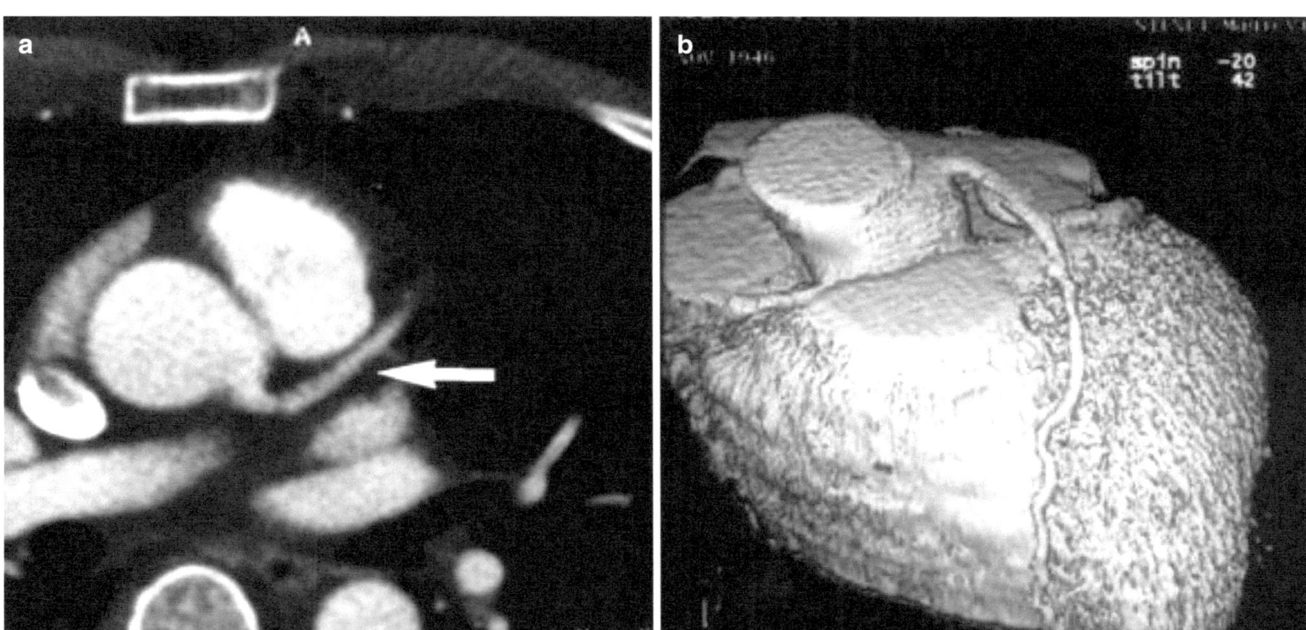

Fig. 6.2 Axial image of a contrast-enhanced EBCT scan, showing the left main and left anterior descending coronary artery (arrow) (**a**). Surface-rendered view of the heart by visualizing only voxels above a certain threshold (**b**) (From Achenbach et al. [35], with permission)

enabled [38], this relevant specification parameter for coronary CT imaging was already matched by 16-slice CT systems at the end of 1990s and then outperformed substantially by the introduction of 64-slice MDCT systems providing routinely submillimeter image resolution in the early 2000s. In addition, volume scanning, the ability to apply modern dose reduction techniques such as low kV scanning, utilization of shaped filters, or patient-specific tube current modulation never became available or were technically impossible to implement on an EBCT system.

Multi-detector Row CT Setup (MDCT)

The basic CT system design of modern MDCT system is shown in Fig. 6.3. Today, all manufacturers use the same fan-beam CT design, characterized by an X-ray tube and an opposing detector which are mounted on a rotating gantry ring. The detector is a two-dimensional array, consisting of 2–320 element rows aligned in the *z*-axis direction (the *z*-axis is the length axis of the patient) and around 650–1000 detector elements in each row. The fan angle of the detector is wide enough (approximately 45–55°) to cover a whole-body scan field of view (SFOV) of typically 50 cm in diameter. In a CT scan, the detector array measures the X-ray attenuation profile of the patient at 1000–5000 different angular positions depending on the rotation time, during a full gantry rotation. All measurement values acquired at the same angular position of the measurement system are called a "projection" or "view." Slip ring designs which pass the electrical signals across sliding contacts allow for continuous rotation of the measurement system.

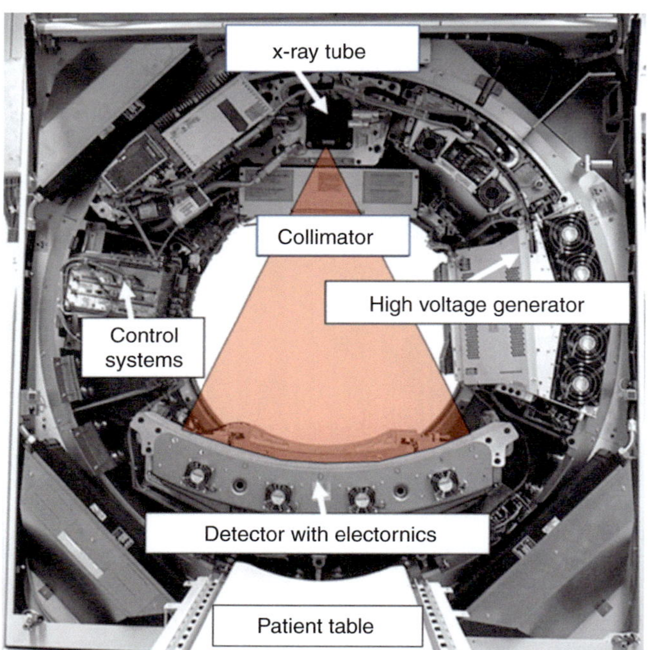

Fig. 6.3 Main components of a modern MDCT system. The X-ray fan beam is indicated in red; it covers a SFOV of typically 50 cm in diameter. The data measurement system consists of detector and detector electronics. The patient is positioned within the gantry using a dedicated patient table

State-of-the-art X-ray tubes are powered by onboard generators and provide peak powers of 60–120 kW at different user-selectable voltages ranging from 70 to 150 kV. Scanning at low tube voltage is favorable for dose-efficient scans, such as pediatric CT [39, 40] or CT angiographic scanning [16, 41–43], because the X-ray attenuation of iodine significantly increases at lower kV [40].

All modern MDCT systems use solid-state scintillation detectors. The incident X-rays interact with a radiation-sensitive crystal or ceramic (such as gadolinium oxide, gadolinium oxysulfide, or garnets) with suitable doping. They are absorbed, and their energy is converted into visible light which is detected by a silicon photodiode attached to the backside of the scintillation detector. The resulting electrical current is then converted into a digital signal. Key requirements for a detector material are good detection efficiency, i.e., high atomic number, very good signal linearity, and very short afterglow time to enable fast readout at the high gantry rotation speeds that are essential for cardiothoracic CT.

The image noise in a CT image is caused by the quantum noise of the X-ray photons and the electronic noise of the detection system. In high-dose scanning situations, the image noise is dominated by quantum noise, whereas when larger patients are scanned or in examinations at low radiation dose, e.g., in low-dose thorax scans, electronic noise is more dominant. In addition, electronic noise degrades image quality and the stability of CT values. Recently, detector systems with integrated electronics were commercially introduced (e.g., Stellar, Siemens Healthcare, Forchheim, Germany; NanoPanel Elite, Philips Healthcare, Amsterdam, Netherlands), with the goal of reducing electronic noise and detector cross talk. In these designs, photodiodes and analog-to-digital converters (ADC) are combined and directly attached to the ceramic scintillators, without the need for noise-sensitive analog connection cables (Fig. 6.4). In a recent study, for a 30 cm phantom corresponding to an average abdomen, reduction of image noise by up to 40% was demonstrated with the use of an integrated electronic detector at 80 kV [44]. According to the authors, this noise reduction translated into a dose reduction of up to 50% while achieving equivalent image noise.

In early MDCT detectors, ADC electronics and data transmission were a limiting factor and a strong contributor to the total cost of a system. An efficient way of enabling higher scan speeds based on a larger *z*-axis collimation was through the development of detector elements with a larger number of detector rows. The total beam width in the *z*-

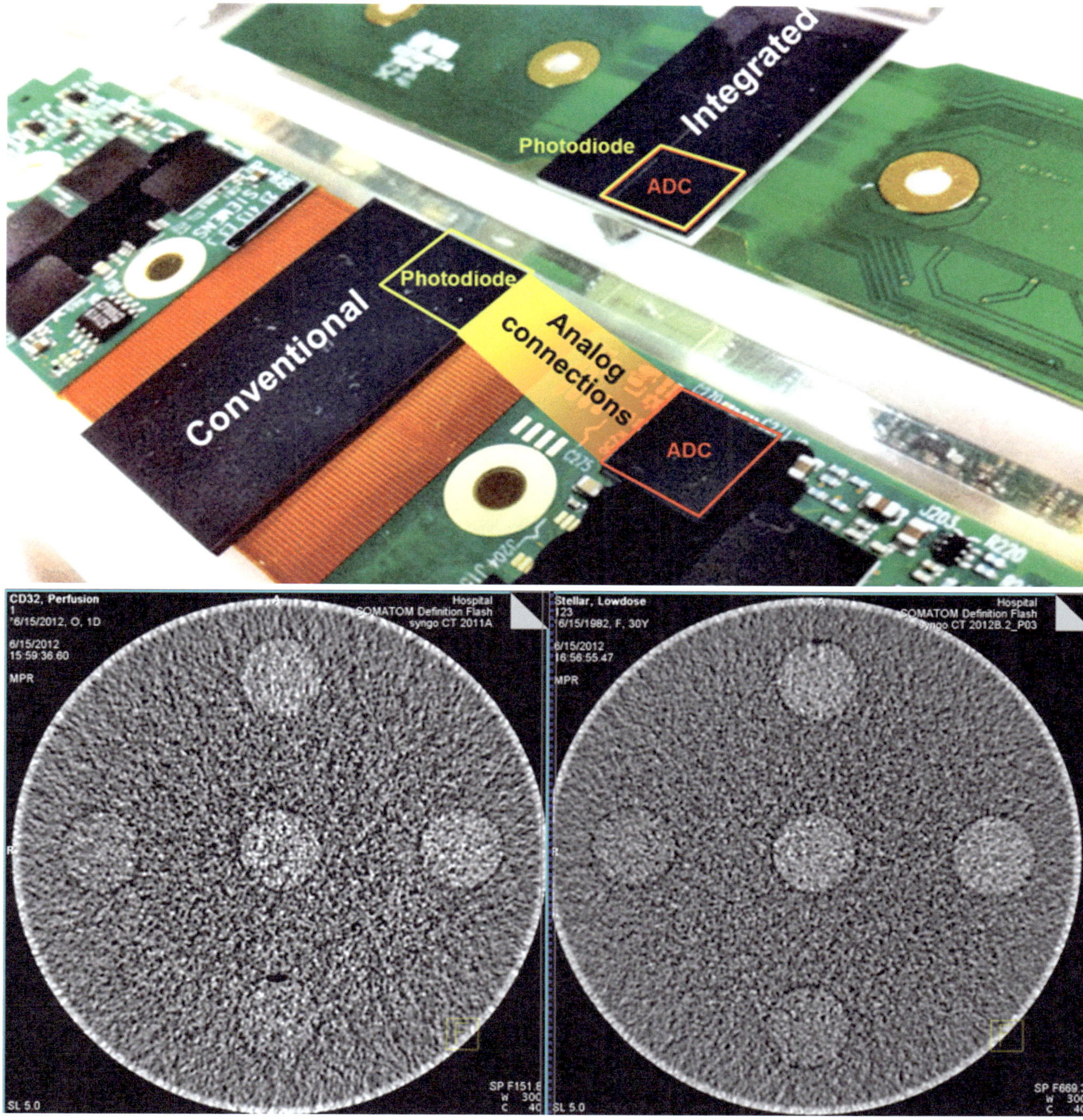

Fig. 6.4 Comparison of the Si-tile without scintillator ceramics – with and without integrated electronics (top) (Siemens Healthcare). At the bottom CT images of a 30 cm water phantom acquired at same dose (80 kV, 30 mA) are illustrated. The integrated design leads to substantially lower noise values (right bottom image)

direction is subsequently adjusted by pre-patient collimation at the expense of fusing two (or more) detectors along the *z*-axis electronically into thicker slices.

The detector of a 16-slice CT (Siemens SOMATOM Emotion 16) as an example comprises 16 central rows, each with 0.6 mm collimated slice width, and 4 outer rows on either side, each with 1.2 mm collimated slice width – in total, 24 rows with a *z*-width of 19.2 mm at isocenter (Fig. 6.5). By adjusting the X-ray beam width such that only the central detector rows are illuminated, the system provides 16 collimated 0.6 mm slices. By illuminating the entire detector, reading out all rows and electronically combining the signals of every 2 central rows, the system provides 16 collimated 1.2 mm slices. The 16-slice detectors of other

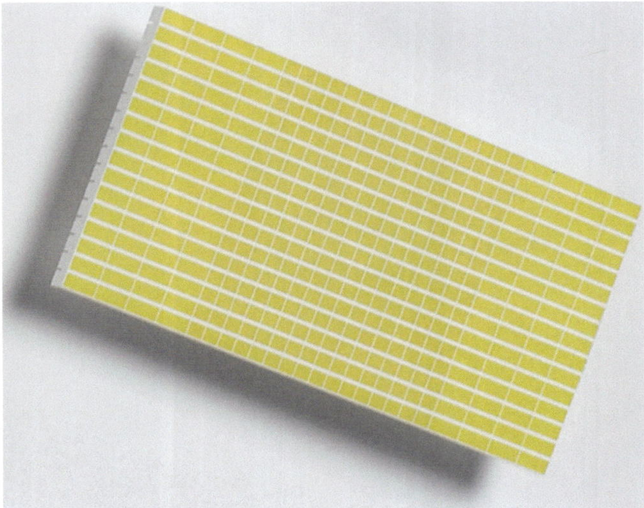

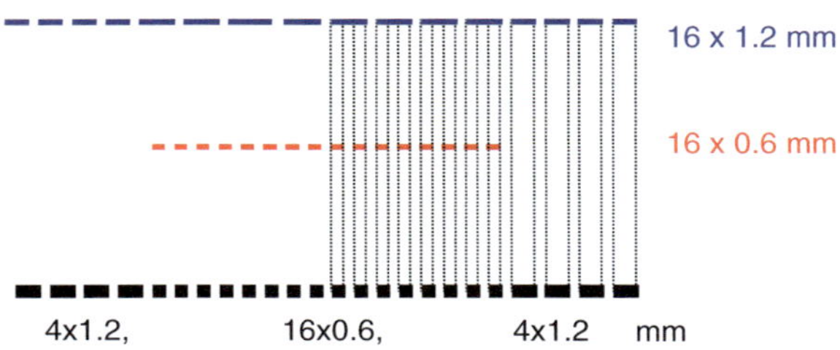

Fig. 6.5 Example of a 16-slice detector, which consists of 24 detector rows and provides either 16 collimated 0.6 mm slices or – by combination of the signals of every 2 central rows – 16 collimated 1.2 mm slices

manufacturers are similarly designed, with slightly different collimated slice widths (0.5 mm, 0.6 mm, or 0.625 mm, depending on the manufacturer).

With the introduction of MDCT detectors with 64 or more detector rows and a vendor-dependent minimal slice width of 0.5 mm, 0.6 mm, or 0.625 mm, the detector row fusing mechanisms described above was no longer necessary. As of today a wide variety of detector row configurations exist (e.g., 96 × 0.6 mm, *z*-width 6 cm at the isocenter; 128 × 0.625 mm, *z*-width 8 cm at the isocenter) up to the widest commercially available CT detectors covering 16 cm at isocenter. The acquisition is either based on 320 collimated 0.5 mm slices (Aquilion ONE, Toshiba Medical, Japan) or 256 collimated 0.625 mm slices (Revolution, GE Healthcare, USA).

All modern MDCT scanners enable reconstruction of images with different image slice widths from the same raw data according to the clinical needs (e.g., 3 mm or 5 mm for initial viewing and additional submillimeter slices or 1 mm slices for post processing).

Some CT systems employ a hardware-based oversampling scheme effectively doubling the number of simultaneously acquired slices by means of a *z*-flying focal spot [45, 46] (Z-FFS, Siemens Healthcare, Forchheim, Germany; Ingenuity DAS, Philips Healthcare, Amsterdam, Netherlands). The focal spot in the X-ray tube is periodically moved between two *z*-positions on the anode plate by electromagnetic deflection. As a consequence, the measurement rays of two readings are shifted by half a collimated slice width at isocenter and can be interleaved to one projection with double the number of slices but half the *z*-sampling distance (Fig. 6.6). Two 64-slice readings with 0.6 mm slice width and 0.6 mm *z*-sampling distance, as an example, are combined to one projection with 128 overlapping 0.6 mm slices at 0.3 mm *z*-sampling distance. The *z*-flying focal spot provides improved data sampling in the *z*-direction for better through-plane resolution, reconstruction of thinner slices, and reduced spiral windmill artifacts (Fig. 6.7).

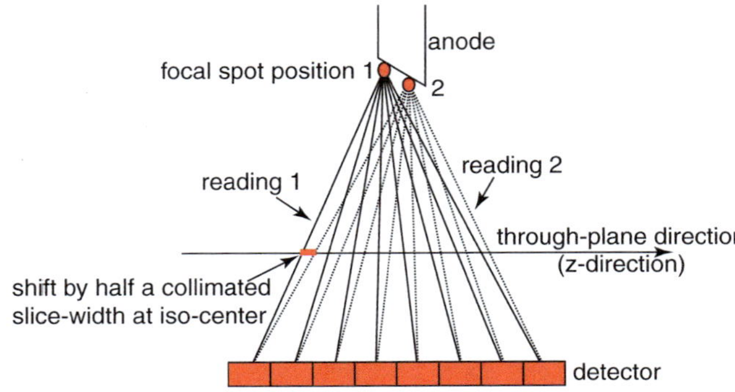

Fig. 6.6 Basic principle of a *z*-flying focal spot. Consecutive readings are shifted periodically by half a slice width on the anode plate. Every two readings are interleaved to one projection with double the number of slices and half the *z*-sampling distance

ECG-Based Imaging with MDCT

To acquire images of the heart, recording of the ECG signal is mandatory. On one hand one wants to be able to process and view a dedicated phase of the cardiac cycle which requires a time stamp-based link between the cardiac phase of the patient and the acquired CT data. On the other hand, in the case of limited detector coverage, data from multiple heart beats is acquired over time and then stitched together to allow the reconstruction and display of the whole heart. For MDCT with 64 or more detector rows, typically two different acquisition modes are used – ECG-gated spiral/helical and prospective ECG-triggered sequence acquisition. More details about data acquisition and reconstruction are provided in Chaps. 6 and 11. However, to illuminate recent technical developments in CT technology, a short summary of the acquisition techniques and influencing parameters on coverage and temporal resolution is provided.

During the first years of routine clinical integration of coronary CT angiography, retrospectively ECG-gated spiral (helical) scanning was the most widely used data acquisition

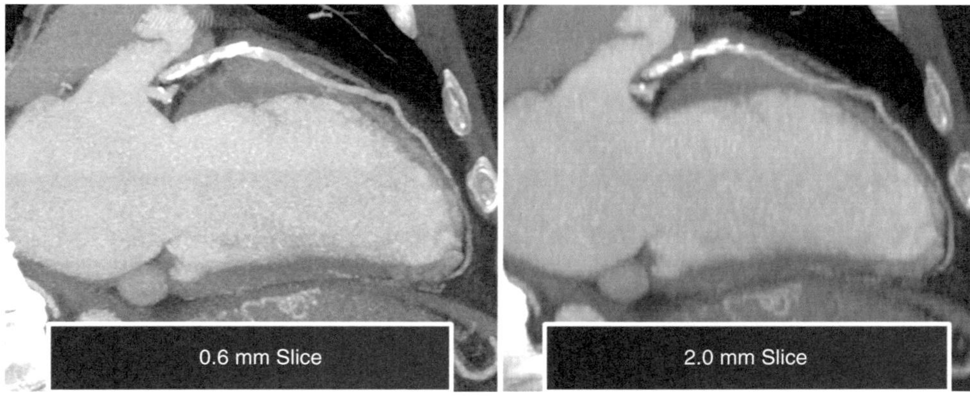

Fig. 6.7 Impact of slice thickness on resolution. Z-flying focal spot techniques allow for the reconstruction of thinner slices and this sharper delineation of anatomical structures

technique. A spiral CT scan with continuous data acquisition and table movement at low table feed (low spiral pitch of approximately 0.2) is performed to examine the patient's heart. Simultaneously, the patient's ECG is recorded. Following data acquisition, the ECG serves as guidance to select those data intervals in the spiral CT data set that describe the same user-selected cardiac phase, measured in different cardiac cycles. Those data are then used for phase-consistent image reconstruction of the coronary anatomy. The upper part of Fig. 6.8 shows the principle of retrospectively ECG-gated spiral scanning. This scan mode is very versatile because it allows for retrospective optimization of the reconstruction window and image reconstruction in different cardiac phases.

As a downside, retrospectively ECG-gated spiral scanning of the heart requires strongly overlapping spiral data acquisition at low table feed for phase-consistent imaging and is therefore associated with relatively high radiation dose to the patient, which can be somewhat reduced by using ECG-controlled dose modulation approaches ("ECG-pulsing"). Many modern CT scanners are equipped with such versatile ECG-pulsing algorithms which react flexibly to arrhythmia and ectopic beats and have the potential to extend the clinical application spectrum of ECG-synchronized dose modulation to patients with irregular heart rates.

As an alternative scan mode, prospectively ECG-triggered sequential scanning in a "step-and-shoot" technique is more commonly used with newer generations of CT systems. During the CT examination, the patient's ECG is used to trigger the start time for the acquisition of axial (sequential) CT images; see lower part of Fig. 6.8. The patient table is moved to its defined start position: with a user-selectable temporal distance from an R-wave, an axial CT scan without table movement is performed. The CT system acquires scan data covering a sub-volume of the patient's cardiac anatomy which corresponds to around 90% of the total *z*-width for a 64-row detector and is reduced for CT systems with large detectors in the *z*-axis direction which have to cope more with cone-beam effects. The table is then moved to the next *z*-position, and the next axial CT scan is performed at the corresponding temporal distance from the next R-wave. This way, the heart volume is sequentially covered by axial scans.

ECG-triggered axial scanning is a very dose-efficient scan technique. In a simple technical realization, a partial scan data interval – the minimum amount of data necessary for image reconstruction – is acquired in a user-selected phase of the patient's cardiac cycle. Then, however, neither retrospective reconstruction in a slightly different phase of the patient's cardiac cycle to minimize motion artifacts is possible nor are multiphase reconstructions for evaluation of cardiac function. Furthermore, due to the fact that incomplete data is acquired, the temporal offset of scan data acquisition to the next R-wave is based on a prospective estimate of the previous cycle's length. This is a challenge in patients with irregular heart beat and arrhythmia, unless the acquisition strategy is properly tailored and aimed at an end-systolic cardiac phase [47].

From 4 cm MDCT CT Systems to Area Detector and Dual-Source CT

Area Detector CT

ECG-synchronized CT volume imaging of the heart acquired by the abovementioned MDCT systems typically results in 3–4 sub-volumes reconstructed from data measured over multiple consecutive heart beats (Fig. 6.9) [48]. Variations of heart motion from one cardiac cycle to the next, as well as contrast media dynamics between the cycles, can result in these image sub-volumes being shifted relative to each other and, as a consequence, resulting in stairstep or slab registration artifacts in multi-planar reformations (MPRs) or volume rendered images (VRTs). Recently, 128-row, 256-slice CT systems with 80 mm *z*-axis coverage were commercially introduced (Philips ICT, Philips Healthcare, Best, the Netherlands). They facil-

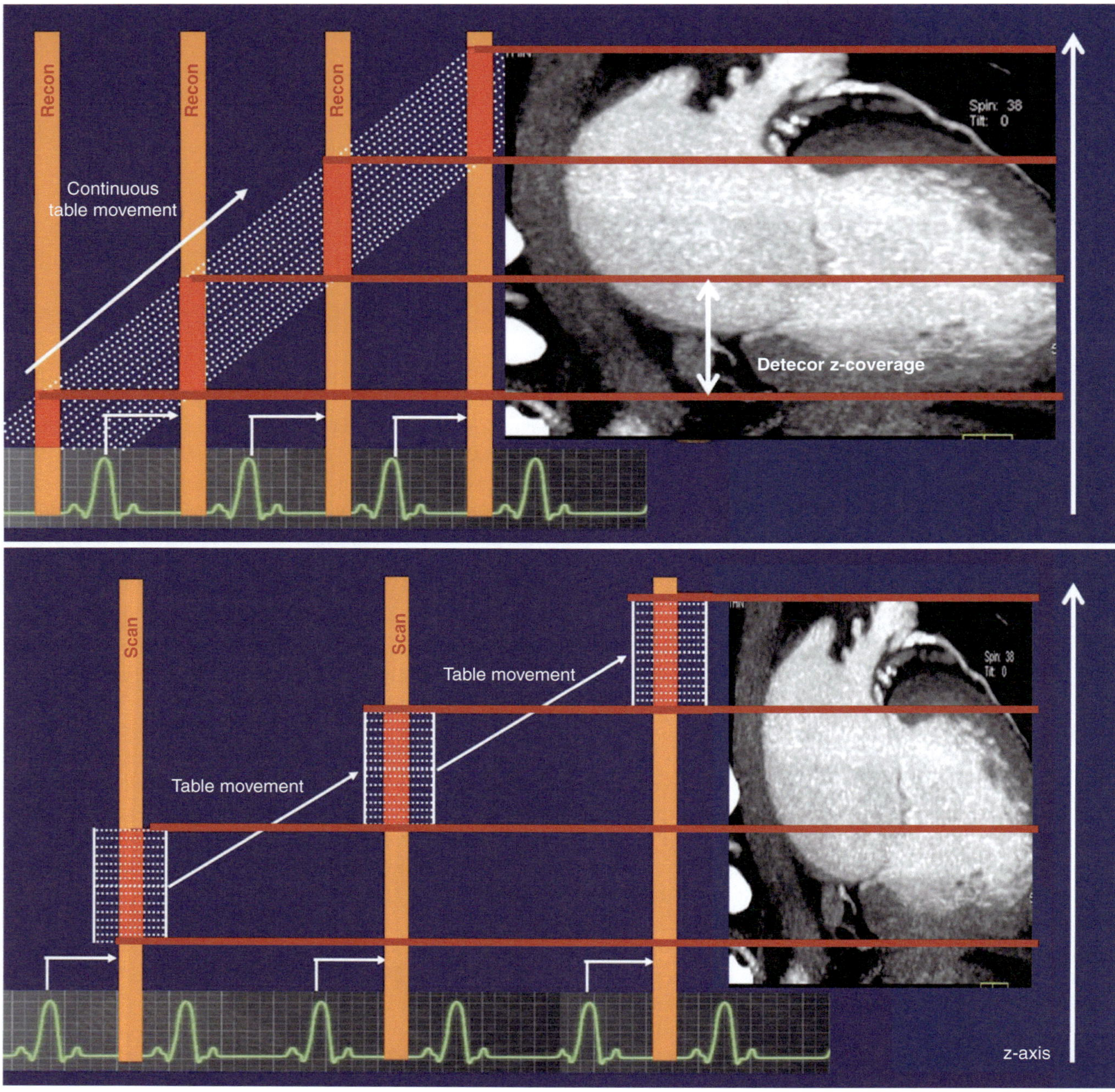

Fig. 6.8 Established acquisition modes for cardiac scanning with CT systems up to 4 cm coverage: In retrospective ECG-gated scan mode (upper part), a helical scan with a comparatively small, fixed heart rate-dependent table feed is performed. For higher heart rates, table feed is increased. In case of a 4 cm system, after 3–4 heart beats, the heart is covered. Similar scan times are accomplished in prospectively ECG-triggered axial (sequential) scanning of the heart (lower part). Based on the user-selected phase position of ECG signal, an axial scan is performed. After each axial scan, the table moves to the next *z*-position. This acquisition technique is also called "step-and-shoot"

itate examinations of the heart with two axial scans, thereby reducing the number of potential "steps" in the volume image to one [49]. In a study with 160 consecutive patients, prospectively triggered axial coronary CTA performed on 256-slice CT provided significantly improved and more stable image quality at an equivalent effective radiation dose compared with 64-slice CT [50].

As of today, two CT vendors provide single-source CT systems with large area detectors capable of imaging the entire heart in one beat, using one axial scan without table movement. With 320 × 0.5 mm collimation at 0.28 s rotation time (Toshiba Aquilion ONE, Toshiba Medical Systems Corporation, Tokyo, Japan) and 256 × 0.625 mm collimation at 0.28 s rotation time (GE Revolution, GE Healthcare,

Waukesha, USA), these systems can cover 16 cm in the *z*-axis direction at isocenter, large enough to cover the entire heart in one beat and hence avoid stairstep and slab registration artifacts, as well as problems related to inconsistent contrast enhancement in different sub-volumes [51].

A possible consequence of the large cone-beam angle that those systems have compared to systems with smaller *z*-coverage can be limitations in the field of view available for reconstruction (Fig. 6.10). In addition, due to this effect also dose efficiency is compromised since not all acquired data can be utilized fully for the reconstruction of the images. Another challenge of larger detector *z*-coverage is increased X-ray scatter. Scattered radiation may cause hypo-dense cupping or streaking artifacts, and the scatter-induced noise may reduce the contrast-to-noise ratio (CNR) in the images [52]. To reduce scatter – in this case forward scatter – some vendors have added scatter grids. While anti-scatter grids are a well-known topic for dual-source CT systems, it is important to note that anti-scatter grids are also recommended in the case of single-source system with wide detectors. A study by Engel et al. showed that the contribution of scatter for a 16 cm single-source system is even higher than in the case of an 8 cm dual-source system, which again motivates the need for anti-scatter grids (ASG) even for single-source systems in case of wide detectors [53]. The requirements were intensely evaluated by Vogtmeier et al. [54]. Figure 6.11 shows the impact on scatter for 1D and 2D scatter grids, for different collimations. In particular, for collimations between 8 and 16 cm coverage, the 2D grids performed substantially better.

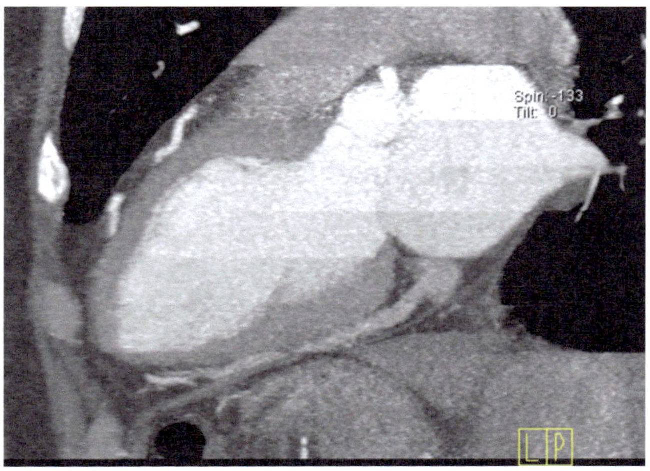

Fig. 6.9 Non-axial view of a cardiac examination performed with ECG-gated spiral mode. Due to the limited coverage, slab artifacts are pronounced due to contrast dynamics and a slight phase mismatch between different acquired heart beats combined with limited temporal resolution

Another challenge of area detectors are the often necessary changes to the tube design. In order to compensate for the so-called Heel effect and to accomplish a homogeneous intensity on the detector along the scan direction (Fig. 6.12), the anode angle is often flatted [55]. The intensity profile is improved, however, at the price of reduced tube power. This consequence can also be seen when looking at the maximum

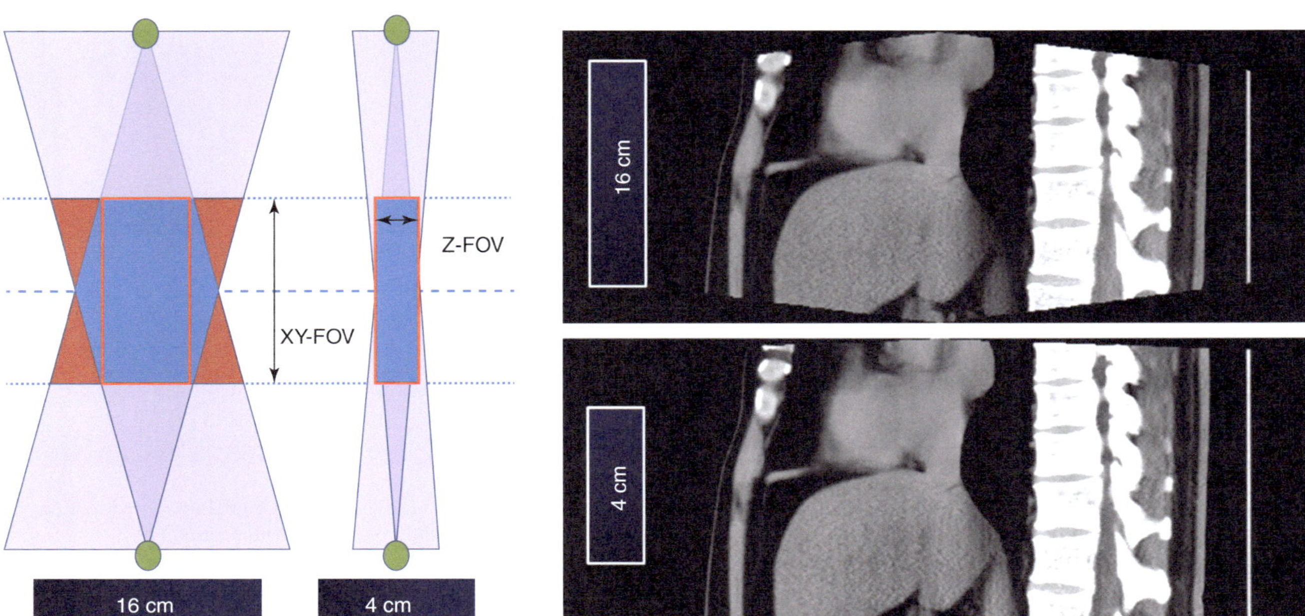

Fig. 6.10 Comparison of systems with 16 cm and 4 cm detector coverage in axial scan mode. Left side: view from the side. The area of full FOV is substantially reduced in case of wide detector systems. Although regions are exposed (highlighted in red), they cannot be reconstructed with traditional reconstruction techniques. As a consequence distorted regions are often cropped in the reconstructed images (see right side)

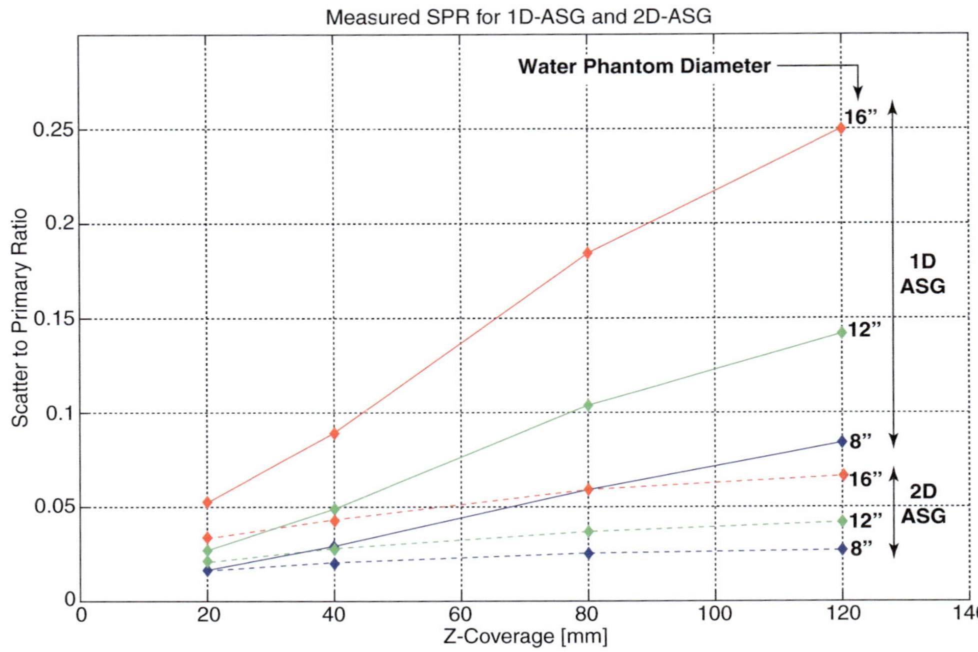

Fig. 6.11 Contribution of scatter to the primary signal for different collimations and designs of anti-scatter grid (ASG). (From Engel et al. [53], with permission)

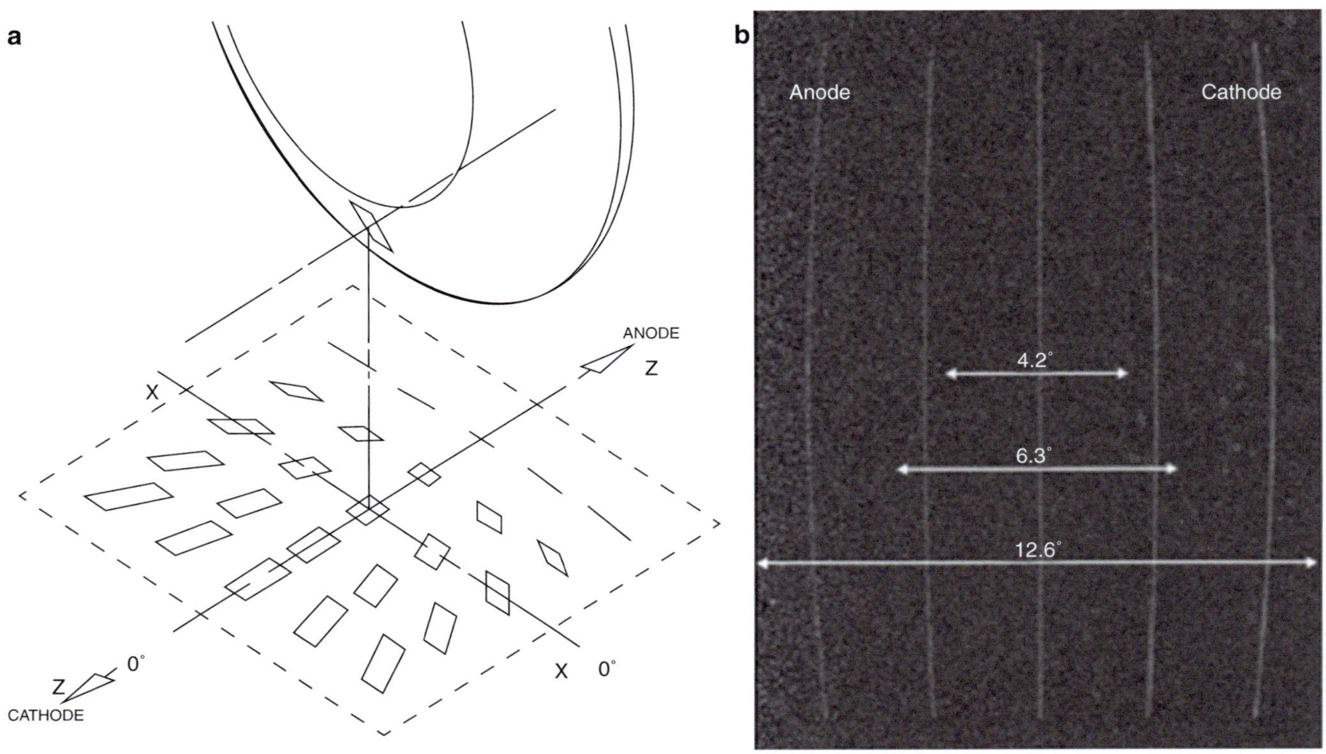

Fig. 6.12 Due to the Heel effect, the footprint of the projected focal spot becomes much narrower on the anode side. To compensate and have a more homogeneous intensity, typically the anode angle is changed to a flatter design. The drawback might be a reduced power output of the tube. (From Li et al. [55], with permission)

tube currently available on high-end CTs. For non-16 cm systems, tube currents up to 1000 mA (Philips) and 1300 mA (Siemens) are enabled, whereas the 16 cm systems have maximum mA values of 735 mA (GE) and 600 mA (Toshiba).

Despite all the abovementioned challenges, successful use of CT systems with 16 cm detector coverage for coronary CTA has been demonstrated [53, 56, 57]. The application spectrum has been extended to scanning of patients with atrial fibrillation [58] and coronary CTA combined with first pass perfusion evaluation [59, 60]. The second generation of 320-row CT scanners has been shown to enable coronary CTA at reduced radiation dose compared to the first generation [52, 56].

As a second benefit, CT systems with wide-area detectors can acquire dynamic volume data by repeatedly scanning the same anatomical range without table movement. This is useful in dynamic CT angiographic examinations or for whole heart functional data acquisition. So et al. published first results on phantoms and an animal model, demonstrating general feasibility for the quantitative evaluation of the myocardial blood flow [61].

As discussed above in detail, systems with 16 cm detectors suffer multiple limitations. Some of the challenges are related to the X-ray source. To compensate for some of the effects, multiple sources in *z*-direction have been proposed (Fig. 6.13). Fast alternating switching is realized between two X-ray tubes during data acquisition. Due to the improved geometry setup, this approach does not suffer, for example, from cone-beam artifacts compared to traditional wide-area 16 cm CT systems. A commercially available system of this kind was introduced in 2016 (SpotLight CT, Arineta Ltd., Israel). Optimized for a small footprint, the system has a diagnostic field of view limited to 250 mm, 192 detector rows with *z*-coverage of 140 mm and a fast gantry rotation time of 0.24 s [62]. One can derive from these specifications that the system comprises a highly specialized cardiac CT system in contrast to the above-described multipurpose full-body scanners.

Dual-Source CT

A dual-source CT (DSCT) is a CT system with two X-ray tubes and two detectors at an angle of approximately 90° (Fig. 6.14). Both measurement systems acquire CT scan data simultaneously at the same anatomical level of the patient (same *z*-position).

The first generation of DSCT scanners with 2 × 64 slices using *z*-flying focal spot (19.2 mm detector coverage) and 0.33 s gantry rotation time was introduced in 2006 (SOMATOM Definition, Siemens Healthcare, Forchheim, Germany), the second generation with 2 × 128 slices

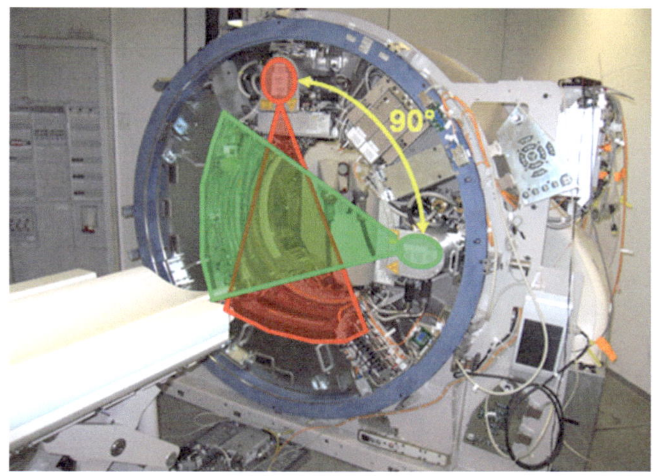

Fig. 6.14 DSCT with two independent measurement systems. The image shows the first-generation DSCT with an angle of 90° between both measurement systems. To increase the SFOV of detector B, an angle of 95° was chosen for the second- and third-generation systems

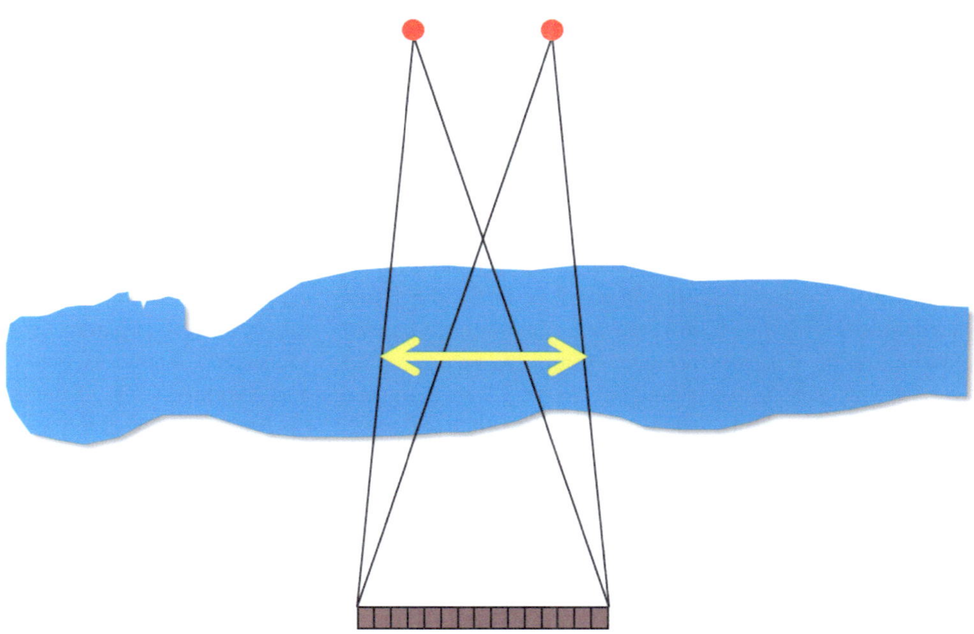

Fig. 6.13 Setup of CT system in so-called inverse geometry

(38.4 mm detector coverage) and 0.28 s gantry rotation time in 2009 (SOMATOM Definition Flash, Siemens Healthcare, Forchheim, Germany), and the third generation with 2 × 192 slices (57.6 mm detector coverage) and 0.25 s gantry rotation time in 2014 (SOMATOM Definition Force, Siemens Healthcare, Forchheim, Germany).

DSCT systems provide significantly improved temporal resolution for cardiothoracic imaging. The shortest data acquisition time for an image corresponds to a quarter of the gantry rotation time. Close to the isocenter, 180° of scan data is the minimum needed for image reconstruction. Due to the 90° angle between both X-ray tubes, each of the measurement systems needs to acquire only 90° of scan data. The two 90° segments at the same anatomical level are put together to form the 180° scan. Using this technique, a temporal resolution of 83 ms, 75 ms, and 66 ms, respectively, is achieved for the three generations of DSCT systems. With the dual-source approach, temporal resolution is independent of the patient's heart rate, because data from only one cardiac cycle are used to reconstruct an image. This is a major difference to single-source MDCT systems, which can provide similar temporal resolution by combining data from several heart cycles to an image in a multi-segment reconstruction. Then, however, temporal resolution strongly depends on the relation of heart rate and gantry rotation time. Meanwhile, several clinical studies have demonstrated the potential of DSCT to reliably perform coronary CT angiographic studies in patients with high and even irregular heart rates (e.g., [63–65]). DSCT is sufficiently accurate to diagnose clinically significant coronary artery disease in difficult to image patients [66, 67]. The high temporal resolution is also beneficial for reducing motion artifacts in cardiothoracic studies (e.g., [68]).

With a DSCT system, both X-ray tubes can also be operated at different kV settings, e.g., 80 and 140 kV, to acquire dual-energy CT data. The advantages and disadvantages of different techniques to acquire dual-energy CT data as well as clinically relevant applications will be discussed substantially more in detail in Chap. 4.

While the maximum spiral pitch in single-source CT images is limited to about 1.5 to ensure gapless volume coverage, DSCT systems can be operated at twice the pitch. Data acquired with the second measurement system a quarter rotation after the first measurement system can be used to fill the sampling gaps up to a pitch of about 3.2 in a limited SFOV that is covered by both detectors [69, 70]. At maximum pitch, no redundant data are acquired, and a quarter rotation of data per measurement system is used for image reconstruction. Temporal resolution is then a quarter of the gantry rotation time. At decreasing pitch, temporal resolution decreases because of the increasing angular data segment that corresponds to an image. At a pitch of 2, for example, temporal resolution is about 0.4 times the rotation time – this is 100 ms with the second-generation DSCT [70].

With the high-pitch scan mode, very high scan speed is achieved – up to 450 mm/s with the second-generation DSCT (38.4 mm detector coverage, 0.28 s gantry rotation time) and up to 737 mm/s with the third-generation DSCT (57.6 mm detector coverage, 0.25 s gantry rotation time). This is beneficial for the examination of larger anatomical ranges in very short scan times, e.g., for chest CTA at high temporal resolution [24], for the evaluation of pulmonary embolism and visualization of most cardiac structures and proximal coronary arteries [71], for fast CTA scans of the aorta at low radiation and contrast dose [72], or when the patient has limited ability to cooperate, such as in pediatric radiology [73–76].

The high-pitch scan mode can also be used in combination with ECG-triggering – the patient's ECG triggers both table motion and data acquisition. The patient table is positioned, and table acceleration is started in a way that the table arrives at the prescribed start z-position (e.g., the base or the apex of the heart) at the requested cardiac phase after full table speed has been reached (Fig. 6.15). Then data acquisition begins. The scan data for images at adjacent z-positions are acquired at slightly different – typically diastolic – phases of the cardiac cycle. Meanwhile, several clinical studies have demonstrated the successful use of the high-pitch scan technique for coronary CT angiography in patients with sufficiently low and stable heart rate (<62 bpm with the second-generation DSCT, <70 bpm with the third-generation DSCT), with the potential to scan the entire heart in one beat at very low radiation dose [23, 77–80].

ECG-triggered high-pitch scans can be used also for comprehensive thorax examinations in the emergency room and in the planning of TAVR procedures, because they provide adequate visualization of the coronary arteries, the aorta, and the iliac arteries in one scan at low radiation dose and high temporal resolution. The very short total scan time may potentially allow for a reduction of the amount of contrast agent; see, e.g., [27, 81]. Figure 6.15 shows an ECG-triggered high-pitch CTA of the aorta as an example.

Despite their clinical benefits, DSCT systems have to cope with some challenges. One challenge is the presence of cross-scattered radiation, i.e., scattered radiation from X-ray tube B detected by detector A and vice versa. Cross-scattered radiation – if not corrected for – can result in image artifacts and degraded CNR of the images [69]. Another challenge is the limited SFOV of the second detector, which was increased from 25 cm in the first-generation DSCT to 35.5 cm in the third-generation DSCT.

The most straightforward correction approach is to directly measure the cross-scattered radiation in detectors A and B and to subtract it from the measured signal. This technique was first implemented in the second-generation

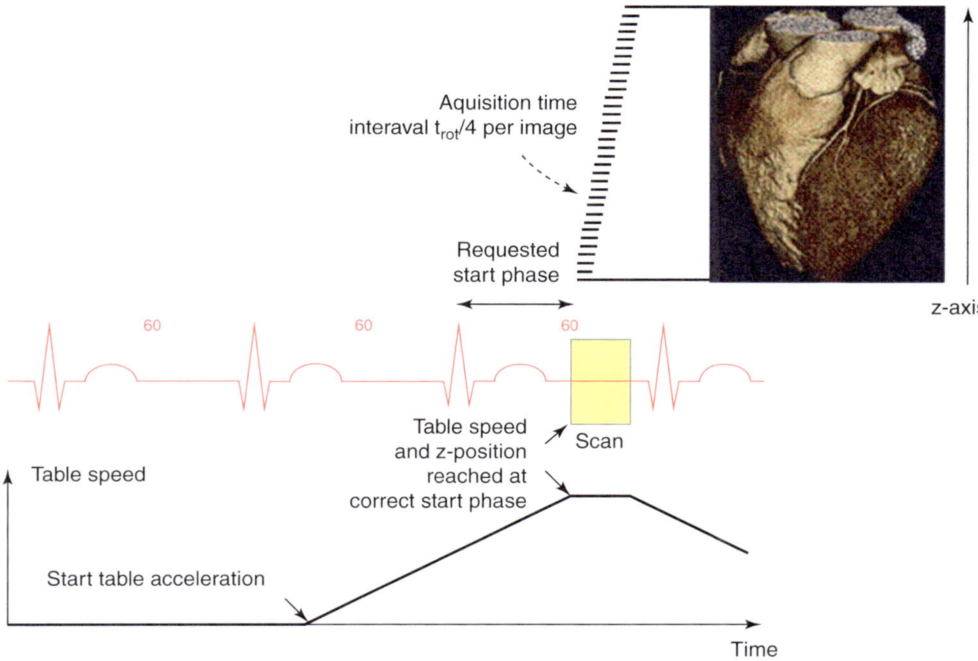

Fig. 6.15 ECG-triggered start of table movement and data acquisition for the high-pitch DSCT spiral

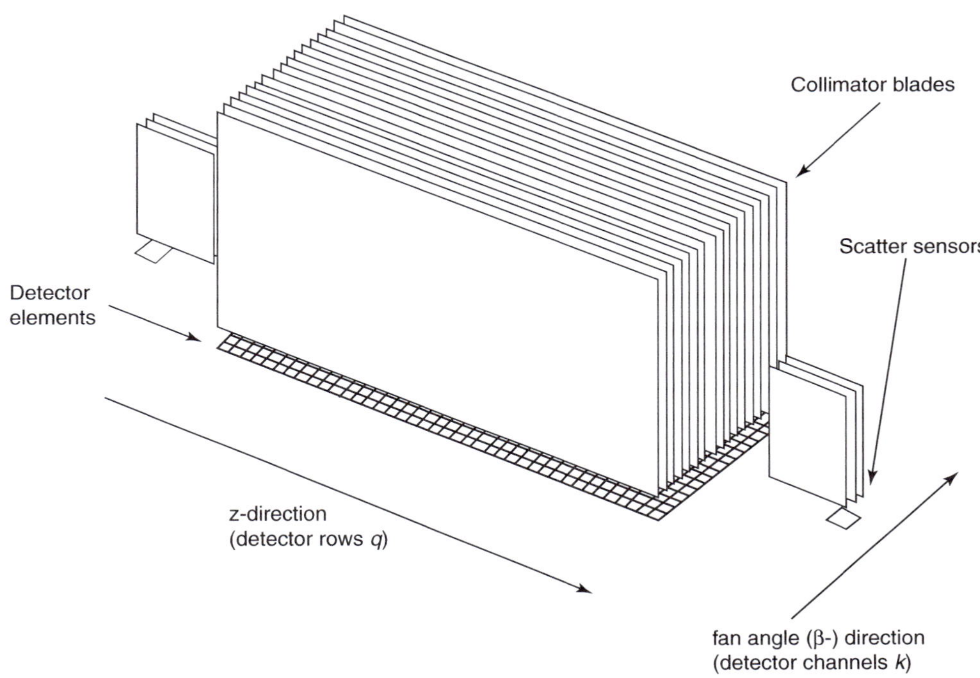

Fig. 6.16 Schematic diagram of a detector module with scatter sensors outside the direct beam. The center region consists of the primary detector pixels, positioned below the collimator blades of the anti-scatter collimator. The scattered radiation sensors, placed on both sides of the primary detector module, are equipped with collimator blades as well. The arrows indicate the *z*-direction (row direction) and the fan-angle direction (channel direction)

DSCT. It requires additional detector elements on each detector outside the direct beam (Fig. 6.16). An alternative to direct measurement is a model-based cross-scatter correction. The primary source of cross-scattered radiation is Compton scatter at the object surface. In the first-generation DSCT, pre-stored cross-scatter tables for objects with similar surface shape are used for an online correction of the cross-scattered radiation in each measured projection. In the third-generation DSCT, an iterative cross-scatter correction based on a simplified Monte Carlo simulation is applied.

While image artifacts caused by cross-scattered radiation can be significantly reduced by either model-based or measurement-based correction approaches, these corrections are often considered to come at the expense of increased image noise and reduced contrast-to-noise ratio (CNR) in the images. It has been demonstrated, however, that careful low pass filtering of the scatter correction term can efficiently mitigate the image noise increase without visually affecting image detail resolution or image contrast. CNR can in fact be increased beyond the values achieved without cross-scatter correction, and it approaches or sometimes even surpasses the CNR performance of a comparable single-source scan using these techniques.

Another – evitable – challenge of dual-source dual-energy CT (DE) is the 90° offset of projections acquired by both X-ray tubes at the same z-position. Because high-energy and low-energy projections are not simultaneously acquired at the same projection angle, raw data-based DE algorithms are difficult to realize. DE algorithms are therefore image based – which has the huge advantage of avoiding the limited and sensitive calibration of raw data-based methods. It is often claimed that image-based methods are strongly limited by the problem of beam hardening. However, under certain conditions – which are typically fulfilled in modern CT scanners – image-based methods are practically equivalent for clinical tasks. A prerequisite for image-based material decomposition is the validity of the thin absorber model. For example, if one uses water and iodine as the basis materials for image-based dual-energy decomposition, the maximum X-ray attenuation of the iodine along any measured ray path is expected to be so small that it is valid to assume a linear contribution to the total attenuation. In clinical practice, this prerequisite is typically fulfilled. If necessary, still dedicated established single energy-based methods for beam-hardening corrections can be applied to allow for respective data correction. As a second prerequisite, both the CT value of water and the CT values of small iodine samples are expected to be independent from their position within the scanned object. DSCT scanners are therefore equipped with an optimized bowtie filter of sufficient beam hardening, and the approximately cylindrical patient cross-section has to be centered within the SFOV – typically being fulfilled in case of clinical CT systems. Anyhow, in practice, electronic noise, scanner calibration, stability of emitted spectra, cone-beam effects, and scattered radiation can have a larger impact on the obtained results than the raw data or image-based analysis method itself. Further on, the ability for an optimized, independent selection of X-ray voltage and spectral filtration – but still dose-wise well and optimally balanced high and low energy beam – and therefore an optimal spectral separation enables robust dual-energy imaging at a huge variety for applications and thus compensates for potential limitations and challenges. Further details are provided in Chap. 4, dedicated to dual-energy imaging of the heart.

A third challenge is the fact that moving objects, such as the heart, are seen by both detectors with an angular offset of about 90°. Motion artifacts in the corresponding A and B images can therefore be slightly different, which can affect the material decomposition of the dual-energy images. In practice, however, this problem is not relevant thanks to the good temporal resolution of DSCT, and it can be further mitigated by nonrigid registration of A and B images.

References

1. Kalender WA, Seissler W, Klotz E, Vock P. Spiral volumetric CT with single-breath-hold technique, continuous transport, and continuous scanner rotation. Radiology. 1990;176(1):181–3.
2. Achenbach S, Ulzheimer S, Baum U, et al. Noninvasive coronary angiography by retrospectively ECG-gated multi-slice spiral CT. Circulation. 2000;102:2823–8.
3. Becker C, Knez A, Ohnesorge B, Schöpf U, Reiser M. Imaging of non calcified coronary plaques using helical CT with retrospective EKG gating. AJR. 2000;175:423–4.
4. Knez A, Becker C, Leber A, Ohnesorge B, Reiser M, Haberl R. Noninvasive assessment of coronary artery stenoses with multidetector helical computed tomography. Circulation. 2000;101:e221–2.
5. Ohnesorge B, Flohr T, Becker C, Kopp A, Schoepf U, Baum U, Knez A, Klingenbeck Regn K, Reiser M. Cardiac imaging by means of electro- cardiographically gated multisection spiral CT – initial experience. Radiology. 2000;217:564–71.
6. Nieman K, Oudkerk M, Rensing B, van Oijen P, Munne A, van Geuns R, de Feyter P. Coronary angiography with multi-slice computed tomography. Lancet. 2001;357:599–603.
7. Hoffmann MHK, Shi H, Schmitz BL, Schmid FT, Lieberknecht M, Schulze R, Ludwig B, Kroschel U, Jahnke N, Haerer W, Brambs H-J, Aschoff AJ. Noninvasive coronary angiography with multislice computed tomography. JAMA. 2005;293:2471–8.
8. Leschka S, Wildermuth S, Boehm T, Desbiolles L, Husmann L, Plass A, Koepfli P, Schepis T, Marincek B, Kaufmann PA, Alkadhi H. Noninvasive coronary angiography with 64-section CT: effect of average heart rate and heart rate variability on image quality. Radiology. 2006;241(2):378–85.
9. Leber AW, Knez A, Ziegler F, Becker A, Nikolaou K, Paul S, Wintersperger B, Reiser MF, Becker CR, Steinbeck G, Boekstegers P. Quantification of obstructive and nonobstructive coronary lesions by 64-slice computed tomography – a comparative study with quantitative coronary angiography and intravascular ultrasound. J Am Coll Cardiol. 2005;46(1):147–54.
10. Raff GL, Gallagher MJ, O'Neill WW, Goldstein JA. Diagnostic accuracy of non-invasive coronary angiography using 64-slice spiral computed tomography. J Am Coll Cardiol. 2005;46(3):552.
11. Salem R, Remy-Jardin M, Delhaye D, Khalil C, Teisseire A, Delannoy-Deken V, Duhamel A, Remy J. Integrated cardio-thoracic imaging with ECG-gated 64-slice multidetector-row CT: initial findings in 133 patients. Eur Radiol. 2006;16(9):1973–81.
12. Bruzzi JF, Rémy-Jardin M, Delhaye D, Teisseire A, Khalil C, Rémy J. When, why, and how to examine the heart during thoracic CT: part 1, basic principles. AJR Am J Roentgenol. 2006;186(2):324–32.
13. Bruzzi JF, Rémy-Jardin M, Delhaye D, Teisseire A, Khalil C, Rémy J. When, why, and how to examine the heart during thoracic CT: part 2, clinical applications. AJR Am J Roentgenol. 2006;186(2):333–41.
14. Delhaye D, Remy-Jardin M, Salem R, Teisseire A, Khalil C, Delannoy-Deken V, Duhamel A, Remy J. Coronary imaging quality in routine ECG-gated multidetector CT examinations of the entire

thorax: preliminary experience with a 64-slice CT system in 133 patients. Eur Radiol. 2007;17(4):902–10.
15. Flohr T, Ohnesorge B. Heart rate adaptive optimization of spatial and temporal resolution for electrocardiogram-gated multislice spiral CT of the heart. J Comput Assist Tomogr. 2001;25(6):907–23.
16. Hausleiter J, Martinoff S, Hadamitzky M, et al. Image quality and radiation exposure with a low tube voltage protocol for coronary CT angiography: results of the PROTECTION II trial. JACC Cardiovasc Imaging. 2010;3(11):1113–23.
17. Flohr TG, McCollough CH, Bruder H, Petersilka M, Gruber K, Süß C, Grasruck M, Stierstorfer K, Krauss B, Raupach R, Primak AN, Küttner A, Achenbach S, Becker C, Kopp A, Ohnesorge BM. First performance evaluation of a dual-source CT (DSCT) system. Eur Radiol. 2006;16(2):256–68.
18. Johnson TR, Nikolaou K, Busch S, Leber AW, Becker A, Wintersperger BJ, Rist C, Knez A, Reiser MF, Becker CR. Diagnostic accuracy of dual-source computed tomography in the diagnosis of coronary artery disease. Investig Radiol. 2007;42(10):684–91.
19. Pontana F, Faivre JB, Remy-Jardin M, Flohr T, Schmidt B, Tacelli N, Pansini V, Remy J. Lung perfusion with dual-energy multidetector-row CT (MDCT): feasibility for the evaluation of acute pulmonary embolism in 117 consecutive patients. Acad Radiol. 2008;15(12):1494–504.
20. Thieme SF, Becker CR, Hacker M, Nikolaou K, Reiser MF, Johnson TR. Dual energy CT for the assessment of lung perfusion--correlation to scintigraphy. Eur J Radiol. 2008;68(3):369–74.
21. Achenbach S, Marwan M, Ropers D, et al. Coronary computed tomography angiography with a consistent dose below 1 mSv using prospectively electrocardiogram-triggered high-pitch spiral acquisition. Eur Heart J. 2010;31(3):340–6.
22. Alkadhi H, Stolzmann P, Desbiolles L, Baumueller S, Goetti R, Plass A, Scheffel H, Feuchtner G, Falk V, Marincek B, Leschka S. Low-dose, 128-slice, dual-source CT coronary angiography: accuracy and radiation dose of the high-pitch and the step-and-shoot mode. Heart. 2010;96(12):933–8. https://doi.org/10.1136/hrt.2009.189100.
23. Lell M, Hinkmann F, Anders K, Deak P, Kalender WA, Uder M, Achenbach S. High-pitch electrocardiogram-triggered computed tomography of the chest: initial results. Investig Radiol. 2009;44(11):728–33.
24. Tacelli N, Remy-Jardin M, Flohr T, Faivre JB, Delannoy V, Duhamel A, Remy J. Dual-source chest CT angiography with high temporal resolution and high pitch modes: evaluation of image quality in 140 patients. Eur Radiol. 2010;20(5):1188–96.
25. Schulz B, Jacobi V, Beeres M, Bodelle B, Gruber T, Lee C, Bauer R, Kerl M, Vogl T, Zangos S. Quantitative analysis of motion artifacts in high-pitch dual-source computed tomography of the thorax. J Thorac Imaging. 2012;27(6):382–6.
26. Beeres M, Schell B, Mastragelopoulos A, Herrmann E, Kerl JM, Gruber-Rouh T, Lee C, Siebenhandl P, Bodelle B, Zangos S, Vogl TJ, Jacobi V, Bauer RW. High-pitch dual-source CT angiography of the whole aorta without ECG synchronisation: initial experience. Eur Radiol. 2012;22(1):129–37.
27. Wuest W, Anders K, Schuhbaeck A, May MS, Gauss S, Marwan M, Arnold M, Ensminger S, Muschiol G, Daniel WG, Uder M, Achenbach S. Dual source multidetector CT-angiography before Transcatheter Aortic Valve Implantation (TAVI) using a high-pitch spiral acquisition mode. Eur Radiol. 2012;22(1):51–8.
28. Plank F, Friedrich G, Bartel T, Mueller S, Bonaros N, Heinz A, Klauser A, Cartes-Zumelzu F, Grimm M, Feuchtner G. Benefits of high-pitch 128-slice dual-source computed tomography for planning of transcatheter aortic valve implantation. Ann Thorac Surg. 2012;94(6):1961–6.
29. Hsiao EM, Rybicki FJ, Steigner M. CT coronary angiography: 256-slice and 320-detector row scanners. Curr Cardiol Rep. 2010;12(1):68–75. https://doi.org/10.1007/s11886-009-0075-z.
30. Ohno Y, Koyama H, Matsumoto K, Onishi Y, Takenaka D, Fujisawa Y, Yoshikawa T, Konishi M, Maniwa Y, Nishimura Y, Ito T, Sugimura K. Differentiation of malignant and benign pulmonary nodules with quantitative first-pass 320-detector row perfusion CT versus FDG PET/CT. Radiology. 2011;258(2):599–609.
31. Willems PW, Taeshineetanakul P, Schenk B, Brouwer PA, Terbrugge KG, Krings T. The use of 4D-CTA in the diagnostic work-up of brain arteriovenous malformations. Neuroradiology. 2012;54(2):123–31.
32. Motosugi U, Ichikawa T, Sou H, Morisaka H, Sano K, Araki T. Multi-organ perfusion CT in the abdomen using a 320-detector row CT scanner: preliminary results of perfusion changes in the liver, spleen, and pancreas of cirrhotic patients. Eur J Radiol. 2012;81(10):2533–7.
33. US Patent X-Ray transmission scanning system and method and electron beam X-ray scan tube for use therewith. US 4352021. 1982.
34. Agatston AS, Janowitz WR, Hildner FJ, et al. Quantification of coronary artery calcium using ultrafast computed tomography. J Am Coll Cardiol. 1990;15(4):827–32.
35. Achenbach S, Ropers D, Regenfus M, Muschiol G, Daniel WG, Moshage W. Contrast enhanced electron beam computed tomography to analyse the coronary arteries in patients after acute myocardial infarction. Heart. 2000;84(5):489–93.
36. Rumberger JA, Sheedy PF, Breen JF. Use of ultrafast (cine) x-ray computed tomography in cardiac and cardiovascular imaging. In: Giuliani ER, Gersh BJ, McGoon MD, Hayes DL, Schaff HF, editors. Mayo clinic practice of cardiology. 3rd ed. St. Louis: Mosby; 1996. p. 303–24.
37. Bell MR, Lerman LO, Rumberger JA. Validation of minimally invasive measurement of myocardial perfusion using electron beam computed tomography and application in human volunteers. Heart. 1999;81:628–35.
38. Lu B, Zhuang N, Mao S, Bakhsheshhi H, Liu S, Budoff M. Image quality of three-dimensional electron beam coronary angiography. J Comput Assist Tomogr. 2002;26:202–9.
39. Niemann T, Henry S, Duhamel A, Faivre JB, Deschildre A, Colas L, Santangelo T, Remy J, Remy-Jardin M. Pediatric chest CT at 70 kVp: a feasibility study in 129 children. Pediatr Radiol. 2014;44(11):1347–57.
40. Durand S, Paul JF. Comparison of image quality between 70 kVp and 80 kVp: application to paediatric cardiac CT. Eur Radiol. 2014;24(12):3003–9.
41. LaBounty TM, Leipsic J, Poulter R, et al. Coronary CT angiography of patients with a normal body mass index using 80 kVp versus 100 kVp: a prospective, multicenter, multivendor randomized trial. AJR Am J Roentgenol. 2011;197(5):W860–7.
42. Oda S, Utsunomiya D, Funama Y, et al. A low tube voltage technique reduces the radiation dose at retrospective ECG-gated cardiac computed tomography for anatomical and functional analyses. Acad Radiol. 2011;18(8):991–9.
43. Nakagawa M, Ozawa Y, Sakurai K, Shimohira M, Ohashi K, Asano M, Yamaguchi S, Shibamoto Y. Image quality at low tube voltage (70 kV) and sinogram-affirmed iterative reconstruction for computed tomography in infants with congenital heart disease. Pediatr Radiol. 2015;45(10):1472–9.
44. Duan X, Wang J, Leng S, Schmidt B, Allmendinger T, Grant K, Flohr T, McCollough CH. Electronic noise in CT detectors: impact on image noise and artifacts. AJR Am J Roentgenol. 2013;201(4):W626–32.
45. Flohr T, Stierstorfer K, Raupach R, Ulzheimer S, Bruder H. Performance evaluation of a 64-slice CT-system with z-flying focal spot. Rofo. 2004;176:1803–10.
46. Flohr TG, Stierstorfer K, Ulzheimer S, Bruder H, Primak AN, McCollough CH. Image reconstruction and image quality

evaluation for a 64-slice CT scanner with z-flying focal spot. Med Phys. 2005;32(8):2536–47.
47. Lee AM, Beaudoin J, Engel LC, Sidhu MS, Abbara S, Brady TJ, Hoffmann U, Ghoshhajra BB. Assessment of image quality and radiation dose of prospectively ECG-triggered adaptive dual-source coronary computed tomography angiography (cCTA) with arrhythmia rejection algorithm in systole versus diastole: a retrospective cohort study. Int J Cardiovasc Imaging. 2013;29(6):1361–70.
48. Flohr TG, Schoepf UJ, Ohnesorge BM. Chasing the heart: new developments for cardiac CT. J Thorac Imaging. 2007;22(1):4–16.
49. Muenzel D, Noel PB, Dorn F, Dobritz M, Rummeny EJ, Huber A. Coronary CT angiography in step-and-shoot technique with 256-slice CT: impact of the field of view on image quality, craniocaudal coverage, and radiation exposure. Eur J Radiol. 2012;81(7):1562–8.
50. Klass O, Walker M, Siebach A, Stuber T, Feuerlein S, Juchems M, Hoffmann MH. Prospectively gated axial CT coronary angiography: comparison of image quality and effective radiation dose between 64- and 256-slice CT. Eur Radiol. 2010;20(5):1124–31.
51. Rybicki FJ, Otero HJ, Steigner ML, Vorobiof G, Nallamshetty L, Mitsouras D, Ersoy H, Mather RT, Judy PF, Cai T, Coyner K, Schultz K, Whitmore AG, Di Carli MF. Initial evaluation of coronary images from 320-detector row computed tomography. Int J Cardiovasc Imaging. 2008;24(5):535–46.
52. Tomizawa N, Maeda E, Akahane M, Torigoe R, Kiryu S, Ohtomo K. Coronary CT angiography using the second-generation 320-detector row CT: assessment of image quality and radiation dose in various heart rates compared with the first-generation scanner. Int J Cardiovasc Imaging. 2013;29(7):1613–8.
53. Engel KJ, Herrmann C, Zeitler G. X-ray scattering in single- and dual-source CT. Med Phys. 2008;35(1):318–32.
54. Vogtmeier G, Dorscheida R, Engela KR, Luhtab K, Mattsonb R, Harwoodb B, Applebyc M, Randolphc B, KlingerVogtmeier J, et al. Two-dimensional anti-scatter grids for computed tomography detectors. Medical imaging. International Society for Optics and Photonics. 2008.
55. Li B, Toth TL, Hsieh J, et al. Simulation and analysis of image quality impacts from single source, ultra-wide coverage CT scanner. J Xray Sci Technol. 2012;20(4):395–404.
56. Chen MY, Shanbhag SM, Arai AE. Submillisievert median radiation dose for coronary angiography with a second-generation 320-detector row CT scanner in 107 consecutive patients. Radiology. 2013;267(1):76–85.
57. Nasis A, Leung MC, Antonis PR, Cameron JD, Lehman SJ, Hope SA, Crossett MP, Troupis JM, Meredith IT, Seneviratne SK. Diagnostic accuracy of noninvasive coronary angiography with 320-detector row computed tomography. Am J Cardiol. 2010;106(10):1429–35.
58. Kondo T, Kumamaru KK, Fujimoto S, Matsutani H, Sano T, Takase S, Rybicki FJ. Prospective ECG-gated coronary 320-MDCT angiography with absolute acquisition delay strategy for patients with persistent atrial fibrillation. AJR Am J Roentgenol. 2013;201(6):1197–203.
59. George RT, Mehra VC, Chen MY, Kitagawa K, Arbab-Zadeh A, Miller JM, Matheson MB, Vavere AL, Kofoed KF, Rochitte CE, Dewey M, Yaw TS, Niinuma H, Brenner W, Cox C, Clouse ME, Lima JA, Di Carli M. Myocardial CT perfusion imaging and SPECT for the diagnosis of coronary artery disease: a head-to-head comparison from the CORE320 multicenter diagnostic performance study. Radiology. 2015;274(2):626.
60. Sharma RK, Arbab-Zadeh A, Kishi S, Chen MY, Magalhães TA, George RT, Dewey M, Rybicki FJ, Kofoed KF, de Roos A, Tan SY, Matheson M, Vavere A, Cox C, Clouse ME, Miller JM, Brinker JA, Arai AE, Di Carli MF, Rochitte CE, Lima JA. Incremental diagnostic accuracy of computed tomography myocardial perfusion imaging over coronary angiography stratified by pre-test probability of coronary artery disease and severity of coronary artery calcification: the CORE320 study. Int J Cardiol. 2015;201:570–7.
61. So A, Imai Y, Nett B, Jackson J, Nett L, Hsieh J, Wisenberg G, Teefy P, Yadegari A, Islam A, Lee TY. Technical Note: Evaluation of a 160-mm/256-row CT scanner for whole-heart quantitative myocardial perfusion imaging. Med Phys. 2016;43(8):4821. https://doi.org/10.1118/1.4957389.
62. FDA, 510k Summary Document https://www.accessdata.fda.gov/cdrh_docs/pdf16/K161066.pdf
63. Sun ML, Lu B, Wu RZ, Johnson L, Han L, Liu G, Yu FF, Hou ZH, Gao Y, Wang HY, Jiang S, Yang YJ, Qiao SB. Diagnostic accuracy of dual-source CT coronary angiography with prospective ECG-triggering on different heart rate patients. Eur Radiol. 2011;21(8):1635–42.
64. Lee AM, Engel LC, Shah B, Liew G, Sidhu MS, Kalra M, Abbara S, Brady TJ, Hoffmann U, Ghoshhajra BB. Coronary computed tomography angiography during arrhythmia: radiation dose reduction with prospectively ECG-triggered axial and retrospectively ECG-gated helical 128-slice dual-source CT. J Cardiovasc Comput Tomogr. 2012;6(3):172–183.e2.
65. Paul JF, Amato A, Rohnean A. Low-dose coronary-CT angiography using step and shoot at any heart rate: comparison of image quality at systole for high heart rate and diastole for low heart rate with a 128-slice dual-source machine. Int J Cardiovasc Imaging. 2013;29(3):651–7.
66. Westwood ME, Raatz HD, Misso K, Burgers L, Redekop K, Lhachimi SK, Armstrong N, Kleijnen J. Systematic review of the accuracy of dual-source cardiac CT for detection of arterial stenosis in difficult to image patient groups. Radiology. 2013;267(2):387–95.
67. Sidhu MS, Venkatesh V, Hoffmann U, et al. Advanced adaptive axial-sequential prospectively electrocardiogram-triggered dual-source coronary computed tomographic angiography in a patient with atrial fibrillation. J Comput Assist Tomogr. 2011;35(6):747–8.
68. Hutt A, Tacelli N, Faivre JB, Flohr T, Duhamel A, Remy J, Remy-Jardin M. Is bronchial wall imaging affected by temporal resolution? Comparative evaluation at 140 and 75 ms in 90 patients. Eur Radiol. 2016;26(2):469–77.
69. Petersilka M, Stierstorfer K, Bruder H, Flohr T. Strategies for scatter correction in dual source CT. Med Phys. 2010;37(11):5971–92.
70. T G F, Leng S, Yu L, Allmendinger T, Bruder H, Petersilka M, Eusemann CD, Stierstorfer K, Schmidt B, McCollough C. Dual-source spiral CT with pitch up to 3.2 and 75 ms temporal resolution: image reconstruction and assessment of image quality. Med Phys. 2009;36(12):5641–53.
71. Hou DJ, Tso DK, Davison C, Inacio J, Louis LJ, Nicolaou S, Reimann AJ, Hou DJ, Tso DK, Davison C, Inacio J, Louis LJ, Nicolaou S, Reimann AJ. Clinical utility of ultra high pitch dual source thoracic CT imaging of acute pulmonary embolism in the emergency department: are we one step closer towards a non-gated triple rule out? Eur J Radiol. 2013;82(10):1793–8.
72. Apfaltrer P, Hanna EL, Schoepf UJ, Spears JR, Schoenberg SO, Fink C, Vliegenthart R. Radiation dose and image quality at high-pitch CT angiography of the aorta: intraindividual and interindividual comparisons with conventional CT angiography. AJR Am J Roentgenol. 2012;199(6):1402–9.
73. Han BK, Overman DM, Grant K, et al. Non-sedated, free breathing cardiac CT for evaluation of complex congenital heart disease in neonates. J Cardiovasc Comput Tomogr. 2013;7(6):354–60.
74. Lee JH, Han D, Danad I, et al. Multimodality imaging in coronary artery disease: focus on computed tomography. J Cardiovasc Ultrasound. 2016;24(1):7–17.
75. Lell MM, May M, Deak P, Alibek S, Kuefner M, Kuettner A, Köhler H, Achenbach S, Uder M, Radkow T. High-pitch spiral computed tomography: effect on image quality and radiation dose in pediatric chest computed tomography. Investig Radiol. 2011;46(2):116–23.

76. Bridoux A, Hutt A, Faivre JB, Flohr T, Duhamel A, Pagniez J, Remy J, Remy-Jardin M. Coronary artery visibility in free-breathing young children on non-gated chest CT: impact of temporal resolution. Pediatr Radiol. 2015;45(12):1761–70.
77. Achenbach S, Marwan M, Schepis T, Pflederer T, Bruder H, Allmendinger T, Petersilka M, Anders K, Lell M, Kuettner A, Ropers D, Daniel WG, Flohr T. High-pitch spiral acquisition: a new scan mode for coronary CT angiography. J Cardiovasc Comput Tomogr. 2009;3:117–21.
78. Leschka S, Stolzmann P, Desbiolles L, Baumueller S, Goetti R, Schertler T, Scheffel H, Plass A, Falk V, Feuchtner G, Marincek B, Alkadhi H. Diagnostic accuracy of high-pitch dual-source CT for the assessment of coronary stenoses: first experience. Eur Radiol. 2009;19(12):2896–903.
79. Gordic S, Husarik DB, Desbiolles L, Leschka S, Frauenfelder T, Alkadhi H. High-pitch coronary CT angiography with third generation dual-source CT: limits of heart rate. Int J Cardiovasc Imaging. 2014;30(6):1173–9.
80. Morsbach F, Gordic S, Desbiolles L, Husarik D, Frauenfelder T, Schmidt B, Allmendinger T, Wildermuth S, Alkadhi H, Leschka S. Performance of turbo high-pitch dual-source CT for coronary CT angiography: first ex vivo and patient experience. Eur Radiol. 2014;24(8):1889–95.
81. Azzalini L, Abbara S, Ghoshhajra BB. Ultra-low contrast computed tomographic angiography (CTA) with 20-mL total dose for transcatheter aortic valve implantation (TAVI) planning. J Comput Assist Tomogr. 2014;38(1):105–9.

Principles of Cardiac CT Image Acquisition

7

Thomas Henzler, Patricia Carrascosa, Brian S. Ko, and Ronen Rubinshtein

Ongoing technical developments in CT have established cardiac CT angiography (cCTA) as a robust noninvasive imaging test of the heart and coronary arteries, with ever-improving image quality and diagnostic accuracy [1–3]. However, concerns have been raised (with the first- and second-generation scanners) regarding radiation exposure from cCTA, which has traditionally been comparatively high relative to other CT applications, although the dose levels compare well with other longer established cardiac imaging tests such as radionuclide-based myocardial perfusion imaging. Considering the increasing number of cCTA investigations around the globe, however, and expected sustained growth, the contribution of cCTA to the radiation exposure of the general population is not negligible. While there is no evidence that the level of radiation that is ordinarily applied at cCTA bestows any kind of risk, the current uncertainties regarding the biological effects of radiation, our commitment to the ALARA (As Low As Reasonably Achievable) principles, and increasing public radiation awareness behoove us to keep radiation dose at medical imaging to a minimum.

Over the past years, several acquisition techniques for cCTA have been developed in order to minimize patients' radiation exposure including prospective ECG gating, high-pitch cCTA, and single-heartbeat cCTA using large detectors that allow whole-heart coverage. Moreover, the last years have also seen significant progress in novel iterative reconstruction techniques that allow further dose reduction for cCTA as well as improved image quality [4, 5]. However, all CT vendors have slightly different approaches within their cCTA protocols that make it difficult to provide a universal overview on cCTA acquisition principles. Therefore, this chapter separately describes cCTA acquisition protocols for the major vendors from the perspective of experienced users in order to provide the readership with a practical approach that can be directly transferred into their own clinical routine.

General Principles for Cardiac CT Image Acquisition

Scan Coverage Optimization

The scan coverage is planned using the topogram or "scout" view identical to other CT acquisitions. As the total radiation dose delivered is directly proportional to the scan coverage, precise collimation is important to minimize the DLP (dose length product = scan length × $CTDI_{vol}$). With the improved capabilities of CT systems, there is a general tendency to increase the area of coverage, due to faster acquisition and less limitation of tube power. If the *z*-axis of the scan is too long, for example, including the upper part of the abdomen or the neck, there will be unnecessary radiation delivered to abdominal organs or the thyroid gland. However, if the scan length is too short, excluding a portion of the coronary artery tree, the examination would not be complete and repeat scanning would be required, resulting in increased radiation and contrast media volume to the patient. For dedicated coronary artery imaging (i.e., excluding coronary artery bypass and "triple-rule-out" acute chest pain studies to rule out aortic dissection or pulmonary embolism in addition to coronary disease), scanning should begin at the level of the bifurcation of the trachea in most cases, but the exact starting position is dependent on individual anatomy. For example, in thin

T. Henzler (✉)
Institute of Clinical Radiology and Nuclear Medicine, University Medical Center Mannheim, Medical Faculty Mannheim, Heidelberg University, Heidelberg, Germany
e-mail: thomas.henzler@me.com

P. Carrascosa
Department of Cardiovascular Imaging, Diagnóstico Maipú, Buenos Aires, Argentina

B. S. Ko
Department of Medicine Monash Medical Centre (MMC), Monash Cardiovascular Research Centre, MonashHEART, Monash Health and Monash University, Melbourne, Australia

R. Rubinshtein
Department of Cardiovascular Medicine, Lady Davis Carmel Medical Center, The Ruth and Bruce Rappaport School of Medicine, Technion-Israel Institute of Technology, Haifa, Israel

U. J. Schoepf (ed.), *CT of the Heart*, Contemporary Medical Imaging, https://doi.org/10.1007/978-1-60327-237-7_7

patients with a small, vertically oriented heart, scanning may start lower than the carina without the risk of missing the proximal coronary artery tree. It is also important to be able to stop the scan during the acquisition once the entire cardiac anatomy is covered, so as to avoid unnecessary radiation to the upper abdomen. Thus, adjustment of scan length, and thus optimization of the radiation dose, requires the careful attention of the CT technologist. Scan length optimization solely based on the topogram may be difficult, as the heart position may vary with diaphragmatic motion, and some patients may have difficulty keeping the same respiratory state for successive acquisitions. If a noncontrast calcium scoring scan is acquired preceding cCTA, as it is practice at many institutions, the landmarks obtained at calcium scoring can be advantageously used for more exact planning of the scan range of the contrast-enhanced study.

Retrospective Versus Prospective ECG Synchronization

Retrospective ECG gating has been the traditional method of ECG synchronization with mechanical CT scanners, which comprises simultaneous acquisition of the ECG signal combined with constant X-ray emission during slow-pitch spiral/helical scan acquisitions [6–10]. Because of this constant, slow-pitch application of radiation, which enables the acquisition of oversampled data sets that allow interrogation of the entire cardiac anatomy across the RR interval, cardiac CT has traditionally been considered radiation dose-intensive, especially in light of the small volume covered (i.e., only approximately 12–13 cm in the *z*-axis for adult hearts) (Fig. 6.1). The relatively high radiation dose is the result of the particular requirements of this imaging test, where, more than with other applications, diagnostic evaluation of the small and rapidly moving coronary arteries depends on the combination of high temporal resolution, spatial resolution, and signal-to-noise ratio [7]. Image noise is mainly influenced by the number of X-ray photons reaching the detector, which in turn is a factor of the object attenuation and tube voltage and is proportional to the slice width, tube current, and amount of time required to acquire the projection data needed for image reconstruction [11]. For cCTA, the best possible temporal resolution is required to minimize artifacts resulting from cardiac motion. This goal is achieved by using only projections gathered in a defined, short time window for image reconstruction, which in turn requires relatively high X-ray tube settings to ensure sufficient photon flux during this narrow acquisition window. High temporal resolution is ordinarily achieved by fast gantry rotation times [8]; however, in most available CT scanners, this necessitates the use of a slower pitch to avoid discontinuities in the anatomic coverage of the heart. A slow pitch in turn yields a higher radiation dose. Thus, the high temporal, spatial, and contrast resolution required for retrospectively ECG-gated cCTA is obtained at the expense of an increase in radiation exposure. Increased awareness of these relationships has prompted the development of a variety of strategies aimed at improving the efficiency of ECG-synchronized acquisition techniques. With appropriate application of these techniques, a more efficient utilization of X-ray photons does not necessarily sacrifice the image quality of a cCTA study [12]. Choice of the ECG synchronization method at cCTA should be informed by various factors, such as patients' heart rate or rhythm, and the clinical question. Until a few years, the most frequently used scan technique for ECG synchronization at cCTA has been retrospective ECG gating. The ECG signal is continuously recorded, while a low-pitch spiral/helical CT scan with continuous emission of X-rays is acquired. Because the spiral/helical pitch used for this technique is very low compared to a standard CT examination (usually around 0.2), the radiation exposure may be up to three times higher than that of a standard (non-ECG-gated) CT examination of the same anatomic region (Fig. 7.1). This scan technique is still commonly employed in patients with an irregular heart rhythm or in whom functional assessment of the myocardium or the valves is desired. However, the increased radiation burden with use of this technique has to be individually justified by the additional diagnostic benefit of functional assessment, particularly if other radiation-free tests such as echocardiography or MRI are available.

Prospective ECG triggering, also in jargon referred to as "step-and-shoot mode" [13], has developed to be the most frequently used technique for cCTA over the last years. This scan mode eliminates redundant radiation that occurs from low-pitch cardiac spiral/helical scanning, since radiation is exclusively applied during a defined, predetermined phase of the cardiac cycle (typically during diastole with slower heart rates and during systole with faster heart rates), while the X-ray tube is completely shut off or turned down by approximately 80% during the remainder of the cardiac cycle (Fig. 7.1). With this technique, the effective radiation dose equivalent can be an order of magnitude lower than with traditional retrospective ECG gating. However, prospective ECG triggering may suffer from image degradation as more heartbeats are necessary for the acquisition of the entire scan volume. Accordingly, prospective ECG triggering will only provide adequate image quality if the detector of the CT system is wide enough to scan the entire heart within a limited number of cardiac cycles (around four steps with a detector of 4 cm), as is the case with 64-slice and higher CT systems. More importantly, the use of prospective ECG triggering has traditionally been restricted to patients with regular sinus rhythm, while this acquisition technique has been considered unsuitable for patients with an arrhythmia, because the occurrence of the desired cardiac phase for image acquisition

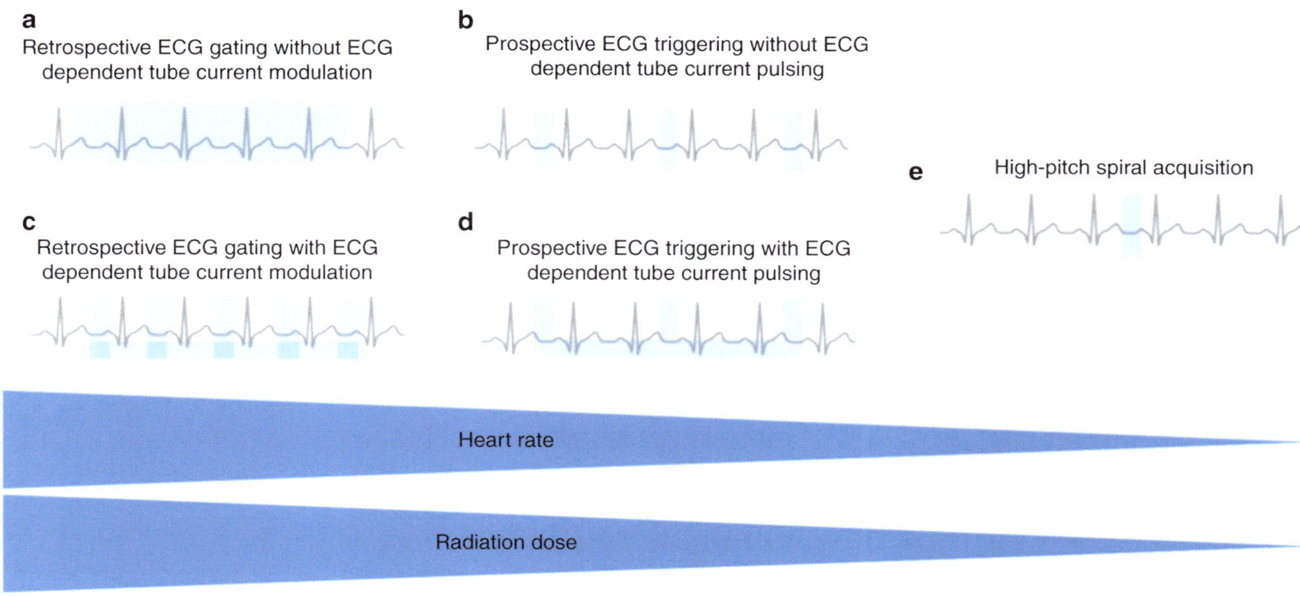

Fig. 7.1 General principles of cardiac CT angiography acquisition protocols. The light blue bars represent the time and intensity of the tube current during the different ECG phases

becomes increasingly unpredictable with varying length RR intervals. Accordingly, patients with an arrhythmia have traditionally not benefited from this radiation protection strategy and had to be imaged with conventional retrospective ECG gating, which leaves the operator with more flexibility to choose the portion of the cardiac cycle with the least cardiac motion for image reconstruction.

There are various technical attempts at improving the robustness of prospective ECG triggering vis-à-vis faster and more irregular heart rates. These include prolonging the acquisition interval during the RR cycle ("ECG padding") to provide more flexibility in choosing the most suitable phase of image reconstruction. While ECG padding provides greater flexibility and improves the robustness to account for variations in heart rhythm, it also increases radiation exposure by widening the temporal window ("tolerance") during which the X-ray tube is turned on. A more sophisticated method to account for heart rate variability is adaptive online monitoring of the ECG. This technique detects the occurrence of extrasystoles and automatically rejects arrhythmic beats in order to ensure that image acquisition occurs only during the desired cardiac phase. Last, recent developments have successfully addressed the inability of obtaining functional information with prospective ECG triggering. Hybrid acquisition techniques use a short, prospectively ECG-triggered pulse of nominal tube output radiation to supply morphological data flanked by phases of low-radiation image acquisition covering end-systole and end-diastole, which enables functional evaluation (Fig. 7.1). However, again, since this involves exposure through a longer period of the cardiac cycle, this approach is associated with an increase in radiation compared with traditional prospective ECG triggering albeit with dose levels that are still substantially lower than with conventional retrospectively ECG-triggered techniques and ECG-based tube current modulation.

High Pitch Versus Broad Detector Coverage

Dual-source CT (DSCT) was introduced in 2005 and provides particularly high temporal resolution for cCTA. The system uses two X-ray tubes and two detectors arranged at an angle of 90° (95° in the second and third generation). Therefore, only one-quarter rotation of the gantry is necessary to acquire the X-ray data for one cross-sectional image. This effectively doubles the temporal resolution when compared with single-source CT at the same rotation speed. With the introduction of second-generation DSCT, so-called high-pitch single-heartbeat acquisition became feasible. In early reports, the ability to perform ECG-triggered spiral data acquisition using very high-pitch values (around 3.2) has been described for DSCT [14, 15]. The high pitch allows image acquisition of the entire volumetric data set of the heart within a single cardiac cycle. Since with high-pitch acquisitions no redundant data is acquired, this scan mode is associated with approximately 1/10 the exposure of a retrospectively gated spiral scan and 1/2 to 1/3 the dose of a prospectively ECG-triggered scan. In combination with low tube voltage techniques, effective radiation doses of 1 mSv or less can be routinely obtained [16]. When applied to the entire chest for the purpose of "triple-rule-out" acute chest pain studies, the effective radiation dose equivalent still remains at below 2 mSv, depending on the X-ray tube setting. However, since the heart must remain motion-free for the entire scan time, this mode has been predominantly applied in patients with slow heart rates below 65–75 beats per minute [15, 16]. Similar to second- and third-generation DSCT, broad detector 320-row CT scanners allow image acquisition of the entire heart within a single heartbeat. With this technology, the entire *z*-axis of the heart is covered by a broad (i.e., 16 cm) detector, allowing for the single-heartbeat acquisition.

ECG-Based Tube Current Modulation

ECG-based tube current modulation is currently the most widely used technical tool to reduce radiation dose without sacrificing image quality at retrospectively ECG-gated acquisitions as well as during prospective ECG triggering with a second low-dose pulsing window. Radiation may be reduced by up to 60% by the application of a simple principle: radiation dose is decreased during phases of the cardiac cycle that are not anticipated to be useful for morphological evaluation, and the full dose is delivered only during the cardiac phase which is expected to yield diagnostic results for morphological evaluation [17]. Some CT manufacturers allow adjustment of the temporal window receiving full dose, which can be beneficial for optimizing the performance of ECG-dependent tube current modulation. For example, if the cardiac rhythm is regular, sinusoidal, and slow, there is a high probability that the most suitable phase for reconstruction will be found in diastole. In such cases it is advisable to apply the full dose during end-diastole, representing a temporal window of only 20% of the full RR interval. The remaining 80% of the cardiac cycle receives reduced tube current. For faster heart rates, the most suitable phase for reconstruction becomes more difficult to predict and may vary from 30% to 80%. In this scenario, it is possible to set the full-dose period from 30% to 80% (or less), which increases the likelihood of including the optimal reconstruction phase in the full-dose window, albeit with reduced radiation savings. Future developments should aim at providing operators with the ability to adjust the temporal amplitude of the modulation more flexibly across the RR cycle. For example, with faster heart rates, it may be desirable to have available both mid-diastolic and end-systolic images at full dose.

It is also important to remember that the effectiveness of ECG-based tube current modulation varies with heart rate: the slower the heart rate, the more efficient the modulation, because the full-dose phase is proportionally shorter within the RR interval. Consequently, the use of rate-controlling agents for lowering the heart rate will lengthen the diastolic phase and thus enhance the effectiveness of ECG-based tube current modulation with lower incident radiation doses.

ECG-based dose modulation is activated prospectively, according to an automated analysis of the preceding heartbeats. One drawback associated with the use of ECG-based dose modulation is that, similar to prospective ECG triggering, the exact occurrence of systolic and/or diastolic phases cannot be reliably predicted in patients with arrhythmia or frequent premature ventricular contractions. In these cases, there is a risk of incurring image reconstructions during a low-radiation dose phase, with consequent increases in image noise and loss of image quality within the *z*-extent of the data acquired during the arrhythmic beat. Thus, in cases of cardiac arrhythmia, the use of ECG-based tube current modulation should be used with caution. Similar as with automated online ECG monitoring techniques for prospective ECG triggering, however, this limitation is increasingly addressed by the recent availability of sophisticated algorithms that automatically detect premature contraction of the heart and suspend ECG-based tube current modulation mid-scan in a real-time fashion. Despite these current limitations, ECG-based tube current modulation has become one of the most successful and widely used techniques for radiation protection in clinical routine [18].

Tube Voltage

Lowering the X-ray tube voltage is one of the most effective and simplest methods for radiation dose reduction, since the radiation dose roughly changes with the square of the tube voltage [19–21]. However, reduced tube voltage causes an increase in image noise [19, 22]; thus, use of low tube voltage protocols requires an increase in the tube current and performs best with state-of-the-art iterative reconstruction techniques in order to maintain a diagnostic contrast-to-noise ratio [21, 23]. With further development of X-ray tubes, a wider variety of tube voltage options has become available in cCTA with potential benefits considering luminal contrast and radiation exposure. X-ray photon absorption of a particular object is dependent on the object's material composition. Different materials show different mass attenuation coefficients, dependent on the photon energy. In addition, the photon energy itself is dependent on the particular X-ray tube and tube voltage. Iodine molecules effectively absorb photons with photon energies ranging from 33.2 to 43.3 keV with the highest absorption at 33.2 keV (k-edge). However clinical CT systems' X-ray tubes always generate a polychromatic X-ray beam with resulting mean photon energy. This limits the capability to generate photons in the range of iodine k-edge to some extent. In recent years the X-ray tubes with 80 kV were the method of choice to get close to iodine k-edge. 80kV tube voltage has been successfully used in chest CTA with beneficial effects on image quality and improved vascular attenuation. A further decrease in tube voltage to 70 kV, which is equivalent to mean photon energy of approximately 53,5 keV, stresses these benefits. However, until recently the applicability of 70 kV was limited by the maximum tube current output of 500 mA in previous CT systems. This issue has been overcome with the introduction of new-generation scanners allowing higher tube output (such as the third-generation DSCT with a potential maximum tube current of up to 1300 mA) which enables routine cCTA at 70 kV tube voltage in patients with BMI <26 kg/m^2. Moreover, higher tube output (higher mA) and low tube voltage (lower kV) allow better tissue penetrance and may be suitable for obese patients thus allowing better image quality without significant increase in image noise.

Iterative Reconstruction

Iterative reconstruction (IR) techniques were developed almost two decades ago, and their advantages over traditional filtered back projection (FBP) reconstruction have long been recognized. However, only a few years ago, the increasing performance of mainframe computers enabled their entry into clinical CT routine. IR methods substantially reduce image noise and thereby may also allow substantial reduction of radiation dose. Modern IR algorithms are all vendor specific leading to slight differences in the image appearance. By now every big vendor (e.g., General Electric, Philips, Toshiba, and Siemens) offers and develops different IR algorithms with increasing capabilities considering image quality and noise reduction. While early algorithms mainly relied on statistical IR, increasingly sophisticated and complex full or partially raw data domain-based methods are implemented and available with the latest scanner technology.

The use of IR algorithms results in reduced image noise thus enabling primary acquisition with decreased tube voltage and/or tube current while maintaining or even improving diagnostic image quality with cCTA. Besides lower radiation exposure, a reduction in tube voltage has other beneficial effects on vessel-to-tissue contrast as explained in the tube voltage section. In addition, IR is a possibility for noise reduction in obese patients where other measures of noise reduction, like increased tube voltage and tube current, might be limited by the specific CT system used. Since use of IR means a tremendous change to the image generation process, there have been concerns this might alter image characteristics such as degree of stenosis or plaque composition. At this juncture it is uncontroversial that the use of IR techniques results in fewer blooming artifacts on cCTA which induces less overestimation of degree of stenosis, especially in heavily calcified vessels and stents [24, 25]. Consecutively there is a tendency to lower percentage of high attenuation plaque if compared to FBP. Studies evaluating the effect on plaque volume and plaque composition assessment have shown minimal effect in quantified plaque volume [26]. Besides improvements in image quality, IR has a great impact on radiation exposure in cCTA by two different means. In general IR enables reduction of tube current during primary image acquisition with preserved image quality compared to FBP. This is caused by IR inherently better denoising capabilities and results in dose savings of around 50% [4]. Furthermore the lower image noise enables reduction of tube voltage in the latest CT systems with potential for further reduction of radiation exposure [16].

Overview of Cardiac CT Acquisition Platforms and Techniques Used by the Various CT Vendors

Siemens

CT Systems for cCTA

Nowadays, robust cCTA imaging vendor independently requires CT systems with 64 slices or higher. In general, Siemens CT systems have to be divided into single-source CT systems (SSCT) and dual-source CT systems (DSCT). DSCT systems are equipped with two X-ray tubes and two corresponding detectors that are oriented in the gantry with an angular offset of 90° (Fig. 7.2). The two X-ray source/detector systems rotate simultaneously capturing image data in half the time required with conventional technology which is of significant importance in patients with high heart rates and or arrhythmia. Using this technology, DSCT systems have been the leader in temporal resolution when compared to other manufacturers over the last 10 years. Moreover, the temporal resolution continuously decreased from first-, second-, to third- generation DSCT from 83 ms, 75 ms, to 66 ms. DSCT was also the first technology that allowed dual-energy CT (DECT) without a temporal offset. DECT means that the system uses two X-ray sources simultaneously at different energy levels. This makes it possible to differentiate not only between fat, soft tissue, and bone but also between calcifications and iodinated contrast material on the basis of their unique energy-dependent attenuation profiles. For cCTA, DECT allows to quantitatively measure the myocardial iodine concentration as a surrogate of myocardial perfusion at a single time point ("snapshot" perfusion during peak enhancement) [27, 28]. Moreover, novel DECT approaches from Siemens also allow subtraction of coronary calcifications using the spectral differences between iodine and calcium. This approach has the potential to further improve the specificity of cCTA which was traditionally hampered by blooming artifacts in patients with severe calcifications leading to false-positive test results. The selective visualization of iodinated contrast material does also allow the calculation of so-called virtual noncontrast images which could be used for coronary artery calcium scoring based on a single cCTA acquisition [29]. However, although DECT

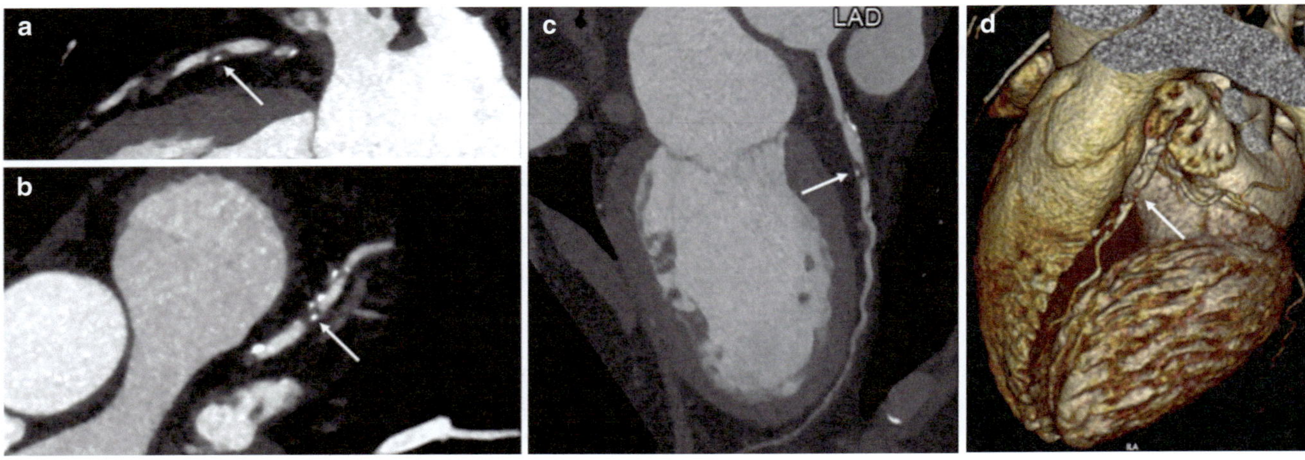

Fig. 7.2 Retrospective ECG-gated cardiac CT angiography (cCTA) of a 52-year-old male patient with acute chest pain performed on a third-generation dual-source CT. The retrospective cCTA protocol was chosen due to the high irregular heart rate of the patient 95 bpm. In order to save radiation dose, the protocol was performed at 70 kVp tube voltage resulting in a total radiation dose of 3.2 mSv. The case demonstrates the high potential of radiation dose reduction due to low tube voltage imaging even in adult normal weight patients in which retrospective ECG gating was necessary

offers several advantages for cCTA, it is important to keep in mind that the inherent high temporal resolution of DSCT systems is reduced by 50% using DECT settings. However, novel advantages in image reconstruction that are currently under investigation have the potential to virtually save the high temporal resolution during raw data reconstruction using iterative reconstructions that require less than 180° of projections [30]. State-of-the-art SSCT systems from Siemens also provide a high temporal resolution for cCTA up to 142 ms (e.g., SOMATOM Edge) due to a high gantry rotation time of 0.28 s.

Scan Acquisition

Siemens recognized early the general need for low tube voltage imaging in cardiovascular CT. Today, all cardiac CT systems from Siemens provide sufficient tube current output to perform low tube voltage cCTA studies dependent on patients' BMI. With the introduction of third-generation DSCT, routine cCTA at 70 kVp has become a reality even in adult patients with a high BMI. Technically, routine 70 kVp imaging was realized by the integration of two Vectron tubes that both provide a tube current of up to 1300 mA, utilizing power reserves from two 120 kW generators. One of the main breakthroughs related to this technology is the possibility to have full tube voltage setting flexibilities since the system allows the tube voltage modification from 70 to 150 kVp in 10 kVp intervals. Siemens also integrated automated tube voltage selection into all of their novel CT systems. Automated tube voltage selection interacts with the well-known automated tube current modulation and automatically selects the optimal tube voltage tube current combination based on patients' anatomy detected with the topogram.

Likewise, to other manufacturers Siemens continuously developed and improved IR techniques over the past 6 years. Whereas the first-generation of IR (IRIS) was slightly hampered by a so-called plastic-like appearance of the CT images compared to traditional FBP, this issue was solved by the two following generations of IR techniques (SAFIRE/ADMIRE). IR is of paramount importance for low kVp imaging since image noise significantly increases with decreased tube voltage. Thus, it is recommended to use IR techniques in all cCTA studies acquired with a tube voltage below 100 kVp. Lowering the tube voltage in combination with IR has the advantage to simultaneously reduce radiation dose and the amount of contrast material. A recently published study demonstrated the total amount of contrast material can be reduced from 80 cc for a cCTA performed at 100 kVp to 50 cc for a cCTA performed at 70 kVp, recommending a reduction of 10 cc per 10 kVp tube voltage reduction [31].

Acquisition Protocol Selection

Selection of the scan acquisition protocols (retrospective gating, prospective gating, high-pitch acquisition) should be based on patient's heart rate and rhythm and the clinical scenario (high-risk elderly patient = robust imaging; low risk young patient = robust but as gently as possible; LV function required = no high-pitch acquisition). Generally, high-pitch acquisitions deliver high diagnostic image quality in patients with regular heart rates of up to 70 bpm (up to 75 with third-generation DSCT) (Fig. 7.3). With Siemens CT systems above 64 slices, prospective ECG triggering has become the most frequently used technique for cCTA especially since the technique also enabled LV function analysis. Traditionally, evaluation of cardiac function with cCTA was restricted to

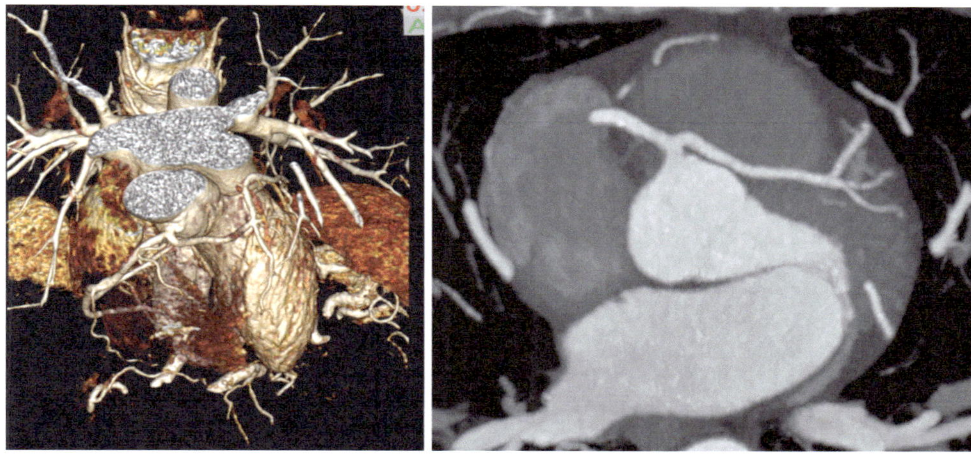

Fig. 7.3 High-pitch (3.2) cardiac CT acquisition of a 59-year-old female patient with chest pain. The study was performed with 70 kVp using automated tube voltage selection in combination with automated tube current modulation resulting in a radiation dose of 0.2 mSv. The heart rate of the patient was regular with 73 bpm

retrospective ECG gating with or without ECG-dependent tube current modulation which resulted in high radiation dose levels. Using the concept of ECG-dependent tube current modulation, Siemens introduced low-dose imaging of the whole cardiac cycle also for prospective ECG gating. By using this so-called adaptive cardiac sequence, the tube voltage is reduced to 20% of the maximum tube current output during the desired phase of the cardiac cycle before moving to the next table position. However, this technique should only be used with CT systems that allow to cover the heart in only three single steps in order to minimize contrast inhomogeneities throughout the coronary arteries in the z-axis direction. Based on our experience, the full tube current should be applied throughout a larger part of the cardiac cycle (30–80%) in patients with heart rated above 80 bpm in order to obtain both systolic and diastolic images at full dose. Table 7.1 provides an overview on basic characteristics of three typical CT systems from Siemens.

General Electric

GE Healthcare with the Revolution CT family offers three options to perform these studies: (1) Revolution CT, (2) Revolution HD (with /without GSI), and (3) Revolution EVO.

All of them operate with any of the two contrast injection protocols: (a) bolus timing scan (BTS) or SmartPrep (SM) also known as automatic bolus tracking system.

There are differences between each of the three scanners regarding coverage, temporal resolution, and number of slices among other issues that are shown in Table 7.2.

Revolution CT is GE's newest CT scanner, also known as volume high definition (VHD).

It has a wide coverage detector width of 160 mm allowing to scan a complete organ as the heart in a single gantry rotation. Revolution CT offers uncompromised image quality and clinical skills through the junction of coverage, spatial and temporal resolution: all in one system [32]. This scanner has been built using the new Gemstone Clarity detector of 256 detector rows of 0.625 mm thickness. The z coverage extends up to 160 mm width achieving up to 512 slices with 280 ms of gantry rotation and temporal resolution of 140 ms (Fig. 7.4).

Cardiac Protocols

Calcium Score The technical parameters to perform this study in this scanner are 120 Kv, 300 mA, 0.28 s gantry rotation, noise index 20, and ASIR 50%.

Coronary CT Angiography Revolution CT has a wide coverage thus allowing to scan the heart in a single gantry rotation.

It has a wide cone cardiac axial (WCCA) that provides an approximately 35% dose reduction with constant mA profile for single-phase acquisition, generating a great dose advantage compared to Revolution HD and Revolution EVO.

If the region to be covered is larger such as patients with bypass grafts, two axial volumes have to be selected for optimal visualization.

It is recommended to scan the heart at least an additional 1 cm in all directions because there is excellent temporal and spatial resolution in the center of the selected region but reduction of both at the outer margins. The first and last images will have reduced field of view and will be more susceptible to motion artifacts.

Revolution CT has a tool called "auto-gating" that automatically determines the heart rate-dependent settings for triggered acquisition and gated reconstructions. In this way the scanner automatically establishes the best scan mode for that patient: snapshot pulse or cardiac helical. With regard to patients' heart rate, it will also establish the

Table 7.1 Basic characteristics of Siemens CT scanners

Model	Source	Coverage	Slice	Detection	Rotation time	Acquisition mode	Recon mode	Recon algorithm
Definition edge	Single source, with dual focal spot, 100 kW	38.4 mm	2 × 64 × 0.6	Single layer	0.28 s	Sequential (step-and-shoot), helical	Standard, second gen. Iterative (SAFIRE)	Sequential: multi-cycle, single cycle Helical: multi-cycle, single cycle
Definition flash	Dual source, with dual focal spot, 2 × 100 kW	38.4 mm	2 × 64 × 0.6 per source/ detector pair	Single layer	0.28 s	High pitch (flash mode), sequential (step-and-shoot), helical	Standard, second gen. Iterative (SAFIRE)	High pitch: single cycle Sequential: multi-cycle, single cycle Helical: multi-cycle, single cycle
Definition force	Dual source, with dual focal spot, 2 × 120 kW	52.2 mm	2 × 96 × 0.6 per source/ detector pair	Single layer	0.25 s	High pitch (flash mode), sequential (step-and-shoot), helical	Standard, third gen. Iterative (ADMIRE)	High pitch: Single cycle Sequential: multi-cycle, single cycle Helical: multi-cycle, single cycle

Table 7.2 Comparison between GE scanners for cardiac studies

Technical parameters and tools	Revolution CT	Revolution HD	Revolution EVO
Detector row (N°)	128	64	64
Slices per rotation (N°)	512	128	128
Gantry rotation (ms)	280	350	350
Temporal resolution (ms)	140	175	175
Iterative reconstruction	ASIR V	ASIR	ASIR V
Snapshot freeze	✓(Intelligent)	✓	✓
Dual energy mode	Work in progress	✓optional	x
Other cardiac tools	Cardiac auto-gating	Cardiac assist	Cardiac assist

cardiac phase range to acquire, which phase needs to be reconstructed, and when snapshot freeze should be applied. Regarding patients' beat-to-beat HR variation, it will determine how much additional padding may be needed, whether +ms-based trigger should be used instead of % of the RR interval or if retrigger double scan is appropriate in patients with irregular rhythm such as arrhythmias or preventricular contraction.

For functional evaluation, regardless of the heart rate, the tube current will be 100% power at 40% and 75% and only 20% at the other phases. In this acquisition mode, additional phases every 10% will be reconstructed to show the complete heartbeat and allow ejection fraction calculation.

Parameter settings such as pitch and ECG modulation are also determined automatically. Based on patient size observed in a scout view, kV assist will provide with optimal mA and kVp. Cardiac modulation of mA is available allowing to provide the adequate exposure to the patient in order to attain the best image quality with the lowest radiation dose in keeping with the ALARA principle (as low as reasonably achievable). This new tool admits simplification and robustness pressing only one button and no longer in need of heart rate-specific protocols.

Revolution CT applies new iterative reconstruction algorithm called ASIR-V that enables up to 80% radiation dose reduction compared to standard filtered back projection (FBP) with similar reconstruction speed. It also improves low-contrast detectability up to 135% at the same dose, spatial resolution, and image noise and can reduce low-signal artifacts such as streak artifacts.

Snapshot freeze (SSF) can be used to reduce coronary artery motion artifacts in high-definition or in standard cardiac studies. A three-phase image series is generated for subsequent motion correction processing on the AW workstation or AW server [33].

1. *Revolution HD (with/without GSI):* consists in a high-definition scanner that works in single energy (SE) or dual energy (DE) using Gemstone Spectral Imaging (GSI).

This scanner is 64-row detectors and has coverage of 4 cm. Other technical information: collimation width 0.625 mm, gantry rotation 0.35 s, and temporal resolution 175 ms.

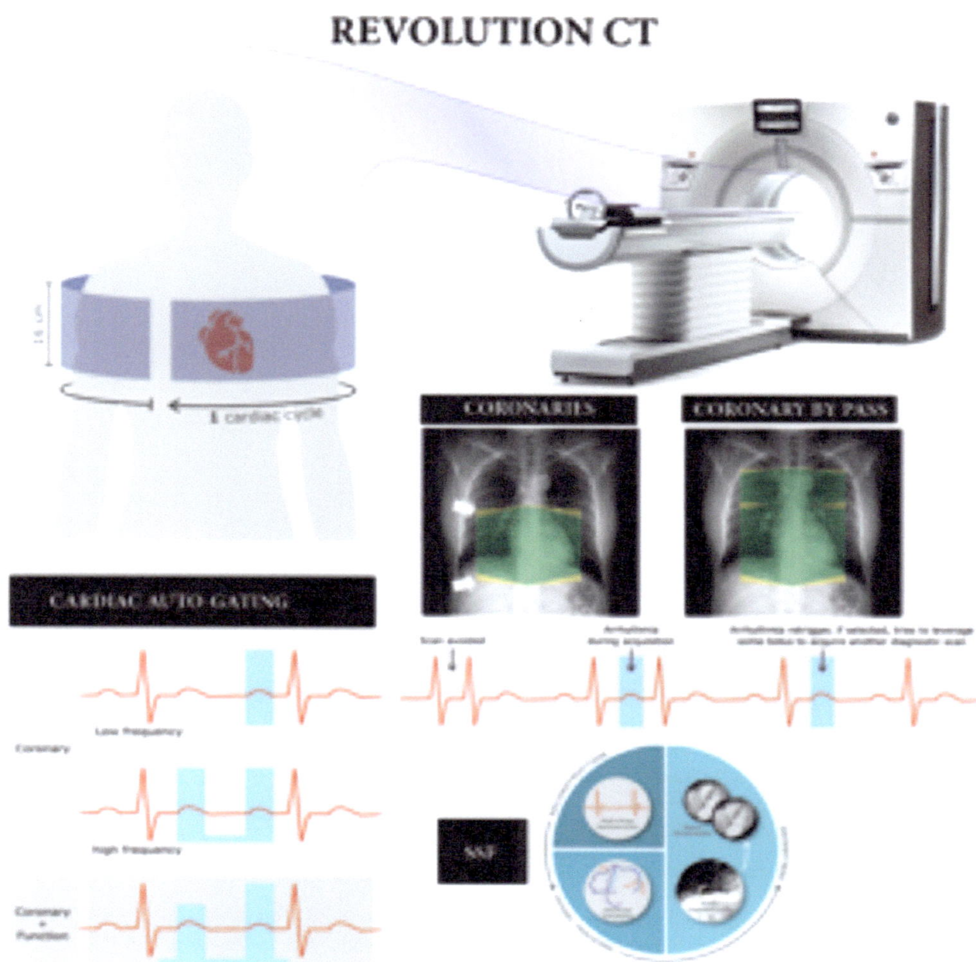

Fig. 7.4 The newest CT scanner with wide coverage of 160 mm that allows scanning the complete heart in one gantry rotation. In cases of patients with bypass grafts, two volumes need to be acquired. The fast gantry rotation of 0.28 ms gives an ideal temporal resolution to scan patients even with high heart rates and obtains excellent image quality. Cardiac auto-gating tool automatically determines the best scan mode for that patient (snapshot pulse or cardiac helical), the cardiac phase range to acquire, which phase needs to be reconstructed, and when snapshot freeze should be applied making the scan very simple. Also it determines if retrigger double scan is necessary in patients with irregular rhythm such as arrhythmias or pre-ventricular contraction

It operates with Smart Dose technologies such as kV assist, dosed organ modulation, 3D dose modulation, and dose check among others. It also operates with ASIR.

Single Energy Single energy works in standard or high-definition mode allowing to improve spatial resolution to 0.28 mm [34]. Snapshot assist (SSA) helps the user to determine the acquisition mode according to the patient's heart rate, beat-to-beat variation, and size. SSF can be applied in prospective or retrospective techniques. For intermediate heart rates (65–74 bpm), especially with moderate to high variability, SSF has to be prescribed at 75% phase (mid-diastole) and 45% RR interval (end-systole), and in cases with high HR > 75 bpm, only 45% phase is needed [35]. Appropriate cardiac phase selection is mandatory for optimal performance. Excellent contrast opacification is essential for ideal SSF correction [36].

Dual-Energy GSI It operates exclusively in prospective mode for all cardiac studies. It acquires the information performing rapid switching (0.3–0.5 ms) between low and high tube potentials (80–140 kVp) using only one source [37]. According to the patient's heart rate and variability, different phases and additional padding could be necessary. For patients with (a) <65 bpm, center phase at 75%. Additional padding of 100 ms can be complemented if the rhythm is unstable: (b) 65–74 bpm center phase at 60%, padding 150–200 ms, and (c) >75 bpm center phase at 40%, padding 100 ms. SSF can be applied to improve temporal resolution with similar results with single energy [38]. ASIR is actually available in GSI in all energy levels (40–140 keV) admitting to reduce noise mainly at 40–60 keV (levels with highest noise). Dual-energy CT significantly reduces *blooming* in patients with severe calcification of the coronary arteries and beam-hardening artifacts improving combined anatomo-functional evaluation present with single-energy CT in determined population (Fig. 7.5) [39].

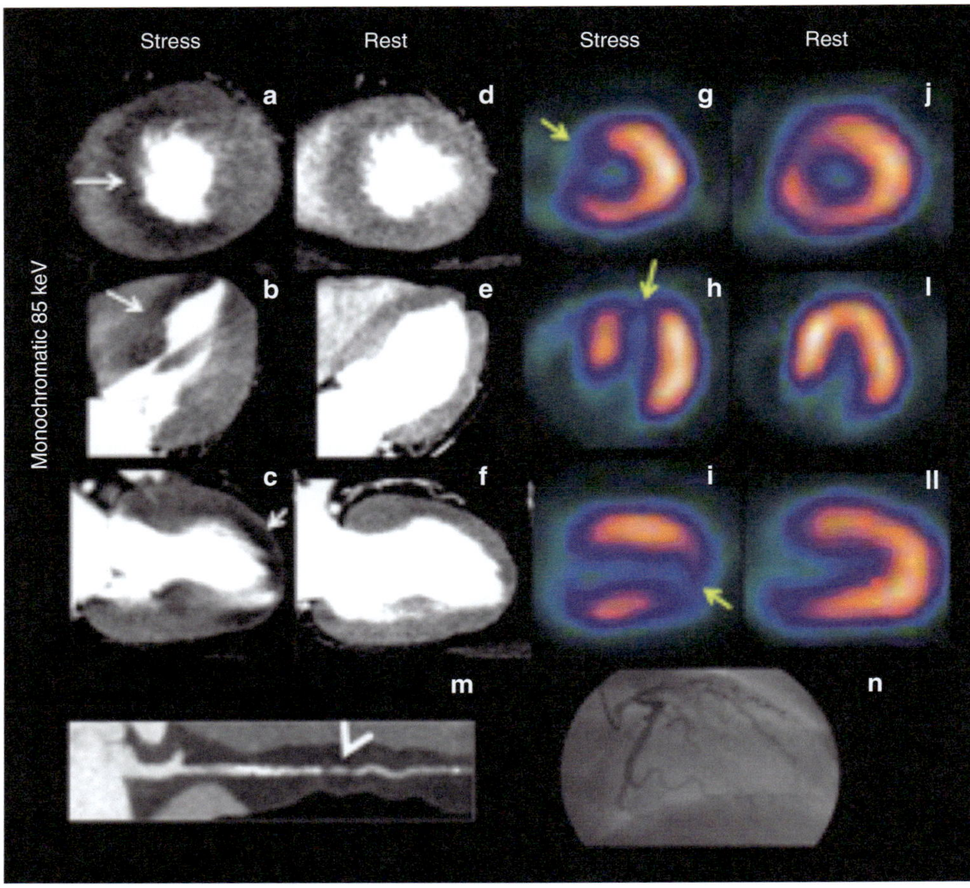

Fig. 7.5 A 75-year-old female with cardiovascular risk factors such as hypertension, dyslipidemia, and diabetes. She presents with angina and dyspnea FC II–III. A combined anatomo-functional evaluation was performed with dual-energy CT (GSI) to assess coronary stenosis and myocardial perfusion with reduction of booming and beam-hardening artifacts. Monochromatic evaluation at medium energy levels (85 keV) was used for the analysis. (**a–c**) Stress CT at short-axis, four-chamber, and long-axis views, respectively, showing severe hypoperfusion in septal, anteroseptal, apical, and inferior walls (white arrows). (**d–f**) Rest CT in the same views demonstrating normal perfusion stress (**g**, **h**, **l**) and rest (**j**, **l**, **ll**) SPECT images show the same findings than dual-energy CT confirming an anteroseptal, septal, apical, and inferior ischemia. (**m**) CTCA of the left anterior descendent (LAD) artery exhibiting a severe stenosis in the midportion (arrow head). (**n**) Invasive coronary angiography showing the same lesion in the LAD

2. *Revolution EVO:* this scanner has a coverage of 4 cm, gantry rotation of 0.35 ms, collimation width of 0.625 mm, and clarity detector that improves dose efficiency and signal-to-noise ratio.

It operates with ASIR V and applies Smart Dose technologies, snapshot assist, snapshot pulse, ECG dose modulation, 3D mA modulation, and pre-scan dose estimates.

Philips

Several CT scanners from Philips Medical Systems are currently available (Table 7.3). Those include the 64-slice version (Brilliance 64) which was the first 64-slice scanner offered for clinical use in October 2004. The later 64- and 128-slice scanners using a dual focal spot correction, therefore allowing for 128-row and 256-row acquisition (Brilliance iCT-SP (128), and Brilliance iCT (256)) were introduced in 2008 for clinical use and underwent several iterations until its current configuration. Philips takes special care toward its detector technology and rapid gantry rotation time. Image analysis may be performed via dedicated software available on their Extended Brilliance Workstation (EBW) and also via a PC-based portal that allows most analysis processes to be performed on raw data accessed from a laptop or office-/home-based personal computer.

Recently, Philips introduced a new version of the 64-slice scanner equipped with their new detector technology (NanoPanel Prism) allowing separation between low- and high-energy raw data resulting in spectral imaging. This new spectral CT scanner (IQon) technology will not be discussed here. The IQon gantry rotation speed is higher than the conventional Brilliance 64 and similar to the Brilliance iCT-SP,

Table 7.3 Basic characteristics of Philips CT scanners

Model	Source	Coverage	Slice	Detection	Rotation time	Acquisition mode	Recon mode	Recon algorithm
Br64/ Inginuity64	Single source, with dual focal spot, 80 kW	40 mm	64 × 0.625	Single layer	0.42 s/rot	Axial (step-and-shoot), helical	Standard, iDose4, IMR	Helical: multi-cycle, single cycle Axial: single cycle
iCT-SP (128)	Single source, with dual focal spot, 120 kW	40 mm	128 × 0.625	Single layer	0.27 s/rot	Axial (step-and-shoot), helical	Standard, iDose4, IMR	Helical: multi-cycle, single cycle Axial: single cycle
iCT-SP (256)	Single source, with dual focal spot, 120 kW	80 mm	256 × 0.625	Single layer	0.27 s/rot	Axial (step-and-shoot), helical	Standard, iDose4, IMR	Helical: multi-cycle, single cycle Axial: single cycle
IQon	Single source, with dual focal spot, 120 kW	40 mm	128 × 0.625	Dual layer	0.27 s/rot	Axial (step-and-shoot), helical	Standard, iDose4, IMR	Helical: multi-cycle, single cycle Axial: single cycle

and most acquisition parameters are similar too. The fundamentals of dual energy and spectral imaging are presented elsewhere in this textbook. Additionally, all Philips platforms allow for the use of iterative reconstruction (either conventional "iDose" or the model-based "iMR").

Brilliance 64: Typical Image Acquisition and Commonly Used Protocols

Calcium Score Acquisition The coronary artery calcium score (Agatston units) may be measured on a non-enhanced scan using prospective ECG triggering. Typical scan parameters include a tube voltage of 120 kV, tube current of 55 mAs, gantry rotation time of 0.42/s, and collimation of 64 × 0.625 mm. Reconstruction is performed with a CB filter with 2.5 mm or 3 mm slice thickness without overlap. Coronary CT angiography when using the 60 kW tube of the scanner may be performed with retrospective electrocardiographic (ECG) gating or with prospective ECG triggering (step-and-shoot mode). The contrast-enhanced scan is performed using a bolus of approximately 70 (range 40–120) ml of contrast media injected into an antecubital vein at a flow rate of 5–7 ml/s, followed by a 50 ml saline chaser bolus. Scanning is typically performed at 120 kV, effective tube current 600–1000 mAs, slice collimation of 64 × 0.625 mm acquisition, 0.42 s gantry rotation time, and pitch 0.2 as a standard. ECG-based tube current modulation for retrospective gating ("DoseRight Cardiac") may be used to decrease radiation when possible. Reconstruction is performed using a window centered at 75% of the RR interval as default (to coincide with ventricular diastasis). For heart rates above 70 beats/min, an earlier reconstruction phase (usually 45% or less) is frequently used (coinciding with isovolumic relaxation). Typically a multi-cycle scan image reconstruction with XCC filter (Philips) and slice thickness reconstruction of 0.67 mm with 50% overlap is used (allowing spatial resolution of 10–24 lp/cm depending on scanner version). If movement artifacts are apparent, additional reconstruction windows may be analyzed. A dedicated cardiac gating algorithm is used that identified the same physiologic phases of the cardiac cycle while taking into account the nonlinear changes in the individual cardiac states with the heart rate variations during CT acquisition. As mentioned above cardiac adaptive multi-cycle (or multi-segment) reconstruction technique is typically used that combined data from consecutive cardiac cycles, thus improving temporal resolution. Dedicated software (Arrhythmia Editing, Philips Medical Systems, Cleveland, OH) allowed correction for R wave irregularity after data acquisition in patients with marked sinus arrhythmia or frequent premature beats. Local "phase point" editing is also available post acquisition (not only R-tag detection).

Brilliance iCT (256)

cCTA is performed on this 256-row scanner which has a longitudinal coverage of 8 cm, offers options for different rotation times which can be as fast as 0.27/s, and has a 120 kW generator. cCTA is performed either as prospectively triggered "step-and-shoot" mode or with helical retrospective ECG gating. ECG-based tube current modulation can be used when possible with retrospective gating (DoseRight Cardiac).

The coronary artery calcium score (Agatston units) may be measured on a non-enhanced scan using prospective ECG triggering. Typical scan parameters include a tube voltage of 120 kV, tube current of 55 mAs, and gantry rotation time of 0.27/s, and autocollimation is frequently 128 × 0.625 mm. Reconstruction is performed with a XCB filter with 2.5 mm or 3 mm slice thickness without overlap.

Contrast-enhanced scan is performed on the iCT using a bolus of 65 (range 50–100) ml contrast media injected into an antecubital vein at a flow rate of 5–7 ml/s, followed by a mixed 50% contrast/saline injection and then a 20–30 ml saline chaser bolus. Contrast media dose with Philips scanners is calculated according to the following formula: [(predicted scan time in seconds +5) × IV contrast flow rate]. Scans are performed at 120 kV [or 80/100/140 kV depending on body mass index (BMI)] with a slice collimation of 128 × 0.625 mm, with dual *z*-focal spot positions (which leads to a double number of simultaneous imaged slices per gantry rotation, therefore 256-row acquisition) and a rotation time of 0.27 or 0.33 s. For low kV scans (80 or 100 kV), a slower injection rate (4 ml/s) is frequently used resulting in an overall lower volume of contrast thus maintaining a relatively stable contrast to noise ratio. The helical scans (retrospective ECG gating) are performed with an effective tube current (rotation time product normalized by the pitch) in the range of 900–1500 mAs (effective) depending on BMI and body habitus and a pitch of 0.14–0.18. The step-and-shoot (prospective triggering) scans are performed in patients with stable heart rhythm and heart rate < 65 beats per minute with a tube current X-ray ON time product of 160–300 mAs. The scanner provides several predefined protocols which determines the pitch and rotation time in each protocol according to scanning mode, heart rate, and whether a "bariatric mode"(high mA) is used (to allow optimal temporal resolution at all settings). Reconstruction is again performed using a window centered at 75% of the RR interval as default. For heart rates above 70 BPM, an earlier reconstruction phase (usually 45% or less) is frequently used with retrospective gating. Typical filter used for reconstruction is XCC and same 0.67 mm slice thickness with 50% overlap (Fig. 7.6).

Toshiba

Toshiba manufactures both narrow (80 detectors) and wide detector (320 detectors) CT scanners (Table 7.4), the latter is the focus of the chapter. Wide detector scanners with 320 detector rows and up to 16 cm of craniocaudal coverage uniquely enable whole-heart coverage in an axial (not helical) scan mode with one gantry rotation typically within a single heartbeat in as little as 0.138 s. The short duration required for scan acquisition makes the technique applicable even in patients with atrial fibrillation [40] and reduces the time required for patient breath hold (1–2 seconds) hence rendering the technique very convenient for the patient while minimizing potential artifacts secondary to respiratory motion [41].

Image data is reconstructed using a half-scan reconstruction algorithm, typically with a 512 × 512 matrix and 0.5 mm thick sections. Wide detector imaging eliminates "stair-step" or misalignment artifacts and permits uniform attenuation when evaluating the coronary arteries, when analyzing myocardial defects [42, 43], or when measuring contrast attenuation gradients across atherosclerotic lesions [44] (Figs. 7.7, 7.8, and 7.9). The ability to cover the entire heart in one shot permits dynamic volume assessment including of left ventricular function and assessment of absolute myocardial blood flow [45]. Radiation doses are lower with wide detector scanners owing to shorter scan times and reduction of redundant radiation from either overlapping of sequential axial scans or helical oversampling [46]. In addition, total iodinated contrast volume can be decreased to as low as 40 ml at 5 ml/s in patients with normal cardiac output [47].

There have been three generations of 320 detectors CT (Aquilion ONE, Aquilion VISION, and Aquilion GENESIS). Despite equivalent spatial resolution (0.5 mm), the gantry speed for the VISION and GENESIS generation scanner is faster than that of the first-generation scanner (275 vs. 350 ms), with a temporal resolution of 138 vs. 175 ms, respectively. In patients with elevated heart rates, in order to improve the temporal resolution, data from two or three cardiac cycles can be used for image reconstruction, which is called multi-segment reconstruction. Accordingly, in the first-generation scanner, the temporal resolution of multi-segment reconstruction can be theoretically improved to 88 or 58 ms, using two- and three-beat reconstruction. With its improved temporal resolution, the newer-generation scanners have been demonstrated to permit single-beat imaging in vast majority (93%) in those with heart rates of up to

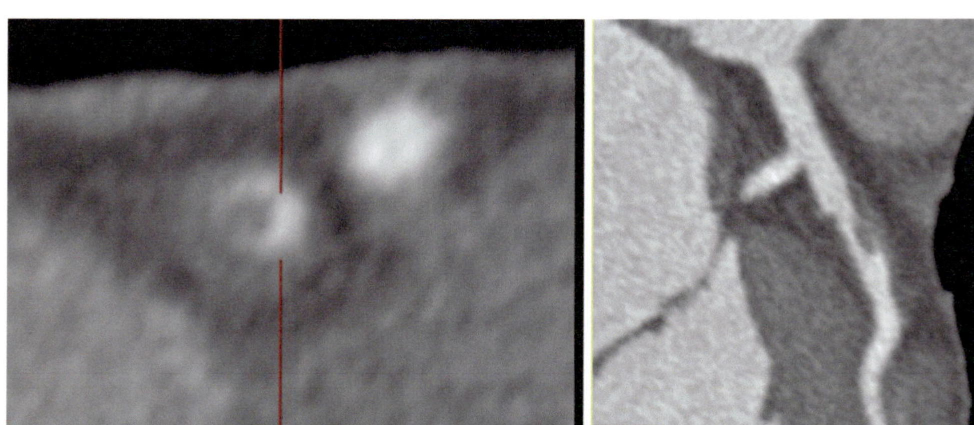

Fig. 7.6 High-risk/ruptured plaque (napkin-ring sign) (right panel-long axis, left panel-short axis) in the proximal left anterior descending coronary artery demonstrating the high-resolution image that may be acquired with Brilliance iCT

Table 7.4 Basic characteristics of Toshiba cardiac CT scanners

		Aquilion PRIME	Aquilion ONE	Aquilion ONE vision	Aquilion ONE GENESIS
Basic performance	No. of detectors	80	320	320	320
	Thickness of detectors	0.5 mm	0.5 mm	0.5 mm	0.5 mm
	No. of slices acquirable	160 using double-slice technology	640 using double-slice technology	640 using double-slice technology	640 using double-slice technology
	Cranial caudal coverage	4 cm	16 cm	16 cm	16 cm
	Gantry rotation speed	350 ms	350 ms	275 ms	275 ms
	Opening size	78	78 cm	78 cm	78 cm
	Tilt angle	30	22	30	30
	Acquisition mode	Prospective or retrospective helical	Axial volume	Axial volume	Axial volume
	Single beat cardiac CT acquisition	No, 4–5 beats	Yes – up to 65BPM	Yes up to 65 bpm	Yes – up to 75BPM
Tube and generator	Generator capacity	72 kW	72 kW	100 kW	100 kW
	Tube voltage	80/100/120/135 kV	80/100/120/135 kV	80/100/120/135 kV	80/100/120/135 kV
	Tube current	10–600 mA	10–600 mA	10-10-900 mA	10–900 mA
Computer system	Iterative reconstruction	AIDR 3D hybrid	AIDR 3D hybrid		AIDR 3D hybrid/ FIRST model based
	Reconstruction speed	30 ips	50 ips		80 ips

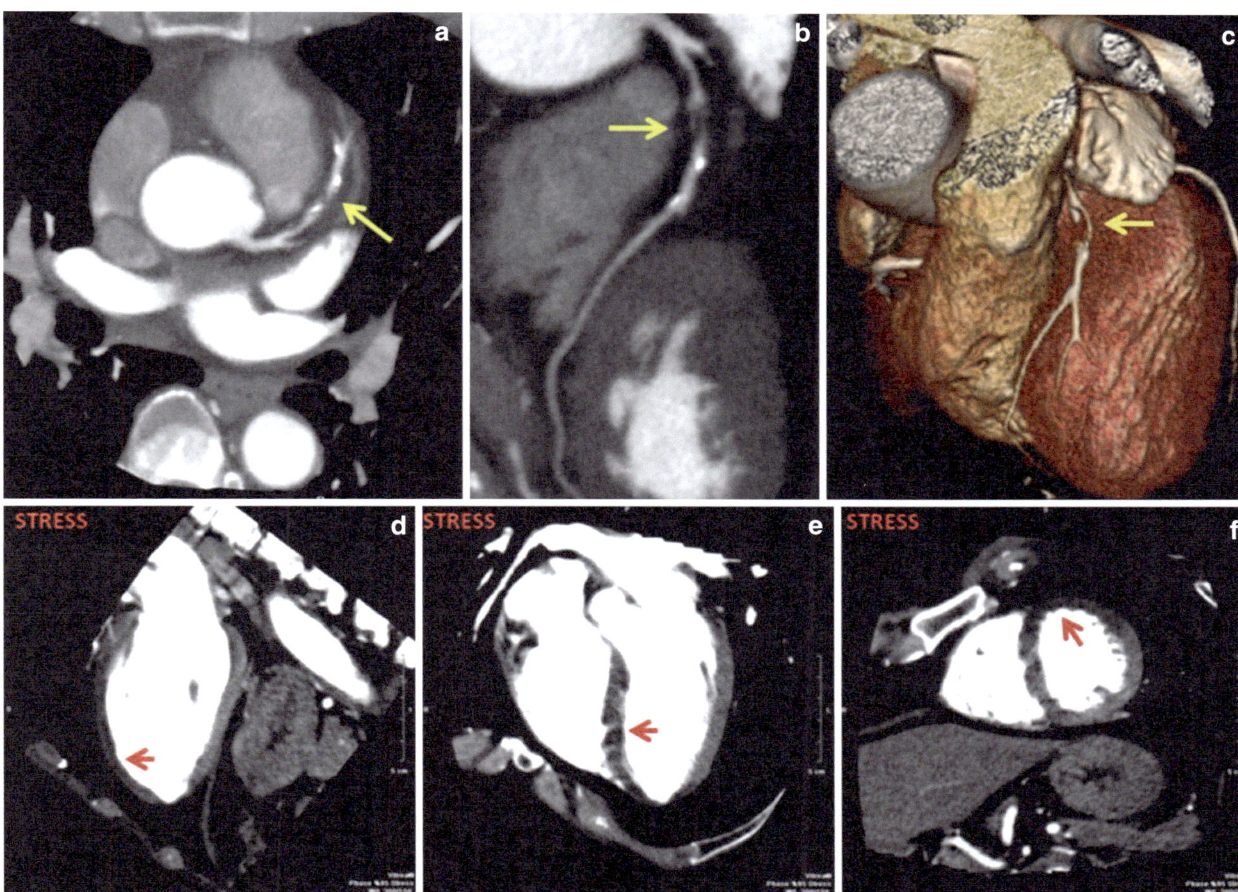

Fig. 7.7 Wide detector CT examination of a patient with critical stenosis in the proximal left anterior descending artery secondary to mixed calcified and noncalcified atherosclerotic plaque as demonstrated on axial, curved planar reformat and volume-rendered images on CTCA (**a**–**c**). There are corresponding perfusion defects in the basal, mid-, and distal anteroseptal, anterior, and anterolateral myocardial segments (red arrows) observed during CT stress myocardial perfusion imaging (**d**–**f**), which are also present but to a much less extent on the corresponding rest images (**g**–**i**). This case highlights volumetric assessment providing both coronary anatomy and perfusion using single-beat imaging. (Adapted from Ko et al. [42], with permission.)

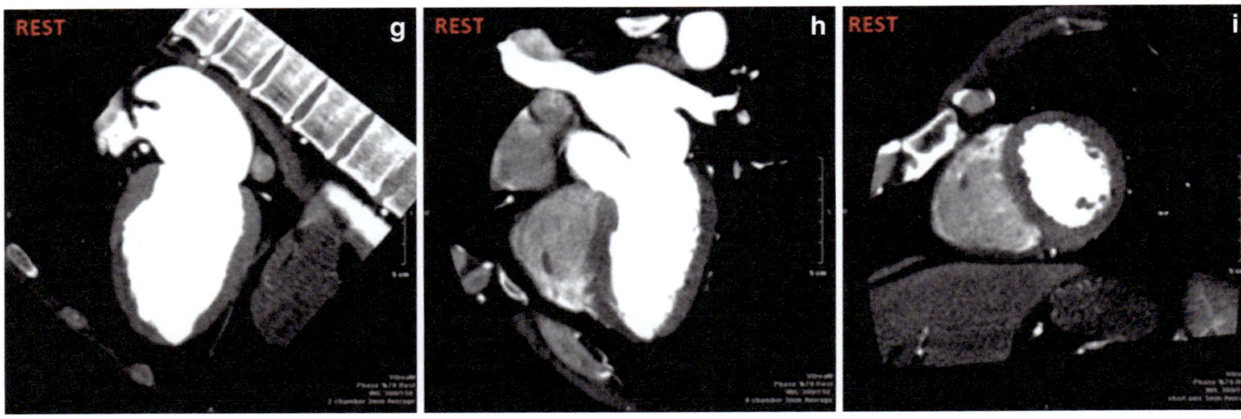

Fig. 7.7 (continued)

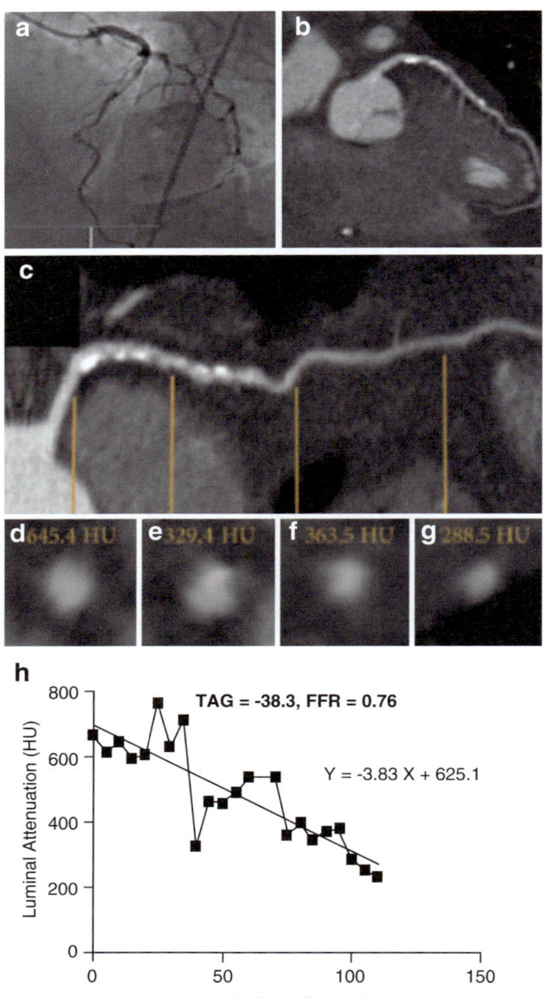

Fig. 7.8 Left anterior descending artery (LAD) with significant obstructive plaque burden imaged by invasive angiography (**a**) and 320-detector CTCA (**b**). Curved planar reformat and representative cross-sectional views with corresponding luminal attenuation on CCTA (**c–g**), which permitted the calculation of the intraluminal attenuation gradient (**h**) across a single heartbeat. The gradient was considered significant (−38.3); the corresponding invasive fractional flow reserve value was 0.76 in the distal LAD. (Adapted from Wong et al. [44], with permission.)

75 bpm [48]. When compared with the first-generation scanner in patients with elevated heart rates, it has been demonstrated to provide superior image quality with 35% radiation dose reduction [49, 50].

Until recently, body weight or body mass index (BMI) has been used to manually select the tube voltage and tube current for cardiac CT applications. Based on observations that attenuation and body habitus over the thorax can be discrepant from BMI or weight, Toshiba scanners are currently equipped with automated exposure control (SureExposure 3D) which determine a tube potential on the basis of the X-ray attenuation on anterior-posterior and lateral scout images, body profile of the individual patient and the reconstruction kernel [51]. SureExposure 3D adopts the standard deviation noise as a measure of image quality and aims to match the image noise to the targeted standard deviation [52]. This has demonstrated to reduce radiation exposure by up to 42% [51], without significant impairment of image quality compared to the results obtained using a BMI-based protocol.

Similar to other CT vendors, as part of a dose reduction strategy, Toshiba scanners are equipped with adaptive iterative dose reduction (AIDR 3D), a reconstruction algorithm which is uniquely adapted for large cone-beam CT examinations and wide-volume acquisitions. The AIDR algorithm can be applied to all acquisition modes for routine clinical use including CTCA and calcium scores [53] and efficiently eliminates noise and streak artifact due to photon starvation with a statistical noise and scanner model considering both photon and electronic noise in the raw data domain. The raw data are reconstructed with filtered back projection (FBP), and then a sophisticated iterative technique which optimizes reconstructions for the particular regions is applied in the image domain, resulting in noise reduction while preserving spatial resolution and image texture [54]. It enables the elimination of up to 50% of image noise [55], compared with FBP reconstruction, and may reduce the radiation dose up to 22–65% [56, 57].

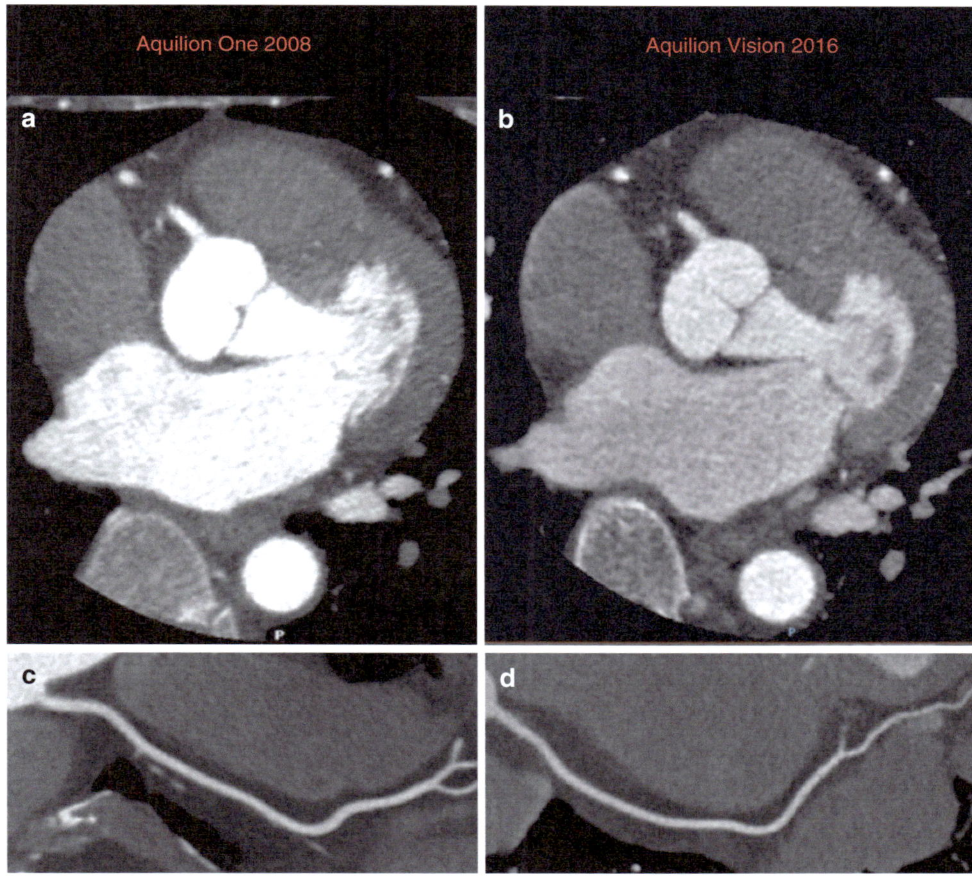

Fig. 7.9 The same patient underwent CTCA with Toshiba Acquilion ONE scanner in 2008 using retrospective ECG gating and standard filter back projection reconstruction (**a**, **b**) and again with the Toshiba Vision scanner in 2016 using prospective ECG gating and AIDR3D iterative reconstruction (**c**, **d**). The representative right coronary arteries are displayed, respectively (**b**, **d**). The heart rate acquired in both scans was 58 bpm. DLP has reduced by 60% from 440 to 176 mGy-cm

Arineta Inc. SpotLight CT, Cesarea, Israel

A new type of "stereo" CT with a compact size and high gantry rotation speed intended specifically for cardiovascular imaging was recently introduced and received FDA approval. This new scanner has two overlapping cone beams facing a single detector array rotating around the patient. It has a coverage (14 cm) sufficient for whole heart scanning in a single beat (acquisition time of 120 ms). This scanner has the fastest CT gantry rotation time currently available (0.24 s). Default acquisition is with prospective ECG triggering. This 280-slice CT scanner (192 detector rows) with a temporal resolution of 120 ms is of small size (60 cm gantry), compatible with small rooms, and was designed for optimal spatial and temporal resolution at a lower cost. The initial clinical assessment is promising with this scanner.

References

1. Bastarrika G, Lee YS, Huda W, Ruzsics B, Costello P, Schoepf UJ. CT of coronary artery disease. Radiology. 2009;253:317–38.
2. Meijboom WB, Weustink AC, Pugliese F, et al. Comparison of diagnostic accuracy of 64-slice computed tomography coronary angiography in women versus men with angina pectoris. Am J Cardiol. 2007;100:1532–7.
3. Roberts WT, Bax JJ, Davies LC. Cardiac CT and CT coronary angiography: technology and application. Heart. 2008;94:781–92.
4. Moscariello A, Takx RA, Schoepf UJ, et al. Coronary CT angiography: image quality, diagnostic accuracy, and potential for radiation dose reduction using a novel iterative image reconstruction technique-comparison with traditional filtered back projection. Eur Radiol. 2011;21:2130–8.
5. Den Harder AM, Willemink MJ, De Ruiter QM, et al. Dose reduction with iterative reconstruction for coronary CT angiography: a systematic review and meta-analysis. Br J Radiol. 2016;89:20150068.
6. Brenner D, Elliston C, Hall E, Berdon W. Estimated risks of radiation-induced fatal cancer from pediatric CT. AJR Am J Roentgenol. 2001;176:289–96.
7. Brenner DJ. Radiation risks potentially associated with low-dose CT screening of adult smokers for lung cancer. Radiology. 2004;231:440–5.
8. Brenner DJ, Hall EJ. Risk of cancer from diagnostic X-rays. Lancet. 2004;363:2192; author reply –3.
9. Brenner DJ, Hall EJ. Computed tomography – an increasing source of radiation exposure. N Engl J Med. 2007;357:2277–84.
10. Einstein AJ, Moser KW, Thompson RC, Cerqueira MD, Henzlova MJ. Radiation dose to patients from cardiac diagnostic imaging. Circulation. 2007;116:1290–305.

11. Primak AN, McCollough CH, Bruesewitz MR, Zhang J, Fletcher JG. Relationship between noise, dose, and pitch in cardiac multi-detector row CT. Radiographics. 2006;26:1785–94.
12. Hausleiter J, Meyer T, Hermann F, et al. Estimated radiation dose associated with cardiac CT angiography. JAMA. 2009;301:500–7.
13. Efstathopoulos EP, Kelekis NL, Pantos I, et al. Reduction of the estimated radiation dose and associated patient risk with prospective ECG-gated 256-slice CT coronary angiography. Phys Med Biol. 2009;54:5209–22.
14. Flohr TG, Leng S, Yu L, et al. Dual-source spiral CT with pitch up to 3.2 and 75 ms temporal resolution: image reconstruction and assessment of image quality. Med Phys. 2009;36:5641–53.
15. Achenbach S, Marwan M, Ropers D, et al. Coronary computed tomography angiography with a consistent dose below 1 mSv using prospectively electrocardiogram-triggered high-pitch spiral acquisition. Eur Heart J. 2010;31:340–6.
16. Meyer M, Haubenreisser H, Schoepf UJ, et al. Closing in on the K edge: coronary CT angiography at 100, 80, and 70 kV-initial comparison of a second- versus a third-generation dual-source CT system. Radiology. 2014;273:373–82.
17. Poll LW, Cohnen M, Brachten S, Ewen K, Modder U. Dose reduction in multi-slice CT of the heart by use of ECG-controlled tube current modulation ("ECG pulsing"): phantom measurements. Rofo. 2002;174:1500–5.
18. Hausleiter J, Meyer T, Hadamitzky M, et al. Radiation dose estimates from cardiac multislice computed tomography in daily practice: impact of different scanning protocols on effective dose estimates. Circulation. 2006;113:1305–10.
19. Huda W, Scalzetti EM, Levin G. Technique factors and image quality as functions of patient weight at abdominal CT. Radiology. 2000;217:430–5.
20. Niemann T, Henry S, Duhamel A, et al. Pediatric chest CT at 70 kVp: a feasibility study in 129 children. Pediatr Radiol. 2014;44:1347–57.
21. Leschka S, Stolzmann P, Schmid FT, et al. Low kilovoltage cardiac dual-source CT: attenuation, noise, and radiation dose. Eur Radiol. 2008;18:1809–17.
22. Stolzmann P, Leschka S, Scheffel H, et al. Dual-source CT in step-and-shoot mode: noninvasive coronary angiography with low radiation dose. Radiology. 2008;249:71–80.
23. Hsieh J, Londt J, Vass M, Li J, Tang X, Okerlund D. Step-and-shoot data acquisition and reconstruction for cardiac x-ray computed tomography. Med Phys. 2006;33:4236–48.
24. Renker M, Nance JW Jr, Schoepf UJ, et al. Evaluation of heavily calcified vessels with coronary CT angiography: comparison of iterative and filtered back projection image reconstruction. Radiology. 2011;260:390–9.
25. Renker M, Ramachandra A, Schoepf UJ, et al. Iterative image reconstruction techniques: applications for cardiac CT. J Cardiovasc Comput Tomogr. 2011;5:225–30.
26. Naoum C, Blanke P, Leipsic J. Iterative reconstruction in cardiac CT. J Cardiovasc Comput Tomogr. 2015;9:255–63.
27. Meinel FG, De Cecco CN, Schoepf UJ, et al. First-arterial-pass dual-energy CT for assessment of myocardial blood supply: do we need rest, stress, and delayed acquisition? Comparison with SPECT. Radiology. 2014;270:708–16.
28. Weininger M, Schoepf UJ, Ramachandra A, et al. Adenosine-stress dynamic real-time myocardial perfusion CT and adenosine-stress first-pass dual-energy myocardial perfusion CT for the assessment of acute chest pain: initial results. Eur J Radiol. 2012;81:3703–10.
29. Schwarz F, Nance JW Jr, Ruzsics B, Bastarrika G, Sterzik A, Schoepf UJ. Quantification of coronary artery calcium on the basis of dual-energy coronary CT angiography. Radiology. 2012;264:700–7.
30. Apfaltrer P, Schoendube H, Schoepf UJ, et al. Enhanced temporal resolution at cardiac CT with a novel CT image reconstruction algorithm: initial patient experience. Eur J Radiol. 2013;82:270–4.
31. Mangold S, Wichmann JL, Schoepf UJ, et al. Automated tube voltage selection for radiation dose and contrast medium reduction at coronary CT angiography using 3(rd) generation dual-source CT. Eur Radiol. 2016;26:3608–16.
32. Latif MA, Sanchez FW, Sayegh K, et al. Volumetric single-beat coronary computed tomography angiography: relationship of image quality, heart rate, and body mass index. Initial patient experience with a new computed tomography scanner. J Comput Assist Tomogr. 2016;40:763–72.
33. Pontone G, Andreini D, Bertella E, et al. Impact of an intra-cycle motion correction algorithm on overall evaluability and diagnostic accuracy of computed tomography coronary angiography. Eur Radiol. 2016;26:147–56.
34. Pontone G, Bertella E, Mushtaq S, et al. Coronary artery disease: diagnostic accuracy of CT coronary angiography – a comparison of high and standard spatial resolution scanning. Radiology. 2014;271:688–94.
35. Andreini D, Pontone G, Mushtaq S, et al. Low-dose CT coronary angiography with a novel IntraCycle motion-correction algorithm in patients with high heart rate or heart rate variability. Eur Heart J Cardiovasc Imaging. 2015;16:1093–100.
36. Carrascosa P, Deviggiano A, Capunay C, De Zan MC, Goldsmit A, Rodriguez-Granillo GA. Effect of intracycle motion correction algorithm on image quality and diagnostic performance of computed tomography coronary angiography in patients with suspected coronary artery disease. Acad Radiol. 2015;22:81–6.
37. So A, Lee TY, Imai Y, et al. Quantitative myocardial perfusion imaging using rapid kVp switch dual-energy CT: preliminary experience. J Cardiovasc Comput Tomogr. 2011;5:430–42.
38. Carrascosa P, Deviggiano A, Leipsic JA, et al. Dual energy imaging and intracycle motion correction for CT coronary angiography in patients with intermediate to high likelihood of coronary artery disease. Clin Imaging. 2015;39:1000–5.
39. Rodriguez-Granillo GA, Carrascosa P, Cipriano S, et al. Beam hardening artifact reduction using dual energy computed tomography: implications for myocardial perfusion studies. Cardiovasc Diagn Ther. 2015;5:79–85.
40. Xu L, Yang L, Fan Z, Yu W, Lv B, Zhang Z. Diagnostic performance of 320-detector CT coronary angiography in patients with atrial fibrillation: preliminary results. Eur Radiol. 2011;21:936–43.
41. Kang EJ, Lee J, Lee KN, Kown H, Ha DH, Kim RB. An initial randomised study assessing free-breathing CCTA using 320-detector CT. Eur Radiol. 2013;23:1199–209.
42. Ko BS, Cameron JD, Leung M, et al. Combined CT coronary angiography and stress myocardial perfusion imaging for hemodynamically significant stenoses in patients with suspected coronary artery disease: a comparison with fractional flow reserve. JACC Cardiovasc Imaging. 2012;5:1097–111.
43. Rochitte CE, George RT, Chen MY, et al. Computed tomography angiography and perfusion to assess coronary artery stenosis causing perfusion defects by single photon emission computed tomography: the CORE320 study. Eur Heart J. 2014;35(17):1120–30.
44. Wong DT, Ko BS, Cameron JD, et al. Transluminal attenuation gradient in coronary computed tomography angiography is a novel noninvasive apporach to the identification of functionally significant coronary artery stenosis: a comparison with fractional flow reserve. J Am Coll Cardiol. 2013;61:1271–9.
45. Kikuchi Y, Oyama-Manabe N, Naya M, et al. Quantification of myocardial blood flow using dynamic 320-row multi-detector CT as compared with (1)(5)O-H(2)O PET. Eur Radiol. 2014;24:1547–56.
46. Hsiao EM, Rybicki FJ, Steigner M. CT coronary angiography: 256-slice and 320-detector row scanners. Curr Cardiol Rep. 2010;12:68–75.

47. Kim R, Park EA, Lee W, Chung JW. Feasibility of 320-row area detector CT coronary angiography using 40 mL of contrast material: assessment of image quality and diagnostic accuracy. Eur Radiol. 2016;26(11):3802–10.
48. Chen MY, Shanbhag SM, Arai AE. Submillisievert median radiation dose for coronary angiography with a second-generation 320-detector row CT scanner in 107 consecutive patients. Radiology. 2013;267:76–85.
49. Wong DT, Soh SY, Ko BS, et al. Superior CT coronary angiography image quality at lower radiation exposure with second generation 320-detector row CT in patients with elevated heart rate: a comparison with first generation 320-detector row CT. Cardiovasc Diagn Ther. 2014;4:299–306.
50. Tomizawa N, Maeda E, Akahane M, Torigoe R, Kiryu S, Ohtomo K. Coronary CT angiography using the second-generation 320-detector row CT: assessment of image quality and radiation dose in various heart rates compared with the first-generation scanner. Int J Cardiovasc Imaging. 2013;29:1613–8.
51. Lim J, Park EA, Lee W, Shim H, Chung JW. Image quality and radiation reduction of 320-row area detector CT coronary angiography with optimal tube voltage selection and an automatic exposure control system: comparison with body mass index-adapted protocol. Int J Cardiovasc Imaging. 2015;31(Suppl 1):23–30.
52. Lee CH, Goo JM, Ye HJ, et al. Radiation dose modulation techniques in the multidetector CT era: from basics to practice. Radiographics. 2008;28:1451–9.
53. Choi AD, Leifer ES, Yu J, et al. Prospective evaluation of the influence of iterative reconstruction on the reproducibility of coronary calcium quantification in reduced radiation dose 320 detector row CT. J Cardiovasc Comput Tomogr. 2016;10:359–63.
54. Tatsugami F, Higaki T, Fukumoto W, et al. Radiation dose reduction for coronary artery calcium scoring at 320-detector CT with adaptive iterative dose reduction 3D. Int J Cardiovasc Imaging. 2015;31:1045–52.
55. Gervaise A, Osemont B, Lecocq S, et al. CT image quality improvement using Adaptive Iterative Dose Reduction with wide-volume acquisition on 320-detector CT. Eur Radiol. 2012;22:295–301.
56. Yoo RE, Park EA, Lee W, et al. Image quality of adaptive iterative dose reduction 3D of coronary CT angiography of 640-slice CT: comparison with filtered back-projection. Int J Cardiovasc Imaging. 2013;29:669–76.
57. Chen MY, Steigner ML, Leung SW, et al. Simulated 50% radiation dose reduction in coronary CT angiography using adaptive iterative dose reduction in three-dimensions (AIDR3D). Int J Cardiovasc Imaging. 2013;29:1167–75.

Dual Energy and Spectral CT Techniques in Cardiovascular Imaging

8

B. Krauss and C. H. McCollough

The terms "Dual Energy CT" and "spectral CT" or "spectral imaging" [1, 2] refer to X-ray computed tomography scanners that image a patient using two or more X-ray spectra so that differences in the chemical composition of body materials can be analyzed. At the moment all commercially available CT scanners of this type work with only two X-ray spectra, and therefore the term Dual Energy CT will be used for all of them in the following. Several technologies can be used to either generate different spectra at the side of the X-ray source or to measure two different spectra at the side of the detector [3]. Effectively, all of these technologies generate similar information, but they differ in terms of dose efficiency, sensitivity to motion, and effectiveness for specific applications. One of the most important clinical applications of Dual Energy CT is the selective [4], quantitative [5], and possibly enhanced visualization [6] of iodinated contrast material, which is enabled by the special X-ray attenuation properties of iodine. In contrast to soft body tissues, the X-ray attenuation of iodine decreases strongly with energy within the spectral range that is commonly used for clinical CT scanners. This is a consequence of the high atomic number of iodine ($Z = 53$), which results in a dominance of the photoelectric effect. For water and soft body tissues, the decrease of the attenuation coefficient with energy is much less pronounced due to a dominance of Compton scattering. Since the definition of the Hounsfield unit uses water as reference material, the CT number of these tissues in Hounsfield units (HU) is almost independent of the X-ray spectrum.

Dual Energy CT has a long history and is almost as old as single energy CT. In the 1970s, it was demonstrated that Dual Energy CT could be used to make CT images more quantitative and to differentiate materials with low atomic numbers from materials with high atomic numbers [7, 8]. In contrast to some other imaging modalities, CT is not sensitive to chemical binding but mainly depends on the total number of electrons in a given volume (electron density) and the atomic number of the atoms (effective atomic number). The same applies also to Dual Energy CT, which also allows for explicitly measuring these two quantities [9, 10]. One of the earliest clinical applications of Dual Energy was related to the detection of calcium. In the 1980s, the first commercially available Dual Energy CT scanner was introduced, which could measure bone mineral density in the spine with improved accuracy [11]. However, at that time multi-slice spiral CT scanning was not yet invented, limiting the clinical capabilities of the technique. Dual Energy CT disappeared again from the market, until it was revived in 2005, when the first clinical Dual-Source Dual Energy CT scanner was introduced [12].

Since then, there has been an increasing interest in this technology, indicated by the several hundred peer-reviewed clinical publications on this topic. Each of the large manufacturers of CT scanners is currently offering Dual Energy CT scanners, and many new diagnostic applications have been identified [1]. Some of them are related to oncological questions [3], but there are also benefits for other fields like urology [13], rheumatology [14], and pulmonology [15]. As with single energy CT, most of the cardiovascular applications require high-speed arterial phase imaging and are therefore mainly feasible with CT scanners that have at least 64 data channels along the z-axis and rotation times no greater than 0.3 s. A power injector is needed, and for pulmonary CT angiography (CTA), it may be advantageous if the injector allows for several injection phases with different saline admixtures within the same bolus [16].

B. Krauss (✉)
Siemens Healthcare GmbH, Forchheim, Germany
e-mail: bernhard.krauss@siemens-healthineers.com

C. H. McCollough
Department of Radiology, Mayo Clinic, Rochester, MN, USA

U. J. Schoepf (ed.), *CT of the Heart*, Contemporary Medical Imaging, https://doi.org/10.1007/978-1-60327-237-7_8

Dual Energy CT Technology

Scanner Types

Dual Energy CT scanning can be realized in two very different ways, as the measured X-ray spectrum depends on the X-ray spectrum emitted by the X-ray source as well as the energy-dependent measurement response of the detector. Hence, energy separation can take place either at the side of the X-ray source or at the side of the detector. Under these two main categories exist several subcategories representing different technical implementations.

Because of the requirement for high scan speed, not all of the currently available Dual Energy CT scanners are suitable for cardiovascular imaging. This refers, for example, to the case of Dual Spiral (also called single-source helical) Dual Energy CT, where two independent spiral scans, each at a different X-ray tube voltage, are performed one after the other [17]. In this case, the time delay between measuring the same anatomic region with the two different spectra is in the order of several seconds, so that arterial phase iodine concentrations in the vessels change considerably. For non-contrast Dual Spiral scans, effects from patient motion can be reduced by appropriate motion correction algorithms. This is not possible, however, if CT numbers change due to changing concentrations of the iodinated contrast material. Under these conditions, an approach that scans a non-contrast phase and a contrast-enhanced phase, and subtracts the two resulting image sets, may be more promising for measuring or isolating iodine enhancement [18].

Lower sensitivity to patient motion or contrast agent dynamics is realized with slow kV-switching (also called single-source sequential) Dual Energy CT scanners [19] and split-filter (also called single-source twin beam) Dual Energy CT scanners [20]. For slow kV-switching, data are acquired during one gantry rotation using one tube voltage, and for the following gantry rotation, data are acquired at a different tube voltage. Since the minimum amount of projection data that are needed for image reconstruction of the scanned anatomy is less than one rotation (i.e., 180° + fan angle), these data can be acquired during a portion of the first gantry rotation, and the remaining time in the rotation can be used to switch the tube voltage and tube current before the next rotation. This can be done in a sequential or spiral acquisition mode; in both cases there is a delay of approximately one rotation between the projection data acquired with different spectra for the same anatomic region.

For split-filter scanners, two different filter materials separate the fan beam into two different spectra so that half of the detector (along the z-axis) is exposed to one spectrum and the other half to the other spectrum. This acquisition mode is only possible with spiral CT scanning, when the same anatomic region of the patient is translated through both beams. Data acquisition at both spectra is simultaneous, as well as continuous, so that motion artifacts can be suppressed by conventional motion correction algorithms [21]. However, there is less freedom in the choice of spectra, and the delay between the acquisition of data for the same anatomic region with the low and high beam spectra is about one rotation. Because of this one rotation delay, slow kV-switching scanners and split-filter scanners are in principle suitable for Dual Energy CTA of the head-neck area [22] or of the abdomen. Even pulmonary angiography has been shown to be feasible [23], but cardiac scanning is likely not feasible. Both methods appear to be most useful for cooperative patients and relatively static situations (body parts that do not move quickly or iodine concentrations that do not change quickly).

The lowest sensitivity to patient motion is obtained with Fast kV-switching (also called single-source rapid-switching) [24], Dual-Layer [25], and Dual-Source [26] Dual Energy CT technologies. With Fast kV-switching, the tube voltage is switched after each acquisition of an individual "frame" of the X-ray projection data. Switching speed is reported to be below one millisecond so that corresponding projection data frames obtained with the two spectra are well aligned. In addition, gantry rotation times of 0.28 s have been achieved. Possible disadvantages of the technology are a reduced frame rate (number of projections acquired per unit time) at each energy, finite switching time which reduces spectral separation, and limitations concerning the combination of this technique with fast and automatic tube current modulation.

Dual-Layer detectors have the advantage that no special technology is needed on the side of the X-ray tube. Conventional tube voltages such as 120 kV or 140 kV can be used, and the fairly wide spectrum is decomposed into two effective energy spectra by the detector. Technically this is achieved by using a detector consisting of two layers of scintillators. While low-energy photons are typically stopped in the top layer, high-energy photons are typically stopped in the bottom layer. Due to the statistical nature of photon absorption in the scintillator material, energy discrimination in such a setup is less than for other methods [27].

Dual-Source Dual Energy configurations have the advantage that no modification is needed for the X-ray tube or for the detector. In order to increase spectral separation, the available X-ray spectra are modified by applying additional filtration to the high kV spectra. Because the two tube/detector systems are separate, the tube potential and tube current settings, and also tube current modulation, are independent. While spectral quality and the potential for low radiation dose [28] are the strengths of this technique, fast and substantial motion can lead to false iodine enhancement at air/tissue boundaries because of lower temporal coherence (as will be discussed below).

All three of the discussed techniques are suitable for vascular imaging in all contrast phases and also pulmonary angiography. For cardiac imaging at higher heart rates, there are limitations with all three methods because of potentially rapid motion during data acquisition. As a conclusion, not all Dual Energy CT scanners can be used for vascular imaging, and even fewer can be used for cardiac imaging.

Special Requirements for Cardiovascular Imaging

For cardiovascular Dual Energy CT, strong iodine enhancement is required in the CT images so that vessel anatomy can be assessed. This means that the average photon energy of the applied X-ray spectra should be rather low, which is in conflict with the idea that a wide spectral separation is needed for best post-processing results. Typically, the noise-optimized weighted average of the low- and high-energy images has similar iodine enhancement as a conventional 120 kV image, but techniques like iterative reconstruction or nonlinear image filter algorithms can be used to further increase the iodine contrast-to-noise ratio.

In spite of good iodine contrast, there are other effects that can impede the spectral evaluation of small vessels. In order to demonstrate this, the cross-sectional view of a partly calcified vessel will be considered. Under ideal conditions it looks like as shown in Fig. 8.1a.

One important effect is spatial resolution of the images (Fig. 8.1b), which must be sufficient to see the vascular anatomy of interest [29]. Spatial resolution depends on the size of the detector pixels, the use of flying focal spot techniques [30], and the reconstruction kernel. A typical clinical case is the question of in-stent restenosis in coronary arteries, where the typical diameter of the vessel is less than 5 mm. In this situation, improved spatial resolution helps to reduce the size of blooming artifacts, which are caused by the high CT numbers of metal [31]. If spatial resolution is not sufficient to separate the plaque from the blooming, visualization of vessel anatomy cannot really be improved by using spectral information. Similar problems arise when plaque composition is assessed on contrast-enhanced images; for both spectra the neighboring dense iodine in the vessel may contaminate the measured attenuation values of the plaque due to its close proximity [32]. In general, a quantitative interpretation of CT numbers often requires structures that are considerably larger than the nominal spatial resolution of a CT scanner, which is usually assessed based on the visibility of high-contrast features. Moreover, depending on the technique, the Dual Energy or spectral scan mode may offer poorer spatial resolution than the corresponding single energy scan mode. In reality, one additional complication is that there is image noise in addition to finite spatial resolution. The effect of reduced resolution in combination with realistic noise is shown in Fig. 8.1c.

Good temporal resolution and coherence are essential for cardiac imaging and have already been mentioned in the context of different scanner technologies. Typically, temporal resolution is defined by the time interval that is needed in order to collect all projection data for the reconstruction of at least one image. On single-source systems and especially in cardiac mode, it is assumed to be gantry rotation time divided by two. If some structure moves faster than this, motion artifacts will be present in both projection data sets, so that vessel blurring or false stenosis may be seen on the resulting images. For cardiac scanning the three fastest Dual Energy methods have similar temporal resolution, with Dual-Source Dual Energy being the fastest with its 0.25 s gantry rotation time. The effect of low temporal resolution on spectral data is schematically shown in Fig. 8.1d.

Temporal coherence denotes the time over which motion leads to a displacement between object contours in the low- and high-energy projection data set. Here the Dual-Source Dual Energy scan mode has a temporal coherence that is about a factor of 2 better than its temporal resolution, while Fast kV-switching and Dual-Layer detectors have almost perfect temporal coherence. The occurrence of motion artifacts depends on both time components, temporal resolution and coherence. As a consequence, the visual appearance of motion artifacts may differ between the three CT scanner types, but all of them are sensitive to motion that occurs on a time scale of less than 150 ms. The combined effect of fast vessel motion and non-zero temporal coherence is schematically shown in Fig. 8.1e.

Another criterion to be considered is spectral resolution [33]: in order to separate, e.g., calcium from iodine with high spatial resolution, the original spatial resolution of the low- and high-energy images is not the only concern. For most body materials, low- and high-energy images only show small differences. For Dual Energy CT, these small differences have to be amplified, and this leads to an enormous increase in image noise if, e.g., iodine enhancement is to be selectively visualized. There are different strategies to reduce noise: radiation dose can be increased – which may not be appropriate for each patient – or spectral resolution can be increased. In both cases, dedicated denoising algorithms are also needed. However, for very small structures, the effectiveness of such algorithms may be limited. The effect of increased spectral resolution in the absence of motion is shown in Fig. 8.1f, which can be compared directly to Fig. 8.1c.

In addition to these properties of Dual Energy technologies, there are several effects in cardiac imaging that can decrease image quality, although they may be difficult to avoid [34]. The first limitation arises as a consequence of scattered radiation: all multi-slice CT scanners that are fast

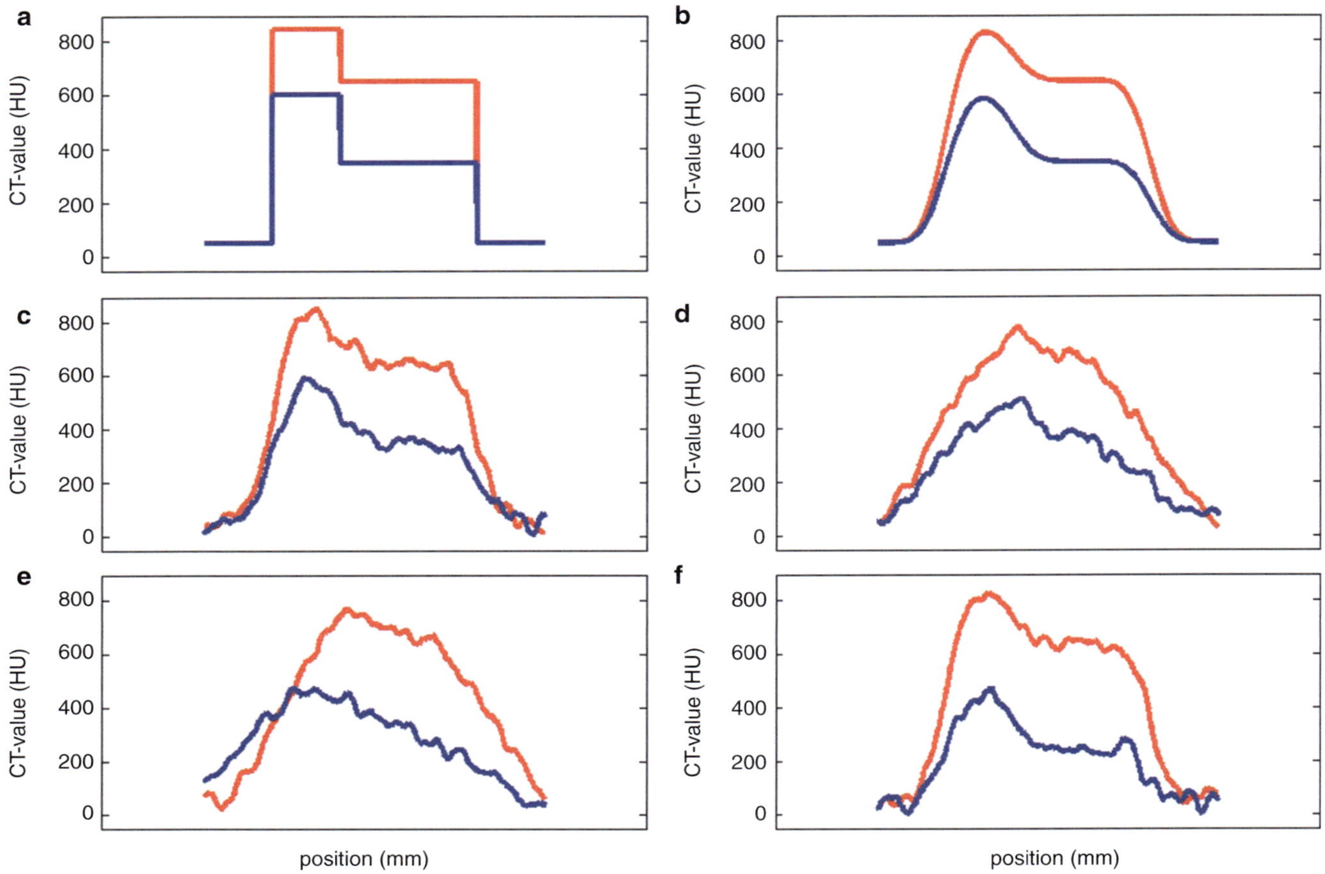

Fig. 8.1 Schematic cross-section of a cardiac vessel that contains a calcified plaque (high CT values on the left side) as well as highly concentrated iodine (plateau on the right side). The low-energy profile is shown in red; the high-energy profile is shown in blue. (**a**) Ultrahigh spatial resolution at infinite radiation dose; (**b**) effect of finite spatial resolution; (**c**) finite spatial resolution and image noise; (**d**) finite spatial resolution, image noise, and patient motion (high temporal coherence); (**e**) finite spatial resolution, image noise, and patient motion (lower temporal coherence); (**f**) finite spatial resolution, image noise, and improved spectral resolution

enough for cardiac imaging either use a wide collimation or a Dual-Source configuration. In both cases the amount of scattered radiation relative to transmitted radiation increases and can lead to a potential distortion of CT numbers in both spectral channels. This effect is more prominent if only half a rotation of raw data is collected instead of a full rotation, as is commonly done for cardiac CT [35]. Strategies against scattered radiation include improved anti-scatter grids as well as the subtraction of a simulated or measured scatter signal [36].

In addition, beam-hardening artifacts may originate from the large amount of dense contrast material inside the ventricles, which may exceed an enhancement-length product of 5000 HU-cm along certain directions. Apart from the enhancement-length product, the strength of the observed artifacts also depends on the tube voltage and prefiltration and thus on the scanner type. The generated artifacts can be especially problematic for the detection of iodine in the myocardium and the assessment of blood clots inside the ventricles. Beam-hardening artifacts may either be reduced by projection data Dual Energy processing [37] or by projection data-based iterative beam-hardening correction [38]. Strong iodine enhancement of ventricles and vessels may also cause cone-beam artifacts related to these structures.

Finally there may be step artifacts, if the detector is not wide enough to cover the heart in a single heartbeat. All effects together imply that high-quality quantitative CT imaging of the beating heart is a much more challenging task than Dual Energy imaging of the abdomen.

Data and Image Processing

Dual Energy CT data contain a wealth of additional information, and the analysis of this information can be performed in different ways. The traditional approach starts with a projection data-based base material decomposition that converts the measured X-ray attenuations at low and high energy into base material column densities from which material density images are reconstructed. Typical base materials for this approach are aluminum and Lucite or iodine and water. Because of the dominance of the photoelectric effect and the Compton effect, all naturally occurring body materials will receive meaningful equivalent water and iodine densities [7]. However, contrast agents with high effective atomic number – like gadolinium – will not be handled consistently in this approach. The generated base material images can be used to perform further material differentiation and quantification or to calculate beam-hardening free CT images (monoenergetic images). Alternatively, images can first be corrected for beam-hardening using an iterative projection data-based method and the following analysis performed in CT number space. In both cases, image-based analysis can be used once the beam-hardening effects are removed.

In image space, the concept of base material decomposition can be understood by considering a CT number diagram (Fig. 8.2) that plots the low-energy CT number against the high-energy CT number. Different body materials are located at different positions in this diagram. Most soft body tissues are located on one of two lines: the air-water line or the fat-soft tissue line. Adding iodine or calcium to soft body tissues simply shifts their CT values in a characteristic direction. If this direction is known, it is mathematically possible to reverse this shift by means of simple geometrical projection. In this way the CT numbers of the underlying body material can be obtained from the measured CT numbers. At the same time, the contrast material concentration in mg/ml or the iodine enhancement in HU can be calculated.

One feature of base material decomposition is that the user has to make assumptions about the chemical composition of the body materials that are present in the image. For example, a three-material decomposition into air, water, and iodine will show false-negative enhancement in body fat, while a three-material decomposition into fat, soft tissue, and iodine will be corrected in fat and liver tissue but not in the lungs. It is therefore important to choose the correct material decomposition or post-processing application for the clinical question that has to be answered. The image obtained after iodine subtraction is commonly known as "virtual non-contrast" image, since it shows similar CT numbers as a true non-contrast scan. The deviation between the two images depends on the calibration of the scanner and the post-processing software and can be in the order of ±10 Hounsfield units. This has to be compared with deviations between different scanners and scan modes in single energy mode, which may also be in the order of several HU [39].

Base material decomposition is also the first step for the calculation of monoenergetic or monochromatic images. These images show the same CT numbers as images that have been acquired with a real monochromatic X-ray source such as a synchrotron. After measuring the equivalent water and iodine concentrations with Dual Energy CT, the tabulated iodine attenuation for each X-ray energy can be used to derive the monoenergetic CT number at the selected energy.

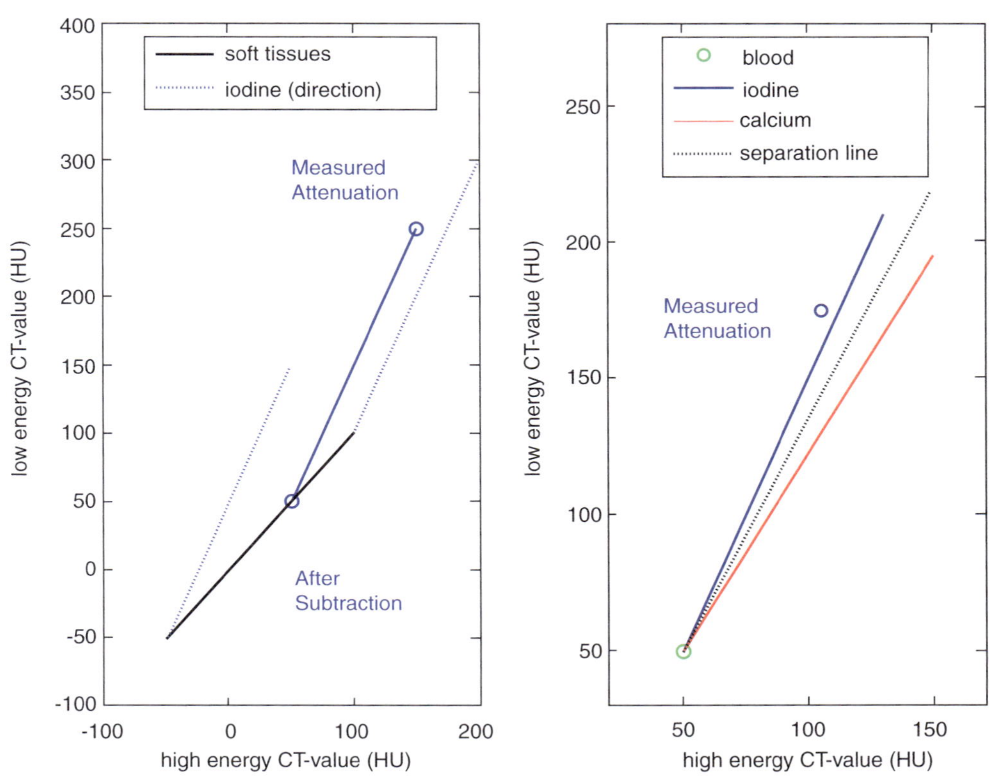

Fig. 8.2 Base material decomposition (left) and material classification or labeling (right). In case of base material decomposition, the measured attenuation is projected to the soft tissue line in order to obtain the virtual non-contrast image and the iodine concentration. In case of material classification, the measured CT value is above the separation line (blue dot) so that the voxel is classified as iodine

Due to the dominance of photoelectric effect and Compton effect, this works not only for mixtures of these base materials but also for all other body tissues.

An alternative method for the analysis of Dual Energy results is material classification or material labeling. In this case two or more body materials have to be distinguished, which are embedded in the same body tissue. The in vivo differentiation of various kidney stone types is a typical application of Dual Energy CT, but also the differentiation between calcified plaques and contrast agent belongs into this category. Separation between the various materials is typically achieved by using separation lines in the CT value diagram (Fig. 8.2). In the right side of Fig. 8.2, calcifications are located below the separation line, while iodine contrast material is located above the separation line. For low concentrations of iodine and calcium, it is not possible to distinguish the two materials because of the small distance between the two lines.

Denoising

Image noise is one of the known limitations of Dual Energy CT. Even for iodine, the difference between the low-energy and the high-energy image is typically much smaller than the iodine enhancement in the low kV image. So the spectral differences to be evaluated are relatively small, and image noise in virtual non-contrast images is strongly increased relative to the original images. This means that a straightforward base material decomposition is usually too noisy to be clinically useful. Different strategies have been developed to compensate for this effect. An example is shown in Fig. 8.3.

Some methods exploit the anticorrelation [40] of iodine and water images after base material decomposition to distinguish between image noise and image features. Other researchers have proposed to tailor iterative reconstruction techniques specifically for Dual Energy data [41] or to use spectral denoising [42]. Another noise reduction method uses frequency band decomposition to extract the high spatial frequencies from the low noise average of the original images [43]. For all techniques, it is important to note that nonlinear processing can modify image resolution, as well as noise texture, depending on the image content. On clinical products, denoising is usually applied as part of the base material decomposition, which may be accomplished in one step during image reconstruction or post-processing.

Radiation Dose

The question of radiation dose and radiation dose efficiency is important for all new techniques in medical imaging, including Dual Energy [44]. First it must be clarified whether, for the same applied dose, images that emulate conventional single energy CT images can be obtained with no loss in information from Dual Energy CT examinations. At least in the absence of major beam-hardening effects by bone or iodine, this is indeed the case. Virtual monoenergetic images that are generated without additional denoising algorithms have been shown to have the same CT number values as single energy CT images for naturally occurring body materials as long as the correct virtual monoenergetic energy level is selected [45]. The same image can also be generated by calculating the appropriately weighted average of the original low- and high-energy images.

Thus, two CT data sets, acquired with different spectra and reduced radiation dose levels relative to a standard clinic CT exam, can be combined into one conventional CT image that uses all of the applied dose, which is typically set at the level of a standard clinical exam. As noted as early as 1979 [46], it is in general not true that radiation dose must increase with the usage of Dual Energy techniques to obtain the same diagnostic value. It is true, however, that the average dose efficiency of the low- and the high-energy spectra can be worse than the dose efficiency of some optimum spectrum in the middle. Hence, the dose efficiency of a Dual Energy scan mode depends on the selected spectra but also on patient size, electronic noise of the detector, and specifications of the Dual Energy scan mode, such as a different gantry rotation time or a different exposure time per reading.

For example, low noise readout electronics [47] and additional filtration for the high-energy spectrum [48] can be combined, so that similar image noise and iodine contrast can be generated at the same radiation dose as with a conventional 120 kV spectrum [49]. A similar behavior can be expected from split-filter scanners [19] and scanners with energy-sensitive detectors that are operated at 120 kV [50]. For other techniques, differences in dose efficiency may also be small depending on protocol optimization and patient diameter. One major consideration is the extent to which the approach supports automatic tube current modulation and whether the minimum and maximum dose levels for a given patient and protocol can actually be achieved. Software modifications such as iterative reconstruction [51] may help to improve dose efficiency, although the change in diagnostic image quality is hard to assess in terms of simple metrics such as image noise or contrast-to-noise ratio [52].

A very different criterion to measure dose efficiency is the quality of the resultant Dual Energy images. For example, the best dose efficiency of weighted average images may be obtained with one scan mode, but the best quality of virtual non-contrast (VNC) images may be obtained with another scan mode [33]. In general, the use of extra radiation for a Dual Energy CT scan (relative to a single energy technique) is only justified if the additional information cannot otherwise be obtained or if competing methods have similar risks and benefits.

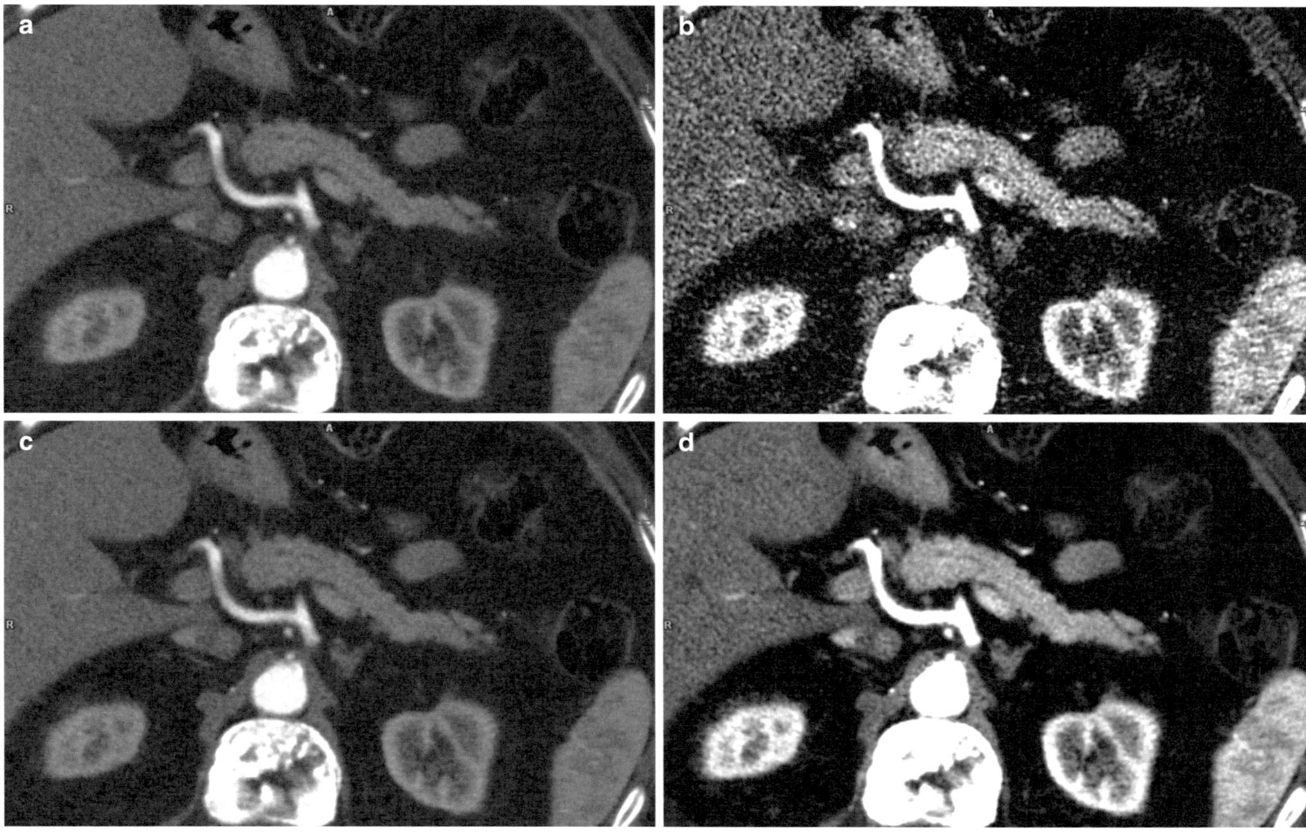

Fig. 8.3 Image-based processing was used to generate virtual monoenergetic images (**a** and **b**). These are in comparison to virtual monoenergetic images with an applied denoising algorithm (bottom row). Although there is negligible difference between the 70 keV images (**c**), noise is substantially reduced by the denoising algorithm for the 40 keV images (**d**). This makes, for example, structures in the contrast-enhanced pancreas clearer

In summary, the dose efficiency of Dual Energy CT depends on the comparison that is made: typical approaches include the comparison of single energy and Dual Energy reference protocols on the same scanner, the comparison of protocols on different scanners that are designed to accomplish the same diagnostic task, or the comparison between Dual Energy and highly optimized single energy protocols. Because results differ depending on the approach, published studies have shown mixed results [53–56]. The observed differences between Dual Energy and single energy dose results also have to be compared with the significant dose variations that have been observed between different single energy scanners for the same diagnostic task [57].

Clinical Applications for Cardiovascular Imaging

Vascular Imaging

Dual Energy CT has numerous applications in the field of vascular imaging [58]. Probably the most obvious application is the automatic removal of the bone from CTA images. The iodine and bone can have similar high CT number values, but because they are chemically different, they can be distinguished using Dual Energy CT and a material classification approach. This method can be compared with single energy techniques, which try to differentiate between the bone and iodine based on anatomical and morphological criteria. Both approaches can achieve high-quality results, but especially on scanners with good spectral separation, the Dual Energy method provides superior results for unusual vessel anatomy or aneurysms close to the bone [59]. One feature of Dual Energy bone removal is that hard plaques and bones are both removed, since both contain large amounts of calcium. In order to display the calcified plaques without displaying the bone, morphological algorithms are used to identify plaques. An example for this is shown in Fig. 8.4. Also, trabecular bone containing yellow bone marrow requires special processing, as its Dual Energy behavior is similar to iodinated contrast media in the blood and Dual Energy techniques alone therefore cannot remove all of the bone.

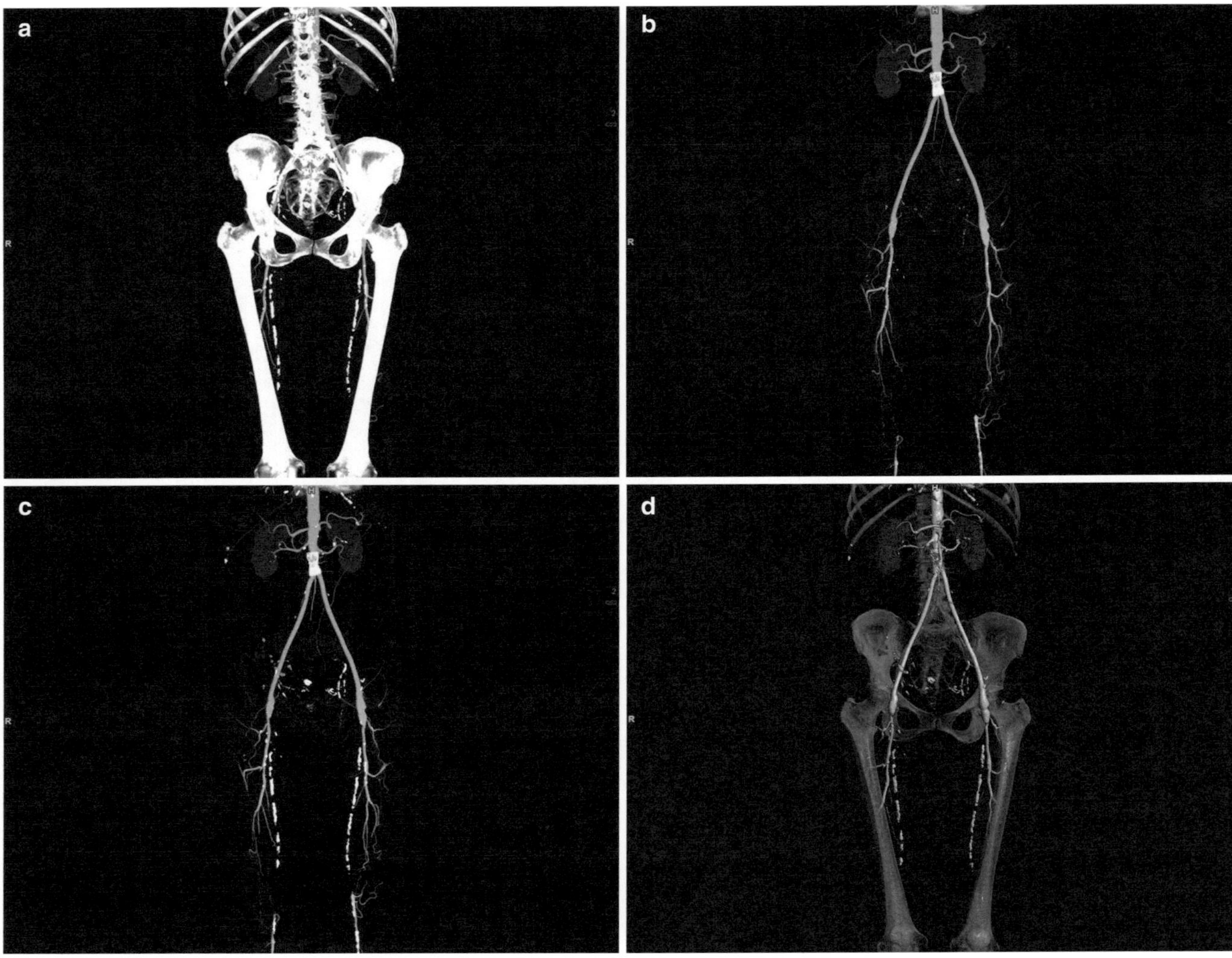

Fig. 8.4 Four views of the same patient: original CTA image (maximum intensity projection (MIP), **a**); after Dual Energy-based calcium subtraction (MIP, **b**); after adding plaques and other calcifications based on morphological criteria (MIP, **c**); combined visualization with different coloring of bone and vessels (bottom right, **d**). No manual editing was applied

However, material classification may not be the best approach to remove calcified plaques in small vessels. Due to the finite spatial resolution of CT images, there is a transition range (one or more voxels) between the plaque and the vessel lumen (e.g., see Fig. 8.1). Segmentation algorithms that try to preserve the vessel lumen will typically differentiate between plaque and lumen at the middle of this transition region, but this may leave a bright rim surrounding the lumen. At the expense of increased image noise, this can be avoided by explicitly performing a base material decomposition [60]. That is, by decomposing the imaging into the blood, calcium hydroxyapatite, and iodine, the calcium hydroxyapatite signal can be subtracted from the image, which also subtracts all blooming effects. However, since this approach does not simultaneously increase image resolution, quantification of the remaining lumen may still be a challenge.

Virtual monoenergetic imaging can be helpful for assessing the vessel lumen; the CT number values of iodinated contrast media change more quickly with energy than do the CT number values of calcium. In this way, the relative contrast between the lumen and plaques can be optimized [61]. Monoenergetic images can also be used to reduce metal artifacts and blooming from stents [62], so that an optimum balance can be found between artifact strength, which decreases with energy, and iodine contrast-to-noise ratio, which also decreases with energy, but not necessarily at the same rate. At the lower photon energies, virtual monoenergetic imaging can also be used to enhance the contrast-to-noise ratio of iodinated vessels. This may be especially helpful for the visualization of small vessels on maximum intensity projection (MIP) images. Energy levels of 40–55 keV are usually recommended for this purpose, provided that state-of-the-art denoising methods are implemented in the software [63].

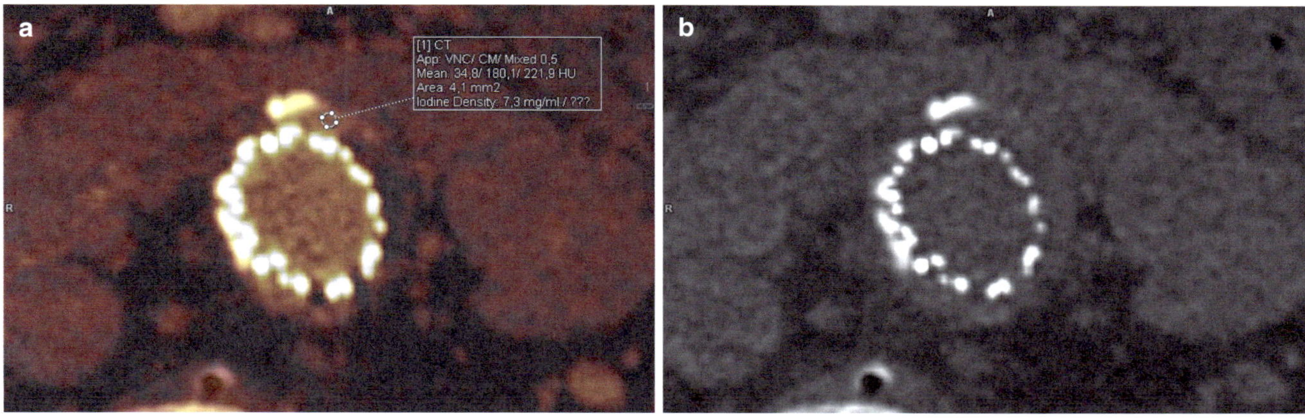

Fig. 8.5 Endoleak detection with Dual-Source Dual Energy. (**a**) The leakage of contrast agent is seen as an orange area outside the stent (circled region of interest). In this fused image, the virtual non-contrast (VNC) image is displayed in gray, and the iodine base material image is shown in red and orange colors; the measured iodine density is 7.3 mg/ml. (**b**) At the same position, the VNC image alone does not show increased CT number values; hence, calcium and hemorrhage can be excluded

On scanners with wide spectral separation, similar effects can also be obtained from nonlinear image blending of the low- and high-energy images, where the low-energy image receives a higher weight in vessels, such that the iodine contrast is increased [64–66]. Also, the optimization of linear blending can lead to improved contrast-to-noise ratio of iodinated vessels and differentiation of plaque from the lumen [67].

Analysis of the vessel wall [68] and plaques attached to it is a challenging task. Diagnostic tasks such as the detection of intramural hemorrhage [69] are very sensitive to the use of different noise reduction algorithms and may also be difficult to answer if the dense contrast agent in the vessel lumen is not fully subtracted. In this context, it is important to note that the subtraction of iodine enhancement is usually easier at low concentrations than at high concentrations, so that VNC images tend to be less reliable in the vessels during arterial phase than during portal venous phase [70]. Attempts have been made to look for chemical anomalies, such as the presence of iron in soft plaques [71] or iodine uptake in soft plaques [72]. The results of these studies suggest a possible clinical value, but more research is necessary before such methods can be used for routine imaging of human patients under realistic conditions.

It has been convincingly demonstrated that patients who have undergone endovascular repair may benefit from the application of Dual Energy CT techniques. Acute leakage of contrast agent after such a procedure (referred to as an endoleak) is not always easily distinguishable from previous bleedings or calcifications in the same area. With single energy CT, multiphase examinations are usually performed including a non-contrast phase, so that false-positive findings can be avoided. Alternatively, it has been shown that a single-phase Dual Energy CT scan achieves very high sensitivity and specificity for this diagnostic task [73, 74]. An example for this application is shown in Fig. 8.5. In addition, endoleaks may be more conspicuous on low-energy virtual monoenergetic images [75].

The lungs are especially interesting for Dual Energy techniques, since they represent a highly movable and compressible organ with a strong air/soft tissue contrast and delicate structures. One limitation of single energy CT is the difficulty to assess the iodine content of lung vessels below 1–2 mm in diameter because of partial volume effects with the neighboring low-density lung tissue. Dual Energy CT can be used to visualize the iodine content in such small vessels, as it is possible to calculate a ratio which is almost independent of the partial volume effects. This technique has been used for the detection of peripheral emboli [76].

Another popular method for the visualization of pulmonary embolism with Dual Energy CT is the measurement of the iodine uptake in the lung parenchyma [77, 78]. After a good arterial injection, iodine enhancement in the lung parenchyma can reach values of more than 30 HU. But with single energy CT, a reduction of iodine uptake is not easily distinguished from variation in parenchymal density, which can produce effects on a similar scale. With Dual Energy CT, the iodine uptake can be selectively visualized so that perfusion defects can be readily recognized. Depending on the analysis software, iodine enhancement in the lungs may be displayed in the parenchyma only or together with the enhancement of the vessels. Results can be compared with other methods to quantify lung perfusion such as scintigraphy, SPECT [79], and MR [80]. Because of the different contrast agent kinetics, scintigraphy and Dual Energy CT may not agree in all cases.

Cardiac Applications

Dual Energy CT techniques can also be applied to the moving heart [81], provided that the scanner is fast enough. Similarly to other vessels in the human body, virtual monoenergetic imaging can be used for the coronary arteries to either optimize iodine contrast-to-noise ratio [82] or to reduce calcium blooming and metal artifacts [83–85]. Vessel segments that are subject to very rapid motion may have to be excluded from the evaluation in the same way as for single energy CT. There are also sources of metal artifacts, which are only found for cardiac CT scans, such as valve implants, pacemakers, and sternal wires. Especially for the less massive metal objects such as clips and sternal wires, Dual Energy-based metal artifact reduction has been reported to be helpful [86].

Other artifact patterns, however, are not completely reduced. For example, projection- as well as image-based Dual Energy CT approaches show limited improvement for artifacts associated with dense contrast media in the superior vena cava [87]. These artifacts are related to a combination of effects, including motion, beam-hardening, and scattered radiation. By removing only the beam-hardening component, the artifact pattern may not improve substantially.

Beam-hardening artifacts are more prominent in other situations. In coronary CTA, beam-hardening is often seen along the axis of the left ventricle, the aorta, and the spine as a dark shadow in the soft tissue between these areas. The dark shadow may also extend beyond the tip of the ventricle into the myocardium. Such a feature can cause difficulties in the assessment of myocardial enhancement; Dual Energy CT [88] as well as single energy iterative methods [38] can be used to improve image quality. Beam-hardening correction also appears to be relevant when measuring the attenuation properties of ventricular thrombi.

Dual Energy CT can be used to extract first-pass enhancement of the myocardium [89], as shown in Fig. 8.6. Compared to other imaging techniques, this method has been demonstrated to achieve high sensitivity and specificity for the detection of relevant reduction of myocardial perfusion. In order to stabilize the measured CT number values, full rotation reconstructions, instead of half rotation reconstructions, tend to be more suitable for this application.

Dual Energy CT has also been used in stress testing, where patients receive adenosine before the coronary CTA exam [90]. One side effect of this approach is that – after the application of adenosine – the heart rate can increase; consequently it may not be possible to reconstruct motion-free images. Motion will have a bigger effect on the iodine-only images than on the low- or high-energy images or weighted CT images. Thus, a failure of the iodine/tissue decomposition process does not automatically imply a waste of radiation dose.

Due to the absence of dense contrast media in the ventricle, image quality appears to be better later after the injection of iodinated contrast media. In particular, late enhancement scans have been proposed, which can highlight contrast media in an infarcted area several minutes after application of the contrast agent. Promising results have been obtained for chronic myocardial infarction [91].

VNC imaging has also been studied to determine whether VNC images can be used for calcium scoring. This approach has been confirmed by several studies [92, 93] and may be close to clinical routine.

The analysis of soft cardiac plaque composition is a challenging task. Currently, single energy CT has limitations concerning quantitative assessment and correlation with clinical symptoms [94], and it is not clear if Dual Energy can add any additional relevant information [95]. At very high spatial resolution, Dual Energy could potentially be useful to detect diffuse calcium accumulation or iodine uptake inside

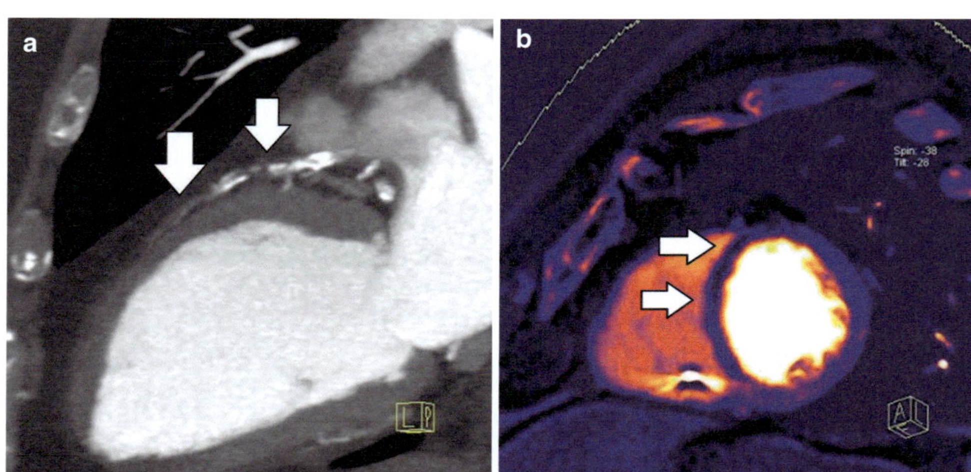

Fig. 8.6 Dual Energy CT for the detection of reduced myocardial perfusion. Occluded left anterior descending coronary artery (**a**) and resulting perfusion defect in the anterior wall and septum in a patient with acute myocardial infarction (**b**). The reduced iodine uptake (dark area) is visualized by using three-material decomposition (Courtesy of R. Bauer, University Hospital Frankfurt, Frankfurt, Germany)

the plaque [96]. Neither technique has yet been verified in vivo with existing clinical CT scanners.

Finally, the use of Dual Energy CT has been suggested in order to detect chemical anomalies in soft tissues. For example, Dual Energy CT can be used for the detection of iron in the myocardium [97]. It may also reveal iodine deposition from amiodarone in the liver [98]. Both indications require non-contrast Dual Energy CT scans.

Future Directions: Multi-energy CT

For true spectral CT imaging, referred to as multi-energy CT, more than two X-ray spectra have to be measured simultaneously [99]. This is feasible with energy-sensitive detectors, where the individual energy of each X-ray photon can be measured. In this way, X-ray spectroscopy becomes possible, which is potentially useful to separate K-edge contrast agents, such as gadolinium or gold, from iodine and body tissues.

Technically, multi-energy CT is realized by using a high atomic number semiconductor like CdTe or CdZnTe, which can stop X-ray photons within a short range due to a strong photoelectric effect. A rather large voltage is applied to the semiconductor so that the generated charges drift toward the top and bottom electrodes. In this way, a voltage pulse is created at the input of the readout electronics, and its height correlates with the energy of the original photon. Technically, large photon fluence rates of the order of 10^9 photons/mm^2/second have to be accurately measured, which has been one of the biggest obstacles in developing such CT scanners. For this reason, it is not possible to measure and store the energy of each photon. Instead, a number of counters are implemented in the readout electronics so that each counter counts the number of photons above a preset energy threshold. X-ray attenuation is measured as a fractional reduction of the photon fluence rate for each energy threshold.

So far, there is no commercially available clinical scanner of this type. However, prototype installations have been reported in literature [100, 101], and these have shown promising results for phantoms, animals, and a limited number of patients. The advantage of such photon-counting detectors is that very good spectral resolution can be combined with perfect temporal coherence, which has advantages for vascular as well as cardiac imaging.

The analysis of multi-energy data with more than two spectral channels is much more involved [27]. If K-edge contrast agents such as gadolinium or gold are to be used, a corresponding multi-material decomposition is needed to measure the concentrations of these contrast agents in addition to the CT number values of body tissues or iodine. The efficient calibration of a projection-based multi-material decomposition is not a trivial task. Additionally, noise propagation and systematic uncertainties have to be carefully evaluated and addressed.

Conclusions

More and more clinical CT scanners have Dual Energy CT capabilities, and routine usage of this technique, as well as the number of scientific publications on this topic, is increasing rapidly. At the moment, several technical approaches are commercially available that have different strengths and weaknesses. Also, post-processing features differ considerably between different software products. However, the need for a certain degree of standardization has already been recognized by the community [2].

For cardiovascular imaging, the main focus of Dual Energy CT is on the visualization and quantification of iodinated contrast media in vessels. Virtual monoenergetic images allow for an interactive optimization of iodine contrast relative to soft tissue, calcium, or stent material. Virtual monoenergetic CT number values are independent of the patient or the prefiltration of the used scanner; they are in this way more objective and reproducible. Additional diagnostic information is available through the calculation of iodine maps for the heart and lungs. While some of the discussed applications are at the very early stage of feasibility studies, others, such as bone removal, virtual monoenergetic imaging, or the visualization of iodine uptake in the lung parenchyma, are already now widely used.

There are also other opportunities for the future. As automatic segmentation algorithms will have access to chemical information as well as X-ray attenuation information, increased automation based on Dual Energy data may be possible. In addition, further technological improvements such as better temporal resolution can be expected on the scanner side, so that new clinical applications may become feasible.

References

1. McCollough CH, Leng S, Yu L, Fletcher JG. Dual- and multi-energy CT: principles, technical approaches, and clinical applications. Radiology. 2015;276(3):637–53.
2. Siegel MJ, Kaza RK, Bolus DN, Boll DT, Rofsky NM, De Cecco CN, Foley WD, Morgan DE, Schoepf UJ, Sahani DV, Shuman WP, Vrtiska TJ, Yeh BM, Berland LL. White paper of the society of computed body tomography and magnetic resonance on dual-energy CT, part 1: technology and terminology. J Comput Assist Tomogr. 2016;40(6):841–5.
3. Johnson TR. Dual-energy CT: general principles. AJR Am J Roentgenol. 2012;199(5 Suppl):S3–8.
4. De Cecco CN, Darnell A, Rengo M, Muscogiuri G, Bellini D, Ayuso C, Laghi A. Dual-energy CT: oncologic applications. AJR Am J Roentgenol. 2012;199(5Suppl):S98–S105.
5. Koonce JD, Vliegenthart R, Schoepf UJ, Schmidt B, Wahlquist AE, Nietert PJ, Bastarrika G, Flohr TG, Meinel FG. Accuracy of dual-energy computed tomography for the measurement of iodine concentration using cardiac CT protocols: validation in a phantom model. Eur Radiol. 2014;24(2):512–8.
6. Caruso D, De Cecco CN, Schoepf UJ, Schaefer AR, Leland PW, Johnson D, Laghi A, Hardie AD. Can dual-energy computed

tomography improve visualization of hypoenhancing liver lesions in portal venous phase? Assessment of advanced image-based virtual monoenergetic images. Clin Imaging. 2016;41:118–24.
7. Alvarez RE, Macovski A. Energy-selective reconstructions in X-ray computerized tomography. Phys Med Biol. 1976;21(5):733–44.
8. Hünemohr N, Krauss B, Tremmel C, Ackermann B, Jäkel O, Greilich S. Experimental verification of ion stopping power prediction from dual energy CT data in tissue surrogates. Phys Med Biol. 2014;59(1):83–96.
9. Goodsitt MM, Christodoulou EG, Larson SC. Accuracies of the synthesized monochromatic CT numbers and effective atomic numbers obtained with a rapid kVp switching dual energy CT scanner. Med Phys. 2011;38(4):2222–32.
10. Kalender WA, Klotz E, Suess C. Vertebral bone mineral analysis: an integrated approach with CT. Radiology. 1987;164(2):419–23.
11. Flohr TG, McCollough CH, Bruder H, Petersilka M, Gruber K, Süss C, Grasruck M, Stierstorfer K, Krauss B, Raupach R, Primak AN, Küttner A, Achenbach S, Becker C, Kopp A, Ohnesorge BM. First performance evaluation of a dual-source CT (DSCT) system. Eur Radiol. 2006;16(2):256–68.
12. Stolzmann P, Kozomara M, Chuck N, Müntener M, Leschka S, Scheffel H, Alkadhi H. In vivo identification of uric acid stones with dual-energy CT: diagnostic performance evaluation in patients. Abdom Imaging. 2010;35(5):629–35.
13. Choi HK, Burns LC, Shojania K, Koenig N, Reid G, Abufayyah M, Law G, Kydd AS, Ouellette H, Nicolaou S. Dual energy CT in gout: a prospective validation study. Ann Rheum Dis. 2012;71(9):1466–71.
14. Hoffman EA, Lynch DA, Barr RG, van Beek EJ, Parraga G. IWPFI investigators. Pulmonary CT and MRI phenotypes that help explain chronic pulmonary obstruction disease pathophysiology and outcomes. J Magn Reson Imaging. 2016;43(3):544–57.
15. Kerl JM, Bauer RW, Renker M, Weber E, Weisser P, Korkusuz H, Schell B, Larson MC, Kromen W, Jacobi V, Vogl TJ. Triphasic contrast injection improves evaluation of dual energy lung perfusion in pulmonary CT angiography. Eur J Radiol. 2011;80(3):e483–7.
16. Leng S, Shiung M, Ai S, Qu M, Vrtiska TJ, Grant KL, Krauss B, Schmidt B, Lieske JC, McCollough CH. Feasibility of discriminating uric acid from non-uric acid renal stones using consecutive spatially registered low- and high-energy scans obtained on a conventional CT scanner. AJR Am J Roentgenol. 2015;204(1):92–7.
17. Tomandl BF, Hammen T, Klotz E, Ditt H, Stemper B, Lell M. Bone-subtraction CT angiography for the evaluation of intracranial aneurysms. AJNR Am J Neuroradiol. 2006;27(1):55–9.
18. Diekhoff T, Ziegeler K, Feist E, Kiefer T, Mews J, Hamm B, Hermann KG. First experience with single-source dual-energy computed tomography in six patients with acute arthralgia: a feasibility experiment using joint aspiration as a reference. Skelet Radiol. 2015;44(11):1573–7.
19. Euler A, Parakh A, Falkowski AL, Manneck S, Dashti D, Krauss B, Szucs-Farkas Z, Schindera ST. Initial results of a single-source dual-energy computed tomography technique using a split-filter: assessment of image quality, radiation dose, and accuracy of dual-energy applications in an in vitro and in vivo study. Investig Radiol. 2016;51(8):491–8.
20. Sotiras A, Davatzikos C, Paragios N. Deformable medical image registration: a survey. IEEE Trans Med Imaging. 2013;32(7):1153–90.
21. Kaemmerer N, Brand M, Hammon M, May M, Wuest W, Krauss B, Uder M, Lell MM. Dual-energy computed tomography angiography of the head and neck with single-source computed tomography: a new technical (split filter) approach for bone removal. Investig Radiol. 2016;51(10):618–23.
22. Cai XR, Feng YZ, Qiu L, Xian ZH, Yang WC, Mo XK, Wang XB. Iodine distribution map in dual-energy computed tomography pulmonary artery imaging with rapid kVp switching for the diagnostic analysis and quantitative evaluation of acute pulmonary embolism. Acad Radiol. 2015;22(6):743–51.
23. Zhang D, Li X, Liu B. Objective characterization of GE discovery CT750 HD scanner: gemstone spectral imaging mode. Med Phys. 2011;38(3):1178–88.
24. Hidas G, Eliahou R, Duvdevani M, Coulon P, Lemaitre L, Gofrit ON, Pode D, Sosna J. Determination of renal stone composition with dual-energy CT: in vivo analysis and comparison with x-ray diffraction. Radiology. 2010;257(2):394–401.
25. Johnson TR, Krauss B, Sedlmair M, Grasruck M, Bruder H, Morhard D, Fink C, Weckbach S, Lenhard M, Schmidt B, Flohr T, Reiser MF, Becker CR. Material differentiation by dual energy CT: initial experience. Eur Radiol. 2007;17(6):1510–7.
26. Faby S, Kuchenbecker S, Sawall S, Simons D, Schlemmer HP, Lell M, Kachelrieß M. Performance of today's dual energy CT and future multi energy CT in virtual non-contrast imaging and in iodine quantification: a simulation study. Med Phys. 2015;42(7):4349–66.
27. Siegel MJ, Curtis WA, Ramirez-Giraldo JC. Effects of dual-energy technique on radiation exposure and image quality in pediatric body CT. AJR Am J Roentgenol. 2016;4:1–10. [Epub ahead of print].
28. Ulrich A, Burg MC, Raupach R, Bunck A, Schuelke C, Maintz D, Heindel W, Seifarth H. Coronary stent imaging with dual-source CT: assessment of lumen visibility using different convolution kernels and postprocessing filters. Acta Radiol. 2015;56(1):42–50.
29. Flohr TG, Stierstorfer K, Ulzheimer S, Bruder H, Primak AN, McCollough CH. Image reconstruction and image quality evaluation for a 64-slice CT scanner with z-flying focal spot. Med Phys. 2005;32(8):2536–47.
30. Gassenmaier T, Petri N, Allmendinger T, Flohr T, Weng AM, Kunz AS, Petritsch B, Voelker W, Bley TA. In vitro comparison of second- and third-generation dual-source CT for coronary stent visualization at different tube potentials. Acad Radiol. 2016;23(8):961–8.
31. Horiguchi J, Fujioka C, Kiguchi M, Shen Y, Althoff CE, Yamamoto H, Ito K. Soft and intermediate plaques in coronary arteries: how accurately can we measure CT attenuation using 64-MDCT? AJR Am J Roentgenol. 2007;189(4):981–8.
32. Krauss B, Grant KL, Schmidt BT, Flohr TG. The importance of spectral separation: an assessment of dual-energy spectral separation for quantitative ability and dose efficiency. Investig Radiol. 2015;50(2):114–8.
33. Kalisz K, Buethe J, Saboo SS, Abbara S, Halliburton S, Rajiah P. Artifacts at cardiac CT: physics and solutions. Radiographics. 2016;36(7):2064–83.
34. Stenner P, Schmidt B, Bruder H, Allmendinger T, Haberland U, Flohr T, Kachelriess M. Partial scan artifact reduction (PSAR) for the assessment of cardiac perfusion in dynamic phase-correlated CT. Med Phys. 2009;36(12):5683–94.
35. Ohnesorge B, Flohr T, Klingenbeck-Regn K. Efficient object scatter correction algorithm for third and fourth generation CT scanners. Eur Radiol. 1999;9(3):563–9.
36. Carrascosa PM, Cury RC, Deviggiano A, Capunay C, Campisi R, López de Munain M, Vallejos J, Tajer C, Rodriguez-Granillo GA. Comparison of myocardial perfusion evaluation with single versus dual-energy CT and effect of beam-hardening artifacts. Acad Radiol. 2015;22(5):591–9.
37. Bucher AM, Wichmann JL, Schoepf UJ, Wolla CD, Canstein C, McQuiston AD, Krazinski AW, De Cecco CN, Meinel FG, Vogl TJ, Geyer LL. Quantitative evaluation of beam-hardening artefact correction in dual-energy CT myocardial perfusion imaging. Eur Radiol. 2016;26(9):3215–22.
38. Birnbaum BA, Hindman N, Lee J, Babb JS. Multi-detector row CT attenuation measurements: assessment of intra- and

interscanner variability with an anthropomorphic body CT phantom. Radiology. 2007;242(1):109–19.
39. Kalender WA, Klotz E, Kostaridou L. An algorithm for noise suppression in dual energy CT material density images. IEEE Trans Med Imaging. 1988;7(3):218–24.
40. Dong X, Niu T, Zhu L. Combined iterative reconstruction and image-domain decomposition for dual energy CT using total-variation regularization. Med Phys. 2014;41(5):051909.
41. Leng S, Yu L, Fletcher JG, McCollough CH. Maximizing iodine contrast-to-noise ratios in abdominal CT imaging through use of energy domain noise reduction and virtual monoenergetic dual-energy CT. Radiology. 2015;276(2):562–70.
42. Grant KL, Flohr TG, Krauss B, Sedlmair M, Thomas C, Schmidt B. Assessment of an advanced image-based technique to calculate virtual monoenergetic computed tomographic images from a dual-energy examination to improve contrast-to-noise ratio in examinations using iodinated contrast media. Investig Radiol. 2014;49(9):586–92.
43. Foley WD, Shuman WP, Siegel MJ, Sahani DV, Boll DT, Bolus DN, De Cecco CN, Kaza RK, Morgan DE, Schoepf UJ, Vrtiska TJ, Yeh BM, Berland LL. White paper of the society of computed body tomography and magnetic resonance on dual-energy CT, part 2: radiation dose and iodine sensitivity. J Comput Assist Tomogr. 2016;40(6):846–50.
44. Yu L, Leng S, McCollough CH. Dual-energy CT-based monochromatic imaging. AJR Am J Roentgenol. 2012;199(5 Suppl):S9–S15.
45. Alvarez R, Seppi E. A comparison of noise and dose in conventional and energy selective computed tomography. IEEE Trans Nucl Sci. 1979;NS-26:2853–6.
46. Christe A, Heverhagen J, Ozdoba C, Weisstanner C, Ulzheimer S, Ebner L. CT dose and image quality in the last three scanner generations. World J Radiol. 2013;5(11):421–9.
47. Primak AN, Giraldo JC, Eusemann CD, Schmidt B, Kantor B, Fletcher JG, McCollough CH. Dual-source dual-energy CT with additional tin filtration: dose and image quality evaluation in phantoms and in vivo. AJR Am J Roentgenol. 2010;195(5):1164–74.
48. Uhrig M, Simons D, Kachelrieß M, Pisana F, Kuchenbecker S, Schlemmer HP. Advanced abdominal imaging with dual energy CT is feasible without increasing radiation dose. Cancer Imaging. 2016;16(1):15.
49. Gutjahr R, Halaweish AF, Yu Z, Leng S, Yu L, Li Z, Jorgensen SM, Ritman EL, Kappler S, McCollough CH. Human imaging with photon counting-based computed tomography at clinical dose levels: contrast-to-noise ratio and cadaver studies. Investig Radiol. 2016;51(7):421–9.
50. Ohana M, Labani A, Jeung MY, El Ghannudi S, Gaertner S, Roy C. Iterative reconstruction in single source dual-energy CT pulmonary angiography: is it sufficient to achieve a radiation dose as low as state-of-the-art single-energy CTPA? Eur J Radiol. 2015;84(11):2314–20.
51. Kofler JM, Yu L, Leng S, Zhang Y, Li Z, Carter RE, McCollough CH. Assessment of low-contrast resolution for the American College of Radiology Computed Tomographic Accreditation Program: what is the impact of iterative reconstruction? J Comput Assist Tomogr. 2015;39(4):619–23.
52. Schick D, Pratap J. Radiation dose efficiency of dual-energy CT benchmarked against single-source, kilovoltage-optimized scans. Br J Radiol. 2016;89(1058):20150486.
53. Purysko AS, Primak AN, Baker ME, Obuchowski NA, Remer EM, John B, Herts BR. Comparison of radiation dose and image quality from single-energy and dual-energy CT examinations in the same patients screened for hepatocellular carcinoma. Clin Radiol. 2014;69(12):e538–44.
54. Dubourg B, Caudron J, Lestrat JP, Bubenheim M, Lefebvre V, Godin M, Tron C, Eltchaninoff H, Bauer F, Dacher JN. Single-source dual-energy CT angiography with reduced iodine load in patients referred for aortoiliofemoral evaluation before transcatheter aortic valve implantation: impact on image quality and radiation dose. Eur Radiol. 2014;24(11):2659–68.
55. Takrouri HS, Alnassar MM, Amirabadi A, Babyn PS, Moineddin R, Padfield NL, BenDavid G, Doria AS. Metal artifact reduction: added value of rapid-kilovoltage-switching dual-energy CT in relation to single-energy CT in a piglet animal model. AJR Am J Roentgenol. 2015;205(3):W352–9.
56. Cody DD, Kim HJ, Cagnon CH, Larke FJ, McNitt-Gray MM, Kruger RL, Flynn MJ, Seibert JA, Judy PF, Wu X. Normalized CT dose index of the CT scanners used in the National Lung Screening Trial. AJR Am J Roentgenol. 2010;194(6):1539–46.
57. Machida H, Tanaka I, Fukui R, Shen Y, Ishikawa T, Tate E, Ueno E. Dual-energy spectral CT: various clinical vascular applications. Radiographics. 2016;36(4):1215–32.
58. Watanabe Y, Uotani K, Nakazawa T, Higashi M, Yamada N, Hori Y, Kanzaki S, Fukuda T, Itoh T, Naito H. Dual-energy direct bone removal CT angiography for evaluation of intracranial aneurysm or stenosis: comparison with conventional digital subtraction angiography. Eur Radiol. 2009;19(4):1019–24.
59. Andreini D, Pontone G, Mushtaq S, Bertella E, Conte E, Segurini C, Giovannardi M, Baggiano A, Annoni A, Formenti A, Petullà M, Beltrama V, Volpato V, Bartorelli AL, Trabattoni D, Fiorentini C, Pepi M. Diagnostic accuracy of rapid kilovolt peak-switching dual-energy CT coronary angiography in patients with a high calcium score. JACC Cardiovasc Imaging. 2015;8(6):746–8.
60. Mannelli L, MacDonald L, Mancini M, Ferguson M, Shuman WP, Ragucci M, Monti S, Xu D, Yuan C, Mitsumori LM. Dual energy computed tomography quantification of carotid plaques calcification: comparison between monochromatic and polychromatic energies with pathology correlation. Eur Radiol. 2015;25(5):1238–46.
61. Mangold S, De Cecco CN, Schoepf UJ, Yamada RT, Varga-Szemes A, Stubenrauch AC, Caruso D, Fuller SR, Vogl TJ, Nikolaou K, Todoran TM, Wichmann JL. A noise-optimized virtual monochromatic reconstruction algorithm improves stent visualization and diagnostic accuracy for detection of in-stent restenosis in lower extremity run-off CT angiography. Eur Radiol. 2016;26(12):4380–9.
62. Beeres M, Trommer J, Frellesen C, Nour-Eldin NE, Scholtz JE, Herrmann E, Vogl TJ, Wichmann JL. Evaluation of different keV-settings in dual-energy CT angiography of the aorta using advanced image-based virtual monoenergetic imaging. Int J Cardiovasc Imaging. 2016;32(1):137–44.
63. Apel A, Fletcher JG, Fidler JL, Hough DM, Yu L, Guimaraes LS, Bellemann ME, McCollough CH, Holmes DR 3rd, Eusemann CD. Pilot multi-reader study demonstrating potential for dose reduction in dual energy hepatic CT using non-linear blending of mixed kV image datasets. Eur Radiol. 2011;21(3):644–52.
64. Li S, Wang C, Jiang X, Xu G. Effects of dual-energy CT with non-linear blending on abdominal CT angiography. Korean J Radiol. 2014;15(4):430–8.
65. Paul J, Tan MM, Farhang M, Beeres M, Vogl TJ. Dual-energy CT spectral and energy weighted data sets: carotid stenosis and plaque detection. Acad Radiol. 2013;20(9):1144–51.
66. Jorgensen SM, Korinek MJ, Vercnocke AJ, Anderson JL, Halaweish A, Leng S, McCollough CH, Ritman EL. Arterial wall perfusion measured with photon counting spectral X-ray CT. Proc SPIE Int Soc Opt Eng. 2016;28:9967.
67. Lemos AA, Pezzullo JC, Fasani P, Gullo M, Giannitto C, Lo Gullo R, Biondetti PR. Can the unenhanced phase be eliminated from dual-phase CT angiography for chest pain? Implications for diagnostic accuracy in acute aortic intramural hematoma. AJR Am J Roentgenol. 2014;203(6):1171–80.

68. Toepker M, Moritz T, Krauss B, Weber M, Euller G, Mang T, Wolf F, Herold CJ, Ringl H. Virtual non-contrast in second-generation, dual-energy computed tomography: reliability of attenuation values. Eur J Radiol. 2012;81(3):e398–405.
69. Wang J, Garg N, Duan X, Liu Y, Leng S, Yu L, Ritman EL, Kantor B, McCollough CH. Quantification of iron in the presence of calcium with dual-energy computed tomography (DECT) in an ex vivo porcine plaque model. Phys Med Biol. 2011;56(22):7305–16.
70. Shinohara Y, Sakamoto M, Kuya K, Kishimoto J, Iwata N, Ohta Y, Fujii S, Watanabe T, Ogawa T. Assessment of carotid plaque composition using fast-kV switching dual-energy CT with gemstone detector: comparison with extracorporeal and virtual histology-intravascular ultrasound. Neuroradiology. 2015;57(9):889–95.
71. Stolzmann P, Frauenfelder T, Pfammatter T, Peter N, Scheffel H, Lachat M, Schmidt B, Marincek B, Alkadhi H, Schertler T. Endoleaks after endovascular abdominal aortic aneurysm repair: detection with dual-energy dual-source CT. Radiology. 2008;249(2):682–91.
72. Flors L, Leiva-Salinas C, Norton PT, Patrie JT, Hagspiel KD. Endoleak detection after endovascular repair of thoracic aortic aneurysm using dual-source dual-energy CT: suitable scanning protocols and potential radiation dose reduction. AJR Am J Roentgenol. 2013;200(2):451–60.
73. Maturen KE, Kaza RK, Liu PS, Quint LE, Khalatbari SH, Platt JF. "Sweet spot" for endoleak detection: optimizing contrast to noise using low keV reconstructions from fast-switch kVp dual-energy CT. J Comput Assist Tomogr. 2012;36(1):83–7.
74. Lee CW, Seo JB, Song JW, Kim MY, Lee HY, Park YS, Chae EJ, Jang YM, Kim N, Krauss B. Evaluation of computer-aided detection and dual energy software in detection of peripheral pulmonary embolism on dual-energy pulmonary CT angiography. Eur Radiol. 2011;21(1):54–62.
75. Pontana F, Faivre JB, Remy-Jardin M, Flohr T, Schmidt B, Tacelli N, Pansini V, Remy J. Lung perfusion with dual-energy multidetector-row CT (MDCT): feasibility for the evaluation of acute pulmonary embolism in 117 consecutive patients. Acad Radiol. 2008;15(12):1494–504.
76. Apfaltrer P, Bachmann V, Meyer M, Henzler T, Barraza JM, Gruettner J, Walter T, Schoepf UJ, Schoenberg SO, Fink C. Prognostic value of perfusion defect volume at dual energy CTA in patients with pulmonary embolism: correlation with CTA obstruction scores, CT parameters of right ventricular dysfunction and adverse clinical outcome. Eur J Radiol. 2012;81(11):3592–7.
77. Yang GF, Yang X, Zhang LJ, Zhu H, Chai X, Hu XB, Hu YX, Lu GM. Pulmonary enhancement imaging with dual energy CT for the detection of pulmonary embolism in a rabbit model: comparison to perfusion planar scintigraphy, SPECT and SPECT-CT modalities. Acad Radiol. 2011;18(5):605–14.
78. Zhang LJ, Lu L, Bi J, Jin LX, Chai X, Zhao YE, Chen B, Lu GM. Detection of pulmonary embolism comparison between dual energy CT and MR angiography in a rabbit model. Acad Radiol. 2010;17(12):1550–9.
79. Danad I, Ó Hartaigh B, Min JK. Dual-energy computed tomography for detection of coronary artery disease. Expert Rev Cardiovasc Ther. 2015;13(12):1345–56.
80. Raju R, Thompson AG, Lee K, Precious B, Yang TH, Berger A, Taylor C, Heilbron B, Nguyen G, Earls J, Min J, Carrascosa P, Murphy D, Hague C, Leipsic JA. Reduced iodine load with CT coronary angiography using dual-energy imaging: a prospective randomized trial compared with standard coronary CT angiography. J Cardiovasc Comput Tomogr. 2014;8(4):282–8.
81. Mangold S, Cannaó PM, Schoepf UJ, Wichmann JL, Canstein C, Fuller SR, Muscogiuri G, Varga-Szemes A, Nikolaou K, De Cecco CN. Impact of an advanced image-based monoenergetic reconstruction algorithm on coronary stent visualization using third generation dual-source dual-energy CT: a phantom study. Eur Radiol. 2016;26(6):1871–8.
82. Halpern EJ, Halpern DJ, Yanof JH, Amin-Spector S, Fischman D, Aviram G, Sosna J. Is coronary stent assessment improved with spectral analysis of dual energy CT? Acad Radiol. 2009;16(10):1241–50.
83. Stehli J, Clerc OF, Fuchs TA, Possner M, Gräni C, Benz DC, Buechel RR, Kaufmann PA. Impact of monochromatic coronary computed tomography angiography from single-source dual-energy CT on coronary stenosis quantification. J Cardiovasc Comput Tomogr. 2016;10(2):135–40.
84. Secchi F, De Cecco CN, Spearman JV, Silverman JR, Ebersberger U, Sardanelli F, Schoepf UJ. Monoenergetic extrapolation of cardiac dual energy CT for artifact reduction. Acta Radiol. 2015;56(4):413–8.
85. Geyer LL, Scherr M, Körner M, Wirth S, Deak P, Reiser MF, Linsenmaier U. Imaging of acute pulmonary embolism using a dual energy CT system with rapid kVp switching: initial results. Eur J Radiol. 2012;81(12):3711–8.
86. So A, Hsieh J, Imai Y, Narayanan S, Kramer J, Procknow K, Dutta S, Leipsic J, Min JK, Labounty T, Lee TY. Prospectively ECG-triggered rapid kV-switching dual-energy CT for quantitative imaging of myocardial perfusion. JACC Cardiovasc Imaging. 2012;5(8):829–36.
87. Vliegenthart R, Pelgrim GJ, Ebersberger U, Rowe GW, Oudkerk M, Schoepf UJ. Dual-energy CT of the heart. AJR Am J Roentgenol. 2012;199(5 Suppl):S54–63.
88. Ko SM, Song MG, Chee HK, Hwang HK, Feuchtner GM, Min JK. Diagnostic performance of dual-energy CT stress myocardial perfusion imaging: direct comparison with cardiovascular MRI. AJR Am J Roentgenol. 2014;203(6):W605–13.
89. Wichmann JL, Arbaciauskaite R, Kerl JM, Frellesen C, Bodelle B, Lehnert T, Monsefi N, Vogl TJ, Bauer RW. Evaluation of monoenergetic late iodine enhancement dual-energy computed tomography for imaging of chronic myocardial infarction. Eur Radiol. 2014;24(6):1211–8.
90. Schwarz F, Nance JW Jr, Ruzsics B, Bastarrika G, Sterzik A, Schoepf UJ. Quantification of coronary artery calcium on the basis of dual-energy coronary CT angiography. Radiology. 2012;264(3):700–7.
91. Yamada Y, Jinzaki M, Okamura T, Yamada M, Tanami Y, Abe T, Kuribayashi S. Feasibility of coronary artery calcium scoring on virtual unenhanced images derived from single-source fast kVp-switching dual-energy coronary CT angiography. J Cardiovasc Comput Tomogr. 2014;8(5):391–400.
92. Sudarski S, Fink C, Sueselbeck T, Kayed H, Schoenberg SO, Borggrefe M, Vliegenthart R, Oudkerk M, Henzler T. Quantitative analysis of coronary plaque composition by dual-source CT in patients with acute non-ST-elevation myocardial infarction compared to patients with stable coronary artery disease correlated with virtual histology intravascular ultrasound. Acad Radiol. 2013;20(8):995–1003.
93. Henzler T, Porubsky S, Kayed H, Harder N, Krissak UR, Meyer M, Sueselbeck T, Marx A, Michaely H, Schoepf UJ, Schoenberg SO, Fink C. Attenuation-based characterization of coronary atherosclerotic plaque: comparison of dual source and dual energy CT with single-source CT and histopathology. Eur J Radiol. 2011;80(1):54–9.
94. Barreto M, Schoenhagen P, Nair A, Amatangelo S, Milite M, Obuchowski NA, Lieber ML, Halliburton SS. Potential of dual-energy computed tomography to characterize atherosclerotic plaque: ex vivo assessment of human coronary arteries in comparison to histology. J Cardiovasc Comput Tomogr. 2008;2(4):234–42.
95. Hazirolan T, Akpinar B, Unal S, Gümrük F, Haliloglu M, Alibek S. Value of dual energy computed tomography for detection of

myocardial iron deposition in Thalassaemia patients: initial experience. Eur J Radiol. 2008;68(3):442–5.
96. Suzuki H, Imafuji A, Kato M, Omiya H. Dual energy CT assessment of amiodarone induced liver damage. SOMATOM Sessions Online. 2014. https://health.siemens.com/ct_applications/somatomsessions/index.php/dual-energy-ct-assessment-of-amiodarone-induced-liver-damage/.
97. Schlomka JP, Roessl E, Dorscheid R, Dill S, Martens G, Istel T, Bäumer C, Herrmann C, Steadman R, Zeitler G, Livne A, Proksa R. Experimental feasibility of multi-energy photon-counting K-edge imaging in pre-clinical computed tomography. Phys Med Biol. 2008;53(15):4031–47.
98. Yu Z, Leng S, Jorgensen SM, Li Z, Gutjahr R, Chen B, Halaweish AF, Kappler S, Yu L, Ritman EL, McCollough CH. Evaluation of conventional imaging performance in a research whole-body CT system with a photon-counting detector array. Phys Med Biol. 2016;61(4):1572–95.
99. Pourmorteza A, Symons R, Sandfort V, Mallek M, Fuld MK, Henderson G, Jones EC, Malayeri AA, Folio LR, Bluemke DA. Abdominal imaging with contrast-enhanced photon-counting CT: first human experience. Radiology. 2016;279(1):239–45.
100. Holmes DR 3rd, Fletcher JG, Apel A, Huprich JE, Siddiki H, Hough DM, Schmidt B, Flohr TG, Robb R, McCollough C, Wittmer M, Eusemann C. Evaluation of non-linear blending in dual-energy computed tomography. Eur J Radiol. 2008;68(3):409–13.
101. Zatz LM. The effect of the kVp level on EMI values. Radiology. 1976;119:683–8.

Drugs in Cardiac CT

9

Sebastian Rogowski, Virginia W. Lesslie, and Ullrich Ebersberger

In spite of the advances in scanner technology in coronary CT angiography (CCTA), image quality is still influenced by heart rate (HR) and the consistency of the cardiac cycle. Additionally, HR is related to the diagnostic value and level of radiation exposure of CCTA [1–3].

The reason for pharmaceutical intervention in patients' CCTA examinations for the assessment of coronary disease (CAD) and myocardial perfusion is the reduction of HR and the instigation of coronary vasodilatation in order to achieve maximal coronary flow. The current guidelines propose a HR of <65 bpm before imaging [4].

Pharmacological Interventions to Lower the Heart Rate

The use of medication to lower HR in cardiac CT is common in clinical practice. In many centers, the intravenous (IV) and oral administration of β-blockers is used to reduce HR [5, 6]. However, there is no widely accepted protocol for this practice. Furthermore, the use of non-dihydropyridine calcium channel blockers (CCBs), nitrates, and ivabradine is described.

Role of β-Blockers in Controlling Heart Rate

At many centers, clinicians control HR by administering a cardio-selective β-adrenergic antagonist [7]. Metoprolol has become the standard agent (Table 9.1). It is safe to use in patients with congestive heart failure as well as in patients with significant chronic obstructive pulmonary disease. In addition, the agent is low cost and reliable [8]. The most common oral approach involves a dose of 100 mg of metoprolol. Hence, one possible protocol is to give 100 mg orally 1 h before the scan (slow-release forms should not be used). If HR remains >60 bpm, additional metoprolol may be given intravenously to expedite HR reduction. Atenolol may be chosen for patients with significant hepatic dysfunction because of its renal route of clearance.

Beta-blockers have the potential to cause a variety of side effects related to their β1-receptor activity. At high one-off doses, the risk of β2-receptor-mediated adverse effects increases. Potential adverse events include bradycardia, atrioventricular block, hypotension, bronchospasm, Raynaud phenomenon, and anaphylaxis [9]. The half-life of IV metoprolol is approximately 3–7 h; therefore, an adverse effect may debilitate the patient for an extended period of time [10].

In such cases, esmolol may be used as an alternative. Esmolol is an ultrashort-acting cardio-selective IV β-receptor blocking agent with rapid onset (within 2–3 min) and ultrashort duration of action (mean half-life 9 min) [10, 11]. In contrast to the longer-acting β-receptor antagonists, the activity of

Table 9.1 β-Blockers

Administration	Drug	Dose	Onset	Half-life
Oral	Metoprolol	50–100 mg	1 h	3–7 h
	Atenolol	50–100 mg	2 h	6–10 h
Intravenous	Metoprolol	2.5–5.0 mg (up to 15 mg)	1 min	3–4 h
	Atenolol	2.5–5.0 mg (up to 10 mg)	1 min	6–10 h
	Esmolol	0.5 mg/kg (25–50 mg)	1–2 min	9 min

S. Rogowski
Department of Cardiology and Intensive Care Medicine, Heart Center Munich-Bogenhausen, Munich, Germany

V. W. Lesslie
Division of Cardiovascular Imaging, Department of Radiology and Radiological Science, Medical University of South Carolina, Charleston, SC, USA

U. Ebersberger (✉)
Department of Cardiology and Intensive Care Medicine, Heart Center Munich-Bogenhausen, Munich, Germany

Division of Cardiovascular Imaging, Department of Radiology and Radiological Science, Medical University of South Carolina, Charleston, SC, USA
e-mail: ebersberger@gmx.net

U. J. Schoepf (ed.), *CT of the Heart*, Contemporary Medical Imaging, https://doi.org/10.1007/978-1-60327-237-7_9

Table 9.2 Side effects of B-blockers

Drug class	Cardiac adverse effects	Non-cardiovascular side effects
Ivabradine	Dizziness, weakness (symptomatic bradycardia)	Eyesight problems: Increased brightness Phosphenes (bright spots) Blurred vision
Metoprolol, esmolol, and other beta-blockers	Hypotension Bradycardia Adrenergic-mediated coronary spasm on sudden withdrawal	Fatigue Erectile dysfunction Insomnia Hyperlipidemia Depression Airway disease Raynaud's phenomenon
CCB	Hypotension Bradycardia	Constipation Drowsiness

esmolol is short with a fast onset and short duration of activity, which constitutes a major safety factor [12]. Efficient HR control is crucial during CCTA; therefore, esmolol might be an effective alternative to the standard of care metoprolol. At present, esmolol is routinely used in intensive care treatment of acute supraventricular arrhythmias; however, administration before CCTA for HR reduction is an "off-label" indication. In an observational study, Degertekin et al. [13] reported that 65% of patients achieved a HR of <65 bpm using 50 mg of oral β-blocker (atenolol) combined with 1–2 mg/kg of IV esmolol (range, 50–300 mg).

More evidence is needed regarding the safety and efficiency of IV esmolol administered in a stepwise bolus protocol. Furthermore, no direct comparison of esmolol and metoprolol administration for HR control during CCTA is available (Table 9.2).

Active bronchospastic disease is considered a contraindication to treatment with β-blockers. Another medical treatment option for these patients is the use of short-acting CCBs or ivabradine. However, there is no robust data available in the literature. Caution is advised in the use of β-blockers in patients with the following: known or suspected sick sinus syndrome, unexplained pre-syncope or collapse, current use of other antiarrhythmic medications (including but not limited to CCBs, digoxin, or amiodarone), depressed left or right ventricular function, or allergy to β-blockers.

Role of Calcium Channel Blockers (CCBs) in Controlling Heart Rate

When β-blockers are contraindicated, CCBs can be an alternative method to control HR (Fig. 9.1). Phenylalkylamine non-dihydropyridine, verapamil, and diltiazem are the only CCBs used for this purpose; however, poor HR control with CCBs and benzodiazepines was reported in a recent trial [14].

Role of Ivabradine in Controlling Heart Rate

Ivabradine is another attractive option for reducing patient HR for CCTA. It selectively inhibits the I_f-current, which is a mixed K^+-Na^+-inward current activated by hyperpolarization, and contributes to the activity of the sinoatrial node [15, 16]. It slows the diastolic depolarization phase of the sinoatrial cells and slows the HR at rest and during exercise without affecting myocardial contractility [17, 18]. Therefore, it can be administered in patients in sinus rhythm but not other rhythms such as atrial fibrillation. Guaricci et al. showed that the administration of ivabradine over a 5-day period prior to CCTA is successful in reducing HR for CCTA [19].

A recently published trial with administration of an IV bolus of ivabradine achieved rapid, safe, and sustained HR reduction during CCTA, increased procedural convenience, and reduced radiation exposure when compared to the placebo [20, 21].

There is not yet a consensus about the protocol for ivabradine administration. In a recent study, a larger number of patients achieved a HR under 65 bpm by oral administration of a 7.5 mg dose of ivabradine in comparison with a 5 mg dose [21].

Pharmacological Interventions for Vasodilatation

Reducing motion artifact alone may not be enough to achieve the best possible image results. The diameter of coronary arteries can be increased significantly by coronary vasodilatation. Administration of sublingual nitrate can dilate the coronary arteries by approximately 15%. Administration of nitrates also increases the visualization of side branches including septal branches.

Nitroglycerin leads to the release of nitric oxide, which in turn initiates smooth muscle relaxation independent of endothelial function [22] and reduces the likelihood of coronary artery vasospasm. The administration of nitrates was recommended by the American College of Cardiology/American Heart Association (ACC/AHA) in 1999 for a reliable assessment of the extent of coronary stenosis [23, 24]. Nitroglycerin is also used for dilatation of coronary arteries in CCTA examinations, optimizing visualization of the vessel lumen and improving stenosis assessment [25].

Administration in the form of a sublingual spray (0.4–0.8 mg) is the most efficacious method with the least amount of side effects. The most common side effect is dizziness caused by nitroglycerin-induced hypotension or headaches, which are of short duration and self-limiting [9].

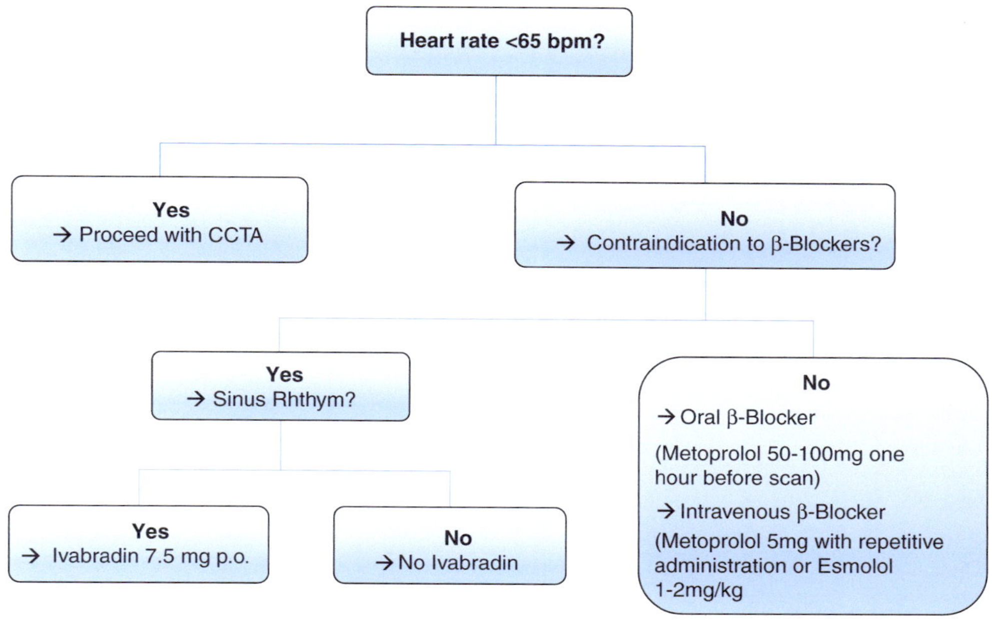

Fig. 9.1 Heart rate control in CCTA

Another point of concern with the administration of nitroglycerin is the potential decrease in blood pressure or reflex tachycardia, which can result in more motion artifacts on CCTA [26]. Furthermore nitroglycerin should never be used in patients taking erectile dysfunction medications like sildenafil or patients with severe anemia. In patients with severe aortic stenosis, nitroglycerin should also be administered with extreme caution.

Pharmacological Interventions for Stress Perfusion Evaluation

The diagnostic accuracy for CAD is similar for all vasodilators, which have a higher cardiac uptake than catecholamines and improve the heart/background contrast ratios. In combination with exercise, dobutamine may double coronary perfusion as compared to coronary flow at rest. However, vasodilators may even quadruple the flow.

Pharmacological stress agents most extensively validated by feasibility trials include adenosine and dipyridamole [27, 28]. Dipyridamole blocks adenosine reuptake. Adenosine dilates coronary arteries by interaction with adenosine A2 receptors.

Adenosine

The main effect of adenosine consists of a coronary arteriolar vasodilation by specific activation of the A2A receptor and leads to a 3.5- to 4-fold increase in myocardial blood flow. If perfusion is limited by coronary stenosis, there is a diminished hyperemic response.

Adenosine has a short half-life (<10 s) and is rapidly removed from the body upon administration. Thus, it has a rapid onset and short duration of action. Continuous infusion of 140 mcg/kg/min is required for the purpose of CT myocardial perfusion (CT-MPI). At the 3-minute mark, the stress radiopharmaceutical is injected and the infusion is continued for 3 additional minutes. Due to the short duration of the treatment with adenosine, medication is not expected to be associated with prolonged side effects (Tables 9.3, 9.4, and 9.5).

Absolute contraindications for adenosine stress testing include asthma, second- or third-degree AV block, sick sinus syndrome, or the recent use of dipyridamole.

Dipyridamole

Dipyridamole increases the level of endogenous adenosine by decreasing the level of reuptake by endothelial cells [28]. Both adenosine and dipyridamole have good sensitivity and specificity for the detection of myocardial perfusion defect with stress CT-MPI (Table 9.5). They have similar side effects, including reflex tachycardia, and are similarly contraindicated in patients with asthma, COPD, and high-grade atrioventricular block in the absence of a pacemaker. The standard dose of dipyridamole (0.142 mg/kg/min) is infused over 4 min. However, its effects last longer than 4 min. If side effects occur, administering aminophylline – an adenosine receptor antagonist – might be necessary to reverse the effects of dipyridamole. Both dipyridamole and adenosine require weight-based dosing.

Table 9.3 Adenosine receptor activation

A1 receptor	AV block
A2B receptor	Peripheral vasodilation, bronchospasm
A3 receptor	Bronchospasm

Table 9.4 Adenosine side effects

Symptoms	Incidence (%)
Flushing	35–40
Chest pain*	25–30
Dyspnea	20
Dizziness	7
Nausea	5
Symptomatic hypotension	5

*Chest pain is nonspecific and is not necessarily indicative of CAD

Table 9.5 Stress perfusion drug evaluation

Adenosine	Good sensitivity and specificity
Dipyridamole	Good sensitivity and specificity, inexpensive
Regadenoson	Easier dosing (10-s bolus), fewer side effects
Dobutamine	Physiological mechanism – increase oxygen consumption in the myocardium

Regadenoson

Another A2A adenosine receptor agonist is regadenoson. Similar to adenosine, it induces selective coronary vasodilation by binding to A2A adenosine receptors in the walls of the heart blood vessels.

The recommended dose of regadenoson is a single injection of 400 micrograms (5 mL), without dose adjustment according to the body weight. Regadenoson is injected into a peripheral vein for 10 s. The injection should be immediately followed by a 5 mL saline flush. The same contraindications must be observed as with adenosine.

Dobutamine

Another option for the medical stress test is the administration of a synthetic catecholamine - dobutamine. It raises blood pressure, myocardial contractility, and HR by unselective stimulation of the β-receptor.

According to protocol, it should be given at a starting dose of 5 mcg/kg/min for 3 min with subsequent increases (10, 20, 30, and 40 mcg/kg/min) until the stress endpoint is achieved. The endpoints are reaching target HR or the experience of chest pain, ECG changes, or hypotension. In case of adverse side effects, administration should be stopped immediately and can be reversed using 0.5 mg/kg of IV esmolol.

The application of medications in CCTA enables demonstrably improved results by means of better image quality and dose reduction. Practitioners should be aware of the dose, half-life, and effects of medications as well as their indications, contraindications, and interaction with other medications.

References

1. Stolzmann P, Goetti RP, Maurovich-Horvat P, et al. Predictors of image quality in high-pitch coronary CT angiography. AJR Am J Roentgenol. 2011;197:851e858.
2. Matt D, Scheffel H, Leschka S, et al. Dual-source CT coronary angiography: image quality, mean heart rate, and heart rate variability. AJR Am J Roentgenol. 2007;189:567e573.
3. Dewey M, Zimmermann E, Deissenrieder F, et al. Noninvasive coronary angiography by 320-row computed tomography with lower radiation exposure and maintained diagnostic accuracy: comparison of results with cardiac catheterization in a head-to-head pilot investigation. Circulation. 2009;120:867e875.
4. Abbara S, Arbab-Zadeh A, Callister T, et al. SCCT guidelines for performance of coronary computed tomographic angiography: a report of the Society of Cardiovascular Computed Tomography Guidelines Committee. J Cardiovasc Comput Tomogr. 2009;3:190–204.
5. Groen JM, Greuter MJ, van Ooijen PM, Willems TP, Oudkerk M. Initial results on visualization of coronary artery stents at multiple heart rates on a moving heart phantom using 64-MDCT. J Comput Assist Tomogr. 2006;30:812–7.
6. Pannu H, Alvarez W, Fishman E. Beta-blockers for cardiac CT: a primer for the radiologist. Am J Roentgenol. 2006;186:S341–5.
7. Mahabadi AA, Achenbach S, Burgstahler C, et al. Safety, efficacy, and indications of beta-adrenergic receptor blockade to reduce heart rate prior to coronary CT angiography. Radiology. 2010;257:614e623.
8. Le Jemtel TH, Padeletti M, Jelic S. Diagnostic and therapeutic challenges in patients with coexistent chronic obstructive pulmonary disease and chronic heart failure. J Am Coll Cardiol. 2007;49:171–82.
9. López-Sendón J, Swedberg K, McMurray J, et al. Expert consensus document on beta-adrenergic receptor blockers. Eur Heart J. 2004;25:1341–62.
10. Westfall TC, Westfall DP. Beta adrenergic receptor antagonists. In: Brunton LL, editor. Goodman & Gilman's the pharmacological basis of therapeutics. New York: The McGraw-Hill; 2011.
11. Wiest D. Esmolol. A review of its therapeutic efficacy and pharmacokinetic characteristics. Clin Pharmacokinet. 1995;28:190e202.
12. Wiest DB, Haney JS. Clinical pharmacokinetics and therapeutic efficacy of esmolol. Clin Pharmacokinet. 2012;51:347e356.
13. Degertekin M, Gemici G, Kaya Z, et al. Safety and efficacy of patient preparation with intravenous esmolol before 64-slice computed tomography coronary angiography. Coron Artery Dis. 2008;19:33e36.
14. Maffei E, Palumbo AA, Martini C, et al. "In-house" pharmacological management for computed tomography coronary angiography: heart rate reduction, timing and safety of different drugs used during patient preparation. Eur Radiol. 2009;19:2931e2940.
15. Bois P, Bescond J, Renaudon B, Lenfant J. Mode of action of bradycardic agent, S 16257, on ionic currents of rabbit sinoatrial node cells. Br J Pharmacol. 1996;118:1051–7.
16. DiFrancesco D. Characterization of single pacemaker channels in cardiac sino-atrial node cells. Nature. 1986;324:470–3.
17. Gardiner SM, Kemp PA, March JE, Bennett T. Acute and chronic cardiac and regional haemodynamic effects of the novel bradycardic agent, S16257, in conscious rats. Br J Pharmacol. 1995;115:579–86.

18. Ragueneau I, Laveille C, Jochemsen R, Resplandy G, Funck-Brentano C, Jaillon P. Pharmacokinetic-pharmacodynamic modeling of the effects of ivabradine, a direct sinus node inhibitor, on heart rate in healthy volunteers. Clin Pharmacol Ther. 1998;64:192–203.
19. Guaricci AI, Schuijf JD, Cademartiri F, et al. Incremental value and safety of oral ivabradine for heart rate reduction in computed tomography coronary angiography. Int J Cardiol. 2012;156(1):28–33.
20. Cademartiri F, Garot J, Tendera M, et al. Intravenous ivabradine for control of heart rate during coronary CT angiography: a randomized, double-blind, placebo-controlled trial. J Cardiovasc Comput Tomogr. 2015;9(4):286–94.
21. Guaricci AI, et al. Heart rate control with oral ivabradine in computed tomography coronary angiography: a randomized comparison of 7.5 mg vs 5 mg regimen. Int J Cardiol. 2012;168(1):362–8. more.
22. Ignarro LJ, Napoli C, Loscalzo J. Nitric oxide donors and cardiovascular agents modulating the bioactivity of nitric oxide: an overview. Circ Res. 2002;90:21–8.
23. Jost S, Rafflenbeul W, Reil GH, et al. Reproducible uniform coronary vasomotor tone with nitrocompounds: prerequisite of quantitative coronary angiographic trials. Catheter Cardiovasc Diagn. 1990;20:168–73.
24. Scanlon PJ, Faxon DP, Audet AM, et al. ACC/AHA guidelines for coronary angiography. A report of the American College of Cardiology/American Heart Association task force on practice guidelines (committee on coronary angiography). Developed in collaboration with the Society for Cardiac Angiography and Interventions. J Am Coll Cardiol. 1999;33:1756–824.
25. Johnson PT, Eng J, Pannu HK, Fishman EK. 64-MDCT angiography of the coronary arteries: nationwide survey of patient preparation practice. AJR Am J Roentgenol. 2008;190:743–7.
26. Khan M, Cummings KW, Gutierrez FR, Bhalla S, Woodard PK, Saeed IM. Contraindications and side effects of commonly used medications in coronary CT angiography. Int J Cardiovasc Imaging. 2011;27:441–9.
27. Blankstein R, Shturman LD, Rogers IS, et al. Adenosine-induced stress myocardial perfusion imaging using dual-source cardiac computed tomography. J Am Coll Cardiol. 2009;54:1072–84.
28. Cury RC, Magalhaes TA, Borges AC, et al. Dipyridamole stress and rest myocardial perfusion by 64-detector row computed tomography in patients with suspected coronary artery disease. Am J Cardiol. 2010;106:310–5.

Contrast Media Injection Protocols in CT Coronary Angiography

10

Casper Mihl, Madeleine Kok, Joachim E. Wildberger, and Marco Das

Optimal contrast enhancement of the coronary arteries is of pivotal importance for the proper assessment of coronary artery disease (CAD). Despite the degree of intravascular enhancement, overall image quality in coronary computed tomography angiography (CCTA) will depend on patient- and scan-related parameters. Previous studies have demonstrated that at a tube voltage of 120 kV enhancement levels in the coronary arteries above 325 Hounsfield units (HU) are necessary for optimal diagnosis [1, 2]. Attenuation values >500 HU may lead to underestimation of the degree of stenosis [3]. This necessitates synchronization of contrast material (CM) administration protocols with the scanning protocol offering individual timing based on the patient-specific situation [4, 5]. Technological advances in CCTA including shortening of the overall acquisition time and the broad availability of advanced reconstruction techniques (iterative reconstruction, [IR]) allow utilization of individual low-dose protocols without compromising image quality parameters in a broad range of patients.

Contrast Material Application

In order to achieve optimal opacification and contrast between vessel lumen and surrounding tissue, respectively, high and constant iodine contrast must be maintained throughout acquisition of the entire dataset. A state-of-the-art CM delivery in CCTA consists of several components, each of which will be addressed separately and linked to a concise recipe for robust clinical use.

C. Mihl (✉) · M. Kok · J. E. Wildberger · M. Das
Department of Radiology and Nuclear Medicine, Maastricht University Medical Center, Maastricht, The Netherlands

CARIM School for Cardiovascular Diseases, Maastricht University Medical Center, Maastricht, The Netherlands

Concentration

Different CM concentrations are used in CCTA and vary between 240 and 400 mg iodine per millilitre (mgI/ml). In terms of the degree of intravascular enhancement, all concentrations can be comparably used in the clinical setting, as long as the iodine delivery rate (IDR) or iodine flux (gI/s) remains constant.

Flow Rate

Contrast material will be intravenously delivered at a dedicated speed of injection. Flow rates <5 ml/s are most commonly used in clinical practice. Higher flow rates (up to 8.8 ml/s), however, can also be used safely [6]. Injections with high flow rates lead to a shorter and steeper peak enhancement and thus a proportional increase in vascular and parenchymal enhancement at the expense of a shorter time window in which these high enhancement levels are available [5, 7].

Volume

The overall iodine volume is the key determinant for solid organ imaging. In general, shorter acquisition times may to some extent reduce the total amount of CM required. For CCTA, this aspect is of minor importance. However, fixed CM volumes show large variation between different weight groups. Diagnostic attenuation of the coronary arteries can be acquired with total injected CM volumes varying between 50 ml and 94 ml (tube voltage: 100 kV, concentration: 300 mgI/ml), depending on weight of the patient (39–109 kg) and scan duration [8].

U. J. Schoepf (ed.), *CT of the Heart*, Contemporary Medical Imaging, https://doi.org/10.1007/978-1-60327-237-7_10

Saline Chaser

A saline chaser pushes the tail of the injected CM bolus into the central blood volume. Otherwise, approximately 20–30 ml of CM will be retained in the "dead space" between the brachial vein and the superior vena cava [9]. Consequently, saline flushing improves arterial enhancement and reduces the amount of contrast needed for a diagnostic examination. Therefore, the use of dual-head power injectors and a saline chaser is highly recommended. The latter should be injected at the same flow rate as used for the CM bolus.

Preheating

There is an exponential relationship between iodine concentration and viscosity. In general, the higher the iodine concentration, the higher the viscosity. High viscosity increases the friction resistance and the pressure needed for the same flow rate [10]. In addition, viscosity is directly influenced by temperature and can be lowered by preheating [11–13]. Low viscosity can be advantageous in several ways and has a direct influence on different aspects in CM injection: accelerated CM distribution, sustaining mixing of CM with blood as well as lower injection pressure [14, 15]. Therefore, standardized preheating of CM should be a prerequisite for clinical CM administration (Fig. 10.1).

Iodine Delivery Rate (IDR)

The IDR is the decisive factor for attenuation of the coronary arteries and can easily be calculated by multiplying the iodine concentration of the CM used (mg/ml) by the flow rate of the injector (ml/s). Injection of lower concentrated CM will provide identical attenuation of the coronary arteries in comparison to higher concentrated CM when keeping IDR identical [16, 17]. As a rule of thumb, an IDR of 2 gI/s is reasonable for CCTA applications at 120 kV. This can be done by either using a higher flow rate or using a higher concentration of CM. This implies a flow rate of approximately 6.7 ml/s for a CM concentration of 300 mgI/ml, and a flow rate of 5 ml/s for a CM concentration of 400 mgI/ml would produce identical attenuation. Normalizing IDR is a straightforward means of making different injection protocols comparable. At first glance, it seems obvious that the choice of high iodine-concentration contrast agents permits the use of lower flow rates. However, as already outlined, it should be kept in mind that the relationship between iodine concentration and viscosity is exponential. It follows that pressure created by the power injector, resulting pressures at the site of injection, and subsequent pressures inside the patient's veins can even be higher with high iodine-concentration agents than with low iodine-concentration agents. The benefits of preheated CM (to a mean body temperature of 37 °C) in order to reduce viscosity are obvious. As technical advances are aimed at scanning with lower tube voltages, which leads to an increase in attenuation, IDR will have to be modified (e.g. lowered) accordingly.

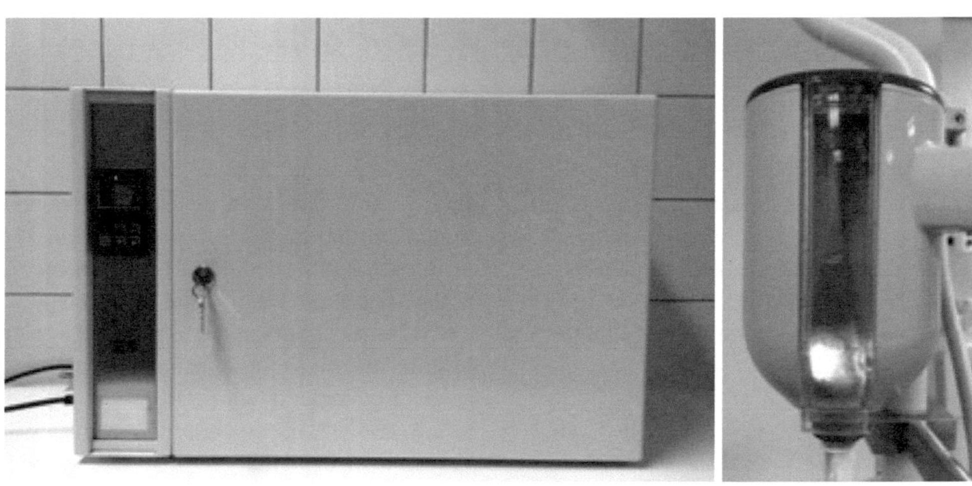

Fig. 10.1 Standardized preheating of CM should be a prerequisite for clinical CM administration. Left: Heating cabinet for storage of CM bottles up to 500 ml in the preparation room. CM will be heated to 38 °C (100°F), in order to ensure that the CM is injected at body temperature. Right: Small incubator in the scanner room, accommodating one CM bottle of up to 500 ml, to prevent temperature drop on site. Note: the small warming pads regularly delivered with the power injector are usually not capable of maintaining a constant temperature of 37 °C (99 °F)

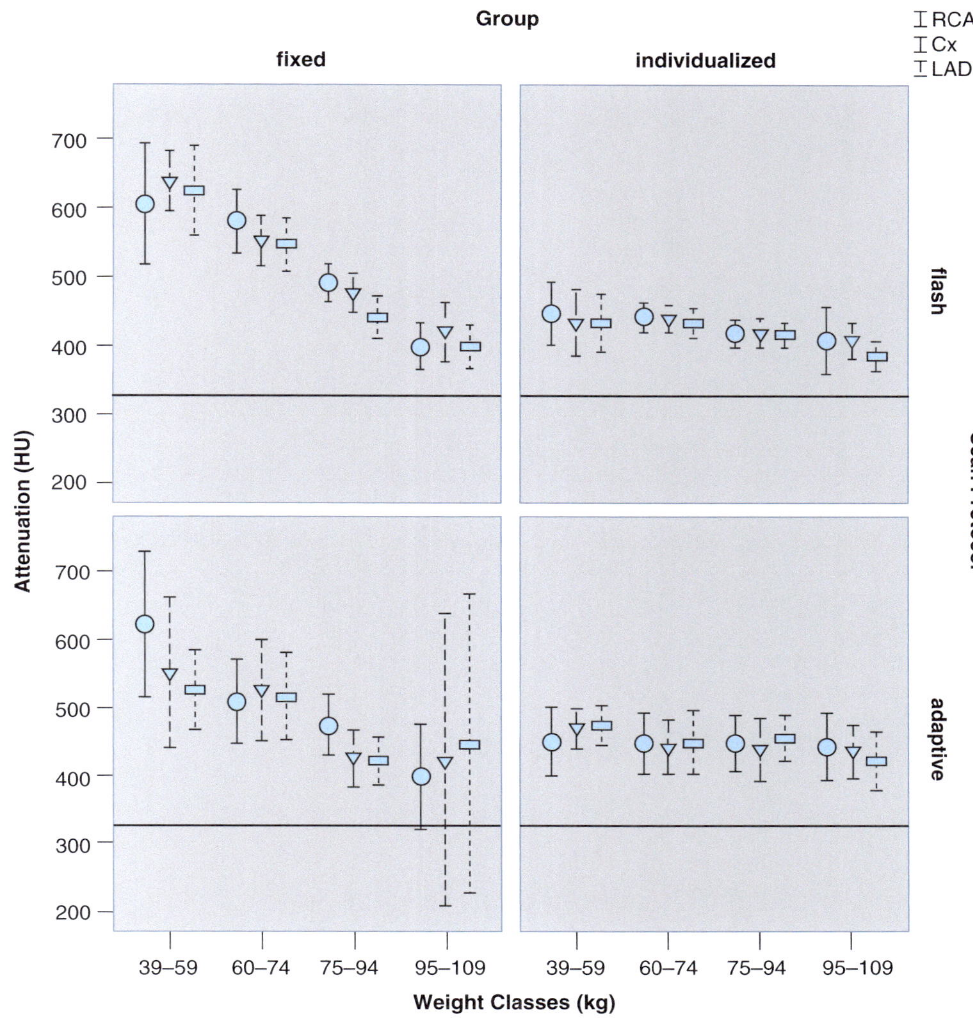

Fig. 10.2 Comparison between fixed CM injection (left) and individualized injection protocol (right) based on CCTA protocols on a third-generation dual-source scanner. Two different protocols are presented with acquisition times of around 1 s and 7 s, respectively. Error bars show the mean attenuation values with standard errors for all coronary arteries in both injection protocols and all weight classes. Reference line for attenuation was set to 325 HU

Total Iodine Load (TIL)

The TIL can easily be calculated by multiplying the iodine concentration of the CM used (mgI/ml) by the overall volume of CM to be delivered (ml) and is mostly relevant for organ studies and, as a minor factor, as a weight-related aspect in CCTA.

In summary, all concentrations can be used in the clinical setting, as long as the IDR remains constant. However, in terms of injection pressure, the use of lower concentrations is advantageous as viscosity increases exponential with higher concentrations of CM. The latter results in higher pressures created by the power injector despite usage of lower flow rates.

Patient Care

Injection Site

The preferred site for CM injection is the right antecubital vein. The administrated CM will drain into the basilic vein or a forearm vein that subsequently drains into the deep venous circulation of the elbow or the subclavian vein through the cephalic vein. The clinical effect of different flow rates and CM viscosities on the incidence of paravasation is not fully understood due to the absence of prospective large population studies. Large-access lines (e.g. 18G needles) are recommended for CCTA. When experiencing difficulties, due to impairment of peripheral veins (e.g. old patients, patients under chemotherapy or who are receiving corticosteroids), consider using 20G needles and bring down IDR accordingly (e.g. 1.5 gI/s max.).

Comfort

Results from the EICAR trial nicely show that a broad range of flow rates, up to 8.3 ml (at 240 mgI/ml) can be applied without an increased risk of extravasation and without the presence of negative side effects such as discomfort, pain or stress [6]. Injection with higher flow rates should not be considered a drawback in clinical practice. Furthermore, this creates a final doorway towards applicability of a broad

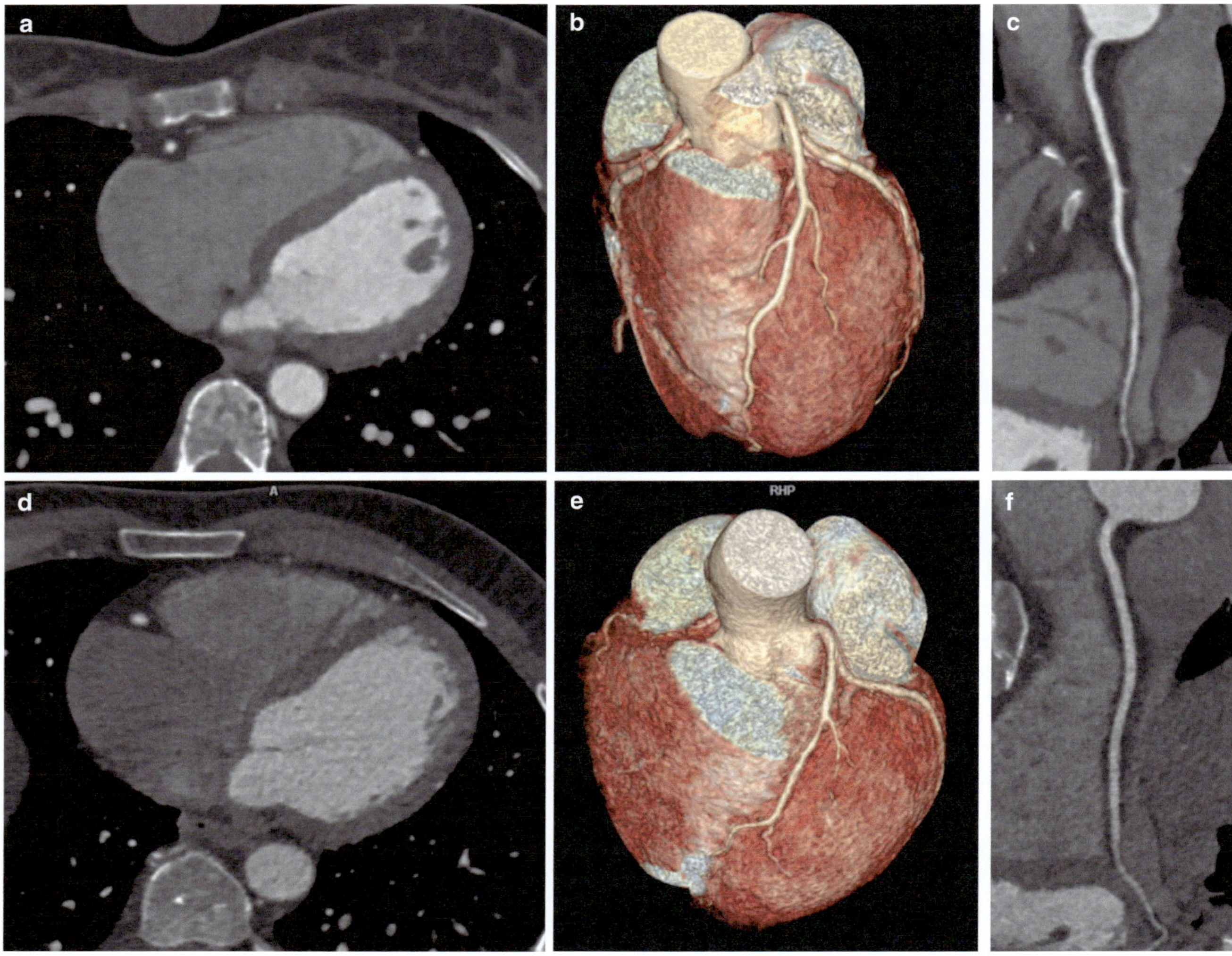

Fig. 10.3 Example of individualized CM injection protocol tailored to patient's weight. Patient 1 (**a–c**): body weight, 59 kg; length, 162 cm; BMI, 22.5; total injected CM volume, 71 ml. Patient 2 (**d–f**): body weight, 95 kg; length, 182 cm; BMI, 28.7; total injected CM volume, 100 ml. Note an equal homogeneous attenuation in RCA in both patients

variety in flow rates and IDR's and subsequently more individually tailored injection protocols.

Weight and Body Mass Index

Body weight and body mass index (BMI) are known to have a substantial impact on vascular attenuation and time to peak in CCTA. A fixed injection protocol causes a large variation between different weight groups indicating suboptimal use of CM in different patient weight groups, ranging from high contrast levels in patients with low body weight (as a result of too much contrast) to low contrast levels in heavy patients (e.g. not enough contrast) [8]. Individually tailored CM injections are beneficial in terms of individual adaptation of the IDR and the overall volume based upon a non-linear relationship between patient weight and scan duration in order to achieve diagnostic and comparable intravascular enhancement in all patients (Fig. 10.2). For a CCTA acquisition at 100 kV and patients weighing between 39 and 109 kg, a graded IDR between 1.6 and 2.2 gI/s and TIL between 15 and 28 gI are recommended (Fig. 10.3) [8].

Cardiac Output

Physical factors such as cardiac output may cause variability of vascular enhancement as well. The patient's cardiovascular circulation critically affects CM bolus transit time which needs to be considered when determining individualized scan timing [7, 18]. Empiric scan delays can no longer be recommended. Test bolus technique and bolus tracking technique are both proper techniques for calculation of the CM bolus transit time in routine clinical practice and the total amount of CM which is needed. The use of test bolus technique can overcome suboptimal attenuation due to timing-related issues. Alternatively, the scan delay can be determined individually by acquisition of a single-level dynamic CT series (automated bolus tracking). In this mode, a pre-monitoring scan is performed within the target volume to localize the target vessel for contrast timing; a low-dose scanning technique (e.g. 120 kVp; 20 $mAs_{eff.}$) is usually applied for this purpose. A region of interest (ROI) is then placed in the target vessel (ascending aorta), and attenuation values (in HU) are measured every 2 s during the contrast injection. When the predefined trigger threshold level is reached (e.g. 140 HU; range 50–150 HU based on the current literature) [7], an automated start of the CT scan is initialized. In this mode the additional transition delay has to be considered, defined as the delay between reaching the threshold and the start of the actual CT scan (e.g. 6–7 s; usually ranging between 0 and 18 s).

Scanner

Bolus Geometry

Bolus geometry is the pattern of enhancement plotted on a time (s)/attenuation (Hounsfield units [HU]) curve measured in the ROI [19]. A physiological time enhancement curve shows a rapid rise in aortic contrast enhancement followed by a very short steady state plateau and a steady decline in enhancement due to recirculation and hemodynamic perturbation [5, 19]. Bi- and multiphasic protocols aim to create a longer plateau of enhancement during scan time by means of a higher injection rate at the beginning of the injection and a lower rate in the second part [20]. Sixty-four-slice systems provide a scan time of approximately 7–12 s for a spiral CCTA. As the acquisition time is rather in the range of 1–5 s for latest equipment, these (complex) injection protocols are no longer needed and a monophasic injection protocol is appropriate for clinical routine.

Tube Voltage

Technical developments of CT technique have also made the use of lower tube voltage (kVp) feasible. The use of lower kVp settings is accompanied by higher contrast enhancement; this is explained by the fact that lower tube voltage translates into lower effective photon energy (effective photon energy being approximately half the kVp), bringing the latter closer to the K-edge of iodine (33.2 keV) [21, 22]. However, if lower tube voltages will be used without concordantly increasing tube-current-time product (mAs), image noise will increase and invariably the signal-to-noise ratio (SNR) will decrease as a result of radiation dose reduction. Therefore, low tube voltage settings should only be used in combination with an adaptation of the tube-current-time product (mAs) to higher levels.

Practically, when the selection of lower tube voltage is possible by the available scanner, the total amount of iodine can be reduced accordingly. In general, 12% reduction of iodine dose is diagnostically acceptable for a 100 kV scan compared to a 120 kV scan. For 80 kV and 70 kV, reduction percentages of 45% and 56% might be considered, respectively [21].

Reconstruction Technique

Newly available reconstruction technologies such as IR reduce image noise and significantly improve image quality in terms of SNR and contrast-to-noise ratio (CNR) compared to routinely used filtered back projection

Table 10.1 Checklist for various parameters in CM injection protocol in CCTA, based on a tube voltage of 100 kVp

Parameters	Range	Factors influencing range
CM concentration (mgI/ml)	240–400	Supplier
Flow rate (ml/s)	2.5–8.8	Based on IDR CM concentration Acquisition time Needle size Needle position
Volume (ml)	50–94	Based on TIL CM concentration Acquisition time
Saline chaser (ml)	~30–50[a] volume	Flow rate
Preheating	Body temperature (37 °C)	
IDR (gI/s)	1.6–2.2	Tube voltage Patient size/ weight
TIL (gI)	15–28	Tube voltage Patient size/ weight
Injection site	Right antecubital vein	Patient condition
Needle size (G)	18	Needle position Vessel size
Timing	Bolus tracking Test bolus	Cardiac output (Ir)regular heart rate
Reconstruction technique	IR (preferred)	Scanner technique
Tube voltage (kVp)	70–120[b]	Patient size/ weight Scanner technique

[a]Make sure the flow rate is identical to the flow rate used for main bolus
[b]All values estimated for this CM injection protocol are based on a tube voltage of 100 kVp. For lower kVp settings, reductions of TIL and IDR can be applied [21]. If so, please go through the checklist (again)

Table 10.2 CM injection parameters based upon body weight adapted CM injection software, currently used in our clinical routine, using second-generation as well as third-generation dual-source CT for clinical CCTA

Weight classes	Scan protocol (100 kV)	CM volume (ml)	TIL (gI)	Saline flush (ml)	Flow rate (ml/s)	IDR (gI/s)
39–59 kg	Sequential/ spiral	~60	~18	30	5.3	1.6
	High pitch	~50	~15			
60–74 kg	Sequential/ spiral	~70	~21	30	5.6	1.7
	High pitch	~60	~18			
75–94 kg	Sequential/ spiral	~80	~24	30	6.7	2.0
	High pitch	~70	~21			
95–109 kg	Sequential/ spiral	~90	~27	30	7.3	2.2
	High pitch	~80	~24			

Data from references [8, 27]

(FBP) in contrast-enhanced CT [23–26]. When available, the use of IR and dedicated cardiac reconstruction kernels are recommended to ensure diagnostic image quality whilst using reduced radiation dose.

In summary, optimal CM injection during CCTA is key. Many parameters influence attenuation patterns and overall image quality of CCTA. A thorough understanding of the underlying principles and their interaction is necessary to provide the full picture on the interplay of the various CM aspects, scanner-related factors as well as patient-related aspects. The ultimate goal is to create a personalized CM injection protocol, where all these parameters are tailored individually in order to provide adequate diagnostic attenuation values and image quality, based on a standardized concept. Table 10.1 is provided to serve as a checklist, where recommended values and ranges of all parameters stated above are briefly addressed. In addition, Table 10.2 states the CM injection parameters based upon body weight adapted CM injection software, currently used in our clinical routine.

References

1. Isogai T, Jinzaki M, Tanami Y, Kusuzaki H, Yamada M, Kuribayashi S. Body weight-tailored contrast material injection protocol for 64-detector row computed tomography coronary angiography. Jpn J Radiol. 2011;29(1):33–8.
2. Cademartiri F, Maffei E, Palumbo AA, Malago R, La Grutta L, Meijjboom WB, et al. Influence of intra-coronary enhancement on diagnostic accuracy with 64-slice CT coronary angiography. Eur Radiol. 2008;18(3):576–83.
3. Fei X, Du X, Yang Q, Shen Y, Li P, Liao J, et al. 64-MDCT coronary angiography: phantom study of effects of vascular attenuation on detection of coronary stenosis. Am J Roentgenol. 2008;191(1):43–9.
4. Budoff MJ, Dowe D, Jollis JG, Gitter M, Sutherland J, Halamert E, et al. Diagnostic performance of 64-multidetector row coronary computed tomographic angiography for evaluation of coronary artery stenosis in individuals without known coronary artery disease: results from the prospective multicenter ACCURACY (assessment by coronary computed tomographic angiography of individuals undergoing invasive coronary angiography) trial. J Am Coll Cardiol. 2008;52(21):1724–32.
5. Bae KT. Optimization of contrast enhancement in thoracic MDCT. Radiol Clin N Am. 2010;48(1):9–29.
6. Kok M, Mihl C, Hendriks BM, Altintas S, Eijsvoogel NG, Kietselaer BL, et al. Patient comfort during contrast media injection in coronary computed tomographic angiography using varying contrast media concentrations and flow rates: results from the EICAR trial. Investig Radiol. 2016;51(12):810–5.
7. Bae KT. Intravenous contrast medium administration and scan timing at CT: considerations and approaches. Radiology. 2010;256(1):32–61.
8. Mihl C, Kok M, Altintas S, Kietselaer BL, Turek J, Wildberger JE, et al. Evaluation of individually body weight adapted contrast media injection in coronary CT-angiography. Eur J Radiol. 2016;85(4):830–6.
9. Schoellnast H, Tillich M, Deutschmann HA, Deutschmann MJ, Fritz GA, Stessel U, et al. Abdominal multidetector row computed tomography: reduction of cost and contrast material dose using saline flush. J Comput Assist Tomogr. 2003;27(6):847–53.
10. Kok M, Mihl C, Mingels AA, Kietselaer BL, Muhlenbruch G, Seehofnerova A, et al. Influence of contrast media viscosity and temperature on injection pressure in computed tomographic angiography: a phantom study. Investig Radiol. 2014;49(4):217–23.
11. Halsell RD. Heating contrast media: role in contemporary angiography. Radiology. 1987;164(1):276–8.
12. Halsell RD. Heating contrast media in a microwave oven. Radiology. 1987;163(1):279–80.
13. Schwab SA, Kuefner MA, Anders K, Adamietz B, Heinrich MC, Baigger JF, et al. Peripheral intravenous power injection of iodinated contrast media: the impact of temperature on maximum injection pressures at different cannula sizes. Acad Radiol. 2009;16(12):1502–8.
14. Bae KT, Tran HQ, Heiken JP. Uniform vascular contrast enhancement and reduced contrast medium volume achieved by using exponentially decelerated contrast material injection method. Radiology. 2004;231(3):732–6.
15. Muhlenbruch G, Behrendt FF, Eddahabi MA, Knackstedt C, Stanzel S, Das M, et al. Which iodine concentration in chest CT? a prospective study in 300 patients. Eur Radiol. 2008;18(12):2826–32.
16. Mihl C, Wildberger JE, Jurencak T, Yanniello MJ, Nijssen EC, Kalafut JF, et al. Intravascular enhancement with identical iodine delivery rate using different iodine contrast media in a circulation phantom. Investig Radiol. 2013;48(11):813–8.
17. Mihl C, Kok M, Wildberger JE, Altintas S, Labus D, Nijssen EC, et al. Coronary CT angiography using low concentrated contrast media injected with high flow rates: feasible in clinical practice. Eur J Radiol. 2015;84(11):2155–60.
18. Bae KT, Heiken JP, Brink JA. Aortic and hepatic contrast medium enhancement at CT. Part I. Prediction with a computer model. Radiology. 1998;207(3):647–55.
19. Cademartiri F, van der Lugt A, Luccichenti G, Pavone P, Krestin GP. Parameters affecting bolus geometry in CTA: a review. J Comput Assist Tomogr. 2002;26(4):598–607.
20. Fleischmann D, Rubin GD, Bankier AA, Hittmair K. Improved uniformity of aortic enhancement with customized contrast medium injection protocols at CT angiography. Radiology. 2000;214(2):363–71.

21. Mahesh M. MDCT physics: the basics: technology, image quality and radiation dose. 1st ed. Philadelphia: Lippincott Williams and Wilkins; 2009.
22. Brooks RA. A quantitative theory of the Hounsfield unit and its application to dual energy scanning. J Comput Assist Tomogr. 1977;1(4):487–93.
23. Renker M, Nance JW Jr, Schoepf UJ, O'Brien TX, Zwerner PL, Meyer M, et al. Evaluation of heavily calcified vessels with coronary CT angiography: comparison of iterative and filtered back projection image reconstruction. Radiology. 2011;260(2):390–9.
24. Wang R, Schoepf UJ, Wu R, Nance JW Jr, Lv B, Yang H, et al. Diagnostic accuracy of coronary CT angiography: comparison of filtered back projection and iterative reconstruction with different strengths. J Comput Assist Tomogr. 2014;38(2):179–84.
25. Pontana F, Pagniez J, Duhamel A, Flohr T, Faivre JB, Murphy C, et al. Reduced-dose low-voltage chest CT angiography with sinogram-affirmed iterative reconstruction versus standard-dose filtered back projection. Radiology. 2013;267(2):609–18.
26. Wang R, Schoepf UJ, Wu R, Reddy RP, Zhang C, Yu W, et al. Image quality and radiation dose of low dose coronary CT angiography in obese patients: sinogram affirmed iterative reconstruction versus filtered back projection. Eur J Radiol. 2012;81(11):3141–5.
27. Seifarth H, Puesken M, Kalafut JF, Wienbeck S, Wessling J, Maintz D, et al. Introduction of an individually optimized protocol for the injection of contrast medium for coronary CT angiography. Eur Radiol. 2009;19(10):2373–82.

Cardiovascular CT: Image Reconstruction

11

Annemarie M. den Harder, Arnold M. R. Schilham, and Martin J. Willemink

Image reconstruction is the formation of images based on CT projection data. This process has undergone tremendous improvements in recent years. This chapter focuses on the different types of image reconstructions. First, the steps before the actual reconstruction can take place will be explained, including calibration of the CT system, formation of raw data, z-interpolation for spiral acquisitions, and ECG editing. Subsequently, the most common reconstruction techniques filtered back projection (FBP) and iterative reconstruction and their applications in cardiac CT will be discussed.

Calibration

Low-energy x-ray photons attenuate more easily than high-energy photons. Therefore, the fraction of low-energy photons decreases more than the fraction of high-energy photons when passing through different tissues. This results in beam hardening: an increased mean energy of the beam, which can cause artifacts. This is especially the case when dense materials are imaged (e.g., bone or metal implants). The CT system is calibrated to correct for beam hardening and inhomogeneities based on assumptions of tissue attenuation and x-ray photon energy [1, 2]. Inhomogeneities can, for example, be caused by a defective detector element or low attenuation in air. Calibration phantoms with known attenuation profiles are used to compare known attenuation properties to acquired attenuations.

A. M. den Harder · A. M. R. Schilham · M. J. Willemink (✉)
Department of Radiology, University Medical Center Utrecht, Utrecht, The Netherlands

Raw Data

X-ray photons travel from the CT tube to the detector. Once they hit the detector, x-ray photons are converted to light photons which are converted to an electrical signal that scales with the number of light photons and thus the intensity of the detected x-rays. Those electrical signals have certain intensities. The detector will receive multiple signals with different intensities. This can be used to create a signal intensity profile, which displays the number of signals with a specific intensity. All signals received from a certain beam angle form a projection. The signal intensity profiles of each projection are transformed into x-ray attenuation values. If an object is placed between the CT tube and the detector, a decreased electrical signal is measured, which reflects an increase of the total x-ray attenuation along the line between the detector and the tube.

Projection data can be stored in a two-dimensional image, which is called a sinogram because of its sinusoid shape. A sinogram is a set of projections for certain orientations using line integrals (Fig. 11.1). The x-axis represents the distance along the projection direction, and the y-axis represents the angle of the projection. The intensity in the sinogram represents the attenuation values; more attenuation results in lower signal and vice versa. The collection of projection data in a sinogram is called the raw data set, which can be used to reconstruct an image.

Z-Interpolation

In spiral CT acquisitions, the x-ray beam rotates continuously with simultaneous movement of the table. The table movement per rotation divided by collimator width is defined as the pitch. A pitch below 1 results in beam overlap, while a pitch above 1 results in gaps (Fig. 11.2). In cases of the latter, data from different projections have to be interpolated to form transverse slices of projection data. Interpolation is the

U. J. Schoepf (ed.), *CT of the Heart*, Contemporary Medical Imaging, https://doi.org/10.1007/978-1-60327-237-7_11

computation of an unknown value by using known values on either side. The distance between the values on either side is the z-spacing. A higher pitch results in an increased distance, which can result in interpolation artifacts [3]. Values can be separated by a full rotation (360° interpolation) or a half rotation (180° interpolation). 180 degrees interpolation can be performed by synthesizing data using projections from opposite directions. Linear interpolation of 180° is often preferred, since this will result in improved resolution and thinner slices because the values used are closer to the desired plane. It also offers the possibility to increase the pitch to 2 without sampling gaps. However, images are noisier compared to 360° interpolation [4].

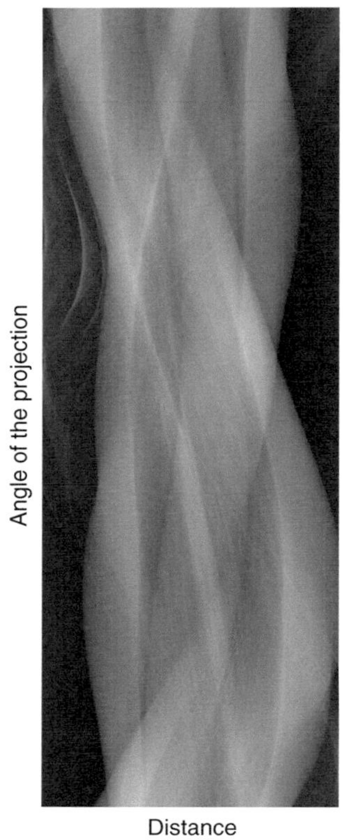

Fig. 11.1 Sinogram of a cardiac CT acquisition

ECG Editing

With retrospective electrocardiography (ECG)-gated acquisitions, images can be reconstructed at different time intervals. R-waves are automatically detected, and images can be reconstructed throughout the entire cardiac cycle, usually at an increment of 5–10%. The most optimal reconstruction phase can be selected in the post-processing phase. Although usually the end-diastolic phase is used for reconstruction (approximately 75% of the R-R interval), occasionally a different phase might result in better image quality, for example, in patients with atrial fibrillation [5]. The most optimal phase can be selected manually by evaluating reconstructions of all R-R intervals; however this is a very time-consuming process. To overcome this drawback, algorithms are available which automatically reconstruct the entire cardiac cycle and select the best reconstruction based on motion [6].

Due to irregular or high heart rates, the detection of R waves might be incorrect, leading to artifacts, or the temporal window can be too short leading to a lack of data. As illustrated in Fig. 11.3, the affected temporal window can be deleted, and additional windows can be added in the next heartbeat. If there are long pauses, additional windows can also be added [7].

Back Projection

Images are created from projection data using a technique called back projection. Every projection contains the sum of the single attenuation values of each pixel along the line of projection. The total sum of attenuation values is known; however the exact positions of those values along the

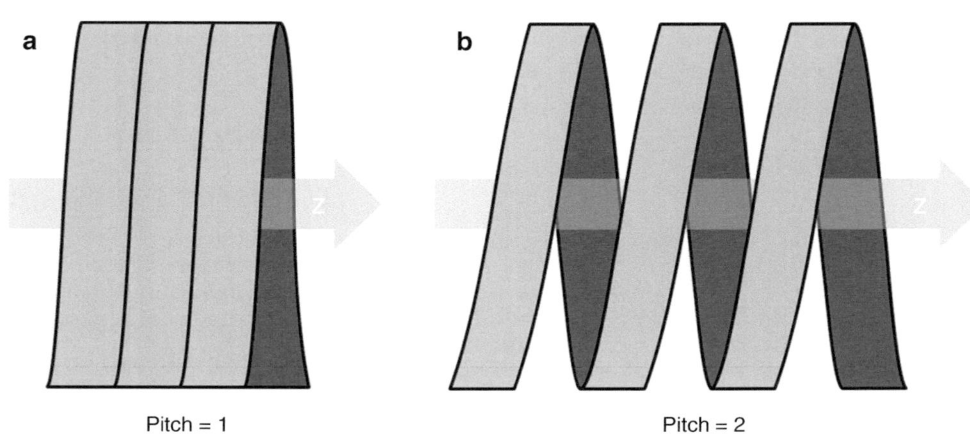

Fig. 11.2 Schematic illustration of z-interpolation. An acquisition with a pitch of 1 (**a**) and a pitch of 2 (**b**) is shown. Using 360° interpolation, a pitch of 2 will result in sampling gaps. With 180° interpolation it is still possible to use a pitch of 2 without sampling gaps, because the spaces between the rotations are filled by synthesizing data using projections from opposite directions

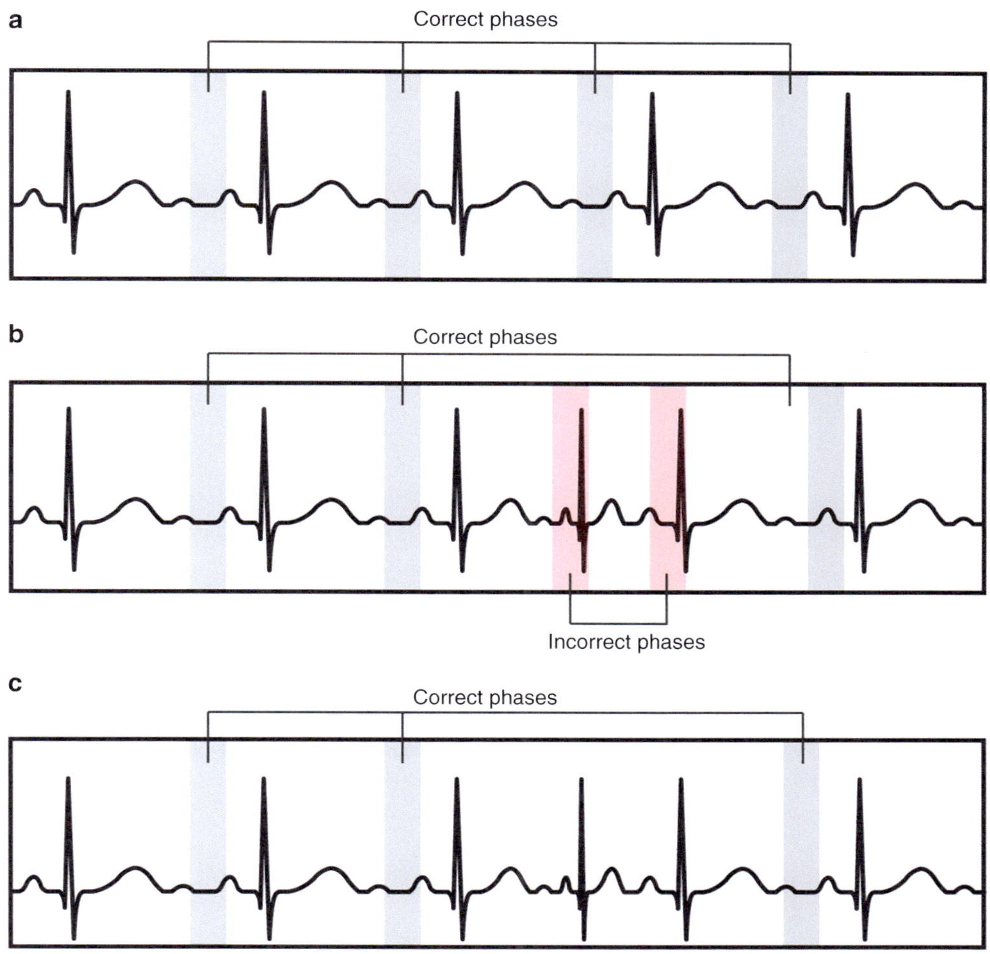

Fig. 11.3 Schematic illustration of ECG editing. The first ECG signal (**a**) represents a normal sinus rhythm resulting in correct phase detection. The second ECG signal (**b**) is arrhythmic resulting in incorrect phase detections. With ECG editing the wrongly detected phases can be deleted (**c**), and images are based on correct phases

projection are unknown. To compute an image from those values, the total sum of attenuations is averaged over the different pixels on the projection line. This is explained in Fig. 11.4. In Fig. 11.4a, an image is shown with four pixels (a). The number in the left upper matrix represents the attenuation value of a pixel. P_1 to P_4 show the total measured attenuation values from different projections acquired from the true object. It is possible to get an approximation of the numbers based on the total sum of attenuation values. To this aim, the values are smeared out across the projection, and the different projections are summed and renormalized by dividing the total amount by the number of projections (in this example 4). Increasing the number of projections will lead to a better approximation of the true object. However, even with hundreds of projections, the image will still remain an approximation, and with simple back projection, the final image will be blurred (Fig. 11.4b). A convolution kernel is necessary for mathematical filtering to improve the approximation.

Convolution Kernels

Because back projection alone results in blurred images, a convolution kernel is applied. The kernel is also called a filter. Convolution takes the values of neighboring pixels into account with certain weights based on the distance. Depending on the kernel, this can result in a smooth or a sharp image and everything in between (Fig. 11.5). All manufacturers developed their own kernels with different names. After the convolution kernel is applied to the projection data, back projection is performed to create an image.

The choice of convolution kernel will influence the amount of noise and the spatial resolution. A smooth kernel will result in reduced noise at the cost of spatial resolution, while a sharper kernel results in improved spatial resolution at the cost of increased noise. In cardiac CT this can, for example, influence quantification of coronary plaques [8]. Sharper kernels will reduce blooming and are therefore preferred when stents are present or for heavily calcified arteries.

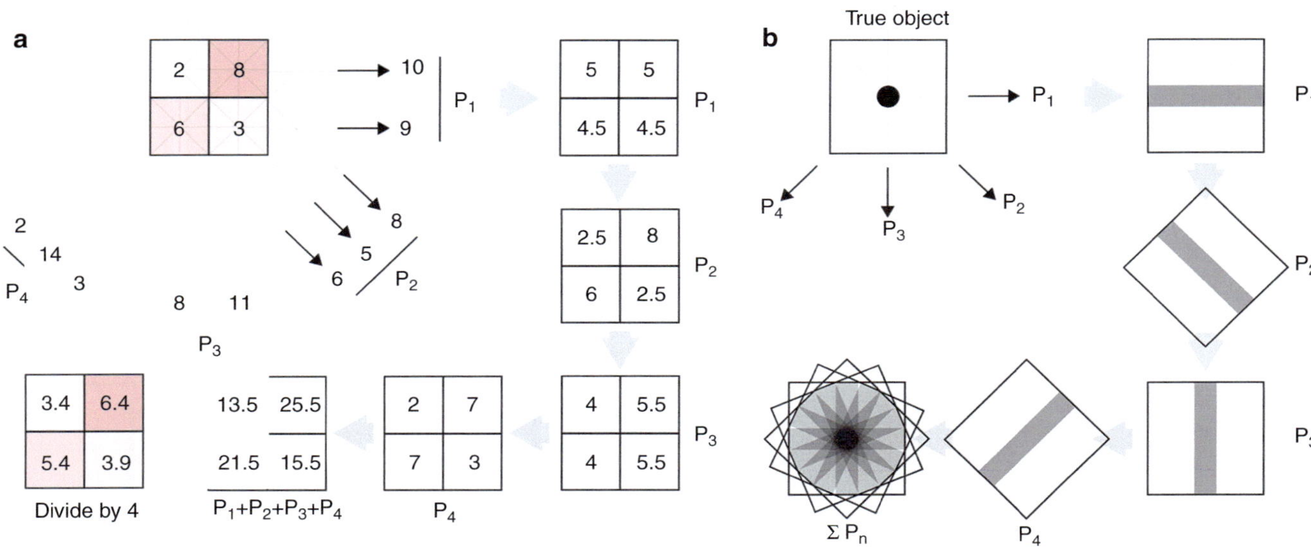

Fig. 11.4 Back projection schematically explained (**a**). The upper left matrix indicates the measured attenuation values of the true object. In this example there are four pixels, and four projections are acquired at different angles (P_1 to P_4). The first projection (P_1) shows the measured attenuation from left to right, and the other projections (P_2 to P_4) are rotated by 45°. The values are smeared out across the projection. For example, the 10 in P_1 is divided by two (number of pixels); therefore a 5 is allocated to each pixel. While in P_2 the 8 and 6 are not divided because these are projections of a single pixel. Subsequently the projections are summed. Finally the numbers are divided by the number of projections, which is 4 in this case. The final reconstruction is shown in the left lower corner. Increasing numbers of projections improve the quality of the approximated final reconstruction. However, even with a large number of projections, the reconstructed image will be blurred with simple back projection (**b**)

Fig. 11.5 Example of different convolution kernels. A convolution kernel uses the value of neighboring pixels to smoothen the image or to enhance the edges. The use of a convolution kernel will result in a filtered profile, which can be used for back projection

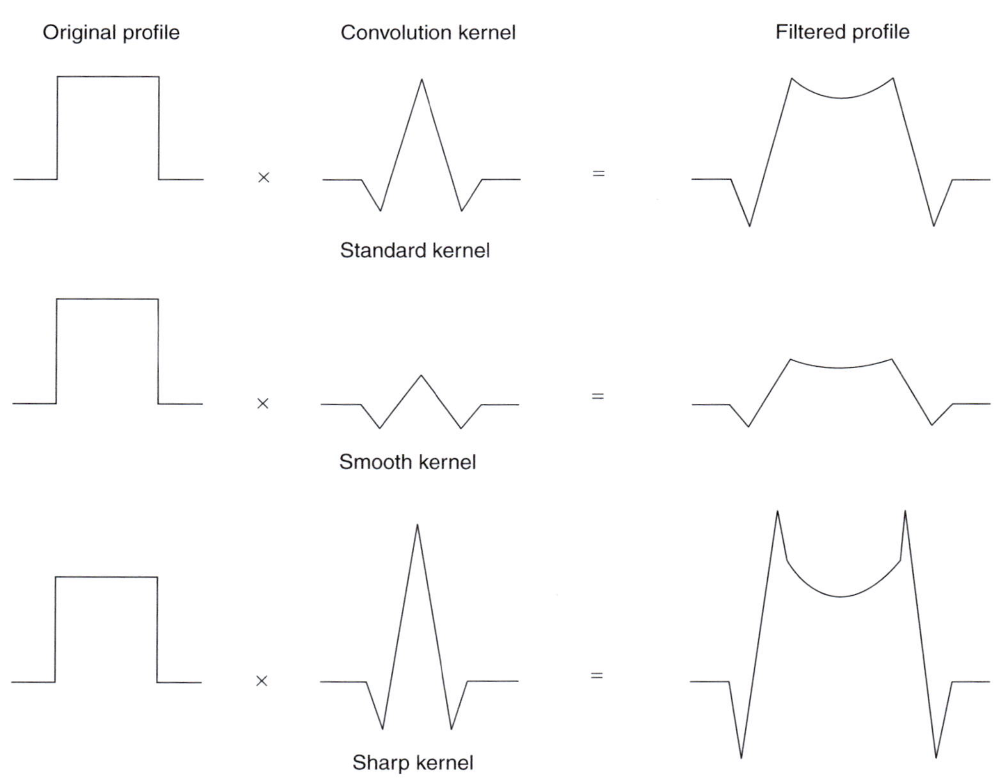

However, smooth kernels will result in less noise, which will improve lumen visualization. Usually medium-smooth kernels are used for cardiac CT angiography, while sharper kernels are applied for coronary calcium scoring.

Iterative Reconstruction

A commonly used reconstruction method is FBP, in which a convolution kernel is applied to the projection data, followed by a back projection as explained above. This method works well in most situations; however at low-radiation doses and in large patients, FBP produces noisy images. To reduce the amount of noise, iterative reconstruction algorithms have been developed [9]. A form of iterative reconstruction was first described in the 1970s under the name algebraic reconstruction [10]. Due to the limited computational power at that time, it was not suitable for clinical practice.

The first step of iterative reconstruction is a FBP. From the images derived from the FBP, new projection data are generated based on prior information concerning the scanner geometry, the x-ray spectrum, the detector characteristics, and a noise model. Subsequently the new projection data are compared to the original projection data, and corrections in noise modeling are performed. This process is repeated (iterated) several times. Each time the newly generated projection data will represent a closer match to the original projection data. This iteration process can be repeated until the differences are very small or until a certain number of iterations are reached. This process is also called model-based iterative reconstruction. A simplified, less time-consuming method is hybrid iterative reconstruction. In hybrid iterative reconstruction, noise is iteratively filtered in the projection domain and in the image domain without multiple iterations in forward and backward projection steps (Fig. 11.6). In image-based iterative recon-

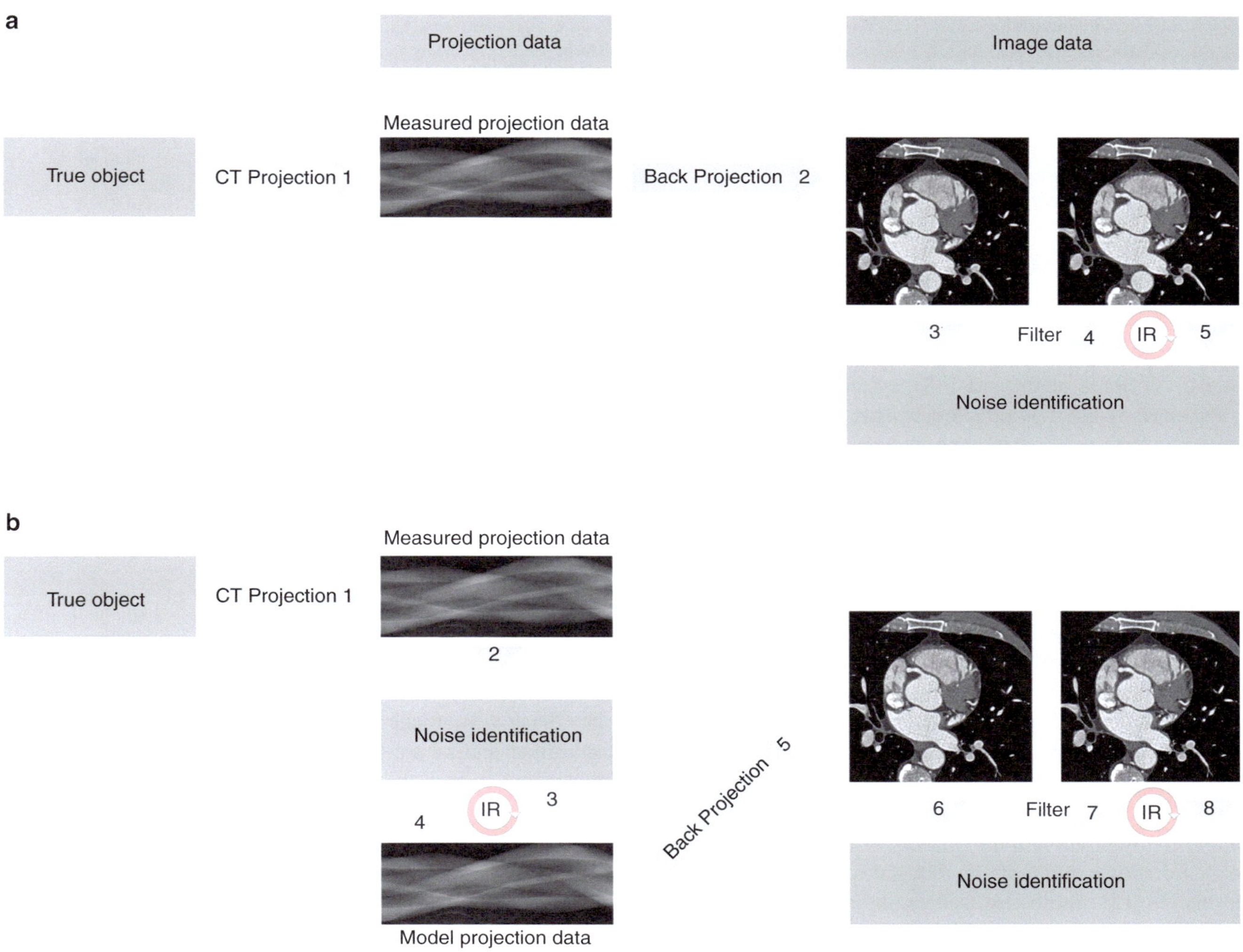

Fig. 11.6 Image-based (**a**), hybrid (**b**), and model-based (**c**) iterative reconstruction schematically explained. The numbers represent the subsequent steps undertaken. In image-based iterative reconstruction (**b**), a FBP is performed after which noise is reduced in the image domain (steps 5–6). Hybrid iterative reconstruction (**c**) reduces noise both in the projection domain (steps 3–4) and in the image domain (steps 7–8). Model-based iterative reconstruction (**a**) is more advanced and compares and corrects the modeled projection data to the true projection data (step 4) after which a new back projection is performed. This process is iterated several times to acquire model projection data that are a close match to the measured projection data

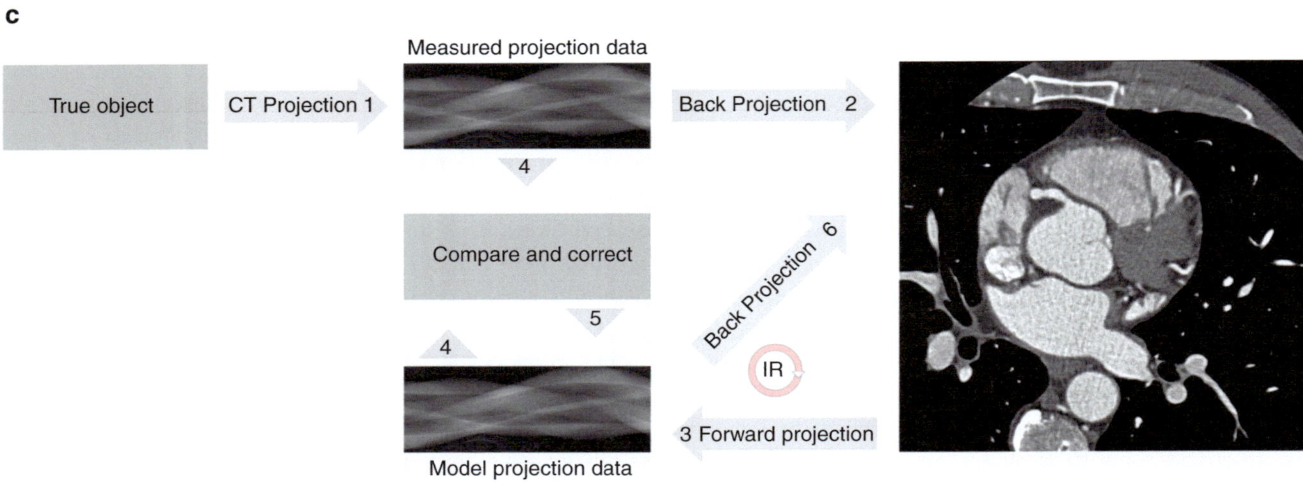

Fig. 11.6 (continued)

struction, noise is only reduced in the image domain. In both hybrid and image-based iterative reconstruction, no forward projection steps are performed based on the acquired image resulting in less computational demanding algorithms.

The current clinically available iterative reconstruction algorithms are provided in Table 11.1. Most current clinically available algorithms have several levels or percentages indicating the amount of noise reduction. A larger level or percentage implies more noise reduction, which can, for example, be achieved by a higher number of iterations.

Iterative reconstruction is nowadays widely implemented and used. Some of the latest CT systems do not offer FBP anymore but only use iterative reconstruction. Iterative reconstruction has several advantages and disadvantages. The main advantage is noise reduction, which results in two major applications. First, image quality is improved compared to FBP at a similar dose level. Second, it also offers the opportunity to acquire images at lower radiation dose levels with comparable image quality compared to FBP at routine dose levels. The reported achievable dose reduction for cardiac CT acquisitions using iterative reconstruction varies widely and is dependent on several factors including the reconstruction algorithm, CT system, and study population. Recent studies have shown that iterative reconstruction allowed for coronary CT angiography at radiation dose levels of 2–3 mSv, while with FBP doses up to 10 mSv are used [11]. Using iterative reconstruction, non-contrast-enhanced acquisitions for coronary calcium scoring can be reduced to submillisievert dose levels [12, 13]. These results are mainly based on hybrid iterative reconstruction algorithms. Further dose reduction is expected using model-based iterative reconstruction. Reported disadvantages of iterative reconstruction are longer reconstruction times and a different, smoother image appearance. Iterative reconstruction requires more computational power, and therefore reconstruction times can be prolonged. The delay with image-based and hybrid iterative algorithms is limited and is not likely to result in clinically relevant delays, not even in the emergency setting [14]. Model-based algorithms initially required several hours for image reconstruction, but advancements in reconstruction algorithms and computational power have reduced this to less than half an hour and for some algorithms to only a few minutes [15]. It is likely that the reconstruction time will be reduced even further in the future and therefore will not be a barrier anymore. The second commonly mentioned disadvantage is the different image appearance, also described as "plastic," "blotchy," or "artificial" (Fig. 11.7). This is caused by low noise levels

Table 11.1 Overview of current clinically used iterative reconstruction algorithms

Algorithm	Vendor	Type
Iterative Reconstruction in Image Space (IRIS)	Siemens	Image-based
Adaptive Iterative Dose Reduction 3D (AIDR 3D)	Toshiba	Hybrid
Adaptive Statistical Iterative Reconstruction (ASiR)	General Electric	Hybrid
Adaptive Statistical Iterative Reconstruction (ASiR – V)	General Electric	Hybrid
Advanced Modeled Iterative Reconstruction (ADMIRE)	Siemens	Hybrid
iDose[4]	Philips	Hybrid
Sinogram-Affirmed Iterative Reconstruction (SAFIRE)	Siemens	Hybrid
Model-Based Iterative Reconstruction (MBIR-Veo)	GE	Model-based
Iterative Model Reconstruction (IMR)	Philips	Model-based
Forward projected model-based Iterative Reconstruction SoluTion (FIRST)	Toshiba	Model-based

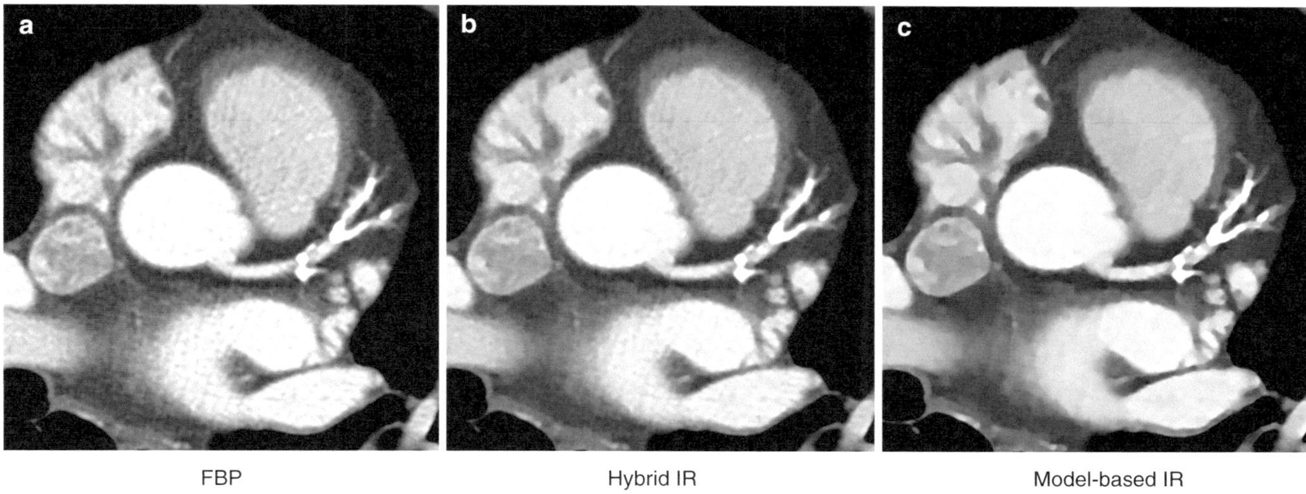

Fig. 11.7 Contrast-enhanced CT acquisition of the heart in a 56-year-old male with a heart rate of 59 beats/minute and a weight of 80 kilograms. Reconstructed with FBP (**a**), hybrid iterative reconstruction (**b**, iDose level 4, Philips), and model-based iterative reconstruction (**c**, IMR level 2, Philips). Note the smoother image appearance with model-based iterative reconstruction, due to low noise levels

and is more pronounced in higher noise reduction settings for hybrid iterative reconstruction algorithms and for all model-based iterative reconstruction algorithms. There are concerns that this will result in decreased diagnostic accuracy; however this has not been investigated yet.

References

1. Ketcham RA, Hannah RD. Beam hardening correction for X-ray computed tomography of heterogeneous materials. Comput Geosci. 2014;67:49–61.
2. Boas FE, Fleischmann D. CT artifacts: causes and reduction techniques. Imaging Med. 2012;4:229–40.
3. Goldman LW. Principles of CT: multislice CT. J Nucl Med Technol. 2008;36(2):57,68; quiz 75–6.
4. Brink JA, Heiken JP, Wang G, McEnery KW, Schlueter FJ, Vannier MW. Helical CT: principles and technical considerations. Radiographics. 1994;14(4):887–93.
5. Matsumoto H, Kondo T, Watanabe S, et al. ECG-edited middiastolic phase reconstruction improves image quality at 64-MDCT coronary angiography of patients with atrial fibrillation. AJR Am J Roentgenol. 2008;191(6):1659–66.
6. Cademartiri F, Mollet NR, Runza G, et al. Improving diagnostic accuracy of MDCT coronary angiography in patients with mild heart rhythm irregularities using ECG editing. AJR Am J Roentgenol. 2006;186(3):634–8.
7. Kruger BL, Lee F, Bruesewitz MR, Primak A, Williamson EE, McCollough CH. Quality recovery in cardiac CT angiography: how to edit an ECG trace to improve image quality. Abstract Archives of the RSNA 2007(LL-PH5183).
8. Cademartiri F, La Grutta L, Runza G, et al. Influence of convolution filtering on coronary plaque attenuation values: observations in an ex vivo model of multislice computed tomography coronary angiography. Eur Radiol. 2007;17(7):1842–9.
9. Willemink MJ, de Jong PA, Leiner T, et al. Iterative reconstruction techniques for computed tomography part 1: technical principles. Eur Radiol. 2013;23(6):1623–31.
10. Fleischmann D, Boas FE. Computed tomography–old ideas and new technology. Eur Radiol. 2011;21(3):510–7.
11. Den Harder AM, Willemink MJ, De Ruiter QM, et al. Dose reduction with iterative reconstruction for coronary CT angiography: a systematic review and meta-analysis. Br J Radiol. 2015;89:20150068.
12. Hecht HS, de Siqueira ME, Cham M, et al. Low- vs. standard-dose coronary artery calcium scanning. Eur Heart J Cardiovasc Imaging. 2015;16(4):358–63.
13. van Osch JA, Mouden M, van Dalen JA, et al. Influence of iterative image reconstruction on CT-based calcium score measurements. Int J Cardiovasc Imaging. 2014;30(5):961–7.
14. Willemink MJ, Schilham AM, Leiner T, Mali WP, de Jong PA, Budde RP. Iterative reconstruction does not substantially delay CT imaging in an emergency setting. Insights Imaging. 2013;4(3):391–7.
15. Oda S, Weissman G, Vembar M, Weigold WG. Cardiac CT for planning redo cardiac surgery: effect of knowledge-based iterative model reconstruction on image quality. Eur Radiol. 2015;25(1):58–64.

The Challenging Patient

12

Damiano Caruso, Domenico De Santis, Taylor M. Duguay, Sheldon E. Litwin, and Carlo N. De Cecco

In the past decade, coronary CT angiography (CCTA) has established itself as a robust imaging technique for the exclusion of coronary artery disease (CAD) in patients presenting with acute chest pain [1, 2] and moderate cardiovascular risk [3–5] due to its high sensitivity and negative predictive value in detecting significant coronary artery stenosis [6]. Noninvasive CCTA has become a reliable alternative to invasive angiography [7] and, thanks to recent technical innovations, has raised its power from just a morphological evaluation to a more comprehensive morphological and functional assessment [2, 8]. Specifically, novel CT technological advancements such as CT myocardial perfusion imaging (CT-MPI) provide a reliable functional analysis of the heart capable of accurately presenting hemodynamically significant coronary artery stenosis [9–11]. CCTA coupled with CT-MPI could raise CT as the stand-alone image modality for a comprehensive evaluation of CAD and direct assessment of myocardial ischemia in a single examination [12].

Technically speaking, CCTA presents a greater challenge and is more demanding than other CT applications due to the nature of its target, the continuously moving heart [13, 14]. Thus, higher spatial and temporal resolutions are mandatory for a proper visualization of small-caliber vessels such as coronary arteries. In addition, image acquisition should be synchronized with the patient's electrocardiogram (ECG) in order to achieve optimal image quality. Due to its technical complexity, the accurate selection and preparation of the patient are mandatory for obtaining a high-level examination [15].

Despite the continuous technological advances that have unleashed the diagnostic power of CCTA and allowed accurate diagnoses even in difficult clinical scenarios, some minor limitations should still be taken into account when performing CCTA examinations. The comprehensive definition of *a challenging patient* embraces some clinical conditions that should be investigated in order to always guarantee a safe and accurate CT examination.

The Ideal Patient

Due to the technical limitations of CT in its early years, CCTA had to be reserved to a select population in order to achieve diagnostic results [16–18]. On one hand, the accurate selection of patients who can benefit from a CCTA is important in order to avoid unnecessary invasive procedures such as coronary angiography, while on the other hand, it is necessary to ensure that all CCTA examinations provide diagnostic input. The most important factors that allow successful CCTA examinations are a heart rate less than 60 beats per minute (bpm) and a sinus rhythm [19, 20]. Additionally, sufficient renal function is also mandatory for patients undergoing CCTA due to the need for IV iodinated contrast media.

The main goal of CCTA is to obtain high-quality images while delivering the lowest reasonably achievable radiation

D. Caruso
Department of Radiological Sciences, Oncological and Pathological Sciences, University of Rome "Sapienza", Latina, Italy

D. De Santis
Department of Radiological Sciences, Oncological and Pathological Sciences, University of Rome "Sapienza", Latina, Italy

Division of Cardiovascular Imaging, Department of Radiology and Radiological Science, Medical University of South Carolina, Charleston, SC, USA

T. M. Duguay (✉)
Division of Cardiovascular Imaging, Department of Radiology and Radiological Science, Medical University of South Carolina, Charleston, SC, USA
e-mail: duguay@musc.edu

S. E. Litwin
Division of Cardiology, Department of Medicine, Medical University of South Carolina, Charleston, SC, USA

C. N. De Cecco (✉)
Department of Radiology and Radiological Science, Medical University of South Carolina, Charleston, SC, USA
e-mail: dececco@musc.edu

U. J. Schoepf (ed.), *CT of the Heart*, Contemporary Medical Imaging, https://doi.org/10.1007/978-1-60327-237-7_12

dose to the patient [21, 22]. Generally speaking, image quality and radiation dose are intrinsically linked – high-dose examinations return higher perceived image quality. However, radiation dose is not the only contributing factor to the quality of images. Patient weight has been shown to affect image quality [23, 24]; and in fact the diagnostic quality of CCTA images of obese patients is often severely limited. In addition, the ideal patient must be hemodynamically stable, able to perform a sufficient breath-hold of 15 s, and able to lay in a supine position with their arms extended behind their head. The administration of beta-blockers and/or sublingual nitroglycerine is common in clinical practice in order to achieve an optimal heart rate less than 60 bpm and sufficient vasodilation, both of which have been shown to provide superior image quality [25, 26]. However, patients contraindicated for beta-blockers and/or sublingual nitroglycerine *(discussed further in subsequent sections)* also present a challenge in terms of producing optimal image quality [27].

The Challenging Patient

Elevated Heart Rates and Arrhythmias

The accuracy of CCTA is highly dependent on the image quality of the dataset, and robust heart rate control, ideally less than 60 bpm, is essential for optimizing image quality and minimizing radiation dose [28]. Beta-blockers are routinely administered in clinical practice for heart rate reduction and cardiac rhythm stabilization. Drugs classified as beta-blockers are grouped based on the β1 selectivity, lipid solubility, and partial agonistic activity [28]. Dedicated guidelines have been established in order to avoid complications with the administration of beta-blockers. These contraindications are as follows: severe chronic obstructive pulmonary disease, asthma, sensitivity to beta-blockers, second- or third-degree heart block, and sinus bradycardia with systolic blood pressure less than 100 mmHg [29].

Patients who have a heart rate < 60 bpm during pre-scan monitoring do not require beta-blockers, whereas patients with irregular rhythms or a heart rate > 60 bpm require beta-blockers to avoid any motion artifacts. Despite having several cardio-selective beta-blockers, metoprolol tartrate (5 mg) is typically chosen due to its availability and cardio-selectivity. Metoprolol tartrate (5 mg) is typically intravenously administered in order for the drug to take effect quickly (5–10 min), whereas metoprolol oral tablets need to be administered 60–90 min before the scan. In the absence of contraindications, an initial bolus of 5 mg is usually injected once the patient is lying on the scanner table. In cases of unsatisfactory heart rate response, a maximum 15 mg of metoprolol tartrate can be administered.

The most commonly seen heart rate irregularity is atrial fibrillation. In order to overcome the irregular heart rhythm, CCTA image acquisition is usually performed using a retrospective acquisition protocol. CCTA has been described to have a high diagnostic accuracy in patient affected by atrial fibrillation, as reported in a recent meta-analysis [30]; however, the retrospective acquisition protocol often results in an increased radiation dose. A recent study evaluated the feasibility of prospective ECG-triggered sequential acquisition in patients affected by atrial fibrillation and reported an excellent diagnostic accuracy (around 90%) [20].

Ivabradine, a selective inhibitor of I_f channels located in the sinus node, is an alternative choice to metoprolol tartrate for heart rate reduction. Unfortunately, it is recommended that ivabradine only be administered to patients with a sinus rhythm [31]. On the other hand, ivabradine has a good safety profile and does not lower left ventricle contractility. Moreover, no rebound effects were reported after drug cessation nor was there an onset of tolerance reported after prolonged use. Ivabradine is administered orally and generally allows for a heart rate reduction of around 10 bpm at the recommended dosage (no more than 15 mg/day). Several trials have demonstrated the efficacy of ivabradine in lowering the heart rate [27, 32–36] and established it as a single-dose premedication proven to be effective and safe in heart rate reduction prior to CCTA [27, 35].

The most recent generation of CT scanners have provided superior image quality and improved diagnostic performance that is less dependent on heart rate. These scanners allow for the acquisition of the entire heart in a single heartbeat, providing great image quality with a lower radiation dose and administered contrast media amount [37].

Reduced Renal Function

Patients with a reduced renal function present a unique challenge as they are limited to the amount of intravenous contrast media they can be administered. Contrast-induced acute kidney injury (CI-AKI) is an iatrogenic disease that occurs within 3 days of the intravascular injection of iodinated contrast media in absence of an alternative etiology. It is defined as an absolute increase in serum creatinine concentration of ≥0.5 mg/dL or a relative increase of ≥25% above baseline. CI-AKI has received significant public attention which has resulted in the administration of iodinated contrast media being considered a general risk factor for worsening renal function [38].

Estimated glomerular filtration rate (eGFR), calculated from the serum creatinine, is the preeminent method of estimating renal function prior to contrast media administration. The Chronic Kidney Disease Epidemiology Collaboration (CKD-EPI) formula gives the most accurate eGFR. An eGFR value below 45 ml/min/1.73m^2 is considered a risk factor for contrast-induced nephropathy (CIN) as reported from dedicated guidelines [39], and preventive measures are required in such patients.

Hydration is considered the common strategy for CIN prevention. In patients with eGFR between 30 and 45 mL/min/1.73m^2, intravenous hydration should be arranged before and after the administration of contrast media. ESUR guidelines suggest intravenous protocol of 1.0–1.5 mL/kg/h for at least 6 h before and after contrast media administration [38, 40]. If intravenous hydration cannot be appropriately performed, oral hydration should be prescribed.

Contrast media volume has also been shown to be associated with CIN [41]. As such, reducing contrast media volume used during CCTA is a reliable option in reducing the risk of CIN. The ability to lower contrast media volume is directly related to reducing the tube current. Low tube energies are closer to the iodine k-edge (33.2 keV), and thus, lower energy levels maximize iodine attenuation allowing a substantial reduction contrast media [42]. Recent studies confirm the possibility to use low volumes of contrast media (30 mL) in CCTA by using prospectively ECG-triggered high-pitch gated acquisition at 70 kVp without any lack of image quality in selected patients with BMIs <23 kg/m^2 and heart rates <65 bpm [43]. Unfortunately, high BMI values significantly limit the image quality when low tube voltages are applied.

The Obese Patient

Obese patients are considerable challenges for CCTA, as the higher image noise generated by the photon starvation phenomenon [44] degrades both contrast and spatial resolution causing a poor evaluation of small vessels and noncalcified atherosclerotic plaques. With previous generations of CT scanners, increasing the tube voltage to 140 kVp was considered one of the most effective solutions for improving the image quality in obese patients [45]. Although this increases photon flux, higher tube voltage returns lower attenuation and consequently lowers the signal of iodinated contrast media, all while bearing the cost of an increased radiation dose.

In such patients, slower gantry rotation speeds may be advisable to enhance photon flux and improve the signal-to-noise ratio. In addition, the use of a high iodine concentration contrast medium at a faster flow rate could be helpful in compensating for the increased levels of image noise that limit contrast resolution. Moreover, dedicated iterative reconstructions, by using different strategies and mathematical algorithms, allow for a reduced image noise and an improved image quality compared to standard filtered back projection [46, 47].

The introduction of the latest generation of dual-source CT scanner overcame the need to increase the tube voltage to 140 kV. These new CT scanners, equipped with the latest technical developments, are able to improve the image quality even in obese patients thanks to the increased power of the tubes, a higher spatial resolution related to a smaller focal spot, and an improved temporal resolution due to shorter gantry times, along with a fully integrated circuit detector system for noise reduction. Mangold et al. have demonstrated that even severe obese patients with a BMI greater than 40 kg/m^2 can be imaged at 120 kVp if high amperage and dedicated iterative reconstructions are available. This technical approach led to satisfactory objective and subjective CCTA image quality and adequate coronary intravascular attenuation with an approximate contrast media dose of 80 mL [24]. In addition, automated tube voltage selection (ATVS) technology and the most recent generation of iterative reconstructions can be reliably used to assess coronary artery disease in obese patients returning an excellent diagnostic accuracy at a reduced radiation dose compared to standard 120 kV CCTA examinations. ATVS individually selects the tube voltage based on the patient's habitus, system specifics, and the clinical task. With the implementation of this technology, even obese patients can undergo CCTA examination with tube voltages less than 120 kV and maintain adequate diagnostic accuracy [48].

The Anxious Patient

Beta-blockers are administered in CCTA in order to achieve low and stable heart rates that are mandatory for obtaining diagnostic image quality at the lowest radiation dose. However, not all patients respond to beta-blocker treatment, which is sometimes due to patient anxiety [49]. Different strategies have been considered to reduce patient anxiety such as the use of benzodiazepines. Even if benzodiazepines are not significantly involved in the mechanism for lowering the heart rate, they can be useful in reducing the physiological burden of the examination [50]. According to one study, benzodiazepines are usually used when beta-blockers are required but contraindicated. A comprehensive overlook of different challenging scenarios and related countermeasures are summarized in Table 12.1.

How to Manage Angina Onset During Stress Cardiac CT

With the use of pharmacological stress agent, patients can experience common side effects such as flushing, chest pain, dyspnea, headache, and gastrointestinal discomfort. The most common pharmacological stress agents used

Table 12.1 Challenging scenarios and related strategies

Challenge	Strategy	Drug	Dose	Peak	Side effects	Contraindications
Elevated heart rates and arrhythmias	Beta-blockers	Metoprolol (IV)	5 mg (up to 15 mg)	5–10 min	LV contraction depression, arteriolar and bronchiolar constriction	Sinus bradycardia, heart block greater than first degree, systolic blood pressure < 100 mmHg
		Metoprolol (oral)	100 mg	60–90 min		
		Atenolol (IV)	5 mg	5 min		
	Selective I_f channel inhibitor	Ivabradine (oral)	15 mg	60 min	Luminous phenomenon (phosphenes); enhanced brightness in visual field	Acute decompensated heart failure, blood pressure < 90/50 mmHg, sick sinus syndrome
eGFR <45 mL/min/1.73 m^2	Hydration	Saline or bicarbonate	Saline: IV injection1.0–1.5 mL/kg/h for at least 6 h before and after CM Bicarbonate: 154 mEq/L in dextrose (5% water): 3 mL/kg/h for 1 h before CM and 1 mL/kg/h for 6 h after CM	–	–	–
	Lower the CM amount					
Obese patient	ATVS Iterative reconstruction	–	–	–	–	Increased radiation exposure
Anxious patient	Benzodiazepines	Lorazepam (oral)	0.5–1 mg (20–40 drops)	60 min	Sedation, tremor, agitation, dizziness, hypersomnia	Acute narrow-angle glaucoma
		Diazepam (oral)	2 mg (10 drops)	30–120 min		
Heart ischemia	Methylxanthines	Aminophylline (IV)	50–250 mg at slow rate (50–100 mg over 30–60 s)	1–2 min	Abdominal pain, blurred vision, fainting	Not to be used in case of seizures
	Nitrates	Nitroglycerine (SL)	0.4 mg	5 min	Headache, blurred vision, fainting	Severe anemia, increased intracranial pressure, hypersensitivity to nitroglycerin
	Cardiopulmonary resuscitation maneuvers Transfer the patient to the emergency department					

Abbreviations: LV Left ventricle, *eGFR* estimated glomerular filtration rate, *CM* contrast media, *ATVS* automatic tube voltage selection

during CT-MPI are regadenoson and adenosine. Regadenoson has been shown to have a lower incidence of flushing and chest pain and higher incidence of abdominal discomfort and headache compared to adenosine [51]. Both stress agents have reported extremely rare but serious side effects such as seizures and myocardial infarction [52]. In cases where a patient experiences pharmacological stressor-induced seizures, the use of methylxanthines (aminophylline, theophylline, and caffeine) is not recommended [53, 54]. Moreover, it should be pointed out that some seizures can be prolonged and may require anticonvulsive therapy.

Patients affected by angina during a stress cardiac CT are somewhat fortunate in the sense that they are already hospitalized and can receive treatment almost immediately, avoiding the common delay of 1.5–2 h reported for patients that develop stress-induced angina outside of a hospital setting [55, 56]. Since the patient is ECG-monitored during the exam, any suspicious change in the baseline ECG, even if non-specific for myocardial ischemia, is immediately identifiable. Intravenous injection of aminophylline (50–250 mg) at a slow rate (50–100 mg over 30–60 s) is the first choice in cases of adverse side effects [57] and usually leads to resolution of the patient's symptoms.

Cases of asystole following regadenoson administration have been reported [58]. In such rare scenarios, CT personnel must be prepared to perform immediate cardiopulmonary resuscitation and medical stabilization. Rare cases of acute myocardial infarct up to 15 min after pharmacological stress test were also reported [59, 60] and are typically treated with sublingual nitroglycerine and intravenous administration of heparin and saline. IV atropine administration (0.5–1 mg) should also be considered. It is highly recommended that in the CT section, there is an availability of transcutaneous pacing for bradyarrhythmias or heart block associated with regadenoson or adenosine. Most importantly, patients suffering from rare but serious side effects must be transferred to the emergency department for comprehensive monitoring and further medical management.

Summary

The aforementioned scenarios represent just some of the challenges that can be observed around the CT scanner in everyday practice. Despite being coined a "challenge," the *challenging patient* represents an objective issue in clinical management. However, with the continuous technological and pharmacological advances in addition to an effective training of CT personnel, we are nowadays able to effectively face and overcome many of these issues, all in an effort to guarantee safe and adequate examinations for all patients.

References

1. Meinel FG, et al. Coronary computed tomographic angiography in clinical practice: state of the art. Radiol Clin N Am. 2015;53(2):287–96.
2. Takx RA, et al. Computed tomography-derived parameters of myocardial morphology and function in black and white patients with acute chest pain. Am J Cardiol. 2016;117(3):333–9.
3. Hoffmann U, et al. ACR appropriateness criteria acute nonspecific chest pain-low probability of coronary artery disease. J Am Coll Radiol. 2015;12(12 Pt A):1266–71.
4. Bastarrika G, et al. CT of coronary artery disease. Radiology. 2009;253(2):317–38.
5. Bastarrika G, Schoepf UJ. Evolving CT applications in ischemic heart disease. Semin Thorac Cardiovasc Surg. 2008;20(4):380–92.
6. von Ballmoos MW, et al. Meta-analysis: diagnostic performance of low-radiation-dose coronary computed tomography angiography. Ann Intern Med. 2011;154(6):413–20.
7. De Cecco CN, et al. Beyond stenosis detection: computed tomography approaches for determining the functional relevance of coronary artery disease. Radiol Clin N Am. 2015;53(2):317–34.
8. Ruzsics B, et al. Comparison of dual-energy computed tomography of the heart with single photon emission computed tomography for assessment of coronary artery stenosis and of the myocardial blood supply. Am J Cardiol. 2009;104(3):318–26.
9. Varga-Szemes A, et al. CT myocardial perfusion imaging. AJR Am J Roentgenol. 2015;204(3):487–97.
10. Caruso D, et al. Dynamic CT myocardial perfusion imaging. Eur J Radiol. 2016;85(10):1893–9.
11. Jin KN, et al. Myocardial perfusion imaging with dual energy CT. Eur J Radiol. 2016;85(10):1914–21.
12. Pelgrim GJ, et al. The dream of a one-stop-shop: meta-analysis on myocardial perfusion CT. Eur J Radiol. 2015;84(12):2411–20.
13. Flohr TG, et al. Computed tomographic assessment of coronary artery disease: state-of-the-art imaging techniques. Radiol Clin N Am. 2015;53(2):271–85.
14. Flohr TG, et al. Pushing the envelope: new computed tomography techniques for cardiothoracic imaging. J Thorac Imaging. 2010;25(2):100–11.
15. Taylor CM, Blum A, Abbara S. Patient preparation and scanning techniques. Radiol Clin N Am. 2010;48(4):675–86.
16. Schussler JM, Grayburn PA. Non-invasive coronary angiography using multislice computed tomography. Heart. 2007;93(3):290–7.
17. Kopp AF, et al. Coronary arteries: retrospectively ECG-gated multidetector row CT angiography with selective optimization of the image reconstruction window. Radiology. 2001;221(3):683–8.
18. Nieman K, et al. Coronary angiography with multi-slice computed tomography. Lancet. 2001;357(9256):599–603.
19. Fuchs TA, et al. Impact of a new motion-correction algorithm on image quality of low-dose coronary CT angiography in patients with insufficient heart rate control. Acad Radiol. 2014;21(3):312–7.
20. Yang L, et al. Prospectively ECG-triggered sequential dual-source coronary CT angiography in patients with atrial fibrillation: influence of heart rate on image quality and evaluation of diagnostic accuracy. PLoS One. 2015;10(7):e0134194.
21. Yin WH, et al. Detection of coronary artery stenosis with submilliSievert radiation dose by prospectively ECG-triggered high-pitch spiral CT angiography and iterative reconstruction. Eur Radiol. 2013;23(11):2927–33.
22. Zhang LJ, et al. Feasibility of prospectively ECG-triggered high-pitch coronary CT angiography with 30 mL iodinated contrast agent at 70 kVp: initial experience. Eur Radiol. 2014;24(7):1537–46.
23. Cecco CN, Schoepf UJ. Future of cardiac computed tomography. World J Radiol. 2015;7(12):421–3.
24. Mangold S, et al. Coronary CT angiography in obese patients using 3(rd) generation dual-source CT: effect of body mass index on image quality. Eur Radiol. 2016;26(9):2937–46.
25. Takx RA, et al. Sublingual nitroglycerin administration in coronary computed tomography angiography: a systematic review. Eur Radiol. 2015;25(12):3536–42.
26. Shim SS, Kim Y, Lim SM. Improvement of image quality with beta-blocker premedication on ECG-gated 16-MDCT coronary angiography. AJR Am J Roentgenol. 2005;184(2):649–54.
27. Celik O, et al. Single dose ivabradine versus intravenous metoprolol for heart rate reduction before coronary computed tomography angiography (CCTA) in patients receiving long-term calcium channel-blocker therapy. Acta Radiol. 2014;55(6):676–81.
28. Sabarudin A, Sun Z. Beta-blocker administration protocol for prospectively ECG-triggered coronary CT angiography. World J Cardiol. 2013;5(12):453–8.
29. Pannu HK, Alvarez W Jr, Fishman EK. Beta-blockers for cardiac CT: a primer for the radiologist. AJR Am J Roentgenol. 2006;186(6 Suppl 2):S341–5.
30. Vorre MM, Abdulla J. Diagnostic accuracy and radiation dose of CT coronary angiography in atrial fibrillation: systematic review and meta-analysis. Radiology. 2013;267(2):376–86.
31. National Institute for Health and Care Excellence (NICE). Ivabradine for treating chronic heart failure (NICE website). 2012. Published online at https://www.nice.org.uk/guidance/ta267/resources/ivabradine-for-treating-chronicheart-failure-pdf-82600557030853

32. Adile KK, et al. Safety and efficacy of oral ivabradine as a heart rate-reducing agent in patients undergoing CT coronary angiography. Br J Radiol. 2012;85(1016):e424–8.
33. Guaricci AI, et al. Incremental value and safety of oral ivabradine for heart rate reduction in computed tomography coronary angiography. Int J Cardiol. 2012;156(1):28–33.
34. Lambrechtsen J, Egstrup K. Pre-treatment with a sinus node blockade, ivabradine, before coronary CT angiography: a retrospective audit. Clin Radiol. 2013;68(10):1054–8.
35. Pichler P, et al. Ivabradine versus metoprolol for heart rate reduction before coronary computed tomography angiography. Am J Cardiol. 2012;109(2):169–73.
36. Bayraktutan U, et al. Efficacy of ivabradin to reduce heart rate prior to coronary CT angiography: comparison with beta-blocker. Diagn Interv Radiol. 2012;18(6):537–41.
37. Morsbach F, et al. Performance of turbo high-pitch dual-source CT for coronary CT angiography: first ex vivo and patient experience. Eur Radiol. 2014;24(8):1889–95.
38. Tao SM, et al. Contrast-induced nephropathy in CT: incidence, risk factors and strategies for prevention. Eur Radiol. 2016;26(9):3310–8.
39. Stacul F, et al. Contrast induced nephropathy: updated ESUR Contrast Media Safety Committee guidelines. Eur Radiol. 2011;21(12):2527–41.
40. Ohno I, et al. Guidelines on the use of iodinated contrast media in patients with kidney disease 2012: digest version: JSN, JRS, and JCS Joint Working Group. Clin Exp Nephrol. 2013;17(4):441–79.
41. Nozue T, et al. Contrast medium volume to estimated glomerular filtration rate ratio as a predictor of contrast-induced nephropathy developing after elective percutaneous coronary intervention. J Cardiol. 2009;54(2):214–20.
42. Yuan R, et al. Reduced iodine load at CT pulmonary angiography with dual-energy monochromatic imaging: comparison with standard CT pulmonary angiography–a prospective randomized trial. Radiology. 2012;262(1):290–7.
43. Zhang LJ, et al. High-pitch coronary CT angiography at 70 kVp with low contrast medium volume: comparison of 80 and 100 kVp high-pitch protocols. Medicine (Baltimore). 2014;93(22):e92.
44. Barrett JF, Keat N. Artifacts in CT: recognition and avoidance. Radiographics. 2004;24(6):1679–91.
45. Lee AM, et al. Coronary computed tomography angiography at 140 kV versus 120 kV: assessment of image quality and radiation exposure in overweight and moderately obese patients. Acta Radiol. 2014;55(5):554–62.
46. Gebhard C, et al. Image quality of low-dose CCTA in obese patients: impact of high-definition computed tomography and adaptive statistical iterative reconstruction. Int J Cardiovasc Imaging. 2013;29(7):1565–74.
47. Geyer LL, et al. State of the art: iterative CT reconstruction techniques. Radiology. 2015;276(2):339–57.
48. Mangold S, et al. Diagnostic accuracy of coronary CT angiography using 3rd-generation dual-source CT and automated tube voltage selection: clinical application in a non-obese and obese patient population. Eur Radiol. 2017 Jun;27(6):2298–308.
49. Jimenez-Juan L, et al. Failed heart rate control with oral metoprolol prior to coronary CT angiography: effect of additional intravenous metoprolol on heart rate, image quality and radiation dose. Int J Cardiovasc Imaging. 2013;29(1):199–206.
50. Maffei E, et al. "In-house" pharmacological management for computed tomography coronary angiography: heart rate reduction, timing and safety of different drugs used during patient preparation. Eur Radiol. 2009;19(12):2931–40.
51. Cerqueira MD, et al. Effects of age, gender, obesity, and diabetes on the efficacy and safety of the selective A2A agonist regadenoson versus adenosine in myocardial perfusion imaging integrated ADVANCE-MPI trial results. JACC Cardiovasc Imaging. 2008;1(3):307–16.
52. Kitt T, Jiang J. Serious complications associated with regadenoson administration for myocardial perfusion imaging. J Nucl Cardiol. 2015;22(2):395.
53. Agarwal V, DePuey EG. Regadenoson and seizures: a real clinical concern. J Nucl Cardiol. 2014;21(5):869–70.
54. Adenoscan [package insert]. Northbrook: I.A., Inc.; 1995. Updated in 2014.
55. Goldberg RJ, et al. Prehospital delay in patients with acute coronary syndromes (from the global registry of acute coronary events [GRACE]). Am J Cardiol. 2009;103(5):598–603.
56. Spencer FA, et al. Delay to reperfusion in patients with acute myocardial infarction presenting to acute care hospitals: an international perspective. Eur Heart J. 2010;31(11):1328–36.
57. Grady EC, Barron JT, Wagner RH. Development of asystole requiring cardiac resuscitation after the administration of regadenoson in a patient with pulmonary fibrosis receiving n-acetylcysteine. J Nucl Cardiol. 2011;18(3):521–5.
58. AlJaroudi WA, et al. Safety and tolerability of regadenoson in 514 SPECT MPI patients with and without coronary artery disease and submaximal exercise heart rate response. Eur J Nucl Med Mol Imaging. 2013;40(3):341–8.
59. Hsi DH, et al. Regadenoson induced acute ST-segment elevation myocardial infarction and multivessel coronary thrombosis. J Nucl Cardiol. 2013;20(3):481–4.
60. Shah S, Parra D, Rosenstein RS. Acute myocardial infarction during regadenoson myocardial perfusion imaging. Pharmacotherapy. 2013;33(6):e90–5.

13 Cardiac CT: Contemporary Clinical Image Data Display, Analysis, and Quantification

Moritz H. Albrecht, Marwen Eid, and Pal Spruill Suranyi

Why Do We Need "Advanced Visualization" and Quantification?

One of the most significant breakthroughs in cardiac CT imaging was being able to acquire isotropic resolution datasets with sufficient temporal resolution to take "snapshots" of this dynamic, ever-moving organ. Isotropic three-dimensional (3D) datasets acquired with either prospective triggering or retrospective gating, and further complicated by the dimension of time within the cardiac cycle, effectively yielding four-dimensional (4D) datasets, allow for a variety of post-processing techniques useful for advanced visualization of cardiovascular anatomy and pathology. Some of these techniques are fancy, colorful, and eye-pleasing or just serve as an aid to student or patient education, but others have become a crucial part of our clinical routine when evaluating cardiac CT images and discussing findings with non-radiology physicians.

Secondly, in the era of "precision medicine" and "imaging biomarkers," it is paramount to strive for more quantitative analysis of our findings. Thus, teasing out objective numbers and values from our large datasets is becoming increasingly important. Initially calcium scoring was the pioneer in quantitative cardiac evaluation. Since then various workstations and algorithms have been developed for routine clinical use to measure myocardial mass and function, to evaluate cardiac chamber sizes, and to assess coronary plaques and stenoses.

Lastly, as we are striving to understand the correlation between pathophysiology, qualitative and quantitative image findings, and patient outcomes, multiple investigational methods are still being developed, holding the promise of future clinical utility for myocardial perfusion imaging and analysis of coronary hemodynamics. In this chapter, we will briefly touch on each of these methods and will try to elucidate their diagnostic value and potential future clinical implementation.

Clinical Image Data Display and Analysis

3D Volume Rendering Techniques (VRT)

Although initially developed by the animation movie industry, 3D VRT reconstructions have been rapidly adopted in clinical medical imaging [1]. While the exact technical details are beyond the scope of this chapter, the general idea is that interactive probability-based algorithms and workstations build virtual 3D models of an organ using the 3D matrix of enhancement values by deciding whether a given volume element, i.e., voxel, belongs to an adjacent structure or not.

To stay on focus, this chapter will include all of these techniques under the umbrella of 3D VRT. However, it should be noted that there are fine nuances differentiating the various surface rendering techniques, e.g., shaded realistic surface displays (Fig. 13.1), and volume rendering approaches which can be further manipulated to generate fly-through or fly-around views of various organs [2]. Using creative display colors for different tissue types as well as various lighting methods and depth shading, these techniques enable the analysis of a dataset from any desired angle, including from within the vessel lumen. By changing the attenuation level-based visualization thresholds, one can hide or accentuate certain organs and tissue types or even make them semitransparent. In order to simplify the selection

M. H. Albrecht
Department of Diagnostic and Interventional Radiology, University Hospital Frankfurt, Frankfurt am Main, Germany

M. Eid
Division of Cardiovascular Imaging, Department of Radiology and Radiological Science, Medical University of South Carolina, Charleston, SC, USA

P. S. Suranyi (✉)
Division of Cardiovascular Imaging, Department of Radiology and Radiological Science, Medical University of South Carolina, Charleston, SC, USA

Division of Cardiology, Department of Medicine, Medical University of South Carolina, Charleston, SC, USA
e-mail: suranyi@musc.edu

U. J. Schoepf (ed.), *CT of the Heart*, Contemporary Medical Imaging, https://doi.org/10.1007/978-1-60327-237-7_13

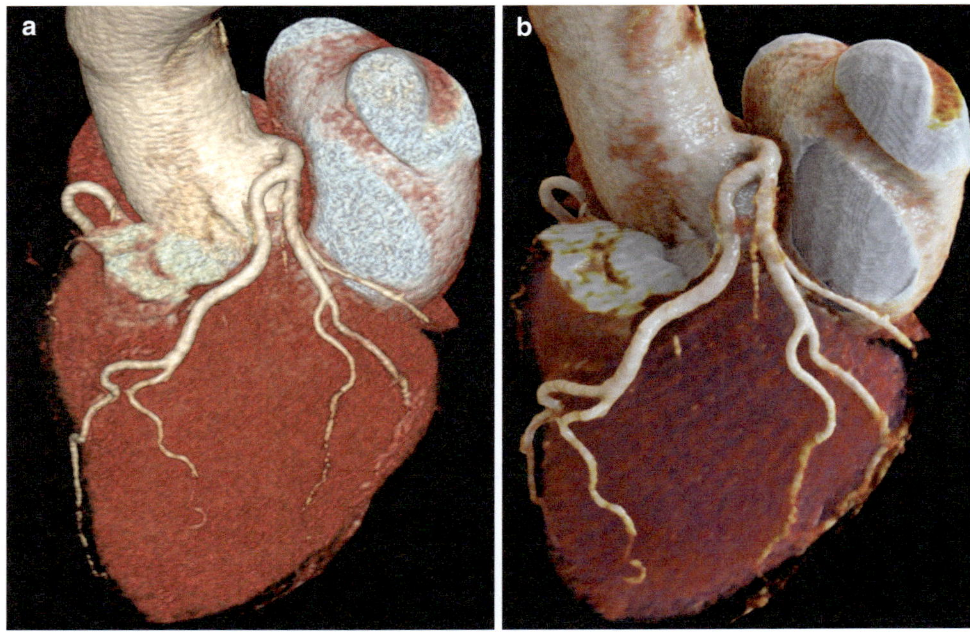

Fig. 13.1 Several approaches exist for 3D visualization of the heart and coronaries. While traditional 3D volume rendering technique (VRT) images (**a**) facilitate the orientation and anatomical relations to adjacent organs, novel cinematic rendering (**b**) allows furthermore for a photo-realistic appearance and analysis of the organ surfaces

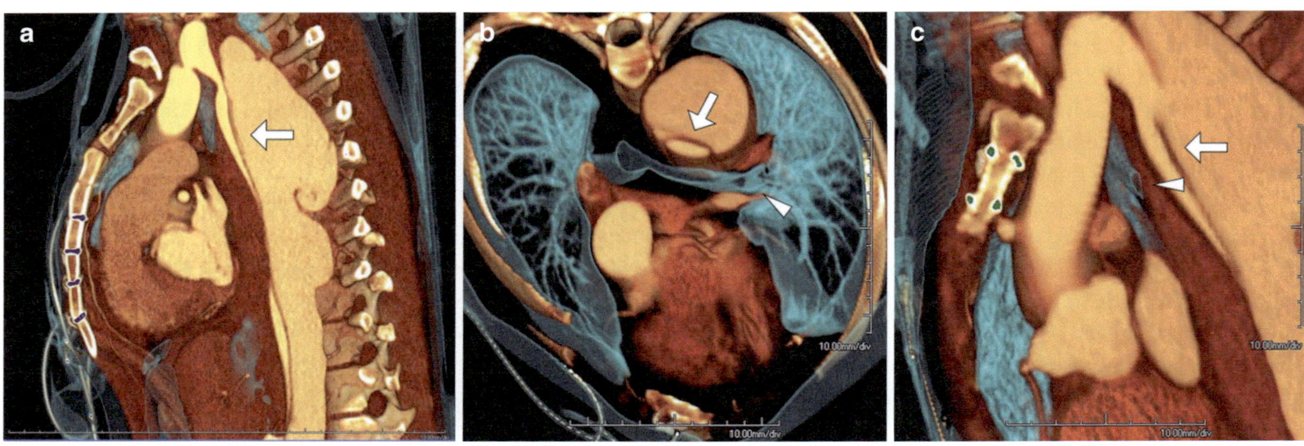

Fig. 13.2 3D reconstruction images displaying the utility of 3D VRT images in a patient with Marfan syndrome with prior history of ascending aorta repair (note sternal wires highlighted in purple, **a**), presenting with acute chest pain and shortness of breath. The sagittal image (**a**) shows a type-B aortic dissection (*arrow*). The oblique axial (**b**) and sagittal (**c**) images show the aneurysmal descending aorta (*arrow*) compressing on the left main bronchus (*arrowhead*). The various tissue types and metallic sternal wires can be clearly delineated by assigning different colors based on CT attenuation enabling us to demonstrate the relationship of airways to great vessels and the proximity of anterior structures to sternal wires

of the best technique for a given indication, workstations have presets stored for various purposes which often require further interactive manual adjustment by the reader.

Volume rendering of the heart and adjacent anatomic structures is helpful to obtain an overall understanding of the spatial relationship between organs, airways, the chest wall, and vascular pathologies (Fig. 13.2). 3D VRT is also beneficial in providing an overview of the quality of our datasets, especially in the case of arrhythmias or misregistrations, also called “step-offs,” which can be easily spotted in a 3D view.

When emphasizing vessels, however, one must understand that the goal of contrast media administration in cardiac CT is to improve the visualization of the vascular lumen rather than its surface. Also, when analyzing vessels with stents, 3D VRT shows the presence of the stent but does not show its content. Thus, 3D VRT cannot determine whether a stented vessel lumen is patent, occluded, or if it has intimal hyperplasia.

Further shortcomings of 3D VRT include locating the presence of calcifications, which may appear to be located on the surface of the vessel when in fact they are in the vessel wall. It is also important to note that motion artifacts and streak artifacts may cause artifactual vessel stenosis on 3D VRT, which may be misleading for beginners in cardiac CT. Therefore, experts do not recommend making diagnoses solely based on VRT reconstructions but advise using 3D VRT as an auxiliary technique to supplement standard cross-sectional images when making a diagnosis.

Automated, Semiautomated, or Manual Segmentation of the Heart

Sophisticated workstations offer the option for automatic segmentation of the heart, which virtually "removes" the rib-cage and the lungs to allow for 360-degree visualization of the heart's chambers and vessels. Such automated segmentation simplifies the visualization of routine cases, but semiautomated or manual segmentation is preferred when trying to analyze more challenging postsurgical cases or patients with unusual anatomies.

Unfortunately, automated segmentation algorithms may "remove" venous bypass grafts, the internal mammary arteries, or parts thereof, which may lead to the erroneous diagnosis of occluded bypass grafts. Similarly, human observers may inadvertently "remove" vessel segments or create "nicks" in vessels during post-processing when generating the volume-rendered segmented heart, thus causing potential problems for interpretation. This is why most experts strongly emphasize looking at the "source images" whenever a 3D VRT image suggests abnormal pathology.

The alternative to segmenting out the heart is to look at the entire 3D dataset using a cut plane or a slab, which allows the user to scroll through the organs in the chest in 3D while also making sure that no structures remain hidden due to erroneous segmentation (Fig. 13.3).

Dedicated Cardiac Planes, MPR, and Thick-MPR

Multi-planar reformatting (MPR) images represent the standard cross-sectional reconstructions in cardiac CT. A 3D or 4D dataset with essentially isotropic resolution allows one to arbitrarily choose the ideal plane when studying the heart. Whether it is one of the standard long- and short-axis planes (Fig. 13.4) or a more dedicated view such as one showing the aortic valve leaflets or any other structure of interest, this can be performed at a workstation in a matter of seconds using MPR of the original source imaging data. Thus, a "simple" MPR image shows the reconstructed data in arbitrary non-axial planes with a thickness of one voxel. These views are useful in performing anatomic measurements in vessels or valves or within the chambers.

Most workstations also offer the option of generating "thick-MPRs," which consist of virtually thickened CT slices that improve the signal-to-noise ratio in compromised datasets and help visualize structures that may be moving in and out of the imaging plane during the cardiac cycle (e.g., aortic valve). Furthermore, thick-MPRs are also useful if structures have both high- and low-density components, e.g., a sclerotic aortic valve with superimposed vegetation or thrombus (Fig. 13.5).

Curved MPR, Stretched MPR, and MAR

The basic principle of curved MPR (cMPR) is similar to that of linear MPR in that it uses the reconstructed dataset without additional manipulation of the Hounsfield units (HU) but still allows for the close-up analysis of vessels. The key feature of cMPR is the "centerline," which is either automatically or semiautomatically predetermined. Subsequently, the dataset is reformatted with resulting images showing data that is perpendicular to this centerline. It is paramount that the centerline should go through the vessel lumen, because otherwise the vessel may appear artifactually stenosed. Thus, before actually examining the cMPRs, one must carefully check – and if needed, adjust – the centerline. Normally there are two cMPR images displayed next to each other, where one is perpendicular to the other and both are perpendicular to the centerline. This dataset can then be manually "swiveled" about the centerline to look at all possible aspects of a vessel and take a closer look at any particular vessel segment of interest (Fig. 13.6).

In this context, it is important to emphasize the relevance of the window/level settings when studying vessels with stenosis, especially with the presence of calcifications or implanted stents. The apparent size of the calcified lesions greatly depends on the window/level settings, as shown in Fig. 13.7. Therefore, when stents or calcifications are present and cause blooming artifacts, it is important to take a second look at the vessel after "darkening" the image prior to making a diagnosis. This can be achieved by widening the window settings, which reduces the influence of blooming artifacts that can potentially lead to an overestimation of luminal narrowing.

A second caveat to remember is that stents and calcified vessel segments are better evaluated using a sharper reconstruction kernel and iterative reconstruction techniques. Unfortunately, these need to be applied at the time of reconstructing the axial datasets from the raw imaging data [3] (Figs. 13.8 and 13.9).

Another capability of the above technique is that the centerline's natural curves can be virtually stretched, resulting in sMPR images ("s" for stretched or straight). However, some experts consider this method too unnatural and vulnerable to over manipulation. Additionally, multiple aligned reformats can be generated by combining the cMPRs of multiple vessels. This technique uses

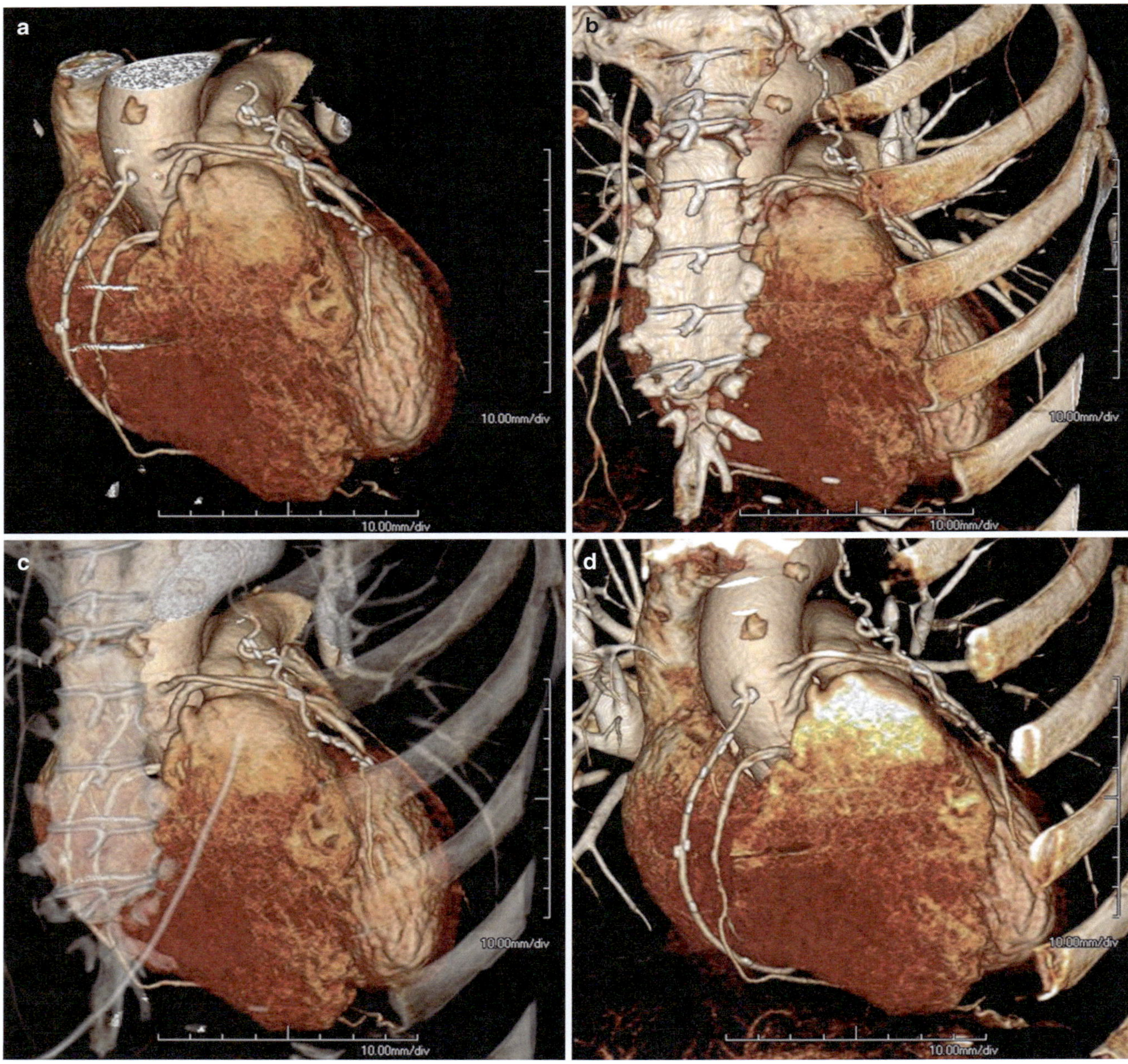

Fig. 13.3 3D reconstruction of the heart in a patient after coronary arterial bypass graft (CABG) surgery. The heart can be automatically segmented (**a**) and isolated from the remaining structures; however, this technique sometimes artificially removes important parts of the anatomy, like the proximal aspect of the LIMA graft in this case. Unfortunately, the heart and grafts cannot be seen in their entirety on the full volume either, due to overlying ribs and sternum. (**b**) The solution is a semitransparent (**c**) rib cage or a clip plane/slab, which both can visualize structures obscured by the chest wall (**d**), without losing information, thus reducing the likelihood of misinterpretation

the same principles as cMPR but aims to depict several vessel paths simultaneously by taking into account the multiple centerlines of multiple vessels. This technique provides an overview of the coronary anatomy and may prove useful in planning the placement of multiple stents near bifurcations.

The efficient segmentation of the coronary tree can provide us with a quick overall understanding of the blood supply routes of the myocardium. The coronary tree may then be projected onto polar maps of regional function or perfusion (Fig. 13.10), which has the added benefit of being able to "pair" vessel-specific stenosis with corresponding regional myocardial dysfunction or perfusion abnormality.

Projection Techniques

Maximum and minimum intensity projections are obtained when a 3D slab of the original reconstructed dataset is taken (more than one voxel in thickness) and a single two-

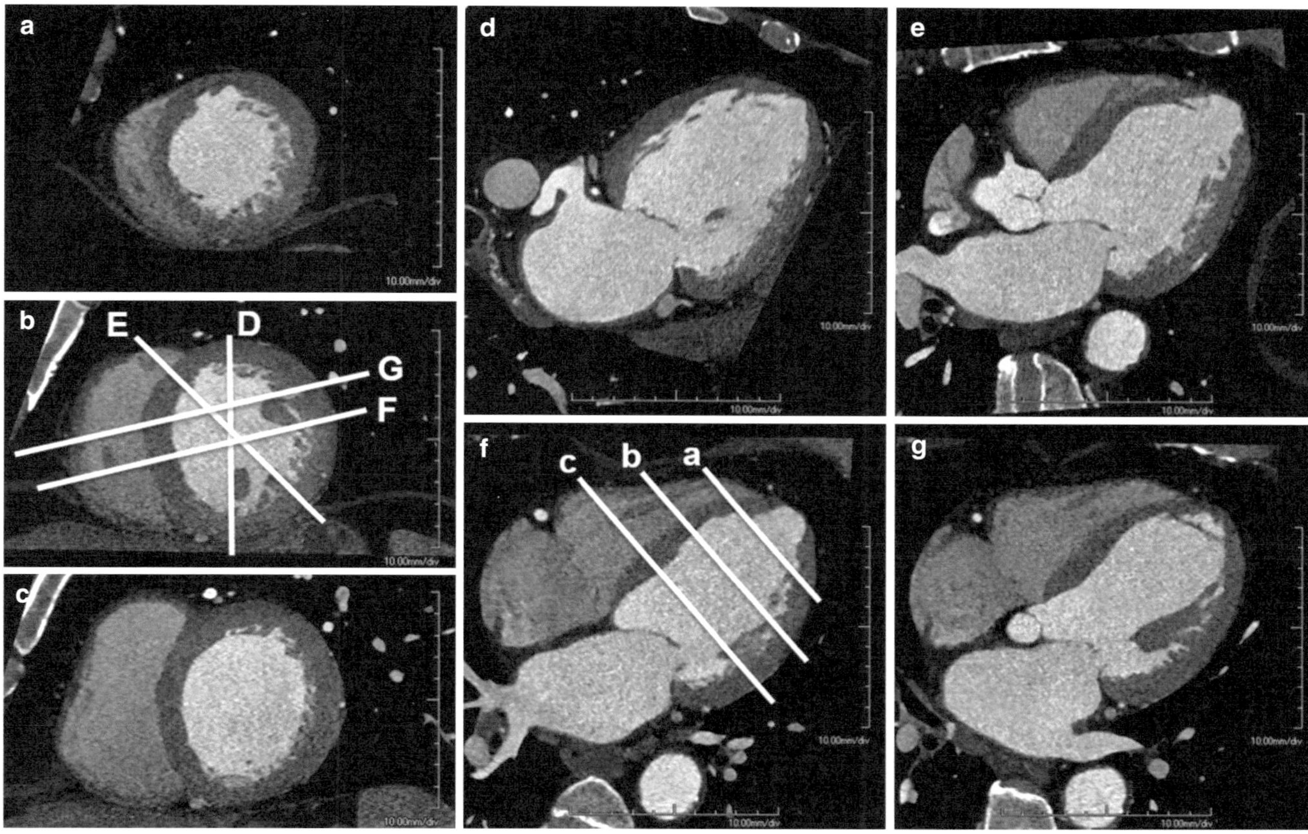

Fig. 13.4 This figure shows the standard planes for cardiac CT evaluation. As the cardiac axis is highly variable in every individual, conventional radiological axial, sagittal, and coronal images are not optimal for assessment of the heart. Manual adjustment on a 3D workstation is necessary to define true long and short axes of the heart. The spatial correlation among the short-axis (**a**, apical; **b**, mid; **c**, basal), 2-chamber (**d**), 3-chamber (**e**), 4-chamber (**f**), and 5-chamber views (**g**) is demonstrated here by white reference lines

dimensional image is generated. This can be performed by either taking only the lowest (minimum intensity projection (MINIP)) or only the highest attenuation (maximum intensity projection (MIP)) across the slab. An additional technique called average intensity projection (AIP), also called "thick-MPR" as previously described, uses the average attenuation values of all voxels across the slab.

MIP

Thin (<10 mm) and thick (>10 mm) MIPs are most useful for the assessment of vessels or bypass grafts when the contrast medium-filled lumen is of high interest. MIPs facilitate the tracking of the vessel paths, bifurcation analysis, and the evaluation of the length of stenotic segments. It is worth mentioning that some workstations have the capability to generate curved MIP images (cMIP), which uses the same principles as cMPR except that the end result is a MIP that is perpendicular to the centerline throughout the length of a given vessel. Although MIP is very useful for the aforementioned purposes, care must be taken when using it to assess the severity of vessel stenosis due to its potential to mislead the observer and cause over- or underestimation of stenosis. Thus, for the quantification of stenosis, it is most appropriate to use either the source images or cMPR images. An additional shortcoming of only using MIPs is the potential to "miss" low-density lesions such as small emboli, intimal flaps, abnormal valve apparatus (e.g., ruptured chordae), or even myocardial hypoattenuation.

MINIP

When the structures of interest are of low attenuation, it is helpful to use MINIPs, which may reveal pathologies that would be too subtle, if not invisible when using MPRs or MIPs. Examples include ischemic regions of the myocardium, infarcted areas, fatty infiltration of the myocardium, valves, chordae tendineae, papillary muscles, vegetations, thrombi or dissection membranes, and even airways. Figure 13.11 provides an example where MINIP, MPR, and MIP are compared side by side.

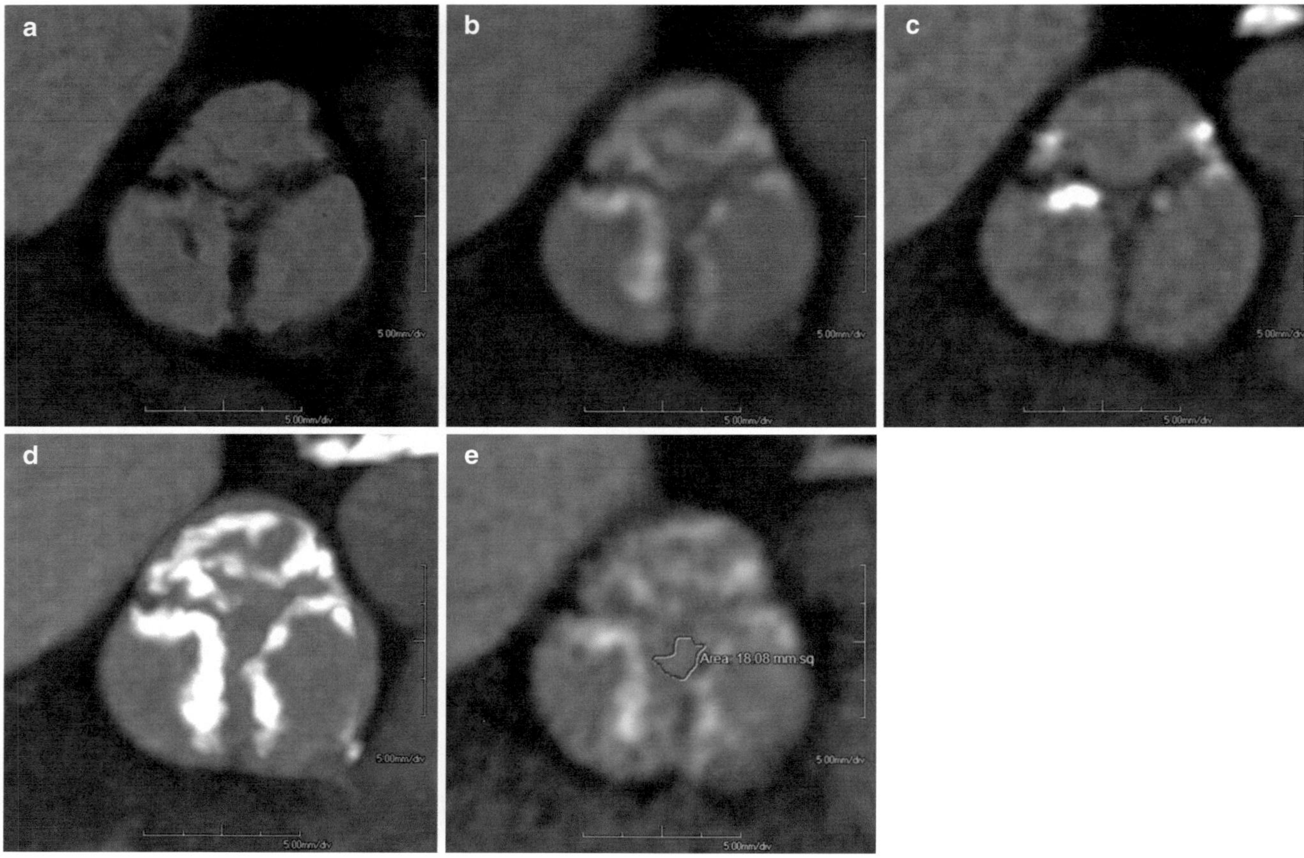

Fig. 13.5 Varying cross-sectional visualization techniques lead to different depictions of a calcified and stenotic aortic valve. (**a**) Minimum intensity projection (MINIP), showing only low-density portions of the valve. (**b**) Thick multi-planar reformat (thick-MPR) shows all portions of the valve but is blurry due to volume averaging. (**c**) Standard MPR, with high spatial resolution, does not show the entirety of the valve and the true extent of disease. (**d**) Maximum intensity projection (MIP) highlighting calcifications but hiding noncalcified portions of the valve. (**e**) Valve orifice measurement on the thick-MPR

Quantification

In addition to the relatively well-established contemporary clinical image data display and analyzing techniques, the field of objective image quantification is rapidly growing and represents the most investigated topic in state-of-the-art cardiac CT.

Calcium Scoring

Coronary artery calcium scoring, also known as Agatston scoring, is the most validated method for the prediction of patient outcome and risk stratification and has substantially enhanced the utility of cardiac CT imaging. In a standardized fashion, the Agatston score is semiautomatically calculated based on two parameters: the area of calcified coronary plaques with an attenuation greater than 130 HU on an ECG-synchronized noncontrast cardiac CT and a density factor which is based on the maximal attenuation of the same plaque. Using an online calculator based on the Multi-Ethnic Study of Atherosclerosis (MESA) study (https://www.mesa-nhlbi.org/Calcium/input.aspx), patients can be assigned to standardized risk categories with a low user-dependent variability compared to purely subjective or qualitative CT analysis. More advanced quantitative methods include calcium volume and density scores, and the hope is that fully automated Agatston scoring may be available in the near future [4]. Further details regarding Agatston scoring are discussed in another chapter of this book.

Coronary Stenosis Quantification/Fractional Flow Reserve

Workstations have evolved to the point where algorithms based on attenuation levels within the coronary lumen allow us to quantitatively evaluate vessel stenosis [5, 6]. Currently, this is performed in a semiautomated fashion in which the observer defines the segment of interest by placing a mark just proximal to the starting point of the plaque and another just beyond the distal end of the plaque using cMPR images

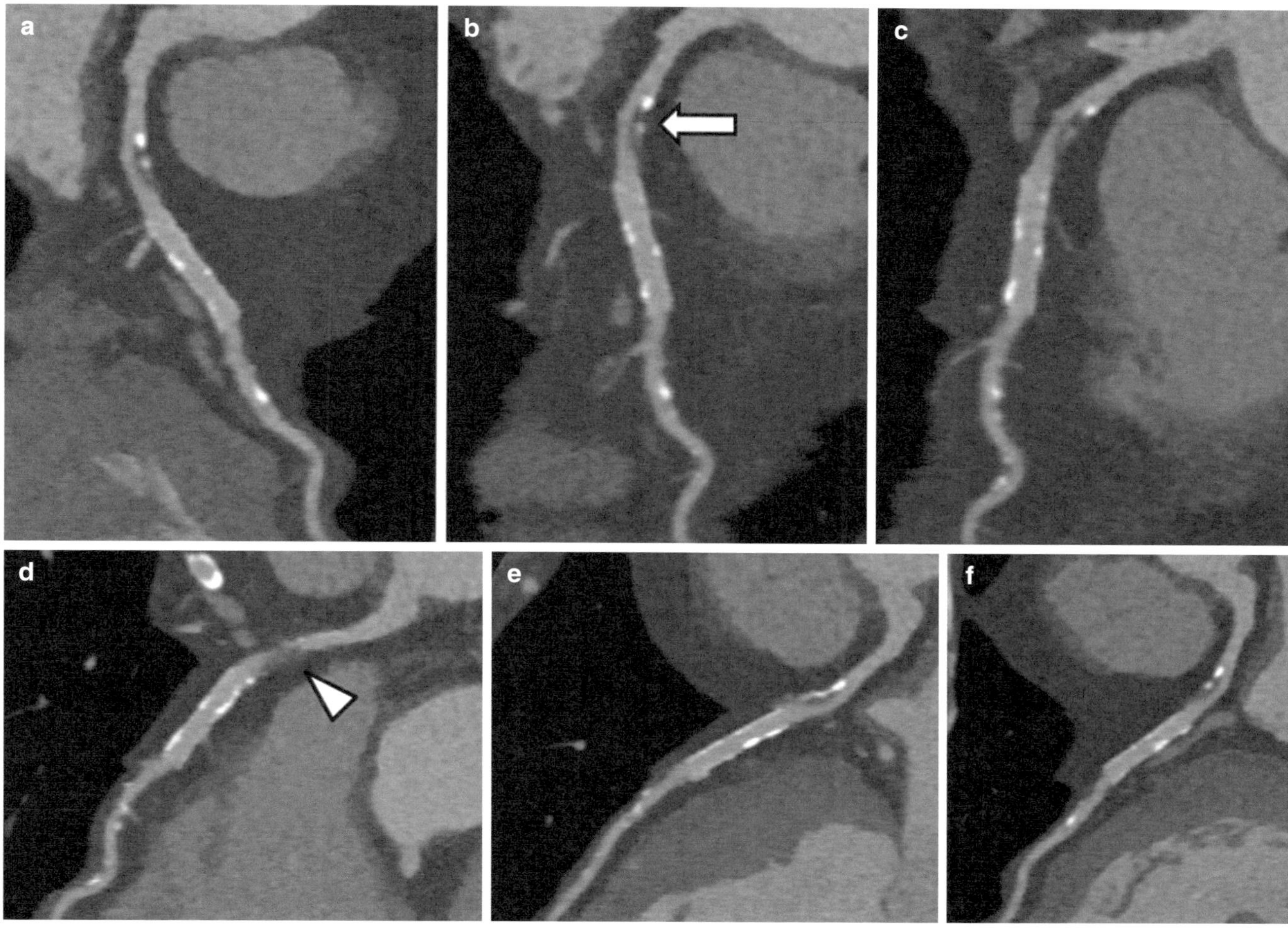

Fig. 13.6 The assessment of curved multi-planar reformat (cMPR) images from multiple views is crucial for accurate coronary artery evaluation. Varying angulations, achieved by manual swiveling around the coronary centerline, reveal different details of a coronary stenosis (*arrow*) with mixed calcified and soft-plaque of the LAD proximal to an implanted stent. Note that the severity of luminal narrowing could be over- or underestimated by only examining one cMPR image (**d**, *arrowhead*). The full extent of this mixed calcified-noncalcified plaque, and its effect on the lumen, is best understood when all different projections are considered. Figure (**d**) accentuates the noncalcified portion (*arrowhead*) and makes the stenosis appear more severe than it really is. (**a**), (**b**), (**c**), (**e**), and (**f**) demonstrate the mixed nature of the plaque and less severe stenosis

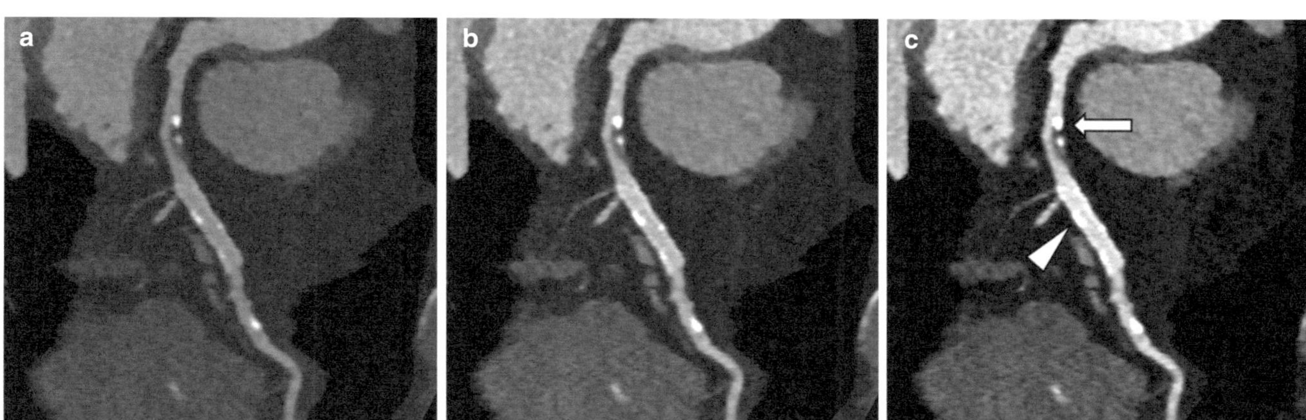

Fig. 13.7 cMPR images of a diseased LAD show the effect of adjusted window/level settings on the apparent size of calcifications within a significant stenotic lesion. Both window width decreases and level increases from image (**a**) to (**c**). The calcifications are overestimated using narrower and brighter window settings due to blooming artifacts (**c**, *arrow*). The same effect can be observed for an implanted stent (*arrowhead*). This highlights the necessity of widening preset settings for improved luminal visualization in the presence of calcified plaque or stents

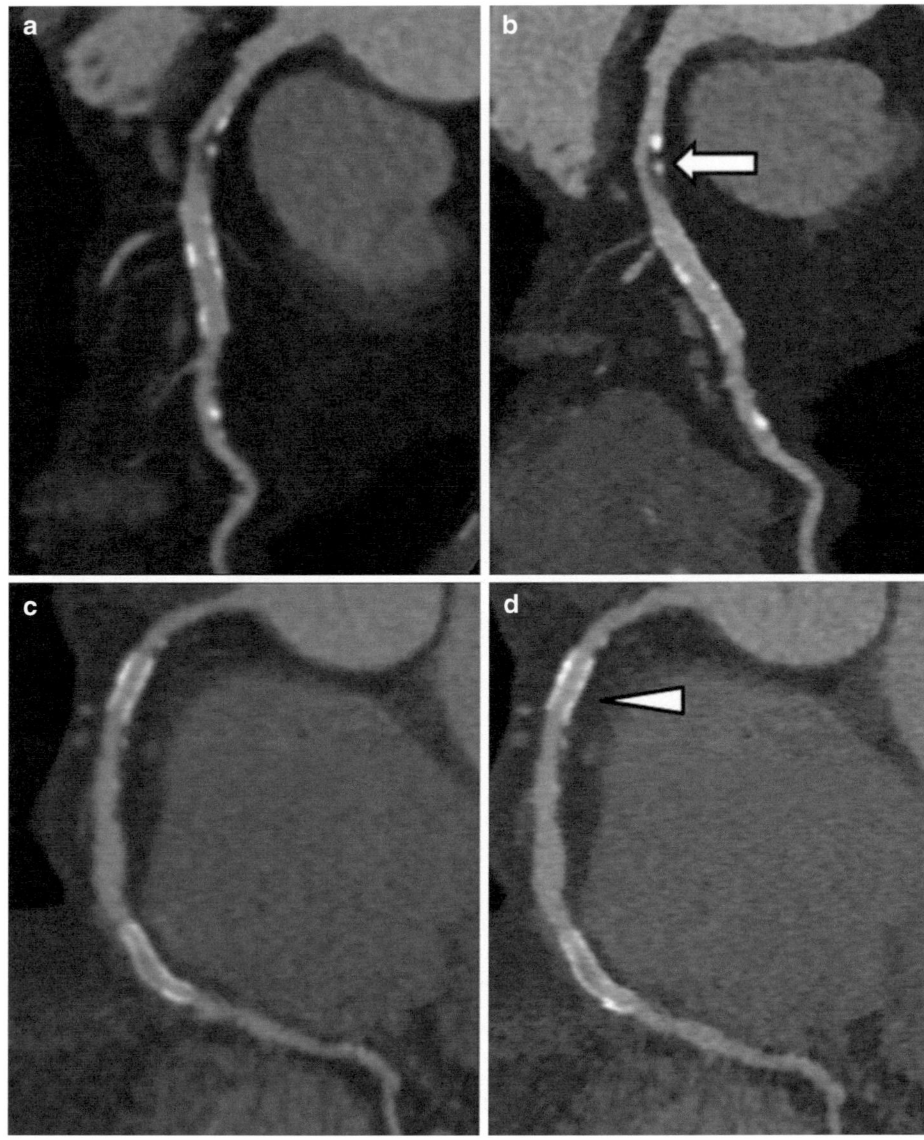

Fig. 13.8 In this patient, post-processing was performed using filtered back projection (**a** and **c**), as well as with iterative reconstruction (**b** and **d**). A mixed stenosing plaque of the LAD (*arrow*) and a coronary stent in the RCA (*arrowhead*) are more sharply depicted by means of iterative reconstruction, whereas filtered back projection images show a grainier image appearance and blurry coronary lumen

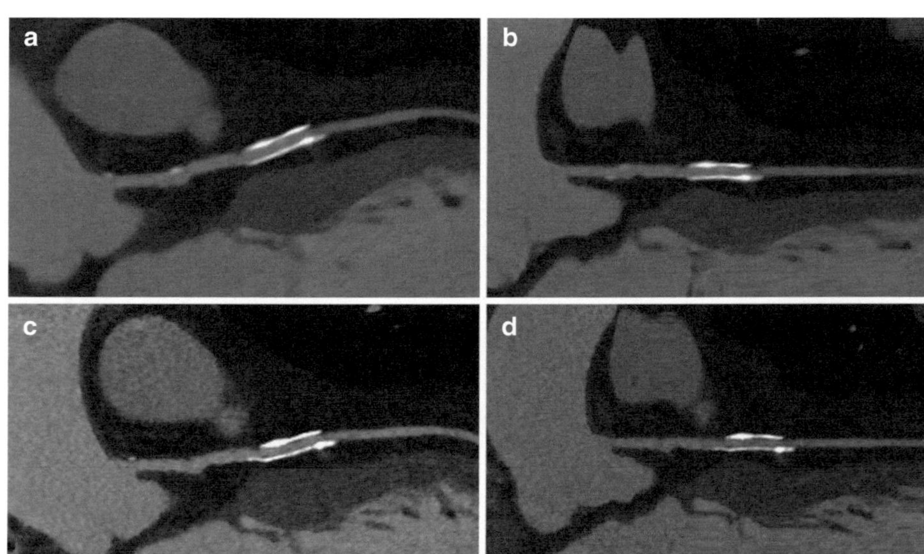

Fig. 13.9 In this patient, an LAD stent is visualized on a cMPR (**a**) and a sMPR (**b**), both of which are based on *soft tissue kernel* reconstructions. The same coronary is then depicted using a dataset reconstructed with *stent (sharp) kernel* on cMPR (**c**) and sMPR (**d**). The coronary stent is more sharply depicted by means of the stent kernel reducing blooming artifacts and increasing our ability to detect subtle intimal hyperplasia in the midportion of the stent

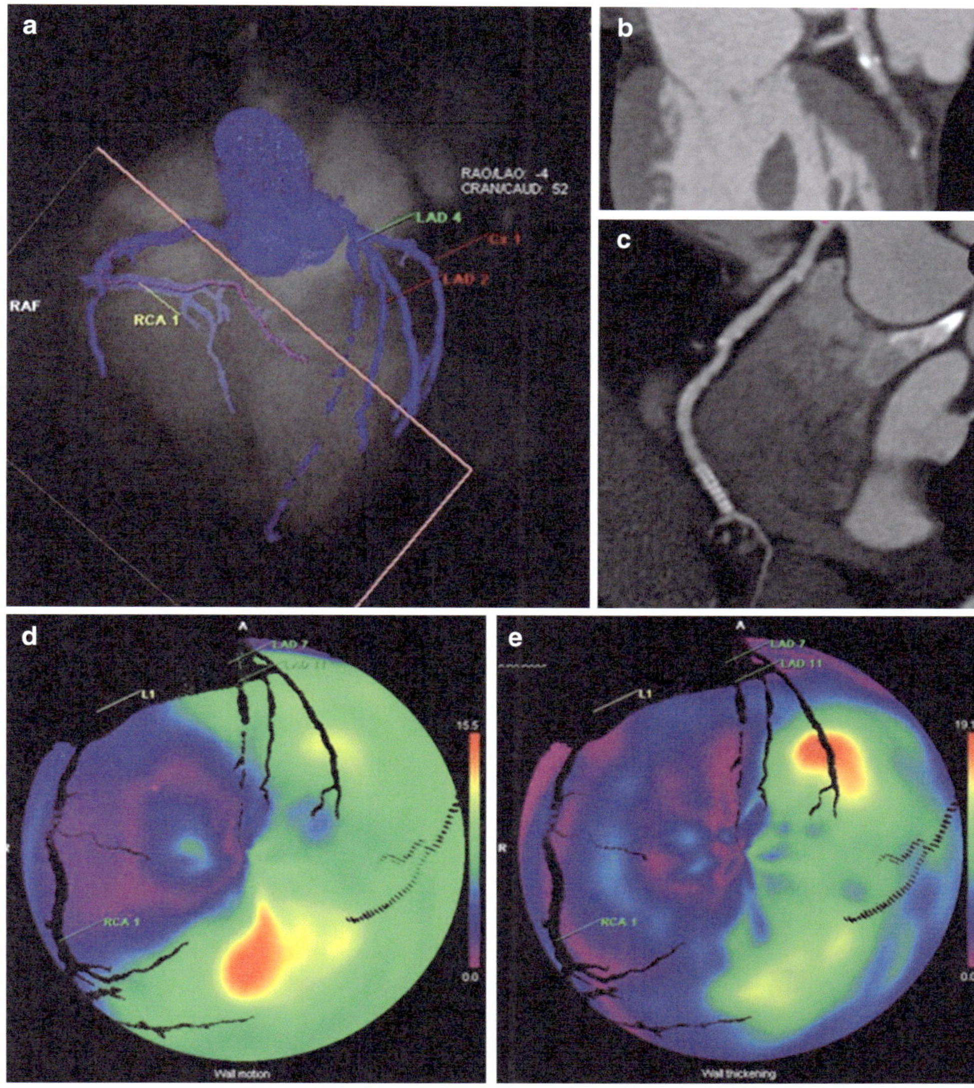

Fig. 13.10 Segmentation and evaluation of the coronary tree (**a**) of this patient revealed subtotal occlusion of the LAD (cMPR, **b**) and severely diseased, stented RCA (cMPR, **c**). By projecting the coronary tree onto polar maps of regional function obtained from the functional CT dataset (wall motion, **d**; wall thickening, **e**), the significance of coronary disease and consequent functional impairment (shown in cold colors) becomes apparent

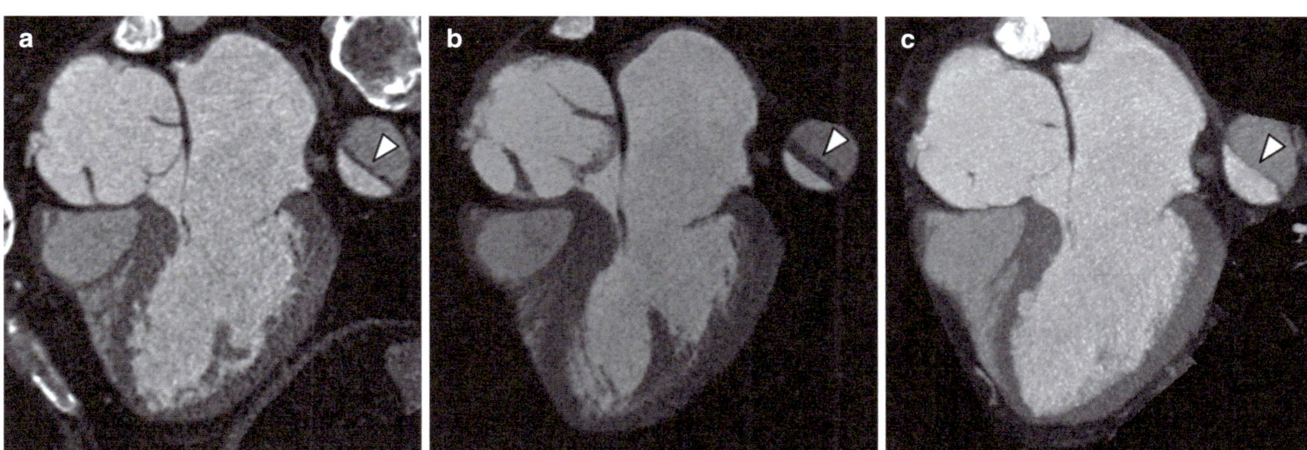

Fig. 13.11 (**a**–**c**) Three-chamber views applying MPR (0.75 mm), MINIP (10 mm), and MIP (10 mm) algorithms of the same location of a patient with aortic dissection. Note that hypoattenuating structures such as valves or dissection membranes (*arrowheads*) are best visualized with MINIP while they are almost invisible on MIP images

(see above). Some workstations will also ask for the user to mark the point of maximal stenosis in the vessel of interest. However, defining the point of maximal stenosis is often difficult due to the presence of bifurcations, calcifications, and potentially motion artifacts that may cause erroneous measurements.

Therefore, automated stenosis quantification using cardiac multi-detector CT (MDCT) data is a controversial issue, despite the fact that some investigators have shown that specialized software may be just as efficient as visual grading or invasive coronary angiography with regard to quantitative analysis [6, 7]. Many studies have demonstrated the outstanding negative predictive value of MDCT [8, 9]. However, the accurate determination of whether a stenotic lesion causes myocardial ischemia remains a challenge. Even if our images and anatomic stenosis quantification methods were impeccable, simulating the hemodynamic characteristics over a narrowed coronary is incredibly complex and is dependent on numerous additional factors beyond the extent of stenosis. For example, stenosis length, lesion geometry, blood viscosity, blood pressure, heart rate, myocardial mass, and peripheral resistance in the capillary bed are all contributing factors to determining the hemodynamic significance of a lesion. In an effort to standardize stenosis-severity reporting, a new reporting system (CAD-RADS) has just been published [10]. This system stratifies patients into risk categories and provides the probability that the source of observed chest pain is visible in the epicardial coronary arteries using CTA. The current consensus is that a radiologist – whose decision is based solely on anatomic imaging – is unable to definitively assess the hemodynamic significance of a lesion and should defer their diagnosis to the treating clinicians who should ultimately exercise clinical judgment to decide between discharge, observation, functional stress testing, and invasive catheterization.

An emerging technique of CT-derived fractional flow reserve (CT-FFR) is gaining increasing interest by using computational fluid dynamic models to quantify stenosis severity and to "simulate" how a coronary would respond to vasodilator stress testing. In general, FFR describes the decrease of blood pressure over a coronary stenosis and thus indicates the hemodynamic relevance of a lesion. Notably, current CT-FFR algorithms are based on normal static CCTA datasets and can be retrospectively employed in addition to the standard examination when more information is required [11]. To date, CT-FFR is performed mainly by outsourcing CCTA images to off-site, specialized core labs. This method takes the purely anatomic imaging a step further to virtual physiologic testing but is still highly dependent on the quality of anatomic data acquired (Fig. 13.12).

Plaque Composition Analysis

Current approaches to plaque composition analysis are still mainly investigational tools used in research projects; however, these techniques hold great promise for future CCTA evaluation and subsequent risk stratification [12]. Using threshold limits for various plaque components allows for the differentiation and volumetric determination of calcified, dominantly fibrous, and lipid-rich plaque components and provides the cardiac imager with quantitative measurements (Fig. 13.13). Analogous to the quantification of total calcified plaque burden in the context of calcium/Agatston scoring described above, these techniques may allow for more comprehensive and robust

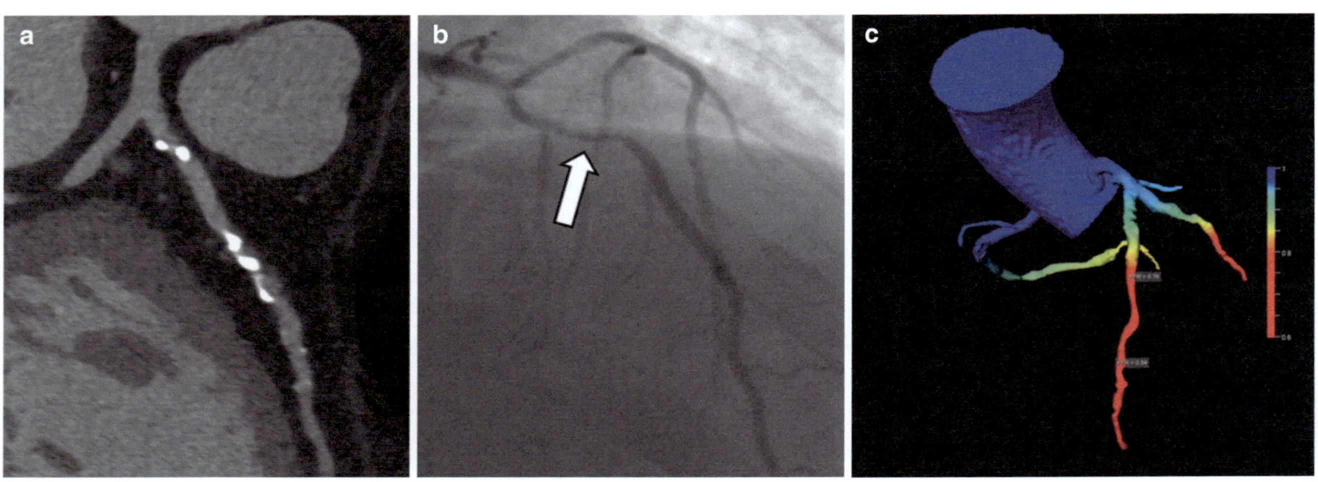

Fig. 13.12 While a stenotic calcified lesion of the LAD is clearly depicted using only cMPR images (**a**) and invasive catheterization (*arrow* in **b**), the assessment of its hemodynamic relevance remains uncertain. By means of retrospective CT-FFR calculation (**c**), this limitation can be overcome. A CT-FFR of 0.76 was shown, with almost perfect agreement to invasive FFR measurement of 0.75, an indication of a flow-restrictive coronary stenosis. (Courtesy of Christian Tesche, MD, Medical University of South Carolina, Charleston, SC, USA)

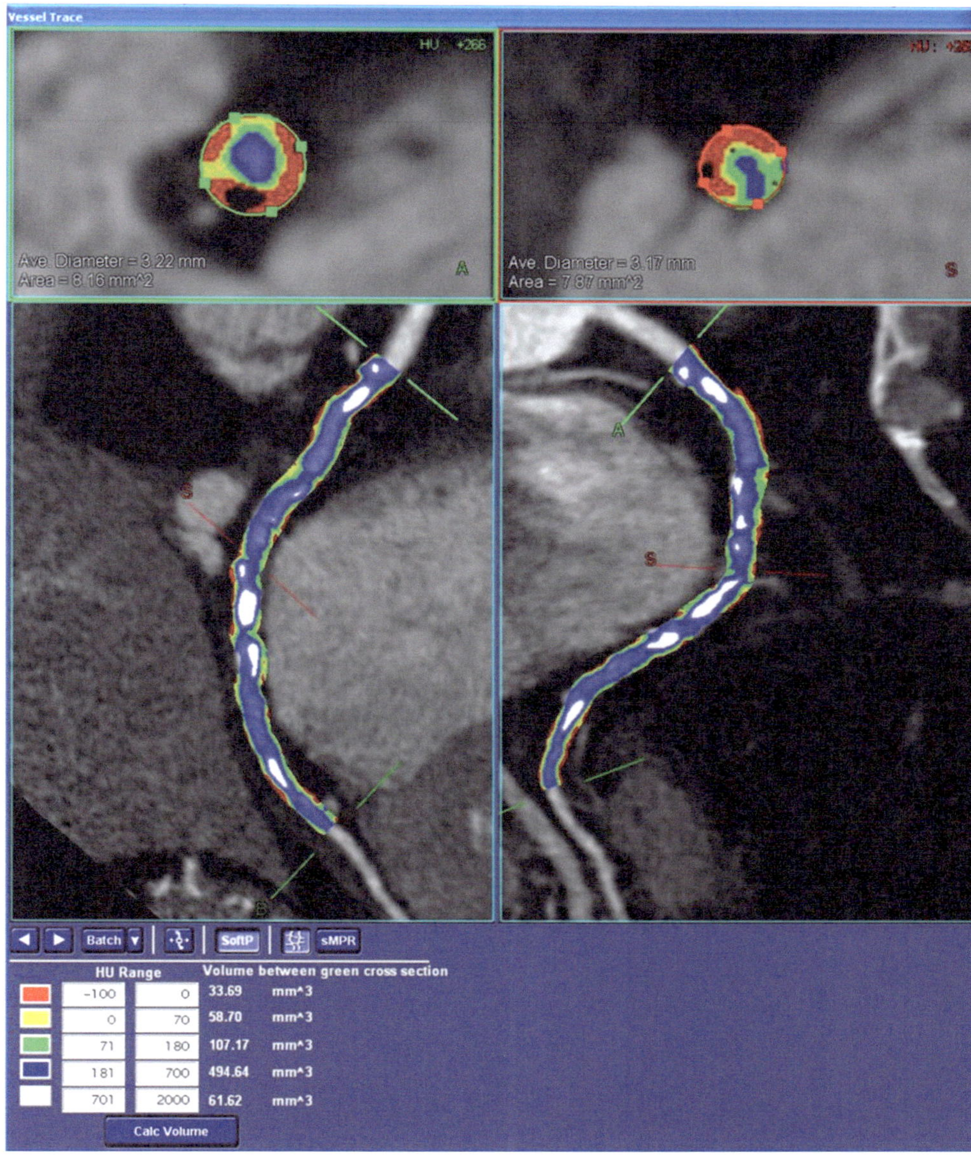

Fig. 13.13 Entire vessel plaque burden measurement using user-defined thresholds for lumen (blue), lipid-rich plaques (yellow), fibrous plaques (green), and calcifications (white). Epicardial fat and severely fatty plaques appear red

evaluation of CCTA examinations by providing quantitative results on the total lipid-rich versus fibrous plaque burden. Figure 13.13 demonstrates the processing steps of VRT, MIP, cMPR, and plaque analysis in a patient with calcified and noncalcified plaque components. Other than quantitative approaches, qualitative criteria for plaque composition and vulnerability have also been described in the literature [13].

Chamber Volumes and Ejection Fraction

The assessment of cardiac chamber dimensions and ejection fraction is an important diagnostic tool for managing patients with heart disease and making clinical decisions regarding device implantation and catheter-based or surgical interventions. Although the temporal resolution of cardiac CTA is sub-par relative to MRI or echocardiography, in patients where the first-line modalities fail or are contraindicated, CTA becomes an important surrogate to assess biventricular size and function. Various post-processing software which offer semiautomated and automated applications for volumetric analysis of cardiac chambers have become widely adopted in clinical workflows (Fig. 13.14). Most software use a combination of thresholding and contour-detection algorithms to delineate the actual complex shape of cardiac chambers, offering a tremendous advantage over conventional 2D echocardiography which mainly uses geometrical assumptions.

Quantification of ventricular chamber volumes is not only useful in assessing global systolic function and ventricular dilation but can also be utilized in assessing regurgitant frac-

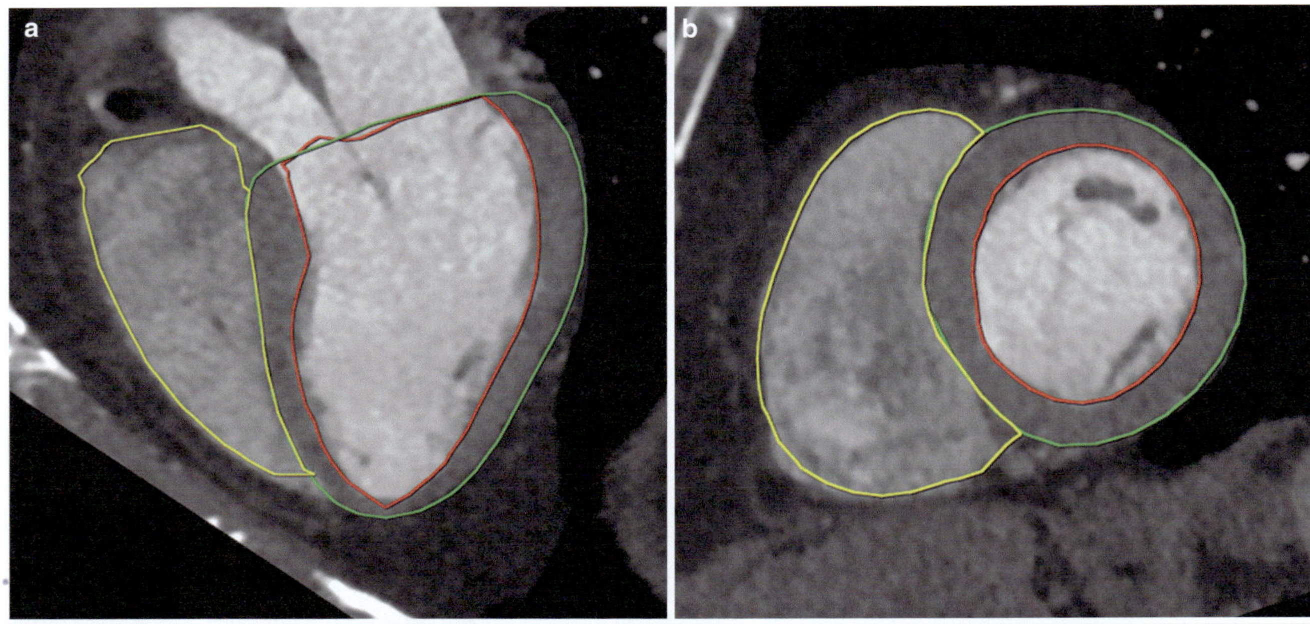

c Blood Vol. Mode		LV	RV	Normal Values
Ejection Fraction	%	64	47	47 - 80
Myocardial Mass ED	g	119.57	-	24 - 55
Stroke Volume	ml	60.03	60.05	33 - 98
ED Volume	ml	93.92	127.64	58 - 154
ES Volume	ml	33.89	67.6	23 - 103
Cursor Volume	ml	93.92	127.64	
Cardiac Output	(l/min)	5.7	5.7	2.82 - 8.82

Height:	165	cm	5	ft	5	in	Sex:	Female
Weight:	75	kg	165	lbs			BSA / m²	1.85

Fig. 13.14 Myocardial function analysis. Long- (**a**) and short-axis (**b**) views of the heart showing the segmentation of the right ventricle (yellow line) and left ventricle (red and green lines) for function analysis. Subsequently, a table with the different volumetric values is generated (**c**), providing the cardiac imager with quantitative data to assess global cardiac function, myocardial mass, and ventricular volumes

tion or pulmonic to systemic flow (Qp/Qs) in patients with valve disease or shunts.

As with any other post-processing technique, there are certain caveats one should bear in mind before "blindly" accepting the automatically generated results. The data are only as good as the source images, and the results will be influenced by overall image quality, i.e., temporal resolution, partial coverage of the cardiac cycle, signal-to-noise and contrast-to-noise relationships, streak artifacts from devices, motion artifacts, misregistrations due to arrhythmia, or patient motion. Moreover, erroneous segmentation of the chamber vs. myocardium, inclusion of atria or outflow tracts, and the faulty delineation of valve levels can all lead to an incorrect estimation of cardiac volumes (Fig. 13.15).

Assessment of the Myocardium, Regional Function, and Epicardial Fat

Hypertrophic cardiomyopathy, hypertension, and aortic stenosis are the most common causes of myocardial "overgrowth." By delineating endo- and epicardial contours, the total left ventricular myocardial mass can be determined, which can be helpful to assess disease severity and prognosis. If the contouring is performed for both end-diastole and end-systole, objective and quantitative parameters of regional function can be obtained (such as wall thickening, wall motion, segmental ejection fraction), which may help in identifying vessel territories with impaired blood supply (Fig. 13.16). However, in routine clinical practice, the traditional subjective, visual inspection of regional wall motion

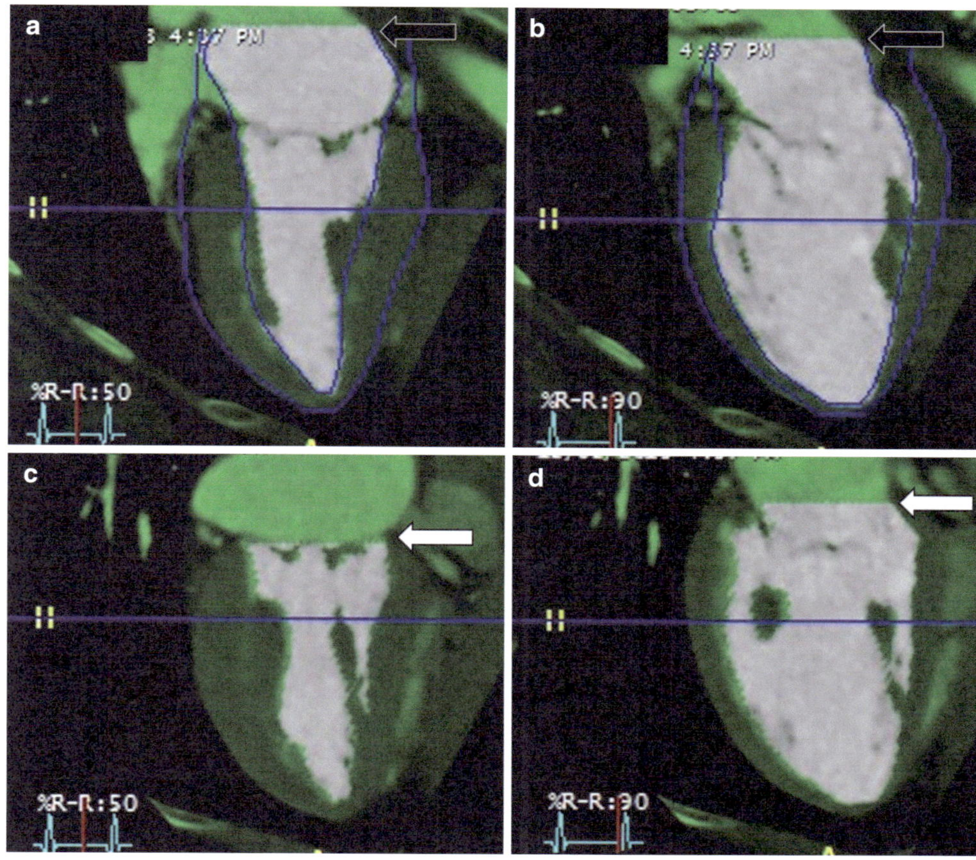

Fig. 13.15 It is crucial to visually assess the segmentation provided by automated software algorithms to avoid erroneous functional measurements. Automatically segmented images are demonstrated in systole (**a** and **c**) and diastole (**b** and **d**). In this particular case, the initial segmentation (**a** and **b**) included large parts of the left atrium (*black arrows*), and this leads to marked underestimation of the ejection fraction (38%). After manual adjustment of the mitral valve level (*white arrows*), the ejection fraction was calculated to be 70%, within normal range

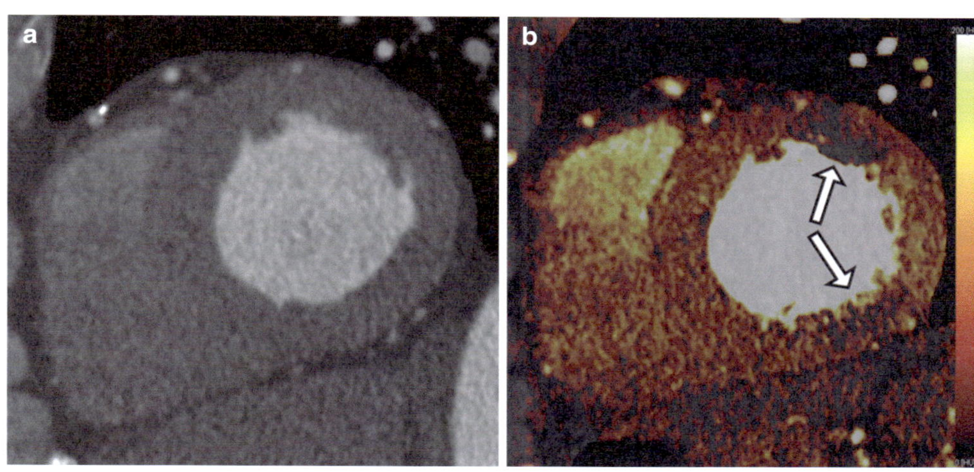

Fig. 13.16 Dual-energy CT myocardial iodine maps. This figure shows a short-axis MPR image of the heart (**a**) where the myocardium appears normal. Post-processing of the dual-energy CT dataset allowed the generation of an iodine map of the myocardium (**b**) which helped detect areas of subtle hypoperfusion (*arrows*)

remains the standard method of choice and is performed using dedicated cardiac planes in the long and short axis, as discussed above.

While contrast-enhanced MRI remains the gold standard for myocardial viability assessment, the phenomenon of delayed hyperenhancement has also been described as useful in delineating subacute infarcts and fibrosis with cardiac CT [14, 15]. Extracellular volume fraction (ECVF) calculations can also be performed to quantify and assess myocardial fibrosis [16]. ECVF is calculated based on attenuation characteristics on unenhanced and contrast-enhanced CT images, taking the patient's hematocrit into account. These techniques are discussed in more detail elsewhere in this book, but are not currently part of routine clinical evaluation.

Several studies have quantified epicardial fat in both semi-automated and automated fashions and suggested an added value for predicting patient outcome and risk stratification [17]. The most sophisticated, cutting-edge post-processing to date is using CTA-derived data to depict infiltrating myocardial fat and delayed hyperenhancing infarcts/fibrosis fused with electrophysiological mapping data [18]. This method holds the promise to potentially guide radiofrequency ablation for ventricular or atrial arrhythmias.

Dual-Energy CT/Perfusion Imaging

Another rapidly growing field in cardiac CT is the development of gated dual-energy cardiac scans, which is further detailed in other chapters of this book. One method to generate these images is to use two different tube currents (e.g., 80 kV and 140 kV) in two tubes of a dual-source scanner, which acquires two accurately co-registered image sets with a temporal resolution of a single-source 64-slice CT scanner. In many cases, this is sufficient for simultaneous CCTA. The mAs setting is usually adjusted so that the noise levels are similar in the two image sets. Thus, the trade-off is temporal resolution (for instance, 165 ms vs. 83 ms), but the benefit is the ability to identify, localize, and quantify the amount of iodine present in varying tissues. This value is correlated with tissue perfusion, which can be quantified in mg/ml, and may be beneficial in cases of suspected perfusion deficits and myocardial tissue characterization. Using dedicated filtering (D kernels) for reconstruction is essential, and various color codes can be used to visualize hypoperfused regions of the myocardium (Fig. 13.17).

CT myocardial perfusion during vasodilator stress, based on principles similar to MRI-based first-pass perfusion, is yet another exciting field emerging and receiving growing acceptance from the radiology community. One approach provides a "subtraction" dataset, depicting areas of differential perfusion between rest and stress datasets (Fig. 13.17). While other chapters in this book will discuss the various ways of acquiring these images, we wanted to include an example of a post-processed dataset where myocardial blood flow is quantitatively mapped over time with dynamic, also known as time-resolved, perfusion CT technique (Fig. 13.18).

Fusion with Other Modalities

The volumetric data from cardiac CTA is also being used to enhance visualization and provide guidance for several additional modalities. While a comprehensive overview of this topic is beyond the scope of our current chapter, CT has been fused with nuclear medicine SPECT or PET myocardial perfusion imaging [19], where the power of anatomic detail with CT is paired with the physiologic information from SPECT or PET. CT has also been instrumental in the developments of electrophysiology, where surface mapping fused with CT data helps identify the substrate for ventricular arrhythmia and 3D visualization of pulmonary venous anatomy can aid in radiofrequency ablations for atrial fibrillation [20].

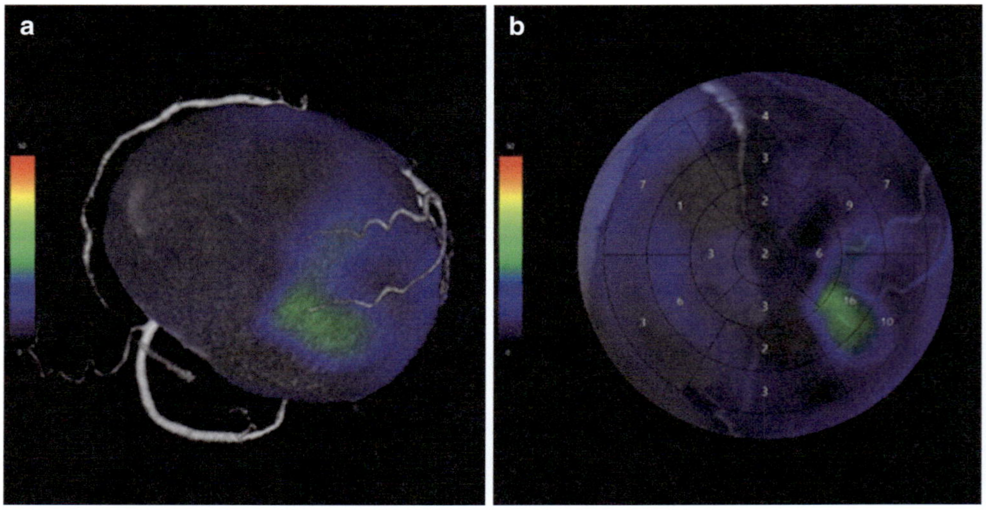

Fig. 13.17 Myocardial stress perfusion images can be subtracted from the rest dataset. The resulting 3D VRT (**a**) and superimposed polar map (**b**) show green areas of stress-induced ischemia. (Courtesy of FUJIFILM Medical Systems USA, Inc.)

Outsourcing, Web Clients, and the "Cloud"

Outsourcing of the post-processing steps – whether to the well-trained CT technologist in the department or to dedicated 3D-workstation experts overseas – has become somewhat of a routine in some centers. This approach is meant to speed up interpretation by providing the interpreting physician with snapshots of MIPs, 3D VRTs, and cMPRs of the heart and allowing them to "flip through" the pictures, which clearly has advantages in terms of workflow and throughput. Still, we firmly believe that in complex or challenging cases, the ability to interact with the post-processed dataset firsthand is crucial for avoiding errors in interpretation. The clinician needs to be able to adjust the window/level settings, rotate the 3D VRT heart, swivel around the entire vessel when using cMPR, and adjust the thickness of a MIP or a MINIP to fully assess and understand the true extent of the pathology. Thus, interpreters of cardiac CT need to train themselves and become comfortable with applying these techniques to allow for a comprehensive analysis of CT images of the heart (Fig. 13.19). A great aid for this are "web-client"-based systems, allowing simultaneous use of a 3D workstation by multiple users from anywhere, at any time, provided they have a computer and a reasonable internet connection. In addition, ongoing and future research is needed to investigate the clinical value and cost-effectiveness of various existing visualization and quantification techniques. Workflow optimization remains a major concern as we strive to adopt these novel approaches into the routine clinical workflow of cardiac imaging.

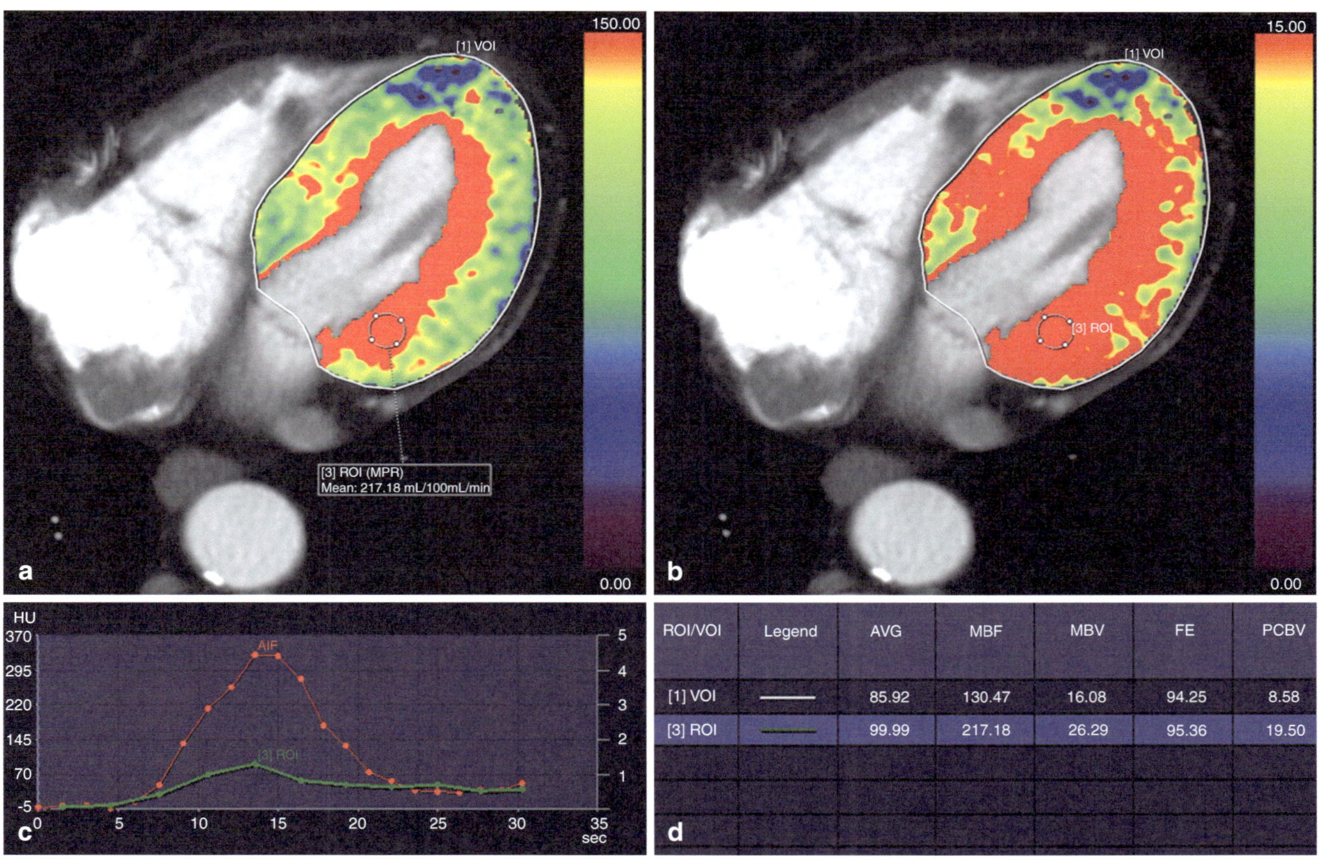

Fig. 13.18 Quantitative myocardial perfusion analysis. Color-coded maps of myocardial blood flow (**a**) and myocardial blood volume (**b**) illustrating myocardial perfusion. Note the apical area of hypoperfusion (blue area). ROIs can be placed to generate arterial input functions (AIF) and perfusion curves (**c**), where each point indicates the attenuation during the dynamic sequential image acquisition. As a result, a table of objective calculated values (**d**), such as myocardial blood flow (MBF) and myocardial blood volume (MBV), can be generated for quantitative myocardial perfusion analysis

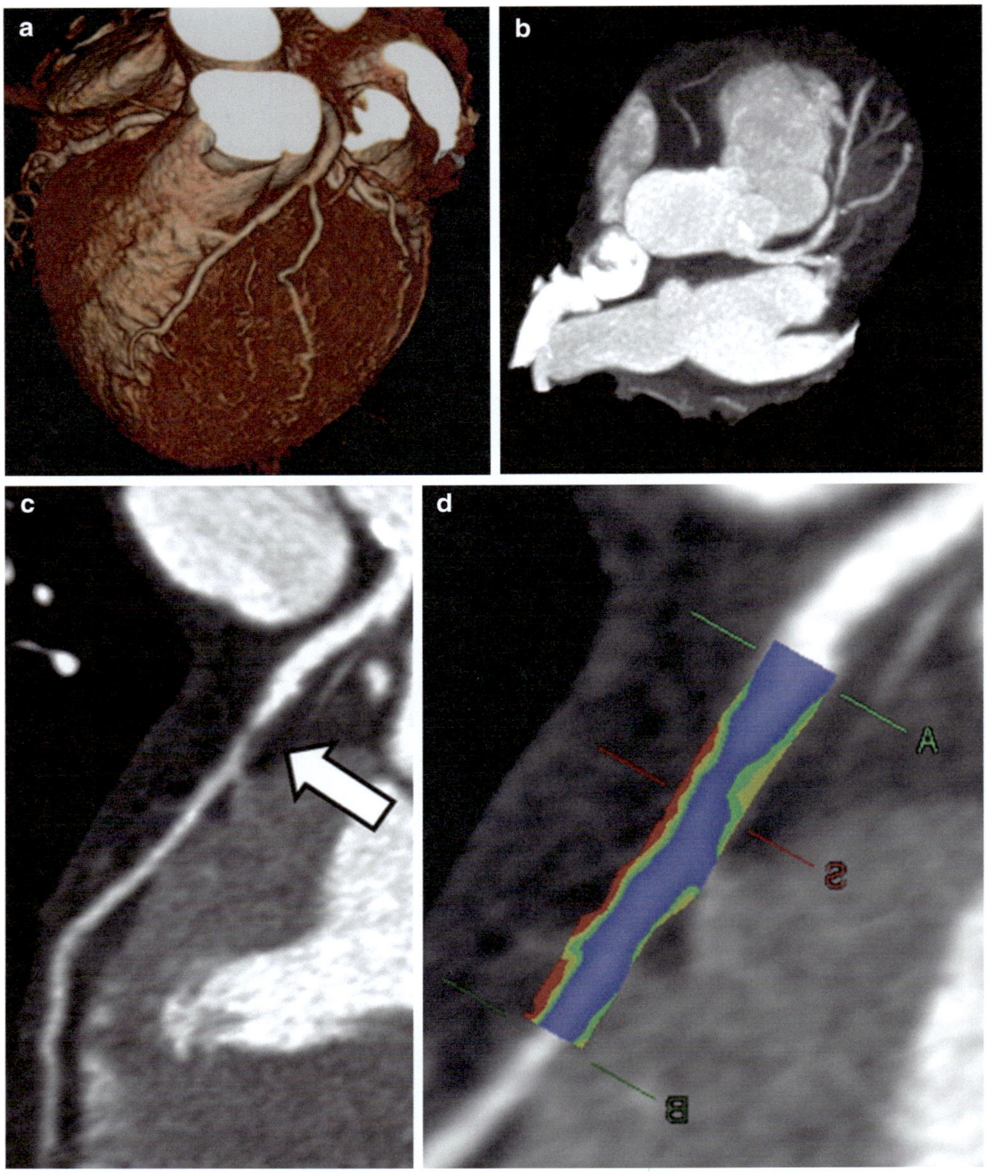

Fig. 13.19 Working up a case: 3D VRT showed a suspicious bifurcation of the LAD and the first diagonal (**a**). MIP showed the presence of mixed, calcified and noncalcified components (**b**). cMPRs of the LAD (**c**) and color-coded plaque analysis (**d**) showed the lipid-rich nature of the noncalcified portions of the lesion

References

1. Fishman EK, Ney DR, Heath DG, et al. Volume rendering versus maximum intensity projection in CT angiography: what works best, when, and why. Radiographics. 2006;26:905–22.
2. van Ooijen PMA, Ho KY, Dorgelo J, Oudkerk M. Coronary artery imaging with multidetector CT: visualization issues. Radiographics. 2003;23:e16.
3. Geyer LL, Glenn GR, De Cecco CN, et al. CT evaluation of small-diameter coronary artery stents: effect of an integrated circuit detector with iterative reconstruction. Radiology. 2015;276:706–14.
4. Hecht HS. Coronary artery calcium scanning. JACC Cardiovasc Imaging. 2015;8:579–96.
5. Busch S, Johnson TRC, Nikolaou K, et al. Visual and automatic grading of coronary artery stenoses with 64-slice CT angiography in reference to invasive angiography. Eur Radiol. 2007;17:1445–51.
6. Arbab-Zadeh A, Hoe J. Quantification of coronary arterial stenoses by multidetector CT angiography in comparison with conventional angiography. JACC Cardiovasc Imaging. 2011;4:191–202.
7. Boogers MJ, Schuijf JD, Kitslaar PH, et al. Automated quantification of stenosis severity on 64-slice CT. JACC Cardiovasc Imaging. 2010;3:699–709.
8. Stein PD, Yaekoub AY, Matta F, Sostman HD. 64-slice CT for diagnosis of coronary artery disease: a systematic review. Am J Med. 2008;121:715–25.
9. Janne d'Othée B, Siebert U, Cury R, et al. A systematic review on diagnostic accuracy of CT-based detection of significant coronary artery disease. Eur J Radiol. 2008;65:449–61.
10. Cury RC, Abbara S, Achenbach S, et al. CAD-RADS™: coronary artery disease – reporting and data system. J Am Coll Radiol. 2016;13(12 Pt A):1458–1466.e9.
11. Gaur S, Taylor CA, Jensen JM, et al. FFR derived from coronary CT angiography in nonculprit lesions of patients with recent STEMI. JACC Cardiovasc Imaging. 2016;10:424–33.

12. Gitsioudis G, Schüssler A, Nagy E, et al. Combined assessment of high-sensitivity troponin T and noninvasive coronary plaque composition for the prediction of cardiac outcomes. Radiology. 2015;276:73–81.
13. Maurovich-Horvat P, Schlett CL, Alkadhi H, et al. The napkin-ring sign indicates advanced atherosclerotic lesions in coronary CT angiography. JACC Cardiovasc Imaging. 2012;5:1243–52.
14. Lardo AC. Contrast-enhanced multidetector computed tomography viability imaging after myocardial infarction: characterization of myocyte death, microvascular obstruction, and chronic scar. Circulation. 2006;113:394–404.
15. Gerber BL. Characterization of acute and chronic myocardial infarcts by multidetector computed tomography: comparison with contrast-enhanced magnetic resonance. Circulation. 2006;113:823–33.
16. Bandula S, White SK, Flett AS, et al. Measurement of myocardial extracellular volume fraction by using equilibrium contrast-enhanced CT: validation against histologic findings. Radiology. 2013;269:396–403.
17. Spearman JV, Meinel FG, Schoepf UJ, et al. Automated quantification of epicardial adipose tissue using CT angiography: evaluation of a prototype software. Eur Radiol. 2014;24:519–26.
18. Truong QA, Thai W, Wai B, et al. Myocardial scar imaging by standard single-energy and dual-energy late enhancement CT: comparison with pathology and electroanatomic map in an experimental chronic infarct porcine model. J Cardiovasc Comput Tomogr. 2015;9:313–20.
19. Thilo C, Schoepf UJ, Gordon L, et al. Integrated assessment of coronary anatomy and myocardial perfusion using a retractable SPECT camera combined with 64-slice CT: initial experience. Eur Radiol. 2009;19:845–56.
20. Cochet H, Dubois R, Sacher F, et al. Cardiac arrhythmias: multimodal assessment integrating body surface ECG mapping into cardiac imaging. Radiology. 2014;271:239–47.

Workflow Optimization

14

Thomas Allmendinger, Andrew N. Primak, and Christian D. Eusemann

Cardiac CT imaging is considered to be complicated due to a wide variety of rules, recommendations, and different guidelines in combination with a rapid technological development in the last 15 years. However, the primary underlying acquisition challenge stems from the fact that cardiac imaging is a patient-dependent optimization problem with diagnostic image quality being the first and X-ray radiation dose the second important degree of freedom which need to be balanced against each other. If there were absolutely no concern for radiation dose, cardiac CT acquisition would most likely be identical to the approach 15 years back – a retrospective ECG-gated spiral scanning without any tube current modulation enabling maximum freedom for image reconstruction based on the acquired data. However, as this approach conflicts with the ALARA principle, today's approaches are more finely tuned.

This chapter has two parts. The first part focuses on acquisition strategy recommendations applicable to a broad spectrum of state-of-the-art CT systems. In the second part, specific key elements of the patient preparation, important for a successful cardiac workflow, are discussed – patient positioning, ECG, and breath-hold training.

T. Allmendinger (✉)
Department of Computed Tomography, Siemens Healthcare GmbH, Forchheim, Germany
e-mail: thomas.allmendinger@siemens.com

A. N. Primak
Department of Diagnostic Imaging, Siemens Healthineers, Malvern, PA, USA

C. D. Eusemann
Department of Collaborations, Siemens Medical Solutions USA, Inc., Malvern, PA, USA

A Brief Recap of the Available Tools for Cardiac CT Data Acquisition

A detailed technical description of the state-of-the-art cardiac CT technology and the different acquisition modes was provided in Chap. 6. Therefore, only a brief summary and refresher of the technical nomenclature is provided here.

From a cardiac CT point of view, the oldest most widely used scanning technique is retrospective ECG-gated spiral scanning also called helical scanning. The scan is characterized by a continuous data acquisition in combination with a continuous table motion at relatively low table feed (low spiral pitch) with simultaneous recording of the patient's ECG. After the data acquisition, the recorded ECG is utilized as guidance to select those data intervals in the CT data set that were measured in different heartbeats in the same user-selected cardiac phase, subsequently building a consistent image volume. Over the years the dose efficiency and comfort of this "straight-forward" approach were improved by technological features like the tube current modulation during the individual cardiac cycles [1, 2], automatic calculation of the optimal spiral pitch based on the patient's heart rate [3], and algorithms for optimized reconstruction with minimal cardiac motion [4, 5].

In contrast to the spiral acquisition, the sequence technique, also called a step-and-shoot acquisition, was developed from the opposite direction. In its earliest form, an axial CT scan without table movement was performed in a single prospectively ECG-triggered cardiac phase. The CT system acquired scan data covering a sub-volume of the patient's cardiac anatomy corresponding roughly to the total z-width of the CT detector. The duration of such a sub-volume acquisition was limited to a quick-scan range to enable the reconstruction of a single set of images at this position corresponding to around three quarters of a rotation. Afterwards the table is moved to the next z-position, and the next axial CT scan is performed at the same cardiac phase in a later cardiac cycle. This way, the heart volume is sequentially covered by multiple axial scans. By design the table feed of such a sequential

U. J. Schoepf (ed.), *CT of the Heart*, Contemporary Medical Imaging, https://doi.org/10.1007/978-1-60327-237-7_14

scan is only determined by geometrical factors of the CT system and independent of the patient's heart, which contributes already significantly to the improved dose efficiency of this scan acquisition. By further limiting the data acquisition to a single cardiac phase as it was done in the early years, the sequence technique was considered optimized for "low-dose scanning" however at the cost of a limited robustness. Technological developments of later years vastly increased the flexibility and robustness of sequential techniques by introducing features like arrhythmia rejection and recovery scanning [6, 7], a flexible definition of the desired cardiac phase acquisition window and an automatic adjustment of this acquisition based on the cardiac rhythm [8].

A common remaining challenge for both acquisition techniques described above is the proper alignment and registration of the images acquired and reconstructed in stacks over multiple cardiac cycles. A hardware-based system solution to this "last" challenge of cardiac imaging, which is currently available in the form of several high-end CT systems from different manufacturers, is provided in two rather fundamentally different ways – single-source volume scanning with wide-area detector systems [9, 10] and ECG-triggered high-pitch scanning with dual-source systems [11].

As of today, cardiac volume scanning is offered by two vendors. With a detector collimation of 320 × 0.5 mm at 0.28 s rotation time (Toshiba Aquilion One, Toshiba Medical Systems Corporation, Tokyo, Japan) and 256 × 0.625 mm detector collimation at 0.28 s rotation time (GE Revolution, GE Healthcare, Waukesha, USA), these systems are capable of a 16-cm volume coverage in the z-axis direction at the isocenter, large enough to scan the entire heart in one beat in most of the clinical cases, therefore avoiding stair-step and banding artifacts and problems with inconsistent contrast enhancement in different sub-volumes. Even if these wide-area detector CT systems do not need to answer the basic scan mode acquisition technique question, the planning of the suitable cardiac phases and the width of the acquisition window remain. Therefore, these systems are also discussed as a part of the single-source discussion below.

As an alternative, single-heartbeat volume scanning can also be achieved with dual-source CT systems by means of a spiral acquisition at high pitch values of around 3.2–3.4. Depending on the generation of the CT system, this approach yields table feeds of 450 mm/s (SOMATOM Definition Flash, Siemens Healthineers) or 736 mm/s (SOMATOM Force, Siemens Healthineers) enabling the coverage of an entire cardiac volume in the diastolic rest phase by controlling the acquisition in a prospective ECG-triggered fashion. The prospective nature of the scan mode limits the application of the scan mode in patients with irregular heart rate, as discussed below; however the possibility to cover an extended range beyond the heart anatomy in a single acquisition makes it a clinical valuable tool for CABG or TAVI scans [12, 13].

Customizing Cardiac Data Acquisition to the Individual Patient

Whether to scan in a retrospective gated spiral mode or a prospectively triggered sequence mode is considered the basic first decision step for a cardiac CT acquisition. As described above, the very steep, near steplike, transition from a retrospective spiral without tube current modulation to a prospective sequence limited to a single cardiac phase should be a thing of the past. Basically all modern CT systems enhanced the capabilities of their respective sequence acquisition modes with an automatic heart rate rhythm-dependent acquisition window adjustment, the possibility to manually select wide acquisition windows, which allow coverage of end-systole and end-diastole phases, combined with mechanisms for handling extra-systolic events (PVCs, SVC). The reasons for sticking to retrospective spiral acquisitions are a possible lack of some of those features in sequence mode on some scanner platforms and an improved shorter total scan time for high heart rates due to the commonly applied heart rate-dependent automatic pitch adaptation. This shortening of the total scan time is important for higher heart rates as it counters the effect of increased cardiac throughput, which would otherwise trigger a necessary increase of the contrast injection time as it is the case in high heart rate sequence acquisitions.

Besides the scan mode, the second decision to be made is the targeted cardiac phase, typically choosing between end-diastole, end-systole, or both and whether the phase target is limited to a single time point or if a slightly wider acquisition window is configured to enable the possibility to search locally for the best image reconstruction time. In addition, due to the nature of the contraction and filling of the cardiac chambers throughout the cardiac cycle, the question whether to make the phase definition in a relative fashion (in units of percent relative to the 100% of a cardiac cycle RR interval) or in an absolute millisecond-based parameter setting needs to be answered. A more detailed discussion on the acquisition and reconstruction consequences of the phase unit selection is done further below.

Finally, similar to the desired cardiac acquisition phase and unit, the target for the image reconstruction needs to be defined as well. However, this decision is secondary to the acquisition as one can add multiple reconstructions within the available acquired data set or utilize motion-optimized image reconstructions [4, 5]. Nevertheless, a manual selection of the target phase unit is, in most cases, still required, which could potentially have significant effects on the final image quality.

A "correct" level of tuning and separation into individual scan parameter sets or classes cannot be easily specified due to the fact that a very detailed description into many individual classes based on clinical question, heart rate, cardiac rhythm, patient size, age, sex, and possible other additional factors might be desirable from an academic point of view. However, such a detailed approach is not feasible in a daily routine, if the protocol adjustments are made by manual parameter modifications. As a consequence, the approach discussed below is, to some extent, a compromise with a limited amount of individual classes still maintaining a certain high level of detail.

Of note, the subgroups described below can be combined if further simplification is desired.

The first selection step is indication-driven, based on the required diagnostic image quality level. Even if there is a very wide range of clinical questions, the two most common applications on opposite sides of the image quality spectrum are coronary calcium scoring (CaSc) and coronary CT angiography (CCTA). CaSc, applied since the early 1990s and originally driving cardiac CT system development with dedicated designs (e.g., EBCT [14]), has nowadays become a "screening-like test" focusing primarily on limiting X-ray radiation dose. The image quality requirements for accurate calculation of a calcium score are rather relaxed even allowing the evaluation in non-ECG-gated scans [15]. In contrast to this, the image quality requirements for CCTA were relatively high to begin with, in terms of spatial resolution, visible contrast, and absence of cardiac motion. These requirements tightened in recent years, due to the fact that the reporting of additional coronary plaque features, beyond a "simple" stenosis quantification, became clinically relevant, driving the image quality needs even further [16].

Besides this obvious clinical choice, a characterization of the individual patient's cardiac heart rate and rhythm needs to take place in order to adjust the scan parameters appropriately.

The determination of an average heart rate is rather straightforward and often provided automatically by the attached ECG system. One should however be mindful that these values are typically derived during a free-breathing patient state, while the CT exam is normally done with the patient holding his/her breath. Patient heart rates typically drop by an average of 4–6 BPM during a breath-hold and often in combination with a reduction of the overall heart rate variability. In general, this behavior is beneficial for the CT acquisition. One still needs to pay attention in cases of an automatic pitch selection with retrospectively gated spiral scans, as the heart rate determining the pitch value is measured during the free-breathing state of the patient and is set prior to the scan, with a safety reserve of around 8–10 BPM. In rare cases, the heart rate of patients can drop below these values during breath-hold, requiring a manual pitch selection in order to avoid image artifacts from data gaps.

A standardized method of calculation or classification of cardiac rhythm, comparable to a mean or median value for the heart rate, is not established and agreed on a wide basis with a necessary focus on the requirements of cardiac CT imaging. The established clinical classifications of cardiac arrhythmia are too detailed and therefore not really suitable for this kind of application. A simple, robust, and mostly descriptive classification scheme which can be applied is the utilization of the three different cardiac rhythm groups – *regular, unstable, and arrhythmic*. A regular heart rate is classified as a normal sinus rhythm with minimal variation in correlation with the breathing rate of the patient. An unstable rhythm is characterized by continuous beat-to-beat variation of up to 8–10 BPM or multiple extra beats within a few cycles. An arrhythmic cardiac rhythm, as it is used in this context, is characterized by the fact that the determination of a valid average heart rate is already difficult if looking at 10–15 cardiac cycles. Typical examples of ECG yielding a classification like that would be a bigeminy rhythm or atrial fibrillation.

In addition to the clinical and physiological grouping detailed above, the CT hardware itself needs to be clustered, to some extent, to allow the development of a practical decision guide. The solution chosen here splits the guidance into four different blocks illustrated by Figs. 14.1, 14.2, 14.3, and 14.4. These blocks are separated according to the clinical indication, CCTA (Figs. 14.1 and 14.2) and CaSc (Figs. 14.3 and 14.4), and one key technical differentiator, the temporal resolution for cardiac imaging. Based on this temporal resolution difference, the guidance is also separated into single-source (Figs. 14.1 and 14.3) and dual-source technologies (Figs. 14.2 and 14.4).

Illustrated in Fig. 14.1 is a CCTA classification scheme for single-source CT systems. The classification assumes that the prospective sequence has modern features, which can handle extra beats properly and allow a separate definition of the start and end of a cardiac phase. To provide some guidance despite the wide range of available rotation times, ranging from 0.27 s to 0.35 s [17], and detector collimations, ranging from 2 cm to 8 cm, the cutoff values for the classification into low, moderate, and high heart rates are made system dependent as shown on the left side of Fig. 14.1. As a general pattern, one can explain the approach as follows, starting in the bottom left with a regular low rhythm, which enables the utilization of an end-diastolic single-phase cardiac sequence acquisition. With increasing heart rate or variability, the uncertainty of where to image optimally is mitigated by increasing the acquisition window, slightly in the unstable direction or considerably in the elevated heart rate region, as it is undetermined if an end-diastolic or an end-systolic image reconstruction provides the more diagnostic images. For high heart rates, the full transition into a solely end-systolic acquisition is natural as diastole simply becomes too short for imaging. The explanation for the strategy of end-systolic imaging, based on an absolute millisecond phase definition, can be found in the next section

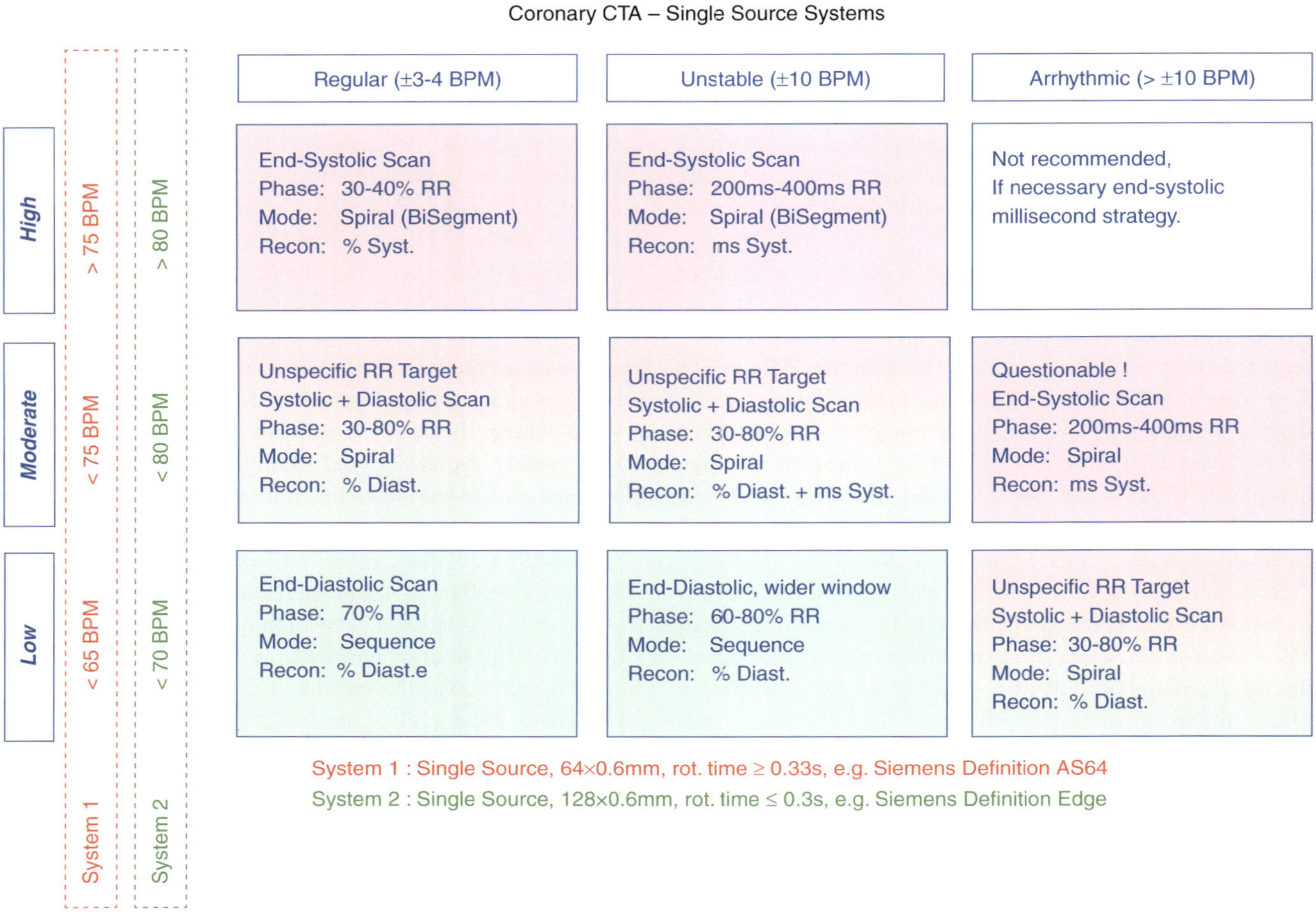

Fig. 14.1 Practical decision guide – coronary CT angiography using a single-source imaging system. The cutoff values for the different heart rate ranges depend on the capabilities of the CT scanner system, illustrated for a mid-range and high-end single-source scanner system with different temporal resolution and detector coverage

as it is a clinically proven concept established for dual-source CT. Even though this concept can be applied to single-source systems, it does (as all end-systolic approaches) depend on a very good temporal resolution and, therefore, is more suitable for dual-source systems.

Handling the heart rate rhythm in dedicated separate groups with specific measures, switching between percentage diastolic or millisecond systolic acquisitions, is to a large extent attributed to the previously described stack alignment and the registration challenge of systems acquiring only a part of the heart anatomy in single detector z-coverage. With wide-area detector systems, the dedicated handling of the cardiac rhythm can be neglected to some extent and the scan parametrization can be solely based on the regular heart rate in combination with the average heart rate determined by the ECG.

Figure 14.2 illustrates the CCTA selection scheme for dual-source systems. The grouping into the three different heart rate levels (low, moderate, and high) is also system dependent reflecting the technical advancement between the second and third dual-source generations. The most noticeable difference compared to the single-source approach is the lack of an undetermined region, which would require both end-systolic and end-diastolic combined acquisitions, but a rather sharp transition from a diastolic to a systolic approach at a certain heart rate. The change of the cardiac phase unit toward absolute milliseconds is an effective measure to limit the radiation dose despite an increasing irregular heart rate. The reason for this behavior is simply the fact that all percent-based definitions are relative with respect to the best guess time point into the future where the R-peak closing the current cardiac cycle should appear. If the quality or precision of this estimate deteriorates due to an irregular rhythm, nearly all modern CT systems react with an automatic widening of the acquisition window, which can lead to a greatly increased radiation dose. If the cardiac target phase is configured by an absolute millisecond approach, aiming at the end-systole, no prospective estimate is required, and the necessary X-ray control time points are derived in a stopwatch-like manner, without any effect on the width of the

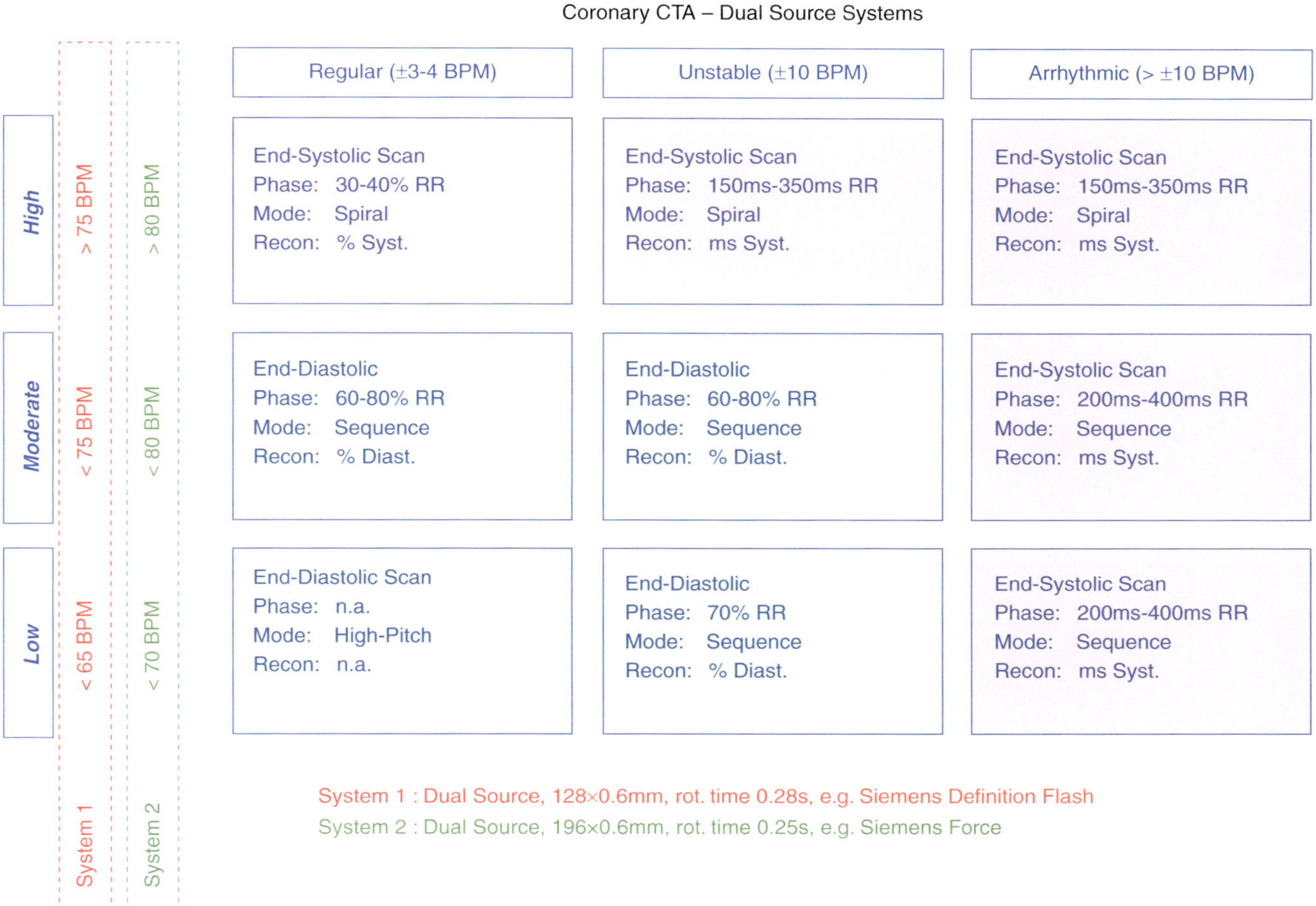

Fig. 14.2 Practical decision guide – coronary CT angiography using a dual-source imaging system. The cutoff values for the different heart rate ranges depend on the capabilities of the dual-source scanner generation. This is especially important for the definition of the "low heart rate" category, where second- and third-generation systems differ in their upper limits for dual-source high-pitch scanning

acquisition window. A detailed description of this approach including its clinical results in terms of dose and image quality can be found here [18–20].

The approaches for CaSc illustrated in Figs. 14.3 and 14.4 can be summarized as single-phase limited acquisitions focusing primarily on radiation dose in combination with a simplified grouping and classification scheme for easy application.

Future: Fully Automated Cardiac CT Systems?

In the advent of self-driving cars and deep learning technologies which are rapidly evolving, one can raise the question if such a manual set of recommendations as presented above are still state of the art and will be relevant in a few years. So far, initial steps have been undertaken by different manufacturers to support the user in their decision and selection process. Examples are the FlashCheck [21] for high-pitch scanning, the FAST Phase feature on Siemens systems with syngo CT VB10 [22] or the Auto Gating feature on GE Revolution CT [23].

However, a truly intelligent system would need to include way more patient- and indication-specific input factors in order to reach a dedicated tailored scan and reconstruction solution, which would lead to a dramatic increase in the level of details in the decision tree. While such a system can easily handle a finely tuned classification scheme from a technical point of view, the user operating the system still needs to be empowered to understand the underlying reasoning of the system (i.e., "why will this patient be scanned and reconstructed in this specific way?") beyond the actual displaying of all scan and reconstruction parameters ("what will be done?"), as he/she still bears the full responsibility for the CT scan and therefore for patient image quality and radiation dose. This "trust in automation" challenge is well known [24, 25], and a satisfying answer needs to be provided in the context of CT systems by the manufacturers to enable the widespread acceptance of partially or fully automated CT scanners.

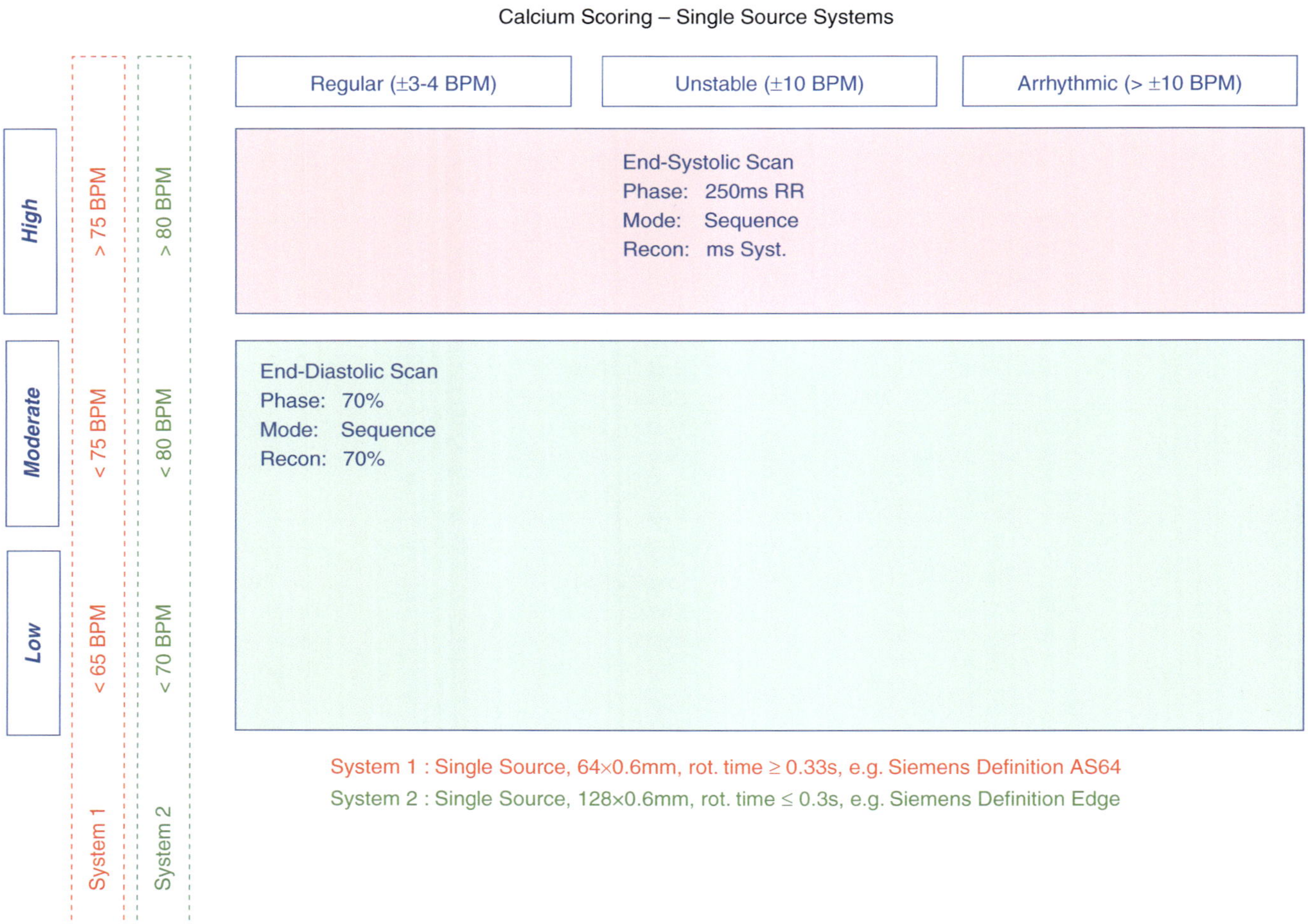
Calcium Scoring – Single Source Systems
Regular (±3-4 BPM)
Unstable (±10 BPM)
Arrhythmic (> ±10 BPM)
High
Moderate
Low
> 75 BPM
< 75 BPM
< 65 BPM
> 80 BPM
< 80 BPM
< 70 BPM
System 1
System 2
End-Systolic Scan
Phase: 250ms RR
Mode: Sequence
Recon: ms Syst.
End-Diastolic Scan
Phase: 70%
Mode: Sequence
Recon: 70%
System 1 : Single Source, 64×0.6mm, rot. time ≥ 0.33s, e.g. Siemens Definition AS64
System 2 : Single Source, 128×0.6mm, rot. time ≤ 0.3s, e.g. Siemens Definition Edge

Fig. 14.3 Practical decision guide – coronary calcium scoring using a single-source imaging system. The primary focus of calcium scoring exams is the minimization of X-ray dose therefore accepting a somewhat reduced overall image quality. This approach is reflected by a guide, which is drastically simplified compared to the CTA approach limiting it to a single decision point

Patient Positioning, ECG, and Breath-Hold Training

Preparing the patient prior to the CT scan includes multiple steps, typically performed by the technologist staff, prior to the actual scan, ranging from communicating to the patient about the upcoming exam, checking laboratory values up to the management of contrast media administration. From this wide range of responsibilities, three are discussed in greater detail here as they are an integral part of a successful cardiac CT examination – patient positioning, ECG acquisition, and breath-hold training.

Patient Positioning

When positioning the patient on the CT table, one question arising in cardiac exams is whether to put the heart itself, as anatomic organ of interest, into the isocenter of the CT system or if the entire chest should be placed in the system isocenter. Depending on the individual patient anatomy, the two approaches can yield different table height settings, between 5 cm and 10 cm, and can significantly influence the results of the exam. Unfortunately, a decisive answer to this question is difficult as both approaches have their merits and limitations. A suitable approach needs to be picked individually based on the available CT hardware, requested clinical procedure, and body habitus.

Some CT systems, e.g., GE VCT scanners [26], enable the manual selection of a dedicated cardiac bowtie filter, which limits the X-ray radiation to a smaller scan field of view (SFOV). This selection needs to be done prior to the scan and therefore, if selected, mandates the positioning of the heart into the isocenter of the system as it leads to a limitation of the reconstruction field of view to values ranging from 32 cm to 40 cm. On the other hand, the benefit of such an aggressive bowtie filter approach is a possible lowering of the radiation dose of up to 40% [26]. The routine use of small

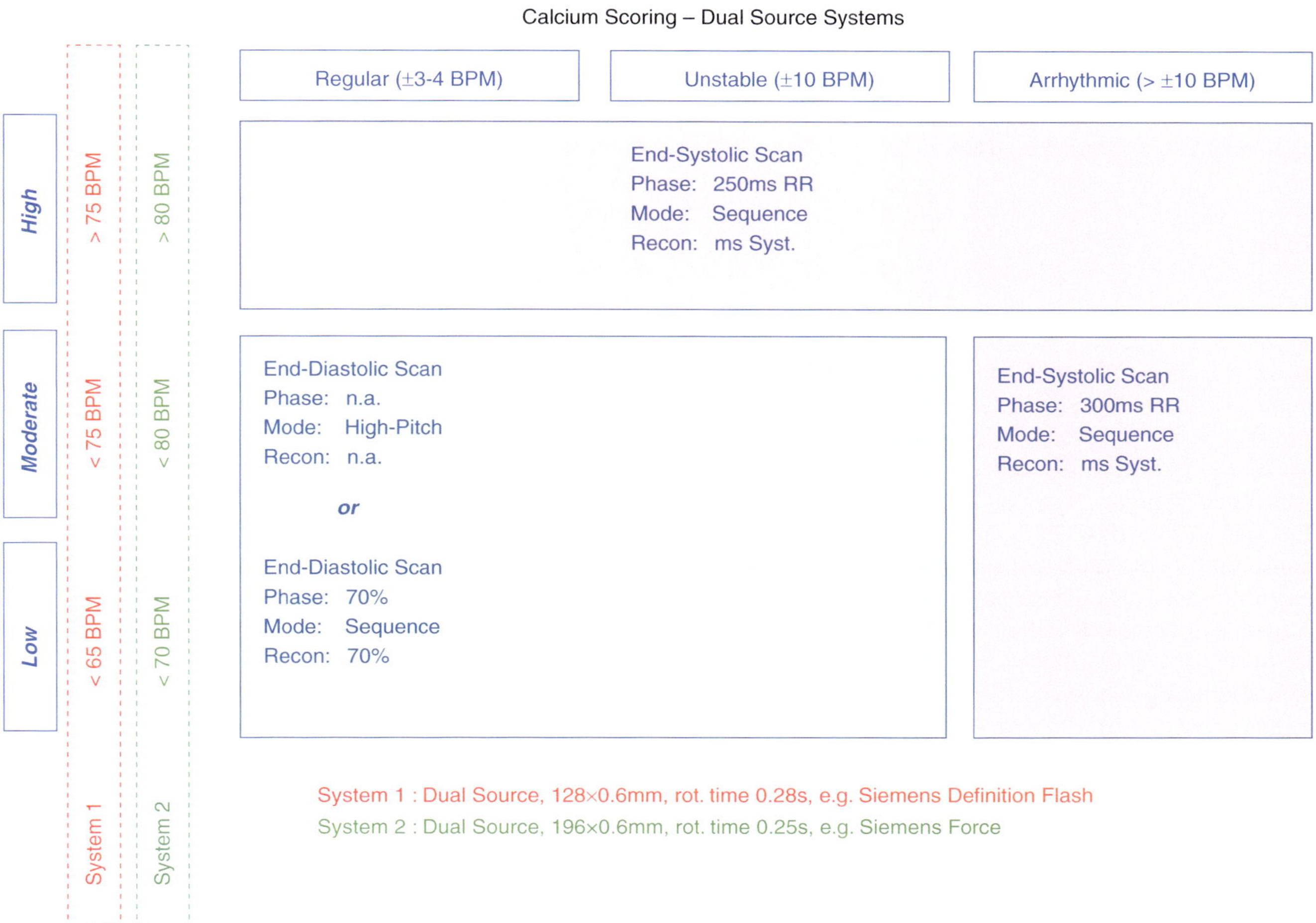
Calcium Scoring – Dual Source Systems
Regular (±3-4 BPM)
Unstable (±10 BPM)
Arrhythmic (> ±10 BPM)
High
> 75 BPM
> 80 BPM
Moderate
< 75 BPM
< 80 BPM
Low
< 65 BPM
< 70 BPM
End-Systolic Scan
Phase: 250ms RR
Mode: Sequence
Recon: ms Syst.
End-Diastolic Scan
Phase: n.a.
Mode: High-Pitch
Recon: n.a.
or
End-Diastolic Scan
Phase: 70%
Mode: Sequence
Recon: 70%
End-Systolic Scan
Phase: 300ms RR
Mode: Sequence
Recon: ms Syst.
System 1 : Dual Source, 128×0.6mm, rot. time 0.28s, e.g. Siemens Definition Flash
System 2 : Dual Source, 196×0.6mm, rot. time 0.25s, e.g. Siemens Force
System 1
System 2

Fig. 14.4 Practical decision guide – coronary calcium scoring using a dual-source imaging system. The guide is drastically simplified reflecting the lowered image quality expectations for this kind of exam while at the same time optimizing the acquisition in the direction of an overall low X-ray dose

bowtie filters and small FOV will both reduce radiation dose and limit incidental findings related to non-cardiac disease (primarily non-cancerous lung nodules). Whether these incidental findings improve outcomes is still debated in the scientific literature [27–29].

Other CT systems, e.g., Siemens scanners, do utilize cardiac bowtie filters focusing the radiation dose more strongly to the isocenter of the scanner yet still enable the reconstruction images in the full field of view (on most scanner systems 50 cm) at the price of slightly elevated image noise in the periphery. The achievable dose reduction comparing to a standard body bowtie setting with the corresponding cardiac settings is approximately 20–30% in this approach [3, 30]. This freedom naturally leads to the recommendation to position the chest into the isocenter as it enables the reconstruction of the heart and lung anatomy in separate reconstruction jobs in its entirety. An important benefit of this approach can be derived from the fact that, on some systems, the automatic exposure control (AEC) of a scanner is due to user preference relying on a single AP topogram (or scout) for the estimation of the necessary scan exposure settings. If in this case the positioning of the patient is chosen systematically off-center, the image aberration introduced in the topogram image due to the fan beam nature of the CT system could yield an unwanted bias in the AEC estimation. In case of a personal preference for the heart isocenter placement approach, it is recommended to add a second lateral topogram to the exam, which provides the full attenuation information to the AEC system, therefore removing all possible bias [31].

Another quite interesting, more specialized technique is the less known so-called breast displacement technique for female patients. The idea is simply to push the breasts up so they are covering a smaller portion of the scan range. A recent publication describes this approach in a cardiac CT practice, which is accomplished by using the Velcro patient positioning strap attached to the scanner table. This “reshaping” of the patient anatomy prior to the acquisition of the topogram (or scout) images supports overall dose reduction by keeping the more radiation-sensitive breast tissue partially outside of the cardiac scan range in combination with the reduced patient chest attenuation, which leads to an improved image quality or alternatively a lowered exposure [32].

ECG

The acquisition of quality ECG data is critical to provide a reliable and resilient signal for controlling the X-ray exposure during a cardiac CT examination. This statement is valid for all acquisition strategies, a retrospective spiral with ECG pulsing, which modulates the tube current, based on the phase in the cardiac cycle and all prospectively triggered acquisitions, which determine the X-ray on and off time points from the ECG information. Poor ECG quality can result in the CT system's inability to recognize the R-wave, thus affecting X-ray exposure with a high likelihood of increasing the patient dose substantially combined with a potentially detrimental effect on the final image quality of the exam. This section only provides a brief summary of essential elements; more detailed guidance can be found in these white papers [33, 34].

Citing a relatively old article from 1984, in Critical Care Nursing, this statement discussing ECG artifacts still holds true despite advancements in ECG devices: "Improvement in electrode preparation techniques and a better understanding of the sources of artifact can enhance equipment performance, resulting in improved patient assessment, more effective utilization of nursing time, and reduced operating costs" [35]. Improving ECG quality is an important factor built on the following key elements: correct placement, good skin preparation, use of quality electrodes, proper electrode application, good electrode-to-patient contact, and proper lead selection.

When positioning ECG electrodes, it is important to avoid bony protuberances and scar tissue and keep enough distance between the individual electrodes. Bones and scar tissue can interfere with the electrical impulse transmission. Larger distances between the electrodes typically provide signals with larger amplitude. One should avoid, if possible, positioning electrodes in the scan field, i.e., near or at the level of the heart, because ECG trace artifacts may be generated when electrodes are hit by the X-ray beam.

The skin is a poor conductor of electricity, and artifacts from the outer layer of the skin (epidermis) are more troublesome than other types of artifacts because it is difficult to filter electronically, and its amplitude is often larger than the ECG signal [36]. Unfortunately, clinical studies have shown that the electrode-skin interface is frequently overlooked as a major source of artifacts affecting many electrophysiological recordings [37]. Although skin preparation can add a little time, the extra effort may reduce the time spent dealing with a poor CT examination. To prepare the skin for electrode placement, dry, dead epidermal layers of the skin must be removed, along with any natural oils and dirt that impede electrical flow and thus create a resistance to signal quality. Prepare the skin by cleaning the area for application of electrodes. This can be done with soap and water. Alcohol may only be used on particularly oily skin as alcohol dries out the skin while removing the oil. Wipe the skin area multiple times with gentle pressure and an abrasive skin prep pad (e.g., 3M 2236 One Step Skin Prep).

The use of suitable quality electrodes is an important part of the overall monitoring process. When selecting electrodes the following simple guidelines apply:

1. All electrodes selected should be of the same brand and type to help minimize noise.
2. Adhere to all instructions for use found on the electrode packaging (e.g., 'Use by' date).
3. Electrodes that are packaged together in large quantities should be used shortly after the packaging is open or the packaging should be tightly resealed since extended exposure to air will dry out electrodes prematurely and reduce their adhesive and conductive properties.
4. Using wet gel electrodes (e.g., 2700 Cleartrace 2) is beneficial for the needs of a short-term ECG in combination with a CT exam.

Recent technological developments support the efforts of the clinicians at this critical patient-machine interface in the form of an automated ECG electrode impedance measurement combined with reporting the result in real-time on the gantry display of the CT system (ECG Monitor, Siemens Drive, Siemens Force). The example of Fig. 14.5 illustrates such a support mechanism yielding, in case of a poor critical left arm electrode connection, a very high electrical impedance and a red warning triangle (Fig. 14.5a), and an acceptable, but not very good, "yellow" warning (Fig. 14.5b). In case of good electrode connections, the patient view is replaced by a display of the current heart rate, the overall ECG signal strength, and the selected ECG lead channel (Fig. 14.5c).

Breath-Hold: Training Prior to the Scan and Image Analysis After the Scan

It is well known that the suspension of the respiration during scan acquisition is of great importance for a successful and high-quality CT of the upper chest area such as a cardiac CT exam. On the other hand, one could get the impression that this topic is treated as the "annoying poor cousin" of cardiac CT. For example, an otherwise very good book on technologist training devotes only few lines of text to this crucial topic [38].

The first part of the section provides a comprehensive summary of respiratory instructions based on this excellent detailed publication [39]. In the second part, illustrations of breathing

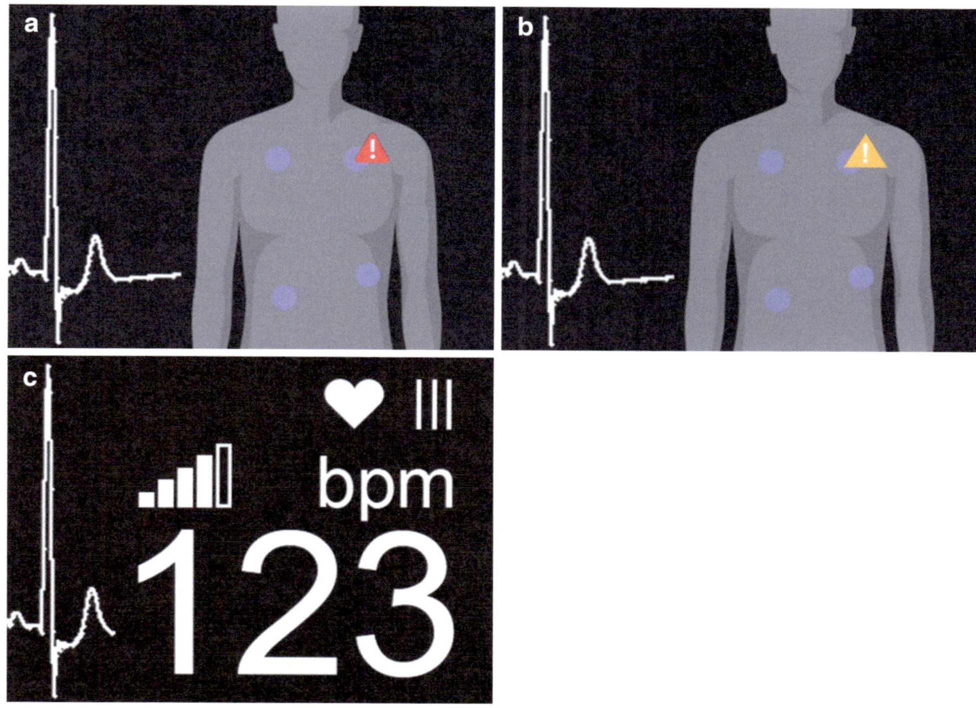

Fig. 14.5 Example of a poor and acceptable ECG electrode connection indicated on the gantry display either by (**a**) red ("bad impedance") or (**b**) yellow ("weak impedance") warning signs. A proper high-quality electrode connection is indicated by (**c**) displaying average heart rate, overall ECG signal strength, and ECG lead channel

artifacts in cardiac exams are shown. They provide some image analysis strategies answering the question: "How to distinguish breathing artifacts from cardiac motion artifacts?"

Breath-Hold Training

All explanations to the patient should be as simple and figurative as possible. A cardiac CT exam might be a simple routine task for a radiologist or technologist; however, it can be an unusual and potentially alienating experience for most patients. Using brief, simple, and figurative sentences explaining the procedure and what is expected from the patient serves as framework for the following steps.

The breathing instructions should be performed in the same body position as the CT exam that is typically supine and with the arms extended behind the head. Ideally, training should be performed with the patient positioned on the CT table simulating the experience of the later CT scan. The technologist or radiologist should proactively demonstrate the breathing maneuver as many patients are not properly instructed or have never seen a demonstration on how maneuvers are supposed to be performed. One should carefully check if the training is successful and the patient adheres to the instructions by closely monitoring motion of the chest during the breath-hold or if there is a considerable delay between the breath-hold command and the actual breath-hold state of the patient.

Almost all CT systems provide digitally recorded voice commands, a convenient solution with a consistent level of repeatability. However, it needs to be checked initially if the available built-in breath-hold commands are suitable for the specific needs of a cardiac exam as they tend to be quite short in order to minimize effects on the inter-scan delay of automatically coupled scan ranges. A possible solution, which is offered by most modern CT systems, is the possibility to record and save an individual breath-hold command of the technologist during the setup of the scan protocol, which can be applied if the need for such a dedicated command arises.

Finally, there are often additional CT scans occurring prior to the more critical contrast-enhanced cardiac exam (e.g., topogram, a test bolus series scan, CaSc scan). Briefly reviewing these images for the presence of breathing motion artifacts can prevent a failed exam by reinstructing the patient.

Breathing Artifacts in Cardiac Images

In Fig. 14.6 one can see examples of curved planar reformat (CPR) images of the main coronaries with clear indications of stack registration and misalignment artifact of the underlying prospectively triggered cardiac sequence. In case of this kind of artifact, a question arises, whether these alignment issues are due to cardiac motion, which could potentially be fixed by alternative reconstructions at different cardiac phase points, or if the misalignment is due to an incomplete breath-hold of the patient.

Figure 14.7 shows coronal and sagittal reconstructions of the lung. The original thin-slice axial reconstructions were chosen with an option that limits each individual image

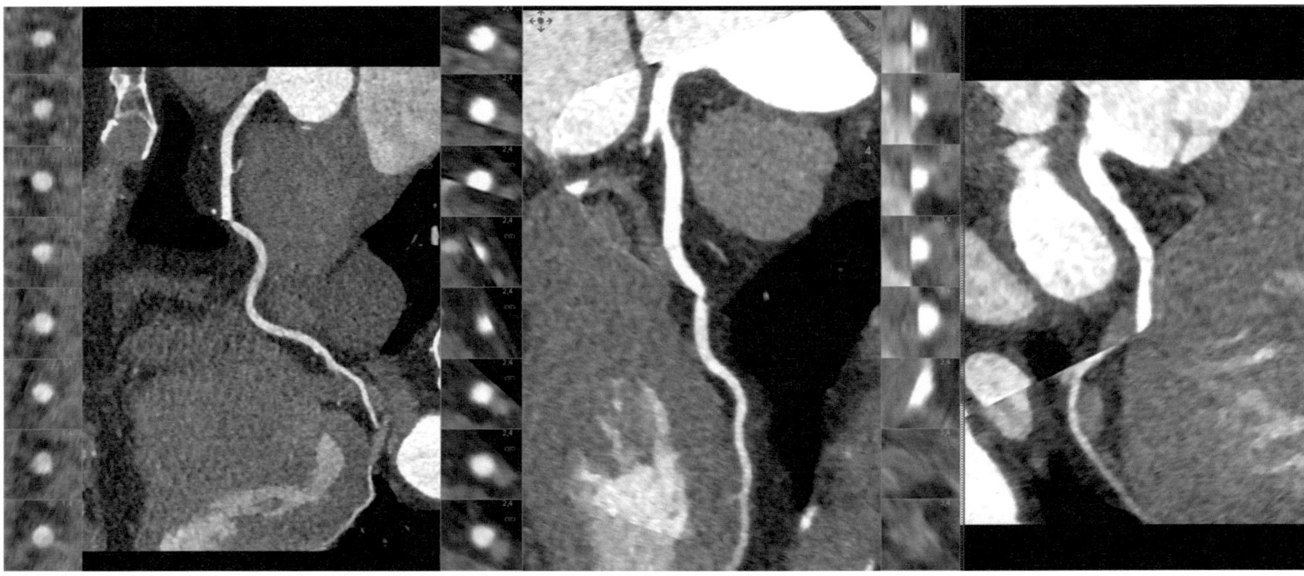

Fig. 14.6 Examples of curved planar reformat (CPR) images of the RCA (left), LCA (middle), and CX (right) coronaries. The reconstructions were derived from a prospectively triggered cardiac sequence and stack misalignment artifacts are clearly visible

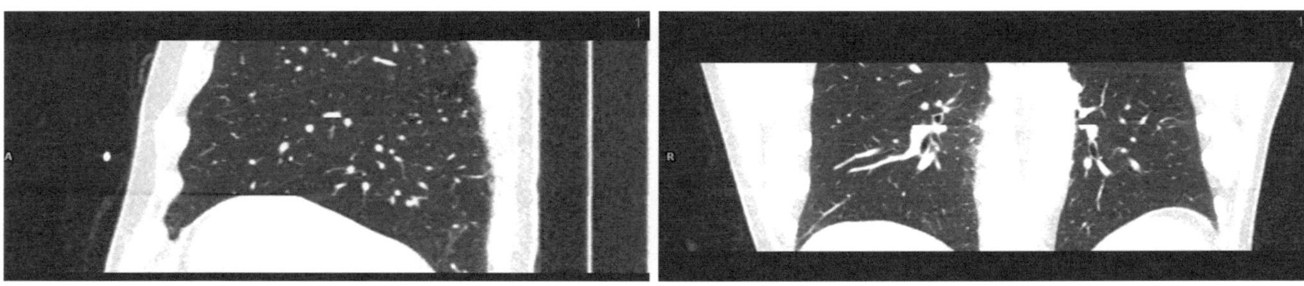

Fig. 14.7 Coronal (left) and sagittal (right) MPR images of the lung. The misalignment of the different stacks is clearly visible in the lung vessels with a considerable gap between the structures shown in these images and any fast-moving cardiac structures. A characteristic signature of breathing through the diaphragm can be seen as the misalignment is limited to the lung vessels in combination with the flat liver dome and no misalignment is visible for the thorax surface or ribs

source data to a single cardiac cycle without allowing any data stack overlap (TrueStack, Siemens Healthineers). The location of the coronal and sagittal image planes were set at a deliberate distance of a few centimeters away from the heart minimizing the influence of residual cardiac motion on these images. The misalignment of the individual stacks is clearly visible in these image views, indicating breathing motion as the root cause of the image artifacts. In addition, as a characteristic sign of breathing through the diaphragm, one can see that the misalignment is limited to the lung vessels including the flat liver dome and no signs of misalignment or steps are present in the ribs or thorax surface of the patient. Due to the good alignment of the outer thorax and ribs, this kind of diaphragm breathing-induced artifact is often wrongfully attributed to cardiac motion.

A viable alternative for the identification of these kinds of artifacts to the MPR reconstructions of Fig. 14.8 are thick-slice MIP images with a slice thickness of 40–50 mm illustrated in Fig. 14.8. Breathing motion artifacts through the diaphragm can also be easily demonstrated if visualized using thick-slice MIP images. Two additional cases of insufficient breath-hold and subsequent breathing artifacts are illustrated in Fig. 14.9, both visualized as thick 40-mm MIP images in the coronal view making the root cause of the problem easily identifiable.

Conclusion

In this chapter key workflow elements that are crucial for a successful cardiac CT examination were described. Ignoring any of them can easily result in a suboptimal or non-diagnostic exam. Since the described workflow is quite complex, a dedicated cardiac CT training of the technologists is highly desirable. Keeping

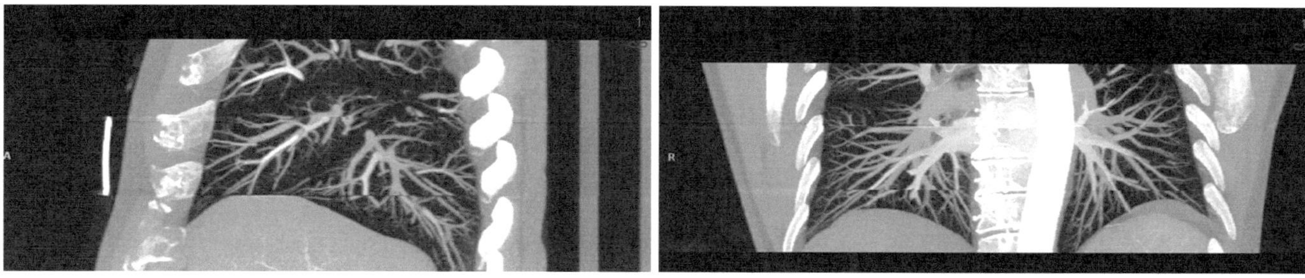

Fig. 14.8 Coronal (left) and sagittal (right) 40-mm thick MIP images of the lung. These are from the same case as above illustrating the improved visibility of the breathing artifacts by switching from a MPR to a MIP display

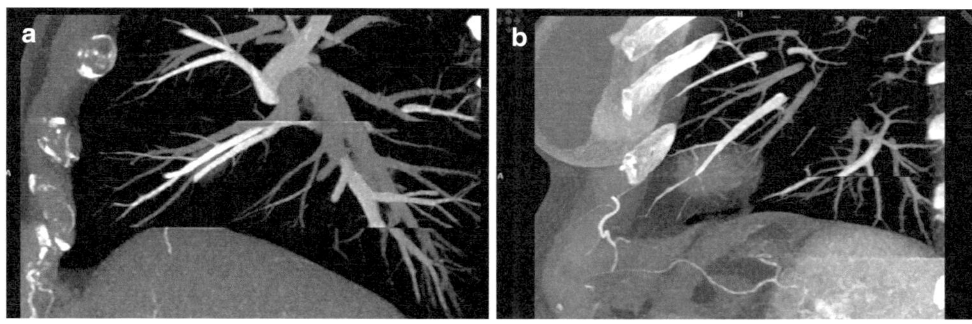

Fig. 14.9 (**a**, **b**) Additional case examples of breathing artifacts visualized as thick-slice MIP images in a coronal image view

in mind that cardiac CT technology is quickly evolving, such training should occur on a regular basis. Clinical practices with well-trained dedicated cardiac CT technologists perform exceptionally well. For example, a recent publication from one of such practices reports only one non-diagnostic CCTA in 1022 consecutive examinations [40]. This example clearly proves that cardiac CT can (and should) be successfully performed when all the key workflow instructions are followed. This chapter at hand only focused on two major aspects of the cardiac CT workflow: patient preparation and selection of the most appropriate acquisition mode. Other important aspects such as use of beta-blockers, contrast injection, dealing with difficult-to-image patients (e.g., morbidly obese or with poor renal function), and cardiac CT post-processing were deliberately omitted here because they are described in other chapters of this book.

References

1. Jakobs TF, Becker CR, Ohnesorge B, et al. Multislice helical CT of the heart with retrospective ECG gating: reduction of radiation exposure by ECG-controlled tube current modulation. Eur Radiol. 2002;12(5):1081–6.
2. Weustink AC, Mollet NR, Pugliese F, et al. Optimal electrocardiographic pulsing windows and heart rate: effect on image quality and radiation exposure at dual-source coronary CT angiography. Radiology. 2008;248(3):792–8.
3. McCollough CH, Primak AN, Saba O, et al. Dose performance of a 64-channel dual-source CT scanner. Radiology. 2007;243(3):775–84.
4. Ruzsics B, Gebregziabher M, Lee H, Brothers RL, Allmendinger T, Vogt S, Costello P, Schoepf UJ. Coronary CT angiography: automatic cardiac-phase selection for image reconstruction. Eur Radiol. 2009;19:1906–13.
5. Hoffmann MH, Lessick J, Manzke R, Schmid FT, Gershin E, Boll DT, Rispler S, Aschoff AJ, Grass M. Automatic determination of minimal cardiac motion phases for computed tomography imaging: initial experience. Eur Radiol. 2006;16:365–73.
6. Lee AM, Engel LC, Shah B, Liew G, Sidhu MS, Kalra M, Abbara S, Brady TJ, Hoffmann U, Ghoshhajra BB. Coronary computed tomography angiography during arrhythmia: radiation dose reduction with prospectively ECG-triggered axial and retrospectively ECG-gated helical 128-slice dual-source CT. J Cardiovasc Comput Tomogr. 2012;6(3):172–183.e2.
7. Lee AM, Beaudoin J, Engel LC, Sidhu MS, Abbara S, Brady TJ, Hoffmann U, Ghoshhajra BB. Assessment of image quality and radiation dose of prospectively ECG-triggered adaptive dual-source coronary computed tomography angiography (cCTA) with arrhythmia rejection algorithm in systole versus diastole: a retrospective cohort study. Int J Cardiovasc Imaging. 2013;29(6):1361–70.
8. Siemens data sheet: Flex: http://www.neocoil.com/docs/16CH_Flex_Siemens_MRI/NC00S007%20Rev%20A%2016ch%20Siemens%20Flex%20Data%20Sheet.pdf.
9. Williams MC, Weir NW, Mirsadraee S, Scott AE, Uren NG, McKillop G, van Beek EJ, Reid JH, Newby DE. Image quality with single-heartbeat 320-multidetector computed tomographic coronary angiography. J Comput Assist Tomogr. 2014;38(3):444–50.
10. Latif MA, Sanchez FW, Sayegh K, Veledar E, Aziz M, Malik R, Haider I, Agatston AS, Batlle JC, Janowitz W, Peña C, Ziffer JA, Nasir K, Cury RC. Volumetric single-beat coronary computed tomography angiography: relationship of image quality, heart rate, and body mass index. Initial patient experience with a new computed tomography scanner. J Comput Assist Tomogr. 2016;40(5):763–72.
11. Meyer M, Haubenreisser H, Schoepf UJ, Vliegenthart R, Leidecker C, Allmendinger T, Lehmann R, Sudarski S, Borggrefe M,

Schoenberg SO, Henzler T. Closing in on the K edge: coronary CT angiography at 100, 80, and 70 kV-initial comparison of a second- versus a third-generation dual-source CT system. Radiology. 2014 Nov;273(2):373–82.
12. Felmly LM, De Cecco CN, Schoepf UJ, Varga-Szemes A, Mangold S, McQuiston AD, Litwin SE, Bayer RR 2nd, Vogl TJ, Wichmann JL. Low contrast medium-volume third-generation dual-source computed tomography angiography for transcatheter aortic valve replacement planning. Eur Radiol. 2017;27(5):1944–53.
13. Koplay M, Guneyli S, Akbayrak H, Demir K, Sivri M, Avci A, Erdogan H, Paksoy Y. Diagnostic accuracy and effective radiation dose of high pitch dual source multidetector computed tomography in evaluation of coronary artery bypass graft patency. Wien Klin Wochenschr. 2016;128(13–14):488–94.
14. Budoff MJ, Georgiou D, Brody A, Agatston AS, Kennedy J, Wolfkiel C, Stanford W, Shields P, Lewis RJ, Janowitz WR, Rich S, Brundage BH. Ultrafast computed tomography as a diagnostic modality in the detection of coronary artery disease: a multicenter study. Circulation. 1996;93:898–904.
15. Hecht HS, Cronin P, Blaha MJ, Budoff MJ, Kazerooni EA, Narula J, Yankelevitz D, Abbara S. 2016 SCCT/STR guidelines for coronary artery calcium scoring of noncontrast noncardiac chest CT scans: a report of the Society of Cardiovascular Computed Tomography and Society of Thoracic Radiology. J Cardiovasc Comput Tomogr. 2017;32(5):W54–66.
16. Cury RC, Abbara S, Achenbach S, Agatston A, Berman DS, Budoff MJ, Dill KE, Jacobs JE, Maroules CD, Rubin GD, Rybicki FJ, Schoepf UJ, Shaw LJ, Stillman AE, White CS, Woodard PK, Leipsic JA. CAD-RADS(TM) Coronary Artery Disease – Reporting and Data System. An expert consensus document of the Society of Cardiovascular Computed Tomography (SCCT), the American College of Radiology (ACR) and the North American Society for Cardiovascular Imaging (NASCI). Endorsed by the American College of Cardiology. J Cardiovasc Comput Tomogr. 2016;10(4):269–81.
17. Halliburton S, Arbab-Zadeh A, De D, Einstein AJ, Gentry R, et al. State-of-the-art in CT hardware and scan modes for cardiovascular CT. J Cardiovasc Comput Tomogr. 2012;6:154–63.
18. Celeng C, Vadvala H, Puchner S, Pursnani A, Sharma U, Kovacs A, Maurovich-Horvat P, Hoffmann U, Ghoshhajra B. Defining the optimal systolic phase targets using absolute delay time for reconstructions in dual-source coronary CT angiography. Int J Cardiovasc Imaging. 2016;32(1):91–100.
19. Srichai MB, Barreto M, Lim RP, Donnino R, Babb JS, Jacobs JE. Prospective-triggered sequential dual-source end-systolic coronary CT angiography for patients with atrial fibrillation: a feasibility study. J Cardiovasc Comput Tomogr. 2013;7(2):102–9.
20. Kondo T, Kumamaru KK, Fujimoto S, Matsutani H, Sano T, Takase S, Rybicki FJ. Prospective ECG-gated coronary 320-MDCT angiography with absolute acquisition delay strategy for patients with persistent atrial fibrillation. AJR Am J Roentgenol. 2013;201(6):1197–203.
21. Siemens data sheet: FlashCheck.
22. Siemens syngo CT VB10 data sheet.
23. GE lookup tables. http://www3.gehealthcare.com/en/education/product_education_clinical/tip_applications/computed_tomography_hq_class/revolution_ct.
24. Lee JD, See KA. Trust in automation: designing for appropriate reliance. Hum factors. Spring. 2004;46(1):50–80.
25. Parasuraman R, Sheridan TB, Wickens CD. A model for types and levels of human interaction with automation. IEEE Trans Syst Man Cybern Syst Hum. 2000;30(3):286–97.
26. Budoff MJ. Maximizing dose reductions with cardiac CT. Int J Cardiovasc Imaging. 2009;25(Suppl 2):279–87.
27. Budoff MJ. Ethical issues related to lung nodules on cardiac CT. AJR Am J Roentgenol. 2009;192(3):W146.
28. Budoff MJ, Gopal A. Incidental findings on cardiac computed tomography. Should we look? J Cardiovasc Comput Tomogr. 2007;1(2):97–105.
29. Goehler A, McMahon PM, Lumish HS, Wu CC, Munshi V, Gilmore M, Chung JH, Ghoshhajra BB, Mark D, Truong QA, Gazelle GS, Hoffmann U. Cost-effectiveness of follow-up of pulmonary nodules incidentally detected on cardiac computed tomographic angiography in patients with suspected coronary artery disease. Circulation. 2014;130(8):668–75.
30. Co SJ, Mayo J, Liang T, Krzymyk K, Yousefi M, Nicolaou S. Iterative reconstructed ultra high pitch CT pulmonary angiography with cardiac bowtie-shaped filter in the acute setting: effect on dose and image quality. Eur J Radiol. 2013;82(9):1571–6.
31. Franck C, Bacher K. Influence of localizer and scan direction on the dose-reducing effect of automatic tube current modulation in computed tomography. Radiat Prot Dosim. 2016;169(1–4):136–42.
32. Vadvala H, Kim P, Mayrhofer T, Pianykh O, Kalra M, Hoffmann U, Ghoshhajra B. Coronary CTA using scout-based automated tube potential and current selection algorithm, with breast displacement results in lower radiation exposure in females compared to males. Cardiovasc Diagn Ther. 2014 Dec;4(6):470–9.
33. http://www.mysupplies.philips.com/Documents/lit/453564119681.pdf.
34. http://multimedia.3m.com/mws/media/358372O/proper-skin-prep-ecg-trace-quality-white-paper.pdf.
35. Smith M. Rx for ECG monitoring artifact. Crit Care Nurse. 1984;4:64–6.
36. Odma S, Oberg P. Movement-induced potentials in surface electrodes. Med Biol Eng Comput. 1982;20:159–66.
37. Adams-Hamoda MG, Caldwell MA, Stotts NA, Drew BJ. Factors to consider when analyzing 12-lead electrocardiograms for evidence of acute myocardial ischemia. Am J Crit Care. 2003;12:9–18.
38. Romans LE. Computed tomography for technologists: exam review. Lippincott Williams & Wilkins. 2010. https://www.amazon.com/Computed-Tomography-Technologists-Lippincott-Williams/dp/0781777968.
39. Bankier AA, O'Donnell CR, Boiselle PM. Quality initiatives. Respiratory instructions for CT examinations of the lungs: a hands-on guide. Radiographics. 2008;28:919–31.
40. Ghoshhajra BB, Takx RA, Staziaki PV, Vadvala H, Kim P, Neilan TG, Meyersohn NM, Bittner D, Janjua SA, Mayrhofer T, Greenwald JL, Truong QA, Abbara S, Brown DF, Januzzi JL, Francis S, Nagurney JT, Hoffmann U, MGH Emergency Cardiac CTA Program Contributors. Clinical implementation of an emergency department coronary computed tomographic angiography protocol for triage of patients with suspected acute coronary syndrome. Eur Radiol. 2017;27(7):2784–93.

Defining the Role and Benefits of a 3D Laboratory for Cardiovascular CT

15

Laura J. Pierce, Daniel T. Boll, and Geoffrey D. Rubin

In addition to understanding methods for successfully acquiring and interpreting computed tomographic angiogram (CTA) images of the heart and cardiovascular structures, cardiovascular (CV) radiologists and cardiologists must also be facile with the creation and evaluation of post-processed three- and four-dimensional images and analyses of these structures. Particularly for assessing cardiovascular structure and function across modalities and over time for longitudinal comparisons, CT post-processing is essential (Fig. 15.1). The primary interpreter of the CTA should be capable of exploring the CT data using three- and four-dimensional analysis tools and performing a full spectrum of assessments including the creation of volume renderings, curved planar reformations (CPR), maximum intensity projections (MIP), and the measurement of the cardiac and vascular dimensions, quantitation of coronary calcium, and assessing myocardial function through qualitative review of regional wall motion and quantitation of ventricular ejection fraction [1]. This work is most often accomplished separately from the CT scanner, using independent 3D workstations or client applications to remotely interact with server-based analytical tools over a network. While physicians bear primary responsibility for fully interpreting the CT data, there are compelling reasons for physicians to partner with technologists within a formal "3D laboratory" to facilitate the creation, communication, and curation of post-processed images and measurements and, in collaboration with radiologists and referring clinicians, facilitate structured reporting. This chapter focuses on the rationale for establishing a 3D laboratory for managing CV CTA workflows and on some of the operational aspects to consider to assure consistently high-quality output and service.

L. J. Pierce · G. D. Rubin (✉)
Department of Radiology, Duke University School of Medicine, Durham, NC, USA
e-mail: grubin@duke.edu

D. T. Boll
Department of Radiology, University of Basel, Basel, Switzerland

Developing a 3D/CV Service to Meet Needs of the Medical Community

When performing 3D analyses of CT data, there are many priorities that imaging practices and hospitals may have. These include the creation of consistently high-quality visualizations and measurements, operations and results that comply with regulations for payment and communication of the results, efficient operations to off-load tasks from physicians, freeing them to engage in higher value activities, enhanced and intuitive communication with patients and referring providers, marketing of clinical programs, facilitation of clinical research protocols, and education and training of medical staff (Fig. 15.2).

Assessing Community Needs and Priorities

Cardiovascular 3D image post-processing can be very time-consuming for physicians, especially when the CTA dataset contains several thousand images from multiple time points throughout the cardiac cycle. If the local medical community has a large population with cardiovascular imaging needs, it may be prudent and more efficient for physicians to centralize the CV image post-processing in a 3D Laboratory, staffed by 3D radiologic technologists who have received advanced training in cardiovascular image post-processing and supervised by radiologists to grow and evolve offerings according to the needs of referring clinicians and their patients.

Because the source datasets are very large and present the anatomy from perspectives that may not be intuitive to referrers and their patients, cardiologists, cardiovascular surgeons, and other medical specialists rely on 3D images to understand a patient's anatomy and pathologies, to plan interventions, and to communicate these details to their

U. J. Schoepf (ed.), *CT of the Heart*, Contemporary Medical Imaging, https://doi.org/10.1007/978-1-60327-237-7_15

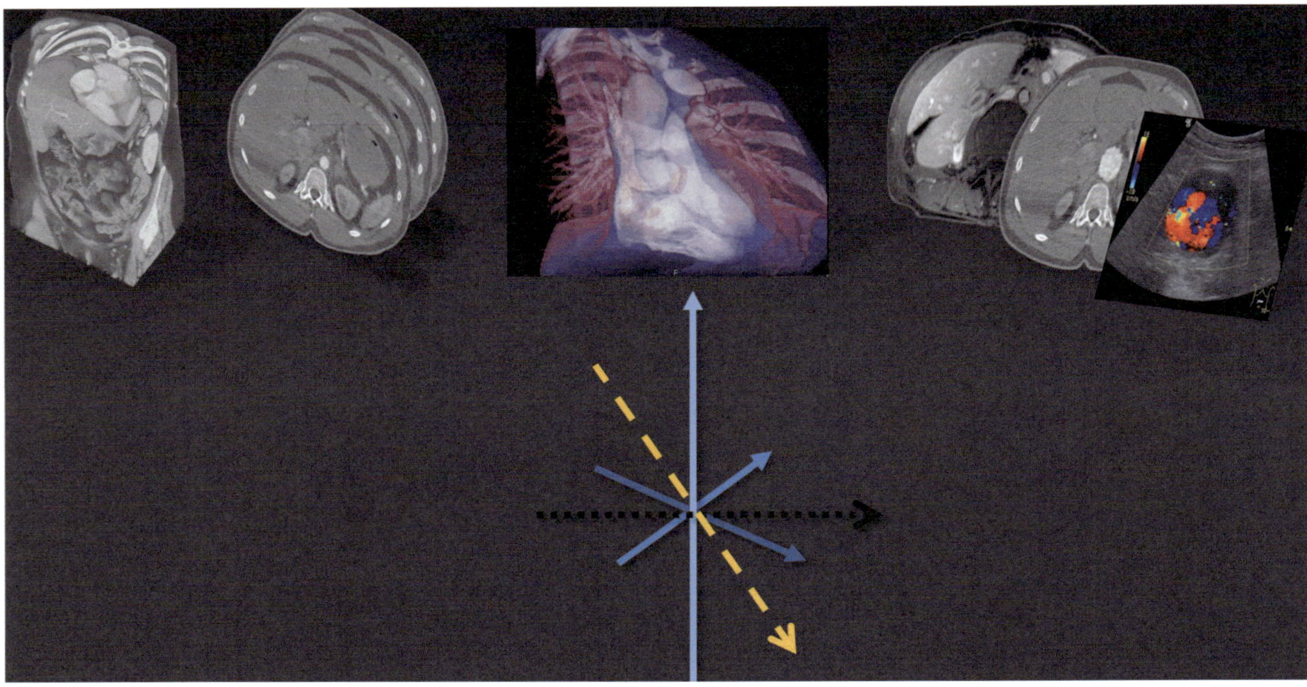

Fig. 15.1 Schematic emphasizing the multidimensionality of imaging data. High-resolution isometric-voxel acquisitions (left pictogram) are acquired either days, weeks, or years apart as follow-up examinations (pictogram second from left) or only milliseconds apart (middle pictogram) and then compared in an intermodal approach (right pictogram)

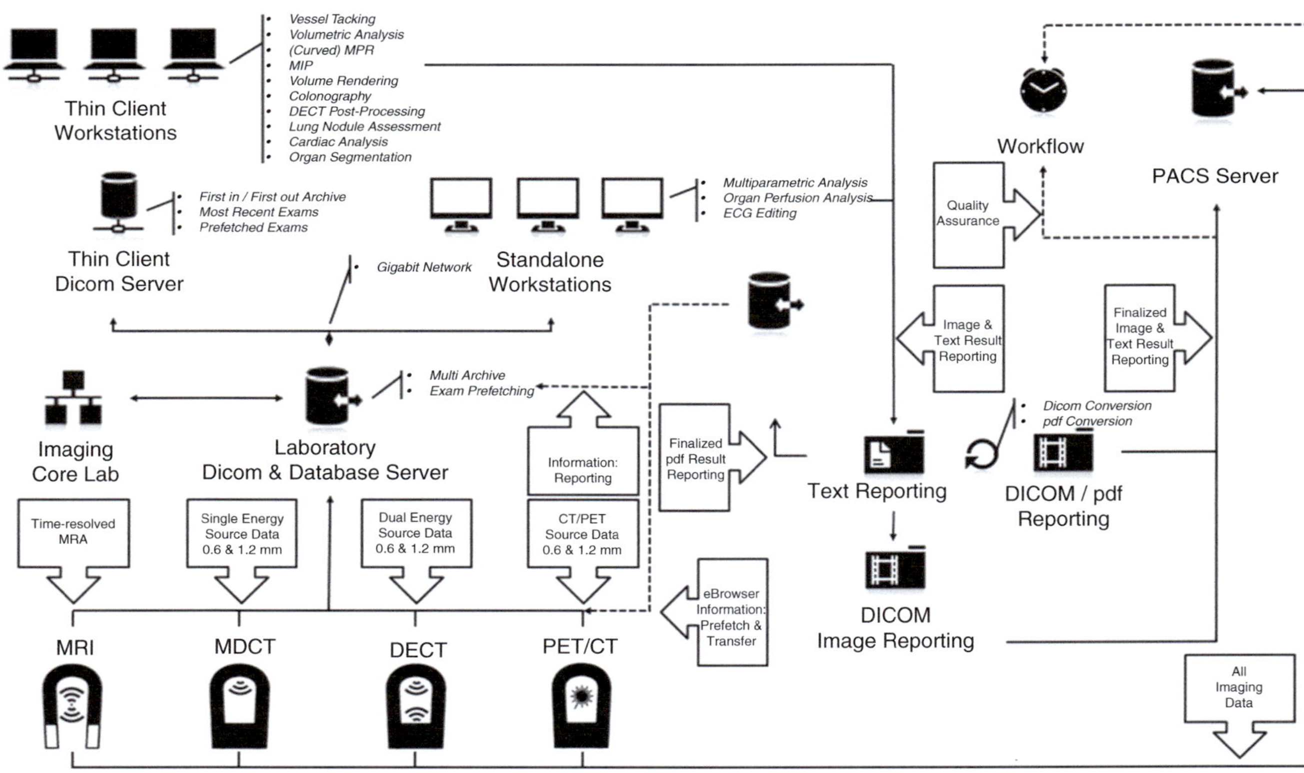

Fig. 15.2 Flowchart highlighting the complex workflows of a post-processing laboratory. Following the source data acquisition (lower left-hand corner), various forms of post-processing and creation of structured reporting are performed on different types of post-processing solutions. Every workflow step is logged and thereby lends itself to continuous workflow optimization procedures

patients. When interpreting CTA scans, radiologists and cardiologists are principally focused upon the interpretation and its narrative report and less on the creation of images for the referrers. Even when considering the needs of referring providers, physicians interpreting the scans rarely take an organized approach to image creation, preferring to capture a few views analogous to "spot views" captured during other real-time imaging explorations such as with gastrointestinal fluoroscopy or sonography. While a couple of well-positioned and annotated images can be valuable for referring physicians and their patients, most prefer a standard set of views similar to those that are routinely acquired by sonographers and radiologic technologists following upper or lower gastrointestinal tract contrast studies. The task of creating reliably formatted and labeled standard views is an excellent task for a 3D technologist. Labeled standard views of previous imaging can be easily incorporated to document longitudinal assessments of cardiovascular atherosclerosis and cardiac function, for example.

Establishing these standard views is best done in partnership with the physicians who need to use them to manage their patients. Understanding and assessing referring physicians' needs and expectations for CV imaging is an important first step in the development of a 3D laboratory service. The optimal approach for extracting this information is to identify and interview key referring cardiovascular physicians in the local community. Significant insights may be extracted from these interviews, which will assist a radiology group in establishing a service that reflects the voice of its customers [2] (Fig. 15.3). Some physicians may be principally focused on standard image creation, while other may need detailed measurements recorded on standardized forms. Structured reporting facilitates reports that are targeted to the specific needs of referring clinicians and their patients. Some referring physicians may express an interest in manipulating and constructing the post-processed images themselves, thus requiring remote access to the 3D server software in the clinical or surgical environment. Remote access would require additional technical and training support that may be provided by the 3D laboratory staff. Workflow prioritization, reporting of quantitative analysis, and coordination of image review between cardiothoracic surgery and radiology services are also services that may be facilitated by a 3D laboratory.

In a large medical center where many surgical specialists may practice, protocol standardization is imperative for efficient workflows and reliable results. The development of five different 3D coronary CTA protocols for a group of five different cardiothoracic surgeons is a recipe for errors and unhappy referrers, particularly when cross-covering one another. A physician champion in the role of 3D laboratory director may need to intervene with the group of referrers to help them organize themselves and create a single consensus-driven solution. Regardless of the nuances and idiosyncrasies encountered, a fundamental approach to a successful system-wide 3D lab resource is outreach to referrers and regular engagement to maximize the value of the lab's output and enhance dependencies between the referrers and the lab.

Quality, Efficiency, and Compliance

According to the American College of Radiology [3] practice parameters for cardiac CT, 3D post-processing should be performed by a physician, a registered radiologic technologist, or other experienced personnel who

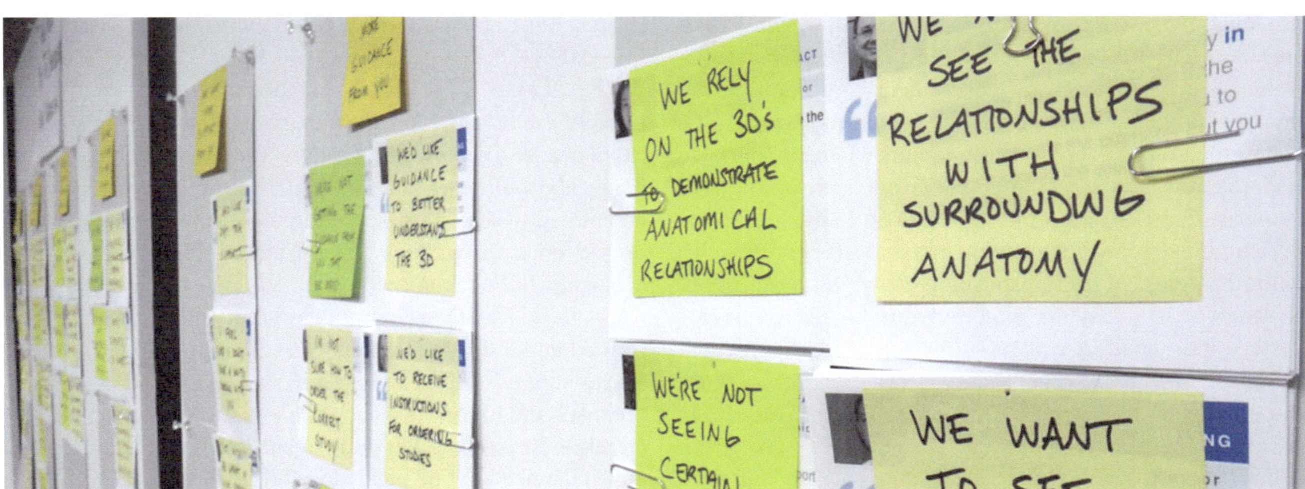

Fig. 15.3 Example of an affinity chart analysis performed to learn wants and needs from referring clinicians. Which type of post-processing and reporting is desired as part of a "voice of the customer" service improvement initiative

have sufficient knowledge of cardiovascular anatomy and pathophysiology [3]. Because 3D post-processing for large cardiac CT datasets can be very time-consuming, it may be cost-efficient to off-load most of the 3D tasks to a trained 3D technologist, rather than an MD. Assigning the bulk of the creation and quantitation of 3D images to a technologist allows the radiologist or cardiologist to focus upon interpretation and reporting of the examination. Because 3D technologists devote all their time to post-processing and quantitative data analysis, they can become very efficient at these tasks. 3D lab staffing models ideally should be flexible and responsive to variations in demand to assure that turnaround time goals are met. In the event of after-hours emergencies, 3D technologists may be given access to the 3D processing server to process urgent CTA studies remotely.

Quantitative analyses of cardiovascular structures and pathology are important measures of disease progress. Key management decisions may be based on subtle changes in vascular dimensions. However, 3D cardiovascular structure measurement results vary with operator experience, intra- and interobserver inconsistencies, CT acquisition, and differences among 3D software tools and algorithms [4].

3D technologists can provide baseline presurgical and follow-up postsurgical aortic diameters, areas, volumes, angles, and lengths, as well as coronary artery stenosis and cardiac chamber function measurements (Fig. 15.4). A qualified 3D Laboratory will provide oversight and established consistency in cardiac and aortic measurements, permanently store measurement images on a radiology imaging archive, and record quantitative findings into the electronic CTA examination report for review and signature by the interpreting radiologist or cardiologist. Preoperative measurements may be useful for screening for patient candidacy for aortic stent graft or aortic valve replacement, as well as for stent/valve sizing selection. When follow-up exams come through, 3D technologists can recall the prior measurements and assure that measurements are made in the same location and with the same techniques, providing greater reliability of serial measurements when compared to standard clinical reading. Graphical displays of variations in key measurements over time can be useful adjuncts to the standard images and measurement tables (Fig. 15.5). To reduce the potential for transposition errors in transcription, quantitative data may be exported directly from the 3D interface into the CTA text report or stored in a permanent database where it may be accessed for comparison with postoperative or follow-up CTA studies. The measurements may also be programmed to be automatically exported from the database into the CTA report for confirmation and final signature by the attending radiologist or cardiologist. When quantitative results are outside normal value, they may be flagged automatically for review.

Beyond the creation and curation of 3D images and measurements, a 3D laboratory can act as a central point of communication with the medical center to address any 3D post-processing requests or questions. A consistent point of contact built into the imaging workflow facilitates follow-through and accountability to assure that the required processing is completed and that exams do not slip through the cracks.

Compliance

Beyond assuring that images are created consistently, the 3D lab can assure that necessary requirements are met to comply with requirements for billing. When scheduling a CTA study of the heart in the United States, the correct Current Procedural Terminology (CPT) code must be assigned to ensure that the correct bill is released to the payer. Radiology CPT codes are maintained by the American Medical Association (AMA) and uniformly describe diagnostic services. CPT codes for cardiac CT range from 75571 to 75574, varying in complexity from a non-contrast CT of the coronary arteries to a postoperative pre-/post-intravenous contrast CTA of the heart that includes arterial and/or venous structures. Reimbursement is not only dependent on valid medical indication but also correct documentation of the procedure performed. All cardiac CT CPT codes include some type of 3D post-processing. Because the 3D service is bundled with the CTA charges, there is not a separate charge for 3D imaging. To compliantly bill for the cardiac CT examination, 3D imaging must be performed, and the 3D results must be included in the final report. The American College of Radiology [3] also recommends that the post-processed images be labeled with patient and facility identification, examination date, and anatomic location depicted. The 3D images must be saved and archived with the CTA sectional images [3].

The 3D lab is excellently positioned to serve as a single point of contact to confirm billing compliance by reviewing exam charges, proofreading reports for proper technique verbiage, and validating that the 3D images are labeled correctly and stored in the proper CT examination folder for viewing in the enterprise PACS. The Centers for Medicare and Medicaid Services (CMS) state that if a technologist performs the CTA 3D examination, the procedure must be performed under the direct supervision of a physician (level 2). Direct supervision means the physician must be present on premises and immediately available to furnish assistance and direction throughout the performance of the procedure. The physician need not be present in the room when a 3D procedure is performed [5]. For audit purposes, a 3D laboratory administrator can confirm documentation of physician supervision for 3D examinations.

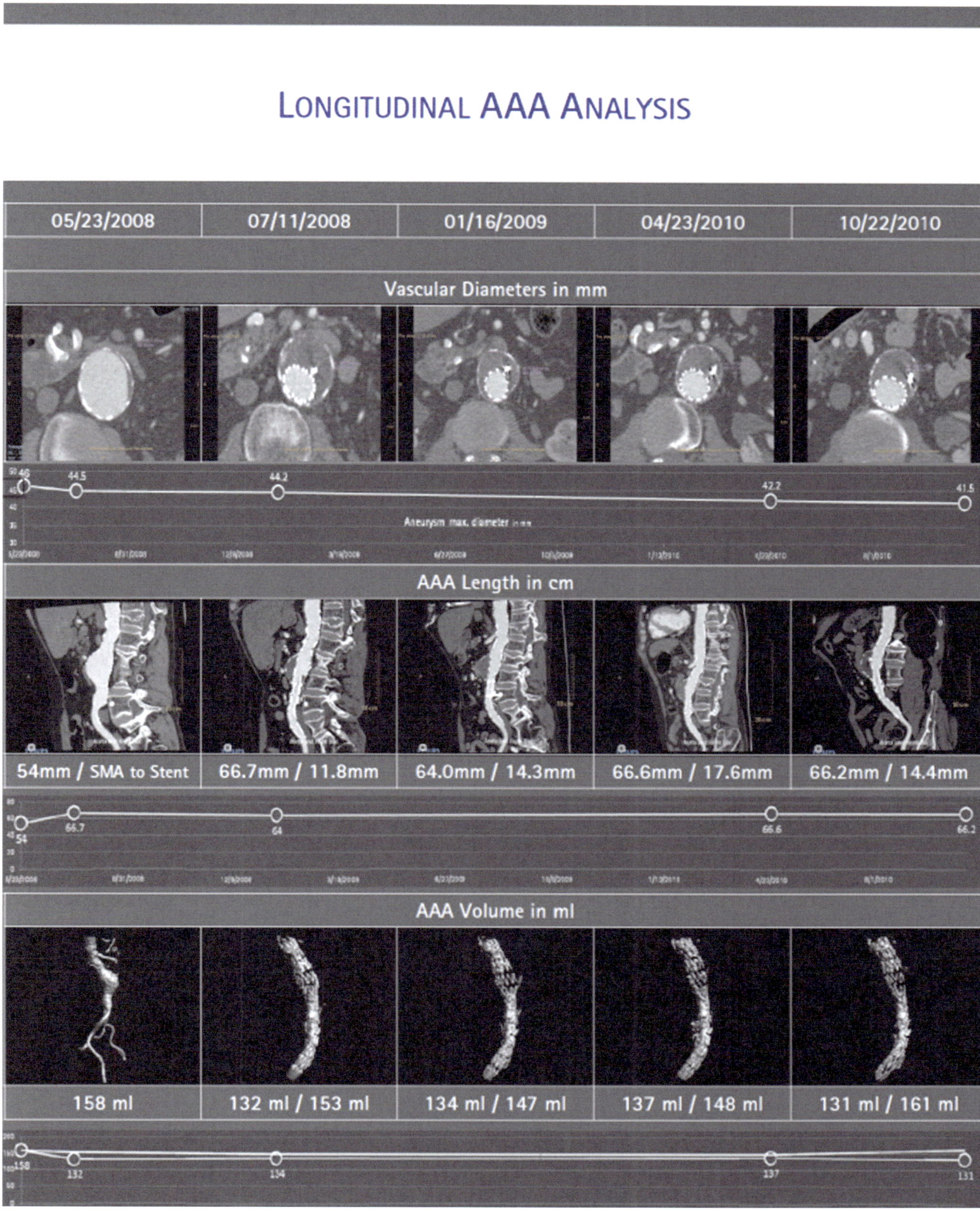

Fig. 15.4 Longitudinal report describing the evolution of a treated aortic aneurysm over time following endovascular treatment as a function of cross-sectional diameter (upper row of thumbnail images and corresponding graphical chart), aneurysms' craniocaudal extension (middle row of thumbnail images and corresponding graphical chart) and configuration of the implanted endograft over time with a volumetric assessment of aneurysm size (lower role of thumbnail images and corresponding graphical chart)

Category	Measurement Name	Major	Minor
Orthogonal Diameter in mm(wall to wall, including calcium)	Left ventricular outflow tract	28.8	18.2
	Major Aortic Annulus diameter (systole)	27.9	
	Perpendicular Minor Aortic annulus diameter (systole)	26.0	
	Aortic annulus in diastole	27.7	25.1
	Sinus of Valsalva diameter, right coronary	32.0	
	Sinus of Valsalva diameter, left coronary	33.7	
	Sinus of Valsalva diameter, non-coronary	32.3	
	Sinotubular junction	30.6	60.4
	Aorta 4 cm distal to annulus	32.4	30.6
	Descending thoracic aorta distal to the LSA	27.6	25.8
	Descending thoracic aorta at the level of diaphragm	23.4	22.5
Orthogonal Diameter in mm(flowlumen, within calcium)	Rightsubclavian artery minimum lumen diameter (MLD)	5.2	
	Rightsubclavian artery diameter perpendicular to MLD	7.0	
	Left subclavian artery minimum lumen diameter	5.8	
	Left subclavian artery diameter perpendicular to MLD	5.2	
	Abdominal aorta proximal to renal arteries	20.9	18.1
	Abdominal aorta distal to renal arteries	16.2	14.9
	Minimum abdominal aortic diameter	12.5	
	Perpendicular abdominal aortic diameter at minimum	14.2	
	Distal abdominal aortic proximal to aortic bifurcation	13.6	12.8
	Right common iliac artery proximal	10.0	8.2
	Right common iliac artery minimum lumen diameter	7.7	
	Right common iliac artery perpendicular to MLD	9.0	
	Right common iliac artery distal	9.0	7.7
	Right external iliac artery minimum lumen diameter	6.5	
	Right external iliac artery perpendicular to MLD	7.0	
	Right common femoral artery minimum lumen diameter	6.5	
	Right common femoral artery perpendicular to MLD	7.4	
	Left common iliac artery proximal	10.3	10.0
	Left common iliac artery minimum lumen diameter	8.6	
	Left common iliac artery perpendicular to MLD	9.6	
	Left common iliac artery distal	9.5	8.8
	Left external iliac artery minimum lumen diameter	7.8	
	Left external iliac artery perpendicular to MLD	7.8	
	Left common femoral artery minimum lumen diameter	7.8	
	Left common femoral artery perpendicular to MLD	7.9	
Angle in degrees	Aortic Root Angulation (diastole)	41.6	
	Angle of SOV leaflets, RAO	7.0	
	Angle of SOV leaflets, CAU	3.0	
Length in mm	Annulus to RCA origin	14.2	
	Annulus to Lt main origin	11.8	
	Sinus of Valsalva height, Right coronary (diastole)	22.0	
	Sinus of Valsalva height, Left coronary (diastole)	19.7	
	Sinus of Valsalva height, Non coronary (diastole)	21.9	
	Average Sinuses of Valsalva height	21.2	
Circumference in mm	Aortic annulus perimeter systole including mural calcium	76.0	
Ejection Fraction in Percentage	LV Ejection Fraction	58.0	

Fig. 15.5 Tabulated measurements (**a**) and corresponding measurement locations (**b**) as desired by referring clinicians for planning prior to TAVR procedure

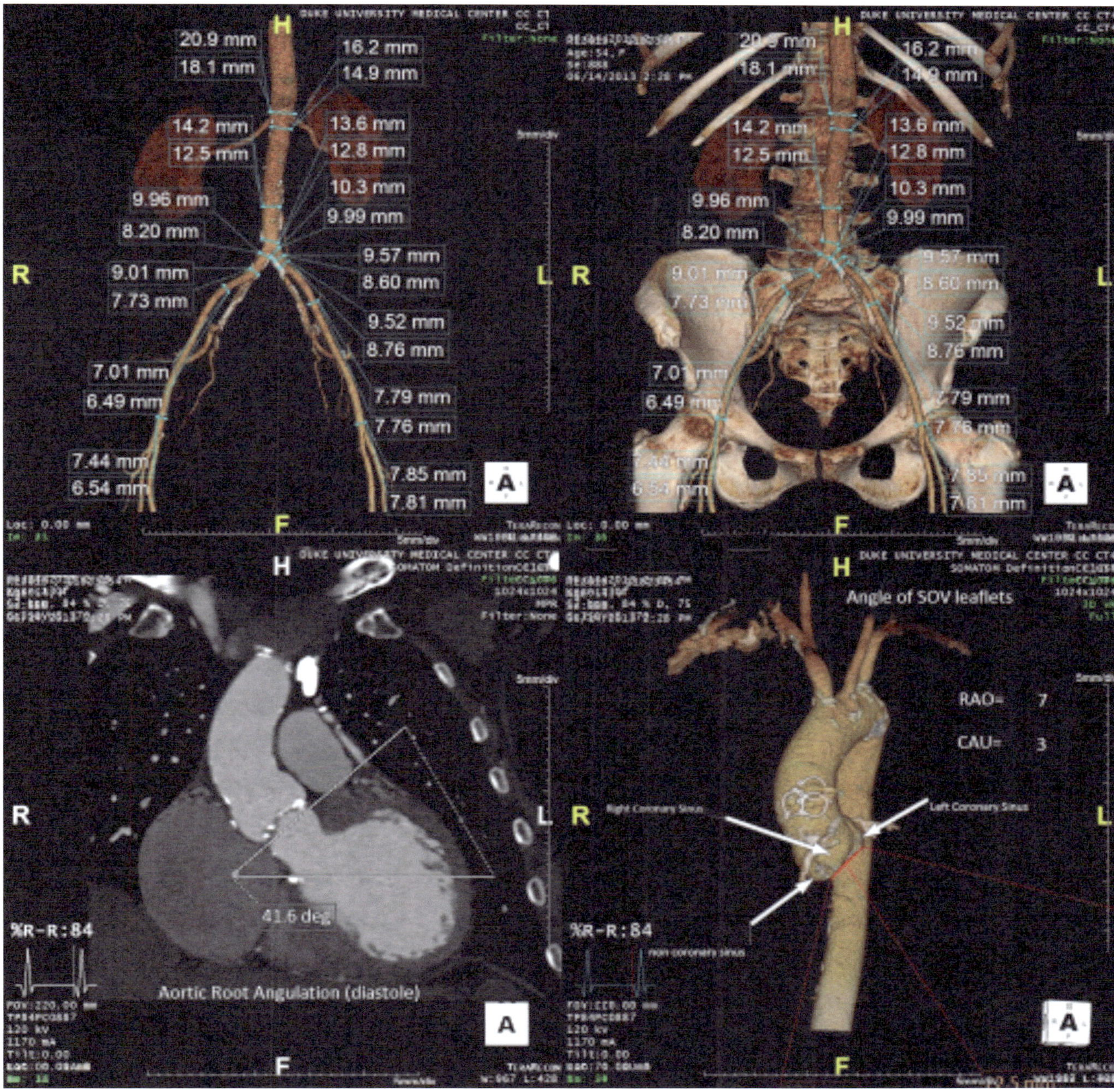

Fig. 15.5 (continued)

Another critical compliance need in the United States centers around confidentiality of medical information and personal records. All staff in the 3D lab must follow protocol to maintain compliance with the Health Information Portability and Accountability Act (HIPAA). Training for HIPAA compliance is mandatory for all 3D staff. To ensure confidentiality, when 3D images are exported for education or research purposes, the 3D technologist can anonymize or de-identify the images electronically, stripping the 18 HIPAA Privacy Rule identifiers from the Digital Imaging and Communications in Medicine (DICOM) image header. 3D laboratory policies and procedures should contain language about the need to access only needed patient information, not sharing passwords, not emailing confidential images or information outside the institution, and not sharing patient information with unauthorized personnel. Lab policies must also include HIPAA protections for the enterprise-wide 3D software that resides on central servers. Rules must limit access to the 3D software to currently trained staff, with strong passwords and time-out limits to assure that 3D computers are not left unattended when patient accounts are open and active. This becomes even more important as users can access the 3D server remotely from off-site locations. Analogously and particularly for patients who are enrolled in clinical trials, the ability to de-identify or anonymize complex source data and processed imaging series may represent another important type of "post-processing" if imaging data needs to be sent to an external facility.

Outreach Facilitated by 3D Imaging

Patient Centricity

The formal creation of 3D images provides benefits beyond those derived by referring physicians and interpreting physicians directly. When surgeons are discussing options for cardiothoracic surgery with their patients, 3D images that display aberrant anatomy or abnormal conditions may be very helpful for demonstrating the gravity of a newly diagnosed condition or to explain a surgical approach. Patients are better able to understand the benefits of a pending intervention after seeing a lifelike 3D model of their anatomy, compared with viewing the hundreds of stacked axial images that are produced in a CTA. Engaging patients in their treatment and diagnosis benefits the patient and the referring physicians. Many referring physicians relish the opportunity to show beautiful 3D reformations to their patients who provide word-of-mouth endorsements that may enhance future referrals.

Enhancing Referrals

3D images can also be used by the imaging practice or the hospital to support a strategy that promotes referrals for specialized cardiovascular procedures, such as an atrial fibrillation treatment program or a percutaneous trans-aortic valve replacement for aortic stenosis. 3D images in brochures, websites, and advertisements can highlight the technical expertise of an institution, which the public may find attractive when compared with other regional or international competitors. A 3D laboratory can prepare and anonymize high-resolution 3D static images and 4D temporal videos that highlight institution offerings for marketing or educational purposes.

Benefits for Research and Education

When an institution performs clinical research, a 3D laboratory with trained technologists can ensure that consistency, quality, and integrity are built into the data collection for the research protocol. With proper documentation of training, performance, policies, and procedures, a 3D laboratory can assure compliance to the Food and Drug Administration (FDA) and research sponsors.

Within a large medical center, the 3D laboratory can act as a centralized 3D imaging training center for technologists, radiologists, fellows, residents, clinicians, researchers, and students. The completion of formalized training may be required prior to qualifying users for secure access to enterprise-wide 3D servers. If a remote user has any difficulty with any 3D software, a 3D laboratory technologist may be made available for on-the-spot instruction.

Training protocols may be tailor-made for each group's clinical 3D post-processing needs. This is important for consistency and quality in imaging throughout an institution, as there is the potential for variation in 3D imaging depending on a user's abilities and training. After completing and being signed off for training in the 3D laboratory, cardiovascular or radiology residents and fellows may be utilized for any real-time post-processing needs during emergency or clinical readout of CTA cardiac/thoracic studies. In addition, researchers from other medical departments who are trained in the 3D laboratory may in turn develop collaborations with radiologists and exchange valuable information regarding the latest advances in surgical technology. This increased communication between departments has been shown to be advantageous to diminishing organizational silos [2].

Operational Considerations for an Effective 3D Laboratory

Establishment of Proper Communication Channels

One of the most challenging and important functions of a 3D laboratory is the establishment of proper communication channels between all stakeholders in the cardiovascular imaging service line. A key component of 3D laboratory procedures is the establishment of two-sided communication channels. Examples include communication of initial imaging orders between the radiology information system and the 3D laboratory, exchange of relevant clinical information between the referring MD and the responsible radiologist, assignment of proper scanning and post-processing protocols from the radiologist to the CT and 3D technologists, requesting retrospective image reconstructions between the 3D laboratory and CT technologists, and communication of CT and 3D results to the referring MD.

Because 3D post-processing is often performed on equipment that is located apart from the CT scanners, communication between the scanners and the 3D laboratory is particularly critical to the acquisition and processing of clinically effective imaging exams. Procedures should be developed within the 3D laboratory to collect and then review problematic CT acquisitions with the CT technologists. Mutual respect and regular communication between these two key groups is critical to assuring effective cardiac CT performance. Imaging workflow map should be developed and monitored starting from the generation of the CT examination request in the clinical arena to the finalized report in the medical record. This will assist in identifying and addressing key points of communication failure which is inherent in a system with several healthcare personnel addressing a patient's clinical data in separate geographical locations.

A solution to assure effective communication may utilize customized workflow software that may be integrated with the institution's electronic medical records. Continuous HL7 data streams containing timestamped updates of clinical information may be transmitted from the electronic health record to the 3D laboratory workflow software, assisting with workflow prioritizations. The real-time 3D laboratory worklist may be accessed remotely by authorized 3D technologists, radiologists, and referring clinicians. Users may electronically convey any updated quantitative imaging needs or additional clinical information. Radiologists and clinicians may electronically request priority processing of urgent CTA examinations and may view the post-processing status of a CTA examination in real time [2].

Managing Source Image Flow Across the Enterprise

Following the imaging workflow map, 3D laboratory personnel can instruct enterprise information technology services to automatically route all thin-section CTA images from the CT scanners to a server serving as a central repository, where the images may then be accessed throughout the enterprise. If desired, the images may be routed to the 3D server before being routed to PACS to allow preliminary 3D viewing and post-processing to begin immediately. After reviewing the initial imaging, the radiologist or 3D technologist may contact the CT technologist directly for any additional image reconstructions to be performed retrospectively. For example, another series may be needed from a cardiac phase with less motion to improve the visualization of the coronary arteries or the cardiac valves on the 3D post-processed images.

In addition to 3D laboratory output, 3D images may be produced throughout the enterprise by physicians and their trainees. It is important to monitor which 3D images become a permanent part of the patient's medical record in the PACS. It is easy for someone with insufficient training to create a 3D image that falsely represents the patient's anatomy. The 3D laboratory can validate all 3D images that arrive on PACS and remove any 3D images that contain errors in imaging. This is an important quality control function that should be built into 3D laboratory workflow.

3D Laboratory Technologist Creates Protocolled Images/Reports

As discussed previously, input from requesting physicians is critical to the creation of clinically valuable post-processing protocols. 3D laboratory personnel must also work with the radiologists and cardiologists to formalize and harmonize standardized 3D imaging protocols and reports in a manner that attempts to accommodate the preference of requesting physicians as much as possible. All 3D technologists should be trained to produce the specific 3D images and standardized measurements contained within each protocol in a consistent manner to reduce output variability. 3D lab report formatting is another key target for formalization to assure consistency. One important source of flexibility to be built into the protocols is an opportunity for 3D technologists to include additional 3D images that demonstrate unexpected pathologies.

Segmentation of CT Data for Surgical Planning and Guidance Programs

With their advanced knowledge of anatomy and pathology, 3D technologists have the capability to segment anatomical structures from a CTA dataset by using a combination of automatic and manual segmentation tools (Fig. 15.6). These segmented CT images can be exported as a new series, either in a standard radiology image format (Digital Imaging and Communications in Medicine (DICOM)) or in a format that is specific to an external application that might be used by the referring physicians to plan or guide procedures. For example, a segmented CT dataset of the aorta may be fused with live fluoroscopic images in surgery for catheter and device implantation guidance (Vessel Navigator, Philips Healthcare, Cleveland, Ohio). The segmented images may also be exported as stereolithography files for rapid prototyping of 3D models or to create life-sized models of anatomical structures using a 3D printer. These models may be used for presurgical planning or creation of tailor-made anatomical implants [6].

Software Upgrades

3D software companies release frequent patches (bug fixes) and updates with new features and functionalities. Although these software upgrades are tested by the manufacturers in their development environment, they cannot duplicate the typical clinical environment where the software will actually

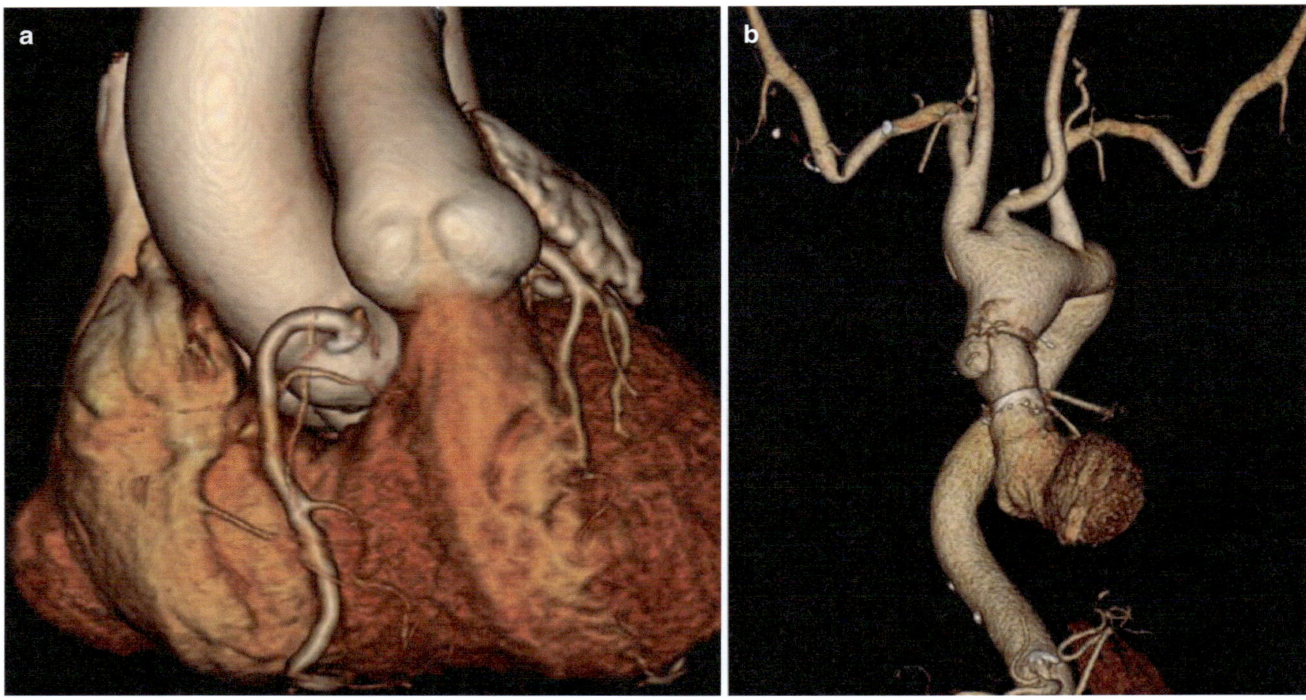

Fig. 15.6 Volume renderings showing (**a**) the proximal and mid-right coronary artery and (**b**) ascending aortic repair with distal anastomotic pseudoaneurysm and residual aortic arch aneurysm. The clear anatomical depiction shown in both views is the result of detailed segmentation by 3D laboratory technologists

be performing. Therefore, it is advisable to thoroughly assess and validate new releases in a test environment at each clinical site, using anonymized clinical datasets and running predetermined 3D imaging and quantitative functions on each dataset. This will ensure that each 3D software application accurately, reliably, and consistently fulfills its intended purpose. This time-consuming validation task may be performed by 3D personnel who will in turn feedback to the manufacturer any performance issues *before* the software upgrade is released into the clinical environment. This validation process can help prevent the consequences of software failures in the clinical environment, which could potentially have a negative impact on patient care and clinical workflow [7].

Training and Quality Control of Technologists

The success of a 3D laboratory depends on the selection and training of qualified radiologic technologists. Candidates should have several years of experience in CT or MRI scanning and have completed a formal in-house training program in a radiology 3D laboratory. A valuable component of training includes mentorship by a cardiovascular radiologist, including case review of cardiovascular anatomy and pathology, recognition of image artifacts, and preferred techniques for acquiring quantitative analysis. Technologists in training should participate in a quality control process that is specified within a 3D laboratory's quality assurance policy and should include peer review of 3D images and measurements before they are submitted for interpretation. Offering a fellowship-like training program for external technologists may also increase the reputation of the local post-processing laboratory and provide a source for external referrals.

Quality Assurance

A quality assurance (QA) program is critical for optimizing reliability and credibility in 3D imaging and measurements. Key components of a QA program include outlining procedures for communication, following standardized protocols, quality control, obtaining and documenting measurements, reviewing reports, rectifying exam billing or scheduling errors, validating 3D software and upgrades, monitoring performance of personnel, and assuring that all 3D operators receive consistent and updated training and mentoring [5, 8].

Documentation and Archive of Results

Numerical results from 3D measurements should be included in the body of the formal CT report, but an institution's electronic medical records (EMR) system may also have the capability to store screen captures of key 3D images and videos associated with the examination. The 3D laboratory can validate and insert these images along with text into the final report within the RIS prior to sign-off by the attending radiologist or cardiologist. This mixed media presentation can enhance the clinical value of the CT reports.

Clinical Protocols

The creation of specific post-processed images and measurements are guided by standardized protocols, which as discussed previously will be institution specific and informed by the preferences of referring and interpreting physicians. Broad classes of cardiac CT applications that are commonly implemented in 3D laboratories are as follows:

- Coronary CT angiography: depiction of native vessel disease, bypass grafts, and stents.
- Coronary calcium measurement: risk assessment of coronary heart disease.
- Pulmonary vein mapping: planning and guiding pulmonary vein ablation in the management of atrial fibrillation.
- Transarterial aortic valve implantation: preprocedural planning for aortic valve replacement. Results are used to plan delivery route, device type, and device size.
- Thoracic aortic CT angiography: depiction and measurement of aortic aneurysm, traumatic injury, acute aortic syndrome, vasculitis, or congenital abnormality [9].
- Central vein mapping: assessment of stenoses, occlusions, or thrombi within the superior vena cava and its primary supplying veins.
- Myocardial function: measurement of right or left ventricular ejection fraction. Assessment of reginal wall motion abnormalities.
- Pulmonary artery CT angiography: while 3D assessment is not routine in the setting of suspected acute thromboembolism, 3D assessment can be very helpful in mapping congenital lesions of the central pulmonary arteries and assessing anatomical relationships and graft status in the pre- or postoperative assessment of congenital heart disease.
- Cardiac CT in congenital heart disease: depiction of the heart before or after repair of congenital heart disease.

An example of a pulmonary vein mapping protocol is illustrated in Table 15.1.

Table 15.1 Sample pulmonary vein mapping protocol

Task	Number of images	Notes
Curved planar reformations (two planes)		Create curved images in two planes through each major coronary artery. Also, create curved planar reformations through the entire aorta and any takeoff vessels in the neck and abdomen, if included in the scan
All coronary arteries (gated or not per LH)	6–8	
Aorta and takeoff vessels	~11	
Multiplanar reformations		
Three transverse images of the left atrium to demonstrate the esophagus	3	
Volume rendering		Create a volume rendered image of the left atrium, left atrial appendage, and several cm of pulmonary vein branches. Save as horizontal and vertical movies, ~36 images each. Also save horizontal and vertical movies as avi files, 72 images each, for PDFs
Horizontal and vertical left atrium movie including the left atrial appendage	36 × 2	
Horizontal and vertical left atrium movie including the left atrial appendage, avi files for pdf	72 × 2	
Measurements		
Pulmonary mapping measurement protocol		Perform measurements per PV measurement template: Orthogonal diameters and areas of the origins of each pulmonary vein. Measure only the contrast-filled flow lumen. Screen capture corresponding 2D image in two planes to demonstrate the location of your measurement. In 3D, screen capture a posterior VR reference image of the left atrium showing location of diameter measurements Measure the left atrium volume including the left atrial appendage Include Sup/inf and Ant/post diameters of the left atrium, measured on true sagittal image Measure centerline distance between LSPV and RSPV If patient has a prior study, look at prior measurements and try to duplicate the cardiac phase and positioning for comparison

Conclusion

Post-processing CT images is mandatory for many cardiac CT acquisitions. While the interpreting physician should always assess the images using an interface that provides ready access to multiplanar reformations, maximum intensity projections, curved planar reformations, volume renderings, and measurement tools, a 3D laboratory is a key adjunct for an effective workflow. Staffed by technologists with administrative support, 3D laboratories offer consistent, high-quality image and measurement preparations and archive. They provide a reliable interface with referring physicians and are better positioned to address special processing needs as they might arise. By serving as the primary resource for creating archival images for cardiac CT exams, they off-load work from interpreting radiologists and cardiologists, allowing them to shift their focus away from record keeping and increase their focus on the interpretation of imaging studies.

References

1. Kramer CM, Budoff MJ, Fayad ZA, et al. ACCF/AHA 2007 clinical competence statement on vascular imaging with computed tomography and magnetic resonance. A report of the American College of Cardiology Foundation/American Heart Association/American College of Physicians Task Force on Clinical Competence and Training. J Am Coll Cardiol. 2007;50:1097–114.
2. Boll DT. Affinity chart analysis: a method for structured collection, aggregation, and response to customer needs in radiology. Am J Roentgenol. 2017 Apr;208(4):W134–45.
3. ACR–NASCI–SPR practice parameter for the performance and interpretation of cardiac computed tomography (CT). Amended 2016 (Resolution 21). Accessed 21 Nov 2016.
4. Cayne NS, Veith FJ, Lipsitz EC, et al. Variability of maximal aortic aneurysm diameter measurements on CT scan: significance and methods to minimize. J Vasc Surg. 2004;39:811–5.
5. Physician supervision of diagnostic tests. In: cms.gov; 2001. Accessed 15 Jul 2016.
6. Rengier F, Mehndiratta A, Tengg-Kobligk von H, Zechmann CM, Unterhinninghofen R, Kauczor H-U, Giesel FL. 3D printing based on imaging data: review of medical applications. Int J Comput Assist Radiol Surg. 2010;5:335–41.
7. Center for Devices, Radiological Health, Center for Biologics Evaluation, Research. Guidance documents (medical devices and radiation-emitting products) – general principles of software validation; Final guidance for industry and FDA staff; 2002.
8. Pierce L, Raman K, Rosenberg J, Rubin GD. Quality Improvement in 3D Imaging. AJR Am J Roentgenol. 2012;198:150–5.
9. Budoff MJ, Cohen MC, Garcia MJ, et al. ACCF/AHA clinical competence statement on cardiac imaging with computed tomography and magnetic resonance: a report of the American College of Cardiology Foundation/American Heart Association/American College of Physicians Task Force on Clinical Competence and Training. J Am Coll Cardiol. 2005;46:383–402.

Structured Reporting for Cardiac CT

16

Anil Attili and Ella A. Kazerooni

The cardiac CT report is an important document that first and foremost communicates the findings and their clinical implications to the consumers of the report, including the referring physician, the patient and their families, and the cardiovascular specialists who use the information to make decisions about procedural intervention appropriateness, eligibility, and approach. The report also serves as the documentation of the imaging episode of care and services rendered, used for medical record documentation, billing, and compliance. The structure of a report can also be used to enable quality improvement, outcomes tracking, and research. To these ends, a comprehensive, consistent easily readable cardiac CT report using standardized descriptive terminology and quantitative metrics where relevant is recommended [1–4].

Structured reports assure quality and consistency within and across practices, providing information in a consistent, predictable manner to those who consume it. Important elements are less likely to be omitted using a structured report template assembled using systematically defined and arranged elements. Standardized reports reduce the variability of individual communication styles that may result in the same findings being perceived differently by the consumers. Specifically, the use of structured reporting has been shown to improve clinician's comprehension of coronary CT angiography (CCTA) reports [5]. This structure also facilitates research through the use of uniform data fields for data extraction and use of standard definitions. Educators will find structured reports aid trainees in learning the important elements of study description, clinical elements, definitions, and terminology. As cardiac CT has matured and now recommended in numerous clinical guidelines, ranging from stable and acute chest pain syndromes to structural heart disease, reporting templates can be tailored to specific study protocols and to disease states [6–11]. Finally, structured reporting ensures the elements required for billing and billing compliance are documented, including adequate information to support clinical necessity, and a sufficient description of exam technique for accurate first time Current Procedural Terminology (CPT) coding. While the final output and format do not need to be the same from practice to practice, inclusion of standard elements, terminology, and definitions are essential to meet the needs of those who consume the reports. We will share our report formats with you. Details of how to obtain, analyze, and interpret examinations are covered in chapters throughout this text.

A. Attili · E. A. Kazerooni (✉)
Department of Radiology, Division of Cardiothoracic Radiology, University of Michigan, Ann Arbor, MI, USA
e-mail: ellakaz@med.umich.edu

Components of a Structured Report

A structured report begins with an organization of the key components. Each of the following key components will be discussed in detail.

- Clinical indications
- Review of prior cardiac imaging examination images and/or reports
- Study technique
- Image quality
- Findings
- Impression and management recommendations when appropriate

Clinical Indications

The specific reason(s) for the examination should be reviewed and documented, including the relevant clinical signs and symptoms, physical examination findings, and medical and surgical history, and should be sufficient for applicable ICD-10 coding. Cardiovascular risk factors and the inclusion of demographic information such as patient age, gender, body mass index, procedure date, and referring physician are recommended. Clinical history should include

U. J. Schoepf (ed.), *CT of the Heart*, Contemporary Medical Imaging, https://doi.org/10.1007/978-1-60327-237-7_16

coronary risk factors, nature and status of cardiac symptoms, prior tests and procedures (such as the location and extent of ischemia on stress testing), and the nature of any future planned procedures following the cardiac CT.

The major indications for cardiac CT include [11]:

1. Coronary artery calcium scoring in asymptomatic patients with a low to intermediate risk of coronary artery disease (CAD)
2. Evaluation of suspected or known coronary artery anomalies
3. Evaluation of low to intermediate risk stable patients with chest pain or suspected acute coronary syndrome
4. Discordant or inconclusive stress tests
5. Evaluation of non-coronary pathology, including the great vessels, veins, cardiac chambers, myocardium, valves, and pericardium
6. Evaluation of cardiac chamber function
7. Evaluation of cardiac structure and morphology in the setting of congenital heart disease

Study Technique

The procedure section of the CT report describes both image acquisition and image reconstruction.

Elements of image acquisition that should be documented include:

- Examination type or protocol, such as:
  - Coronary calcium score
  - Coronary CTA
  - Cardiac structural exam, such as for cardiac mass or congenital heart disease
  - Left atrium and pulmonary vein assessment
  - Left atrial appendage occluder planning
  - Transcatheter aortic valve planning (TAVR) or mitral valve planning
- Technical acquisition parameters, including collimation, mA and kVp
- Scanner type, such as detector configuration and single or dual source
- ECG gating used: prospective and at what phases of the cardiac cycle or retrospective
- Anatomic region scanned (e.g., carina to the base of the heart for routine CCTA)
- Contrast administration:
  - Volume, type, and rate
  - Timing method—bolus tracking or test bolus
  - Uni-, bi-, or triphasic
- Additional medications administered, such as nitroglycerin and heart rate-reducing agents
- Radiation exposure (such as dose length product) and use of any dose-reduction strategies
- Clinical parameters if relevant, such as heart rate and rhythm
- Any complications, such as a contrast reaction or extravasation

Elements of image reconstruction that should be documented include:

- Slice thickness
- Slice increment
- Phase of cardiac cycle reconstructed
- Display field of view (DFOV)
- Additional elements to consider include:
  - Reconstruction filter
  - Reconstructed imaging planes
  - Post-processing methods used, such as multiplanar reformats (MPR), maximum intensity projections (MIP), and 3D volume-rendered reformations

Image Quality

Overall image quality, contributing factors to reduced image quality, and the presence of artifacts should be reported. These variables impact both the reader as they interpret the study and the confidence in their findings and are used by the consumer report in their assessment of their confidence in the interpretation. Image quality may be degraded by technical factors and patient-related factors, and these impact the ability to obtain a better-quality examination in the future. While there are no standard statements to describe overall study quality, terms such as excellent, good, or diagnostic when there is a mild reduction in quality or minor artifacts that do not limit the interpretation, acceptable when there are further artifacts or reductions in quality that may limit a part of the interpretation, and nondiagnostic represent a scale of quality. The factors that contribute to any reduction in quality, particularly when it reduces diagnostic quality or confidence, should be specifically mentioned. For example, when segments of the coronary tree are not interpretable, which segments and the reason(s) why should be clearly stated.

Patient-related factors to reduced image quality include:

- Large patient size which may reduce quality by an increase in image noise
- Metal implants or extensive calcification that may create beam hardening artifact
- Motion of the body in general, respiratory motion due to breathing, and cardiac motion due to a rapid and/or irregular heart rate

- Poor contrast enhancement, due to poor cardiac output, hemodilution with increased circulating blood volume, intracardiac shunts including opening of a patent foramen ovale, and large patient size

Technical factors that may contribute to reduced image quality include:

- Insufficient signal to noise due to low photon number (mA)
- Insufficient image contrast due to inappropriate photon energy selection (kVp)
- Insufficient contrast volume or rate
- Inappropriate gating technique
- Insufficient or lack of heart rate-lowering medications or use of nitroglycerin

Findings

The finding section should be tailored to the specific type of cardiac examination type; within a practice, consistency across templates is recommended where possible. A coronary calcium CT report will have a different findings section than a coronary CTA or a TAVR planning examination. Sample reporting templates and reporting checklists are provided.

Coronary Artery Calcium Scoring

Table 16.1 summarizes the reporting elements for a coronary calcium CT. This may be an independent exam or included with as part of a coronary CT in patients who have not previously undergone coronary artery stent(s) placement or bypass surgery. The most frequently used measure for coronary calcium scoring remains the Agatston score (AJ-130 score) which has been validated with outcome studies, histological studies, and available nomograms [12, 13]. The AJ-130 score measures the amount of calcium based on voxels which exceed 130 HU and reach a size threshold. Software programs measure each calcification and sum the score for each major vessel and for all vessels together, the latter representing the total calcium score. Each of these values should be reported, as well as the percentile rank by the patients' age and gender as established on nomograms [14]. The newer scores such as the volume score and mass score for each vessel and total score by these methods may also be reported, as they have the advantage of greater reproducibility but have less data in aggregate behind them [15–18].

The presence of calcium in other portions of the heart such as the aortic valve, aorta, myocardium, mitral valve, and pericardium should be noted and reported semiquantitatively as mild, moderate, or severe. Evaluation of the cardiac chambers is limited on non-contrast exams, however if abnormally dilated should be reported. Low attenuation of blood due to anemia reduces the density of blood in the cardiac chambers relative to myocardium and may serve as internal contrast by which to separate myocardium from the chamber cavities. Coronary anomalies may be evident and should be described (see section on CCTA). Finally, all non-cardiac structures in the field of view should be reviewed and reported on (see section on non-cardiac findings).

A standardized reporting and data classification system for coronary artery calcification scoring known as CAC-RADS for the Coronary Artery Calcification Reporting and Data System was developed by the Society of Cardiovascular Computed Tomography (SCCT) and the Society of Thoracic Radiology and is applicable for the reporting of coronary artery calcification on non-contrast, non-gated CT examinations [19] and may be used when non-gated exams are obtained as part of a cardiac CT.

Table 16.1 Components of a coronary calcium non-contrast CT report

Section	Specific component(s)
Clinical data	
General	Indication or reason for test, procedure date
Demographics	Name, date of birth, sex, referring clinician, height, weight
History	Symptoms, risk factors, relevant diagnostic tests
Procedure data	
Equipment	Scanner type: Number of detectors, rotation time
Acquisition	Gating method
	Tube voltage
	Estimated radiation dose
Reconstruction	Slice thickness
	Slice increment, reconstruction filter, phases of cardiac cycle
Results	
Technical quality	Overall quality
	Presence and type of artifact and effect on interpretation
Coronary	Agatston score for individual vessels and total Agatston score
	Agatston score percentile for age and sex
	Volume score and mass score
Non-coronary cardiac	Presence of calcium in aortic wall, pericardium, myocardium, and valves Dilated chambers or total heart enlargement Presence of pericardial effusion or thickening
Non-cardiac	Abnormalities in the lungs, mediastinum, esophagus, chest wall, and upper abdomen if present
Impressions and conclusions	Total Agatston score and percentile
	Correlation to other or prior cardiac studies
	Documentation of communication to referring physician for urgent finding(s)
	Clinical recommendations

Coronary CT Angiography (CCTA)

Coronary findings: There are several sections that are important to a structured report with respect to the coronary arteries, including:

- Coronary artery dominance
- Coronary artery anatomy, specifically
  - Course:
    - Normal
    - Normal variants
    - Anomalies, including origin; course; relationship to cardiac relevant anatomy including cardiac chambers, the ascending aorta, pulmonary artery, and ventricular septum; anomalous artery lumen caliber; shape and evidence of dynamic narrowing or occlusion during the cardiac cycle; and any intramural course
  - Myocardial bridging
- Coronary artery atherosclerotic stenosis: by location, severity, plaque composition, and morphology
- Coronary artery aneurysms
- Coronary artery bypass grafts
- Coronary artery stents

The location of stenosis should be described for each major epicardial coronary artery using a standardized scheme the American Heart Association (AHA) segmentation developed for catheter-based coronary angiography; initially proposed in 1975, this schema has stood the test of time and been used in many long-term outcome studies relating the location of stenosis to major adverse cardiac events (MACE) [20]. An axially based version of this standard model has been adapted for CCTA by the Society of Cardiac Computed Tomography (SCCT) and more closely emulates CCTA views than those obtained during invasive angiography [4], as illustrated in Fig. 16.1 and described in Table 16.2. Each major epicardial coronary arteries is divided into proximal, mid, and distal segments. The proximal right coronary artery (RCA) extends from the ostium to one-half the distance to the acute margin of the heart, mid RCA from the end of proximal RCA to the acute margin of the heart, and distal segment from the end of mid RCA to PDA. The proximal left anterior descending (LAD) artery extends from the end of the left main to the origin of the first large diagonal or septal perforator, the mid LAD extends from the end of the proximal LAD to one-half the distance to the apex, and the distal LAD extends from the end of the mid LAD to the end of the LAD. The proximal left circumflex coronary artery (LCx) is the segment between the end of the left main and the origin of the first obtuse marginal branch (OM1), and the mid and distal LCx are the segments distal to the OM1 to the end of the vessel or the origin of a left PDA.

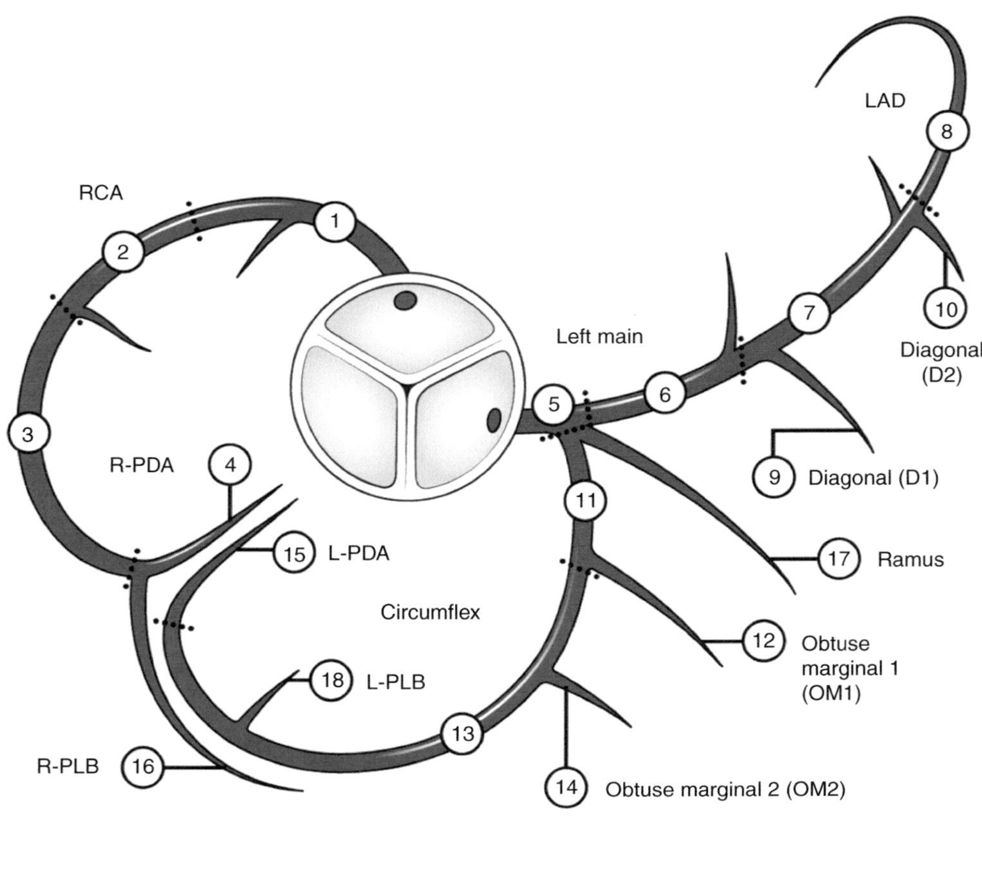

Fig. 16.1 SCCT coronary segmentation diagram. The abbreviation and description for each segment can be found in Table 16.2. (From Leipsic et al. [4], with permission)

Table 16.2 Axial coronary anatomy legend

Segment	Abbreviation	Description
1. Proximal right coronary artery (RCA)	pRCA	Ostium of the RCA to one-half the distance to the acute margin of the heart
2. Mid RCA	mRCA	End of proximal RCA to the acute margin of heart
3. Distal RCA	dRCA	End of mid RCA to origin of the PDA (posterior descending artery)
4. PDA-R	R-PDA	PDA from RCA
5. Left main (LM)	LM	Ostium of LM to bifurcation of LAD (left anterior descending artery) and LCx (left circumflex artery)
6. Proximal LAD	pLAD	End of LM to the first large septal or D1 (first diagonal; >1.5 mm in size) whichever is most proximal
7. Mid LAD	mLAD	End of proximal LAD to one-half the distance to the apex
8. Distal LAD	dLAD	End of mid LAD to end of LAD
9. D1	D1	First diagonal branch D1
10. D2	D2	Second diagonal branch D2
11. Proxiaml LCx	pLAD	End of LM to the origin of the OM1 (first obtuse marginal)
12. OM1	OM1	First OM1 traversing the lateral wall of the left ventricle
13. Mid and distal LCx	LCx	Traveling in the atrioventricular groove, distal to the OM1 branch to the end of the vessel or origin of the L-PDA (left PDA)
14. OM2	OM2	Second marginal OM2
15. PDA-L	L-PDA	PDA from LCx
16. PLB-R	R-PLB	PLB from RCA
17. Ramus intermedius	RI	Vessel originating from the left main between the LAD and LCx in case of a trifurcation
18. PLB-L	L-PLB	PLD from LCx

From Leipsic et al. [4], with permission
Additional nomenclature may be added, for example, D3, R-PDA2, saphenous vein graft, and mLAD
PLB posterior-lateral branch

Quantification of luminal stenosis, area stenosis, and plaque content may be done using analysis software; however current technology has not demonstrated sufficient reproducibility or accuracy in predicting invasive coronary angiography findings to make such measurements a routine clinical practice [21]. Studies have reported that visual CCTA quantification of lesion severity by percent maximal diameter stenosis has good correlation with quantitative invasive angiography and intravascular ultrasound, but with a relatively large standard deviation [21–25]. These comparative studies suggest that at a 95% confidence limit, CCTA currently predicts invasive quantitative angiography to within ±25%. The term "normal" in reference to the coronary arteries should be used only when there is no evidence of any coronary artery disease (i.e., normal lumen and no calcified and non-calcified plaque). Segments containing nonobstructive atherosclerotic plaque should not be described as normal. The following stenosis grading is recommended based on a visual semiquantitative maximal diameter stenosis assessment [4, 21]:

- Normal: Absence of plaque; no luminal stenosis
- Minimal: Plaque with <25% stenosis
- Mild: Plaque with 25–49% stenosis
- Moderate: Plaque with 50–69% stenosis
- Severe: 7 plaque with 0–99% stenosis
- Occlusion

Plaque composition should be described as calcified when the entire plaque appears as calcium by attenuation, non-calcified when the entire plaque is devoid of calcium, or partially calcified when both elements are present [26]. Very low attenuation within plaque, indicating lipid-rich plaque, should also be described. Plaque morphology can be used to identify vulnerable plaque, with some features independently associated with future acute coronary events [27, 28]. These include positive remodeling (the ratio of outer vessel diameter at the site of plaque divided by the average outer diameter of the proximal and distal vessel greater than 1.1), low-attenuation plaque (less than 30 HU), spotty calcium defined as punctate calcium within a plaque, and the napkin-ring sign, defined as central low attenuation with a peripheral rim of higher CT attenuation. The presence of any of these high-risk features should be evaluated and reported. Other morphological descriptors including bifurcation or ostial involvement, plaque ulceration, dissection, or fissuring should be reported. Arterial occlusion should be described by location and length. Several features indicative of lesions that are less amenable to successful percutaneous coronary intervention should be reported if present, including stenosis length >3 cm, ostial or bifurcation location, calcification particularly at the proximal cap, and the degree of collateralization [29–32]. CAD-RADS is a structured reporting tool for CCTA that uses stenosis severity and plaque composition to grade the severity of disease and is discussed in detail later on in this chapter.

If bypass grafts are present, the type and number of grafts and their origin and insertion should be reported. There is extensive evidence validating the accuracy of CCTA for evaluation of graft patency [33]. Patency of the proximal and distal anastomosis of each graft as well as the distal runoff vessels should be documented. Graft stenosis should be reusing the same schema use for native coronary arteries. Review of the surgical report from bypass surgery is critical to identifying grafts. With chronic graft occlusion, grafts become markedly atretic and may be identified as occlusion by the inability to identify them. In the event of planned redo cardiac surgery, a detailed description of graft location relative to the chest wall is important for operative planning; CT has been shown to reduce the rate of reentry injury and improved perioperative outcomes in redo cardiac surgery [34–36]. The relationship of the brachiocephalic vessels, aorta, right ventricle, and pericardium to the midline sternum should be assessed in axial or reconstructed sagittal and volume-rendered CT images. High-risk CT findings include <10 mm distance between the right ventricle and aorta to the chest wall or a graft crossing the midline within 10 mm of the sternum in the anteroposterior direction. In addition, extensive atherosclerotic calcification of the ascending aorta, known as a "porcelain" aorta, is associated with a high risk of plaque dislodgement during cannulation for cardiopulmonary bypass that may result in cerebrovascular accidents. Calcification of the thoracic aorta should be described with respect to location and extent (e.g., mild, moderate, severe, or porcelain) and may be demonstrated on maximum intensity 3D reconstructions as a calcium map.

Coronary stents should be described with respect to location, quality of interpretability, and the presence of obstruction. Evaluation of lumen patency inside stents is possible in most cases, though evaluation of in-stent stenosis is dependent on stent size and composition [37–39]. In general, 64-slice and newer-generation CT scanners exclude in-stent restenosis with a high negative predictive value; however, precise quantification of the in-stent restenosis is not accurate. CT is considered appropriate for risk assessment after revascularization in asymptomatic patients with a history of left main coronary artery stenting and a stent diameter of 3 mm or larger [11]. When interpretable, stents should generally be reported as patent, with mild in-stent stenosis (<50%), significant in-stent stenosis (50–99%), or occlusion.

Non-coronary Cardiac Findings

All structures within the field of view should be reviewed and reported on. For CCTA, this includes the pericardium, cardiac chambers, atrial and ventricular septum, atrioventricular and ventriculoarterial valves, pulmonary arteries and veins, systemic veins, and portions of the thoracic aorta. Depending on the contrast infusion protocol, typically, the left-sided chambers and sometimes the right-sided are suitable for interpretation. Reconstruction of the axial source data in the standard cardiac planes (short axis, four-chamber, two-chamber, and three-chamber/LVOT view) should be performed. A description of the non-coronary cardiac structures should be provided in the report to include the following:

- Thoracic vasculature:
  - Aorta include diameters of the aortic root, ascending and descending aorta
  - Superior and inferior vena cava
  - Pulmonary arteries
  - Pulmonary veins
- Cardiac chambers:
  - Size and morphology, including aneurysms, diverticula
  - Myocardium: hypertrophy, thinning, fatty replacement, lack of enhancement
  - Masses
  - Congenital anomalies
  - Wall motion and function if full cardiac cycle data is obtained
- Cardiac valves:
  - Atrioventricular and semilunar valve thickening, calcification, or structural abnormalities such as a bicuspid aortic valve
  - Valvular stenosis or regurgitation if full cardiac cycle data is obtained, including planimetry of the open aortic valve at early/mid-systole
- Pericardium: thickening, calcification, or effusion

Shunting between the atria and ventricles may be visible depending on the contrast injection protocol and should be mentioned. The interatrial and interventricular septum should be anatomically evaluated for integrity. Measurement and reporting of chamber diameter and wall thickness are considered optional. Most contemporary scan protocols do not include the true end-diastolic phase and mid-diastolic or end-systolic measures of ventricular cavity size, and wall thickness may not be representative.

Multiphase reconstruction of these structures may be available with retrospective ECG-gated protocols permitting dynamic display of segmental wall motion and quantitative evaluation of size and function. In such cases, left and right ventricular end-diastolic volumes, end-systolic volumes, stroke volumes, and ejection fractions referenced to body surface area can be measured and reported providing additional important information for patient management [40, 41]. Regional wall motion abnormalities should be reported using the AHA 17-segment format and assigned to each of the major coronary artery distributions [42]. Wall motion may be reported as normal, hypokinetic, akinetic or dyskinetic, and aneurysmal.

Myocardial CT enhancement patterns should be assessed. During the arterial, hypodense areas of myocardium may represent decreased myocardial perfusion as a result of prior myocardial infarction or severe obstructive CAD. Old myocardial infarcts are characterized by hypoenhancement with wall thinning and/or fat replacement, ventricular remodeling, and/or the presence of calcifications and thrombi. 5–8-mm-thick averaged MPR reconstructions, a narrow width and level, and the application of minimum intensity projection techniques improve detection of low-attenuation myocardial areas due to hypoperfusion and infarction. Perfusion defects and myocardial abnormalities should be described using the AHA 17-segment model used for wall motion abnormalities. Aortic valve planimetry measurement has been shown to correlate with the severity of aortic stenosis on transesophageal and transthoracic echocardiography [43, 44].

CAD-RADS: The Coronary Artery Disease Reporting and Data System

A standardized reporting and data classification system for CCTA, called CAD-RADS, has been recently developed and reported as an expert consensus document of the Society of Cardiovascular Computed Tomography (SCCT), the American College of Radiology (ACR), and the North American Society for Cardiovascular Imaging (NASCI) [45]. The intent of CAD-RADS is to create a standardized method to communicate CCTA findings in order to facilitate decision-making regarding patient management. The CAD-RADS classification is applied at the patient level, based on the highest-grade coronary lesion. CAD-RADS codes range from 0 in the absence of stenosis and plaque to CAD-RADS 5 in the presence of at least one totally occluded coronary artery. The CAD-RADS reporting and data system for patients with stable and acute chest pain is shown in Tables 16.3 and 16.4, respectively. The grading scale for stenosis severity suggested

Table 16.3 CAD-RADS reporting and data system for patients presenting with stable chest pain

	Degree of maximal coronary stenosis	Interpretation	Further cardiac investigation	Management
CAD-RADS 0	0% (no plaque or stenosis)	Documented absence of CAD	None	Reassurance. Consider non- atherosclerotic causes of chest pain
CAD-RADS 1	1–24%—minimal stenosis or plaque with no stenosis[a]	Minimal nonobstructive CAD	None	Consider non-atherosclerotic causes of chest pain Consider preventive therapy and risk factor modification
CAD-RADS 2	25–49% mild stenosis	Mild non-obstructive CAD	None	Consider non-atherosclerotic causes of chest pain Consider preventive therapy and risk factor modification, particularly for patients with non-obstructive plaque in multiple segments
CAD-RADS 3	50–69% stenosis	Moderate stenosis	Consider functional assessment	Consider symptom-guided anti-ischemic and preventative pharmacotherapy as well as risk factor modification per guideline-directed care[b] Other treatments should be considered per guideline-directed care[b]
CAD-RADS 4	70–99% stenosis or B—left main >50% or three-vessel obstructive (≥70%) disease	Severe stenosis	A: Consider ICA or functional assessment B: ICA is recommended	Consider symptom-guided anti-ischemic and preventative pharmacotherapy as well as risk factor modification per guideline-directed care[b] Other treatments (including options of revascularization) should be considered per guideline-directed care[b]
CAD-RADS 5	100% (total occlusion)	Total coronary occlusion	Consider ICA and/or viability assessment	Consider symptom-guided anti-ischemic and preventative pharmacotherapy as well as risk factors modification per guideline-directed care[b] Other treatments (including options of revascularization) should be considered per guideline-directed care[b]
CAD-RADS N	Nondiagnostic study	Obstructive CAD cannot be excluded	Additional or alternative evaluation may be needed	

From Cury et al. [45], with permission

Note: The CAD-RADS classification should be applied on a per-patient basis for the clinically most relevant (usually highest-grade) stenosis. All vessels greater than 1.5 mm in diameter should be graded for stenosis severity. CAD-RADS will not apply for smaller vessels (<1.5 mm in diameter)

Modifiers: If more than one modifier is present, the symbol "/" (slash) should follow each modifier in the following order:

First: modifier N (non-diagnostic)
Second: modifier S (stent)
Third: modifier G (graft)
Fourth: modifier V (vulnerability)

CAD coronary artery disease, *ICA* invasive coronary angiography

[a]CAD-RADS 1—This category should also include the presence of plaque with positive remodeling and no evidence of stenosis

[b]Guideline-directed care per ACC Stable Ischemic Heart Disease Guidelines [46]

Table 16.4 CAD-RADS reporting and data system for patients presenting with acute chest pain, negative first troponin, negative or nondiagnostic electrocardiogram, and low to intermediate risk (TIMI risk score < 4) (emergency department or hospital setting)

	Degree of maximal coronary stenosis	Interpretation	Management
CAD-RADS 0	0%	ACS highly unlikely	No further evaluation of ACS is required Consider other etiologies
CAD-RADS 1	1–24%[a]	ACS highly unlikely	Consider evaluation of non-ACS etiology, if normal troponin and no ECG changes Consider referral for outpatient follow-up for preventive therapy and risk factor modification
CAD-RADS 2	25–49%[b]	ACS unlikely	Consider evaluation of non-ACS etiology, if normal troponin and no ECG changes Consider referral for outpatient follow-up for preventive therapy and risk factor modification If clinical suspicion of ACS is high or if high-risk plague features are noted, consider hospital admission with cardiology consultation
CAD-RADS 3	50–69%	ACS possible	Consider hospital admission with cardiology consultation, functional testing, and/or ICA for evaluation and management Recommendation for anti-ischemic and preventive management should be considered as well as risk factor modification. Other treatments should be considered if there is presence of a hemodynamically significant lesion
CAD-RADS 4	A: 70–99% B: Left main >50% or three-vessel obstructive disease	ACS likely	Consider hospital admission with cardiology consultation. Further evaluation with ICA and revascularization as appropriate Recommendation for anti-ischemic and preventive management should be considered as well as risk factor modification
CAD-RADS 5	100% (total occlusion)	ACS very likely	Consider expedited ICA on a timely basis and revascularization if appropriate if acute occlusion.[c] Recommendation for anti-ischemic and preventive management should be considered as well as risk factor modifications
CAD-RADS N	Nondiagnostic study	ACS cannot be excluded	Additional or alternative evaluation for ACS is needed

From Cury et al. [45], with permission

Note: The CAD-RADS classification should be applied on a per-patient basis for the clinically most relevant (usually highest-grade) stenosis. All vessels greater than 1.5 mm in diameter should be graded for stenosis severity. CAD-RADS will not apply for smaller vessels (<1.5 mm in diameter)

Modifiers: If more than one modifier is present, the symbol "/" (slash) should follow each modifier in the following order:

First: modifier N (non-diagnostic)
Second: modifier S (stent)
Third: modifier G (graft)
Fourth: modifier V (vulnerability)

ACS acute coronary syndrome, *ICA* invasive coronary angiography

[a]CAD-RADS 1—This category should also include the presence of plaque with positive remodeling and no evidence of stenosis

[b]CAD-RADS 2—Modifier 2/V can be used to indicate vulnerable/high-risk plaque

[c]Unless the total coronary occlusion can be identified as chronic (through CT and clinical characteristics or patient history)

by the SCCT is used. All vessels greater than 1.5 mm in diameter should be graded for stenosis severity; CAD-RADS does not apply for vessels less than 1.5 mm in diameter. CAD-RADS categories can be complimented by modifiers to indicate that a study is not fully evaluable or nondiagnostic (N) or to indicate the presence of stents (S), grafts (G), and vulnerable plaques (V). Specific recommendations are provided for further management of patients with stable or acute chest pain based on the CAD-RADS classification and code. These suggestions for further patient management should always be considered in light of the full clinical information available to the treating physician. The basic structure of a CCTA report incorporating CAD-RADS is as described in this chapter and in accordance with professional society guidelines. A CAD-RADS code ranging from 0 to 5 is assigned in the impression section based on the highest-grade coronary stenosis along with corresponding management recommendations. CAD-RADS reinforces the objective of structured reporting in communicating findings in a clear consistent manner, facilitating education, research, peer review, and quality assurance.

Examples of CAD lesions categorized using the CAD-RADS system are shown in Figs. 16.2, 16.3, 16.4, 16.5, and 16.6.

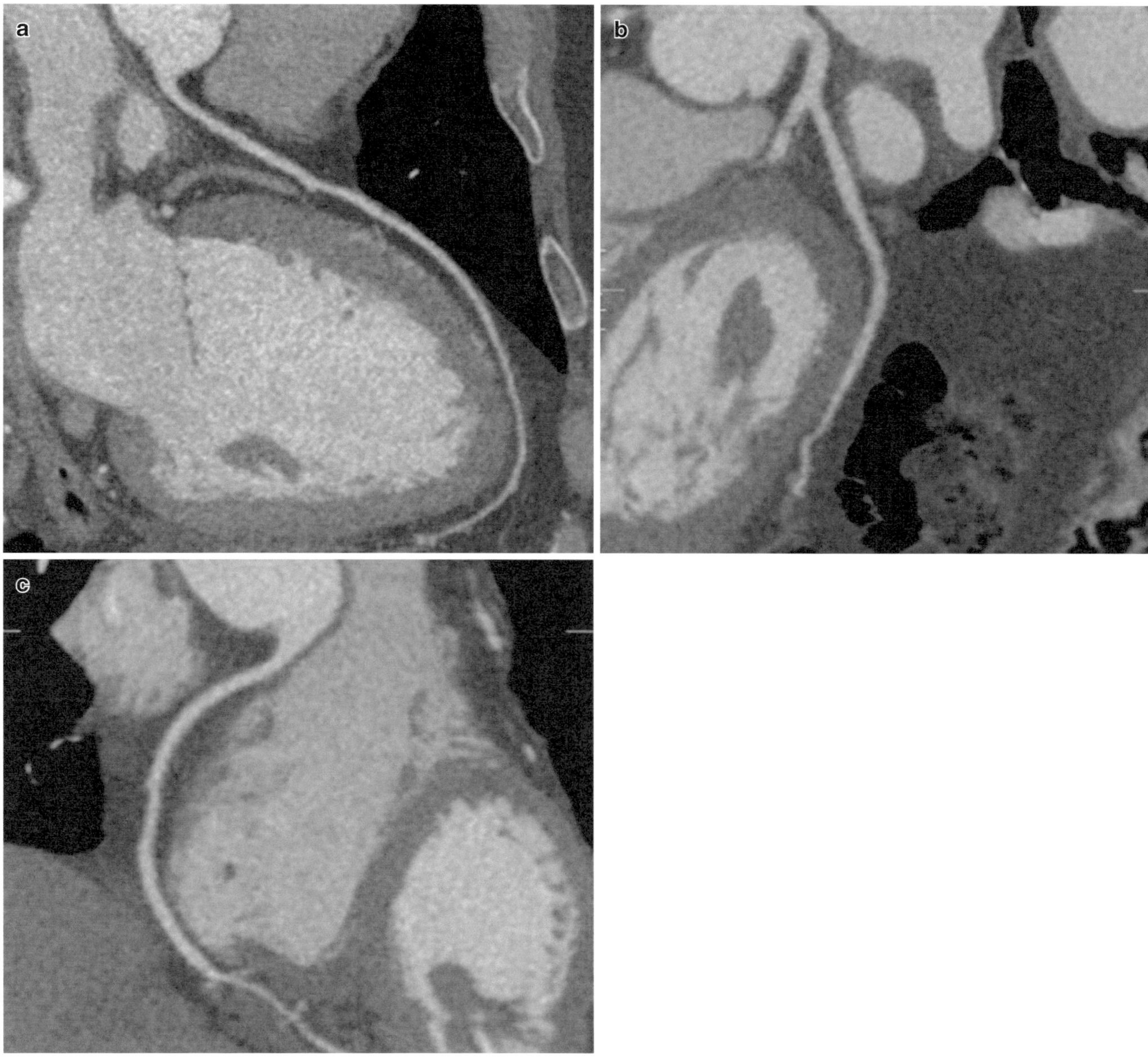

Fig. 16.2 (**a**–**c**) CAD-RADS 0. Normal left main and LAD, LCX, and RCA without plaque or stenosis

Cardiac CT for Electrophysiology Applications

Pre-procedural cardiac CT imaging provides information about cardiac structure and anatomy that may be crucial for successful atrial and ventricular ablation for arrhythmias and structural interventions in electrophysiology. Pre-procedural CT combined with imaging obtained during EP interventions enhances procedural safety, reduces exposure to ionizing radiation from fluoroscopy, reduces exposure time, and may improve outcomes.

Pre-procedural CT Imaging for Left Atrial Ablation

Pre-procedural left atrial (LA) imaging by CT focuses on determining atrial and pulmonary venous anatomy, ruling out atrial thrombi, and identifying adjacent structures. Knowledge of patient-specific anatomy of the pulmonary veins facilitates guiding catheter manipulation and delivery of radiofrequency energy at antral or ostial locations, thereby reducing the risk of pulmonary vein stenosis [47, 48]. In patients with paroxysmal AF, circumferential PV isolation

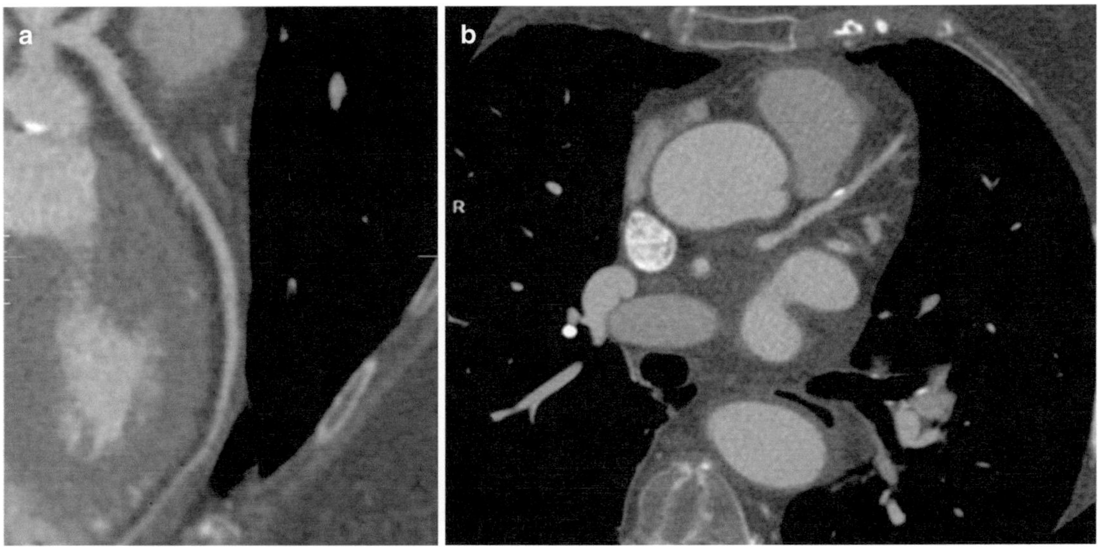

Fig. 16.3 (**a**, **b**) CAD-RADS 1. Calcified plaque in the mid LAD with minimal luminal narrowing (less than 25% diameter stenosis)

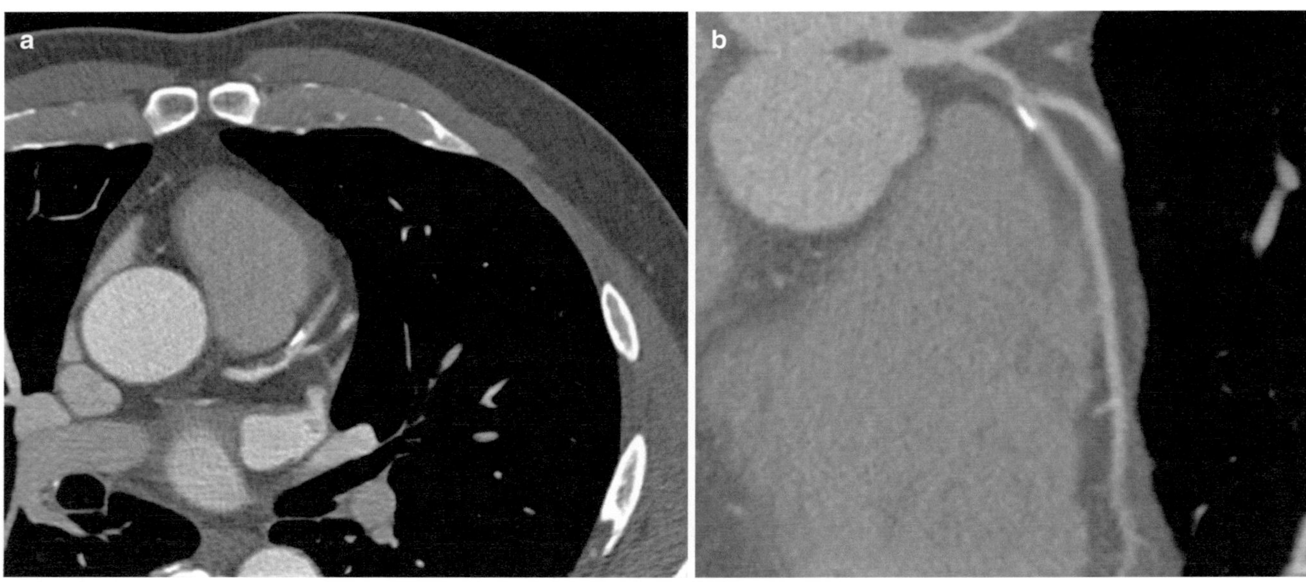

Fig. 16.4 (**a**, **b**) CAD-RADS 3. Predominantly non-calcified plaque in the proximal LAD with 50–69% diameter stenosis

guided by image integration significantly improves clinical outcome in comparison with both circumferential PV isolation guided by 3D mapping alone and with segmental electrophysiologically guided PV isolation [49]. The preprocedural CT report should include:

- Pulmonary veins:
  - Anatomy: number of veins and any anatomic variants and accessory or anomalous veins
  - Ostial diameter of each vein in long and short axis
  - Distance to first-order branch of each vein
- Left atrial dimensions and size
- Presence of absence of left atrial appendage thrombus
- Adjacent structures: esophagus and phrenic nerve

Conventional pulmonary venous anatomy is defined as the presence of single right and left superior and inferior pulmonary veins that drain into the LA without any accessory veins. The most common variants are a common or conjoined vein when the superior and inferior veins combine proximal to the LA, resulting in only one atriopulmonary venous junction on the involved side, as most commonly

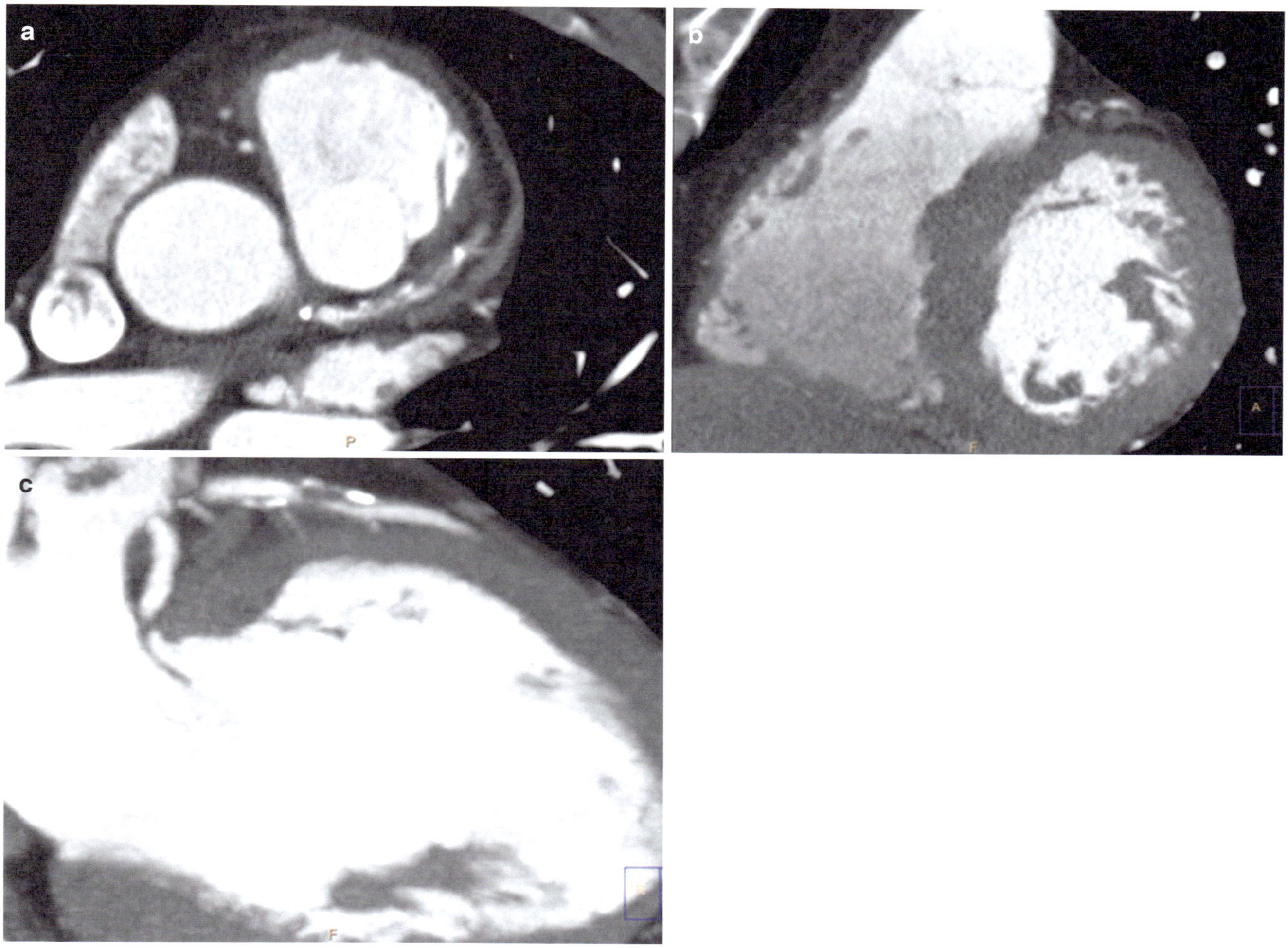

Fig. 16.5 (a–c) CAD-RADS 4A. Non-calcified and calcified plaque in the mid LAD causing 70–99% diameter stenosis

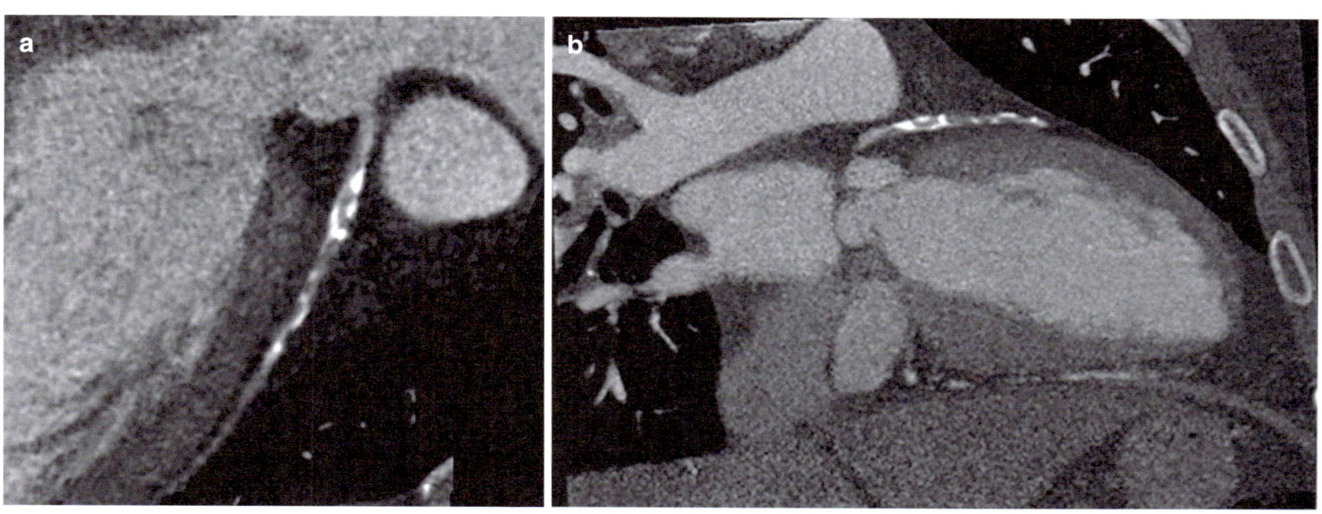

Fig. 16.6 (a, b) CAD-RADS 5. Complete occlusion of the LAD

seen on the left. Supernumerary or accessory pulmonary veins are extra veins with independent atriopulmonary venous junctions separate from the superior and inferior pulmonary veins and are named for the pulmonary lobe or segment that they drain, sometimes crossing pulmonary lobar fissures before emptying into the left atrium. Common examples include an additional right middle lobe vein. Anomalous pulmonary venous anatomy occurs when pulmonary veins drain into a structure other than the left atrium.

A variety of post-processing methods are used to display left atrial and pulmonary venous anatomy including 3D volume rendering (extra-atrial surface views and intra-atrial endoscopic views) MPR, CPR, and MIP views. To obtain the correct measurement of ostial diameter of each PV, both MPR and CPR images should be selected to show the en face ostial image. Then, ostial diameter should be measured as minor and major axis diameter by orthogonal angles and reported [23, 50].

LA size is related to the chronicity of AF and the likelihood of success for achieving sinus rhythm following ablation procedures. Reference normal and indexed values for LA size, volumes, and function have been published for ECG-gated MDCT [51]. The LA diameter can be measured and reported as a single anterior-posterior measurement on a three-chamber reconstruction in end-systole. However due to the complex shape of the LA and asymmetrical remodeling in AF, 2D measurements may not reflect the true size of the structure. LA function and volume can be calculated and reported using a modified method of Simpson with manual tracing of the endocardial borders on successive slices at both end-systole and end-diastole [52, 53]. An incremental predictive value has been shown for LA volumes by CT over echocardiographic dimensions in predicting the outcome of AF ablations.

The presence of LAA thrombus should be identified and reported. Poor contrast opacification of the LAA is often caused by slow flow and a delayed acquisition 1–2 min after the initial scan increases the accuracy for thrombus detection [54]. Phrenic nerve (PN) injury is a known complication of RF catheter ablation of AF. The right cardiophrenic artery can be visualized by CT and serves as a landmark to identify the adjacent phrenic nerve [55]. The anatomic path of the right cardiophrenic artery consistently runs anterior to the right superior pulmonary vein within the pericardial tissue anterior and adjacent to the right superior pulmonary vein and the SVC. Although the CT tissue density of the right phrenic nerve remains the same as tissue densities of the surrounding structures, the right cardiophrenic artery enhanced with contrast can be identified on the pre-procedural CT. During LA catheter ablation, an atrioesophageal fistula can develop as a result of thermal injury of the esophagus during ablation along the posterior LA. The esophagus and its relationship to the left atrium, pulmonary vein ostia, and pulmonary veins can be delineated on CT [56]; however it must be noted that the esophagus is a mobile structure and can shift by ≥2 cm in patients undergoing AF ablation under conscious sedation. Therefore real-time fluoroscopic imaging during the procedure is preferable [57].

Pre-procedural CT for Ventricular Ablation

Late gadolinium enhancement cardiac MR (CMR) is the reference standard for detection of myocardial scar and is used to guide and target arrhythmogenic tissue with catheter ablation in ischemic and nonischemic cardiomyopathies. However, many patients with ventricular tachycardia (VT) have a cardiac implanted electronic device (CIED), with cardiac MR services not widely available to these patients, or artifacts from the CIED may preclude assessment of scar tissue on the CMR exam. Regional wall thinning and hypoperfusion on cardiac CT have been found to correlate with the arrhythmogenic substrate in postinfarction VT [58]. Both epicardial fat and scar tissue result in low epicardial voltage on EP mapping procedures. Cardiac CT can differentiate epicardial fat from scar or muscle on the basis of their distinct attenuation, with epicardial ablations at sites with >10 mm of fat found to be ineffective [59]. The thickness of the epicardial fat over areas of scar and low voltage on electroanatomic mapping is therefore relevant to patient selection and the success of epicardial ablation procedures. Multiplanar and 3D images of epicardial fat generated from the pre-procedural CT examination are co-registered with the electroanatomic voltage map. Other relevant imaging features on pre-procedural CT include the relationship and proximity of the site of the arrhythmic focus to the coronary venous system, coronary arteries, and phrenic nerve [60]. Evaluation and reporting of these measurements require close collaboration with referring electrophysiologists and knowledge of the abnormalities on electroanatomic voltage maps.

Cardiac CT for Structural Heart Disease

CT offers high spatial resolution 3D anatomic assessment, with the temporal resolution enabled by gating permitting focused assessment at specific phases of the cardiac cycle, all important for patient selection, device eligibility, and pre-procedural planning for interventions in structural heart disease. This includes planning for transaortic valve replacement (TAVR), trans-mitral valve implantation, and left atrial appendage occlusion.

Transcatheter Aortic Valve Replacement (TAVR)

TAVR has become the treatment of choice for symptomatic severe aortic stenosis in both high-risk and intermediate-risk patients. CT plays an important role in the workup of patients who are candidates for implantation of a transcatheter aortic valve [61]. Essential elements of a TAVR CT report include detailed information about the aortic outflow, annulus, root, and proximal ascending aorta for valve sizing and assessment of common access vessels for appropriateness, the latter usually being the iliofemoral arteries but may also include the upper extremity arteries as well. Details of each structure are provided below. For a detailed description of the use of CT in pre-procedural planning of a TAVR procedure, please refer to Chap. 40.

Elements of a structured report for TAVR planning include:

- Aortic valve:
  - Number of leaflets
  - Presence and severity of aortic valve leaflet calcification (none, mild, moderate, or severe
- Aortic root:
  - Aortic annulus diameter (maximum and minimum)
  - Aortic annulus perimeter
  - Aortic annulus area
  - Sinus of Valsalva height for the right, left, and non-coronary sinuses
  - Sinus of Valsalva diameter for the right, left, and non-coronary sinuses
  - Height from annulus to left main and right coronary artery origins
  - Ascending aorta maximum diameter, including 4 cm above the aortic annulus
  - Aortic root angulation in degrees
- Access vessel assessment with minimum diameter (maximum and minimum diameter at this location), tortuosity and calcification assessment of each segment, and if present any aneurysm (including maximum diameter and location), stent, endograft or anatomic variant:
  - Thoracic aorta
  - Abdominal aorta
  - Left common iliac artery, including high-riding bifurcation
  - Left external iliac artery
  - Left femoral artery
  - Right common artery, including high-riding bifurcation
  - Right external artery
  - Right femoral artery
  - Left subclavian artery
  - Right subclavian artery
  - Right innominate artery

Mitral Valve Interventions

Transmitral valve implantation (TMVI) is an evolving treatment strategy for patients with mitral regurgitation, requiring detailed pre-procedural imaging for evaluation of annulus shape and dimensions, the valve leaflets, coronary sinus anatomy, and papillary muscle structure. The geometry of the mitral valve and supporting structures is more complex and variable than the aortic valve and annulus, making real-time assessment with echocardiography more critical in decision-making. CT plays a complementary role to 3D echocardiography in determining patient suitability by 3D anatomical quantification and landing zone characterization [62]. Specific items for a structured report should include the details listed below. Currently, TMVI devices in use and development are typically placed by a transapical route, less often transeptal or transatrial route; therefore aortic and arterial measurements are not required [63]. Leaflet length is generally measured using echocardiography and not CT.

- Mitral annulus calcification (none, mild, moderate, or severe)
- Mitral annulus diameter across each commissure
- Mitral annulus circumference
- Mitral annulus area
- Angle between coronary sinus and the mitral annulus
- Presence of leaflet prolapse if cine imaging obtained
- Subvalvular apparatus evaluation for unfavorable anatomy, including:
  - Irregular papillary muscle head branching or fused heads
  - Chordae tendinae extending to the subannular groove of the mitral valve
  - Large strut chordae
- Left ventricle:
  - End-diastolic diameter
  - Presence of basal septal bulging, hypertrophy, or thinning

Left Atrial Appendage Occlusion

Percutaneous closure of the left atrial appendage (LAA) is an effective and safe alternative for treating patients with atrial fibrillation and contraindication for oral anticoagulants [64]. The Watchman LAA occlusion device is FDA approved in the United States for patients with nonvalvular atrial fibrillation with acceptable anatomy who are at increased risk for stroke and would be candidates for anticoagulation in whom there is concern about the risk/benefit ratio of chronic anticoagulation [65]. Preimplantation cardiac CT can provide crucial information for safe device planning and selection and has been shown to be more accurate than echocardiography for LAA measurements and overall geometry of this complex eccentric structure [66]. Important preimplantation considerations to be mentioned in the structured report include the following:

- Left atrial appendage:
  - Morphology and shape: windsock, cactus, chicken wing, or broccoli [66, 67]

  - Length and diameter
  - Volume
  - Presence or absence of thrombus
  - Relationship to the left superior pulmonary vein
  - Relationship to the adjacent pulmonary artery
- Atrial appendage ostium
  - Ostium shape: oval, foot-like, triangular, water drop-like, or round
  - Maximum and minimum diameter
  - Perimeter
- Relationship of LAA to adjacent left upper lobe pulmonary vein and pulmonary artery

There are four types of LAA shape. The windsock type has a dominant central lobe allowing straightforward insertion of the occlusion device. The cactus type has a dominant central lobe, with secondary lobes arising from the central lobe, however does not contraindicate insertion. The chicken wing type has a dominant central lobe with a sharp kink. A kink very proximal to the ostium creates a small usable length that may complicate insertion. The broccoli or cauliflower type is the least common with multiple lobes and a short length, generally considered unsuitable for occlusion.

The LAA ostium has a variable shape and may be classified into five types including oval, foot-like, triangular, water drop-like, and round. The shape has implications for device placement as the ostium has to adapt to the shape of the round device. The measured maximal diameter of a very flat ostium will not be reflective of the diameter at device insertion. The perimeter and a perimeter-based ostial diameter have been reported to be the best parameters for sizing the LAA occlusion device due to the variable shape and morphology of the ostium [68]. The approximate LAA length is measured as the distance from the LAA ostial plane to the LAA apex in the primary lobe. LAA thrombus is a contraindication to implantation, and its presence or absence should be reported. The LAA ridge is a barrier between the LAA orifice and the adjacent left upper lobe pulmonary vein (LUPV). The width of the LAA ridge and proximity of the LAA to the LUPV could also affect a safe occlusion. For example, the expansion of an occluder may markedly compress the pulmonary vein when a LAA orifice is extremely flat and in close proximity to the LUPV. Perforation of the pulmonary artery and consequent hemopericardium is a recognized complication of LAA occluder insertion. If the ostium is very close to the main pulmonary artery, this should be described.

Myocardial Perfusion Imaging and Delayed Enhancement CT

Technologic improvements allowing for faster lower radiation exposure imaging facilitate the ability to perform CT myocardial perfusion imaging at rest and stress. Myocardial stress perfusion CT imaging is performed during the administration of a pharmacological vasodilator such as adenosine, regadenoson, or dipyridamole. Several single-center and multicenter trials indicate that stress CT perfusion is noninferior to SPECT and FFR to detect myocardial ischemia and hemodynamically relevant stenosis [69–71]. CT assessment of myocardial perfusion is based on the distribution of iodinated contrast material during its first pass through the myocardium. Contrast material distribution is dependent on the arterial supply; hence myocardial perfusion deficits are identified as hypoattenuating areas. Details of exam acquisition technique are covered in Chap. 62.

A stepwise approach to combined visual interpretation and reporting of CCTA and CT perfusion imaging is recommended [72] and should include (1) coronary CTA interpretation as covered earlier in this chapter, (2) reconstruction and processing of myocardial CT perfusion images, (3) image quality assessment and the identification of potentially confounding artifacts, (4) rest and stress image interpretation for enhancement patterns and areas of hypoattenuation, and (5) correlation of coronary anatomy and myocardial perfusion deficits.

CT perfusion images should be reconstructed in the three traditional cardiac views: short axis, horizontal long axis, and vertical long axis that allow for evaluation of each myocardial perfusion territory in more than two planes and viewed at a narrow window width and level (300/150 or 200/100). The data set should be examined for image quality and artifacts such as poor signal to noise, misalignment, and beam hardening. Typical locations for artifacts due to beam hardening are the basal inferior lateral wall and the left ventricular apex. Multiphase data sets should be used if available to differentiate true perfusion defects from artifacts, the former persisting over several cycles and are in the distribution of a coronary artery. Rest and stress perfusion images are read serially and compared, to assess for ischemia and infarction. The content of a structured report should include:

- Quality of myocardial perfusion images and presence of any artifacts
- Visual assessment of the perfusion to each myocardial segment at rest and stress:
  - 0 = normal myocardial perfusion
  - 1 = mild, perfusion deficit is less than one-third transmurality
  - 2 = moderate, ≤50% transmurality
  - 3 = severe, >50% transmurality
  - 4 = thinned chronic infarct
- Reversibility of each defect
- Transmyocardial perfusion ratio when relevant
- Whether each defect corresponds to an anatomic lesion on CCTA
- Absolute myocardial blood flow if dynamic CT perfusion technique is used

A reversible perfusion deficit consistent with inducible myocardial ischemia will show normal resting perfusion and abnormal stress perfusion. A predominately fixed perfusion deficit may have two different appearances: (1) rest perfusion deficit may persist on stress imaging and remain the same size, or (2) a rest perfusion deficit may partially hyperenhance to differing degrees due to relative hyperenhancement of an infarct. The transmyocardial perfusion ratio (TPR) is a semiquantitative perfusion metric representing the ratio of subendocardial attenuation and the entire subepicardial attenuation within a myocardial segment. TPR reflects the normal relation between subendocardial and subepicardial blood flow, which is normally higher in the subendocardium and is also the area compromised first during coronary stenosis [72, 73]. In subjects with no coronary disease, the mean TPR is 1.12 ± 0.13, and it is considered potentially abnormal when it is <0.99 or more than 1 SD below the mean normal TPR. In case of dynamic CT perfusion, a calculation of absolute blood flow in the myocardium can be performed and has been shown to have a good correlation to invasive fractional flow reserve [69, 74].

Delayed enhancement CT allows accurate visualization of myocardial infarction and viability and can be performed with a second CT scan performed 5–10 min after coronary CTA to demonstrate hyperenhancement [75–79]. The regional extent of delayed enhancement is assessed using a 17-segment model. MinIP and thick MPR detect infarcted myocardium with greater visibility and definition than MIP and thin MPR [80]. Each segment is described and reported as involved or healthy and the percentage of transmural extent of enhancement graded using a 4-point scale (1–4): 0–25%, 26–50%, 51–75%, or 76–100%.

Congenital Heart Disease

Improved CT scanner technology and reconstruction methods allowing rapid, high spatial and temporal resolution imaging of the heart with low radiation doses make CT an attractive and increasingly used imaging modality for congenital heart disease (CHD) in both pediatric and adult patients. The use of cardiac CT for CHD is a guideline recommended in specific circumstances, such as inability to undergo MRI due to claustrophobia, nondiagnostic MRI due to metallic artifacts, and when higher spatial resolution anatomical imaging is required [81–83].

Imaging targets and reporting elements of CT for CHD depend on the nature of the lesion and prior surgical interventions, e.g., right ventricular size, function, right ventricular outflow tract anatomy and branch pulmonary arteries after tetralogy of Fallot repair, recoarctation or pseudoaneurysm formation after coarctation repair, and patency of baffles and conduits after blood flow redirection surgery. Structured reporting for CHD should follow a sequential segmental approach with a systematic description as below and include a detailed description of lung parenchyma, airways, and chest wall given the association of other congenital abnormalities.

- Visceral and atrial situs
- Position and location of the apex
- Systemic and pulmonary venous connections
- Atrioventricular connections
- Ventriculoarterial connections
- Atrial size and interatrial septum
- Ventricular size, function, and interventricular septum
- Relationship of the great vessels
- Outflow tracts and semilunar valves
- Patency, size, and branching of the aorta and pulmonary arteries
- Origins and course of the coronary arteries
- Functional and volumetric data relative to body surface area and available normal values

Extracardiac Structures

Dedicated cardiac CT data sets include portions of noncardiovascular thoracic and upper abdominal anatomy, which should be reviewed and reported for two important reasons: recognizing associated primary and secondary comorbid pathology and identification of abnormalities that may lead to alternative cause for symptoms (e.g., pulmonary embolism or pneumonia in the acute setting). A full field of view reconstruction should be performed, and all the extracardiac structures in the field of view should be examined and abnormalities reported [4].

Impressions and Management Recommendations

The concluding section should summarize the major findings in a clear concise manner, answer the specific clinical questions posed, and guide further clinical management. In the context of CCTA for ischemic symptoms, the major findings regarding coronary artery and cardiac structure and function should be concisely stated. Additional tests may be recommended if the significance of scan findings is uncertain, e.g., nuclear medicine or other functional ischemia tests to analyze borderline stenosis. The results of the CCTA can be broadly described in the conclusion as normal coronary arteries (no plaque or stenosis), nonobstructive CAD (1–49% stenosis), or significant CAD (>/=50% or >/=70% stenosis) with further qualification on the location and extent of disease. If the CAD-RADS reporting and data system is used, the specific CAD-RADS code for the findings and recommendations for further workup should be mentioned in the impressions.

Table 16.5 Components of comprehensive cardiac CT report

	Specific component(s)	Necessity
Clinical data		
General	Indication or reason for test, procedure date	Required
Demographics	Name, date of birth, sex, referring clinician height, weight, BMI	Required
History	Symptoms, risk factors, relevant diagnostic tests	Recommended
Procedure data		
Description	Test type (e.g., coronary CT angiography, calcium scoring, ventricular function, pulmonary vein, others)	Required
Equipment	Scanner type: Number of detectors, rotation time, number of X-ray sources	Recommended
Acquisition	Gating method: Retrospective vs prospective ECG synchronization	Required
	Tube voltage, tube current, dose modulation (if used)	Recommended
	Estimated radiation dose, e.g., dose length product	Recommended
Reconstruction	Scanned or reconstructed phase of cardiac cycle	Recommended
	Slice thickness, increment, reconstruction filter	Required
Medications	Contrast type, volume, β-blockers, nitroglycerin, or any other, if given	Required
	Contrast rate	Recommended
Patient parameters	Complication(s), if present	Required
	Heart rate, arrhythmia, if present	Recommended
Results		
Technical quality	Overall quality	Required
	Presence and type of artifact and effect on interpretation	Required
Coronary	Calcium score (if calcium scan performed)	Required
	Coronary anatomy: anomalies (origins and course), dominance, dilatation/aneurysms, anatomical variance, bridging	Required
	Stenosis location and severity	Required
	Uninterpretable segments, arteries, or overall study	Required
	Stenosis plaque type: Calcified, non-calcified, or partially calcified	Required
	Stenosis extent and vulnerable features: length, ostial or branch involvement, positive remodeling, low-attenuation plaque, napkin-ring sign, spotty calcifications, tortuosity	Recommended
	Use of SCCT stenosis severity classification	Required
	Use of SCCT axial coronary segmentation model	Recommended
	Calcium score percentile (if calcium scan performed)	Required
Prior cardiac procedures	Stents: Location, interpretability, patency Prior CABG: Type, location, course and anastomosis, interpretability, patency, stenosis	Required
Non-coronary cardiac structures		
Vessels	Abnormalities of the aorta, vena cava, pulmonary arteries, and pulmonary veins, if present	Required
	Pulmonary vein morphology and ostia sizes (required for pre-ablation studies)	Required
Cardiac chambers	Abnormal chamber dilation, hypertrophy, masses, thrombus, shunts, and other structural diseases, if present	Required
	Left ventricular size, EF, and volume (if function data is obtained)	Required
	Left atrial volume (for pre-ablation studies)	Recommended
	Right ventricular size and volume (if functional data obtained)	Required
	Left ventricular wall motion (17-segment model) and EF (if functional data obtained)	Required
Myocardium	Evidence of prior MI (hypoperfusion, wall thinning, fat, calcification, aneurysms)	Required
	End-diastolic left ventricular wall thickness	Recommended
	Perfusion defects and abnormal enhancement using a 17-segment model (if performed)	Required
Pericardium	Abnormal thickness, calcification, effusion if present	Required
Valves	Abnormal aortic and mitral valve calcification, thickness, stenosis, morphology Prosthetic valves: type, location, pannus, thrombus, mobility	Required
Non-cardiac	Abnormalities in the lungs, mediastinum, esophagus, bony structures, chest wall, etc., if present	Required
Impressions and conclusions	Coronary interpretation	Required
	Abnormal non-coronary cardiac findings	Required
	Abnormal non-cardiac findings	Required
	Correlation to other or prior cardiac studies	Recommended
	Documentation of communication to referring physician for urgent finding(s)	Recommended
	Clinical recommendations	Recommended
	CAD-RADS code	Recommended

In case of extracardiac findings, their relevance and any recommendations for further workup should be stated. The components of a comprehensive cardiac CT report are summarized in Table 16.5. A sample standardized reporting template for CCTA with calcium scoring (normal examination) is provided below in Table 16.6.

Table 16.6 A sample standardized reporting template for CCTA (normal examination)

Procedure: CT cardiac (without and with contrast, with 3D reformatting)—coronary CTA protocol including coronary calcium CT
Clinical history: [ ]
Comparison: [ ]
Technique: Using a [*scanner type*], a preliminary scout study was obtained, followed by coronary artery calcium protocol. Following administration of [x] ml iodinated intravenous contrast [contrast name], [*0.5*] mm collimated images were obtained from the carina to the base of the heart. [*Prospective*; *Retrospective*>] ECG triggering was used. Heart rate at the time of acquisition was approximately [ ] bpm.
Multiplanar and 3D reformatted images were rendered and reviewed on an advanced processing workstation to further define anatomy and possible pathology (DFOV = 25/cm)
Medications: [*100 mg of oral metoprolol and x mg IV metoprolol was administered prior to scanning*]. [0.*4 mg sublingual nitroglycerine was administered immediately prior to scanning*]
Technical quality: [*excellent, with no artifacts*; *good, with minor artifact but good diagnostic quality; acceptable, with moderate artifacts; poor/suboptimal, with severe artifacts*]
Findings
CT coronary calcium scoring
LMA =
LAD =
LCX =
RCA =
PDA =
Total calcium score = [ ] using the AJ-130 method. This score is in the percentile rank for age and gender, meaning that [ ] % of patients of the same age and gender will have a higher score. The total volume score is [ ]
Coronary CT angiography
The coronary artery origins and proximal course are normal. There is ____ (right/left/co) coronary artery dominance
Note: Stenoses are reported as maximum percentage diameter stenosis
Stenosis grading is reported using the following scheme:
Normal: no plaque
Minimal: negligible impact on the lumen (<25% stenosis)
Mild: no flow-limiting stenosis (25–49% stenosis)
Moderate: possible flow-limiting disease (50–69% stenosis)
Severe: probable flow-limiting disease (70–99% stenosis)
Occluded
Left main: The left main coronary artery is a _____ (short/medium/large) size vessel and (bifurcates in LAD and LCX/or trifurcates in LAD, LCX, and a ramus branch). It is patent with no evidence of plaque or stenosis
LAD: The left anterior descending artery is patent with no evidence of plaque or stenosis. It gives off ____ patent diagonal branches
LCX: The left circumflex artery is patent with no evidence of plaque or stenosis. It gives off ____ patent obtuse marginal branches
RCA: The right coronary artery is patent with no evidence of plaque or stenosis. It gives off a patent posterior descending artery and a patent posterior left ventricular branch
Cardiac structure and morphology
Cardiac chambers: Non-enlarged. No myocardial hypertrophy
Cardiac valves: There is no thickening or calcifications in the aortic and mitral valves
Pericardium: No effusion, thickening, or calcifications
Chest
Within the imaged field of view, evaluation of the visualized thoracic and upper abdominal structures demonstrates no additional abnormalities; specifically, there are no pulmonary nodules or enlarged lymph nodes. There is a three-leaflet aortic valve with no aortic leaflet calcification. The aortic root is normal in diameter, measuring – cm. The central pulmonary arteries are unremarkable
Impression
1. Total coronary calcium score = [ ] and is at the [ ] percentile for age and gender
2. Normal coronary arteries
3. Normal cardiac chamber size
4. Unremarkable aortic valve and aortic root
5. Unremarkable pericardium

Time Line for Report Distribution

To expedite patient flow in the emergency department (ED), cardiac CT studies for acute chest pain should be interpreted and reported within 60 min of reconstruction. It is also recommended that all emergency scans including normal studies be reported verbally to the ED providers and that all exams with moderate- or high-grade stenosis be communicated in all clinical settings, with documentation of the verbal communication in the report. Physicians should be notified immediately of life-threatening critical findings, such as pulmonary embolism or aortic dissection. Similarly, incidental unexpected findings requiring follow-up that may lead to later downstream medical problems, such as lung nodules requiring follow-up CT exams to ensure their lack of growth, should be communicated and documented. Elective studies should be reported within 1–2 working days of the procedure.

Conclusion

The use of structured reporting in cardiac CT is recommended to improve communication of results to referring physicians. Furthermore structured reporting benefits research, education, peer review, and quality assurance and results in improved quality of care. The structured report should contain adequate information to support the clinical necessity for the procedure and a comprehensive description of the findings and their significance using standardized terminology to enable proper clinical management.

References

1. Sundaram B, Patel S, Bogot N, Kazerooni EA. Anatomy and terminology for the interpretation and reporting of cardiac MDCT: part 1, Structured report, coronary calcium screening, and coronary artery anatomy. AJR Am J Roentgenol. 2009;192(3):574–83.
2. Sundaram B, Patel S, Agarwal P, Kazerooni EA. Anatomy and terminology for the interpretation and reporting of cardiac MDCT: part 2, CT angiography, cardiac function assessment, and noncoronary and extracardiac findings. AJR Am J Roentgenol. 2009;192(3):584–98.
3. Stillman AE, Rubin GD, Teague SD, White RD, Woodard PK, Larson PA. Structured reporting: coronary CT angiography: a white paper from the American College of Radiology and the North American Society for Cardiovascular Imaging. J Am Coll Radiol JACR. 2008;5(7):796–800.
4. Leipsic J, Abbara S, Achenbach S, Cury R, Earls JP, Mancini GJ, Nieman K, Pontone G, Raff GL. SCCT guidelines for the interpretation and reporting of coronary CT angiography: a report of the Society of Cardiovascular Computed Tomography Guidelines Committee. J Cardiovasc Comput Tomogr. 2014;8(5):342–58.
5. Ghoshhajra BB, Lee AM, Ferencik M, Elmariah S, Margey RJ, Onuma O, Panagia M, Abbara S, Hoffmann U. Interpreting the interpretations: the use of structured reporting improves referring clinicians' comprehension of coronary CT angiography reports. J Am Coll Radiol JACR. 2013;10(6):432–8.
6. Litt HI, Gatsonis C, Snyder B, Singh H, Miller CD, Entrikin DW, Leaming JM, Gavin LJ, Pacella CB, Hollander JE. CT angiography for safe discharge of patients with possible acute coronary syndromes. N Engl J Med. 2012;366(15):1393–403.
7. Goldstein JA, Chinnaiyan KM, Abidov A, Achenbach S, Berman DS, Hayes SW, Hoffmann U, Lesser JR, Mikati IA, O'Neil BJ, Shaw LJ, Shen MY, Valeti US, Raff GL, Investigators C-S. The CT-STAT (coronary computed tomographic angiography for systematic triage of acute chest pain patients to treatment) trial. J Am Coll Cardiol. 2011;58(14):1414–22.
8. Investigators S-H. CT coronary angiography in patients with suspected angina due to coronary heart disease (SCOT-HEART): an open-label, parallel-group, multicentre trial. Lancet. 2015;385(9985):2383–91.
9. Douglas PS, Hoffmann U, Patel MR, Mark DB, Al-Khalidi HR, Cavanaugh B, Cole J, Dolor RJ, Fordyce CB, Huang M, Khan MA, Kosinski AS, Krucoff MW, Malhotra V, Picard MH, Udelson JE, Velazquez EJ, Yow E, Cooper LS, Lee KL, Investigators P. Outcomes of anatomical versus functional testing for coronary artery disease. N Engl J Med. 2015;372(14):1291–300.
10. Raff GL, Chinnaiyan KM, Cury RC, Garcia MT, Hecht HS, Hollander JE, O'Neil B, Taylor AJ, Hoffmann U, Society of Cardiovascular Computed Tomography Guidelines C. SCCT guidelines on the use of coronary computed tomographic angiography for patients presenting with acute chest pain to the emergency department: a report of the Society of Cardiovascular Computed Tomography Guidelines Committee. J Cardiovasc Comput Tomogr. 2014;8(4):254–71.
11. Taylor AJ, Cerqueira M, Hodgson JM, Mark D, Min J, O'Gara P, Rubin GD. ACCF/SCCT/ACR/AHA/ASE/ASNC/NASCI/SCAI/SCMR 2010 appropriate use criteria for cardiac computed tomography. A report of the American College of Cardiology Foundation Appropriate Use Criteria Task Force, the Society of Cardiovascular Computed Tomography, the American College of Radiology, the American Heart Association, the American Society of Echocardiography, the American Society of Nuclear Cardiology, the North American Society for Cardiovascular Imaging, the Society for Cardiovascular Angiography and Interventions, and the Society for Cardiovascular Magnetic Resonance. J Cardiovasc Comput Tomogr. 2010;4(6):407 e1–33.
12. Greenland P, Bonow RO, Brundage BH, Budoff MJ, Eisenberg MJ, Grundy SM, Lauer MS, Post WS, Raggi P, Redberg RF, Rodgers GP, Shaw LJ, Taylor AJ, Weintraub WS, Harrington RA, Abrams J, Anderson JL, Bates ER, Grines CL, Hlatky MA, Lichtenberg RC, Lindner JR, Pohost GM, Schofield RS, Shubrooks SJ Jr, Stein JH, Tracy CM, Vogel RA, Wesley DJ, American College of Cardiology Foundation Clinical Expert Consensus Task F, Society of Atherosclerosis I, Prevention, Society of Cardiovascular Computed T. ACCF/AHA 2007 clinical expert consensus document on coronary artery calcium scoring by computed tomography in global cardiovascular risk assessment and in evaluation of patients with chest pain: a report of the American College of Cardiology Foundation Clinical Expert Consensus Task Force (ACCF/AHA Writing Committee to Update the 2000 Expert Consensus Document on Electron Beam Computed Tomography). Circulation. 2007;115(3):402–26.
13. Agatston AS, Janowitz WR, Hildner FJ, Zusmer NR, Viamonte M Jr, Detrano R. Quantification of coronary artery calcium using ultrafast computed tomography. J Am Coll Cardiol. 1990;15(4):827–32.
14. Detrano R, Guerci AD, Carr JJ, Bild DE, Burke G, Folsom AR, Liu K, Shea S, Szklo M, Bluemke DA, O'Leary DH, Tracy R, Watson K, Wong ND, Kronmal RA. Coronary calcium as a predictor of coronary events in four racial or ethnic groups. N Engl J Med. 2008;358(13):1336–45.

15. Rutten A, Isgum I, Prokop M. Coronary calcification: effect of small variation of scan starting position on Agatston, volume, and mass scores. Radiology. 2008;246(1):90–8.
16. Hong C, Becker CR, Schoepf UJ, Ohnesorge B, Bruening R, Reiser MF. Coronary artery calcium: absolute quantification in nonenhanced and contrast-enhanced multi-detector row CT studies. Radiology. 2002;223(2):474–80.
17. Rumberger JA, Kaufman L. A rosetta stone for coronary calcium risk stratification: agatston, volume, and mass scores in 11,490 individuals. AJR Am J Roentgenol. 2003;181(3):743–8.
18. Callister TQ, Cooil B, Raya SP, Lippolis NJ, Russo DJ, Raggi P. Coronary artery disease: improved reproducibility of calcium scoring with an electron-beam CT volumetric method. Radiology. 1998;208(3):807–14.
19. Hecht HS, Cronin P, Blaha MJ, Budoff MJ, Kazerooni EA, Narula J, Yankelevitz D, Abbara S. 2016 SCCT/STR guidelines for coronary artery calcium scoring of noncontrast noncardiac chest CT scans a report of the Society of Cardiovascular Computed Tomography and Society of Thoracic Radiology. J Cardiovasc Comput Tomogr. 2017;11(1):74–84.
20. Austen WG, Edwards JE, Frye RL, Gensini GG, Gott VL, Griffith LS, McGoon DC, Murphy ML, Roe BB. A reporting system on patients evaluated for coronary artery disease. Report of the Ad Hoc Committee for Grading of Coronary Artery Disease, Council on Cardiovascular Surgery, American Heart Association. Circulation. 1975;51(4 Suppl):5–40.
21. Cheng V, Gutstein A, Wolak A, Suzuki Y, Dey D, Gransar H, Thomson LE, Hayes SW, Friedman JD, Berman DS. Moving beyond binary grading of coronary arterial stenoses on coronary computed tomographic angiography: insights for the imager and referring clinician. JACC Cardiovasc Imaging. 2008;1(4):460–71.
22. Achenbach S, Moselewski F, Ropers D, Ferencik M, Hoffmann U, MacNeill B, Pohle K, Baum U, Anders K, Jang IK, Daniel WG, Brady TJ. Detection of calcified and noncalcified coronary atherosclerotic plaque by contrast-enhanced, submillimeter multidetector spiral computed tomography: a segment-based comparison with intravascular ultrasound. Circulation. 2004;109(1):14–7.
23. Miller JM, Rochitte CE, Dewey M, Arbab-Zadeh A, Niinuma H, Gottlieb I, Paul N, Clouse ME, Shapiro EP, Hoe J, Lardo AC, Bush DE, de Roos A, Cox C, Brinker J, Lima JA. Diagnostic performance of coronary angiography by 64-row CT. N Engl J Med. 2008;359(22):2324–36.
24. Raff GL, Gallagher MJ, O'Neill WW, Goldstein JA. Diagnostic accuracy of noninvasive coronary angiography using 64-slice spiral computed tomography. J Am Coll Cardiol. 2005;46(3):552–7.
25. Budoff MJ, Dowe D, Jollis JG, Gitter M, Sutherland J, Halamert E, Scherer M, Bellinger R, Martin A, Benton R, Delago A, Min JK. Diagnostic performance of 64-multidetector row coronary computed tomographic angiography for evaluation of coronary artery stenosis in individuals without known coronary artery disease: results from the prospective multicenter ACCURACY (Assessment by Coronary Computed Tomographic Angiography of Individuals Undergoing Invasive Coronary Angiography) trial. J Am Coll Cardiol. 2008;52(21):1724–32.
26. Weigold WG, Abbara S, Achenbach S, Arbab-Zadeh A, Berman D, Carr JJ, Cury RC, Halliburton SS, McCollough CH, Taylor AJ, Society of Cardiovascular Computed T. Standardized medical terminology for cardiac computed tomography: a report of the Society of Cardiovascular Computed Tomography. J Cardiovasc Comput Tomogr. 2011;5(3):136–44.
27. Puchner SB, Liu T, Mayrhofer T, Truong QA, Lee H, Fleg JL, Nagurney JT, Udelson JE, Hoffmann U, Ferencik M. High-risk plaque detected on coronary CT angiography predicts acute coronary syndromes independent of significant stenosis in acute chest pain: results from the ROMICAT-II trial. J Am Coll Cardiol. 2014;64(7):684–92.
28. Motoyama S, Sarai M, Harigaya H, Anno H, Inoue K, Hara T, Naruse H, Ishii J, Hishida H, Wong ND, Virmani R, Kondo T, Ozaki Y, Narula J. Computed tomographic angiography characteristics of atherosclerotic plaques subsequently resulting in acute coronary syndrome. J Am Coll Cardiol. 2009;54(1):49–57.
29. Hsu JT, Kyo E, Chu CM, Tsuji T, Watanabe S. Impact of calcification length ratio on the intervention for chronic total occlusions. Int J Cardiol. 2011;150(2):135–41.
30. Martin-Yuste V, Barros A, Leta R, Ferreira I, Brugaletta S, Pujadas S, Carreras F, Pons G, Cinca J, Sabate M. Factors determining success in percutaneous revascularization of chronic total coronary occlusion: multidetector computed tomography analysis. Rev Esp Cardiol. 2012;65(4):334–40.
31. Yokoyama N, Yamamoto Y, Suzuki S, Suzuki M, Konno K, Kozuma K, Kaminaga T, Isshiki T. Impact of 16-slice computed tomography in percutaneous coronary intervention of chronic total occlusions. Catheter Cardiovasc Interv. 2006;68(1):1–7.
32. Luo C, Huang M, Li J, Liang C, Zhang Q, Liu H, Liu Z, Qu Y, Jiang J, Zhuang J. Predictors of interventional success of antegrade PCI for CTO. J Am Coll Cardiol Img. 2015;8(7):804–813.8.
33. Chan M, Ridley L, Dunn DJ, Tian DH, Liou K, Ozdirik J, Cheruvu C, Cao C. A systematic review and meta-analysis of multidetector computed tomography in the assessment of coronary artery bypass grafts. Int J Cardiol. 2016;221:898–905.
34. Kamdar AR, Meadows TA, Roselli EE, Gorodeski EZ, Curtin RJ, Sabik JF, Schoenhagen P, White RD, Lytle BW, Flamm SD, Desai MY. Multidetector computed tomographic angiography in planning of reoperative cardiothoracic surgery. Ann Thorac Surg. 2008;85(4):1239–45.
35. Aviram G, Sharony R, Kramer A, Nesher N, Loberman D, Ben-Gal Y, Graif M, Uretzky G, Mohr R. Modification of surgical planning based on cardiac multidetector computed tomography in reoperative heart surgery. Ann Thorac Surg. 2005;79(2):589–95.
36. Imran Hamid U, Digney R, Soo L, Leung S, Graham AN. Incidence and outcome of re-entry injury in redo cardiac surgery: benefits of preoperative planning. Eur J Cardiothorac Surg. 2015;47(5):819–23.
37. de Graaf FR, Schuijf JD, van Velzen JE, Boogers MJ, Kroft LJ, de Roos A, Reiber JH, Sieders A, Spano F, Jukema JW, Schalij MJ, van der Wall EE, Bax JJ. Diagnostic accuracy of 320-row multidetector computed tomography coronary angiography to noninvasively assess in-stent restenosis. Investig Radiol. 2010;45(6):331–40.
38. Kumbhani DJ, Ingelmo CP, Schoenhagen P, Curtin RJ, Flamm SD, Desai MY. Meta-analysis of diagnostic efficacy of 64-slice computed tomography in the evaluation of coronary in-stent restenosis. Am J Cardiol. 2009;103(12):1675–81.
39. Carrabba N, Schuijf JD, de Graaf FR, Parodi G, Maffei E, Valenti R, Palumbo A, Weustink AC, Mollet NR, Accetta G, Cademartiri F, Antoniucci D, Bax JJ. Diagnostic accuracy of 64-slice computed tomography coronary angiography for the detection of in-stent restenosis: a meta-analysis. J Nucl Cardiol. 2010;17(3):470–8.
40. Stojanovska J, Prasitdumrong H, Patel S, Sundaram B, Gross BH, Yilmaz ZN, Kazerooni EA. Reference absolute and indexed values for left and right ventricular volume, function and mass from cardiac computed tomography. J Med Imaging Radiat Oncol. 2014;58(5):547–58.
41. Lin FY, Devereux RB, Roman MJ, Meng J, Jow VM, Jacobs A, Weinsaft JW, Shaw LJ, Berman DS, Callister TQ, Min JK. Cardiac chamber volumes, function, and mass as determined by 64-multidetector row computed tomography: mean values among healthy adults free of hypertension and obesity. JACC Cardiovasc Imaging. 2008;1(6):782–6.
42. Cerqueira MD, Weissman NJ, Dilsizian V, Jacobs AK, Kaul S, Laskey WK, Pennell DJ, Rumberger JA, Ryan T, Verani MS, American Heart Association Writing Group on Myocardial S, Registration for Cardiac I. Standardized myocardial segmentation and nomenclature for tomographic imaging of the heart. A

statement for healthcare professionals from the Cardiac Imaging Committee of the Council on Clinical Cardiology of the American Heart Association. Circulation. 2002;105(4):539–42.
43. Feuchtner GM, Dichtl W, Friedrich GJ, Frick M, Alber H, Schachner T, Bonatti J, Mallouhi A, Frede T, Pachinger O, zur Nedden D, Muller S. Multislice computed tomography for detection of patients with aortic valve stenosis and quantification of severity. J Am Coll Cardiol. 2006;47(7):1410–7.
44. LaBounty TM, Sundaram B, Agarwal P, Armstrong WA, Kazerooni EA, Yamada E. Aortic valve area on 64-MDCT correlates with transesophageal echocardiography in aortic stenosis. AJR Am J Roentgenol. 2008;191(6):1652–8.
45. Cury RC, Abbara S, Achenbach S, Agatston A, Berman DS, Budoff MJ, Dill KE, Jacobs JE, Maroules CD, Rubin GD, Rybicki FJ, Schoepf UJ, Shaw LJ, Stillman AE, White CS, Woodard PK, Leipsic JA. CAD-RADS: Coronary Artery Disease – Reporting and Data System: an expert consensus document of the Society of Cardiovascular Computed Tomography (SCCT), the American College of Radiology (ACR) and the North American Society for Cardiovascular Imaging (NASCI). Endorsed by the American College of Cardiology. J Am Coll Radiol JACR. 2016;13(12 Pt A):1458–1466 e1459.
46. Fihn SD, Gardin JM, Abrams J, Berra K, Blankenship JC, Dallas AP, Douglas PS, Foody JM, Gerber TC, Hinderliter AL, King SB III, Kligfield PD, Krumholz HM, Kwong RYK, Lim MJ, Linderbaum JA, Mack MJ, Munger MA, Prager RL, Sabik JF, Shaw LJ, Sikkema JD, Smith CR Jr, Smith SC Jr, Spertus JA, Williams SV. ACCF/AHA/ACP/AATS/PCNA/SCAI/STS guideline for the diagnosis and management of patients with stable ischemic heart disease: a report of the American College of Cardiology Foundation/American Heart Association Task Force on, American Association for Thoracic Surgery, Preventive Cardiovascular Nurses Association, Society for Cardiovascular Angiography and Interventions, and Society of Thoracic Surgeons. J Am Coll Cardiol. 2012;60:e44–164.
47. Ang R, Hunter RJ, Baker V, Richmond L, Dhinoja M, Sporton S, Schilling RJ, Pugliese F, Davies C, Earley M. Pulmonary vein measurements on pre-procedural CT/MR imaging can predict difficult pulmonary vein isolation and phrenic nerve injury during cryoballoon ablation for paroxysmal atrial fibrillation. Int J Cardiol. 2015;195:253–8.
48. Cronin P, Kelly AM, Desjardins B, Patel S, Gross BH, Kazerooni EA, Morady F, Oral H, Carlos RC. Normative analysis of pulmonary vein drainage patterns on multidetector CT with measurements of pulmonary vein ostial diameter and distance to first bifurcation. Acad Radiol. 2007;14(2):178–88.
49. Bertaglia E, Bella PD, Tondo C, Proclemer A, Bottoni N, De Ponti R, Landolina M, Bongiorni MG, Coro L, Stabile G, Dello Russo A, Verlato R, Mantica M, Zoppo F. Image integration increases efficacy of paroxysmal atrial fibrillation catheter ablation: results from the CartoMerge Italian Registry. Europace. 2009;11(8):1004–10.
50. Cronin P, Sneider MB, Kazerooni EA, Kelly AM, Scharf C, Oral H, Morady F. MDCT of the left atrium and pulmonary veins in planning radiofrequency ablation for atrial fibrillation: a how-to guide. AJR Am J Roentgenol. 2004;183(3):767–78.
51. Stojanovska J, Cronin P, Patel S, Gross BH, Oral H, Chughtai K, Kazerooni EA. Reference normal absolute and indexed values from ECG-gated MDCT: left atrial volume, function, and diameter. AJR Am J Roentgenol. 2011;197(3):631–7.
52. Parikh SS, Jons C, McNitt S, Daubert JP, Schwarz KQ, Hall B. Predictive capability of left atrial size measured by CT, TEE, and TTE for recurrence of atrial fibrillation following radiofrequency catheter ablation. Pacing Clin Electrophysiol PACE. 2010;33(5):532–40.
53. Stojanovska J, Cronin P, Gross BH, Kazerooni EA, Tsodikov A, Frank L, Oral H. Left atrial function and maximum volume as determined by MDCT are independently associated with atrial fibrillation. Acad Radiol. 2014;21(9):1162–71.
54. Romero J, Husain SA, Kelesidis I, Sanz J, Medina HM, Garcia MJ. Detection of left atrial appendage thrombus by cardiac computed tomography in patients with atrial fibrillation: a meta-analysis. Circ Cardiovasc Imaging. 2013;6(2):185–94.
55. Horton R, Di Biase L, Reddy V, Neuzil P, Mohanty P, Sanchez J, Nguyen T, Mohanty S, Gallinghouse GJ, Bailey SM, Zagrodzky JD, Burkhardt JD, Natale A. Locating the right phrenic nerve by imaging the right pericardiophrenic artery with computerized tomographic angiography: implications for balloon-based procedures. Heart Rhythm. 2010;7(7):937–41.
56. Lemola K, Sneider M, Desjardins B, Case I, Han J, Good E, Tamirisa K, Tsemo A, Chugh A, Bogun F, Pelosi F Jr, Kazerooni E, Morady F, Oral H. Computed tomographic analysis of the anatomy of the left atrium and the esophagus: implications for left atrial catheter ablation. Circulation. 2004;110(24):3655–60.
57. Good E, Oral H, Lemola K, Han J, Tamirisa K, Igic P, Elmouchi D, Tschopp D, Reich S, Chugh A, Bogun F, Pelosi F Jr, Morady F. Movement of the esophagus during left atrial catheter ablation for atrial fibrillation. J Am Coll Cardiol. 2005;46(11):2107–10.
58. Komatsu Y, Cochet H, Jadidi A, Sacher F, Shah A, Derval N, Scherr D, Pascale P, Roten L, Denis A, Ramoul K, Miyazaki S, Daly M, Riffaud M, Sermesant M, Relan J, Ayache N, Kim S, Montaudon M, Laurent F, Hocini M, Haissaguerre M, Jais P. Regional myocardial wall thinning at multidetector computed tomography correlates to arrhythmogenic substrate in postinfarction ventricular tachycardia: assessment of structural and electrical substrate. Circ Arrhythm Electrophysiol. 2013;6(2):342–50.
59. Desjardins B, Morady F, Bogun F. Effect of epicardial fat on electroanatomical mapping and epicardial catheter ablation. J Am Coll Cardiol. 2010;56(16):1320–7.
60. Njeim M, Desjardins B, Bogun F. Multimodality imaging for guiding EP ablation procedures. J Am Coll Cardiol Img. 2016;9(7):873–86. 9.
61. Achenbach S, Delgado V, Hausleiter J, Schoenhagen P, Min JK, Leipsic JA. SCCT expert consensus document on computed tomography imaging before transcatheter aortic valve implantation (TAVI)/transcatheter aortic valve replacement (TAVR). J Cardiovasc Comput Tomogr. 2012;6(6):366–80.
62. Blanke P, Dvir D, Cheung A, Levine RA, Thompson C, Webb JG, Leipsic J. Mitral annular evaluation with CT in the context of transcatheter mitral valve replacement. J Am Coll Cardiol Img. 2015;8(5):612–5.
63. Natarajan N, Patel P, Bartel T, Kapadia S, Navia J, Stewart W, Tuzcu EM, Schoenhagen P. Peri-procedural imaging for transcatheter mitral valve replacement. Cardiovasc Diagn Ther. 2016;6(2):144–59.
64. Xu H, Xie X, Wang B, Ma S, Wang F. Efficacy and safety of percutaneous left atrial appendage occlusion for stroke prevention in nonvalvular atrial fibrillation: a meta-analysis of contemporary studies. Heart Lung Circ. 2016;25(11):1107–17.
65. Holmes DR Jr, Reddy VY. Left atrial appendage and closure: who, when, and how. Circ Cardiovasc Interv. 2016;9(5):e002942.
66. Kwong Y, Troupis J. Cardiac CT imaging in the context of left atrial appendage occlusion. J Cardiovasc Comput Tomogr. 2015;9(1):13–8.
67. Di Biase L, Santangeli P, Anselmino M, Mohanty P, Salvetti I, Gili S, Horton R, Sanchez JE, Bai R, Mohanty S, Pump A, Cereceda Brantes M, Gallinghouse GJ, Burkhardt JD, Cesarani F, Scaglione M, Natale A, Gaita F. Does the left atrial appendage morphology correlate with the risk of stroke in patients with atrial fibrillation? Results from a multicenter study. J Am Coll Cardiol. 2012;60(6):531–8.
68. Wang Y, Di Biase L, Horton RP, Nguyen T, Morhanty P, Natale A. Left atrial appendage studied by computed tomography to help planning for appendage closure device placement. J Cardiovasc Electrophysiol. 2010;21(9):973–82.

69. Bamberg F, Becker A, Schwarz F, Marcus RP, Greif M, von Ziegler F, Blankstein R, Hoffmann U, Sommer WH, Hoffmann VS, Johnson TR, Becker HC, Wintersperger BJ, Reiser MF, Nikolaou K. Detection of hemodynamically significant coronary artery stenosis: incremental diagnostic value of dynamic CT-based myocardial perfusion imaging. Radiology. 2011;260(3):689–98.
70. Blankstein R, Shturman LD, Rogers IS, Rocha-Filho JA, Okada DR, Sarwar A, Soni AV, Bezerra H, Ghoshhajra BB, Petranovic M, Loureiro R, Feuchtner G, Gewirtz H, Hoffmann U, Mamuya WS, Brady TJ, Cury RC. Adenosine-induced stress myocardial perfusion imaging using dual-source cardiac computed tomography. J Am Coll Cardiol. 2009;54(12):1072–84.
71. Rochitte CE, George RT, Chen MY, Arbab-Zadeh A, Dewey M, Miller JM, Niinuma H, Yoshioka K, Kitagawa K, Nakamori S, Laham R, Vavere AL, Cerci RJ, Mehra VC, Nomura C, Kofoed KF, Jinzaki M, Kuribayashi S, de Roos A, Laule M, Tan SY, Hoe J, Paul N, Rybicki FJ, Brinker JA, Arai AE, Cox C, Clouse ME, Di Carli MF, Lima JA. Computed tomography angiography and perfusion to assess coronary artery stenosis causing perfusion defects by single photon emission computed tomography: the CORE320 study. Eur Heart J. 2014;35(17):1120–30.
72. Mehra VC, Valdiviezo C, Arbab-Zadeh A, Ko BS, Seneviratne SK, Cerci R, Lima JA, George RT. A stepwise approach to the visual interpretation of CT-based myocardial perfusion. J Cardiovasc Comput Tomogr. 2011;5(6):357–69.
73. George RT, Silva C, Cordeiro MA, DiPaula A, Thompson DR, McCarthy WF, Ichihara T, Lima JA, Lardo AC. Multidetector computed tomography myocardial perfusion imaging during adenosine stress. J Am Coll Cardiol. 2006;48(1):153–60.
74. Rossi A, Dharampal A, Wragg A, Davies LC, van Geuns RJ, Anagnostopoulos C, Klotz E, Kitslaar P, Broersen A, Mathur A, Nieman K, Hunink MG, de Feyter PJ, Petersen SE, Pugliese F. Diagnostic performance of hyperaemic myocardial blood flow index obtained by dynamic computed tomography: does it predict functionally significant coronary lesions? Eur Heart J Cardiovasc Imaging. 2014;15(1):85–94.
75. Mahnken AH, Koos R, Katoh M, Wildberger JE, Spuentrup E, Buecker A, Gunther RW, Kuhl HP. Assessment of myocardial viability in reperfused acute myocardial infarction using 16-slice computed tomography in comparison to magnetic resonance imaging. J Am Coll Cardiol. 2005;45(12):2042–7.
76. Boussel L, Ribagnac M, Bonnefoy E, Staat P, Elicker BM, Revel D, Douek P. Assessment of acute myocardial infarction using MDCT after percutaneous coronary intervention: comparison with MRI. AJR Am J Roentgenol. 2008;191(2):441–7.
77. Habis M, Capderou A, Ghostine S, Daoud B, Caussin C, Riou JY, Brenot P, Angel CY, Lancelin B, Paul JF. Acute myocardial infarction early viability assessment by 64-slice computed tomography immediately after coronary angiography: comparison with low-dose dobutamine echocardiography. J Am Coll Cardiol. 2007;49(11):1178–85.
78. Jacquier A, Boussel L, Amabile N, Bartoli JM, Douek P, Moulin G, Paganelli F, Saeed M, Revel D, Croisille P. Multidetector computed tomography in reperfused acute myocardial infarction. Assessment of infarct size and no-reflow in comparison with cardiac magnetic resonance imaging. Investig Radiol. 2008;43(11):773–81.
79. Paul JF, Wartski M, Caussin C, Sigal-Cinqualbre A, Lancelin B, Angel C, Dambrin G. Late defect on delayed contrast-enhanced multi-detector row CT scans in the prediction of SPECT infarct size after reperfused acute myocardial infarction: initial experience. Radiology. 2005;236(2):485–9.
80. Rogers IS, Cury RC, Blankstein R, Shapiro MD, Nieman K, Hoffmann U, Brady TJ, Abbara S. Comparison of postprocessing techniques for the detection of perfusion defects by cardiac computed tomography in patients presenting with acute ST-segment elevation myocardial infarction. J Cardiovasc Comput Tomogr. 2010;4(4):258–66.
81. Han BK, Rigsby CK, Leipsic J, Bardo D, Abbara S, Ghoshhajra B, Lesser JR, Raman SV, Crean AM, Nicol ED, Siegel MJ, Hlavacek A. Computed tomography imaging in patients with congenital heart disease, part 2: technical recommendations. An expert consensus document of the Society of Cardiovascular Computed Tomography (SCCT): endorsed by the Society of Pediatric Radiology (SPR) and the North American Society of Cardiac Imaging (NASCI). J Cardiovasc Comput Tomogr. 2015;9(6):493–513.
82. Han BK, Rigsby CK, Hlavacek A, Leipsic J, Nicol ED, Siegel MJ, Bardo D, Abbara S, Ghoshhajra B, Lesser JR, Raman S, Crean AM. Computed tomography imaging in patients with congenital heart disease part I: rationale and utility. An expert consensus document of the Society of Cardiovascular Computed Tomography (SCCT): endorsed by the Society of Pediatric Radiology (SPR) and the North American Society of Cardiac Imaging (NASCI). J Cardiovasc Comput Tomogr. 2015;9(6):475–92.
83. Bhatt AB, Foster E, Kuehl K, Alpert J, Brabeck S, Crumb S, Davidson WR Jr, Earing MG, Ghoshhajra BB, Karamlou T, Mital S, Ting J, Tseng ZH, American Heart Association Council on Clinical C. Congenital heart disease in the older adult: a scientific statement from the American Heart Association. Circulation. 2015;131(21):1884–931.

Integration of CT Data into Clinical Workflows: Role of Modern IT Infrastructure Including Cloud Technology

17

Paul Schoenhagen and Mathis Zimmermann

Since its introduction to medical imaging in the 1970s [1, 2], CT has developed into a central imaging modality in a wide array of clinical conditions. In cardiovascular medicine, this includes emergent indication (e.g., acute aortic syndromes [AAS], pulmonary embolism [PE]), many elective indications, and novel indications (e.g., structural and valvular heart disease). Its use has increased exponentially, supported by rapid developments of scanner technology and software applications [3, 4].

Initial developments of cardiovascular CT technology were focused on scanner hardware and image generation. A critical step was ECG-synchronized imaging acquisition, which allowed to minimize cardiac motion artifacts. Subsequent, consecutive generations of scanners with increased cranio-caudal coverage and speed of acquisition expanded cardiovascular applications. Initially the acquired series of CT images were printed on film sheets and reviewed on film boxes (Figs. 17.1 and 17.2). This was subsequently replaced by digital review on expensive workstations in "reading rooms" close to the CT scanner. The true potential of CT lies in the ability to combine multiple thin-slice axial images into a 3-D dataset and digital manipulation. This was realized with development of increasingly powerful workstations and software allowing post-processing resulting in unlimited image planes oblique to the acquisition plane (Fig. 17.3). The ability of 3-D reconstruction has been a key element for the modern use of cardiovascular CT. Importantly, complex image reconstruction is performed by several users, including imaging specialist/radiologist and clinical interventionalist/surgeon. Review by these users is typically separated by time and location.

Imaging and image review/reconstruction are increasingly part of a stepwise decision-making process, transforming traditional single-observer reading and reporting to a process involving a team of interdisciplinary clinical specialists. This trend is observed in several subspecialties including oncology (e.g., "tumor board" for cancer treatment planning) and cardiovascular medicine (e.g., "heart team" in the context of transcatheter aortic valve replacement, TAVR). These developments require a new level of data accessibility and performance of imaging systems, including ability to share data beyond the "reading room" in large healthcare systems. It is supported by novel developments of IT architecture, allowing sharing of a centrally stored dataset between multiple peripheral workstations (client-server). Connection of scanners and workstations into a network or "cloud" with integration into the entire electronic health record (EHR) allows exchange of information across healthcare systems and supports multidisciplinary teams working on defined clinical workflows. It has been adopted rapidly for CT imaging. In this chapter we will review these developments and discuss the impact on clinical workflows involving CT imaging.

Computed Tomography: CT Scanner and Review Software/Workstation

The diagnostic use of computed tomography (CT) is based on developments in the field of physics during the 1970s [1, 2]. Since then CT has developed into an established diagnostic modality in cardiovascular medicine. The diagnostic spectrum includes routine indications such as the assessment of aortic, pulmonary, and coronary vascular disease, as well as novel applications, including the evaluation in the context of minimally invasive cardiothoracic surgery and transcatheter interventions.

Initially used electron-beam technology (EBCT) has almost completely been replaced by multi-detector CT (MDCT) systems. In MDCT systems, the gantry (X-ray tube and detector) rotates rapidly around the patient [5, 6].

P. Schoenhagen (✉)
Imaging Institute, Cleveland Clinic, Lerner College of Medicine, Cleveland, OH, USA
e-mail: Schoenp1@ccf.org

M. Zimmermann
Digital Health Services, Siemens Healthineers, Malvern, PA, USA

U. J. Schoepf (ed.), *CT of the Heart*, Contemporary Medical Imaging, https://doi.org/10.1007/978-1-60327-237-7_17

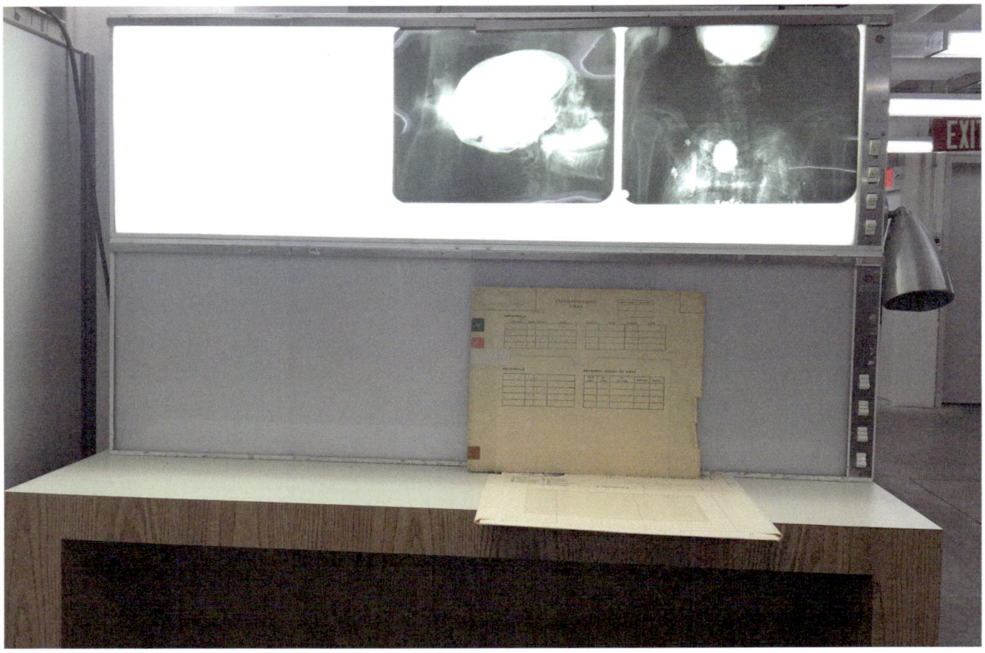

Fig. 17.1 This figure shows an old-fashioned viewing station. The X-ray films show images obtained from an ancient mummy

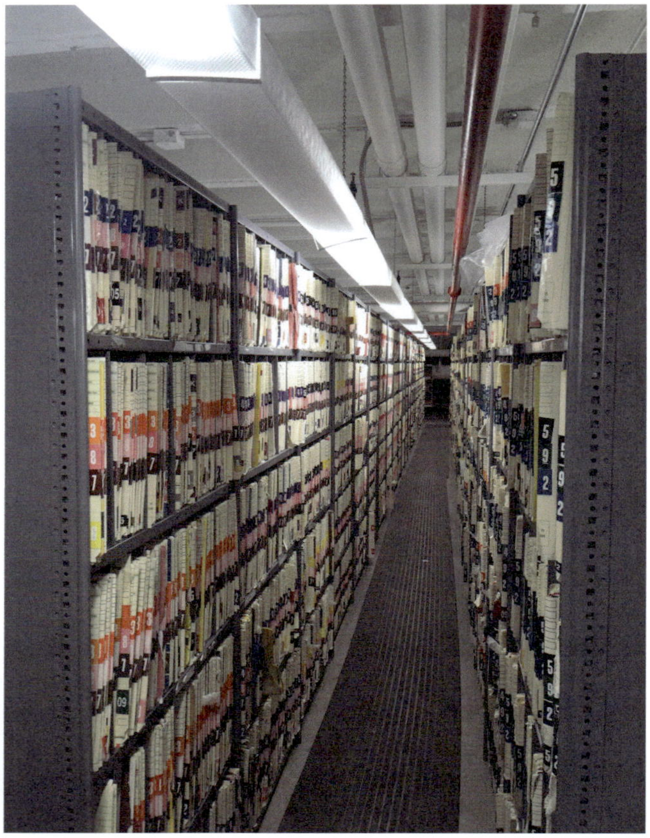

Fig. 17.2 This figure shows a traditional film library where X-ray images are archived and retrieved if necessary

Subsequent generations of multi-slice scanners with 8, 16, 64, 256, and 320 slice acquisition per rotation were introduced in rapid progression over the last two decades [7–10]. Modern systems with fast gantry rotation and thin collimated detector rows with ECG-synchronized acquisition of multiple slices per gantry rotation are optimized for cardiovascular imaging. Dual-source scanners, with two X-ray tubes/ detector systems, allow further reduction in temporal resolution [11, 12]. Today, high-end scanners permit rotation times as low as 250 ms, with resulting temporal resolution of 135 ms (single source) and 66 ms (dual source). Modern systems acquire data with a minimum collimated detector row width of 0.5 mm resulting in isotropic spatial resolution of around 0.5 × 0.5 × 0.5 mm. The acquired raw data is reconstructed at the scanner and then sent to workstations and/or storage systems (PACS).

Early generations of workstations were local systems with powerful local graphics hardware for 3-D reconstruction. The complete data from individual studies was transferred to the workstations as DICOM data, either directly from the scanner or via the PACS system. Because of the high cost of such workstations, only a few would be available, typically in the "reading room" close to the scanner. Sharing of data was limited to a few reconstructed images (printed or saved on CD or sent by e-mail). If a clinician wanted to directly review images, this was only possible in the reading room.

Subsequent generations of local client-server systems combine a central server with local access stations at several locations. In these systems, storage of the complete data and

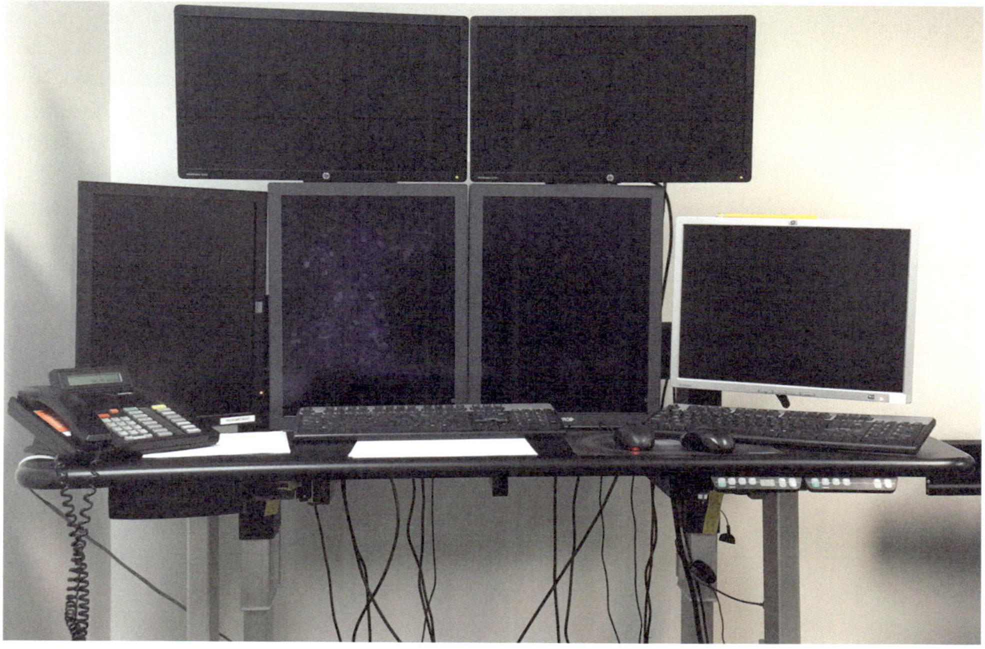

Fig. 17.3 This figure shows a modern workstation with multiple monitors. The workstation is connected to the central data center, where the imaging data is archived and processed

data reconstruction is performed at the central server level ("remote rendering"). The reconstructed images are displayed at the local client workstation, allowing use of less expensive computer systems, such as those used for access of the EHR. The central storage of images in a clinical data center facilitates the creation of a network of connected workstations but requires sufficient bandwidth for enterprise-wide data transfer (Fig. 17.4). This approach protects clinical data because data is maintained within the hospital IT network. It enables shared access to the same imaging study for different clinical groups, e.g., surgeons or referring physicians at multiple locations contributing diagnostic or interventional information.

The most recent approach is the use of "cloud servers." Advantages are use of readily available cheaper cloud storage and almost unlimited processing power. It allows new applications, e.g., retrospective and even prospective (predictive) data analytics, specifically in the context of integration into the EHR. However, it introduces new challenges and requirements, e.g., data security aspects of storing patient health information in the cloud on third-party servers (Fig. 17.5).

Integration of CT/Imaging Data and EHR

The digital availability of data and ability to share as part of the EHR support enhanced integration of imaging data into clinical pathways. Integration of CT data and EHR servers allows to consider the CT data in the context of the clinical pathway of the patient. Enterprise-wide access has the potential to streamline the ordering process (e.g., avoiding unnecessary repeat studies, tracking of cumulative radiation exposure) and allows collaborative reading and reporting. Data transfer of discrete values enables structured reporting and data mining/ analytics for clinical research and administrative purposes.

In large healthcare systems, this requires a complex infrastructure/network spanning across multiple locations. A central data center connects a large number of servers ("server farm"), with integration between EHR, PACS systems, and additional 3-D/4-D analysis tools (Figs. 17.4 and 17.5). The core storage provides access to all data generated in the healthcare system, which can be visualized in a patient-centric fashion through the electronic health record (EHR), PACS, or more dedicated systems. These systems already are a form of cloud computing, described as a "private medical-grade cloud." Hospital systems may be able to maintain a "private cloud" or alternatively use third-party data service, but issues of reliable patient identification and data security need to be clarified. While technically complex, the benefit of "online" sharing of data files between professionals at multiple locations within a treatment network appears to be obvious [13, 14].

"Smart" computer systems are not limited to data storage but also contribute to its collection and analysis. Examples are computer-aided detection (CAD) systems in diagnostic imaging/radiology and automatic data analysis. A recent

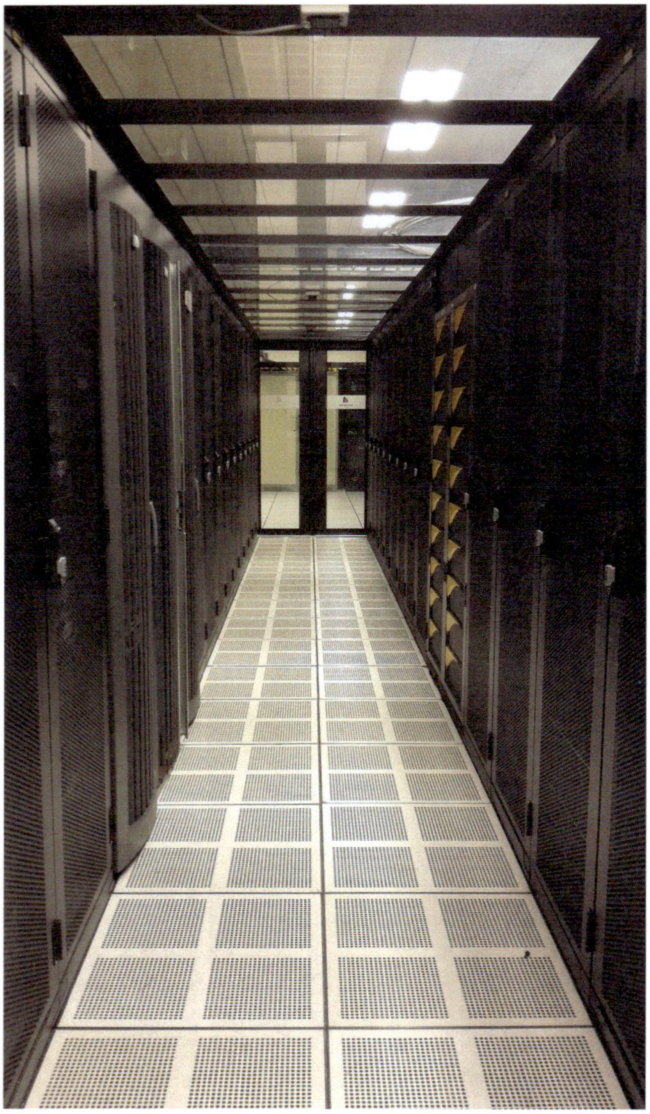

Fig. 17.4 This figure shows a server farm in a data center

paper examined the usefulness of CAD for the diagnosis of lung nodules on CT scans [15]. CAD systems detected lung cancers that were initially missed by a radiologist but failed to detect other lung lesions identified by the radiologist, suggesting a complementary role of CAD systems. Automatic analysis ("data mining") of large datasets can be performed with minimal human input. This process is called "machine learning" (ML) and is used for various applications including weather forecasting or recommending items of interest to consumers while using online search engines [16–18]. Machine learning uses algorithms to identify expected and unexpected patterns and can consider a greater number and complexity of variables than traditional methods of predictive analysis. ML techniques are increasingly applied to large amounts of imaging and other discrete data in healthcare in order to build predictive models, both for individual patients and larger populations [19–21].

While these approaches are exciting, it is important to consider potential limitations. The tremendous amount and complexity of patient-related data accumulating in large healthcare institutions require advanced software and hardware and a dedicated group of IT professionals for maintenance [22]. Data has to be available 24/7, and there are mandated requirements for long-term data storage. A particular challenge is unequivocal patient identification, in particular if data is to be shared across large healthcare systems and with other institutions. Complex issues related to data security and ownership (hospital system or patient) have to be addressed. Because of the complexity and associated cost of maintaining such "data clouds", healthcare systems may consider external providers for data management, further complicating oversight and regulation (Fig. 17.5).

Impact on Clinical Management

The potential clinical value of systems combining imaging data and the EHR can be studied using clinical scenarios, where CT imaging is central, e.g., transcatheter aortic valve replacement (TAVR) and acute aortic syndromes (AAS).

In the case of AAS, regional treatment networks have been established, which coordinate diagnosis, triage, and treatment between local emergency rooms as the initial point of contact, and central specialized centers, experienced in definitive pharmacological, interventional, or surgical treatment [23–27]. In contrast to acute myocardial infarction (MI), AAS lacks simple diagnostic biomarkers. Triage of patients with suspected AAS requires definitive imaging. Computed tomography is typically performed and interpreted at the initial point of access in the local ED, where subspecialized expertise is often lacking. As such, false-positive transfer activation is not uncommon, especially in the setting of complex prior endovascular repair [28–30]. The large image data files have traditionally been transferred with the patient either in film or CD format. At the tertiary referral center, the images were then downloaded and subsequently reinterpreted to form the basis for definitive treatment. The availability of imaging data within a shared EHR would allow proactive triage prior or during patient transfer by specialists available within the network at different locations [31, 32]. Modern IT network structures and specifically "cloud" technology allow upload of data from multiple sites onto central "cloud servers" and subsequent access and review from anywhere within network [13, 14]. Mobile online access to the central electronic health record including imaging and

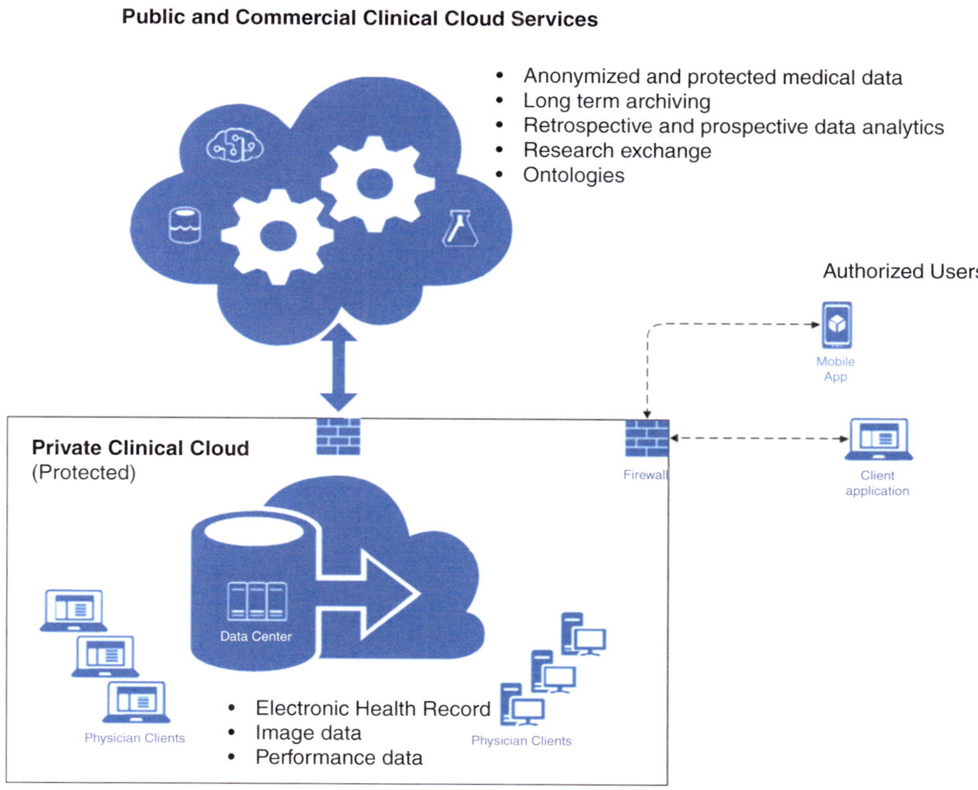

Fig. 17.5 Schematic state-of-the-art cloud services in context of reading and reporting

non-imaging data from tablet computers and smartphones allows review without limitations to place and time and enables surveillance and online communication within a network of specialists [33].

The process of CT image acquisition and analysis in the context of TAVR has evolved and is increasingly standardized [34–37]. After initial general review including noncardiac structures, the cardiovascular analysis is focused on the access site/route and aortic root deployment zone. The peripheral access arteries (iliac and axillary arteries) are evaluated for luminal size, calcified and non-calcified atherosclerotic plaque of the vessel wall, and vessel tortuosity [38–43]. Because TAVR stent/valve prostheses are available in limited size ranges, precise measurement of the aortic annulus is critical. Specifically, the annulus is measured as the plane at the lowest insertion point of the aortic valve leaflets and minimal/maximal diameter, circumference, and area are described. In addition, the spatial relation of the coronary ostia to the annulus and the angiographic plane orthogonal to the valve plane is defined to ensure optimal positioning/alignment of the prosthesis with the vessel axis. The analysis process is best organized into a multistep workflow, which involves manual or semiautomated aortic root segmentation, centerline reconstruction of the aorta and iliac arteries, and additional 4-D functional analysis of ventricular and valvular function. While manual analysis with standard, basic 3-D software is possible, it is time-intensive and operator-dependent. Increasingly, semiautomated software systems pre-analyze the data, providing the evaluating physician with a structured template for final analysis and documentation/reporting [44, 45].

In most clinical centers, selection of patients suitable for the TAVR procedure involves an interdisciplinary team of physicians, including cardiologists, cardiothoracic surgeons, and imaging specialists/radiologists. After an initial clinical appointment, subsequent testing including imaging is performed. The imaging specialist analyzes the data and prepares a report including saved key images and presentation states. The interventional cardiologist and surgeon review the accumulated data, which is used for decision-making and planning of the procedure. All these single steps do not necessarily happen at the same place and time, they may be performed independently at different places in the hospital at different time points. Therefore, organization of the huge amount of accumulated data in a centralized archive and customized reading software models optimized for the workflow of individual groups of clinicians support the clinical pathway.

The examples of TAVR and AAS demonstrate the impact of an integrated EHR including imaging data on clinical workflows in acute and elective clinical scenarios involving CT imaging. Other clinical examples including those involving other imaging modalities, e.g., echocardiography or MRI, can be readily identified [46, 47].

Conclusion

Following hard- and software development to optimize image acquisition and analysis of individual scanner/workstation systems, recent and future developments increasingly create networks of systems integrated into the EHR. These "cloud" systems are transforming clinical workflows, exemplified by the examples of acute aortic syndromes (AAS) and transcatheter aortic valve replacement (TAVR), where CT imaging has a central role. However, experience is limited, and further evaluation of the appropriate infrastructure including requirement for reliable patient identification between provider organizations and data safety is critical. Further the potential clinical impact needs to be evaluated in clinical trials. The widespread use of CT and its standardized data structure makes CT a perfect example, but other imaging modalities including echocardiography and MRI are also evaluated extensively.

References

1. Ambrose J, Hounsfield G. Computerized transverse axial tomography. Br J Radiol. 1973;46:148–9.
2. Hounsfield GN. Computed medical imaging. Science. 1980;210:22–8.
3. Mettler FA Jr, Bhargavan M, Faulkner K, Gilley DB, Gray JE, Ibbott GS, Lipoti JA, Mahesh M, McCrohan JL, Stabin MG, Thomadsen BR, Yoshizumi TT. Radiologic and nuclear medicine studies in the United States and worldwide: frequency, radiation dose, and comparison with other radiation sources – 1950-2007. Radiology. 2009;253:520–31.
4. Brenner DJ, Hall EJ. Computed tomography – an increasing source of radiation exposure. N Engl J Med. 2007;357:2277–84.
5. Kalendar WA, Seissler W, Klotz E, Vock P. Spiral volumetric CT with single-breath-hold technique, continuous transport, and continuous scanner rotation. Radiology. 1990;176:181–3.
6. Klingenbeck-Regn K, Schaller S, Flohr T, Ohnesorge B, Kopp A, Baum U. Subsecond multi-slice computed tomography: basics and applications. Eur J Radiol. 1999;31:110–24.
7. Nieman K, Cademartiri F, Lemos PA, Raaijmakers R, Pattynama PMT, de Feyter PJ. Reliable noninvasive coronary angiography with fast submillimeter multislice spiral computed tomography. Circulation. 2002;106:2051–4.
8. Chao SP, Law WY, Kuo CJ, Hung HF, Cheng JJ, Lo HM, Shyu KG. The diagnostic accuracy of 256-row computed tomographic angiography compared with invasive coronary angiography in patients with suspected coronary artery disease. Eur Heart J. 2010;31:1916–23.
9. Einstein AJ, Elliston CD, Arai AE, Chen MY, Mather R, Pearson GD, Delapaz RL, Nickoloff E, Dutta A, Brenner DJ. Radiation dose from single-heartbeat coronary CT angiography performed with a 320-detector row volume scanner. Radiology. 2010;254:698–706.
10. George RT, Arbab-Zadeh A, Miller JM, Vavere AL, Bengel FM, Lardo AC, Lima JA. Computed tomography myocardial perfusion imaging with 320-row detector computed tomography accurately detects myocardial ischemia in patients with obstructive coronary artery disease. Circ Cardiovasc Imaging. 2012;5:333–40.
11. Flohr TG, CH MC, Bruder H, Petersilka M, Gruber K, Suss C, Grasruck M, Stierstorfer K, Krauss B, Raupach R, Primak AN, Kuttner A, Achenbach S, Becker C, Kopp A, Ohnesorge BM. First performance evaluation of a dual-source CT (DSCT) system. Eur Radiol. 2006;16:256–68.
12. Achenbach S, Ropers D, Kuettner A, Flohr T, Ohnesorge B, Bruder H, Theessen H, Karakaya M, Daniel WG, Bautz W, Kalender WA, Anders K. Contrast-enhanced coronary artery visualization by dual-source computed tomography – initial experience. Eur J Radiol. 2006;57:331–5.
13. Schoenhagen P, Zimmermann M, Falkner J. Advanced 3-D analysis, client-server systems, and cloud computing-Integration of cardiovascular imaging data into clinical workflows of transcatheter aortic valve replacement. Cardiovasc Diagn Ther. 2013;3:80–92.
14. Schoenhagen P, Falkner J, Piraino D. Transcatheter aortic valve repair, imaging, and electronic imaging health record. Curr Cardiol Rep. 2013;15:319.
15. Liang M, Tang W, Xu DM, Jirapatnakul AC, Reeves AP, Henschke CI, Yankelevitz D. Low-dose CT screening for lung cancer: computer-aided detection of missed lung cancers. Radiology. 2016;281:279–88.
16. Waljee AK, Higgins PDR. Machine learning in medicine: a primer for physicians. Am J Gastroenterol. 2010;105:1224–6.
17. Deo RC. Machine learning in medicine. Circulation. 2015;132:1920–30.
18. Dietterich TG. Ensemble methods in machine learning. Lect Notes Comput Sci. 2000;1857:1–15.
19. Waljee AK, Joyce JC, Wang S, Saxena A, Hart M, Zhu J, Higgins PD. Algorithms outperform metabolite tests in predicting response of patients with inflammatory bowel disease to thiopurines. Clin Gastroenterol Hepatol. 2010;8:143–50.
20. Singal AG, Mukherjee A, Elmunzer BJ, Higgins PD, Lok AS, Zhu J, Marrero JA, Waljee AK. Machine learning algorithms outperform conventional regression models in identifying risk factors for hepatocellular carcinoma in patients with cirrhosis. Am J Gastroenterol. 2013;108:1723–30.
21. Motwani M, Dey D, Berman DS, Germano G, Achenbach S, Al-Mallah M. Machine learning for prediction of all-cause mortality in patient with suspected coronary artery disease: a 5-year multicenter prospective registry analysis. Eur Heart J. 2017;38(7):500–7.
22. Drowning in big data? Reducing information technology complexities and costs for healthcare organizations. http://www.emc.com/collateral/analyst-reports/frost-sullivan-reducing-information-technology-complexities-ar.pdf.
23. Boyd DR, Dunea MM, Flashner BA. The Illinois plan for a statewide system of trauma centers. J Trauma. 1973;13:24–31.
24. Cowley RA, Hudson F, Scanlan E, Gill W, Lally RJ, Long W, et al. An economical and proved helicopter program for transporting the emergency critically ill and injured patient in Maryland. J Trauma. 1973;13:1029–38.
25. Harris KM, Strauss CE, Duval S, Unger BT, Kroshus TJ, Inampudi S, et al. Multidisciplinary standardized care for acute aortic dissection: design and initial outcomes of a regional care model. Circ Cardiovasc Qual Outcomes. 2010;3:424–30.
26. Henry TD, Sharkey SW, Burke MN, Chavez IJ, Graham KJ, Henry CR, et al. A regional system to provide timely access to percutaneous coronary intervention for ST-elevation myocardial infarction. Circulation. 2007;116:721–8.
27. Jollis JG, Roettig ML, Aluko AO, Anstrom KJ, Applegate RJ, Babb JD, et al., Reperfusion of Acute Myocardial Infarction in North Carolina Emergency Departments (RACE) Investigators. Implementation of a statewide system for coronary reperfusion for ST-segment elevation myocardial infarction. JAMA. 2007;298:2371–80.
28. Aggarwal B, Raymond CE, Randhawa MS, Roselli E, Jacob J, Eagleton M, Kralovic DM, Kormos K, Holloway D, Menon

V. Transfer metrics in patients with suspected acute aortic syndrome. Circ Cardiovasc Qual Outcomes. 2014;7:780–2.
29. Raymond CE, Aggarwal B, Schoenhagen P, Kralovic DM, Kormos K, Holloway D, Menon V. Prevalence and factors associated with false positive suspicion of acute aortic syndrome: experience in a patient population transferred to a specialized aortic treatment center. Cardiovasc Diagn Ther. 2013;3:196–204.
30. Aggarwal B, Raymond C, Jacob J, Kralovic D, Kormos K, Holloway D, Menon V. Transfer of patients with suspected acute aortic syndrome. Am J Cardiol. 2013;112:430–5.
31. Schoenhagen P, Mehta N. Big data, smart computer systems, and doctor-patient relationship. Eur Heart J. 2017;38(7):508–10.
32. Cowie MR, Chronaki CE, Vardas P. E-health innovation: time for engagement with the cardiology community. Eur Heart J. 2013;34:1864–8.
33. Matar R, Renapurkar R, Obuchowski N, Menon V, Piraino D, Schoenhagen P. Utility of hand-held devices in diagnosis and triage of cardiovascular emergencies. Observations during implementation of a PACS-based system in an acute aortic syndrome (AAS) network. J Cardiovasc Comput Tomogr. 2015;9:524–33.
34. Leon MB, Piazza N, Nikolsky E, et al. Standardized endpoint definitions for transcatheter aortic valve implantation clinical trials: a consensus report from the valve academic research consortium. Eur Heart J. 2011;32:205–17.
35. Vahanian A, Alfieri OR, Al-Attar N, et al. Transcatheter valve implantation for patients with aortic stenosis: a position statement from the European Association of Cardio-Thoracic Surgery (EACTS) and the European Society of Cardiology (ESC), in collaboration with the European Association of Percutaneous Cardiovascular Interventions (EAPCI). Eur J Cardiothorac Surg. 2008;34:1–8.
36. Achenbach S, Delgado V, Hausleiter J, et al. SCCT expert consensus document on computed tomography imaging before transcatheter aortic valve implantation (TAVI)/transcatheter aortic valve replacement (TAVR). J Cardiovasc Comput Tomogr. 2012;6:366–80.
37. Schoenhagen P, Hausleiter J, Achenbach S, et al. Computed tomography in the evaluation for transcatheter aortic valve implantation (TAVI). Cardiovasc Diagn Ther. 2011;1:44–56.
38. Kurra V, Kapadia SR, Tuzcu EM, et al. Pre-procedural imaging of aortic root orientation and dimensions comparison between X-ray angiographic planar imaging and 3-dimensional multidetector row computed tomography. JACC Cardiovasc Interv. 2010;3:105–13.
39. Gurvitch R, Wood DA, Leipsic J, et al. Multislice computed tomography for prediction of optimal angiographic deployment projections during transcatheter aortic valve implantation. JACC Cardiovasc Interv. 2010;3:1157–65.
40. da Gama RV, Vouga L, Markowitz A, et al. Vascular access in transcatheter aortic valve implantation. Int J Cardiovasc Imaging. 2011;27:1235–43.
41. Petronio AS, De Carlo M, Bedogni F, et al. Safety and efficacy of the subclavian approach for transcatheter aortic valve implantation with the CoreValve revalving system. Circ Cardiovasc Interv. 2010;3:359–66.
42. Svensson LG, Dewey T, Kapadia S, et al. United States feasibility study of transcatheter insertion of a stented aortic valve by the left ventricular apex. Ann Thorac Surg. 2008;86:46–54; discussion 54–5.
43. Walther T, Simon P, Dewey T, et al. Transapical minimally invasive aortic valve implantation: multicenter experience. Circulation. 2007;116:I240–5.
44. Schoenhagen P, Tuzcu EM, Kapadia SR, Desai MY, Svensson LG. Three-dimensional imaging of the aortic valve and aortic root with computed tomography: new standards in an era of transcatheter valve repair/implantation. Eur Heart J. 2009;30:2079–86.
45. Schoenhagen P, Numburi U, Halliburton SS, Aulbach P, von Roden M, Desai MY, Rodriguez LL, Kapadia SR, Tuzcu EM, Lytle BW. Three-dimensional imaging in the context of minimally invasive and transcatheter cardiovascular interventions using multidetector computed tomography: from pre-operative planning to intra-operative guidance. Eur Heart J. 2010;31:2727–40.
46. Cavalcante JL, Lalude OO, Schoenhagen P, Lerakis S. Cardiovascular magnetic resonance imaging for structural and valvular heart disease interventions. JACC Cardiovasc Interv. 2016;9(5):399–425.
47. Natarajan N, Patel P, Bartel T, Kapadia S, Navia J, Stewart W, Tuzcu EM, Schoenhagen P. Peri-procedural imaging for transcatheter mitral valve replacement. Cardiovasc Diagn Ther. 2016;6(2):144–59.

Thoughts on Coding and Reimbursement

18

Adefolakemi Babatunde and Pamela K. Woodard

Accurate Current Procedural Terminology (CPT) [1] and International Classification of Diseases (ICD) coding [2] along with documentation within the report are critical parts of the reporting and billing processes. Errors in coding ultimately lead to denial of claims from Medicaid and Medicare and insurance payers. CPT codes provide third-party payers with information about the procedure that was performed, while ICD codes provide them with the indication for the procedure.

In reporting cardiac computed tomography (CT) examinations, as with any imaging study, the report should clearly document the examination performed and the volume of contrast, and the title of the study performed in the report should match the CPT code. In addition, information on any 3D processing that was performed on a dedicated workstation (apart from standard 3D reconstructions at the scanner) should be reported. Documenting processing performed is important in reporting cardiac CT scans as the processing component of the examination is included within the CPT code description. It is important to note that no additional 3D processing code should be added to the cardiac CT codes. Other information important to include is the indication for the examination, for the purposes of ICD-10 coding.

It is also important to note whether or not the insurance provider requires precertification or preauthorization for the study. For cardiac CT studies, most insurance providers do require preauthorization. Ensuring that the referring physician's office has obtained insurance company preauthorization prior to the examination and not afterwards significantly increases the likelihood of reimbursement for the procedure.

A. Babatunde
Cardiovascular Division, Department of Medicine, Washington University School of Medicine, St. Louis, MO, USA

P. K. Woodard (✉)
Mallinckrodt Institute of Radiology, Washington University School of Medicine, St. Louis, MO, USA
e-mail: woodardp@wustl.edu

CPT Codes

In late 2009 four cardiac CPT codes were released by the American Medical Association (AMA) as category I codes to be used for all cardiac CT billing purposes. CPT codes are standardized codes published by the AMA for medical procedures [1]. There are four CPT codes for cardiac CT:

- 75571: computed tomography, heart, without contrast material, with quantitative evaluation of coronary calcium
- 75572: computed tomography, heart, with contrast material, for evaluation of cardiac structure and morphology (this includes 3D image post-processing, assessment of cardiac function, and evaluation of venous structures, if performed)
- 75573: computed tomography, heart, with contrast material, for evaluation of cardiac structure and morphology in the setting of congenital heart disease (this includes 3D image post-processing, assessment of LV cardiac function, RV structure and function and evaluation of venous structures, if performed)
- 75574: computed tomographic angiography, heart, coronary arteries, and bypass grafts (when present), with contrast material, including 3D image post-processing (including evaluation of cardiac structure and morphology, assessment of cardiac function, and evaluation of venous structures, if performed) [1]

These codes are used with ICD-9 codes for indications for scan use.

Indications for Calcium Scoring

The coronary artery calcium (CAC) scan is a non-contrast prospectively gated cardiac CT scan used to define coronary calcium in the epicardial coronary arteries. Its indications are coronary artery disease screening and further patient risk

U. J. Schoepf (ed.), *CT of the Heart*, Contemporary Medical Imaging, https://doi.org/10.1007/978-1-60327-237-7_18

stratification in asymptomatic patients of intermediate risk [3]. It is rarely if ever appropriate for asymptomatic patients with low global risk for CAD and for symptomatic patients. The code 75571 should be billed alone and should not be billed with either codes 75572 or 75574.

The first coronary calcium score was developed by Arthur Agatston and is defined as the product of calcified plaque area and weighted density score given to the highest attenuation value (HU) in the area of calcium [4]. The threshold for selection of calcium for Agatston scoring is any coronary calcium that is greater than 130 Hounsfield units (HU) [4].

Calcium score ranges from 0 for absence of calcium, 1–10 for minimal plaque, 11–100 for mild plaque, 101–400 for moderate plaque, and >400 for severe plaque [5]. The calcium volume score, defined as volume of calcium greater than 130 HU in the epicardial coronary system, may also be reported and is thought to be more reproducible than the Agatston score and thus a better indicator to be followed in patients to determine disease progression [6].

CAC score is currently a class of recommendation (COR) IIb with the principal indication for CAC scoring further risk stratification of individuals that are at intermediate risk after formal risk assessment [2].

The CAC scan (CPT code 75571), as a screening tool, initially was not covered by either the Center for Medicaid and Medicare Services (CMS) or private insurance companies, and most patients who underwent the examination paid out of pocket. Currently some CMS carriers and insurance companies cover the cost of this examination.

Indications for Coronary CTA

Indications for coronary CT angiography include both acute and chronic angina as well as newly diagnosed heart failure in order to determine whether the etiology is ischemic or nonischemic. It is important to note that coronary CT angiography is not a screening examination. The CPT code 75574, at present, is used whether or not the study is performed alone as a dedicated coronary CT angiogram, or with a stress agent such as adenosine or regadenoson for perfusion, and whether or not the CT data is sent for fractional flow reserve (FFR) calculation. The single code of 75574 should also be billed if the study is performed with calcium scoring (the code 75571 should not also be billed). The code 75574 should also be billed alone in the performance of a "triple rule-out" for coronary CTA, aortic dissection, and pulmonary embolism assessment, although the entirety of the chest is covered. If billing for coronary CTA rest/stress perfusion, the 75574 code should be billed only once (*not* twice – once for coronary assessment/rest and once for stress). It is possible, depending upon the insurance company, to bill for the stress supervision component of a CT perfusion examination and the adenosine and/or regadenoson stress agent separately using a J code. The dose of stress agent, along with the dose of iodinated contrast agent, should be reported.

Acute Chest Pain

Because of its high negative predictive value, use of coronary CT angiography (CTA) (CPT code 75574) has shown to be useful in the emergency department. Several studies have supported the early use of cardiac CT in the emergency department in patients that present with acute chest pain concerning for acute coronary syndrome [7–9]. The Rule Out Myocardial Infarction using Computer-Assisted Tomography (ROMICAT) trial was an observational cohort study of patients with chest pain that demonstrated low-to-intermediate risk patients with a negative CCTA were unlikely to be diagnosed with ACS [9]. These findings resulted in a follow-up trial, ROMICAT II, which randomized patients who presented with symptoms of ACS to the emergency department to either early coronary CTA or standard of care. This study further supported the use of early coronary CTA in chest pain evaluation. Early coronary CTA led to decreased length of stay with no missed ACS events [7]. Also supporting the use of coronary CTA in the emergency department for early acute chest pain triage in low-to-intermediate risk patients is the ACRIN 4005 trial (CT Angiography for Safe Discharge of Patients with Possible Acute Coronary Syndromes) [8]. This study was a similar study of patients presenting to the emergency department with possible ACS but with the primary end point of safety. In ACRIN 4005, there was a higher rate of detection of CAD than in ROMICAT II; however, the high negative predictive value of CCTA still allowed patients to be safely discharged from the ED [8].

Chronic Stable Chest Pain

While there is less evidence for use of coronary CT angiography in patients with chronic stable angina, there are studies that suggest its utility [10].

The Prospective Multicenter Imaging Study for Evaluation of Chest Pain (PROMISE) trial evaluated ambulatory patients with stable chest pain using coronary CTA compared to functional testing. Patients who received coronary CTA had a better correlation with cardiac catheterization results. Coronary CTA again demonstrated excellent negative predictive value and, unlike functional testing, led to fewer invasive coronary angiograms (ICAs) that showed no obstructive CAD. This led to the finding of less radiation exposure with coronary CTA, if the comparative functional testing included radiation because there would be an elimination of many unnecessary cardiac catheterizations. Coronary CTA has the advantage over other functional testing, in that it provides anatomy. Although coronary CTA does not change clinical outcomes, it appears to reduce the number of unnecessary invasive studies [10].

In addition, investigators in the Randomized Evaluation of patients with Stable angina Comparing Utilization of non-invasive Examinations (RESCUE) trial sought to use coronary CTA to specifically determine which patients had left main disease and which did not, directing patients without left main disease to optimal medical therapy (OMT) alone and those with left main disease to OMT plus ICA and intervention [11]. This trial design was based on the results of the Clinical Outcomes Utilizing Revascularization and Aggressive Drug Evaluation (COURAGE) trial which showed that in stable coronary artery disease percutaneous coronary intervention does not reduce the risk of death, MI, or other major cardiovascular events when compared to OMT [12]. Whether CCTA will ultimately be used to triage patients to ICA and intervention, or OMT alone, will depend upon the results of larger CCTA trials designed in the manner of the COURAGE and RESCUE trials.

Other Indications

Coronary CTA is appropriate for assessing newly diagnosed systolic heart failure in determining whether its etiology is ischemic or nonischemic and may be appropriate in newly diagnosed diastolic heart failure and syncope with intermediate for high global CAD risk. Coronary CTA can be used in patients with arrhythmia, especially in diagnosing the etiology of sustained ventricular tachycardia (VT), ventricular fibrillation, exercised induced VT, or nonsustained VT, and prior to initiation of anti-arrhythmia therapy in high global CAD risk patients [3].

Coronary CTA can be used as follow-up imaging procedure to further assess a prior abnormal test or uncertain prior results. This might include abnormal imaging studies such as an abnormal echocardiogram or nuclear medicine stress test but may also be used to further assess abnormal rest ECG findings in patients with low, intermediate, or high global CAD risk. Lastly, coronary CTA may be appropriate for assessing symptomatic patients post revascularization. Coronary CTA is rarely appropriate for follow-up testing in asymptomatic patients [3].

Indications for Anatomic Assessment

The code 75572 should be used for routine anatomic assessment, such as in pulmonary vein anatomy assessment for radiofrequency (RF) ablation, whereas 75573 should be used in patients being assessed for congenital heart disease.

Pulmonary Vein Assessment Pre-RF Ablation

Atrial fibrillation is the most common arrhythmia and is associated with significant morbidity. Prevalence increases with age. In the United States, an estimated 5% of patients over the age of 65 are affected by atrial fibrillation [13]. One important mechanism described in the initiation and maintenance of atrial fibrillation is the rapidly discharging triggers that arise in the smooth muscle of the pulmonary veins. Electrophysiologists try to isolate the pulmonary veins to prevent propagation of the rapid discharge from the musculature lining the pulmonary veins to the endocardium [14]. An indication for cardiac CT is the mapping of pulmonary vein anatomy prior to pulmonary vein isolation during atrial fibrillation RF ablation as it can be time consuming when done with traditional angiography. In addition to mapping, cardiac CT can be used to assess for the presence of pulmonary stenosis as a complication of RF ablation [15].

Assessment of Prosthetic Valves

The two main types of prosthetic heart valves (PHVs) are biologic and mechanical. Biological valves have the advantage of not requiring anticoagulation but over time deteriorate. Multiple imaging modalities exist to monitor the integrity of PHVs. ACC/AHA guidelines recommend TTE for the initial evaluation of bioprosthetic valve hemodynamics and then an annual TTE after the first 10 years, even in the absence of a change in clinical status [16].

Mechanical PHV dysfunction is rare but should be suspected if there is a change in a patient's clinical status. The estimated prevalence of mechanical valve dysfunction is 0.01%–6% [17–20]. Because there are limitations in anatomical visualization with TTE, cardiac CT provides an attractive alternative as it is quick and can allow for multiple cardiac phase reconstruction to assess for valve leaflet mobility. Mechanical valves have reference guides that describe opening and closing angles and the interpreting physician can consult these to determine if there is a change in the opening or closing leaflet angle. Moreover, contrast-enhanced cardiac CT can help to diagnose pannus formation, thrombus, paravalvular leak, endocarditis, or mycotic aneurysm [21–23] as well as provide information about adjacent structures including coronary arteries, distance from the sternum, and involvement of the aorta, all of which may be important for surgical planning [24].

Congenital Heart Disease

CT can play a role in the assessment of congenital heart disease. When used for this purpose, cardiac CT has its own CPT code, 75563. This study can be performed with prospective gating to define anatomy or retrospective gating in order to diagnose functionality (ventricular function and valve mobility), realizing retrospective gating techniques will provide the patient with greater radiation dose exposure. Regardless of the gating technique, the same CPT code is used.

Some centers provide 3D printing services as part of pre-surgical planning for congenital heart patients. At present there is no code to cover the added costs associated with 3D printing.

Transcatheter Aortic Valve Replacement: A New Indication

Aortic stenosis leads to progressive left ventricular outflow obstruction. Symptoms include angina, dyspnea, syncope, and heart failure. Transcatheter aortic valve replacement (TAVR) is an alternative to surgical aortic valve replacement for patients with severe aortic stenosis and high surgical risk because of age and comorbidities. Significant pre-procedural planning must occur, and computed tomographic angiography is becoming a more central piece in planning. Information is needed regarding aortic root anatomy, aortic valve annulus (measured in systole), coronary arteries, deployment angle, abdominal aorta and iliofemoral artery diameters, tortuosity, and extent of calcification [25, 26]. Patient eligibility for TAVR depends upon annular size, location of coronary arteries, and peripheral access. Precise and accurate deployment of the valve is crucial for safety [25]. If the valve is too low, there is increased risk of heart block, paravalvular regurgitation, and mitral valve regurgitation. If deployment is too high, risks of valve embolization, aortic root injury, and paravalvular regurgitation are increased. CT when used with 2D echo reduces paravalvular regurgitation, as more information can be gathered regarding aortic annulus size, geometry, and anatomy. Specific protocols have been designed for TAVR assessment. Heart rate is marginally less important in data acquisition for TAVR and beta blockers can be detrimental in severe AS given the risk of low cardiac output in these patients with a fixed left ventricular outflow tract obstruction [26]. The cardiac CT CPT code usually used for this purpose is 75572 rather than 75574 since the goal of this study is not coronary atherosclerosis assessment but rather anatomic evaluation. An additional CPT code of 74174 is required when this study is performed along with CTA of the abdomen and pelvis for aorta and iliofemoral artery assessment.

Summary

In short, following the above rules when coding for cardiac CT examinations will increase accuracy in coding and increase likelihood of reimbursement.

References

1. American Medical Association Current Procedural Technology Professional Edition; 2013.
2. International Classification of Diseases (ICD), 11th Revision (ICD-11) [Cited 2018 October 30]. Available from: http://www.who.int/classifications/icd/en/
3. Wolk MJ, Bailey SR, Doherty JU, Douglas PS, Hendel RC, Kramer CM, et al. ACCF/AHA/ASE/ASNC/HFSA/HRS/SCAI/SCCT/SCMR/STS 2013 multimodality appropriate use criteria for the detection and risk assessment of stable ischemic heart disease: a report of the American College of Cardiology Foundation Appropriate Use Criteria Task Force, American Heart Association, American Society of Echocardiography, American Society of Nuclear Cardiology, Heart Failure Society of America, Heart Rhythm Society, Society for Cardiovascular Angiography and Interventions, Society of Cardiovascular Computed Tomography, Society for Cardiovascular Magnetic Resonance, and Society of Thoracic Surgeons. J Am Coll Cardiol. 2014;63(4):380–406.
4. Agatston AS, Janowitz WR, Hildner FJ, Zusmer NR, Viamonte M Jr, Detrano R. Quantification of coronary artery calcium using ultrafast computed tomography. J Am Coll Cardiol. 1990;15(4):827–32.
5. Hecht HS. Coronary artery calcium scanning: past, present, and future. J Am Coll Cardiol Img. 2015;8(5):579–96.
6. Kopp AF, Ohnesorge B, Becker C, Schroder S, Heuschmid M, Kuttner A, et al. Reproducibility and accuracy of coronary calcium measurements with multi-detector row versus electron-beam CT. Radiology. 2002;225(1):113–9.
7. Hoffmann U, Truong QA, Schoenfeld DA, Chou ET, Woodard PK, Nagurney JT, et al. Coronary CT angiography versus standard evaluation in acute chest pain. N Engl J Med. 2012;367(4):299–308.
8. Litt HI, Gatsonis C, Snyder B, Singh H, Miller CD, Entrikin DW, et al. CT angiography for safe discharge of patients with possible acute coronary syndromes. N Engl J Med. 2012;366(15):1393–403.
9. Hoffmann U, Bamberg F, Chae CU, Nichols JH, Rogers IS, Seneviratne SK, et al. Coronary computed tomography angiography for early triage of patients with acute chest pain: the ROMICAT (Rule Out Myocardial Infarction using Computer Assisted Tomography) trial. J Am Coll Cardiol. 2009;53(18):1642–50.
10. Douglas PS, Hoffmann U, Patel MR, Mark DB, Al-Khalidi HR, Cavanaugh B, et al. Outcomes of anatomical versus functional testing for coronary artery disease. N Engl J Med. 2015;372(14):1291–300.
11. Stillman AE, Gatsonis C, Lima JA, Black WC, Cormack J, Gareen I, et al. Rationale and design of the Randomized Evaluation of patients with Stable angina Comparing Utilization of noninvasive Examinations (RESCUE) trial. Am Heart J. 2016;179:19–28.
12. Boden WE, O'Rourke RA, Teo KK, Hartigan PM, Maron DJ, Kostuk WJ, et al. Optimal medical therapy with or without PCI for stable coronary disease. N Engl J Med. 2007;356(15):1503–16.
13. Sellers MB, Newby LK. Atrial fibrillation, anticoagulation, fall risk, and outcomes in elderly patients. Am Heart J. 2011;161(2):241–6.
14. Friedman PA, Asirvatham SJ, Grice S, Glikson M, Munger TM, Rea RF, et al. Noncontact mapping to guide ablation of right ventricular outflow tract tachycardia. J Am Coll Cardiol. 2002;39(11):1808–12.
15. Cronin P, Sneider MB, Kazerooni EA, Kelly AM, Scharf C, Oral H, et al. MDCT of the left atrium and pulmonary veins in planning radiofrequency ablation for atrial fibrillation: a how-to guide. AJR Am J Roentgenol. 2004;183(3):767–78.
16. Nishimura RA, Otto C. 2014 ACC/AHA valve guidelines: earlier intervention for chronic mitral regurgitation. Heart. 2014;100(12):905–7.
17. Khan S. Long-term outcomes with mechanical and tissue valves. J Heart Valve Dis. 2002;11(Suppl 1):S8–14.
18. Hammermeister K, Sethi GK, Henderson WG, Grover FL, Oprian C, Rahimtoola SH. Outcomes 15 years after valve replacement with a mechanical versus a bioprosthetic valve: final report of the veterans affairs randomized trial. J Am Coll Cardiol. 2000;36(4):1152–8.
19. Grunkemeier GL, Li HH, Naftel DC, Starr A, Rahimtoola SH. Long-term performance of heart valve prostheses. Curr Probl Cardiol. 2000;25(2):73–154.
20. Cannegieter SC, Rosendaal FR, Briet E. Thromboembolic and bleeding complications in patients with mechanical heart valve prostheses. Circulation. 1994;89(2):635–41.

21. Symersky P, Budde RP, Prokop M, de Mol BA. Multidetector-row computed tomography imaging characteristics of mechanical prosthetic valves. J Heart Valve Dis. 2011;20(2):216–22.
22. Konen E, Goitein O, Feinberg MS, Eshet Y, Raanani E, Rimon U, et al. The role of ECG-gated MDCT in the evaluation of aortic and mitral mechanical valves: initial experience. AJR Am J Roentgenol. 2008;191(1):26–31.
23. Habets J, Symersky P, van Herwerden LA, de Mol BA, Spijkerboer AM, Mali WP, et al. Prosthetic heart valve assessment with multidetector-row CT: imaging characteristics of 91 valves in 83 patients. Eur Radiol. 2011;21(7):1390–6.
24. Habets J, Mali WP, Budde RP. Multidetector CT angiography in evaluation of prosthetic heart valve dysfunction. Radiographics Rev Publ Radiological Soc North Am Inc. 2012;32(7):1893–905.
25. Litmanovich DE, Ghersin E, Burke DA, Popma J, Shahrzad M, Bankier AA. Imaging in Transcatheter Aortic Valve Replacement (TAVR): role of the radiologist. Insights Imaging. 2014;5(1):123–45.
26. Blanke P, Schoepf UJ, Leipsic JA. CT in transcatheter aortic valve replacement. Radiology. 2013;269(3):650–69.

Part IV

Where We Are: Cardiac CT Fundamentals

Pathology and Pathophysiology of Coronary Atherosclerotic Plaques

19

Hiroyoshi Mori, Frank D. Kolodgie, Aloke V. Finn, and Renu Virmani

The death rate from coronary artery disease has declined in the past few decades through greater understanding of risk factors of coronary heart disease as well as through better treatment, including the creation of coronary care units. However, because of the lack of an animal model of unstable plaque, our understanding of atherosclerotic plaque morphology comes only from static histology of lesion morphology in patients dying of acute coronary syndromes [1]. Although transgenic models of atherosclerosis have markedly enhanced our understanding of certain aspects of plaque progression and regression, they have failed thus far to explain the relationship of the coagulation parameters and plaque morphology that precipitate coronary thrombosis [1]. Until we are able to create a better model or study plaque morphology prospectively and determine the mechanisms and the anatomic markers of progression, we will make progress very slowly. This review is based on the examination of human coronary artery pathology in patients dying a sudden coronary death, in order to ascertain the pathologic lesion morphologies that are linked to plaque progression and thrombosis, which will be necessary for us to be able to recognize by invasive or noninvasive means the prospective lesions that are likely to produce symptoms.

Classification of Atherosclerosis

Our understanding of atherosclerosis has been enhanced by the development of the various classifications that have come from the insights of scientists like Virchow, who was a pioneer in pathology. Systematic studies of lesion development, described by the giants of atherosclerosis including Robert Wissler, Herbert Stary, Henry McGill, and Michael Davies in the last century, have made enormous contributions to the better understanding of early lesions, the influence of risk factors on plaque progression, and the role of plaque rupture in the occurrence of luminal thrombosis.

The cellular participants of atherosclerosis include smooth muscle cells, endothelial cells, macrophages, T- and B-lymphocytes, red cells, platelets, neutrophils, and basophils. The noncellular components include lipid, proteoglycans, collagen, elastic fibers, calcium, iron (hemosiderin), and blood components, including fibrin and factor VIII. These various components help to form the various lesions that are recognized as part of the atherosclerotic process. These include adaptive intimal thickening (AIT), intimal xanthomas, pathological intimal thickening (PIT), fibroatheroma, thin-cap fibroatheroma, plaque rupture, plaque erosion, calcified nodule, fibrocalcific plaque, healed plaque rupture, and fibrous plaque (either from healed plaque erosion or propagated thrombus).

The best known of the classifications is the American Heart Association (AHA) reported by Stary et al. [2]. However, this classification missed two important clinical etiologies of coronary thrombus that are distinct from rupture. One is surface erosion, which accounts for 25–30% of thrombosis, and the other is calcified nodule, which occurs in <5% of patients. Furthermore, plaque fissure which is another form of communication between the lumen and underlying necrotic core was not included to the AHA classification [3]. Another important concept missing in the AHA classification was the recognition of precursor lesions to plaque rupture, known as "thin-cap fibroatheroma" or "vulnerable plaque." Table 19.1 shows our modified AHA classification [4]. AHA lesion types I–IV were replaced by descriptive terms of adaptive intimal thickening, intimal xanthoma (fatty streak), pathological intimal thickening, and fibroatheroma. AHA categories V and VI were discarded because it doesn't explain three etiologies of coronary thrombosis (rupture, erosion, and calcified nodule). The concept of healed plaque rupture and healed erosion was also added, which can lead to increases in plaque burden, luminal narrowing, or even silent or symptomatic chronic total occlusion.

H. Mori · F. D. Kolodgie · R. Virmani (✉)
CVPath Institute, Gaithersburg, MD, USA
e-mail: rvirmani@cvpath.org

A. V. Finn
CVPath Institute, University of Maryland, Gaithersburg, MD, USA

U. J. Schoepf (ed.), *CT of the Heart*, Contemporary Medical Imaging, https://doi.org/10.1007/978-1-60327-237-7_19

Table 19.1 Updated classification of atherosclerotic lesions based on morphology

Type of lesion	Subtype of lesion	Morphological description
Nonatherosclerotic intimal lesions	Intimal thickening	Natural accumulation of neointimal smooth muscle cells in the absence of lipid, macrophage foam cells, and thrombosis
	Intimal xanthoma	Superficial accumulation of foam cells without a necrotic core, fibrous cap, or thrombosis
Progressive atherosclerotic lesions	Pathological intimal thickening	Plaque rich in smooth muscle cells, with hyaluronan and proteoglycan matrix and focal accumulation of extracellular lipid. Absence of thrombosis
	Fibroatheroma	During early necrosis: focal macrophage infiltration into areas of lipid pools with an overlying fibrous cap. During late necrosis: loss of matrix and extensive cellular debris with an overlying fibrous cap. With or without calcification. Absence of thrombosis
	Intraplaque hemorrhage or plaque fissure	Large necrotic core (size >10% to plaque area) with hemorrhage, and plaque area shows the presence of angiogenesis. Necrotic core communicates with the lumen through a fissure. Minimal tear without obvious thrombus
	Thin-cap fibroatheroma	A thin, fibrous cap (<65 μm) infiltrated by macrophages and lymphocytes, with rare or no smooth muscle cells and relatively large underlying necrotic core (size >10% to plaque area). Intraplaque hemorrhage and/or fibrin might be present. Absence of thrombosis
Lesions with acute thrombi	Plaque rupture	Thin-cap fibroatheroma with cap disruption. Thrombosis is present and may or may not be occlusive. The luminal thrombus communicates with the underlying necrotic core
	Plaque erosion	Can occur on pathological intimal thickening or on a fibroatheroma. Thrombosis is present and may or may not be occlusive. No communication of the thrombus with the necrotic core.
	Calcified nodule	Eruptive (shedding) of calcified nodule with an underlying fibrocalcific plaque with minimal or no necrosis. Thrombosis is usually not occlusive
Healed lesions	Healed plaque rupture, erosion, or calcified nodule	Healed lesion composed of smooth muscle cells, proteoglycans, and type III collagen with or without underlying disrupted fibrous cap, necrotic core, or nodular calcification. Lesions can contain large areas of calcification with few inflammatory cells and have a small or no necrotic core. The fibrotic or fibrocalcific collagen-rich plaque is associated with significant luminal stenosis. Absence of thrombosis

From Yahagi et al. [4], with permission
An updated version of the modified AHA classification [1, 4], which was based on the original AHA classification published in the mid-1990s [2]

Adaptive Intimal Thickening (AIT)

AIT occurs in most arteries once flow is established in utero or soon after birth, consisting primarily of smooth muscle cells, which are strongly α-actin positive and surrounded by a proteoglycan-rich matrix (Fig. 19.1a). Macrophages are rarely detected. These lesions are most prominent at branch points and are considered by many to be precursor lesions of atherosclerosis [5]. Studies of neonates, adolescents, and young adults have indicated that intimal masses forming near branch points enlarge with advancing age and might be precursors to high-risk plaques [6, 7].

Intimal Xanthomas (Fatty Streak)

We have used the microscopic term intimal xanthoma for fatty streak, the corresponding designation for the lesion as grossly seen in the aorta. We believe intimal xanthoma is not a lesion of atherosclerosis, as it eventually regresses in humans. The Pathobiological Determinants of Atherosclerosis in Youth (PDAY) study showed that fatty streaks are prominent in the third decade in the thoracic aorta but regress later in life [8]. The site of advanced lesions is generally the abdominal aorta, where fatty streaks are relatively uncommon. Fatty streaks are rich in macrophages [9, 10] (hence the term *xanthoma*) but lack necrotic cores or lipid pools (Fig. 19.1b).

Pathological intimal thickening (PIT)

PIT lesion is also rich in smooth muscle cells in a proteoglycan matrix (Fig. 19.2a). However, the area close to the media shows loss of smooth muscle cells and an accumulation of fat as a lipid pool, which stains positive with oil red O. A significant number of smooth muscle cells close to the media show accumulation of intracellular fat and may appear

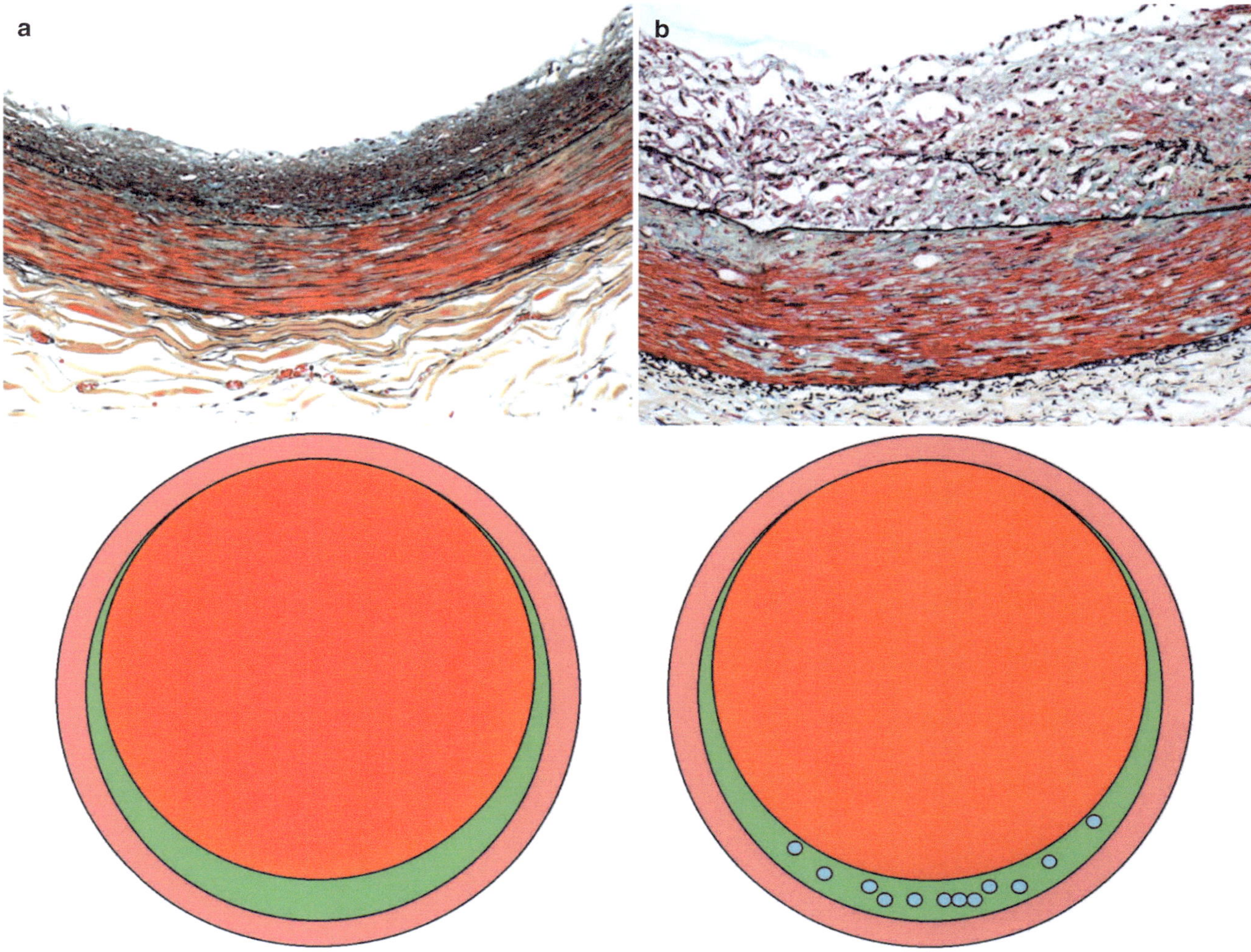

Fig. 19.1 Adaptive intimal thickening (**a**) and intimal xanthoma (**b**). Lesions uniformly present in all populations, although intimal xanthomas are more prevalent with exposure to a Western diet. Intimal xanthomas are commonly produced in animal models; however, they usually do not develop into progressive atherosclerotic lesions. Both lesions occur soon after birth; the intimal xanthoma (otherwise known as a fatty streak) is known to regress. Intimal thickening consists mainly of smooth muscle cells in a proteoglycan-rich matrix, while intimal xanthomas primarily contain macrophage-derived foam cells, T-lymphocytes, and varying degrees of smooth muscle cells. (From Virmani et al. [1], with permission)

foamy, best appreciated by transmission electron microscopy. The smooth muscle cells may appear as ghosts with surrounding thickened basement membrane, which stains strongly periodic acid-Schiff (PAS) positive [11] *(3a)*. The surrounding matrix also stains positive for oil red O and often shows the presence of monohydrate cholesterol, which may appear as cholesterol crystals (lipid pools). There may be macrophage infiltration in the superficial regions of the plaque, but these macrophages are not in proximity to the lipid pools. It is believed that smooth muscle cells are undergoing apoptosis, degeneration, and calcification [12]. We believe that pathological intimal thickening is the precursor lesion of the fibroatheroma.

Fibroatheroma

Fibroatheromas are lesions with a necrotic core and a thick fibrous cap (Fig. 19.2b). The necrotic core is rich in acellular debris and varies in size. The fibrous cap covers the necrotic core completely, is rich in smooth muscle cells within a collagen/proteoglycan matrix, and may contain macrophages and lymphocytes. The thickness of the fibrous cap varies; a thin cap is believed to impart instability and therefore warrants a separate designation of thin-cap fibroatheroma. We recently subcategorized fibroatheromas into "early" and "late" phase [4]. Early fibroatheroma is associated with a decrease in the expression of biglycan, hyaluronan, and

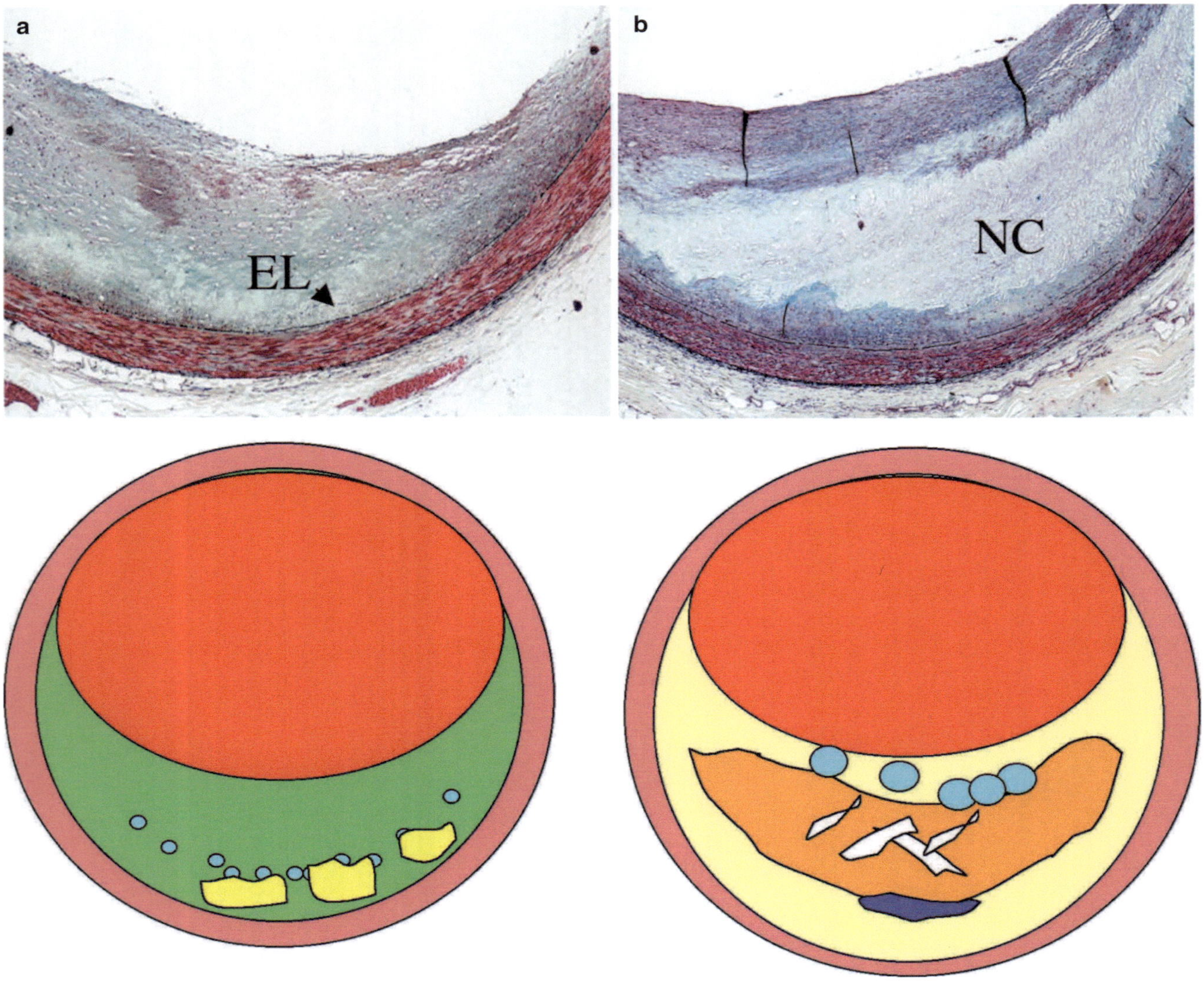

Fig. 19.2 Pathological intimal thickening (**a**) vs. atheroma (**b**). Pathological intimal thickening is a poorly defined entity sometimes referred to in the literature as an "intermediate lesion." True necrosis is not apparent, and there is no evidence of cellular debris; some lipid may be present deep in the lesion near the elastic lamina (EL), but it is dispersed. The fibrous cap overlying the areas of lipid is rich in smooth muscle cells and proteoglycans. Some scattered macrophages and lymphocytes may also be present but are usually sparse. The more definitive lesion or fibrous cap atheroma classically shows a "true" necrotic core (NC), containing cholesterol esters, free cholesterol, phospholipids, and triglycerides. The fibrous cap consists of smooth muscle cells in a proteoglycan-collagenous matrix, with a variable number of macrophages and lymphocytes. The media underneath the plaque is often thin. (From Virmani et al. [1], with permission)

versian within the lipid pool together with infiltrating macrophages, which are undergoing necrosis or apoptosis. Late fibroatheroma is deficient in extracellular matrix and has more cholesterol clefts and calcification [13, 14]. How the necrotic core enlarges and becomes rich in free cholesterol is poorly understood. Hemorrhage into a plaque, either through the leaky vasa vasorum or possibly through plaque fissuring, plays an important role in the enlargement of the necrotic core. Because the vasa vasorum become leaky, allowing fibrinogen to seep into the plaque, especially if pressure within them rises, as they have a poorly developed basement membrane and often lack pericytes and smooth muscle cells. In support of this concept is the frequent finding of fibrin, by immunohistochemical methods, within the necrotic core.

Thin-Cap Fibroatheroma

The original description of AHA classification did not mention the thin-cap fibroatheroma (TCFA) as a precursor lesion of plaque rupture. Partly based on their morphologic resemblance to acute ruptures, we believe that they are the precursor lesions. The TCFA is defined as a lesion with a necrotic core and an overlying fibrous cap that is <65 μm and infil-

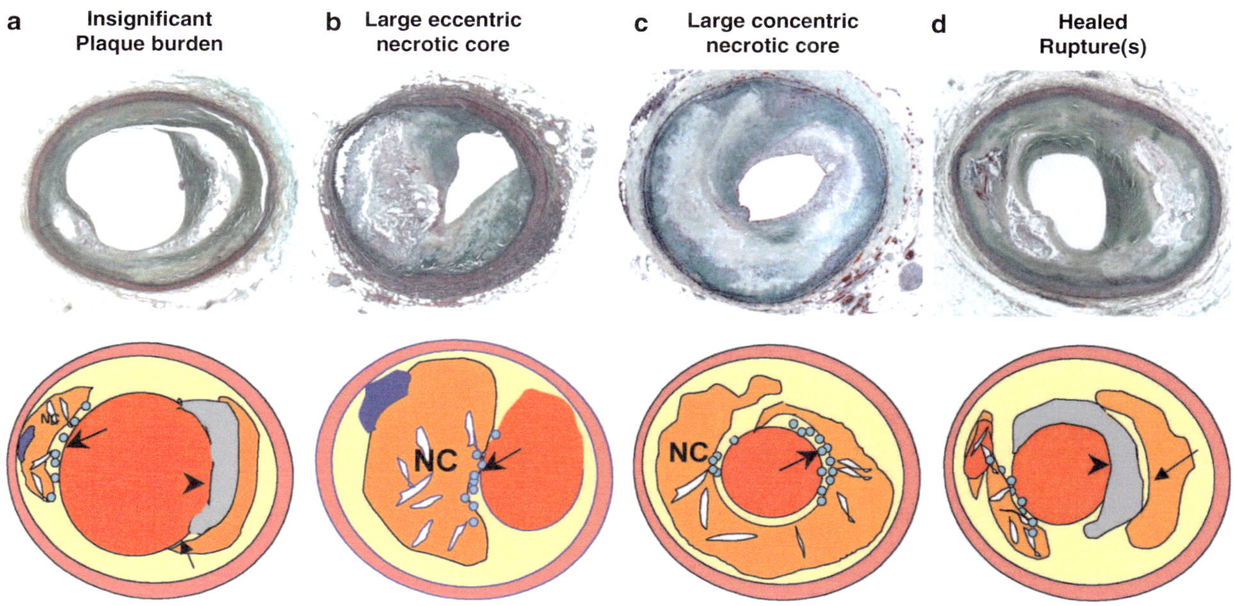

Fig. 19.3 Morphologic variants of the thin-cap atheroma. Thin caps may emerge in fibroatheromas with insignificant plaque burden and insignificant luminal narrowing, in fibroatheromas with large cores that are eccentric or eccentric, and frequently in plaques with evidence of prior rupture. (**a**) In this plaque with insignificant plaque burden, there is an area of proteoglycan-rich smooth muscle cells (arrowheads) suggestive of a prior rupture and multiple areas of thin caps (arrows). (**b**) The necrotic core (NC) is large, with an area of thinned cap (arrow). (**c**) The necrotic core (NC) is concentric with an extensive area of cap thinning (arrow). (**d**) There may be a healed rupture (arrows) with a proteoglycan-rich smooth muscle cell reparative layer (arrowhead)

trated by macrophages (>25 per high-power magnification [0.03 mm diameter field]) [15] (Fig. 19.3). The thickness criterion of TCFA was chosen because 95% of fibrous caps adjacent to acute plaque rupture measured <65 μm, with a mean cap thickness of 23 ± 19 μm. We have also compared other morphologic characteristics between plaque rupture and TCFA. The necrotic core is smaller than that seen in rupture (Table 19.2). In addition, the percent area occupied by the necrotic core is greater in rupture than TCFA, although we were unable to determine any significant differences in length (Table 19.2). The cross-sectional luminal narrowing of TCFA is less than that of acute rupture; nearly 80% of TCFAs had luminal narrowing <75% in contrast to rupture (Fig. 19.4).

Table 19.2 Approximate sizes of necrotic core in fibroatheroma, thin-cap atheroma, and acute rupture

	Plaque type		
Dimension	Fibroatheroma	Thin-cap atheroma	Acute plaque rupture
Length (mm) mean/range	6 mm (range 1–18 mm)	8 mm (range 2–17 mm)	9 mm (range 2.5 ± 22)
Cross-sectional area, mm^2	1.2 ± 2.2	1.7 ± 1.1	4.1 ± 5.5
% Cross-sectional area	15 ± 20%	23 ± 17%	34 ± 17%

From Ref. [45], with permission

Lesions with Thrombi

From studies carried out in patients dying sudden coronary death, we have observed three main causes of luminal thrombi: plaque rupture (the precursor of which is presumably the TCFA), erosion, and calcified nodule (Fig. 19.5). The most frequent cause of thrombosis is plaque rupture (over 60%), plaque erosion is the second most frequent (about 35%), whereas calcified nodule is a rare cause of thrombosis (<5%). These three types of thrombosis occur, respectively, in the setting of a TCFA, fibroatheroma or pathological intimal thickening, and a calcified plaque with or without a necrotic core (Fig. 19.1).

Plaque Rupture

Plaque rupture is defined as a disruption, discontinuous fibrous cap, underlying necrotic core, and superimposed luminal thrombus. Ruptured plaques that result in occlusive luminal thrombi almost invariably have a large necrotic core, which occupies =25% of the plaque area in 80% of cases. Plaque rupture is the major underlying mechanism of luminal thrombosis in sudden death (60%), acute myocardial infarction (75%), and unstable angina (70%) and is

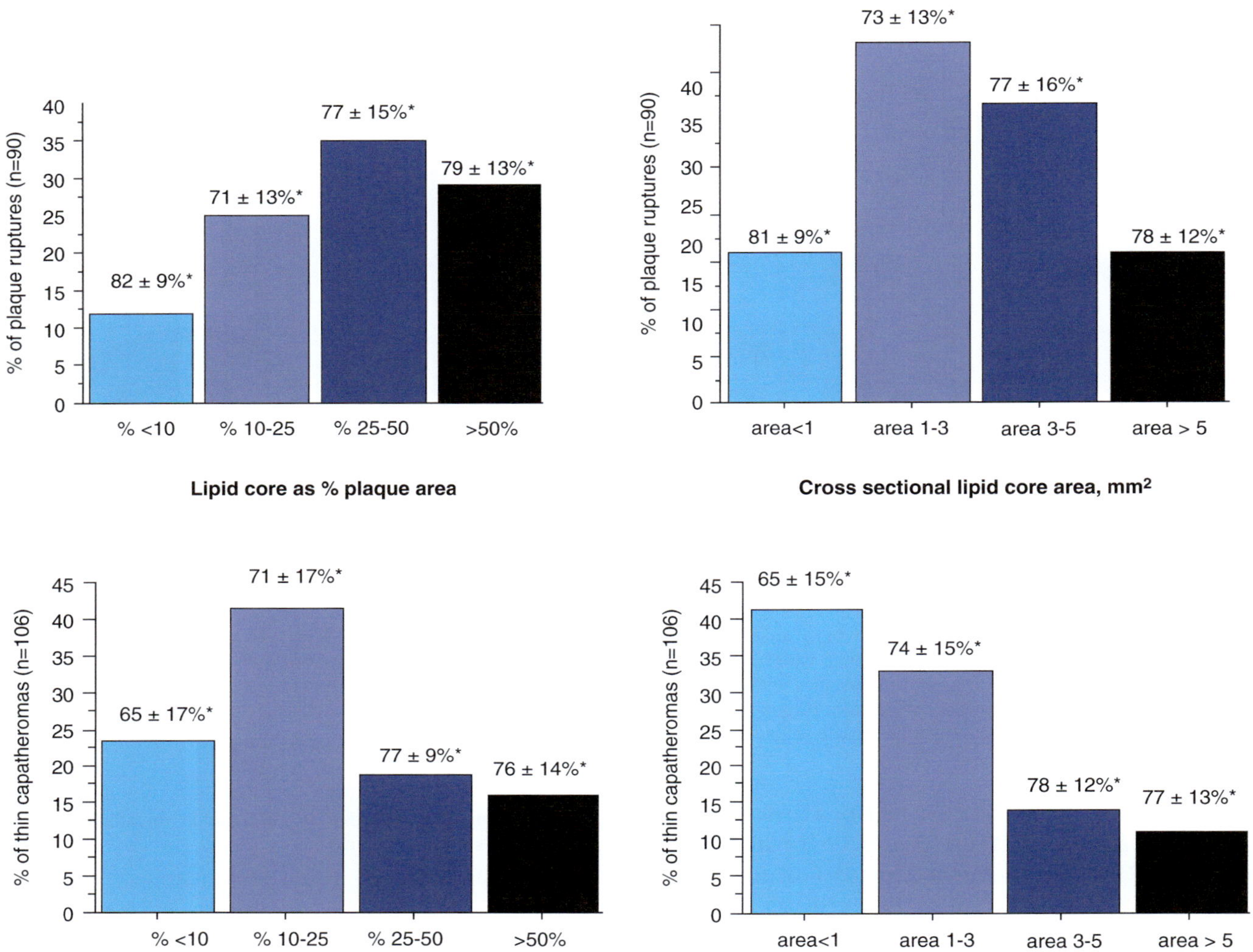

Fig. 19.4 The distribution frequency of plaque ruptures (**a**, **b**) and thin-cap atheromas (**c**, **d**) by size of lipid core or lipid core as a percent of plaque area (*x*-axis). The majority of plaque ruptures occur when lipid core area forms 25% to 50% of plaque area or 1–3 mm^2 lipid core area. In the case of thin-cap atheromas, the degree of cross-sectional area luminal narrowing and area of necrotic core is shifted to the left (lesser or smaller) as compared to plaque ruptures. (From Ref. [45], with permission)

rarely present in stable angina [16–18]. The mechanism of rupture is poorly understood; however, it is generally believed that macrophages infiltrate the cap and release matrix metalloproteinases, which are responsible for the breakdown of the collagens [19, 20]. There is also evidence that macrophage myeloperoxidase may be responsible for the disruption of the fibrous cap by producing the prooxidant species, hypochlorous acid. We have shown that up to 15% of macrophages within ruptured fibrous caps are rich in myeloperoxidase. We have observed that the numbers of plaque hemorrhages in the coronary arteries of patients dying suddenly with acute plaque rupture are greater than in patients with severe coronary disease dying with other forms of thrombosis or without coronary thrombosis [21]. These data suggest that hemorrhage, due to plaque fissure or rupture of vasa vasorum, may be precursors to plaque rupture. Davies has shown that 11% of hearts have plaque fissure with intra-intimal thrombus, 2% have intimal thrombus as the only mechanism of sudden death, while rupture with thrombosis was identified in 74%, and only 5% had no acute coronary lesion [3]. We have observed vasa vasorum to be more prominent in patients dying suddenly during exercise with plaque rupture, compared to patients dying at rest. Also, hemorrhage into a plaque was more frequent in patients dying during exercise than in patients dying at rest [22]. The site of rupture was located at the shoulder more frequently in the cases dying at rest (65%) versus dying during exercise (25%) ($P = 0.02$) [22]. Plaque rupture correlated with high total cholesterol, low HDL cholesterol, and an elevated ratio of total/HDL cholesterol while smoking was found to be a predictor of acute thrombosis regardless of plaque etiology [15].

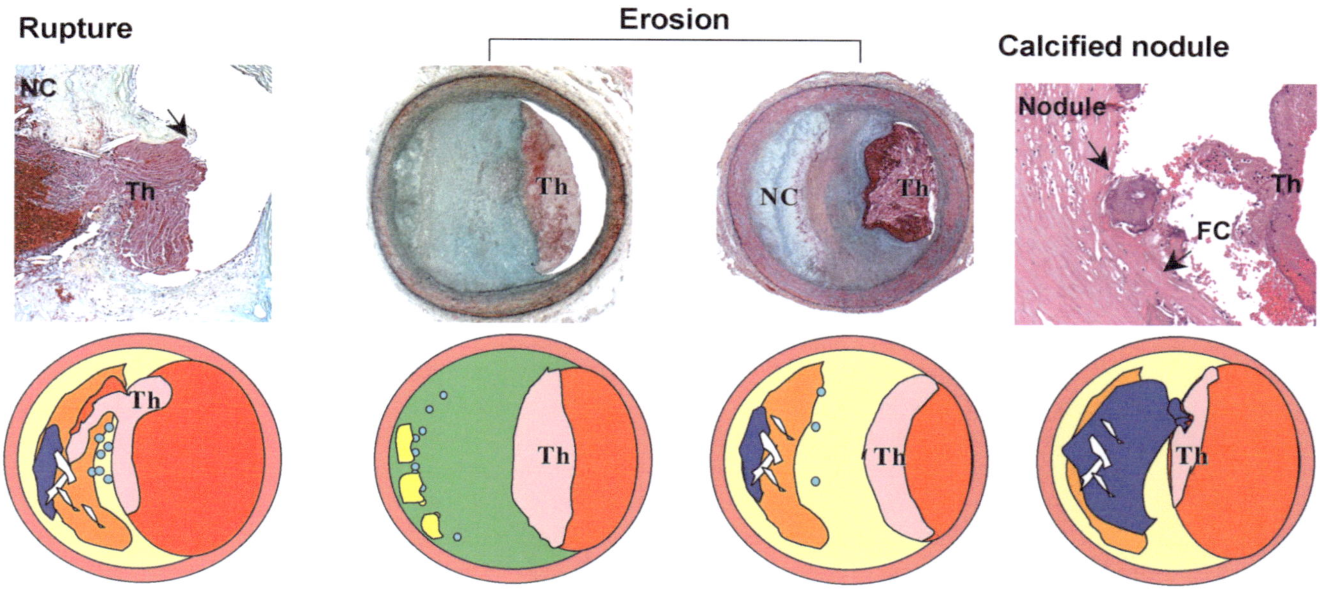

Fig. 19.5 Lesions with thrombi. Ruptured plaques are thin-cap fibroatheroma with luminal thrombi (Th). These lesions usually have an extensive necrotic core containing large numbers of cholesterol crystals and a thin fibrous cap (<65 μm) infiltrated by foamy macrophages and a paucity of T-lymphocytes. The fibrous cap is thinnest at the site of rupture and consists of a few collagen bundles and rare smooth muscle cells. The luminal thrombus is in communication with the lipid-rich necrotic core. Erosions occur over lesions rich in smooth muscle cells and proteoglycans. Luminal thrombi overlay areas lacking surface endothelium. The deep intima of the eroded plaque often shows extracellular lipid pools, but necrotic cores are uncommon; when present, the necrotic core does not communicate with the luminal thrombus. Inflammatory infiltrate is usually absent, but if present, it is sparse and consists of macrophages and lymphocytes. Calcified nodules are plaques with luminal thrombi showing calcific nodules protruding into the lumen through a disrupted thin fibrous cap (FC). There is an absence of endothelium at the site of the thrombus, and inflammatory cells (macrophages, T lymphocytes) are absent. (From Virmani et al. [1], with permission)

Plaque Erosion

Plaque erosion is defined as an acute thrombus in direct contact with intimal plaque rich in smooth muscle cells within a proteoglycan matrix and an absence of endothelium [1, 17]. There are relatively few macrophages and lymphocytes adjacent to the thrombus in the majority of plaque erosions. Plaque erosion accounts for 20% of all sudden coronary deaths and 35% of coronary thrombi in patients dying suddenly with coronary thrombosis [1, 17]. The mean age of patients dying with plaque erosion is less than that of patients dying with acute rupture, and there is less severe narrowing at the sites of thrombosis in plaque erosion. Plaque erosion accounts for over 80% of thrombi occurring in women less than 50 years of age. The lesions tend to be eccentric and are infrequently calcified [17]. Plaque erosions tend to embolize more frequently than plaque rupture (71%, vs. 42%, respectively) [23]. The thrombi of eroded plaques often show at later stage of organization than that of ruptured plaques (88% vs. 54%, respectively, $P < 0.0001$). The risk factors for erosion are poorly understood; similar to acute rupture, there is an increased risk among smokers, but there appears to be a lesser association with dyslipidemia, as compared to plaque rupture [15]. The underlying plaque in erosions is generally the pathological intimal thickening or fibrous cap atheroma (pathological intimal thickening 16%, early fibroatheroma 50%, late fibroatheroma 34%) [24]. Erosion lesions show less calcification with more than half of erosions (56%) showing no calcification, while 40% show microcalcification, while fragmented and sheet of calcification are rarely observed [24]. The most frequent location for both erosion and rupture is the proximal left anterior descending coronary artery (nearly two-thirds of patients) followed by the right coronary artery and the left circumflex. However, patients dying with plaque erosion frequently do not have extensive disease, unlike patients dying with stable plaque or plaque rupture. Over one-half of deaths are seen in patients with single-vessel disease and one-quarter with double-vessel disease. The etiology of plaque erosion is poorly understood; however, it is believed that coronary vasospasm may be involved.

Calcified Nodule

The least frequent lesion that results in coronary luminal thrombus is the calcified nodule, a plaque that contains calcified plates at the site of luminal disruption. The incidence of calcified nodules was only 5% [25]. There may or may not be necrotic core within the plaque, but the characteristic features are the breakage of calcified plates, often with a fibrotic reaction, an interspersed fibrin, a disrupted surface, and an overlying thrombus. Occasionally, bone formation with osteoblasts and osteoclasts is present [1]. Although the precise mechanism is unknown, one hypothesis is that mechanical stress might lead to breakage of the calcified sheets. In between the calcified spicules, fibrin is commonly observed, potentially arising from the surrounding break in the capillaries. Eruptive calcified nodules typically happen in eccentric lesions where protrusion causes disruption of the overlaying cap and endothelium. The lesion is more commonly located in the mid-right coronary artery or left anterior descending artery, generally in a heavily calcified segment [1]. It is more common in older male individuals than women. We have observed these lesions in the carotid arteries as well as the coronaries.

Healed Plaque Ruptures

Not all plaque ruptures result in symptoms; therefore, there should be morphologic hallmarks that could be recognized within plaques that are representative of a previous site of thrombus [26]. Healed ruptures in the coronary vascular bed are readily detected microscopically by the identification of the breaks in the fibrous cap, which is rich in type I collagen, and an overlying repaired lesion, which is richer in type III collagen. The healed lesion can be more easily recognized by Movat's stain (healed site identified by the brilliant blue-green color of the proteoglycan-rich matrix) and confirmed by picrosirius red staining and polarized microscopy. When viewed under polarized light, this stain highlights the breaks in the fibrous cap, which is rich in type I collagen, as yellow-red birefringence with an underlying necrotic core (Fig. 19.6). The plaque overlying the fibrous cap consists of smooth muscle cells in a proteoglycan matrix, which is rich in type

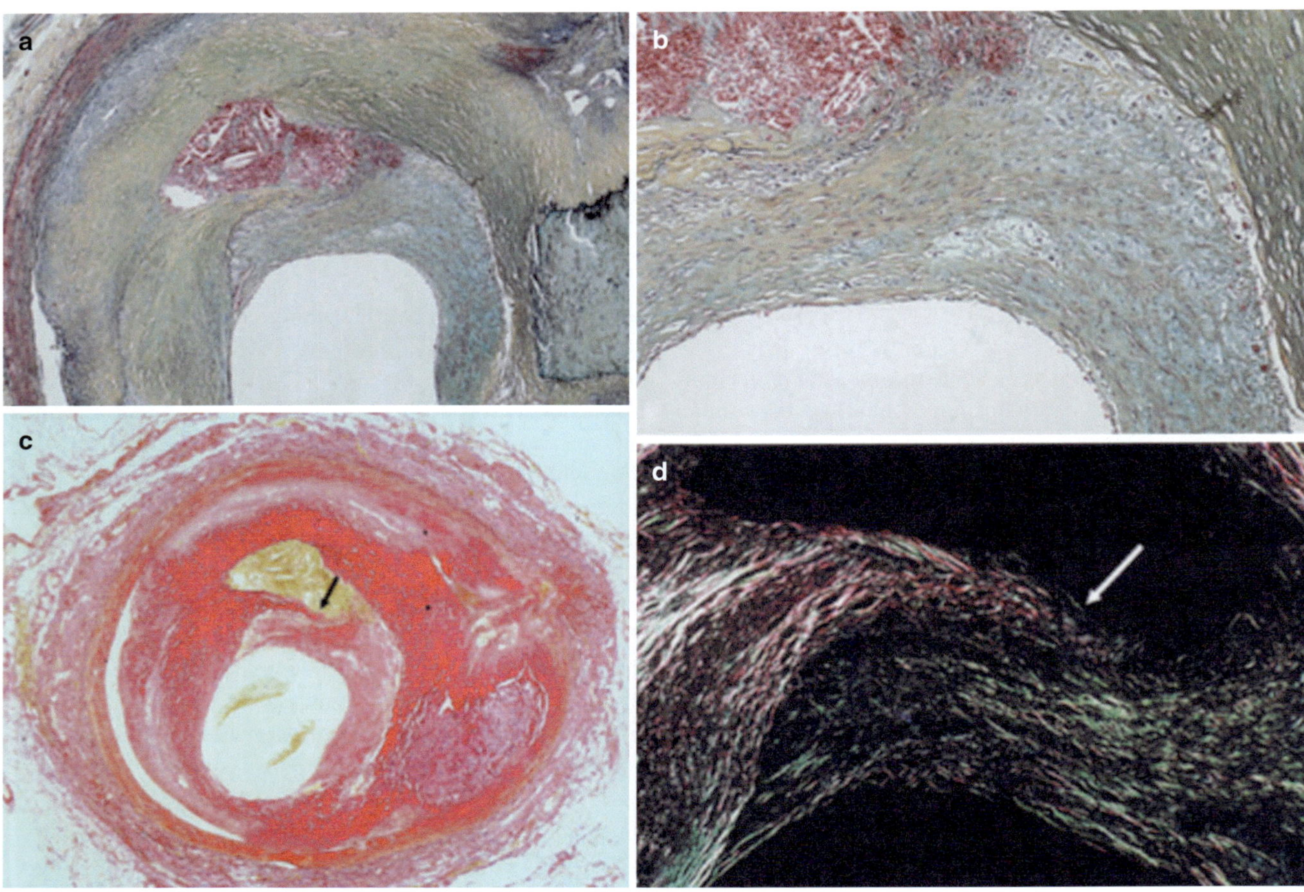

Fig. 19.6 Healed plaque rupture. (**a**) demonstrates areas of intra-intimal lipid-rich core with hemorrhage and cholesterol clefts. (**b**) shows a higher magnification of the looser smooth muscle cell formation within a collagenous proteoglycan-rich neointima showing a clear demarcation with the more fibrous regions of the old plaque to the right. (**c**) and (**d**) demonstrate the layers of collagen by Sirius red staining. In (**c**), note the area of dense dark red collagen surrounding the lipid hemorrhagic cores seen in corresponding view in panel **a**. (**d**) demonstrates an image taken with polarized light. The dense collagen (type 1) which forms the fibrous cap is lighter reddish-yellow and is disrupted (arrow), with the newer greenish type III collagen on the right and above the rupture site (**a** and **b**, Movat's pentachrome). (From Burke et al. [46], with permission)

III collagen and has green birefringence under polarized light (sirius red stained) [22].

We and others believe that healing of a disrupted plaque is the main stimulus for plaque progression beyond 40% cross-sectional area narrowing and is one of the major factors leading to high-grade coronary stenosis [26]. Incidence of healed plaque rupture was 16% in arteries with ≤20% diameter stenosis, 19% with 21–50% diameter stenosis, and 73% for plaque with >50% diameter stenosis [26]. This mechanism would explain the phasic rather than linear progression of coronary disease observed in angiograms carried out annually in patients with chronic ischemic heart disease [26]. However, these are speculations that need to be proven when we can prospectively recognize the sites of vulnerability and follow up the lesional morphologies with advanced imaging techniques. We have also shown that these lesions are the most heavily calcified as compared to acute rupture or thin-cap fibroatheroma, suggesting that healing of a ruptured plaque also results in greater extent of calcification [27].

Total Occlusions

Among patients dying sudden coronary death without prior symptoms, total occlusion is a frequent finding at autopsy (Fig. 19.7). The frequency is as high as 40% when there are no other sites with acute plaque rupture. Healed myocardial infarcts are seen in 90% of patients with a total occlusion [1]. The lumen is composed of dense collagen and/or proteoglycans with interspersed capillaries, arterioles, smooth muscle cells, and macrophages [28]. In the case of total occlusions secondary to thrombi, the proximal and distal ends organize initially, followed by the middle segment, which may demonstrate entrapped red cells and fibrin without cellular ingrowth for long periods. Sites of total occlusion are often associated with negative remodeling of the vessel, probably related to collagen replacement of the thrombus with eventual cross-linking, resulting in artery shrinkage. There is often little calcification within total occlusions, probably because the plaque has formed via organized thrombus, as opposed to successive ruptures of necrotic cores with preserved blood flow.

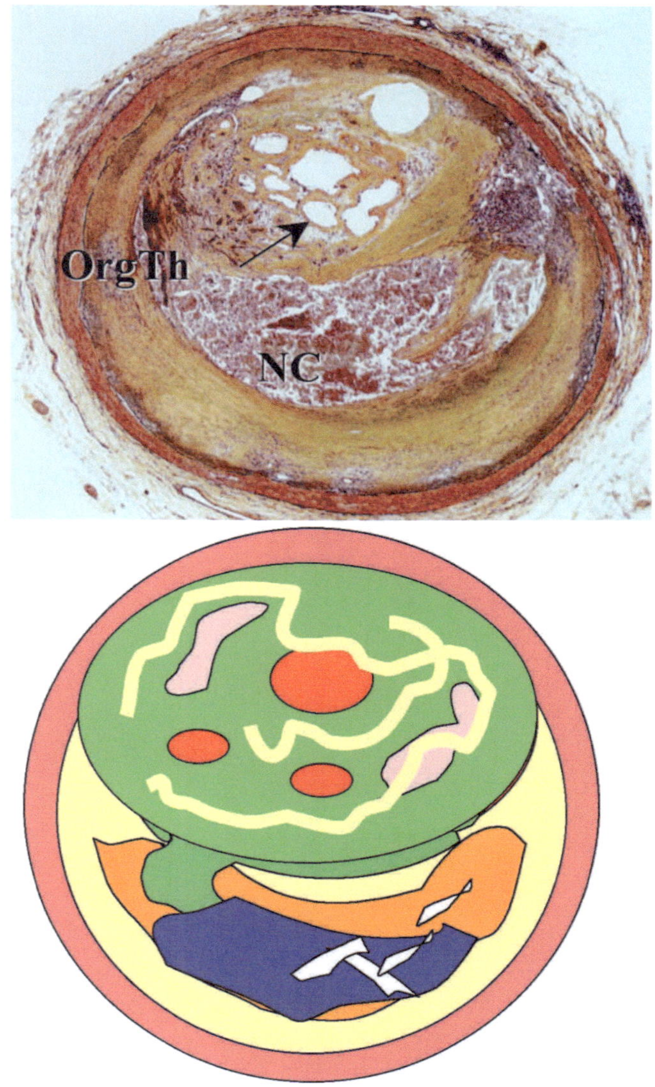

Fig. 19.7 Total occlusion. Plaques with total occlusion from prior thrombi contain mostly smooth muscle cells in a collagen-proteoglycan-rich matrix with capillaries and inflammatory cell infiltrate. This section shows a necrotic core (NC), although this is not always present, and the lumen is filled with an organized thrombus (orgTh) with multiple capillary channels

Fibrous and Fibrocalcific Plaques

A subset of coronary artery plaques have little evidence of lipid pool or necrotic core formation and are designated as fibrous or fibrocalcific plaques, depending on the presence of calcification. The mechanism of plaque enlargement of such plaques is unknown but may be in some cases related to propagated thrombus or healed plaque erosions (Fig. 19.8). These lesions are rich in type I collagen, but type III collagen and proteoglycans may also be present. The calcium deposition may be related to calcified apoptotic smooth muscle cells in the absence of a significant influx of macrophages and other inflammatory cells. The term *fibrous plaque* has not been typically used in formal classifications of coronary artery atherosclerosis, partly because it is a general category that may represent an etiologically diverse set of lesions.

Intraplaque Hemorrhage

As mentioned above, the interrelationship between intraplaque hemorrhage, fibrin, necrotic core, and vasa vasorum has not been fully explained. Most vasa vasorum originate from the parent artery and ramify plexogenically in the

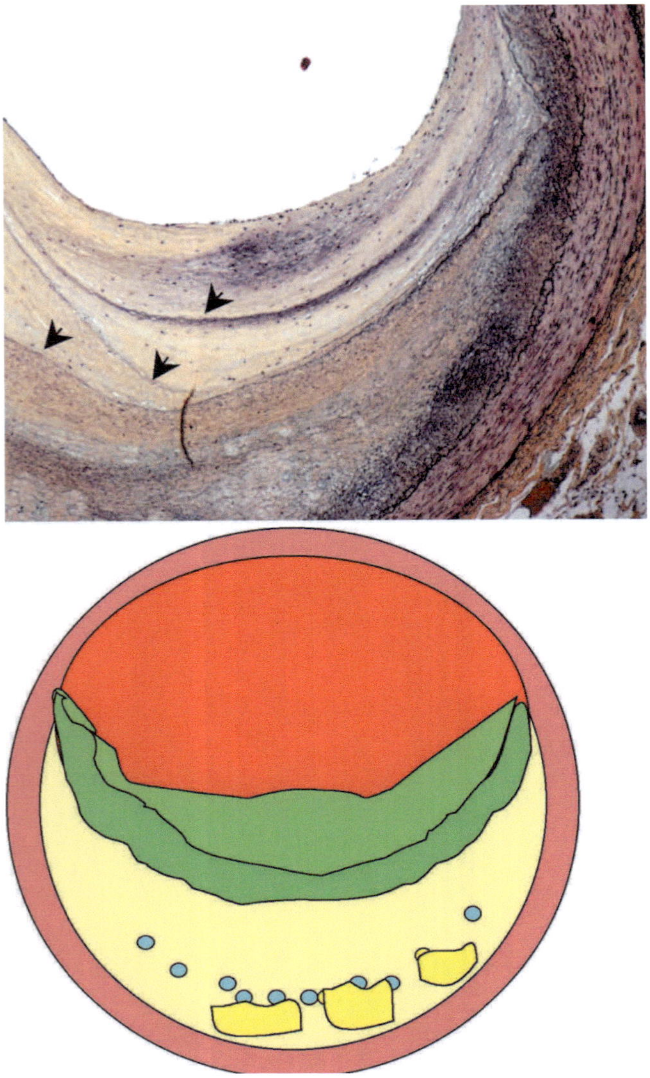

Fig. 19.8 Healed erosion shows deep multilayering of collagen separated by elastin layers (arrowheads) and a paucity of smooth muscle cells. The superficial plaque is rich in smooth muscle cells, collagen, and proteoglycans

adventitia [29]. There is a clear relationship between numbers of vasa vasorum (Fig. 19.9) and blood flow through them and mass of coronary plaque [30]. In addition, increased vasa vasorum are associated with atherosclerotic plaque expansion [29], and plaque regression is paralleled by a decrease in blood flow through the vasa vasorum [31]. Further evidence for a dynamic relationship between vasa vasorum and the atherosclerotic process are the fact that they respond to vasoconstrictor stimuli and that their density is associated with exertional plaque rupture [22].

The mechanisms by which vasa vasorum contribute to plaque growth are poorly understood. Plaque iron content is a surrogate marker of preceding hemorrhage and correlates with plaque neovascularization [29]. The frequency of iron deposition in the coronary plaques is higher in patients with acute coronary syndrome than in those dying of noncardiac causes [32]. Since plaque hemorrhage is a frequent phenomenon, especially in advanced plaques, it is not surprising that some of the free cholesterol may have its origin from the red cell membrane. The increase in iron content correlated with intraplaque hemorrhage is identified by glycophorin A staining, a red-cell specific anion-exchange protein [13].

Rupture of vasa vasorum is not the sole etiology of intraplaque hemorrhage. As Constantinides originally suggested, plaque hemorrhage may occur from cracks or fissures originating from the lumen [33]. Intraplaque hemorrhage, whether from vasa vasorum or the lumen, may be critical to the lesion progression, as it may provide a significant source of nonmetabolic cholesterol [13, 34].

Coronary Calcification

In early coronary atherosclerotic plaques, coronary calcification is identified using sensitive histochemical stains, such as the von Kossa stain. When such tests are applied to fatty streaks, there is little if any calcium is present. However, pathological intimal thickening and fibrous plaques have a high propensity for microscopic calcification, especially when there is evidence of smooth muscle cell apoptosis. The biology of intimal calcification within atherosclerotic regions is complex and involves smooth muscle cell matrix vesicles (related to apoptotic bodies), bone-associated proteins, lipids, and inflammation in the formation of extracellular intimal calcifications [12]. Almost all necrotic cores with apoptotic smooth muscle cells contain calcification (at least 90%), and those cores with predominantly macrophage infiltrates are less likely to initially calcify. The nature of the calcifications differs by cell type, in that fibrous cores contain finely granular calcifications, occasionally coalescing into masses, whereas macrophage "necrotic" cores often contain larger crystalline deposits. Calcification of fibrous plaques in which there is smooth muscle cell death cores progresses to plate-like sheets of calcification and often pipestem-like arteries. However, calcification of necrotic, inflamed, macrophage-rich cores tends to be more irregular, resulting in a radiographic appearance of irregular calcification. Ultrastructural study of coronary plaques will demonstrate calcifications in close contact with dying smooth muscle cells, macrophages, and surrounding cholesterol clefts (Fig. 19.10). In less than 5% of plaques, actual ossification may occur, with osteoblasts, osteoclasts, and even marrow formation (Fig. 19.11).

Calcification does not in itself appear to play a role in the thrombotic process, except under the unusual circumstances of nodular calcification. Successive ruptures or fissures of the fibrous cap result in layering of the plaque, and the deeper

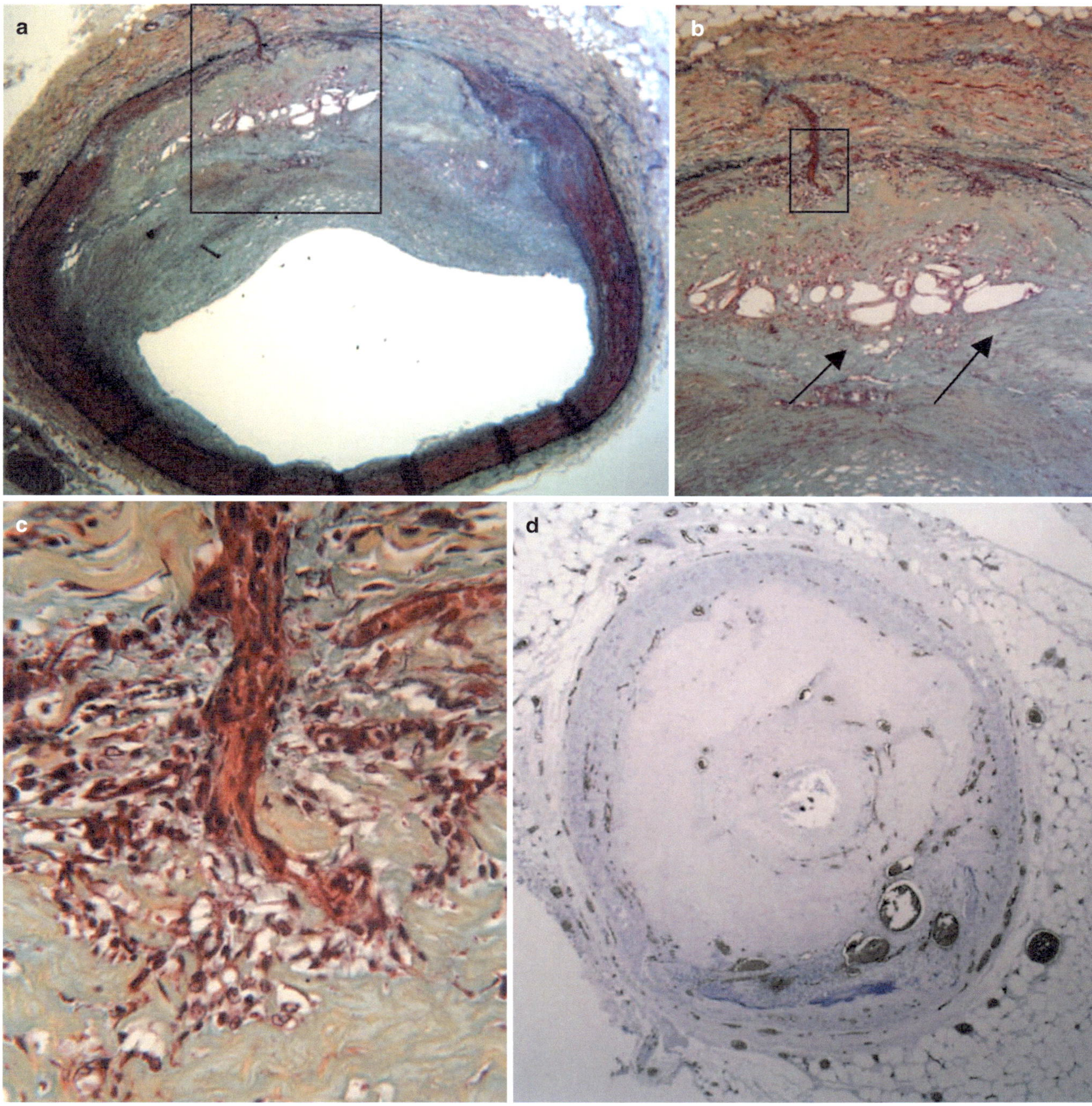

Fig. 19.9 The vasa vasorum within plaque. (**a**) At low magnification, there is thinning of the media with dilated spaces within the plaque. (**b**) A higher magnification of the boxed area in (**a**) shows dilated channels to be blood vessels (arrows). (**c**) A higher magnification of the boxed area in *B* shows a muscular artery feeder vessel traversing the media. (**d**) A different segment of near-total occlusion stained with *Ulex europaeus* lectin highlighting neovessels brown within the adventitia and intima

layers close to the internal elastic lamina typically demonstrate more severe calcification than the surface layers.

We have performed quantitative analysis of calcified matrix in intermediate and later plaque stages, including fibroatheromas, acute and healed plaque ruptures, total occlusions, and plaque erosion. In contrast to rupture, plaque erosion does not expose the contents of the necrotic core to the lumen. Eroded plaques, perhaps partly as a function of their pathogenesis, do not typically occur in calcified arteries and demonstrate far less calcified matrix than acute or healed ruptures. The degree of calcification by plaque type is illustrated in Fig. 19.12.

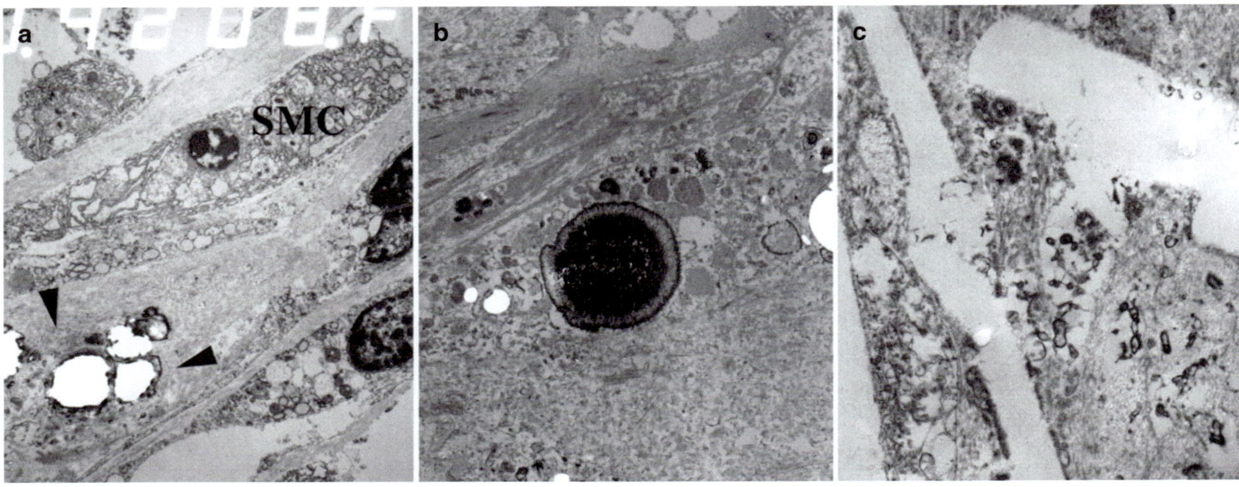

Fig. 19.10 Ultrastructural images of coronary atherosclerotic plaques show extracellular calcifications adjacent to an apoptotic smooth muscle cell (SMC) (**a**), spherical calcification associated with degenerating smooth muscle cell organelles (**b**), and small calcifications surrounding cholesterol clefts in area of macrophage degeneration (**c**)

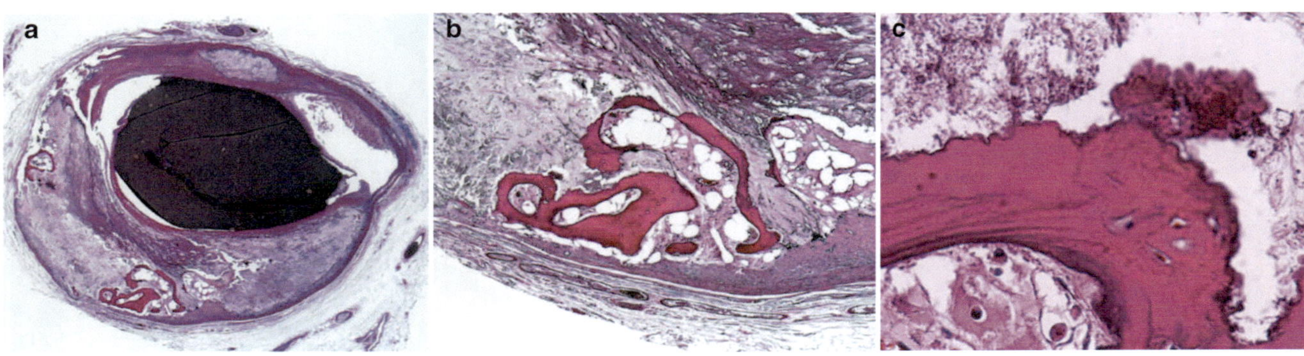

Fig. 19.11 Ossification in coronary plaque. (**a**) demonstrates a low-magnification image of a coronary artery section (proximal left anterior descending artery) in the left anterior descending coronary artery of an obese elderly woman with hypertensive atherosclerotic heart disease. (**a**) is a low magnification of the cross section of the artery; contrast material (black) was injected into the artery postmortem. (**b**) demonstrates the bony trabeculae and (**c**) a higher magnification of lacunae containing osteoblasts

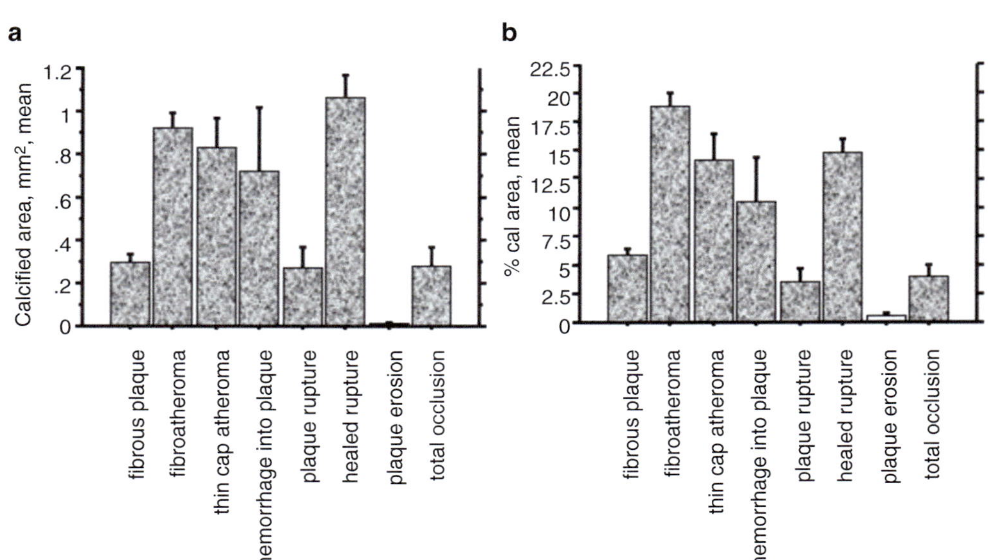

Fig. 19.12 Amount of calcification by plaque morphology. Morphometric measurements were made of calcified matrix in several hundred coronary lesions classified by plaque type. (**a**) Healed ruptures demonstrated the greatest mean area of calcification; plaque erosions demonstrate almost no calcification. (**b**) When expressed as a percentage of the plaque area, total occlusion and plaque ruptures have relatively little calcium and plaque erosions the least. Fibroatheroma and healed ruptures demonstrate the greatest amount of calcified matrix. (From Burke et al. [27], with permission)

Table 19.3 Relationship between calcification and percent luminal narrowing and residual lumen, by arterial section

	Calcified area vs. percent luminal narrowing (simple regression)						Calcified area vs. residual lumen area (simple regression)	
	Men			Women			Men and women (combined)	
Artery	r^a	P	DF	r^a	P	DF	r^b	P
LM	.20	.20	30	.15	.59	14	.14	.58
PLAD	.56	<.0001	122	.15	.27	53	.07	.53
MLAD	.45	<.0001	91	.50	<.0001	66	.10	.29
DLAD	.64	.0003	27	.31	.11	24	.18	28
LD	.59	.001	26	.75	.0004	17	.13	.71
PLC	.30	.01	78	.25	.07	51	.11	.32
MLC	.02	.90	35	.31	.29	13	.21	.40
LOM	.60	.0001	34	72	0.01	11	.13	.30
PRC	.12	.15	143	.09	.54	54	.09	.38
MRC	.29	.001	127	.63	<.0001	68	.09	.37
DRC	.32	.0004	116	.36	.06	27	.17	.29

From Burke et al. [27], with permission

Segments are bolded showing r values >0.4 and a significant correlation $P < 0.05$

Abbreviations: *LM* left main, *PLAD* proximal left anterior descending, *MLAD* mid-left anterior descending, *DLAD* distal left anterior descending, *LD* left diagonal, *PLC* proximal left circumflex, *MLC* mid-left circumflex, *LOM* left obtuse marginal, *PRC* proximal right coronary, *MRC* mid-right coronary, *DRC* distal right coronary, *df* degrees of freedom

[a] *T* values are all positive (positive correlation)

[b] *T* values are negative (PLAD, MRC, DRC, LD) or positive (LM, LOM, MLAD, PLC, MLC, PRC)

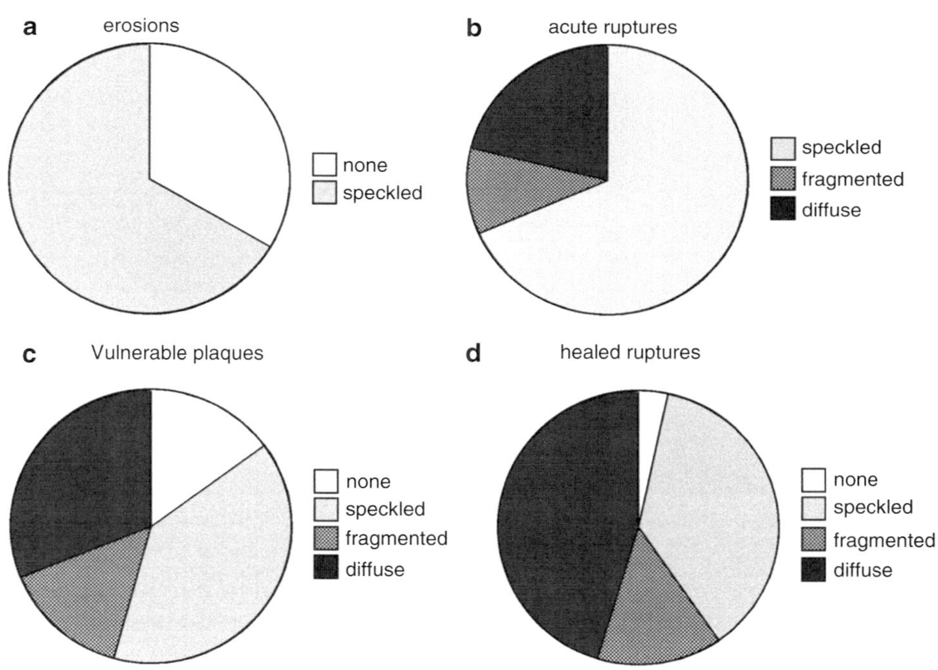

Fig. 19.13 Relationship between plaque morphology and radiographic calcification. Plaque erosions (**a**) were exclusively present in areas with stippled or no calcification. Plaque ruptures (**b**) were most frequently seen in areas of speckled calcification but were also present in blocked or diffuse calcification. Curiously, there were no ruptures in segments devoid of any calcification. Thin-capped atheromas were most frequently present in areas of speckled calcification (**c**) but were also seen in heavily calcified or uncalcified areas, suggesting that calcification pattern is not helpful in diagnosing these lesions. Healed ruptures are almost always seen in areas of calcification and most frequently in diffusely calcified areas (**d**). (From Burke et al. [27], with permission)

The relationship between coronary plaque calcification and plaque instability has been debated. Biomechanical studies have calculated stress at different regions of the plaque. Mathematical models using large-strain finite element analysis have shown that increased lipids are associated with areas of weakness of the fibrous cap, but not calcification [35]. Although calcification is a good marker for plaque burden, absolute calcium scores do not indicate plaques that are unstable or prone to result in clinical events. It has been stated that calcification is a "disease marker" as opposed to a "process marker," unlike markers of inflammation [36]. These findings are corroborated by autopsy studies that demonstrate a good correlation between plaque size and morphometric analysis of calcification, but no correlation between residual lumen and calcification (Table 19.3). Few studies have correlated the radiologic pattern of calcification with plaque instability [37], but there is some suggestion that speckled or fragmented calcification patterns as determined radiologically are most likely associated with unstable plaque types (Fig. 19.13).

Vulnerable Plaque by Computed Tomography

Cardiac computed tomography (CT) imaging is now able to visualize the coronary lumen and atherosclerotic plaques. Motoyama et al. reported that the features of high-risk plaque for acute coronary syndrome were positive remodeling, spotty calcification, and low plaque attenuation (<30 Hounsfield units [HU]) [38]. Other studies have described specific attenuation pattern of atherosclerotic plaques on coronary CT images characterized by a necrotic core with low CT attenuation area surrounded by a rim-like area of higher CT attenuation as "napkin ring" [39–41] (Fig. 19.14). This "napkin-ring" finding has a high specificity and high positive predictive value for the presence of advanced lesions [42, 43]. The noninvasive identification of vulnerable plaque is one of the ultimate goals of coronary imaging because it would improve risk stratification of both symptomatic and asymptomatic patients [44].

Longitudinal Image of CT

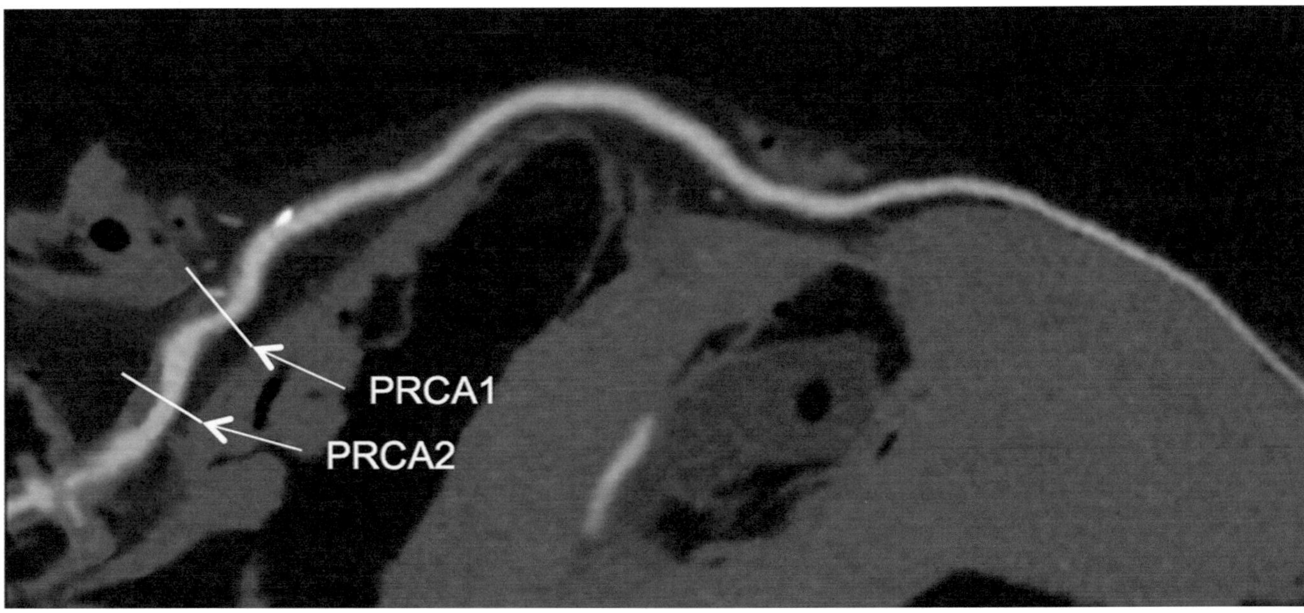

Fig. 19.14 The longitudinal CT image of the RCA demonstrates atherosclerotic plaques with spotty calcification in the proximal segment of the RCA. The bars (*PRCA 1* and *PRCA2*) indicate cross sections within the coronary plaques that were compared with histopathology. The cross-sectional CT images from *PRCA1* show a coronary atherosclerotic plaque cross section with napkin-ring-like attenuation pattern and spotty calcification. The circumferential outer rim (red dashed *line*) of the plaque has a higher CT attenuation in both the noncontrast- (*A*) and contrast-enhanced (*B*) images (61.8 ± 9.3 HU, range 42.4–74.9 HU vs. 67.3 ± 11.6 HU, range 43.4–87.0 HU, respectively) as compared to the attenuation within the central part of the plaque (43.4 ± 7.5 HU, range 35.2–62.9 HU and 43.2 ± 14.0 HU, range 21.2–72.5 HU, on noncontrast- and contrast-enhanced images, respectively). The average noncalcified plaque attenuation on nonenhanced CT was 52.8 ± 10.9 HU versus 58.5 ± 17.1 HU attenuation on the contrast-enhanced image. Histopathology revealed a thin-cap fibroatheroma (*C*, *D*) with spotty calcification (*E*). Again, the necrotic core (*stars*) correlates with the low-attenuation plaque core on the CT images. Similar to the previous figures, the outer-rim attenuation (*red dashed line*) on the noncontrast- and contrast-enhanced CT images corresponds to the fibrous plaque tissue. In addition, the presence of spotty calcification correlates to the CT findings. The CT images from *PRCA2* show a pronounced napkin-ring-like attenuation pattern. The circumferential outer rim (*red dashed line*) of the plaque has a higher CT attenuation in both the noncontrast- (*A*) and contrast-enhanced (*B*) images (57.2 ± 8.8 HU, range 40.0–81.0 HU vs. 57.9 ± 8.7 HU, range 35.0–76.0 HU, respectively) as compared to the attenuation within the central part of the plaque (21.8 ± 4.3 HU, range 13.5–31.6 HU and 26.0 ± 2.0 HU, range 22.0–31.0 HU on noncontrast- and contrast-enhanced images, respectively). The average plaque attenuation on nonenhanced CT was 48.1 ± 14.2 HU versus 52.2 ± 14.0 HU on the contrast-enhanced CT. The corresponding histopathological section (*C*) demonstrates a late fibroatheroma. Again, the plaque contains a necrotic core (*stars*), which correlates to the low-attenuation plaque core on the CT images. The outer portion of the plaque (*red-dashed line*) contains a significant amount of fibrous plaque tissue correlating to the high-attenuation CT rim. Moreover, the histopathological analysis revealed significant vasa vasorum (*C*, *arrowheads*) accompanied by macrophage infiltration in the basal plaque area. (From Maurovich-Horvat et al. [42], with permission)

PRCA 1

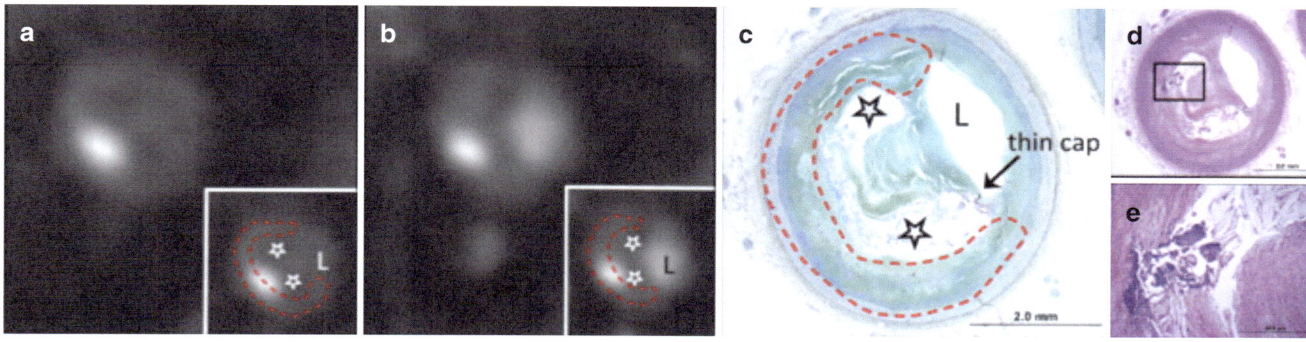

PRCA 2

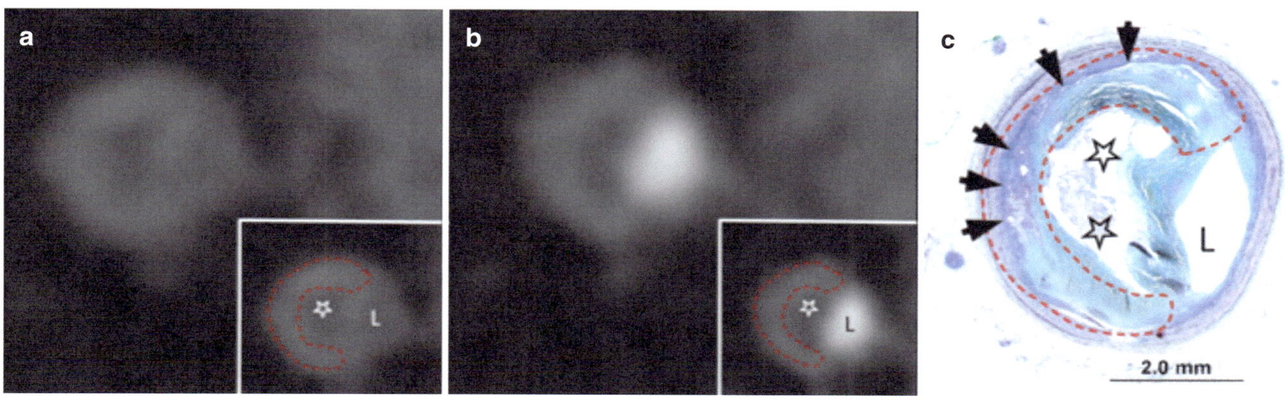

Fig. 19.14 (continued)

References

1. Virmani R, Kolodgie FD, Burke AP, Farb A, Schwartz SM. Lessons from sudden coronary death: a comprehensive morphological classification scheme for atherosclerotic lesions. Arterioscler Thromb Vasc Biol. 2000;20:1262–75.
2. Stary HC, Chandler AB, Dinsmore RE, Fuster V, Glagov S, Insull W, et al. A definition of advanced types of atherosclerotic lesions and a histological classification of atherosclerosis. A report from the Committee on Vascular Lesions of the Council on Arteriosclerosis, American Heart Association. Arterioscler Thromb Vasc Biol. 1995;15:1512–31.
3. Davies MJ, Thomas A. Thrombosis and acute coronary-artery lesions in sudden cardiac ischemic death. N Engl J Med. 1984;310:1137–40.
4. Yahagi K, Kolodgie FD, Otsuka F, Finn AV, Davis HR, Joner M, et al. Pathophysiology of native coronary, vein graft, and in-stent atherosclerosis. Nat Rev Cardiol. 2016;13:79–98. Nature Publishing Group.
5. Nakashima Y, Chen Y-X, Kinukawa N, Sueishi K. Distributions of diffuse intimal thickening in human arteries: preferential expression in atherosclerosis-prone arteries from an early age. Virchows Arch. 2002;441:279–88.
6. Ikari Y, McManus BM, Kenyon J, Schwartz SM. Neonatal intima formation in the human coronary artery. Arterioscler Thromb Vasc Biol. 1999;19:2036–40.
7. Cohn JN, Goldstein SO, Greenberg BH, Lorell BH, Bourge RC, Jaski BE, et al. A dose-dependent increase in mortality with vesnarinone among patients with severe heart failure. Vesnarinone Trial Investigators. N Engl J Med. 1998;339:1810–6.
8. McGill HC, McMahan CA, Herderick EE, Tracy RE, Malcom GT, Zieske AW, et al. Effects of coronary heart disease risk factors on atherosclerosis of selected regions of the aorta and right coronary artery. PDAY Research Group. Pathobiological Determinants of Atherosclerosis in Youth. Arterioscler Thromb Vasc Biol. 2000;20:836–45.
9. Fan J, Watanabe T. Inflammatory reactions in the pathogenesis of atherosclerosis. J Atheroscler Thromb. 2003;10:63–71.
10. Aikawa M, Rabkin E, Okada Y, Voglic SJ, Clinton SK, Brinckerhoff CE, et al. Lipid lowering by diet reduces matrix metalloproteinase activity and increases collagen content of rabbit atheroma: a potential mechanism of lesion stabilization. Circulation. 1998;97:2433–44.
11. Kockx MM, De Meyer GR, Bortier H, de Meyere N, Muhring J, Bakker A, et al. Luminal foam cell accumulation is associated with smooth muscle cell death in the intimal thickening of human saphenous vein grafts. Circulation. 1996;94:1255–62.
12. Proudfoot D, Shanahan CM. Biology of calcification in vascular cells: intima versus media. Herz. 2001;26:245–51.
13. Kolodgie FD, Gold HK, Burke AP, Fowler DR, Kruth HS, Weber DK, et al. Intraplaque hemorrhage and progression of coronary atheroma. N Engl J Med. 2003;349:2316–25.
14. Sluimer JC, Kolodgie FD, Bijnens AP, Maxfield K, Pacheco E, Kutys B, et al. Thin-walled microvessels in human coronary atherosclerotic plaques show incomplete endothelial junctions. Relevance of compromised structural integrity for intraplaque microvascular leakage. J Am Coll Cardiol. 2009;53:1517–27. American College of Cardiology Foundation.

15. Burke AP, Farb A, Malcom GT, Liang YH, Smialek J, Virmani R. Coronary risk factors and plaque morphology in men with coronary disease who died suddenly. N Engl J Med. 1997;336:1276–82.
16. Michel JB, Virmani R, Arbustini E, Pasterkamp G. Intraplaque haemorrhages as the trigger of plaque vulnerability. Eur Heart J. 2011;32:1977–85.
17. Farb A, Burke AP, Tang AL, Liang TY, Mannan P, Smialek J, et al. Coronary plaque erosion without rupture into a lipid core. A frequent cause of coronary thrombosis in sudden coronary death. Circulation. 1996;93:1354–63.
18. Roberts WC, Kragel AH, Gertz SD, Roberts CS, Kalan JM. The heart in fatal unstable angina pectoris. Am J Cardiol. 1991;68:22B–7B.
19. Libby P. Molecular bases of the acute coronary syndromes. Circulation. 1995;91:2844–50.
20. Libby P, Sukhova G, Lee RT, Galis ZS. Cytokines regulate vascular functions related to stability of the atherosclerotic plaque. J Cardiovasc Pharmacol. 1995;25 Suppl 2:S9–12.
21. Virmani R, Kolodgie FD, Burke AP, Finn AV, Gold HK, Tulenko TN, et al. Atherosclerotic plaque progression and vulnerability to rupture: angiogenesis as a source of intraplaque hemorrhage. Arterioscler Thromb Vasc Biol. 2005;25:2054–61.
22. Burke AP, Farb A, Malcom GT, Liang Y, Smialek JE, Virmani R. Plaque rupture and sudden death related to exertion in men with coronary artery disease. JAMA. 1999;281:921–6.
23. Schwartz RS, Burke A, Farb A, Kaye D, Lesser JR, Henry TD, et al. Microemboli and microvascular obstruction in acute coronary thrombosis and sudden coronary death. relation to epicardial plaque histopathology. J Am Coll Cardiol. 2009;54:2167–73. Elsevier Inc.
24. Yahagi K, Zarpak R, Sakakura K, Otsuka F, Kutys R, Ladich E, et al. Multiple simultaneous plaque erosion in 3 coronary arteries. JACC Cardiovasc Imaging. 2014;7:1172–4.
25. Yahagi K, Davis HR, Arbustini E, Virmani R. Sex differences in coronary artery disease: pathological observations. Atherosclerosis. 2015;239:260–7.
26. Mann J, Davies MJ. Mechanisms of progression in native coronary artery disease: role of healed plaque disruption. Heart. 1999;82:265–8.
27. Burke AP, Weber DK, Kolodgie FD, Farb A, Taylor AJ, Virmani R. Pathophysiology of calcium deposition in coronary arteries. Herz. 2001;26:239–44.
28. Sakakura K, Nakano M, Otsuka F, Yahagi K, Kutys R, Ladich E, et al. Comparison of pathology of chronic total occlusion with and without coronary artery bypass graft. Eur Heart J. 2014;35:1683–93.
29. Kumamoto M, Nakashima Y, Sueishi K. Intimal neovascularization in human coronary atherosclerosis: its origin and pathophysiological significance. Hum Pathol. 1995;26:450–6.
30. Heistad DD, Armstrong ML. Blood flow through vasa vasorum of coronary arteries in atherosclerotic monkeys. Arteriosclerosis. 1986;6:326–31.
31. Williams JK, Armstrong ML, Heistad DD. Vasa vasorum in atherosclerotic coronary arteries: responses to vasoactive stimuli and regression of atherosclerosis. Circ Res. 1988;62:515–23.
32. Virmani R, Roberts WC. Extravasated erythrocytes, iron, and fibrin in atherosclerotic plaques of coronary arteries in fatal coronary heart disease and their relation to luminal thrombus: frequency and significance in 57 necropsy patients and in 2958 five mm segments of 224 major epicardial coronary arteries. Am Heart J. 1983;105:788–97.
33. Constantinides P. Coronary thrombosis linked to fissure in atherosclerotic vessel wall. JAMA. 1964;188 Suppl:35–7.
34. Pasterkamp G, Virmani R. The erythrocyte: a new player in atheromatous core formation. Heart. 2002;88:115–6.
35. Huang H, Virmani R, Younis H, Burke AP, Kamm RD, Lee RT. The impact of calcification on the biomechanical stability of atherosclerotic plaques. Circulation. 2001;103:1051–6.
36. Hunt ME, O'Malley PG, Vernalis MN, Feuerstein IM, Taylor AJ. C-reactive protein is not associated with the presence or extent of calcified subclinical atherosclerosis. Am Heart J. 2001;141:206–10.
37. Burke AP, Taylor A, Farb A, Malcom GT, Virmani R. Coronary calcification: insights from sudden coronary death victims. Z Kardiol. 2000;89 Suppl 2:49–53.
38. Motoyama S, Kondo T, Sarai M, Sugiura A, Harigaya H, Sato T, et al. Multislice computed tomographic characteristics of coronary lesions in acute coronary syndromes. J Am Coll Cardiol. 2007;50:319–26.
39. Narula J, Achenbach S. Napkin-ring necrotic cores: defining circumferential extent of necrotic cores in unstable plaques. JACC Cardiovasc Imaging. 2009;2:1436–8.
40. Kashiwagi M, Tanaka A, Kitabata H, Tsujioka H, Kataiwa H, Komukai K, et al. Feasibility of noninvasive assessment of thin-cap fibroatheroma by multidetector computed tomography. JACC Cardiovasc Imaging. 2009;2:1412–9.
41. Tanaka A, Shimada K, Yoshida K, Jissyo S, Tanaka H, Sakamoto M, et al. Non-invasive assessment of plaque rupture by 64-slice multidetector computed tomography – comparison with intravascular ultrasound. Circ J. 2008;72:1276–81.
42. Maurovich-Horvat P, Hoffmann U, Vorpahl M, Nakano M, Virmani R, Alkadhi H. The napkin-ring sign: CT signature of high-risk coronary plaques? JACC Cardiovasc Imaging. 2010;3:440–4.
43. Maurovich-Horvat P, Schlett CL, Alkadhi H, Nakano M, Otsuka F, Stolzmann P, et al. The napkin-ring sign indicates advanced atherosclerotic lesions in coronary CT angiography. JACC Cardiovasc Imaging. 2012;5:1243–52.
44. Narula J, Garg P, Achenbach S, Motoyama S, Virmani R, Strauss HW. Arithmetic of vulnerable plaques for noninvasive imaging. Nat Clin Pract Cardiovasc Med. 2008;5 Suppl 2:S2–10.
45. Can atherosclerosis imaging techniques improve the detection of patients at risk for ischemic heart disease? Proceedings of the 34th Bethesda Conference. Bethesda, Maryland, USA. October 7, 2002. J Am Coll Cardiol. 2003;41:1856–917.
46. Burke AP, Kolodgie FD, Farb A, Weber DK, Malcom GT, Smialek J, et al. Healed plaque ruptures and sudden coronary death: evidence that subclinical rupture has a role in plaque progression. Circulation. 2001;103:934–40.

CT Cardiac Anatomy

20

Michael A. Kadoch and Hans-Christoph R. F. Becker

The heart is a mediastinal structure that rests on the diaphragm and is separated from the lung parenchyma on either side by the pericardium, pleura, and fat. The innermost layer of the ventricle is the endocardium, the bulk of the ventricular wall is comprised of the myocardium, and the outermost layer is the epicardium. The fat layer just beyond the epicardium represents epicardial adipose tissue. The visceral and parietal layers of the pericardium are identified just beyond the epicardial fat. A small amount of pericardial fluid is physiologically present between these layers. The normal thickness of the pericardium is usually 1–2 mm and is considered abnormal when greater than 4 mm. The fat layer just beyond the parietal pericardium represents paracardial adipose tissue. The base of the heart refers to its posterior surface and is formed by the atria, mainly the left atrium, and is separated from the vertebral bodies by the esophagus and aorta. The apex of the heart refers to its inferior tip and is usually formed by the left ventricle.

Coronary Arteries

The coronary arteries (Fig. 20.1) originate normally from the aortic sinuses of Valsalva that face the pulmonary root. The left main coronary artery (LM) arises from the left coronary sinus and courses between the left atrial appendage and the right ventricular outflow tract. The LM usually bifurcates into the left anterior descending (LAD) and left circumflex (LCx) coronary arteries. In approximately 20% of patients, the LM trifurcates with a ramus intermedius (RI) branch identified between the LAD and LCx.

M. A. Kadoch (✉)
Department of Radiology, University of California, Davis, CA, USA
e-mail: mkadoch@ucdavis.edu

H.-C. R. F. Becker
Department of Radiology, Stanford University, Stanford, CA, USA

The LAD courses in the anterior interventricular groove and gives off septal perforator braches that supply the interventricular septum in addition to diagonal branches that supply the anterior and anterolateral walls of the left ventricle. Myocardial bridging is a common congenital anomaly that is seen in approximately 25% of the population and is most commonly identified within the midportion of the LAD. This bridged segment is classically described as being protected from the development of atherosclerotic disease but can occasionally be a cause of anginal symptoms and may predispose to increased plaque development within more proximal portions of the LAD with an associated increased risk of acute coronary events due to rupture of this plaque formation. The LAD typically gives off two diagonal branches (D1 and D2), and its distal end can be seen wrapping around the left ventricular apex in the majority of patients.

The LCx courses in the left atrioventricular groove and contributes obtuse marginal branches (typically two, OM1 and OM2) that supply the lateral and inferolateral walls of the left ventricle. The most common coronary artery anomaly involves the LCx arising from either the right coronary sinus independently or as a branch of the right coronary artery (RCA) before taking a retroaortic course to the left atrioventricular groove. Knowledge of this anomaly is important in patients undergoing aortic valve surgery since its presence can introduce complications during the procedure.

The RCA arises from the right coronary sinus and courses within the right atrioventricular groove. The first branch of the RCA is often the conus artery, which typically supplies the anterior interventricular septum in addition to the conal tissue of the right ventricular outflow tract. Independent origin of the conus artery from the right coronary sinus is a common variant seen in up to 50% of patients. The second branch of the RCA is typically the sinoatrial (SA) nodal artery, which courses posteriorly to supply the SA node. The SA nodal artery is a branch of the LCx as a variant in approximately 40% of patients. The acute marginal branches arise from the mid to distal RCA and are its largest branches,

U. J. Schoepf (ed.), *CT of the Heart*, Contemporary Medical Imaging, https://doi.org/10.1007/978-1-60327-237-7_20

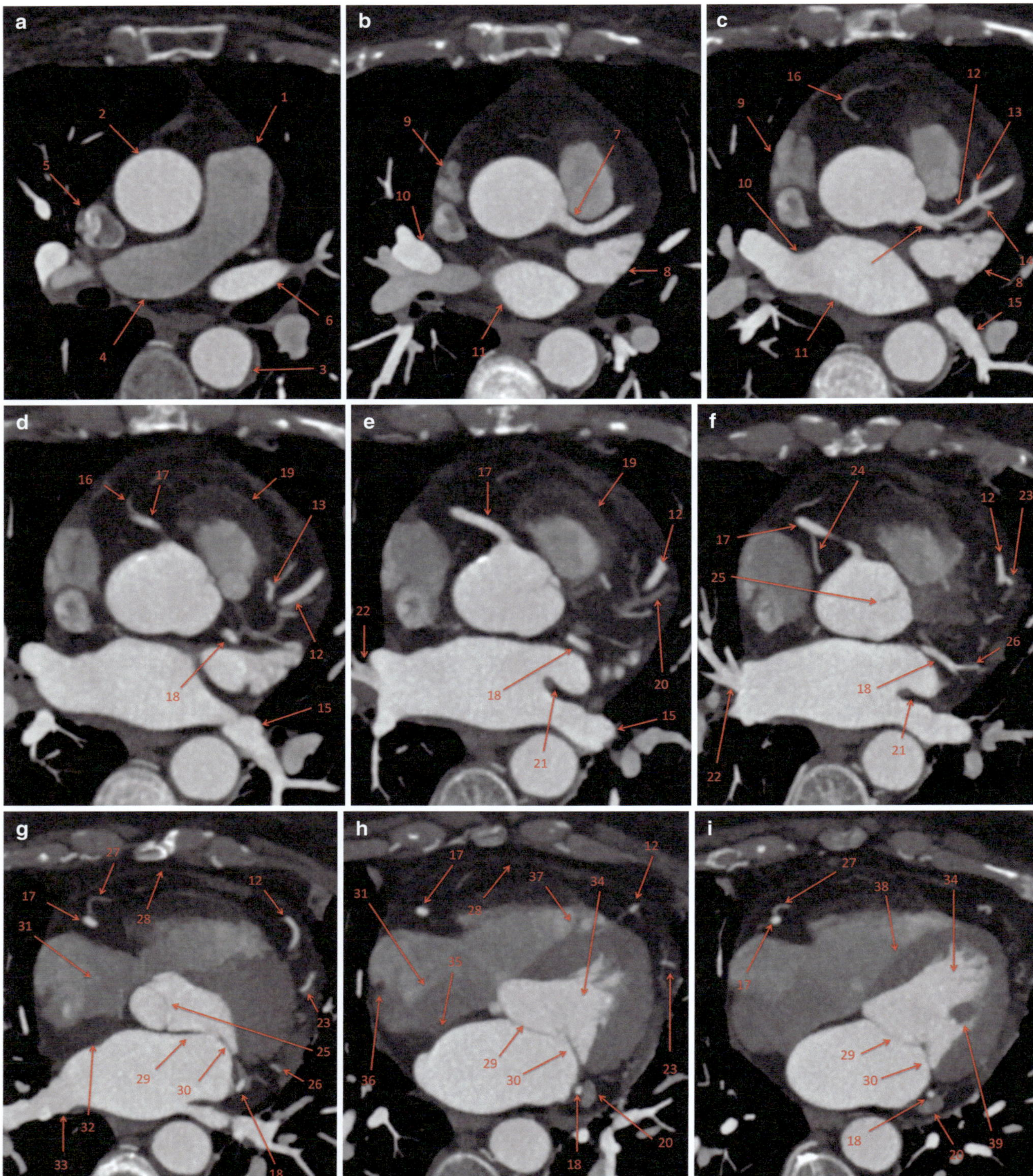

Fig. 20.1 (a–q) Axial CT cardiac anatomy. 1. Main pulmonary artery. 2. Ascending thoracic aorta. 3. Descending thoracic aorta. 4. Right pulmonary artery. 5. Superior vena cava. 6. Left superior pulmonary vein. 7. Left main coronary artery. 8. Left atrial appendage. 9. Right atrial appendage. 10. Right superior pulmonary vein. 11. Left atrium. 12. Left anterior descending coronary artery. 13. First septal perforator. 14. First diagonal branch. 15. Left inferior pulmonary vein. 16. Conus artery. 17. Right coronary artery. 18. Left circumflex coronary artery. 19. Conus. 20. Great cardiac vein. 21. Coumadin ridge. 22. Right middle pulmonary vein. 23. Second diagonal branch. 24. Sinoatrial nodal artery. 25. Aortic valve. 26. First obtuse marginal branch. 27. Acute marginal branch. 28. Pericardium. 29. Anterior leaflet of the mitral valve. 30. Posterior leaflet of the mitral valve. 31. Right atrium. 32. Interatrial septum. 33. Right inferior pulmonary vein. 34. Left ventricle. 35. Fossa ovalis. 36. Crista terminalis. 37. Moderator band. 38. Interventricular septum. 39. Anterior papillary muscle of the left ventricle. 40. Right ventricle. 41. Tricuspid valve. 42. Posterior papillary muscle of the left ventricle. 43. Coronary sinus. 44. Second obtuse marginal branch. 45. Posterolateral branch. 46. Inferior vena cava. 47. Posterior descending coronary artery. 48. Middle cardiac vein

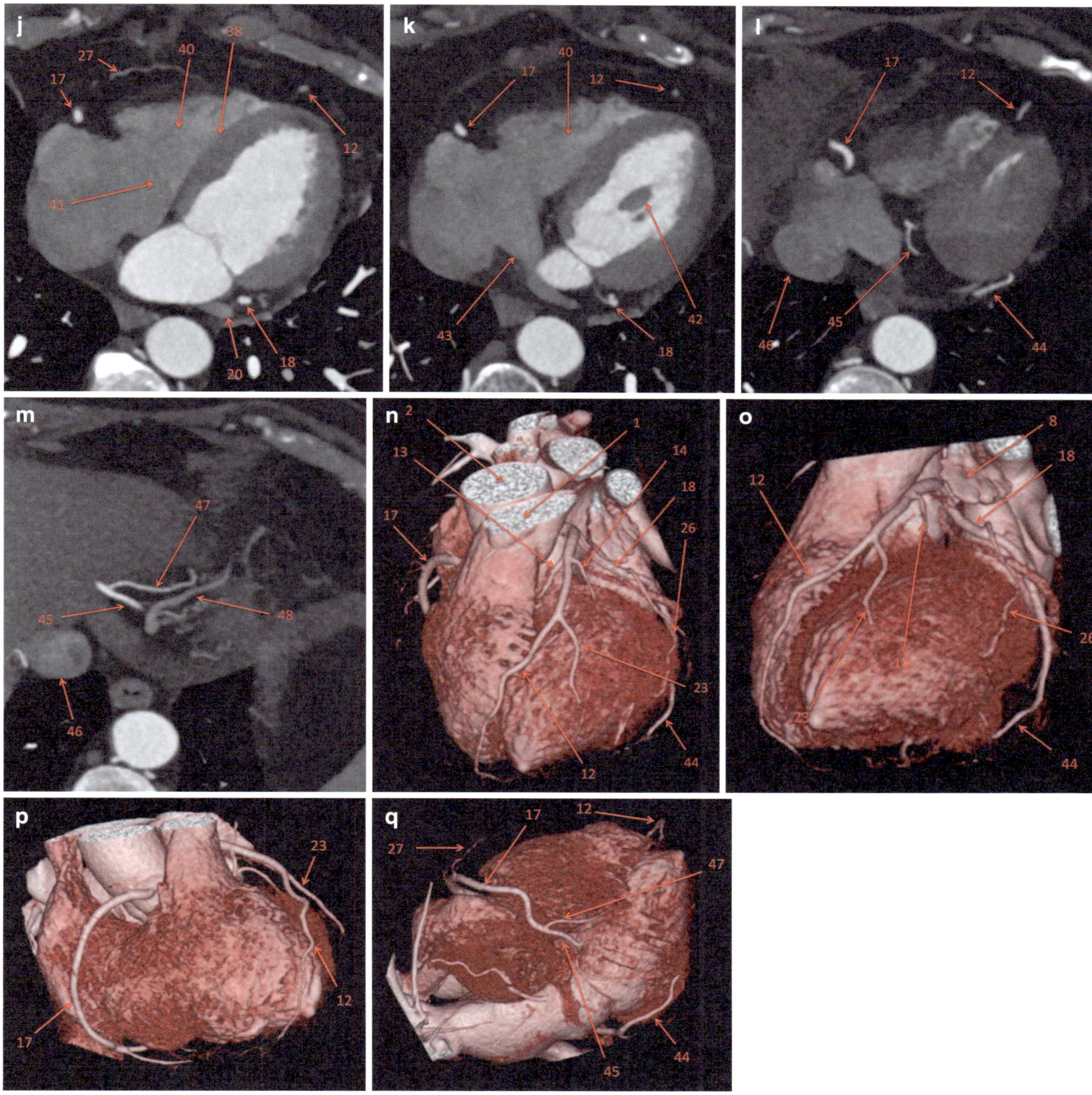

Fig. 20.1 (continued)

which supply the right ventricular free wall. The atrioventricular nodal artery is usually a branch of the RCA at the crux of the heart where it can be seen coursing anteriorly to supply the atrioventricular node. The posterior descending artery (PDA) and the posterolateral branch (PLB) are the terminal branches of the RCA in a right-dominant system supplying the inferior and inferolateral walls of the left ventricle. The PDA courses in the posterior interventricular groove.

Coronary artery dominance is most accurately defined by the coronary artery that supplies the PDA and PLB. In a right-dominant system (approximately 80% of patients), both branches are supplied by the RCA. In a left-dominant system (approximately 15% of patients), both branches are supplied by the LCx. In a codominant system (approximately 5% of patients), the PDA and/or PLB are supplied by branches of both the RCA and LCx.

In 2009, the Society for Cardiovascular Computed Tomography (SCCT) released guidelines for the interpretation and reporting of coronary computed tomographic angiography (CCTA) (Fig. 20.2; Table 20.1) [1]. As part of

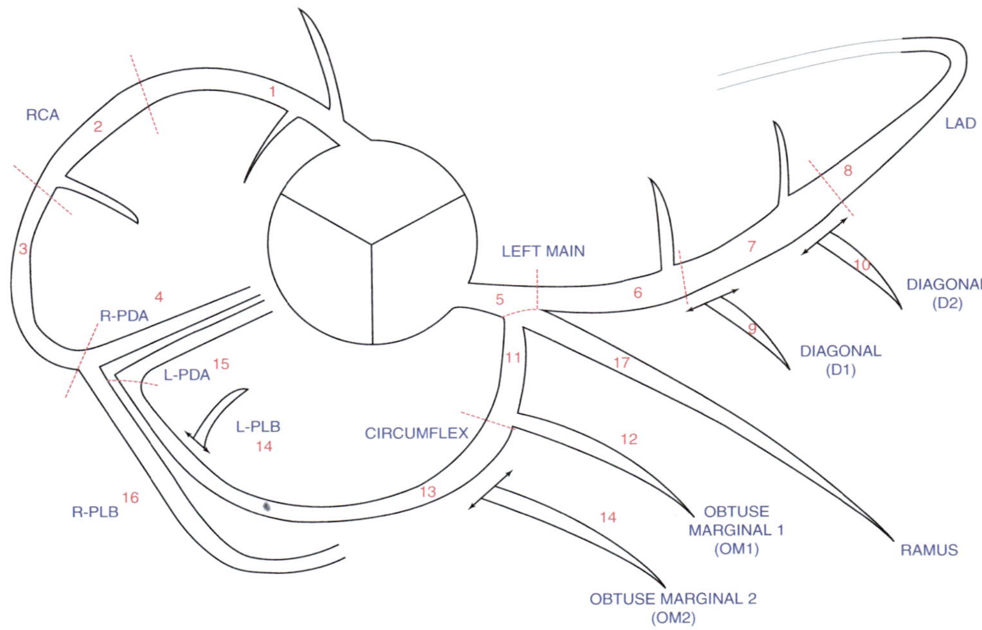

Fig. 20.2 SCCT coronary segmentation diagram. See Table 20.1. (From Raff et al. [1], with permission)

Table 20.1 SCCT segmentation of axial coronary anatomy

Segment	Abbreviation	Description
Proximal RCA	pRCA	Ostium of the RCA (right coronary artery) to one-half the distance to the acute margin of heart
Mid-RCA	mRCA	End of proximal RCA to the acute margin of heart
Distal RCA	dRCA	End of mid-RCA to origin of the PDA (posterior descending artery)
PDA-RCA	R-PDA	PDA from RCA
PLB-RCA	R-PLB	PLB (posterior-lateral branch) from RCA
LM	LM	Ostium of LM (left main) to bifurcation of LAD (left anterior descending artery) and LCx (left circumflex artery)
Proximal LAD	pLAD	End of LM to the first large septal or D1 (first diagonal), whichever is most proximal
Mid LAD	mLAD	End of proximal LAD to one-half the distance to the apex
Distal LAD	dLAD	End of mid-LAD to end of LAD
Diagonal 1	D1	First diagonal branch D1
Diagonal 2	D2	Second diagonal branch D2
Proximal LCx	pCx	End of LM to the origin of the OM1 (first obtuse marginal)
OM1	OM1	First OM1 traversing the lateral wall of the left ventricle
Mid and distal LCx	LCx	Traveling in the AV groove, distal to the first obtuse marginal branch to the end of the vessel or origin of the L-PDA (left posterior descending artery)
OM2	OM2	Second marginal OM2
PDA-LCx	L-PDA	PDA from LCx
Ramus intermedius	RI	Vessel originating from the left main between the LAD and LCx in case of a trifurcation
PLB-L	L-PLB	PLB from LCx
		Dashed lines represent division between RCA, LAD, and LCx and the end of the LMPLB = PLV (posterior left ventricular branch). Additional nomenclature may be added, for example, D3, R-PDA2, SVF (saphenous vein graft), mLAD

See Fig. 20.2 for accompanying diagram. From Raff et al. [1], with permission

that publication, the SCCT advocates for the use of an 18-segment model of the axial coronary anatomy, which more closely emulates the CCTA views of the coronary arteries than the standard views obtained from invasive angiography. Adopting this standardized approach to coronary segmentation can improve the description and communication of findings among radiologists and with referring clinicians.

Coronary Veins

The anatomy of the coronary veins (Fig. 20.1) is not as straightforward as the arterial anatomy since variations are common [2]. However, knowledge of the coronary venous system is increasingly important as more CT imaging is being performed prior to cardiac pacing and transvenous ablation procedures.

The great cardiac vein accompanies the LAD along the anterior interventricular groove and the LCx along the left atrioventricular groove before terminating in the left end of the coronary sinus (CS). The middle cardiac vein accompanies the PDA along the posterior interventricular groove before terminating in the right end of the CS. The small cardiac vein accompanies the RCA along the right atrioventricular groove before terminating in the right end of the CS. The right marginal vein runs along the inferior margin of the heart before terminating in the small cardiac vein. The oblique vein of the left atrium runs along the posterior surface of the left atrium before terminating in the left end of the CS. The posterior vein of the left ventricle runs along the diaphragmatic surface of the left ventricle before terminating in the middle of the CS.

The CS is identified within the posterior atrioventricular groove and is of variable length. A prominent Thebesian valve is occasionally seen at the ostium of the CS, which may pose an obstacle to interventionalists trying to engage the CS.

The anterior cardiac veins of the right ventricle and the smallest cardiac veins (Thebesian veins) terminate directly into the right atrium. The small cardiac vein may also terminate directly into the right atrium.

Cardiac Chambers

The right atrium (RA) receives blood from the superior vena cava (SVC), inferior vena cava (IVC), and the CS. The crista terminalis is a vertically oriented smooth muscle ridge within the superior portion of the right atrium that might occasionally be mistaken for a mass when increased in prominence. The Eustachian valve is occasionally seen at the junction of the IVC and the RA. The right atrial appendage (RAA) is pyramidal in shape and larger in size than the left atrial appendage (LAA).

Blood enters the right ventricle (RV) from the RA via the tricuspid valve (TV). The RV is more coarsely trabeculated than the left ventricle (LV) and can also be distinguished by the presence of the moderator band, which is seen extending from the base of the anterior papillary muscle to the interventricular septum. The TV and pulmonic valve (PV) are separated by the muscular conal tissue of the right ventricular outflow tract (RVOT), which is in distinction to the fibrous continuity of the mitral and aortic valves of the left heart.

Blood returns to the left atrium (LA) via the pulmonary veins. The LAA is variable in shape but can be distinguished from the RAA by its smaller size, finger-like configuration, and corrugated internal surface owing to the presence of parallel pectinate muscles. The atria are separated by the interatrial septum. The fossa ovalis (FO) is an oval-shaped depression on the right atrial side of the interatrial septum, which may be traversed during interventional procedures requiring transseptal puncture. The FO is an important landmark to identify because it may be spared in cases of lipomatous septal hypertrophy, is the location where a patent foramen ovale may be seen, and is the most common region of attachment for cardiac myxomas. Maximum anteroposterior diameter measurements of the LA greater than 4.5 cm at the level of the aortic root on axial images are 91% specific for LA enlargement [3]. LA enlargement is a common finding in patients with atrial fibrillation.

Blood enters the left ventricle (LV) via the mitral valve (MV). The LV lies posterior and to the left of the RV and is distinguished by its smoother wall and two large papillary muscles (anterior and posterior). The left ventricular apical thin point (LVATP) is an important landmark to identify in order to generate the standard cardiac planes. Maximum diameter measurements of the LV greater than 5.5 cm at the level of the papillary muscle tips on axial images are 93% specific for LV enlargement [3].

The American Heart Association (AHA) recommends dividing the heart into 17 segments for assessment of the myocardium and the left ventricular cavity [4]. According to this segmentation system, the heart is divided into equal thirds perpendicular to its long-axis with the basal portion identified at the tips of the mitral valve leaflets, the mid-cavity identified at the level of the papillary muscles, and the apical portion identified beyond the papillary muscles but before the cavity ends (Fig. 20.3). Individual myocardial segments are then assigned to the three major coronary arteries recognizing that there is anatomic variability (Fig. 20.4).

Cardiac Valves

The TV is comprised of anterior, septal, and posterior leaflets. The anterior leaflet is the largest and separates the inflow and outflow tracts of the RV. The septal leaflet has many direct chordal attachments to the interventricular septum, and the posterior leaflet is usually the smallest. The normal TV is slightly displaced apically as compared with the MV. In Ebstein's anomaly, this displacement will exceed 8 mm/m^2 of the body surface area.

The MV is comprised of anterior and posterior leaflets (Fig. 20.1). The large semicircular anterior leaflet separates

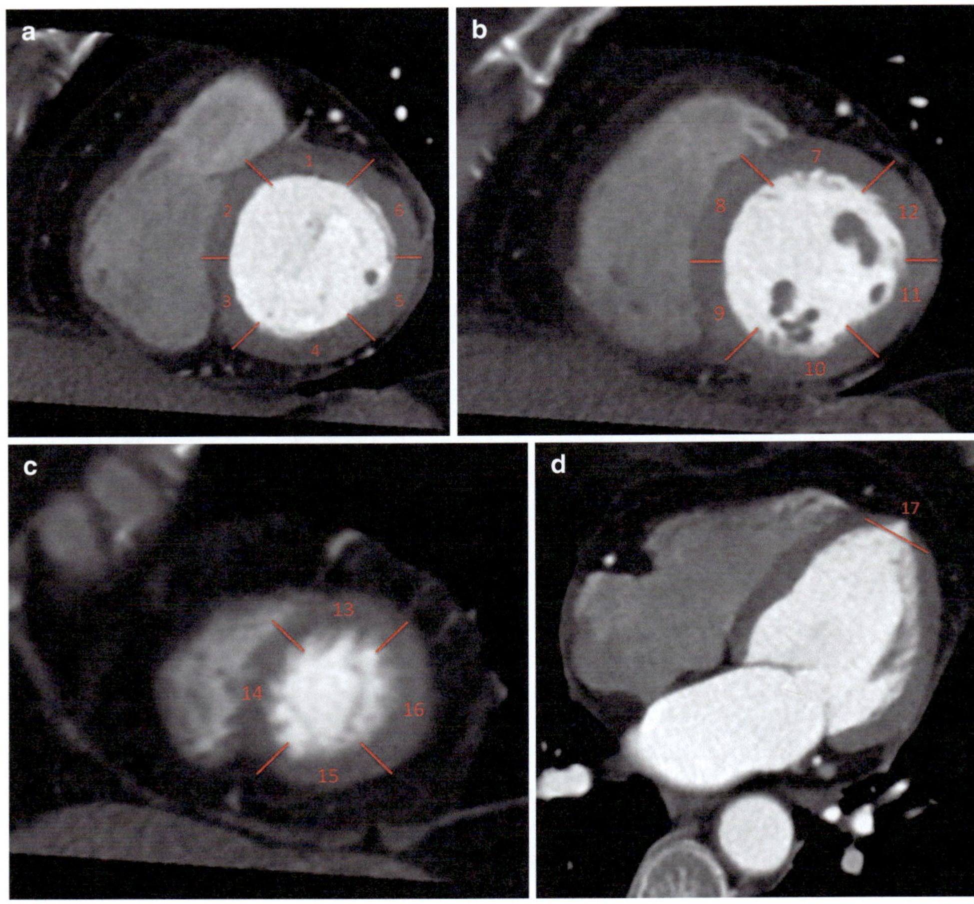

Fig. 20.3 (**a–d**) Short axis view of the heart with AHA 17-segment model of the left ventricle. Segment 1: basal anterior wall. Segment 2: basal anteroseptal wall. Segment 3: basal inferoseptal wall. Segment 4: basal inferior wall. Segment 5: basal inferolateral wall. Segment 6: basal anterolateral wall. Segment 7: mid-anterior wall. Segment 8: mid-anteroseptal wall. Segment 9: mid-inferoseptal wall. Segment 10: mid-inferior wall. Segment 11: mid-inferolateral wall. Segment 12: mid-anterolateral wall. Segment 13: apical anterior wall. Segment 14: apical septal wall. Segment 15: apical inferior wall. Segment 16: apical lateral wall. Segment 17: apex

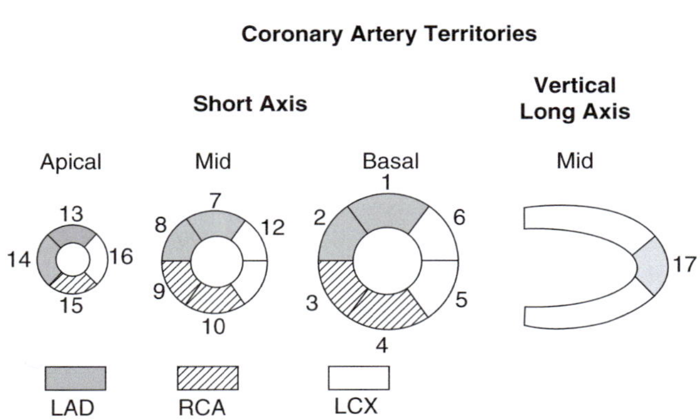

Fig. 20.4 Assignment of the 17 AHA myocardial segments to the coronary artery territories. (LAD left anterior descending coronary artery, RCA right coronary artery, LCX left circumflex coronary artery). (From Cerqueira et al. [4], with permission)

the inflow and outflow tracts of the LV. The anterior and posterior papillary muscles arise from the left ventricular wall and attach to the MV leaflets via fan-like chordae tendineae. Mitral valve prolapse (MVP) is defined by systolic atrial displacement of one or both of the MV leaflets by greater than 2 mm above the mitral annulus in a long-axis view.

The aortic valve (AV) is normally tricuspid and is comprised of semilunar-shaped left, right, and noncoronary cusps and associated commissures extending from the aortic annulus to the sinotubular junction (Fig. 20.5). The noncoronary cusp typically faces the interatrial septum and the right coronary cusp typically faces the sternum. The PV is also normally tricuspid and defines the point of transition from the RVOT to the main pulmonary artery (MPA). The MV and AV are better evaluated with CT than the TV and PV.

Pulmonary Veins

The muscular sleeves of the distal pulmonary veins are a frequent source of ectopic foci in patients with atrial fibrillation. CT is routinely performed for anatomic mapping of the pulmonary veins prior to ablation therapy (Fig. 20.6). The most common configuration of the pulmonary veins includes four separate branches for the right superior, right inferior, left superior, and left inferior pulmonary veins. Common variants include independent drainage of the right middle lobe vein into the left atrium and a single left-sided venous ostium [5, 6]. The "Coumadin ridge" is a ridge of smooth

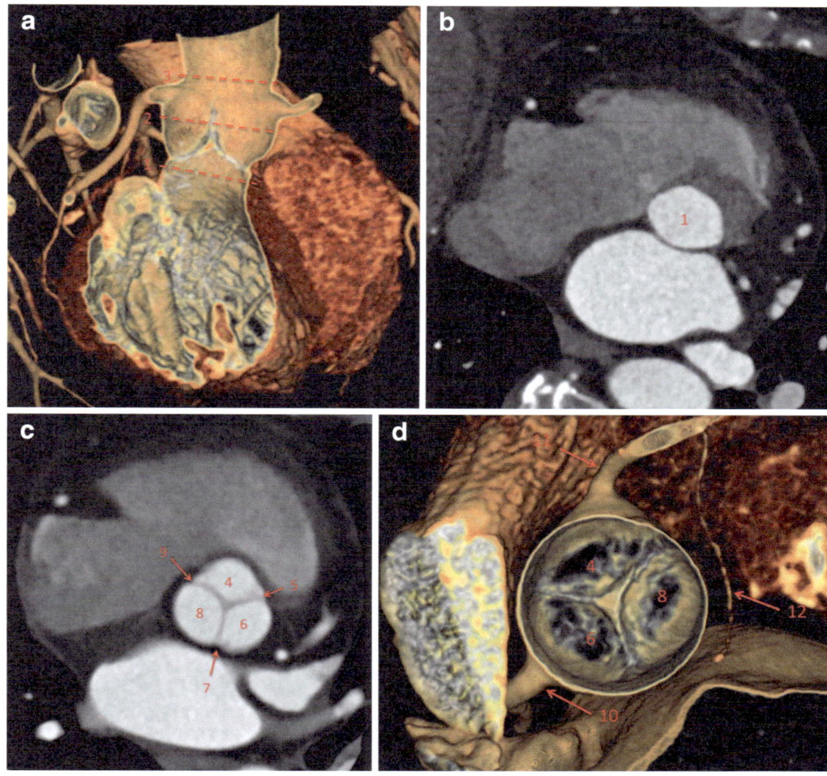

Fig. 20.5 (**a–d**) The aortic root. 1. Aortic annulus. 2. Sinuses of Valsalva. 3. Sinotubular junction. 4. Right coronary sinus. 5. Left-right commissure. 6. Left coronary sinus. 7. Left-noncoronary commissure. 8. Noncoronary sinus. 9. Right-noncoronary commissure. 10. Left main coronary artery. 11. Right coronary artery. 12. Sinoatrial nodal artery

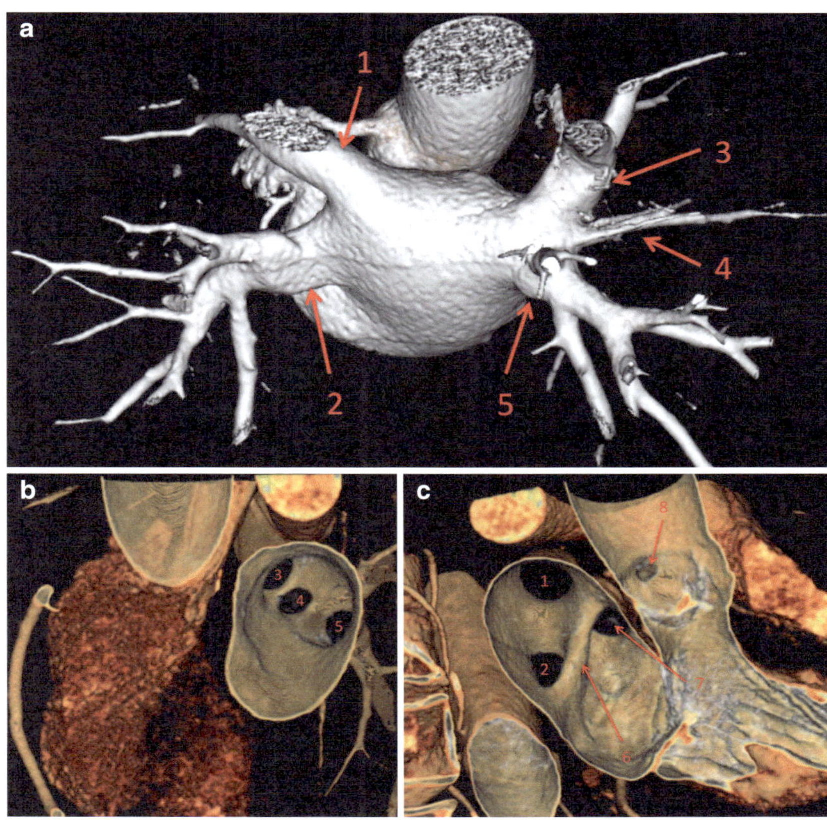

Fig. 20.6 (**a–c**) Pulmonary veins. 1. Left superior pulmonary vein. 2. Left inferior pulmonary vein. 3. Right superior pulmonary vein. 4. Right middle pulmonary vein. 5. Right inferior pulmonary vein. 6. Coumadin ridge. 7. Left atrial appendage. 8. Left main coronary artery

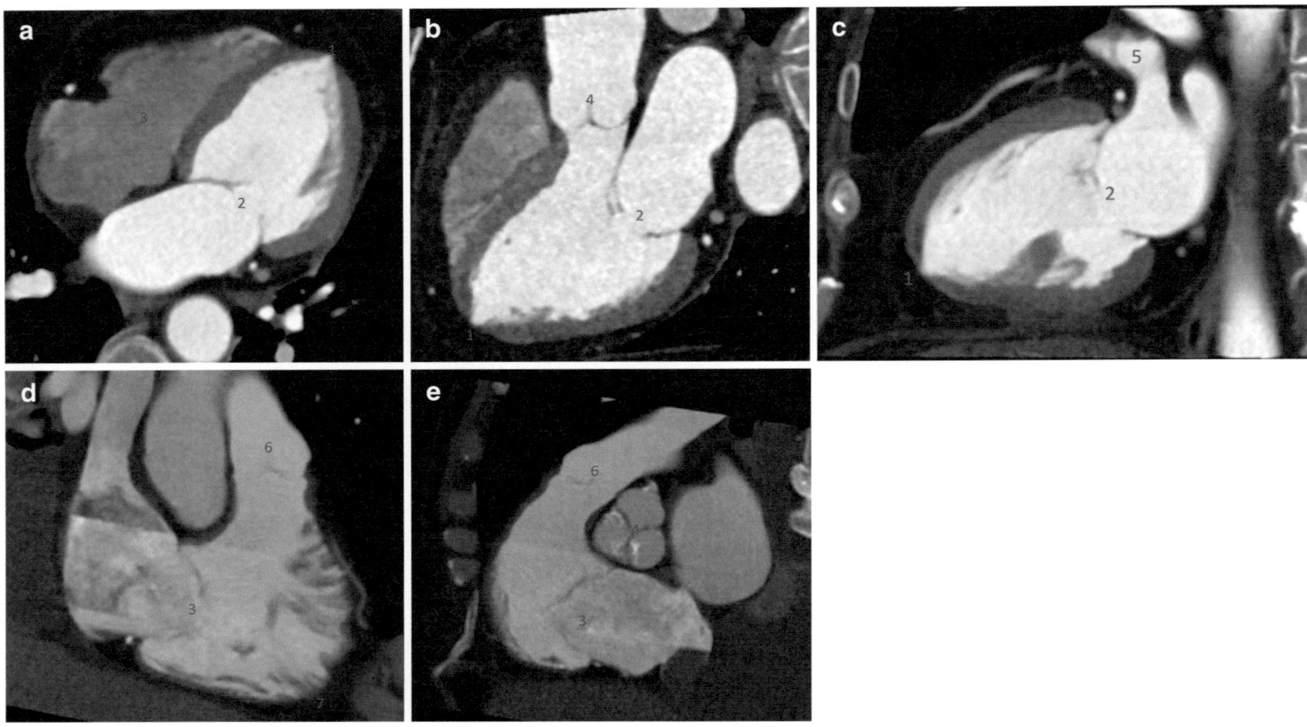

Fig. 20.7 Cardiac planes. (**a**) Horizontal long-axis (HLA) view. (**b**) Left ventricular outflow tract (LVOT) view. (**c**) Vertical long-axis (VLA) view. (**d**) Right ventricular three-chamber view. (**e**) Right ventricular outflow tract (RVOT) view. 1. Left ventricular apical thin point. 2. Mitral valve. 3. Tricuspid valve. 4. Aortic valve. 5. Left atrial appendage. 6. Pulmonic valve. 7. Right ventricular apex

muscle found along the wall of the LA at the junction of the LAA and the entrance of the left superior pulmonary vein. Its name is derived from the fact that it is frequently mistaken for a thrombus (or mass) with subsequent initiation of anticoagulation therapy. Partial anomalous pulmonary venous return is occasionally encountered as an incidental finding in asymptomatic adults with the left upper lobe being the most common site for this abnormality.

Cardiac Planes

In addition to routine axial, sagittal, and coronal planes, standard cardiac planes analogous to those obtained with echocardiography and MRI are often generated from CT data sets for better evaluation of the valves, ventricular walls, and outflow tracts (Fig. 20.7). These planes may be obtained using three points as follows (Fig. 20.7): the horizontal long-axis (HLA, or four-chamber) view using the center of the MV, the center of the TV, and the LVATP; the left ventricular outflow tract (LVOT, or LV three-chamber) view using the center of the MV, the center of the AV, and the LVATP; the vertical long-axis (VLA, or LV two-chamber) view using the center of the MV, the LVATP, and the bifurcation line between the HLA and LVOT views; the RV three-chamber view using the center of the TV, the center of the PV, and the RV apex; and the RVOT view using the center of the TV, the center of the PV, and the bifurcation line of the MPA. The short-axis (SAX) view can then be generated as a stack of perpendicular sections through either of the long-axis views of the heart.

References

1. Raff GL, Abidov A, Achenbach S, et al. SCCT guidelines for the interpretation and reporting of coronary computed tomographic angiography. J Cardiovasc Comput Tomogr. 2009;3(2):122–36.
2. Saremi F, Muresian H, Sánchez-Quintana D. Coronary veins: comprehensive CT-anatomic classification and review of variants and clinical implications. Radiographics. 2012;32(1):E1–32.
3. Huckleberry J, Haltom S, Issac T, et al. Accuracy of non-ECG-gated computed tomography angiography of the chest in assessment of left-sided cardiac chamber enlargement. J Thorac Imaging. 2012;27(6):354–8.
4. Cerqueira MD, Weissman NJ, Dilsizian V, et al. Standardized myocardial segmentation and nomenclature for tomographic imaging of the heart. A statement for healthcare professionals from the Cardiac Imaging Committee of the Council on Clinical Cardiology of the American Heart Association. Circulation. 2002;105(4):539–42.
5. Marom EM, Herndon JE, Kim YH, et al. Variations in pulmonary venous drainage of the left atrium: implications for radiofrequency ablation. Radiology. 2004;230(3):824–9.
6. Ghaye B, Szapiro D, Dacher JN, et al. Percutaneous ablation for atrial fibrillation: the role of cross-sectional imaging. Radiographics. 2003;23(suppl_1):S19–33.

21 Patient Selection: When to Use Cardiac CT Versus Other Imaging or Non-imaging Tests

Pal Spruill Suranyi, Akos Varga-Szemes, Marques L. Bradshaw, Richard R. Bayer II, Salvatore A. Chiaramida, Peter L. Zwerner, and David Gregg

Preamble: The Importance of Appropriateness

Technological advances in imaging may be contributing to the increasing healthcare expenditures as our ability to vividly visualize pathology has skyrocketed the utilization of these imaging techniques. These trends collide with our fears of potentially limited resources in the near future as baby boomers reach old age and healthcare expenditures are cut back. This has led to the crescendoing outcry for cost-effective, precision medicine. Responsible care dictates that we do not perform novel imaging tests just because we can but rather because we are convinced that there is significant benefit in guiding patient management. Heart disease is the leading cause of death in both women and men and consumes a significant amount of advanced imaging. Appropriate utilization of cardiac CT remains a topic of discussion in the evolving healthcare delivery system, and we will need to be mindful in our quest to improve outcomes in all cardiovascular diseases. Numerous societies have joined forces to create and periodically revise guidelines and appropriateness criteria [1–10]; however, our aim here is to give a practical overview of how cardiac CT can complement – rather than compete with – other imaging and non-imaging tests (Table 21.1).

Overview of the Disadvantages of CT When Compared to Other Modalities

The critics of cardiac CT voice concerns over the inherent radiation exposure, the need for iodinated contrast media, the relatively low temporal resolution, the inability to measure flow, the limits on myocardial tissue characterization, and suboptimal viability imaging with CT. Several factors can degrade image quality including arrhythmias, inability to do breath-holds or raise arms, large body habitus, and metallic hardware in the chest. Cardiac CTA is felt to be a more "anatomic" than a "physiologic" test, which is certainly true in the way CT is used clinically today; however, newer advances, such as CT fractional flow reserve (FFR), iodine content mapping, and quantitative CT perfusion for myocardial blood flow during vasodilator stress, are making strides to mitigate those claims. We refer the reader to the respective chapters for further detail on these new approaches. Lastly, the relatively high cost of equipment is a disadvantage when compared to gamma cameras or echo machines.

Overview of the Advantages of CT Relative to Other Modalities

To date, cardiac CT is the most easily accessible, fastest, noninvasive, high spatial resolution (submillimeter) tomographic imaging modality (Table 21.2). Rapid advances in radiation dose reduction are minimizing exposure to a point where, in some patients, sub-milliSievert whole-chest coronary CTAs have become a reality [11]. These low-dose scans are far below the nuclear exposure by SPECT nuclear imaging [12].

P. S. Suranyi (✉) · R. R. Bayer II
Division of Cardiovascular Imaging, Department of Radiology and Radiological Science, Medical University of South Carolina, Charleston, SC, USA

Division of Cardiology, Department of Medicine, Medical University of South Carolina, Charleston, SC, USA
e-mail: suranyi@musc.edu

A. Varga-Szemes
Division of Cardiovascular Imaging, Department of Radiology and Radiological Science, Medical University of South Carolina, Charleston, SC, USA

M. L. Bradshaw
Department of Radiology and Radiological Sciences, Vanderbilt University School of Medicine, Nashville, TN, USA

S. A. Chiaramida · P. L. Zwerner
D. Gregg
Division of Cardiology, Department of Medicine, Medical University of South Carolina, Charleston, SC, USA

U. J. Schoepf (ed.), *CT of the Heart*, Contemporary Medical Imaging, https://doi.org/10.1007/978-1-60327-237-7_21

Table 21.1 Simplified summary for common "appropriate" (ACR appropriateness criteria) indications for cardiac CT

Indication	Patient population	Notes
CAD risk stratification (Ca scoring)	Asymptomatic patient with low to intermediate risk with strong family history	
Preoperative assessment of CAD risk (coronary CTA)	Asymptomatic patients with intermediate probability for CAD, undergoing major noncardiac or valve surgery	
Acute chest pain	Low to intermediate probability with negative or equivocal initial cardiac enzymes and nondiagnostic/equivocal ECG or serial troponins and ECG still negative or borderline for NSTEMI/ACS	In patients with low clinical suspicion of acute aortic syndrome or pulmonary embolism, a cardiac CTA is preferred over an entire chest triple-rule-out
Chronic chest pain	Low-, intermediate-, or high-probability patients (especially following a negative or inconclusive ECG exercise stress or discordant stress ECG and stress imaging results)	
Post-revascularization	Symptomatic (ischemic equivalent) patients after CABG to assess graft patency or location if graft markers not present Asymptomatic patients with prior left main stent or stents ≥3 mm	Whole chest should be covered to include origins of internal mammary arteries
Planning of open heart surgery, (coronary, valve, or congenital)	Minimally invasive valve surgeries Any redo surgery (retrosternal anatomy)	
Native or prosthetic valve disease	Clinically suspected valve dysfunction with inadequate images from other noninvasive methods	CT occasionally may act as an arbitrator if CT and ECHO yield conflicting results
Pre-procedural evaluation for transcatheter valve placement	Most commonly in patients with severe aortic stenosis who are poor surgical candidates Mitral, tricuspid, and pulmonic valve disease (native or bioprosthetic valves) may also be good candidates	The indication may soon be expanded even to patients who would be good surgical candidates Note CT is a one-stop shop also for assessing vascular access, which could be imaged using the same contrast bolus
Known or suspected congenital heart disease	Patients where echocardiography was inconclusive or raised additional questions	Scanning of the entire chest is likely warranted to image all great vessels for potential anomalies
New heart failure (systolic or diastolic), assessment of left or right heart function	Patients where echocardiography was inconclusive and CAD risk is low to intermediate	Adjust injection protocol (longer bolus) when right heart function assessment is needed
Suspected cardiac mass/thrombus	Inadequate images from other methods or contraindications for MRI	Precontrast and delayed scans should also be obtained
Pericardial abnormality	Congenital or acquired diseases of the pericardium	
Arrhythmia/EP procedure, PM/ICD placement	Suspected ARVD/ARVC Planning for RFA – pulmonary vein anatomy Planning RFA to treat potential sources for VF/VTACH Coronary venous mapping	

Table 21.2 Advantages and challenges of cardiac CT

	Advantage	Challenge	Solution on the horizon?
Spatial resolution	High spatial resolution	Spatial resolution still inferior to invasive angiography	Decreasing detector size
Contrast resolution	Depending on body habitus, low-Kv scanning provides improved soft tissue contrast even at low iodine doses	Relatively low soft tissue contrast resolution	Soft tissue contrast improved by iodine mapping with dual energy, ECVF, spectral CT
Temporal resolution		Low effective temporal resolution, dependent on scanner type and scanning mode	Dual source scanners offer highest temporal resolution to date
Anatomic and physiological information gained	Excellent depiction of anatomy	Less information gained on physiology and function	CT-FFR, CT myocardial perfusion
Function	Can assess gross systolic function, wall motion, chamber volumes, and ejection fraction	Relatively low temporal resolution, cannot assess flow, regurgitation, velocity, or diastolic function	Improvements in gantry rotation time and other means of increasing temporal resolution (e.g., dual-source techniques) may make CT competitive for function assessment in the future

Table 21.2 (continued)

	Advantage	Challenge	Solution on the horizon?
Speed	Faster and more easily accessible than MRI, SPECT, PET, and even echo (especially transesophageal)	Difficulties with IV access and need for medications (beta blockers, nitrates) may delay scanning	Scanners with improved temporal and spatial resolution can scan without medications
Radiation	Some techniques allow sub-mSv scanning	Relatively large breast dose; arrhythmic or large patients will receive higher dose	Low kV scanning
Contrast	Peripheral IV access is sufficient	Ideally a power-injectable access is needed; severe allergies or acute renal insufficiency can be contraindications	Low kV scanning can help reduce the contrast volume needed
Equipment cost	Typically cheaper than MRI	More expensive than gamma camera or echo machines	
Implanted medical hardware, electronics, prior intervention/ surgeries	Hardware in patient is never a contraindication	Metallic streak artifact may somewhat degrade image quality	Streak-artifact reduction algorithms, dual-energy scanning
Patient comfort	Claustrophobia is rarely a problem; scan itself lasts only seconds, noninvasive	Need for power injection of contrast, may lead to extravasation	Advanced low kV and dual-energy techniques can reduce contrast amount needed

For a successful cardiac CTA in its current iteration, all one needs is an imaging unit and power-injectable intravenous access. With advances in scanner technology, diagnostic images can be obtained even in patients with high heart rate and arrhythmias. Although prior surgeries, sternal wires, stents, prosthetic valves, and implanted devices may cause some artifacts, it is rare that the entire study is nondiagnostic. Even many bariatric patients can be imaged successfully, as well as those unable to do breath-holds.

Cardiac CT can be useful when contrast cannot be administered. ECG-synchronized non-contrast CT is invaluable for risk stratification of patients for coronary disease and is also able to identify some acute aortic pathologies (e.g., acute intramural hematoma and sometimes dissection).

Additionally, surgeons and most cardiologists – even if imaging is not their primary interest – have become familiar and comfortable with CT images. This ability of clinicians to "look for themselves," especially with web-based intuitive and interactive 3D workstations, has further contributed to the appeal of this modality.

When Should Cardiac CT Be the First Advanced Imaging Test?

Risk Stratification

In very low-risk patients, imaging is likely unwarranted, but calcium scoring is an inexpensive, quick, and effective risk stratification tool. This study can be considered in asymptomatic and low-risk patients, in whom – based on lifestyle, family history of premature CAD, or lab results – advanced or premature coronary atherosclerosis is suspected. Calcium scoring, discussed in detail elsewhere in this book, is most appropriate for intermediate-risk asymptomatic patients, in whom it may provide reassurance of low cardiac risk or, on the other hand, may help guide preventive measures and lipid-lowering therapies [13]. Newer, low-voltage tin filtration protocols allow 75% radiation dose reduction with accurate cardiac risk stratification [14].

An additional indication where CTA may precede or substitute other imaging tests is preoperative assessment of cardiac risk, which can be appropriate in certain patient groups undergoing evaluation for major surgeries (noncardiac surgeries or cardiac valve surgeries) [15, 16].

Acute Chest Pain

Acute chest pain is one indication, where, following a normal CXR and equivocal initial workup in the emergency department (vitals, cardiac enzymes, and ECG), a cardiac CTA (or a whole-chest triple-rule-out) could prove useful for swift and cost-effective patient management [17, 18]. This can be referred to as the "early assessment pathway" [5]. The appropriateness of CTA depends on the pretest probability, which ideally should be low to intermediate, with a TIMI risk score of 0 [19]. CTA is also useful in cases where ischemic symptoms have resolved hours before presenting to the emergency room. Even in patients who undergo the "observational pathway", and serial ECG and troponins remain negative or borderline, CTA is considered an appropriate choice.

There is extensive evidence in the literature that CTA offers an outstanding negative predictive value and low-to intermediate-risk patients can be safely discharged if no or only mild coronary stenosis is found [20]. Moreover, a chest or cardiac CTA will not only visualize coronaries but is very efficient in pointing the clinician to other sources of chest pain, such as acute aortic pathology, pulmonary embolism, lung pathology, chest wall, or gastrointestinal (e.g., hiatal hernia, reflux esophagitis) problems [21]. Admittedly, these findings may lead to increased downstream testing that detracts from the appeal of coronary CTA use in the ER as shown in the ROMICAT II study [17]. These will be further discussed in a separate chapter in this book.

When acute aortic syndrome is included in the differential, ECG-synchronized CTA is preferred over non-gated chest CTA, as ECG gating is crucial when visualizing the aortic root and ascending aorta, with the added benefit of visualizing coronary, aortic valve, and pericardial involvement, when present [22]. Of note, CTA is the only appropriate imaging modality in hemodynamically unstable patients, regardless of whether or not they had prior aorta interventions, since it is "less invasive" than transesophageal echo.

Some have advocated using a negative Ca score scan (NPV 97%) as a means to rule out acute coronary syndrome in the emergency room (ER) setting [23, 24]. However, this approach is certainly not universally accepted, especially because it is possible to have ruptured noncalcified plaques, coronary emboli, thrombosed coronary, or dissected coronaries even in the absence of any calcium.

The last thing to consider in the acute setting is what to do when there are extensive coronary calcifications. The 2010 Appropriateness Criteria warn us that the use of CTA in acutely symptomatic patients with Ca score above 400 is not definitively appropriate. The assessment of "uncertain appropriateness" was rendered due to concerns over poor visualization of the coronaries from beam hardening and "blooming" effects. However, in everyday practice, this is rarely a major problem, especially considering rapidly improving scanner technology. Additionally, performing Ca scoring "on the fly" while the patient is in the scanner is not very practical, as this would require the radiologist to be physically present for every scan. While extensive coronary calcium is certainly a drawback in assessing the coronaries, it does not completely negate the usefulness of a triple-rule-out or coronary CTA in finding the source for chest pain.

Chronic Chest Pain

In the past, guidelines recommended stress ECG to be among the first to evaluate patients with persistent or chronic chest pain, despite the fact that sensitivity and specificity are only a little better than a coin toss, and its accuracy has been shown to be poor in women [25]. Growing evidence suggest that coronary CTA should be the first test when evaluating patients with suspected anginal chest pain [26, 27]. In the United Kingdom, the updated National Institute for Health and Care Excellence (NICE) guidelines have included coronary CT as a first-line test for coronary artery disease, citing its relatively low cost and high sensitivity [28]. CTA has been shown to be at least equivalent in the workup of patients with stable chest pain with good outcomes. CTA's ability to detect nonobstructive coronary disease by way of visualizing not only the lumen but also plaques is very helpful in our efforts trying to understand microvascular disease, plaque erosion, and myocardial infarction with no obstructive coronary artery (MINOCA) [29].

A particularly interesting group is competitive athletes, in whom cardiac CT may prove useful to visualize anomalous coronaries or other cardiac pathologies. Indications in this patient group would include family history of sudden cardiac death, uncertain syncope, post-resuscitation, positive stress ECG without symptoms, and equivocal ischemic symptoms with normal stress ECG [30].

How Can CT Complement Echocardiography?

Echocardiography is likely the first choice for cardiologists to "screen" a patient for suspected congenital heart disease, valvular disease, new heart failure (systolic or diastolic), cardiac embolic source, and pericardial abnormalities [31–34]. Albeit echocardiography is easily accessible and effective in many patients, body habitus and suboptimal acoustic windows may prevent us from reaching a conclusive diagnosis solely with echo in others. Further, echo has clear shortcomings when it comes to visualization of great arteries and veins. The right heart is challenging due to its retrosternal position, the left atrial appendage is faintly seen with transthoracic approach, and the contents of the pericardium can look rather ominous, when there is anything in there, aside from clear serous fluid. The assessment of regional myocardial function and the quantification of chamber volumes and systolic function are known to be operator dependent, subjective, and poorly reproducible when using two-dimensional methods. Lastly, echocardiography is rarely able to visualize the coronaries, and its ability to determine myocardial perfusion and viability is also limited, unless an aggressive stress agent like dobutamine is used. Below we will discuss what cardiac CT can offer when an initial echo is unable to answer the clinical question or when echo raises new questions based on its findings.

Congenital Heart Disease (CHD) and Great Vessel Anomalies/Abnormalities

In newborns and adults alike, CT can prove useful in visualizing anatomic abnormalities of the coronaries, the airways, and the great arteries and veins (anomalous pulmonary veins, left SVC, etc.), aortopulmonary or other systemic to pulmonary collaterals, and pulmonary arteriovenous malformations [35, 36]. Cardiology guidelines emphasize that cardiac CT might be useful in detailed assessment of complex cardiac anatomy, e.g., in unusual VSDs, such as inlet or apical defects, which may be poorly seen by echocardiography [37].

When undetected in childhood, the suspicion of congenital heart disease may be raised in adults due to chamber enlargement or a murmur in the absence of significant valve disease or visible intracardiac shunt, prompting the cardiologist to look for an extracardiac shunt or anomaly.

Although due to its low temporal resolution CT-derived systolic function is not as accurate as cine MRI, functional images can be used to assess regional and global systolic function to provide reasonably accurate volumes of chamber sizes (both the left and right heart) in patients in whom MRI is contraindicated (e.g., unapproved devices or severe claustrophobia).

Chest CTA can be useful in assessment of aortic dimensions (degenerative aortic aneurysms, bicuspid valve, or Marfan-/Ehlers-Danlos-related aneurysms), for which – truthfully – only ECG-synchronized or superfast spiral acquisitions with excellent temporal resolution should be used as only these techniques provide motion-free, accurate measurements of the aortic root and ascending aorta [22].

Cardiac CT is a great tool for postsurgical evaluation and follow-up (anastomoses, baffles, conduits, homografts, shunts, patches, and plasties) and also for preoperative assessment prior to repeat or multistage operations. The ability to visualize retrosternal anatomy in detail is an important benefit before redo sternotomy to plan a safe reentry into the chest.

Valve Disease

When echocardiography is unable to visualize the valves reliably and endocarditis or other acute valve pathology is suspected (e.g., papillary muscle rupture), CTA can be more efficacious. This is especially useful in prosthetic valves, where artifact from the metallic frames often renders echo studies suboptimal. Vegetations, thrombi, pannus, leaflet malfunction, paravalvular leaks, and aneurysms can be beautifully visualized with CT.

Rarely, as a third-line evaluation, when echocardiography and catheter-based pressure measurements disagree and an MRI is contraindicated, CT can act as an arbitrator to measure valve orifice area [38].

Preceding minimally invasive mitral and aortic valve surgeries, CTA can help in planning the best surgical approach and visualizing the complexities of the mitral valve apparatus. For planning percutaneous valve placement, CT is extremely helpful in visualizing the anatomy of the valve annulus, or the potential landing site in a homograft or conduit, as well as calcifications, stenoses, aneurysms, and nearby structures that may be compromised (e.g., coronaries). In addition, the same contrast bolus can be used in some scanners to interrogate also the entire aorta, iliofemoral, and axillary-subclavian access routes to elucidate where the cleanest and safest pathway can be found. For further detail on these, we refer to other chapters of this book.

New Systolic or Diastolic Heart Failure and Regional Wall Motion Abnormalities

Ischemic heart disease is one of the most common reasons for impaired global or regional cardiac function, which can be efficiently ruled out or detected with cardiac CT, if the overall clinician impression about the pretest probability is low to moderate. In patients where ARVD/ARVC is suspected and MRI cannot be done, CT can be performed to evaluate right ventricular function and areas of fatty infiltration.

Cardiac Embolic Source

In patients with embolic events (e.g., strokes, splenic infarct, etc.) where transthoracic echocardiography is unrevealing (e.g., poor acoustic windows) or equivocal (e.g., questionable mass) and transesophageal echo is unavailable (e.g., at night in an understaffed hospital), contraindicated (e.g., unstable/uncooperative patient), or unsuccessful, cardiac CT is a reasonable next step to visualize intracardiac masses. Of note, it is crucial that the imager reviews the images immediately after the scan to decide whether a delayed scan is warranted (i.e., questionable clot in the left atrial appendage). When this is logistically not possible, a low-dose ECG-synchronized delayed scan should be obtained routinely. If a cardiac neoplasm is suspected, a precontrast scan should also be obtained to assess enhancement of the mass, when present. Of the common "normal variants" that can look ominous on echo, CT can usually identify the majority with certainty providing reassurance (lipomatous hypertrophy of the interatrial septum, crista terminalis, prominent Eustachian valve, accessory appendages).

Pericardium

CT can visualize the size of a pericardial effusion but is limited in the ability to detect hemodynamic significance. CT is unable to conclusively demonstrate whether constriction is physiologically present, since ventricular interdependence cannot be demonstrated during a breath-hold. Pericardial enhancement and thickening can only rarely be seen on early arterial phase; therefore it is difficult to decide if active inflammation is present on CTAs; however a delayed prospectively gated scan may highlight pericardial inflammation.

CT is certainly useful in visualizing the extent and distribution of calcification in chronic constrictive pericarditis and may aid in surgical planning for pericardial stripping. When a small pericardial effusion is present, prominent epicardial fat may give the impression of an intrapericardial mass on echocardiograms, which can be easily visualized on CT. In metastatic malignancies, pericardial metastases are also usually well visualized with cardiac CT.

Following Cardiac Devices and Cardiac Surgery

Pacemaker/ICD leads, ventricular assist devices, or other embolized devices (e.g., IVC filters) can best be visualized with CTA. Visualizing retrosternal and great vessel anatomy is crucial prior to LVAD implantation. Following LVAD implantation, CT will be the best modality to visualize thrombus formation in or around the inflow and outflow cannulae or kinking/compression of the non-radiopaque tubing connecting to the ascending aorta.

Following cardiac or aortic surgery, CT can be useful to identify early complications such as anastomotic leaks or pseudoaneurysms. When sternal osteomyelitis and mediastinitis are suspected, a gated cardiac scan will provide better visualization of paracardiac structures to accurately assess the extent of infection, and as a bonus, it also gives superb view of the sternum itself.

Should We Get a Cardiac CT or an MRI Next?

In the United States, between the two major advanced tomographic methods, cardiac CT seems to be preferred, more so than in other parts of the world. When MRI is unavailable or contraindicated (unapproved electronic devices, metallic foreign bodies, severe claustrophobia), CT is obviously a better choice. For some MRI applications, gadolinium-based contrast is crucial, which is contraindicated in pregnancy, end-stage renal failure, or severe allergies to MRI contrast. Nonetheless, for many questions detailed in the above paragraph, cardiovascular MRI is just as efficacious and offers ionizing radiation-free assessment.

In the below paragraphs, we briefly discuss when MRI should be the next step after CT and, vice versa, when a CT might be indicated following cardiac MRI.

Congenital Heart Disease, Great Vessel Abnormalities, Valve Disease, and Biventricular Function

When CHD is suspected based on clinical workup and echo findings, or patients have history of CHD and valve disease of great vessel anomalies, and cardiac CT is chosen as the next step after ECHO, the following questions may remain unanswered even after the CT scan, to which MRI is likely to be able to provide answers:

- What is the Qp/Qs if a shunt is present?
- What is the peak velocity when valvular, subvalvular, or supravalvular stenosis is noted on CT?
- What is the regurgitant fraction in valvular insufficiency?
- What is the pulmonary blood flow to each of the lungs (balanced or unbalanced)?
- Is there a clot in poorly opacified parts of the cardiovascular system, when delayed CT was not obtained to clarify areas of mixing or suboptimal contrast enhancement (e.g., Fontan shunt, when lower extremity is not injected and delays were not obtained)?
- Is there focal myocardial fibrosis/scarring from prior surgery or ischemic event that may lead to arrhythmia?
- Is there stress-inducible ischemia in the myocardium when coronary anomalies/stenoses are detected on CT?
- Depending on the contrast injection protocol, it may be challenging to determine right ventricular function with CT, not to mention that due to its low temporal resolution, CT-derived ventricular volumes are not as accurate as MRI anyways. Thus, MRI might be needed for accurate assessment of biventricular size and systolic function.
- If based on clinical symptoms and CT findings an active vasculitis is suspected, MRI (T2-weighted imaging, dynamic contrast enhancement, and diffusion-weighted imaging) might prove helpful after CTA.
- When an aneurysm is found that needs follow-up in younger patients, it is prudent to schedule routine follow-up with MRI rather than CT to avoid radiation. Of note, if simple sizing is the question, a non-contrast MRA may be sufficient.

When MRI/MRA is ordered first in CHD patients, there may be a number of dilemmas raised that cannot be completely answered without a CT:

- Questionable coronary anomaly, coronary fistula, or stenosis due to postsurgical changes
- Questionable coronary atherosclerosis in older patients
- Calcifications in baffles, patches, shunts, conduits, and homografts
- In-stent intimal hyperplasia
- Stent-graft evaluation where MRI was suboptimal
- Incomplete closure with a closure device
- Suspected artificial valve complications (mechanical failure, clot, pannus, vegetation, small paravalvular aneurysm, or leak)
- Poorly visualized retrosternal anatomy due to artifact from sternal wires

Cardiac Masses

When evaluating a patient with CT for cardiac mass or embolic source, the following issues may arise:

- Visualization of lesions in the right heart (particularly the right atrium) might be compromised due to swirling and mixing of contrasted and non-opacified blood.
- If no precontrast scan is available, it may be difficult to decide if a mass is enhancing.
- Some masses, e.g., fibroma, will only show delayed enhancement and may mimic a thrombus on an arterial phase CT.
- If a thrombus is suspected on CT but delayed images are not available, MRI might be helpful in clarification.

On the other hand, sometimes a mass is detected on MRI, for which further clarification is needed using cardiac CTA:

- Pericardial/paracardiac/mediastinal/pleural/lung mass with suspected coronary or myocardial invasion.
- Suspected calcifications.
- Suspected perivalvular lesion/thrombus/vegetation/pannus/aneurysm adjacent to a prosthetic valve.
- Central line or ICD/pacemaker lead-associated thrombi are better characterized with CT.

Pericardial Disease

As described above, the strength of CT is its ability to visualize calcifications, but differentiating of pericardial thickening from dense fluid is often fraught with difficulty as pericardial enhancement is only rarely visible with CT. CT is also unable to generate real-time deep inspiratory imaging, which is necessary to detect ventricular interdependence, a hallmark of constriction. Further, MRI is the best modality to show pericardial tethering (myocardial tagging) and enhancement (early and delayed).

Ischemic Heart Disease

If based on CT findings and clinical workup the thought of catheterization and revascularization is entertained, it may be prudent to obtain a cardiac MRI stress test, where stress-induced ischemia and viability can be detected with great accuracy. Growing evidence suggests that MRI is superior to nuclear cardiac SPECT myocardial perfusion imaging [39, 40]. It has also been shown that MRI stress is much superior to SPECT in women [41]. The anatomic findings of coronary CTA may be complemented by dual-energy iodine mapping, CT myocardial perfusion assessment, and CT-FFR for a more functional assessment [42]. However, these are currently only practiced at some institutions (detailed in other chapters), and the widespread use of these CT techniques has not yet been implemented. Ultimately it seems that the best diagnostic accuracy will be achieved when anatomic and functional imaging is combined in some form, providing "hybrid cardiac imaging" – as shown in a recent meta-analysis by Rizvi et al. [43].

A currently hot topic of recanalizing chronic total occlusions (CTO) may also benefit from a CTA after MRI establishes viability of the vessel territory: a CTA might be the next best step to serve as a 3D "map" prior to the recanalization procedure.

Transplant-related coronary disease is another realm where CTA may be helpful to rule out epicardial disease, but MRI may be better at picking up on microvascular disease in the peripheral capillary bed. However, to date, neither MRI nor CT is fully reliable in assessing rejection.

Cardiac CT and Nuclear Cardiac Imaging: Friends or Adversaries?

Nuclear cardiac imaging boasts with extensive historical data, tradition, and a vast following. However, SPECT nuclear imaging has been shown to yield particularly low sensitivity and specificity in women, compared to men, seems to struggle demonstrating three-vessel disease and small subendocardial infarcts, and has no ability to visualize epicardial coronary lumens or plaques. In a recent meta-analysis, where invasive angiography and fractional flow reserve were used as the ground truth, SPECT myocardial perfusion was outperformed by cardiac CTA, myocardial perfusion MRI, and even PET perfusion [44]. In another recent meta-analysis, coronary CTA showed higher diagnostic performance than exercise ECG or SPECT testing in stable angina [45].

Since attenuation artifacts have been identified as one of the important causes for false positives, many centers have now implemented an ECG-gated non-contrast CT scan for attenuation correction and used this scan for concurrent calcium scoring for additional risk stratification, which certainly seems like a viable solution for enhancing the accuracy of nuclear imaging.

Cardiac CT has other measurable advantages, namely, that it is able to expedite discharge and has lower radiation exposure and lower cost in the emergency room setting when compared to the standard workup, which – interestingly – is even more pronounced in women vs. men [46]. Additionally, in some institutions, cardiac CT is available 24/7 [47], whereas nuclear imaging is offered typically only during regular work hours. While a complete stress-rest SPECT may take hours and even PET perfusion (where available) will take at least an hour, CT can be done in a matter of minutes. The in-plane spatial resolution of nuclear imaging tests even with the latest improvements is an order of magnitude lower, around 10–5 mm (SPECT vs. PET), as opposed to CT's half a millimeter resolution.

As detailed in other chapters, the radiation dose with cardiac CT has been a downward moving target, and SPECT certainly is unable to keep up with the race. PET perfusion, however, offers relatively lower radiation doses that compete with advanced CT scanners (when function is acquired with tube current modulation) in the 2–5 mSv effective dose range. Thus, depending on the scanners used at one's institution, PET perfusion may be a reasonable option particularly for women in whom quantitative myocardial perfusion measurement may reveal ischemic heart disease where CTA or even conventional angiography cannot find luminal obstruction. Of note, as detailed in another chapter, myocardial perfusion CT has also been getting increasing coverage in the "press." PET imaging has further advantages over CT, especially if MRI is not available in imaging active inflammation, which is particularly useful in sarcoidosis, where CT would be unlikely to detect any changes in the heart.

It is not unusual after an equivocal nuclear cardiac scan – or after a scan when the results are not what the clinician hoped for – that a cardiologist will order a cardiac CTA, to conclusively demonstrate the absence or presence of epicardial disease, before the patient is subjected to an invasive procedure. And indeed, CT has been most helpful in excluding coronary disease when a *false-positive* nuclear result is suspected, given its high negative predictive value [48]. CT has also proven to be helpful in visualizing epicardial coronary disease, positive remodeling, and noncalcified plaques in patients where perfusion defects were absent, but the persistent clinical signs and symptoms prompted the clinician to pursue the disease with further imaging (i.e., clinically deemed *false negatives*). In the recent PROMISE trial, comparing coronary CTA to functional testing, CTA has proven to be a significantly better prognostic indicator than the alternatives, including exercise electrocardiography, exercise or pharmacological nuclear myocardial perfusion imaging, and exercise or pharmacological stress echocardiography [49]. This, again, is particularly important in women, in whom nonobstructive coronary disease (or as some would prefer ischemic heart disease) is more prevalent than in men.

Conclusion: Comprehensive Care, Collaboration, Communication, and Coexistence

There is obviously no simple algorithm for deciding when and how cardiac CT should be used. One has to consider risk factors, pretest probability, clinical presentation, and other noninvasive test results to decide whether cardiac CTA is the best next step in patient management. The question should not be about one modality lording over another but, rather, how we can integrate cardiac CT best into the comprehensive multidisciplinary workup and management of cardiovascular diseases. It is also important to mention that professional society-driven appropriateness criteria cannot keep up with the incredible speed of scanner technology development and rapid advances in novel cardiac device utilization. Therefore, imagers have to maintain flexibility and be ready to take cardiac CTA even to previously uncharted territories for the benefit of our patients.

It seems that cardiac CT is best utilized in an environment where the stakeholders of various modalities communicate and collaborate even before a test is ordered, to ensure that a diversity of opinions is considered and optimal image acquisition is performed, tailored to the specific clinical questions and suspicions, while also keeping individual patient-specific factors in sight. Then, following image acquisition and postprocessing, the team should again reconvene to allow for thorough interpretation involving several subspecialties. This is the only way that cardiac CT will find its rightful place in heart disease management and will provide true value while reducing cost and minimizing risk.

References

1. Taylor AJ, et al. ACCF/SCCT/ACR/AHA/ASE/ASNC/NASCI/SCAI/SCMR 2010 appropriate use criteria for cardiac computed tomography. A report of the American College of Cardiology Foundation Appropriate Use Criteria Task Force, the Society of Cardiovascular Computed Tomography, the American College of Radiology, the American Heart Association, the American Society of Echocardiography, the American Society of Nuclear Cardiology, the North American Society for Cardiovascular Imaging, the Society for Cardiovascular Angiography and Interventions, and the Society for Cardiovascular Magnetic Resonance. J Cardiovasc Comput Tomogr. 2010;4(6):407 e1–33.
2. Expert Panel on Cardiac, I, et al. ACR appropriateness criteria(R) known or suspected congenital heart disease in the adult. J Am Coll Radiol. 2017;14(5S):S166–76.
3. Expert Panel on Cardiac, I, et al. ACR appropriateness criteria(R) chronic chest pain-high probability of coronary artery disease. J Am Coll Radiol. 2017;14(5S):S71–80.
4. Expert Panel on Cardiac, I, et al. ACR appropriateness criteria(R) dyspnea-suspected cardiac origin. J Am Coll Radiol. 2017;14(5S):S127–37.
5. Emergency Department Patients With Chest Pain Writing, P, et al. 2015 ACR/ACC/AHA/AATS/ACEP/ASNC/NASCI/SAEM/SCCT/SCMR/SCPC/SNMMI/STR/STS appropriate utilization of cardiovascular imaging in emergency department patients with chest pain: a joint document of the American College of Radiology Appropriateness Criteria Committee and the American College of Cardiology Appropriate Use Criteria Task Force. J Am Coll Radiol. 2016;13(2):e1–e29.
6. Hoffmann U, et al. ACR appropriateness criteria acute nonspecific chest pain-low probability of coronary artery disease. J Am Coll Radiol. 2015;12(12 Pt A):1266–71.
7. White RD, et al. 2013 ACCF/ACR/ASE/ASNC/SCCT/SCMR appropriate utilization of cardiovascular imaging in heart failure:

an executive summary: a joint report of the ACR Appropriateness Criteria (R) Committee and the ACCF Appropriate Use Criteria Task Force. J Am Coll Radiol. 2013;10(7):493–500.
8. Dill KE, et al. ACR appropriateness criteria imaging for transcatheter aortic valve replacement. J Am Coll Radiol. 2013;10(12):957–65.
9. Earls JP, et al. ACR appropriateness criteria asymptomatic patient at risk for coronary artery disease. J Am Coll Radiol. 2014;11(1):12–9.
10. Mammen L, et al. ACR appropriateness criteria(R) nonischemic myocardial disease with clinical manifestations (ischemic cardiomyopathy already excluded). J Thorac Imaging. 2014;29(4):W44–7.
11. Meinel FG, et al. ECG-synchronized CT angiography in 324 consecutive pediatric patients: spectrum of indications and trends in radiation dose. Pediatr Cardiol. 2015;36(3):569–78.
12. Meinel FG, et al. Radiation risks from cardiovascular imaging tests. Circulation. 2014;130(5):442–5.
13. Vliegenthart R, Morris PB. Computed tomography coronary artery calcium scoring: review of evidence base and cost-effectiveness in cardiovascular risk prediction. J Thorac Imaging. 2012;27(5):296–303.
14. Tesche C, et al. Accuracy and radiation dose reduction using low-voltage computed tomography coronary artery calcium scoring with tin filtration. Am J Cardiol. 2017;119(4):675–80.
15. Hwang JW, et al. Assessment of perioperative cardiac risk of patients undergoing noncardiac surgery using coronary computed tomographic angiography. Circ Cardiovasc Imaging. 2015;8(3):e002582.
16. Morris MF, et al. Computed tomography as an alternative to catheter angiography prior to robotic mitral valve repair. Ann Thorac Surg. 2013;95(4):1354–9.
17. Hoffmann U, et al. Coronary CT angiography versus standard evaluation in acute chest pain. N Engl J Med. 2012;367(4):299–308.
18. Truong QA, et al. Coronary CT angiography versus standard emergency department evaluation for acute chest pain and diabetic patients: is there benefit with early coronary CT angiography? Results of the Randomized Comparative Effectiveness ROMICAT II Trial. J Am Heart Assoc. 2016;5(3):e003137.
19. Rybicki FJ, et al. 2015 ACR/ACC/AHA/AATS/ACEP/ASNC/NASCI/SAEM/SCCT/SCMR/SCPC/SNMMI/STR/ STS appropriate utilization of cardiovascular imaging in emergency department patients with chest pain: a joint document of the American College of Radiology Appropriateness Criteria Committee and the American College of Cardiology Appropriate Use Criteria Task Force. J Am Coll Cardiol. 2016;67(7):853–79.
20. El-Hayek G, et al. Meta-analysis of coronary computed tomography angiography versus standard of care strategy for the evaluation of low risk chest pain: are randomized controlled trials and cohort studies showing the same evidence? Int J Cardiol. 2014;177(1):238–45.
21. Lee HY, Yoo SM, White CS. Coronary CT angiography in emergency department patients with acute chest pain: triple rule-out protocol versus dedicated coronary CT angiography. Int J Cardiovasc Imaging. 2009;25(3):319–26.
22. Hiratzka LF, et al. 2010 ACCF/AHA/AATS/ACR/ASA/SCA/SCAI/SIR/STS/SVM Guidelines for the diagnosis and management of patients with thoracic aortic disease. A Report of the American College of Cardiology Foundation/American Heart Association Task Force on Practice Guidelines, American Association for Thoracic Surgery, American College of Radiology, American Stroke Association, Society of Cardiovascular Anesthesiologists, Society for Cardiovascular Angiography and Interventions, Society of Interventional Radiology, Society of Thoracic Surgeons, and Society for Vascular Medicine. J Am Coll Cardiol. 2010;55(14):e27–e129.
23. Hinzpeter R, Higashigaito K, Morsbach F, et al. Coronary artery calcium scoring for ruling-out acute coronary syndrome in chest pain CT. Am J Emerg Med. 2017;35(10):1565–7.
24. Chaikriangkrai K, et al. Prognostic value of coronary artery calcium score in acute chest pain patients without known coronary artery disease: systematic review and meta-analysis. Ann Emerg Med. 2016;68(6):659–70.
25. Kwok Y, et al. Meta-analysis of exercise testing to detect coronary artery disease in women. Am J Cardiol. 1999;83(5):660–6.
26. Moss AJ, Newby DE. CT coronary angiographic evaluation of suspected anginal chest pain. Heart. 2016;102(4):263–8.
27. Investigators, S.-H. CT coronary angiography in patients with suspected angina due to coronary heart disease (SCOT-HEART): an open-label, parallel-group, multicentre trial. Lancet. 2015;385(9985):2383–91.
28. Moss AJ, et al. The updated NICE guidelines: cardiac CT as the first-line test for coronary artery disease. Curr Cardiovasc Imaging Rep. 2017;10(5):15.
29. Baldassarre LA, et al. Noninvasive imaging to evaluate women with stable ischemic heart disease. JACC Cardiovasc Imaging. 2016;9(4):421–35.
30. Grani C, et al. Multimodality imaging in individuals with anomalous coronary arteries. JACC Cardiovasc Imaging. 2017;10(4):471–81.
31. Baumgartner H, et al. Echocardiographic assessment of valve stenosis: EAE/ASE recommendations for clinical practice. J Am Soc Echocardiogr. 2009;22(1):1–23. quiz 101-2
32. Lang RM, et al. Recommendations for chamber quantification: a report from the American Society of Echocardiography's Guidelines and Standards Committee and the Chamber Quantification Writing Group, developed in conjunction with the European Association of Echocardiography, a branch of the European Society of Cardiology. J Am Soc Echocardiogr. 2005;18(12):1440–63.
33. Group, T.T.A.C.W, et al. ACCF/ASE/ACEP/ASNC/SCAI/SCCT/SCMR 2007 appropriateness criteria for transthoracic and transesophageal echocardiography: a report of the American College of Cardiology Foundation Quality Strategic Directions Committee Appropriateness Criteria Working Group, American Society of Echocardiography, American College of Emergency Physicians, American Society of Nuclear Cardiology, Society for Cardiovascular Angiography and Interventions, Society of Cardiovascular Computed Tomography, and the Society for Cardiovascular Magnetic Resonance. Endorsed by the American College of Chest Physicians and the Society of Critical Care Medicine. J Am Soc Echocardiogr. 2007;20(7):787–805.
34. American College of Cardiology Foundation Appropriate Use Criteria Task, F, et al. ACCF/ASE/AHA/ASNC/HFSA/HRS/SCAI/SCCM/SCCT/SCMR 2011 appropriate use criteria for echocardiography. A report of the American College of Cardiology Foundation Appropriate Use Criteria Task Force, American Society of Echocardiography, American Heart Association, American Society of Nuclear Cardiology, Heart Failure Society of America, Heart Rhythm Society, Society for Cardiovascular Angiography and Interventions, Society of Critical Care Medicine, Society of Cardiovascular Computed Tomography, Society for Cardiovascular Magnetic Resonance American College of chest physicians. J Am Soc Echocardiogr. 2011;24(3):229–67.
35. Han BK, et al. Computed tomography imaging in patients with congenital heart disease part I: rationale and utility. An expert consensus document of the Society of Cardiovascular Computed Tomography (SCCT): Endorsed by the Society of Pediatric Radiology (SPR) and the North American Society of Cardiac Imaging (NASCI). J Cardiovasc Comput Tomogr. 2015;9(6):475–92.
36. Hlavacek AM. Imaging of congenital cardiovascular disease: the case for computed tomography. J Thorac Imaging. 2010;25(3):247–55.
37. Warnes CA, et al. ACC/AHA 2008 guidelines for the management of adults with congenital heart disease: a report of the American College of Cardiology/American Heart Association Task Force on Practice Guidelines (writing committee to develop guidelines on the management of adults with congenital heart disease). Developed in collaboration with the American Society of Echocardiography, Heart Rhythm Society, International Society

for Adult Congenital Heart Disease, Society for Cardiovascular Angiography and Interventions, and Society of Thoracic Surgeons. J Am Coll Cardiol. 2008;52(23):e143–263.
38. Li X, et al. Aortic valves stenosis and regurgitation: assessment with dual source computed tomography. Int J Cardiovasc Imaging. 2009;25(6):591–600.
39. Schwitter J, et al. Superior diagnostic performance of perfusion-cardiovascular magnetic resonance versus SPECT to detect coronary artery disease: the secondary endpoints of the multicenter multivendor MR-IMPACT II (Magnetic Resonance Imaging for Myocardial Perfusion Assessment in Coronary Artery Disease Trial). J Cardiovasc Magn Reson. 2012;14:61.
40. de Jong MC, et al. Diagnostic performance of stress myocardial perfusion imaging for coronary artery disease: a systematic review and meta-analysis. Eur Radiol. 2012;22(9):1881–95.
41. Greenwood JP, et al. Comparison of cardiovascular magnetic resonance and single-photon emission computed tomography in women with suspected coronary artery disease from the Clinical Evaluation of Magnetic Resonance Imaging in Coronary Heart Disease (CE-MARC) Trial. Circulation. 2014;129(10):1129–38.
42. Gonzalez JA, et al. Meta-analysis of diagnostic performance of coronary computed tomography angiography, computed tomography perfusion, and computed tomography-fractional flow reserve in functional myocardial ischemia assessment versus invasive fractional flow reserve. Am J Cardiol. 2015;116(9):1469–78.
43. Rizvi A, Han D, Danad I, et al. Diagnostic performance of hybrid cardiac imaging methods for assessment of obstructive coronary artery disease compared with stand-alone coronary computed tomography angiography: a Meta-analysis. JACC Cardiovasc Imaging. 2018;11(4):589–99.
44. Takx RA, et al. Diagnostic accuracy of stress myocardial perfusion imaging compared to invasive coronary angiography with fractional flow reserve meta-analysis. Circ Cardiovasc Imaging. 2015;8(1):e002666.
45. Nielsen LH, et al. The diagnostic accuracy and outcomes after coronary computed tomography angiography vs. conventional functional testing in patients with stable angina pectoris: a systematic review and meta-analysis. Eur Heart J Cardiovasc Imaging. 2014;15(9):961–71.
46. Truong QA, et al. Sex differences in the effectiveness of early coronary computed tomographic angiography compared with standard emergency department evaluation for acute chest pain: the rule-out myocardial infarction with Computer-Assisted Tomography (ROMICAT)-II Trial. Circulation. 2013;127(25):2494–502.
47. Garrett KG, et al. Residents' performance in the interpretation of on-call "triple-rule-out" CT studies in patients with acute chest pain. Acad Radiol. 2014;21(7):938–44.
48. Chong FY, et al. Negative coronary CT angiography for chest pain assessment predicts low event rate in 5 years. J Med Imaging Radiat Oncol. 2012;56(1):55–7.
49. Hoffmann U, et al. Prognostic value of noninvasive cardiovascular testing in patients with stable chest pain: insights from the PROMISE trial (prospective multicenter imaging study for evaluation of chest pain). Circulation. 2017;135(24):2320–32.

22 Current Guidelines

Kweku Appau and Arthur E. Stillman

In an effort to improve quality, various societies across the globe have developed appropriate use criteria and guidelines for the use of cardiac CT. Imaging guidelines are generally incorporated into various disease conditions or clinical scenarios [1–8] and include qualifications of interpreting physicians, equipment standards, and drugs used for heart rate control and vasodilation [9, 10]. There are two major sources of guidelines in the USA, the American College of Radiology (ACR) and the American College of Cardiology Foundation (ACCF), that discuss the training expectations of physicians for interpretation of cardiac CT. The ACR focuses on radiology training requirements [9], while the ACCF is more focused on cardiologists [11]. The Society of Cardiovascular Computed Tomography (SCCT) has incorporated the training requirements of the ACCF and encourages board certification through the Certification Board of Cardiovascular Computed Tomography (CBCCT) [10]. The ACR offers a Certificate of Advanced Proficiency (CoAP) after passing a rigorous examination [12]. This has greater requirements for experience in interpreting cardiac CT than the minimum ACR requirements. The European Board of Cardiac Radiology and the British Society of Cardiovascular Imaging (BSCI) also provide a diploma confirming competence in performing and interpreting cardiac CT [13, 14]. Tables 22.1 and 22.2 show the differences and similarities between the ACR and the ACCF training requirement guidelines. The ACR and SCCT have helped immensely by providing comprehensive guidelines on optimized image acquisition, image processing, as well as image interpretation and reporting [9, 15, 16]. Recently, both the ACR and SCCT leaders in conjunction with the North American Society for Cardiovascular Imaging (NASCI) have developed a standardized reporting document (CAD-RADS) that not only provides the severity of coronary artery disease (CAD) as detected by cardiac CT but also attempts to guide both patients and ordering physicians on the appropriate interpretation and management of patients based on the degree of CAD stenosis identified on cardiac CT (Tables 22.3 and 22.4) [15].

The ACR and the ACCF have critically evaluated cardiac imaging modalities to guide patients and healthcare providers on the utility of the available cardiac imaging procedures in terms of which are appropriate (A), maybe appropriate (M), or rarely appropriate (R) depending on various cardiac conditions. There are guidelines which discuss the use of imaging for stable coronary heart disease and heart failure [2, 5, 7, 8]. These recommendations are summarized in Tables 22.4, 22.5, 22.6, 22.7, 22.8, 22.9, 22.10, 22.11, 22.12, 22.13, 22.14, 22.15, 22.16, 22.17, 22.18, 22.19, 22.20, 22.21, 22.22, 22.23, 22.24, 22.25, 22.26, 22.27, 22.28, 22.29, 22.30, 22.31, 22.32, 22.33, and 22.34.

There is a strong consensus agreement across the globe with respect to class II and class III indications for the use of cardiac CT [2, 4, 5, 7, 8, 17–19]. Most of the guidelines stress that there are a class II indication for the use of cardiac CT in patients at low to intermediate risk for CAD and a class III indication for patients at high risk. Class I indications for the use of cardiac CT are very limited except in Brazil where there a class I indication for the use of cardiac CT to detect coronary calcium in asymptomatic patients with intermediate risk for CAD [1]. There is also strong consensus agreement among the various cardiac imaging and cardiovascular societies when it comes to appropriate and rarely use criteria for cardiac CT [2, 3, 5, 17, 19–21]. The gray area lies in the maybe appropriate use criteria where clinical judgment (just as in any patient encounter) is strongly advised. In South Korea and most Asian countries, the cardiovascular societies tend to rely heavily on appropriate use criteria alone [19, 20], whereas Western counterparts utilize both appropriate use criteria and guidelines on the use of cardiac CT [2, 3, 5, 7, 8, 22]. Currently, most other countries across the world tend to utilize the ACCF and the

K. Appau
Department of Cardiology, Emory University School of Medicine, Atlanta, GA, USA

A. E. Stillman (✉)
Department of Radiology and Imaging Science, Emory University School of Medicine, Atlanta, GA, USA
e-mail: aestill@emory.edu

U. J. Schoepf (ed.), *CT of the Heart*, Contemporary Medical Imaging, https://doi.org/10.1007/978-1-60327-237-7_22

Table 22.1 Qualifications and responsibilities of personnel: ACR–NASCI–SPR practice parameter for the performance and interpretation of cardiac computed tomography

Cardiac CT procedures must be supervised and interpreted by a physician with one of the following qualifications below:	The supervising physician must also have the following:	Additional qualifications include:
Certification in radiology or diagnostic radiology by the: (a) American Board of Radiology (b) American Osteopathic Board of Radiology (c) Royal College of Physicians and Surgeons of Canada (d) Collège des Médecins du Québec (e) Involvement with the supervision, interpretation, and reporting of 300 CT examinations in the past 36 months	(a) The physician should have documented training in the physics of diagnostic radiology (b) The physician must be familiar with: (a) The principles of radiation protection (b) The hazards of radiation (c) Radiation monitoring requirements as they apply to both patients and personnel	Cardiac CT Category I CME or training in cardiac CT in a training program approved by: (a) The Accreditation Council for Graduate Medical Education (ACGME) (b) The Royal College of Physicians and Surgeons of Canada (RCPSC) (c) The Collège des Médecins du Québec (d) The American Osteopathic Association (AOA)
Completion of a diagnostic radiology residency program approved by: (a) The Accreditation Council for Graduate Medical Education (ACGME) (b) The Royal College of Physicians and Surgeons of Canada (RCPSC) (c) The Collège des Médecins du Québec (d) The American Osteopathic Association (AOA) (e) Involvement with the supervision, interpretation, and reporting of 500 CT examinations in the past 36 months	The physician should be thoroughly acquainted with the many morphologic and pathophysiologic manifestations of artifacts demonstrated on CT. Additionally, supervising physicians should have appropriate knowledge of alternative imaging methods including the use of and indications for general radiography and specialized studies such as: (a) Angiography (b) Ultrasonography (c) Magnetic resonance imaging (d) Nuclear medicine studies	Education in cardiac anatomy, physiology, pathology, and cardiac CT imaging for a time equivalent to at least 30 h of CME
Physicians not board certified in radiology or not trained in a diagnostic radiology residency program who assume the responsibilities for CT imaging exclusively in a specific anatomical area should meet the following criteria: (a) Completion of an ACGME-approved residency program in the specialty practiced plus 200 h of Category I CME in the performance and interpretation of CT in the subspecialty where CT reading occurs (b) Supervision, interpretation, and reporting of 500 cases in that subspecialty area during the past 36 months in a supervised situation	The physician should be familiar with patient preparation for the examination The physician must have training in the recognition and treatment of adverse effects of contrast materials used for these studies (see the ACR Manual on Contrast Media and the ACR–SPR Practice Parameter for the Use of Intravascular Contrast Media)	Supervision, interpretation, or reporting of at least 50 cardiac CT examinations in the last 36 months. Coronary artery calcium scoring does not qualify as meeting these requirements
Completion of an accredited radiology residency in the past 24 months will be presumed to be satisfactory experience for the reporting and interpreting requirement	The physician must have the responsibility for: (a) Reviewing all indications for the examination (b) Specifying the use, dosage, and rate of administration of contrast agents (c) Specifying the imaging technique, including available techniques to reduce radiation dose (d) Interpreting images (e) Generating official/final interpretation reports (f) Maintaining the quality of the images and the interpretations	For any physician or any other physician who assumes responsibilities for cardiac CT imaging, additional qualifications should include: (a) Completion of an ACGME-approved training program in the specialty practice plus 200 h of Category I CME in the performance and interpretation of CT in the subspecialty where CT reading occurs

Table 22.1 (continued)

	The physician's continuing medical education should be in accordance with the ACR Practice Parameter for Continuing Medical Education (CME) of 150 h of approved education every 3 years and should include CME in cardiac CT as is appropriate to the physician's practice needs	Supervision, interpretation, or reporting of 500 cases in cardiothoracic imaging that include at least 50 cardiac CT examinations during the past 36 months in a supervised situation and at least 450 additional thoracic CT or thoracic CT angiography cases Coronary artery calcium scoring does not qualify as meeting these requirements
		Completion of at least 30 h of Category I CME in cardiac imaging, including cardiac CT, anatomy, physiology, and/or pathology, or documented equivalent supervised experience in a facility actively performing cardiac CT

Data from ACR–NASCI–SPR practice parameter for the performance and interpretation of cardiac computed tomography (CT) [9]

Table 22.2 Qualifications and responsibilities of personnel (ACCF: COCATS 4 Task Force 7: training in cardiovascular computed tomographic imaging)

It is required that at least 1 physician should have a minimum of 2 years of clinical experience and/or 300 scan interpretation of coronary CTA	It is recommended that interpretation physicians must have: (a) CBCCT certification (b) ACR board certification (c) Dedicated fellowship training in advanced cardiac imaging
It is required that all other physicians must maintain level 2 coronary CTA certification or equivalent	Cardiac CT fellows must be familiar with cardiovascular: (a) Anatomy (b) Physiology (c) Pathophysiology
Interpreting physicians must be trained in the best-practice protocol selection of the scanner(s) in use	Fellows must also understand the: (a) Clinical application of cardiac CT (b) Principles of cardiac CT physics (c) Radiation generation/exposure
A qualified physician must interpret the non-cardiac anatomy on all scans either as the primary reader or as a consulting physician	To be eligible to sit for the CBCCT examination: (a) US-trained cardiovascular fellows must have undergone training in a program accredited by the ACGME (b) Meet Level II training requirements
Cardiac CT fellows must be familiar with the protocols: (a) For contrast administration and contrast kinetics (b) The potential adverse events resulting from contrast exposure and appropriate treatment	Every cardiovascular fellow should develop familiarity with CCT: (a) Technical performance (b) Strengths (c) Limitations of CCT (d) Gain an understanding of how to effectively use the information provided by CCT
Level II training requirements: (a) Be present in the scanning suite control room and actively participate in the acquisition of 50 cases (b) View a maximum of 50 cases from an educational CD or presentation granting continuing medical education credit that contains CCT data review (c) 150 cases must involve interactive manipulation of reconstructed datasets using a three-dimensional imaging workstation (d) 20 cases must include evaluation of cardiac function (e) 20 cases should involve evaluation of structural and/or congenital heart disease (f) 15 cases must involve evaluation of bypass graft vessels (g) 40 cases should be correlated with invasive angiography and/or myocardial perfusion imaging (h) Be actively involved in acquisition, interpretation, and reporting of 50 cases CCT images	Level III training requirements (in addition to Level II): (a) Additional training and experience beyond the cardiovascular fellowship (b) Acquire specialized knowledge and experience in performing, interpreting, and training others to perform specific procedures or render advanced specialized care at a high level of skill (c) Be involved in the acquisition and interpretation of imaging examinations (d) Participation in research, teaching, and the administrative aspects of laboratory operations (e) Data management, report generation and distribution, quality improvement, and accreditation as well as development of an understanding of evolving multimodality imaging technologies

Data from Garcia et al. [11]

Table 22.3 Equipment specifications (ACR–NASCI–SPR practice parameter for the performance and interpretation of cardiac computed tomography [9])

For diagnostic-quality cardiac CT, the CT scanner should meet or exceed the following specifications:	
ECG synchronization for all scans, with the ability to perform prospective triggering and retrospective gating	Non-contrast-enhanced MDCT for coronary artery calcium scoring may be adequately performed on a scanner with a temporal resolution of 0.50 s using prospectively ECG-triggered "step-and-shoot" sequential acquisition
Setup for bolus tracking of the administered contrast material for appropriate timing of contrast-enhanced cardiac CT exams	Minimum section thickness should be: (a) ≤5 mm (b) ≤3 mm for coronary calcium scoring (c) ≤1.5 mm for CT coronary arteriography
Automated tube modulation during image acquisition for dose reduction	Volumetric computed tomography dose index (CTDI vol) and dose length product (DLP) must be available after each scan for transfer to individual PACS workstations
Contrast-enhanced cardiac CT by MDCT (should meet or exceed a 64-detector scanner), including: (a) CT coronary arteriography (b) A scanner capable of achieving in-plane spatial resolution ≤0.5 × 0.5 mm axial (c) *z*-axis spatial resolution ≤1 mm longitudinal (d) Temporal resolution ≤0.25 s	

Data from ACR–NASCI–SPR practice parameter for the performance and interpretation of cardiac computed tomography (CT) [9]

Table 22.4 CAD-RADS reporting and data system for patients presenting with stable chest pain

Degree of maximal coronary stenosis	Corresponding CAD-RAD classification	Interpretation	Recommendation on further cardiac investigation	Recommendation on management
0% (no plaque or stenosis)	CAD-RADS 0	Documented absence of CAD	None	Reassurance. Consider non-atherosclerotic causes of chest pain
1–24% minimal stenosis or plaque with no stenosis	CAD-RADS 1	Minimal non-obstructive CAD	None	Consider non-atherosclerotic causes of chest pain Consider preventive therapy and risk factor modification
25–49% mild stenosis	CAD-RADS 2	Mild non-obstructive CAD	None	Consider non- atherosclerotic causes of chest pain Consider preventive therapy and risk factor modification particularly for patients with non-obstructive plaque in multiple segments
50–69% stenosis	CAD-RADS 3	Moderate stenosis	Consider functional assessment	Consider symptom-guided anti-ischemic and preventive pharmacotherapy as well as risk factor modification per guideline-directed care Other treatments should be considered per guideline-directed care
A: 70–99% stenosis or B: Left main >50% or 3- vessel obstructive (≥70%) disease	CAD-RADS 4	Severe stenosis	A: Consider ICA or functional assessment B: ICA is recommended	Consider symptom-guided anti-ischemic and preventive pharmacotherapy as well as risk factor modification per guideline-directed care Other treatments (including options of revascularization) should be considered per guideline-directed care
100% (total occlusion)	CAD-RADS 5	Total coronary occlusion	Consider ICA and/or viability assessment	Consider symptom-guided anti-ischemic and preventive pharmacotherapy as well as risk factors modification per guideline-directed care Other treatments (including options of revascularization) should be considered per guideline-directed care
Nondiagnostic study	CAD-RADS N	Obstructive CAD cannot be excluded	Additional or alternative evaluation may be needed	

Data from Cury et al. [15]

Table 22.5 CAD-RADS reporting and data system for patients presenting with acute chest pain, negative first troponin, negative or nondiagnostic electrocardiogram, and low to intermediate risk (TIMI risk score <4) (emergency department or hospital setting)

Degree of maximal coronary stenosis	Corresponding CAD-RAD classification	Interpretation	Recommendation on management
0%	CAD-RADS 0	ACS highly unlikely	No further evaluation of ACS is required Consider other etiologies
1–24%	CAD-RADS 1	ACS highly unlikely	Consider evaluation of non-ACS etiology, if normal troponin and no ECG changes Consider referral for outpatient follow-up for preventive therapy and risk factor modification
25–49%	CAD-RADS 2	ACS unlikely	Consider evaluation of non-ACS etiology, if normal troponin and no ECG changes Consider referral for outpatient follow-up for preventive therapy and risk factor modification If clinical suspicion of ACS is high or if high-risk plaque features are noted, consider hospital admission with cardiology consultation
50–69%	CAD-RADS 3	ACS possible	Consider hospital admission with cardiology consultation, functional testing, and/or ICA for evaluation and management Recommendation for anti-ischemic and preventive management should be considered as well as risk factor modification. Other treatments should be considered if presence of hemodynamically significant lesion
A:70–99% B: Left main >50% or three-vessel obstructive disease	CAD-RADS 4	ACS likely	Consider hospital admission with cardiology consultation. Further evaluation with ICA and revascularization as appropriate Recommendation for anti-ischemic and preventive management should be considered as well as risk factor modification
100% (total occlusion)	CAD-RADS 5	ACS very likely	Consider expedited ICA on a timely basis and revascularization if appropriate if acute occlusion Recommendation for anti-ischemic and preventive management should be considered as well as risk factor modifications
Nondiagnostic study	CAD-RADS N	ACS cannot be excluded	Additional or alternative evaluation for ACS is needed

Data from Cury et al. [15]

Table 22.6 Recommendation on advance imaging in patients with suspected SIHD who require noninvasive testing (ACCF/AHA/ACP/AATS/PCNA/SCAI/STS)

Indications	Class	Level of evidence
CCTA may be reasonable for patients with intermediate pretest probability of IHD	IIb	B
CCTA is reasonable for patients with low to intermediate pretest probability of IHD who are unable to perform moderate physical functioning or have disabling comorbidity	IIa	B
CCTA is reasonable for patients with an intermediate pretest probability of IHD who: (a) Continue to have symptoms despite normal prior test results (b) Have inconclusive results from prior ETT/pharm stress (c) Are unable to undergo stress nuclear MPI or stress echo	IIa	C
For patients with low to intermediate pretest probability of obstructive IHD, non-contrast cardiac CT to determine CAC score may be considered	IIb	C
In asymptomatic adults with diabetes, 40 years of age and older, measurement of CAC is reasonable for cardiovascular risk assessment	IIa	B
Measurement of CAC may be reasonable for cardiovascular risk assessment in persons at low to intermediate risk (6–10% 10-year risk)	IIb	B
Persons at low risk (<6% 10-year risk) should not undergo CAC measurement for cardiovascular risk assessment	III	B
Cardiac CT is not recommended for routine evaluation of LV function in patients who have normal ECG, have no history of MI, have no symptoms, have no signs indicative of heart failure, and have no complex ventricular arrhythmias	III	C
Repeat cardiac CT for LV function evaluation in patients who have had prior LV functional evaluation less than 1 year ago and in whom there has been no change in clinical status or anticipation of a change in therapy is not recommended	III	C

Data from Fihn et al. [2]

Table 22.7 Risk assessment in patients able and unable to exercise (ACCF/AHA/ACP/AATS/PCNA/SCAI/STS)

Indications	Class	Level of evidence
In patients with SIHD who have uninterpretable ECG, CCTA may be reasonable for risk assessment even if they can exercise	IIb	B
In patients who are able to exercise and have interpretable ECG, CCTA is not recommended	III	C
CCTA can be used as a first-line test for cardiovascular risk evaluation in patients with SIHD who are unable to exercise even if they have interpretable ECG	IIa	C
CCTA can be used for cardiovascular risk evaluation in SIHD patients with indeterminate functional test results	IIa	C
CCTA may be used for cardiovascular risk evaluation in SIHD patients who cannot undergo stress imaging tests; or it may be used as an alternative to invasive coronary angiogram in patients with unknown coronary anatomy in whom functional test show moderate- to high-risk result	IIb	C
Performance of stress imaging and CCTA at the same time is not recommended	III	C

Data from Fihn et al. [2]

Table 22.8 Follow-up noninvasive testing in patients with known SIHD who have new, recurrent, or worsening symptoms that is not consistent with unstable angina (ACCF/AHA/ACP/AATS/PCNA/SCAI/STS) [2]

Indications	Class	Level of evidence
In patients with new or worsening symptoms that are not indicative of UA and who have prior stents (with stent diameter of ≥3 mm) or CABG, CCTA can be useful to evaluate for patency of coronary stents and CABG even if they can exercise	IIb	B
In patients with new or worsening symptoms that is not indicative of UA and who have prior stents (with stent diameter of ≥3 mm), CCTA may be useful if there is no evidence of moderate or severe coronary calcifications even if they can exercise	IIb	B
CCTA is not recommended in patients who have evidence of moderate to severe coronary calcifications or prior stents (with stents diameter of less than 3 mm) whether or not they can or cannot exercise	III	B
CCTA is not recommended in asymptomatic patients with prior CABG less than 5 years or prior PCI less than 2 years ago	III	C

Data from Fihn et al. [2]

Table 22.9 Heart failure imaging guidelines (ACCF/ACR/ASE/ASNC/SCCT/SCMR [5])

Recommendations	Class type	Level of evidence
In patients with angina/ischemic equivalent syndrome/angina, noninvasive imaging may be considered to define the likelihood of CAD in patients with HF and LV dysfunction	IIb	C
In patient without angina/ischemic equivalent syndrome/angina, noninvasive imaging may be considered to define the likelihood of CAD in patients with HF and LV dysfunction	IIb	C

Data from Patel et al. [5]

Table 22.10 Stable ischemic heart disease guidelines (ACCF/AHA/ASE/ASNC/HFSA/HRS/SCAI/SCCT/SCMR/STS [8])

Test indications	Calcium scoring	CCTA
Low pretest probability of CAD, ECG interpretable, and able to exercise	R	R
Low pretest probability of CAD, ECG uninterpretable, or unable to exercise	R	M
Intermediate pretest probability of CAD, ECG interpretable, and able to exercise	R	M
Intermediate pretest probability of CAD, ECG uninterpretable, or unable to exercise	R	A
High pretest probability of CAD, ECG interpretable, and able to exercise	R	M
High pretest probability of CAD, ECG uninterpretable, and unable to exercise	R	M

Data from Wolk et al. [8]. A – Appropriate; M – May be appropriate; R – Rarely appropriate; NA – No determination of appropriateness

Table 22.11 Asymptomatic (without symptoms or ischemic equivalent) (ACCF/AHA/ASE/ASNC/HFSA/HRS/SCAI/SCCT/SCMR/STS [8])

Test indications	Calcium scoring	CCTA
Low global CHD risk, regardless of ECG interpretability and ability to exercise	R	R
Intermediate global CHD risk and ECG interpretable and able to exercise	M	R
Intermediate global CHD risk ECG uninterpretable or unable to exercise	M	R
High global CAD risk and ECG interpretable and able to exercise	M	M
High global CAD risk and ECG uninterpretable or unable to exercise	M	M

Data from Wolk et al. [8]. A – Appropriate; M – May be appropriate; R – Rarely appropriate; NA – No determination of appropriateness

Table 22.12 Newly diagnosed heart failure (resting LV function previously assessed but no prior CAD evaluation) (ACCF/AHA/ASE/ASNC/HFSA/HRS/SCAI/SCCT/SCMR/STS [8])

Test indications	Calcium scoring	CCTA
Newly diagnosed systolic heart failure	R	A
Newly diagnosed diastolic heart failure	R	M

Data from Wolk et al. [8]. A – Appropriate; M – May be appropriate; R – Rarely appropriate; NA – No determination of appropriateness

Table 22.14 Syncope without ischemic equivalent (ACCF/AHA/ASE/ASNC/HFSA/HRS/SCAI/SCCT/SCMR/STS [8])

Test indications	Calcium scoring	CCTA
Low global CAD risk	R	R
Intermediate or high global CAD risk	R	M

Data from Wolk et al. [8] A – Appropriate; M – May be appropriate; R – Rarely appropriate; NA – No determination of appropriateness

Table 22.13 Evaluation of arrhythmias without ischemic equivalent (no prior cardiac evaluation) (ACCF/AHA/ASE/ASNC/HFSA/HRS/SCAI/SCCT/SCMR/STS [8])

Test indications	Calcium scoring	CCTA
Sustained VT	R	M
Ventricular fibrillation	R	M
Exercise-induced VT or nonsustained VT	R	M
Frequent PVCs	R	M
Infrequent PVCs	R	R
New-onset atrial fibrillation	R	R
Prior to initiation of anti-arrhythmia therapy in high global CAD risk patients	R	M

Data from Wolk et al. [8]. A – Appropriate; M – May be appropriate; R – Rarely appropriate; NA – No determination of appropriateness

Table 22.15 Prior testing without intervening revascularization (sequential testing (≤90 days): abnormal prior test/study) (ACCF/AHA/ASE/ASNC/HFSA/HRS/SCAI/SCCT/SCMR/STS)

Test indications	Calcium scoring	CCTA
Abnormal rest ECG findings (potentially ischemic in nature such as LBBB, T-wave inversions) and low global CAD risk	R	M
Abnormal rest ECG findings (potentially ischemic in nature such as LBBB, T-wave inversions) and intermediate to high global CAD risk	R	M
Abnormal prior exercise ECG test	R	A
Abnormal prior stress imaging study (assumes not repeat of same type of stress imaging)	R	A
Obstructive CAD on prior CCTA study	NA	NA
Obstructive CAD on prior invasive coronary angiography	R	R
Abnormal prior CCT calcium (Agatston score >100)	NA	M

Data from Wolk et al. [8]. A – Appropriate; M – May be appropriate; R – Rarely appropriate; NA – No determination of appropriateness

Table 22.16 Sequential or follow-up testing (≤90 days): uncertain prior results (ACCF/AHA/ASE/ASNC/HFSA/HRS/SCAI/SCCT/SCMR/STS)

Test indication	Calcium scoring	CCTA
Abnormal rest ECG findings (potentially ischemic in nature such as LBBB, T-wave inversions) and low global CAD risk	R	M
Abnormal rest ECG findings (potentially ischemic in nature such as LBBB, T-wave inversions) and intermediate to high global CAD risk	R	M
Abnormal prior exercise ECG test	R	A
Abnormal prior stress imaging study (assumes not repeat of the same type of stress imaging)	R	A
Obstructive CAD on prior CCTA study	NA	NA
Obstructive CAD on prior invasive coronary angiography	R	R
Abnormal prior CCT calcium (Agatston score >100)	NA	M

Data from Wolk et al. [8]. A – Appropriate; M – May be appropriate; R – Rarely appropriate; NA – No determination of appropriateness

Table 22.17 Sequential or follow-up testing (≤90 days): uncertain prior results – equivocal, borderline, or discordant prior noninvasive evaluation where obstructive CAD remains a concern (ACCF/AHA/ASE/ASNC/HFSA/HRS/SCAI/SCCT/SCMR/STS)

Test indications	Calcium scoring	CCTA
Prior exercise ECG test	R	A
Prior stress imaging study (assumes not repeat of same type of stress imaging)	R	A
Prior CCTA	NA	NA

Data from Wolk et al. [8]. A – Appropriate; M – May be appropriate; R – Rarely appropriate; NA – No determination of appropriateness

Table 22.18 Prior coronary angiography (invasive or noninvasive) (ACCF/AHA/ASE/ASNC/HFSA/HRS/SCAI/SCCT/SCMR/STS [8])

Test indication	Calcium scoring	CCTA
Coronary stenosis or anatomic abnormality of unclear significance found on cardiac CCTA	NA	NA
Coronary stenosis or anatomic abnormality of unclear significance on previous coronary angiography	R	R

Data from Wolk et al. [8]. A – Appropriate; M – May be appropriate; R – Rarely appropriate; NA – No determination of appropriateness

Table 22.19 Follow-up testing (>90 days): asymptomatic or stable symptoms – abnormal prior exercise ECG test asymptomatic or stable symptoms (ACCF/AHA/ASE/ASNC/HFSA/HRS/SCAI/SCCT/SCMR/STS [8])

Test indication	Calcium scoring	CCTA
Last test <2 years ago	R	R
Last test ≥2 years ago	R	R

Data from Wolk et al. [8]. A – Appropriate; M – May be appropriate; R – Rarely appropriate; NA – No determination of appropriateness

Table 22.20 Abnormal prior stress imaging study asymptomatic or stable symptoms (ACCF/AHA/ASE/ASNC/HFSA/HRS/SCAI/SCCT/SCMR/STS [8])

Test indication	Calcium scoring	CCTA
Last study <2 years ago	R	R
Last study ≥2 years ago	R	R

Data from Wolk et al. [8]. A – Appropriate; M – May be appropriate; R – Rarely appropriate; NA – No determination of appropriateness

Table 22.21 Obstructive CAD on prior coronary angiography (invasive or noninvasive) asymptomatic (without ischemic equivalent) or stable symptoms (ACCF/AHA/ASE/ASNC/HFSA/HRS/SCAI/SCCT/SCMR/STS [8])

Test indications	Calcium scoring	CCTA
Last study <2 years ago	R	R
Last study ≥2 years ago	R	R

Data from Wolk et al. [8]. A – Appropriate; M – May be appropriate; R – Rarely appropriate; NA – No determination of appropriateness

Table 22.22 Prior coronary calcium Agatston score asymptomatic (without ischemic equivalent) or stable symptoms (ACCF/AHA/ASE/ASNC/HFSA/HRS/SCAI/SCCT/SCMR/STS [8])

Test indications	Calcium scoring	CCTA
Agatston score <100	R	R
Low to intermediate global CAD risk Agatston score between 100 and 400	R	R
High global CAD risk Agatston score between 100 and 400	R	R
Agatston score >400	R	R

Data from Wolk et al. [8]. A – Appropriate; M – May be appropriate; R – Rarely appropriate; NA – No determination of appropriateness

Table 22.23 Normal prior exercise ECG test asymptomatic (without ischemic equivalent) (ACCF/AHA/ASE/ASNC/HFSA/HRS/SCAI/SCCT/SCMR/STS)

Test indications	Calcium scoring	CCTA
Low global CAD risk	R	R
Intermediate to high global CAD risk and test <2 years ago	R	R
Intermediate to high global CAD risk and test ≥2 years ago	R	R

Data from Wolk et al. [8]. A – Appropriate; M – May be appropriate; R – Rarely appropriate; NA – No determination of appropriateness

Table 22.24 Normal prior stress imaging study or non-obstructive CAD on angiogram (invasive or noninvasive) asymptomatic (without ischemic equivalent) (ACCF/AHA/ASE/ASNC/HFSA/HRS/SCAI/SCCT/SCMR/STS)

Test indications	Calcium scoring	CCTA
Low global CAD risk	R	R
Intermediate to high global CAD risk and study <2 years ago	R	R
Intermediate to high global CAD risk and study ≥2 years ago	R	R

Data from Wolk et al. [8]. A – Appropriate; M – May be appropriate; R – Rarely appropriate; NA – No determination of appropriateness

Table 22.25 Normal prior exercise ECG test stable symptoms (ACCF/AHA/ASE/ASNC/HFSA/HRS/SCAI/SCCT/SCMR/STS)

Test indications	Calcium scoring	CCTA
Low global CAD risk	R	R
Intermediate to high global CAD risk and test <2 years ago	R	R
Intermediate to high global CAD risk and test ≥2 years ago	R	R

Data from Wolk et al. [8]. A – Appropriate; M – May be appropriate; R – Rarely appropriate; NA – No determination of appropriateness

Table 22.26 Normal prior stress imaging study or non-obstructive CAD on angiogram (invasive or noninvasive) stable symptoms (ACCF/AHA/ASE/ASNC/HFSA/HRS/SCAI/SCCT/SCMR/STS)

Test indications	Calcium scoring	CCTA
Low global CAD risk	R	R
Intermediate to high global CAD risk and prior study <2 years ago	R	R
Intermediate to high global CAD risk and prior study ≥2 years ago	R	R

From Wolk et al. [8]. A – Appropriate; M – May be appropriate; R – Rarely appropriate; NA – No determination of appropriateness

Table 22.27 Follow-up testing: new or worsening symptoms (ACCF/AHA/ASE/ASNC/HFSA/HRS/SCAI/SCCT/SCMR/STS)

Test indications	Calcium scoring	CCTA
Normal exercise ECG test	R	A
Non-obstructive CAD on coronary angiography (invasive or noninvasive) or normal prior stress imaging study	R	R
Abnormal exercise ECG test	R	A
Abnormal prior stress imaging study	R	A
Obstructive CAD on CCTA study	R	R
Obstructive CAD on invasive coronary angiography	R	R
Abnormal CCTA calcium (Agatston Score > 100)	R	M

Data from Wolk et al. [8]. A – Appropriate; M – May be appropriate; R – Rarely appropriate; NA – No determination of appropriateness

Table 22.28 Post-revascularization (PCI or CABG) symptomatic (ischemic equivalent) (ACCF/AHA/ASE/ASNC/HFSA/HRS/SCAI/SCCT/SCMR/STS)

Test indication	Calcium scoring	CCTA
Evaluation of ischemic equivalent	R	M

Data from Wolk et al. [8]. A – Appropriate; M – May be appropriate; R – Rarely appropriate; NA – No determination of appropriateness

Table 22.29 Asymptomatic (without ischemic equivalent) (ACCF/AHA/ASE/ASNC/HFSA/HRS/SCAI/SCCT/SCMR/STS)

Test indications	Calcium scoring	CCTA
Incomplete revascularization/additional revascularization feasible	R	R
Prior left main coronary stent	R	M
<5 years after CABG	R	R
≥5 years after CABG	R	R
<2 years after PCI	R	R
≥2 years after PCI	R	R

Data from Wolk et al. [8]. A – Appropriate; M – May be appropriate; R – Rarely appropriate; NA – No determination of appropriateness

Table 22.30 Preoperative evaluation for non-cardiac surgery – Moderate-to-good functional capacity (≥4 METs) or no clinical risk factors (ACCF/AHA/ASE/ASNC/HFSA/HRS/SCAI/SCCT/SCMR/STS)

Test indications	Calcium scoring	CCTA
Any surgery	R	R

Data from Wolk et al. [8]. A – Appropriate; M – May be appropriate; R – Rarely appropriate; NA – No determination of appropriateness

Table 22.31 Asymptomatic and <1 year post any of the following: normal CT or invasive angiogram, normal stress test for CAD, or revascularization (ACCF/AHA/ASE/ASNC/HFSA/HRS/SCAI/SCCT/SCMR/STS)

Test indication	Calcium scoring	CCTA
Any surgery	R	R

Data from Wolk et al. [8]. A – Appropriate; M – May be appropriate; R – Rarely appropriate; NA – No determination of appropriateness

Table 22.32 Poor or unknown functional capacity (<4 METs) (ACCF/AHA/ASE/ASNC/HFSA/HRS/SCAI/SCCT/SCMR/STS)

Test indications	Calcium scoring	CCTA
Low-risk surgery ≥1 clinical risk factor	R	R
Intermediate-risk surgery ≥1 clinical risk factor	R	R
Vascular surgery ≥1 clinical risk factor	R	R
Kidney transplant	R	R
Liver transplant	R	R

Data from Wolk et al. [8]. A – Appropriate; M – May be appropriate; R – Rarely appropriate; NA – No determination of appropriateness

Table 22.33 Determine exercise level prior to initiation of exercise prescription or cardiac rehabilitation exercise prescription (ACCF/AHA/ASE/ASNC/HFSA/HRS/SCAI/SCCT/SCMR/STS)

Test indication	Calcium scoring	CCTA
No prior revascularization	R	R

Data from Wolk et al. [8]. A – Appropriate; M – May be appropriate; R – Rarely appropriate; NA – No determination of appropriateness

Table 22.34 Prior to the initiation of cardiac rehabilitation (as a stand-alone indication): able to exercise (ACCF/AHA/ASE/ASNC/HFSA/HRS/SCAI/SCCT/SCMR/STS)

Test indications	Calcium scoring	CCTA
Post-revascularization (PCI or CABG)	R	R
Heart failure	R	R

Data from Wolk et al. [8]. A – Appropriate; M – May be appropriate; R – Rarely appropriate; NA – No determination of appropriateness

World Health Organization [23, 24] guidelines on the use of cardiac CT. Recommendations from various appropriate use criteria and guidelines are shown in Tables 1-34.

By far, the USA has the most comprehensive set of guidelines and appropriate use criteria, and therefore many other countries tend to utilize the guidelines and the appropriate use criteria found in the USA. Furthermore, the USA is currently shifting from single modality appropriate use criteria to multimodality imaging for various disease scenarios. There is a strong agreement among the guidelines found around the globe with respect to class II and III indications for the use of cardiac CT. There is also a strong agreement among the guidelines across the globe regarding the use of cardiac CT in low- to intermediate- and intermediate-risk patients. There is currently no class I indications for the use of cardiac CT except in Brazil.

References

1. Cesar LA, Ferreira JF, Armaganijan D, Gowdak LH, Mansur AP, Bodanese LC, et al. Guideline for stable coronary artery disease. Arq Bras Cardiol. 2014;103(2 Suppl 2):1–56.
2. Fihn SD, Gardin JM, Abrams J, Berra K, Blankenship JC, Dallas AP, et al. 2012 ACCF/AHA/ACP/AATS/PCNA/SCAI/STS Guideline for the diagnosis and management of patients with stable ischemic heart disease: a report of the American College of Cardiology Foundation/American Heart Association Task Force on Practice Guidelines, and the American College of Physicians, American Association for Thoracic Surgery, Preventive Cardiovascular Nurses Association, Society for Cardiovascular Angiography and Interventions, and Society of Thoracic Surgeons. J Am Coll Cardiol. 2012;60(24):e44–e164.
3. Mancini GB, Gosselin G, Chow B, Kostuk W, Stone J, Yvorchuk KJ, et al. Canadian Cardiovascular Society guidelines for the diagnosis and management of stable ischemic heart disease. Can J Cardiol. 2014;30(8):837–49.
4. Montalescot G, Sechtem U, Achenbach S, Andreotti F, Arden C, Budaj A, et al. 2013 ESC guidelines on the management of stable coronary artery disease: the Task Force on the management of stable coronary artery disease of the European Society of Cardiology. Eur Heart J. 2013;34(38):2949–3003.
5. Patel MR, White RD, Abbara S, Bluemke DA, Herfkens RJ, Picard M, et al. 2013 ACCF/ACR/ASE/ASNC/SCCT/SCMR appropriate utilization of cardiovascular imaging in heart failure: a joint report of the American College of Radiology Appropriateness Criteria Committee and the American College of Cardiology Foundation Appropriate Use Criteria Task Force. J Am Coll Cardiol. 2013;61(21):2207–31.
6. Rybicki FJ, Udelson JE, Peacock WF, Goldhaber SZ, Isselbacher EM, Kazerooni E, et al. 2015 ACR/ACC/AHA/AATS/ACEP/ASNC/NASCI/SAEM/SCCT/SCMR/SCPC/SNMMI/STR/STS Appropriate Utilization of Cardiovascular Imaging in Emergency Department Patients With Chest Pain: A Joint Document of the American College of Radiology Appropriateness Criteria Committee and the American College of Cardiology Appropriate Use Criteria Task Force. J Am Coll Cardiol. 2016;67(7):853–79.
7. White RD, Patel MR, Abbara S, Bluemke DA, Herfkens RJ, Picard M, et al. 2013 ACCF/ACR/ASE/ASNC/SCCT/SCMR appropriate utilization of cardiovascular imaging in heart failure: an executive summary: a joint report of the ACR Appropriateness Criteria (R) Committee and the ACCF Appropriate Use Criteria Task Force. J Am Coll Radiol. 2013;10(7):493–500.
8. Wolk MJ, Bailey SR, Doherty JU, Douglas PS, Hendel RC, Kramer CM, et al. ACCF/AHA/ASE/ASNC/HFSA/HRS/SCAI/SCCT/SCMR/STS 2013 multimodality appropriate use criteria for the detection and risk assessment of stable ischemic heart disease: a report of the American College of Cardiology Foundation Appropriate Use Criteria Task Force, American Heart Association, American Society of Echocardiography, American Society of Nuclear Cardiology, Heart Failure Society of America, Heart Rhythm Society, Society for Cardiovascular Angiography and Interventions, Society of Cardiovascular Computed Tomography, Society for Cardiovascular Magnetic Resonance, and Society of Thoracic Surgeons. J Am Coll Cardiol. 2014;63(4):380–406.
9. ACR–NASCI–SPR practice parameter for the performance and interpretation of cardiac computed tomography (CT). 2016. Available from: http://www.acr.org/~/media/f4720a18f-03b4a26a0c9c3cc18637d87.pdf.
10. Abbara S, Arbab-Zadeh A, Callister TQ, Desai MY, Mamuya W, Thomson L, et al. SCCT guidelines for performance of coronary computed tomographic angiography: a report of the Society of Cardiovascular Computed Tomography Guidelines Committee. J Cardiovasc Comput Tomogr. 2009;3(3):190–204.
11. Garcia MJ, Blankstein R, Budoff MJ, Dent JM, Drachman DE, Lesser JR, et al. COCATS 4 Task Force 7: Training in Cardiovascular Computed Tomographic Imaging. J Am Coll Cardiol. 2015;65(17):1810–21.
12. ACR Cardiac CT Certificate of Advanced Proficiency Cardiac CT: American College of Radiology. Available from: http://www.acr.org/~/media/ACR/Documents/PDF/Education/Exams/CoAP/CoAPBrochure.pdf.
13. European Diploma Cardiac Imaging: European Society of Cardiac Radiology. Available from: http://escr.org/cms/website.php?id=/en/education/diploma.htm.
14. CT Coronary Angiography Service Specification: British Society of Cardiovascular Imaging. 2012. Available from: https://bsci.org.uk/standards-guidelines/ct-coronary-angiography-service-specification.
15. Cury RC, Abbara S, Achenbach S, Agatston A, Berman DS, Budoff MJ, et al. CAD-RADS: Coronary Artery Disease - Reporting and Data System.: An Expert Consensus Document of the Society of Cardiovascular Computed Tomography (SCCT), the American College of Radiology (ACR) and the North American Society for Cardiovascular Imaging (NASCI). Endorsed by the American College of Cardiology. J Am Coll Radiol. 2016;13(12 Pt A):1458–66.e9
16. Leipsic J, Abbara S, Achenbach S, Cury R, Earls JP, Mancini GJ, et al. SCCT guidelines for the interpretation and reporting of coronary CT angiography: a report of the Society of Cardiovascular Computed Tomography Guidelines Committee. J Cardiovasc Comput Tomogr. 2014;8(5):342–58.
17. Beanlands RS, Chow BJ, Dick A, Friedrich MG, Gulenchyn KY, Kiess M, et al. CCS/CAR/CANM/CNCS/CanSCMR joint position statement on advanced noninvasive cardiac imaging using positron emission tomography, magnetic resonance imaging and multidetector computed tomographic angiography in the diagnosis and evaluation of ischemic heart disease--executive summary. Can J Cardiol. 2007;23(2):107–19.
18. Kitagawa K, Choi BW, Chan C, Jinzaki M, Tsai IC, Yong HS, et al. ASCI 2010 appropriateness criteria for cardiac magnetic resonance imaging: a report of the Asian Society of Cardiovascular Imaging cardiac computed tomography and cardiac magnetic resonance imaging guideline working group. Int J Cardiovasc Imaging. 2010;26(Suppl 2):173–86.
19. Tsai IC, Choi BW, Chan C, Jinzaki M, Kitagawa K, Yong HS, et al. ASCI 2010 appropriateness criteria for cardiac computed tomography: a report of the Asian Society of Cardiovascular Imaging

Cardiac Computed Tomography and Cardiac Magnetic Resonance Imaging Guideline Working Group. Int J Cardiovasc Imaging. 2010;26(Suppl 1):1–15.

20. Kim YJ, Yong HS, Kim SM, Kim JA, Yang DH, Hong YJ, et al. Korean guidelines for the appropriate use of cardiac CT. Korean J Radiol. 2015;16(2):251–85.
21. Taylor AJ, Cerqueira M, Hodgson JM, Mark D, Min J, O'Gara P, et al. ACCF/SCCT/ACR/AHA/ASE/ASNC/NASCI/SCAI/SCMR 2010 appropriate use criteria for cardiac computed tomography. A report of the American College of Cardiology Foundation Appropriate Use Criteria Task Force, the Society of Cardiovascular Computed Tomography, the American College of Radiology, the American Heart Association, the American Society of Echocardiography, the American Society of Nuclear Cardiology, the North American Society for Cardiovascular Imaging, the Society for Cardiovascular Angiography and Interventions, and the Society for Cardiovascular Magnetic Resonance. J Am Coll Cardiol. 2010;56(22):1864–94.
22. Greenland P, Alpert JS, Beller GA, Benjamin EJ, Budoff MJ, Fayad ZA, et al. 2010 ACCF/AHA guideline for assessment of cardiovascular risk in asymptomatic adults: a report of the American College of Cardiology Foundation/American Heart Association Task Force on Practice Guidelines. J Am Coll Cardiol. 2010;56(25):e50–103.
23. Global health risks: mortality and burden of disease attributable to selected major risks: World Health Organization. 2009. Available from: http://www.who.int/healthinfo/global_burden_disease/GlobalHealthRisks_report_full.pdf.
24. Global atlas on cardiovascular disease prevention and control: World Health Organization. 2011. Available from: http://www.who.int/cardiovascular_diseases/publications/atlas_cvd/en/.

Part V

Where We Are: Risk Stratification and Management

Clinical Application of the Coronary Artery Calcium Score and Implications for Cardiovascular Disease Prevention

23

Pamela B. Morris and Michael D. Shapiro

Introduction: The Burden of Atherosclerosis

Despite advances in medical technologies and pharmaceutical treatments, the burden of atherosclerotic cardiovascular disease (ASCVD) remains formidable [1]. Applications of evidence-based therapies, including the use of thrombolysis, coronary artery bypass grafting, percutaneous transluminal coronary angioplasty and stents, beta-blockers, angiotensin-converting enzyme inhibitors, spironolactone, and HMG-CoA reductase inhibitors (statins), have contributed to a substantial decline in ASCVD morbidity and mortality in the United States over the past two decades [2]. However, the direct and indirect costs of these treatments for symptomatic heart disease continue to rise, making primary prevention of new onset ASCVD a global priority [1].

To reduce morbidity and mortality from ASCVD, two approaches have been widely implemented: a *population (public health) approach* and a *high-risk (clinical strategy) approach*. The population approach focuses on community-wide education encouraging individuals to maintain an optimal ASCVD risk factor profile, including adoption of a heart healthy dietary pattern, maintenance of optimal weight, regular physical activity, avoidance of tobacco products, and achievement of optimal lipid and blood pressure levels. This approach can be expected to have the greatest long-term impact on reducing the burden of ASCVD across the globe. However, in individuals with established risk factors for atherosclerosis, the high-risk approach intensifies management and specifies evidence-based interventions proven to reduce ASCVD death and disability. The high-risk approach leverages biomarkers that most reliably identify individuals at greatest risk and most likely to benefit from intervention.

More recently, there has been a paradigm shift in the identification of at-risk individuals to include strategies for early detection of ASCVD (the presence of subclinical atherosclerosis), in addition to the use of traditional ASCVD risk factors. Quantification of coronary artery calcification (CAC) with electrocardiographic (ECG)-gated non-contrast cardiac computed tomography (CCT) has emerged as the most effect means to refine ASCVD risk estimation. Studies consistently demonstrate that CAC scores (CACS) provide incremental predictive value above and beyond traditional risk factors and improve the identification of at-risk patients as discussed below.

Global Risk Assessment Tools for ASCVD: Matching Intensity of Intervention with Severity of Risk

Matching intensity of preventive treatments to the severity of risk is based on the concept that high-risk patients receive the greatest benefit from therapeutic intervention, thereby optimizing efficacy, safety, and cost-effectiveness [3]. Risk assessment algorithms have been developed from epidemiologic studies for a variety of populations using conventional ASCVD risk factors to guide selection of candidates for evidence-based preventive drug therapies. The Framingham Risk Score (FRS) algorithms are derived from a predominantly Caucasian population in the USA [4], whereas the *Pro*spective *Ca*rdiovascular *M*unster (PROCAM—Germany) [5] and the Systemic Coronary Risk Evaluation (SCORE) [6] models are derived from European population studies. The 2013 American College of Cardiology (ACC)/American Heart Association (AHA) Cardiovascular (CV) Risk Calculator (based on the Pooled Cohort Equations) is derived from a US population that is composed of primarily Caucasians and blacks [7]. Each algorithm predicts either 10-year risk of coronary heart disease (CHD) events

P. B. Morris (✉)
Seinsheimer Cardiovascular Health Program, Department of Medicine and Cardiology, Medical University of South Carolina, Charleston, SC, USA
e-mail: morrispa@musc.edu

M. D. Shapiro
Department of Medicine, Division of Cardiovascular Medicine, Oregon Health & Science University, Portland, OR, USA

U. J. Schoepf (ed.), *CT of the Heart*, Contemporary Medical Imaging, https://doi.org/10.1007/978-1-60327-237-7_23

(coronary death or myocardial infarction [MI]) or global ASCVD events (fatal or nonfatal MI, fatal or nonfatal stroke, CHD death). The ACC/AHA CV Risk Calculator also provides an estimate of lifetime or 30-year risk of ASCVD events for individuals between the ages of 20 and 59 years.

As cardiovascular risk is most strongly related to age, risk prediction algorithms may underestimate the relative or long-term absolute risk of younger individuals, particularly younger men and middle-aged men and women. Recognizing these limitations, the Reynolds Risk Score was developed to more accurately predict ASCVD risk in men and women before age 60 years [8, 9]. This algorithm includes not only conventional ASCVD risk factors (age, systolic blood pressure, total- and high-density lipoprotein-cholesterol, and tobacco use) but also incorporates hemoglobin A_1C levels, high-sensitivity C-reactive protein (hs-CRP), and family history of premature MI. In a recent analysis of calibration and discrimination among five cardiovascular risk scoring algorithms in the more contemporary MESA population (Multi-Ethnic Study of Atherosclerosis), four of the tools, including the 2013 AHA/ACC CV Risk Calculator, demonstrated overestimation of risk (25% to 115%) in this cohort without baseline clinical ASCVD [10]. The Reynolds Risk Score overestimated risk by 9% in men but underestimated risk by 21% in women.

Nearly 660,000 previously asymptomatic people present annually in the USA with a first MI, and 610,000 people present with a first stroke [1]. This would suggest that although our current risk assessment algorithms are useful for population-based prediction, clinicians evaluating the individual patient may need additional information to accurately identify those at higher risk. While most of the *excess* risk for ASCVD events in a population may be explained by conventional ASCVD risk factors, there is considerable variability in how the disease is expressed in *individuals* within the population. The majority of ASCVD events continue to occur in patients considered either low- or intermediate-risk at baseline assessments, and most individuals are

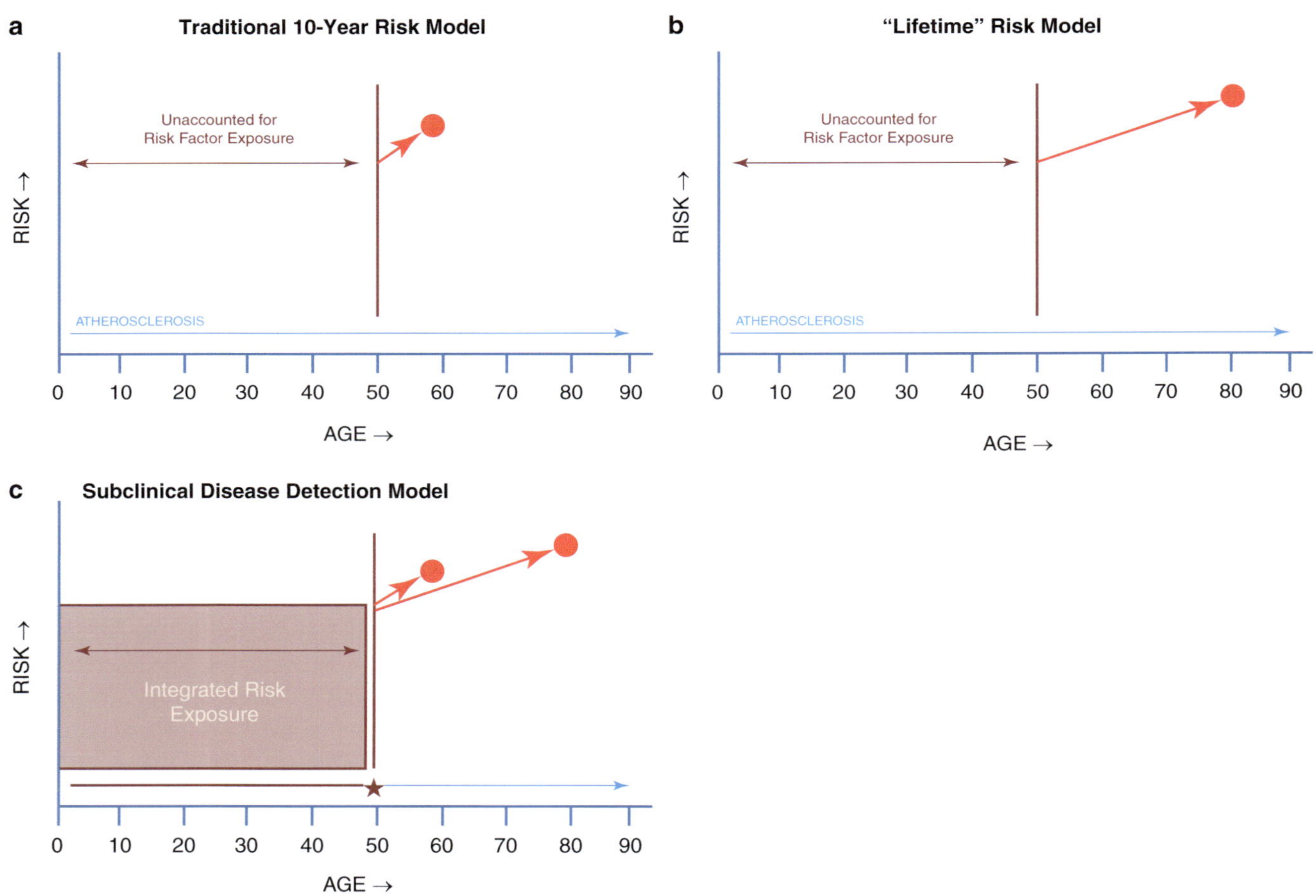

Fig. 23.1 Strategies for risk prediction. Traditional risk models (**a**) use one-time measurements of risk factors taken later in life—in this example at age 50—and project coronary heart disease (CHD) risk during the coming 10 years. Lifetime risk models (**b**) similarly use one-time measurements of risk factors but instead project long-term CHD risk. Subclinical atherosclerosis (**c**), by directly visualizing the accumulated burden of atherosclerosis, integrates lifetime risk exposure and may provide more accurate estimates of near-term and long-term risk. (From Blaha et al. [15], with permission)

not recognized as high-risk prior to first CHD event [11–14]. Previous risk assessment algorithms have focused only on a single measure of traditional risk factors taken at a relatively later stage in adult life and may not accurately capture the risk of cumulative exposure to all risk determinants over a lifetime (Fig. 23.1). This can contribute to over- and underestimation of risk and resultant over- or undertreatment with preventive therapies. To enhance the predictive power in individuals, current interest is focused on the identification of emerging risk factors that influence how the major risk factors affect absolute ASCVD risk, as well as early disease detection strategies such as preventive imaging techniques to identify subclinical atherosclerotic disease. The 2013 ACC/AHA cardiovascular risk assessment guideline suggests consideration of these risk markers if, after quantitative risk assessment, a risk-based treatment decision is uncertain [7]. Recommended risk markers include family history of premature ASCVD, hs-CRP, and measures of subclinical atherosclerotic disease (ankle brachial index [ABI] and CACS).

The presence of subclinical atherosclerosis can inform the treatment decisions (e.g., initiation, intensification) for preventive therapies in carefully selected asymptomatic individuals. CACS directly quantifies the accumulated burden of coronary atherosclerosis and provides a more personalized assessment of risk. As noted by Blaha et al., by integrating the cumulative interaction of early risk determinants (genetic and epigenetic factors) with lifetime exposure to traditional risk factors and other influences (e.g., passive tobacco smoke exposure, air quality), CACS provides a unique measure of the resultant effect on the vasculature [15, 16].

Coronary Artery Calcium: Age, Gender, and Ethnic Differences

The extent of CAC varies with ethnicity, gender, and age as demonstrated in the MESA study [17, 18]. One analysis from MESA included 6110 subjects of which 53% were female. Ethnicity distribution was balanced across gender with 41% white, 11.8% Chinese American, 26.4% black, and 20.9% Hispanic individuals. Men had higher CACS than women in every age group for each ethnicity. Moreover, the extent and severity of CAC increased with age in both men and women. Approximately 62% of women demonstrated no evidence of CAC, whereas only 40% of men had a CACS = 0. Overall, for men, blacks had the lowest, and whites had the highest prevalence of CAC. White women had the highest prevalence of CACS > 0, whereas Hispanic women had the lowest. The prevalence of subclinical atherosclerosis was intermediate in Chinese and black women (Fig. 23.2).

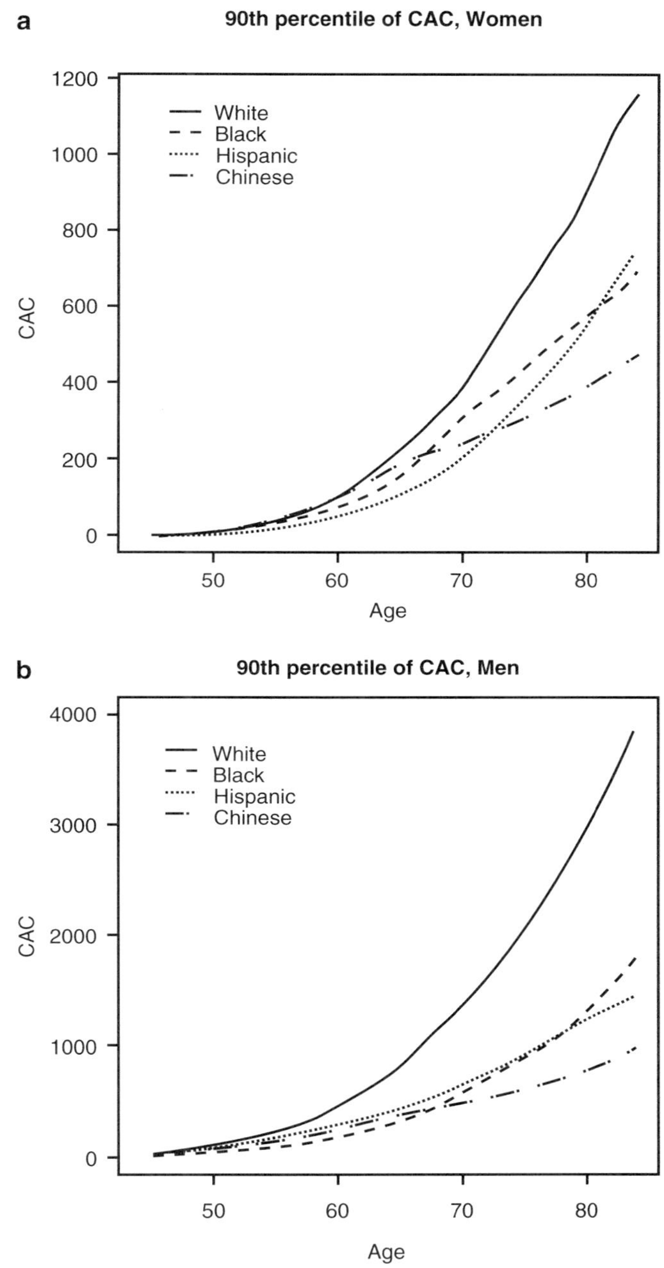

Fig. 23.2 Estimated 90th percentile of the CACS distribution by gender, age, and race/ethnicity. Note that the *y*-axis scales for these two plots are very different, with the scale for the men (**b**) >3 times as large as that for women (**a**). (From McClelland et al. [18], with permission)

Prognostic Implications of CACS and Prognostic Implications of Coronary Artery Calcium in ASCVD Risk Evaluation

Discrimination is a measure of a marker's ability to differentiate between individuals who do and do not have events. The most popular measure of discrimination is the receiver operating characteristic (ROC) curve, a plot of sensitivity vs

1-specificity [19]. The area under the curve (AUC) is also known as the *c*-statistic and can range from 0.5 (no predictive ability) to 1 (perfect discrimination). CACS has been repeatedly demonstrated to be a robust predictor of ASCVD events, including CHD, stroke, and fatal ASCVD and is associated with a significantly better *c*-statistic (improved discrimination) as compared to traditional risk factors, particularly in patients who are deemed to be in the intermediate risk category (Table 23.1) [20–35]. CACS has emerged as the most powerful predictor of risk in asymptomatic individuals as demonstrated in every cohort in which it has been studied. One stunningly consistent observation is the approximate tenfold increased hazard of hard events associated with high CACS compared to CACS = 0 [21, 36]. In a head-to-head comparison of novel risk markers (CACS, ABI, hs-CRP, and family history) for improvement in ASCVD risk assessment in intermediate-risk individuals, all were independent risk markers, but CACS provided markedly superior discrimination and risk reclassification compared to other markers [37]. In MESA, findings suggested that CACS was associated more strongly than carotid intima-media thickness (cIMT) with the risk of incident ASCVD with a *c*-statistic of 0.81 (95% CI 0.78–0.83) for CACS versus 0.78 for cIMT (95% CI 0.75–0.81) [38].

The data from five large prospective, randomized studies provide approximate 10-year event rates associated with increasing levels of CACS (ASCVD events defined in three studies as CHD death, MI, and revascularization and in two studies as CHD death and MI) (Table 23.2) [20, 25, 30, 34, 35, 39, 40]. Asymptomatic patients with CACS 101–400 Agatston had a 10-year event rate of 12.8–16.4%, and patients with CACS 1–100 Agatston had an approximate 10-year event rate between 2.3% and 5.9%. According to the 2018 ACC/AHA Guideline on the Management of Blood Cholesterol, patients with 10-year ASCVD risk of ≥7.5 to <20% are identified as one of four statin benefit groups in primary prevention. Patients with risk from 5% to <7.5 may also be considered for statin therapy in the setting of shared decision making [41, 42]. Thus, the 10-year risk of ASCVD events as estimated by CACS may help to inform the patient clinician discussion regarding preventive therapies.

Historically, duration of follow-up after baseline CACS was only approximately 4–5 years. This is a significant shortcoming given the fact that contemporary risk assessment algorithms, such as the ACC/AHA Pooled Cohort Equations, predict 10-year and lifetime risk of ASCVD events [7]. However, two recent studies have demonstrated that CACS accurately predicts 15-year mortality and support effective long-term risk prediction and reclassification [43, 44].

The net reclassification index (NRI) is used for calibration of risk markers to measure the improvement in risk prediction or risk reclassification when comparing new biomarkers or measures of subclinical atherosclerosis to traditional risk prediction strategies [19]. Several large prospective, population-based studies have demonstrated that CACS improves not only risk stratification and discrimination but also improves accurate reclassification of ASCVD risk beyond traditional risk factors and risk assessment algorithms [37, 40, 45–48]. Though CACS has primarily been recommended for use in patients at intermediate ASCVD risk as determined by conventional risk assessment algorithms, there has also been considerable interest in defining its potential role in individuals at low risk. An early analysis of the MESA study included 2684 women followed for a mean of 3.75 years who were classified as low-risk based on the FRS [33]. The prevalence of any CAC in these low-risk women was 32%. There was a

Table 23.1 Prognostic power of coronary artery calcium in asymptomatic patients

First author (Reference #)	*N*	Mean age (years)	Follow-up (years)	Calcium score cutoff (Agatston)	Comparator group for relative risk calculation	Relative risk ratio
Arad et al. [22]	1172	53	3.6	>160	<160	20.2
Wong et al. [24]	926	54	3.3	Top quartile (>270)	First quartile	8.8
Greenland et al. [29]	1312	66	7.0	>300	CACS = 0	3.9
Shaw et al. [28]	10,377	53	5	≥400	<10	8.4
Arad et al. [30]	4903	59	4.3	≥100	<100	10.7
Taylor et al. [31]	2000	43	3.0	>44	0	11.8
Vliegenthart et al. [25]	2013	71	3.3	>1000 400–1000	<100 <100	8.3 4.6
Budoff et al. [32]	25,503	56	6.8	>400	0	9.2
Lakoski et al. [33]	3601	60	3.75	>0	0	6.5
Becker et al. [34]	1726	57.7	3.4	>400	0	6.8 (men) 7.9 (women)
Detrano et al. [20]	6722	62.2	3.8	>300	0	9.67
Erbel et al. [35]	4129	45–75	5	>75th percentile	<25th percentile	11.1 (men) 3.2 (women)

Adapted from Weber et al. [21], with permission

Table 23.2 Summary of absolute event rates by coronary artery calcium score (CACS) from 14,856 patients in five prospective studies

CACS	FRS equivalent[a]	2013 ACC/AHA statin benefit group[b]	10-year event rate (%)
0	Very low	No	1.1–1.7
1–100	Low	May consider	2.3–5.9
101–400	Intermediate	Yes	12.8–16.4
>400	High	Yes	22.5–28.6
>1000	Very high	Yes	37.0

Adapted from Hecht [39], with permission
[a]FRS indicates Framingham Risk Score (Ref. [4])
[b]2013 ACC/AHA statin benefit group indicates eligibility for statin therapy based on 10-year ASCVD risk as calculated by the Pooled Cohort Equations

sixfold greater risk for a CHD event in women with CACS > 0 compared to women with no evidence of CAC (HR 6.5; 95% CI 2/6–16.4, $p < 0.001$).

Among another cohort of 9715 patients referred for CACS, a total of 2363 asymptomatic men and women were classified as low-intermediate risk using the FRS [47]. After a mean follow-up of 14.6 years, the total mortality ranged from 5.0% for women with a CACS = 0 to 23.5% for those with CACS > 400 ($p < 0.001$). For men, the 15-year mortality ranged from 3.5% among those with CACS = 0 to 18% for those with CACS > 400 ($p < 0.001$). Thus, even among men and women with low-intermediate risk factor burden, the presence of CAC effectively identifies those who are at significantly higher risk than predicted by the FRS alone. Women with CACS > 10 were noted to have higher mortality risk compared to men with similar CACS. The fact that risk assessment based on the traditional risk factor-based algorithm performed poorly in women, suggests that CACS may play an important role to improve risk prediction in women.

More recently, data from MESA was used to calibrate the Pooled Cohort Equations used in the 2013 ACC/AHA cholesterol guideline and to determine whether use of nontraditional risk markers can improve assessment in low-risk individuals who fall below the threshold for statin therapy [49]. During the 10 years of follow-up, 57% of events in the MESA cohort occurred among participants with an estimated 10-year ASCVD risk <7.5%. The presence of significant subclinical atherosclerosis with CACS ≥ 300 reclassified 6.8% as being at higher risk with an event rate of 13.3% and relative risk of 4.0 (95% CI 2.8–5.7, $p < 0.0001$).

A recent meta-analysis assessed the utility of CACS for ASCVD risk estimation among 6739 women with 10-year risk <7.5% by the Pooled Cohort Equations in five large population-based cohorts (the Dallas Heart Study, the Framingham Heart Study, the Heinz Nixdorf Recall study, MESA, and the Rotterdam Study) [50]. The median follow-up period ranged from 7.0 to 11.6 years. CAC was present in 36.1% of these low-risk women. Compared to women with CACS = 0, the presence of any CAC (CACS > 0) was associated with increased risk of ASCVD event (multivariable-adjusted hazard ratio, 2.04 [95% CI, 1.44–2.90]) and modest improvement in prognostic accuracy compared to traditional risk factor-based algorithm (*c*-statistic 0.77 [95% CI, 0.74–0.81] versus 0.73 [95% CI, 0.69–0.77]).

The role of CACS in patients with a low lifetime risk of ASCVD as measured by optimal risk factor status (total cholesterol <180 mg/dL, untreated blood pressure <120/80 mmHg, non-smoking and nondiabetic status) was evaluated in the MESA cohort [51]. At 10.4 years of follow-up, the event rates for CACS = 0, CACS > 0, and CACS > 100 were 0.9/1000, 5.7/1000, and 11.0/1000 person-years, respectively. The presence of CAC was the strongest predictor of incident CHD in this low-risk cohort.

CAC has been found to be predictive of CHD events across all age groups [52]. The MESA cohort ranged in age from 45 to 84 years. With increasing age, there was an increased proportion of the cohort with CACS 1–100 and CACS > 100 and a decreased proportion of patients with CACS = 0 (Fig. 23.3). Compared with CACS = 0, CACS 1–100 and CACS > 100 were associated with a 2-fold and 12-fold increased risk of all CHD events for younger individuals (ages 45–54), respectively. Among patients 75–84 years of age, CACS 1–100 and CACS > 100 were associated with 11-fold and 20-fold increased risk of events compared to those with no evidence of CAC. CACS = 0 in the 75–84 year-old group had an 8.5-year survival of approximately 98% which was comparable to younger patients with no CACS.

In 2015, a novel risk score was derived in the MESA population to estimate 10-year CHD risk using CACS in conjunction with traditional ASCVD risk factors and validated in the Heinz Nixdorf Recall Study (HNR) and the Dallas Heart Study (DHS) [53]. The addition of CACS to the traditional risk factors improved risk prediction significantly (*c*-statistic 0.80 vs. 0.75; $p < 0.0001$) (Fig. 23.4). External validation in both the HNR and DHS populations provided very good discrimination and validation, with Harrell's *c*-statistic of 0.779 in HNR and 0.816 in DHS. The MESA risk score is available online at https://www.mesa-nhlbi.org/MESACHDRisk/MesaRiskScore/RiskScore.aspx and may be used to aid clinicians when communicating risk to patients and as part of the determination of risk-based treatment strategies.

The dominant effect of age on eligibility for statin therapy according to the ACC/AHA cholesterol guideline means that all healthy people, even with optimal risk factors, will automatically qualify for statin therapy between the ages of 63 and 71 years, depending upon sex and ethnicity. A disease-guided approach based upon the presence of subclinical atherosclerosis as assessed by CACS or carotid plaque burden was evaluated in elderly individuals in the BioImage Study

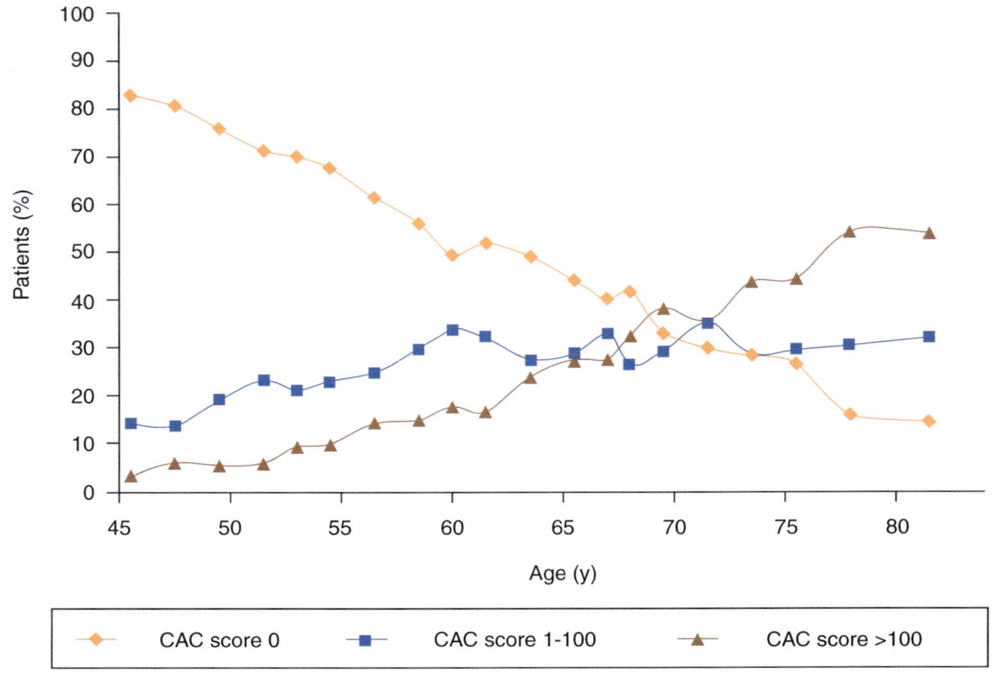

Fig. 23.3 Proportion of patients in each coronary artery calcium (CAC) group with increasing age. (From Tota-Maharaj et al. [52], with permission)

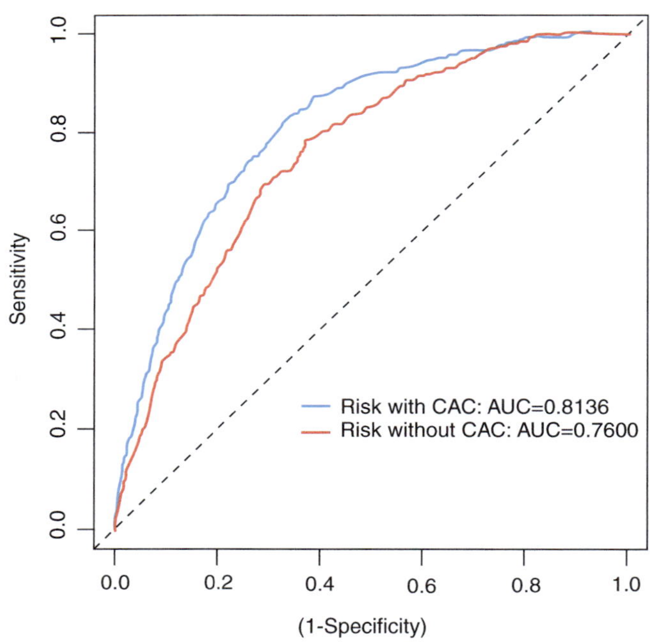

Fig. 23.4 Discrimination of the MESA CHD Risk Score Within the Development Cohort. The area under the survival ROC curve within MESA was 0.81 for the model with CAC, indicating excellent discrimination between events and nonevents. Receiver-operator characteristic (ROC) curves for the risk scores with and without coronary artery calcium (CAC) applied within the MESA (Multi-Ethnic Study of Atherosclerosis) cohort. (Adapted from McClelland et al. [53], with permission)

to more accurately assign statin therapy (Fig. 23.5) [54]. Participants ($N = 5805$) who were mean age 69 years (range 55–80 years) underwent 10-year ASCVD risk assessment by the ACC/AHA Pooled Cohort Equations, as well as CACS and carotid ultrasound imaging to detect and quantify carotid plaque. In the study population, 86% of participants qualified for risk-based statin therapy, but imaging demonstrated that up to one third had no evidence of CAC. The investigators tested the disease-guided reclassification approach to improve specificity (less overtreatment) and sensitivity (less undertreatment) among elderly people. Those individuals with 10-year ASCVD risk ≥7.5% were down-classified from statin eligible to ineligible if there was no evidence of subclinical atherosclerosis. Individuals with intermediate 10-year ASCVD risk (5% to <7.5%) were up-classified from statin optional to statin eligible if CACS ≥ 100 or there was evidence of significant carotid plaque. During the median follow-up of 2.7 years, there were 91 CHD events and 138 CVD events. The specificity for CHD and CVD events improved significantly with CACS-guided reclassification without loss in sensitivity, leading to a binary NRI of 0.20 for CHD and 0.14 for CVD. The positive NRIs were driven primarily by down-classifying the patients with CACS = 0 or no evidence of carotid plaque. The investigators proposed that limiting statin therapy to those with CACS > 0 or evidence of carotid plaque could spare a significant proportion of asymptomatic elderly people from lifelong statin therapy.

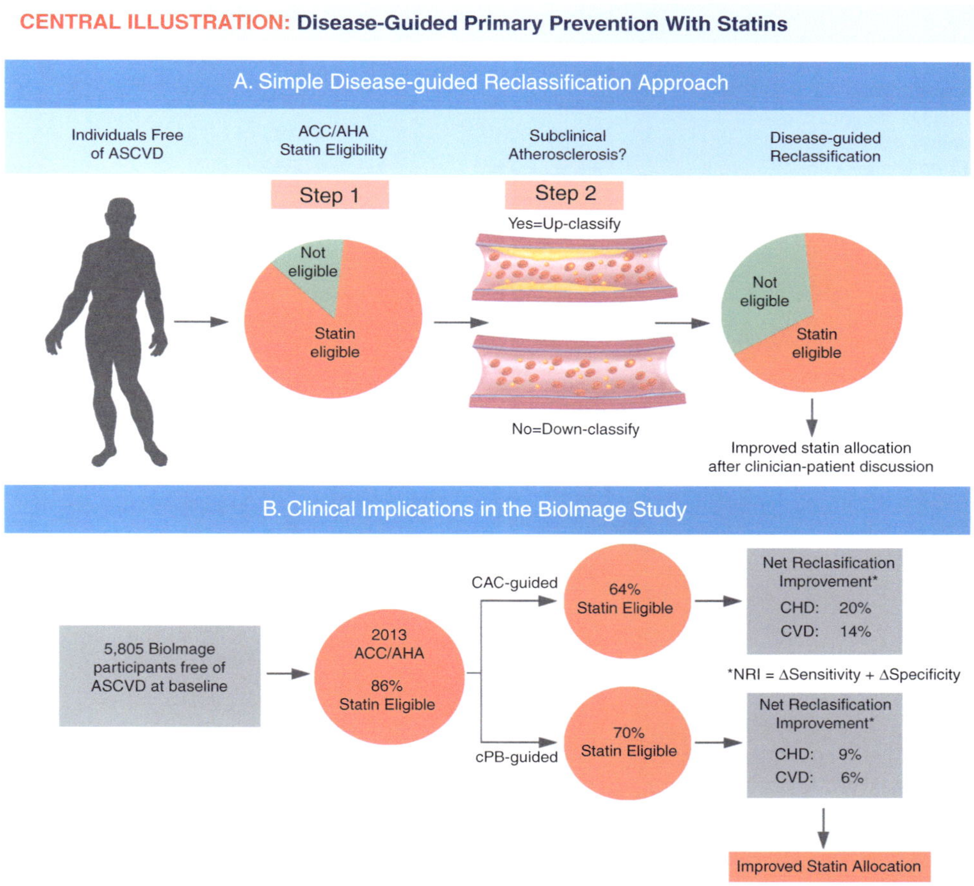

Fig. 23.5 Disease-Guided Primary Prevention With Statins. (**a**) Following guideline-recommended formal risk assessment and atherosclerosis imaging, statin-eligible individuals are down-classified to ineligible in the absence of atherosclerosis and other high-risk features, and statinineligible patients are up-classified to eligible if significant atherosclerosis is present. This principle facilitates an informed clinician-patient discussion, leading to an individualized treatment decision. (**b**) In the BioImage cohort, beneficial reclassification was achieved using coronary artery calcium (CAC) and carotid plaque burden (cPB). ACC/AHA American College of Cardiology/American Heart Association, ASCVD atherosclerotic cardiovascular disease, CHD coronary heart disease, CVD cardiovascular disease, NRI net reclassification index. (From Mortensen et al. [54], with permission)

Diabetes

Asymptomatic individuals with diabetes exhibit more extensive subclinical coronary atherosclerosis than do nondiabetic patients. Moreover, younger patients with diabetes manifest CACS comparable to older individuals without diabetes [55]. Among traditional ASCVD risk factors, diabetes is the strongest correlate for CACS > 0. In a study of young individuals with diabetes (age < 40 years), 3723 asymptomatic patients (4% with diabetes) underwent CACS [56]. Overall, the prevalence of CAC was 43% in young patients with diabetes and was >50% in those aged >35 years. The presence of diabetes was associated with a fourfold higher odds of CACS ≥ 100 when compared to nondiabetic individuals.

In a systematic review and meta-analysis of eight observational studies with a mean follow-up of 5.18 years, including 6521 patients with diabetes, the relative risk for all-cause mortality or CV events, or both, was 5.47 (95% CI, 2.59–11.53, $p < 0.001$) when comparing CACS ≥ 10 compared to CACS < 10 [57]. The relative risk for CV events comparing CACS ≥ 10 to CACS < 10 was 9.22 (95% CI, 2.73–31.07, $p = 0.005$) (Fig. 23.6). The risk of CV events increased with increasing CACS levels of ≥100, ≥400, and ≥1000 compared to patients with diabetes and CACS < 10.

Multiple large prospective studies have demonstrated that baseline CACS is an independent predictor of ASCVD events in patients with diabetes. The prognostic value of CACS in patients with and without diabetes was assessed in 10,377 asymptomatic individuals (903 with diabetes) over an average follow-up of 5.0 years [58]. Overall, mortality was significantly greater in patients with diabetes than in those without diabetes. Mortality increased with increasing CACS for both diabetic and nondiabetic individuals. However, for every increase in CACS, there was a greater increase in mortality for diabetics compared to nondiabetic (Fig. 23.7).

In the MESA population, there were 881 participants (13%) with diabetes [59]. Compared to individuals without diabetes, the adjusted hazard ratios for CHD events in diabetics with CACS 1–99, CACS 100–399, and CACS ≥ 400

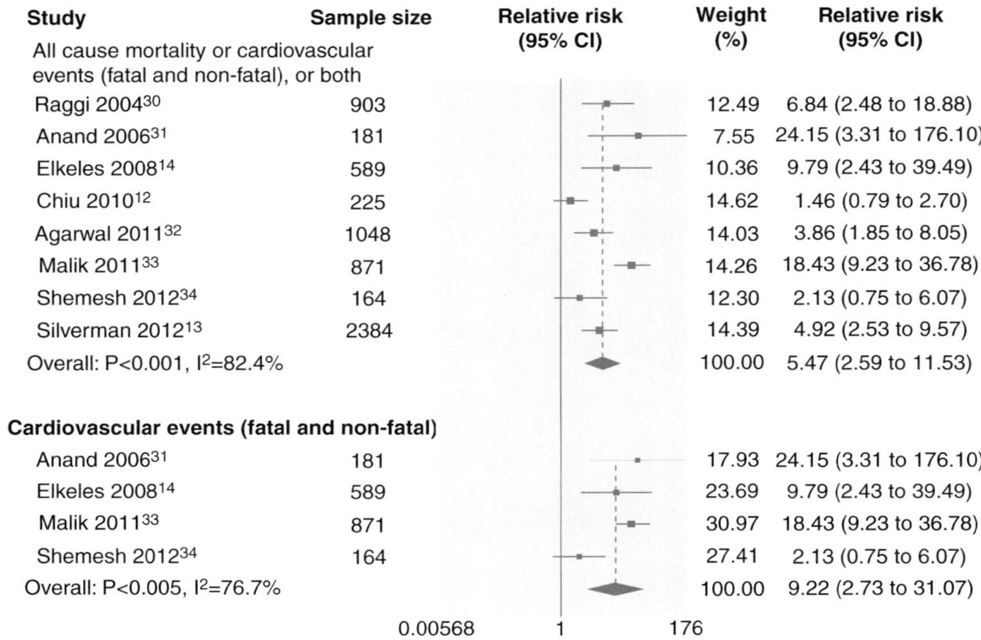

Study	Sample size	Weight (%)	Relative risk (95% CI)
All cause mortality or cardiovascular events (fatal and non-fatal), or both			
Raggi 2004[30]	903	12.49	6.84 (2.48 to 18.88)
Anand 2006[31]	181	7.55	24.15 (3.31 to 176.10)
Elkeles 2008[14]	589	10.36	9.79 (2.43 to 39.49)
Chiu 2010[12]	225	14.62	1.46 (0.79 to 2.70)
Agarwal 2011[32]	1048	14.03	3.86 (1.85 to 8.05)
Malik 2011[33]	871	14.26	18.43 (9.23 to 36.78)
Shemesh 2012[34]	164	12.30	2.13 (0.75 to 6.07)
Silverman 2012[13]	2384	14.39	4.92 (2.53 to 9.57)
Overall: P<0.001, I^2=82.4%		100.00	5.47 (2.59 to 11.53)
Cardiovascular events (fatal and non-fatal)			
Anand 2006[31]	181	17.93	24.15 (3.31 to 176.10)
Elkeles 2008[14]	589	23.69	9.79 (2.43 to 39.49)
Malik 2011[33]	871	30.97	18.43 (9.23 to 36.78)
Shemesh 2012[34]	164	27.41	2.13 (0.75 to 6.07)
Overall: P<0.005, I^2=76.7%		100.00	9.22 (2.73 to 31.07)

Fig. 23.6 Meta-analyses of association between coronary artery calcium score ≥10 and outcome in people with type 2 diabetes. Weights are from random effects analysis. (From Kramer et al. [57], with permission)

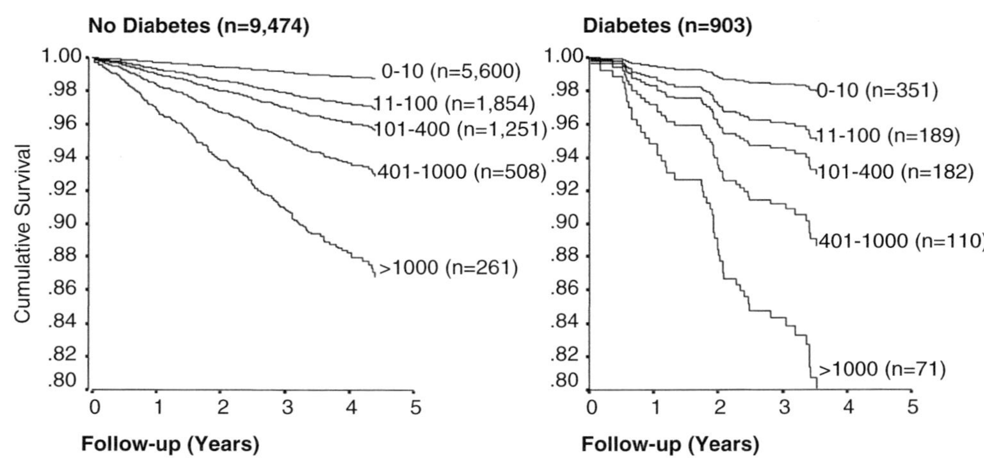

Fig. 23.7 Cox proportional hazards survival (n = 10,377) by electron beam tomography coronary calcium measurements in subjects with and without diabetes (chi-square = 204, $p < 0.0001$). The number of subjects in each calcium score category is in parentheses. (From Raggi et al. [58], with permission)

were 2.9, 3.3, and 6.2, respectively. Thus, although patients with diabetes are at higher ASCVD risk overall, recent evidence does suggest a wide range of risk and supports a role for CACS in selected individuals (particularly in those with diabetes who are younger and with duration of disease of less than 10 years).

The Power of Zero

The focus for integration of CACS into clinical practice for ASCVD risk assessment has largely been on the intermediate-risk patient with evidence of subclinical atherosclerosis to identify higher-risk individuals who may be candidates for more intensive preventive medical therapies. However, multiple population-based studies have clearly demonstrated the favorable prognosis associated with the absence of CAC, leading many experts to suggest that a CACS = 0 may identify patients who could avoid lifelong pharmacotherapy [60, 61]. This is particularly relevant as the 2013 ACC/AHA cholesterol guideline increased the number of US adults eligible for statin therapy from 43 million to 56 million, with the majority of these newly eligible candidates being individuals without clinical ASCVD [62]. Therefore, the value of CACS may now be finding CACS = 0 in a patient with an intermediate 10-year ASCVD risk or uncertainty after consideration of risk estimation to inform clinical decision making when considering the initiation of statin therapy.

Asymptomatic Patients

In a systematic review of 49 studies of the diagnostic and prognostic utility of CACS ($N = 64{,}873$ individuals), 29,312 asymptomatic patients demonstrated a CACS = 0 [45]. Over a mean follow-up period of 50 months, there was a very low event rate (154 ASCVD events; 0.47%) in this cohort. Compared to patients with any CAC, the cumulative relative risk rate for ASCVD events with a CACS = 0 was 0.15 (95% CI: 0.11–0.21, $p < 0.001$).

The absence of CAC and all-cause mortality was assessed in a study of 44,052 consecutive patients referred for CACS [63]. Among the 19,898 patients (45%) with no evidence of CAC, there were 104 deaths (0.52%) over a mean follow-up period of 5.6 years. The annualized all-cause mortality rate for CACS = 0 was 0.87 per 1000 person-years (Table 23.3).

In the MESA population, there were a total of 3415 asymptomatic participants with no detectable CAC [64]. During a median follow-up period of 4.1 years, there were 17 all CHD events (MI, cardiac arrest, fatal CHD, angina, revascularization) and 10 (0.3%) hard CHD events (nonfatal MI and CHD death). Compared to participants with CACS = 0, there was a more than threefold increase in all CHD events (HR, 3.66; p65% CI 1.71–7.85) when even only minimal CAC (CACS 1–10) was present.

The implications of CACS = 0 among statin candidates according to the ACC/AHA cholesterol guideline were also evaluated in the MESA population [65]. Approximately 50% of the 4758 MESA participants in this analysis qualified for statin therapy as per the guidelines, the majority because of an estimated 10-year ASCVD risk ≥7.5% by the Pooled Cohort Equations. Of all participants who were statin eligible (recommend or consider statin therapy per guideline), 44% had CACS = 0 and an event rate of 4.2 per 1000 person-years, which is a lower observed ASCVD risk than the threshold recommended for treatment. Thus, it is suggested that there is significant heterogeneity of risk among patients who are eligible for statin therapy according to the guideline, and the absence of CAC may reclassify approximately half of these individuals to a lower-risk group.

The landmark JUPITER trial demonstrated that healthy patients without clinical ASCVD, normal LDL-C, and elevated hs-CRP benefit from high-intensity statin therapy with a significant reduction in major cardiovascular events [66]. In a subset of MESA participants who met criteria for entry into the JUPITER study, nearly half of the population had no evidence of CAC (47%) [67]. During the mean follow-up period of 5.8 years, the rate of CHD events was 0.8 per 1000 person-years, and there was an unfavorable 5-year number needed to treat (NNT) of 549 (Table 23.4). Most of the events occurred in individuals with CACS > 100 which was associ-

Table 23.3 All-cause mortality rates by CAC scores in overall population ($N = 44{,}052$) of consecutive asymptomatic individuals

	No. of patients	No. of events	Rate/1000 person-years at risk	95% CI for rate
CAC = 0	19,898 (45%)	104 (0.52%)	0.87	0.72–1.05
CAC 1–10	5388 (12%)	58 (1.06%)	1.92	1.48–2.48
CAC > 10	18,766 (43%)	739 (3.96%)	7.48	6.95–8.04
Total	44,052 (100%)	901 (2.05%)	3.62	3.39–3.89

From Blaha et al. [63], with permission

Table 23.4 CHD and CVD events by CAC status in the MESA population eligible for JUPITER

	N (%)	CHD events			CVD events		
		CHD events (%)	Event rate (per 1000 person-years)	Hazard ratio (95% CI)	CVD events (%)	Event rate (per 1000 person-years)	Hazard ratio (95% CI)
CAC 0	444 (47%)	2 (0.5%)	0.8	1* (ref)	9 (2.0%)	3.7	1* (ref)
CAC 1–100	267 (28%)	7 (2.6%)	4.8	4.91 (0.97–24.9)	12 (4.5%)	8.4	1.86 (0.73–4.76)
CAC >100	239 (25%)	25 (10.6%)	20.2	27.8 (5.97–129.8)	32 (13.4%)	26.4	6.16 (2.51–15.1)
Any CAC present	506 (53%)	32 (6.3%)	11.0	11.0 (2.51–48.5)	44 (8.7%)	16.6	3.20 (1.41–7.24)

From Blaha et al. [67], with permission

CHD coronary heart disease, *CVD* cardiovascular disease, *CAC* coronary artery calcium, *MESA* Multi-ethnic Study of Atherosclerosis, *JUPITER* Justification for the Use of statins in Prevention: an Intervention Trial Evaluating Rosuvastatin

*Hazard ratios of 1 were used as a reference

ated with a NNT of only 24. These findings led the authors to suggest that CACS may be used to identify patients most likely to benefit from statin therapy, focusing treatment on those patients with evidence of subclinical atherosclerosis.

One of the most important considerations when using CACS = 0 to reclassify an individual to a lower ASCVD risk category is whether the absence of subclinical atherosclerosis confers long-term protection that is incremental to and independent of traditional risk assessment tools. The "warranty period" (defined as <1% annual mortality) associated with the absence of CAC was evaluated in 9715 consecutive asymptomatic individuals referred for CACS at a single site [44]. Participants were stratified by age and CVD risk (FRS and National Cholesterol Education Program Adult Treatment Panel III [NCEP ATP III] categories) and were followed for a mean of 14.6 years. Among the 4864 patients with CACS = 0, the annual observed rate of mortality remained <1% during the entire follow-up period with a warranty period of 15 years (Fig. 23.8). Compared with the FRS or NCEP ATP III risk assessment tools alone, CACS significantly improved discrimination when added to the models. At all levels of calculated risk, CACS improved risk classification (Table 23.5). Interestingly, a similar study was performed in asymptomatic diabetic subjects who were followed for a mean of 14.7 years. A CACS = 0 in diabetic patients was associated with a favorable 5-year prognosis. However, after 5 years, the risk of mortality increased significantly among diabetics even in the presence of a baseline CACS = 0 [68].

The role of negative risk markers for ASCVD (including CACS = 0, cIMT <25th percentile, absence of carotid plaque, and other risk markers) was also evaluated in recent analysis of the MESA population [48]. The study cohort consisted of 6814 participants who were followed for a mean of 10.3 years. The lowest proportion of total CVD, CHD, and hard CHD events occurred in participants with CACS = 0. Among all negative risk factors, CACS = 0 was the strongest and resulted in the largest, most accurate downward risk reclassification (Fig. 23.9). CACS = 0 was particularly informative in older adults with lower diagnostic likelihood ratios with increasing age, making the test more useful for downgrading disease risk compared to younger adults.

In the BioImage Study of elderly people, the improved sensitivity, specificity, and NRI of a disease-guided approach that incorporates CACS were largely driven by downclassifying, or "de-risking," statin-eligible patients who had a CACS = 0 [54]. CHD and CVD event rates were low in individuals with CACS = 0 and the absence of carotid plaque, even among participants with diabetes. Investigators suggest that withholding statin therapy in older adults without subclinical atherosclerosis could spare patients from lifelong statin therapy that may benefit only a few.

Low- and High-Risk Patients

CACS = 0 has also been demonstrated to provide important prognostic information among asymptomatic individuals without traditional risk factors who are considered to be at low- or high-risk of ASCVD events. In a study cohort of 44,052 individuals referred for assessment of CACS, patients were followed for a mean of 5.6 years [69]. Risk factors were assessed by self-report, and patients were characterized as having 0, 1, 2,

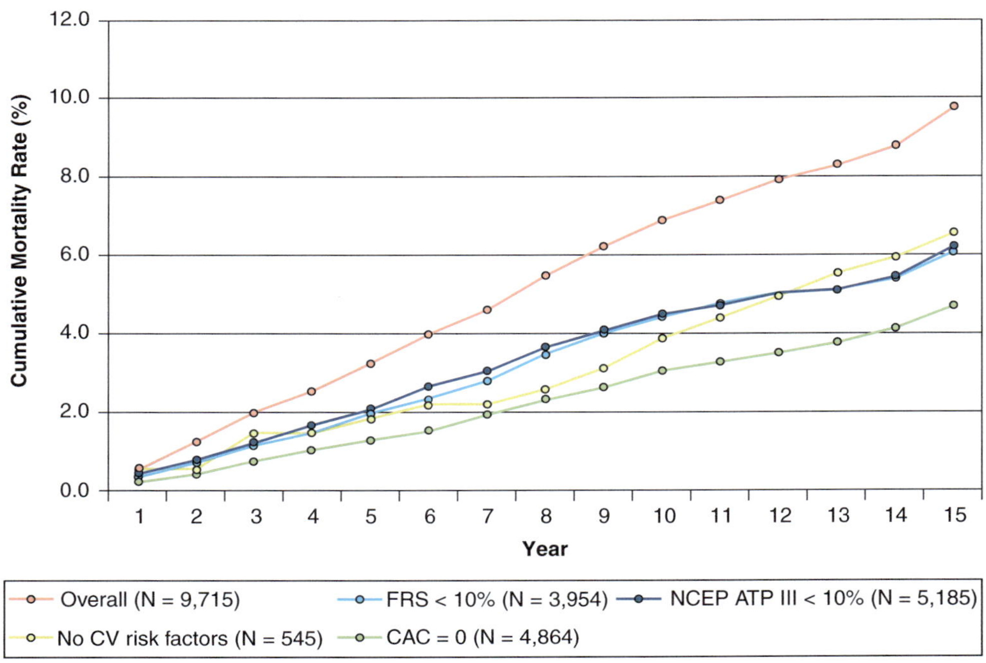

Fig. 23.8 The 15-year cumulative mortality rate for low-risk individuals. (Adapted from Valenti et al. [44], with permission)

Table 23.5 Net reclassification index with the addition of coronary artery calcium (CAC) Scoring to a Model Including the FRS or NCEP ATP III Score

	NRI	95% CI	*p* Value	% of events correctly reclassified	Event *p* value	% of nonevents correctly reclassified	Nonevent*p* value
Overall cohort (*N* = 9715)							
FRS + CAC	0.58966	0.5251–0.6542	<0.0001	29	<0.0001	30	<0.0001
NCEP ATP III + CAC	0.57966	0.5149–0.6444	<0.0001	28	<0.0001	30	<0.0001
Low cardiovascular risk							
FRS + CAC	0.52561	0.3961–0.6551	<0.0001	12	0.07	41	<0.0001
NCEP ATP III + CAC	0.49967	0.3878–0.6116	<0.0001	13	0.02	37	<0.0001
Intermediate cardiovascular risk							
FRS + CAC	0.46417	0.3611–0.5672	<0.0001	23	<0.0001	23	<0.0001
NCEP ATP III + CAC	0.51544	0.3955–0.6354	<0.0001	28	<0.0001	23	<0.0001
High cardiovascular risk							
FRS + CAC	0.58347	0.4709–0.6961	<0.0001	40	<0.0001	18	<0.0001
NCEP ATP III + CAC	0.55956	0.4494–0.6698	<0.0001	37	<0.0001	19	<0.0001

From Valenti et al. [44], with permission
CI confidence interval, *NRI* net reclassification improvement

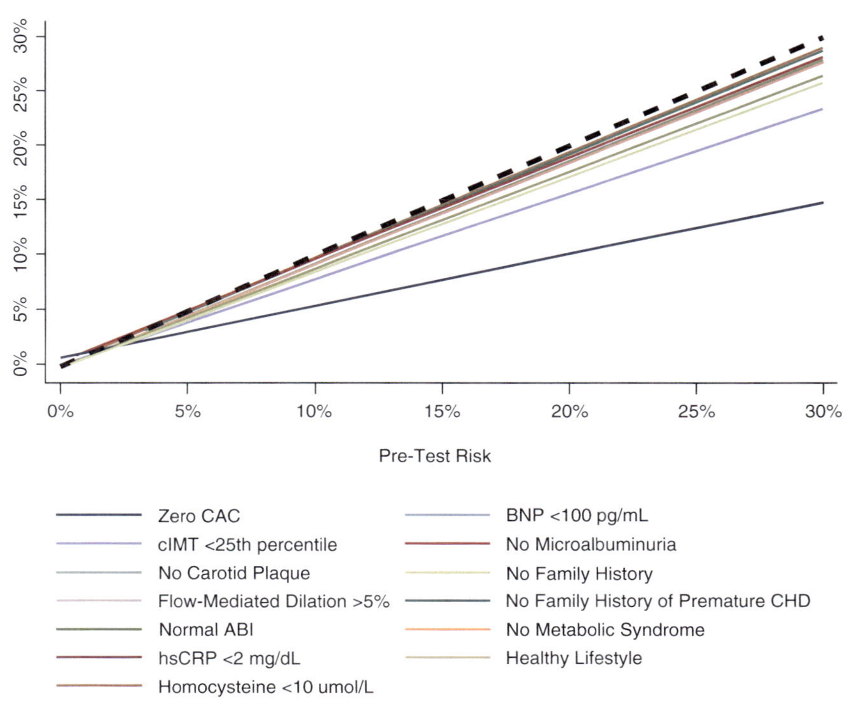

Fig. 23.9 Negative risk markers for cardiovascular disease. Relationship between pretest and posttest cardiovascular disease (CVD) risk after the knowledge of the negative result of each risk marker. The regression lines display the relationship between the pretest predicted 10-year CVD risk (*x* axis) and the posttest risk (*y* axis) after the knowledge of the negative result of each risk marker. A broken back line is displayed as reference (risk shift with no additional testing). Results were obtained by plotting the pretest and posttest risk on the basis of the diagnostic likelihood ratio of each MESA participant and then applying a linear fit. MESA indicates Multi-Ethnic Study of Atherosclerosis, ABI ankle-brachial index, BNP brain natriuretic peptide, CAC coronary artery calcium, CHD coronary heart disease, CIMT carotid intima-media thickness, FMD flow-mediated dilation, hsCRP high-sensitivity C-reactive protein. (From Blaha et al. [48], with permission)

or > 2 risk factors. A total of 19,898 patients (45%) had CACS = 0. As shown in Fig. 23.10, more than half of individuals with no ASCVD risk factors (53%) had evidence of subclinical atherosclerosis with CACS > 0. The lowest all-cause mortality occurred in those with no CAC and no ASCVD risk factors. Of interest, individuals with no risk factors but evidence of significant disease with CACS > 400 had a substantially higher mortality compared to individuals with multiple risk factors but CACS = 0 (16.89 versus 2.72 per 1000 person-years). The authors suggested that the exclusive use of risk assessment tools which rely only upon traditional risk factors may be inadequate in all low- and high-risk patients for guiding the intensity of primary prevention therapies.

The role of CACS in patients at the extremes of calculated ASCVD risk was also evaluated in the MESA cohort [70]. A total of 6698 individuals were followed for a mean of 7.1 years. Fifty percent of the study population had CACS = 0, and only 13% of all CHD events occurred in this group with a total event rate of 1.8 per 1000 person-years (Table 23.6). The annualized event rate increased slightly with increasing risk factors; however, the absolute event rate remained very low at all levels of traditional risk factors. CACS was also able to further risk stratify individuals at the extremes of risk as estimated by the FRS (Fig. 23.11). These findings indicate that assessment of subclinical coronary atherosclerosis may play a role even in patients who are considered to be at low- or high-risk by traditional risk factor assessments.

The MESA cohort was also used to examine two paradigms of risk assessment, in this case dyslipidemia as a risk factor and CACS as a measure of disease burden [71]. Participants (N = 5534) were not on baseline lipid-lowering medications and were classified as having 0–3 lipid abnormalities (including elevated LDL-C, low HDL-C, and/or high triglycerides). Over a median follow-up of 7.6 years, 82% of events occurred in participants with evidence of CAC. However, 65% of events occurred in individuals with only 0–1 lipid abnormality. CACS stratified ASCVD risk across varying levels of dyslipidemia, and when CACS = 0, the absolute rates of ASCVD events were relatively low regardless of the dyslipidemia burden (Fig. 23.12). Even in the presence of three lipid abnormalities, when there was no evidence of subclinical atherosclerosis, the absolute event rate over the 7.6-year follow-up period was <6%. In such individuals, the NNT with statin therapy was 154. The investigators suggested that CACS may help to personalize preventive strategies, especially in individuals with a history of statin-related side effects.

Diabetes

Diabetes was previously considered to be a CHD risk equivalent by the NCEP ATP III guidelines due to the high incidence of ASCVD events among patients with this diagnosis [72]. Patients with diabetes have been shown to have more extensive CAC and an increase in risk of events when compared to nondiabetic as discussed above. However, CACS = 0 is associated with a low short-term risk of death, even in the presence of diabetes [58]. In a study of 10,377 asymptomatic patients (903 diabetics), there are 4800 patients without diabetes and 267 patients with diabetes who had CACS = 0. Over a mean follow-up period of 5.0 years, participants with diabetes and CACS = 0 demonstrated a survival similar to that of individuals without diabetes and CACS = 0 (Fig. 23.13).

Participants in the Diabetes Heart Study (N = 1051) were followed for a mean of 7.4 years [73]. The estimated annual risk of all-cause mortality was lowest in individuals with CACS = 0–9 (0.9%), compared to annual risk of 20.0% in those with CACS ≥ 1000.

Table 23.6 Coronary heart disease events by risk factor burden (A) and coronary artery calcium score (B)

	n (%)	All CHD events (% of total events)	Total CHD event rate (per 1000 person-years)	Hard CHD events (% of total events)	Hard CHD event rate (per 1000 person-years)
A					
0 RF	1067 (16%)	16 (5%)	2.1	11 (5%)	1.4
1 RF	2310 (34%)	82 (24%)	5.0	50 (25%)	3.0
2 RF	2116 (32%)	126 (37%)	8.7	83 (41%)	5.7
≥3 RF	1205 (18%)	115 (34%)	14.6	60 (29%)	7.4
B					
CAC 0	3349 (50%)	44 (13%)	1.8	31 (15%)	1.3
CAC 1–100	1774 (27%)	85 (25%)	6.9	54 (26%)	4.3
CAC 101–300	747 (11%)	73 (22%)	14.4	46 (23%)	8.8
CAC >300	828 (12%)	137 (40%)	26.3	73 (36%)	13.3

From Silverman et al. [70], with permission

RFs considered: high LDL-C, low HDL-C, hypertension, diabetes, current cigarette smoking. Coronary heart disease event rates were significantly different by RF burden ($P < 0.001$). Coronary heart disease event rates were significantly different by CAC score ($P < 0.001$)

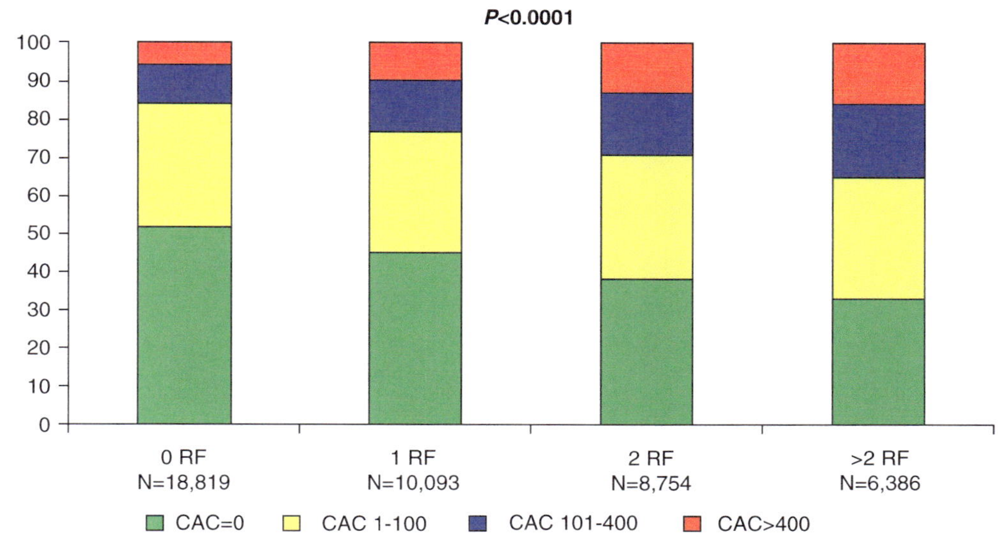

Fig. 23.10 The prevalence and extent of coronary artery calcium (CAC) in asymptomatic patients according to burden traditional risk factors (RFs). (From Nasir et al. [69], with permission)

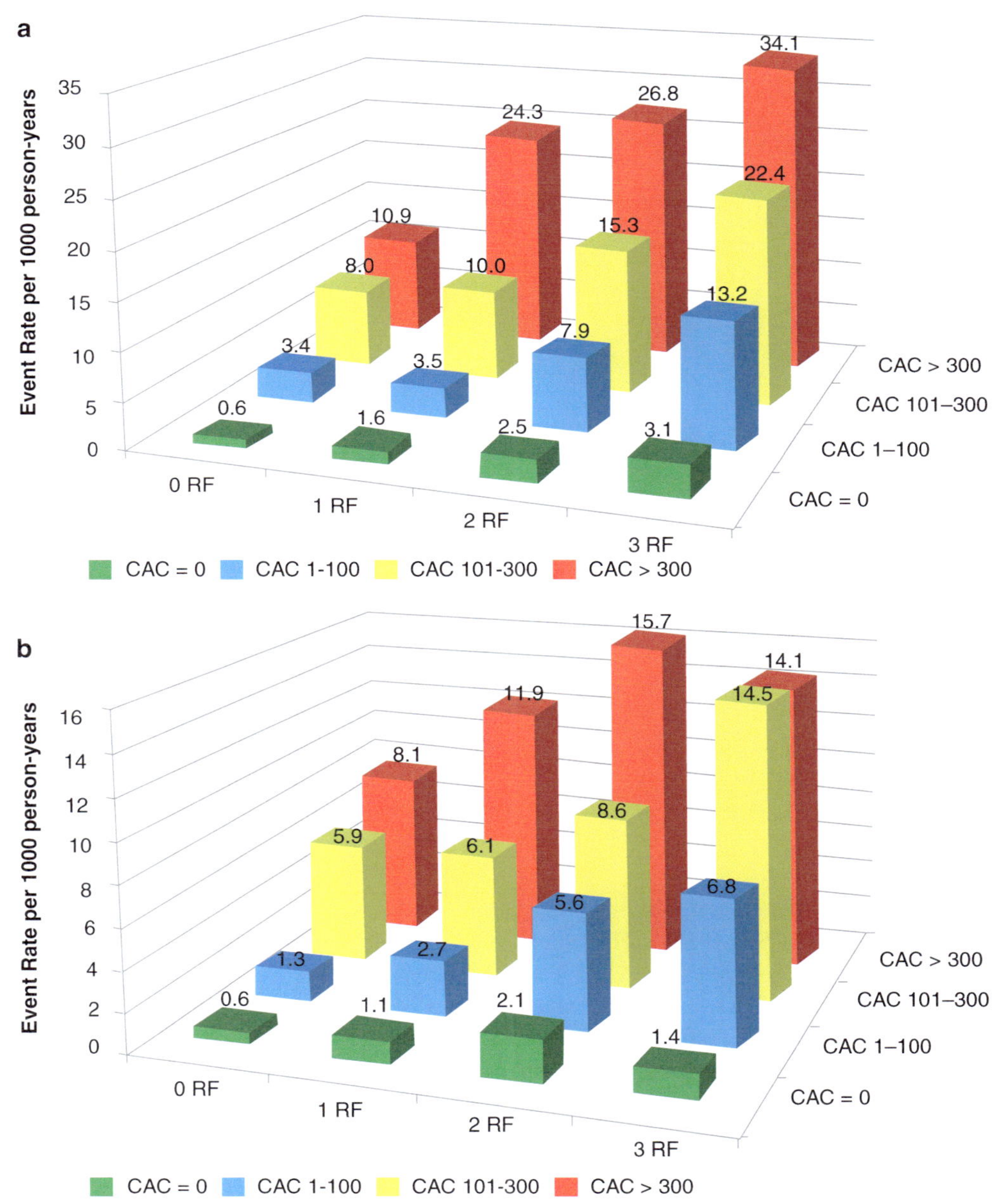

Fig. 23.11 Total (**a**) and hard (**b**) coronary heart disease event rates (per 1000 person-years) with increasing coronary artery calcium scores according to Framingham risk score categories. (From Silverman et al. [70], with permission)

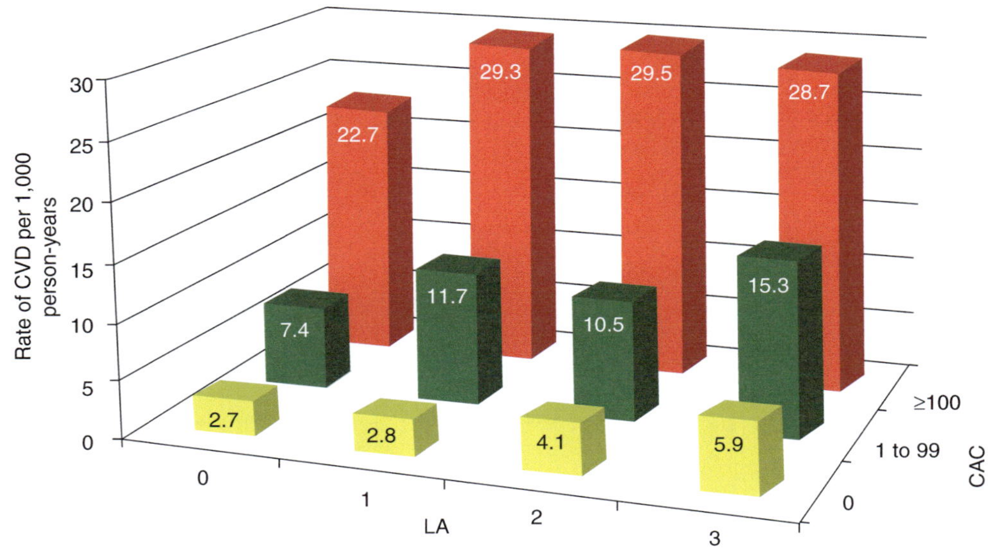

Fig. 23.12 Atherosclerotic cardiovascular disease events per 1000 person-years by strata of coronary artery calcium score (CAC) and lipid abnormality (LA). (From Martin et al. [71], with permission)

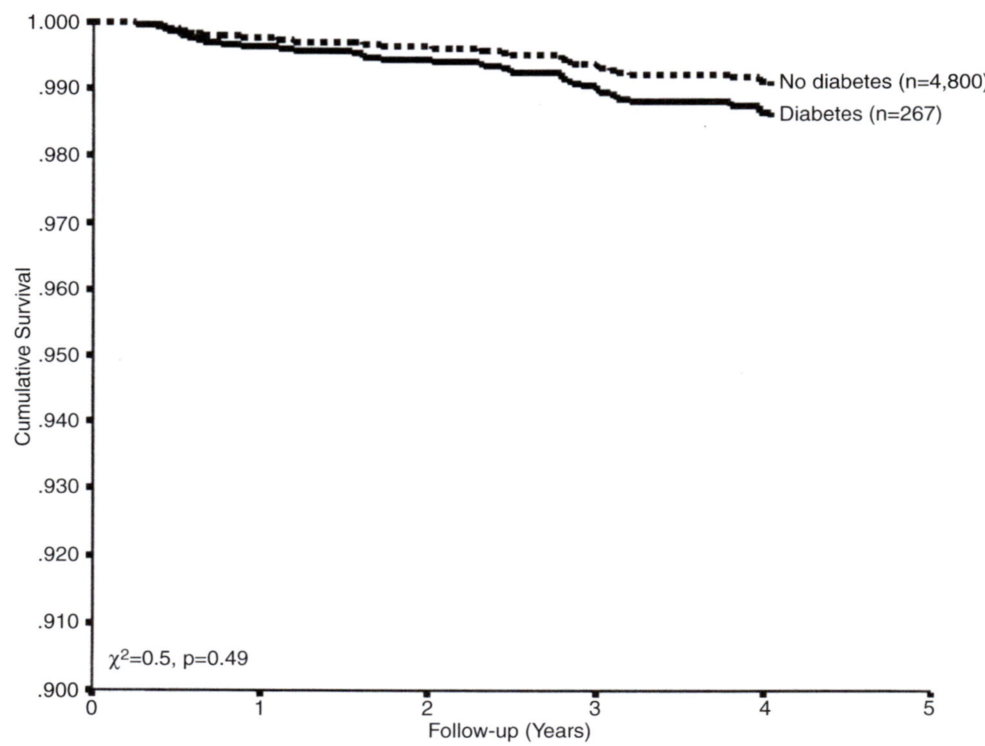

Fig. 23.13 Cox proportional hazards cumulative survival for subjects with and without diabetes mellitus with a calcium score of 0. The number of subjects in each calcium score category is in parentheses. (Raggi et al. [58], with permission)

In the MESA population, 38% of patients with diabetes (n = 881) had CACS = 0 [58]. The annualized CHD and CVD event rates in this group were 0.4% and 0.8%, respectively, compared to CHD and CVD event rates of 4% and 5.1%, respectively, in diabetics with CACS > 400. The tenfold increase in CHD event rates according to the extent of CAC suggests that CACS may play an important role in improvement in risk stratification in patients with diabetes.

Symptomatic Patients: Stable and Acute Chest Pain

Assessment of CAC is primarily recommended for ASCVD risk assessment in asymptomatic individuals, but the prognostic implication of CACS = 0 has also been evaluated in patients presenting with symptoms of suspected CHD [60, 74]. The CONFIRM (Coronary CT Angiography Evaluation for Clinical Outcomes: An International Multicenter) Registry evaluated the prevalence and severity of CAD in relation to prognosis in symptomatic patients who underwent coronary angiography and concomitant CCTA [75]. Among 10,037 individuals, 51% had CACS = 0. Among these patients, CCTA showed no evidence of CAD in 84% of patients. Approximately 13% of patients had nonobstructive CAD, 3.5% had ≥50% stenosis, and 1.4% had ≥70% stenosis. CACS = 0 had a sensitivity and specificity for stenosis ≥50% of 89% and 59%, respectively. The negative and positive predictive values were 96% and 29%, respectively. During the 2.1-year period of follow-up, there was no difference in mortality among patients with CACS = 0 regardless of the presence of obstructive CAD. However, CACS did not add incremental prognostic information compared with extent of CAD at CCTA for the composite endpoint of mortality, MI, or coronary revascularization. Among patients with CACS = 0, the presence of ≥1 coronary stenosis ≥50% was predictive of nonfatal MI and late revascularization.

The CRESCENT (Computed Tomography vs. Exercise Testing in Suspected Coronary Artery Disease) trial evaluated the effectiveness and safety of a CCTA algorithm compared with functional testing with a symptom-limited treadmill stress test in patients with stable angina referred to an outpatient clinic [76]. Myocardial perfusion imaging or stress echocardiography was performed when there was a contraindication to treadmill testing or in cases of noninterpretable or equivocal results. The tiered cardiac CT protocol included CACS followed by CCTA if CACS > 1 to 400. A total of 350 patients with stable angina were prospectively randomized 2:1 to cardiac CT (N = 242) or functional testing (N = 108). In the CT group, 100 patients had CACS = 0 and 2 went on to CCTA due to pretest probability of CAD > 70%. During the mean 1.2-year follow-up period, none of the 98 patients with CACS = 0 underwent further testing, and no adverse events occurred. The authors suggested that a tiered cardiac CT protocol offers an effective and safe alternative to functional testing in patients with stable chest pain.

Among 2088 patients presenting to the hospital with a chest pain syndrome (considered atypical or non-anginal chest pain by clinicians) who underwent CCTA, CACS = 0 was identified in 1114 patients (53%) [77]. Obstructive CAD was found in 48 patients (4.3%), and during the mean 2.8-year follow-up, there were 14 CHD events (1.3%) among the CACS = 0 patients. CAD severity was a strong predictor of events in this group.

The 2013 ACCF/AHA/ASE/ASNC/HFSA/SCAI/SCCT/SCMR/STS Multimodality Appropriate Use Criteria for the Detection and Risk Assessment of Stable Ischemic Heart Disease indicate that CACS is rarely appropriate for evaluation of acute chest pain among patients at any level of baseline ASCVD risk [78]. Preferred diagnostic strategies include myocardial perfusion imaging, stress echocardiography, CCTA, or invasive coronary angiography based on presentation and risk assessment.

Summary

Though there is overwhelming and consistent evidence that the absence of CAC is associated with a low risk of mortality (warranty up to 15 years) and hard CHD events (≥7 years based on MESA) in multiple patient populations, there is not yet clear randomized clinical trial (RCT) evidence that CACS = 0 justifies avoidance of prolonged use of preventive therapies such as statins [79]. Concern remains that ASCVD risk factors have a long latency period of effect and that even though patients with no evidence of CAC are at low near-term risk, they may have significant lifetime risk of events [80]. In addition, in high-risk symptomatic patients, the absence of CAC is not sufficient to rule out the presence of obstructive atherosclerotic coronary artery disease. The 2018 ACC/AHA blood cholesterol guidelines recommend that in individuals at intermediate risk with 10-year ASCVD risk of >7.5% to <20%, if the risk decision is uncertain, calcium scoring may be considered in selected adults [42]. Authors note that a CACS = 0 is useful to reclassify patients to a lower-risk group, often allowing statin therapy to be delayed or witheld unless additional high-risk conditions are present. For patients with a CAC score of 0, it is currently uncertain when follow-up studies should be performed, though many experts consider repeating evaluation at 5–10 years.

CACS-Guided Prevention and Adherence to Therapies

In view of the numerous studies demonstrating that CACS can improve risk assessment in primary prevention, there has been strong interest in understanding whether noninvasive imaging can improve cardiovascular outcomes by guiding the implementation and intensity of preventive strategies and whether knowledge of CACS can increase adherence to preventive therapies [81].

The EISNER (Early Identification of Subclinical Atherosclerosis by Noninvasive Imaging Research) study was a prospective RCT to evaluate the effects of CACS on risk factor management and downstream diagnostic testing [82]. Trial participants (N = 2137) were middle-aged (mean 58.5 years) individuals with established ASCVD risk factors who were randomized 2:1 to undergo CACS or no imaging and followed for a mean of 4 years. All subjects received standardized risk factor counseling. Compared with the no-CACS group, those who underwent CACS had greater improvement in systolic blood pressure, LDL-C, and waist circumference (for those with elevated baseline waist girth). There was no difference in net utilization of downstream diagnostic testing, such as stress tests, carotid ultrasound, invasive coronary angiogram, or revascularization procedures. Approximately two-thirds of subjects with CACS ≥400 underwent some form of noninvasive stress testing, but the frequency of cardiac catheterization and revascularization was substantially lower among patients who underwent CACS compared to those who did not. In patients with CACS = 0, there was a 37% reduction in procedure costs. These results were consistent with the hypothesis that CACS can improve ASCVD risk factor management without significant increases in downstream health-care costs.

A recent systematic review examined the effects of CACS on behavioral or lifestyle modification, perception of risk for CHD, and medication adherence [83]. Of the 15 studies reviewed, 3 were RCTs and 12 were observational. The strongest impact of CACS was found to be improved medication utilization and adherence. The results on lifestyle modification and risk perception were either nonsignificant or inconsistent. In an observational study of 980 asymptomatic patients who underwent assessment of CAC, initiation of aspirin, improvement in dietary habits, and increase in exercise were strongly associated with greater CACS [84]. The prospective incidence of aspirin and statin use was assessed in the PACC (Prospective Army Coronary Calcium) Project [85]. Men ages 40–50 years were screened for CHD risk factors and CACS. Preventive medications were not prescribed by the study investigators. Over the subsequent 6-year follow-up period, patients with evidence of CAC were three times more likely to be prescribed a statin and more likely to receive aspirin than those with CACS = 0. CAC was strongly and independently associated with the use of statin, aspirin, or both (Fig. 23.14). In the largest RCT, the EISNER trial, the CACS group were noted to have high adherence rates for lipid-lowering and antihypertensive medications [83].

The motivational effects of CACS on adherence to statin therapy and behavioral modification for weight loss were retrospectively analyzed in 2608 patients who had underwent baseline study and returned for follow-up at a mean of 4.1 years [86]. Statin adherence was lowest (27.4%) among those with CACS = 0 and increased with increasing levels of CAC to 58.8% adherence among those with CACS > 400. Similarly, behavioral modification resulting in weight loss was lowest (19.8%) among those with CACS = 0 and gradually increased to 33.6% among those with CACS > 400. This study is the largest study to date demonstrating that the CACS results are associated with improved adherence with ASCVD risk reduction behaviors.

Current guidelines have generally only provided a level IIB ("may be considered") endorsement for addition of CACS into risk assessment algorithms. This tepid recommendation is largely due to the lack of large, prospective RCTs of CACS-guided ASCVD prevention strategies [7]. However, there also have not been RCTs demonstrating reduction in ASCVD events based upon risk assessment tools or other biomarkers, such as hs-CRP [87, 88]. In view of the limitations of current risk assessment tools which are strongly influenced by age and the increasing numbers of statin-eligible individuals, there is interest among many stakeholders to conduct such a trial. Recent processes for guideline development have restricted consideration to only large RCTs and have limited the use of observational data, thereby possibly necessitating such a CACS-guided RCT to strengthen recommendations for use of imaging to personal-

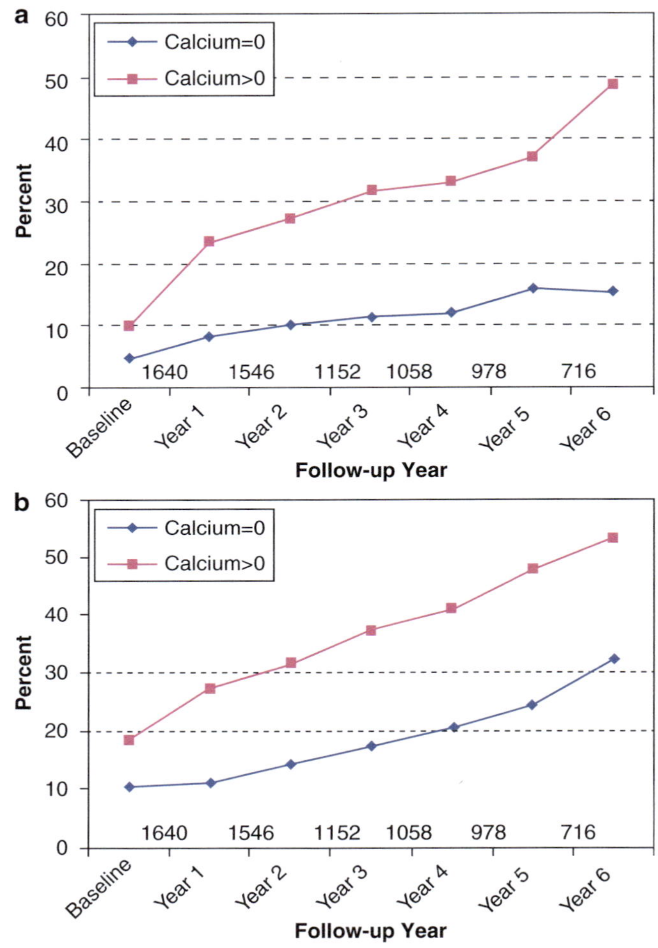

Fig. 23.14 Incidence of statin (**a**) and aspirin (**b**) use during 6-year actuarial follow-up in the PACC Project Cohort. (**a**) Men only; $n = 1640$. Ever use of a statin was noted in 23% of participants, including 48.5% of those with coronary artery calcium and 15.5% of those without coronary artery calcium ($p < 0.001$), which remained significant after controlling for NCEP risk variables (odds ratio 3.53; 95% CI 2.66–4.69). (**b**) Men only; n-1640. Ever-use of aspirin was noted in 31.2% of participants, including 51.5% of those with coronary artery calcium versus 25.3% of those without coronary artery calcium ($p < 0.001$), which remained significant after controlling for NCEP risk variables (odds ratio 3.05; 95% CI 2.30–4.05). (Adapted from Taylor et al. [85], with permission)

ize preventive strategies [89]. The numerous considerations in conducting such a large RCT for CACS are discussed in a recent review and include cost associated with such a trial and previous evidence for cost-effectiveness of CACS, exposure to ionizing radiation, trial feasibility and adequate statistical power, ethical considerations in randomizing patients with extensive CAC to placebo, selection of patients based on the level of risk-based factor risk assessment, and challenges of blinding [82]. Authors also propose consideration of incorporating such a trial into current guideline-based recommendations for low-dose CT screening for lung cancer for persons 55–74 years of age with >30-pack year history of smoking.

The ROBINSCA (Risk Or Benefit IN Screening for Cardiovascular Disease) trial is currently being conducted in Europe and will include 33,000 individuals from the general population [90]. Participants will be randomized (non-blinded) to systematic screening by traditional ASCVD risk factors (SCORE algorithm), systematic screening by CACS, or no intervention (control). Participants in the risk factor-based intervention group with intermediate or high risk for ASCVD are referred to a primary care provider (PCP) for guideline-based preventive management. Participants in the CACS-based intervention group with a high or very high risk for ASCVD based on their CACS are also referred to a PCP and for treatment according to the study protocol. All participants will be followed for 5 years, and the primary study outcome is 5-year fatal and nonfatal CHD. This study is currently enrolling with estimated completion in 2022.

Progression of CACS and Role of Serial Scanning

Multiple retrospective and prospective observational studies have suggested that progression of CAC is associated with increased risk of CHD events and predicts all-cause mortality [91, 92]. In the MESA cohort, the absolute change in CACS was assessed from baseline study to follow-up scan obtained approximately 2.5 years later [93]. Among those individuals with CACS > 0 at baseline, greater change in absolute CACS was associated with higher cumulative proportion of incident CHD events (Fig. 23.15). Those with annual progression of ≥300 had adjusted HRs of 3.8 and 6.3 for total and hard CHD events, respectively, compared to individuals without CAC progression. For patients with CACS = 0 at baseline, compared to those with no increase in CAC, any increase was associated with 1.4- and 1.5-fold greater risks for total and hard CHD events, respectively.

A cohort of 4609 asymptomatic individuals underwent repeat CACS with a mean interscan time of 3.1 years [94]. CAC progression was evaluated as the absolute change in CACS, percent annualized difference between scans, and the difference between square root of the baseline and square root of follow-up CACS > 2.5 (the "SQRT" method). Among patients with baseline CACS > 0, CAC progression added incremental value in predicting all-cause mortality compared to baseline score and traditional risk factors. Progression in the setting of increasing baseline CACS (1–10, 11–100, 101–400, and >400) was associated with increasing risk of all-cause mortality. At all levels of CACS, the risk for all-

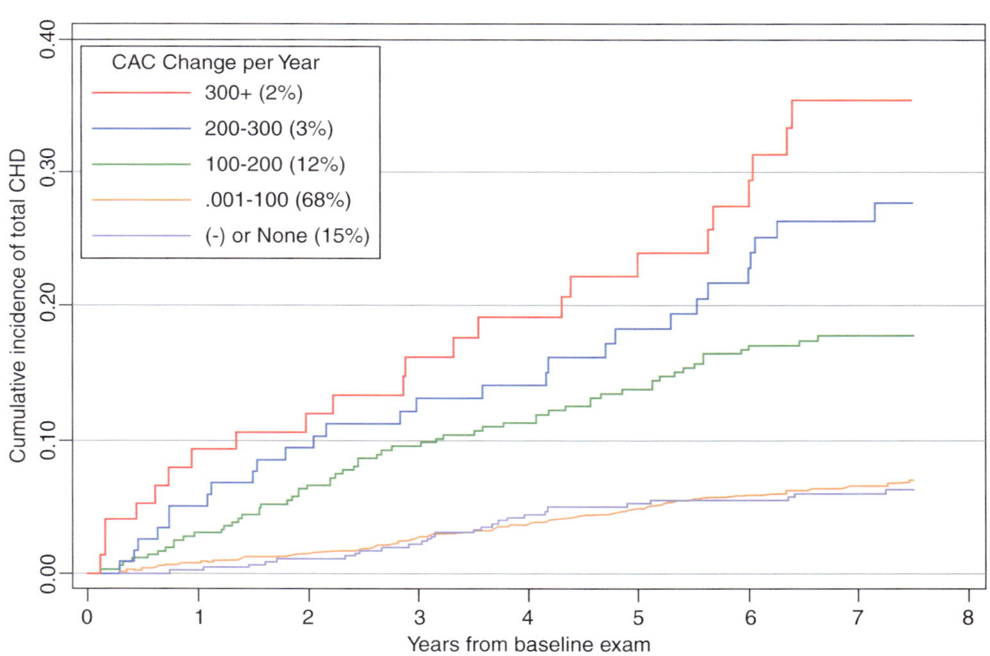

Fig. 23.15 Kaplan-Meier plot of cumulative incidence of total CHD among persons with CAC > 0 at baseline. Numbers in parentheses indicate proportion of subjects in each group. Imputed and nonimputed subjects are included. For log-rank test across CAC change groups, $p < 0.001$. CHD indicates coronary heart disease, CAC coronary artery calcium score. (From Budoff et al. [91], with permission)

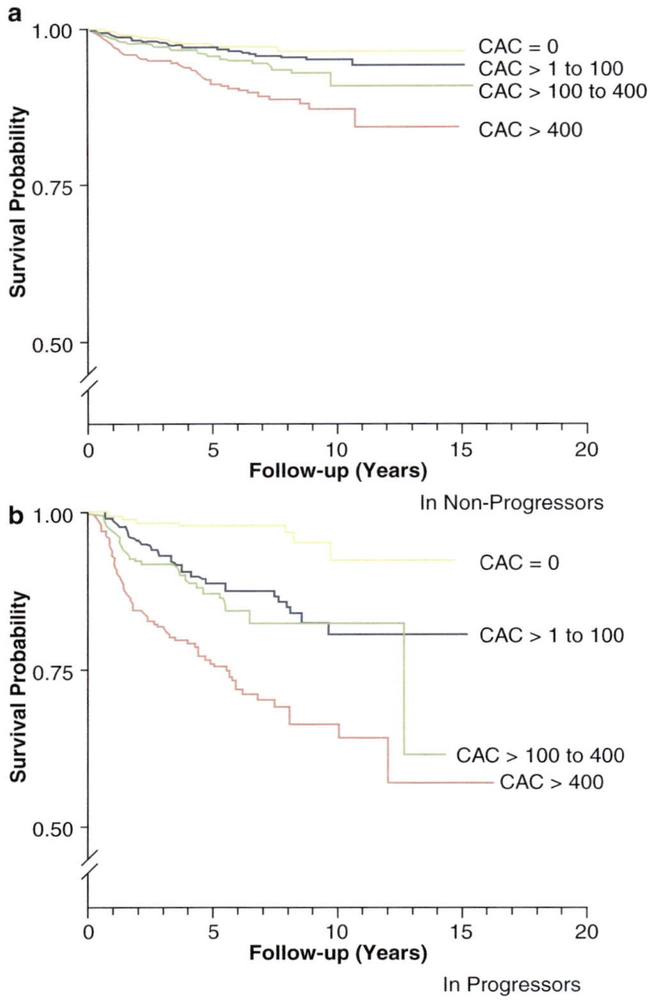

Fig. 23.16 Survival curves demonstrating time to all-cause mortality for nonprogressors and progressors. Cox proportional hazards survival curves demonstrating time to all-cause mortality for patients with a yearly change using survival curve of progression based on our best-fitting model of square root >2.5 according to baseline calcium score: (**a**) nonprogressors and (**b**) outcomes in progressors. CAC indicates coronary artery calcium score. (From Budoff et al. [91], with permission)

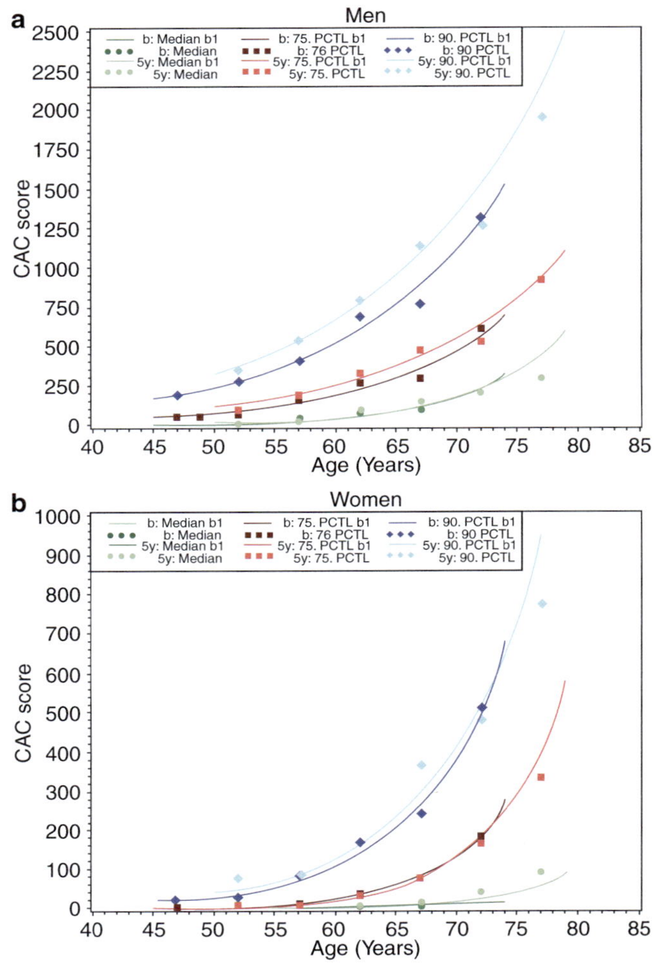

Fig. 23.17 Age- and gender-related percentiles of CAC distribution follow an exponential curvature. Observed and fitted 50th, 75th, and 90th percentile of the CAC distribution for men (n = 1633) (**a**) and women (n = 1848) (**b**) by age categories. In dark colors for the baseline values, when the participants (1633 men) were aged between 45 and 74 years, and in light colors for the 5-year follow-up data, when the cohort was aged 50–79 years. Note the exponential shape of the increase of CAC. Dots represent observed percentile values for each 5-year age category; lines show linear quantile regression on a log scale after retransformation. The y-axis range in (**a**) and (**b**) differs by a factor of 2.5 in men compared with women. (From Erbel et al. [94], with permission)

cause mortality was higher among those with significant progression compared to those with less progression (Fig. 23.16).

In the MESA cohort, individuals with the metabolic syndrome, diabetes, or both were demonstrated to have greater progression of CAC compared to individuals without these conditions. Furthermore, progression predicted CHD events among those in the highest tertile of CAC increase versus no increase [93].

Data from HNR demonstrated that age- and gender-related percentiles of CAC distribution follow an exponential curve, with a nearly indistinguishable shift along the baseline over 5 years of follow-up (Fig. 23.17) [94]. Based on the observed CACS distribution of the cohort, investigators developed a mathematical tool to predict CAC progression for individuals in the study. The model indicated that progression of CAC is nearly inevitable and is only modestly influenced by adjustment for risk factors and lipid lowering and antihypertensive medications.

Continued progression of CAC in patients currently being treated with statin therapy has been shown to be associated with increased risk of MI in patients with and without diabetes [95].

Preventive Therapies and CAC Progression

In a systematic review of trials of preventive therapies and progression of CAC, patients with clinical ASCVD received treatments including statins, antihypertensive agents, or placebo [96]. Patients with chronic kidney disease received interventions including low phosphorous diet, sevelamer hydrochloride, and calcium-based phosphate binders. There was no significant effect of any of these therapies on mean weighted annualized CAC increase in any of these patient populations.

The effects of statin therapy on plaque composition, plaque progression, and the extent and progression of CAC are of specific interest. The dose-dependent beneficial effects of statins on slowing progression of coronary atheroma volume and plaque regression have been well established with intravascular ultrasound (IVUS) [97, 98]. Given the documented correlation between the extent of CAC and total coronary plaque burden, one could hypothesize that statin therapy would be associated with a decrease in progression of CAC [99]. However, despite promising early data, large prospective trials have failed to demonstrate a reduction in CAC with low-, moderate-, or high-intensity statin [100].

Investigators for SALTIRE (Scottish Aortic Stenosis and Lipid Lowering Trial: Impact on Regression) randomized 102 patients with calcific aortic stenosis and CAC to atorvastatin 80 mg or placebo [101]. After a mean follow-up of 2 years, despite significant reductions in LDL-C and hs-CRP, there was a nonsignificant increase in CAC progression in the atorvastatin group (26% per year) compared to the placebo-treated group (18% per year).

The BELLES (Beyond Endorsed Lipid Lowering with EBT Scanning) trial was a randomized, double-blind, multicenter study of atorvastatin 80 mg or pravastatin 40 mg daily in 615 hyperlipidemia women without clinical ASCVD [102]. Women underwent baseline and 12-month CACS to measure percent change in total and single artery calcium volume score from baseline, as well as absolute changes in CACS. Among the 475 women who completed the study, LDL-C was reduced by approximately 47% in those randomized to atorvastatin and 25% in those randomized to pravastatin. Although, high-intensity statin therapy caused a greater reduction in atherogenic lipoproteins, there was no effect upon any measure of CAC progression. In the absence of a placebo group, it was not possible to determine if statin therapy similarly reduced progression of CAC in both treatment groups. In addition, the short duration of the follow-up may have precluded observation of longer-term effects of statin therapy.

The St. Francis Heart Study was a randomized, double-blind, placebo-controlled trial of atorvastatin 20 mg daily, vitamin C, and vitamin E in 1005 asymptomatic individuals on baseline aspirin 81 mg with CACS ≥80th percentile for age and gender [103]. Participants were followed for a mean of 4.3 years. Though treatment reduced LDL-C by 43%, there was no effect on progression of CAC in the treatment group compared to individuals receiving placebo. The mean increase in CACS was 331 ± 421 in the treatment group compared with 323 ± 385 in the control group. Though there were fewer ASCVD events in the overall treatment group, this difference did not achieve statistical significance ($p = 0.08$). However, among those individuals with CACS > 400 (47% of study population), treatment reduced the risk of events by 42% ($p = 0.046$).

Recent serial IVUS studies have provided new insights into the role of statins and plaque composition, progression of calcification, and plaque stability. An analysis of IVUS data from eight large multicenter clinical trials assessing the impact of medical therapies on serial changes in coronary

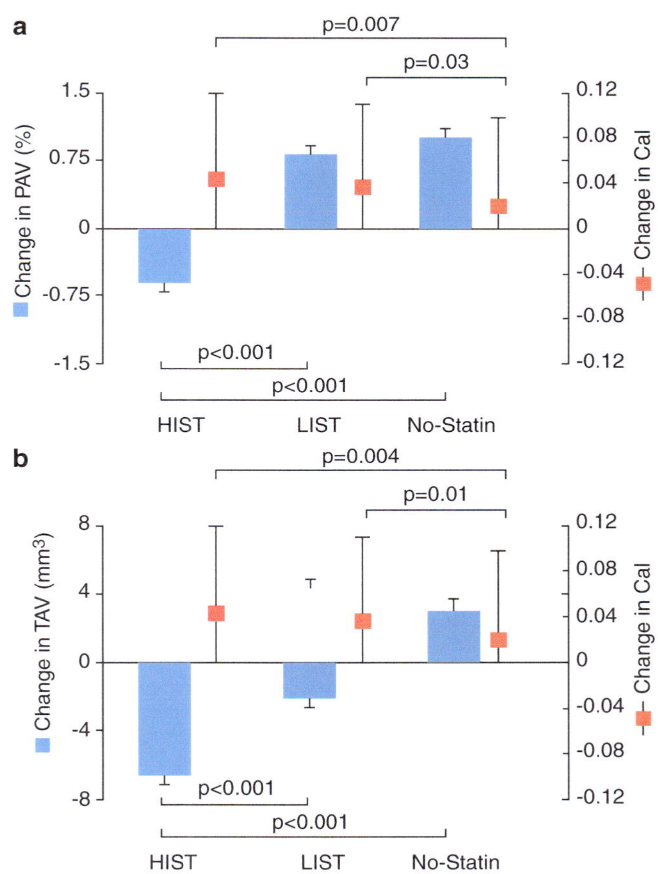

Fig. 23.18 Statins and Coronary Plaque Calcification: Changes in Coronary Atheroma Volume and Calcium Indices According to Therapy. (**a**) Percent atheroma volume (PAV)-adjusted model, depicting corresponding changes in PAV and calcium index (CaI). (**b**) Total atheroma volume (TAV)-adjusted model depicting corresponding changes in TAV and CaI. Changes in PAV and TAV (blue boxes) are reported as least squares mean ± standard error of the mean, whereas the changes in CaI (salmon boxes) are reported as median (interquartile range). CI confidence interval, HIST high-intensity statin therapy, LIST low-intensity statin therapy. (From Puri et al. [104], with permission)

atheroma burden included two trials of intensive lipid lowering with statins (REVERSAL [Reversal of Atherosclerosis with Aggressive Lipid Lowering] and SATURN [the Study of Coronary Atheroma by Intravascular Ultrasound: Effect of Rosuvastatin Versus Atorvastatin]) [104]. High-intensity statin therapy was associated with mean 36.2% reduction in LDL-C and significant regression in percent atheroma volume (PAV) from baseline during 18- to 24-month follow-up, whereas low-intensity statin and no statin therapy were associated with significant PAV progression (Fig. 23.18a). All treatment groups had significant progression of CAC from baseline, and the change in CAC was greatest in the statin-treated groups versus the no-statin group (Fig. 23.18b). The change in CAC was not statistically greater in the high-intensity statin versus low-intensity statin comparison. The greatest increases in CAC were noted in patients on high-intensity statin with significant plaque regression, whereas in patients on no-statin therapy, there was profound progression of coronary atheroma with smaller increases in CAC. Authors suggest that evidence supports the role of statin therapy in de-lipidation of atheroma and probable vascular smooth muscle cell calcification, possibly promoting plaque stability (Fig. 23.19).

The effect of high-intensity statin on plaque composition and plaque burden by serial IVUS was also assessed in 82 patients following non-ST segment elevation MI in IBIS-4 (Integrated Biomarker Imaging Study) [105]. Patients were treated with rosuvastatin 40 mg daily, and IVUS with analysis of matched segments was performed at baseline and 13 months. Statin therapy was associated with significant reductions in percent atheroma volume, percent fibrous plaque volume, and necrotic core volume. The proportion of calcified plaque components was, however, significantly increased (+1.28%; CI 0.66–1.90%; $p < 0.0001$).

Summary

Progression of CAC is clearly associated with an increased risk of future ASCVD events. Despite significant event reduction in patients treated with statin therapy and evidence of reduction in atheroma volume by IVUS, CAC progression

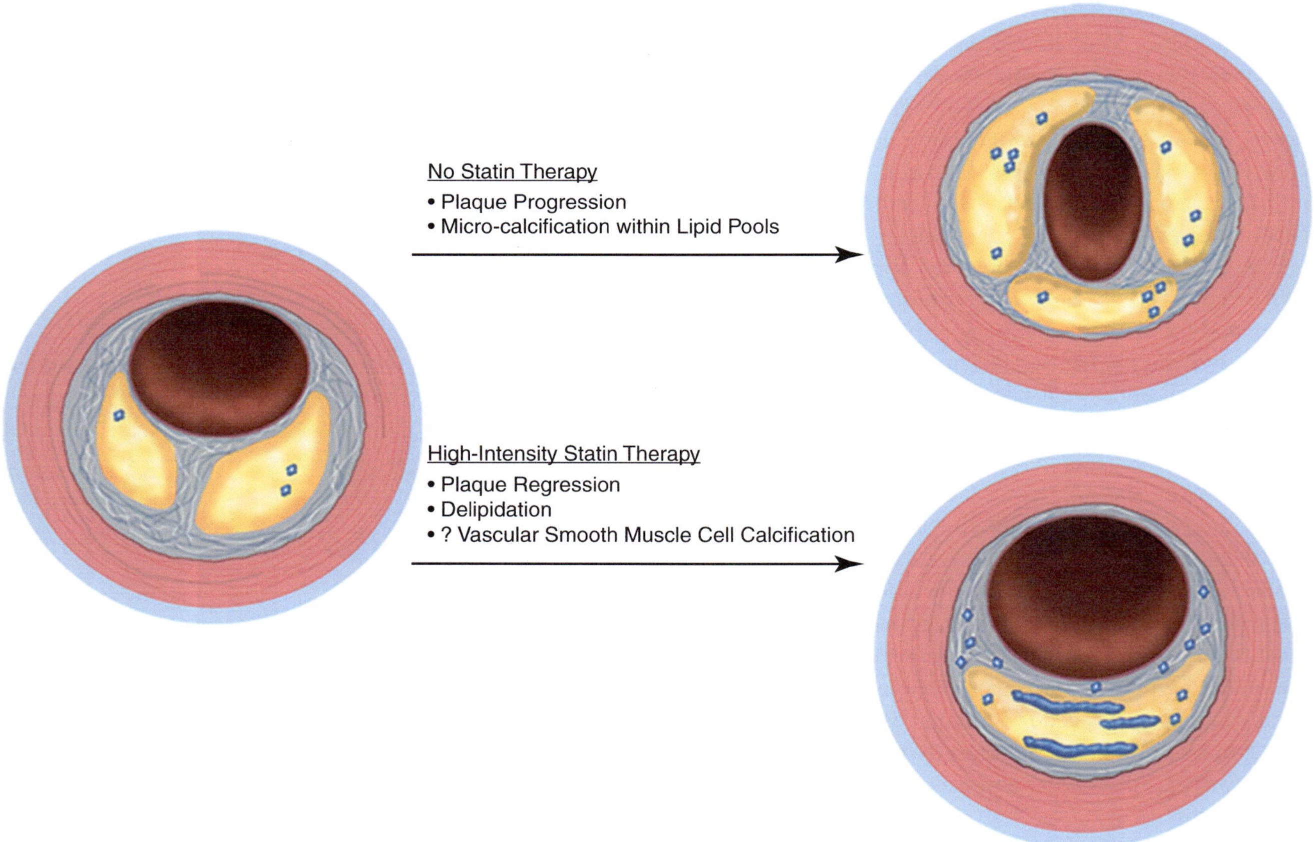

Fig. 23.19 Plaque Calcification in the Setting of No-Statin Therapy or High-Intensity Statin Therapy. Natural plaque progression likely involves lipid-pool expansion coupled with microcalcifications within lipid pools. Following long-term high-intensity statin therapy, plaque regression manifests as delipidation and probable vascular smooth muscle cell calcification, promoting plaque stability. (From Puri et al. [104], with permission)

is not retarded and may even be accelerated on treatment. Greater progression of CAC on statin therapy has been interpreted by many as benign conversion of pre-existing noncalcified to calcified plaque. However, greater progression of CAC on statin therapy has been associated with higher major adverse cardiovascular event rates and does not support this prevailing view. Instead, progression of CAC, irrespective of statin therapy, supports the predominant formation of new atherosclerotic plaque that then becomes calcified. At the current time, there are no medical therapies which have been demonstrated to achieve reductions [98].

The 2013 ACCF/AHA/ASE/ASNC/HFSA/SCAI/SCCT/SCMR/STS Multimodality Appropriate Use Criteria for the Detection and Risk Assessment of Stable Ischemic Heart Disease indicate that repeat CACS is rarely appropriate for patients at any level of ASCVD risk or any baseline level of CAC [79].

Evolution of Guidelines, Recommendations, and Appropriate Use Criteria for Calcium Scoring in ASCVD Risk Assessment

In 2000, the ACC Task Force on Clinical Expert Consensus Documents published the first recommendations for CACS in the diagnosis and prognosis of coronary artery disease [106]. The Writing Group reviewed literature published between 1988 and 1999, which at that time primarily utilized electron beam computed tomography (EBCT). Findings of this meta-analysis demonstrated a high sensitivity of EBCT for the presence of obstructive CHD, a much lower specificity, and an overall accuracy of approximately 70%. Available data at that time did not clarify whether the presence of CAC was additive to the FRS for risk assessment in asymptomatic patients. Additional information was felt to be needed on the value of a positive or negative calcium score in intermediate-risk individuals for risk adjustment. The test was felt to be equivalent but not superior to alternative noninvasive imaging methods such as single- photon emission computed tomography (SPECT) imaging.

The Writing Group III of the American Heart Association (AHA) Prevention Conference V: Noninvasive Tests of Atherosclerotic Burden also considered the role of CACS in assessment of CHD risk in 2000 [107]. While acknowledging CAC as a definitive marker of atherosclerosis, the authors found relatively few prospective studies directly linking CACS to subsequent CHD outcomes. The extent to which CACS predicted events independently of traditional risk factors was also not evident from the data at that time. It was proposed that CAC had the greatest potential for risk adjustment in patients who had an intermediate risk score as calculated by one of the above risk scoring algorithms, but further research was suggested. No definitive recommendations for incorporation of CACS into models of risk assessment and risk reduction were offered in this summary.

The NCEP ATP III released guidelines for detection, evaluation, and treatment of high blood cholesterol levels in 2002 [72]. Authors supported the position of the Prevention V conference writers, recommending against *routine* CACS in asymptomatic persons for risk assessment. However, it was felt that data supported a higher risk of major coronary events in persons with advanced subclinical atherosclerosis. The ATP III guidelines supported the "measurement of coronary calcium as an option for advanced risk assessment in appropriately selected persons, provided the test is ordered by a physician who is familiar with the strengths and weaknesses of noninvasive testing." The guideline writers suggested that the presence of subclinical atherosclerosis could be used to justify intensification of cholesterol therapy in intermediate-risk patients.

The first gender-specific guidelines for the use of noninvasive testing in the evaluation of women with suspected CHD were published in 2005 [108]. Women develop coronary atherosclerosis approximately a decade later than men, and the occurrence of CAC tracks this incidence of clinical events. These differences make it important to consider gender-specific criteria when evaluating the clinical significance of CACS. In the noninvasive testing guidelines for women, CACS was characterized as an "emerging imaging" modality, along with CCTA, magnetic resonance imaging, and carotid intima-media thickness. By the time of this report, a number of studies were available confirming that the presence and severity of CAC have independent and incremental value when added to major ASCVD risk factors in estimation of risk of MI or CHD death. Despite limited data in women, this consensus statement proposed that CACS is useful in risk stratification in women, particularly in women at intermediate CHD risk. Since the publication of these guidelines, MESA has provided a large prospective database for evaluation of age-, gender-, and ethnic-related percentiles for CACS [17, 18].

Given technological advancements and the rapidly evolving literature, the AHA reissued a scientific statement on CCT [109] in 2006 and an expert consensus document on CACS in 2007 [110]. The AHA scientific statement reviewed the most current evidence for the use of CCT for noninvasive imaging of coronary atherosclerosis. Though the authors addressed CCT with and without contrast enhancement, the current discussion focuses on recommendations provided for non-contrast-enhanced CCT for assessment of CAC.

For reproducible and valid measurement of CAC, the 2006 AHA Writing Group established minimum criteria for scanning. Studies comparing measurement of CACS with EBCT and MDCT demonstrate good correlation over a large range of values in large, multiethnic population-based studies [111]. However, to minimize motion artifacts, reduce radiation exposure, and improve intra- and inter-scan reproducibility, it was recommended to use an EBCT or at least four-slice MDCT scanner and to maintain consistency in gating, triggering, and slice thickness parameters. The Agatston score remains the primary tool for risk assessment because of the availability of large prognostic databases that allow clinicians and patients to understand the implication of any given score.

The 2007 ACCF/AHA Clinical Expert Consensus Document on Coronary Artery Calcium Scoring by Computed Tomography in Global Cardiovascular Risk Assessment and in Evaluation of Patients with Chest Pain represented an updated review of scientific data published subsequent to the original ACC/AHA Expert Consensus document on EBCT published in 2000 [112]. The focus of the Writing Committee was on clinical application of CAC quantification by cardiac CT in two areas: (1) CHD risk assessment in the asymptomatic patient to improve selection of candidates for preventive interventions and (2) to improve triage of symptomatic patients, refining selection of candidates for subsequent hospitalization or further diagnostic testing. At the time of this document, significant scientific data was available supporting a directly proportional relationship between risk of CHD death or nonfatal MI, overall CHD events, all-cause mortality, and the extent of CAC, as previously described above. Thus, the measurement of CAC for risk assessment was considered "reasonable" in asymptomatic patients with an intermediate (10–20% absolute 10-year) risk of MI or CHD death by the FRS (Class IIb, Level of Evidence B). The presence of significant CAC in an intermediate-risk individual could appropriately reassign the patient to a higher-risk category and justify more aggressive reduction of CHD risk factors [113]. If an intermediate-risk patient had CACS = 0 or a very low score, the risk stratification may be reduced. The probability of a CHD event in a patient without CAC present was approximately 0.1–0.6% per year (10-year CHD risk of 1.0–6.3%, consistent with FRS low-risk <10%) based on data available at that time. Imaging of CAC was not recommended for patients at low risk of CHD (<10% 10-year risk) or for high-risk (>20% 10-year risk) patients (Class III, Level of Evidence B).

The 2010 ACCF/AHA Guideline for Assessment of Cardiovascular Risk in Asymptomatic Adults evaluated CACS among other emerging risk markers and provided the highest endorsement for its clinical application thus far [114]. CACS was considered reasonable for CVD risk assessment in asymptomatic adults at intermediate risk (10–20% 10-year risk) as defined by the global FRS (Class IIa, Level of Evidence [LOE] B). CACS was also considered reasonable in persons at low to intermediate risk (6–10% 10-year risk) (Class IIb recommendation, LOE B). CACS was not recommended for persons at low risk (<6% 10-year risk) (Class III: No Benefit, LOE B).

As previously noted, the 2013 ACC/AHA Guideline on the Assessment of Cardiovascular Risk indicates that if a risk-based treatment decision is uncertain, CACS may be considered to inform treatment decision making (Class IIb, LOE B) [7].

According to the 2013 ACCF/AHA/ASNC/HFSA/HRS/SCAI/SCCT/SCMR/STS Multimodality Appropriate Use Criteria for the Detection and Risk Assessment of Stable Ischemic Heart Disease, CACS "may be appropriate" in patients with intermediate or high global CHD risk regardless of baseline ECG or ability of patient to exercise [79]. However, CACS is considered "rarely appropriate" for asymptomatic patients with low global CHD risk or in symptomatic patients.

The American College of Radiology Appropriateness Criteria for the Asymptomatic Patient at Risk for Coronary Artery Disease provides a rating scale for CACS as follows: 1,2,3, usually not appropriate; 4,5,6, may be appropriate; and 7,8,9, usually appropriate [115]. For the intermediate-risk patient, CACS is rated 8 or usually appropriate. However, for patients at high and low ASCVD risk, CACS is rated 3 or usually not appropriate.

The 2016 European Society of Cardiology Guidelines on Cardiovascular Disease Prevention in Clinical Practices recommend that "coronary artery calcium scoring may be considered as a risk modifier in CV risk assessment" (Class IIb, LOE B) [116]. However, routine screening with imaging modalities to predict future ASCVD events is generally not recommended in clinical practice.

The 2018 ACC/AHA blood cholesterole guidelines recommend calcium scoring for patients at intermediate risk (>7.5% to <20%) when the risk decision for statin therapy is uncertain (Class IIb, LOE B-NR). For patients with CAC = 0 and no additional high-risk clinical features, consideration may be given to withholding or delaying initiation of statin therapy [42].

Nearly 7.1 million individuals undergo diagnostic non-contrast, non-ECG-gated, chest CT examinations each year in the USA [117]. Recommendations by the 2014 US Preventive Services Task Force for routine lung cancer screening in high-risk individuals (based on age and smoking history) may increase the number of low-dose screening CT scans by another 7–10 million annually [118]. In 2017, the Society of Computed Tomography and the Society of Thoracic Radiology published consensus guidelines for the assessment of CAC from non-contrast chest CT scans [119]. CACS on non-gated CT examinations has been shown to correlate well with scores obtained from conventional ECG-gated scans and provide similar prognostic value in predicting ASCVD events [120–123]. The guidelines recommend incorporation of CACS into *all* non-contrast chest examinations as the appropriate standard of care. This is an extension of the already existing requirement of the American College of Radiology to report "coronary arterial calcification moderate or severe" when present in all lung cancer screening registry patients [124].

Conclusion

Cardiovascular disease continues to be the leading cause of morbidity and mortality around the globe, and CACS is an important tool to readily identify individuals at high risk of events to initiate early lifesaving preventive interventions. The assessment of subclinical coronary atherosclerosis by CACS has been shown to be a robust predictor of both near- and long-term clinical ASCVD events and provides information that outperforms traditional risk factor-based assessments. Current guidelines focus on the consideration of CACS in intermediate-risk patients to inform clinical decision making for initiation of preventive therapies. Knowledge of the subclinical disease can improve adherence to preventive medications and lifestyle interventions.

There is expanding evidence that imaging for subclinical atherosclerosis also provides incremental prognostic information in low- and high-risk individuals. This information may be used to "down-classify" (less overtreatment) or "up-classify" (less undertreatment) patient risk to more accurately evaluate the role of lifelong pharmacotherapy for prevention of ASCVD events. Though there is compelling evidence that the absence of subclinical atherosclerosis by CACS may provide a rationale to de-escalate statins and other preventive therapies, a prospective randomized controlled trial is needed to determine if imaging identifies a lower-risk population and results in accurate assignment of treatments for optimal ASCVD risk reduction. With the expansion of guideline-based low-dose lung cancer screening in high-risk patients and recommendations for simultaneous reporting of CACS, it will be possible to accurately characterize ASCVD risk for millions of individuals.

References

1. Mozaffarian D, Benjamin EJ, Go AS, et al. Heart disease and stroke statistics—2016 update. A report from the American Heart Association. Circulation. 2016;133:e38–e360.
2. Ford ES, Ajani UA, Croft JB, et al. Explaining the decrease in U.S. deaths from coronary disease, 1980-2000. N Engl J Med. 2007;356:2388–98.
3. Greenland P, Bonow RO, Brundage BH, et al. ACCF/AHA 2007 Clinical expert consensus document on coronary artery calcium scoring by computed tomography in global cardiovascular risk assessment and in evaluation of patients with chest pain. Circulation. 2007;115:402–26.
4. Wilson PWF, D'Agostino RB, Levy D, et al. Prediction of coronary heart disease using risk factor categories. Circulation. 1998;97:1837–47.
5. Assmann G, Cullen P, Schulte H. Simple scoring scheme for calculating the risk of acute coronary events based on the 10-year follow-up of the prospective cardiovascular Munster (PROCAM) study. [Erratum: Circulation. 2002;105:900]. Circulation. 2002;105: 310–5.
6. Conroy R, Pylorala K, Fitzgerald AP, et al. The SCORE (Systemic Coronary Risk Evaluation) manuscript. Prediction of ten-year risk of fatal cardiovascular disease in Europe: the SCORE project. Eur Heart J. 2003;24:987–1003.
7. Goff DF, Lloyd-Jones DM, Bennett G, et al. 2013 ACC/AHA guideline on the assessment of cardiovascular risk. J Am Coll Cardiol. 2014;63:2935–57.
8. Ridker PM, Paynter NP, Rifai N, et al. C-reactive protein and parental history improve global cardiovascular risk prediction: the Reynolds risk score for men. Circulation. 2008;118:2243–51.
9. Ridker PM, Buring JE, Firai N, Cook NR. Development and validation of improved algorithms for the assessment of global cardiovascular risk in women: the Reynolds Risk score. JAMA. 2007;297:611–9.
10. DeFilippis AP, Young R, Carrubba CJ, et al. An analysis of calibration and discrimination among multiple cardiovascular risk scores in a modern multiethnic cohort. Ann Intern Med. 2015;162:266–75.
11. Akosah KO, Schaper A, Cogbill C, Schoenfeld P. Preventing myocardial infarction in the young adult in the first place: how do the National Cholesterol Education Panel III guidelines perform? J Am Coll Cardiol. 2003;41:1475–9.
12. Cooney MT, Dudina A, Whincup P, et al., SCORE Investigators. Re-evaluating the Rose approach: comparative benefits of the population and high-risk preventive strategies. Eur J Cardiovasc Prev Rehabil. 2009;16:541–9.
13. Michos ED, Nasir K, Braunstein JB, et al. Framingham risk equation underestimates subclinical atherosclerosis risk in asymptomatic women. Atherosclerosis. 2006;184:2010–6.
14. Schlendorf KH, Nasir K, Blumenthal RS. Limitations of the Framingham risk score are now much clearer. Prev Med. 2009;48:115–6.
15. Blaha MJ, Silverman MG, Budoff MJ. Is there a role for coronary artery calcium scoring for management of asymptomatic patients at risk for coronary artery disease? Circ Cardiovasc Imaging. 2014;7:398–408.
16. Kianoush S, Al Rifai M, Cainzos-Achirica M, et al. An update on the utility of coronary artery calcium scoring for coronary heart disease and cardiovascular disease risk prediction. Curr Atheroscler Rep. 2016;18:13.
17. Bild DE, Detrano R, Peterson D, et al. Ethnic differences in coronary calcification: the Multi-Ethnic Study of Atherosclerosis. Circulation. 2005;111:1313–20.
18. McClelland RL, Chung H, Detrano R, et al. Distribution of coronary artery calcium by race, gender, and age: results from the Multi-Ethnic Study of Atherosclerosis. Circulation. 2006;113:30–7.
19. Cook NR. Statistical evaluation of prognostic versus diagnostic models: beyond the ROC curve. Clin Chem. 2008;54:17–23.
20. Detrano R, Guerci AD, Carr JJ, et al. Coronary calcium as a predictor of coronary events in four racial or ethnic groups. N Engl J Med. 2008;358:1336–45.
21. Weber LA, Cheezum MK, Reese JM, et al. Cardiovascular imaging for the primary prevention of atherosclerotic cardiovascular disease events. Curr Cardiovasc Imaging Rep. 2015;8:36.
22. Arad Y, Spadaro LA, Goodman K, et al. Prediction of coronary events with electron beam computed tomography. J Am Coll Cardiol. 2000;36:1253–60.
23. Raggi P, Callister TQ, Cooil B, et al. Identification of patients at increased risk of first unheralded acute myocardial infarction by electron-beam computed tomography. Circulation. 2000;101:850–5.
24. Wong ND, Hsu JC, Detrano RC, et al. Coronary artery calcium evaluation by electron beam tomography and its relation to new cardiovascular events. Am J Cardiol. 2000;86:495–8.
25. Vliegenthart R, Oudkerk M, Song B, et al. Coronary calcification detected by electron-beam computed tomography and myocardial infraction: the Rotterdam Coronary Calcification Study. Eur Heart J. 2002;23:1596–603.

26. Park R, Detrano RC, Xiang M, et al. Combined use of computed tomography coronary calcium scores and C-reactive protein levels in predicting cardiovascular events in nondiabetic individuals. Circulation. 2002;106:2073–7.
27. Kondos GT, Hoff JA, Sevrukov A, et al. Electron-beam tomography coronary artery calcium and cardiac events. Circulation. 2003;107:2571–6.
28. Shaw LJ, Raggi P, Schisterman E, et al. Prognostic value of cardiac risk factors and coronary artery calcium screening for all-cause mortality. Radiology. 2003;228:826–33.
29. Greenland P, LaBree L, Azen SP, et al. Coronary artery calcium score combined with Framingham score for risk prediction in asymptomatic individuals. JAMA. 2004;291:210–5.
30. Arad Y, Goodman KJ, Roth M, et al. Coronary calcification, coronary disease risk factors, C-reactive protein, and atherosclerotic cardiovascular disease events. J Am Coll Cardiol. 2005;46:158–65.
31. Taylor AJ, Bindeman J, Feuerstein I, et al. Coronary calcium independently predicts incident premature coronary heart disease over measure cardiovascular disease risk factors. J Am Coll Cardiol. 2005;46:807–14.
32. Budoff MJ, Shaw LJ, Liu ST, et al. Long-term prognosis associated with coronary calcification. J Am Coll Cardiol. 2007;49:1860–70.
33. Lakoski SG, Greenland P, Wong ND, et al. Coronary artery calcium scores and risk for cardiovascular events in women classified as "low risk" based on Framingham risk score. Arch Intern Med. 2007;167:2437–42.
34. Becker A, Leber A, Becker C, Knez A. Predictive value of coronary calcifications for future cardiac events in asymptomatic individuals. Am Heart J. 2008;155:154–60.
35. Erbel R, Mohlenkamp S, Moebus S, et al. Coronary risk stratification, discrimination, and reclassification improvement based on quantification of subclinical coronary atherosclerosis. J Am Coll Cardiol. 2010;56:1397–406.
36. Hecht HS, Narula J. Coronary artery calcium scanning in asymptomatic patients with diabetes. J Diabetes. 2012;4:342–50.
37. Yeboah J, McClelland RL, Polonsky TS, et al. Comparison of novel risk markers for improvement in cardiovascular risk assessment in intermediate-risk individuals. JAMA. 2012;308:788–95.
38. Folsom AR, Kronmal RA, Detrano RC, et al. Coronary artery calcification compared with carotid intima-media thickness in the prediction of cardiovascular disease incidence: the Multi-Ethnic Study of Atherosclerosis. Arch Intern Med. 2008;168:1333–9.
39. Hecht HS. Coronary artery calcium scanning: past, present, and future. JACC Cardiovasc Img. 2015;8:580–96.
40. Elias-Smale SE, Vliegenthart R, Koller MT, et al. Coronary calcium score improves classification of coronary heart disease in the elderly. J Am Coll Cardiol. 2010;56:1407–14.
41. Stone NJ, Robinson JG, Lichtenstein AH, et al. The 2013 ACC/AHA guideline on the treatment of blood cholesterol to reduce atherosclerotic cardiovascular risk in adults. J Am Coll Cardiol. 2014;63:2889–934.
42. Grundy SM, Stone NJ, Bailey AL, et al. 2018 ACC/AHA/AACVPR/AAPA/ABC/ACPM/ADA/AGS/APhA/ASPC/NLA/PCNA guideline on the management of blood cholesterol: a report of the American College of Cardiology Foundation and the American Heart Association Task Force on Clinical Practice Guidelines. J Am Coll Cardiol. 2018; https://doi.org/10.1016/j.jacc.2018.11.003.
43. Shaw LJ, Giambrone AE, Blaha MJ, et al. Long-term prognosis after coronary artery calcification testing in asymptomatic patients: a cohort study. Ann Intern Med. 2015;163:14–21.
44. Valenti V, Ó Hartaigh B, Heo R, et al. A 15-year warranty period for asymptomatic individuals without coronary artery calcium: a prospective follow-up of 9,715 individuals. JACC Cardiovasc Imaging. 2015;8:900–9.
45. Sarwar A, Shaw LJ, Shapiro MD, et al. Diagnostic and prognostic value of absence of coronary artery calcification. J Am Coll Cardiol Imaging. 2009;2:678–88.
46. Polonsky TS, McClelland RL, Jorgensen NW, et al. Coronary artery calcium score and risk classification for coronary heart disease prediction. JAMA. 2010;303:1610–6.
47. Kelkar AA, Schultz WM, Khosa F, et al. Long-term prognosis after coronary artery calcium scoring among low-intermediate risk men and women. Circ Cardiovasc Imaging. 2016;9:e003742. https://doi.org/10.1161/circimaging.115.003742.
48. Blaha MJ, Cainzos-Achirica M, Greenland P, et al. Role of coronary artery calcium score of zero and other negative risk markers for cardiovascular disease: the Multi-Ethnic Study of Atherosclerosis (MESA). Circulation. 2016;133:849–58.
49. Yeboah J, Polonsky TS, Young R, et al. Utility of nontraditional risk markers in individuals ineligible for statin therapy according to the 2013 American College of Cardiology/American Heart Association cholesterol guidelines. Circulation. 2015;132:916–22.
50. Kavousi M, Desai CS, Ayers C, et al. Prevalence and prognostic significance of coronary artery calcification in low-risk women: a meta-analysis. JAMA. 2016;316:2126–34.
51. Joshi PH, Patel B, Blaha MJ, et al. Coronary artery calcium predicts cardiovascular events in participants with a low lifetime risk of cardiovascular disease: the Multi-Ethnic Study of Atherosclerosis (MESA). Atherosclerosis. 2016;246:367–73.
52. Tota-Maharaj R, Blaha MJ, Blankstein R, et al. Association of coronary artery calcium and coronary heart disease events in young and elderly participants in the Multi-Ethnic Study of Atherosclerosis: a secondary analysis of a prospective, population-based cohort. Mayo Clin Proc. 2014;89:1350–9.
53. McClelland RL, Jorgensen NW, Budoff M, et al. 10-year coronary heart disease risk prediction using coronary artery calcium and traditional risk factors. J Am Coll Cardiol. 2015;66:1643–53.
54. Mortensen MB, Fuster V, Muntendam P, et al. A simple disease-guided approach to personalize ACC/AHA-recommended statin allocation in elderly people: the BioImage Study. J Am Coll Cardiol. 2016;68:881–91.
55. Hoff JA, Quinn L, Sevrukov A, et al. The prevalence of coronary artery calcium among diabetic individuals without known coronary artery disease. J Am Coll Cardiol. 2003;41:1008–12.
56. Daga N, Nasir K, Hamirani Y, et al. Prevalence and severity of coronary artery calcium in young persons with diabetes. J Cardiovasc Comput Tomogr. 2013;7:241–7.
57. Kramer CK, Ziman B, Gross JL, et al. Coronary artery calcium score prediction of all cause mortality and cardiovascular events in people with type 2 diabetes: systematic review and meta-analysis. BMJ. 2013;346:f1654.
58. Raggi P, Shaw LJ, Berman DS, Callister TQ. Prognostic value of coronary artery calcium screening in subjects with and without diabetes. J Am Coll Cardiol. 2004;43:1663–9.
59. Malik S, Budoff MJ, Katz R, et al. Impact of subclinical atherosclerosis on cardiovascular disease events in individuals with metabolic syndrome and diabetes. Diabetes Care. 2011;34:2285–90.
60. Hecht HS. A zero coronary artery calcium score: priceless. J Am Coll Cardiol. 2010;55:1118–20.
61. Shareghi S, Ahmadi N, Young E, et al. Prognostic significance of zero coronary calcium scores on cardiac computed tomography. J Cardiovasc Comput Tomogr. 2007;1:155–9.
62. Pencina MJ, Navar-Boggan AM, D'Agostino RB Sr, et al. Application of new cholesterol guidelines to a population-based sample. N Engl J Med. 2014;370:1422–31.
63. Blaha M, Budoff MJ, Shaw LJ, et al. Absence of coronary artery calcification and all-cause mortality. J Am Coll Cardiol Img. 2009;2:692–700.

64. Budoff MJ, McClelland RL, Nasir K, et al. Cardiovascular events with absent or minimal coronary calcification: the Multi-Ethnic Study of Atherosclerosis (MESA). Am Heart J. 2009;158:554–61.
65. Nasir K, Bittencourt MS, Blaha MJ, et al. Implications of coronary artery calcium testing among statin candidates according to American College of Cardiology/American Heart Association cholesterol management guidelines. J Am Coll Cardiol. 2015;66:1657–68.
66. Ridker PM, Danielson E, Fonseca FA, et al., for the JUPITER Study Group. Rosuvastatin to prevent vascular events in men and women with elevated C-reactive protein. N Engl J Med. 2008;359:2195–202.
67. Blaha MJ, Budoff MJ, DeFilippis AP, et al. Associations between C-reactive protein, coronary artery calcium, and cardiovascular events: implications for the JUPITER population from MESA, a population-based cohort study. Lancet. 2001;378:684–92.
68. Valenti V, Hartaigh BO, Cho I, et al. Absence of coronary artery calcium identifies asymptomatic diabetic individuals at low near-term but not long-term risk of mortality: a 15-year follow-up study of 9715 patients. Circ Cardiovasc Imaging. 2016;9:e003528. https://doi.org/10.1161/CIRCIMAGING.115.003528.
69. Nasir K, Rubin J, Blaha MJ, et al. Interplay of coronary artery calcification and traditional risk factors for the prediction of all-cause mortality in asymptomatic individuals. Circ Cardiovasc Imaging. 2012;5:467–73.
70. Silverman MG, Blaha MJ, Krumholz HM, et al. Impact of coronary artery calcium on coronary heart disease events in individuals at the extremes of traditional risk factor burden: the Multi-Ethnic Study of Atherosclerosis. Eur Heart J. 2014;35:2232–41.
71. Martin SS, Blaha MJ, Blankstein R, et al. Dyslipidemia, coronary artery calcium, and incident atherosclerotic cardiovascular disease: implications for statin therapy from the Multi-Ethnic Study of Atherosclerosis. Circulation. 2014;129:77–86.
72. National Cholesterol Education Program. Third report of the National Cholesterol Education Program (NCEP) Expert Panel on Detection, Evaluation, and Treatment of High Blood Cholesterol in Adults (Adult Treatment Panel III): final report. Circulation. 2002;106:3149–421.
73. Agarwal S, Morgan T, Herrington DM, et al. Coronary calcium score and prediction of all-cause mortality in diabetes. Diabetes Care. 2001;34:1219–24.
74. Budoff MJ, Diamond GA, Raggi P, et al. Continuous probabilistic prediction of angiographically significant coronary artery disease using electron beam tomography. Circulation. 2002;105:1791–6.
75. Villines TC, Julten EA, Shaw LJ, et al., for the CONFIRM Registry Investigators. Prevalence and severity of coronary artery disease and adverse events among symptomatic patients with coronary artery calcification scores of zero undergoing coronary computed tomography angiography. J Am Coll Cardiol. 2011;58:2533–40.
76. Lubbers M, Dedic A, Coenen A, et al. Calcium imaging and selective computed tomography angiography in comparison to functional testing for suspected coronary artery disease: the multicenter, randomized CRESCENT trial. Eur Heart J. 2016;37:1232. https://doi.org/10.1093/eurheartj/ehv700.
77. Kim YJ, Hur J, Lee HJ, et al. Meaning of zero calcium score in symptomatic patients referred for coronary computed tomography. Eur Heart J Cardiovasc Imaging. 2012;13:776–85.
78. Wolk MJ, Bailey SR, Doherty JU, et al. ACCF/AHA/ASE/ASNC/HFSA/HRS/SCAI/SCCT/SCMR/STS 2103 Multimodality appropriate use criteria for the detection and risk assessment of stable ischemic heart disease. J Am Coll Cardiol. 2014;63:381–406.
79. Greenland P. When nothing is really something. JACC Cardiovasc Imaging. 2015;8:910–2.
80. Taylor AJ, Raggi J, Raggi P. The power of nothing: the zero calcium score. J Cardiovasc Comput Tomogr. 2007;1:160–1.
81. McEvoy JW, Martin SS, Blaha MJ, et al. The case for and against a coronary artery calcium trial. JACC Cardiovasc Imaging. 2016;9:994–1002.
82. Rozanski A, Gransar H, Shaw LJ, et al. Impact of coronary artery calcium scanning on coronary risk factors and downstream testing. The EISNER (Early Identification of Subclinical Atherosclerosis by Noninvasive Imaging Research) prospective randomized trial. J Am Coll Cardiol. 2011;57:1622–32.
83. Mamudu HM, Paul TK, Veeranki SP, Budoff M. The effects of coronary artery calcium screening on behavioral modification, risk perception, and medication adherence among asymptomatic adults. Atherosclerosis. 2014;236:338–50.
84. Orakzai RH, Nasir K, Orakzai SH, et al. Effect of patient visualization of coronary calcium by electron beam computed tomography on changes in beneficial lifestyle changes. Am J Cardiol. 2008;101:999–1002.
85. Taylor AJ, Bindeman J, Feuerstein I, et al. Community-based provision of statin and aspirin after the detection of coronary artery calcium within a community-based screening cohort. J Am Coll Cardiol. 2008;51:1337–41.
86. Kalia NK, Cespedes L, Youssef G, et al. Motivational effects of coronary artery calcium scores on statin adherence and weight loss. Coron Artery Dis. 2015;26:226–30.
87. McEvoy JW, Blaha MJ. Coronary artery calcium testing: exploring the need for a randomized trial. Circ Cardiovasc Imaging. 2014;7:578–80.
88. Kim J, McEvoy JW, Nasir K, et al. Critical review of high-sensitivity C-reactive protein and coronary artery calcium for the guidance of statin allocation. Circ Cardiovasc Imaging. 2014;7:315–22.
89. Institute of Medicine. Clinical practice guidelines we can trust. Available at https://www.nap.edu/read/13058/chapter/1. Accessed 4 Feb 2017.
90. ROBINSCA Study Design. Available at http://www.robinsca.nl/for-researchers/study-design/. Accessed 4 Feb 2017.
91. Budoff MJ, Young R, Lopez VA, et al. Progression of coronary calcium and incident coronary heart disease events: MESA (Multi-Ethnic Study of Atherosclerosis). J Am Coll Cardiol. 2013;61:1231–9.
92. Budoff MJ, Hokanson JE, Nasir K, et al. Progression of coronary artery calcium predicts all-cause mortality. JACC Cardiovas Imaging. 2010;3:1229–36.
93. Wong ND, Nelson JC, Granston T, et al. Metabolic syndrome, diabetes, and incidence and progression of coronary calcium. JACC Cardiovasc Imaging. 2012;5:358–66.
94. Erbel R, Lehmann N, Churzidse S, et al., on behalf of the Heinz Nixdorf Recall Study Investigators. Progression of coronary artery calcification seems to be inevitable, but predictable—results of the Heinz Nixdorf Recall (HNR) study. Eur Heart J. 2014;35:2960–2971.
95. Raggi P, Callister TQ, Shaw LJ. Progression of coronary artery calcium and risk of first myocardial infarction in patients receiving cholesterol-lowering therapy. Arterioscler Thromb Vasc Biol. 2004;24:1272–7.
96. McCullough PA, Chinnaiyan KM. Annual progression of coronary calcification in trials of preventive therapies: a systematic review. Arch Intern Med. 2009;169:2064–70.
97. Nissen SE, Nicholls SJ, Sipahi I, et al. Effects of very high-intensity statin therapy on regression of coronary atherosclerosis: the ASTEROID trial. JAMA. 2006;295:1556–65.
98. Nicholls SJ, Ballantyne CM, Barter PJ, et al. Effect of two intensive statin regimens on progression of coronary disease. N Engl J Med. 2001;365:2078–87.
99. Ferencik M, Chatzizisis YS. Statins and the coronary plaque calcium "paradox": insights from non-invasive and invasive imaging. Atherosclerosis. 2015;241:783–5.

100. McElvoy JW, Blaha MJ, DeFilippis AP, et al. Coronary artery calcium progression: an important clinical measurement? J Am Coll Cardiol. 2010;56:1613–22.
101. Houslay ED, Cowell SJ, Prescott RJ, et al. Progressive coronary calcification despite intensive lipid-lowering treatment: a randomized controlled trial. Heart. 2006;92:1207–12.
102. Raggi P, Davidson M, Callister TQ, et al. Aggressive versus moderate lipid-lowering therapy in hypercholesterolemic postmenopausal women: beyond endorsed lipid lowering with EBT scanning (BELLES). Circulation. 2005;112:563–71.
103. Arad Y, Spadaro LA, Roth M, et al. Treatment of asymptomatic adults with elevated coronary calcium scores with atorvastatin, vitamin C, and vitamin E: the St. Francis Heart Study Randomized Clinical Trial. J Am Coll Cardiol. 2005;46:166–72.
104. Puri R, Nicholls SJ, Shao M, et al. Impact of statin serial coronary calcification during atheroma progression and regression. J Am Coll Cardiol. 2015;65:1273–82.
105. Raber L, Taniwaki M, Zaugg S, et al. Effect of high-intensity statin therapy on atherosclerosis in non-infarct-related coronary arteries (IBIS-4): a serial intravascular ultrasonography study. Eur Heart J. 2015;36:490–500.
106. O'Rourke RA, Brundage BH, Froelicher VF, et al. American College of Cardiology/American Heart Association Expert Consensus Document on electron-beam computed tomography for the diagnosis and prognosis of coronary artery disease. Circulation. 2000;102:126–40.
107. Greenland P, Abrams J, Aurigemma GP, et al. Prevention Conference V. Beyond secondary prevention: identifying the high-risk patient for primary prevention. Noninvasive tests of atherosclerotic burden. Circulation. 2000;101:e16–322.
108. Mieres JH, Shaw LJ, Arai A, et al. Role of noninvasive testing in the clinical evaluation women with suspected coronary artery disease. Consensus Statement from the Cardiac Imaging Committee, Council on Clinic Cardiology, and the Cardiovascular Imaging and Intervention Committee, Council on Cardiovascular Radiology and Intervention, American Heart Association. Circulation. 2005;111:682–96.
109. Budoff MJ, Achenbach S, Blumenthal RS, et al. Assessment of coronary artery disease by cardiac computed tomography. AHA scientific statement from the American Heart Association Committee on Cardiovascular Imaging and Intervention, Council on Cardiovascular Radiology and Intervention, and Committee on Cardiac Imaging, Council on Clinical Cardiology. Circulation. 2006;114:1761–91.
110. Greenland P, Bonow RO, Brundage BH, et al. ACCF/AHA 2007 clinical expert consensus document on coronary artery calcium scoring by computed tomography in global cardiovascular risk assessment and in evaluation of patients with chest pain. A report of the American College of Cardiology Foundation Clinical Expert Consensus Task Force (ACCF/AHA Writing Committee to update the 2000 Expert Consensus Document on electron beam computed tomography). Circulation. 2007;115:402–26.
111. Detrano RC, Anderson M, Nelson J, Wong ND, et al. Coronary calcium measurements: effect of CT scanner type and calcium measure on rescan reproducibility—MESA study. Radiology. 2005;236:477–84.
112. Greenland P, Bonow RO, Brundage BH, et al. ACCF/AHA 2007 clinical expert consensus document on coronary artery calcium scoring by computed tomography in global cardiovascular risk assessment and in evaluation of patients with chest pain: a report of the American College of Cardiology Foundation Clinical Expert Consensus Task Force (ACCF/AHA Writing Committee to Update the 2000 Expert Consensus Document on Electron Beam Computed Tomography) developed in collaboration with the Society of Atherosclerosis Imaging and Prevention and the Society of Cardiovascular Computed Tomography. J Am Coll Cardiol. 2007;49:378–402.
113. Greenland P, Smith SC Jr, Grundy SM. Improving coronary heart disease risk assessment in asymptomatic people: role of traditional risk factors and noninvasive cardiovascular tests. Circulation. 2001;104:1863–7.
114. Greenland P, Alpert JS, Beller GA, et al. 2010 ACCF/AHA guideline for assessment of cardiovascular risk in asymptomatic adults. J Am Coll of Cardiol. 2010;56:e50–103.
115. Earls JP, Woodard PK, Abbara S, et al. ACR appropriateness criteria asymptomatic patient at risk for coronary artery disease. J Am Coll Radiol. 2014;11:12–9.
116. Piepoli MF, Hoes AW, Agewall S, et al. 2016 European guidelines on cardiovascular disease prevention in clinical practice. The Sixth Joint Task Force of the European Society of Cardiology and Other Societies on cardiovascular disease prevention in clinical practice. Eur Heart J. 2016;37:2315–81.
117. Berrington de Gonzalex A, Mahesh M, Kim KP, et al. Projected cancer risks from computed tomographic scans performed in the United States in 2007. Arch Intern Med. 2009;169:2071–7.
118. Moyer VA, on behalf of the U.S. Preventive Services Task Force. Screening for lun cancer: U.S. Preventive Services Task Force recommendation statement. Ann Intern Med. 2014;160:330–8.
119. Hecht HS, Cronin P, Blaha MJ, et al. 2016 SCCT/STR guidelines for coronary artery calcium scoring of noncontrast noncardiac chest CT scans: a report of the Society of Cardiovascular Computed Tomography and Society of Thoracic Radiology. J Cardiovasc Comput Tomogr. 2017; https://doi.org/10.1016/j.jcct.2016.11.003.
120. Budoff MJ, Nasir K, Kinney GL, et al. Coronary artery and thoracic calcium on non-contrast thoracic CT scans: comparison of ungated and gated examinations in patients from the COPD gene cohort. J Cardiovasc Comput Tomogr. 2011;5:113–8.
121. Hughes-Austin JM, Dominquez A, Allison MA, et al. Relationship of coronary artery calcium on standard chest computed tomography scans with mortality. J Am Coll Cardiol Img. 2016;9:152–9.
122. Jacob PC, Prokop M, van der Graaf Y, et al. Comparing coronary artery calcium and thoracic aorta calcium for prediction of all-cause mortality and cardiovascular events on low-dose non-gated computed tomography in high-risk population of heavy smokers. Atherosclerosis. 2010;209:455–62.
123. Mmets OM, Vliegenthart R, Gondrie MJ, et al. Lung cancer screening CT-based prediction of cardiovascular events. J Am Coll Cardiol Img. 2013;6:899–907.
124. Lung Cancer Screening Registry. American College of Radiology. Available at https://www.acr.org/~/media/ACR/Documents/PDF/QualitySafety/NRDR/Lung-Cancer-Screening-Practice-Registry/ACR-LCSR-User-Guide.pdf?la=en. Accessed 1 Apr 2017.

24 The Many Uses of Epicardial Fat Measurements

Mohamed Marwan

The term "epicardial adipose tissue" (EAT) – often called "epicardial fat" – refers to the visceral adipose tissue surrounding the heart and coronary arteries. Along with the pericardial fluid, epicardial adipose tissue creates a smooth surface that facilitates motion of the heart within the pericardium. Notably, both the volume and the distribution of epicardial adipose tissue vary widely between individuals and do not show a strict linear relationship to body weight, body mass index, obesity, or the extent of abdominal visceral fat. In the last years, there has been an increasing interest in imaging and quantification of epicardial adipose tissue. Evidence has so far accumulated showing a significant association between epicardial adipose tissue, risk factors for atherosclerosis, coronary artery disease, and cardiovascular outcome [1–6]. In addition, significant associations have been found between epicardial adipose tissue and non-atherosclerotic diseases, such as atrial fibrillation or left ventricular diastolic dysfunction [7–9]. This chapter summarizes the current data concerning epicardial adipose tissue, its quantification, and its potential use as a novel risk factor for cardiovascular morbidity and mortality.

Fat Stores Surrounding the Heart and Their Development

The nomenclature used in the current literature to define adipose tissue surrounding the heart is heterogeneous. Terms such as "epicardial," "pericardial," "paracardiac," and "intrathoracic" fat have been used [2, 3, 5, 10–15]. "Epicardial adipose tissue" (EAT) refers to the fat between the myocardium and the visceral layer of the pericardial sac, the serous epicardium. Although the simpler term "pericardial fat" has been often used in the imaging literature to refer to adipose tissue enclosed within the pericardial sac, "epicardial adipose tissue" is more accurate. It better describes the location below the epicardium and on the immediate surface of the heart (whereas "pericardial fat" could be on the outside of the pericardium), and "adipose tissue" is more accurate than simply "fat" since the tissue is metabolically active. Adipose tissue on the outer surface of the pericardial is termed "paracardiac fat"(see figure. 24.1). Epicardial fat is a visceral fat depot surrounding the heart similar to intra-abdominal fat, and both evolve embryologically from brown adipose tissue [16]. Vascular supply to epicardial fat is secured through the coronary arteries. Importantly, epicardial fat lies in direct contact with the myocardium with no muscle fascia in between which explains the potential interaction between both the myocardium and epicardial fat both supplied by coronary microcirculation [16].

M. Marwan (✉)
Department of Medicine, Cardiology and Angiology, Universitätsklinikum Erlangen, Erlangen, Germany
e-mail: mohamed.marwan@uk-erlangen.de

Imaging and Quantification of Epicardial Fat

Over the past decade, several imaging modalities have been used to detect and quantify epicardial adipose tissue. They include echocardiography, magnetic resonance, and computed tomography (CT). Surrogate imaging measures to estimate the true volume of epicardial fat include epicardial fat thickness, pericoronary fat thickness or volume, and epicardial fat areas in single cross sections. However, given the considerable inter-individual differences in epicardial fat spatial distribution, it remains questionable whether such surrogate measures correlate well with the absolute amount of epicardial fat. In fact, data indicate that full volume quantification is preferable to surrogate measurements; Bastarrika et al. directly compared volumetric and distance measurements of epicardial fat in relation to coronary artery stenosis in 45 patients who underwent CT imaging and invasive coronary angiography [17]. Patients with significant coronary artery stenosis had greater epicardial fat volumes than those without significant arterial stenosis, while epicardial fat distance failed to show a difference between the two patient groups.

U. J. Schoepf (ed.), *CT of the Heart*, Contemporary Medical Imaging, https://doi.org/10.1007/978-1-60327-237-7_24

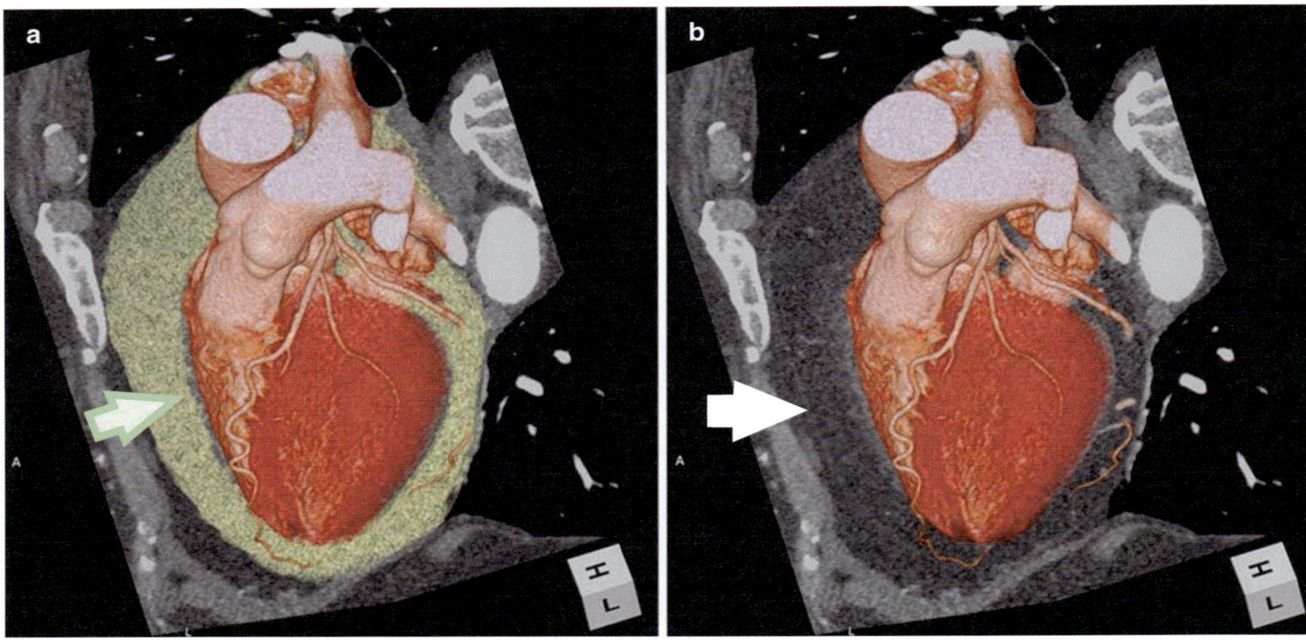

Fig. 24.1 Fifty-two-year-old female patient. (**a**) Three-dimensional reconstruction of the heart within the epicardial adipose tissue depicted in yellow (light green arrow). (**b**) The pericardium is marked by the white arrow. Fat outside the pericardium is termed "paracardiac fat"

Of the noninvasive imaging tools, CT and magnetic resonance tomography offer complete volumetric coverage of the heart. Quantification of epicardial fat from CT is appealing given the high spatial resolution of CT, the full volume coverage of the entire heart in all routinely acquired cardiac scans, and the fact that fat has distinctly lower attenuation values than other tissue types.

Semiautomated software are readily available which allow quantification of epicardial fat volume based on CT attenuation thresholds, after setting the upper and lower boundaries of the heart and tracing the pericardial sac. Fat attenuation thresholds in CT typically range from a lower value of −250 to −190 Hounsfield Units to an upper value of −50 and −30 HU [1, 10, 11, 15, 18]. For non-contrast CT, a typical fat attenuation range of −190 HU to −30 HU has been used. Contrast scans have regularly been used for quantification of epicardial adipose tissue volume in published literature. However, care should be taken that the threshold for detection of epicardial fat needs to be adjusted for contrast scans. In fact, La Grutta et al. recently compared epicardial fat volumes quantified in non-contrast and contrast scans in 76 patients systematically [19]. They observed an underestimation of epicardial adipose tissue volume even after adjustment of post-contrast attenuation.

Anatomical landmarks for measurement of total epicardial fat volumes include the pulmonary artery bifurcation, the mid left atrium, and the aortic root. For the lower boundary, the diaphragm, the left ventricular apex, and a single slice beyond the posterior descending artery have been proposed [2, 7, 11, 15, 18, 20]. Processing time for epicardial fat measurements ranges from 5 to 11 min [11, 20].) Recently, automated EAT volume quantification tools particularly for contrast-enhanced CT are available on some commercial workstations, requiring only minor user interaction, which further decreases the time for EAT volume quantification. EAT volume measurements based on CT are highly reproducible, with reported interobserver variabilities of 7%, 8%, and 15% in three studies [3, 11, 21], with lower variability for volume measurements compared to surrogate markers such as fat thickness [17]. For semiautomated measurements of epicardial and thoracic fat from non-contrast CT, the interscan reproducibility has also been reported to be high, with correlation coefficients ≥0.98 between two separate measurements [22].

Reference Values for Epicardial Fat

A major limitation for widespread clinical use of epicardial fat measurements is the absence of standardized reference values for what is to be considered as "normal" epicardial fat volumes. There is limited data to determine normal limits beyond which epicardial fat volume can be considered abnormally high. In a community-based sample of more than 3000 middle-aged individuals, Thanassouslis et al. quantified

Table 24.1 Summarizes different thresholds and binary cut-off used in literature for epicardial fat quantification

Cohort	Threshold	Outcome/reference
Thanassoulis et al. [10] (healthy reference sample, n = 3312)	139.4 cm³ for men, 119 cm³ for women	Abnormally high epicardial fat volumes on the basis of age and gender-specific 90th percentiles
Iwasaki et al. [23] (n = 197) Sarin et al. [18] (n = 151)	100 cm³	Higher incidence of CAD and higher calcium score
Cheng et al. [20] (n = 232)	125 cm³	MACE on follow-up
Tamarappoo et al. [24] (n = 219)	125 cm³	Ischemia on SPECT
Shmilovich et al. [25] (n = 458)	68 cm³/m²	95th percentile threshold for abnormally high epicardial fat volume, MACE on follow-up
Lee et al. [26] (n = 846)	%EAT >41% (from total body fat)	Obstructive CAD

epicardial and paracardiac fat volumes in participants from the Framingham Heart Study [10]. For the overall sample, the median values for epicardial fat volume were 117.5 cm^3 and 93.9 cm^3, respectively, in men and women and 117.7 cm^3 and 58.4 cm^3 for paracardiac fat, respectively. The authors defined abnormally high epicardial and paracardiac fat volumes on the basis of the age and gender-specific 90th percentiles for these fat depots in a healthy reference sample (139.4 cm^3 in men and 119 cm^3 in women for epicardial fat and 150.5 cm^3 and 73.3 cm^3 for paracardiac fat). Using these thresholds, 29.3% of men and 26.3% of women with coronary artery disease had elevated epicardial fat volumes. In the two studies, a simple threshold of 100 mm^3 for epicardial fat volume was used, and higher epicardial fat volumes were associated with a significantly higher coronary artery calcium score and higher incidence of CAD [18, 23]. Cheng et al. used a threshold of 125 cm^3 and reported that epicardial fat volumes above that threshold were found more frequently in baseline CT scans of asymptomatic patients experiencing MACE on follow-up [20]. Tamarappoo et al. used the same threshold when comparing patients with myocardial ischemia by SPECT to controls [24].

Beyond absolute epicardial fat measurements, several authors suggested to index the volume of epicardial adipose tissue to the body surface area. In a healthy asymptomatic population of 226 subjects, Shmilovich et al. identified a value of 68.1 cm^3/m^2 as the 95th percentile threshold for abnormally high epicardial fat volume [25]. They could show that values exceeding this threshold predicted major adverse cardiovascular events, with a trend to add to standard coronary calcium scoring and Framingham risk score in predicting cardiovascular events. Furthermore, Lee et al. could show recently that percentage epicardial fat and total body fat showed the maximum area under the curve for predicting presence of coronary artery disease and superior discriminative performance compared to epicedial adipose tissue volume and other indexed parameters of EAT [26]. After adjustment for Framingham risk score and calcium score, %EAT >41% was a predictor of obstructive CAD (stenosis >50%) and %EAT >47% for severe CAD (stenosis >70%) Table 24.1.

Function of Epicardial Fat

Epicardial fat not only serves as a mechanical buffer for cardiac motion and coronary artery distension but also has direct metabolic and biochemical effects on the myocardium and coronary vessels. The anatomical, embryological, and biochemical diversity of adipose tissue enclosed within the pericardial sac compared to other adipose tissues, such as paracardiac fat, subcutaneous fat, or visceral adipose tissue, has triggered numerous hypotheses concerning specific metabolic properties of epicardial adipose tissue [13, 14]. Epicardial adipose tissue has greater capacity for release and uptake of free fatty acids than other visceral fat depots. Since free fatty acid oxidation is responsible for about 50–70% of the energy production of the heart, epicardial fat has been proposed to function as a buffer to protect the heart against exposure to excessively high levels of free fatty acids and to provide energy for the myocardium [27]. Furthermore, convincing evidence has emerged confirming the fact that epicardial adipose tissue is metabolically active and serves as a source of several adipokines. This has led numerous authors to assume a direct local influence of epicardial adipose tissue on the neighboring coronary arteries through paracrine and vasocrine mechanisms [13, 14]. This inherent endocrine potential includes the secretion of several pro- and anti-inflammatory mediators and cytokines such as adiponectin, interleukin 6 (Il-6), and tumor necrosis factor (TNF) alpha [1, 28–35]. With increasing amounts of visceral fat, plasma levels of adiponectin decrease [36, 37], which in turn causes an increase in TNF alpha levels and hence to a local increase of inflammation [32]. The resulting imbalance of pro- and anti-inflammatory mediators as well as cytokines secreted by epicardial adipose tissue is thought to contribute to a local influence on the embedded coronary arteries [38].

Epicardial Fat and Cardiovascular Disease

Coronary Atherosclerosis

Two lines of evidence support the "local effect" of epicardial adipose tissue on the coronary arteries and atherosclerosis affecting these vessels. First, the volume of epicardial adipose tissue appears to be relatively independent from overall body adipose tissue but, like intra-abdominal visceral fat, shows an association to the presence and severity of atherosclerosis. Second, histopathological and immunohistochemical studies indicate specific patterns of mediator secretion by epicardial adipose tissue – but not by fatty tissue in remote locations – which correlate to atherosclerosis. In a landmark study, Mazurek et al. analyzed epicardial fat as well as subcutaneous fat of the lower extremity in obese patients referred for coronary artery bypass grafting. They observed an increased expression and secretion of several inflammatory mediators as well as chronic inflammatory cell infiltration with macrophages, lymphocytes, and basophils in epicardial adipose tissue as compared to subcutaneous fat [30]. Along the same line, an increased expression of CD45 mRNA in the epicardial fat of subjects with coronary artery disease has been observed in other studies, with elevated macrophage infiltration [28] and an increase of mast cells in the adventitia of coronary lesions [1, 29]. Moreover, in an immunohistochemical study by Konishi et al., more leucocyte common antigen (LCA)-positive cells were observed in pericoronary fat of autopsy cases with coronary artery disease compared to patients without coronary disease, suggesting inflammation of pericoronary fat in the former group [39]. Hirata et al. analyzed patterns of macrophage polarization in epicardial adipose tissue of patients with and without coronary artery disease (CAD) [40]. They observed a change of the ratio of M1/M2 macrophages with an abundance of the proinflammatory M1-polarized state in patients with CAD [40]. Interestingly, recently Uchida et al. could show in a study using immunohistochemical techniques that pericoronary fat store oxidized low-density lipoproteins (oxLDL) as well as high-density lipoproteins (HDL), both being supplied either by CD 68 (+)- macrophages or through vasa vasorum with the balance between oxLDL and HDL influencing either plaque growth (more oxLDL) or plaque maturation (more HDL) [41].

Clinical observations support a potential direct and local effect of epicardial adipose tissue on the coronary arteries. In an intravascular ultrasound (IVUS) study, Prati et al. suggested a permissive role of epicardial adipose tissue on the positive remodeling of atherosclerotic plaques [42]. Some authors attribute the fact that coronary arteries within myocardial bridges are typically spared from atherosclerosis to the lack of contact to epicardial fat, which may protect the arteries from developing atherosclerosis [43].

In a community-based sample of the Framingham Heart Study (n = 1155), Rosito et al. observed a significant association between epicardial fat, but not intrathoracic fat, with coronary artery calcification quantified by computed tomography (CT) after adjustment for visceral adipose tissue and traditional cardiovascular risk factors [5]. Furthermore, Konishi et al. could show that epicardial fat volume measured in CT, but not waist circumference, was significantly associated with the presence of any coronary plaques, non-stenotic plaques confirmed by coronary angiography, and non-calcified plaques [44]. Moreover, in a study of 214 consecutive patients referred for coronary CT angiography, Alexopoulos et al. observed a significantly larger epicardial fat volume in patients with mixed or non-calcified plaques compared to patients with calcified plaques or no plaques [15]. This relationship remained significant after adjustment for traditional risk factors of coronary artery disease as well as after indexing the epicardial fat volume to body surface area. In an analysis of 402 patients with no prior known CAD, Rajani et al. found that epicardial adipose tissue volume was elevated in patients with calcified plaque, non-calcified plaque, and partially calcified plaque [45]. Furthermore in patients with non-calcified plaque or partially calcified plaque, epicardial fat volume was found to be an independent predictor of coronary stenosis ≥70% even after adjustment of conventional cardiovascular risk factors [45]. Interestingly, in a cross-sectional study of 128 patients with angina undergoing invasive coronary angiography, Gorter et al. observed that the significant association between the severity of coronary atherosclerosis and epicardial as well as pericoronary fat volumes as determined by CT was limited to patients with a low body mass index [12]. The authors assume a potential role of insulin resistance in patients with high body mass index where higher systemic plasma levels of inflammatory cytokines accelerate atherogenesis, so that – in that case – there is little addition to the atherosclerotic process through the local production of adipocytokines in fat surrounding the coronary arteries. In a study by Wang et al., epicardial fat volume and the thickness of epicardial fat in the left atrioventricular groove were found to be associated with the presence and extent of coronary atherosclerosis as defined by four CT-based scores (severity score, extent score, calcium volume score, and number of coronary arteries with ≥50% luminal stenosis) [46]. Interestingly, only epicardial fat thickness in the left atrioventricular groove, but not total epicardial fat volume, was significantly associated with all four parameters of coronary atherosclerosis – in a dose-dependent manner – after adjustment for conventional risk factors, body mass index, waist circumference, C-reactive protein, and intra-abdominal visceral fat area [46]. The authors concluded that measurement of epicardial fat thickness in the left atrioventricular groove may be more predictive concerning atherogenic risk than measurements of the total epicardial fat volume. These data again support the concept that the influence of epicardial adipose tissue on coronary atherosclerosis may be spatially heterogeneous and potentially due to local influence in addition to or instead of a systemic effect. Along the same line, Mahabadi et al. showed in 78 patients and 311 coronary segments that pericoronary fat as quantified by cardiac CT was associated with the presence of calcified or noncalcified coronary lesions in coronary CT angiography. They could demonstrate a 2.5-fold increase of the likelihood to detect plaque in the underlying coronary segment per each doubling of local pericoronary fat volume [1]. As a possible confounder of their observation, it is worth mentioning that, based on anatomical reasons, epicardial fat accumulations are typically more pronounced in some regions of the coronary artery tree, such as the proximal left anterior descending coronary artery. The same regions typically show the first signs of atherosclerosis, so that the association between atherosclerosis and local fat volume may be a coincidence as well as a causal relationship.

Coronary Spasm

Owing to the metabolic activity of epicardial adipose tissue that potentially influences coronary artery morphology by playing a role in the initiation and aggravation of the process of atherosclerosis, evidence is also emerging supporting a possible effect of epicardial adipose tissue on coronary artery function. Ohyama et al. could show recently that coronary perivascular adipose tissue volume measured using CT was significantly higher in patients with vasospastic angina compared to controls [47]. Furthermore, in 97 patients with suspected coronary spastic angina who underwent ergonovine provocation testing, Ito et al. measured epicardial fat volume in CT data sets [48]. In 27 patients with coronary spasm (28%), epicardial fat volume and male gender were significant predictors of coronary spasm. A threshold of 149.4 cm^3 epicardial fat volume was found to be the optimal threshold for identifying patient with coronary spasms (70% sensitivity, 76% specificity, AUC 0.76). These data support a potential role of epicardial fat in inducing endothelial dysfunction.

Acute Coronary Syndromes

The association between epicardial fat and "vulnerable" plaque features potentially leading to acute coronary syndromes (ACS) and future events have been examined in several patient cohorts. Oka et al. assessed coronary plaque components and epicardial fat volume in 357 patients referred for 64-slice CT [49]. They found that a high epicardial fat volume (above 100 cm^3) was associated with vulnerable plaque components (non-calcified plaque, low-density plaque, and positive remodeling) independent of obesity measurements (BMI and visceral adipose tissue) as well as coronary calcium score. Furthermore, Ito et al. measured epicardial adipose tissue in 1308 consecutive symptomatic patients with a zero calcium score [50]. Significant coronary stenoses were present in 7% of the patients, and CT features of vulnerable plaques, specifically positively remodeled plaques with a mean density <30 HU, were found in 5% of the patients. Volume of epicardial adipose tissue was significantly larger both in patients with significant coronary stenoses (mean 124.3 ± 43.2 cm^3) and in patients with CT features of vulnerable plaques (mean 133.0 ± 40.2 cm^3) as compared to controls (mean 95.1 ± 40.3 cm^3). In multivariate analysis, epicardial adipose tissue was found to be a predictor for both significant coronary stenoses and CT features of vulnerable plaque. In an earlier study of patients who underwent both CT and intracoronary optical coherence tomography (OCT), the same authors showed that patients in the highest tertile of epicardial adipose tissue (>130.7 cm^3) were more likely to display thin-capped fibroatheroma in OCT [51]. Harada et al. measured epicardial adipose tissue volume using CT in 80 patients hospitalized for acute coronary syndromes (ST-segment elevation and non-ST-segment elevation infarctions) in comparison to 90 outpatient controls with suspected acute coronary syndrome but in whom CT results were normal [52]. Epicardial fat volume was significantly higher in patients with acute coronary syndromes, and a cutoff value of 100 ml was found to be independently associated with ACS in the multivariate analysis. Recently, in 467 patients enrolled in the ROMICAT II trial, indexed epicardial adipose tissue volume was significantly associated with high-risk plaque features even after adjustment for cardiovascular risk factors, coronary artery calcium score, and obstructive coronary artery disease [53].

Myocardial Ischemia

Earlier studies have investigated the relationship between epicardial fat and inducible myocardial ischemia in SPECT and uniformly report epicardial fat to be associated with an increased likelihood of myocardial perfusion defects [24, 54]. Interestingly in a recent study of 396 consecutive patients undergoing SPECT perfusion imaging, regional thickness, cross-sectional areas, and total epicardial fat volume were quantified using CT. In this study the authors could demonstrate increased regional epicardial fat in patients with reversible perfusion defect compared to patients with normal perfusion or myocardial scars (fixed defects) [55].

Coronary Artery Disease Progression

Regarding the influence of epicardial adipose tissue on coronary artery progression, Nakanishi et al. could show that increase in epicardial fat volume is associated with greater progression of coronary artery calcification in intermediate-risk subjects [56]. Moreover, Yerramasu et al. performed a follow-up study of 333 asymptomatic diabetics referred for a repeat coronary calcium scan at a mean interval of 2.7 years. They observed that epicardial fat volume was an independent predictor for the presence and severity of coronary artery calcification in the baseline scan as well as coronary calcium progression during follow-up [57]. In a long-term CT follow-up study of asymptomatic individual without prior history of coronary artery disease (median 65 months), Hwang et al. observed new development of non-calcified plaque with higher indexed epicardial fat volume at baseline CT (79.9 ± 30.3 cm^3/m^2) compared to patients with no plaque (62.5 ± 24.7 cm^3/m^2) or newly developed calcified plaque (63.7 ± 22.7 cm^3/m^2) [58].

Cardiovascular Outcome

Patient-based cross-sectional analyses provided the first reports of an association between epicardial adipose tissue and prevalent cardiovascular disease. In 2001, Taguchi et al. described an association of epicardial fat determined by cardiac computed tomography, with the presence of CAD in 251 Japanese men [6]. Consecutively, investigators of the Framingham Heart Study described increased epicardial adipose tissue volumes in subjects with prevalent CAD in a cross-sectional analysis in 1267 subjects from the Offspring cohort [10]. Intrathoracic fat, which was defined as fat inside the thorax but outside the pericardial sac, showed no association with cardiac events. While associations of epicardial adipose tissue with CAD were independent of age and gender as well as BMI and waist circumference, no significant association was found after adjusting for traditional cardiovascular risk factors.

For risk stratification purposes, prospective follow-up studies provide more accurate evidence compared to cross-sectional studies. Several prospective analyses have become available for epicardial adipose tissue. In a case-cohort study based on the Multi-Ethnic Study of Atherosclerosis (MESA), intrathoracic fat volume was quantified in the baseline CT of 972 randomly selected individuals with no incident coronary artery disease and compared to the intrathoracic fat volume of 147 MESA participants who developed incident coronary heart disease (myocardial infarction, resuscitated cardiac arrest, angina or fatal coronary heart disease) during follow-up [59]. In unadjusted analysis, and even after adjustment for cardiovascular risk factors, intrathoracic fat volume, but not BMI, was associated with the risk of coronary heart disease. More recently, Cheng et al. confirmed these results in a case-control study based on a registry of 2751 asymptomatic individuals and a 4-year follow-up for major adverse cardiovascular events (MACE), comparing 58 patients with MACE to 174 event-free controls matched for age, risk factors, and coronary calcium score [20]. In this analysis, significantly higher mean epicardial and intrathoracic fat volumes were observed in patients experiencing MACE compared to controls. In agreement with the findings of the Framingham investigators, adding epicardial fat volume and not intrathoracic fat to the coronary calcium score and Framingham risk score improved specificity and overall accuracy in predicting MACE, which supports the hypothesis of a local influence of epicardial adipose tissue on disease development.

In 2013, investigators of the Heinz Nixdorf Recall Study reported the association of epicardial fat volume, quantified from cardiac CT, with incident myocardial infarction in a European, population-based random cohort [60]. The association of epicardial adipose tissue with coronary events was independent of traditional cardiovascular risk factors and remained statistically significant even after further adjustment for the coronary calcium score. This finding was partly explained by a stronger correlation between epicardial adipose tissue and incident events in subjects with low or no coronary calcium. This led the authors to conclude that quantification of epicardial adipose tissue from cardiac CT may complement prognostic information above coronary calcium scoring. In a population of subjects with acute chest pain, however, Forouzandeh et al. found an additional prognostic value of epicardial adipose tissue over coronary calcium only in subjects with calcium scores >400 [61]. In a recent review of 9 studies assessing the prognostic value of epicardial fat volume including 10,252 patients, the majority of the studies suggested that epicardial fat volume is associated with clinical outcomes and provides incremental prognostic value to coronary artery calcium scoring [62]. In this review, the authors observed different thresholds and aggregates of epicardial fat volume used in different studies which renders comparisons between different cohorts difficult. More recently, Oikonomou et al. [63] assessd a novel imaging biomarker – the so-called perivascular fat attenuation index – in two large clincal cohorts from Europe and North America [63]. This index traces spacial changes of pericoronary fat attenuation on coronary CT angiography secondary to coronary inflammation. In 3912 patients from the derivation and validation cohort, the perivascular fat attenuation index around the right coronary artery and the left anterior descending coronary artery were predictive of all-cause and cardiac mortality in a median follow-up of 72 months and 54 months for both cohorts, respectively. These data may potentially help tailoring and intensifying preventive measures in patients deemed to be at high risk of cardiovascular events.

Epicardial Fat and Non-atherosclerotic Cardiovascular Disease

Interestingly the association of epicardial adipose tissue to cardiac disease is not limited to coronary atherosclerosis. A number of studies have shown associations of epicardial fat with non-coronary heart disease. Several studies indicated a link between epicardial adipose tissue and atrial fibrillation which was suggested to be mediated by the inflammatory effects of epicardial fat. Al Chekakie et al. reported higher epicardial adipose tissue volume in subjects with atrial fibrillation compared to subjects with sinus rhythm, and subjects with persistent atrial fibrillation had even higher fat volume than subjects with paroxysmal atrial fibrillation [7]. Wong et al. quantified periatrial, periventricular, and total epicardial fat volume in 110 patients undergoing first-time ablation of atrial fibrillation compared to 20 controls in sinus rhythm. They found a significant association between epicardial fat volume and left atrial volumes, the presence and severity of atrial fibrillation, and poorer outcome after ablation [64]. These data support a potential local effect of adipose tissue as a trigger for atrial fibrillation. Framingham investigators also described a cross-sectional association of epicardial adipose tissue with atrial fibrillation, independent of age, gender, hypertension, and BMI in over 3000 subjects [65]. However, it has to be acknowledged that longitudinal analyses of the role of epicardial adipose tissue regarding the prediction of future atrial fibrillation are lacking. Furthermore, Fox et al. described a significant correlation between epicardial fat – quantified by CT – and left atrial dimension, which by itself is a strong predictor of atrial fibrillation [4].

A potential lipotoxic effect of epicardial adipose tissue on left ventricular function has been suggested in the literature. However, an analysis in participants from the Framingham Heart Study failed to confirm a correlation of epicardial adipose tissue volume and magnetic resonance measures of left ventricular structure or function, independent of general adiposity [4]. In a study in 110 patients from a health screening program without prevalent CAD, Cavalcante et al. described a significant association of EAT with e′ and E/e′ additionally to LA size, suggesting that epicardial adipose tissue may be associated with diastolic dysfunction [9]. Further studies are needed to confirm these results and establish potential mechanisms for the link of epicardial adipose tissue with measures of left ventricular size and function.

Conflicting Evidence

Besides the large body of evidence supporting an association between epicardial fat and coronary artery disease, several studies observed conflicting evidence concerning a causal association between epicardial fat and CAD. In 380 patients enrolled in the CORE320 trial who underwent coronary CT angiography, myocardial perfusion imaging, and clinically driven invasive angiography, no association was found between epicardial fat volume and presence, severity of coronary artery disease, and myocardial perfusion abnormalities [66]. Similarly, in 557 subjects enrolled in the Cardiovascular Risk in Young Finns Study, associations of coronary heart disease risk markers with epicardial fat volume were attenuated after multivariable adjustment with no evidence of increased EFV being independently associated with pre-clinical atherosclerosis [67]. On the same line, Romijn et al., in a study of 122 patients who underwent non-contrast-enhanced CT for quantification of coronary artery calcium and epicardial fat volume as well as invasive angiography with fractional flow reserve measurements, could not demonstrate an incremental value of epicardial fat volume beyond coronary artery calcium score and traditional risk factors for detection of hemodynamically significant coronary artery disease [68].

Summary

In summary, the accumulating evidence over the last years strongly suggests a potential causal relationship between the metabolic and paracrine characteristics of epicardial adipose tissue and cardiovascular disease. Computed tomography is the most accurate imaging method to quantify epicardial adipose tissue. Low-dose, non-contrast acquisitions could potentially be performed specifically to quantify epicardial fat. In addition, the information on individual volume and distribution of epicardial adipose tissue comes for free with the increasing numbers of clinically driven cardiac and coronary CT examinations. Several limitations must be considered: First of all, there may a coincidental co-localization of higher amounts of perivascular adipose tissue and the typical predilection sites of coronary atherosclerotic lesions or vulnerable plaque (such as the proximal left anterior descending coronary artery). Second, the best "threshold" to identify abnormally elevated epicardial fat volumes, probably somewhere around 100–125 cm^3, has not yet been identified, and third, no data is available that would permit to base treatment decisions – specifically, intensification or withholding of risk modifying measures – on the individually determined volume of epicardial adipose tissue. All the same, epicardial fat clearly seems to be more than just a substance to fill empty space, and further prospective investigations will serve to clarify its intriguing association with coronary artery disease and other cardiac disorders.

Further prospective studies are needed to determine age- and gender-specific reference values to help clinicians interpret individual epicardial fat volumes regarding their association with cardiovascular risk and to potentially identify symptomatic and asymptomatic subjects at increased risk who require more intensive risk factor modification.

References

1. Mahabadi AA, Reinsch N, Lehmann N, Altenbernd J, Kalsch H, Seibel RM, et al. Association of pericoronary fat volume with atherosclerotic plaque burden in the underlying coronary artery: a segment analysis. Atherosclerosis. 2010;211(1):195–9.
2. Mahabadi AA, Massaro JM, Rosito GA, Levy D, Murabito JM, Wolf PA, et al. Association of pericardial fat, intrathoracic fat, and visceral abdominal fat with cardiovascular disease burden: the Framingham heart study. Eur Heart J. 2009;30(7):850–6.
3. Greif M, Becker A, von Ziegler F, Lebherz C, Lehrke M, Broedl UC, et al. Pericardial adipose tissue determined by dual source CT is a risk factor for coronary atherosclerosis. Arterioscler Thromb Vasc Biol. 2009;29(5):781–6.
4. Fox CS, Gona P, Hoffmann U, Porter SA, Salton CJ, Massaro JM, et al. Pericardial fat, intrathoracic fat, and measures of left ventricular structure and function: the Framingham Heart Study. Circulation. 2009;119(12):1586–91.
5. Rosito GA, Massaro JM, Hoffmann U, Ruberg FL, Mahabadi AA, Vasan RS, et al. Pericardial fat, visceral abdominal fat, cardiovascular disease risk factors, and vascular calcification in a community-based sample: the Framingham Heart Study. Circulation. 2008;117(5):605–13.
6. Taguchi R, Takasu J, Itani Y, Yamamoto R, Yokoyama K, Watanabe S, et al. Pericardial fat accumulation in men as a risk factor for coronary artery disease. Atherosclerosis. 2001;157(1):203–9.
7. Al Chekakie MO, Welles CC, Metoyer R, Ibrahim A, Shapira AR, Cytron J, et al. Pericardial fat is independently associated with human atrial fibrillation. J Am Coll Cardiol. 2010;56(10):784–8.
8. Zhu W, Zhang H, Guo L, Hong K. Relationship between epicardial adipose tissue volume and atrial fibrillation : a systematic review and meta-analysis. Herz. 2016;41(5):421–7.
9. Cavalcante JL, Tamarappoo BK, Hachamovitch R, Kwon DH, Alraies MC, Halliburton S, et al. Association of epicardial fat, hypertension, subclinical coronary artery disease, and metabolic syndrome with left ventricular diastolic dysfunction. Am J Cardiol. 2012;110(12):1793–8.
10. Thanassoulis G, Massaro JM, Hoffmann U, Mahabadi AA, Vasan RS, O'Donnell CJ, et al. Prevalence, distribution, and risk factor correlates of high pericardial and intrathoracic fat depots in the Framingham heart study. Circ Cardiovasc Imaging. 2010;3(5):559–66.
11. Dey D, Wong ND, Tamarappoo B, Nakazato R, Gransar H, Cheng VY, et al. Computer-aided non-contrast CT-based quantification of pericardial and thoracic fat and their associations with coronary calcium and Metabolic Syndrome. Atherosclerosis. 2010;209(1):136–41.
12. Gorter PM, de Vos AM, van der Graaf Y, Stella PR, Doevendans PA, Meijs MF, et al. Relation of epicardial and pericoronary fat to coronary atherosclerosis and coronary artery calcium in patients undergoing coronary angiography. Am J Cardiol. 2008;102(4):380–5.
13. Sacks HS, Fain JN. Human epicardial adipose tissue: a review. Am Heart J. 2007;153(6):907–17.
14. Iacobellis G, Corradi D, Sharma AM. Epicardial adipose tissue: anatomic, biomolecular and clinical relationships with the heart. Nat Clin Pract Cardiovasc Med. 2005;2(10):536–43.
15. Alexopoulos N, McLean DS, Janik M, Arepalli CD, Stillman AE, Raggi P. Epicardial adipose tissue and coronary artery plaque characteristics. Atherosclerosis. 2010;210(1):150–4.
16. Iacobellis G. Epicardial fat: a new cardiovascular therapeutic target. Curr Opin Pharmacol. 2016;27:13–8.
17. Bastarrika G, Broncano J, Schoepf UJ, Schwarz F, Lee YS, Abro JA, et al. Relationship between coronary artery disease and epicardial adipose tissue quantification at cardiac CT: comparison between automatic volumetric measurement and manual bidimensional estimation. Acad Radiol. 2010;17(6):727–34.
18. Sarin S, Wenger C, Marwaha A, Qureshi A, Go BD, Woomert CA, et al. Clinical significance of epicardial fat measured using cardiac multislice computed tomography. Am J Cardiol. 2008;102(6):767–71.
19. La Grutta L, Toia P, Farruggia A, Albano D, Grassedonio E, Palmeri A, et al. Quantification of epicardial adipose tissue in coronary calcium score and CT coronary angiography image data sets: comparison of attenuation values, thickness and volumes. Br J Radiol. 2016;89(1062):20150773.
20. Cheng VY, Dey D, Tamarappoo B, Nakazato R, Gransar H, Miranda-Peats R, et al. Pericardial fat burden on ECG-gated noncontrast CT in asymptomatic patients who subsequently experience adverse cardiovascular events. JACC Cardiovasc Imaging. 2010;3(4):352–60.
21. Nichols JH, Samy B, Nasir K, Fox CS, Schulze PC, Bamberg F, et al. Volumetric measurement of pericardial adipose tissue from contrast-enhanced coronary computed tomography angiography: a reproducibility study. J Cardiovasc Comput Tomogr. 2008;2(5):288–95.
22. Nakazato R, Shmilovich H, Tamarappoo BK, Cheng VY, Slomka PJ, Berman DS, et al. Interscan reproducibility of computer-aided epicardial and thoracic fat measurement from noncontrast cardiac CT. J Cardiovasc Comput Tomogr. 2011;5(3):172–9.
23. Iwasaki K, Matsumoto T, Aono H, Furukawa H, Samukawa M. Relationship between epicardial fat measured by 64-multidetector computed tomography and coronary artery disease. Clin Cardiol. 2011;34(3):166–71.
24. Tamarappoo B, Dey D, Shmilovich H, Nakazato R, Gransar H, Cheng VY, et al. Increased pericardial fat volume measured from noncontrast CT predicts myocardial ischemia by SPECT. JACC Cardiovasc Imaging. 2010;3(11):1104–12.
25. Shmilovich H, Dey D, Cheng VY, Rajani R, Nakazato R, Otaki Y, et al. Threshold for the upper normal limit of indexed epicardial fat volume: derivation in a healthy population and validation in an outcome-based study. Am J Cardiol. 2011;108(11):1680–5.
26. Lee BC, Lee WJ, Lo SC, Hsu HC, Chien KL, Chang YC, et al. The ratio of epicardial to body fat improves the prediction of coronary artery disease beyond calcium and Framingham risk scores. Int J Cardiovasc Imaging. 2016;32(Suppl 1):117–27.
27. Iacobellis G, Bianco AC. Epicardial adipose tissue: emerging physiological, pathophysiological and clinical features. Trends Endocrinol Metab. 2011;22(11):450–7.
28. Baker AR, Silva NF, Quinn DW, Harte AL, Pagano D, Bonser RS, et al. Human epicardial adipose tissue expresses a pathogenic

profile of adipocytokines in patients with cardiovascular disease. Cardiovasc Diabetol. 2006;5:1.
29. Laine P, Kaartinen M, Penttila A, Panula P, Paavonen T, Kovanen PT. Association between myocardial infarction and the mast cells in the adventitia of the infarct-related coronary artery. Circulation. 1999;99(3):361–9.
30. Mazurek T, Zhang L, Zalewski A, Mannion JD, Diehl JT, Arafat H, et al. Human epicardial adipose tissue is a source of inflammatory mediators. Circulation. 2003;108(20):2460–6.
31. Ouchi N, Kihara S, Arita Y, Okamoto Y, Maeda K, Kuriyama H, et al. Adiponectin, an adipocyte-derived plasma protein, inhibits endothelial NF-kappaB signaling through a cAMP-dependent pathway. Circulation. 2000;102(11):1296–301.
32. Ouchi N, Kihara S, Funahashi T, Nakamura T, Nishida M, Kumada M, et al. Reciprocal association of C-reactive protein with adiponectin in blood stream and adipose tissue. Circulation. 2003;107(5):671–4.
33. Saijo Y, Kiyota N, Kawasaki Y, Miyazaki Y, Kashimura J, Fukuda M, et al. Relationship between C-reactive protein and visceral adipose tissue in healthy Japanese subjects. Diabetes Obes Metab. 2004;6(4):249–58.
34. Wajchenberg BL. Subcutaneous and visceral adipose tissue: their relation to the metabolic syndrome. Endocr Rev. 2000;21(6):697–738.
35. Yatagai T, Nagasaka S, Taniguchi A, Fukushima M, Nakamura T, Kuroe A, et al. Hypoadiponectinemia is associated with visceral fat accumulation and insulin resistance in Japanese men with type 2 diabetes mellitus. Metabolism. 2003;52(10):1274–8.
36. Arita Y, Kihara S, Ouchi N, Maeda K, Kuriyama H, Okamoto Y, et al. Adipocyte-derived plasma protein adiponectin acts as a platelet-derived growth factor-BB-binding protein and regulates growth factor-induced common postreceptor signal in vascular smooth muscle cell. Circulation. 2002;105(24):2893–8.
37. Hajer GR, van Haeften TW, Visseren FL. Adipose tissue dysfunction in obesity, diabetes, and vascular diseases. Eur Heart J. 2008;29(24):2959–71.
38. Tavora F, Kutys R, Li L, Ripple M, Fowler D, Burke A. Adventitial lymphocytic inflammation in human coronary arteries with intimal atherosclerosis. Cardiovasc Pathol. 2010;19(3):e61–8.
39. Konishi M, Sugiyama S, Sato Y, Oshima S, Sugamura K, Nozaki T, et al. Pericardial fat inflammation correlates with coronary artery disease. Atherosclerosis. 2010;213(2):649–55.
40. Hirata Y, Tabata M, Kurobe H, Motoki T, Akaike M, Nishio C, et al. Coronary atherosclerosis is associated with macrophage polarization in epicardial adipose tissue. J Am Coll Cardiol. 2011;58(3):248–55.
41. Uchida Y, Uchida Y, Shimoyama E, Hiruta N, Kishimoto T, Watanabe S. Human pericoronary adipose tissue as storage and possible supply site for oxidized low-density lipoprotein and high-density lipoprotein in coronary artery. J Cardiol. 2017;69(1):236–44.
42. Prati F, Arbustini E, Labellarte A, Sommariva L, Pawlowski T, Manzoli A, et al. Eccentric atherosclerotic plaques with positive remodelling have a pericardial distribution: a permissive role of epicardial fat? A three-dimensional intravascular ultrasound study of left anterior descending artery lesions. Eur Heart J. 2003;24(4):329–36.
43. Ishii T, Asuwa N, Masuda S, Ishikawa Y. The effects of a myocardial bridge on coronary atherosclerosis and ischaemia. J Pathol. 1998;185(1):4–9.
44. Konishi M, Sugiyama S, Sugamura K, Nozaki T, Ohba K, Matsubara J, et al. Association of pericardial fat accumulation rather than abdominal obesity with coronary atherosclerotic plaque formation in patients with suspected coronary artery disease. Atherosclerosis. 2010;209(2):573–8.
45. Rajani R, Shmilovich H, Nakazato R, Nakanishi R, Otaki Y, Cheng VY, et al. Relationship of epicardial fat volume to coronary plaque, severe coronary stenosis, and high-risk coronary plaque features assessed by coronary CT angiography. J Cardiovasc Comput Tomogr. 2013;7(2):125–32.
46. Wang TD, Lee WJ, Shih FY, Huang CH, Chen WJ, Lee YT, et al. Association of epicardial adipose tissue with coronary atherosclerosis is region-specific and independent of conventional risk factors and intra-abdominal adiposity. Atherosclerosis. 2010;213(1):279–87.
47. Ohyama K, Matsumoto Y, Shimokawa H. Impact of epicardial adipose tissue volume quantified by non-contrast electrocardiogram-gated computed tomography on ergonovine-induced epicardial coronary artery spasm. Int J Cardiol. 2017;229:40.
48. Ito T, Fujita H, Ichihashi T, Ohte N. Impact of epicardial adipose tissue volume quantified by non-contrast electrocardiogram-gated computed tomography on ergonovine-induced epicardial coronary artery spasm. Int J Cardiol. 2016;221:877–80.
49. Oka T, Yamamoto H, Ohashi N, Kitagawa T, Kunita E, Utsunomiya H, et al. Association between epicardial adipose tissue volume and characteristics of non-calcified plaques assessed by coronary computed tomographic angiography. Int J Cardiol. 2012;161(1):45–9.
50. Ito T, Suzuki Y, Ehara M, Matsuo H, Teramoto T, Terashima M, et al. Impact of epicardial fat volume on coronary artery disease in symptomatic patients with a zero calcium score. Int J Cardiol. 2013;167(6):2852–8.
51. Ito T, Nasu K, Terashima M, Ehara M, Kinoshita Y, Ito T, et al. The impact of epicardial fat volume on coronary plaque vulnerability: insight from optical coherence tomography analysis. Eur Heart J Cardiovasc Imaging. 2012;13(5):408–15.
52. Harada K, Amano T, Uetani T, Tokuda Y, Kitagawa K, Shimbo Y, et al. Cardiac 64-multislice computed tomography reveals increased epicardial fat volume in patients with acute coronary syndrome. Am J Cardiol. 2011;108(8):1119–23.
53. Lu MT, Park J, Ghemigian K, Mayrhofer T, Puchner SB, Liu T, et al. Epicardial and paracardial adipose tissue volume and attenuation – association with high-risk coronary plaque on computed tomographic angiography in the ROMICAT II trial. Atherosclerosis. 2016;251:47–54.
54. Janik M, Hartlage G, Alexopoulos N, Mirzoyev Z, McLean DS, Arepalli CD, et al. Epicardial adipose tissue volume and coronary artery calcium to predict myocardial ischemia on positron emission tomography-computed tomography studies. J Nucl Cardiol. 2010;17(5):841–7.
55. Khawaja T, Greer C, Thadani SR, Kato TS, Bhatia K, Shimbo D, et al. Increased regional epicardial fat volume associated with reversible myocardial ischemia in patients with suspected coronary artery disease. J Nucl Cardiol. 2015;22(2):325–33.
56. Nakanishi R, Rajani R, Cheng VY, Gransar H, Nakazato R, Shmilovich H, et al. Increase in epicardial fat volume is associated with greater coronary artery calcification progression in subjects at intermediate risk by coronary calcium score: a serial study using non-contrast cardiac CT. Atherosclerosis. 2011;218(2):363–8.
57. Yerramasu A, Dey D, Venuraju S, Anand DV, Atwal S, Corder R, et al. Increased volume of epicardial fat is an independent risk factor for accelerated progression of sub-clinical coronary atherosclerosis. Atherosclerosis. 2012;220(1):223–30.
58. Hwang IC, Park HE, Choi SY. Epicardial adipose tissue contributes to the development of non-calcified coronary plaque: a 5-year computed tomography follow-up study. J Atheroscler Thromb. 2017;24(3):262–74.
59. Ding J, Hsu FC, Harris TB, Liu Y, Kritchevsky SB, Szklo M, et al. The association of pericardial fat with incident coronary heart disease: the Multi-Ethnic Study of Atherosclerosis (MESA). Am J Clin Nutr. 2009;90(3):499–504.
60. Mahabadi AA, Berg MH, Lehmann N, Kalsch H, Bauer M, Kara K, et al. Association of epicardial fat with cardiovascular risk factors and incident myocardial infarction in the general

population: the Heinz Nixdorf Recall Study. J Am Coll Cardiol. 2013;61(13):1388–95.

61. Forouzandeh F, Chang SM, Muhyieddeen K, Zaid RR, Trevino AR, Xu J, et al. Does quantifying epicardial and intrathoracic fat with noncontrast computed tomography improve risk stratification beyond calcium scoring alone? Circ Cardiovasc Imaging. 2013;6(1):58–66.
62. Spearman JV, Renker M, Schoepf UJ, Krazinski AW, Herbert TL, De Cecco CN, et al. Prognostic value of epicardial fat volume measurements by computed tomography: a systematic review of the literature. Eur Radiol. 2015;25(11):3372–81.
63. Oikonomou E, Marwan M, et al. Non-invasive detection of coronary inflammation using computed tomography and prediction of residual cardiovascular risk (the CRISP CT study): a post-hoc analysis of prospective outcome data. Lancet. 2018;392(10151):929–39. https://doi.org/10.1016/S0140-6736(18)31114-0.
64. Wong CX, Abed HS, Molaee P, Nelson AJ, Brooks AG, Sharma G, et al. Pericardial fat is associated with atrial fibrillation severity and ablation outcome. J Am Coll Cardiol. 2011;57(17):1745–51.
65. Thanassoulis G, Massaro JM, O'Donnell CJ, Hoffmann U, Levy D, Ellinor PT, et al. Pericardial fat is associated with prevalent atrial fibrillation: the Framingham Heart Study. Circ Arrhythm Electrophysiol. 2010;3(4):345–50.
66. Tanami Y, Jinzaki M, Kishi S, Matheson M, Vavere AL, Rochitte CE, et al. Lack of association between epicardial fat volume and extent of coronary artery calcification, severity of coronary artery disease, or presence of myocardial perfusion abnormalities in a diverse, symptomatic patient population: results from the CORE320 multicenter study. Circ Cardiovasc Imaging. 2015;8(3):e002676.
67. Hartiala O, Magnussen CG, Bucci M, Kajander S, Knuuti J, Ukkonen H, et al. Coronary heart disease risk factors, coronary artery calcification and epicardial fat volume in the Young Finns Study. Eur Heart J Cardiovasc Imaging. 2015;16(11):1256–63.
68. Romijn MA, Danad I, Bakkum MJ, Stuijfzand WJ, Tulevski II, Somsen GA, et al. Incremental diagnostic value of epicardial adipose tissue for the detection of functionally relevant coronary artery disease. Atherosclerosis. 2015;242(1):161–6.

Part VI

Where We Are: Non-invasive Coronary Artery Imaging

Nonatherosclerotic Coronary Artery Disease

25

Toru Sakuma, Kotaro Ouchi, and Kunihiko Fukuda

Atherosclerotic coronary artery disease (CAD) is not apparent in coronary angiography or necropsy in approximately 4–7% of all patients with acute myocardial infarction (AMI) [1]. Showing only the lumina of arteries, conventional coronary angiography offers very low specificity for diagnosing CAD etiology. However, the temporal and spatial resolution of coronary angiography using computed tomography (CT) allows depiction of the vessel wall and adjacent tissue as well as the arterial lumen that permits the safe and noninvasive detection of various disease manifestations of both nonatherosclerotic and atherosclerotic CAD.

Nonatherosclerotic CAD is rare but can result in severe and life-threatening complications, including coronary artery aneurysm, spasm, dissection, stenosis, and intraluminal thrombosis, that may occur in very young patients and are often silent in the early stages of disease. Accurate diagnosis and proper patient management require that clinicians recognize CT findings associated with the various manifestations of nonatherosclerotic CAD.

We present an overview that includes the pathophysiology, etiology, and findings on coronary CT angiography of coronary artery spasm, dissection, and vasculitis as well as immune-mediated conditions and lymphoproliferative disorder – information that is clinically useful and that can facilitate accurate diagnosis and treatment.

Coronary Artery Spasm

In 1959, Prinzmetal et al. [2] described what they termed a variant form of classic angina pectoris that occurred at rest, was associated with elevation of the ST segment on electrocardiography (ECG), and was not induced by exertion. In the early 1970s, coronary angiography demonstrated spasms of the epicardial coronary artery during such an attack [3]. We now know that coronary artery spasm can lead to arrhythmias and various myocardial ischemic diseases, including the variant angina, which is now described as vasospastic angina, as well as acute coronary syndrome (ACS), acute myocardial infarction, and sudden death [4, 5]. Coronary artery spasm is considered a disease of middle- to old-aged men and postmenopausal women [6]; premenopausal women benefit from the protective effects of estrogen on dilator response in coronary arteries [7].

A recent survey in Japan showed coronary artery spasm in 40.9% of consecutive patients with angina pectoris who underwent coronary angiography [8]. The prominent risk factors for such spasm are age, smoking, and presence in the plasma of high sensitivity C-reactive protein (hsCRP) and remnant lipoproteins, and the rate of smoking is significantly higher among patients with coronary spastic angina than those with stable effort angina [9]. The exact mechanisms of coronary artery spasm remain unknown and may be related to endothelial dysfunction, polymorphisms of the eNOS gene, oxidative stress, chronic low-grade inflammation, hypercontractility of the coronary smooth muscle, and magnesium deficiency [10].

Coronary artery spasm can be reliably diagnosed by provocation test using ergonovine or acetylcholine during coronary angiography, but the test is invasive and can induce severe myocardial ischemia or arrhythmia [11]. As a noninvasive alternative, coronary CT angiography can depict abnormalities of the coronary arteries, but its use does not guarantee visualization of the spasm, which is temporary and rarely occurs during the daytime, and imaging follows sublingual administration of nitroglycerine to dilate the coronary arteries. Nevertheless, Ito's group [12] reported the utility of coronary CT angiography to predict coronary artery spasm, observing noncalcified plaques with intermediate attenuation and negative remodeling of the vessel diameter at spasm sites (Fig. 25.1). Male patients with these characteristic

T. Sakuma (✉) · K. Ouchi · K. Fukuda
Department of Radiology, The Jikei University School of Medicine, Tokyo, Japan
e-mail: sakuma@jikei.ac.jp

U. J. Schoepf (ed.), *CT of the Heart*, Contemporary Medical Imaging, https://doi.org/10.1007/978-1-60327-237-7_25

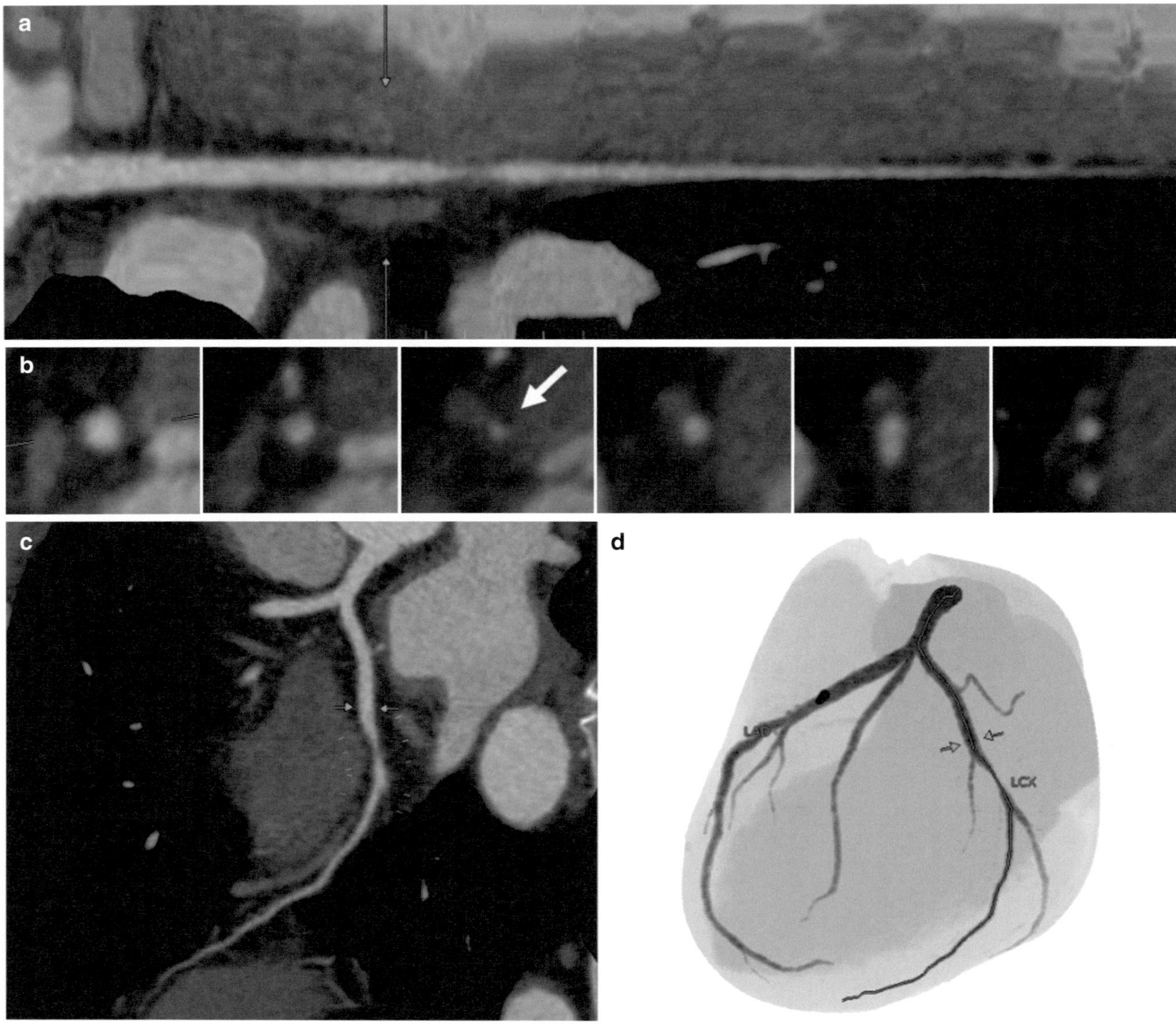

Fig. 25.1 Coronary computed tomography angiography in a 53-year-old man with chest pain at rest in the morning and suspected vasospastic angina. Stretched multiplanar reconstruction (MPR) image (**a**), curved MPR image (**c**) of the left circumflex artery (LCX), and angiographic view of the left coronary artery (**d**) demonstrate stenosis at the middle of the LCX. Cross-sectional images (**b**) at the middle of the LCX show noncalcified plaque with negative remodeling (white arrow). This patient was diagnosed with coronary artery spasm using the provocation test

plaques should be given medication to prevent coronary artery spasm and/or undergo provocation testing to prevent fatal cardiac events. A pilot study by Kang and colleagues [13] demonstrated the safety and feasibility of a protocol using double-acquisition coronary CT angiography with and without intravenous infusion of nitrate as a noninvasive means of depicting vasospastic angina, yielding moderate sensitivity (73%) and high specificity (100%). Nonetheless, sensitivity remained insufficient to rule out vasospastic angina without the provocation test.

Coronary Artery Dissection

Coronary artery dissection has been categorized as either primary, that is, occurring spontaneously, or secondary, occurring after coronary angiography, coronary intervention, cardiac surgery, trauma, or dissection of the aortic root. Spontaneous coronary artery dissection (SCAD) is defined as an idiopathic separation of the coronary arterial wall by intramural hemorrhage that creates a false lumen with or without intimal tear. If the separation occurs in the media,

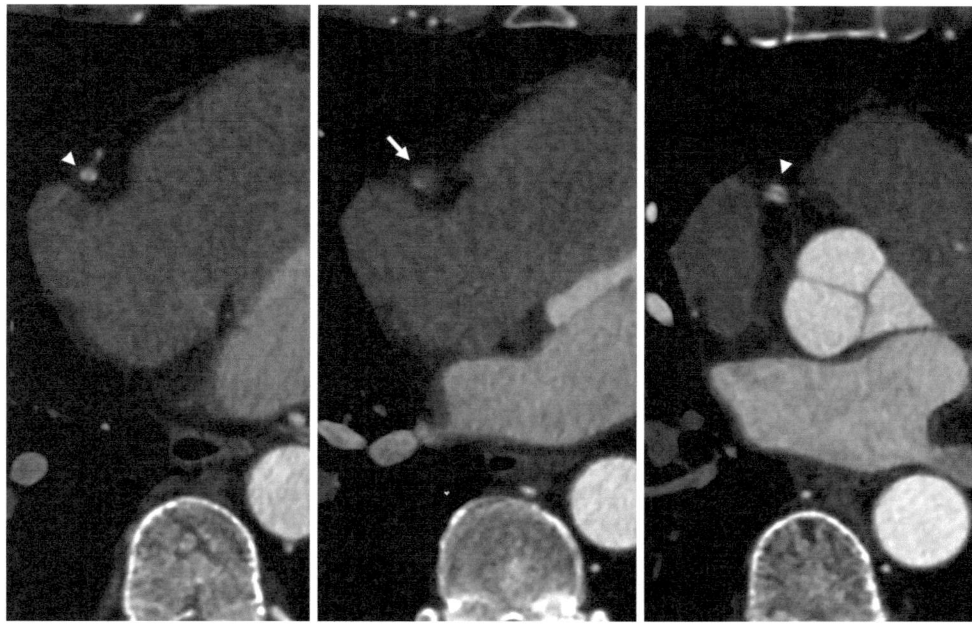

Fig. 25.2 Coronary computed tomography angiography in a 70-year-old man with chest pain during walking and suspected effort angina. Electrocardiography-gated reconstruction images of the right coronary artery (RCA) show dual channels and the intimal flap in the coronary lumen (arrowheads), which represent spontaneous coronary artery dissection (SCAD). The middle part of the SCAD shows aneurysmal dilatation with the thrombosed false lumen and narrowed true lumen (white arrow)

the resulting intramural hematoma or enlarged false lumen compresses the true arterial lumen, thereby compromising blood flow of the coronary artery, and may cause chest pain, subsequent myocardial ischemia, infarction, acute coronary syndrome, ventricular fibrillation, or sudden death. SCAD is atherosclerotic or nonatherosclerotic. Predisposing factors of the nonatherosclerotic type include peripartum state, connective tissue disorders, coronary artery spasm, fibromuscular dysplasia, and systemic inflammatory diseases [14].

In 1931, Pretty [15] first reported the discovery of SCAD at autopsy in a 42-year-old woman who had died suddenly, and Forker's team [16] reported the first angiographic diagnosis in 1973. SCAD has been reported in an estimated 0.07–1.1% of patients undergoing coronary angiography [17], with higher prevalence (3–4%) among patients with acute coronary syndrome than those with stable symptoms (0.3%) and even higher prevalence (8.7%) among women younger than 50 years with ACS [18].

Though coronary angiography is most widely used to diagnose SCAD, the inability of conventional coronary angiography to depict abnormalities of the arterial wall can prevent definitive diagnosis. Thus, the appearance of multiple lumina on conventional coronary angiography demonstrates medial dissection with intimal tear, but stenosis or occlusion of the lumina caused by the dissecting medial hematoma following rupture of the vasa vasorum can be mistaken for stenosis or occlusion due to atherosclerosis. In this setting, intravascular ultrasound (IVUS) or optical coherence tomography (OCT) provides more detailed information about the coronary lumen and vessel wall of the lesion of SCAD [19, 20]. Coronary CT angiography may also be useful in the diagnosis and assessment of SCAD because it allows direct visualization of the coronary wall as well as the arterial lumen without the use of invasive methods like IVUS or OCT (Fig. 25.2).

A large prospective study by Tweet and colleagues [21] suggests initial conservative management as a reasonable strategy for patients with SCAD. Those authors observed a 10-year rate of recurrence after a primary SCAD event of 29.4%, with the median time to a second episode of 2.8 years (range, 3 days–12 years), and a 10-year rate of major adverse cardiac events (death, recurrent SCAD, myocardial infarction, and congestive heart failure) of 47.4% [21]. Although SCAD demonstrates favorable long-term survival, the rate of associated major adverse events is high, and its recurrence is unpredictable. Its management therefore requires both close and long-term follow-up [22]. Noninvasive coronary CT angiography may be the optimal imaging method for the follow-up of patients with SCAD who are initially managed conservatively.

Takayasu Arteritis

Takayasu arteritis (TAK) is an idiopathic systemic granulomatous vasculitis that involves medium and large arteries and is especially prominent in the aortic arch and subclavian and carotid arteries. Mikito Takayasu first described the disease in 1905, when he presented the case of a 21-year-old woman with arteriovenous anastomosis surrounding the papilla of the eyeground. The 2012 revision of the Nomenclature of Vasculitides of the International Chapel

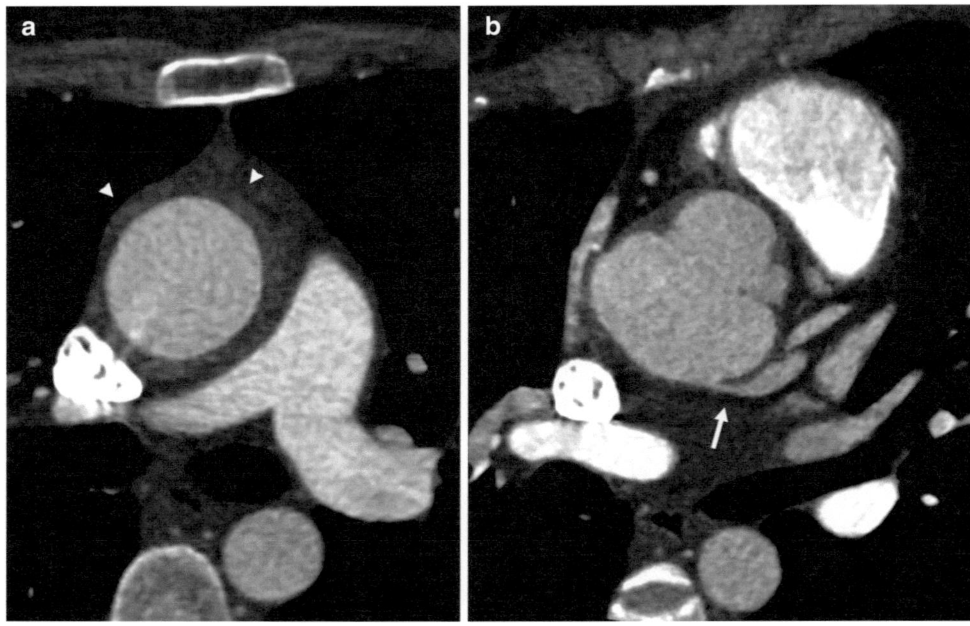

Fig. 25.3 Coronary computed tomography angiography in a 29-year-old woman with active-phase Takayasu arteritis. (**a**) Axial image depicts marked wall thickening of the ascending aorta (arrowheads). (**b**) Cross-sectional multiplanar reconstruction image of the root of the ascending aorta demonstrates constriction of the left main trunk (white arrow) passing through the thickened wall of the sinus of Valsalva

Hill Consensus Conference (CHCC) now categorizes TAK along with giant cell arteritis (GCA) as a vasculitis of large vessels (LVV), defining it as arteritis that is often granulomatous and that predominantly affects the aorta and/or its major branches [23]. Onset usually occurs in patients younger than age 50 but has been observed in older patients. Reported all over the world, TAK is seen more often in Japan, Southeast Asia, Korea, India, China, and Mexico than in the United States and Europe [24]. Its annual incidence is relatively similar in different countries and ranges from 0.4 to 2.6 cases per million in the population [25]. The highest rate is 40 cases per million in the Japanese population. Patients with TAK are predominantly female (82.9–97.0%) and most commonly young women.

Cardiac manifestations of TAK include myocarditis, valvular regurgitation, and coronary involvement that may lead to myocardial infarction, heart failure, or sudden death [26–28]. As minor diagnostic criteria of TAK, Ishikawa included annuloaortic ectasia with aortic regurgitation in 1988 [29], and Sharma's group added the presence of a coronary artery lesion in the absence of risk factors in patients under age 30 in 1995 [30].

Conventional coronary angiography reveals coronary artery disease in approximately 10–30% of cases [27, 31, 32]. In contrast, CT angiography can show abnormalities of the vascular wall as well as luminal information and has been reported to depict coronary involvement in 53.2% of patients with TAK regardless of symptoms and disease activity [24]. An autopsy study of patients with TAK highlighted three abnormal conditions of the coronary artery – stenosis or occlusion of the ostia, diffuse or focal coronary arteritis, and coronary aneurysm [33]. Coronary ostial stenosis in patients with TAK is attributed to the extension of the active inflammatory process from the ascending aorta with thickening and enhancement of the arterial wall in the early and active disease phases (Fig. 25.3). In the later and chronic phases, prolonged inflammation of the coronary vessels may produce diffuse or focal stenosis and the formation of aneurysms (Fig. 25.4). Kang and colleagues [24] observed a lower incidence of non-ostial coronary arterial stenosis in patients with active disease.

Kawasaki Disease

Kawasaki disease (KD) is an acute febrile illness that causes mucosal inflammation, skin rash, and cervical lymphadenopathy, is most often recognized in children younger than 4 years of age, and is of unknown etiology. Dr. Tomisaku Kawasaki described the disease first in the Japanese literature in 1967 [34] and then in English in 1974 [35]. KD produces systemic vasculitis that is most severe in medium-sized arteries and especially prominent in the coronary arteries. The 2012 CHCC nomenclature now categorizes KD along with polyarteritis nodosa (PAN) as a vasculitis of medium vessels (MVV), defining it as arteritis associated with mucocutaneous lymph node syndrome that predominantly affects medium and small arteries. The disease often involves the coronary arteries, may involve the aorta and large arteries, and usually occurs in infants and young children [23].

There is no specific test to identify the presence of KD, so it is diagnosed according to the guidelines of the American

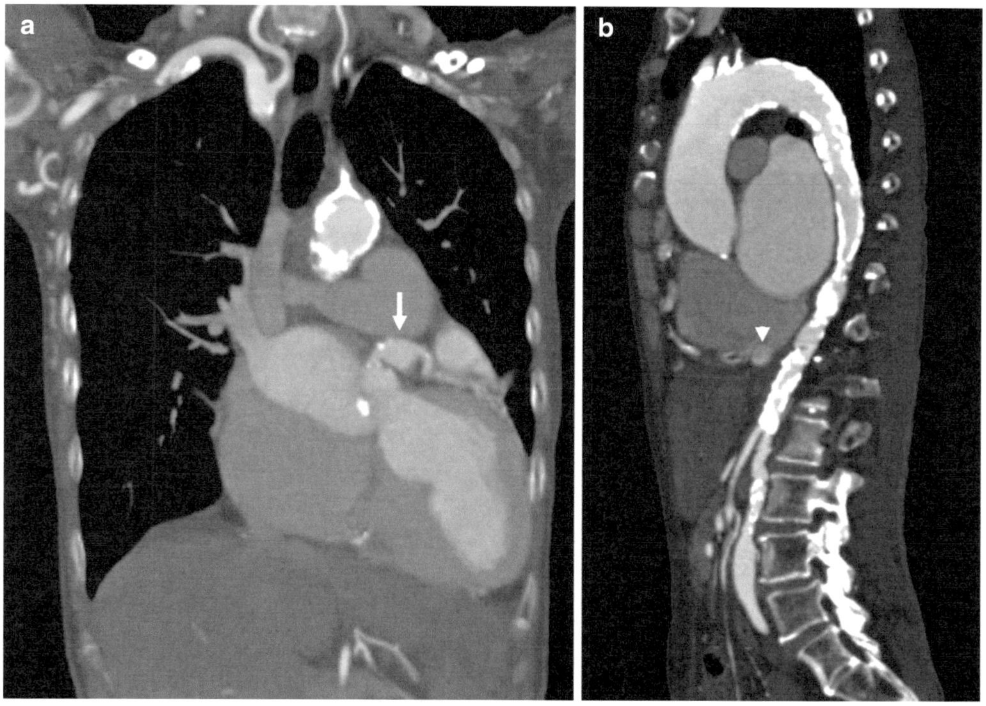

Fig. 25.4 Computed tomography angiography of the thoracic and abdominal aorta in a 72-year-old woman with chronic-phase Takayasu arteritis. (**a**) Coronal image of the chest shows a large coronary artery aneurysm (white arrow) in the left main trunk to the proximal left anterior descending artery. Severe calcification is noted in the aortic arch, and dilated collateral arteries are seen in the right lateral chest wall. (**b**) Sagittal image of the thoracic and abdominal aorta also shows a large aneurysm (arrowhead) in the distal right coronary artery. Severe calcification of the thoracic and abdominal aorta, aneurysmal dilatation of the ascending aorta, and narrowing of the descending and abdominal aorta are also noted with occlusion of the left common carotid and subclavian arteries

Heart Association/American Academy of Pediatrics [36] and JCS Joint Working Group [37]. When coronary aneurysm is recognized on transthoracic echocardiography or coronary angiography (CAG) in patients with fever of at least 5 days' duration, KD can be diagnosed by the observation of four of its five principal clinical features – changes in the extremities, polymorphous exanthem, bilateral bulbar conjunctival injection without exudate, changes in the lips and oral cavity, and cervical lymphadenopathy [36]. Associated morbidity and mortality may be considerable, mostly resulting from myocardial involvement and such coronary artery complications as aneurysm, calcification, and stenosis. KD is a leading cause of acquired heart disease in children in the United States as well as Japan [38].

Prevention of these cardiac abnormalities is the primary goal of its treatment. Though high-dose intravenous immunoglobulin (IVIG) has been administered as the standard therapy in the acute phase of KD, failure of this treatment has been shown in 20.3% of patients, and these patients are at high risk to develop coronary artery complications, particularly aneurysm [39]. A second infusion of IVIG and infliximab is currently used as a follow-up treatment in this group of initial nonresponders.

Orenstein's team [40] reported three linked vasculopathic processes in the arterial wall – necrotizing arteritis, subacute/chronic arteritis, and luminal myofibroblastic proliferation (LMP). Necrosis of the vessel wall in response to the infiltration of neutrophils contributes to aneurysmal formation in the coronary arteries in the acute phase of KD, and in the late phase, LMP narrows the lumina of the arteries [41]. Echocardiography is employed for the initial evaluation and follow-up of lesions of the coronary arteries in KD because it is considered to be the most useful and essential method to evaluate coronary aneurysms. However, as the child grows, visualization of the coronary arteries becomes progressively more difficult by transthoracic echocardiography. Evaluation of aneurysms also becomes more difficult as wall calcification and luminal narrowing progress. For these reasons, coronary CT angiography is the primary modality used in the lifelong surveillance of the coronary arteries.

Medium and giant aneurysms are often associated with thrombotic occlusion in the relatively early stage of KD, but neovascularization can occur. Such development of new vessels has been reported in 15% of patients with coronary artery lesions and on the right coronary artery in 90% of these cases [42] (Fig. 25.5). In addition, localized stenosis,

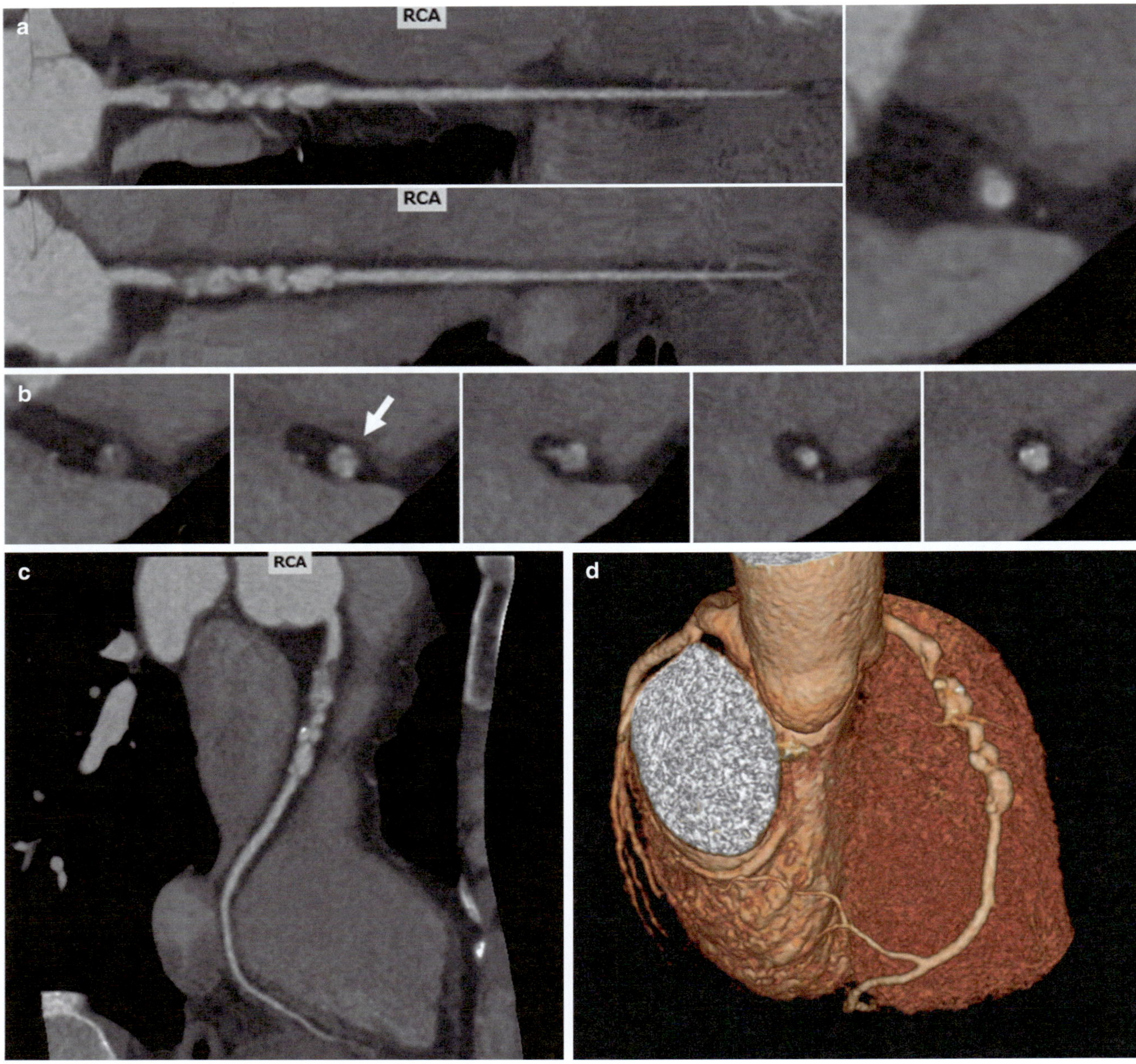

Fig. 25.5 Coronary computed tomography angiography in a 32-year-old man with Kawasaki disease. Stretched multiplanar reconstruction (MPR) image (**a**), curved MPR image (**c**), and volume-rendering image (**d**) of the right coronary artery show a giant aneurysm in its proximal part. Cross-sectional images (**b**) show multiple channels (white arrow) in the coronary lumen, which represent recanalization of the thrombosed aneurysm

particularly at the entrance or exit of an aneurysm, developed in 4.7–12% of patients with coronary artery lesions between 10 and 20 years after onset (Fig. 25.6), and findings of a Japanese multicenter survey reported by Suzuki's group [43] showed that half of patients with giant aneurysms underwent coronary artery bypass grafting (CABG). Coronary CT angiography is also thought to be a promising noninvasive alternative for the assessment of the patency of bypass grafts or residual aneurysms and stenosis.

Immunoglobulin G4-Related Disease (IgG4-Related Disease)

IgG4-related disease is a recently recognized multi-organ, immune-mediated condition characterized by a high concentration of IgG4-positive plasma cells in the site of disease with or without elevation of the serum level of IgG4. Kamisawa and associates [44, 45] first recognized IgG4-related disease as a systemic disorder in 2003, noting

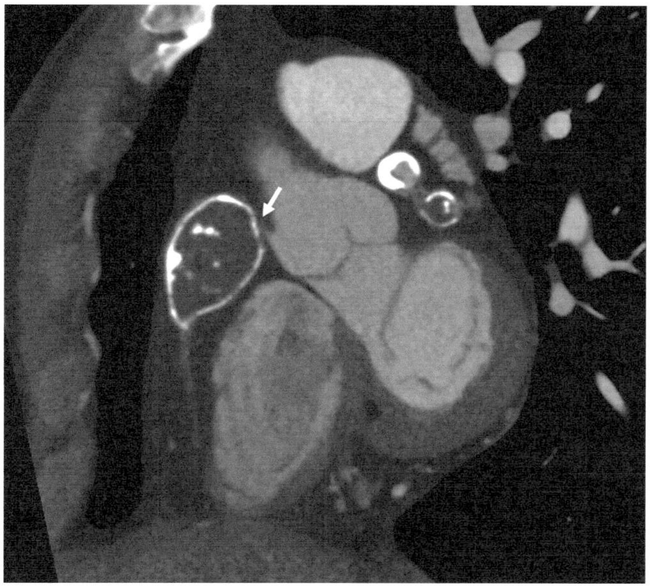

Fig. 25.6 Coronary computed tomography angiography in a 36-year-old man with Kawasaki disease. Short-axis multiplanar reconstruction image shows a giant aneurysm (25 mm in diameter) in the proximal right coronary artery. The entrance of the aneurysm (white arrow) is occluded, and the aneurysm is thrombosed completely. Giant aneurysms are also detected in the proximal left anterior descending artery, which is patent, and the proximal left circumflex artery, which also remains patent despite the large thrombosis

extrapancreatic features in patients with autoimmune pancreatitis. In Japan, the overall prevalence of IgG4-related autoimmune pancreatitis has been estimated as 2.2 cases per 100,000 in the population [46]. Because it affects multiple organs in addition to the pancreas, its true prevalence is unclear and may be underestimated. A national study of autoimmune pancreatitis in Japan [47] showed a greater prevalence of IgG4-related disease among middle- to old-aged men and greater prevalence in male than female patients in a ratio of 2.8 to 1. However, no male predilection is noted in the head and neck lesions. IgG4-related disease has been described in multiple organs – the biliary tree, salivary glands, periorbital tissues, kidneys, lungs, lymph nodes, meninges, aorta, breast, prostate, thyroid, pericardium, and skin. It is also now known to comprise many and various conditions, including autoimmune pancreatitis, eosinophilic angiocentric fibrosis, fibrosing mediastinitis, hypertrophic pachymeningitis, idiopathic hypocomplementemic tubulointerstitial nephritis with extensive tubulointerstitial deposits, inflammatory pseudotumor, Küttner's tumor (chronic sclerosing sialadenitis), Mikulicz syndrome, multifocal fibrosclerosis, periaortitis and periarteritis, inflammatory aortic aneurysm, retroperitoneal fibrosis, Riedel's thyroiditis, and sclerosing mesenteritis [48]. In the late phases after the administration of contrast material on CT, arterial lesions, including inflammatory aneurysm, retroperitoneal fibrosis,

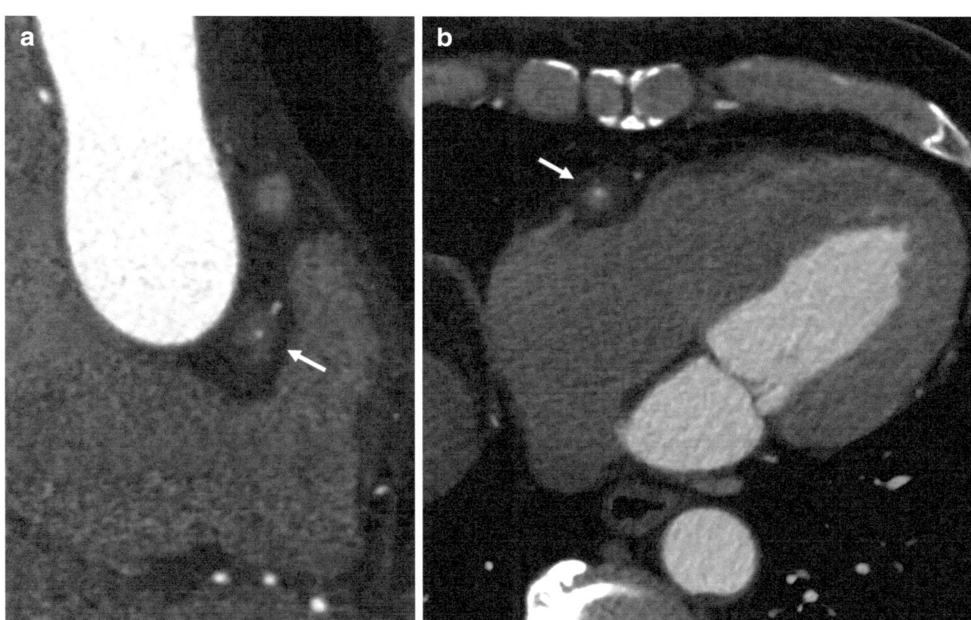

Fig. 25.7 Coronary computed tomography angiography in a 70-year-old man with suspected immunoglobulin G4-related disease. Long-axis multiplanar reconstruction image (**a**) and axial image (**b**) of the proximal right coronary artery (RCA) show periarterial disease (white arrow) of the soft tissue density that causes narrowing of the RCA

periaortitis, and periarteritis, have shown homogeneous wall thickening and enhancement [49]. In contrast to the vasculitis of large vessels – giant cell and Takayasu arteritis – that affects the aortic branches, especially the subclavian arteries, IgG4-related disease often avoids these vessels. Several recent studies have suggested its association with such coronary artery diseases as coronary aneurysm, periarterial pseudotumor (Fig. 25.7), wall calcification, and intimal thickening [50–52]. However, the coronary artery abnormalities of IgG4-related disease have not been fully revealed, and their incidence remains unclear. IgG4-related disease has also been associated with malignant tumor [53]. We must be aware that the pseudotumor of IgG4-related disease resembles the invasion of malignant lymphoma around the coronary artery [54] (Fig. 25.8).

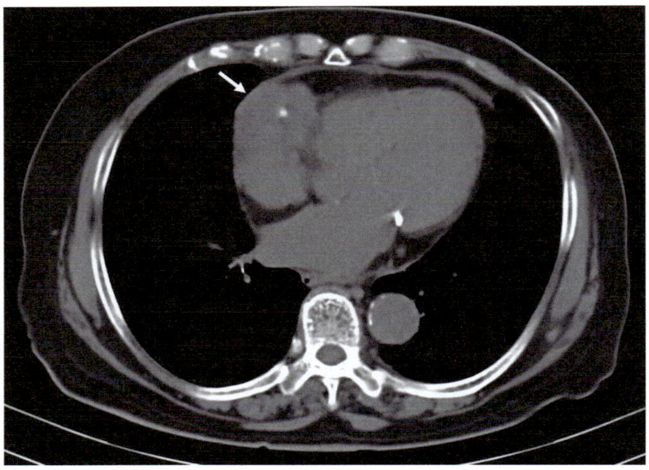

Fig. 25.8 Computed tomography of the chest in a 77-year-old woman with diffuse large B-cell lymphoma reveals a recurrent tumor (white arrow) of the soft tissue density around the calcified right coronary artery. It is sometimes difficult to distinguish immunoglobulin G4-related disease of the coronary artery from malignant lymphoma of the heart

Chronic Active Epstein-Barr Virus Infection

Epstein, Achong, and Barr first discovered the Epstein-Barr virus (EBV) in 1964 within cells cultured from Burkitt's lymphoma tissue [55]. EBV is a herpes virus that infects over 90% of humans and persists throughout life. Primary EBV infection usually occurs in infants and children and is generally asymptomatic or shows nonspecific symptoms. Infections in adolescents and adults frequently result in infectious mononucleosis [56]. EBV directly infects resting B cells of the oropharynx via oral secretions [57]. The infection is controlled by cellular and humoral immune response, but the virus persists in the resting memory B cells [58]. Patients with congenital or acquired immunodeficiency have impaired cellular immunity and are unable to regulate the proliferation of EBV-infected B cells. Their EBV infections result in infectious mononucleosis and localized or disseminated lymphoproliferative disease involving the lymph nodes, liver, lung, kidney, bone marrow, central nervous system, or small intestine [59]. In response to unknown signals, memory B cells may express uncontrolled growth that leads to the development of such tumors as nasopharyngeal carcinoma, Burkitt's lymphoma, and Hodgkin's lymphoma, as well as other cancers [57].

CAEBV demonstrates the clonal expansion of EBV-infected T or natural killer cells. Clinically, patients with CAEBV show persistent and recurrent symptoms that

Fig. 25.9 Coronary computed tomography angiography in a 37-year-old man with chronic active Epstein-Barr virus infection. Volume-rendering image (**a**) and short-axis multiplanar reconstruction image (**b**) show diffuse and inhomogeneous dilatation of the coronary arteries. The anomalous origin of the right coronary artery is also depicted

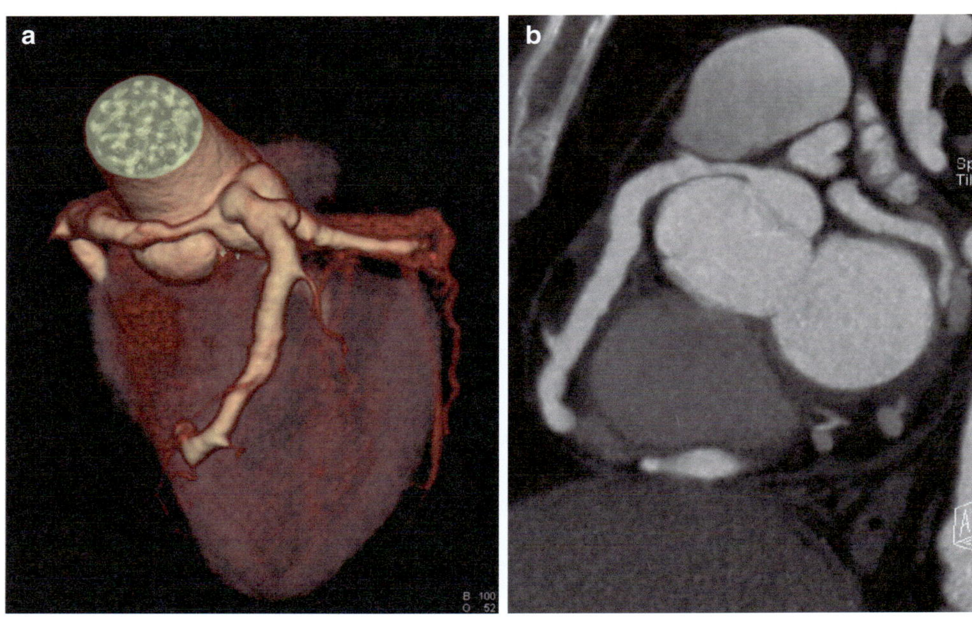

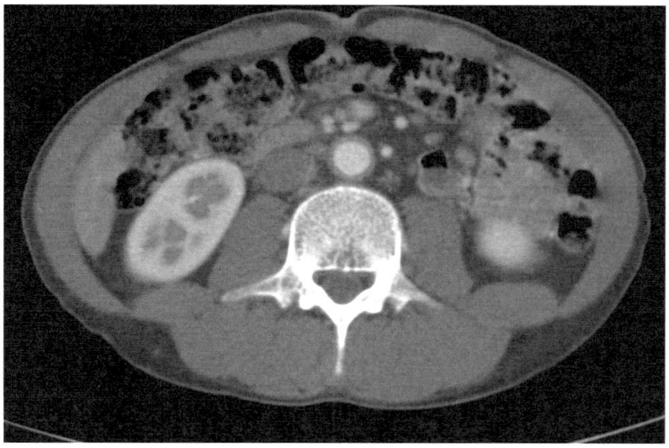

Fig. 25.10 Contrast-enhanced computed tomography of the abdomen in the same patient shown in Fig. 25.9 shows diffuse wall thickening of the abdominal aorta, which represents chronic active arteritis

resemble those of infectious mononucleosis, including fever, lymphadenopathy, and hepatosplenomegaly, and they experience many other complications, such as hematological, digestive tract, neurological, pulmonary, ocular, dermal, and/or cardiovascular disorders (including aneurysm and valvular disease) [60].

First described by Virelizier's group [61] in 1978, CAEBV is now recognized as not only an infectious disease but also as one of the EBV-associated T- and NK-cell lymphoproliferative disorders. Okano and associates [62] proposed a guideline for diagnosing CAEBV in 2005. Patients with CAEBV commonly experience cardiovascular complications because the EBV-infected cells infiltrate the vascular wall and induce vasculitis, and aneurysm of the coronary artery or sinus of Valsalva has been reported [63, 64]. Muneuchi's group [65] reported cardiovascular disease in 60% of patients with CAEBV, which included coronary artery aneurysm (Fig. 25.9), myocarditis, large-vessel arteritis (Fig. 25.10), pulmonary artery hypertension, pericardial effusion, decreased cardiac function, and complete atrioventricular block, and Kimura and colleagues [66] reported coronary artery aneurysm and myocarditis as the complications with the poorest prognoses.

Summary

Nonatherosclerotic CAD is associated with fatal myocardial infarction or sudden cardiac death in all age groups including young age. Cardiologists and radiologists need to be aware of the differential diagnosis of nonatherosclerotic CAD in patients with cardiac symptoms. Coronary CT angiography is a very useful and noninvasive tool to investigate the various manifestations of the nonatherosclerotic CAD and is able to incidentally detect the findings of the disease before the development of life-threatening complications.

References

1. Waller BF. Nonatherosclerotic coronary heart disease. In: Fuster V, Walsh RA, Harrington RA, editors. Hurst's the heart. 13th ed. New York: McGraw-Hill Education; 2011. p. 1257–86.
2. Prinzmetal M, Kennamer R, Merliss R, Wada T, Bor N. Angina pectoris. I. A variant form of angina pectoris; preliminary report. Am J Med. 1959;27:375–88.
3. Oliva PB, Potts DE, Pluss RG. Coronary arterial spasm in Prinzmetal angina. Documentation by coronary arteriography. N Engl J Med. 1973;288:745–51.
4. Nakamura M, Takeshita A, Nose Y. Clinical characteristics associated with myocardial infarction, arrhythmias, and sudden death in patients with vasospastic angina. Circulation. 1987;75:1110–6.
5. Ong P, Athanasiadis A, Hill S, Vogelsberg H, Voehringer M, Sechtem U. Coronary artery spasm as a frequent cause of acute coronary syndrome: the CASPAR (Coronary Artery Spasm in Patients with Acute Coronary Syndrome) study. J Am Coll Cardiol. 2008;52:523–7.
6. Yasue H, Kugiyama K. Coronary spasm: clinical features and pathogenesis. Intern Med. 1997;36:760–5.
7. Williams JK, Adams MR, Klopfenstein HS. Estrogen modulates responses of atherosclerotic coronary arteries. Circulation. 1990;81:1680–7.
8. Yasue H, Sasayama S, Kikuchi K, Okumura K, Matsubara T, Miwa K, et al. The role of coronary spasm in ischemic heart disease among Japanese. In: Annual report of the research on cardiovascular diseases. Osaka: National Cardiovascular Center; 2000. p. 96–7. [in Japanese].
9. Takaoka K, Yoshimura M, Ogawa H, Kugiyama K, Nakayama M, Shimasaki Y, et al. Comparison of the risk factors for coronary artery spasm with those for organic stenosis in a Japanese population: role of cigarette smoking. Int J Cardiol. 2000;72:121–6.
10. Yasue H, Nakagawa H, Itoh T, Harada E, Mizuno Y. Coronary artery spasm--clinical features, diagnosis, pathogenesis, and treatment. J Cardiol. 2008;51:2–17.
11. Szlachcic J, Waters DD, Miller D, Théroux P. Ventricular arrhythmias during ergonovine-induced episodes of variant angina. Am Heart J. 1984;107:20–4.
12. Ito T, Terashima M, Kaneda H, Nasu K, Ehara M, Kinoshita Y, et al. In vivo assessment of ergonovine-induced coronary artery spasm by 64-slice multislice computed tomography. Circ Cardiovasc Imaging. 2012;5:226–32.
13. Kang EJ, Kim MH, De Jin C, Seo J, Kim DW, Yoon SK, et al. Noninvasive detection of coronary vasospastic angina using a double-acquisition coronary CT angiography protocol in the presence and absence of an intravenous nitrate: a pilot study. Eur Radiol. 2016. https://doi.org/10.1007/s00330-016-4476-2.
14. Saw J, Ricci D, Starovoytov A, Fox R, Buller CE. Spontaneous coronary artery dissection: prevalence of predisposing conditions including fibromuscular dysplasia in a tertiary center cohort. JACC Cardiovasc Interv. 2013;6:44–52.
15. Pretty HC. Dissecting aneurysm of coronary artery in a woman aged 42: rupture. Br Med J. 1931;1:667.
16. Forker AD, Rosenlof RC, Weaver WF, Carveth SW, Reese HE. Primary dissecting aneurysm of the right coronary artery with survival. Chest. 1973;64:656–8.
17. Vrints CJ. Spontaneous coronary artery dissection. Heart. 2010;96:801–8.

18. Vanzetto G, Berger-Coz E, Barone-Rochette G, Chavanon N, Bouvaist H, Hacini R, et al. Prevalence, therapeutic management and medium-term prognosis of spontaneous coronary artery dissection: results from a database of 11,605 patients. Eur J Cardiothorac Surg. 2009;35:250–4.
19. Maehara A, Mintz GS, Castagna MT, Pichard AD, Satler LF, Waksman R, et al. Intravascular ultrasound assessment of spontaneous coronary artery dissection. Am J Cardiol. 2002;89:466–8.
20. Alfonso F, Paulo M, Gonzalo N, Dutary J, Jimenez-Quevedo P, Lennie V, et al. Diagnosis of spontaneous coronary artery dissection by optical coherence tomography. J Am Coll Cardiol. 2012;59:1073–9.
21. Tweet MS, Hayes SN, Pitta SR, Simari RD, Lerman A, Lennon RJ, et al. Clinical features, management, and prognosis of spontaneous coronary artery dissection. Circulation. 2012;126:579–88.
22. Alfonso F, Paulo M, Lennie V, Dutary J, Bernardo E, Jiménez-Quevedo P, et al. Spontaneous coronary artery dissection: long-term follow-up of a large series of patients prospectively managed with a "conservative" therapeutic strategy. JACC Cardiovasc Interv. 2012;5:1062–70.
23. Jennette JC, Falk RJ, Bacon PA, Basu N, Cid MC, Ferrario F, et al. 2012 revised International Chapel Hill Consensus Conference Nomenclature of Vasculitides. Arthritis Rheum. 2013;65:1–11.
24. Kang EJ, Kim SM, Choe YH, Lee GY, Lee KN, Kim DK. Takayasu arteritis: assessment of coronary arterial abnormalities with 128-section dual-source CT angiography of the coronary arteries and aorta. Radiology. 2014;270:74–81.
25. de Souza AW, de Carvalho JF. Diagnostic and classification criteria of Takayasu arteritis. J Autoimmun. 2014;48-49:79–83.
26. Subramanyan R, Joy J, Balakrishnan KG. Natural history of aortoarteritis (Takayasu's disease). Circulation. 1989;80:429–37.
27. Park YB, Hong SK, Choi KJ, Sohn DW, Oh BH, Lee MM, et al. Takayasu arteritis in Korea: clinical and angiographic features. Heart Vessels Suppl. 1992;7:55–9.
28. Lee GY, Jang SY, Ko SM, Kim EK, Lee SH, Han H, et al. Cardiovascular manifestations of Takayasu arteritis and their relationship to the disease activity: analysis of 204 Korean patients at a single center. Int J Cardiol. 2012;159:14–20.
29. Ishikawa K. Diagnostic approach and proposed criteria for the clinical diagnosis of Takayasu's arteriopathy. J Am Coll Cardiol. 1988;12:964–72.
30. Sharma BK, Jain S, Suri S, Numano F. Diagnostic criteria for Takayasu arteritis. Int J Cardiol. 1996;54(Suppl):141–7.
31. Amano J, Suzuki A. Coronary artery involvement in Takayasu's arteritis. Collective review and guideline for surgical treatment. J Thorac Cardiovasc Surg. 1991;102:554–60.
32. Endo M, Tomizawa Y, Nishida H, Aomi S, Nakazawa M, Tsurumi Y, et al. Angiographic findings and surgical treatments of coronary artery involvement in Takayasu arteritis. J Thorac Cardiovasc Surg. 2003;125:570–7.
33. Matsubara O, Kuwata T, Nemoto T, Kasuga T, Numano F. Coronary artery lesions in Takayasu arteritis: pathological considerations. Heart Vessels Suppl. 1992;7:26–31.
34. Kawasaki T. Acute febrile mucocutaneous syndrome with lymphoid involvement with specific desquamation of the fingers and toes in children. Allergy. 1967;16:178–222. [in Japanese].
35. Kawasaki T, Kosaki F, Okawa S, Shigematsu I, Yanagawa H. A new infantile acute febrile mucocutaneous lymph node syndrome (MLNS) prevailing in Japan. Pediatrics. 1974;54:271–6.
36. Newburger JW, Takahashi M, Gerber MA, Gewitz MH, Tani LY, Burns JC, et al. Diagnosis, treatment, and long-term management of Kawasaki disease: a statement for health professionals from the Committee on Rheumatic Fever, Endocarditis and Kawasaki Disease, Council on Cardiovascular Disease in the Young, American Heart Association. Circulation. 2004;110:2747–71.
37. JCS Joint Working Group. Guidelines for diagnosis and management of cardiovascular sequelae in Kawasaki disease (JCS 2008)—digest version. Circ J. 2010;74:1989–2020.
38. Taubert KA, Rowley AH, Shulman ST. Nationwide survey of Kawasaki disease and acute rheumatic fever. J Pediatr. 1991;119:279–82.
39. Dajani AS, Taubert KA, Takahashi M, Bierman FZ, Freed M, Ferrieri P, et al. Guidelines for long-term management of patients with Kawasaki disease. Report from the Committee on Rheumatic Fever, Endocarditis, and Kawasaki Disease, Council on Cardiovascular Disease in the Young, American Heart Association. Circulation. 1994;89:916–22.
40. Uehara R, Belay ED, Maddox RA, Holman RC, Nakamura Y, Yashiro M, et al. Analysis of potential risk factors associated with nonresponse to initial intravenous immunoglobulin treatment among Kawasaki disease patients in Japan. Pediatr Infect Dis J. 2008;27:155–60.
41. Orenstein JM, Shulman ST, Fox LM, Baker SC, Takahashi M, Bhatti TR, et al. Three linked vasculopathic processes characterize Kawasaki disease: a light and transmission electron microscopic study. PLoS One. 2012;7(6):e38998.
42. Newburger JW, Takahashi M, Burns JC. Kawasaki disease. J Am Coll Cardiol. 2016;67:1738–49.
43. Suzuki A, Kamiya T, Tsuda E, Tsukano S. Natural history of coronary artery lesions in Kawasaki disease. Prog Pediatr Cardiol. 1997;6:211–8.
44. Kamisawa T, Egawa N, Nakajima H. Autoimmune pancreatitis is a systemic autoimmune disease. Am J Gastroenterol. 2003;98:2811–2.
45. Kamisawa T, Funata N, Hayashi Y, Eishi Y, Koike M, Tsuruta K, et al. A new clinicopathological entity of IgG4-related autoimmune disease. J Gastroenterol. 2003;38:982–4.
46. Kanno A, Nishimori I, Masamune A, Kikuta K, Hirota M, Kuriyama S, et al. Research Committee on Intractable Diseases of Pancreas. Nationwide epidemiological survey of autoimmune pancreatitis in Japan. Pancreas. 2012;41:835–9.
47. Nishimori I, Tamakoshi A, Otsuki M, Research Committee on Intractable Diseases of the Pancreas, Ministry of Health, Labour, and Welfare of Japan. Prevalence of autoimmune pancreatitis in Japan from a nationwide survey in 2002. J Gastroenterol. 2007;42(Suppl 18):6–8.
48. Kamisawa T, Zen Y, Pillai S, Stone JH. IgG4-related disease. Lancet. 2015;385:1460–71.
49. Inoue D, Zen Y, Abo H, Gabata T, Demachi H, Yoshikawa J, et al. Immunoglobulin G4-related periaortitis and periarteritis: CT findings in 17 patients. Radiology. 2011;261:625–33.
50. Matsumoto Y, Kasashima S, Kawashima A, Sasaki H, Endo M, Kawakami K, et al. A case of multiple immunoglobulin G4-related periarteritis: a tumorous lesion of the coronary artery and abdominal aortic aneurysm. Hum Pathol. 2008;39:975–80.
51. Ishizaka N, Sakamoto A, Imai Y, Terasaki F, Nagai R. Multifocal fibrosclerosis and IgG4-related disease involving the cardiovascular system. J Cardiol. 2012;59:132–8.
52. Hourai R, Miyamura M, Tasaki R, Iwata A, Takeda Y, Morita H, et al. A case of IgG4-related lymphadenopathy, pericarditis, coronary artery periarteritis and luminal stenosis. Heart Vessel. 2016;31:1709–13.
53. Yamamoto M, Takahashi H, Tabeya T, Suzuki C, Naishiro Y, Ishigami K, et al. Risk of malignancies in IgG4-related disease. Mod Rheumatol. 2012;22:414–8.
54. Ishizaka N. IgG4-related disease underlying the pathogenesis of coronary artery disease. Clin Chim Acta. 2013;415:220–5.
55. Epstein MA, Achong BG, Barr YM. Virus particles in cultured lymphoblasts from Burkitt's lymphoma. Lancet. 1964;1:702–3.
56. Cohen JI. Epstein-Barr virus infection. N Engl J Med. 2000;343:481–92.

57. Thorley-Lawson DA, Gross A. Persistence of the Epstein-Barr virus and the origins of associated lymphomas. N Engl J Med. 2004;350:1328–37.
58. Babcock GJ, Decker LL, Volk M, Thorley-Lawson DA. EBV persistence in memory B cells in vivo. Immunity. 1998;9:395–404.
59. Cohen JI. Epstein-Barr virus lymphoproliferative disease associated with acquired immunodeficiency. Medicine (Baltimore). 1991;70:137–60.
60. Kimura H. Pathogenesis of chronic active Epstein-Barr virus infection: is this an infectious disease, lymphoproliferative disorder, or immunodeficiency? Rev Med Virol. 2006;16:251–61.
61. Virelizier JL, Lenoir G, Griscelli C. Persistent Epstein-Barr virus infection in a child with hypergammaglobulinaemia and immunoblastic proliferation associated with a selective defect in immune interferon secretion. Lancet. 1978;2:231–4.
62. Okano M, Kawa K, Kimura H, Yachie A, Wakiguchi H, Maeda A, et al. Proposed guidelines for diagnosing chronic active Epstein-Barr virus infection. Am J Hematol. 2005;80:64–9.
63. Kikuta H, Taguchi Y, Tomizawa K, Kojima K, Kawamura N, Ishizaka A, et al. Epstein-Barr virus genome-positive T lymphocytes in a boy with chronic active EBV infection associated with Kawasaki-like disease. Nature. 1988;333:455–7.
64. Sato Y, Tsuboi T, Mikami T, Kurosawa H, Kanou K, Sugita K, et al. Chronic active Epstein-Barr virus infection with dilatation of the Valsalva sinus. Pediatr Int. 2006;48:643–5.
65. Muneuchi J, Ohga S, Ishimura M, Ikeda K, Yamaguchi K, Nomura A, et al. Cardiovascular complications associated with chronic active Epstein-Barr virus infection. Pediatr Cardiol. 2009;30:274–81.
66. Kimura H, Morishima T, Kanegane H, Ohga S, Hoshino Y, Maeda A, et al. Prognostic factors for chronic active Epstein-Barr virus infection. J Infect Dis. 2003;187:527–33.

The Many Faces of Atherosclerosis

26

Nandini (Nina) M. Meyersohn, Jan-Erik Scholtz, and Brian B. Ghoshhajra

Coronary CT angiography (CTA) has been well established as a noninvasive imaging modality for the assessment of coronary artery disease (CAD) and the evaluation of atherosclerotic plaque within the coronary arteries, as reviewed earlier in this volume. While the pathology and pathophysiology of atherosclerosis leading to the development of plaques within the coronary arteries have been covered in earlier chapters, familiarity with the various imaging appearances of coronary artery plaque and their clinical significance is essential for the cardiac imager. In this chapter, the CT imaging features of the range of presentations of atherosclerotic plaque within the coronary arteries will be reviewed and illustrated.

Plaque Calcification

As described in earlier chapters, coronary artery calcification is part of the continuum of development of atherosclerosis [1]. Atherosclerotic plaques may be noncalcified, partially calcified, or predominantly/fully calcified. Of note, noncalcified and partially calcified plaques have been previously referred to as "soft" and "mixed" plaque, respectively; however these terms have fallen out of favor and are no longer used in major society guidelines [2]. Calcification is never normal within the wall of a coronary artery, however the degree of calcification of a plaque is not linked directly to the degree of stenosis.

Heavily calcified plaque can result in minimal or no stenosis, while noncalcified plaque can be obstructive or occlusive. Coronary artery calcium (CAC) is an independent predictor of adverse events, however it remains unclear whether progression of CAC represents true progression of coronary artery disease or rather stabilization and healing of existing plaque [3]. From a technical perspective, the presence of calcification complicates interpretation of CTA due to what is known as "blooming artifact," which is the tendency of calcified objects to appear larger than their true size on CT images because of a complex interaction of volume averaging and beam hardening [4]. Due to the contribution of beam hardening, this artifact is accentuated at lower tube potentials, meaning that dose reduction strategies can often increase the degree of blooming artifact. Care must be taken by the imager to account for blooming artifact when evaluating the degree of luminal stenosis secondary to calcified plaques; examining the degree of remaining contrast-opacified lumen that is visible can help resolve this issue, as can newer technologies such as dual-energy scanning and volume calcium subtraction.

Figure 26.1a depicts a noncalcified plaque in the distal right coronary artery (RCA), which not only demonstrates lack of calcification but also notably low attenuation values as measured by Hounsfield units (HU), a high-risk feature which will be discussed below. Figure 26.1b depicts a partially calcified plaque in the left anterior descending coronary artery (LAD). Partially calcified plaques can lead to diagnostic uncertainty when the density of calcification has a similar attenuation of contrast within the coronary artery lumen. Figure 26.1c demonstrates a fully calcified plaque in the left main coronary artery (LM). Note that in this case, the density of the calcium in this plaque is of significantly higher attenuation than the contrast within the vessel lumen.

N. (N). M. Meyersohn (✉) · B. B. Ghoshhajra
Division of Cardiovascular Imaging, Department of Radiology, Massachusetts General Hospital/Harvard Medical School, Boston, MA, USA

Cardiac MR PET CT Program, Massachusetts General Hospital, Boston, MA, USA
e-mail: nmeyersohn@mgh.harvard.edu

J.-E. Scholtz
Cardiac MR PET CT Program, Massachusetts General Hospital, Boston, MA, USA

U. J. Schoepf (ed.), *CT of the Heart*, Contemporary Medical Imaging, https://doi.org/10.1007/978-1-60327-237-7_26

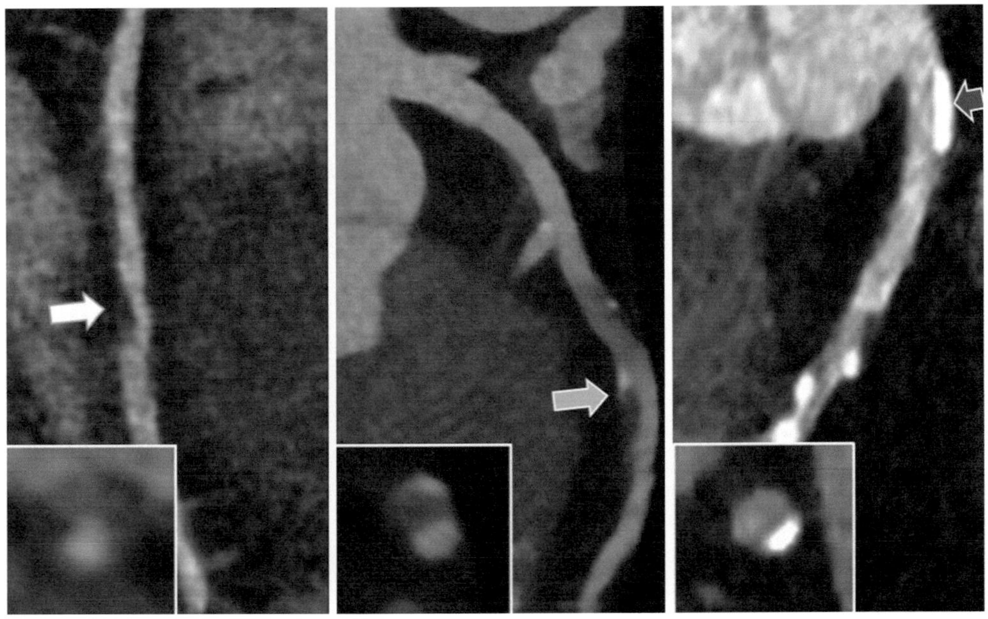

Fig. 26.1 Coronary CT angiography images demonstrating long-axis and short-axis (inset) views of noncalcified plaque with low attenuation (<30 HU) resulting in mild stenosis of the distal RCA (left, white arrow), partially calcified plaque and positive remodeling resulting in mild stenosis of the distal LAD (middle, light gray arrow), and calcified plaque in the wall of the LM resulting in mild stenosis (right, dark gray arrow)

Coronary Artery Stenosis

As coronary CTA evolved from an area of research into a growing clinical subspecialty, the reporting of severity of stenosis resulting from atherosclerotic plaque has also evolved. Reports early on tended to be qualitative in nature and were not necessarily consistent between readers regarding overall burden of atherosclerosis as well as hemodynamic significance of each individual plaque. In 2009, Raff et al. from the Society of Cardiovascular Computed Tomography (SCCT) issued society guidelines on the reporting of coronary CTA that were adopted in clinical practice at many institutions seeking to standardize interpretation [5]. Under this system, if atherosclerotic plaque of any composition was identified in a coronary artery, the stenosis could be graded as minimal (negligible impact on the lumen), mild (less than 49% stenosis), moderate (50–69% stenosis), severe (70–99% stenosis), or occluded. There has been some overlap in the literature with use of the terms “significant” plaque and “obstructive” plaque; one method of resolving this overlap is to reserve the use of “obstructive” for stenoses graded as severe and to use the more general term “significant” for stenosis graded as moderate or higher, as these are of potential but not certain hemodynamic significance.

A more recent multisociety guideline released in 2016 is the CAD-RADS™, or Coronary Artery Disease Reporting and Data System [6]. This system addresses the standardized reporting of degree of coronary artery stenosis in a fashion similar to that described in the 2009 guidelines but with the addition of a numerical score ranging from 0 for no plaque to 5 for complete occlusion. The CAD-RADS system also includes management recommendations to facilitate clinical decision-making authored in collaboration with the American College of Radiology and the North American Society of Cardiovascular Imaging and endorsed by the American College of Cardiology. Separate recommendations exist for patients with acute chest pain and for stable outpatients with chest pain and are meant to integrate evolving clinical experience with the natural history of stenosis found on coronary CTA. Figures 26.2, 26.3, and 26.4 demonstrate atherosclerotic plaques on coronary CTA resulting in mild [CAD-RADS 2), moderate (CAD-RADS 3), and severe stenosis (CAD-RADS 4), respectively, according to these guidelines.

Atherosclerosis in the coronary arteries is also the most common cause of coronary artery aneurysm in adults, defined as abnormal focal dilatation of a vessel with a diameter exceeding the diameter of adjacent unaffected coronary segment by 1.5 times or greater [7]. As in other vessels, an aneurysm is defined as saccular if the transverse diameter exceeds the length of the aneurysm or fusiform if the converse is true. Figure 26.5 demonstrates the CT appearance of a saccular atherosclerotic coronary artery aneurysm.

A specific entity that should be carefully evaluated for on coronary CTA is stenosis of the left main coronary artery. Left main stenosis is important to identify as it is associated with a high rate of complications during catheterization, and patients are often treated instead with coronary artery bypass grafting [8]. Evaluating left main stenosis on coronary CTA mandates the use of multiplanar reformatted images, and it is important for the imager to note that in both classification

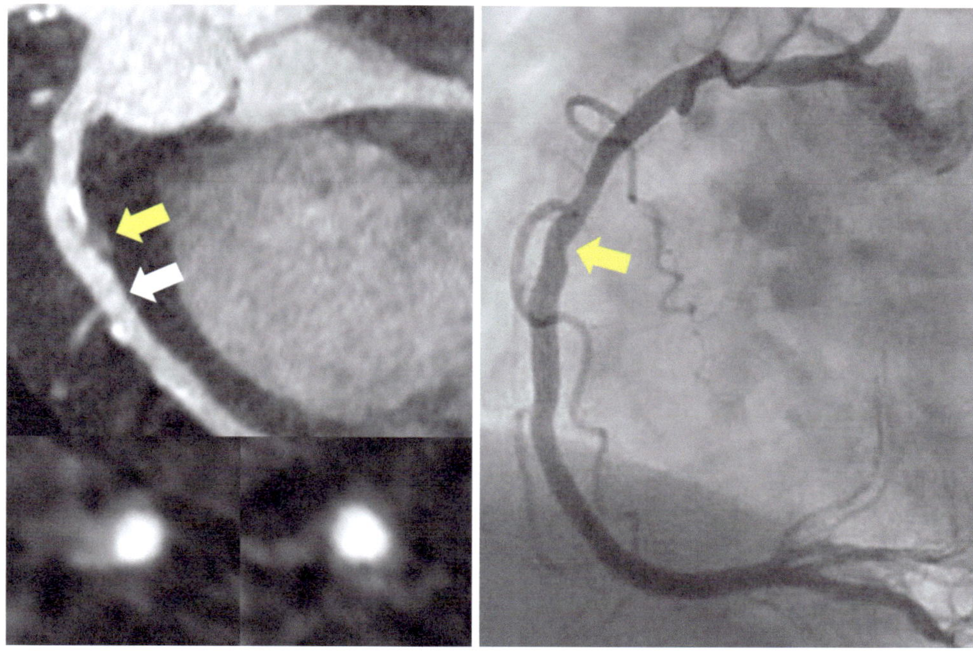

Fig. 26.2 Coronary CT angiography images demonstrate partially calcified plaque in the wall of the proximal RCA resulting in mild (CAD-RADS 2) stenosis (left, yellow arrow). Invasive coronary angiography correlation demonstrating mild stenosis (right, yellow arrow). Comparison of the diameters at the level of mild stenosis (left inset, left panel) and distal to the stenosis (left inset, right panel)

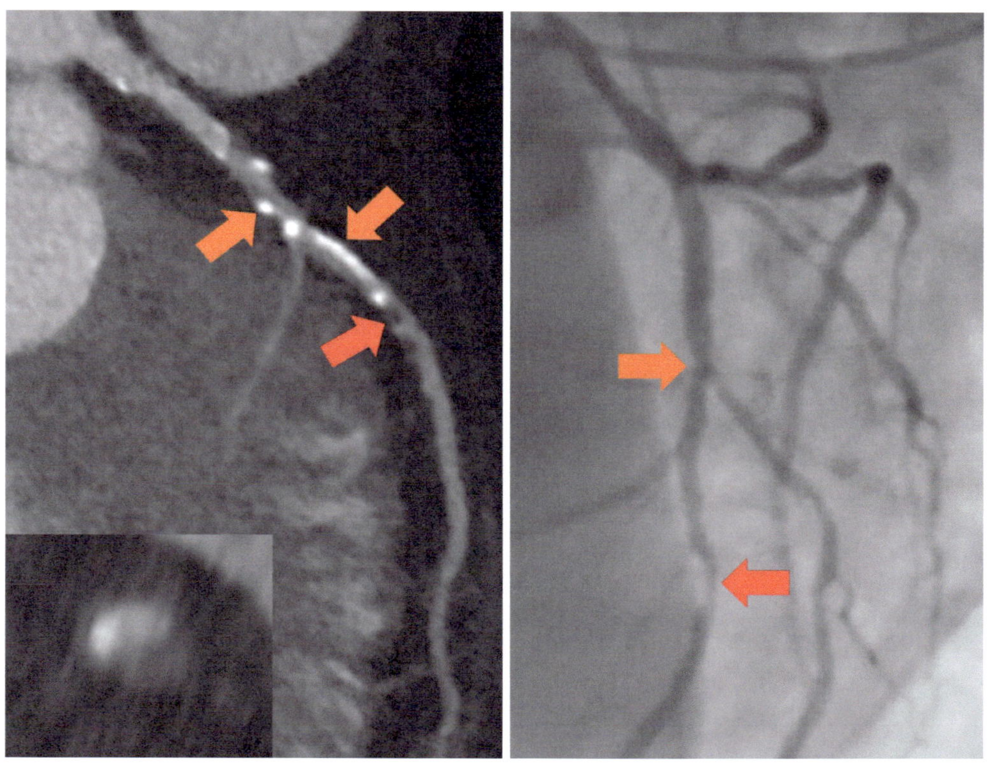

Fig. 26.3 Coronary CT angiography demonstrates partially calcified plaque resulting in moderate luminal narrowing (CAD-RADS 3) at its proximal and mid segment (left and left inset, orange arrows). Coronary angiography confirms diffuse proximal-to-mid vessel calcification in the LAD resulting in focal moderate stenosis (right, orange arrow). Angiography shows additional severe stenosis in the mid LAD (red arrows)

systems described above, stenosis of >50% in the left main coronary artery constitutes a severe (CAD-RADS 4B) lesion. Figure 26.6 demonstrates the CT appearance of a severe left main stenosis.

When describing the overall extent of coronary artery disease burden throughout the entire coronary artery tree as opposed to for a single plaque, two potential commonly used clinical scores are the segment stenosis score and the segment involvement score [9]. The segment involvement score can be calculated as the total number of coronary artery segments demonstrating any degree of plaque, with a minimum of 0 and a maximum of 16 when considering

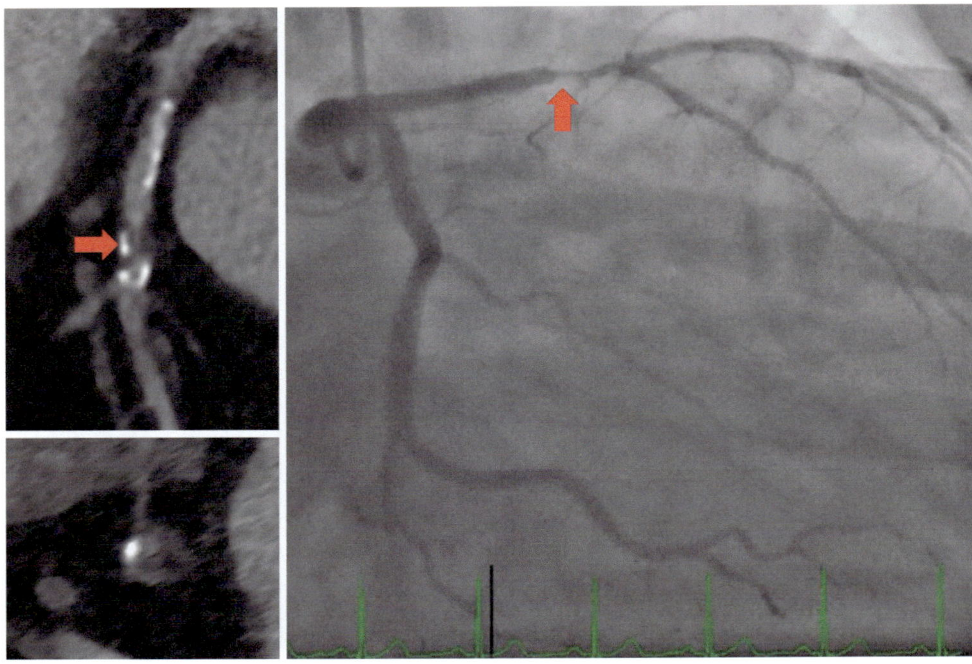

Fig. 26.4 Coronary CT angiography demonstrates partially calcified plaque in the proximal LAD with severe (CAD-RADS 4) luminal narrowing in the long (left top, red arrow) and short axis (left bottom). Coronary angiography confirms 80% stenosis in the proximal LAD (left, red arrow)

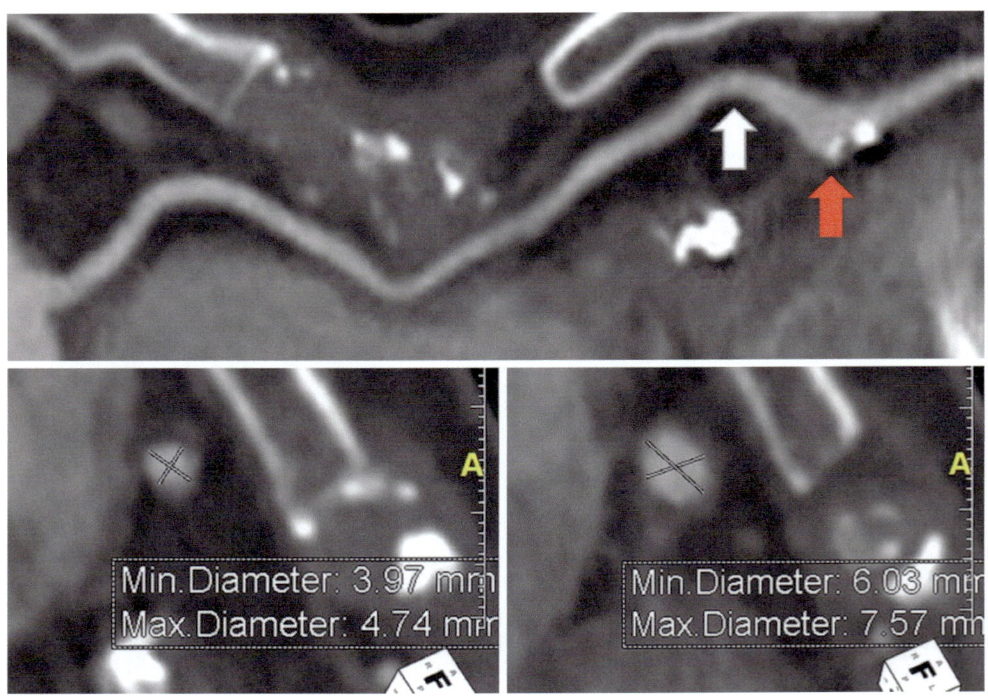

Fig. 26.5 Atherosclerotic aneurysm within the distal RCA in a region of partially calcified plaque (top, red arrow). The diameter within the aneurysm (bottom right) measures >1.5 times that of the vessel proximal to the aneurysm (bottom left, white arrow in top image)

the entire coronary tree. Alternatively, the segment stenosis score grades each coronary segment as demonstrating no to severe plaque (i.e., scores from 0 to 3), which are then summed to yield a total score ranging from 0 to 48. Figure 26.7 demonstrates multi-segment plaque involvement of all three coronary arteries. Given that there is mild stenosis in the left main, mid LAD, and proximal and mid RCA (each 1 point) as well as moderate stenosis in the proximal LAD, proximal LCx, and distal RCA (each 2 points), the segment stenosis score would be 1+1+1+1+2+2+2 for a total of 10. The segment involvement score would be 7, as 7 total coronary artery segments demonstrate plaque.

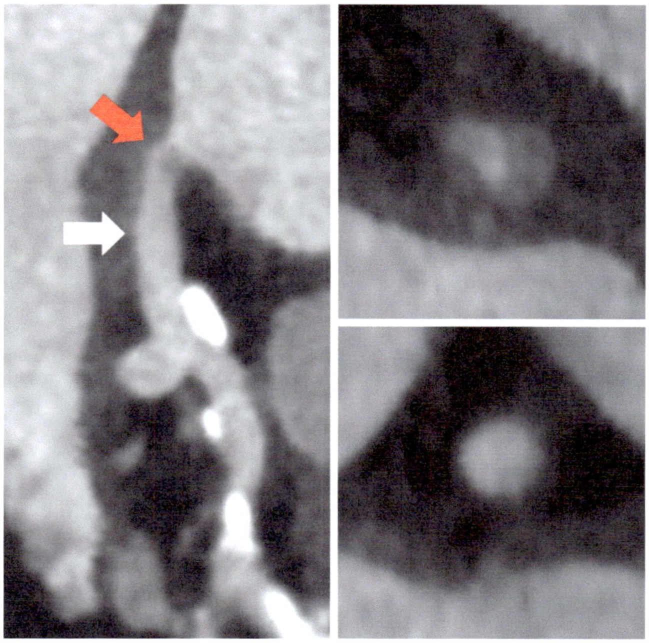

Fig. 26.6 Severe (>50%) stenosis of the LM due to a noncalcified plaque viewed in long axis (left, red arrow). Short-axis images demonstrate the vessel appearance at the level of the stenosis (top right) and distal to the stenosis (bottom right, white arrow in long-axis image)

Chronic Total Occlusion

On the spectrum of coronary artery stenosis secondary to atherosclerotic plaque, the most extreme manifestation is chronic total occlusion (CTO). This entity is defined as complete occlusion of a coronary artery for greater than 3 months [10] and in some situations can be clinically silent for an extended period of time before coming to attention after an acute event in another vessel. In recent years, techniques have been developed to attempt percutaneous coronary intervention (PCI) for revascularization of CTOs, although they remain quite technically challenging. Factors for which the imager should evaluate that are correlated with a lower chance of technical success during revascularization include a blunt stump, lesion calcification, a CTO that is in a vessel other than the left anterior descending coronary artery, and lesion length $\geq$20 mm [11]. Detailed reporting of these factors may assist the referring interventional physician in understanding the likelihood of technical success and determining appropriate candidates. Figure 26.8 demonstrates the CTA appearance of a chronic total occlusion of the left anterior descending coronary artery.

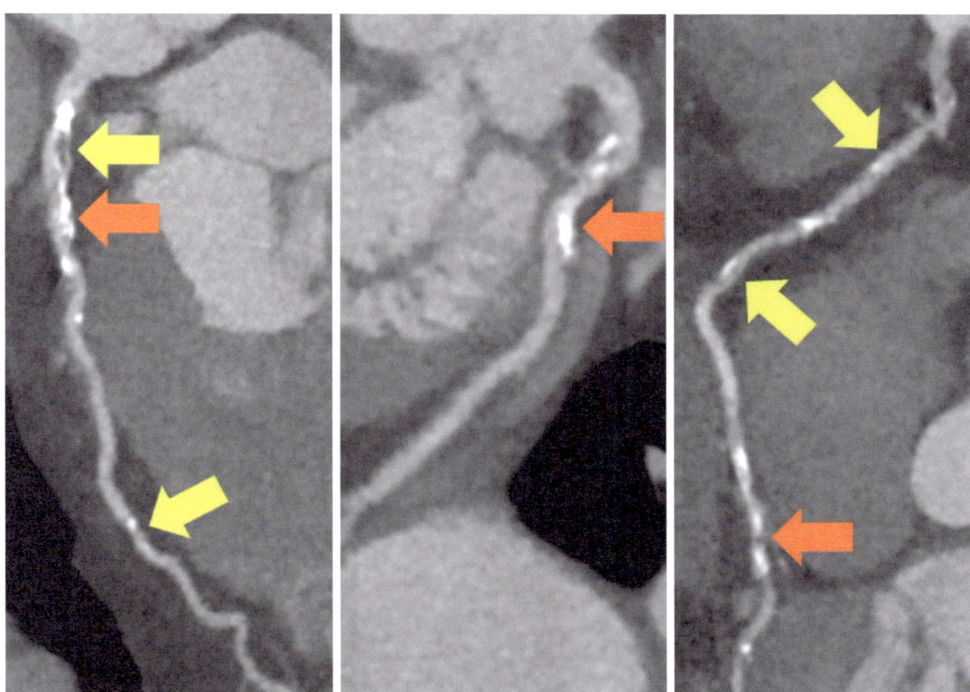

Fig. 26.7 Multi-segment plaque involvement of all three coronary arteries (LM and LAD, left; LCx, middle; RCA, right). Curved planar reformats demonstrate mild luminal narrowing (yellow arrows) in the LM, mid LAD, and proximal and mid RCA. Moderate luminal stenoses (orange arrows) are in the proximal LAD, proximal LCx, and distal RCA

High-Risk Plaque Features

Multiple coronary artery plaque features have been identified that are independently linked with adverse outcomes. These have been termed high-risk plaque (HRP) features and are important to recognize clinically. The four most commonly referenced are low-attenuation plaque, spotty calcium, positive remodeling, and the "napkin-ring" sign. Low-attenuation plaque has been defined as attenuation less than 30 Hounsfield units (HU) in three regions of interest (ROIs) within the noncalcified portion of a plaque [12, 13]. Low-attenuation plaque is thought to reflect lipid-rich plaque which is histologically vulnerable to rupture. Spotty calcium has been defined as the presence of calcified plaque with a diameter of less than 3 mm in direction, length less than 1.5 times the vessel diameter, and width less than two-thirds of the vessel diameter [14–16]. Positive remodeling is generally defined as a ratio of outer vessel diameter in the region of plaque to uninvolved vessel of 1.1 or greater [17, 18]. The "napkin-ring" sign is defined as a noncalcified portion of coronary artery plaque with a higher attenuation peripheral ring and a lower attenuation core [19–21]. The "napkin-ring" sign is thought to correspond by histology to a thin-cap fibroatheroma which may be vulnerable to rupture. Figures 26.9, 26.10, 26.11, and 26.12 demonstrate the CT appearance of these four high-risk plaque features.

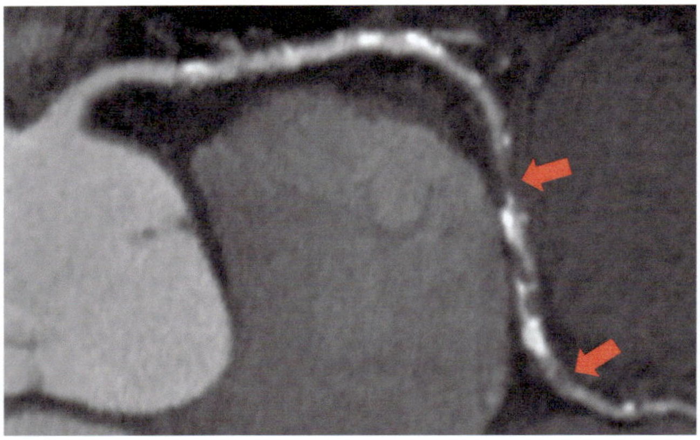

Fig. 26.8 Curved planar reformat demonstrates chronic total occlusion of approximately 30 mm length (red arrows demarcate full length) of the mid RCA with following additional characteristics: tapered stump and calcification greater than 50%

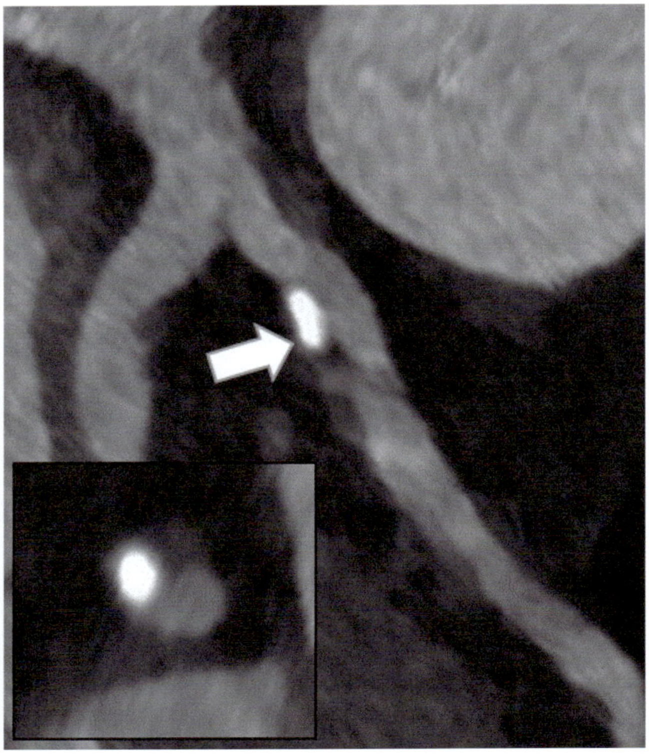

Fig. 26.9 Coronary CT angiography images demonstrating mild stenosis with positive remodeling (ratio of plaque to uninvolved vessel >1.1) due to a partially calcified plaque in the wall of the proximal LAD (white arrow) with corresponding short-axis view (inset)

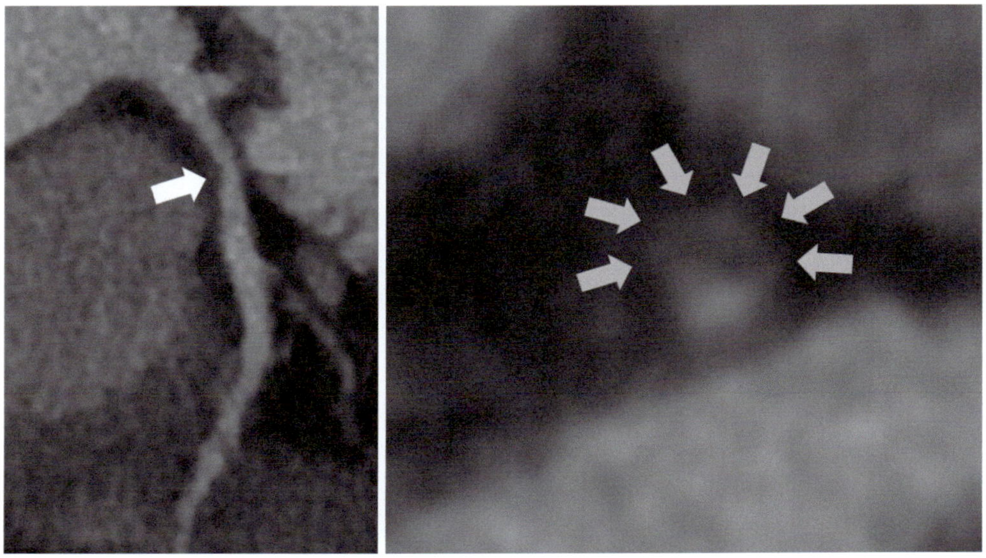

Fig. 26.10 Coronary CT angiography images in long- and short-axis views demonstrating focal noncalcified plaque causing moderate luminal narrowing in the proximal LAD (left, white arrow). This plaque exhibits high-risk plaque features including low attenuation, positive remodeling, and napkin-ring sign (right, light gray arrows)

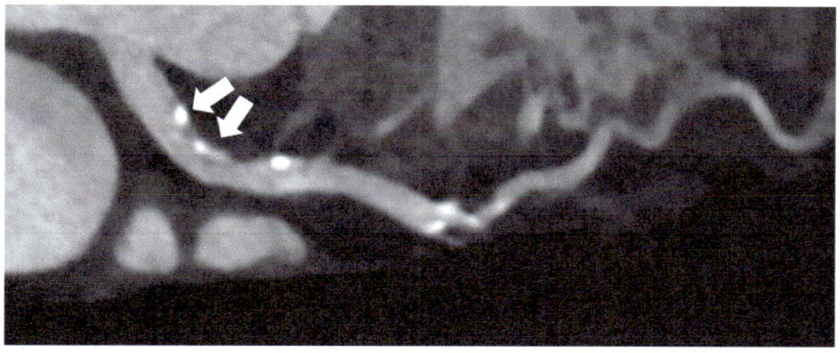

Fig. 26.11 Curved planar reformat demonstrates spotty calcification in the proximal LAD (white arrows)

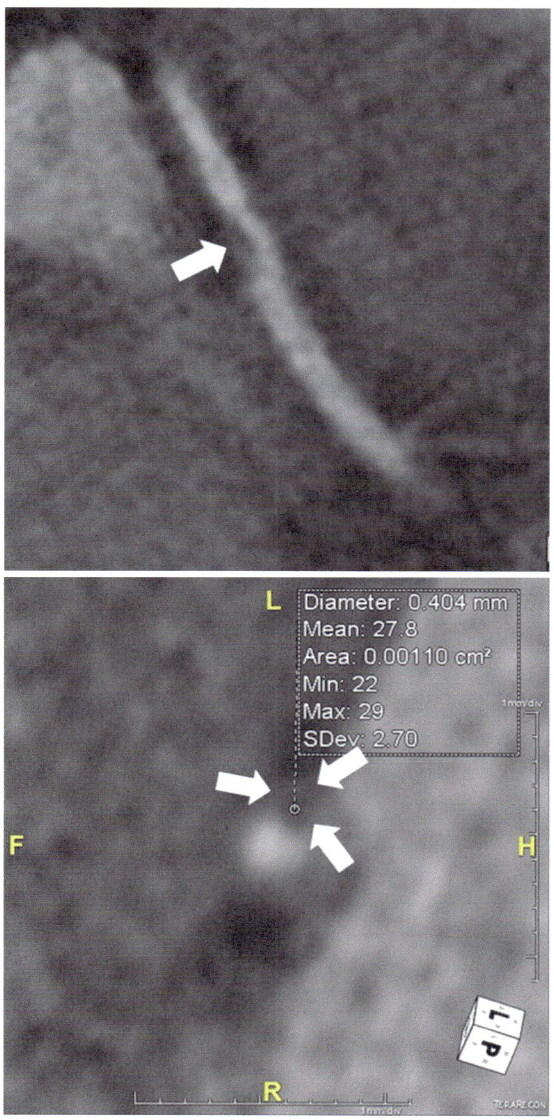

Fig. 26.12 Coronary CT angiography images in long-axis (left) and short-axis (right) views demonstrating noncalcified plaque with low attenuation (<30 HU) in the wall of the distal RCA (white arrows and ROI)

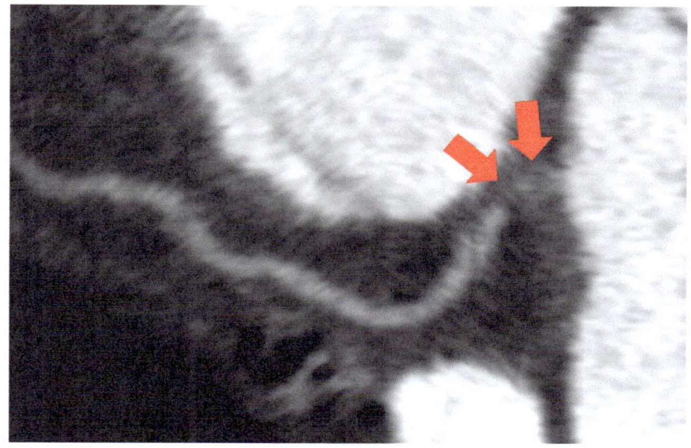

Fig. 26.13 Coronary CT angiography curved planar reformat demonstrating short-segment atherothrombotic occlusion of the RCA at its ostium (red arrows)

High-risk plaque features increase the rate of plaque rupture, which can be responsible for acute coronary syndrome (ACS) secondary to atherothrombosis, which is the development of coronary thrombosis superimposed on a ruptured plaque. Atherothrombosis is a main cause of unstable angina and acute myocardial infarction [22]. Figure 26.13 demonstrates the CT appearance of an atherothrombotic occlusion of a coronary artery.

Perivascular fat stranding has been identified as a sign of plaque rupture, which is an important entity to identify in the emergency setting. Figure 26.14 demonstrates the CT appearance of perivascular stranding adjacent to an acute plaque rupture [23].

After a percutaneous intervention has been performed and a stent has been placed across a stenosis felt to be hemodynamically significant, subsequent in-stent stenosis can develop over time due to neointimal hyperplasia. Challenges in imaging in-stent restenosis include beam hardening and partial volume averaging artifacts, which can be mitigated in part by the use of scanners with high spatial resolution and iterative reconstruction [24]. Figure 26.15 demonstrates the CT appearance of in-stent restenosis in a diagonal branch coronary artery.

A final entity which should not be confused for atherosclerotic plaque is a myocardial bridge, where a segment of coronary artery travels through the myocardium (Fig. 26.16). Plaque within a bridge is unusual, although plaque can form proximally, perhaps due to unusual shear stress at the entry point to the myocardium.

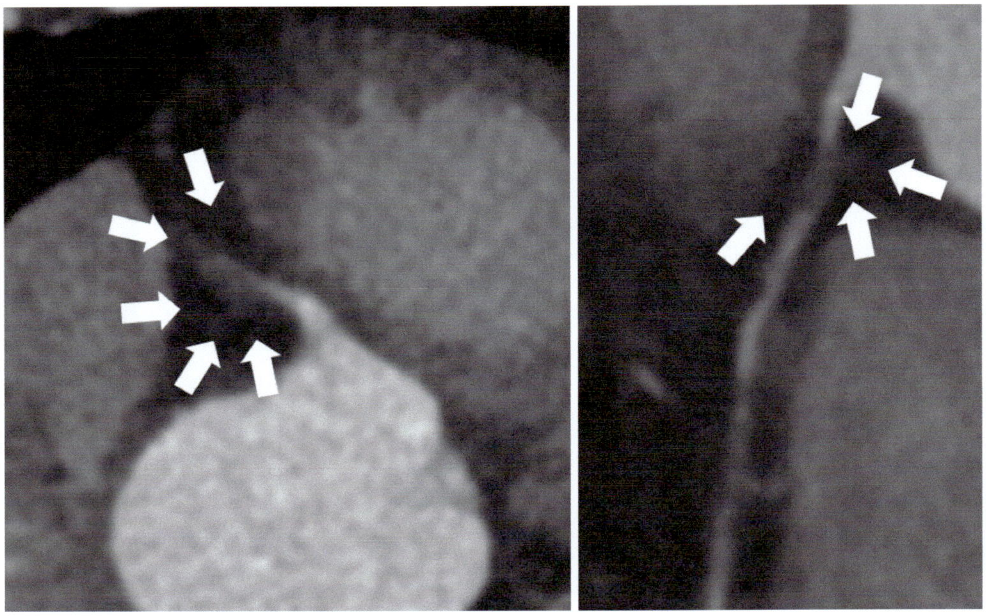

Fig. 26.14 Coronary CT angiography demonstrating perivascular fat stranding (white arrows) adjacent to an acute plaque rupture within the proximal RCA in axial view (left) and curved planar reformat (right)

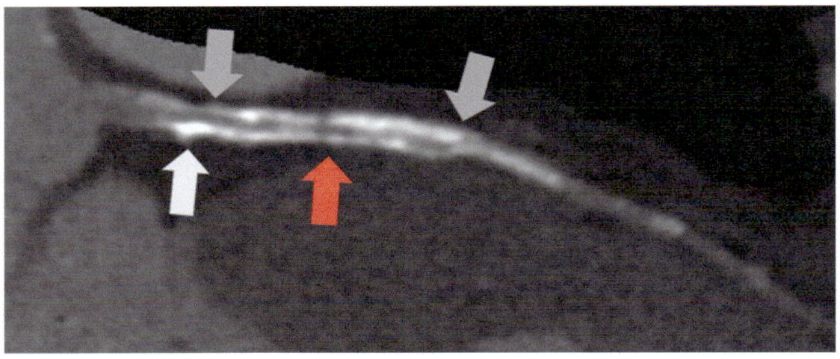

Fig. 26.15 Curved planar reformat of the LAD with a partially calcified plaque (white arrow) and a stent that spans approximately 40 mm from the distal LM to the mid LAD (light gray arrows) with segments of in-stent restenosis (red arrow)

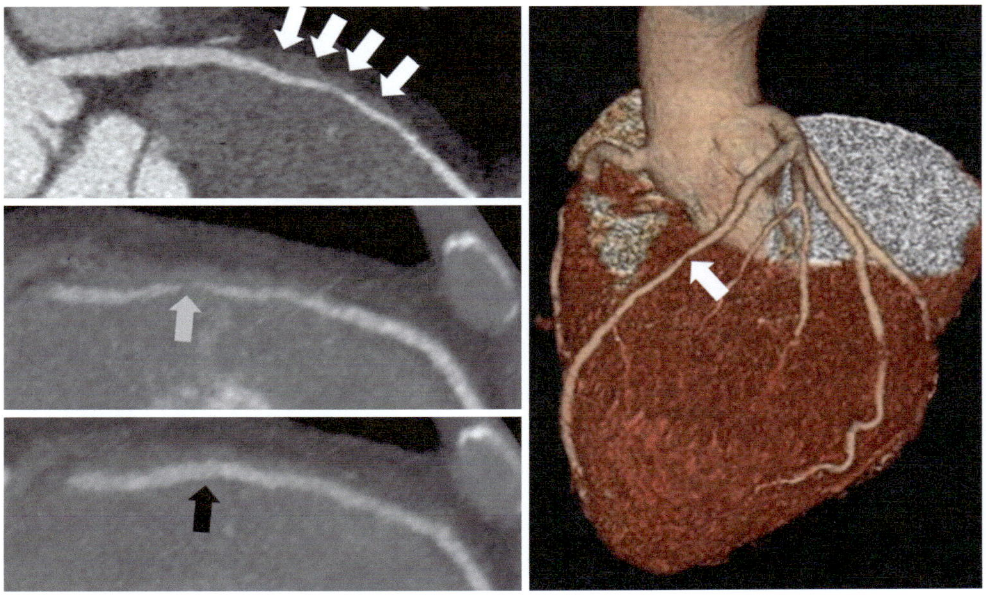

Fig. 26.16 Coronary CT angiography demonstrating myocardial bridge in the mid LAD with myocardium overlying the vessel (top left, white arrows). Evidence of systolic compression (middle left, gray arrow; right, white arrow) and diastolic decompression (bottom left, black arrow)

Conclusion

Atherosclerosis in the coronary arteries can have many faces and take on a wide variety of appearances on CT. Familiarity with the characteristic types of plaque composition as well as the degrees of stenosis in which they result is at the core of cardiac CT imaging. Knowledge of the appearance of chronic total occlusions and the relationship with PCI, as well as of the role of specific plaque features in conferring an elevated risk of adverse events, is also an essential component of a high-quality practice of acquiring and interpreting CT of the heart.

References

1. O'Rourke RA, Brundage BH, Froelicher VF, Greenland P, Grundy SM, Hachamovitch R, et al. American College of Cardiology/American Heart Association Expert Consensus document on electron-beam computed tomography for the diagnosis and prognosis of coronary artery disease. Circulation. 2000;102(1):126–40.
2. Weigold WG, Abbara S, Achenbach S, Arbab-Zadeh A, Berman D, Carr JJ, et al. Standardized medical terminology for cardiac computed tomography: a report of the Society of Cardiovascular Computed Tomography. J Cardiovasc Comput Tomogr. 2011;5(3):136–44.
3. Rodriguez-Granillo GA, Carrascosa P, Bruining N. Progression of coronary artery calcification at the crossroads: sign of progression or stabilization of coronary atherosclerosis? Cardiovasc Diagn Therapy. 2016;6(3):250–8.
4. Andrew M, John H. The challenge of coronary calcium on coronary computed tomographic angiography (CCTA) scans: effect on interpretation and possible solutions. Int J Cardiovasc Imaging. 2015;31(Suppl 2):145–57.
5. Raff GL, Abidov A, Achenbach S, Berman DS, Boxt LM, Budoff MJ, et al. SCCT guidelines for the interpretation and reporting of coronary computed tomographic angiography. J Cardiovasc Comput Tomogr. 2009;3(2):122–36.
6. Abbara S, Blanke P, Maroules CD, Cheezum M, Choi AD, Han BK, et al. SCCT guidelines for the performance and acquisition of coronary computed tomographic angiography: a report of the society of Cardiovascular Computed Tomography Guidelines Committee: endorsed by the North American Society for Cardiovascular Imaging (NASCI). J Cardiovasc Comput Tomogr. 2016;10(6):435–49.
7. Diaz-Zamudio M, Bacilio-Perez U, Herrera-Zarza MC, Meave-Gonzalez A, Alexanderson-Rosas E, Zambrana-Balta GF, et al. Coronary artery aneurysms and ectasia: role of coronary CT angiography. Radiographics Rev Publ Radiol Soc North Am Inc. 2009;29(7):1939–54.
8. Virani SS, Mendoza CE, Ferreira AC, de Marchena E. Left main coronary artery stenosis: factors predicting cardiac events in patients awaiting coronary surgery. Tex Heart Inst J. 2006;33(1):23–6.
9. Min JK, Shaw LJ, Devereux RB, Okin PM, Weinsaft JW, Russo DJ, et al. Prognostic value of multidetector coronary computed tomographic angiography for prediction of all-cause mortality. J Am Coll Cardiol. 2007;50(12):1161–70.
10. Stone GW, Kandzari DE, Mehran R, Colombo A, Schwartz RS, Bailey S, et al. Percutaneous recanalization of chronically occluded coronary arteries. A consensus document: part I. Circulation. 2005;112(15):2364–72.
11. Alessandrino G, Chevalier B, Lefevre T, Sanguineti F, Garot P, Unterseeh T, et al. A clinical and angiographic scoring system to predict the probability of successful first-attempt percutaneous coronary intervention in patients with total chronic coronary occlusion. JACC Cardiovasc Interv. 2015;8(12):1540–8.
12. Motoyama S, Sarai M, Harigaya H, Anno H, Inoue K, Hara T, et al. Computed tomographic angiography characteristics of atherosclerotic plaques subsequently resulting in acute coronary syndrome. J Am Coll Cardiol. 2009;54(1):49–57.
13. Motoyama S, Kondo T, Sarai M, Sugiura A, Harigaya H, Sato T, et al. Multislice computed tomographic characteristics of coronary lesions in acute coronary syndromes. J Am Coll Cardiol. 2007;50(4):319–26.
14. van Velzen JE, de Graaf FR, de Graaf MA, Schuijf JD, Kroft LJ, de Roos A, et al. Comprehensive assessment of spotty calcifications on computed tomography angiography: comparison to plaque characteristics on intravascular ultrasound with radiofrequency backscatter analysis. J Nucl Cardiol Off Publ Am Soc Nucl Cardiol. 2011;18(5):893–903.
15. Kitagawa T, Yamamoto H, Horiguchi J, Ohhashi N, Tadehara F, Shokawa T, et al. Characterization of noncalcified coronary plaques and identification of culprit lesions in patients with acute coronary syndrome by 64-slice computed tomography. J Am Coll Cardiol Img. 2009;2(2):153–60.
16. Kashiwagi M, Tanaka A, Kitabata H, Tsujioka H, Kataiwa H, Komukai K, et al. Feasibility of noninvasive assessment of thin-cap fibroatheroma by multidetector computed tomography. J Am Coll Cardiol Img. 2009;2(12):1412–9.
17. Gauss S, Achenbach S, Pflederer T, Schuhback A, Daniel WG, Marwan M. Assessment of coronary artery remodelling by dual-source CT: a head-to-head comparison with intravascular ultrasound. Heart. 2011;97(12):991–7.
18. Hoffmann U, Moselewski F, Nieman K, Jang IK, Ferencik M, Rahman AM, et al. Noninvasive assessment of plaque morphology and composition in culprit and stable lesions in acute coronary syndrome and stable lesions in stable angina by multidetector computed tomography. J Am Coll Cardiol. 2006;47(8):1655–62.
19. Ito T, Terashima M, Kaneda H, Nasu K, Matsuo H, Ehara M, et al. Comparison of in vivo assessment of vulnerable plaque by 64-slice multislice computed tomography versus optical coherence tomography. Am J Cardiol. 2011;107(9):1270–7.
20. Otsuka K, Fukuda S, Tanaka A, Nakanishi K, Taguchi H, Yoshikawa J, et al. Napkin-ring sign on coronary CT angiography for the prediction of acute coronary syndrome. J Am Coll Cardiol Img. 2013;6(4):448–57.
21. Maurovich-Horvat P, Hoffmann U, Vorpahl M, Nakano M, Virmani R, Alkadhi H. The napkin-ring sign: CT signature of high-risk coronary plaques? J Am Coll Cardiol Img. 2010;3(4):440–4.
22. Fuster V, Moreno PR, Fayad ZA, Corti R, Badimon JJ. Atherothrombosis and high-risk plaque: part I: evolving concepts. J Am Coll Cardiol. 2005;46(6):937–54.
23. Laine P, Kaartinen M, Penttila A, Panula P, Paavonen T, Kovanen PT. Association between myocardial infarction and the mast cells in the adventitia of the infarct-related coronary artery. Circulation. 1999;99(3):361–9.
24. Andreini D, Pontone G, Mushtaq S, Bartorelli AL, Bertella E, Trabattoni D, et al. Coronary in-stent restenosis: assessment with CT coronary angiography. Radiology. 2012;265(2):410–7.

Chronic Chest Pain

27

Richard A. P. Takx and Csilla Celeng

Chronic chest pain is a multifactorial clinical problem, and the diagnosis is based on patients' history. It is characterized by recurrent episodes of chest pain occurring in a relatively stable pattern. About four million cardiac stress tests (in 87% of cases combined with imaging) are performed annually in the United States [1] for chest pain evaluation. There is concern regarding the rising healthcare costs, inappropriate utilization, and patient safety of diagnostic testing, with approximately one-third of cardiac stress tests being likely inappropriately requested [1]. In addition, around 25% of invasive coronary angiography is performed among asymptomatic patients [2].

The primary diagnostic consideration in patients with chronic chest pain is coronary artery disease (CAD). The prevalence of stable angina increases with age for both sexes, from 5–7% at 45–64 years to 10–12% at 65–84 years in females and from 4–7% at 45–64 years to 12–14% at 65–84 in males [3]. Of note is that angina is more prevalent in middle-aged females than in males, most likely due to microvascular disease, while at older age angina is more prevalent in males [4, 5]. There is no accurate epidemiological data on the frequency of microvascular angina and vasospastic angina. However, recent clinical data suggest that coronary microvascular spasm is present in two-third of patients with normal angiograms [6]. Conventional cardiovascular risk factors such hypertension, hyperlipidemia, diabetes, physical inactivity, obesity, smoking and family history facilitate the progression of CAD. Patients with diabetes mellitus have a similar risk for myocardial infarction as patients without diabetes with prior myocardial infarction [7]. Nevertheless, the occurrence of chest pain in this patient population is less frequent due to a high threshold for pain. Diabetes and hypertension might be accompanied by renal dysfunction, which has a negative impact on the prognosis of patients with stable angina. In patients with chronic kidney disease (CKD), symptoms of chest pain are often misleading due to diabetic and uremic neuropathy [8]. Besides CAD, coronary artery anomalies can also lead to the development of chronic chest pain. Myocardial bridging is one of the most common coronary anomalies. The reported prevalence of myocardial bridging depends on the diagnostic method used. Autopsy studies report a wide prevalence of 5–86% [9], coronary angiography studies 0.4–15.8% [10], and in CT studies numbers range between 4% and 58% [11].

Pathophysiology of Stable Chest Pain

Stable CAD is typically characterized by recurrent episodes of myocardial ischemia due to a mismatch between oxygen demand and supply, which can be induced by exercise, emotion, or other forms of stress, but it may also occur spontaneously. These ischemic/hypoxic episodes are commonly associated with transient chest discomfort (i.e. angina pectoris). The occurrence of angina can be attributable to various pathological conditions including (1) plaque-related coronary artery stenosis, (2) focal or diffuse spasm of the coronary arteries, (3) microvascular disease, (4) ischemic cardiomyopathy/left ventricular dysfunction, and (5) coronary anomalies. These mechanisms may act separate but can also overlap in the same patient, and some may change over time [4]. The clinical manifestation of angina may be specific for the underlying pathology. Effort-induced angina is associated with coronary artery stenosis and/or local vasoconstriction at the site of the stenosis and/or microvascular dysfunction, while rest angina is related to focal or diffuse vasospasm of the epicardial vessels or the microvasculature. Hypoxia-induced metabolic changes initiate the ischemic cascade, and the consequences occur in a predefined temporal manner (Fig. 27.1):

R. A. P. Takx (✉)
Department of Radiology, University Medical Center Utrecht, Utrecht, The Netherlands
e-mail: r.a.p.takx@umcutrecht.nl

C. Celeng
Department of Radiology, Heart and Vascular Center, Semmelweis University, Budapest, Hungary

U. J. Schoepf (ed.), *CT of the Heart*, Contemporary Medical Imaging, https://doi.org/10.1007/978-1-60327-237-7_27

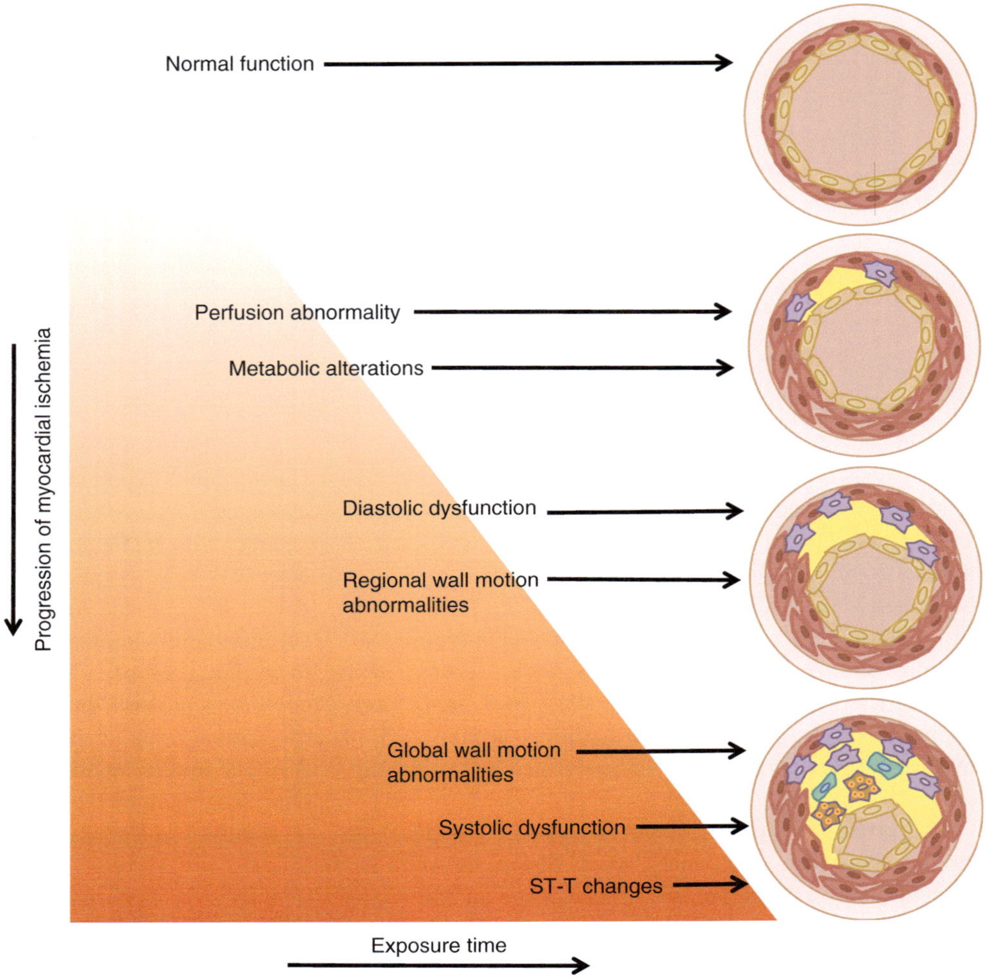

Fig. 27.1 The ischemic cascade; perfusion abnormality caused by reduced coronary blood flow initiates the ischemic cascade, and the consequences occur in a predefined temporal manner

1. During ischemia, the anaerobic conditions prevail, which results in a decrease of cell pH. To balance the accumulation of hydrogen ions, the Na^+/H^+ exchanger excretes excess hydrogen ions, which entails a large influx of sodium ions. Hypoxia also depletes the cellular concentration of ATP, which leads to the decreased function of Na^+/K^+-ATPase pump and K-ATP channels. These mechanisms lead to accumulation of extracellular K^+ and membrane depolarization, which inactivates the Na^+ channels. Decreased action potential upstroke leads to reduced conduction velocity, which can result in the development of arrhythmias. Furthermore, ATP pump dysfunction reduces the active efflux of Ca^{2+} and its reuptake to the endoplasmic reticulum, thus causing intracellular Ca^{2+} overload, which induces Ca^{2+}-dependent apoptotic cascade and tissue damage [12].
2. Perfusion abnormalities lead to metabolic changes and abnormal myocardial performance that involves diastolic dysfunction (slowed ventricular relaxation) and systolic dysfunction with regional and later global wall motion abnormalities (reduced ejection fraction).
3. These mechanisms result in the development of ST-T segment changes on the ECG.
4. Finally myocardial ischemia manifests in chest pain [13]. Other "angina equivalent" symptoms such as dyspnea, fatigue, palpitations, or syncope can be also present in addition to or instead of angina.

Histological Characteristics of Atherosclerotic Plaques

Previous investigations revealed that atherosclerotic plaques in patients with stable chest pain show different histological characteristics than those with acute coronary syndrome: stable plaques are associated with smaller necrotic core and a thicker cap (>84 μm) [14] made up of smooth muscle cells and contain less macrophages [15–17]. In contrast plaques that are prone to rupture usually have a large necrotic core with an overlying thin fibrous cap (between 55 μm and 84 μm), which is infiltrated by macrophages [14]. The presence of calcification as a marker of plaque stability is still unclear. Unstable plaques detected in patients in their fourth decade tend to contain more calcification than stable plaques; however, with increasing age this difference disappears and more calcification is observed in stable plaques compared to unstable plaques [18]. Coronary computed tomography angiography (CTA) provides a noninvasive approach for the detection of coronary atherosclerotic lesions. Beyond the visualization of the coronary artery lumen, the submillimeter spatial resolution of CTA allows for detailed characterization as well as quantification of coronary plaques. Similar to histology, stable and unstable plaques on CTA show different characteristics: stable plaques have smaller plaque volume and area, lower remodeling indices, and lower proportion of non-calcified material [19, 20]. In contrast unstable lesions have higher plaque volume and area, higher remodeling indices and contain a greater proportion of non-calcified component representing the necrotic core (Fig. 27.2) [19, 20].

Focal or Diffuse Spasm of the Coronary Arteries

Vasospastic angina (often called as variant or Prinzmetal's angina) is determined as a focal and/or diffuse narrowing of normal or diseased epicardial artery that can result in the reduction of coronary blood flow [21]. Focal spasm is typically characterized by ST-segment elevation, while diffuse vasoconstriction is usually followed by ST depression.

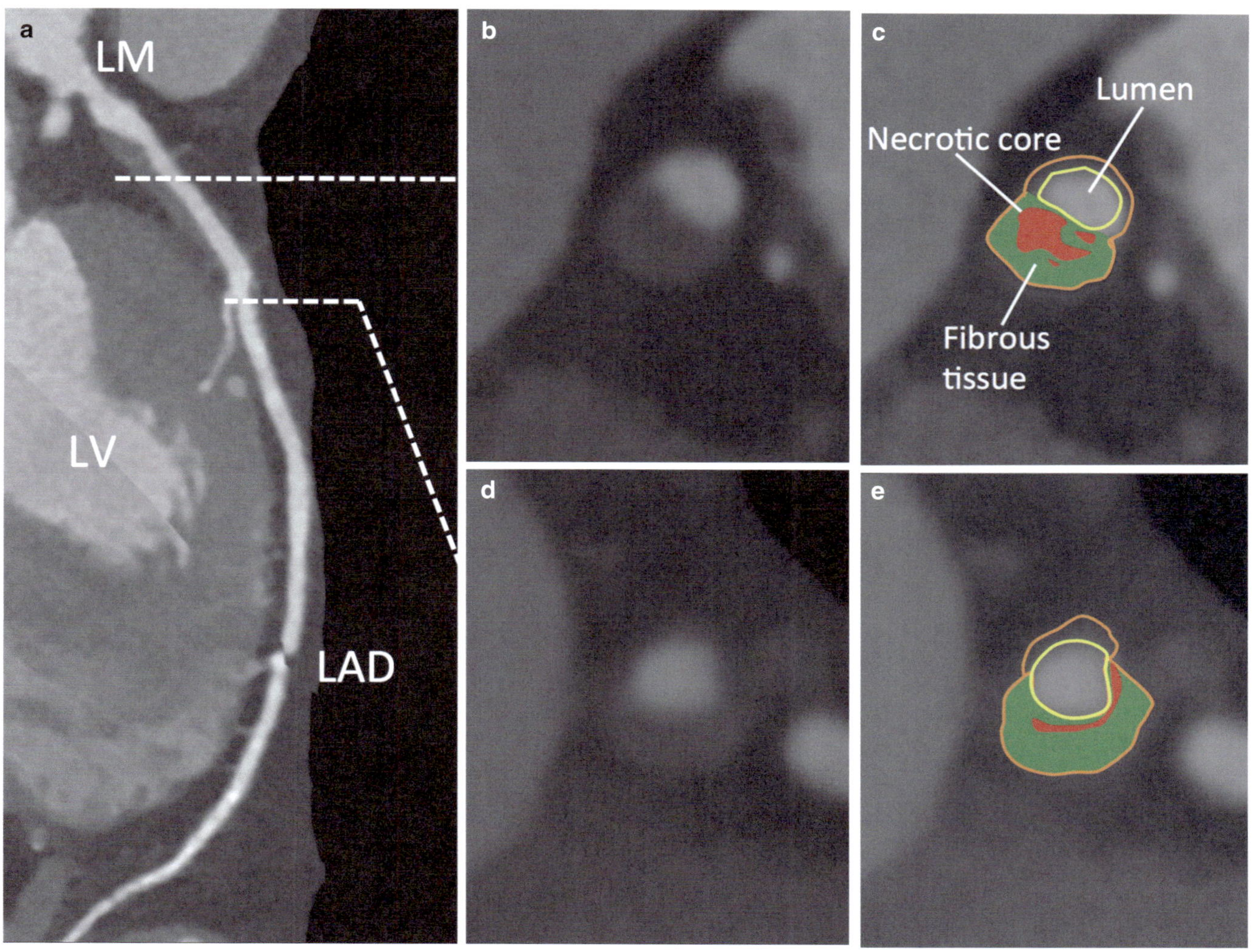

Fig. 27.2 Curved multiplanar reconstruction (**a**) of the LM-LAD with the presence of non-calcified plaques. Horizontal lines represent two different plaque types. Cross-sectional images of the first plaque without (**b**) and with color overlay (**c**) represent an unstable plaque, with positive remodeling, large necrotic core (red), and smaller amount of fibrous tissue (green). Cross-sectional images of the second plaque without (**d**) and with (**e**) color overlay show a stable plaque with a smaller necrotic core and more pronounced fibrous tissue

Coronary spasm can result in myocardial ischemia, arrhythmias, and heart failure and may even lead to myocardial infarction [22]. Spastic motion can be frequently found in the coronary microvasculature alone (microvascular angina) and might suggest the presence of the underlying microvascular disease [6]. The pathogenesis of abnormal coronary vasomotion is heterogeneous and involves several contributing factors such as increased kinase activity, which induces the phosphorylation of myosin light chain and consequently the contraction of smooth muscle cells [23]; endothelial dysfunction that results in an altered paracrine signaling as well as in enhanced release of vasoactive substances such as endothelin [24]; hyperreactivity of the autonomic nervous system, in which imbalances in both sympathetic and parasympathetic neurotransmitters can induce coronary artery spasm; smoking that results in the exposure of toxic agents, which can cause damage of the vascular system, thus increasing the risk of coronary spasm; and a high prevalence of coronary vasospasm that was observed in Asian people [25]. Also, in a recent European cohort, microvascular spasm was found in two-third of patients with normal coronary arteriograms and was shown to occur more frequently in females [6]. Currently, vasospasm is demonstrated using invasive provocation tests (ergonovine or acetylcholine). In the future coronary CTA might become a useful tool for the diagnosis of vasospasm in the absence of provocation tests, for example, by performing double-acquisition coronary CTA in the absence and presence of intravenous infusion of nitrate [26].

Microvascular Dysfunction

Stable microvascular angina (often referred to as cardiac syndrome X) is described as effort-induced chest pain that is attributable to abnormal circulation in small coronary arteries (<500 μm) [27]. Similar to epicardial stenosis, microvascular dysfunction is also characterized by the reduction of coronary blood flow; however, the pattern of myocardial ischemia is substantially different. Flow-limiting stenosis in epicardial arteries results in a homogenously distributed perfusion defect and is accompanied by impairment of segmental ventricular contraction. In contrast, microvascular dysfunction is characterized by a more scattered manner of perfusion defects and preserved segmental ventricular contraction, due to the presence of normal myocardial cells. This phenomenon might explain the arising difficulties when trying to identify the presence of microvascular ischemia by standard imaging methods (Fig. 27.3). Microvascular dysfunction can be associated with various pathological mechanisms. Impaired bioactivity of the endothelium-dependent nitric oxide is the most common cause of reduced vascular relaxation. Abnormal

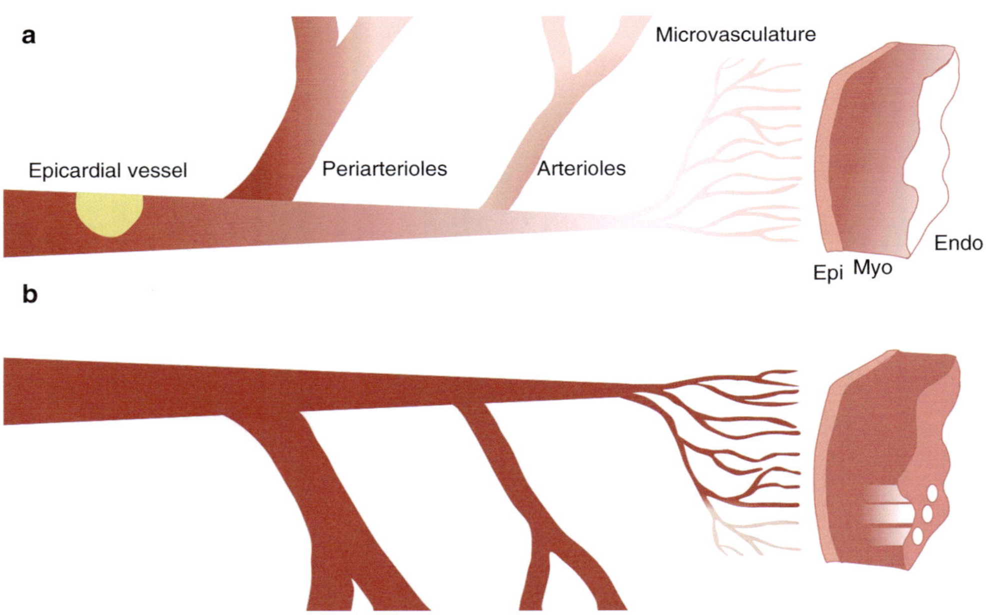

Fig. 27.3 Epicardial stenosis (**a**) and attributable gradual decreasing of coronary blood flow within myocardial layers covering the epicardial-endocardial axis. Homogenous distribution of the perfusion defect results in detectable segmental impairment of contractile function. Microvascular dysfunction (**b**) involves small myocardial areas and leads to the development of more localized perfusion defects. Patchy distribution of ischemic territories hampers the detection of abnormal contractile function due to the presence of normal contractile myocardial cells within the same myocardial segment. Epi: epicardium, myo: myocardium, endo: endocardium

endothelial function in patients with higher cholesterol level leads to reduced release of nitric oxide [28]. Similarly, decreased level of estradiol in postmenopausal females is associated with increased breakdown of nitric oxide [29]. In the *W*omen's *I*schemia *S*yndrome *E*valuation (WISE) study during a 5.4-year follow-up period, a significant association was found between lower coronary flow reserve (due to microvascular dysfunction) and major adverse outcomes in females of whom the majority (81%) had either no CAD or non-obstructive CAD on invasive angiography [30]. Other conditions including hypertension, diabetes, and ventricular hypertrophy can also contribute to the development of microvascular dysfunction. Reduced vasodilator response of the diseased small vessels supports the development of coronary steal phenomenon by normal microvessels, thus leading to myocardial ischemia. The spatial resolution of current CT scanners (≈400 μm) limits the precise detection of microvascular disease; however, future technical advances in stress-induced CT myocardial perfusion might serve as a noninvasive imaging method for detecting microvascular disease [31].

Ischemic Cardiomyopathy

Chronic chest pain can be a clinical manifestation of ischemic cardiomyopathy, which has been defined as left ventricular systolic dysfunction with a history of prior myocardial infarction or revascularization, or ≥75% stenosis of left main or proximal LAD, or ≥75% stenosis of two or more epicardial vessels [32]. The development of chronic dysfunction is of particular interest due to the observation that chronically hypoperfused myocardium (i.e., hibernating myocardium) after revascularization can recover [33]. The pathophysiological background of this phenomenon is characterized by a spectrum of adaptive mechanism (including myocardial stunning, hibernation, and scarring) in which the "smart heart" reduces the myocardial demand by a loss in contractile apparatus [34]. Myocardial stunning evolves after 15–20 min of reduced perfusion and is most probably caused by the abnormal function of the sarcoplasmic reticulum due to oxygen radicals [35]. After restoration of blood flow, impaired contractility can persist up to several hours, but eventually it leads to full recovery. More prolonged periods of ischemia lead to the development of myocardial hibernation where besides metabolic alterations several structural changes in the contractile material occur (e.g., loss of sarcoplasmic reticulum and t-tubules). The hibernated myocardium represents the hallmarks of left ventricular remodeling; however, at early stages no scarring mechanism is present. In case of chronic hibernation, structural changes such as diffuse fibrosis and expansion of extracellular matrix stay fixed and eventually result in myocardial scarring. The ability of delayed contrast-enhanced CTA to differentiate viable and nonviable myocardium has been already established in animal studies, where both acute and chronic infarction appeared as hyperenhanced areas on CTA ≈5 min after the contrast injection [36]. Since the method is accompanied by only a slight increase in radiation dose in the future, its application might be relevant in the comprehensive evaluation of patients with advanced cardiovascular disease.

Coronary Anomaly

Myocardial bridging may also be associated with exertional angina. It is characterized by the presence of cardiac muscle overlying part of a coronary artery [37] and usually involves the left descending artery [38] (Fig. 27.4). Ultrasound studies showed that during early diastole, when coronary blood flow is highest, myocardial bridging results in delayed relaxation, thus limiting coronary flow [39]. Coronary lesions

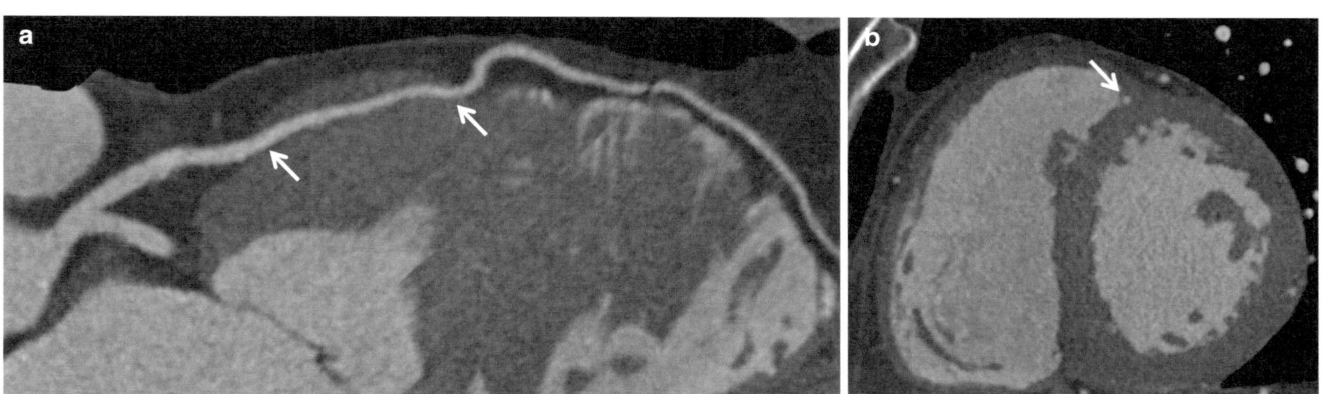

Fig. 27.4 Myocardial bridge in a 53-year-old male with chronic chest pain. Curved multiplanar reconstruction of the LM-LAD (**a**) with the presence of a myocardial bridge in the middle part of the LAD (arrows). Short-axis reconstruction (**b**) and cross section of the LAD (arrow) with an overlying myocardial tissue

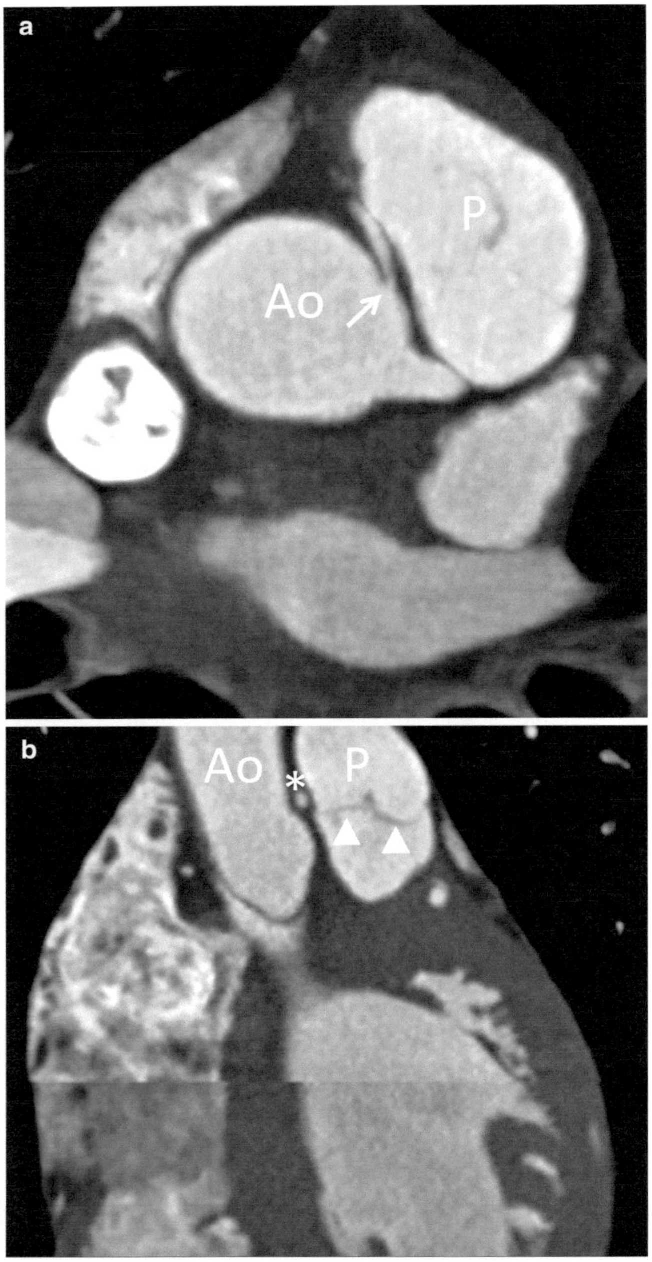

Fig. 27.5 Axial (**a**) and coronal (**b**) reconstructions of a patient without CAD but with an abnormal origin of the right coronary artery (arrow) with a malignant course (*) between the aorta (Ao) and the pulmonary trunk (P) above the pulmonary valve (arrowheads)

usually evolve proximal to the bridge [40]. Anomalous origin of a coronary artery arising from the opposite sinus can be also a cause of chronic chest pain. A course between the pulmonary trunk and aorta is considered malignant or interarterial course (Fig. 27.5). The 3D nature of CTA allows for precise characterization of the myocardial bridge and enables accurate visualization of the anomalous origin and course of the coronary artery.

Diagnosing CAD in Patients with Chronic Chest Pain

All patients suspected of chronic chest pain without an obvious noncardiac cause should undergo 12-lead resting ECG [4, 41]. Though a normal resting ECG does not exclude the presence of myocardial ischemia, it may demonstrate signs of prior myocardial infarction and is useful as a baseline reference. Prior to diagnostic imaging, estimation of pre-test probability may assist in the decision on appropriate imaging technique and help to avoid unnecessary invasive procedures [42]. The pre-test probability can be determined using risk calculators such as ASCVD risk (https://tools.acc.org/ASCVD-Risk-Estimator/) or SCORE (https://www.escardio.org/Guidelines-&-Education/Practice-tools/CVD-prevention-toolbox/SCORE-Risk-Charts). Patients with a pre-test probability between 15 and 85% are recommended to undergo noninvasive testing (Table 27.1) [4]. Exercise ECG can be used as an initial test for diagnosing stable coronary artery disease, with a good specificity of 85–90% and a limited sensitivity of 45–50% [43, 44]. Prior to exercise ECG patients should temporarily stop taking anti-ischemic medication and have a relative normal ECG at baseline. Nonetheless the test may be inconclusive in some patients (usually when 85% of maximum heart rate is not reached) [4]. Therefore if available (i.e. equipment and expertise), myocardial perfusion imaging (MPI) or coronary CTA is recommended [4]. MPI can be performed using single-photon emission computed tomography (SPECT), echocardiography (i.e., wall motion abnormality), magnetic resonance imaging (MRI), positron emission tomography (PET), and computed tomography (CT). In a meta-analysis [45], the diagnostic accuracy of the various MPI techniques was compared to invasive coronary angiography (ICA) with fractional flow reserve (FFR) for the diagnosis of hemodynamically significant CAD. PET, CT, and MRI demonstrated superior diagnostic accuracy compared to SPECT and echocardiography (Fig. 27.6). Considering that MRI does not expose the patient to ionizing radiation and has good diagnostic performance [46], MRI could be regarded as the technique of choice, with CT being an appropriate alternative in those who have contraindications for undergoing MRI. Adenosine stress-rest cardiac CT is able to identify stress-induced myocardial perfusion defects and as such is capable of reducing the number of false-positive CTA findings [47, 48]. Using dual-source CT ventricular function and wall motion abnormalities can be obtained by prospectively ECG-triggered (80% reduced mAs) dual-step pulsing [49] or full radiation using retrospective ECG-gated CTA.

Coronary CTA is an increasingly popular alternative for ruling out CAD. The examination traditionally consists of two diagnostic parts: first a non-contrast scan is made for

Table 27.1 Pre-test probability of CAD in patients with chest pain split on sex

	Non-cardiac chest pain		Atypical chest pain		Typical chest pain	
Age (y)	Female	Male	Female	Male	Female	Male
30 - 39		Intermediate	Low	Intermediate	Intermediate	Intermediate
40 - 49		Intermediate	Low	Intermediate	Intermediate	High
50 - 59	Low	Intermediate	Intermediate	Intermediate	Intermediate	High
60 - 69	Intermediate	Intermediate	Intermediate	Intermediate	Intermediate	High
70 - 79	Intermediate	Intermediate	Intermediate	High	High	Very high
>80	Intermediate	Intermediate	Intermediate	High	High	Very high

Low: <15% pre-test probability no further testing needed
Intermediate: 15–65% pre-test probability additional testing is warranted, consider MPI
High: 66-85% pre-test probability additional testing is warranted, consider coronary CTA or MPI
Very high: >85% pre-test probability CAD is assumed to be present.
Pre-test probability based on data from Genders et al. [80]

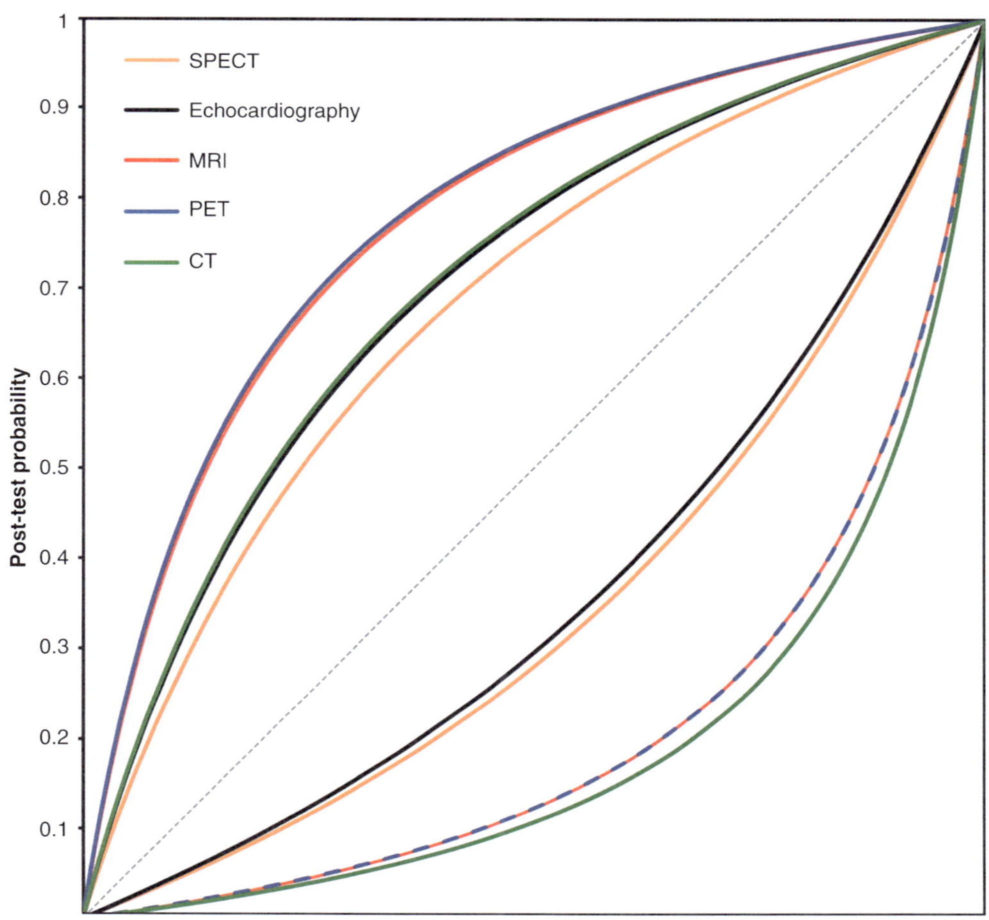

Fig. 27.6 Diagram relating pre- and posttest probability of hemodynamically significant coronary artery disease for the various techniques, with the upper left half representing a positive test and the lower right half a negative test. (From Takx et al. [45], with permission)

measuring coronary artery calcification (CAC); second, iodine-containing contrast agent is administered intravenously to visualize the coronary lumen, in combination with nitroglycerin [50] and depending on heart rate and site policy short-acting β-blockers. Examinations should be performed using modern hardware (≥64 slice).

CAC is defined as pixels above a threshold of 130 Hounsfield units (HU) and is traditionally quantified using the Agatston score [51], which is calculated by multiplying the lesion area (mm^2) by a density factor (between 1 and 4 based on the voxel with the highest density). However, recent research suggests that density might be inversely related to cardiovascular events [52]. In addition, a CAC score of zero does not exclude the presence of a significant non-calcified stenosis [53]. Novel automated and semiautomated software algorithms enable the quantification of CAC score using contrast-enhanced CTA series. Several studies demonstrated good correlations (above 0.95) and kappa values (above 0.87) for the quantification of CAC score using ECG-gated contrast-enhanced CTA series compared to standard ECG-gated unenhanced CT, suggesting that the use of quantification tools might allow for a lower radiation dose in the future by omitting the non-contrast CAC scan from the scan protocol [54, 55].

Some centers use high CAC scores (≥400 Agatston score) as a threshold for not performing coronary CTA; however, modern scanners demonstrate good diagnostic performance even in cases with high CAC scores [56]. A 64-row or higher coronary CTA has an excellent sensitivity of 95.6% and good specificity of 81.5%; nondiagnostic scans occur in 2.5% of patients with CAD and 7.5% without CAD [57]. A significant stenosis on coronary CTA requires verification to confirm the hemodynamic severity of CAD (angiography optionally with FFR), nondiagnostic coronary CTA requires alternative imaging (e.g., MPI), and a negative CTA reliably excludes significant CAD. Of note is that majority of CTA studies define obstructive CAD as ≥50% stenosis degree, while ICA studies usually consider ≥70% stenosis degree. Lesion characterization by stenosis degree alone on ICA might not be sufficient for intermediate stenosis (40–70%); therefore FFR measurement is recommendable [58]. In addition, FFR values have a continuous and independent relationship with cardiac events (i.e., the lower the FFR value, the more cardiac events occur) [59]. Even so, there is an ongoing debate on the true reference standard for the quantification of myocardial ischemia, and this question might be answered by results as obtained in the *I*nternational *S*tudy of *C*omparative *H*ealth *E*ffectiveness with *M*edical and *I*nvasive *A*pproaches (ISCHEMIA) trial (ClinicalTrials.gov Identifier: NCT01471522). Furthermore advances in computational fluid dynamics allow for the modeling of FFR from coronary CTA datasets (FFR_{CT}) [60]; as such the role of CTA is expected to increase in therapy guidance [61].

Prognostic Value of CTA

A meta-analysis on the prognostic value of coronary CTA demonstrated that 50% stenosis degree is a strong independent predictor of cardiovascular events [62]. In detail, the presence of significant coronary stenosis was associated with a sixfold increased hazard ratio (HR) for death, myocardial infarction, and unstable angina pectoris independent of CAC score. Also, in patients with diabetes, no CAD on coronary CTA allows for safely ruling out future events, and the detection of CAD is associated with a higher risk for events [63]. In patients with CKD, a clear increase is seen in annualized event rates (myocardial infarction, cerebrovascular accident, and death) when patients have both moderate CKD and obstructive CAD on CTA (3.7% for both vs. 2.5% for only moderate CKD or obstructive CAD) [64]. Multivariate Cox models demonstrated that both moderate CKD (HR 2.4, 95%CI 1.1–5.2, $p = 0.03$) and obstructive CAD (HR 2.8, 95%CI 1.4–5.4, $p < 0.01$) are independent predictors of events [64]. Recently two large randomized controlled trials investigated the effect of coronary CTA on survival compared to standard-of-care treatment. The *PRO*spective *M*ulticenter *I*maging *S*tudy for *E*valuation of Chest Pain (PROMISE) trial randomized 10,003 symptomatic patients with suspected CAD to an initial strategy of either coronary CTA or to functional testing during a median follow-up period of 25 months [65]. The PROMISE trial showed no significant difference between the CTA strategy and functional testing in respect to cardiovascular events (HR 1.04, 95%CI 0.83–1.29, $p = 0.75$). These results are partly influenced by the fact that CTA images were read at nonexpert centers and the limited statistical power (actual event rate 3.0% vs. 8.0% estimated). However the trial showed a reduction in the number of invasive angiograms with non-obstructive disease in the CTA group vs. functional testing group (3.4% vs. 4.3%, respectively, $p = 0.02$). The *S*cottish *CO*mputed *T*omography of the *HEART* (SCOT-HEART) trial randomly assigned 4146 patients with stable chest pain due to suspected coronary heart disease to standard of care plus CTA and standard of care alone group [66]. During a median follow-up of 1.7 years, the SCOT-HEART trial showed a considerable, though nonsignificant reduction of 38% in fatal and nonfatal myocardial infarction in standard of care plus CTA vs. standard of care alone group (HR 0.62, 95%CI 0.38–1.01, $p = 0.053$). Combined, these data demonstrate that coronary CTA is at least equivalent to conventional functional testing, and with growing experience, it is expected that it will be applied more widely in clinical practice.

Sex Differences

Despite improvements in healthcare, hospitalization rates for acute myocardial infarction have not declined in people younger than 55 years old, besides young females have more comorbidity and higher in-hospital mortality than young males [67]. Females commonly present with atypical chest pain (i.e. less exertional symptoms) [68]. In addition, risk scores poorly categorize females for pre-test CAD probability [69]. Traditionally, the goal of coronary CTA is focused on diagnosing obstructive CAD, while in females non-obstructive CAD is relatively common [30, 70]. Also, positive remodeling, plaque erosion, and microvascular embolization are more prevalent in females [71]. The importance of non-obstructive plaque in females is stressed by the finding that the number of non-obstructive plaques is predictive of mortality in females even after adjusting for the presence of obstructive CAD [72]. Results from the PROMISE trial found evidence that CTA yields more prognostic information in females than stress testing compared to males [73], while the *Co*ronary CT Angiography Evaluatio*n f*or Clinical Outcomes: An *i*nte*r*national *m*ulticenter (CONFIRM) registry observed no difference in prognostic value of CTA between both sexes with a similar disease extent [74]. As such there is still equipoise considering the role of non-obstructive CAD on coronary CTA in females.

Therapy of Patients with Stable CAD

The *C*linical *O*utcomes *U*tilizing *R*evascularization and *A*ggressive Dru*g E*valuation (COURAGE) trial [75] randomized 1149 patients with stable chest pain to percutaneous coronary intervention (PCI) plus optimal medical therapy (OMT) and 1138 for OMT alone. The trial demonstrated that during a median follow-up of 4.6 years, the addition of PCI to OMT reduced the occurrence of angina, but it did not reduce the risk of mortality, myocardial infarction, and hospitalization for acute coronary syndromes compared to OMT alone [75]. Coronary artery bypass graft (CABG) surgery should be considered in patients with two- or three-vessel disease (complex CAD), while in less complex cases and in patients with high operative risk, PCI is recommended [76]. In patients with diabetes and significant coronary disease (≥50% stenosis on coronary angiography with a positive stress test or ≥70% stenosis with classic angina pectoris), CABG is preferred over OMT [77].

CTA has the potential to improve the identification and monitoring of high-risk patients who would benefit from lipid-lowering therapy. A recent study demonstrated that the use of statins results in the reduction of non-calcified plaque volume and low-attenuation plaque volume on coronary CTA [78]. Guidelines on secondary prevention could be interpreted as supporting aggressive statin treatment in patients with obstructive CAD. However, in case of non-obstructive CAD and high-risk plaque features, guidelines are unclear, despite literature showing that extensive non-obstructive CAD (≥4 involved coronary segments) yields similar event rates as obstructive CAD [79]. Also, high-risk plaque features (low-attenuation plaque and positive remodeling) result in a significant higher risk over >50% stenosis degree [80]. The available data suggest that coronary CTA-guided therapy is expected to be incorporated in future guidelines.

Conclusions

In the past years, coronary CTA has become an integral part of strategies for evaluation of chronic chest pain. It allows for quick and reliable ruling out of the presence of CAD; furthermore it is capable to perform perfusion imaging and has the potential to guide and monitor therapy. In patients with diabetes mellitus and CKD, CAD on CTA remains an independent predictor of events. In females coronary CTA also adds prognostic information, though the exact differences between CAD findings on CTA between the sexes still have to be elucidated. Advances in quantification algorithms as well as modeling of FFR from coronary CTA datasets have the potential to increase the role of CTA in decision-making and therapy guidance.

References

1. Ladapo JA, Blecker S, Douglas PS. Physician decision making and trends in the use of cardiac stress testing in the United States: an analysis of repeated cross-sectional data. Ann Intern Med. 2014;161:482–90.
2. Bradley SM, Spertus JA, Kennedy KF, et al. Patient selection for diagnostic coronary angiography and hospital-level percutaneous coronary intervention appropriateness: insights from the National Cardiovascular Data Registry. JAMA Intern Med. 2014;174:1630–9.
3. National Institutes of Health NHL, and Blood Institute. Morbidity & mortality: 2012 chart book on cardiovascular, lung, and blood diseases. Bethesda: National Heart, Lung, and Blood Institute; 2012.
4. Task Force M, Montalescot G, Sechtem U, et al. 2013 ESC guidelines on the management of stable coronary artery disease: the Task Force on the management of stable coronary artery disease of the European Society of Cardiology. Eur Heart J. 2013;34:2949–3003.
5. Crea F, Camici PG, Bairey Merz CN. Coronary microvascular dysfunction: an update. Eur Heart J. 2014;35:1101–11.
6. Ong P, Athanasiadis A, Borgulya G, Mahrholdt H, Kaski JC, Sechtem U. High prevalence of a pathological response to acetylcholine testing in patients with stable angina pectoris and unobstructed coronary arteries. The ACOVA Study (Abnormal COronary VAsomotion in patients with stable angina and unobstructed coronary arteries). J Am Coll Cardiol. 2012;59:655–62.

7. Haffner SM, Lehto S, Ronnemaa T, Pyorala K, Laakso M. Mortality from coronary heart disease in subjects with type 2 diabetes and in nondiabetic subjects with and without prior myocardial infarction. N Engl J Med. 1998;339:229–34.
8. Cai Q, Mukku VK, Ahmad M. Coronary artery disease in patients with chronic kidney disease: a clinical update. Curr Cardiol Rev. 2013;9:331–9.
9. Mohlenkamp S, Hort W, Ge J, Erbel R. Update on myocardial bridging. Circulation. 2002;106:2616–22.
10. Ishikawa Y, Kawawa Y, Kohda E, Shimada K, Ishii T. Significance of the anatomical properties of a myocardial bridge in coronary heart disease. Circ J. 2011;75:1559–66.
11. Wirianta J, Mouden M, Ottervanger JP, et al. Prevalence and predictors of bridging of coronary arteries in a large Indonesian population, as detected by 64-slice computed tomography scan. Neth Heart J. 2012;20:396–401.
12. Sanada S, Komuro I, Kitakaze M. Pathophysiology of myocardial reperfusion injury: preconditioning, postconditioning, and translational aspects of protective measures. Am J Physiol Heart Circ Physiol. 2011;301:H1723–41.
13. Detry JM. The pathophysiology of myocardial ischaemia. Eur Heart J. 1996;17(Suppl G):48–52.
14. Narula J, Nakano M, Virmani R, et al. Histopathologic characteristics of atherosclerotic coronary disease and implications of the findings for the invasive and noninvasive detection of vulnerable plaques. J Am Coll Cardiol. 2013;61:1041–51.
15. Virmani R, Burke AP, Farb A, Kolodgie FD. Pathology of the vulnerable plaque. J Am Coll Cardiol. 2006;47:C13–8.
16. Celeng C, Takx RA, Ferencik M, Maurovich-Horvat P. Noninvasive and invasive imaging of vulnerable coronary plaque. Trends Cardiovasc Med. 2016;26:538–47.
17. Tarkin JM, Dweck MR, Evans NR, et al. Imaging atherosclerosis. Circ Res. 2016;118:750–69.
18. Otsuka F, Finn AV, Virmani R. Do vulnerable and ruptured plaques hide in heavily calcified arteries? Atherosclerosis. 2013;229:34–7.
19. Hoffmann U, Moselewski F, Nieman K, et al. Noninvasive assessment of plaque morphology and composition in culprit and stable lesions in acute coronary syndrome and stable lesions in stable angina by multidetector computed tomography. J Am Coll Cardiol. 2006;47:1655–62.
20. Pflederer T, Marwan M, Schepis T, et al. Characterization of culprit lesions in acute coronary syndromes using coronary dual-source CT angiography. Atherosclerosis. 2010;211:437–44.
21. Maseri A, Chierchia S. Coronary artery spasm: demonstration, definition, diagnosis, and consequences. Prog Cardiovasc Dis. 1982;25:169–92.
22. Hao PP, Shang R, Liu YP, et al. Cardiogenic shock from acute ST-segment elevation myocardial infarction induced by severe multivessel coronary vasospasm. Eur Heart J. 2014;35:146.
23. Amano M, Ito M, Kimura K, et al. Phosphorylation and activation of myosin by Rho-associated kinase (Rho-kinase). J Biol Chem. 1996;271:20246–9.
24. Toyo-oka T, Aizawa T, Suzuki N, et al. Increased plasma level of endothelin-1 and coronary spasm induction in patients with vasospastic angina pectoris. Circulation. 1991;83:476–83.
25. Shimokawa H, Nagasawa K, Irie T, et al. Clinical characteristics and long-term prognosis of patients with variant angina. A comparative study between western and Japanese populations. Int J Cardiol. 1988;18:331–49.
26. Kang EJ, Kim MH, De Jin C, et al. Noninvasive detection of coronary vasospastic angina using a double-acquisition coronary CT angiography protocol in the presence and absence of an intravenous nitrate: a pilot study. Eur Radiol. 2016. https://doi.org/10.1007/s00330-016-4476-2.
27. Lanza GA. Cardiac syndrome X: a critical overview and future perspectives. Heart. 2007;93:159–66.
28. Casino PR, Kilcoyne CM, Quyyumi AA, Hoeg JM, Panza JA. The role of nitric oxide in endothelium-dependent vasodilation of hypercholesterolemic patients. Circulation. 1993;88:2541–7.
29. Collins P, Rosano GM, Sarrel PM, et al. 17 beta-estradiol attenuates acetylcholine-induced coronary arterial constriction in women but not men with coronary heart disease. Circulation. 1995;92:24–30.
30. Pepine CJ, Anderson RD, Sharaf BL, et al. Coronary microvascular reactivity to adenosine predicts adverse outcome in women evaluated for suspected ischemia results from the National Heart, Lung and Blood Institute WISE (Women's Ischemia Syndrome Evaluation) study. J Am Coll Cardiol. 2010;55:2825–32.
31. de Roos A. Myocardial perfusion imaging with multidetector CT: beyond lumenography. Radiology. 2010;254:321–3.
32. Felker GM, Shaw LK, O'Connor CM. A standardized definition of ischemic cardiomyopathy for use in clinical research. J Am Coll Cardiol. 2002;39:210–8.
33. Rahimtoola SH. A perspective on the three large multicenter randomized clinical trials of coronary bypass surgery for chronic stable angina. Circulation. 1985;72:V123–35.
34. Rahimtoola SH. The hibernating myocardium. Am Heart J. 1989;117:211–21.
35. Poole-Wilson PA, Holmberg SR, Williams AJ. A possible molecular mechanism for 'stunning' of the myocardium. Eur Heart J. 1991;12(Suppl F):25–9.
36. Lardo AC, Cordeiro MA, Silva C, et al. Contrast-enhanced multidetector computed tomography viability imaging after myocardial infarction: characterization of myocyte death, microvascular obstruction, and chronic scar. Circulation. 2006;113:394–404.
37. De Giorgio F, Grassi VM, Polacco M, Pascali VL, d'Aloja E, Arena V. Myocardial bridging and sudden cardiac death: is the actual classification exhaustive? Int J Cardiol. 2014;172:e383–4.
38. Loukas M, Curry B, Bowers M, et al. The relationship of myocardial bridges to coronary artery dominance in the adult human heart. J Anat. 2006;209:43–50.
39. Yamada R, Tremmel JA, Tanaka S, et al. Functional versus anatomic assessment of myocardial bridging by intravascular ultrasound: impact of arterial compression on proximal atherosclerotic plaque. J Am Heart Assoc. 2016;5:e001735.
40. Corban MT, Hung OY, Eshtehardi P, et al. Myocardial bridging: contemporary understanding of pathophysiology with implications for diagnostic and therapeutic strategies. J Am Coll Cardiol. 2014;63:2346–55.
41. Fihn SD, Gardin JM, Abrams J, et al. 2012 ACCF/AHA/ACP/AATS/PCNA/SCAI/STS Guideline for the diagnosis and management of patients with stable ischemic heart disease: a report of the American College of Cardiology Foundation/American Heart Association Task Force on Practice Guidelines, and the American College of Physicians, American Association for Thoracic Surgery, Preventive Cardiovascular Nurses Association, Society for Cardiovascular Angiography and Interventions, and Society of Thoracic Surgeons. J Am Coll Cardiol. 2012;60:e44–e164.
42. Diamond GA, Forrester JS. Analysis of probability as an aid in the clinical diagnosis of coronary-artery disease. N Engl J Med. 1979;300:1350–8.
43. Morise AP, Diamond GA. Comparison of the sensitivity and specificity of exercise electrocardiography in biased and unbiased populations of men and women. Am Heart J. 1995;130:741–7.
44. Froelicher VF, Lehmann KG, Thomas R, et al. The electrocardiographic exercise test in a population with reduced workup bias: diagnostic performance, computerized interpretation, and multivariable prediction. Veterans Affairs Cooperative Study in Health Services #016 (QUEXTA) Study Group. Quantitative exercise testing and angiography. Ann Intern Med. 1998;128:965–74.
45. Takx RA, Blomberg BA, El Aidi H, et al. Diagnostic accuracy of stress myocardial perfusion imaging compared to invasive coronary angiography with fractional flow reserve meta-analysis. Circ Cardiovasc Imaging. 2015;8(1). pii: e002666.
46. Morton G, Chiribiri A, Ishida M, et al. Quantification of absolute myocardial perfusion in patients with coronary artery disease: comparison between cardiovascular magnetic resonance and positron emission tomography. J Am Coll Cardiol. 2012;60:1546–55.

47. Feuchtner G, Goetti R, Plass A, et al. Adenosine stress high-pitch 128-slice dual-source myocardial computed tomography perfusion for imaging of reversible myocardial ischemia: comparison with magnetic resonance imaging. Circ Cardiovasc Imaging. 2011;4:540–9.
48. De Cecco CN, Harris BS, Schoepf UJ, et al. Incremental value of pharmacological stress cardiac dual-energy CT over coronary CT angiography alone for the assessment of coronary artery disease in a high-risk population. AJR Am J Roentgenol. 2014;203:W70–7.
49. Takx RA, Moscariello A, Schoepf UJ, et al. Quantification of left and right ventricular function and myocardial mass: comparison of low-radiation dose 2nd generation dual-source CT and cardiac MRI. Eur J Radiol. 2012;81:e598–604.
50. Takx RA, Sucha D, Park J, Leiner T, Hoffmann U. Sublingual nitroglycerin administration in coronary computed tomography angiography: a systematic review. Eur Radiol. 2015;25:3536–42.
51. Agatston AS, Janowitz WR, Hildner FJ, Zusmer NR, Viamonte M Jr, Detrano R. Quantification of coronary artery calcium using ultrafast computed tomography. J Am Coll Cardiol. 1990;15:827–32.
52. Criqui MH, Denenberg JO, Ix JH, et al. Calcium density of coronary artery plaque and risk of incident cardiovascular events. JAMA. 2014;311:271–8.
53. Akram K, O'Donnell RE, King S, Superko HR, Agatston A, Voros S. Influence of symptomatic status on the prevalence of obstructive coronary artery disease in patients with zero calcium score. Atherosclerosis. 2009;203:533–7.
54. Ebersberger U, Eilot D, Goldenberg R, et al. Fully automated derivation of coronary artery calcium scores and cardiovascular risk assessment from contrast medium-enhanced coronary CT angiography studies. Eur Radiol. 2013;23:650–7.
55. Schuhbaeck A, Otaki Y, Achenbach S, et al. Coronary calcium scoring from contrast coronary CT angiography using a semiautomated standardized method. J Cardiovasc Comput Tomogr. 2015;9:446–53.
56. Westwood ME, Raatz HD, Misso K, et al. Systematic review of the accuracy of dual-source cardiac CT for detection of arterial stenosis in difficult to image patient groups. Radiology. 2013;267:387–95.
57. Menke J, Kowalski J. Diagnostic accuracy and utility of coronary CT angiography with consideration of unevaluable results: a systematic review and multivariate Bayesian random-effects meta-analysis with intention to diagnose. Eur Radiol. 2016;26:451–8.
58. Tobis J, Azarbal B, Slavin L. Assessment of intermediate severity coronary lesions in the catheterization laboratory. J Am Coll Cardiol. 2007;49:839–48.
59. Johnson NP, Toth GG, Lai D, et al. Prognostic value of fractional flow reserve: linking physiologic severity to clinical outcomes. J Am Coll Cardiol. 2014;64:1641–54.
60. Celeng C, Leiner T, Maurovich-Horvat P, et al. Anatomical and functional computed tomography for diagnosing hemodynamically significant coronary artery disease. J Am Coll Cardiol Img. 2018:S1936-878X(18)30681–8.
61. Taylor CA, Fonte TA, Min JK. Computational fluid dynamics applied to cardiac computed tomography for noninvasive quantification of fractional flow reserve: scientific basis. J Am Coll Cardiol. 2013;61:2233–41.
62. Bamberg F, Sommer WH, Hoffmann V, et al. Meta-analysis and systematic review of the long-term predictive value of assessment of coronary atherosclerosis by contrast-enhanced coronary computed tomography angiography. J Am Coll Cardiol. 2011;57:2426–36.
63. Celeng C, Maurovich-Horvat P, Ghoshhajra BB, Merkely B, Leiner T, Takx RA. Prognostic value of coronary computed tomography angiography in patients with diabetes: a meta-analysis. Diabetes Care. 2016;39:1274–80.
64. Yiu KH, de Graaf FR, Schuijf JD, et al. Prognostic value of renal dysfunction for the prediction of outcome versus results of computed tomographic coronary angiography. Am J Cardiol. 2011;108:968–72.
65. Douglas PS, Hoffmann U, Patel MR, et al. Outcomes of anatomical versus functional testing for coronary artery disease. N Engl J Med. 2015;372:1291–300.
66. investigators S-H. CT coronary angiography in patients with suspected angina due to coronary heart disease (SCOT-HEART): an open-label, parallel-group, multicentre trial. Lancet. 2015;385:2383–91.
67. Gupta A, Wang Y, Spertus JA, et al. Trends in acute myocardial infarction in young patients and differences by sex and race, 2001 to 2010. J Am Coll Cardiol. 2014;64:337–45.
68. Bugiardini R. Women, 'non-specific' chest pain, and normal or near-normal coronary angiograms are not synonymous with favourable outcome. Eur Heart J. 2006;27:1387–9.
69. Cheng VY, Berman DS, Rozanski A, et al. Performance of the traditional age, sex, and angina typicality-based approach for estimating pretest probability of angiographically significant coronary artery disease in patients undergoing coronary computed tomographic angiography: results from the multinational coronary CT angiography evaluation for clinical outcomes: an international multicenter registry (CONFIRM). Circulation. 2011;124:2423–32. 2421-2428
70. Pepine CJ, Ferdinand KC, Shaw LJ, et al. Emergence of nonobstructive coronary artery disease: a woman's problem and need for change in definition on angiography. J Am Coll Cardiol. 2015;66:1918–33.
71. Bairey Merz CN, Shaw LJ, Reis SE, et al. Insights from the NHLBI-sponsored Women's Ischemia Syndrome Evaluation (WISE) study: Part II: gender differences in presentation, diagnosis, and outcome with regard to gender-based pathophysiology of atherosclerosis and macrovascular and microvascular coronary disease. J Am Coll Cardiol. 2006;47:S21–9.
72. Shaw LJ, Min JK, Narula J, et al. Sex differences in mortality associated with computed tomographic angiographic measurements of obstructive and nonobstructive coronary artery disease: an exploratory analysis. Circ Cardiovasc Imaging. 2010;3:473–81.
73. Pagidipati NJ, Hemal K, Coles A, et al. Sex differences in functional and CT angiography testing in patients with suspected coronary artery disease. J Am Coll Cardiol. 2016;67:2607–16.
74. Schulman-Marcus J, ó Hartaigh B, Gransar H, et al. Sex-specific associations between coronary artery plaque extent and risk of major adverse cardiovascular events: the CONFIRM long-term registry. JACC Cardiovasc Imaging. 2016;9:364–72.
75. Boden WE, O'Rourke RA, Teo KK, et al. Optimal medical therapy with or without PCI for stable coronary disease. N Engl J Med. 2007;356:1503–16.
76. Deb S, Wijeysundera HC, Ko DT, Tsubota H, Hill S, Fremes SE. Coronary artery bypass graft surgery vs percutaneous interventions in coronary revascularization: a systematic review. JAMA. 2013;310:2086–95.
77. Group BDS, Frye RL, August P, et al. A randomized trial of therapies for type 2 diabetes and coronary artery disease. N Engl J Med. 2009;360:2503–15.
78. Zeb I, Li D, Nasir K, et al. Effect of statin treatment on coronary plaque progression – a serial coronary CT angiography study. Atherosclerosis. 2013;231:198–204.
79. Bittencourt MS, Hulten E, Ghoshhajra B, et al. Prognostic value of nonobstructive and obstructive coronary artery disease detected by coronary computed tomography angiography to identify cardiovascular events. Circ Cardiovasc Imaging. 2014;7:282–91.
80. Yamamoto H, Kitagawa T, Ohashi N, et al. Noncalcified atherosclerotic lesions with vulnerable characteristics detected by coronary CT angiography and future coronary events. J Cardiovasc Comput Tomogr. 2013;7:192–9.
81. Genders TS, Steyerberg EW, Alkadhi H, et al. A clinical prediction rule for the diagnosis of coronary artery disease: validation, updating, and extension. Eur Heart J. 2011;32:1316–30.

Coronary CT Angiography for Evaluation of Acute Coronary Syndrome in the Emergency Department

28

Nam Ju Lee and Harold Litt

There is nearly one death from heart disease every 38 s in the United States [1]. Acute chest pain is the single most common complaint of patients older than 15 years of age presenting to the emergency department (ED) [2] and accounts for about 4% of ED visits in the United States [3]. Origins of chest pain include diseases of the heart, aorta, pulmonary system, esophagus, upper abdomen, and chest wall and even psychiatric disorders. Determination of the etiology of the chest pain is often difficult, although different types of chest pain are classically ascribed to different corresponding diseases. Acute coronary syndrome (ACS) is estimated to be responsible for 20% of all clinical encounters for acute chest pain [4]. Patients with ACS present with unstable angina, acute myocardial infarction, or sudden cardiac death [5]; therefore, timely triage of ACS is important as it affects treatment and prognosis. Also timely triage may save significant costs. Using coronary CTA to evaluate patients instead of admitting patients for a rule-out approach with serial troponin has the potential to save significant costs to the healthcare system.

Risk Assessment

The initial step in evaluation of potential ACS in the ED is assessment of patient risk; this may be performed using scales such as the thrombosis in myocardial infarction (TIMI) score, including clinical and medical history, coronary artery disease risk factors, electrocardiogram (ECG) results, and serum cardiac enzyme levels [6]. In approximately 10% of all ED chest pain patients, with a TIMI risk score of zero combined with negative serial cardiac biomarker testing, the patient may be considered at low risk and discharged directly from the ED [7]. The presence or absence of specific symptoms is not reliable when used to rule out myocardial ischemia [8], and risk factors (hypercholesterolemia, hypertension, family history, and tobacco use) remain poor predictors of ACS [9, 10]. The standard 12-lead ECG cannot exclude ACS conclusively because diagnostic ECG findings are present only in a minority of patients, although it is the single best test to identify ST-segment elevation MI (STEMI) [11, 12]. Despite improvements in cardiac biomarkers (creatine kinase, CK-MB, myoglobin, troponin I, troponin T) for early diagnosis and risk stratification of acute MI [13–16], they are not universally elevated in patients with unstable angina or transient myocardial ischemia [17]. Therefore, negative markers cannot exclude ACS entirely, and evaluation is still needed according to their clinical presentations.

Patients with low–intermediate TIMI score without initial enzyme level elevation or ECG changes are typically admitted for complete evaluation with further enzyme analysis and often for myocardial stress imaging, whereas patients with a high-risk score are referred for intravenous (IV) heparin and further investigation with catheterization for intervention [18].

The HEART score in another risk classification system is based on history, ECG, age, risk factors, and troponin. In the initial derivation cohort, MACE occurred in 1.7% of those with low HEART scores (values 0–3), which was 36.4% of patients; therefore low HEART scores (0–3) exclude short-term MACE with >98% certainty. Conservative evaluation policies might be considered for those patients compared to more aggressive evaluation in patients with high HEART scores (7–10) who have a higher risk of MACE [19]. The c-statistic of the HEART score (0.83) is significantly higher than the c-statistic of TIMI (0.75) and GRACE (0.70), respectively ($p < 0.0001$) [19].

Weinstock et al. showed in adult patients with chest pain admitted with two negative serial biomarkers, no concerning vital signs, and nonischemic ECG findings, short-term clinically relevant adverse cardiac events were rare and commonly iatrogenic and suggested that routine inpatient admission may not be a beneficial strategy for this group [20].

N. J. Lee
Department of Radiology, Mayo Clinic, Rochester, MN, USA

H. Litt (✉)
Department of Radiology, Perelman School of Medicine of the University of Pennsylvania, Philadelphia, PA, USA
e-mail: harold.litt@uphs.upenn.edu

U. J. Schoepf (ed.), *CT of the Heart*, Contemporary Medical Imaging, https://doi.org/10.1007/978-1-60327-237-7_28

However, the reported 2–4% rate of missed diagnosis of ACS [21–23] may expand the number of tests and hospitalizations in relatively low-risk populations with chest pain without definite evidence of ACS [24].

CCTA for ACS Patients in ER

Patients with a low to intermediate risk of ACS are usually judged clinically according to initial risk assessment data including clinical history, ECG, biomarkers, and TIMI score of 0–2. CCTA may be performed for patients with prior negative stress test or even for those with TIMI score 3–4, which would allow cardiac CTA to be ordered for approximately 60–70% of patients [25–27]. Recently, appropriate use of criteria for the imaging of ED patients presenting with chest pain has been published [28, 29].

Most international guidelines suggest that the least expensive and most widely available stress test, treadmill ECG, should be the first-line test for patients at intermediate risk for acute coronary syndrome [30]. However, Hermann et al. demonstrated that routine provocative cardiac testing generated a small therapeutic yield with new diagnoses of coronary artery disease being uncommon, but many false-positive results in an emergency department-based chest pain unit [31]. In their study, routine provocative testing was positive for coronary ischemia in 470/4181 (11.2%) patients, of whom 123 underwent coronary angiography. Obstructive disease was confirmed in 63 of 123 (51.2% true positive), and 28 (0.7% overall) had findings consistent with the potential benefit from revascularization (American Heart Association class I or IIa) [31].

The application of CCTA in the ED is based on trial data and observation from a limited number of centers [32–37], and CCTA is now seen as a viable alternative to functional testing in the evaluation of patients with acute chest pain in the ED [38–40].

Early utilization of CCTA in the ED for appropriately selected patients with a low to intermediate risk of ACS identifies low-risk patients quickly without the added delay of serial biomarkers or prolonged observation. It facilitates more rapid discharge from the ED compared to those undergoing non-CCTA standard care including serial ECGs, cardiac biomarkers, and subsequent cardiac testing such as exercise testing, stress perfusion imaging, or cardiac catheterization without a statistically significant difference in major adverse cardiac events (MACE) [34, 38–43]. In a prospective cohort trial of 568 patients in the ED with low TIMI score, 84% of patients were discharged based on a negative CCTA without adverse outcomes in 30 days with only one potential cardiac death at 1-year follow-up [36].

ACRIN PA 4005 was a randomized controlled study of CCTA versus usual care for low-to-intermediate-risk patients presenting with a possible acute coronary syndrome. Of 640 patients with a negative CCTA examination, none died or had a myocardial infarction within 30 days, and patients in the CCTA group had a higher rate of direct discharge from the ED (49.6% vs. 22.7%), a shorter length of stay (LOS) (median, 18.0 h vs. 24.8 h), and a higher rate of detection of coronary disease (9.0% vs. 3.5%) compared with patients receiving traditional care [39].

CCTA is comparable to myocardial stress perfusion imaging in terms of safety and accuracy for excluding or diagnosing ACS [33].

The Computed Tomographic Angiography for the Systematic Triage of Acute Chest Pain Patients to Treatment (CT-STAT) trial showed that CCTA and stress SPECT myocardial perfusion imaging led to a similar number of patients referred to invasive coronary angiography, 6.9% and 6.2%, respectively, similar to findings in ACRIN PA 4005. Time to diagnosis and hospital costs were significantly reduced with CCTA, to an average of 3 h compared with 7 h for those who received stress SPECT MPI; direct costs were reduced by 38%, from roughly $3500 to $2000. However, Salerno et al. pointed out that there was lack of stress ECG as a comparator [44].

CCTA also reduces cost in addition to reduction in diagnostic time in the intermediate-risk population [32, 45]. Recent randomized controlled trials in acute ED patients that compared CCTA to nuclear SPECT [39] or to a mixed standard of care showed lower length of stay at lower cost [38, 40].

In the ROMICAT II trial, 1000 patients with symptoms suggestive of ACS were randomized to an early CCTA or standard ED evaluation. Similar to the other studies, ROMICAT II demonstrated a shorter length of stay (LOS) for patients who underwent CCTA than standard evaluation, and ED costs were lower. However, catheterization and revascularization rates were higher in the CCTA arm, leading to higher inpatient costs and overall cost neutrality. Women in the CCTA arm had greater reduction in LOS, lower hospital admission rates, and a smaller increase in cumulative radiation dose than men when comparing ED strategies (p-interactions ≤ 0.02) [46]. While women had lower ACS rates than men, sex differences in LOS persisted after adjustment for baseline differences including ACS rate (p-interaction < 0.03). LOS was similar between sexes with normal CCTA findings ($p = 0.11$). However, there was limitation of the lack of stress ECG as a comparator.

The recent CT Coronary Angiography Compared to Exercise ECG (CT-COMPARE) study represents the largest prospective, randomized trial of CCTA comparing to treadmill exercise ECG as part of the standard of care in low–intermediate risk possible ACS patients presenting to the ED to evaluate diagnostic performance measures and the hospital-based costs of CCTA-based care as compared to

ECG-based care [30]. The data showed that CCTA-based evaluation is 35% faster and 20% less expensive than ExECG in patients at low–intermediate risk of acute coronary syndrome. These results suggest that coronary CT angiography is faster and less expensive, with improved diagnostic performance compared to exercise treadmill ECG-based care in symptomatic patients at low–intermediate risk for acute coronary syndrome presenting to the emergency department [30]. These data add additional proof that protocols using CCTA rather than stress testing-based care in emergency departments should be considered [30].

CCTA has shown its safety and efficiency in excluding coronary artery disease or relevant stenosis for advanced risk stratification over the past decade in the setting of ambiguous acute chest pain of a low to intermediate risk of ACS with 86–100% sensitivity, 92–98% specificity, 93–100% negative predictive value, and 50–90% positive predictive value [32, 47–50]. However, patients with indeterminate lesions or nondiagnostic CCTA will be referred for stress testing to evaluate the physiologic relevance of intermediate lesions. There are minority of uninterpretable cases due to patient's motion or unexpected variability of heart rate, with a goal to be below 5% of total studies.

Performing CCTA

Patients with a serum creatinine level of greater than 1.5 mg/dL or a severe allergy to iodinated contrast material and those who are pregnant are not eligible for CCTA. Conditions that may be not suitable for CCTA are active asthma or other contraindications to β-blocker administration, irregular heart rhythms such as atrial fibrillation, and weight more than 150 kg, depending on the specific CT technology in use. Heart rate control to less than 70 bpm is required for high-quality CCTA, depending upon the technology in use [51]. A fast-acting β-blocker with a short half-life, typically oral metoprolol, is given at least 1 h before imaging for patients with fast heart rates when there is no contraindications, e.g., active or unstable small airways disease, hypotension, sinus bradycardia, or recent cocaine use. The initial dose is 50–100 mg with additional doses up to 200 mg if needed [52]. IV metoprolol can be administered in the CT suite, and the effect occurs typically in 5–10 min; 5 mg IV can be given initially, with additional doses up to 20 mg if required. For patients with contraindications to β-blockers, calcium channel blockers, preferably diltiazem with the least negative inotropic effect, can be considered as an alternative (initial IV bolus of up to 0.25 mg/kg). Careful monitoring of vital signs is required with IV medication. Utilizing sublingual nitroglycerin before contrast-enhanced images is valuable for improving the contrast-to-noise ratio and vessel visualization by vasodilation of the coronary arteries [53, 54]. Contraindications to nitroglycerin include recent phosphodiesterase inhibitor therapy, commonly used for erectile dysfunction or pulmonary hypertension, hypotension, and critical aortic stenosis.

Cardiovascular computed tomography angiography (CCTA) had been associated with considerable radiation doses, with previous studies reporting high average radiation doses of >10 mSv [55]. Retrospective electrocardiographically (ECG)-gated CCTA was used in which radiation is applied during the entire cardiac cycle with 100% tube current. A substantial reduction in radiation dose was achieved with the introduction of prospective ECG-triggered CCTA in which radiation is only administered during a predefined phase of the cardiac cycle and the tube current is turned off or reduced outside that phase [56]. Although retrospective ECG-triggering yields functional information during the cardiac cycle, its use exposes patients to more radiation, whereas prospective ECG-triggering provides fewer cardiac phases for interpretation but reduces the radiation dose. A meta-analysis comparing retrospective and prospective ECG-triggering found that an almost fourfold reduction in radiation dose (11.3–3.5 mSv) was possible using prospective ECG-triggering, while image quality remained comparable [57]. Therefore, prospective ECG-triggering is now widely used for the majority of CCTA acquisitions. Despite these advances, the ability to lower dose in CCTA by prospective ECG-triggering alone remains problematic in patients with high heart rates or arrhythmias [58].

Conventionally, a low pitch is used for retrospectively gated CCTA acquisitions to ensure adequate data sampling; however, with second- and third-generation dual-source scanners, high-pitch acquisitions are possible in which the entire chest including the heart is covered within a single heartbeat. This is possible because the second detector fills in the gaps in data sampling from the first detector. It is possible to maintain image quality using high-pitch spiral prospective ECG-triggering in patients with a regular heart rhythm up to 70 beats/min [56]. Wide area or volume detector scanners are not constrained by pitch because the whole heart can be imaged within a single heartbeat [57].

Blooming artifact from densely calcified plaque limits the accurate evaluation of stenosis, and the degree of stenosis is often overestimated [59]. Despite concerns about image quality in patients with calcium score over 400, a study showed that only a small percentage of these scans in ED patients are uninterpretable [60]. Newer dual-energy technology using simultaneous or alternating imaging at two different X-ray tube potentials allows improved quantification of calcified plaque by reducing tissue blooming and beam hardening beyond single-energy MDCT [61]. Imagers may decide to proceed with scanning based on the likelihood of a diagnostic study even in patients with high calcium score. Evaluation of coronary stent patency is limited due to blooming artifacts similar to dense calcium [62]. However, stents are unlikely to be present in a patient with low to intermediate risk of ACS presenting to the ED.

Triple-rule-out (TRO) CT examines the coronary arteries, the thoracic aorta, and the pulmonary arteries simultaneously [63]. For the diagnosis of coronary artery disease, TRO CT has a sensitivity of 94.3%, a specificity of 97.4%, and a negative predictive value of 99%, findings that are similar to those obtained with the use of dedicated coronary CTA [64]. Compared with dedicated CCTA, TRO CT has greater anatomic coverage, including the structures above the carina, leading to a higher radiation dose [65]. Therefore, TRO CT requires a slightly higher IV contrast load to opacify both the right- and left-side circulations [64, 65]. TRO CT is thought to be beneficial in the evaluation of patients with chest pain for whom additional diagnoses other than ACS are considered in addition to a low to intermediate risk for ACS at baseline, such as pulmonary embolism or aortic dissection [66]. Because of the relatively low prevalence of pulmonary embolism and aortic dissection in this patient population [64], appropriate patient selection is important for the effective application of TRO CT [63].

Coronary Calcium Evaluation

Coronary artery calcification (CAC) can be seen in most patients with ACS or sudden cardiac death, and it has been established as a quantitative marker and indicator of atherosclerosis using the Agatston score [67–70]. The Agatston scoring scale calculates an area for all pixels above a threshold of 130 HU, in contiguous 3 mm slices, (the slice thickness and spacing used by Agatston et al), and multiplies it by a density factor. The score is the summed or total "score" for the entire epicardial coronary system. Prospective ECG-triggering is the current mode for measuring coronary calcium at most centers.

A study of 1031 patients with a median CACS of 0 (61% with CACS of 0) showed a majority of patients evaluated for chest pain of uncertain cardiac cause have a CACS of 0, which predicts both a normal SPECT result and an excellent short-term outcome [71]. Only 2 events occurred in 625 patients with a CACS of 0 (0.3%, 95% confidence interval 0.04–1.1%). Both of these patients developed increased troponin levels during their index visit but had normal serial ECG and SPECT study results and no cardiac events at 6-month follow-up [71].

However, a lack of coronary calcium does not definitely exclude coronary stenosis, and a high amount of calcium does not necessarily correlate with angiographic luminal stenosis or vulnerability of plaques [72, 73]. The role of calcium scoring in ED patients with suspected ACS continues to be debated, because it has been shown that calcium scores alone cannot be used to determine risk in patients presenting with potential ACS in the ED and does not add prognostic value for acute events although it may be useful for long-term management of cardiac risk in outpatients. One study showed that a significant number of patients with a zero CAC had CTA findings [74]; therefore, CTA is better than CAC scoring in determining the atheroma burden, especially in patients with risk factors.

However, higher Agatston score is correlated with increased risk of cardiac events and worse overall prognosis [75]. Framingham risk score combined with coronary calcium score can improve 10-year risk stratification of asymptomatic people, especially those with intermediate risk (Framingham risk score 10–20%) [76]. Calcium scoring may be recommended in this group to support clinical decision-making, particularly whether to start aggressive medical therapy. The risk is highest when the Agatston score is above 400. Cardiovascular risk increases proportionally to the amount of calcium, and an annual progression of more than 15% enhances the risk of myocardial infarctions although positive predictive value of CAC progression is low as a marker of risk [77–79]. After myocardial infarction, patients have higher CAC progression than event-free subjects [80]. CAC scoring does not necessarily add relevant information in high- or low-risk populations [47]. While an unenhanced series may be useful to customize the CCTA scan field and other parameters to reduce doses, the effective dose of a calcium scoring acquisition is now similar to CCTA doses obtained with lower tube voltage technique, and therefore its value in the ED is uncertain [81].

Coronary Stenosis

There is a very low MACE rate (0.5%) in the 30 days after ED presentation in patients with a stenosis of 25–50% on cardiac CTA [82], although one study reported that 2.6% of ED patients with visible atherosclerosis but less than 50% stenosis at CCTA experienced ACS as identified by serial cardiac markers but not by stress testing [37]. All patients had small vessel disease, which is associated with a low incidence of adverse events and mortality, and is not generally amenable to revascularization [83–87]. Nonetheless, small vessels are a limitation of CCTA evaluation [88], and therefore, serial cardiac makers may be beneficial in patients with less than 50% stenosis on CCTA, but further evaluation such as stress testing is not indicated during the index visit [82]. Short-interval outpatient follow-up is important to establish strategies for primary prevention.

The ROMICAT I trial demonstrated a 77% sensitivity of a stenosis ≥50% for detection of ACS [37]. In the ROMICAT II study, a stenosis ≥50% was detected in 78% of patients with ACS, which is similar to invasive angiography studies that observed an absence of significant stenosis in 12–14% of patients with ACS [89]. A clinical registry by Velzen et al. showed sensitivity, specificity, and positive and negative predictive values to detect significant CAD on CTA were 100, 87, 93, and 100%, respectively [90]. During mean follow-up of 13.7 months, no cardiovascular events occurred in patients with a normal CTA examination. In patients with nonsignificant CAD on CTA, no cardiac deaths or myocardial infarctions occurred and only one patient underwent revascularization due to unstable angina. In patients presenting with acute chest pain, an excellent clinical performance for the noninvasive assessment of significant CAD was demonstrated using CTA. Normal or nonsignificant CAD on CTA predicted a low rate of adverse cardiovascular events and favorable outcome during follow-up [90]. ROMICAT I demonstrated limited positive value of a stenosis >50% at CCTA for ACS because matching perfusion abnormalities on SPECT MPI testing were seen in only 46% of these patients [91]. The optimal management of patients with intermediate lesions at CCTA remains uncertain and may result in an increased frequency of downstream testing and interventions [38–40, 92]. However, patients with significant stenosis on CTA cannot be discharged from the ED after initial troponin and ECG [38–40, 92].

Coronary Atherosclerotic Plaques

Atherosclerotic lesions can be characterized as calcified, non-calcified, and partially calcified (mixed plaques) on CT (Fig. 28.1). On a cellular basis, atherosclerotic changes can be classified in to six types (I–VI). Type III is the border where atherosclerotic changes become visible to the eyes [93]. Types IV, V, and VI are classified as advanced plaques [94]. The entire vessel grows with increasing plaque volume so that the lumen diameter is maintained; therefore, type IV lipid core atheroma and type V fibroatheroma (atheroma with fibrous tissue) can be asymptomatic with adaptive change of the arteries [95]. When thrombus or hemorrhage develops in type IV–V lesions, patients can be symptomatic (type VI, complicated). Most ACS are thought to be the result of sudden luminal thrombosis, which occurs from plaque rupture, plaque erosion, or calcified nodules [5, 96–100]. Plaque rupture refers to luminal thrombosis occurring when the highly necrotic core of a ruptured thin-cap fibroatheroma contracts with platelets. Hemodynamically nonsignificant plaque may be prone to rupture depending on the morphology and biochemical structure [89, 101–105]. Thin-cap fibroatheroma is often seen pathologically in plaque rupture with myocardial infarctions, where speckled calcification

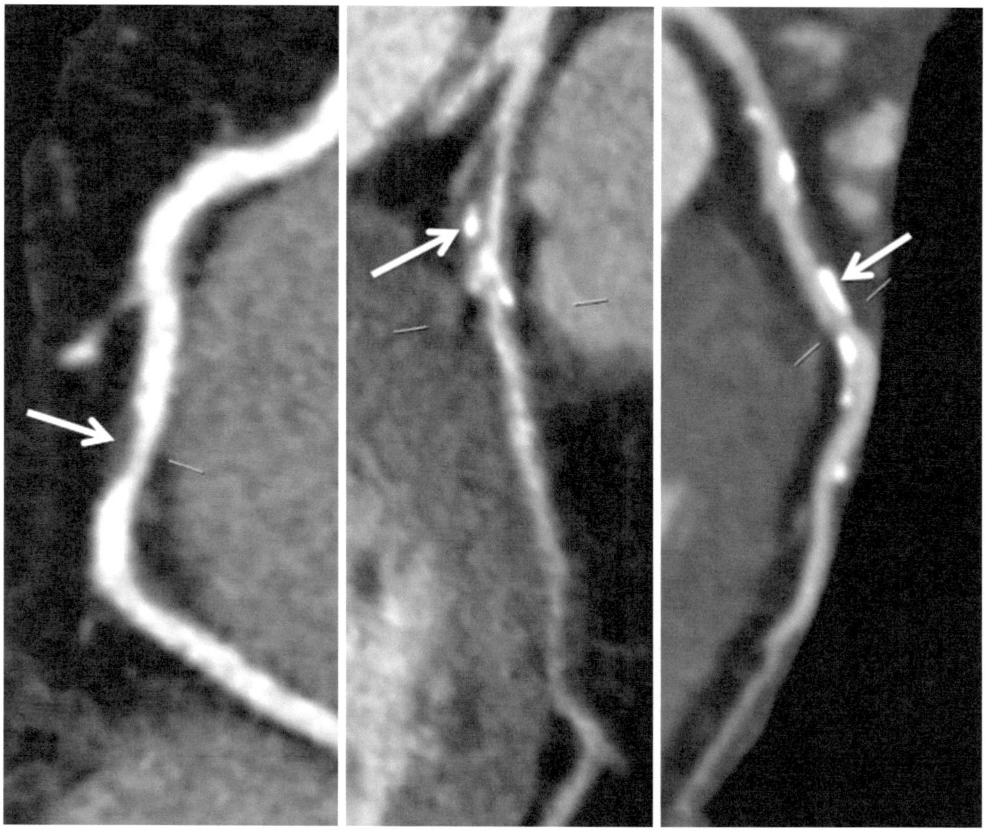

Fig. 28.1 Characterization of atherosclerotic plaques by CT. Curved planar reformatted images from coronary CT studies performed on ED chest pain patients demonstrate non-calcified (left), mixed (center), and calcified (right) plaques

can be visualized [5]. Luminal thrombus from plaque erosion occurs when there is minimal inflammation of an underlying base rich in proteoglycans and smooth muscle cells, in which plaque is mostly devoid of necrotic core or the necrotic core dose not communicate with the lumen due to a thick fibrous cap. Calcified nodules are the least common in luminal thrombosis, and their effect on instability is less evident although coronary calcification correlates highly with plaque burden [5].

ACS develops frequently from relatively mild or moderate lesions angiographically in the early stage of atherosclerosis [104, 106, 107]. Coronary artery plaque features may assist in further stratifying risk beyond that obtained using percent stenosis [108–110]. Reported features of high-risk plaque (Fig. 28.2) are large plaque volume, positive remodeling, spotty calcium, greater proportion of non-calcified plaque, low mean and minimal CT attenuation value (Hounsfield units, HU), and a contrast-enhanced rim seen around the central filling defect (napkin-ring sign) [109, 111–117], which are similar to high-risk findings on intravascular imaging (positive remodeling, larger plaque area, spotty calcium, and large necrotic core) [118, 119] as well as histology. These changes can directly be visualized on CCTA but will not appear on invasive angiography because the vessel wall is not visualized [47]. Multi-energy imaging techniques may assess plaque composition [61], and myocardial perfusion provides prognostic information [120]. Dual-energy CT may assist in distinguishing densely calcified plaques from other plaque types although further plaque discrimination such as fibrous vs. lipid-rich plaque is not currently possible [121].

High-risk plaque features have been associated with an increased risk for future cardiovascular events in patients with stable chest pain syndromes [110, 122, 123]. These findings are more often seen with culprit lesions in patients with ACS compared with similarly stenotic plaques in patients with stable angina [63]. Studies reported 5–15% prevalence of high-risk plaque features in the acute chest pain population, in patients undergoing invasive coronary angiography, and in non-culprit vessels of patients with ACS (Providing Regional Observations to Study Predictors of Events in the Coronary Tree, PROSPECT trial) [92, 108–110, 114, 115]. The value of high-risk plaque features for the diagnosis of ACS in patients with significant stenosis was demonstrated in the ROMICAT I trial [124]. In the ROMICAT II trial, high-risk plaques on coronary CTA increased the likelihood of ACS independent of stenotic CAD and clinical risk assessment (age, sex, and number of cardiovascular risk factors) in patients presenting to the ED with acute chest pain but negative initial electrocardio-

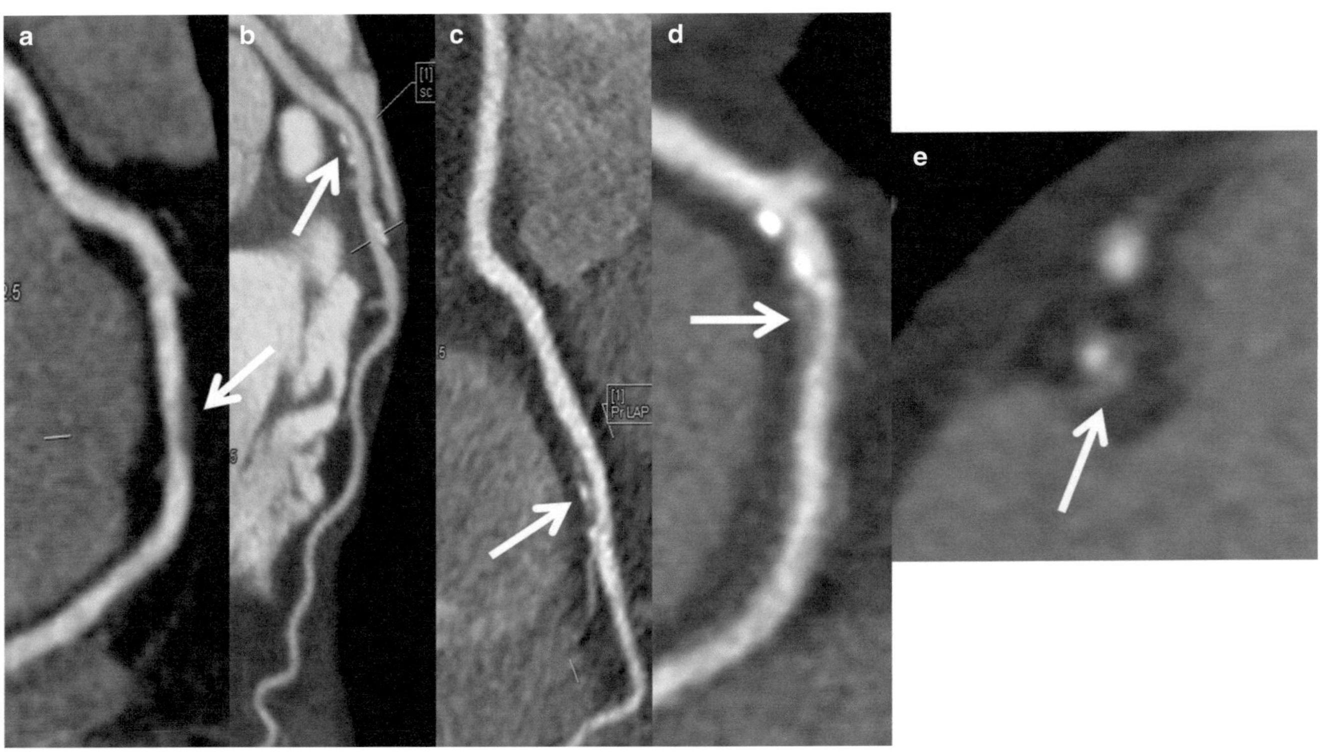

Fig. 28.2 High-risk plaque features. Curved planar and MPR images from coronary CT studies performed on ED chest pain patients show various high-risk plaque features including (**a**) low attenuation plaque and positive remodeling, (**b**) spotty calcification, (**c**) low attenuation plaque, positive remodeling, and spotty calcification, and (**d, e**) the napkin-ring sign

gram and troponin [92]. The ROMICAT score derived from semiautomated quantitative measurements of high-risk plaque features (volume of <60HU plaque, remodeling index, spotty calcium, plaque length) was an independent predictor of ACS during the index hospitalization and was incremental to gender and presence of ≥50% stenosis [125]. When applying the ROMICAT score derived from the ROMICAT I trial to the patient population of the ROMICAT II trial, the ROMICAT score (OR 2.9, 95% CI 1.4–6.0, $p = 0.003$) was a predictor of ACS after adjusting for gender and ≥50% stenosis [125]. The AUC of the model containing ROMICAT score, gender, and ≥50% stenosis was 0.91 (95% CI 0.86–0.96) and was better than with a model that included only gender and ≥ 50% stenosis (AUC 0.85, 95% CI 0.77–0.92, $p = 0.002$) [125].

Interestingly, nonalcoholic fatty liver disease (NAFLD) was reported to be associated with advanced high-risk coronary plaque, independent of traditional cardiovascular risk factors and the extent and severity of coronary artery disease [126].

Patients with remaining obstructive non-culprit plaques and higher plaque burden index had a higher risk of MACE. In multivariate analysis, with diabetes, dyslipidemia, and plaque burden index, obstructive non-culprit plaques remained an independent predictor of MACE [127]. Almost a quarter of the study population experienced a new event arising from a non-culprit plaque during a follow-up of almost 5 years. ACS patients with remaining obstructive non-culprit plaques or high plaque burden have an increased risk of future MACE [127].

Advanced Application of CCTA

In the presence of coronary stenosis, fractional flow reserve (FFR) can be measured angiographically to determine the coronary blood volume. Typically FFR over 0.75–0.8 has been associated with more positive outcomes and decreased ischemia after revascularization [128]. CT-FFR adds functional aspects to stenosis assessment and reduces false-positive test results, which leads to improved specificity [129]. A recent meta-analysis [129] suggests that noninvasive CT-FFR offers improved specificity without noticeably altering the sensitivity of CCTA in detecting hemodynamically relevant lesions in patients with suspected or known coronary artery disease over anatomic interpretation by CCTA alone [129]. At this time, three large prospective clinical trials have demonstrated the diagnostic value of a noninvasive FFR (fractional flow reserve from coronary computed tomographic angiography [CT-FFR]) algorithm (HeartFlow, Inc., Redwood City, CA) [130–132]. Furthermore, an initial study presented results on the diagnostic performance of an alternative on-site algorithm (Siemens Healthineers, Forchheim, Germany); these results were subsequently corroborated by a larger study [133, 134]. These investigations have demonstrated that algorithm-based noninvasive FFR derivation from CCTA compares favorably to the diagnostic gold standard of invasive FFR.

CT myocardial perfusion is growing as a new technique that provides a functional assessment of the myocardium along with a comprehensive evaluation of coronary artery disease within a single modality [135]. The addition of dynamic CT myocardial perfusion to standard coronary CTA can provide insightful information on significant coronary stenosis, particularly for hemodynamically relevant lesions, which may be helpful for patient management [135]. Recently, CT myocardial perfusion studies have been performed with promising results [136–138]. Although results are promising, this technique comes at the price of additional radiation exposure and contrast media along with the need for pharmacologic stress agents [139].

CCTA Reporting

CAD-RADS categories depend on stenosis severity, and a classification system suggested by the Society of Cardiovascular Computed Tomography is used to grade stenosis severity [140–142]. They range from CAD-RADS 0 (absence of atherosclerosis) to CAD-RADS 5 (presence of at least one total occlusion) (Table 28.1) (Fig. 28.3). Categories should reflect the clinically most relevant finding per patient and be complementary to the final impression of the report to provide specific information regarding the location and extent of coronary plaque and stenosis.

Table 28.1 Grading scale for stenosis severity and CAD-RADS

CAD-RADS	Degree of luminal diameter stenosis (%)	Terminology	interpretation
N	Nondiagnostic		ACS cannot be excluded
1	0	No visible stenosis	ACS highly unlikely
2	1–24	Minimal stenosis	ACS highly unlikely
3	25–49	Mild stenosis	ACS unlikely
4	50–69	Moderate stenosis	ACS possible
5	70–99	Severe stenosis	ACS likely
6	100	Occluded	ACS very likely

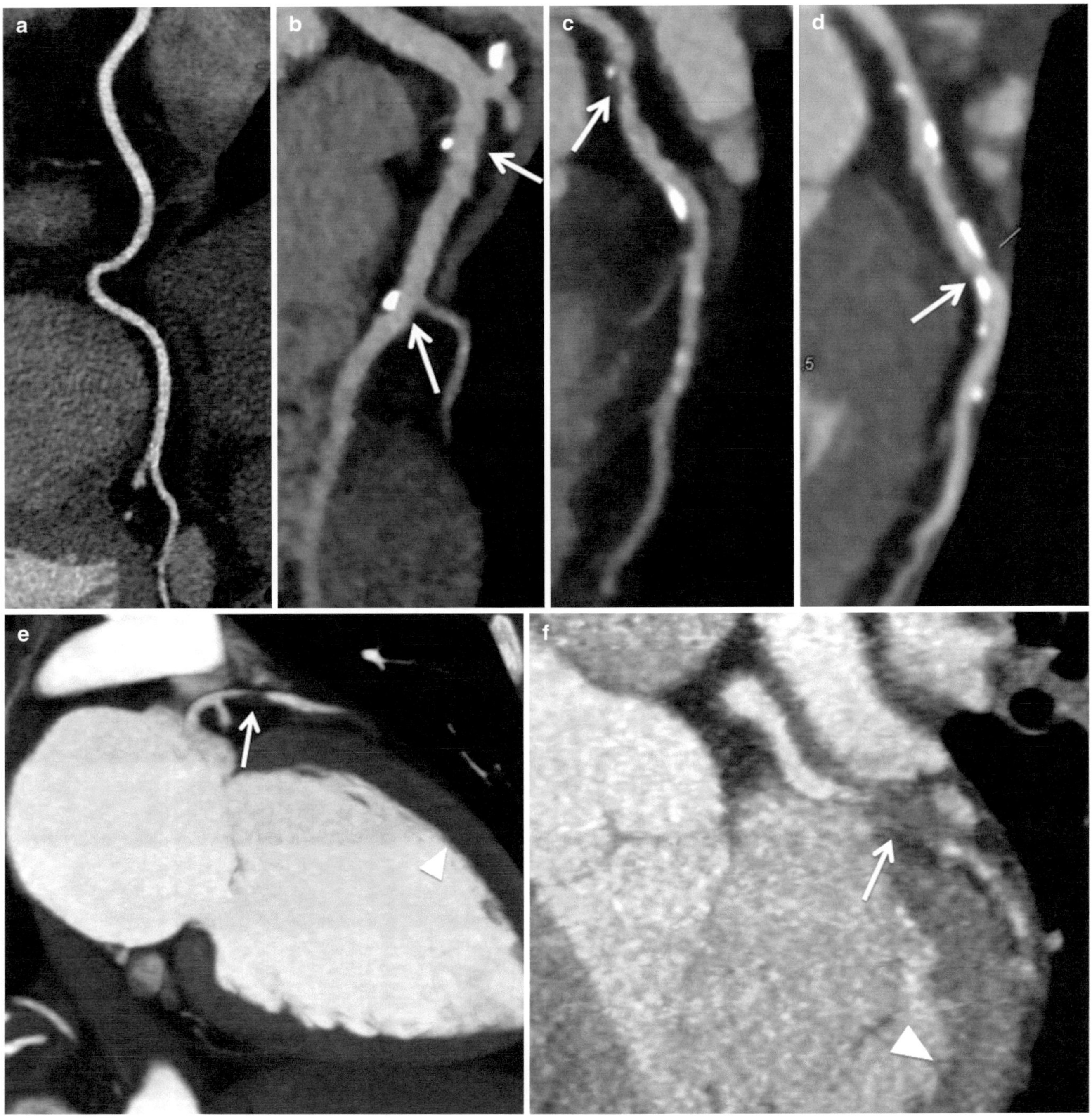

Fig. 28.3 CAD-RADS reporting categories. Curved planar and MPR images from coronary CT studies performed on ED chest pain patients show (**a**) CAD-RADS1, no luminal stenosis in the RCA; (**b**) CAD-RADS2, calcified and non-calcified plaque causing 1–24% stenosis of the LAD; (**c**) CAD-RADS3, mixed plaque causing 25–49% stenosis of the LAD; (**d**) CAD-RADS4, calcified plaque causing 50–69% stenosis of the LAD; (**e**) CAD-RADS5, non-calcified plaque causing 70–99% stenosis of the LAD (arrow) and a corresponding subendocardial perfusion defect in the anterior wall (arrowhead); (**f**) CAD-RADS6, occlusion of the circumflex artery (arrow) and a corresponding subendocardial perfusion defect in the lateral wall (arrowhead)

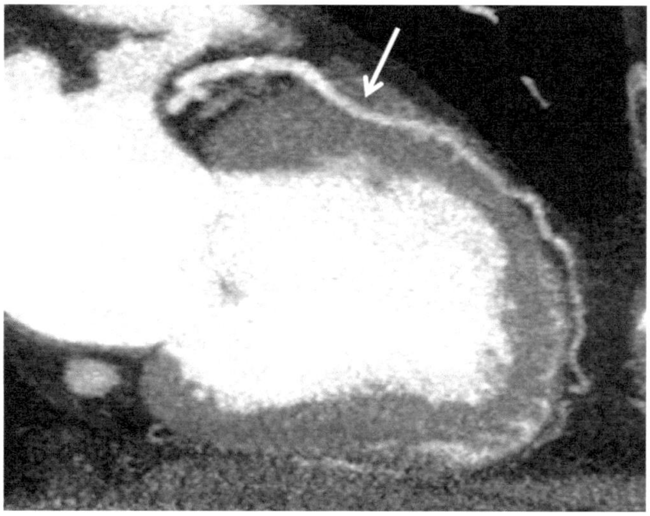

Fig. 28.4 Myocardial bridging. MPR image from a coronary CT study performed on an ED patient with chest pain demonstrates long intramyocardial course of the mid-LAD, without narrowing of the bridged segment

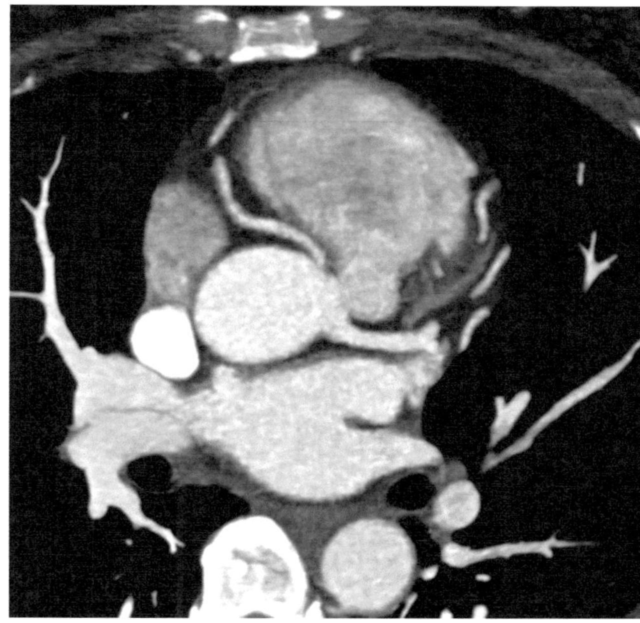

Fig. 28.5 Coronary anomalies. Thin-slab MIP image from a coronary CT study performed on an ED patient with chest pain demonstrates anomalous origin of the right coronary artery from the left cusp with interarterial course. This course has been associated with arrhythmia and sudden cardiac death

Non-atherosclerotic Causes of Chest Pain

Myocardial bridging (Fig. 28.4), a segment of an epicardial coronary artery coursing within the myocardium, is present in about one third of adults [143]. In the majority of cases, systolic compression of the tunneled segment remains clinically silent. With provocative testing in patients with angiographically normal coronary arteries, myocardial bridges are revealed in ≤40% of cases by increasing systolic compression [144]. Rare complications of myocardial bridging include angina, myocardial ischemia, myocardial infarction, left ventricular dysfunction, myocardial stunning, paroxysmal AV blockade, exercise-induced ventricular tachycardia, and sudden cardiac death [145–148]. The likelihood of ischemia also increases with the intramyocardial depth of the tunneled segment; however, there is no consistent association between the patient's symptom and the length and depth of the tunneled segment or the degree of systolic compression [149, 150].

CCTA is ideal to demonstrate the anatomic course of coronaries and caliber change throughout the cardiac cycle when retrospectively ECG-gated CCTA is employed. About 80% of coronary artery anomalies are benign and incidental findings at the time of catheterization [151]. Although the significance of coronary anomalies is mostly unclear, potentially serious anomalies (Fig. 28.5) which include ectopic coronary origin from the pulmonary artery or opposite aortic sinus, single coronary artery, and large coronary fistulae can result in angina pectoris, myocardial infarction, heart failure, arrhythmias, and sudden cardiac arrest [151]. Younger patients in their first three decades with isolated coronary artery anomalies are at risk of dying, especially with exercise [152]. Sudden cardiac arrest (SCA) secondary to congenital anomalous coronary artery disease occurs due to insufficient coronary flow by the anomalous LCA to meet elevated left ventricular myocardial metabolic demand, usually during exertion or exercise. In a majority of previously reported cases, SCA was triggered by exertion, and most of these patients have a positive exercise stress test [153]. Contributing factors to an increased resistance in the LCA include compression between the great vessels, a slit-like ostium, myocardial bridging, or unfavorable geometry [154]. High-risk defects include those involved with the proximal coronary artery or coursing of the anomalous artery between the aorta and pulmonary trunk [152]. Left anterior descending coronary arteries arising from the right cusp with an interarterial course have been considered malignant (Fig. 28.6), and anomalous coronary origins can be associated with acute chest pain [152].

High-sensitivity Troponin Assays (Hs–Troponins)

The introduction of high-sensitivity troponin (hs-troponin) assays has changed standard optimal care (SOC) considerably, and measurement has become standard practice in many institutions, allowing for more accurate and faster

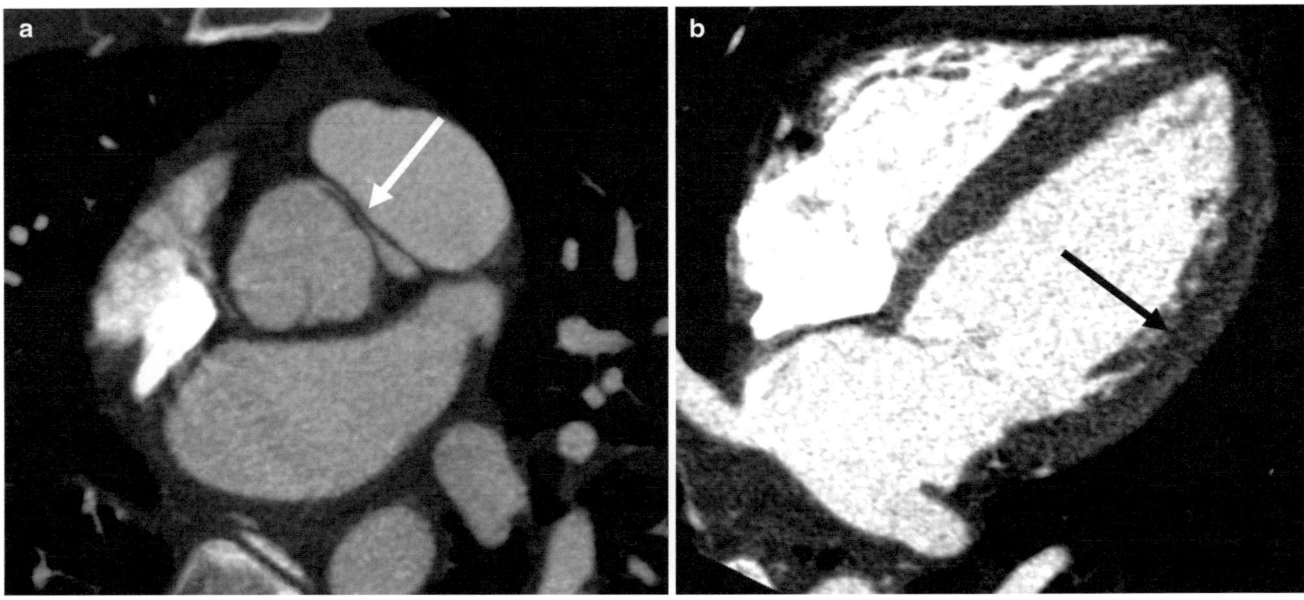

Fig. 28.6 Malignant coronary anomaly. (**a**) Thin-slab MIP image from a coronary CT performed on an ED patient with chest pain demonstrates anomalous origin of the LAD from the right cusp, with an interarterial course. The LAD is markedly narrowed in the interarterial segment, leading to a large subendocardial perfusion defect seen on a four-chamber MPR image (**b**)

rule-out of ACS [15, 16]. These new assays are more sensitive and reach negative predictive values of >97% for myocardial infarction within 3 h [15, 16]. Early observations indicated that hs-troponins would allow fast and accurate exclusion of ACS in a substantial proportion of low- to intermediate-risk patients, obviating the need for prolonged observation and in-hospital diagnostic testing in the absence of elevated high-sensitivity cardiac biomarkers or precarious ECG abnormalities [155–157].

The BEACON (Better Evaluation of Acute Chest Pain with Coronary Computed Tomography Angiography) trial is a European randomized trial comparing a diagnostic strategy supplemented by early CCTA with SOC for patients suspected of ACS in the era of hs-troponins [158]. In their study, CCTA applied early in the work-up of suspected ACS is safe and associated with less outpatient testing and lower costs. However, CCTA does not identify more patients with significant CAD requiring coronary revascularization, shorten hospital stay, or allow for more direct discharge from the ED in the era of hs-troponins [158]. Discharge from the ED was not more frequent after CCTA (65% vs. 59%, $p = 0.16$), and length of stay was similar (6.3 h in both groups, $p = 0.80$). The CCTA group had lower direct medical costs (€337 vs. €511, $p < 0.01$) and less outpatient testing after the index ED visit (10 [4%] vs. 26 [10%], $p < 0.01$). There was no difference in incidence of undetected ACS [158].

Korley FK et al. showed that no subjects with undetectable hsTnI or zero calcium score (CACS) had a MACE. A strategy of avoiding further testing in subjects with undetectable initial hsTnI, performing CACS on subjects with detectable initial hsTnI but nonincreased hsTnI (less than 99th percentile), and obtaining CTA in subjects with Agatston greater than 0 will have a negative predictive value of 100.0% (95% confidence interval, 98.2%–100.0%). The addition of CACS to hsTnI improves the identification of low-risk subjects in whom CTA might be avoided [159].

A cohort study in patients with suspected ACS enrolled in the ROMICAT II trial and randomized to coronary CTA who also had hsTnI measurement at the time of the emergency department presentation assessed coronary CTA for traditional (no CAD, nonobstructive CAD, ≥50% stenosis) and advanced features of CAD (≥50% stenosis, high-risk plaque features: positive remodeling, low <30-Hounsfield units plaque, napkin-ring sign, spotty calcium) [160]. hsTnI at the time of presentation followed by early advanced coronary CTA assessment improved the risk stratification and diagnostic accuracy for ACS as compared to conventional troponin and traditional coronary CTA assessment [160]. The study showed absence of ≥50% stenosis and high-risk plaque ruled out ACS in patients with intermediate hsTnI ($n = 87$, 54.4%; ACS rate 0%), whereas patients with both ≥50% stenosis and high-risk plaque were at high risk ($n = 13$, 8.1%; ACS rate 69.2%) and patients with either ≥50% stenosis or high-risk plaque were at intermediate risk for ACS ($n = 39$, 24.4%; ACS rate 7.7%) [160].

Alternative Tests

In patients with low to intermediate pretest probability, other tests with high negative predictive value to rule in or rule out ACS or myocardial infarct (MI) to enable early discharge include rest CMR, echocardiography, and SPECT MPI, though these must be performed while the patient is experiencing chest pain. Resting SPECT MPI with technetium-99m sestamibi is useful in the setting of suspected ACS [161–164], and its use in the ED setting resulted in earlier discharge, lower cost, and fewer unnecessary admissions [165–167]. Observational studies demonstrated its high negative predictive value to rule out MI or short-term cardiac events. However, a considerable limitation of resting SPECT MPI in ED patients is the limited availability of tracers and interpreting personnel as well as decreased accuracy when not performed during an episode of chest pain. Resting two-dimensional (2D) echocardiography provides information by evaluating wall motion and ejection fraction rapidly and noninvasively [168, 169]. However, the positive predictive value is only 0–44% [168, 170, 171] with difficulty distinguishing acute from chronic ischemia. In addition, coronary stenosis cannot be evaluated unless the patient has a wall motion abnormality; as with multiphase CCTA, rest echo may be useful for evaluation of nonischemic causes of chest pain. Cardiac MR (CMR) can image coronary anatomy, ventricular function, myocardial perfusion, and myocardial fibrosis/scar. In observational studies, CMR has a sensitivity of 70–85% to detect ischemic heart disease [172–174], and coronary MR angiography showed 72% accuracy detecting stenosis. Although a normal CMR is associated with good prognosis and a very low risk, lower spatial resolution and limited availability compared to CCTA limit its clinical application in the ED setting [175]. Conventional catheter angiography, considered a gold standard for diagnosis of coronary artery disease, should be reserved for use as a confirmative test and for intervention for patients with significant stenosis or occlusion who will undergo intervention with certain likelihood rather than for initial evaluation of patients at less than high risk for ACS. Hence, invasive catheterization should be a purely therapeutic option.

Future Direction: More or Less

Data suggest that the management of low- to intermediate-risk chest pain patients is changing to enable safe discharge and reduced testing at the index visit [19, 20]. With mounting evidence that early objective testing rarely changes management [31] and that hospitalization provides no benefit in patients with timely and appropriate follow-up [20] and may incur harm [176], care should be taken to avoid unnecessary diagnostic interventions and resource use for low- to intermediate-risk populations [177, 178]. Applying risk stratification tools (such as the HEART score), combined with normal ECG findings and negative cardiac biomarker level results, is sufficient to identify a low- to intermediate-risk patient population who will not benefit from the addition of coronary CT angiography or other means of objective assessment [178, 179].

Also, at least one study has shown that patients who did not undergo initial noninvasive testing were no more likely to experience an MI than were those who did receive testing [177]. Compared with no testing, exercise electrocardiography, myocardial perfusion scintigraphy, and coronary computed tomography angiography were associated with significantly higher odds of cardiac catheterization and revascularization procedures without a concomitant improvement in the odds of experiencing an MI [177]. Patients with chest pain evaluated in the ED who do not have an MI are at very low risk of experiencing an MI during short- and longer-term follow-up in a cohort of privately insured patients. This low risk does not appear to be affected by the initial testing strategy. Deferral of early noninvasive testing appears to be reasonable [177].

References

1. Lloyd-Jones D, Adams RJ, Brown TM, et al. Heart disease and stroke statistics--2010 update: a report from the American Heart Association. Circulation. 2010;121(7):e46–e215. https://doi.org/10.1161/CIRCULATIONAHA.109.192667.
2. Pitts SR, Niska RW, Xu J, Burt CW. National Hospital Ambulatory Medical Care Survey: 2006 emergency department summary. Natl Health Stat Report. 2008;7:1–38.
3. McCaig LF, Burt CW. National Hospital Ambulatory Medical Care Survey: 2002 emergency department summary. Adv Data. 2004;340:1–34.
4. Pozen MW, D'Agostino RB, Selker HP, Sytkowski PA, Hood WB Jr. A predictive instrument to improve coronary-care-unit admission practices in acute ischemic heart disease. A prospective multicenter clinical trial. N Engl J Med. 1984;310(20):1273–8.
5. Virmani R, Burke AP, Farb A, Kolodgie FD. Pathology of the vulnerable plaque. J Am Coll Cardiol. 2006;47(8 Suppl):C13–8.
6. Antman EM, Cohen M, Bernink PJ, McCabe CH, Horacek T, Papuchis G, Mautner B, Corbalan R, Radley D, Braunwald E. The TIMI risk score for unstable angina/non-ST elevation MI: a method for prognostication and therapeutic decision making. JAMA. 2000;284(7):835–42.
7. Than M, Cullen L, Reid CM, et al. A 2-h diagnostic protocol to assess patients with chest pain symptoms in the Asia-Pacific region (ASPECT): a prospective observational validation study. Lancet. 2011;377(9771):1077–84.
8. Hickam DH, Sox HC Jr, Sox CH. Systematic bias in recording the history in patients with chest pain. J Chronic Dis. 1985;38(1):91–100.
9. Jayes RL Jr, Beshansky JR, D'Agostino RB, Selker HP. Do patients' coronary risk factor reports predict acute cardiac ischemia in the emergency department? A multicenter study. J Clin Epidemiol. 1992;45(6):621–6.

10. Han JH, Lindsell CJ, Storrow AB, Luber S, Hoekstra JW, Hollander JE, Peacock WF, Pollack CV, Gibler WB. The role of cardiac risk factor burden in diagnosing acute coronary syndromes in the emergency department setting. Ann Emerg Med. 2007;49(2):145–52. 152 e141.
11. Lloyd-Jones DM, Camargo CA Jr, Lapuerta P, Giugliano RP, O'Donnell CJ. Electrocardiographic and clinical predictors of acute myocardial infarction in patients with unstable angina pectoris. Am J Cardiol. 1998;81(10):1182–6.
12. Chase M, Brown AM, Robey JL, Pollack CV Jr, Shofer FS, Hollander JE. Prognostic value of symptoms during a normal or nonspecific electrocardiogram in emergency department patients with potential acute coronary syndrome. Acad Emerg Med. 2006;13(10):1034–9.
13. Green GB, Beaudreau RW, Chan DW, DeLong D, Kelley CA, Kelen GD. Use of troponin T and creatine kinase-MB subunit levels for risk stratification of emergency department patients with possible myocardial ischemia. Ann Emerg Med. 1998;31(1):19–29.
14. Newby LK. The emerging role of myoglobin for risk stratification. Am Heart J. 2001;142(1):4–6.
15. Reichlin T, Hochholzer W, Bassetti S, Steuer S, Stelzig C, Hartwiger S, Biedert S, Schaub N, Buerge C, Potocki M, Noveanu M, Breidthardt T, Twerenbold R, Winkler K, Bingisser R, Mueller C. Early diagnosis of myocardial infarction with sensitive cardiac troponin assays. N Engl J Med. 2009;361(9):858–67.
16. Keller T, Zeller T, Peetz D, et al. Sensitive troponin I assay in early diagnosis of acute myocardial infarction. N Engl J Med. 2009;361(9):868–77.
17. Januzzi JL Jr, Bamberg F, Lee H, Truong QA, Nichols JH, Karakas M, Mohammed AA, Schlett CL, Nagurney JT, Hoffmann U, Koenig W. High-sensitivity troponin T concentrations in acute chest pain patients evaluated with cardiac computed tomography. Circulation. 2010;121(10):1227–34.
18. Braunwald E, Antman EM, Beasley JW, et al. ACC/AHA guideline update for the management of patients with unstable angina and non-ST-segment elevation myocardial infarction--2002: summary article: a report of the American College of Cardiology/ American Heart Association Task Force on Practice Guidelines (Committee on the Management of Patients With Unstable Angina). Circulation. 2002;106(14):1893–900.
19. Backus BE, Six AJ, Kelder JC, et al. A prospective validation of the HEART score for chest pain patients at the emergency department. Int J Cardiol. 2013;168(3):2153–8.
20. Weinstock MB, Weingart S, Orth F, VanFossen D, Kaide C, Anderson J, Newman DH. Risk for clinically relevant adverse cardiac events in patients with chest pain at hospital admission. JAMA Intern Med. 2015;175(7):1207–12.
21. Pope JH, Aufderheide TP, Ruthazer R, et al. Missed diagnoses of acute cardiac ischemia in the emergency department. N Engl J Med. 2000;342(16):1163–70.
22. Goldberg A, Litt HI. Evaluation of the patient with acute chest pain. Radiol Clin N Am. 2010;48(4):745–55.
23. Lee TH, Rouan GW, Weisberg MC, et al. Clinical characteristics and natural history of patients with acute myocardial infarction sent home from the emergency room. Am J Cardiol. 1987;60(4):219–24.
24. Fineberg HV, Scadden D, Goldman L. Care of patients with a low probability of acute myocardial infarction. Cost effectiveness of alternatives to coronary-care-unit admission. N Engl J Med. 1984;310(20):1301–7.
25. Galperin-Aizenberg M, Cook TS, Hollander JE, Litt HI. Cardiac CT angiography in the emergency department. AJR Am J Roentgenol. 2015;204(3):463–74.
26. Hollander JE, Chang AM, Shofer FS, Collin MJ, Walsh KM, McCusker CM, Baxt WG, Litt HI. One-year outcomes following coronary computerized tomographic angiography for evaluation of emergency department patients with potential acute coronary syndrome. Acad Emerg Med. 2009;16(8):693–8.
27. Lee NJ, Litt H. Cardiac CT angiography for evaluation of acute chest pain. Int J Cardiovasc Imaging. 2016;32(1):101–12.
28. Rybicki FJ, Udelson JE, Peacock WF, Goldhaber SZ, Isselbacher EM, Kazerooni E, Kontos MC, Litt H, Woodard PK. 2015 ACR/ ACC/AHA/AATS/ACEP/ASNC/NASCI/SAEM/SCCT/SCMR/ SCPC/SNMMI/STR/STS appropriate utilization of cardiovascular imaging in emergency department patients with chest pain: a joint document of the American College of Radiology Appropriateness Criteria Committee and the American College of Cardiology Appropriate use Criteria Task Force. J Am Coll Radiol. 2016;13(2):e1–e29.
29. Rybicki FJ, Udelson JE, Peacock WF, Goldhaber SZ, Isselbacher EM, Kazerooni E, Kontos MC, Litt H, Woodard PK. 2015 ACR/ ACC/AHA/AATS/ACEP/ASNC/NASCI/SAEM/SCCT/SCMR/ SCPC/SNMMI/STR/STS appropriate utilization of cardiovascular imaging in emergency department patients with chest pain: a joint document of the American College of Radiology Appropriateness Criteria Committee and the American College of Cardiology Appropriate Use Criteria Task Force. J Am Coll Cardiol. 2016;67(7):853–79.
30. Hamilton-Craig C, Fifoot A, Hansen M, Pincus M, Chan J, Walters DL, Branch KR. Diagnostic performance and cost of CT angiography versus stress ECG--a randomized prospective study of suspected acute coronary syndrome chest pain in the emergency department (CT-COMPARE). Int J Cardiol. 2014;177(3):867–73.
31. Hermann LK, Newman DH, Pleasant WA, Rojanasarntikul D, Lakoff D, Goldberg SA, Duvall WL, Henzlova MJ. Yield of routine provocative cardiac testing among patients in an emergency department-based chest pain unit. JAMA Intern Med. 2013;173(12):1128–33.
32. Rubinshtein R, Halon DA, Gaspar T, Jaffe R, Karkabi B, Flugelman MY, Kogan A, Shapira R, Peled N, Lewis BS. Usefulness of 64-slice cardiac computed tomographic angiography for diagnosing acute coronary syndromes and predicting clinical outcome in emergency department patients with chest pain of uncertain origin. Circulation. 2007;115(13):1762–8.
33. Goldstein JA, Gallagher MJ, O'Neill WW, Ross MA, O'Neil BJ, Raff GL. A randomized controlled trial of multi-slice coronary computed tomography for evaluation of acute chest pain. J Am Coll Cardiol. 2007;49(8):863–71.
34. Hoffmann U, Nagurney JT, Moselewski F, Pena A, Ferencik M, Chae CU, Cury RC, Butler J, Abbara S, Brown DF, Manini A, Nichols JH, Achenbach S, Brady TJ. Coronary multidetector computed tomography in the assessment of patients with acute chest pain. Circulation. 2006;114(21):2251–60.
35. Gallagher MJ, Ross MA, Raff GL, Goldstein JA, O'Neill WW, O'Neil B. The diagnostic accuracy of 64-slice computed tomography coronary angiography compared with stress nuclear imaging in emergency department low-risk chest pain patients. Ann Emerg Med. 2007;49(2):125–36.
36. Hollander JE, Chang AM, Shofer FS, McCusker CM, Baxt WG, Litt HI. Coronary computed tomographic angiography for rapid discharge of low-risk patients with potential acute coronary syndromes. Ann Emerg Med. 2009;53(3):295–304.
37. Hoffmann U, Bamberg F, Chae CU, Nichols JH, Rogers IS, Seneviratne SK, Truong QA, Cury RC, Abbara S, Shapiro MD, Moloo J, Butler J, Ferencik M, Lee H, Jang IK, Parry BA, Brown DF, Udelson JE, Achenbach S, Brady TJ, Nagurney JT. Coronary computed tomography angiography for early triage of patients with acute chest pain: the ROMICAT (Rule Out Myocardial Infarction using Computer Assisted Tomography) trial. J Am Coll Cardiol. 2009;53(18):1642–50.
38. Hoffmann U, Truong QA, Schoenfeld DA, Chou ET, Woodard PK, Nagurney JT, Pope JH, Hauser TH, White CS, Weiner SG,

Kalanjian S, Mullins ME, Mikati I, Peacock WF, Zakroysky P, Hayden D, Goehler A, Lee H, Gazelle GS, Wiviott SD, Fleg JL, Udelson JE. Coronary CT angiography versus standard evaluation in acute chest pain. N Engl J Med. 2012;367(4):299–308.
39. Litt HI, Gatsonis C, Snyder B, Singh H, Miller CD, Entrikin DW, Leaming JM, Gavin LJ, Pacella CB, Hollander JE. CT angiography for safe discharge of patients with possible acute coronary syndromes. N Engl J Med. 2012;366(15):1393–403.
40. Goldstein JA, Chinnaiyan KM, Abidov A, Achenbach S, Berman DS, Hayes SW, Hoffmann U, Lesser JR, Mikati IA, O'Neil BJ, Shaw LJ, Shen MY, Valeti US, Raff GL. The CT-STAT (coronary computed tomographic angiography for systematic triage of acute chest pain patients to treatment) trial. J Am Coll Cardiol. 2011;58(14):1414–22.
41. Cook TS, Galperin-Aizenberg M, Litt HI. Coronary and cardiac computed tomography in the emergency room: current status and future directions. J Thorac Imaging. 2013;28(4):204–16.
42. Cury RC, Feuchtner GM, Batlle JC, Pena CS, Janowitz W, Katzen BT, Ziffer JA. Triage of patients presenting with chest pain to the emergency department: implementation of coronary CT angiography in a large urban health care system. AJR Am J Roentgenol. 2013;200(1):57–65.
43. Hoffmann U, Pena AJ, Moselewski F, Ferencik M, Abbara S, Cury RC, Chae CU, Nagurney JT. MDCT in early triage of patients with acute chest pain. AJR Am J Roentgenol. 2006;187(5):1240–7.
44. Salerno M, Bourque JM, Beller GA. Coronary angiographic evaluation of low-risk chest pain in the emergency department CT-STAT, or maybe not quite that fast? J Am Coll Cardiol. 2011;58(14):1423–5.
45. Rubinshtein R, Halon DA, Gaspar T, Jaffe R, Goldstein J, Karkabi B, Flugelman MY, Kogan A, Shapira R, Peled N, Lewis BS. Impact of 64-slice cardiac computed tomographic angiography on clinical decision-making in emergency department patients with chest pain of possible myocardial ischemic origin. Am J Cardiol. 2007;100(10):1522–6.
46. Truong QA, Hayden D, Woodard PK, Kirby R, Chou ET, Nagurney JT, Wiviott SD, Fleg JL, Schoenfeld DA, Udelson JE, Hoffmann U. Sex differences in the effectiveness of early coronary computed tomographic angiography compared with standard emergency department evaluation for acute chest pain: the rule-out myocardial infarction with Computer-Assisted Tomography (ROMICAT)-II Trial. Circulation. 2013;127(25):2494–502.
47. Eckert J, Schmidt M, Magedanz A, Voigtlander T, Schmermund A. Coronary CT angiography in managing atherosclerosis. Int J Mol Sci. 2015;16(2):3740–56.
48. Fazel P, Peterman MA, Schussler JM. Three-year outcomes and cost analysis in patients receiving 64-slice computed tomographic coronary angiography for chest pain. Am J Cardiol. 2009;104(4):498–500.
49. Romero J, Husain SA, Holmes AA, Kelesidis I, Chavez P, Mojadidi MK, Levsky JM, Wever-Pinzon O, Taub C, Makani H, Travin MI, Pina IL, Garcia MJ. Non-invasive assessment of low risk acute chest pain in the emergency department: a comparative meta-analysis of prospective studies. Int J Cardiol. 2015;187:565–80.
50. Beigel R, Oieru D, Goitein O, Chouraqui P, Konen E, Shamiss A, Hod H, Or J, Matetzky S. Usefulness of routine use of multidetector coronary computed tomography in the "fast track" evaluation of patients with acute chest pain. Am J Cardiol. 2009;103(11):1481–6.
51. Shim SS, Kim Y, Lim SM. Improvement of image quality with beta-blocker premedication on ECG-gated 16-MDCT coronary angiography. AJR Am J Roentgenol. 2005;184(2):649–54.
52. Abbara S, Arbab-Zadeh A, Callister TQ, Desai MY, Mamuya W, Thomson L, Weigold WG. SCCT guidelines for performance of coronary computed tomographic angiography: a report of the Society of Cardiovascular Computed Tomography Guidelines Committee. J Cardiovasc Comput Tomogr. 2009;3(3):190–204.
53. Dewey M, Hoffmann H, Hamm B. Multislice CT coronary angiography: effect of sublingual nitroglycerine on the diameter of coronary arteries. Rofo. 2006;178(6):600–4.
54. Decramer I, Vanhoenacker PK, Sarno G, Van Hoe L, Bladt O, Wijns W, Parizel PM. Effects of sublingual nitroglycerin on coronary lumen diameter and number of visualized septal branches on 64-MDCT angiography. AJR Am J Roentgenol. 2008;190(1):219–25.
55. Hausleiter J, Meyer T, Hermann F, Hadamitzky M, Krebs M, Gerber TC, McCollough C, Martinoff S, Kastrati A, Schomig A, Achenbach S. Estimated radiation dose associated with cardiac CT angiography. JAMA. 2009;301(5):500–7.
56. Earls JP, Berman EL, Urban BA, Curry CA, Lane JL, Jennings RS, McCulloch CC, Hsieh J, Londt JH. Prospectively gated transverse coronary CT angiography versus retrospectively gated helical technique: improved image quality and reduced radiation dose. Radiology. 2008;246(3):742–53.
57. Menke J, Unterberg-Buchwald C, Staab W, Sohns JM, Seif Amir Hosseini A, Schwarz A. Head-to-head comparison of prospectively triggered vs retrospectively gated coronary computed tomography angiography: meta-analysis of diagnostic accuracy, image quality, and radiation dose. Am Heart J. 2013;165(2):154–63. e153.
58. den Harder AM, Willemink MJ, de Jong PA, Schilham AM, Rajiah P, Takx RA, Leiner T. New horizons in cardiac CT. Clin Radiol. 2016;71(8):758–67.
59. Lau GT, Ridley LJ, Schieb MC, Brieger DB, Freedman SB, Wong LA, Lo SK, Kritharides L. Coronary artery stenoses: detection with calcium scoring, CT angiography, and both methods combined. Radiology. 2005;235(2):415–22.
60. Chang AM, Le J, Matsuura AC, Litt HI, Hollander JE. Does coronary artery calcium scoring add to the predictive value of coronary computed tomography angiography for adverse cardiovascular events in low-risk chest pain patients? Acad Emerg Med. 2011;18(10):1065–71.
61. Boll DT, Merkle EM, Paulson EK, Mirza RA, Fleiter TR. Calcified vascular plaque specimens: assessment with cardiac dual-energy multidetector CT in anthropomorphically moving heart phantom. Radiology. 2008;249(1):119–26. https://doi.org/10.1148/radiol.2483071576.
62. Boll DT, Merkle EM, Paulson EK, Fleiter TR. Coronary stent patency: dual-energy multidetector CT assessment in a pilot study with anthropomorphic phantom. Radiology. 2008;247(3):687–95.
63. Wnorowski AM, Halpern EJ. Diagnostic yield of triple-rule-out CT in an emergency setting. AJR Am J Roentgenol. 2016;207(2):295–301.
64. Ayaram D, Bellolio MF, Murad MH, Laack TA, Sadosty AT, Erwin PJ, Hollander JE, Montori VM, Stiell IG, Hess EP. Triple rule-out computed tomographic angiography for chest pain: a diagnostic systematic review and meta-analysis. Acad Emerg Med. 2013;20(9):861–71.
65. Burris AC 2nd, Boura JA, Raff GL, Chinnaiyan KM. Triple rule out versus coronary CT angiography in patients with acute chest pain: results from the ACIC consortium. JACC Cardiovasc Imaging. 2015;8(7):817–25.
66. Takakuwa KM, Halpern EJ. Evaluation of a "triple rule-out" coronary CT angiography protocol: use of 64-Section CT in low-to-moderate risk emergency department patients suspected of having acute coronary syndrome. Radiology. 2008;248(2):438–46.
67. Pohle K, Ropers D, Maffert R, Geitner P, Moshage W, Regenfus M, Kusus M, Daniel WG, Achenbach S. Coronary calcifications in young patients with first, unheralded myocardial infarction: a risk factor matched analysis by electron beam tomography. Heart. 2003;89(6):625–8.

68. Schmermund A, Schwartz RS, Adamzik M, Sangiorgi G, Pfeifer EA, Rumberger JA, Burke AP, Farb A, Virmani R. Coronary atherosclerosis in unheralded sudden coronary death under age 50: histo-pathologic comparison with 'healthy' subjects dying out of hospital. Atherosclerosis. 2001;155(2):499–508.
69. Budoff MJ, Achenbach S, Blumenthal RS, Carr JJ, Goldin JG, Greenland P, Guerci AD, Lima JA, Rader DJ, Rubin GD, Shaw LJ, Wiegers SE. Assessment of coronary artery disease by cardiac computed tomography: a scientific statement from the American Heart Association Committee on cardiovascular imaging and intervention, council on cardiovascular radiology and intervention, and committee on cardiac imaging, council on clinical cardiology. Circulation. 2006;114(16):1761–91.
70. O'Rourke RA, Brundage BH, Froelicher VF, Greenland P, Grundy SM, Hachamovitch R, Pohost GM, Shaw LJ, Weintraub WS, Winters WL Jr. American College of Cardiology/American Heart Association expert consensus document on electron-beam computed tomography for the diagnosis and prognosis of coronary artery disease. J Am Coll Cardiol. 2000;36(1):326–40.
71. Nabi F, Chang SM, Pratt CM, Paranilam J, Peterson LE, Frias ME, Mahmarian JJ. Coronary artery calcium scoring in the emergency department: identifying which patients with chest pain can be safely discharged home. Ann Emerg Med. 2010;56(3):220–9.
72. Marwan M, Ropers D, Pflederer T, Daniel WG, Achenbach S. Clinical characteristics of patients with obstructive coronary lesions in the absence of coronary calcification: an evaluation by coronary CT angiography. Heart. 2009;95(13):1056–60. https://doi.org/10.1136/hrt.2008.153353.
73. Davies MJ. The composition of coronary-artery plaques. N Engl J Med. 1997;336(18):1312–4.
74. Ergun E, Kosar P, Ozturk C, Basbay E, Koc F, Kosar U. Prevalence and extent of coronary artery disease determined by 64-slice CTA in patients with zero coronary calcium score. Int J Cardiovasc Imaging. 2011;27(3):451–8.
75. Sarwar A, Shaw LJ, Shapiro MD, Blankstein R, Hoffmann U, Cury RC, Abbara S, Brady TJ, Budoff MJ, Blumenthal RS, Nasir K. Diagnostic and prognostic value of absence of coronary artery calcification. JACC Cardiovasc Imaging. 2009;2(6):675–88.
76. Greenland P, LaBree L, Azen SP, Doherty TM, Detrano RC. Coronary artery calcium score combined with Framingham score for risk prediction in asymptomatic individuals. JAMA. 2004;291(2):210–5.
77. Raggi P, Cooil B, Ratti C, Callister TQ, Budoff M. Progression of coronary artery calcium and occurrence of myocardial infarction in patients with and without diabetes mellitus. Hypertension. 2005;46(1):238–43.
78. Greenland P, Bonow RO, Brundage BH, Budoff MJ, Eisenberg MJ, Grundy SM, Lauer MS, Post WS, Raggi P, Redberg RF, Rodgers GP, Shaw LJ, Taylor AJ, Weintraub WS. ACCF/AHA 2007 clinical expert consensus document on coronary artery calcium scoring by computed tomography in global cardiovascular risk assessment and in evaluation of patients with chest pain: a report of the American College of Cardiology Foundation Clinical Expert Consensus Task Force (ACCF/AHA Writing Committee to Update the 2000 Expert Consensus Document on Electron Beam Computed Tomography) developed in collaboration with the Society of Atherosclerosis Imaging and Prevention and the Society of Cardiovascular Computed Tomography. J Am Coll Cardiol. 2007;49(3):378–402.
79. Budoff MJ, Hokanson JE, Nasir K, Shaw LJ, Kinney GL, Chow D, Demoss D, Nuguri V, Nabavi V, Ratakonda R, Berman DS, Raggi P. Progression of coronary artery calcium predicts all-cause mortality. JACC Cardiovasc Imaging. 2010;3(12):1229–36.
80. Raggi P, Callister TQ, Shaw LJ. Progression of coronary artery calcium and risk of first myocardial infarction in patients receiving cholesterol-lowering therapy. Arterioscler Thromb Vasc Biol. 2004;24(7):1272–7.
81. Herzog C, Britten M, Balzer JO, Mack MG, Zangos S, Ackermann H, Schaechinger V, Schaller S, Flohr T, Vogl TJ. Multidetector-row cardiac CT: diagnostic value of calcium scoring and CT coronary angiography in patients with symptomatic, but atypical, chest pain. Eur Radiol. 2004;14(2):169–77.
82. Miller CD, Litt HI, Askew K, Entrikin D, Carr JJ, Chang AM, Kilkenny J, Weisenthal B, Hollander JE. Implications of 25% to 50% coronary stenosis with cardiac computed tomographic angiography in ED patients. Am J Emerg Med. 2012;30(4):597–605.
83. Wu E, Ortiz JT, Tejedor P, Lee DC, Bucciarelli-Ducci C, Kansal P, Carr JC, Holly TA, Lloyd-Jones D, Klocke FJ, Bonow RO. Infarct size by contrast enhanced cardiac magnetic resonance is a stronger predictor of outcomes than left ventricular ejection fraction or end-systolic volume index: prospective cohort study. Heart. 2008;94(6):730–6.
84. Miller TD, Christian TF, Hopfenspirger MR, Hodge DO, Gersh BJ, Gibbons RJ. Infarct size after acute myocardial infarction measured by quantitative tomographic 99mTc sestamibi imaging predicts subsequent mortality. Circulation. 1995;92(3):334–41.
85. Elezi S, Kastrati A, Neumann FJ, Hadamitzky M, Dirschinger J, Schomig A. Vessel size and long-term outcome after coronary stent placement. Circulation. 1998;98(18):1875–80.
86. Togni M, Eber S, Widmer J, Billinger M, Wenaweser P, Cook S, Vogel R, Seiler C, Eberli FR, Maier W, Corti R, Roffi M, Luscher TF, Garachemani A, Hess OM, Wandel S, Meier B, Juni P, Windecker S. Impact of vessel size on outcome after implantation of sirolimus-eluting and paclitaxel-eluting stents: a subgroup analysis of the SIRTAX trial. J Am Coll Cardiol. 2007;50(12):1123–31.
87. Schunkert H, Harrell L, Palacios IF. Implications of small reference vessel diameter in patients undergoing percutaneous coronary revascularization. J Am Coll Cardiol. 1999;34(1):40–8.
88. Herzog C, Zwerner PL, Doll JR, Nielsen CD, Nguyen SA, Savino G, Vogl TJ, Costello P, Schoepf UJ. Significant coronary artery stenosis: comparison on per-patient and per-vessel or per-segment basis at 64-section CT angiography. Radiology. 2007;244(1):112–20.
89. Roe MT, Harrington RA, Prosper DM, Pieper KS, Bhatt DL, Lincoff AM, Simoons ML, Akkerhuis M, Ohman EM, Kitt MM, Vahanian A, Ruzyllo W, Karsch K, Califf RM, Topol EJ. Clinical and therapeutic profile of patients presenting with acute coronary syndromes who do not have significant coronary artery disease. The platelet glycoprotein IIb/IIIa in unstable angina: receptor suppression using integrilin therapy (PURSUIT) trial investigators. Circulation. 2000;102(10):1101–6.
90. van Velzen JE, de Graaf FR, Kroft LJ, de Roos A, Reiber JH, Bax JJ, Jukema JW, Schuijf JD, Schalij MJ, van der Wall EE. Performance and efficacy of 320-row computed tomography coronary angiography in patients presenting with acute chest pain: results from a clinical registry. Int J Cardiovasc Imaging. 2012;28(4):865–76.
91. Ahmed W, Schlett CL, Uthamalingam S, Truong QA, Koenig W, Rogers IS, Blankstein R, Nagurney JT, Tawakol A, Januzzi JL, Hoffmann U. Single resting hsTnT level predicts abnormal myocardial stress test in acute chest pain patients with normal initial standard troponin. JACC Cardiovasc Imaging. 2013;6(1):72–82.
92. Puchner SB, Liu T, Mayrhofer T, Truong QA, Lee H, Fleg JL, Nagurney JT, Udelson JE, Hoffmann U, Ferencik M. High-risk plaque detected on coronary CT angiography predicts acute coronary syndromes independent of significant stenosis in acute chest pain: results from the ROMICAT-II trial. J Am Coll Cardiol. 2014;64(7):684–92.
93. Stary HC, Chandler AB, Glagov S, Guyton JR, Insull W Jr, Rosenfeld ME, Schaffer SA, Schwartz CJ, Wagner WD, Wissler RW. A definition of initial, fatty streak, and intermediate lesions of

atherosclerosis. A report from the committee on vascular lesions of the council on arteriosclerosis, American Heart Association. Arterioscler Thromb. 1994;14(5):840–56.

94. Stary HC, Chandler AB, Glagov S, Guyton JR, Insull W Jr, Rosenfeld ME, Schaffer SA, Schwartz CJ, Wagner WD, Wissler RW. A definition of initial, fatty streak, and intermediate lesions of atherosclerosis. A report from the Committee on Vascular Lesions of the Council on Arteriosclerosis, American Heart Association. Circulation. 1994;89(5):2462–78.
95. Glagov S, Weisenberg E, Zarins CK, Stankunavicius R, Kolettis GJ. Compensatory enlargement of human atherosclerotic coronary arteries. N Engl J Med. 1987;316(22):1371–5.
96. Burke AP, Farb A, Malcom GT, Liang YH, Smialek J, Virmani R. Coronary risk factors and plaque morphology in men with coronary disease who died suddenly. N Engl J Med. 1997;336(18):1276–82.
97. Burke AP, Farb A, Malcom GT, Liang Y, Smialek J, Virmani R. Effect of risk factors on the mechanism of acute thrombosis and sudden coronary death in women. Circulation. 1998;97(21):2110–6.
98. Farb A, Tang AL, Burke AP, Sessums L, Liang Y, Virmani R. Sudden coronary death. Frequency of active coronary lesions, inactive coronary lesions, and myocardial infarction. Circulation. 1995;92(7):1701–9.
99. Virmani R, Kolodgie FD, Burke AP, Farb A, Schwartz SM. Lessons from sudden coronary death: a comprehensive morphological classification scheme for atherosclerotic lesions. Arterioscler Thromb Vasc Biol. 2000;20(5):1262–75.
100. Kolodgie FD, Burke AP, Farb A, Gold HK, Yuan J, Narula J, Finn AV, Virmani R. The thin-cap fibroatheroma: a type of vulnerable plaque: the major precursor lesion to acute coronary syndromes. Curr Opin Cardiol. 2001;16(5):285–92.
101. Burke AP, Taylor A, Farb A, Malcom GT, Virmani R. Coronary calcification: insights from sudden coronary death victims. Z Kardiol. 2000;89:Suppl 2:49–53.
102. Wallentin L. Non-ST-elevation acute coronary syndrome: fuel for the invasive strategy. Lancet. 2002;360(9335):738–9.
103. Burke AP, Kolodgie FD, Farb A, Weber DK, Malcom GT, Smialek J, Virmani R. Healed plaque ruptures and sudden coronary death: evidence that subclinical rupture has a role in plaque progression. Circulation. 2001;103(7):934–40.
104. Nakamura M, Nishikawa H, Mukai S, Setsuda M, Nakajima K, Tamada H, Suzuki H, Ohnishi T, Kakuta Y, Nakano T, Yeung AC. Impact of coronary artery remodeling on clinical presentation of coronary artery disease: an intravascular ultrasound study. J Am Coll Cardiol. 2001;37(1):63–9.
105. Maehara A, Mintz GS, Bui AB, Walter OR, Castagna MT, Canos D, Pichard AD, Satler LF, Waksman R, Suddath WO, Laird JR Jr, Kent KM, Weissman NJ. Morphologic and angiographic features of coronary plaque rupture detected by intravascular ultrasound. J Am Coll Cardiol. 2002;40(5):904–10.
106. Ambrose JA, Tannenbaum MA, Alexopoulos D, Hjemdahl-Monsen CE, Leavy J, Weiss M, Borrico S, Gorlin R, Fuster V. Angiographic progression of coronary artery disease and the development of myocardial infarction. J Am Coll Cardiol. 1988;12(1):56–62.
107. Giroud D, Li JM, Urban P, Meier B, Rutishauer W. Relation of the site of acute myocardial infarction to the most severe coronary arterial stenosis at prior angiography. Am J Cardiol. 1992;69(8):729–32.
108. Stone GW, Maehara A, Lansky AJ, de Bruyne B, Cristea E, Mintz GS, Mehran R, McPherson J, Farhat N, Marso SP, Parise H, Templin B, White R, Zhang Z, Serruys PW. A prospective natural-history study of coronary atherosclerosis. N Engl J Med. 2011;364(3):226–35.
109. Pflederer T, Marwan M, Schepis T, Ropers D, Seltmann M, Muschiol G, Daniel WG, Achenbach S. Characterization of culprit lesions in acute coronary syndromes using coronary dual-source CT angiography. Atherosclerosis. 2010;211(2):437–44.
110. Motoyama S, Sarai M, Harigaya H, Anno H, Inoue K, Hara T, Naruse H, Ishii J, Hishida H, Wong ND, Virmani R, Kondo T, Ozaki Y, Narula J. Computed tomographic angiography characteristics of atherosclerotic plaques subsequently resulting in acute coronary syndrome. J Am Coll Cardiol. 2009;54(1):49–57.
111. Hoffmann U, Moselewski F, Nieman K, Jang IK, Ferencik M, Rahman AM, Cury RC, Abbara S, Joneidi-Jafari H, Achenbach S, Brady TJ. Noninvasive assessment of plaque morphology and composition in culprit and stable lesions in acute coronary syndrome and stable lesions in stable angina by multidetector computed tomography. J Am Coll Cardiol. 2006;47(8):1655–62.
112. Gauss S, Achenbach S, Pflederer T, Schuhback A, Daniel WG, Marwan M. Assessment of coronary artery remodelling by dual-source CT: a head-to-head comparison with intravascular ultrasound. Heart. 2011;97(12):991–7.
113. Motoyama S, Kondo T, Sarai M, Sugiura A, Harigaya H, Sato T, Inoue K, Okumura M, Ishii J, Anno H, Virmani R, Ozaki Y, Hishida H, Narula J. Multislice computed tomographic characteristics of coronary lesions in acute coronary syndromes. J Am Coll Cardiol. 2007;50(4):319–26.
114. Kashiwagi M, Tanaka A, Kitabata H, Tsujioka H, Kataiwa H, Komukai K, Tanimoto T, Takemoto K, Takarada S, Kubo T, Hirata K, Nakamura N, Mizukoshi M, Imanishi T, Akasaka T. Feasibility of noninvasive assessment of thin-cap fibroatheroma by multidetector computed tomography. JACC Cardiovasc Imaging. 2009;2(12):1412–9.
115. Kitagawa T, Yamamoto H, Horiguchi J, Ohhashi N, Tadehara F, Shokawa T, Dohi Y, Kunita E, Utsunomiya H, Kohno N, Kihara Y. Characterization of noncalcified coronary plaques and identification of culprit lesions in patients with acute coronary syndrome by 64-slice computed tomography. JACC Cardiovasc Imaging. 2009;2(2):153–60.
116. Obaid DR, Calvert PA, Gopalan D, Parker RA, Hoole SP, West NE, Goddard M, Rudd JH, Bennett MR. Atherosclerotic plaque composition and classification identified by coronary computed tomography: assessment of computed tomography-generated plaque maps compared with virtual histology intravascular ultrasound and histology. Circ Cardiovasc Imaging. 2013;6(5):655–64. https://doi.org/10.1161/CIRCIMAGING.112.000250.
117. Pundziute G, Schuijf JD, Jukema JW, Decramer I, Sarno G, Vanhoenacker PK, Reiber JH, Schalij MJ, Wijns W, Bax JJ. Head-to-head comparison of coronary plaque evaluation between multislice computed tomography and intravascular ultrasound radiofrequency data analysis. JACC Cardiovasc Interv. 2008;1(2):176–82.
118. Hong MK, Mintz GS, Lee CW, Suh J, Kim JH, Park DW, Lee SW, Kim YH, Cheong SS, Kim JJ, Park SW, Park SJ. Comparison of virtual histology to intravascular ultrasound of culprit coronary lesions in acute coronary syndrome and target coronary lesions in stable angina pectoris. Am J Cardiol. 2007;100(6):953–9.
119. Pundziute G, Schuijf JD, Jukema JW, Decramer I, Sarno G, Vanhoenacker PK, Boersma E, Reiber JH, Schalij MJ, Wijns W, Bax JJ. Evaluation of plaque characteristics in acute coronary syndromes: non-invasive assessment with multi-slice computed tomography and invasive evaluation with intravascular ultrasound radiofrequency data analysis. Eur Heart J. 2008;29(19):2373–81.
120. Ruzsics B, Lee H, Zwerner PL, Gebregziabher M, Costello P, Schoepf UJ. Dual-energy CT of the heart for diagnosing coronary artery stenosis and myocardial ischemia-initial experience. Eur Radiol. 2008;18(11):2414–24.
121. Barreto M, Schoenhagen P, Nair A, Amatangelo S, Milite M, Obuchowski NA, Lieber ML, Halliburton SS. Potential of dual-energy computed tomography to characterize atherosclerotic

plaque: ex vivo assessment of human coronary arteries in comparison to histology. J Cardiovasc Comput Tomogr. 2008;2(4):234–42.
122. Yamamoto H, Kitagawa T, Ohashi N, Utsunomiya H, Kunita E, Oka T, Urabe Y, Tsushima H, Awai K, Kihara Y. Noncalcified atherosclerotic lesions with vulnerable characteristics detected by coronary CT angiography and future coronary events. J Cardiovasc Comput Tomogr. 2013;7(3):192–9.
123. Versteylen MO, Kietselaer BL, Dagnelie PC, Joosen IA, Dedic A, Raaijmakers RH, Wildberger JE, Nieman K, Crijns HJ, Niessen WJ, Daemen MJ, Hofstra L. Additive value of semiautomated quantification of coronary artery disease using cardiac computed tomographic angiography to predict future acute coronary syndrome. J Am Coll Cardiol. 2013;61(22):2296–305.
124. Ferencik M, Schlett CL, Ghoshhajra BB, Kriegel MF, Joshi SB, Maurovich-Horvat P, Rogers IS, Banerji D, Bamberg F, Truong QA, Brady TJ, Nagurney JT, Hoffmann U. A computed tomography-based coronary lesion score to predict acute coronary syndrome among patients with acute chest pain and significant coronary stenosis on coronary computed tomographic angiogram. Am J Cardiol. 2012;110(2):183–9.
125. Ferencik M, Mayrhofer T, Puchner SB, Lu MT, Maurovich-Horvat P, Liu T, Ghemigian K, Kitslaar P, Broersen A, Bamberg F, Truong QA, Schlett CL, Hoffmann U. Computed tomography-based high-risk coronary plaque score to predict acute coronary syndrome among patients with acute chest pain--results from the ROMICAT II trial. J Cardiovasc Comput Tomogr. 2015;9(6):538–45.
126. Puchner SB, Lu MT, Mayrhofer T, Liu T, Pursnani A, Ghoshhajra BB, Truong QA, Wiviott SD, Fleg JL, Hoffmann U, Ferencik M. High-risk coronary plaque at coronary CT angiography is associated with nonalcoholic fatty liver disease, independent of coronary plaque and stenosis burden: results from the ROMICAT II trial. Radiology. 2015;274(3):693–701.
127. Dedic A, Kurata A, Lubbers M, Meijboom WB, van Dalen BM, Snelder S, Korbee R, Moelker A, Ouhlous M, van Domburg R, de Feijter PJ, Nieman K. Prognostic implications of non-culprit plaques in acute coronary syndrome: non-invasive assessment with coronary CT angiography. Eur Heart J Cardiovasc Imaging. 2014;15(11):1231–7.
128. Pijls NH, Sels JW. Functional measurement of coronary stenosis. J Am Coll Cardiol. 2012;59(12):1045–57.
129. Baumann S, Renker M, Hetjens S, Fuller SR, Becher T, Lossnitzer D, Lehmann R, Akin I, Borggrefe M, Lang S, Wichmann JL, Schoepf UJ. Comparison of coronary computed tomography angiography-derived vs invasive fractional flow reserve assessment: meta-analysis with subgroup evaluation of intermediate stenosis. Acad Radiol. 2016; https://doi.org/10.1016/j.acra.2016.07.007.
130. Min JK, Leipsic J, Pencina MJ, Berman DS, Koo BK, van Mieghem C, Erglis A, Lin FY, Dunning AM, Apruzzese P, Budoff MJ, Cole JH, Jaffer FA, Leon MB, Malpeso J, Mancini GB, Park SJ, Schwartz RS, Shaw LJ, Mauri L. Diagnostic accuracy of fractional flow reserve from anatomic CT angiography. JAMA. 2012;308(12):1237–45.
131. Koo BK, Erglis A, Doh JH, Daniels DV, Jegere S, Kim HS, Dunning A, DeFrance T, Lansky A, Leipsic J, Min JK. Diagnosis of ischemia-causing coronary stenoses by noninvasive fractional flow reserve computed from coronary computed tomographic angiograms. Results from the prospective multicenter DISCOVER-FLOW (diagnosis of ischemia-causing stenoses obtained via noninvasive fractional flow reserve) study. J Am Coll Cardiol. 2011;58(19):1989–97.
132. Norgaard BL, Leipsic J, Gaur S, Seneviratne S, Ko BS, Ito H, Jensen JM, Mauri L, De Bruyne B, Bezerra H, Osawa K, Marwan M, Naber C, Erglis A, Park SJ, Christiansen EH, Kaltoft A, Lassen JF, Botker HE, Achenbach S. Diagnostic performance of noninvasive fractional flow reserve derived from coronary computed tomography angiography in suspected coronary artery disease: the NXT trial (analysis of coronary blood flow using CT angiography: next steps). J Am Coll Cardiol. 2014;63(12):1145–55.
133. Renker M, Schoepf UJ, Wang R, Meinel FG, Rier JD, Bayer RR 2nd, Mollmann H, Hamm CW, Steinberg DH, Baumann S. Comparison of diagnostic value of a novel noninvasive coronary computed tomography angiography method versus standard coronary angiography for assessing fractional flow reserve. Am J Cardiol. 2014;114(9):1303–8.
134. Coenen A, Lubbers MM, Kurata A, Kono A, Dedic A, Chelu RG, Dijkshoorn ML, Gijsen FJ, Ouhlous M, van Geuns RJ, Nieman K. Fractional flow reserve computed from noninvasive CT angiography data: diagnostic performance of an on-site clinician-operated computational fluid dynamics algorithm. Radiology. 2015;274(3):674–83.
135. Caruso D, Eid M, Schoepf UJ, Jin KN, Varga-Szemes A, Tesche C, Mangold S, Spandorfer A, Laghi A, De Cecco CN. Dynamic CT myocardial perfusion imaging. Eur J Radiol. 2016;85(10):1893–9.
136. De Cecco CN, Varga-Szemes A, Meinel FG, Renker M, Schoepf UJ. Beyond stenosis detection: computed tomography approaches for determining the functional relevance of coronary artery disease. Radiol Clin North Am. 2015;53(2):317–34.
137. Varga-Szemes A, Meinel FG, De Cecco CN, Fuller SR, Bayer RR 2nd, Schoepf UJ. CT myocardial perfusion imaging. AJR Am J Roentgenol. 2015;204(3):487–97.
138. Cury RC, Magalhaes TA, Borges AC, Shiozaki AA, Lemos PA, Junior JS, Meneghetti JC, Rochitte CE. Dipyridamole stress and rest myocardial perfusion by 64-detector row computed tomography in patients with suspected coronary artery disease. Am J Cardiol. 2010;106(3):310–5.
139. Techasith T, Cury RC. Stress myocardial CT perfusion: an update and future perspective. JACC Cardiovasc Imaging. 2011;4(8):905–16.
140. Cury RC, Abbara S, Achenbach S, Agatston A, Berman DS, Budoff MJ, Dill KE, Jacobs JE, Maroules CD, Rubin GD, Rybicki FJ, Schoepf UJ, Shaw LJ, Stillman AE, White CS, Woodard PK, Leipsic JA. CAD-RADS(TM) coronary artery disease - reporting and data system. An expert consensus document of the Society of Cardiovascular Computed Tomography (SCCT), the American College of Radiology (ACR) and the North American Society for Cardiovascular Imaging (NASCI). Endorsed by the American College of Cardiology. J Cardiovasc Comput Tomogr. 2016;10(4):269–81.
141. Cury RC, Abbara S, Achenbach S, Agatston A, Berman DS, Budoff MJ, Dill KE, Jacobs JE, Maroules CD, Rubin GD, Rybicki FJ, Schoepf UJ, Shaw LJ, Stillman AE, White CS, Woodard PK, Leipsic JA. CAD-RADS: coronary artery disease - reporting and data system.: an expert consensus document of the Society of Cardiovascular Computed Tomography (SCCT), the American College of Radiology (ACR) and the North American Society for Cardiovascular Imaging (NASCI). Endorsed by the American College of Cardiology. J Am Coll Radiol. 2016;13(12 Pt A):1458–66.
142. Cury RC, Abbara S, Achenbach S, Agatston A, Berman DS, Budoff MJ, Dill KE, Jacobs JE, Maroules CD, Rubin GD, Rybicki FJ, Schoepf UJ, Shaw LJ, Stillman AE, White CS, Woodard PK, Leipsic JA. Coronary artery disease - reporting and data system (CAD-RADS): an expert consensus document of SCCT, ACR and NASCI: endorsed by the ACC. JACC Cardiovasc Imaging. 2016;9(9):1099–113.
143. Mohlenkamp S, Hort W, Ge J, Erbel R. Update on myocardial bridging. Circulation. 2002;106(20):2616–22.
144. Iversen S, Hake U, Mayer E, Erbel R, Diefenbach C, Oelert H. Surgical treatment of myocardial bridging causing coronary artery obstruction. Scand J Thorac Cardiovasc Surg. 1992;26(2):107–11.

145. Noble J, Bourassa MG, Petitclerc R, Dyrda I. Myocardial bridging and milking effect of the left anterior descending coronary artery: normal variant or obstruction? Am J Cardiol. 1976;37(7):993–9.
146. Lee SS, Wu TL. The role of the mural coronary artery in prevention of coronary atherosclerosis. Arch Pathol. 1972;93(1):32–5.
147. Endo M, Lee YW, Hayashi H, Wada J. Angiographic evidence of myocardial squeezing accompanying tachyarrhythmia as a possible cause of myocardial infarction. Chest. 1978;73(3):431–3.
148. Tauth J, Sullebarger T. Myocardial infarction associated with myocardial bridging: case history and review of the literature. Catheter Cardiovasc Diagn. 1997;40(4):364–7.
149. Ferreira AG Jr, Trotter SE, Konig B Jr, Decourt LV, Fox K, Olsen EG. Myocardial bridges: morphological and functional aspects. Br Heart J. 1991;66(5):364–7.
150. Roberts WC, Dicicco BS, Waller BF, Kishel JC, McManus BM, Dawson SL, Hunsaker JC 3rd, Luke JL. Origin of the left main from the right coronary artery or from the right aortic sinus with intramyocardial tunneling to the left side of the heart via the ventricular septum. The case against clinical significance of myocardial bridge or coronary tunnel. Am Heart J. 1982;104(2 Pt 1):303–5.
151. Yamanaka O, Hobbs RE. Coronary artery anomalies in 126,595 patients undergoing coronary arteriography. Catheter Cardiovasc Diagn. 1990;21(1):28–40.
152. Taylor AJ, Rogan KM, Virmani R. Sudden cardiac death associated with isolated congenital coronary artery anomalies. J Am Coll Cardiol. 1992;20(3):640–7.
153. Basso C, Maron BJ, Corrado D, Thiene G. Clinical profile of congenital coronary artery anomalies with origin from the wrong aortic sinus leading to sudden death in young competitive athletes. J Am Coll Cardiol. 2000;35(6):1493–501.
154. Bartoli CR, Wead WB, Giridharan GA, Prabhu SD, Koenig SC, Dowling RD. Mechanism of myocardial ischemia with an anomalous left coronary artery from the right sinus of Valsalva. J Thorac Cardiovasc Surg. 2012;144(2):402–8.
155. Reichlin T, Schindler C, Drexler B, Twerenbold R, Reiter M, Zellweger C, Moehring B, Ziller R, Hoeller R, Rubini Gimenez M, Haaf P, Potocki M, Wildi K, Balmelli C, Freese M, Stelzig C, Freidank H, Osswald S, Mueller C. One-hour rule-out and rule-in of acute myocardial infarction using high-sensitivity cardiac troponin T. Arch Intern Med. 2012;172(16):1211–8.
156. Haaf P, Reichlin T, Twerenbold R, Hoeller R, Rubini Gimenez M, Zellweger C, Moehring B, Fischer C, Meller B, Wildi K, Freese M, Stelzig C, Mosimann T, Reiter M, Mueller M, Hochgruber T, Sou SM, Murray K, Minners J, Freidank H, Osswald S, Mueller C. Risk stratification in patients with acute chest pain using three high-sensitivity cardiac troponin assays. Eur Heart J. 2014;35(6):365–75.
157. Body R, Carley S, McDowell G, Jaffe AS, France M, Cruickshank K, Wibberley C, Nuttall M, Mackway-Jones K. Rapid exclusion of acute myocardial infarction in patients with undetectable troponin using a high-sensitivity assay. J Am Coll Cardiol. 2011;58(13):1332–9.
158. Dedic A, Lubbers MM, Schaap J, Lammers J, Lamfers EJ, Rensing BJ, Braam RL, Nathoe HM, Post JC, Nielen T, Beelen D, le Cocq d'Armandville MC, Rood PP, Schultz CJ, Moelker A, Ouhlous M, Boersma E, Nieman K. Coronary CT angiography for suspected ACS in the era of high-sensitivity troponins: randomized multicenter study. J Am Coll Cardiol. 2016;67(1):16–26.
159. Korley FK, George RT, Jaffe AS, Rothman RE, Sokoll LJ, Fernandez C, Falk H, Post WS, Saheed MO, Gerstenblith G, Berkowitz SA, Hill PM. Low high-sensitivity troponin I and zero coronary artery calcium score identifies coronary CT angiography candidates in whom further testing could be avoided. Acad Radiol. 2015;22(8):1060–7.
160. Ferencik M, Liu T, Mayrhofer T, Puchner SB, Lu MT, Maurovich-Horvat P, Pope JH, Truong QA, Udelson JE, Peacock WF, White CS, Woodard PK, Fleg JL, Nagurney JT, Januzzi JL, Hoffmann U. hs-Troponin I followed by CT angiography improves acute coronary syndrome risk stratification accuracy and work-up in acute chest pain patients: Results from ROMICAT II trial. JACC Cardiovasc Imaging. 2015;8(11):1272–81.
161. Hilton TC, Fulmer H, Abuan T, Thompson RC, Stowers SA. Ninety-day follow-up of patients in the emergency department with chest pain who undergo initial single-photon emission computed tomographic perfusion scintigraphy with technetium 99m-labeled sestamibi. J Nucl Cardiol. 1996;3(4):308–11.
162. Conti A, Gallini C, Costanzo E, Ferri P, Matteini M, Paladini B, Francois C, Grifoni S, Migliorini A, Antoniucci D, Pieroni C, Berni G. Early detection of myocardial ischaemia in the emergency department by rest or exercise (99m)Tc tracer myocardial SPET in patients with chest pain and non-diagnostic ECG. Eur J Nucl Med. 2001;28(12):1806–10.
163. Schaeffer MW, Brennan TD, Hughes JA, Gibler WB, Gerson MC. Resting radionuclide myocardial perfusion imaging in a chest pain center including an overnight delayed image acquisition protocol. J Nucl Med Technol. 2007;35(4):242–5.
164. Kontos MC, Haney A, Ornato JP, Jesse RL, Tatum JL. Value of simultaneous functional assessment in association with acute rest perfusion imaging for predicting short- and long-term outcomes in emergency department patients with chest pain. J Nucl Cardiol. 2008;15(6):774–82.
165. Radensky PW, Hilton TC, Fulmer H, McLaughlin BA, Stowers SA. Potential cost effectiveness of initial myocardial perfusion imaging for assessment of emergency department patients with chest pain. Am J Cardiol. 1997;79(5):595–9.
166. Udelson JE, Beshansky JR, Ballin DS, Feldman JA, Griffith JL, Handler J, Heller GV, Hendel RC, Pope JH, Ruthazer R, Spiegler EJ, Woolard RH, Selker HP. Myocardial perfusion imaging for evaluation and triage of patients with suspected acute cardiac ischemia: a randomized controlled trial. JAMA. 2002;288(21):2693–700.
167. Kontos MC, Schmidt KL, McCue M, Rossiter LF, Jurgensen M, Nicholson CS, Jesse RL, Ornato JP, Tatum JL. A comprehensive strategy for the evaluation and triage of the chest pain patient: a cost comparison study. J Nucl Cardiol. 2003;10(3):284–90.
168. Kontos MC, Arrowood JA, Paulsen WH, Nixon JV. Early echocardiography can predict cardiac events in emergency department patients with chest pain. Ann Emerg Med. 1998;31(5):550–7.
169. Muscholl MW, Oswald M, Mayer C, von Scheidt W. Prognostic value of 2D echocardiography in patients presenting with acute chest pain and non-diagnostic ECG for ST-elevation myocardial infarction. Int J Cardiol. 2002;84(2–3):217–25.
170. Lim SH, Sayre MR, Gibler WB. 2-D echocardiography prediction of adverse events in ED patients with chest pain. Am J Emerg Med. 2003;21(2):106–10.
171. Weston P, Alexander JH, Patel MR, Maynard C, Crawford L, Wagner GS. Hand-held echocardiographic examination of patients with symptoms of acute coronary syndromes in the emergency department: the 30-day outcome associated with normal left ventricular wall motion. Am Heart J. 2004;148(6):1096–101.
172. Kwong RY, Schussheim AE, Rekhraj S, Aletras AH, Geller N, Davis J, Christian TF, Balaban RS, Arai AE. Detecting acute coronary syndrome in the emergency department with cardiac magnetic resonance imaging. Circulation. 2003;107(4):531–7.
173. Ingkanisorn WP, Kwong RY, Bohme NS, Geller NL, Rhoads KL, Dyke CK, Paterson DI, Syed MA, Aletras AH, Arai AE. Prognosis of negative adenosine stress magnetic resonance in patients presenting to an emergency department with chest pain. J Am Coll Cardiol. 2006;47(7):1427–32.

174. Cury RC, Shash K, Nagurney JT, Rosito G, Shapiro MD, Nomura CH, Abbara S, Bamberg F, Ferencik M, Schmidt EJ, Brown DF, Hoffmann U, Brady TJ. Cardiac magnetic resonance with T2-weighted imaging improves detection of patients with acute coronary syndrome in the emergency department. Circulation. 2008;118(8):837–44.
175. Kim WY, Danias PG, Stuber M, Flamm SD, Plein S, Nagel E, Langerak SE, Weber OM, Pedersen EM, Schmidt M, Botnar RM, Manning WJ. Coronary magnetic resonance angiography for the detection of coronary stenoses. N Engl J Med. 2001;345(26):1863–9.
176. James JT. A new, evidence-based estimate of patient harms associated with hospital care. J Patient Saf. 2013;9(3):122–8.
177. Foy AJ, Liu G, Davidson WR Jr, Sciamanna C, Leslie DL. Comparative effectiveness of diagnostic testing strategies in emergency department patients with chest pain: an analysis of downstream testing, interventions, and outcomes. JAMA Intern Med. 2015;175(3):428–36.
178. Finnerty NM, Weinstock MB. Coronary computed tomography angiography for low-risk chest pain. Ann Emerg Med. 2016;68(5):645.
179. Redberg RF. Coronary CT angiography for acute chest pain. N Engl J Med. 2012;367(4):375–6.

The Role of Cardiac CT in Patients with Metabolic Disorders

29

Gianluca Pontone, Giuseppe Muscogiuri, and Mark Rabbat

Diabetes

Diabetes mellitus (DM) is a complex and heterogeneous disorder that can be classified in two subtypes [1]. Type 1 has a juvenile onset and is caused by autoimmune destruction of the pancreatic beta cell and subsequent insulin deficiency. Type 2 is typically characterized by adult onset and associated with being overweight, a sedentary lifestyle, and a diet high in fat and/or calories [1]. Oftentimes, diabetes is associated with the presence of cardiovascular disease. Therefore, optimal cardiovascular risk stratification is needed for an optimal therapeutic approach [2].

Before the institution of contemporary coronary care, the mortality for myocardial infarction (MI) in diabetic patients was higher than 40% and at least double compared with patients without diabetes [3]. In a large cohort of patients, Haffner et al. demonstrated that comparing patients with prior myocardial infarction, patients with DM had poor outcomes with a higher probability of developing a myocardial infarction compared to nondiabetics [4].

Although diabetes has been associated with coronary artery disease (CAD), recently, some data suggests that it should not be considered a CAD equivalent. Indeed, associating imaging findings, functional tests and severity of diabetes have reclassified the therapeutic approach and risk stratification to better identify and predict ischemic event in patients with DM [5].

A coronary artery calcium (CAC) score is easily acquired using cardiac CT and provides a wealth of diagnostic and prognostic information. The association of CAC scores with atherosclerotic plaque burden has been well described [6]. Hence, patients with high CAC are more likely to develop inducible ischemia [7]. In the CACTI study, Dabelea et al. showed that CAC is more extensive and prevalent in patients with type 1 DM compared to sex-matched controls [8]. Therefore, if the threshold of calcium scores associated with a high prevalence of ischemia in nondiabetic patients is >400, in diabetics the threshold maybe lower [9, 10].

Despite the CACTI study demonstrating an increased CAC value in patients with diabetes, a large portion of patients with DM show a very low or CAC score of 0 [5]. This finding supports the evidence that diabetes by itself is not a CAD equivalent.

Additionally, diabetics with a low CAC score have a low short-term risk of death similar to nondiabetic patients and do not appear to benefit from aspirin and statin use [11–13]. Extending the follow-up to 5 years, Valenti et al. support the theory that patients with a calcium score of 0 maintain low cardiovascular risk [14].

Although a large portion of diabetics have very low or CAC scores of 0, those with elevated CAC scores appear to have poor mid- and long-term outcome compared to nondiabetics [11, 14]. Therefore the evaluation of CAC scores in patients with DM is extremely important to help determine the best therapeutic approach and risk stratification. In fact, CAC scoring demonstrated a specificity and sensitivity of diagnosing CAD in patients with asymptomatic type 2 diabetes mellitus of 100% and 88%, respectively [15].

Taking into account the importance of CAC for risk stratification of patients, McClelland et al. suggested the use of a new algorithm that combines the CAC score with clinical information such as presence of diabetes, total cholesterol, HDL cholesterol, smoking, and systolic blood pressure in order to better predict the 10-year risk of developing coronary heart disease [16].

In addition to CAC, many papers in the literature have studied the role of coronary computed angiography (cCTA) for the assessment of CAD in patients with DM. In diabetics, although cCTA has high sensitivity for early identification of significant CAD, its diagnostic performance is reduced compared to nondiabetics [17, 18]. In several studies, risk stratification in patients with diabetes using cCTA has demonstrated greater extent, severity, and prevalence of

G. Pontone (✉) · G. Muscogiuri
Centro Cardiologico Monzino, IRCCS, Milan, Italy
e-mail: gianluca.pontone@ccfm.it

M. Rabbat
Department of Medicine, Division of Cardiology, Loyola University Chicago, Chicago, IL, USA

Department of Medicine, Division of Cardiology, Edward Hines Jr. VA Hospital, Hines, IL, USA

U. J. Schoepf (ed.), *CT of the Heart*, Contemporary Medical Imaging, https://doi.org/10.1007/978-1-60327-237-7_29

CAD, leading to an increased risk of mortality [19]. Kim et al. demonstrated that a longer duration of diabetes in asymptomatic patients is associated with increased major adverse cardiac and cerebrovascular events in 10 years of follow-up. Another study by Min et al. demonstrated similar results despite shorter-term follow-up of 3 years [20, 21]. In addition, other studies have demonstrated that diabetics had worse prognosis at both 5 and 7 years [22, 23].

Despite the strong evidence of a real impact in prognosis and risk stratification of cCTA, currently, its use for screening of CAD is not recommended. In the FACTOR-64 trial, at mean follow-up of 4 years, the primary composite end point of all-cause mortality, nonfatal myocardial infarction and hospitalization for unstable angina did not differ for DM patients compared to the control group. Furthermore, the secondary end point of ischemic major adverse cardiovascular events was similar [24]. Thus, the findings from FACTOR-64 do not support cCTA for screening of CAD.

However the lack of significant improvement for both primary and secondary outcomes observed in the FACTOR-64 trial may be explained by the low-risk study population and by the lack of benefit from an invasive therapeutic approach based solely on the anatomical evaluation of coronaries [24].

Studies comparing invasive fractional flow reserve (FFR) to anatomical imaging, including quantitative coronary angiography (QCA), cCTA, or intravascular ultrasound (IVUS), have consistently demonstrated an unreliable relationship between anatomic measures of stenosis and lesion-specific ischemia [25, 26]. In addition, overestimation of stenosis in calcified plaque is a well-known limitation, and some vendors have adopted technical strategies to reduce blooming artifact [27].

To overcome these limitations, CT perfusion (CTP) and fractional flow reserve CT (FFR-CT) have developed to bridge the anatomic evaluation of CAD to the functional relevance of stenosis [28, 29]. While the current guidelines state a level IIa recommendation for CAC scoring and level III recommendation for routine cCTA for risk stratification, the novel noninvasive approach based on CTP, FFR-CT, and plaque analysis will likely expand and broaden the indication for cCTA in order to accurately risk stratify patients with DM (Table 29.1) [30, 31]. In fact, Vliegenthart et al. recently identified early abnormal CTP in patients with diabetes which may improve CAD risk stratification [32].

In conclusion, both CAC scoring and cCTA may be helpful in risk stratification and management of asymptomatic patients with DM. Moreover, a combined approach utilizing FFR-CT, CTP, and plaque characteristics may play a key role in future CAD risk stratification (Table 29.2).

Table 29.1 Current guidelines in patients with diabetes mellitus [5]

Risk factor assessment	Class I
Coronary artery calcium scanning	Class IIa
Hemoglobin A1c for risk assessment	Class IIb
Not supported	
Carotid intima media thickness	Class III
Routine functional testing	Class III

Data from Budoff et al. [5]
Class III

Table 29.2 Computed tomography in metabolic disorders

Metabolic disorders	Role of CT
Diabetes	CAC Extent and severity of CAD Possible functional evaluation of CAD 1. FFR-CT 2. CTP
Gaucher disease	Calcifications of valves and thoracic aorta
Mucopolysaccharidoses	Evaluation of valve morphology Narrowing of coronary arteries
Alkaptonuria	CAC Myocardial, valve, vascular calcification
Cystinosis	CAC
Obesity	CAC EAT

CT computed tomography, *CAC* coronary artery calcium, *CAD* coronary artery disease, *FFR-CT* fractional flow reserve computed tomography, *CTP* computed tomography perfusion, *EAT* epicardial adipose tissue

Gaucher Disease

Gaucher disease (GD) is the most common lysosomal storage disorder. It is characterized by the loss of function of the catabolic lysosomal enzyme acid beta-glucocerebrosidase causing accumulation of sphingolipid glycosylceramide in lysosomes. Different types of genetic mutations involving the GBA gene are responsible for the diminished function of the enzyme [33, 34].

Clinical manifestation of GD can be very heterogeneous but can be divided into three types [34].

- Type 1: Characterized by hepatosplenomegaly, anemia, thrombocytopenia, and bone disease.
- Type 2: Typical onset in infancy with neurologic and visceral manifestations associated with arrest of growth and death in early childhood.
- Type 3: Characterized by neurologic involvement usually with onset in early childhood. Based upon the involvement of visceral disease and neurological signs, type 3 GD can be further divided into three subgroups: 3a, 3b, and 3c.

Cardiac involvement in GD is manifested as calcification of the myocardium and mitral and aortic valve [35–37]. Few case reports describe the role of CT for the evaluation of patients with GD. The papers do not use ECG-gated acquisition and describe the appearance of calcified valves and thoracic aorta in patients with GD [38, 39].

Mucopolysaccharidoses

Mucopolysaccharidoses (MPS) is a genetic disease due to a lysosomal storage disorder that causes impaired degradation of glycosaminoglycans (GAG) [40, 41]. There are nine different subtypes of MPS depending on the enzyme deficit with heterogeneous clinical manifestations [40].

MPS is a multivisceral disease and involves the musculoskeletal system, heart, lung, eyes, liver, spleen, and occasionally the cerebral nervous system [41].

Cardiac involvement in MPS is caused by the accumulation of GAG. Thickening of the cardiac valves, intramyocardial deposition of GAG, patchy interstitial fibrosis, coronary artery narrowing from myointimal proliferation, and systemic hypertension may all contribute to the development of heart failure [42].

Left-sided cardiac valves are commonly affected in MPS and these individuals typically have MPS subtypes I, II, and IV [43]. The mitral valve leaflets are usually thickened, the chordae tendineae are short, and the papillary muscles are dysmorphic. The abnormal morphologic changes of the valves result in pathologic valvular function and the development of stenosis and insufficiency.

Transthoracic two-dimensional echocardiography is the first-line noninvasive technique that allows reliable evaluation of valvular function and morphology. However, in patients with poor acoustic windows or in cases where transesophageal echocardiography cannot be performed, cCTA represents an alternative diagnostic technique. While cCTA can provide key information regarding valvular morphology, it is important and good practice to consider the radiation exposure to patients [43].

Narrowing of coronaries is described in all subtypes of MPS; however, it is more common in subtypes I and II. A decrease in coronary lumen diameter is caused by the deposition of GAG that leads to a progressive diffuse intimal proliferation [43–45].

It is debatable whether cCTA is useful and maintains high diagnostic performance in patients with MPS mainly from the diffuse involvement of the vessels [43]. However, Felice et al. describe a case of a 30-year-old patient with MPS, aortic stenosis, and left ventricular hypertrophy who underwent cCTA and successfully ruled out involvement of coronary narrowing [46].

Alkaptonuria

Alkaptonuria is an autosomal recessive metabolic disorder caused by a deficient activity of homogentisate 1, 2-dioxygenase (HGO), an enzyme involved in the metabolism of tyrosine. The decreased function of HGO leads to an increase of homogentisic acid (HGA). Excessive production of HGA is eliminated in the urine or accumulates in connective tissue causing ochronosis and subsequent darkening of bones and cartilage, arthritis, joint destruction, and degeneration of cardiac valves [47].

In alkaptonuria, ochronosis seems to be upstream cause of cardiac valvular deterioration. The deposits of HGA manifest a classic pigmentation to the cardiac valves that subsequently undergo a gradual progression to valvular calcification [48]. The association of degenerative aortic stenosis and alkaptonuria has been described [49–51]. As in GD, cCTA can be useful for the evaluation of myocardial, valve, or vascular calcification [52]. CAC is commonly found in patients with alkaptonuria and can be quantified using the Agatston score [47, 52].

Cystinosis

Cystinosis is a rare, autosomal recessive disease in which cystine is accumulated in the lysosomes. The biallelic mutation of the cystinosin, lysosomal cystine transporter (CTNS) gene, leads to deficient cystinosin (which is a cystine-proton cotransporter) and consequently cystine is accumulated in the lysosomes [53].

Cystinosis is the most common cause of Fanconi syndrome. Typically onset of symptoms occurs in early childhood. Polyuria, polydipsia, vomiting, constipation, growth retardation, rickets, dehydration, and acidosis have been associated with the disease [54]. Photophobia and blepharospasm are common in patients with cystinosis as result of corneal cystine crystals accumulation. Loss of thyroid function is caused by the gradual cystine accumulation and crystal formation in thyroid follicular cells [53, 55]. Other extrarenal manifestations include pancreatic and pulmonary dysfunction, muscle atrophy or weakness, and rarely impairment of the central nervous system [54].

The progressive renal impairment in patients with cystinosis may lead to kidney failure and eventual kidney transplantation.

Ueda et al. observed the increase of coronary artery and vascular calcification in patients with cystinosis after kidney transplantation [56]. They report that increased values of CAC were associated with to the onset of diabetes and/or abnormalities of calcium and phosphate homeostasis [56]. Furthermore, in one cystinosis patient with significant CAC noted on CT, coronary angiography was performed to evaluate the severity of CAD [56]. However, it is yet to be determined whether patients with cystinosis may benefit from the evaluation of CAC scoring and severity of CAD using cCTA.

Obesity

Obesity is characterized by a body mass index (BMI) higher than 30 Kg/m^2 in adults and above the 95th percentile in the pediatric population. The development of obesity results from the complex interaction between genetic, socioeconomic, and cultural influences [57].

Obesity represents an important and serious health problem in developed and developing countries which greatly influence the cost to healthcare system [58]. Furthermore, obesity is associated with several comorbidities that may adversely affect the clinical condition of patients, resulting in poor outcomes. The combination of being overweight and obese in 2010 was estimated to cause 3.4 million deaths [59, 60].

Comorbidities often associated with an obese body habitus include but not limited to obstructive sleep apnea, female infertility, diabetes, and coronary heart disease [59, 61]. The relationship between obesity and development of CAC is debatable. In 2005, Cassidy et al. showed a positive correlation between CAC and waist circumference, waist-to-hip ratio, and BMI [62]. In 2010, the CARDIA study demonstrated that baseline BMI was associated positively and linearly with CAC at year 20 of follow-up [63]. In contrast to the above results, Kovacic et al. found an inverse correlation between BMI and CAC, while other studies report the lack of significant association [64–66].

The conflicting results regarding the association of CAC and BMI were further investigated by two large studies. Analysis performed on the CONFIRM registry found that obese patients have a statistically significant higher CAC compared to normal weight patients [67]. Similar results were observed by Fujiyoshi et al. where after adjusting for age, smoking, alcohol, hypertension, lipids, and diabetes mellitus, CAC was independently and positively associated with prevalent CAC in a large population of 1212 patients [68].

Another finding that can be evaluated in obese and nonobese patients is the amount of epicardial adipose tissue (EAT). EAT, the visceral adipose tissue located between the myo-epicardium and visceral pericardium, is an independent risk factor for CAD. EAT plays a local homeostatic role in management of lipid and energy. In particular, it is responsible for free fatty acid release and uptake [69]. The amount of EAT is correlated with components of metabolic syndrome, and the increase in EAT has been associated with the progression of CAC [70, 71]. In addition, Spearman et al. report that there may be incremental prognostic value of EAT over CAC alone [72].

Although cardiac CT can be useful in obese patients for the evaluation of CAC, EAT, and CAD extent and severity, image quality may be limited if tube potential and current are not adequately adjusted according to the individuals BMI [73].

However, one must be cognizant that the increase of tube voltage and current leads to increased radiation dose to the patient. Hence, several strategies have been developed by the vendors in order to overcome this issue. Mangold et al. report high diagnostic image quality in obese patients with third-generation dual-source CT using a tube voltage of 120-kV. In fact, diagnostic accuracy between obese and nonobese patients showed no significant difference in image quality even when 44% of the obese patients underwent cCTA with tube voltage <120 kV [74, 75].

References

1. Polonsky KS. The past 200 years in diabetes. N Engl J Med. 2012;367(14):1332–40.
2. Inzucchi SE. Diagnosis of diabetes. N Engl J Med. 2013;368(2):193.
3. Nesto RW, Zarich S. Acute myocardial infarction in diabetes mellitus: lessons learned from ACE inhibition. Circulation. 1998;97(1):12–5.
4. Haffner SM, Lehto S, Ronnemaa T, Pyorala K, Laakso M. Mortality from coronary heart disease in subjects with type 2 diabetes and in nondiabetic subjects with and without prior myocardial infarction. N Engl J Med. 1998;339(4):229–34.
5. Budoff MJ, Raggi P, Beller GA, Berman DS, Druz RS, Malik S, et al. Noninvasive cardiovascular risk assessment of the asymptomatic diabetic patient: the imaging council of the American College of Cardiology. JACC Cardiovasc Imaging. 2016;9(2):176–92.
6. Rumberger JA, Simons DB, Fitzpatrick LA, Sheedy PF, Schwartz RS. Coronary artery calcium area by electron-beam computed tomography and coronary atherosclerotic plaque area. A histopathologic correlative study. Circulation. 1995;92(8):2157–62.
7. Bavishi C, Argulian E, Chatterjee S, Rozanski A. CACS and the frequency of stress-induced myocardial ischemia during MPI: a meta-analysis. JACC Cardiovasc Imaging. 2016;9(5):580–9.
8. Dabelea D, Kinney G, Snell-Bergeon JK, Hokanson JE, Eckel RH, Ehrlich J, et al. Effect of type 1 diabetes on the gender difference in coronary artery calcification: a role for insulin resistance? The Coronary Artery Calcification in Type 1 Diabetes (CACTI) Study. Diabetes. 2003;52(11):2833–9.
9. He ZX, Hedrick TD, Pratt CM, Verani MS, Aquino V, Roberts R, et al. Severity of coronary artery calcification by electron beam computed tomography predicts silent myocardial ischemia. Circulation. 2000;101(3):244–51.
10. Wong ND, Rozanski A, Gransar H, Miranda-Peats R, Kang X, Hayes S, et al. Metabolic syndrome and diabetes are associated with an increased likelihood of inducible myocardial ischemia among patients with subclinical atherosclerosis. Diabetes Care. 2005;28(6):1445–50.
11. Raggi P, Shaw LJ, Berman DS, Callister TQ. Prognostic value of coronary artery calcium screening in subjects with and without diabetes. J Am Coll Cardiol. 2004;43(9):1663–9. https://doi.org/10.1016/j.jacc.2003.09.068.

12. Silverman MG, Blaha MJ, Budoff MJ, Rivera JJ, Raggi P, Shaw LJ, et al. Potential implications of coronary artery calcium testing for guiding aspirin use among asymptomatic individuals with diabetes. Diabetes Care. 2012;35(3):624–6.
13. Nasir K, Bittencourt MS, Blaha MJ, Blankstein R, Agatson AS, Rivera JJ, et al. Implications of coronary artery calcium testing among statin candidates according to American College of Cardiology/American Heart Association cholesterol management guidelines: MESA (Multi-Ethnic Study of Atherosclerosis). J Am Coll Cardiol. 2015;66(15):1657–68.
14. Valenti V, Hartaigh BO, Cho I, Schulman-Marcus J, Gransar H, Heo R, et al. Absence of coronary artery calcium identifies asymptomatic diabetic individuals at low near-term but not long-term risk of mortality: a 15-year follow-up study of 9715 patients. Circ Cardiovasc Imaging. 2016;9(2):e003528.
15. Rassi CH, Churchill TW, Tavares CA, Fahel MG, Rassi FP, Uchida AH, et al. Use of imaging and clinical data to screen for cardiovascular disease in asymptomatic diabetics. Cardiovasc Diabetol. 2016;15:28.
16. McClelland RL, Jorgensen NW, Budoff M, Blaha MJ, Post WS, Kronmal RA, et al. 10-year coronary heart disease risk prediction using coronary artery calcium and traditional risk factors: derivation in the MESA (Multi-Ethnic Study of Atherosclerosis) with validation in the HNR (Heinz Nixdorf Recall) study and the DHS (Dallas Heart Study). J Am Coll Cardiol. 2015;66(15):1643–53.
17. Andreini D, Pontone G, Bartorelli AL, Agostoni P, Mushtaq S, Antonioli L, et al. Comparison of the diagnostic performance of 64-slice computed tomography coronary angiography in diabetic and non-diabetic patients with suspected coronary artery disease. Cardiovasc Diabetol. 2010;9:80.
18. Ulimoen GR, Ofstad AP, Endresen K, Gullestad L, Johansen OE, Borthne A. Low-dose CT coronary angiography for assessment of coronary artery disease in patients with type 2 diabetes--a cross-sectional study. BMC Cardiovasc Disord. 2015;15:147.
19. Rana JS, Dunning A, Achenbach S, Al-Mallah M, Budoff MJ, Cademartiri F, et al. Differences in prevalence, extent, severity, and prognosis of coronary artery disease among patients with and without diabetes undergoing coronary computed tomography angiography: results from 10,110 individuals from the CONFIRM (COronary CT Angiography EvaluatioN For Clinical Outcomes): an InteRnational Multicenter Registry. Diabetes Care. 2012;35(8):1787–94.
20. Kim JJ, Hwang BH, Choi IJ, Choo EH, Lim S, Kim JK, et al. Impact of diabetes duration on the extent and severity of coronary atheroma burden and long-term clinical outcome in asymptomatic type 2 diabetic patients: evaluation by Coronary CT angiography. Eur Heart J Cardiovasc Imaging. 2015;16(10):1065–73.
21. Min JK, Labounty TM, Gomez MJ, Achenbach S, Al-Mallah M, Budoff MJ, et al. Incremental prognostic value of coronary computed tomographic angiography over coronary artery calcium score for risk prediction of major adverse cardiac events in asymptomatic diabetic individuals. Atherosclerosis. 2014;232(2):298–304.
22. Andreini D, Pontone G, Mushtaq S, Bertella E, Conte E, Baggiano A, et al. Prognostic value of multidetector computed tomography coronary angiography in diabetes: excellent long-term prognosis in patients with normal coronary arteries. Diabetes Care. 2013;36(7):1834–41.
23. Halon DA, Azencot M, Rubinshtein R, Zafrir B, Flugelman MY, Lewis BS. Coronary computed tomography (CT) angiography as a predictor of cardiac and noncardiac vascular events in asymptomatic type 2 diabetics: a 7-year population-based cohort study. J Am Heart Assoc. 2016;5(6):e003226.
24. Muhlestein JB, Lappe DL, Lima JA, Rosen BD, May HT, Knight S, et al. Effect of screening for coronary artery disease using CT angiography on mortality and cardiac events in high-risk patients with diabetes: the FACTOR-64 randomized clinical trial. JAMA. 2014;312(21):2234–43.
25. Pontone G, Andreini D, Baggiano A, Bertella E, Mushtaq S, Conte E, et al. Functional relevance of coronary artery disease by cardiac magnetic resonance and cardiac computed tomography: myocardial perfusion and fractional flow reserve. Biomed Res Int. 2015;2015:297696.
26. Pontone G, Muscogiuri G, Andreini D, Guaricci AI, Guglielmo M, Mushtaq S, et al. The new frontier of cardiac computed tomography angiography: fractional flow reserve and stress myocardial perfusion. Curr Treat Options Cardiovasc Med. 2016;18(12):74.
27. Pontone G, Bertella E, Mushtaq S, Loguercio M, Cortinovis S, Baggiano A, et al. Coronary artery disease: diagnostic accuracy of CT coronary angiography--a comparison of high and standard spatial resolution scanning. Radiology. 2014;271(3):688–94.
28. Wang R, Renker M, Schoepf UJ, Wichmann JL, Fuller SR, Rier JD, et al. Diagnostic value of quantitative stenosis predictors with coronary CT angiography compared to invasive fractional flow reserve. Eur J Radiol. 2015;84(8):1509–15.
29. Ko BS, Cameron JD, Leung M, Meredith IT, Leong DP, Antonis PR, et al. Combined CT coronary angiography and stress myocardial perfusion imaging for hemodynamically significant stenoses in patients with suspected coronary artery disease: a comparison with fractional flow reserve. JACC Cardiovasc Imaging. 2012;5(11):1097–111.
30. Nakazato R, Park HB, Gransar H, Leipsic JA, Budoff MJ, Mancini GB, et al. Additive diagnostic value of atherosclerotic plaque characteristics to non-invasive FFR for identification of lesions causing ischaemia: results from a prospective international multicentre trial. EuroIntervention. 2016;12(4):473–81.
31. Gaur S, Ovrehus KA, Dey D, Leipsic J, Botker HE, Jensen JM, et al. Coronary plaque quantification and fractional flow reserve by coronary computed tomography angiography identify ischaemia-causing lesions. Eur Heart J. 2016;37(15):1220–7.
32. Vliegenthart R, De Cecco CN, Wichmann JL, Meinel FG, Pelgrim GJ, Tesche C, et al. Dynamic CT myocardial perfusion imaging identifies early perfusion abnormalities in diabetes and hypertension: insights from a multicenter registry. J Cardiovasc Comput Tomogr. 2016;10(4):301–8.
33. Horowitz M, Elstein D, Zimran A, Goker-Alpan O. New directions in Gaucher disease. Hum Mutat. 2016;37:1121.
34. Bendikov-Bar I, Horowitz M. Gaucher disease paradigm: from ERAD to comorbidity. Hum Mutat. 2012;33(10):1398–407.
35. Shah S, Misri A, Bhat M, Maheshwari S. Gaucher's disease type III C: unusual cause of intracardiac calcification. Ann Pediatr Cardiol. 2008;1(2):144–6.
36. Chabas A, Cormand B, Grinberg D, Burguera JM, Balcells S, Merino JL, et al. Unusual expression of Gaucher's disease: cardiovascular calcifications in three sibs homozygous for the D409H mutation. J Med Genet. 1995;32(9):740–2.
37. Abrahamov A, Elstein D, Gross-Tsur V, Farber B, Glaser Y, Hadas-Halpern I, et al. Gaucher's disease variant characterised by progressive calcification of heart valves and unique genotype. Lancet. 1995;346(8981):1000–3.
38. Ceyhan M, Celik FK, Elmali M, Gurmen N. An unusual form of Gaucher's disease: pulmonary and cardiovascular involvement and cholelitiasis. Cent Eur J Med. 2010;5(4):495–8.
39. Altunbas G, Ercan S, Inanc IH, Ozer O, Kervancioglu S, Davutoglu V. Extensive vascular and valvular involvement in Gaucher disease. Asian Cardiovasc Thorac Ann. 2015;23(4):446–8.
40. Coutinho MF, Lacerda L, Alves S. Glycosaminoglycan storage disorders: a review. Biochem Res Int. 2012;2012:471325.
41. Valayannopoulos V, Wijburg FA. Therapy for the mucopolysaccharidoses. Rheumatology (Oxford). 2011;50(Suppl 5):v49–59.

42. Braunlin E, Wang R. Cardiac issues in adults with the mucopolysaccharidoses: current knowledge and emerging needs. Heart. 2016;102(16):1257–62.
43. Braunlin EA, Harmatz PR, Scarpa M, Furlanetto B, Kampmann C, Loehr JP, et al. Cardiac disease in patients with mucopolysaccharidosis: presentation, diagnosis and management. J Inherit Metab Dis. 2011;34(6):1183–97.
44. Brosius FC 3rd, Roberts WC. Coronary artery disease in the hurler syndrome. Qualitative and quantitative analysis of the extent of coronary narrowing at necropsy in six children. Am J Cardiol. 1981;47(3):649–53.
45. Kettles DI, Sheppard M, Liebmann RD, Davidson C. Left ventricular aneurysm, aortic valve disease and coronary narrowing in a patient with Hunter's syndrome. Cardiovasc Pathol. 2002;11(2):94–6.
46. Felice T, Murphy E, Mullen MJ, Elliott PM. Management of aortic stenosis in mucopolysaccharidosis type I. Int J Cardiol. 2014;172(3):e430–1.
47. Phornphutkul C, Introne WJ, Perry MB, Bernardini I, Murphey MD, Fitzpatrick DL, et al. Natural history of alkaptonuria. N Engl J Med. 2002;347(26):2111–21.
48. Butany JW, Naseemuddin A, Moshkowitz Y, Nair V. Ochronosis and aortic valve stenosis. J Card Surg. 2006;21(2):182–4.
49. Ffolkes LV, Brull D, Krywawych S, Hayward M, Hughes SE. Aortic stenosis in cardiovascular ochronosis. J Clin Pathol. 2007;60(1):92–3.
50. Hiroyoshi J, Saito A, Panthee N, Imai Y, Kawashima D, Motomura N, et al. Aortic valve replacement for aortic stenosis caused by alkaptonuria. Ann Thorac Surg. 2013;95(3):1076–9.
51. Fisher AA, Davis MW. Alkaptonuric ochronosis with aortic valve and joint replacements and femoral fracture: a case report and literature review. Clin Med Res. 2004;2(4):209–15.
52. Hannoush H, Introne WJ, Chen MY, Lee SJ, O'Brien K, Suwannarat P, et al. Aortic stenosis and vascular calcifications in alkaptonuria. Mol Genet Metab. 2012;105(2):198–202.
53. Elmonem MA, Veys KR, Soliman NA, van Dyck M, van den Heuvel LP, Levtchenko E. Cystinosis: a review. Orphanet J Rare Dis. 2016;11:47.
54. Emma F, Nesterova G, Langman C, Labbe A, Cherqui S, Goodyer P, et al. Nephropathic cystinosis: an international consensus document. Nephrol Dial Transplant. 2014;29(Suppl 4):iv87–94.
55. Nesterova G, Gahl WA. In: Pagon RA, Adam MP, Ardinger HH, Wallace SE, Amemiya A, LJH B, et al., editors. Cystinosis. Seattle: GeneReviews; 1993.
56. Ueda M, O'Brien K, Rosing DR, Ling A, Kleta R, McAreavey D, et al. Coronary artery and other vascular calcifications in patients with cystinosis after kidney transplantation. Clin J Am Soc Nephrol. 2006;1(3):555–62.
57. Apovian CM. Obesity: definition, comorbidities, causes, and burden. Am J Manag Care. 2016;22(7 Suppl):s176–85.
58. Finkelstein EA, Trogdon JG, Cohen JW, Dietz W. Annual medical spending attributable to obesity: payer-and service-specific estimates. Health Aff (Millwood). 2009;28(5):w822–31.
59. Haslam D. Obesity: a medical history. Obes Rev. 2007;8(Suppl 1):31–6.
60. Ng M, Fleming T, Robinson M, Thomson B, Graetz N, Margono C, et al. Global, regional, and national prevalence of overweight and obesity in children and adults during 1980-2013: a systematic analysis for the Global Burden of Disease Study 2013. Lancet. 2014;384(9945):766–81.
61. Mitchell A, Fantasia HC. Understanding the effect of obesity on fertility among reproductive-age women. Nurs Womens Health. 2016;20(4):368–76.
62. Cassidy AE, Bielak LF, Zhou Y, Sheedy PF 2nd, Turner ST, Breen JF, et al. Progression of subclinical coronary atherosclerosis: does obesity make a difference? Circulation. 2005;111(15):1877–82.
63. Lee DH, Steffes MW, Gross M, Park K, Holvoet P, Kiefe CI, et al. Differential associations of weight dynamics with coronary artery calcium versus common carotid artery intima-media thickness: The CARDIA Study. Am J Epidemiol. 2010;172(2):180–9.
64. Kovacic JC, Lee P, Baber U, Karajgikar R, Evrard SM, Moreno P, et al. Inverse relationship between body mass index and coronary artery calcification in patients with clinically significant coronary lesions. Atherosclerosis. 2012;221(1):176–82.
65. Bild DE, Detrano R, Peterson D, Guerci A, Liu K, Shahar E, et al. Ethnic differences in coronary calcification: the Multi-Ethnic Study of Atherosclerosis (MESA). Circulation. 2005;111(10):1313–20.
66. Taylor AJ, Feuerstein I, Wong H, Barko W, Brazaitis M, O'Malley PG. Do conventional risk factors predict subclinical coronary artery disease? Results from the Prospective Army Coronary Calcium Project. Am Heart J. 2001;141(3):463–8.
67. Labounty TM, Gomez MJ, Achenbach S, Al-Mallah M, Berman DS, Budoff MJ, et al. Body mass index and the prevalence, severity, and risk of coronary artery disease: an international multicentre study of 13,874 patients. Eur Heart J Cardiovasc Imaging. 2013;14(5):456–63.
68. Fujiyoshi A, Sekikawa A, Shin C, Masaki K, David Curb J, Ohkubo T, et al. A cross-sectional association of obesity with coronary calcium among Japanese, Koreans, Japanese Americans, and U.S. whites. Eur Heart J Cardiovasc Imaging. 2013;14(9):921–7.
69. Iacobellis G, Malavazos AE, Corsi MM. Epicardial fat: from the biomolecular aspects to the clinical practice. Int J Biochem Cell Biol. 2011;43(12):1651–4.
70. Yorgun H, Canpolat U, Hazirolan T, Ates AH, Sunman H, Dural M, et al. Increased epicardial fat tissue is a marker of metabolic syndrome in adult patients. Int J Cardiol. 2013;165(2):308–13.
71. Nakanishi R, Rajani R, Cheng VY, Gransar H, Nakazato R, Shmilovich H, et al. Increase in epicardial fat volume is associated with greater coronary artery calcification progression in subjects at intermediate risk by coronary calcium score: a serial study using non-contrast cardiac CT. Atherosclerosis. 2011;218(2):363–8.
72. Spearman JV, Renker M, Schoepf UJ, Krazinski AW, Herbert TL, De Cecco CN, et al. Prognostic value of epicardial fat volume measurements by computed tomography: a systematic review of the literature. Eur Radiol. 2015;25(11):3372–81.
73. Halliburton SS, Abbara S, Chen MY, Gentry R, Mahesh M, Raff GL, et al. SCCT guidelines on radiation dose and dose-optimization strategies in cardiovascular CT. J Cardiovasc Comput Tomogr. 2011;5(4):198–224.
74. Mangold S, Wichmann JL, Schoepf UJ, Litwin SE, Canstein C, Varga-Szemes A, et al. Coronary CT angiography in obese patients using 3(rd) generation dual-source CT: effect of body mass index on image quality. Eur Radiol. 2016;26(9):2937–46.
75. Mangold S, Wichmann JL, Schoepf UJ, Caruso D, Tesche C, Steinberg DH, et al. Diagnostic accuracy of coronary CT angiography using 3rd-generation dual-source CT and automated tube voltage selection: clinical application in a non-obese and obese patient population. Eur Radiol. 2017;27(6):2298–308.

Use of Coronary Computed Tomography Angiography in Cardiac Risk Assessment for Non-cardiac Surgery

30

Gregory Jackson and Richard R. Bayer II

It has been estimated that approximately 900,000 patients each year will suffer a major adverse cardiac event in the postoperative period [1]. As such preoperative cardiac risk stratification is an important aspect in the clincal practice of internal medicine physicians, cardiologists, anesthesiologists, and surgeons alike. Traditional risk assessment models utilize patient-specific comorbidities to allow estimation of perioperative cardiac risk. Such models have historically included the Multifactorial Cardiac Risk Index, Revised Cardiac Risk Index (RCRI), and Detsky's Modified Cardiac Risk Index [2–4]. Once a patient-specific risk has been estimated, the practitioner must not only determine the appropriateness of further testing but if the results of subsequent testing would alter treatment plans [5]. Traditionally, if further testing was deemed appropriate, this was accomplished utilizing stress treadmill electrocardiography (ECG), single-photon emission computed tomography (SPECT), or stress echocardiography [6]. In recent years, coronary computed tomography angiography (CCTA) has become an alternative method for the evaluation of coronary artery disease. CCTA has repeatedly demonstrated the ability to exclude significant coronary artery disease with an extremely high sensitivity and negative predictive value [7, 8]. However, to date its use in the evaluation of preoperative cardiac risk stratification has not been well established [6].

Preoperative Risk Assessment

The Revised Cardiac Risk Index (RCRI) is a multifactorial risk index developed in 1999 by Lee et al. which stratifies patients based upon specific medical comorbidities [3]. Both the American Heart Association (AHA) and the American College of Cardiology (ACC) have emphasized the use of the RCRI for preoperative cardiac risk evaluation [9]. This risk model utilizes patient-specific clinical risk factors including chronic kidney disease with a creatinine greater than 2.0, insulin dependent diabetes mellitus, history of cerebrovascular accident (CVA), history of ischemic heart disease, and history of congestive heart failure (Table 30.1) [9]. In combination with assessing the risk of surgery itself, a patient's risk of major adverse cardiac events can and should also be estimated. This can range from a very low risk of 0.4% to high risk with an 11% risk of perioperative cardiac complications (Table 30.2) [10]. In addition to clinical risk factors, any assessment of preoperative risk also includes a functional assessment (Table 30.3) [5]. Utilizing both the RCRI risk score and patient's functional capacity, the ACC and AHA have issued a stepwise algorithm for preoperative cardiac risk assessment (Fig. 30.1) [9]. The highlighted

Table 30.1 Clinical risk factors utilized in preoperative cardiac risk assessment via the Revised Cardiac Risk Index (RCRI)

Revised Cardiac Risk Index (RCRI)
History of ischemic heart disease
History of congestive heart failure
History of cerebrovascular accident
Chronic kidney disease with creatinine >2.0
History of insulin dependent diabetes mellitus

Table 30.2 Risk of perioperative complications based on number of RCRI risk factors

Risk class	# of risk factors	Risk of complications
Very low risk	0	0.4%
Low risk	1	0.9%
Moderate risk	2	7.0%
High risk	≥3	11.0%

G. Jackson
Department of Cardiology, Medical University of South Carolina, Charleston, SC, USA

R. R. Bayer II (✉)
Division of Cardiovascular Imaging, Department of Radiology and Radiological Science, Medical University of South Carolina, Charleston, SC, USA

Division of Cardiology, Department of Medicine, Medical University of South Carolina, Charleston, SC, USA
e-mail: bayer@musc.edu

U. J. Schoepf (ed.), *CT of the Heart*, Contemporary Medical Imaging, https://doi.org/10.1007/978-1-60327-237-7_30

Table 30.3 Physical activity and corresponding metabolic equivalents (METs)

Physical activity	METs
Sleeping	0.9
Watching television	1.0
Walking slowly on level ground (1.7 mph)	2.3
Walking 3.0 miles per hour	3.3
Vacuuming, sweeping floor	3.3
Bicycling <10 miles per hour	4.0
Climb two flights of stairs	4.0
Washing car	4.5
Golf (carrying clubs)	4.5
Walking 4.0 miles per hour	5.0
Weightlifting	6.0
Jogging	7.0
Basketball	8.0
Jump roping	10.0
Running (9 min/mile)	11.0

sections represent situations where further testing may be appropriate.

With patients unable to complete ≥4 METs or who have an unknown functional capacity and are intermediate to high risk, further noninvasive testing may be appropriate. This of course is with the caveat that it will alter management prior to proceeding with surgery [5]. In accordance with the appropriate use criteria, only SPECT and stress echocardiography receive scores of "appropriate" [9]. Additionally exercise stress ECG and stress cardiac magnetic resonance (CMR) imaging earn scores of "may be appropriate" [9]. Conversely, in all situations CCTA is deemed "rarely appropriate" [9]. These recommendations stem largely from the lack of current evidence for the use of CCTA in the setting of preoperative risk stratification [11].

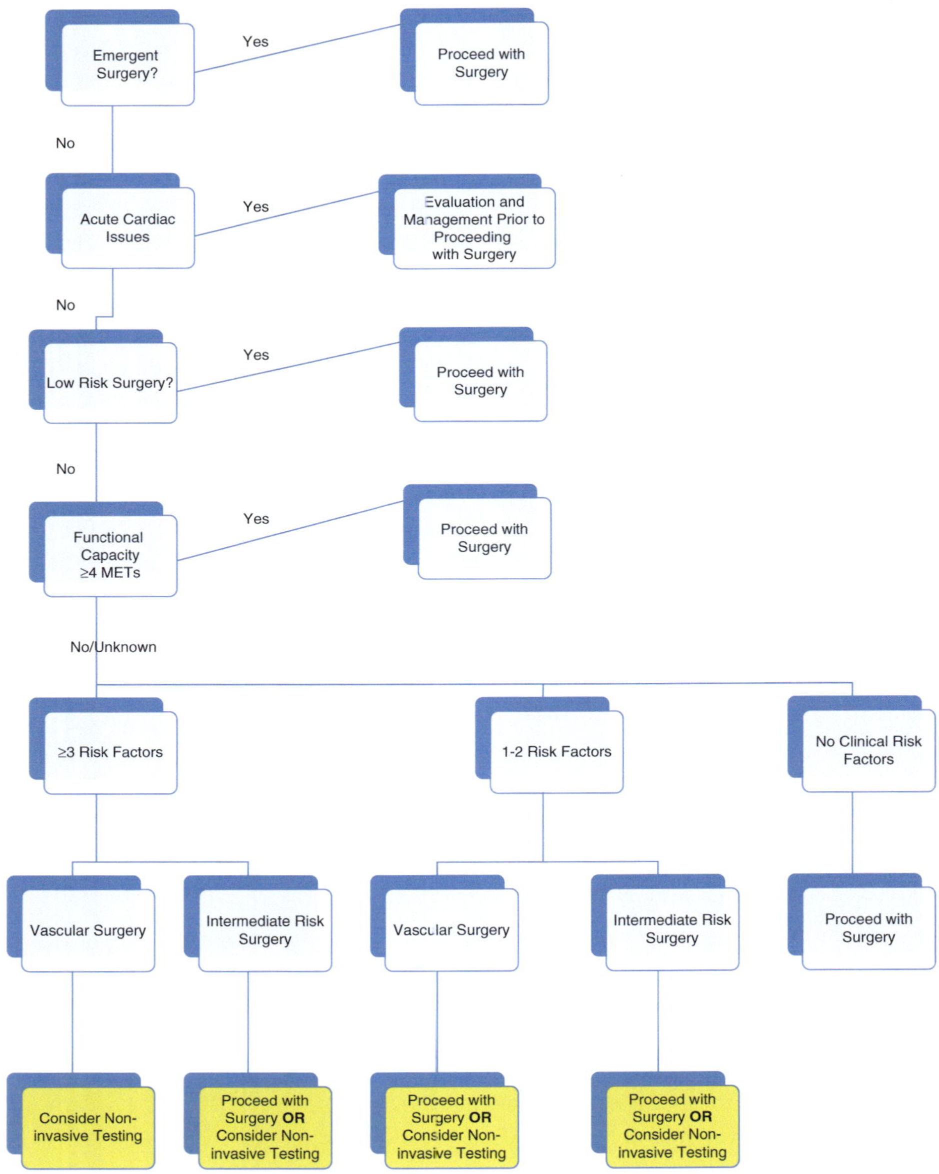

Fig. 30.1 Stepwise approach to preoperative risk stratification prior to undergoing non-cardiac surgery

CCTA for Preoperative Risk Assessment

Although the indication for CCTA as part of preoperative evaluation has not been well defined, the excellent sensitivity and negative predictive value provides the rational for its use as a screening test to exclude significant coronary disease prior to non-cardiac surgery. While the volume of data is insufficient to allow recommendation for the use of CCTA as a noninvasive method in existing preoperative risk assessment models, there does exist several small studies investigating its utility.

The first study included 100 patients whom underwent CCTA prior to undergoing scheduled non-cardiac surgery [12]. Patients whom were found to have significant coronary artery stenoses or in whom motion artifact or significant calcification prevented luminal assessment were referred for invasive angiography and excluded from analysis [12]. Significant stenosis was defined as luminal narrowing >50% [12]. Of the 100 patients enrolled, CCTA was able to exclude significant coronary artery disease in 81 patients and subsequently proceeded to surgery without further cardiac testing [12]. These patients were followed for the onset of any major adverse cardiac events (MACE) during the perioperative period and for 3 months postoperatively [12]. MACE was defined as death due to cardiac causes, acute myocardial infarction, cardiac arrest, or nonelective coronary revascularization [12]. In these 81 patients, no MACE were noted during either the observed perioperative nor the postoperative follow-up period [12].

A second study evaluated consecutive patients undergoing intermediate risk non-cardiac surgery [6]. RCRI scores were calculated in all patients [6]. Additionally, patients were not only evaluated with CCTA but also underwent coronary artery calcium scoring (CACS) [6]. While CACS alone is unable assess the degree of coronary artery stenosis or the precise location of potentially stenotic lesions, elevated CACS portends an increased risk of major cardiovascular events [13]. In one study of over 6500 asymptomatic patients who underwent calcium scoring, the baseline calcium score and the number of vessels involved were each independent predictors of future coronary revascularizations during an 8.5-year follow-up period [13]. In another large observational registry of more than 25,000 patients, unadjusted survival over the follow-up period was 97.4% for patients with calcium scores ranging from 11 to 100 and 73% for patients with calcium scores ≥1000 [14]. Conversely, the absence of coronary artery calcification was associated with extremely low rates adverse cardiac events [15]. In the aforementioned study, 239 patients underwent evaluation with CACS and 234 with CCTA [6]. Coronary stenoses were graded as minimal (<30%) (Fig. 30.2), nonsignificant (>30% but <50%), and significant (>50%) (Fig. 30.3) [6]. Patients were then subsequently followed for 30 days postoperatively for the presence of MACE, defined as cardiac death, unstable angina, nonfatal myocardial infarction, pulmonary edema, ventricular fibrillation/tachycardia, and complete heart block [6]. MACE was seen in 3.5% of patients with minimal coronary artery disease and 7.1% of patients with nonsignificant disease [6]. However, in patients with significant coronary artery disease, the rate of adverse events increased dramatically to 17.2% [6]. The presence of multivessel disease increased rates of adverse events above that of single-vessel disease, and higher CACS also resulted in higher rates of adverse cardiac events [6]. In patients with a CACS ≥113, the odds ratio (OR) for adverse cardiac events was 5.84 [6]. This difference persisted when stratified based on RCRI scores. In patients with CACS <113 compared to CACS ≥113, event rates in the RCRI score of 0 were 1.4% vs. 15.2%, 3.6% vs. 4.7% with a risk score of 1, 0% vs. 21.1% with a risk score of 2, and 50% vs. 66.7% with a risk score of 3 or more [6].

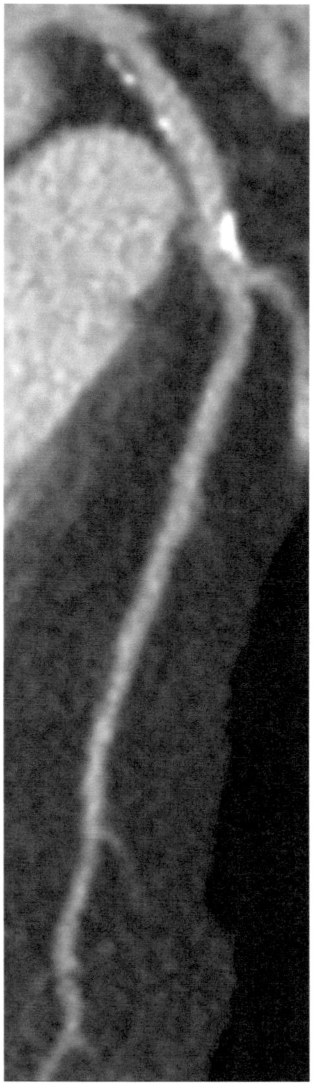

Fig. 30.2 Calcified lesion in the left anterior descending (LAD) artery with resultant mild stenosis

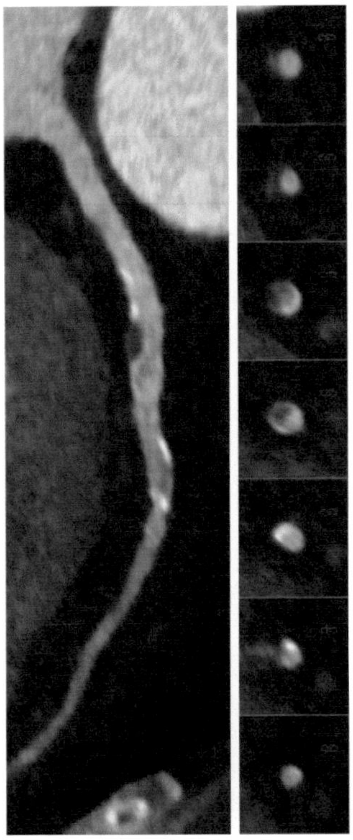

Fig. 30.3 Calcified and non-calcified plaque in the LAD with moderate stenosis

Finally, the third and largest study included 844 patients undergoing CCTA prior to elective non-cardiac surgery [16]. Similar to prior studies, patients were followed for 30 days postoperatively for the development of MACE, defined as pulmonary edema, myocardial infarction, or cardiac death [16]. As expected patients with a higher RCRI risk index had increasing postoperative MACE, an event rate of 1.2% with an RCRI score of 1 compared to a 5.8% event rate with a RCRI score of ≥3 [16]. With respect to CCTA findings, regardless of RCRI score patients with nonsignificant coronary stenosis (<50%) had fewer events that those with significant stenosis (≥50%), 1.7% vs. 8%, respectively [16]. When the two measures were combined, CCTA demonstrated the ability to reclassify patients within the same RCRI score group. In patients with an RCRI score of 2 or 3, the presence of any significant coronary artery stenosis increased postoperative risk of MACE 3–17 times [16].

The previous studies would suggest that in patients without significant coronary artery stenosis on preoperative CCTA, there is a low rate of postoperative MACE. Furthermore, positive and negative predictive values with CCTA were on par with those of myocardial perfusion imaging and dobutamine stress echocardiography published within the European Society of Cardiology (ESC), AHA, and ACC guidelines [16–18].

Additional Considerations

At present when additional noninvasive testing is indicated prior to non-cardiac surgery, guidelines recommend the use of functional testing (myocardial perfusion imaging, stress echocardiography, stress CMR). However, these modalities do not provide anatomic assessment of the coronary arteries nor identify potential non-flow limiting stenosis, the latter of which could pose risk for plaque rupture and subsequent adverse clinical outcomes. Indeed it has been demonstrated that many postoperative MACE are a result of nonobstructive coronary lesions that may be more prone to plaque rupture in the increased inflammatory setting of the operative period [19–21]. The ability to diagnose the presence of any coronary artery disease may allow for modification of medical management in the preoperative period resulting in mitigation of risk postoperatively. It has been observed that the addition of statins in patients undergoing surgery reduces rates of atrial fibrillation, myocardial infarction, as well as length of hospital stay [22]. Additionally, while data regarding beta-blockade in the perioperative period is conflicting, there is data to support improved patient outcomes if beta-blockade is initiated early enough in the preoperative period [23–25]. Apart from the anatomical assessment of the coronaries themselves, CCTA has the ability to provide additional clinically relevant information pertaining to the lung parenchyma, pleura, mediastinum, and great vessels [26, 27].

Conversely, while myocardial perfusion imaging, stress ECG, stress echocardiography, and stress CMR do not provide anatomical assessment of the coronary arteries, CCTA does not provide functional assessment. However, with the advent of computed tomography-derived fractional flow reserve measurements (FFR_{CT}), the ability to assess the hemodynamic significance of lesions identified on CCTA noninvasively exists [28–30]. Coupling CCTA with FFR_{CT} would allow not only for anatomical assessment of the coronary arteries as well as surrounding cardiac structures but also functional assessment as to the presence of ischemia. In a recent meta-analysis, the sensitivity for FFR_{CT} was on par with that of stress CMR (90% and 90%, respectively) and surpassed that of both SPECT and stress echocardiography (70% and 77%, respectively) [31]. Specificity was similar between FFR_{CT}, SPECT, and stress echocardiography at 71%, 78%, and 75%, respectively [31].

Clinical Challenges

A significant challenge in the decision-making process of preoperative evaluation is the timing and appropriateness of pursuing intervention if significant coronary artery disease is discovered. One must balance these findings against additional aspects of surgical planning, such as delay of nonemergent surgery to pursue revascularization, duration of dual antiplatelet therapy, and further evaluation of extracardiac findings (such as previously undiagnosed malignancies or incidental findings warranting further workup). Regardless of modality, preoperative noninvasive cardiac testing should be reserved for appropriate patients as determined by risk assessment and in whom results of testing would alter preoperative management [5].

Conclusions

CCTA has proven to be a highly sensitive and reliable modality for the exclusion of significant coronary artery disease. When utilized in conjunction with techniques such as noninvasive fractional flow reserve, it yields excellent sensitivity – on par with that of stress CMR – as well as good specificity, similar to that of SPECT and stress echocardiography. Despite these data, a paucity of data exists for the use of CCTA in preoperative cardiac risk assessment. As such current guidelines and appropriate use criteria classify CCTA as "rarely appropriate" as it pertains to preoperative testing. While CCTA holds promise to be a valuable modality for preoperative risk assessment, further investigation and larger studies will be needed prior to its adoption into this arena.

References

1. Devereaux PJ, Goldman L, Cook DJ, Gilbert K, Leslie K, Guyatt GH. Perioperative cardiac events in patients undergoing noncardiac surgery: a review of the magnitude of the problem, the pathophysiology of the events and methods to estimate and communicate risk. CMAJ. 2005;173:627–34.
2. Goldman L, Caldera DL, Nussbaum SR, et al. Multifactorial index of cardiac risk in noncardiac surgical procedures. N Engl J Med. 1977;297:845–50.
3. Lee TH, Marcantonio ER, Mangione CM, et al. Derivation and prospective validation of a simple index for prediction of cardiac risk of major noncardiac surgery. Circulation. 1999;100:1043–9.
4. Detsky AS, Abrams HB, McLaughlin JR, et al. Predicting cardiac complications in patients undergoing non-cardiac surgery. J Gen Intern Med. 1986;1:211–9.
5. Fleisher LA, Beckman JA, Brown KA, et al. ACC/AHA 2007 guidelines on perioperative cardiovascular evaluation and care for noncardiac surgery: executive summary: a report of the American College of Cardiology/American Heart Association Task Force on Practice Guidelines (Writing Committee to Revise the 2002 Guidelines on Perioperative Cardiovascular Evaluation for Noncardiac Surgery) Developed in Collaboration With the American Society of Echocardiography, American Society of Nuclear Cardiology, Heart Rhythm Society, Society of Cardiovascular Anesthesiologists, Society for Cardiovascular Angiography and Interventions, Society for Vascular Medicine and Biology, and Society for Vascular Surgery. J Am Coll Cardiol. 2007;50:1707–32.
6. Ahn JH, Park JR, Min JH, et al. Risk stratification using computed tomography coronary angiography in patients undergoing intermediate-risk noncardiac surgery. J Am Coll Cardiol. 2013;61:661–8.
7. Achenbach S, Schuhbaeck A, Marwan M, et al. Multicenter evaluation of dual source ct coronary angiography in patients with intermediate likelihood of coronary artery stenoses (medic): accuracy for the detection of individuals with significant coronary artery stenoses. J Am Coll Cardiol. 2012;59:E1337.
8. Meijboom WB, Meijs MF, Schuijf JD, et al. Diagnostic accuracy of 64-slice computed tomography coronary angiography: a prospective, multicenter, multivendor study. J Am Coll Cardiol. 2008;52:2135–44.
9. Ronan G, Wolk MJ, Bailey SR, et al. ACCF/AHA/ASE/ASNC/HFSA/HRS/SCAI/SCCT/SCMR/STS 2013 multimodality appropriate use criteria for the detection and risk assessment of stable ischemic heart disease: a report of the American College of Cardiology Foundation Appropriate Use Criteria Task Force, American Heart Association, American Society of Echocardiography, American Society of Nuclear Cardiology, Heart Failure Society of America, Heart Rhythm Society, Society for Cardiovascular Angiography and Interventions, Society of Cardiovascular Computed Tomography, Society for Cardiovascular Magnetic Resonance, and Society of Thoracic Surgeons. J Nucl Cardiol. 2014;21:192–220.
10. Lee SP, Jang EJ, Kim YJ, et al. Cost-effectiveness of coronary CT angiography in patients with chest pain: Comparison with myocardial single photon emission tomography. J Cardiovasc Comput Tomogr. 2015;9:428–37.
11. Taylor AJ, Cerqueira M, Hodgson JM, et al. ACCF/SCCT/ACR/AHA/ASE/ASNC/NASCI/SCAI/SCMR 2010 appropriate use criteria for cardiac computed tomography. A report of the American College of Cardiology Foundation appropriate use criteria task force, the society of cardiovascular computed tomography, the American College of Radiology, the American Heart Association, the American Society of Echocardiography, the American Society of Nuclear Cardiology, the North American Society for Cardiovascular Imaging, the society for cardiovascular angiography and interventions, and the society for cardiovascular magnetic resonance. Circulation. 2010;122:e525–55.
12. Buffa V, De Cecco CN, Cossu L, et al. Preoperative coronary risk assessment with dual-source CT in patients undergoing noncoronary cardiac surgery. Radiol Med. 2010;115:1028–37.
13. Silverman MG, Harkness JR, Blankstein R, et al. Baseline subclinical atherosclerosis burden and distribution are associated with frequency and mode of future coronary revascularization: multi-ethnic study of atherosclerosis. JACC Cardiovasc Imaging. 2014;7:476–86.
14. Budoff MJ, Shaw LJ, Liu ST, et al. Long-term prognosis associated with coronary calcification: observations from a registry of 25,253 patients. J Am Coll Cardiol. 2007;49:1860–70.
15. Kelkar AA, Schultz WM, Khosa F, et al. Long-term prognosis after coronary artery calcium scoring among low-intermediate risk women and men. Circ Cardiovasc Imaging. 2016;9:e003742.
16. Hwang JW, Kim EK, Yang JH, et al. Assessment of perioperative cardiac risk of patients undergoing noncardiac surgery using coronary computed tomographic angiography. Circ Cardiovasc Imaging. 2015;8:e002582.
17. Wijeysundera DN, Duncan D, Nkonde-Price C, et al. Perioperative beta blockade in noncardiac surgery: a systematic review for the 2014 ACC/AHA guideline on perioperative cardiovascular evaluation and management of patients undergoing noncardiac surgery: a report of the American College of Cardiology/American Heart Association Task Force on Practice Guidelines. Circulation. 2014;130:2246–64.
18. Kristensen SD, Knuuti J, Saraste A, et al. 2014 ESC/ESA Guidelines on non-cardiac surgery: cardiovascular assessment and management: The Joint Task Force on non-cardiac surgery: cardiovascular assessment and management of the European Society of Cardiology (ESC) and the European Society of Anaesthesiology (ESA). Eur Heart J. 2014;35:2383–431.

19. Cohen MC, Aretz TH. Histological analysis of coronary artery lesions in fatal postoperative myocardial infarction. Cardiovasc Pathol. 1999;8:133–9.
20. Dawood MM, Gutpa DK, Southern J, Walia A, Atkinson JB, Eagle KA. Pathology of fatal perioperative myocardial infarction: implications regarding pathophysiology and prevention. Int J Cardiol. 1996;57:37–44.
21. Duvall WL, Sealove B, Pungoti C, Katz D, Moreno P, Kim M. Angiographic investigation of the pathophysiology of perioperative myocardial infarction. Catheter Cardiovasc Interv. 2012;80:768–76.
22. Chopra V, Wesorick DH, Sussman JB, et al. Effect of perioperative statins on death, myocardial infarction, atrial fibrillation, and length of stay: a systematic review and meta-analysis. Arch Surg. 2012;147:181–9.
23. Andersson C, Merie C, Jorgensen M, et al. Association of beta-blocker therapy with risks of adverse cardiovascular events and deaths in patients with ischemic heart disease undergoing noncardiac surgery: a Danish nationwide cohort study. JAMA Intern Med. 2014;174:336–44.
24. Group PS, Devereaux PJ, Yang H, et al. Effects of extended-release metoprolol succinate in patients undergoing non-cardiac surgery (POISE trial): a randomised controlled trial. Lancet. 2008;371:1839–47.
25. Chopra V, Plaisance B, Cavusoglu E, Flanders SA, Eagle KA. Perioperative beta-blockers for major noncardiac surgery: Primum Non Nocere. Am J Med. 2009;122:222–9.
26. Akhtar NJ, Markowitz AH, Gilkeson RC. Multidetector computed tomography in the preoperative assessment of cardiac surgery patients. Radiol Clin N Am. 2010;48:117–39.
27. Bastarrika G, Thilo C, Headden GF, Zwerner PL, Costello P, Schoepf UJ. Cardiac CT in the assessment of acute chest pain in the emergency department. AJR Am J Roentgenol. 2009;193:397–409.
28. Koo BK, Erglis A, Doh JH, et al. Diagnosis of ischemia-causing coronary stenoses by noninvasive fractional flow reserve computed from coronary computed tomographic angiograms. Results from the prospective multicenter DISCOVER-FLOW (Diagnosis of Ischemia-Causing Stenoses Obtained Via Noninvasive Fractional Flow Reserve) study. J Am Coll Cardiol. 2011;58:1989–97.
29. Min JK, Leipsic J, Pencina MJ, et al. Diagnostic accuracy of fractional flow reserve from anatomic CT angiography. JAMA. 2012;308:1237–45.
30. Norgaard BL, Leipsic J, Gaur S, et al. Diagnostic performance of noninvasive fractional flow reserve derived from coronary computed tomography angiography in suspected coronary artery disease: the NXT trial (Analysis of Coronary Blood Flow Using CT Angiography: Next Steps). J Am Coll Cardiol. 2014;63:1145–55.
31. Danad I, Szymonifka J, Twisk JW, et al. Diagnostic performance of cardiac imaging methods to diagnose ischaemia-causing coronary artery disease when directly compared with fractional flow reserve as a reference standard: a meta-analysis. Eur Heart J. 2017;38(13):991–8.

CT for Guiding Successful Revascularization

31

Maksymilian P. Opolski

Both percutaneous coronary intervention (PCI) and coronary computed tomography angiography (coronary CTA) belong to the most evolving fields in modern cardiology. In parallel to the expanding indications for coronary CTA, a continually increasing number of patients undergo PCI following coronary CTA examination [1, 2]. In this regard, the abundance of anatomic, morphological, and physiological data incorporated from a one-stop-shop computed tomographic study can aid to optimize PCI strategy [3, 4]. The purpose of this chapter is to highlight contemporary and future advancements of coronary CTA that might help guide PCI.

Interventional Applications

Once a patient has been identified as having a flow-limiting plaque in need of stenting (Fig. 31.1), coronary CTA data can be used to better plan percutaneous strategy, particularly in angiographically demanding lesions such as coronary chronic total occlusions (CTO), bifurcation lesions, or coronary anomalies. Below a number of potential applications of coronary CTA for PCI have been described.

Selection of Stent Size and Length

Numerous studies in the drug-eluting stent era have repeatedly identified greater residual reference segment disease and stent underexpansion as independent predictors of subsequent stent edge restenosis and thrombosis [5, 6]. Hence, complete lesion coverage and well-matched vessel diameters are paramount to decrease the risk of stent failure and improve clinical outcomes. Invasive coronary angiography (ICA) represents a two-dimensional technique that cannot reliably visualize the atherosclerotic involvement of the arterial wall [2]. Consequently, it often underestimates lesion length and vessel size compared with intravascular ultrasound (IVUS) and coronary CTA (specifically when diffuse disease or negative remodeling are present) [7]. Whereas IVUS is still the current gold standard to optimize stent implantation [1], there is compelling evidence that measurements of lumen area and diameter performed with coronary CTA and IVUS are well correlated [8], and noninvasive CTA is the only imaging technique to quantify lesion length and vessel size before the procedure has even started. The concept of CTA-guided stent sizing was first reported in a simulation study by LaBounty et al. who reevaluated 18 patients with 24 coronary lesions and pre-procedural CTA datasets [9]. Interestingly, by using CTA operators selected longer stents with larger stent diameters than with ICA. In another small pilot study of 17 patients with 26 native coronary lesions, Kass et al. indicated relatively good agreement between CTA- and IVUS-derived stent sizes [10]. These findings were subsequently replicated in 22 saphenous vein graft lesions, wherein both coronary CTA and IVUS demonstrated similar measurements of the proximal and distal reference lumen diameters as well as lesion length [11] Additionally, the assessment of stent length by coronary CTA but not invasive coronary angiography (ICA) dictates the exact actual length of the implanted stent as reported by the stent's manufacturer [12]. Of particular interest, in the prospective randomized single-center study of 71 patients, Pregowski et al. investigated whether the addition of coronary CTA to PCI planning could affect immediate procedural results as defined by IVUS endpoints [13]. To this end, angiography plus CTA-guided PCI versus angiography-guided PCI was compared, wherein computed tomographic criteria for lumen area >4.5 mm^2 in the reference segments were used to determine the optimal landing zone for stent implantation. Notably, coronary stents selected under CTA guidance were significantly longer with a trend toward larger nominal stent diameter compared with angiography-guided strategy alone (Fig. 31.2). This further translated into more complete lesion coverage and larger stent expansion as con-

M. P. Opolski (✉)
Department of Interventional Cardiology and Angiology, Institute of Cardiology, Warsaw, Poland

U. J. Schoepf (ed.), *CT of the Heart*, Contemporary Medical Imaging, https://doi.org/10.1007/978-1-60327-237-7_31

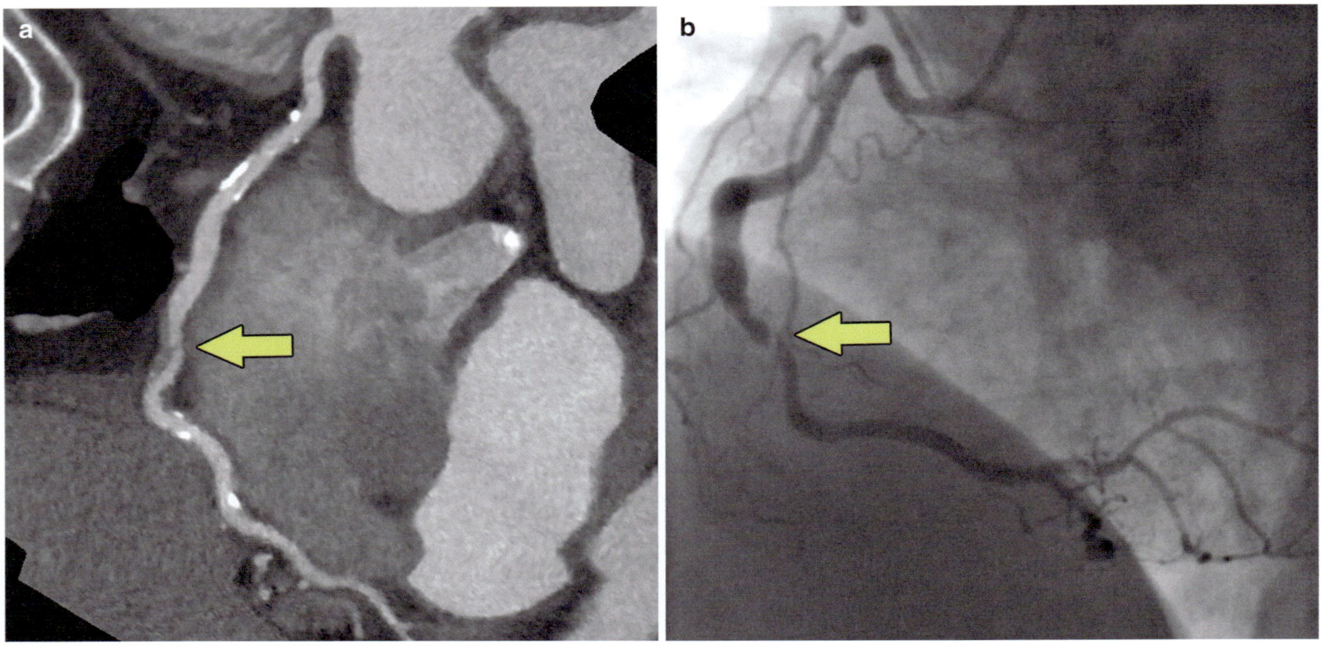

Fig. 31.1 High-grade stenosis in coronary computed tomography angiography. (**a**) Curved multiplanar reconstruction showing high-grade lesion in the mid-segment of the right coronary artery (arrow). (**b**) Corresponding invasive angiographic view

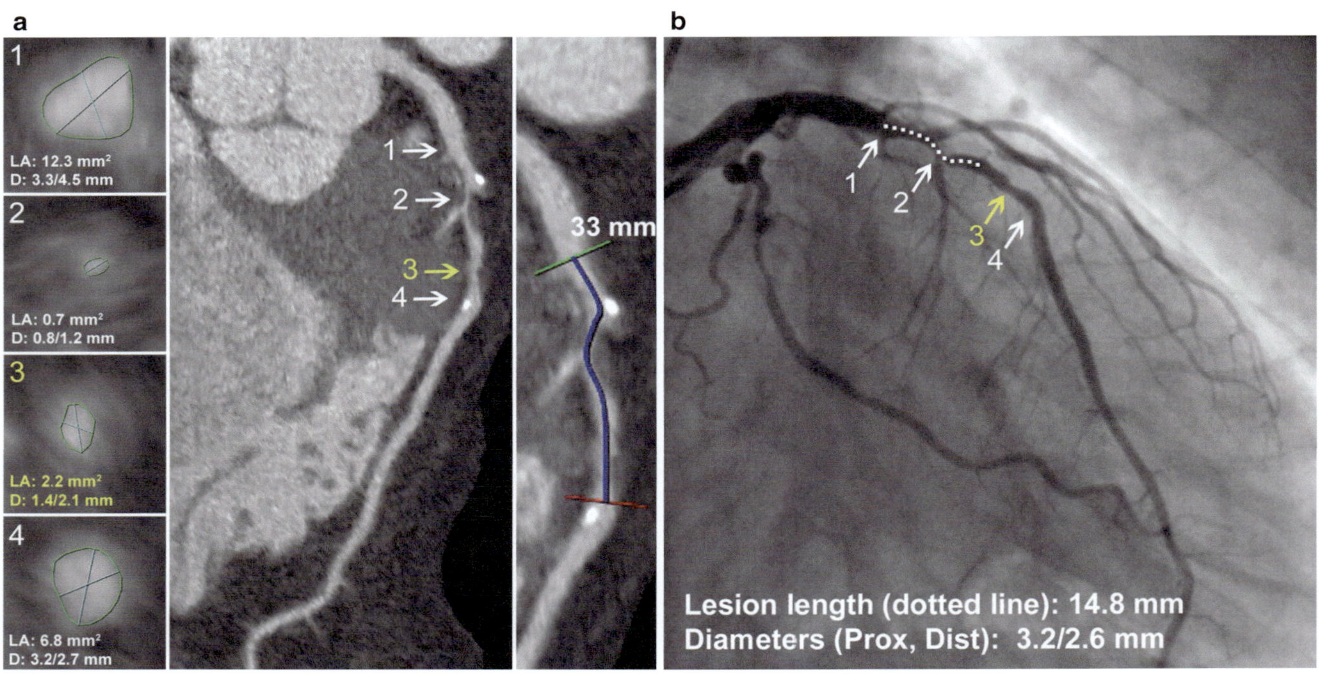

Fig. 31.2 Computed tomography angiography-assisted planning of percutaneous coronary intervention. (**a**) Curved multiplanar reconstructions of the high-grade stenosis in the mid-segment of the left anterior descending artery with corresponding cross-sectional areas (1 to 4). Based on computed tomographic data the planned stent length is 33 mm with proximal and distal stent diameters of 4.0 mm (cross section 1) and 3.0 mm (cross section 4), respectively. (**b**) Corresponding invasive angiographic view. In the angiography-guided strategy, the significant reference plaque burden (cross section 3) would likely be overlooked and stent diameters underestimated

firmed by smaller peri-stent plaque burden and larger minimal stent area in the CTA group. Lately Wolny et al. evaluated the value of CTA in planning PCI strategy in bifurcation lesions in a prospective randomized study of 93 patients [14]. Whereas CTA-assisted bifurcation PCI was equally safe (with similar rate of periprocedural myocardial infarction, amount of contrast and radiation dose during PCI) compared with angiography-guided revascularization, it prompted PCI operators to choose simpler PCI technique with higher use of single-stent procedures and proximal optimization technique along with less frequent side-branch stenting. Possible explanation of this observation is that angiography-defined lesion length is often underestimated, leading to a selection of too short a stent – a phenomenon that may be occasionally associated with suboptimal immediate angiographic result (i.e., stent edge dissection or plaque protrusion caused by stent placement in a region with high plaque burden) – and thus requires additional stent implantation. Whether the anatomic approach for CTA-guided stent implantation may also improve lesion-specific ischemia compared to the standard-of-care angiography-guided PCI is yet to be determined. Until these trials are completed, selection of stent size and length based on CTA data will likely be slowly incorporated into clinical practice, notwithstanding the absence of clear guideline recommendation.

Ischemia-Guided PCI by Computerized Tomography Fractional Flow Reserve

Given the ascendancy of ischemia-guided intervention over anatomic-guided intervention [15], the ability of computerized tomography fractional flow reserve (FFR-CT) to detect lesion-specific ischemia opens a door for FFR-CT-guided PCI. In the RIPCORD study, 200 consecutive patients from the NXT trial underwent sequential decision-making for the most optimal treatment strategy (optimal medical therapy alone, PCI, coronary artery bypass grafting, or more information required) based on coronary CTA alone or the hybrid anatomic-physiological approach of coronary CTA plus FFR-CT [16]. The decision was made by consensus of three experienced interventional cardiologists reporting on the changes in their management plan after disclosure of FFR-CT. Overall, there was a change in management in 36% of patients, with a 23% increase in the use of optimal medical therapy alone, a 5% decrease in PCI, and a 0.5% increase in CABG. Among patients assigned to PCI, in 18% the target vessel for PCI was changed, whereas 30% were reallocated to optimal medical therapy. Not surprisingly, FFR-CT can also optimize PCI by dictating the landing zone for stent implantation necessary to resolve ischemia (Fig. 31.3). In a pilot study of 48 ischemia-causing stenoses with post-PCI invasive FFR data, the ability of FFR-CT to predict the functional benefit of coronary revascularization by "virtual stenting" was tested [17]. Specifically, "virtual stenting" was performed by modification of the computational model in the region of the virtual stent according to the proximal and distal reference areas, and the diagnostic accuracy of FFR-CT to predict ischemia after stenting was 96%. Whether FFR-CT could determine which method of coronary revascularization maximally reduces ischemia ("virtual stenting" versus "virtual bypass surgery") based on patient-specific anatomy is to be elucidated.

Plaque Assessment for Planning PCI Interventions

Several CT studies have consistently confirmed the close relationship between high-risk features of coronary plaques and invasive FFR [18–21]. In the study by Nakazato et al. in 58 patients with 58 intermediate coronary lesions, percent aggregate plaque volume (cumulative plaque volume as a function of total vessel volume) showed the highest predictive value for identification, discrimination, and reclassification of ischemic lesions compared with anatomic measurements of coronary stenosis [18]. In the larger multicenter evaluation of 407 stenoses in 252 patients from the DeFACTO study, positive remodeling was an independent predictor of ischemia across all coronary lesions, whereas percent aggregate plaque volume and low-attenuation plaque were associated with ischemia in obstructive lesions (≥50%) only [19]. Further, in the substudy of the NXT trial of 254 patients with 484 vessels employing semiautomated CT software, low-density noncalcified plaque volume ≥30 mm^3 was the only independent determinant of ischemia with incremental predictive value over CTA stenosis >50% [20].

The presence, location, and extent of calcification on CTA might potentially affect the results of catheter-based interventions. For example, for lesions with severe calcium (mostly defined as calcification >50% of vessel cross section), plaque modification with rotablation, intravascular lithotripsy or high-pressure balloons may be required to achieve complete stent expansion [22]. Whereas coronary dissections are often encountered at the junction of calcified and noncalcified plaque, the optimal landing zone for stent implantation in calcium-free vessel segments should be considered. The potential difficulties in calcified lesions have been emphasized in a study showing that hard plaques with CT density >120 Hounsfield units were associated with occurrence of dissection or perforation during PCI [23]. Moreover, plaques with a higher calcium score had larger reference plaque burden following stent implantation and were more likely to require balloon post-dilation under IVUS guidance [24].

Assessment of plaque composition by coronary CTA can also predict the occurrence of distal emboli during PCI that may ultimately result in periprocedural myocardial infarction [25–29]. In the study by Harigaya et al. including 78 patients with acute coronary syndrome or stable angina, the presence of CTA-derived low-attenuation plaque with a length >4.7 mm was an independent predictor of the no-reflow phenomenon [27]. Consequently, Kodama et al. found that low-attenuation plaque surrounded by circumferential plaque calcification conferred a higher risk of slow-flow phenomenon after PCI in a series of 40 patients [28]. Also, a larger prospective study of 189 stable patients corroborated the decisive role of low-attenuation plaque in predicting periprocedural myocardial injury as confirmed by positive troponin-T at 18 h post-PCI [26]. Ultimately, large analysis of 180

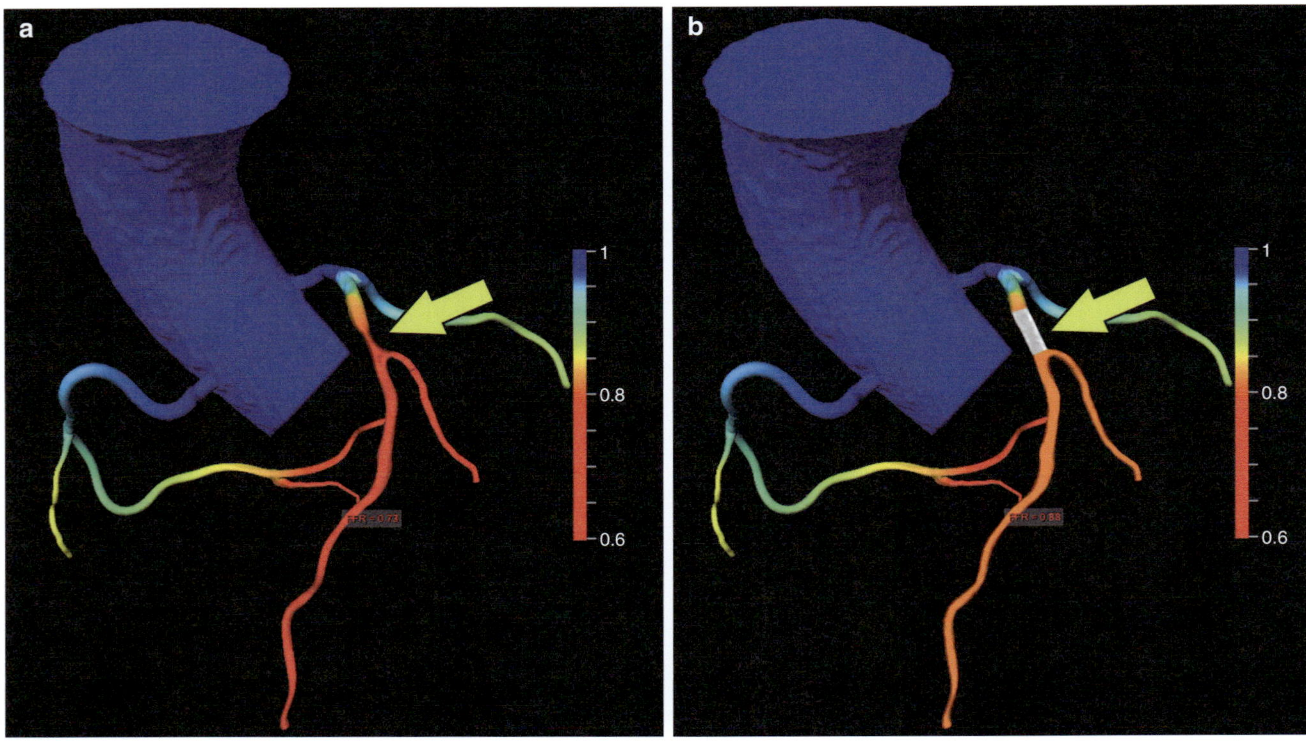

Fig. 31.3 Noninvasive treatment planning using fractional flow reserve derived from computed tomographic data with virtual stenting algorithm. (**a**) Computerized tomography fractional flow reserve demonstrating functionally significant stenosis in the proximal segment of the left anterior descending artery (arrow). (**b**) Computerized tomography fractional flow reserve showing resolution of ischemia in the left anterior descending coronary artery after virtual stenting (arrow)

patients with non-ST-segment elevation acute coronary syndrome and pre-procedural CTA yielded low-attenuation plaque and napkin-ring sign as independent predictors of slow-flow phenomenon in culprit lesions [29]. All of these studies reinforce the notion that coronary plaques with large lipid area may be prone to being broken down into small atherosclerotic particles following balloon dilatation, with subsequent embolic complications of the distal coronary circulation (Fig. 31.4). In this regard, identification of high-risk plaques on CTA may help in shifting PCI strategy toward the use of direct stenting, distal protection devices, or stronger antithrombotic therapy (e.g., glycoprotein IIb/IIIa receptor inhibitors). Another option might include deferring PCI and starting statin therapy for plaque stabilization. Finally, in patients with multiple high-risk plaques (particularly involving left main or proximal left anterior descending coronary artery), coronary bypass grafting rather than PCI could be considered.

Coronary CTA can also predict mechanical complications of stent implantation. Recently Tesche et al. proposed an elegant method derived from pre-procedural CTA for predicting in-stent restenosis as defined by quantitative ICA [30]. In a retrospective analysis of 74 coronary lesions, their main observation was that lesion length, noncalcified plaque volume, and positive remodeling measured by CTA portended the occurrence of in-stent restenosis with incremental predictive value (sensitivity of 90% and specificity of 84%). Logical explanation for this observation may reside in the inherent properties of a diffusely distributed low-attenuation plaque that could promote inflammatory endothelial response along with exaggerated neointimal proliferation as a reaction to stent strut penetration. In this regard, visualization of a low-attenuation plaque with positive remodeling on CTA should be considered as a "bad omen" (increasing the risk of both slow-flow phenomenon and in-stent restenosis) for PCI operators. Potential solution for mitigating the risk for in-stent restenosis should involve selection of well-expanded drug-eluting stents with minimal late lumen loss that cover the entire length of coronary plaque.

Vulnerable Plaque

The concept of vulnerable plaque is based on the assumption that certain coronary plaques are more prone to rupture than others (Fig. 31.5) [31]. Given the compelling evidence for multifocal nature of vulnerable plaques as well as the strenuous effort for invasive intracoronary imaging of all three

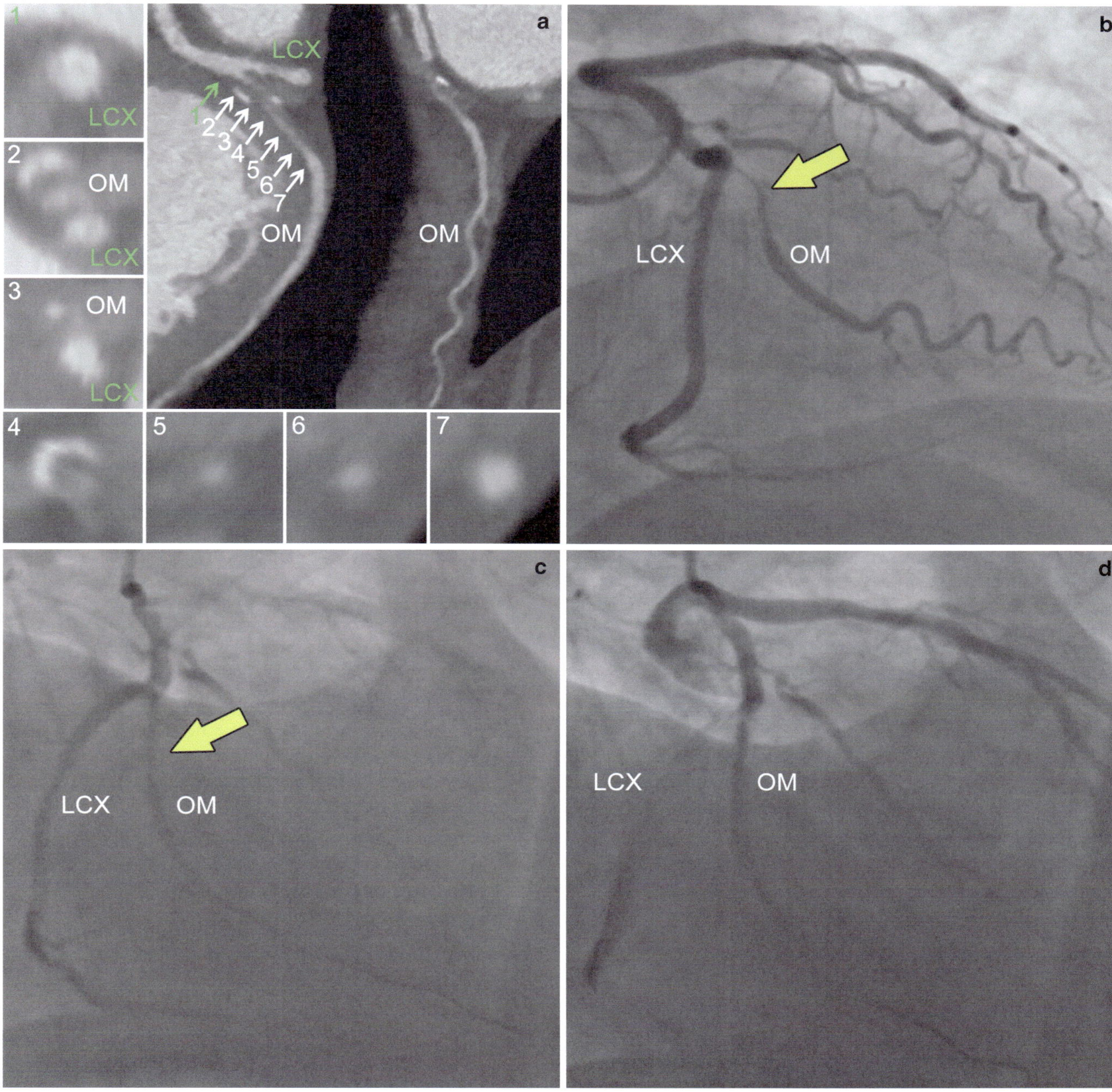

Fig. 31.4 Coronary computed tomography angiography for characterization of a high-risk plaque resulting in a no-reflow phenomenon following percutaneous coronary intervention. (**a**) Curved multiplanar reconstructions along with corresponding cross-sectional areas (1 to 7) show severely stenotic low-attenuation plaque with circumferential calcification in the obtuse marginal branch (arrow). (**b**) Corresponding invasive angiographic view confirming severe stenosis in the obtuse marginal branch (arrow). (**c**) Stent positioning. (**d**) No-reflow in the left circumflex artery and slow-flow in the obtuse marginal branch after stent implantation

coronary vessels, noninvasive CTA has become one of the most versatile techniques for prediction of future coronary events [32]. In a landmark study by Motoyama et al. including 1059 patients with stable chest pain, the presence of low-attenuation plaque and/or positive remodeling conferred a 23% risk for future coronary event during a mean follow-up of 27 months [33]. In a study of 312 patients with non-ST-segment elevation myocardial infarction undergoing coronary CTA, the total amount of noncalcified plaque in nonobstructive coronary lesions was an independent predictor of subsequent coronary events [34]. Moreover, the focus on napkin-ring sign morphology (defined as the presence of a ring of high attenuation around coronary plaque) was undertaken in a prospective study of 895 patients [35]. After

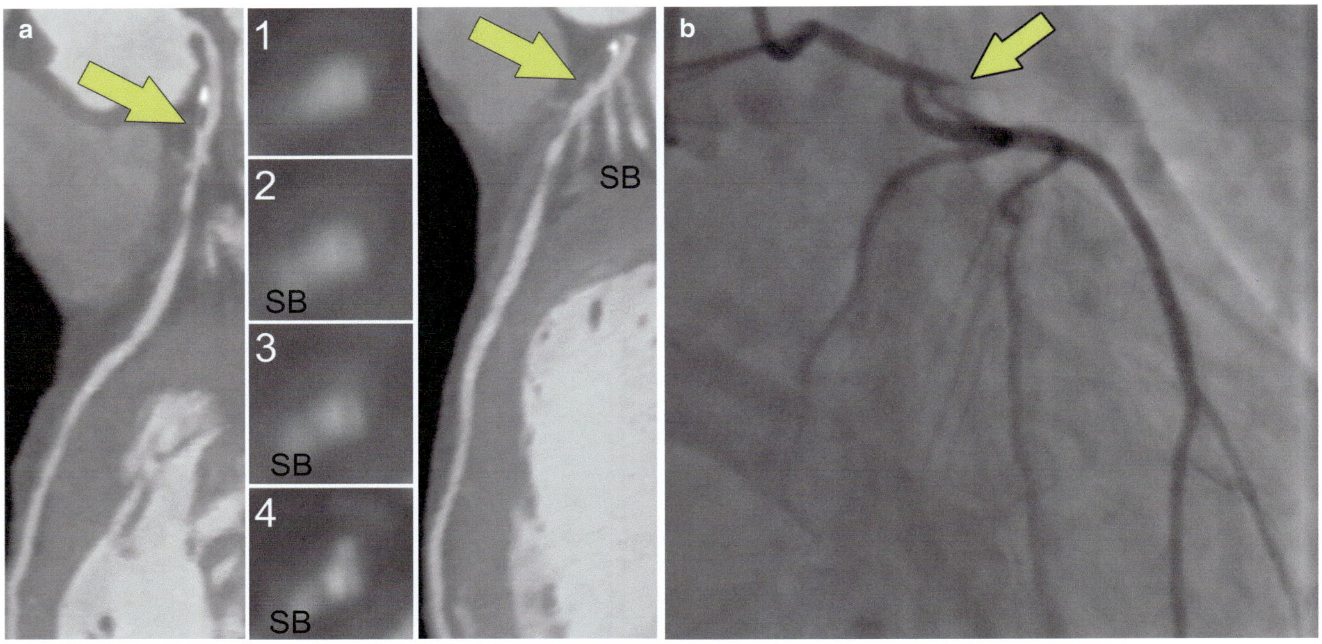

Fig. 31.5 Coronary computed tomography angiography for characterization of a vulnerable plaque causing future ischemic event. (**a**) Curved multiplanar reconstructions of the left anterior descending artery with corresponding cross-sectional areas (1 to 4) at the site distal to the origin of the first diagonal branch demonstrate low-attenuation plaque with positive remodeling and a napkin-ring sign (cross sections 1 to 3) along with isolated circumferential contrast accumulation that might correspond to plaque ulceration (cross section 4). (**b**) Invasive angiogram showing acute occlusion of the proximal left anterior descending artery at follow-up (arrowhead). *SB* side-branch

a mean of 2.3 years, both the napkin-ring sign along with positive remodeling and low-attenuation plaque showed an independent relationship with future episodes of acute coronary syndrome. Finally, in the latest meta-analysis across six CT studies, the risk of future coronary event was significantly higher in high-risk plaques (defined by at least one of the following criterions: low attenuation, increased remodeling index, or the presence of spotty calcification) versus low-risk plaques with odds ratio of 12.14 [36]. On a practical level, the potential clinical use of CTA to detect vulnerable plaques would require the development of effective preventive measures mitigating the risk of subsequent plaque rupture [31]. Futuristic approaches may involve vulnerable plaque sealing with coronary stents or biodegradable vascular scaffolds.

Coronary Chronic Total Occlusions

A CTO may be incidentally identified on a diagnostic coronary CTA, or CTA may be specifically performed for a better characterization of CTO (usually in cases with a previously failed recanalization attempt) [22]. In the former case, the prevalence of CTO is non-negligible and may reach up to 6.2% in patients with obstructive coronary artery disease [37]. Although CTO are defined based on the angiographic criterion of antegrade blood flow interruption of ≥3 months' duration, CTA reproducibly demonstrates a complete lack of contrast opacification within the occlusion site with subsequent contrast enhancement in the distal vessel segment (Fig. 31.6) [22].

Unlike ICA, coronary CTA allows for complete visualization of the occlusion site and distal vessel segment [22, 38]. This is particularly apparent in long and tortuous CTO lesions or when the distal CTO segment cannot be entirely visualized in ICA (e.g., patients after coronary artery bypass grafting) [22, 39]. Furthermore, it has been consistently established in several trials that CTA reliably quantifies morphological (i.e., calcification, number of occlusion sites) [39–42] and anatomical (e.g., tortuosity, length) [40, 41, 43] features of CTO. Three-dimensional reconstructions enable the visualization of the exact vessel trajectory with accurate measurement of the occlusion length avoiding calibration limitations or lesion foreshortening [7]. Also, CTA can be used for providing guidance for the location of ostial CTO and multiple occlusion sites, characteristics usually missed in ICA [39, 42].

All features described above have been used in a number of CT studies predicting the procedural outcome with CTO PCI (Table 31.1) [38, 40, 42–52]. Mollet et al. were the first to show that calcifications involving >50% of the vessel cross-sectional area along with an occlusion length >15 mm were independent predictors of guidewire crossing failure in a series of 47 CTO lesions [43]. In a study by Ehara et al.

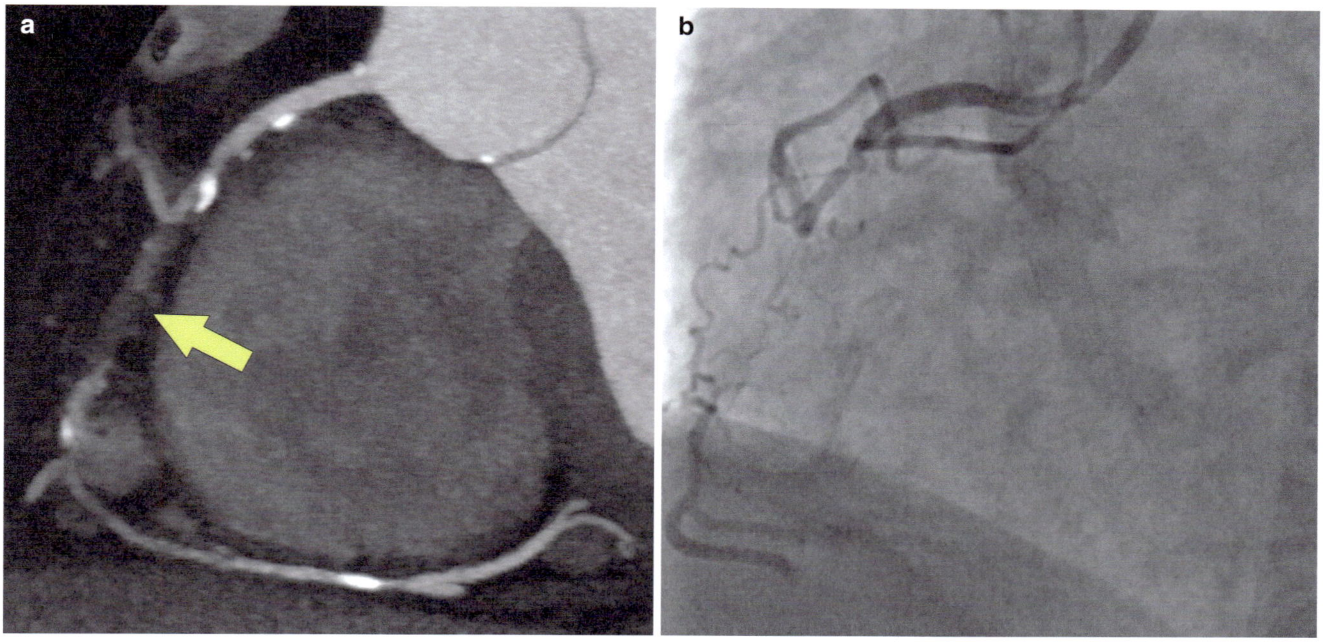

Fig. 31.6 Chronic total occlusion in coronary computed tomography angiography. (**a**) Multiplanar reformation demonstrating noncalcified occlusion that lacks contrast opacification in the mid-segment of the right coronary artery (arrow). The vessel distal to the occluded segment is opacified with contrast. (**b**) Corresponding invasive angiographic view. (From Opolski and Achenbach [22], with permission)

Table 31.1 Studies investigating the ability of computed tomography angiography to predict successful percutaneous coronary intervention in chronic total occlusion

Author, year	Type of CT	No of CTO	Study endpoint	Success rate	Independent predictors of PCI failure
Mollet et al. 2005 [43]	16-slice	47	Guidewire crossing	55%	Calcium >50% CSA Occlusion length >15 mm
Soon et al. 2007 [40]	16-slice	43	Guidewire crossing with stenting (TIMI 3 flow and <25% stenosis)	56%	Calcium ≥50% CSA
Ehara et al. 2009 [44]	64-slice	110	Guidewire crossing	85%	Bending (>45°) Shrinkage (<1 mm in vessel diameter) Severe calcium (~360° CSA)
García-García et al. 2009 [38]	16/64-slice	142	Guidewire crossing (TIMI 2–3 flow and <50% stenosis)	63%	Calcium >50% CSA
Cho et al. 2010 [45]	64-slice	72	Guidewire crossing with stenting (TIMI 3 flow)	76%	%Calcium area/CSA
Li et al. 2010 [46]	64-slice dual source	74	Guidewire crossing (TIMI 2–3 flow and <20% stenosis)	77%	Occlusion length Severity of calcification (noncalcified, spot-calcified, arc-calcified, circular-calcified)
Hsu et al. 2011 [47]	64-slice	82	Guidewire crossing (TIMI 2–3 flow and <30% stenosis)	89%	Calcification length ratio (calcification length/occlusion length) >0.5
Choi et al. 2011 [48]	64-slice	186	Guidewire crossing (TIMI 3 flow and <30% stenosis)	77%	Occlusion length >18 mm Segmental density >139HU CTO duration >12 months or unknown
Martín-Yuste et al. 2012 [49]	64-slice	77	Guidewire crossing	62%	Calcium arc/CSA
Li et al. 2013 [50]	64-slice dual source	88	Guidewire crossing (TIMI 3 flow and <25% stenosis)	58%	Linear intrathrombus enhancement
Opolski et al. 2015 [42]	64/128-slice dual source	240	Guidewire crossing within 30 min	62%	Calcium >50% CSA Bending (>45°) Multiple occlusion sites Blunt stump CTO duration ≥12 months or unknown Previously failed PCI at CTO

(continued)

Table 31.1 (continued)

Author, year	Type of CT	No of CTO	Study endpoint	Success rate	Independent predictors of PCI failure
Luo et al. 2015 [51]	256-slice	108	Guidewire crossing (TIMI 3 flow and <20% stenosis without MACE)	74%	Negative remodeling Occlusion length ≥32 mm
Chen et al. 2015 [52]	64-slice	281	Guidewire crossing (TIMI 3 flow and <25% stenosis)	85%	Attenuation of proximal CTO segment Occlusion length Total coronary calcium score

CSA cross-sectional area, *CT* computed tomography, *CTO* chronic total occlusion, *MACE* major adverse cardiac events, *PCI* percutaneous coronary intervention, *TIMI* thrombolysis in myocardial infarction

including 110 CTO lesions, bending (defined as an angle >45°) was the most powerful predictor of wire failure (followed by vessel shrinkage and severe calcium) [44]. Subsequently, García-García et al. found that calcification >50% of vessel cross section was the only independent correlator of failed PCI among 142 CTO, conferring an almost sixfold higher risk for procedural failure [38]. Consistent findings were consequently replicated by other authors, highlighting the deleterious role of severe calcium in hampering successful guidewire passage [40, 45, 46–49]. There are conflicting data regarding the impact of CTA-derived occlusion length on PCI result. Whereas some studies repeatedly indicated that long CTO (defined as either >15 mm or >18 mm or ≥32 mm or continuous variable) confer a higher risk for procedural failure [43, 46, 48, 50–52], others failed to demonstrate any relationship between occlusion length and PCI outcome [38, 40, 42, 44, 45, 47, 49]. In lieu of these findings, the relevance of CT-derived severe calcification and occlusion length cannot be overemphasized as both of these features (along with minimal vessel area) are associated with adverse clinical outcomes after PCI of CTO [53]. More recently, the CT-RECTOR score was introduced as a noninvasive robust prediction tool to predict successful guidewire crossing through CTO within 30 min [42]. It was derived from 240 consecutive CTO lesions from a multicenter European registry, and the outcome variable was specifically set to represent the difficulty level intrinsic to CTO rather than operator skills and perseverance. Of note, the CT-RECTOR score is calculated by assigning one point for each of the independent predictors (multiple occlusions, blunt stump, severe calcification, bending, CTO age ≥12 months, previously failed PCI) and adding them per CTO lesion (Fig. 31.7). With an increasing score, the likelihood of guidewire crossing ≤30 min decreased, ranging from 95% for a CT-RECTOR score of 0 to 22% for a CT-RECTOR score of ≥3. As an alternative, the noninvasive counterpart of the commonly used angiographic J-CTO score (the so called J-CTOCT score) has been shown high predictive value for predicting guidewire crossing ≤30 min [54].

In summary, the entirety of information proffered by CTA can affect the technique of PCI for CTO. For example, identification of severe and diffuse calcium at the entry site, together with a good retrograde collateral flow, makes intuitive sense for choosing the retrograde approach. Furthermore, by showing a highly tortuous, calcified and/or long CTO, the "knuckle-wire" technique can be recommended for easier tracking of the curved path of occluded vessel segments. Finally, CT-derived scores may be used to assess CTO difficulty level, both to allocate resources and improve training programs (e.g. by assigning less experienced operators to simple CTO lesions) (Fig. 31.8).

Coronary Anomalies

Although coronary anomalies are uncommon, they constitute a major diagnostic puzzle for most of the cardiologists interpreting ICA results and may thus mislead clinicians into employing inappropriate therapeutic decisions. This issue is further complicated because anomalous arteries significantly increase the difficulty level of coronary revascularization (not to mention high contrast and radiation loads) – a phenomenon that keeps awake most of the interventional cardiologists and cardiac surgeons. Fortunately, CTA comes as a "release" for accurate characterization of the origin, course, and termination of coronary anomalies in a one-stop-shop examination [55]. In a prospective study by Pregowski et al., ostial anomalies comprised 24% of all nondiagnostic catheterizations, all of which were readily seen on coronary CTA [56]. Specifically, CTA can be used to locate coronary ostia (e.g., anomalous origin from the opposite aortic sinus, high origin of the coronary artery) and overcome hurdles related to failed catheter placement [55]. Also, CTA can depict the exact position of the coronary artery in relation to the aorta and pulmonary artery for accurate differentiation between the potentially malignant and benign courses of the anomalous artery originating from the opposite aortic sinus [55]. To some extent, multiplanar and three-dimensional volume-rendered CT reconstructions can identify the high-risk features of the interarterial course (e.g., slitlike ostium, acute angle of takeoff, or stretch of the intramural segment within the aortic wall) and thus help guide revascularization strategies [57]. To date, only single case reports have reported the modification of interventional treatment strategies in coronary anomalies based on CTA datasets [58, 59].

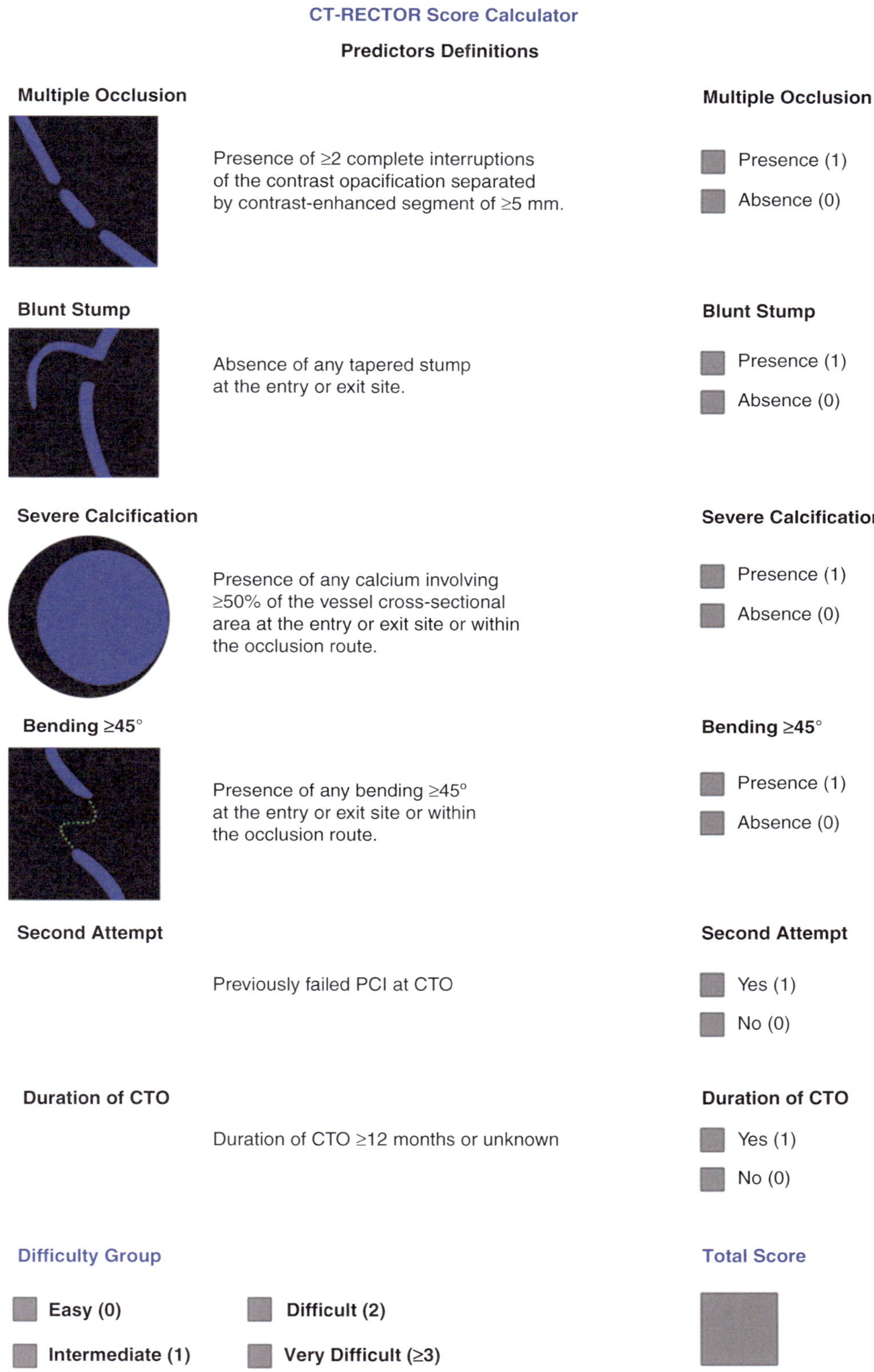

Fig. 31.7 Calculation sheet for the CT-RECTOR score with illustrated definitions of each variable and listing of the difficulty groups. (From Opolski et al. [42], with permission)

Coronary CTA for Periprocedural Guidance of PCI

Coronary CTA can be directly used in the catheterization laboratory for periprocedural guidance of PCI. To date, one approach has been to project three-dimensional CTA data onto separate monitors in the catheterization laboratory. This application allows operators to simultaneously display CTA

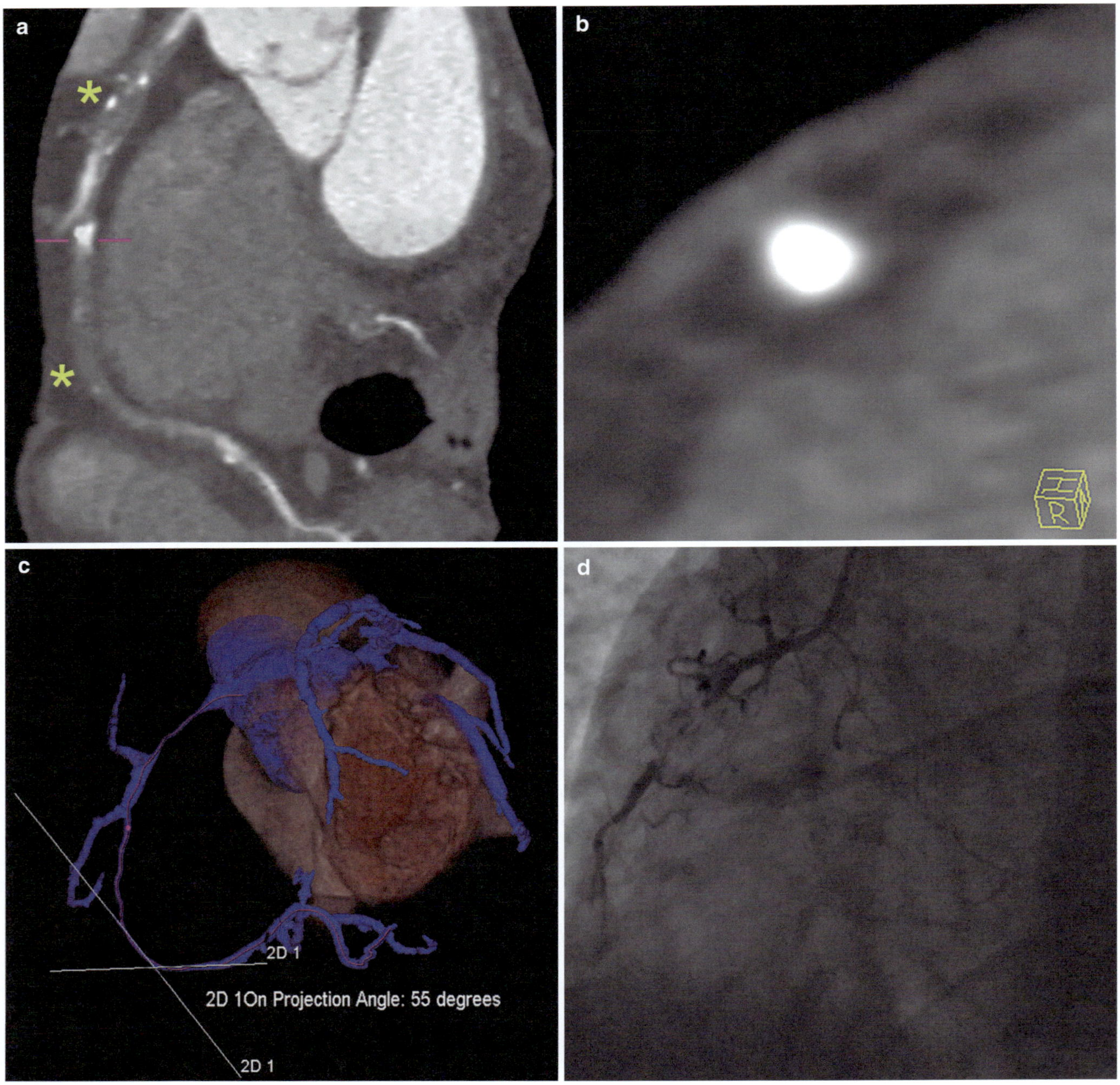

Fig. 31.8 Very difficult lesion from the guidewire-failure group. (**a**) Curved multiplanar reconstruction displaying two occlusion sites (yellow asterisks) and severe calcification in the mid-segment of the right coronary artery. (**b**) Cross-sectional view of the calcification occupying ≥50% vessel area. (**c**) Three-dimensional reconstruction displaying bending of 55° within the occlusion route. (**d**) Coronary angiography after failed attempt of guidewire crossing within 55 min. (From Opolski et al. [42], with permission)

projections and fluoroscopic angulations for identification of the most optimal working angles without foreshortening and can be particularly used during guidewire advancement in CTO with suboptimal visualization in ICA [22]. Indeed, this has been affirmed in a study by Rolf et al. who showed significantly higher success rates for CTO PCI with periprocedural CTA monitors compared with PCI without CTA overlay [41]. Alternatively, the concept of wearable head-mounted devices superimposing augmented reality data onto the user's field of view has garnered particular attention in the context of periprocedural planning for PCI. The advantage of wearable computers relies on limitless display and intuitive manipulation of multiple imaging data using simple hand gestures, voice commands, or motion tracking [60]. Indeed, recently Google Glass worn by cardiologists in the catheterization laboratory has been used for successful CTO PCI by

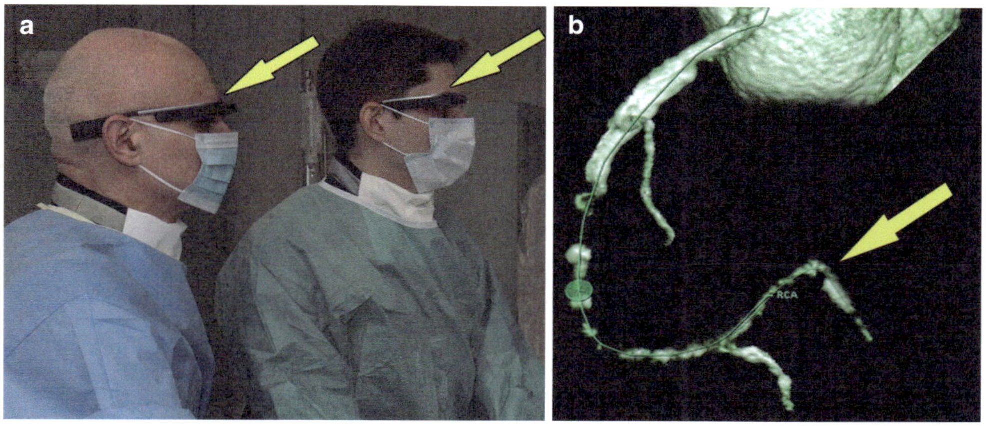

Fig. 31.9 Computed tomography data displayed in a wearable computer during recanalization attempt of a chronic total occlusion. (**a**) Interventional cardiologists viewing computed tomographic images in the upper right visual field on Google Glass (Google Inc., Mountain View, CA) (arrows). (**b**) Three-dimensional computed tomographic reconstruction projected directly onto the Google Glass showing the exact trajectory of the right coronary artery (arrow). (From Opolski et al. [61], with permission)

providing access to a three-dimensional CTA "roadmap" of the occluded vessel (Fig. 31.9) [61].

Alternatively, a more computationally intense approach of real-time fusion of three-dimensional coronary CTA with X-ray fluoroscopy has been introduced (Fig. 31.10). In a small series of 43 CTO patients who underwent attempted PCI based on CTA data in combination with magnetic navigation, only a moderate success rate of 44% was achieved [62]. This may reflect the essential shortcomings of the fusion techniques (such as patient, cardiac, and respiratory motion artifacts) resulting in a relatively wide margin of registration errors that consequently compromise the submillimetric precision required for CTO PCI (e.g., differentiating intraluminal versus subintimal guidewire location). Nevertheless, recently Ghoshhajra et al. raised hope for a wider adoption of coupling CTA and angiographic data for CTO PCI by showing that CTA-derived extent and localization of coronary calcification along with vessel tortuosity may influence the strategy of antegrade dissection reentry technique [63]. This however did not translate into higher success rates compared with PCI without CTA overlay.

Most likely, the best "remedy" for real-time integration of CTA datasets with fluoroscopic environment is to bring CT scanner directly to the catheterization laboratory. Although it might appear to be a herculean task, Kim et al. installed an advanced CTA system in the catheterization room (allowing for interchangeable CT scanning and invasive fluoroscopy) to investigate its role for the identification of guidewire location during CTO PCI in a series of 61 patients [64]. By onsite review of the CT images in a 360-degree view, the exact position of the guidewire tip was classified as intraluminal, subintimal, or outside the vessel wall. Interestingly, this study demonstrated that successful prediction of the guidewire location by intraprocedural CTA is not only feasible but also associated with a numerically higher recanalization rates compared with cases in which the position of the guidewire was indeterminate (83% vs 63%). However, not every CTA result provided adequate information about guidewire location (not to mention potentially higher labor input, time, and radiation dose of intraprocedural CTA scanning).

Future Perspectives

Most likely, future advancements for guiding revascularization procedures by coronary CTA would evolve into further validation and wider adoption of FFR-CT, steady improvements in CT technology for better characterization of coronary plaque, and ongoing technical developments for mobile display of CTA datasets in the catheterization laboratory. Specifically, coupling the anatomical and physiological information by coronary CTA may be the best approach for accurate stent selection. Also, the accuracy of CTA is a "moving target" and could be further enhanced by wider adoption of automated plaque assessment tools, machine learning algorithms, and computational fluid dynamics to provide time-saving multidimensional information on individual plaques prior to PCI. Finally, the value of wearable computers for projection of CTA data to the catheterization laboratory has yet to receive widespread attention.

Conclusions

The ability of coronary CTA to show and characterize atherosclerotic plaque can assist interventional cardiologists with planning percutaneous coronary intervention strategies. This is particularly salient in cases where noninvasive

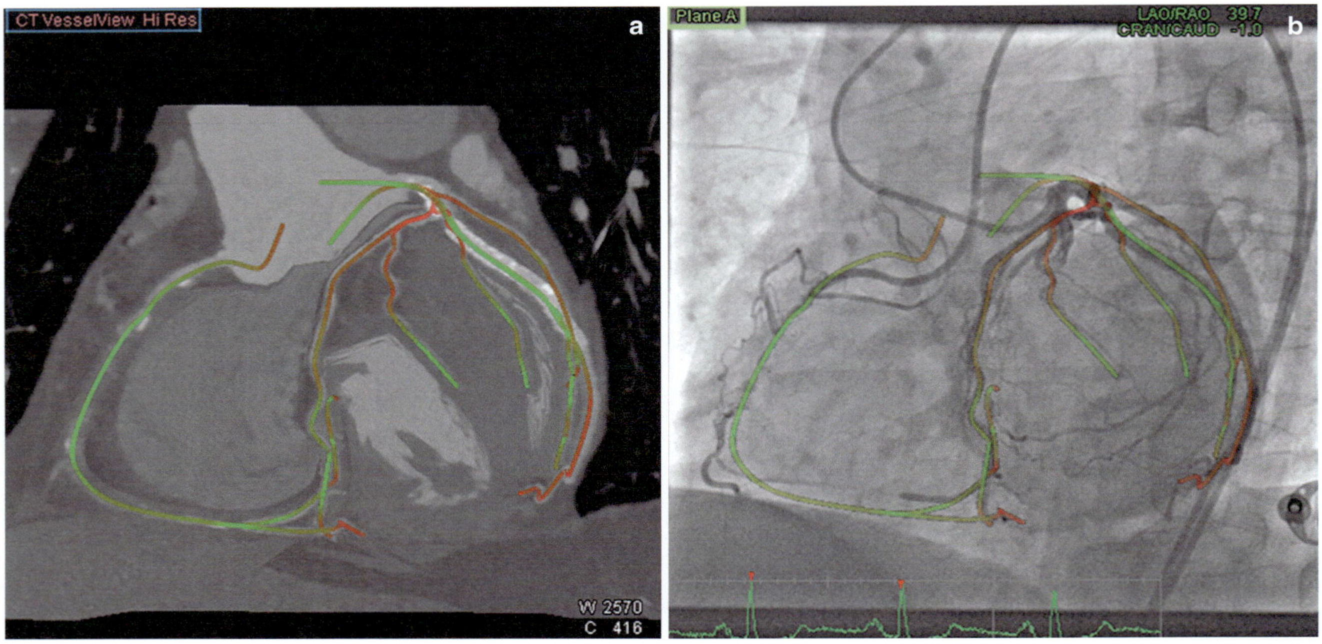

Fig. 31.10 Image fusion of coronary computed tomography angiography and fluoroscopic images. (**a**) Three-dimensional anatomy of the coronary arteries derived from computed tomography angiography facilitates identification of projections without foreshortening for each respective vessel segment. (**b**) Computed tomography angiography and fluoroscopic data are combined to show coronary segments in green (no foreshortening) or red (substantial foreshortening). Prototype, Siemens Healthcare, Erlangen, Germany. (From Opolski and Achenbach [22], with permission)

CTA exceeds the characterization of coronary lesions compared to invasive angiogram (e.g., coronary chronic total occlusions, bifurcation lesions, or coronary anomalies) [22]. Moreover, the importance of noninvasive CTA detection of "adverse plaque characteristics" (mainly low-attenuation plaque) that confer a higher risk for periprocedural complications cannot be overemphasized in the context of tailored catheter interventions [25–29]. Of particular interest, the ability of FFR-CT to pinpoint lesion-specific ischemia goes far beyond enhancing diagnostic performance of coronary CTA and may aid in ischemia-guided "virtual stenting" procedures – a phenomenon not evaluable by any other single imaging technique [17]. In this context, if coronary CTA is available prior to percutaneous intervention, it would be desirable that the operator takes good note of all the information provided starting from lesion-specific ischemia and ending up with optimal viewing angles, true lesion length (most often underestimated in ICA), reference vessel diameters, and morphological plaque characteristics. Noteworthy, this task may be substantially simplified by projection of CTA datasets directly to the catheterization laboratory. Although more data are clearly needed to uncover the full potential of CTA for planning PCI, coronary CTA is already gaining recognition as the only imaging tool for crossing the borders between noninvasive and invasive management of coronary artery disease.

References

1. Windecker S, Kolh P, Alfonso F, et al. 2014 ESC/EACTS Guidelines on myocardial revascularization. Eur Heart J. 2014;35:2541–619.
2. Achenbach S. Coronary CTA and percutaneous coronary intervention - a symbiosis waiting to happen. J Cardiovasc Comput Tomogr. 2016;10:384–5.
3. Min JK, Chandrashekhar Y, Narula J. Diagnosis of coronary disease and icing on the cake. JACC Cardiovasc Imaging. 2015;8:1117–20.
4. Wink O, Hecht HS, Ruijters D. Coronary computed tomographic angiography in the cardiac catheterization laboratory: current applications and future developments. Cardiol Clin. 2009;27:513–29.
5. Sonoda S, Morino Y, Ako J, et al. Impact of final stent dimensions on long-term results following sirolimus-eluting stent implantation: serial intravascular ultrasound analysis from the sirius trial. J Am Coll Cardiol. 2004;43:1959–63.
6. Sakurai R, Ako J, Morino Y, et al. Predictors of edge stenosis following sirolimus-eluting stent deployment (a quantitative intravascular ultrasound analysis from the SIRIUS trial). Am J Cardiol. 2005;96:1251–3.
7. van Velzen JE, de Graaf MA, Ciarka A, et al. Non-invasive assessment of atherosclerotic coronary lesion length using multidetector computed tomography angiography: comparison to quantitative coronary angiography. Int J Cardiovasc Imaging. 2012;28:2065–71.
8. Leber AW, Knez A, von Ziegler F, et al. Quantification of obstructive and nonobstructive coronary lesions by 64-slice computed tomography: a comparative study with quantitative coronary angiography and intravascular ultrasound. J Am Coll Cardiol. 2005;46:147–54.
9. LaBounty T, Sundaram B, Chetcuti S, et al. Stent size selection using 64-detector coronary computed tomography angiography: a comparison to invasive coronary angiography. Acad Radiol. 2008;15:820–6.

10. Kass M, Glover CA, Labinaz M, So DY, Chen L, Yam YCB. Lesion characteristics and coronary stent selection with computed tomographic coronary angiography: a pilot investigation comparing CTA, QCA and IVUS. J Invasive Cardiol. 2010;22:328–34.
11. Pregowski J, Kepka C, Kalinczuk L, et al. Comparison of intravascular ultrasound, quantitative coronary angiography, and dual-source 64-slice computed tomography in the preprocedural assessment of significant saphenous vein graft lesions. Am J Cardiol. 2016;107:1453–9.
12. Ciszewski M, Zalewska J, Pregowski J, et al. Comparison of stent length reported by the stent's manufacturer to that determined by quantitative coronary angiography at the time of implantation versus that determined by coronary computed tomographic angiography at a later time. Am J Cardiol. 2013;111:1111–6.
13. Pregowski J, Kepka C, Kruk M, et al. Comparison of usefulness of percutaneous coronary intervention guided by angiography plus computed tomography versus angiography alone using intravascular ultrasound end points. Am J Cardiol. 2011;108:1728–34.
14. Wolny R, Pregowski J, Kruk M, et al. Computed tomography angiography versus angiography for guiding percutaneous coronary interventions in bifurcation lesions – A prospective randomized pilot study. J Cardiovasc Comput Tomogr. 2017;11:119–28.
15. Tonino PAL, De Bruyne B, Pijls NHJ, et al. Fractional flow reserve versus angiography for guiding percutaneous coronary intervention. N Engl J Med. 2009;360:213–24.
16. Curzen NP, Nolan J, Zaman AG, et al. Does the routine availability of CT–derived FFR influence management of patients with stable chest pain compared to CT angiography alone?: the FFRCT RIPCORD study. JACC Cardiovasc Imaging. 2016;9:1188–94.
17. Kim K-H, Doh J-H, Koo B-K, et al. A novel noninvasive technology for treatment planning using virtual coronary stenting and computed tomography-derived computed fractional flow reserve. JACC Cardiovasc Interv. 2014;7:72–8.
18. Nakazato R, Shalev A, Doh J-H, et al. Aggregate plaque volume by coronary computed tomography angiography is superior and incremental to luminal narrowing for diagnosis of ischemic lesions of intermediate stenosis severity. J Am Coll Cardiol. 2013;62:460–7.
19. Park H-B, Heo R, ó Hartaigh B, et al. Atherosclerotic plaque characteristics by CT angiography identify coronary lesions that cause ischemia: a direct comparison to fractional flow reserve. JACC Cardiovasc Imaging. 2015;8:1–10.
20. Gaur S, Øvrehus KA, Dey D, et al. Coronary plaque quantification and fractional flow reserve by coronary computed tomography angiography identify ischaemia-causing lesions. Eur Heart J. 2016;37:1220–7.
21. Tesche C, De Cecco CN, Caruso D, et al. Coronary CT angiography derived morphological and functional quantitative plaque markers correlated with invasive fractional flow reserve for detecting hemodynamically significant stenosis. J Cardiovasc Comput Tomogr. 2016;10:199–206.
22. Opolski MP, Achenbach S. CT angiography for revascularization of CTO: crossing the borders of diagnosis and treatment. JACC Cardiovasc Imaging. 2015;8:846–58.
23. Kinohira Y, Akutsu Y, Li H-L, et al. Coronary arterial plaque characterized by multislice computed tomography predicts complications following coronary intervention. Int Heart J. 2007;48:25–33.
24. Pregowski J, Jastrzebski J, Kępka C, et al. Relation between coronary plaque calcium deposits as described by computed tomography coronary angiography and acute results of stent deployment as assessed by intravascular ultrasound. Postepy Kardiol Interwencyjnej. 2013;9:115–20.
25. Nakazawa G, Tanabe K, Onuma Y, et al. Efficacy of culprit plaque assessment by 64-slice multidetector computed tomography to predict transient no-reflow phenomenon during percutaneous coronary intervention. Am Heart J. 2008;155:1150–7.
26. Uetani T, Amano T, Kunimura A, et al. The association between plaque characterization by CT angiography and post-procedural myocardial infarction in patients with elective stent implantation. JACC Cardiovasc Imaging. 2010;3:19–28.
27. Harigaya H, Motoyama S, Sarai M, et al. Prediction of the no-reflow phenomenon during percutaneous coronary intervention using coronary computed tomography angiography. Heart Vessel. 2011;26:363–9.
28. Kodama T, Kondo T, Oida A, et al. Computed tomographic angiography–verified plaque characteristics and slow-flow phenomenon during percutaneous coronary intervention. JACC Cardiovasc Interv. 2012;5:636–43.
29. Miura K, Kato M, Dote K, et al. Association of nonculprit plaque characteristics with transient slow flow phenomenon during percutaneous coronary intervention. Int J Cardiol. 2015;181:108–13.
30. Tesche C, De Cecco CN, Vliegenthart R, et al. Coronary CT angiography-derived quantitative markers for predicting in-stent restenosis. J Cardiovasc Comput Tomogr. 2016;10:377–83.
31. Opolski MP, Kepka C, Ruzyłło W. Computed tomography for detection of vulnerable coronary plaque - a Cassandra's dream? Postepy Kardiol Interwencyjnej. 2014;10:147–52.
32. Maurovich-Horvat P, Ferencik M, Voros S, et al. Comprehensive plaque assessment by coronary CT angiography. Nat Rev Cardiol. 2014;11:390–402.
33. Motoyama S, Sarai M, Harigaya H, et al. Computed tomographic angiography characteristics of atherosclerotic plaques subsequently resulting in acute coronary syndrome. J Am Coll Cardiol. 2009;54:49–57.
34. Kristensen TS, Kofoed KF, Kühl JT, et al. Prognostic implications of nonobstructive coronary plaques in patients with non–ST-segment elevation myocardial infarction: a multidetector computed tomography study. J Am Coll Cardiol. 2011;58:502–9.
35. Otsuka K, Fukuda S, Tanaka A, et al. Napkin-ring sign on coronary CT angiography for the prediction of acute coronary syndrome. JACC Cardiovasc Imaging. 2013;6:448–57.
36. Thomsen C, Abdulla J. Characteristics of high-risk coronary plaques identified by computed tomographic angiography and associated prognosis: a systematic review and meta-analysis. Eur Heart J Cardiovasc Imaging. 2016;17:120–9.
37. Opolski MP, ó Hartaigh B, Berman DS, et al. Current trends in patients with chronic total occlusions undergoing coronary CT angiography. Heart. 2015;101:1212–8.
38. García-García HM, Van Mieghem H, Gonzalo N, et al. Computed tomography in total coronary occlusions (CTTO registry): radiation exposure and predictors of successful percutaneous intervention. EuroIntervention. 2009;4:607–16.
39. Opolski MP, Kepka C, Achenbach S, et al. Coronary computed tomographic angiography for prediction of procedural and intermediate outcome of bypass grafting to left anterior descending artery occlusion with failed visualization on conventional angiography. Am J Cardiol. 2012;109:1722–8.
40. Soon KH, Cox N, Wong A, et al. CT coronary angiography predicts the outcome of percutaneous coronary intervention of chronic total occlusion. J Interv Cardiol. 2007;20:359–66.
41. Rolf A, Werner GS, Schuhbäck A, et al. Preprocedural coronary CT angiography significantly improves success rates of PCI for chronic total occlusion. Int J Cardiovasc Imaging. 2013;29:1819–27.
42. Opolski MP, Achenbach S, Schuhbäck A, et al. Coronary computed tomographic prediction rule for time-efficient guidewire crossing through chronic total occlusion: insights from the CT-RECTOR multicenter registry (computed tomography registry of chronic total occlusion revascularization). JACC Cardiovasc Interv. 2015;8:257–67.
43. Mollet NR, Hoye A, Lemos PA, et al. Value of preprocedure multislice computed tomographic coronary angiography to predict the outcome of percutaneous recanalization of chronic total occlusions. Am J Cardiol. 2005;95:240–3.

44. Ehara M, Terashima M, Kawai M, et al. Impact of multislice computed tomography to estimate difficulty in wire crossing in percutaneous coronary intervention for chronic total occlusion. J Invasive Cardiol. 2009;21:575–82.
45. Cho JR, Kim YJ, Ahn C-M, et al. Quantification of regional calcium burden in chronic total occlusion by 64-slice multi-detector computed tomography and procedural outcomes of percutaneous coronary intervention. Int J Cardiol. 2010;145:9–14.
46. Li P, Gai L, Yang X, et al. Computed tomography angiography-guided percutaneous coronary intervention in chronic total occlusion. J Zhejiang Univ Sci B. 2010;11:568–74.
47. Te HJ, Kyo E, Chu CM, et al. Impact of calcification length ratio on the intervention for chronic total occlusions. Int J Cardiol. 2011;150:135–41.
48. Choi J-H, Bin SY, Hahn J-Y, et al. Three-dimensional quantitative volumetry of chronic total occlusion plaque using coronary multidetector computed tomography. Circ J. 2011;75:366–75.
49. Martín-Yuste V, Barros A, Leta R, et al. Determinantes del éxito de la revascularización de las oclusiones coronarias crónicas: estudio mediante tomografía computarizada con multidetectores. Rev Española Cardiol. 2012;65:334–40.
50. Li M, Zhang J, Pan J, Lu Z. Coronary total occlusion lesions: linear intrathrombus enhancement at CT predicts better outcome of percutaneous coronary intervention. Radiology. 2013;266:443–51.
51. Luo C, Huang M, Li J, et al. Predictors of interventional success of antegrade PCI for CTO. JACC Cardiovasc Imaging. 2015;8:804–13.
52. Chen Y, Lu B, Hou Z, et al. Predicting successful percutaneous coronary intervention in patients with chronic total occlusion: the incremental value of a novel morphological parameter assessed by computed tomography. Int J Cardiovasc Imaging. 2015;31:1263–9.
53. Ito T, Tsuchikane E, Nasu K, et al. Impact of lesion morphology on angiographic and clinical outcomes in patients with chronic total occlusion after recanalization with drug-eluting stents: a multislice computed tomography study. Eur Radiol. 2015;25:3084–92.
54. Li Y, Xu N, Zhang J, et al. Procedural success of CTO recanalization: comparison of the J-CTO score determined by coronary CT angiography to invasive angiography. J Cardiovasc Comput Tomogr. 2015;9:578–84.
55. Earls JP. Coronary artery anomalies. Tech Vasc Interv Radiol. 2006;9:210–7.
56. Pregowski J, Kepka C, Kruk M, et al. The clinical significance and management of patients with incomplete coronary angiography and the value of additional computed tomography coronary angiography. Int J Cardiovasc Imaging. 2014;30:825–32.
57. Opolski MP, Pregowski J, Kruk M, et al. Prevalence and characteristics of coronary anomalies originating from the opposite sinus of valsalva in 8,522 patients referred for coronary computed tomography angiography. Am J Cardiol. 2013;111:1361–7.
58. Jo Y, Uranaka Y, Iwaki H, et al. Sudden cardiac arrest associated with anomalous origin of the right coronary artery from the left main coronary artery. Tex Hear Inst J. 2011;38:539–43.
59. Kiefer TL, Vavalle J, Halim S, et al. Anterograde percutaneous coronary–cameral fistula closure employing a guide-in-guide technique. JACC Cardiovasc Interv. 2013;6:1105–7.
60. Dugas CM, Schussler JM. Advanced technology in interventional cardiology: a roadmap for the future of precision coronary interventions. Trends Cardiovasc Med. 2016;26:466–73.
61. Opolski MP, Debski A, Borucki BA, et al. First-in-man computed tomography-guided percutaneous revascularization of coronary chronic total occlusion using a wearable computer: proof of concept. Can J Cardiol. 2016;32:829.e11–3.
62. Ramcharitar S, van der Giessen W, van der Ent M, et al. The feasibility and safety of applying the magnetic navigation system to manage chronically occluded vessels: a single Centre experience. EuroIntervention. 2011;6:711–6.
63. Ghoshhajra BB, Takx RAP, Stone LL, et al. Real-time fusion of coronary CT angiography with x-ray fluoroscopy during chronic total occlusion PCI. Eur Radiol. 2017;27:2464–73.
64. Kim B-K, Cho I, Hong M-K, et al. Usefulness of intraprocedural coronary computed tomographic angiography during intervention for chronic total coronary occlusion. Am J Cardiol. 2016;117:1868–76.

Stent Assessment

32

Junjie Yang, Christian Tesche, Taylor M. Duguay, Lucas L. Geyer, and Yundai Chen

Percutaneous coronary intervention (PCI) with stent placement is a standard therapy for myocardial revascularization of hemodynamically significant coronary artery disease (CAD). Although PCI procedures are being performed at increasing rates, in-stent restenosis (ISR) after stent placement remains a frequent complication [1, 2]. Three generations of stents have been introduced, which include bare-metal stents, durable polymer drug-eluting stents, and biodegradable-polymer drug-eluting stents. An appropriate noninvasive imaging technique to serve as a post-procedural follow-up strategy and for the evaluation of stent patency has been desired for some time. Coronary CT angiography (CCTA) has been studied extensively for this purpose and has been incorporated into current accepted guidelines for the evaluation of larger coronary stents (≥3 mm) [3]. Recent technical refinements have improved the accuracy of CCTA stent evaluation, showing negative predictive values >90% for exclusion of in-stent restenosis (ISR) [4–6]. However, blooming and beam-hardening artifacts caused by stent struts and stents with diameters <3 mm are existing challenges that limit the diagnostic accuracy of CCTA in the evaluation on stent patency [7, 8]. Improvements in image acquisition and post-processing, including several new approaches to enhance the evaluation of stent patency, ISR, and stent structure, have been developed. Iterative reconstruction techniques, use of high convolution kernels, and dual-energy CT (DECT) acquisitions have shown promising results [9–12].

In-Stent Restenosis and Stent Fracture

The introduction of bare-metal stents in the mid-1980s was a milestone in the evolution of PCI. However, the appearance of ISR with related increased morbidity and mortality was a drawback of this technique. Incidences of ISR up to 20–30% after bare-metal stenting leading to repeated target vessel revascularization have been reported [13]. Newer-generation drug-eluting stents have decreased the incidence of ISR significantly as compared to bare-metal stents; however ISR rates between 5% and 30% are still observed [14, 15]. Several procedural factors, lesion-related characteristics, and patient attributes are related to the development of ISR [16, 17]. Angiographic factors such as vessel size, lesion length, location, and plaque burden as well as clinical factors such as smoking status, diabetes mellitus, and inflammatory status attribute to ISR. Furthermore, stent characteristics like strut thickness and mechanical problems associated with stent deployment contribute to ISR. Stent fracture is a well-established cause of ISR typically observed after drug-eluting stent implantation due to the reduced stent strut thickness and fewer stent cell connections. These characteristics have led to weaker longitudinal strength in the new-generation DES [18]. A representative example of in-stent restenosis is illustrated in Fig. 32.1.

J. Yang · Y. Chen
Division of Cardiovascular Imaging, Department of Radiology and Radiological Science, Medical University of South Carolina, Charleston, SC, USA

Department of Cardiology, People's Liberation Army General Hospital, Beijing, China

C. Tesche (✉)
Division of Cardiovascular Imaging, Department of Radiology and Radiological Science, Medical University of South Carolina, Charleston, SC, USA

Department of Cardiology and Intensive Care Medicine, Heart Center Munich-Bogenhausen, Munich, Germany

T. M. Duguay
Division of Cardiovascular Imaging, Department of Radiology and Radiological Science, Medical University of South Carolina, Charleston, SC, USA

L. L. Geyer
Division of Cardiovascular Imaging, Department of Radiology and Radiological Science, Medical University of South Carolina, Charleston, SC, USA

Institute for Clinical Radiology, Ludwig-Maximilians-University Hospital Munich, Munich, Germany

U. J. Schoepf (ed.), *CT of the Heart*, Contemporary Medical Imaging, https://doi.org/10.1007/978-1-60327-237-7_32

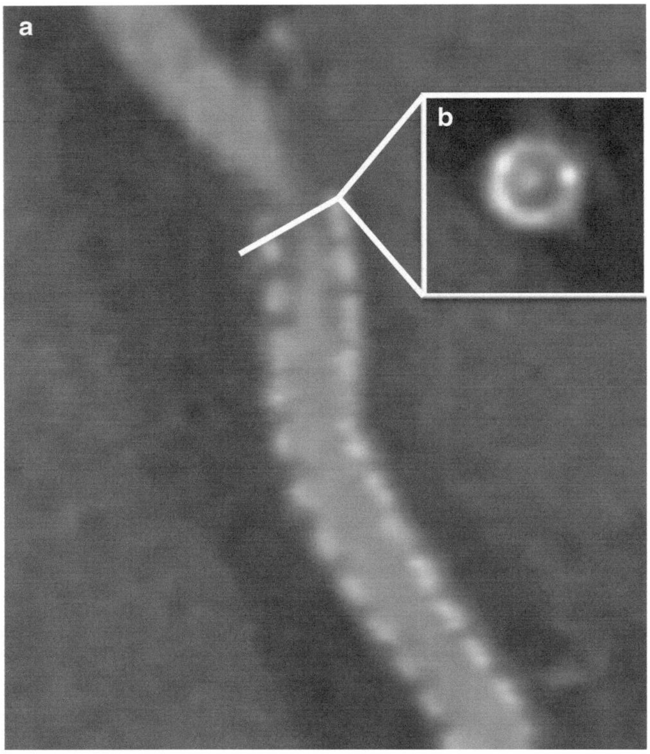

Fig. 32.1 A 55-year-old man presenting with chest pain. (**a**) CCTA using curved multi-planar reconstruction with sinogram-affirmed iterative reconstruction demonstrates presence of in-stent restenosis in the 3.5 mm diameter drug-eluting stent of the right coronary artery (arrow). (**b**) Boxed area clarifies the cross-section view

CT Assessment of Coronary Stents

Contrast Enhancement

Sufficient intravascular contrast enhancement is a prerequisite for adequate delineation of lumen and stent visibility. High contrast is crucial as factors like image noise (due to sharp convolution kernels in the presence of stents) reduce the contrast-to-noise ratio. Furthermore, appropriate window setting requires optimal intravascular attenuation to allow correct identification of vessel lumen, intimal hyperplasia within the stent, and stent struts. To achieve high-contrast concentration in the coronary vessel, appropriate contrast agents and injection protocols with bolus tracking or test bolus application are essential.

Motion Artifacts

Coronary artery and respiratory motions and irregular or high heart rates deteriorate CCTA image quality. As stent assessment is challenging, per se, the importance of following acquisition practice according to current guidelines for the best possible image quality is imperative. The implementation of ECG-synchronized acquisition protocols and the use of CT scanners with high temporal resolution, e.g., dual-source CT (DSCT) systems providing up to 75 ms, are the foundation of current cardiac CT imaging. In addition to these features, optimal patient preparation is required, including the appropriate use of beta-blockers for heart rate control and nitroglycerin for optimal coronary artery visualization and reduction of motion artifacts. However, residual coronary motion remains a major problem as it causes blurring and, as stents are high-contrast objects, it intensifies the adverse effect of blooming on the images.

Blooming Artifacts

Beam-hardening and partial-volume artifacts are the main causes of the artificial thickening of stent struts with CCTA. This phenomenon is more commonly known as a "blooming artifact." This blooming effect results in significant luminal narrowing and an underestimation of the stent lumen. The impact and degree of blooming artifacts are influenced by image acquisition and reconstruction parameters as well as stent type and diameter. Blooming artifacts increase with strut thickness and the corresponding density of the strut material. Furthermore, overlapping stents and additional calcifications in the stent segment aggravate beam-hardening effects resulting in further impairment of CT stent assessment. With current state-of-the-art CT systems, visualization of stent lumen diameter ranges between 50% and 80% [19, 20]. Newly biodegradable-polymer drug-eluting stents may overcome the limitation of blooming artifacts caused by stent struts and may allow for sufficient stent assessment. A representative example of a biodegradable-polymer drug-eluting stent is shown in Fig. 32.2.

Tube Potential

The appropriate use of a high kV acquisition is another approach to reduce blooming artifacts and thus improve stent visualization [21]. However, the increase in kV level results in a significantly higher radiation exposure to the patient and is therefore not recommended. In an in vitro study, Sirineni et al. investigated the impact of different kV settings on the visualization of stent luminal diameter and showed no significant improvement in stent lumen visibility when increasing from 120 to 140 kV [22].

Reconstruction Kernels

The applied convolution kernel for image reconstruction has the greatest impact of stent lumen visualization and the appropriate ability for stent patency evaluation. For the visualization

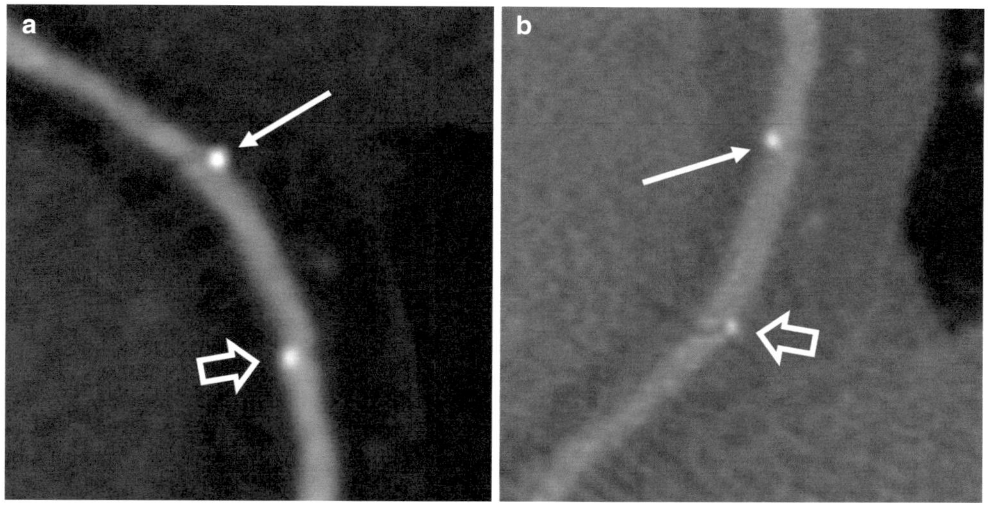

Fig. 32.2 A 43-year-old male patient with a biodegradable-polymer drug-eluting stent in the right coronary artery 15 months after stent implantation. Curved planar reconstruction for both B26 kernel (**a**) and B46 kernel (**b**) illuminated the presence of remaining biodegradable stent markers. The long arrow indicates the proximal end of the biodegradable-polymer drug-eluting stent, and short arrow points to the distal end

and assessment of coronary artery plaques, a medium smooth convolution kernel is recommended while an edge-enhancing kernel is necessary for the delineation of the stent lumen. These vendor-specific dedicated sharp convolution kernels (high-spatial-frequency reconstruction algorithms) for stent evaluation lead to an enhancement of edges in high-attenuation structures like stents. This results in a significant reduction in blooming artifact severity; however adversely increased image noise is observed hindering the evaluation of coronary plaques in non-stented coronary segments [23]. Recently, a combined approach using both kernels for image reconstruction that were post-processed with a corresponding filter algorithm investigated lumen visibility, intraluminal attenuation, and image noise. However, the use of edge-enhanced post-processing filter failed to compensate the pronounced blooming artifacts caused by stent struts and was proven inferior to the dedicated edge-enhancing kernel [24].

Spatial Resolution

Technical improvements in CT technology leading to ongoing improved spatial resolution are the main key for sufficient stent assessment. Third-generation dual-source CT (DSCT) provides isotropic submillimeter resolution to visualize the coronary arteries. These improvements of spatial resolution also result in an optimized in-stent assessment with changes of in-stent lumen visibility from 30% to 60% with the use of 16-slice and 64-slice CT systems, respectively, and up to 80% with third-generation DSCT systems [19].

Iterative Reconstruction

Although blooming artifacts are mainly caused by beam-hardening and partial-volume effects, the reduction of image noise allows for significantly improved stent visualization and is vital due to the fact that increased image noise is the main drawback of technical solutions such as high-resolution kernels or submillimeter data acquisition. In recent years, iterative reconstruction algorithms have been introduced and have successively replaced filtered back projection as the standard method of data reconstruction in routine CT imaging [25]. Concerning image quality, iterative reconstruction techniques focus on reducing artifacts, such as streak artifacts caused by dense objects and image noise. As a result, iterative reconstruction has shown significant improvements in CT stent imaging. Besides a potential dose reduction, the key feature is a more accurate assessment of the stent lumen resulting in a more precise detection of in-stent stenosis [4]. Furthermore, iterative reconstruction facilitates the implementation of integrated circuit detectors offering a minimal section thickness of 0.5 mm without increasing image noise. Therefore, the visualization of small-diameter stents (< 3 mm) can be improved [5].

Monoenergetic Reconstruction with DECT

DECT offers another approach to reduce beam-hardening artifacts which occur if polychromatic X-ray energy spectra are used for image reconstruction. In contrast, image generation from monochromatic (or monoenergetic) X-rays will not lead to such artifacts. Mathematical methods allow the calculation of virtual monoenergetic images at different levels of kiloelectron volt (keV) from DECT data. As a consequence, artifacts caused by metallic objects, e.g., implants, can be significantly reduced [10]. CT stent assessment can also benefit from virtual monoenergetic imaging. Although luminal CT numbers decrease at high keV levels, the overall in-stent visualization and accuracy of diameter measurements increase remarkably due to the reduction of blooming artifacts. Even the lumen visualization of small stents (<3 mm) can be improved by using advanced methods of virtual monoenergetic imaging when compared to standard, polychromatic CT imaging [12].

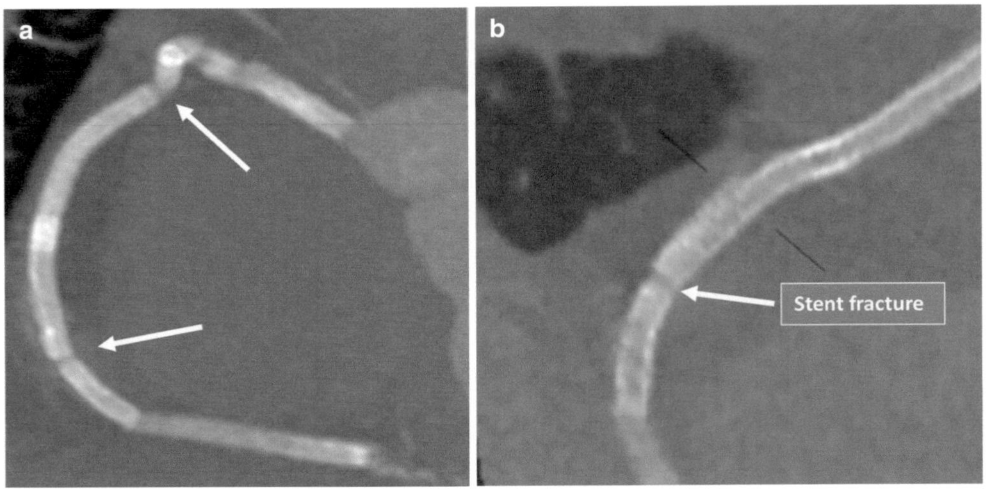

Fig. 32.3 A 46-year-old male patient with new onset of dyspnea and angina 22 months after placement of overlapping stents in the right coronary artery. (**a**) Maximum intensity projection and (**b**) curved planar reconstruction reveal stent fracture (white arrows) with stent malposition. Hypodensity indicates in-stent restenosis mainly observed at the stent gaps

Clinical Evidence

With the introduction of four-slice CT systems by all major vendors in 1998 and gating techniques for multi-slice CT in 2000, CT became more important as a noninvasive imaging technique for stent evaluation (Figs. 32.3 and 32.4). However, the limited spatial and temporal resolution did not allow for appropriate visualization of stent lumen visibility; thus stent patency was assessed indirectly by evaluating the visual assessment of the distal runoff [26]. Stent lumen visibility ranged between 20% and 40% with an unacceptable high number of excluded stents (up to 80–90% due to insufficient lumen visibility) [27]. When 16-slice CT systems enabled direct visualization of the stent lumen with improved temporal resolution and submillimeter spatial resolution, CT became more accepted for the assessment of ISR. Studies using 16-slice CT reported sensitivities and specificities of 54–100% and 88–100%, respectively [28]. However, a major drawback was the high number of unevaluable stents resulting in an exclusion rate up to 14%. With the introduction 64-slice CT systems, noninvasive stent assessment with CT was widely accepted. In a recent meta-analysis, the diagnostic value of 64-slice CT for the detection of ISR was significantly higher than that of 16-slice CT angiography (91 vs 81%) as a result of the increased spatial and temporal resolution [6]. Pooled sensitivity and specificity of 87% and 95% were reported. The diagnostic accuracy of ISR detection is highly dependent on stent diameter. For stents with a diameter of ≤3 mm, sensitivity was 54%, whereas for stent diameter with ≥3 mm, sensitivity increased up to 86%. Thus, based on the results of 64-slice CT systems, current guidelines recommend CCTA for the assessment of stents ≥3 mm.

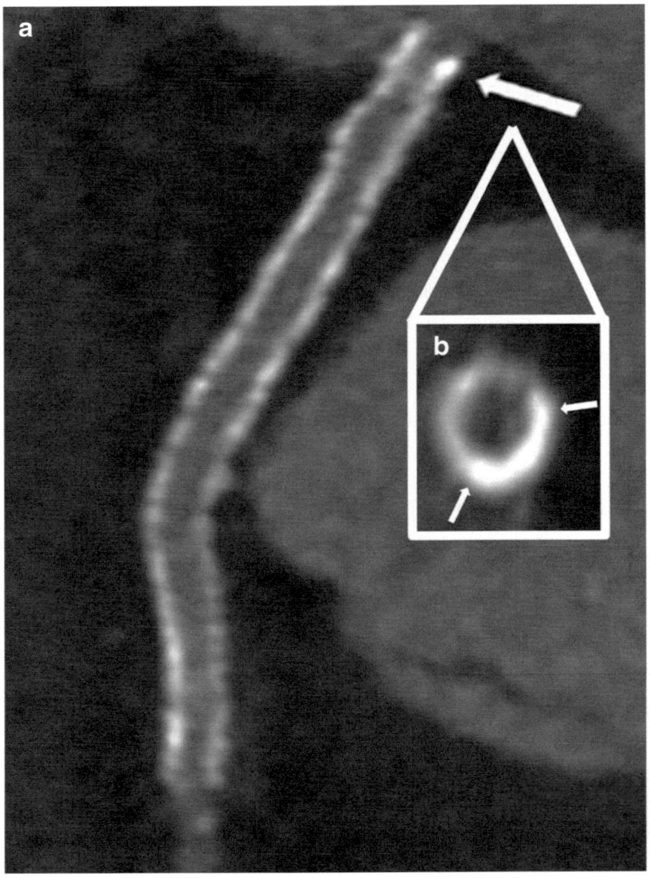

Fig. 32.4 A 65-year-old male with a drug-eluting stent in the left main to proximal left anterior descending artery. (**a**) Curved multi-planar reconstruction shows uneven shortening of the stent strut in in the proximal portion of the stent (arrow) due to longitudinal compression. (**b**) Cross-sectional image demonstrates diffuse in-stent restenosis

References

1. Smith SC Jr, Dove JT, Jacobs AK, et al. ACC/AHA guidelines for percutaneous coronary intervention (revision of the 1993 PTCA guidelines)-executive summary: a report of the American College of Cardiology/American Heart Association task force on practice guidelines (Committee to revise the 1993 guidelines for percutaneous transluminal coronary angioplasty) endorsed by the Society for Cardiac Angiography and Interventions. Circulation. 2001;103:3019–41.
2. Kim LK, Feldman DN, Swaminathan RV, et al. Rate of percutaneous coronary intervention for the management of acute coronary syndromes and stable coronary artery disease in the United States (2007 to 2011). Am J Cardiol. 2014;114:1003–10.
3. Raff GL, Abidov A, Achenbach S, et al. SCCT guidelines for the interpretation and reporting of coronary computed tomographic angiography. J Cardiovasc Comput Tomogr. 2009;3:122–36.
4. Ebersberger U, Tricarico F, Schoepf UJ, et al. CT evaluation of coronary artery stents with iterative image reconstruction: improvements in image quality and potential for radiation dose reduction. Eur Radiol. 2013;23:125–32.
5. Geyer LL, Glenn GR, De Cecco CN, et al. CT evaluation of small-diameter coronary artery stents: effect of an integrated circuit detector with iterative reconstruction. Radiology. 2015;276:706–14.
6. Sun Z, Almutairi AM. Diagnostic accuracy of 64 multislice CT angiography in the assessment of coronary in-stent restenosis: a meta-analysis. Eur J Radiol. 2010;73:266–73.
7. Sheth T, Dodd JD, Hoffmann U, et al. Coronary stent assessability by 64 slice multi-detector computed tomography. Catheter Cardiovasc Interv. 2007;69:933–8.
8. Chung SH, Kim YJ, Hur J, et al. Evaluation of coronary artery in-stent restenosis by 64-section computed tomography: factors affecting assessment and accurate diagnosis. J Thorac Imaging. 2010;25:57–63.
9. Eisentopf J, Achenbach S, Ulzheimer S, et al. Low-dose dual-source CT angiography with iterative reconstruction for coronary artery stent evaluation. JACC Cardiovasc Imaging. 2013;6:458–65.
10. Bamberg F, Dierks A, Nikolaou K, Reiser MF, Becker CR, Johnson TR. Metal artifact reduction by dual energy computed tomography using monoenergetic extrapolation. Eur Radiol. 2011;21:1424–9.
11. Meinel FG, Bischoff B, Zhang Q, Bamberg F, Reiser MF, Johnson TR. Metal artifact reduction by dual-energy computed tomography using energetic extrapolation: a systematically optimized protocol. Investig Radiol. 2012;47:406–14.
12. Mangold S, Cannao PM, Schoepf UJ, et al. Impact of an advanced image-based monoenergetic reconstruction algorithm on coronary stent visualization using third generation dual-source dual-energy CT: a phantom study. Eur Radiol. 2016;26:1871–8.
13. Chen MS, John JM, Chew DP, Lee DS, Ellis SG, Bhatt DL. Bare metal stent restenosis is not a benign clinical entity. Am Heart J. 2006;151:1260–4.
14. Palmerini T, Biondi-Zoccai G, Della Riva D, et al. Clinical outcomes with bioabsorbable polymer- versus durable polymer-based drug-eluting and bare-metal stents: evidence from a comprehensive network meta-analysis. J Am Coll Cardiol. 2014;63:299–307.
15. Cohen DJ, Van Hout B, Serruys PW, et al. Quality of life after PCI with drug-eluting stents or coronary-artery bypass surgery. N Engl J Med. 2011;364:1016–26.
16. Holmes DR Jr, Kereiakes DJ, Garg S, et al. Stent thrombosis. J Am Coll Cardiol. 2010;56:1357–65.
17. Mehran R, Dangas G, Abizaid AS, et al. Angiographic patterns of in-stent restenosis: classification and implications for long-term outcome. Circulation. 1999;100:1872–8.
18. Park KW, Park JJ, Chae IH, et al. Clinical characteristics of coronary drug-eluting stent fracture: insights from a two-center des registry. J Korean Med Sci. 2011;26:53–8.
19. Gassenmaier T, Petri N, Allmendinger T, et al. In vitro comparison of second- and third-generation dual-source CT for coronary stent visualization at different tube potentials. Acad Radiol. 2016;23:961–8.
20. Gebhard C, Fiechter M, Fuchs TA, et al. Coronary artery stents: influence of adaptive statistical iterative reconstruction on image quality using 64-HDCT. Eur Heart J Cardiovasc Imaging. 2013;14:969–77.
21. Suzuki S, Furui S, Kuwahara S, et al. Assessment of coronary stent in vitro on multislice computed tomography angiography: improved in-stent visibility by the use of 140-kV tube voltage. J Comput Assist Tomogr. 2007;31:414–21.
22. Sirineni GK, Kalra MK, Pottala K, Waldrop S, Syed M, Tigges S. Effect of contrast concentration, tube potential and reconstruction kernels on MDCT evaluation of coronary stents: an in vitro study. Int J Cardiovasc Imaging. 2007;23:253–63.
23. Seifarth H, Raupach R, Schaller S, et al. Assessment of coronary artery stents using 16-slice MDCT angiography: evaluation of a dedicated reconstruction kernel and a noise reduction filter. Eur Radiol. 2005;15:721–6.
24. Ulrich A, Burg MC, Raupach R, et al. Coronary stent imaging with dual-source CT: assessment of lumen visibility using different convolution kernels and postprocessing filters. Acta Radiol. 2015;56:42–50.
25. Geyer LL, Schoepf UJ, Meinel FG, et al. State of the art: iterative CT reconstruction techniques. Radiology. 2015;276:339–57.
26. Kruger S, Mahnken AH, Sinha AM, et al. Multislice spiral computed tomography for the detection of coronary stent restenosis and patency. Int J Cardiol. 2003;89:167–72.
27. Maintz D, Grude M, Fallenberg EM, Heindel W, Fischbach R. Assessment of coronary arterial stents by multislice-CT angiography. Acta Radiol. 2003;44:597–603.
28. Sun Z, Davidson R, Lin CH. Multi-detector row CT angiography in the assessment of coronary in-stent restenosis: a systematic review. Eur J Radiol. 2009;69:489–95.

Multidetector CT Angiography for Coronary Bypass Graft Assessment and Reoperative Cardiac Surgery

33

Lloyd M. Felmly

Coronary Bypass Grafting

Coronary artery bypass grafting (CABG) is a surgical method of treating coronary artery disease that involves the harvest of conduits from the patient's own vasculature, followed by myocardial revascularization by the implantation of these autologous grafts into the coronary arteries distal to known obstructions. While the number of CABGs has steadily declined in recent years, it remains the most common cardiac surgery and one of the most common surgeries worldwide, with approximately 800,000 CABGs performed yearly [1]. The decline in CABG volume can be correlated with improved medical management and the proliferation of percutaneous coronary intervention (PCI), but it continues to be a relevant method of treating coronary disease. Radiographic assessment of the coronary arteries is integral to the ability to perform bypass surgery.

Proximally, graft blood flow may originate from the vessel's native takeoff as for in situ right (RIMA) and left internal mammary arteries (LIMA), and less commonly the gastroepiploic artery, or from a proximal aortic anastomosis in the case of saphenous vein, radial artery, or pedicled IMA grafts. The LIMA was originally used as the primary graft early in the history of CABG, especially for bypassing the left anterior descending artery (LAD); however it fell from favor due to the larger lumens of saphenous vein graft and greater technical ease of implanting these grafts. However the LIMA re-emerged as a critical aspect of any CABG operation after a landmark paper from Loop et al. at the Cleveland Clinic demonstrated improved patency and long-term survival when this graft was used to bypass the LAD [2]. CABG can be conducted with the use of cardiopulmonary bypass (CPB) and cardioplegic arrest or on a beating heart with the aid of stabilizing devices. This "off-pump" approach allows the surgeon to avoid the systemic inflammatory response, coagulopathy, and temporary myocardial dysfunction associated with CPB and may decrease the risk of stroke associated with aortic cross-clamping. However it is important to note that distal anastomotic patency may be compromised due to the increased technical difficulty of these anastomoses [3], especially in the hands of a surgeon who does not routinely perform off-pump surgery. Minimally invasive techniques have been employed in an on- or off-pump fashion to avoid sternotomy while bypassing certain coronary territories. More recently, studies on bypass grafting using all-arterial bypass grafts have shown improved patency rates and outcomes [4]. Reoperative CABG is undertaken in a similar fashion to primary CABG but with important differences. Entry to the chest is typically via redo sternotomy, which can be time-consuming and hazardous. In addition, choice of grafts may be limited due to prior graft harvesting. However its conduct, CABG as an operation is highly dependent on imaging to define the course and stenoses of the coronary vasculature and in reoperative surgery, to define the mediastinal anatomy and course of prior bypass grafts.

Historical Comment on CT for the Evaluation of Coronary Bypass Grafts

Computed tomography (CT) has been used to radiographically characterize cardiac disease since the 1970s. The excellent temporal resolution of electron beam computed tomography (EBCT), approximately 100 ms, allowed the accurate detection of coronary artery calcium, a useful tool to assess disease and predict the risk of adverse events such as heart attack or stroke. Coronary calcium scanning is still a useful risk-predictive tool; however the data it provides is limited to assessment of calcific plaque load. CT imaging of the coronaries combined with concurrent administration of iodinated contrast media in the arterial phase, known as coronary computed tomographic angiography (CCTA), allows for a more detailed analysis of vessel lumens as well as non-calcific plaque characteristics. Conventional CT with con-

L. M. Felmly (✉)
Department of Surgery, Division of Cardiothoracic Surgery, Medical University of South Carolina, Charleston, SC, USA
e-mail: felmly@musc.edu

U. J. Schoepf (ed.), *CT of the Heart*, Contemporary Medical Imaging, https://doi.org/10.1007/978-1-60327-237-7_33

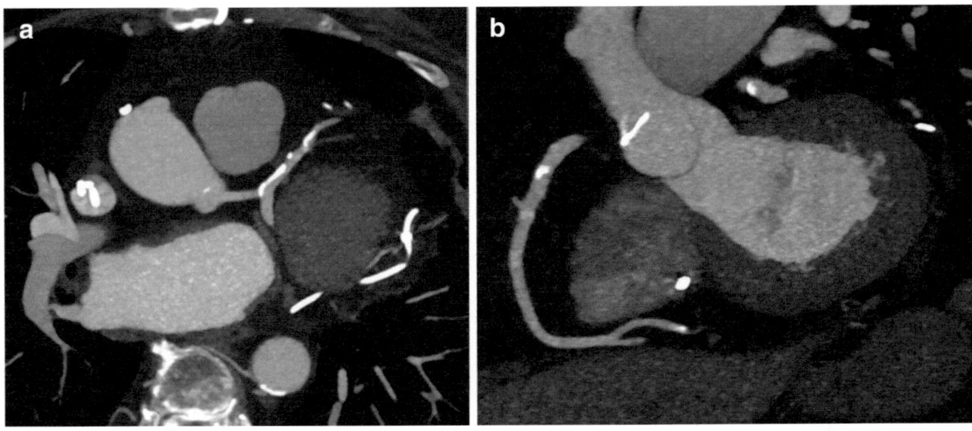

Fig. 33.1 Occluded bypass grafts imaged on a 3rd generation DSCT scanner with high fidelity. The takeoff of the occluded vein graft to the left circumflex artery and distally occluded LIMA graft can be visualized (**a**), as can the proximally occluded vein graft to the right coronary artery (**b**)

trast attenuation was able to image venous grafts; however this was limited to basic binary assessment of patency versus occlusion [5–7]. The introduction of spiral CT, which reduced motion artifact, allowed adequate assessment of venous bypass grafts, but visualizing distal anastomotic sites as well as arterial grafts remained a challenge [8]. While the temporal resolution of EBCT was far superior to that of conventional and spiral CT scanners at the time of its introduction, it failed to achieve widespread use, mostly due to high cost and lack of indications outside of cardiac scanning. Technological advances in the more commonplace spiral CT, specifically subsecond rotation time, the addition of detector rows to acquire multiple slices simultaneously, and the development of electrocardiogram (ECG) synchronization, allowed for spiral CT to take a larger role in the evaluation of cardiac pathology. Decreases in acquisition time in single-slice CT improved visualization of graft patency for both arterial and venous grafts [9], but the progression from single-slice spiral scanners to multidetector computed tomography (MDCT) represented a critical jump in CT scanner technology. Early 4-slice scanners had improved temporal resolution compared to single-slice scanners, between 125 and 250 ms at a 0.5 s gantry rotation time, and brought MDCT of the coronaries to a broad audience. There have been great advances in multi-row detector technology since this time, related to increasing detector rows and therefore greater simultaneous slice acquisition, dual-source acquisition which reduces gantry rotation time, and improved reconstructive algorithms. Coronary arteries can now be reliably followed out to third-order segmental coronary arteries with MDCT [10], and temporal resolution now compares favorably to EBCT. Recent generations of dual-source CT (DSCT) scanners allow acquisition of 384 slices with a gantry rotation time of 0.25 s, producing a temporal resolution of 66 ms and a spatial resolution of 0.24 mm [11]. Third-generation DSCT has been shown to diagnose significant coronary stenoses with sensitivity, specificity, positive predictive value, negative predictive value (NPV), and accuracy of 96.9%, 95.5%, 93.9%, 97.7%, and 96.1%, respectively [12] (Fig. 33.1).

These hardware advances in MDCT have contributed to the reduction in motion artifact. Changes in technique have allowed reductions in iodinated contrast medium volume and radiation exposure, allowing for safer scanning. Software innovations such as new reconstructive techniques have also improved image quality. Taken together these advances have allowed MDCT to overtake EBCT as the dominant cross-sectional and 3D imaging modality for coronary arteries and bypass grafts. Future directions will likely focus on improved reconstructive algorithms to further decrease artifact from motion, ECG dyssynchrony, and objects with high attenuation, as well as continued development of detector technology.

Preoperative Applications

CCTA is a useful methodology for the diagnosis and assessment of CAD. The validity of CCTA as an initial diagnostic test for CAD has been studied extensively and is covered in previous chapters. Instead we will focus on the use of CCTA in the context of preoperative CABG planning. In the last several years, there have been several studies evaluating CCTA as a sole diagnostic test with which to proceed with CABG [13, 14], showing sensitivities and specificities as high as 98.5% and 99.1% in detecting significant stenoses [15]. Despite advances in MDCT technology allowing CT to approach the spatial and temporal resolutions of typical fluoroscopy systems, at 0.16mm and 30 ms [16], respectively, invasive coronary angiography (ICA) remains the test of choice among interventionalists and cardiac surgeons in proceeding CABG, likely with some of this preference due to familiarity [17]. However, as the accuracy of CCTA improves with newer generations of scanners, functional flow data becomes more available, and surgeon familiarity with CCTA increases, it is possible that CT may become the "gatekeeper" to not only the catheterization lab but the operating room as well.

Computed tomography fractional flow reserve (CT-FFR) is a new technique that determines the hemodynamic significance of coronary artery stenoses via flow dynamics and computational algorithms. This is in comparison to invasive catheter FFR, the current gold standard, which relies on proximal and distal stenosis pressure measurements to determine whether a lesion is flow-limiting and therefore a likely source of ischemia. CT-FFR is discussed in detail elsewhere in this text, and therefore we will only briefly make note of its applications to CABG. CT-FFR is currently not widely available due to the complexity of the employed algorithms, which require transfer of data to an off-site supercomputer; however multiple studies have shown that it compares favorably to invasive FFR. Invasive FFR has been studied in the context of CABG and has revealed that less significant lesions are associated with decreased graft patency [18], likely due to competitive flow, and that certain lesion characteristics, such as diffuse instead of focal disease, are also associated with decreased graft patency [19], likely due to impaired runoff. CT-FFR has not been extensively studied in the context of planning for CABG; however Curzen et al. demonstrated that providing CT-FFR data changed management plans in more than one third of patients with significant CAD when compared to CCTA data alone [20]. While decisions to proceed to CABG are not routinely based on CCTA data, as CCTA for bypass planning evolves and CT-FFR becomes more widespread, CT-FFR may become more important in these management decisions.

While CCTA has not been widely adopted as the sole imaging test before coronary surgery, it offers more information on cardiac and mediastinal anatomy than ICA, which is limited in this regard due to its application being confined almost exclusively to evaluation of the vessel lumen. CCTA of the chest further delineates coronary artery course, as well as the anatomy of the subclavian and mammary arteries. While calcium can be seen on fluoroscopy and ICA, accurate and extensive assessment of calcium load, which may influence choice of bypass target sites, is limited [21]. CCTA adequately visualizes calcium and clearly defines coronary artery course, revealing vessels that take an intramyocardial course or run deep within the epicardial fat. This can predict success in minimally invasive CABG as well as bypass distal to a total coronary occlusion which may not be well visualized on ICA [22]. In addition to anatomic information, CT can also provide information regarding cardiac function [23] and myocardial viability [24].

The LIMA is often used as a graft without preoperative evaluation; however it has been shown that angiographic visualization may change surgical strategy. In a series of 262 patients, anomalies in the origin, course, branching, or atherosclerotic lesions resulted in a more meticulous dissection of the artery in 26% of patients and a complete modification in surgical strategy in 4% of patients [25]. Subclavian artery anatomy has also been studied preoperatively using angiography, and identification of stenosis proximal to the LIMA origin, which carries a prevalence of 2–7% [26, 27], allows for adaptive strategies such as stenting of the subclavian arteries or use of alternative bypass grafts [28]. While CCTA has not been extensively studied in this respect, it has the benefit over catheter evaluation of being noninvasive. In addition, routine preoperative catheter evaluation of the IMAs and/or subclavian arteries may not be common in some practices, and therefore abnormalities of this vascular tree may be missed. As CCTA offers comprehensive evaluation of the thoracic vasculature, it is reasonable to assume that this modality would have a higher sensitivity for detecting abnormalities due to a more consistent technique. The author's institution recently performed a reoperative CABG in which the initial operation had been an all-saphenous vein graft CABG at another hospital, with the LIMA still in its native position. Prior operative reports and notes were not available; however as we perform preoperative CCTA before all redo cases, we identified a proximal left subclavian artery stenosis that was not identified on preoperative catheterization, allowing us to change our operative strategy and use alternative grafts (Fig. 33.2).

While the majority of CABG procedures in the USA are performed in an open fashion through a median sternotomy,

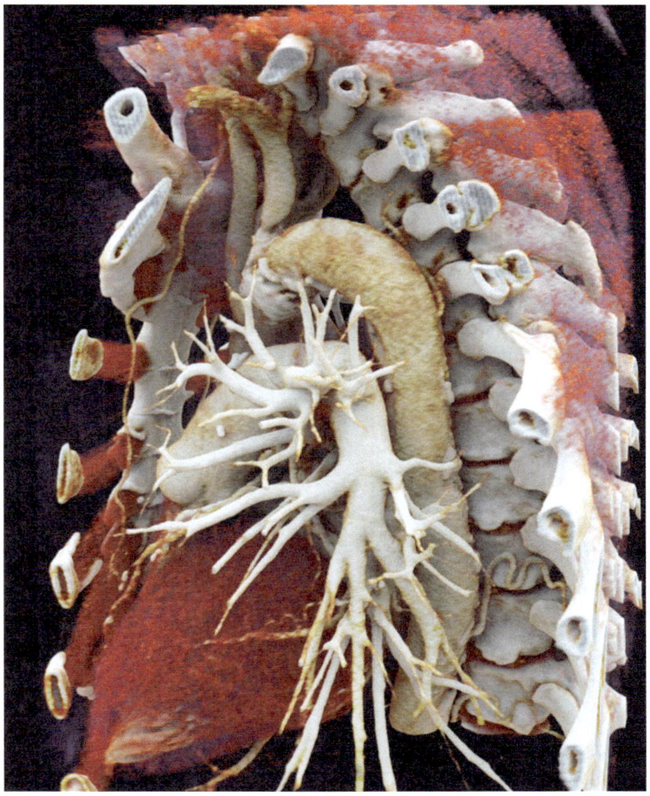

Fig. 33.2 3D reconstruction of a patient with three-vessel disease presenting for repeat CABG. Preoperative CT scan identified a subclavian artery stenosis proximal to the LIMA origin, and therefore the LIMA was not used as a bypass grafting

it is possible to perform bypass grafting via non-sternotomy approaches. Minimally invasive direct coronary artery bypass (MIDCAB) utilizes an approach via a left anterior minithoracotomy, whereas total endoscopic coronary artery bypass (TECAB) is a robotic procedure that allows a complete closed-chest approach to revascularization [29]. These approaches offer the benefits of avoiding a sternotomy and in many cases the need for cardiopulmonary bypass, providing an "off-pump" procedure. These approaches may offer a less morbid procedure and a more appealing cosmetic result; however they have several limitations, leading to less widespread adoption than might be expected. Firstly, access to these procedures may be limited to specific centers and surgeons with the technology and expertise to perform them. Secondly, the ability to achieve a full revascularization may be limited by coronary anatomy, especially when adopting an off-pump approach, as the cardiac manipulation required to reach specific targets in the right coronary or left circumflex distributions may cause intraoperative hemodynamic instability. MIDCAB offers only visualization of the left side of the heart, limiting its application to two-vessel coronary disease on the left side of the heart. TECAB allows better visualization of the posterior aspect of the heart; however a full revascularization then requires the application of cardiopulmonary bypass via femoral cannulation with aortic "clamping" via endo-aortic balloon occlusion. Either one of these techniques may be applied in concert with percutaneous intervention to achieve full revascularization via a hybrid approach.

In cases in which minimally invasive CABG is pursued, preoperative planning is paramount in order to determine appropriate vessel anatomy and relationships. EBCT has been successfully used to determine appropriate incision placement based on coronary anatomy and desired targets [30]; however MDCT may also be employed successfully. Distances between the LIMA and LAD as assessed by 16-slice MDCT have been shown to correlate with operative time in TECAB [31]. This has been confirmed in other studies, which have in addition shown that assessing soft-tissue thickness around the mammary as well as the pericardial fat pad around the LAD assists in operative planning [32]. Importantly, an intramyocardial vessel course or a course deep within the epicardial fat is important to delineate preoperatively. In open CABG, appropriate anastomotic targets, free of calcific plaque, are often determined by digital palpation. If it is necessary to graft to an intramyocardial segment, myocardial dissection can be carried out safely, especially with the assistance of CPB and cardioplegic arrest. Dissection and palpation of intramyocardial vessels may be difficult but still possible in MIDCAB. Vessel palpation is impossible in TECAB, and therefore intramyocardial vessel course is a contraindication to TECAB. In addition, accurate vessel course may be difficult to appreciate or dissect out from minimally invasive approaches if it is deep in the epicardial fat, especially if an off-pump strategy is employed. For this reason preoperative CCTA is an important aspect of preoperative planning for minimally invasive CABG, particularly in TECAB, as a robotic approach precludes tactile feedback and makes extensive dissection hazardous.

Off-pump CABG via sternotomy suffers from some of the same limitations of minimally invasive CABG, in that coronary arterial courses deep into the cardiac muscle or fat may make bypass challenging or impossible. While off-pump surgery through a traditional sternotomy retains the option of converting to an on-pump surgery for better visualization, planning with CCTA delineates coronary anatomy and may lead to a change in bypass target site or a wholesale change in surgical strategy to on-pump surgery. This is significant, as intraoperative conversion from off-pump to on-pump surgery has been associated with worsened outcomes [33]. In addition, CT allows the identification of patients with a "porcelain aorta," or aorta with extensive circumferential calcification. Under these circumstances the application of an aortic cross-clamp may represent a prohibitive risk of stroke [7], and appropriate locations for the placement of proximal aortocoronary anastomoses may not be present.

As mentioned before, CCTA allows evaluation of both mammary arteries to determine their suitability as bypass grafts. This is significant, as there has been a trend toward bypass grafting using all-arterial grafts due to higher demonstrated patencies, which may lead to better long-term outcomes [4]. An all-arterial strategy is also attractive in that it is conducive to an off-pump approach due to the reduced need for aortocoronary anastomoses (Fig. 33.3). While minimally invasive CABG is useful in select populations, a minimally invasive approach may preclude use of the right internal mammary artery (RIMA) as a graft, which has at least equal patency as compared to the radial artery and may be higher in some circumstances [34]. This may be another reason that there has not been widespread adoption of minimally invasive techniques. Regardless, preoperative CT is useful in planning minimally invasive CABG, off-pump CABG, and all-arterial bypasses.

Postoperative Applications

Invasive catheter angiography (ICA) has been the traditional method of evaluating bypass graft patency postoperatively; however contrast-enhanced coronary CT offers an appealing, noninvasive method of evaluation, with the additional ability to offer plaque characterization in late postoperative assessments. Initial studies were ungated, and while this allows evaluation of proximal and mid-vessel aspects of the graft, which tend to demonstrate less motion in the cardiac cycle than the coronary vasculature, an ungated approach

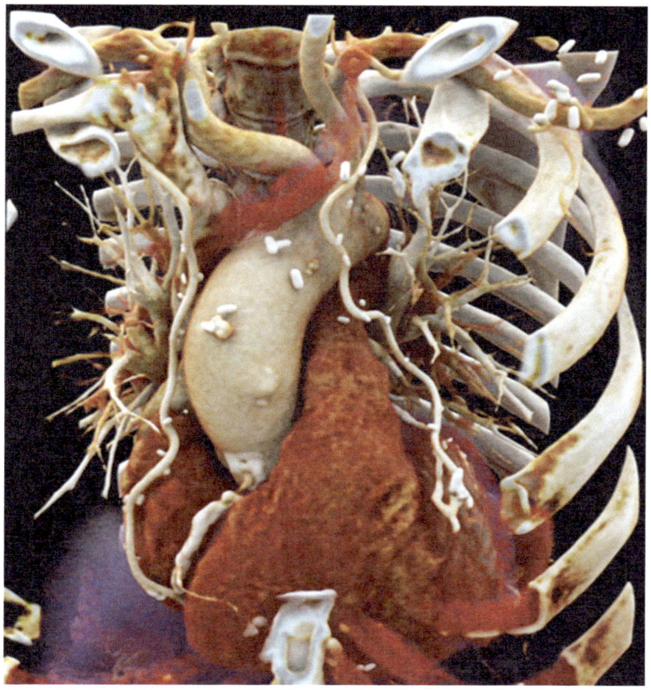

Fig. 33.3 3D reconstruction of a patient with two-vessel disease now status post a two-vessel CABG with bilateral IMA grafts. This approach can obviate the need for aortocoronary anastomoses and is a useful technique in patients with porcelain aorta in which avoiding aortic manipulation is desirable

does not allow assessment of distal anastomoses [35]. Prospective ECG-triggering was also found to be inadequate early on [36]; however retrospective ECG-gating has been found to be highly successful in evaluating grafts, including their distal anastomoses, albeit at the cost of a higher radiation dose [37, 38]. More recent studies have shown prospective ECG synchronization to be equal to retrospective gating, however, allowing either of these methods to be employed for diagnostic image quality [39].

Assessment of bypass grafts has improved as newer generations of CT scanners have added additional detector rows. Stein et al. published a systematic review in 2005 comparing results of single-slice, 4-slice, and 16-slice scanning in assessing bypass grafts in a pooled review comprising 1570 total patients [40]. They found that single-slice CT was not sensitive for detecting occlusion, with a sensitivity of 81%, compared to 93% with 4-slice CT and 99% with 16-slice CT. While the differences in occlusion detection were nonsignificant between 4- and 16-slice CT, the ability to detect significant stenoses was significantly different, with a sensitivity of 74% for 4-slice CT and 88% for 16-slice CT. Multiple studies have furthered the validation of 16-slice CT as a useful tool to assess bypass graft patency, with sensitivities as high as 100% for detecting occlusion [41]. One caveat that remained was with regard to the number of evaluable grafts; multiple studies reported high sensitivities for assessment of significant stenosis in evaluable grafts; however the percentage varies between studies, with reports of 78–92% of grafts being completely evaluable [41–43]. An interesting study of 64-slice CT for bypass assessment found that CCTA demonstrated perfect sensitivity in determining graft occlusion or distal anastomotic stenosis when compared to ICA; however, CCTA tended to overcall both [44]. The authors attributed the false positives for occlusion to "string sign" visualized on ICA, suggesting a lack of adequate spatial resolution, and to competitive flow at distal anastomotic sites. While this study did identify some shortcomings with CCTA, it is important to note that all grafts were evaluable by 64-slice CCTA and that performance overall was excellent. A recent meta-analysis comparing 64-slice CCTA to ICA in the evaluation of graft occlusion and stenosis also yielded excellent results for CCTA [45]. This meta-analysis by Chan et al. comprised 31 studies with 1975 total patients and demonstrated a sensitivity of 96.3% for identifying stenosis or occlusion compared to ICA. They did note, however, that CCTA was significantly better ($p = 0.004$) for identifying abnormalities of saphenous vein grafts compared to arterial grafts, indicating once again spatial resolution as a potential limiting factor.

CCTA has not been specifically studied for the evaluation of all-arterial bypass grafting; however there are plenty of data regarding the evaluation of arterial grafts in combined arterial and venous bypass. Arterial grafts have traditionally been more challenging to image than venous grafts – due to surgical technique, they tend to have more clip artifacts than venous grafts, and their smaller lumens require high spatial resolution to visualize. Early studies gave conflicting results on the accuracy of CT evaluation of arterial grafts as compared to venous grafts; however as CT technology has improved, this difference has become less significant. One study of single-slice CT gave accuracies of 96.4%, 65.7%, and 45.5% for evaluating patency in venous, IMA, and radial artery grafts, respectively [46]. However a contemporaneous study comparing IMA grafts to venous grafts resulted in accuracies of 88% and 96%, respectively, with no significant difference [9]. The evaluation of arterial grafts on a 4-slice system rendered similar results, with a sensitivity, specificity, and overall accuracy of 100%, 98.7%, and 98.9%, respectively, for evaluating patency versus obstruction in arterial grafts, as compared to 81.8%, 93.7%, and 88.9% in venous grafts [47]. Data from 64-slice CT showed a sensitivity, specificity, and accuracy of 100% for evaluating venous graft occlusion versus 83.3%, 100%, and 98.9% for evaluating arterial graft occlusion, respectively [48]. This study also evaluated severity of stenosis in patent grafts and found a sensitivity, specificity, and accuracy of 94.4%, 98.4%, and 96.9% in evaluating significant stenoses in venous grafts versus 100%, 97.7%, and 98% in arterial grafts, respectively. More recently, 320-slice CT evaluation for the detection of

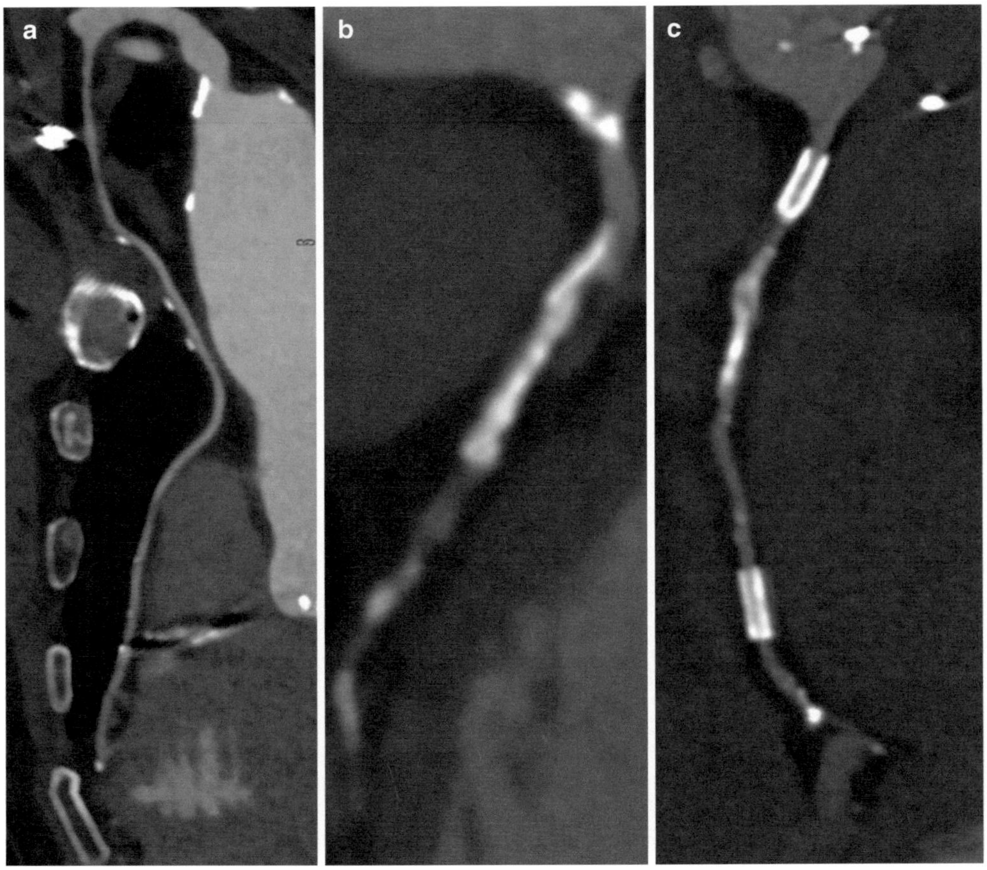

Fig. 33.4 Artifact can be introduced by metallic objects in and around coronaries and bypass grafts such as surgical clips adjacent to the LIMA (**a**), extensive calcification in a native coronary artery (**b**), and coronary stents (**c**)

significant stenoses gave sensitivity, specificity, and diagnostic accuracy of 95%, 93%, and 93% for venous grafts versus 100%, 91%, and 93% for arterial grafts [49]. Taken with the results of the preceding study by Chan et al., it is important to note that there is still conflict in the literature with regard to the evaluation of arterial grafts. However, the overall body of evidence indicates that CCTA is a useful modality for evaluating arterial grafts and with current results would be acceptable as a first-line evaluation of patients with an all-arterial bypass to avoid the complications of ICA in patients who do not require further investigation or intervention.

While invasive catheter FFR has applications in the assessment of bypass graft stenoses, CT-FFR has yet to be studied in this context but may eventually find utility in certain types of grafts. Saphenous vein grafts in particular tend to develop atherosclerosis at an aggressive rate compared to arterial grafts, and the resultant plaques are very friable and subject to rupture with distal embolization of contents when manipulated. Therefore, CT-FFR may provide added value to the analysis of these lesions, as it avoids the risks of manipulation associated with invasive assessment, namely, distal embolization and resultant periprocedural myocardial infarction.

Currently, CCTA is a useful modality to assess previous bypass grafts. Continued limitations besides spatial resolution include the performance of CCTA in the presence of metallic artifact such as clips, stents, or heavy calcification (Fig. 33.4), which may also cause overestimation of stenoses. However newer generations of CT scanners may overcome these limitations, especially with software advances in reconstructive techniques. With continued improvement in MDCT design, it is likely that CCTA may serve as a first step in evaluating CABG grafts, ideally allowing ICA to be reserved for those requiring procedural intervention.

Reoperative Surgery

Reoperative surgery is an important aspect of cardiac surgical practice, and one in which MDCT plays an increasingly important role. Due to the progressive nature of coronary artery disease, as well as the effect of atherosclerosis on previously placed bypass grafts, a certain percentage of CABG patients will require repeat surgical revascularization in their lifetime. In addition to revascularization, patients who have undergone valvular or other cardiac surgeries, with or without concomitant bypass grafting, may require repeat cardiac surgical intervention.

Decreased graft patency with time, leading to symptoms and cardiovascular events, is the major determinant for proceeding to PCI or reoperative CABG. It is important to note that different grafts demonstrate different patencies. A large series published in 1996 demonstrated SVG patency of 81% at 1 year, 75% at 5 years, and 50% at 15 years [50]. This translates into a need for reoperative CABG of 2% at 5 years, 12% at 10 years, and 20% at 12 years, in addition to patients undergoing percutaneous interventions [51]. Arterial grafts demonstrate much higher patency, however, with the 10-year LIMA graft patency of 94.6% when grafted to the LAD [52]. Long-term RIMA and radial artery patencies are less than that of the LIMA but still superior to SVG [53]. Therefore adoption of an "all-arterial" strategy as noted before may lead to improved long-term graft patency with decreased need for reintervention, and has been linked to improved outcomes [4].

The frequency of reoperative cardiac surgery is evolving, and the incidence of reoperation depends on the indication of the initial operation. There has been a steady decrease in reoperative CABG in the past several decades, likely due to improved medical management and the proliferation of PCI. Conversely, there has been an increased need for valvular reintervention, as this patient population have experienced greater longevity, along with increasing usage of bioprosthetic valves [54], which have limited long-term durability. Reports on regional or institutional trends regarding reoperative volume are subject to local practice patterns, but national databases are useful in determining general trends. Ghanta et al. reported in a Society of Thoracic Surgeons (STS) database analysis that between 2000 and 2009, redo CABG decreased from 6.0% to 3.4% of overall national CABG volume [55]. 5.9% of aortic valve procedures nationally were redo operations in the period between 2011 and 2013 [56]. While need for aortic valve intervention may be increasing, the number of redo surgeries will likely see a decrease as transcatheter aortic valve implantation (TAVI) is used more commonly in a "valve-in-valve" fashion to treat bioprosthetic aortic valve stenosis. CT is indispensable in the planning of TAVI; however that topic is covered in detail elsewhere in this text and will not be discussed here. Conversely, reoperation for mitral valve pathology is increasing, with more than 10% of mitral operations being redo operations, 35% of whom had undergone prior CABG [57]. Due to a current lack of robust transcatheter mitral valve therapies, this number is likely to increase in the near future.

Reoperative cardiac surgery has traditionally been associated with significantly higher morbidity and mortality than primary cardiac surgery, with perioperative mortality traditionally being reported in the 4–9% range, although mortality can exceed 20% in selected populations [55, 58]. This can be attributed to several reasons, such as older age, increased medical comorbidities, and damage to substernal structures on reentry. Redo sternotomy can be a hazardous procedure, as the inflammatory and scar responses from primary sternotomy result in dense mediastinal adhesions. The aorta, right coronary artery, right ventricle, and anteriorly located bypass grafts may be in close proximity, if not adhered, to the posterior table of the sternum, making them susceptible to injury. The location of patent bypass grafts is of particular importance, as myocardial dependence on these sources of blood flow may be increased from the primary operation due to progression of native coronary disease, and injury sustained during reentry may be difficult if not impossible to repair. Specific difficult situations include a RIMA used to bypass a left coronary territory or SVGs that come anteriorly off the aorta to bypass left-sided territories, as both of these graft pat-

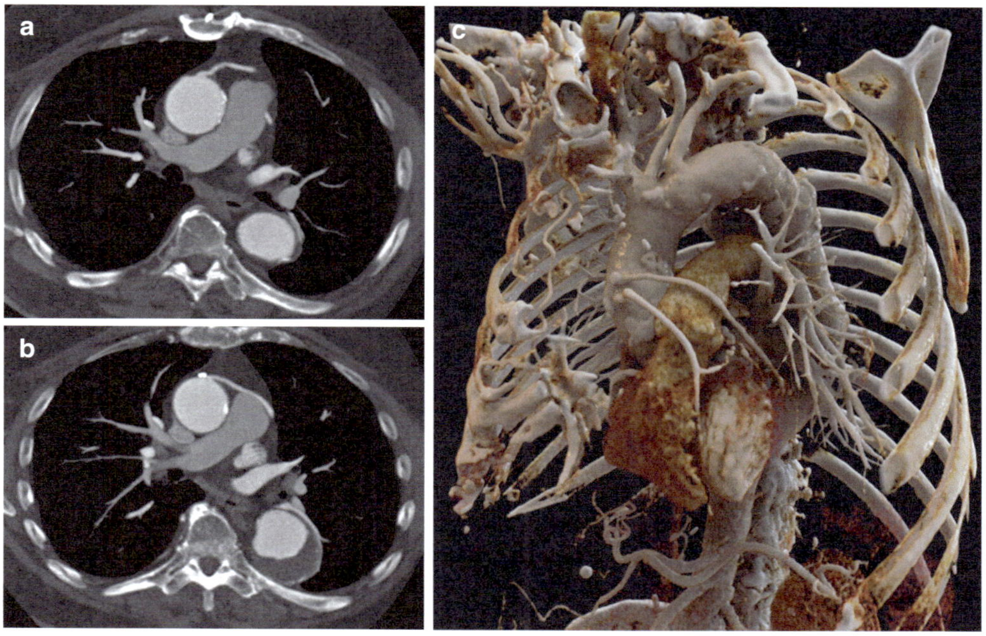

Fig. 33.5 Preoperative CT is critical prior to redo sternotomy, as bypass grafts may be vulnerable to injury on reentry. In this particular instance, there are two venous grafts that arise anteriorly from the aorta and cross the midline to supply the left circumflex artery and a diagonal branch of the LAD. Grafts that cross midline can be at risk for damage; however in this instance they are a safe distance away from the sternum

terns cross midline and may be in close proximity to the site of re-sternotomy (Fig. 33.5). Regardless of sternal proximity, it is always important to localize the LIMA, as control of this graft is critical for myocardial protection. SVGs are placed on the proximal aorta and therefore can carry cold, high-potassium cardioplegia to their supplied territories after cross-clamping distally on the ascending aorta. However an in situ LIMA to LAD graft obligatorily originates past the aortic cross-clamp and if not controlled and occluded during cardioplegic arrest will carry warmer, lower-potassium blood from the bypass circuit to the LAD and any collateralized territories, compromising myocardial protection.

Despite the difficulties associated with reoperative CABG and other cardiac surgeries, outcomes have improved in recent years and approach if not match outcomes of primary surgery in some contemporary reports [55, 57]. The reason for this is multifactorial, with improvements in anesthesia, medical management of comorbidities, and postoperative care contribution. However, the importance of preoperative MDCT cannot be understated. Preoperative CT is a prerequisite for redo surgery in the context of previous bypass grafts in allowing appropriate planning with which many injuries upon reentry can be avoided. Three-dimensional reconstructions are particularly useful in visualizing the mediastinal anatomy. It is standard practice to acquire preoperative CT for all reoperative adult cardiac surgeries at the author's institution. Multiple studies have shown that preoperative CT often changes management, with a high rate of adoption of protective strategies such as alternate incision sites, exposure of peripheral vascular access sites, and preemptive initiation of cardiopulmonary bypass prior to redo sternotomy [59–61]. It has been demonstrated that preoperative CCTA is associated with at least a trend toward decreased complications after redo surgery [62, 63], which would likely be significant in larger series. In addition, preoperative CCTA appears cost-effective in reoperative cardiac surgery, as it may prevent the cost of treating complications, although this must be balanced with the cost of the additional OR time and equipment necessary for protective maneuvers [64]. As CT technology improves, so does this ability to plan for reoperative cardiac surgery. Improved spatial and temporal resolution affords accurate localization of substernal structures, as do improved reconstructive models [65].

Conclusion

Multidetector CCTA is a useful tool for diagnosing and evaluating coronary artery disease, as well as elucidating mediastinal anatomy pertinent to coronary artery bypass grafting. Multiple developments in hardware, software, and technique have contributed to improved spatial and temporal resolution while imaging the heart, giving high-quality information on native coronary arteries and bypass grafts. While CCTA is not routinely used as a sole test to proceeding with CABG, it provides more information on mediastinal anatomy than ICA and is indispensable for minimally invasive CABG and off-pump CABG and for evaluating potential arterial grafts for all-arterial bypass. In addition, CCTA has been shown to accurately assess coronary artery bypass grafts for stenosis and overall patency, in both venous and arterial grafts. CCTA is indispensable to reoperative surgery in determining the location of bypass grafts and other mediastinal structures in order to avoid damage during sternal reentry. The current status of MDCT for use with CABG is promising, and advances in newer-generation CT scanners may lead to it becoming the "gatekeeper" to the catheterization lab and the operating room.

References

1. Roach GW, et al. Adverse cerebral outcomes after coronary bypass surgery. Multicenter Study of Perioperative Ischemia Research Group and the Ischemia Research and Education Foundation Investigators. N Engl J Med. 1996;335(25):1857–63.
2. Loop FD, et al. Influence of the internal-mammary-artery graft on 10-year survival and other cardiac events. N Engl J Med. 1986;314(1):1–6.
3. Zhang B, et al. Comparison of graft patency between off-pump and on-pump coronary artery bypass grafting: an updated meta-analysis. Ann Thorac Surg. 2014;97(4):1335–41.
4. Locker C, et al. Multiple arterial grafts improve late survival of patients undergoing coronary artery bypass graft surgery: analysis of 8622 patients with multivessel disease. Circulation. 2012;126(9):1023–30.
5. Arad Y, et al. Predictive value of electron beam computed tomography of the coronary arteries. 19-month follow-up of 1173 asymptomatic subjects. Circulation. 1996;93(11):1951–3.
6. Godwin JD, et al. Clinical value of coronary bypass graft evaluation with CT. AJR Am J Roentgenol. 1983;140(4):649–55.
7. Daniel WG, et al. Value and limitations of computed tomography in assessing aortocoronary bypass graft patency. Circulation. 1983;67(5):983–7.
8. Tello R, et al. Spiral CT evaluation of coronary artery bypass graft patency. J Comput Assist Tomogr. 1993;17(2):253–9.
9. Engelmann MG, et al. Accuracy of spiral computed tomography for identifying arterial and venous coronary graft patency. Am J Cardiol. 1997;80(5):569–74.
10. Becker CR, et al. Current development of cardiac imaging with multidetector-row CT. Eur J Radiol. 2000;36(2):97–103.
11. Flohr T, Schmidt B. Technical aspects of dual energy CT with dual source CT systems. In: Carrascosa PM, Cury RC, Garcia MJ, Leipseic JA, editors. Dual-energy CT in cardiovascular imaging. New York: Springer International Publishing; 2015. p. 11–32.
12. Mangold S, et al. Diagnostic accuracy of coronary CT angiography using 3rd-generation dual-source CT and automated tube voltage selection: clinical application in a non-obese and obese patient population. Eur Radiol. 2017;27:2298.
13. Treede H, et al. Multidetector computed tomography (MDCT) in coronary surgery: first experiences with a new tool for diagnosis of coronary artery disease. Ann Thorac Surg. 2002;74(4):S1398–402.
14. Plass A, et al. Sixteen-channel multidetector row computed tomography versus coronary angiography in a surgical view. Heart Surg Forum. 2006;9(2):E572–8.

15. Bedi HS, Gill JA, Bakshi SS. Can we perform coronary artery bypass grafting on the basis of computed tomographic angiography alone? A comparison with conventional coronary angiography. Eur J Cardiothorac Surg. 2008;33(4):633–8.
16. Otero HJ, Steigner ML, Rybicki FJ. The "post-64" era of coronary CT angiography: understanding new technology from physical principles. Radiol Clin N Am. 2009;47(1):79–90.
17. Sadigh G, et al. Impact of coronary CT angiography on surgical decision-making for coronary artery bypass graft surgery. Acad Radiol. 2013;20(9):1083–90.
18. Botman CJ, et al. Does stenosis severity of native vessels influence bypass graft patency? A prospective fractional flow reserve-guided study. Ann Thorac Surg. 2007;83(6):2093–7.
19. Shiono Y, et al. Impact of functional focal versus diffuse coronary artery disease on bypass graft patency. Int J Cardiol. 2016;222:16–21.
20. Curzen NP, et al. Does the routine availability of CT-derived FFR influence management of patients with stable chest pain compared to CT angiography alone?: The FFRCT RIPCORD Study. JACC Cardiovasc Imaging. 2016;9(10):1188–94.
21. Alexopoulos D, Moulias A. In the search of coronary calcium. Int J Cardiol. 2013;167(2):310–7.
22. Kepka C, et al. Computed tomography to predict surgical revascularization of a left anterior descending artery occlusion incompletely visualized by conventional angiography. J Thorac Imaging. 2012;27(3):184–93.
23. Jones CM, et al. Multi-slice computed tomography in coronary artery disease. Eur J Cardiothorac Surg. 2006;30(3):443–50.
24. Hsiao EM, Rybicki FJ, Steigner M. CT coronary angiography: 256-slice and 320-detector row scanners. Curr Cardiol Rep. 2010;12(1):68–75.
25. Bauer EP, et al. Internal mammary artery anomalies. Thorac Cardiovasc Surg. 1990;38(5):312–5.
26. Prasad A, et al. Prevalence and treatment of proximal left subclavian artery stenosis in patients referred for coronary artery bypass surgery. Int J Cardiol. 2009;133(1):109–11.
27. Byrne C, et al. Ten-year experience in subclavian revascularisation. A parallel comparative observational study. Vascular. 2016;24(4):378–82.
28. Rigatelli G, Rigatelli G. Simultaneous preoperative brachiocephalic angiography and coronary angiography to prevent coronary-subclavian steal syndrome in coronary surgery candidates. Heart Surg Forum. 2005;8(3):E175–7.
29. Holzhey DM, Rastan AJ, Falk V, Mohr FW. Minimally invasive myocardial revascularization. In: Cohn LH, editor. Cardiac surgery in the adult. 4th ed. New York: McGraw-Hill Education; 2012. p. 553–66.
30. Gulbins H, et al. Preoperative 3D-reconstructions of ultrafast-CT images for the planning of minimally invasive direct coronary artery bypass operation (MIDCAB). Heart Surg Forum. 1998;1(2):111–5.
31. Schachner T, et al. Does preoperative multislice computed tomography predict operative times in total endoscopic coronary artery bypass grafting? Heart Surg Forum. 2005;8(5):E314–8.
32. Wehman B, et al. Patient anatomy predicts operative time in robotic totally endoscopic coronary artery bypass surgery. Interact Cardiovasc Thorac Surg. 2014;19(4):572–6.
33. Stevens LM, et al. Conversion after off-pump coronary artery bypass grafting: the CORONARY trial experience. Eur J Cardiothorac Surg. 2017 Mar 1;51(3):539–46.
34. Benedetto U, et al. Searching for the second best graft for coronary artery bypass surgery: a network meta-analysis of randomized controlled trialsdagger. Eur J Cardiothorac Surg. 2015;47(1):59–65; discussion 65.
35. Yamaguchi A, et al. Three-dimensional computed tomographic angiography as preoperative evaluation of a patent internal thoracic artery graft. J Thorac Cardiovasc Surg. 2000;120(4):811–2.
36. von Smekal A. The potential of cardio-computed tomography. Multislice CT: a practical guide. Proceedings of the 5th International Somatom CT User Conference, Zurich, June 2000.
37. Nieman K, et al. Coronary angiography with multi-slice computed tomography. Lancet. 2001;357(9256):599–603.
38. Ropers D, et al. Investigation of aortocoronary artery bypass grafts by multislice spiral computed tomography with electrocardiographic-gated image reconstruction. Am J Cardiol. 2001;88(7):792–5.
39. Lee JH, et al. Prospective versus retrospective ECG-gated 64-detector coronary CT angiography for evaluation of coronary artery bypass graft patency: comparison of image quality, radiation dose and diagnostic accuracy. Int J Cardiovasc Imaging. 2011;27(5):657–67.
40. Stein PD, et al. Usefulness of 4-, 8-, and 16-slice computed tomography for detection of graft occlusion or patency after coronary artery bypass grafting. Am J Cardiol. 2005;96(12):1669–73.
41. Anders K, et al. Coronary artery bypass graft (CABG) patency: assessment with high-resolution submillimeter 16-slice multidetector-row computed tomography (MDCT) versus coronary angiography. Eur J Radiol. 2006;57(3):336–44.
42. Yamamoto M, et al. Noninvasive assessment of off-pump coronary artery bypass surgery by 16-channel multidetector-row computed tomography. Ann Thorac Surg. 2006;81(3):820–7.
43. Houslay ES, et al. Non-invasive assessment of coronary artery bypass graft patency using 16-slice computed tomography angiography. J Cardiothorac Surg. 2007;2:27.
44. Tochii M, et al. Accuracy of 64-slice multidetector computed tomography for diseased coronary artery graft detection. Ann Thorac Surg. 2010;89(6):1906–11.
45. Chan M, et al. A systematic review and meta-analysis of multidetector computed tomography in the assessment of coronary artery bypass grafts. Int J Cardiol. 2016;221:898–905.
46. Ueyama K, et al. Evaluation of coronary artery bypass grafts using helical scan computed tomography. Catheter Cardiovasc Interv. 1999;46(3):322–6.
47. Marano R, et al. Non-invasive assessment of coronary artery bypass graft with retrospectively ECG-gated four-row multi-detector spiral computed tomography. Eur Radiol. 2004;14(8):1353–62.
48. Romagnoli A, et al. Diagnostic accuracy of 64-slice CT in evaluating coronary artery bypass grafts and of the native coronary arteries. Radiol Med. 2010;115(8):1167–78.
49. de Graaf FR, et al. Diagnostic performance of 320-slice multidetector computed tomography coronary angiography in patients after coronary artery bypass grafting. Eur Radiol. 2011;21(11):2285–96.
50. Fitzgibbon GM, et al. Coronary bypass graft fate and patient outcome: angiographic follow-up of 5,065 grafts related to survival and reoperation in 1,388 patients during 25 years. J Am Coll Cardiol. 1996;28(3):616–26.
51. Weintraub WS, et al. Frequency of repeat coronary bypass or coronary angioplasty after coronary artery bypass surgery using saphenous venous grafts. Am J Cardiol. 1994;73(2):103–12.
52. Zeff RH, et al. Internal mammary artery versus saphenous vein graft to the left anterior descending coronary artery: prospective randomized study with 10-year follow-up. Ann Thorac Surg. 1988;45(5):533–6.
53. Achouh P, et al. Reappraisal of a 20-year experience with the radial artery as a conduit for coronary bypass grafting. Eur J Cardiothorac Surg. 2012;41(1):87–92.
54. Javadzadegan H, Javadzadegan A, Mehdizadeh Baghbani J. Factors influencing mortality after bioprosthetic valve replacement; a midterm outcome. J Cardiovasc Thorac Res. 2013;5(4):163–5.
55. Ghanta RK, et al. Evolving trends of reoperative coronary artery bypass grafting: an analysis of the Society of Thoracic Surgeons Adult Cardiac Surgery Database. J Thorac Cardiovasc Surg. 2013;145(2):364–72.

56. Kaneko T, et al. Contemporary outcomes of repeat aortic valve replacement: a benchmark for transcatheter valve-in-valve procedures. Ann Thorac Surg. 2015;100(4):1298–304; discussion 1304.
57. Ghoreishi M, et al. Repeat sternotomy: no longer a risk factor in mitral valve surgical procedures. Ann Thorac Surg. 2013;96(4):1358–65.
58. Christenson JT, Schmuziger M, Simonet F. Reoperative coronary artery bypass procedures: risk factors for early mortality and late survival. Eur J Cardiothorac Surg. 1997;11(1):129–33.
59. Gasparovic H, et al. Three dimensional computed tomographic imaging in planning the surgical approach for redo cardiac surgery after coronary revascularization. Eur J Cardiothorac Surg. 2005;28(2):244–9.
60. Imran Hamid U, et al. Incidence and outcome of re-entry injury in redo cardiac surgery: benefits of preoperative planning. Eur J Cardiothorac Surg. 2015;47(5):819–23.
61. Kamdar AR, et al. Multidetector computed tomographic angiography in planning of reoperative cardiothoracic surgery. Ann Thorac Surg. 2008;85(4):1239–45.
62. Aviram G, et al. Open heart reoperations after coronary artery bypass grafting: the role of preoperative imaging with multidetector computed tomography. Isr Med Assoc J. 2009;11(8):465–9.
63. den Harder AM, et al. Effect of computed tomography before cardiac surgery on surgical strategy, mortality and stroke. Eur J Radiol. 2016;85(4):744–50.
64. Gada H, Desai MY, Marwick TH. Cost-effectiveness of computed tomographic angiography before reoperative coronary artery bypass grafting: a decision-analytic model. Circ Cardiovasc Qual Outcomes. 2012;5(5):705–10.
65. Oda S, et al. Cardiac CT for planning redo cardiac surgery: effect of knowledge-based iterative model reconstruction on image quality. Eur Radiol. 2015;25(1):58–64.

Cardiac CT in the Setting of Heart Transplantation

34

Gorka Bastarrika and Gregorio Rábago

Heart transplantation is a definitive treatment option for patients with end-stage heart failure. According to the 28th report of the International Society for Heart and Lung Transplantation (ISHLT) transplant registry, in the last decade, between 3600 and 3850 heart transplants were registered every year [1].

Prognosis and long-term survival after heart transplantation has significantly improved in the last decades particularly due to effective antirejection therapy and infection control. The first year after transplant represents the period with the highest risk of death, mainly due to graft failure, infection, multiple organ failure, and rejection. Conversely, long-term mortality is related to cardiac allograft vasculopathy (CAV), renal failure, and malignancy [1].

In fact, CAV is a well-known factor limiting the successful long-term outcome of heart transplantation. Because of the allograft denervation occurring after transplantation, this entity is frequently asymptomatic. Clinical manifestations of CAV vary from arrhythmia to congestive heart failure or sudden cardiac death.

Nowadays, conventional coronary angiography is the standard of reference to rule out CAV, although intravascular ultrasound is the most sensitive tool for early detection of the disease. Due to the fact that these two techniques carry a relatively high cost and risk, there has been vigorous research on imaging modalities allowing noninvasive detection, characterization, and follow-up of CAV. In the last decade, cardiac computed tomography (CT) has emerged as a very useful imaging test in this clinical setting.

In the field of cardiac transplantation, CT allows to assess the typical appearance of the transplanted heart and to detect complications. Advances in CT technology and improvement in spatial and temporal resolution also allow visualization of the coronary artery lumen and wall with unprecedented anatomical detail. Further, ECG-triggered acquisition enables to evaluate cardiac function using the same CT datasets, without the need of additional contrast media or radiation dose. Moreover, CT is helpful in detecting transplant-related ancillary findings that may influence patient outcome. In this chapter the usefulness of CT to provide an integrative approach to the transplanted heart is reviewed.

Cardiovascular Anatomy After Heart Transplantation

Orthotopic Heart Transplantation

The first surgical technique for orthotopic heart transplantation was described by Shumway and Lower in 1966 [2]. The so-called biatrial approach consists in leaving posterior right and left atrial cuffs to facilitate the reimplantation of the donor heart. The donor's superior vena cava cuff is fixed above the right atrium, and the donor's inferior vena cava is included in the right atrial anastomosis.

More recently, the standard biatrial technique was modified to launch the so-called bicaval approach [3, 4]. With this surgical approach, the donor's left atrium is sutured to the posterior cuff of the recipient's native left atrium containing pulmonary vein insertion, the donor's inferior and superior vena cava are sutured to the corresponding recipient cuffs, and the intervention is finalized with anastomosis of the ascending aorta and main pulmonary artery. The bicaval technique allows better preservation of the right atrial morphology and function, thus reducing the incidence of arrhythmias, right atrial dilatation, and tricuspid regurgitation [5].

CT imaging shows characteristic findings that will allow to differentiate between the two surgical techniques. In patients undergoing heart transplantation with the biatrial surgical technique, CT will show enlargement of both atrial cavities, particularly of the left atrium (Fig. 34.1), whereas

G. Bastarrika (✉)
Cardiothoracic Imaging Division, Department of Radiology, Clínica Universidad de Navarra, Pamplona, Spain
e-mail: bastarrika@unav.es

G. Rábago
Department of Cardiac Surgery, Clínica Universidad de Navarra, Pamplona, Spain

U. J. Schoepf (ed.), *CT of the Heart*, Contemporary Medical Imaging, https://doi.org/10.1007/978-1-60327-237-7_34

patients undergoing heart transplantation with the bicaval approach show a clockwise-rotated heart with normal size atria (Fig. 34.2). The anastomotic sutures of the aorta and main pulmonary artery are easily depicted, particularly when there is size discrepancy between recipient and donor arteries. In these cases, postsurgical changes may show the appearance of perivascular soft tissue, redundancy, stenosis, or aneurysmal dilatation [6] (Fig. 34.3).

Graft outcome will depend on variables such as enlargement of the atria, asynchronous contraction of the donor and recipient atria, tendency for thrombus formation, conduction disturbances, and residual atrioventricular valve regurgitation [7–9]. Cardiac CT will also detect potential complications of the procedure early after surgery or during the surveillance (Fig. 34.4), emphasizing its role in the comprehensive evaluation of the transplanted heart.

Heterotopic Heart Transplantation

Heterotopic heart transplantation is reserved for patients with irreversible high pulmonary vascular resistance and body weight mismatch (over 20%) between recipient and donor or for patients with potentially reversible myocardial dysfunction. The donor heart is positioned side by side with the recipient heart. Surgeons perform anastomosis of right atria, left atria, aorta, and main pulmonary arteries [10]. In heterotopic heart transplantation, the native right ventricle

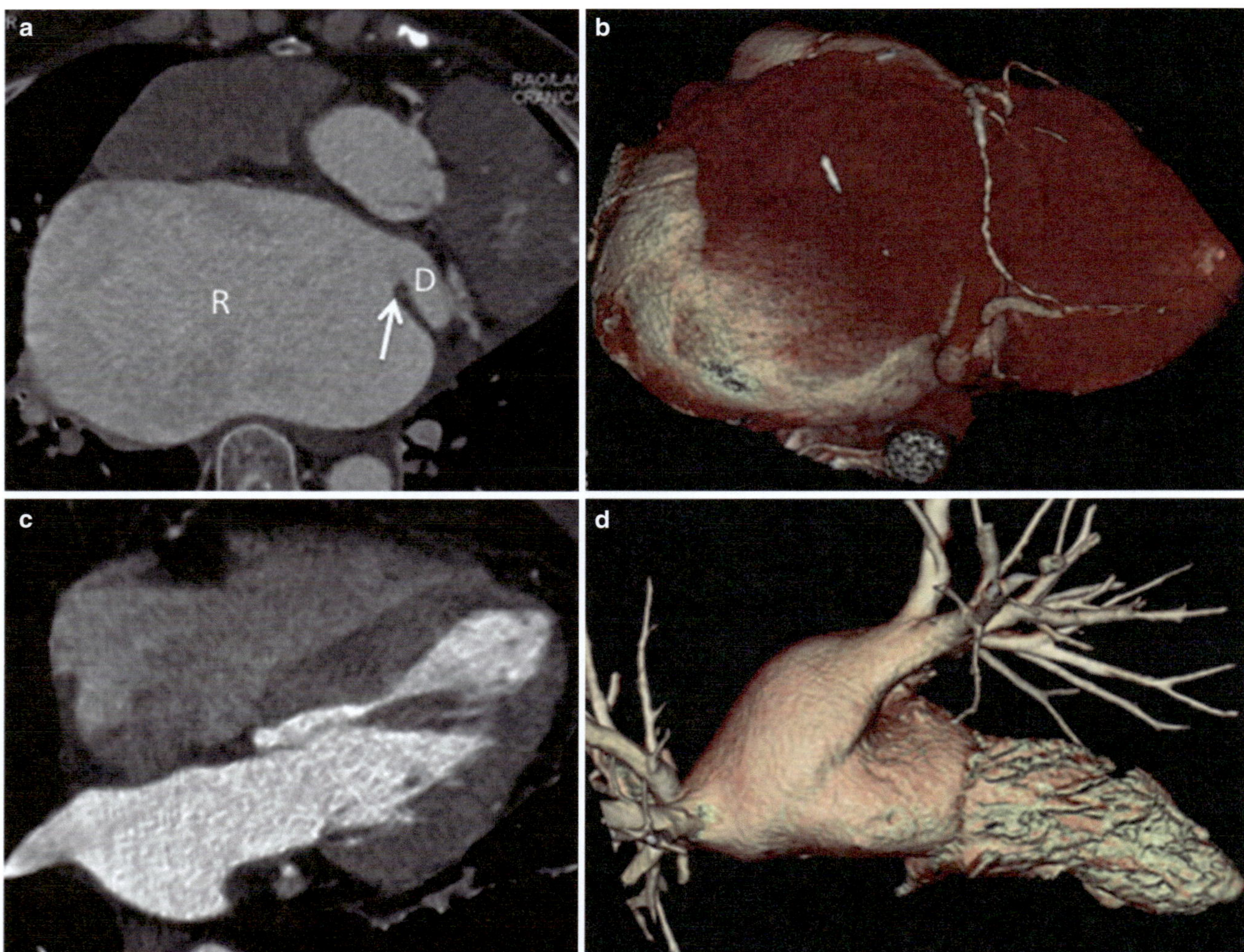

Fig. 34.1 Orthotopic heart transplantation. (**a**, **b**) Biatrial technique. In this 63-year-old woman who underwent heart transplantation with the biatrial surgical technique, CT imaging demonstrated enlargement of both atrial cavities, particularly of the left atrium. Note that most of the left atrial cavity is provided by the receptor (R), whereas only a small portion is provided by the donor (D). The site of the anastomosis is clearly depicted (arrow). (**c**, **d**) Bicaval technique. CT exam of a 61-year-old man who underwent heart transplantation with the bicaval approach. In this technique the donor's left atrium is sutured to the posterior cuff of the recipient's native left atrium containing pulmonary vein insertion. As a result, there is no significant enlargement of atrial cavities

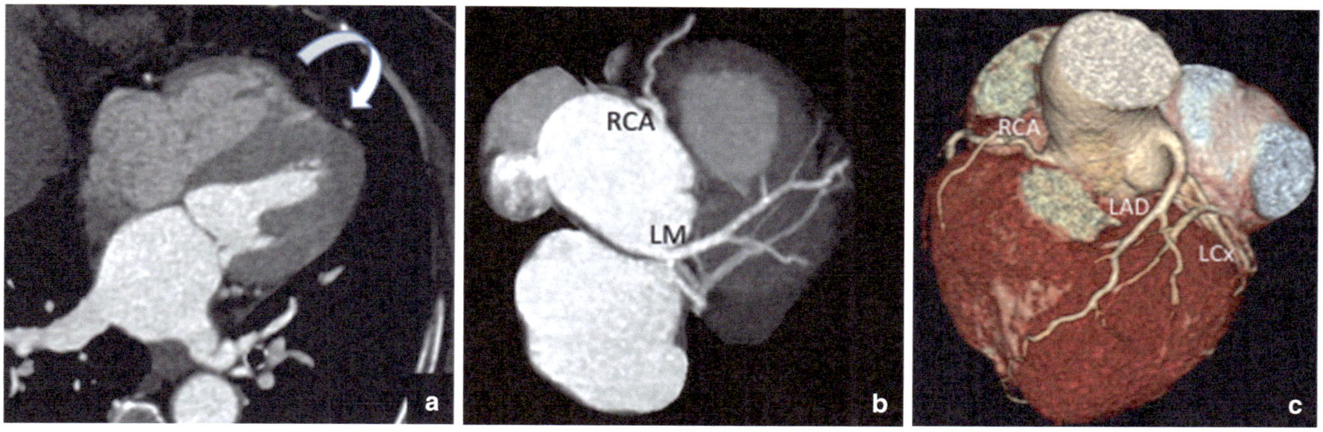

Fig. 34.2 CT appearance of the graft in a patient with orthotopic heart transplantation operated with the bicaval technique. (**a**) Axial image. (**b**) Maximum intensity projection (MIP) image. (**c**) Volume-rendered image. The heart is clockwise-rotated (curved arrow in **a**). Note clockwise rotation of the origin of the coronary vessels (**b**, left main, LM; right coronary artery, RCA). Despite this, the volumetric image is similar to that of a non-transplanted heart (**c**). (*LAD* left anterior descending coronary artery, *LCx* left circumflex, *RCA* right coronary artery)

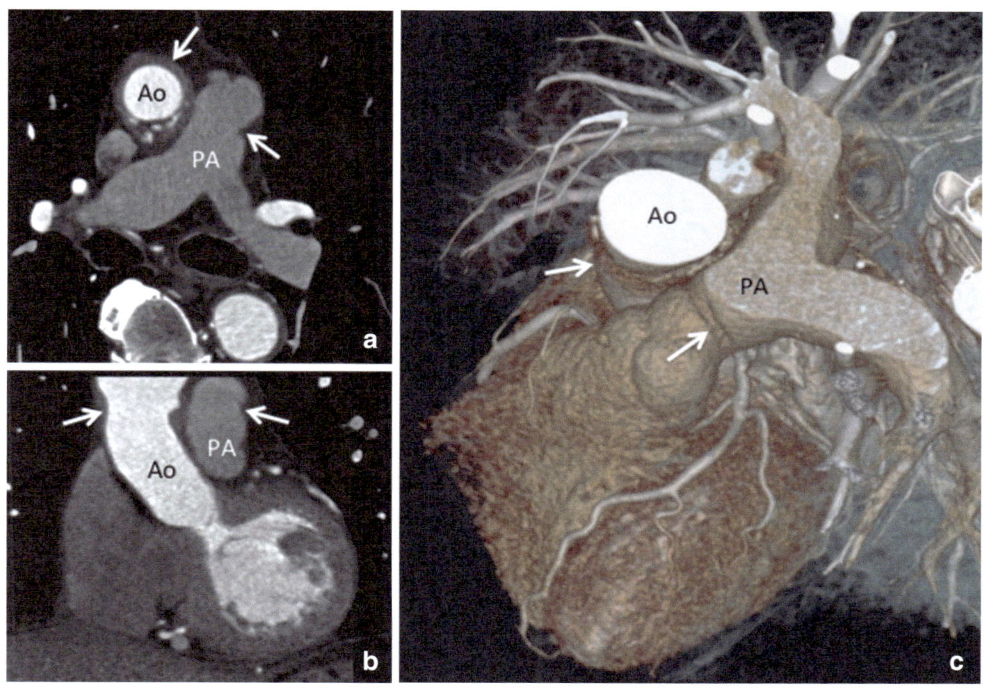

Fig. 34.3 Postsurgical CT appearance of vascular anastomoses in a 68-year-old male after heart transplantation. (**a**) Axial image. (**b**) Coronal image. (**c**) Volume-rendered image. The anastomotic sutures of the aorta (Ao) and main pulmonary artery (PA) after transplantation are clearly depicted (arrows)

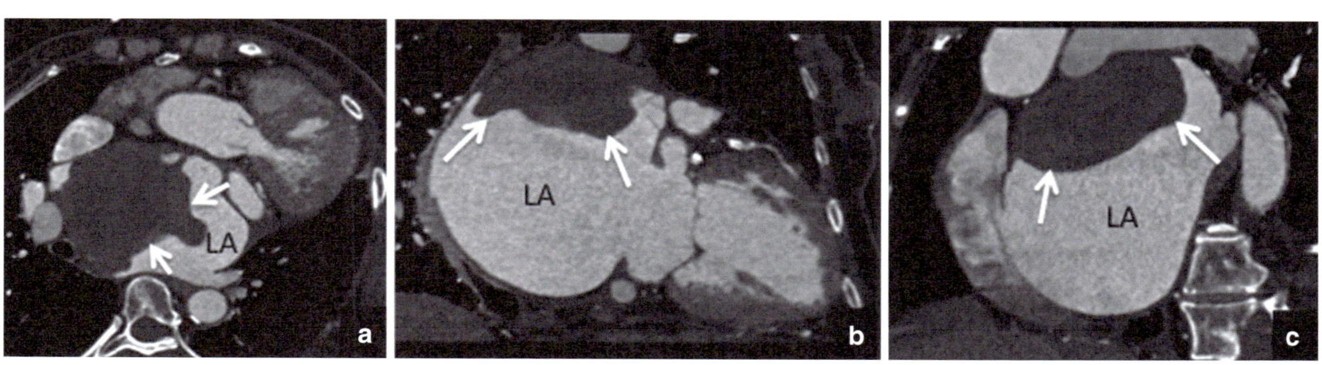

Fig. 34.4 Cardiac CT in a 65-year-old woman after heart transplantation with the biatrial technique. (**a**) Axial image. (**b**) Two-chamber view. (**c**) Short-axis view. The exam showed a large intracavitary thrombus within the left atrium (LA, arrows)

provides most of right-side cardiac output, and the donor left ventricle delivers the majority of left-side cardiac output [6]. Complications of this surgical technique include native heart angina, ventricular fibrillation, and thromboembolic events [11]. Graft stenosis is a frequent complication when grafts are interposed between the recipient and donor pulmonary arteries and may lead to pulmonary hypertension [10].

Cardiac Allograft Vasculopathy

Cardiac allograft vasculopathy (CAV) is a progressive fibroproliferative process that extensively affects the coronary arteries of a transplanted heart and is likely the consequence of cumulative endothelial injuries [12]. As said, this entity is responsible for a significant proportion of deaths after transplant. According to recent ISHLT data, the prevalence of CAV remains high: 20% at 3 years, 30% at 5 years, and 45% at 8 years after transplant. The disease is present in approximately 54% of survivors 10 years after heart transplantation [1].

Risk factors of CAV development depend on donor and recipient characteristics. Donor characteristics include old donor age, male sex, high body surface area, history of hypertension, history of infection, and cause of death, whereas recipient characteristics related with CAV comprise history of ischemic heart disease, ventricular assist device implant before transplant, and history of infection [1]. Other factors, such as the number of HLA-DR mismatches and the use of certain type of immunosuppression before discharge, also increase the risk of CAV.

The pathophysiology of CAV entails endothelial dysfunction and vascular injury. Adaptive and innate immune responses, alloantigen-independent factors, and endothelial replacement in the transplanted heart have been suggested to play a role in the pathophysiology of the disease [12]. Persistent inflammatory response results in concentric intimal hyperplasia causing diffuse luminal narrowing of the coronary vasculature. This will ultimately lead to myocardial ischemia and ventricular dysfunction.

Pathophysiological similarities and differences between CAV and atherosclerosis are reviewed by Rahmani et al. [13]. As opposed to conventional atherosclerotic disease, CAV typically affects distal segments and progresses to proximal segments. Vessel involvement is concentric, longitudinal, and diffuse. Collateral vasculature is generally absent. In contrast, conventional atherosclerosis usually involves the proximal coronary segments and progresses distally. Atherosclerotic plaques are commonly focal and noncircumferential and show calcification more frequently than CAV. Thus, early after heart transplantation, focal and noncircumferential thickening may be observed, usually transmitted by the donor and representing conventional atherosclerotic disease (Fig. 34.5). Late after transplant, however, focal atherosclerotic plaques and/or diffuse intimal thickening may be seen representing CAV (Fig. 34.6).

As mentioned, CAV is one of the main factors that will influence the prognosis and long-term survival after heart transplantation. Thus, early detection of the disease becomes mandatory [14]. This is generally performed using diverse imaging modalities.

Diagnosis of Cardiac Allograft Vasculopathy

According to the ISHLT guidelines for the care of heart transplant recipients, annual or biannual coronary angiography should be considered to assess the development of CAV. Patients free of CAV at 3–5 years after heart transplantation, especially those with renal insufficiency, may undergo less frequent invasive evaluation (recommendation Class I, Level of Evidence: C) [15]. Recommendations for the use of imaging modalities for the diagnosis and management of CAV are shown in Table 34.1.

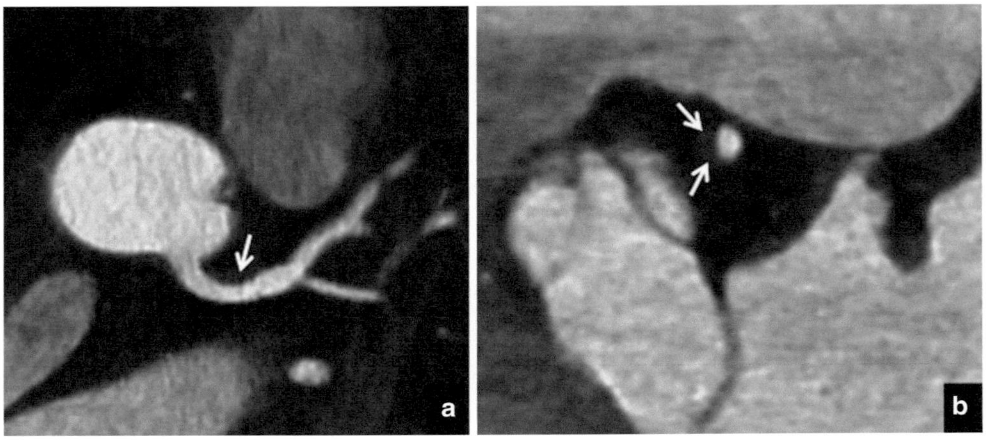

Fig. 34.5 Coronary CT angiography in a 64-year-old man 2 years after heart transplantation. (**a**) Axial image. (**b**) Perpendicular cross-sectional image. The study demonstrated a non-calcified plaque in the left main coronary vessel (arrow). Note that the plaque is focal, eccentric, and non-circumferential (arrows in **b**), likely representing atherosclerotic disease transmitted by the donor

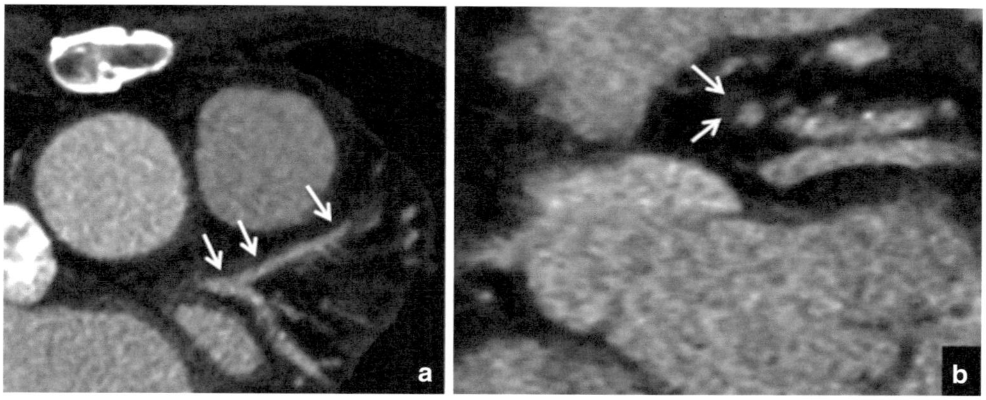

Fig. 34.6 Coronary CT angiography in a 75-year-old asymptomatic man 12 years after heart transplantation. (**a**) Axial image. (**b**) Perpendicular cross-sectional image. Note the almost concentric, longitudinal, and diffuse involvement of the left anterior descending coronary artery caused by cardiac allograft vasculopathy (arrows)

Table 34.1 Recommendations for the diagnosis and management of cardiac allograft vasculopathy (CAV) according to the International Society for Heart and Lung Transplantation (ISHLT) guidelines for the care of heart transplant (HT) recipients

Class I
Annual or biannual coronary angiography should be considered to assess the development of CAV. Patients free of CAV at 3 to 5 years after HT, especially those with renal insufficiency, may undergo less frequent invasive evaluation *(Level of Evidence: C)*
Selective coronary angiography is the investigation of choice for the diagnosis of CAV in pediatric HT recipients. It should be performed at yearly or biannual intervals *(Level of Evidence: C)*
Class IIa
A baseline coronary angiogram at 4 to 6 weeks after HT may be considered to exclude donor coronary artery disease *(Level of Evidence: C)*
Intravascular ultrasound (IVUS) in conjunction with coronary angiography with a baseline study at 4 to 6 weeks and at 1 year after HT is an option to exclude donor coronary artery disease, to detect rapidly progressive CAV, and to provide prognostic information *(Level of Evidence: B)*
IVUS can be safely used in older pediatric HT recipients to assess CAV *(Level of Evidence: C)*
Evaluation of coronary flow reserve in conjunction with coronary angiography may be useful for the detection of small-vessel coronary disease, which is a manifestation of CAV *(Level of Evidence: C)*
Treadmill or dobutamine stress echocardiography and myocardial perfusion imaging may all be useful for the detection of CAV in HT recipients unable to undergo invasive evaluation. Noninvasive testing for CAV is technically possible in children *(Level of Evidence: B)*
Class IIb
Ultrafast computed tomography (CT) for the detection of coronary calcium has been used mostly as an investigational tool for assessing CAV in HT recipients but is being superseded by advances in CT angiography *(Level of Evidence: C)*
CT coronary angiography shows promise in the evaluation of CAV in HT recipients, although higher resting heart rates in these patients limit the technical quality of this study *(Level of Evidence: C)*

Modified from Costanzo et al. [15], with permission

Conventional Coronary Angiography

Conventional coronary angiography remains the standard of care for the screening and surveillance of CAV. Recent data show that angiographic findings are able to guide management and possess prognostic significance for graft survival, patient survival, and adverse cardiac events [16]. However, there is concern about the limited sensitivity of conventional coronary angiography for the detection of early stage CAV and about its accuracy to establish the presence and extent of the disease, particularly when compared with intravascular ultrasound (IVUS) [17, 18], optical coherence tomography (OCT) [19, 20], and histopathologic studies [21]. As a major limitation, conventional coronary angiography does not allow to evaluate the arterial wall and to detect early intimal thickening. Thus, this technique can underdiagnose the prevalence as well as the extent of CAV.

IVUS

Due to its ability to define arterial wall layers and to provide accurate quantitative assessment of lumen size, intimal thickening, and vessel wall morphology and composition, IVUS is the most sensitive tool to detect CAV [22, 23]. There are, however, several limitations of this technique that have impeded routine use of IVUS for the surveillance of CAV during regular follow-up of heart transplant recipients, including its high cost, lack of widespread expertise, the relatively large size of currently available IVUS catheters, and the complication rate of multivessel imaging. Similarly, the potential role of OCT in heart transplant recipients, an intravascular imaging technique able to provide detailed information of vessel wall composition, is under active research [24].

Noninvasive Stress Testing

Because of the reduced exercise capacity of heart transplant recipients and the blunted heart rate response to exercise, the accuracy of exercise stress tests for detection of CAV is limited [25].

Imaging modalities performed under pharmacological stress show improved performance. Overall, sensitivity and negative predictive values of noninvasive stress tests are high, whereas their specificity and positive predictive values are low. Therefore, these tests can be employed to rule out significant CAV, and, consequently, some authors recommend their use to avoid the need of annual conventional coronary angiography for surveillance.

In the case of dobutamine stress echocardiography, its sensitivity and specificity to detect CAV range from 65% to 95% and from 55% to 95% when compared to conventional coronary angiography [26, 27] and from 72% to 79% and from 83% to 88% when compared to IVUS [28, 29]. Mastrobuoni et al. showed that coronary CT angiography (CCTA) was able to demonstrate evidence of CAV despite normal dobutamine stress echocardiography [30].

Regarding stress radionuclide myocardial perfusion imaging, Ciliberto et al. showed sensitivity of 92% and specificity of 86% of dipyridamole technetium-99m sestamibi SPECT to detect CAV manifested as angiographic focal stenosis greater than 50% or diffuse disease. The sensitivity dropped to 56% when the technique was used to detect angiographic abnormalities of any grade [31]. Several studies have shown similar sensitivity and specificity values with dobutamine and dipyridamole, despite the fact that according to some authors, the effect of dipyridamole may be limited under microvascular CAV [32].

Less is known about the usefulness of cardiac magnetic resonance (CMR) in the setting of CAV. CMR provides accurate measurements of left and right ventricular volumes, ejection fraction, and mass. Further, late gadolinium-enhanced images [33, 34] and recently developed multiparametric T1 and T2 mapping techniques allow to establish and quantify changes in the myocardial tissue architecture [35–37]. In the field of stress perfusion CMR imaging, studies performed under adenosine demonstrated reduced myocardial blood flow in patients with CAV [38]. In a recent study, Miller et al. demonstrated that CAV, including epicardial and microvascular components, could be detected more accurately using noninvasive CMR-based absolute myocardial blood flow assessment than with conventional coronary angiography [39]. In another study, Chih et al. showed that CMR-derived myocardial perfusion reserve (MPR) index ≤ 1.68 had sensitivity, specificity, negative, and positive predictive values of 100%, 63%, 100%, and 86%, respectively, to detect CAV defined as maximal intimal thickness > 0.5 mm by IVUS of the left anterior descending artery [40].

Coronary CT Angiography and Cardiac Allograft Vasculopathy

Coronary CT angiography (CCTA) has been investigated as a noninvasive alternative to conventional coronary angiography to evaluate coronary artery vasculature and to detect CAV in heart transplant recipients. Being noninvasive, one of the key advantages of this technique is that it provides information about the coronary artery lumen and wall.

Technical Aspects

Despite advances in CT technology and spatial and temporal resolution, heart transplant recipients still represent a challenge for noninvasive coronary artery imaging with CT [41]. The anatomical detail achieved with state-of-the-art technology allows to reliably exclude significant coronary disease involving proximal and mid-coronary segments, but the spatial resolution still remains limited to accurately detect CAV involving more distal and smaller caliber coronary segments.

Another concerning aspect is the temporal resolution of CT systems and the high resting heart rates and the insufficient response to beta-blocker premedication of heart transplant recipients. After heart transplantation there is impairment of the sympathetic and parasympathetic innervations of the graft. As a consequence, patient resting heart rate is high (mean resting heart rates up to 89 beats per minute) [42], and they do not fully respond to different stimuli, such as chronotropic and inotropic medication, including beta-blockers [43–45]. Therefore, the temporal resolution of even 64-multidetector CT scanners with a 0.33-second rotation time remains insufficient to accurately evaluate the coronary vasculature in this patient population, and more advanced CT systems with faster gantry rotation times are required. Dual-source CT systems have shown to provide good image quality of the coronary vasculature in heart transplant recipients [42, 46–48] (Fig. 34.7).

One interesting feature of heart transplant recipients is their low heart rate variability. This allows to optimize cardiac CT acquisition protocols to fully adjust the radiation dose. In this sense, prospectively ECG-triggered protocols may represent a valid alternative to conventional retrospectively ECG-gated acquisition methods [49]. According to recent publications, the mean radiation dose reported for prospectively ECG-triggered CCTA in heart transplant recipients is significantly lower (mean of 4.5 mSv) [46] than the radiation dose reported for the conventional retrospectively ECG-gated acquisition mode (mean of 10.2 mSv) [50]. Of note, triggering the acquisition during the systolic phase of the cardiac cycle has been advocated for the prospective acquisition protocols (Fig. 34.8). Its rationale is based on the observation that the systolic phase has demonstrated to be the optimal reconstruction phase for conventional retrospectively ECG-gated coronary DSCT examinations performed in subjects with high resting heart rates [51] and also in heart transplant recipients [42].

Finally, regarding the use of iodinated intravenous contrast during CCTA acquisition, it is important to note that chronic kidney disease is a common comorbidity in heart transplant recipients. Thus, the amount of contrast should be adjusted to patient weight and scan duration. In most cases, the use of 60 or 70 mL of iodinated contrast should be sufficient to achieve adequate filling of the coronary vasculature.

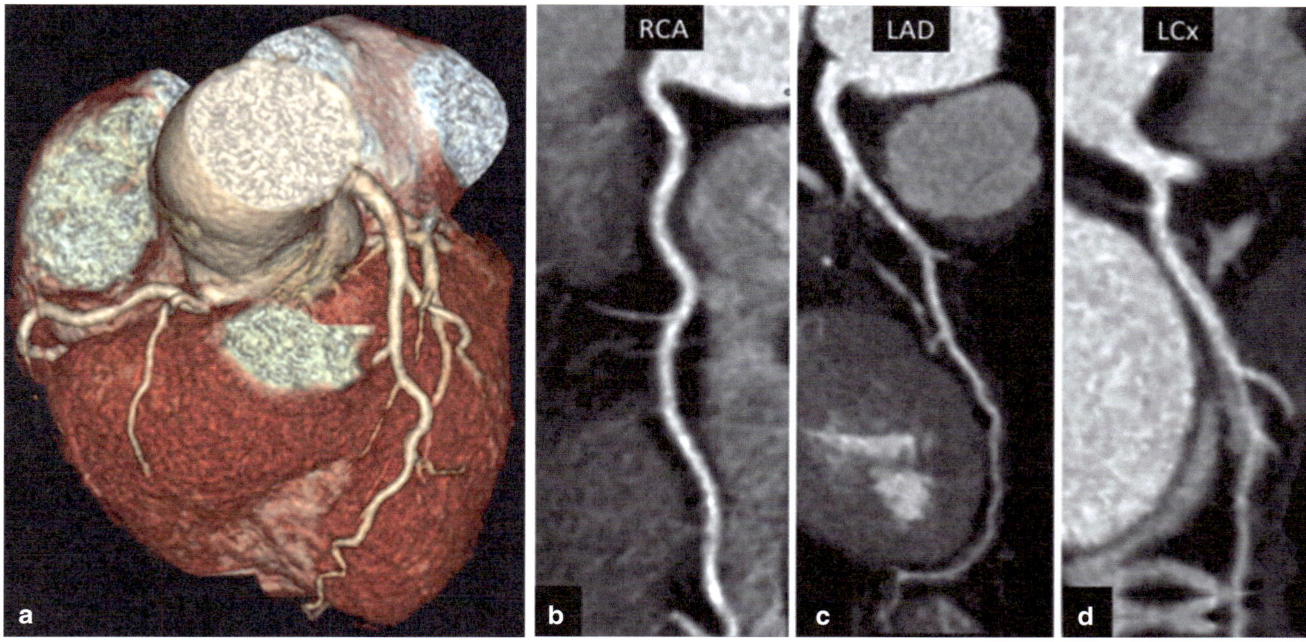

Fig. 34.7 Retrospectively ECG-gated coronary CT angiography in a 63-year-old patient who underwent heart transplantation 5 years earlier. (**a**) Volume-rendered image. (**b–d**) Curved planar reformats of the right coronary artery (RCA), left anterior descending (LAD), and left circumflex (LCx) coronary arteries. The study showed normal coronary arteries, excluding cardiac allograft vasculopathy

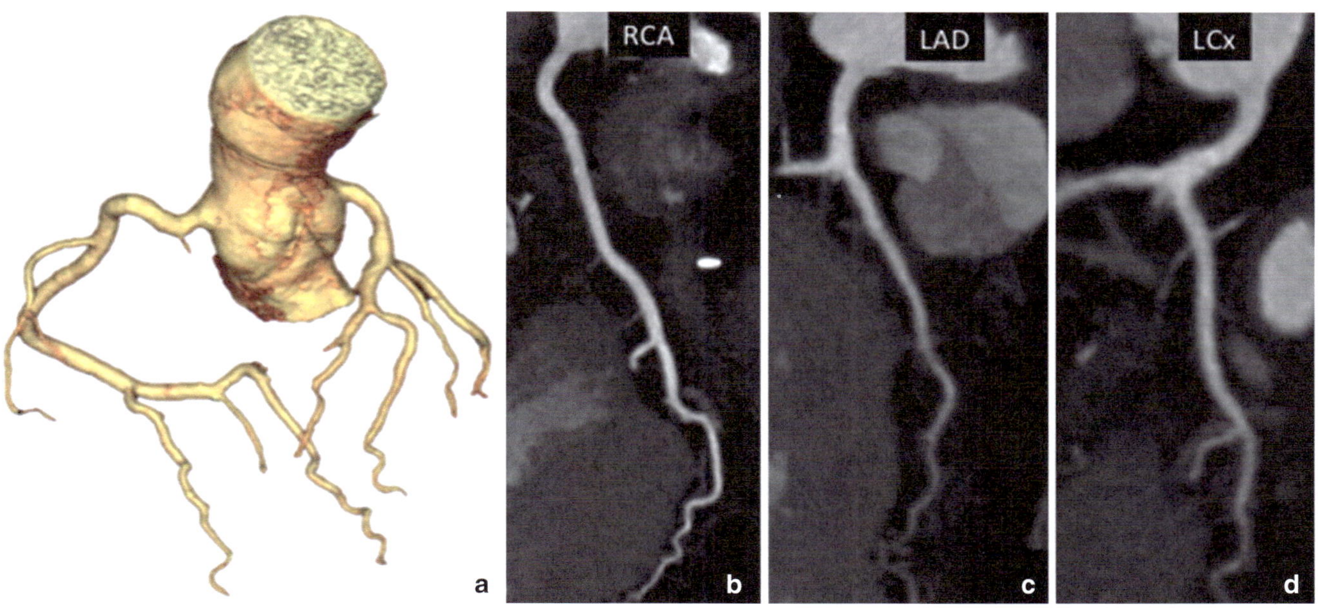

Fig. 34.8 Prospectively ECG-triggered coronary CT angiography in a 56-year-old heart transplant recipient. (**a**) Volume-rendered image. (**b–d**) Curved planar reformats of the right coronary artery (RCA), left anterior descending (LAD), and left circumflex (LCx) coronary arteries. Despite a high resting heart rate (mean of 81 beats per minute) in this patient, the acquisition was prospectively ECG-triggered in systole (35–45% of the R-R´ interval). The exam allowed to reliably exclude cardiac allograft vasculopathy

Detection of Cardiac Allograft Vasculopathy with CCTA

According to the most recent ISHLT guidelines for the care of heart transplant recipients, "CT coronary angiography shows promise in the evaluation of CAV in heart transplant recipients, although higher resting heart rates in these patients limit the technical quality of this study (Class IIb recommendation, *Level of Evidence: C*)." Most recent appropriate use criteria for cardiac computed tomography endorsed by the American College of Cardiology Foundation along with key specialty and subspecialty societies rate as uncertain (score of 6) the routine evaluation of coronary arteries by CCTA following heart transplantation [52].

Coronary Artery Calcification

There is controversy regarding the clinical value of CT-quantified coronary artery calcification as a marker of CAV. In a past publication, Ludman et al. reported that calcium is detected more frequently with CT than would be suggested by studies using intravascular ultrasound [53]. These authors observed that coronary calcium was associated with the presence of angiographic disease and concluded that at follow-up the presence of coronary calcium was associated with an adverse clinical outcome [53]. More recently, after evaluating 161 heart transplant recipients, von Ziegler et al. determined that calcium scoring with dual-source CT is not a valuable noninvasive modality for CAV detection. In fact, these authors suggested that calcium may represent preexisting or de novo traditional coronary atherosclerosis rather than CAV [54].

Coronary CTA Angiography Versus Conventional Coronary Angiography

The potential of CCTA for detecting CAV has been investigated with different generation CT systems. Results of representative studies comparing the diagnostic accuracy of CCTA for the detection of CAV with respect to conventional coronary angiography are shown in Table 34.2 [44, 45, 48, 50, 55–60].

In 2005, Romeo et al. sought to determine if CCTA performed with a 16-row multidetector CT scanner could represent a valid noninvasive alternative to conventional coronary angiography for serial detection and follow-up of coronary stenosis due to CAV [44]. For their study purpose, authors included 50 consecutive heart transplant patients who underwent CCTA within 24 h before or after their annual routine conventional coronary angiography examination. Authors found sensitivity of 83%, specificity of 95%, positive predictive value of 71%, negative predictive value of 95%, and accuracy of 93% for detection of coronary stenosis greater than 50%. They concluded that 16-slice multidetector CT can replace the invasive procedure in de novo heart transplant patients and in patients with strictly normal CCTA at follow-up [44].

In their study, Mittal et al. evaluated the largest heart transplant population published to date with CT [48]. They included 138 heart transplant recipients scheduled for routine conventional coronary angiography who prospectively underwent CT to evaluate coronary artery calcification and retrospectively ECG-gated CCTA with a 64-section scanner to assess vessel status. At the patient level, authors observed that CCTA had an area under the receiver operating characteristic curve of 0.942. Sensitivity, specificity, and positive and negative predictive values of CCTA to detect CAV with 50% or more stenosis were of 96%, 93%, 72%, and 99%, respectively. Interestingly, authors found that none of the 61 patients with normal CCTA angiographic results had CAV on the basis of the invasive procedure, concluding that CCTA compares favorably with conventional coronary angiography in detecting CAV in this patient population and that it may be used as a screening technique [48].

Using a more recent generation dual-source CT scanner, von Ziegler et al. found similar results [59]. In 46 heart transplant recipients undergoing CCTA, authors observed sensitivity of 100%, specificity of 86%, and diagnostic accuracy of 93% on a patient-based evaluation for detection of significant stenosis. Authors concluded that improved image acquisition and robustness of this CT technology allowed to exclude a low number of coronary segments, and, therefore, it could be employed to reliably rule out CAV in heart transplant recipients, avoiding unnecessary conventional coronary angiography for annual follow-up [59].

In a systematic review of the literature performed to determine the accuracy of CCTA in CAV assessment, Khan et al. included three studies performed using 16-row multidetector CT and four studies using 64-row multidetector CT. Per-

Table 34.2 Patient-based diagnostic accuracy of coronary CT angiography for the detection of hemodynamically significant coronary stenosis compared with conventional coronary angiography

CT-system	Author	Number of patients	Sensitivity (%)	Specificity (%)	Positive predictive value (%)	Negative predictive value (%)
MDCT-16	Romeo et al. [44]	50	83	95	71	95
	Sigurdsson et al. [45]	54	94	79	65	97
	Moro et al. [55]	22	50	81	50	81
	Pichler et al. [56]	60	88	97	88	97
MDCT-64	Iyengar et al. [57]	19	100	94	50	100
	von Ziegler et al. [58]	26	100	81	56	100
	Mittal et al. [48]	138	96	78	77	98
DSCT	Schepis et al. [50]	30	93	93	72	99
	von Ziegler et al. [59]	46	100	86	33	100
	Kepka et al. [60]	20	100	94	67	100

Note: *MDCT* multidetector computed tomography, *DSCT* dual-source computed tomography segment analysis revealed pooled estimates for sensitivity, specificity, and negative predictive value for CT ranging from 82% to 89%, 89% to 99%, and 99%, respectively [61].

A recent meta-analysis evaluated the diagnostic accuracy of CCTA for detecting CAV in comparison with conventional coronary angiography, with similar conclusions [62]. After analyzing 13 studies including 615 patients, the patient-based analysis showed mean weighted sensitivity of 97%, specificity of 81%, positive predictive value of 78%, and negative predictive value of 97% for detection of any CAV and mean weighted sensitivity of 94%, specificity of 92%, positive predictive value of 67%, and negative predictive value of 99% for detection of significant CAV (stenosis ≥50%) [62]. Authors concluded that CCTA is a reliable noninvasive imaging alternative to conventional coronary angiography to detect CAV [62].

The outcome of heart transplant recipients using CCTA for serial follow-up was investigated by Rohnean et al. [63]. These authors prospectively enrolled 62 individuals undergoing yearly CCTA for coronary allograft vasculopathy detection. According to their observations, time to stenosis was consistently greater than 3 years, and the mean interval without de novo significant stenosis was 10.31+/−4 years. With these results, authors concluded that CCTA seems to be a safe technique for monitoring heart transplant patients and suggested a follow-up every 2 years with CCTA in patients with normal baseline exams [63].

Coronary CTA Angiography Versus Intravascular Ultrasound

As said, IVUS is the standard of reference to evaluate the vessel wall. As CCTA also allows to assess vessel wall composition, this technique may play a role in the early diagnosis of CAV. Three representative studies have compared the diagnostic accuracy of the latter with respect to IVUS [43, 45, 50] (Table 34.3).

A subset of 54 heart transplant recipients enrolled by Sigurdsson et al. were evaluated with CCTA, conventional coronary angiography, and IVUS [45]. Authors were able to assess a total of 154 coronary segments in 13 individuals. The sensitivity, specificity, and positive and negative predictive values to identify proliferative changes by CCTA with respect to IVUS were 96%, 88%, 80%, and 98%, respectively [45].

In their study, Gregory et al. reported a sensitivity of 70%, specificity of 92%, positive predictive value of 89%, and negative predictive value of 77% for the detection of CAV with CCTA with respect to IVUS, concluding that CCTA has moderate to excellent test characteristics for the detection of CAV [43].

In a third study, Schepis et al. found sensitivity of 85%, specificity of 84%, positive predictive value of 76%, and negative predictive value of 91% for the detection of CAV by DSCT with respect to IVUS [50].

Finally, in a recent meta-analysis, Wever-Pinzon et al. found a mean weighted sensitivity of 81% and specificity of 75% to detect CAV by CCTA compared to IVUS [62].

Therefore, according to most recent literature, CCTA seems to be a robust, reliable, and accurate technique for the diagnosis of CAV (Fig. 34.9). In particular, as in the field of non-transplanted population, CCTA possesses a very high negative predictive value. This allows to reliably exclude CAV in heart transplant patients. As a result, CCTA could be considered as an alternative to conventional coronary angiography in the routine surveillance of heart transplant recipients.

Cardiac Function

The management and follow-up of heart transplant recipients require accurate quantification of ventricular volumes, function, and mass [64]. Evaluation of these parameters is routinely performed with transthoracic echocardiography, although limited acoustic window, postsurgical changes, and elevated body mass indices of heart transplant recipients may represent a limitation to this imaging modality. Further, the limited interobserver reproducibility of echocardiography is well known [65–67]. The reference standard to assess ventricular morphology, volumes, and function is magnetic resonance imaging (MRI) [68–71].

As stated, cardiac CT may be used as an alternative to conventional coronary angiography to detect CAV. Interestingly, when patients are examined with the retrospectively ECG-gated technique, additional reconstructions including all phases of the cardiac cycle provide the ability to evaluate ventricular morphology and function without the need of further acquisitions. Its value in heart transplant patients has been

Table 34.3 Diagnostic accuracy of coronary CT angiography for the detection of hemodynamically significant coronary stenosis compared with intravascular ultrasound (IVUS)

CT-system	Author	Number of patients	Sensitivity (%)	Specificity (%)	Positive predictive value (%)	Negative predictive value (%)
MDCT-16	Sigurdsson et al. [45]	13	96	88	80	98
MDCT-64	Gregory et al. [43]	20	70	92	89	77
DSCT	Schepis et al. [50]	30	85	84	76	91

Note: *MDCT* multidetector computed tomography, *DSCT* dual-source computed tomography

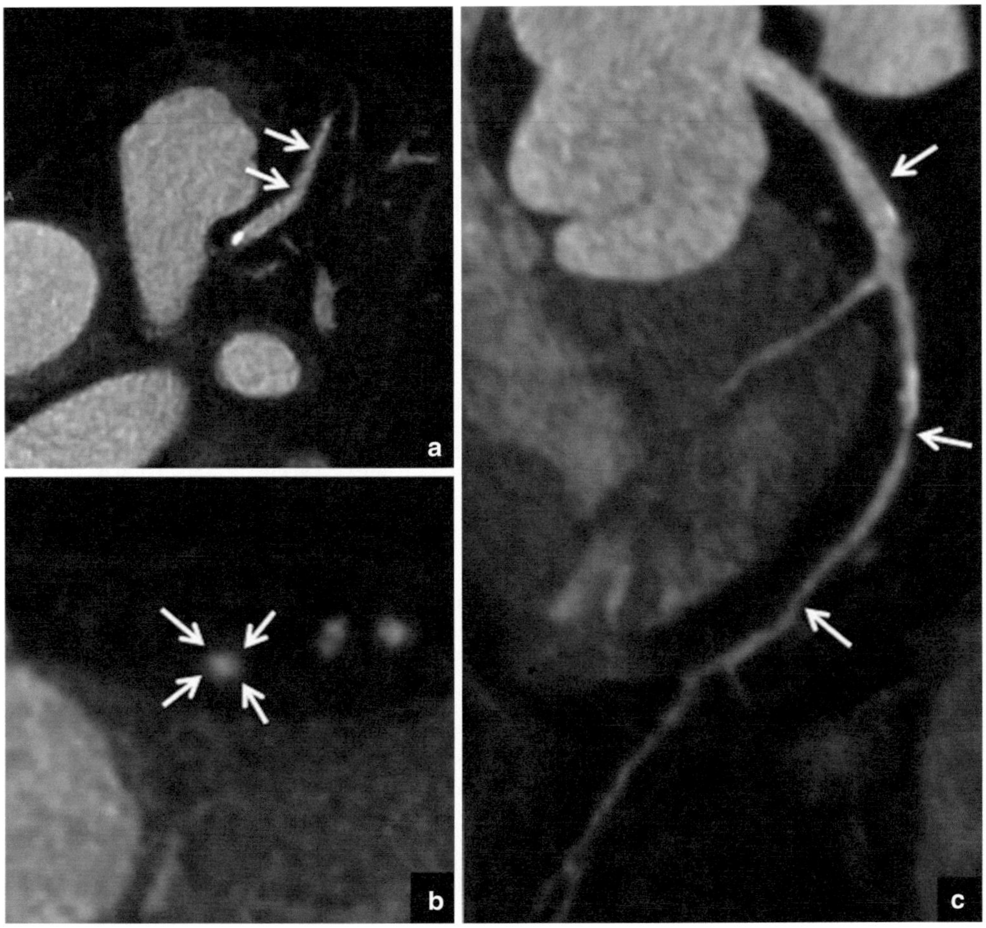

Fig. 34.9 Coronary CT angiography in a 59-year-old asymptomatic patient 15 years after heart transplantation. (**a**) Axial image. (**b**) Perpendicular cross-sectional image. (**c**) Curved planar reformat. The exam demonstrated longitudinal and diffuse involvement of the left anterior descending coronary artery along its course by cardiac allograft vasculopathy (arrows in **a** and **c**). Note the concentric appearance of the disease (arrows in **b**)

shown with 64-row multidetector CT scanners [72], as well as with dual-source CT technology [73, 74] (Fig. 34.10). Usefulness of CT to assess left atrial function in heart transplant recipients has also been demonstrated [75]. According to the results, agreement between echocardiography, CT, and MRI-derived calculations for the assessment of cardiac structure and function seems to be between acceptable limits, suggesting the CT imaging may be used to assess atrial and ventricular parameters in heart transplant recipients.

Transplant-Related Ancillary Findings on Cardiac CT

Cardiac allograft vasculopathy is one of the four major causes of death after heart transplantation. In the first year after transplant, most deaths are related to acute rejection or infection, whereas malignancy is the second most common long-term cause of mortality in heart transplant recipients, likely related to immunosuppression. The carcinogenic consequences of long-term immunosuppression in transplant recipients are well known [76]. In the case of heart transplant patients, skin cancer, solid-organ cancers including gastrointestinal, lung cancer, oral cavity/oropharyngeal cancer, and urologic cancers, as well as hematologic malignancies, such as non-Hodgkin lymphoma, have been described [77].

In general practice, small field-of-view reconstructions limited to the heart are employed to evaluate the coronary vasculature and the cardiac structures. There is discrepancy about the benefit of increasing the field of view to encompass the entire chest and the upper abdomen so as to search for extracardiac findings [78–83]. Of course, the prevalence of extracardiac findings in cardiac CT is directly related to patient's age, clinical symptoms, and risk factors. In non-transplanted patients undergoing CCTA, a variable prevalence of extracardiac findings ranging from 15% to 67% has been reported [84, 85]. Most of these findings do not require further action, whereas occasionally clinically relevant entities are found [86]. Given the relatively high incidence of transplant-related complications that may affect patient survival and the role of CT in their detection and management, full field-of-view reconstructions may be particularly beneficial in this patient population (Fig. 34.11).

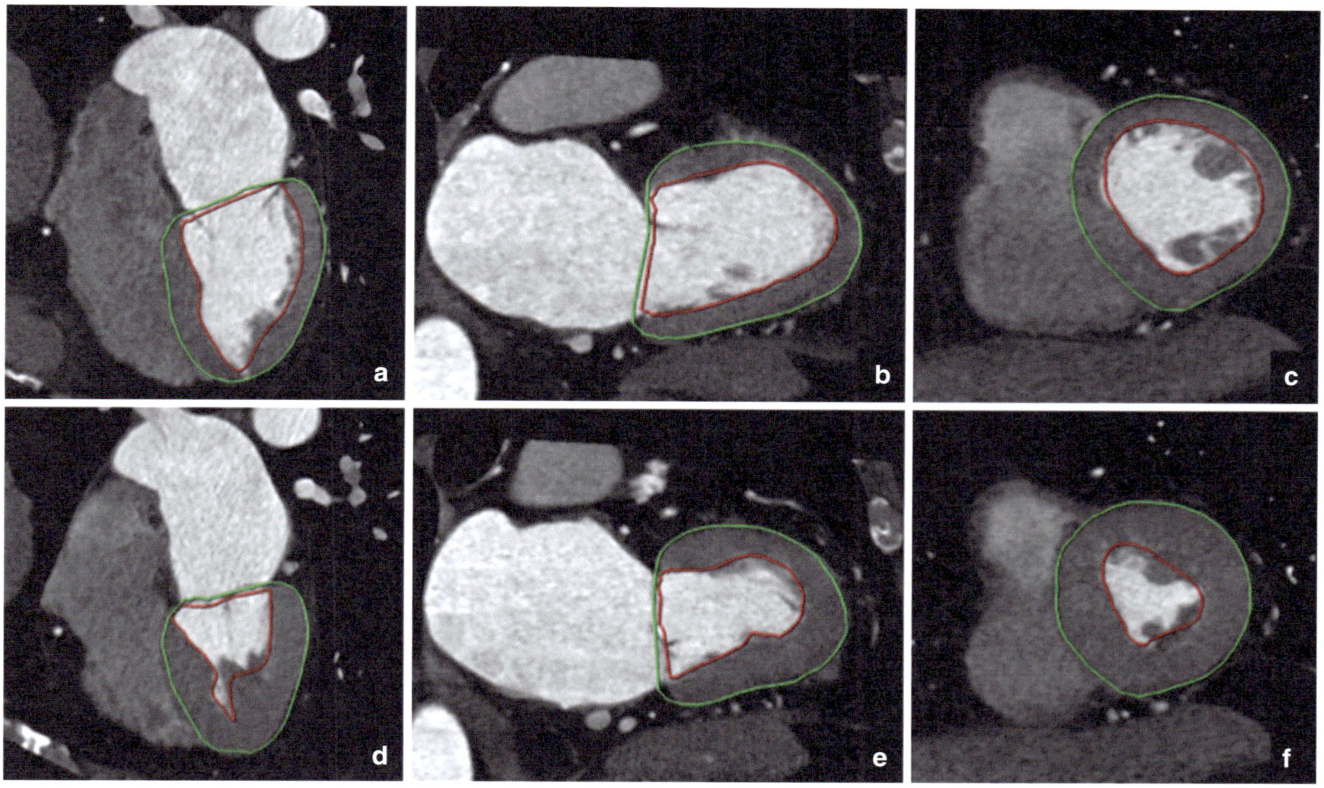

Fig. 34.10 Cardiac CT in a 62-year-old heart transplant recipient. (**a**, **d**) Four-chamber view. (**b**, **e**) Two-chamber view. (**c**, **f**) Short-axis view. (**a**–**c**) Diastole. (**d**–**f**) Systole. Retrospectively ECG-gated cardiac CT protocols allow to assess cardiac function parameters without additional data acquisition. Software solutions automatically generate endocardial (red) and epicardial (green) left ventricular contours to provide left ventricular volumes, ejection fraction, and mass

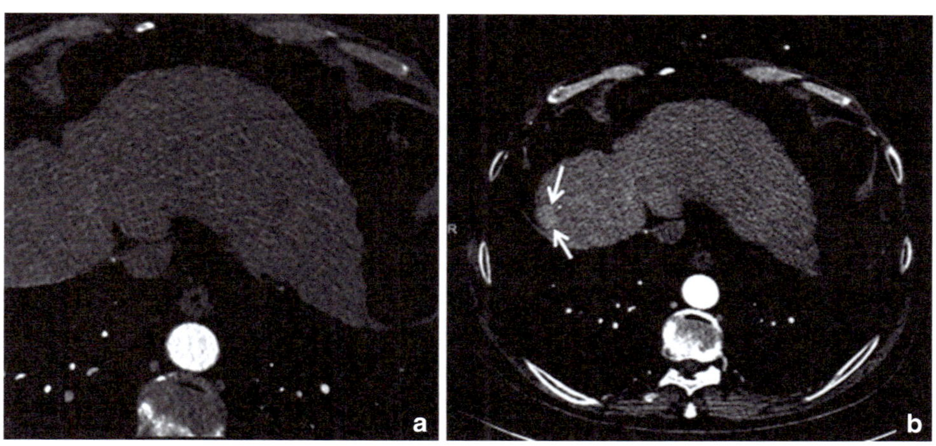

Fig. 34.11 Cardiac CT in 68-year-old patient with heart transplantation 21 years earlier. (**a**) Small field-of-view reconstruction. (**b**) Full field-of-view reconstruction. Small field-of-view reconstructions limited to the heart showed nodular hepatic contours as well as hypertrophy of the left lobe of the liver. These findings were confirmed in full field-of-view reconstructions, which also allowed to depict an arterially hyperenhancing lesion in the right lobe consistent with hepatocellular carcinoma in the setting of cirrhosis

Conclusion

Cardiac transplantation is the treatment of choice for patients with end-stage heart failure. Long-term prognosis and survival after heart transplantation is related to cardiac allograft vasculopathy, renal failure, and malignancy. Cardiac CT, particularly using latest generation equipment, is a unique imaging modality that allows to assess posttransplant anatomy and to detect early and late complications related to the procedure. Coronary artery lumen and wall are now viewed and analyzed with unprecedented anatomical detail, whereas specific CT acquisition modes also enable to evaluate cardiac morphologic and functional parameters in good agreement with established imaging modalities. Although conventional coronary angiography remains the reference standard for the diagnosis of CAV, the results of most recent studies and meta-analysis suggest that CCTA could be considered as an alternative to conventional coronary angiography in the routine surveillance of heart transplant recipients. Still, further research is warranted to determine the impact of this imaging technology in the management and clinical outcomes of this patient population.

References

1. Stehlik J, Edwards LB, Kucheryavaya AY, Benden C, Christie JD, Dobbels F, et al. The registry of the International Society for Heart and Lung Transplantation: twenty-eighth adult heart transplant report – 2011. J Heart Lung Transplant. 2011;30(10):1078–94.
2. Shumway NE, Lower RR, Stofer RC. Transplantation of the heart. Adv Surg. 1966;2:265–84.
3. Dreyfus G, Jebara V, Mihaileanu S, Carpentier AF. Total orthotopic heart transplantation: an alternative to the standard technique. Ann Thorac Surg. 1991;52(5):1181–4.
4. Sievers HH, Weyand M, Kraatz EG, Bernhard A. An alternative technique for orthotopic cardiac transplantation, with preservation of the normal anatomy of the right atrium. Thorac Cardiovasc Surg. 1991;39(2):70–2.
5. Weiss ES, Nwakanma LU, Russell SB, Conte JV, Shah AS. Outcomes in bicaval versus biatrial techniques in heart transplantation: an analysis of the UNOS database. J Heart Lung Transplant. 2008;27(2):178–83.
6. Knisely BL, Mastey LA, Collins J, Kuhlman JE. Imaging of cardiac transplantation complications. Radiographics. 1999;19(2):321–39; discussion 40–1
7. Triposkiadis F, Starling RC, Haas GJ, Sparks E, Myerowitz PD, Boudoulas H. Timing of recipient atrial contraction: a major determinant of transmitral diastolic flow in orthotopic cardiac transplantation. Am Heart J. 1993;126(5):1175–81.
8. Stevenson LW, Dadourian BJ, Kobashigawa J, Child JS, Clark SH, Laks H. Mitral regurgitation after cardiac transplantation. Am J Cardiol. 1987;60(1):119–22.
9. Gorcsan J 3rd, Snow FR, Paulsen W, Arrowood JA, Thompson JA, Nixon JV. Echocardiographic profile of the transplanted human heart in clinically well recipients. J Heart Lung Transplant. 1992;11(1 Pt 1):80–9.
10. Lai HY, Chen JH, Chiu KM, Wang KL, Cheung WK, Li AH, et al. CT of two hearts beating in one chest. AJR Am J Roentgenol. 2008;191(6):1711–6.
11. Roux C, Varnous S, Leprince P, Cluzel P. Two hearts, one soul: heterotopic heart transplantation follow-up with cardiac computed tomography. Eur Heart J. 2016;37:3356.
12. Schmauss D, Weis M. Cardiac allograft vasculopathy: recent developments. Circulation. 2008;117(16):2131–41.
13. Rahmani M, Cruz RP, Granville DJ, McManus BM. Allograft vasculopathy versus atherosclerosis. Circ Res. 2006;99(8):801–15.
14. Lamich R, Ballester M, Marti V, Brossa V, Aymat R, Carrio I, et al. Efficacy of augmented immunosuppressive therapy for early vasculopathy in heart transplantation. J Am Coll Cardiol. 1998;32(2):413–9.
15. Costanzo MR, Dipchand A, Starling R, Anderson A, Chan M, Desai S, et al. The International Society of Heart and Lung Transplantation Guidelines for the care of heart transplant recipients. J Heart Lung Transplant. 2010;29(8):914–56.
16. Mehra MR, Crespo-Leiro MG, Dipchand A, Ensminger SM, Hiemann NE, Kobashigawa JA, et al. International Society for Heart and Lung Transplantation working formulation of a standardized nomenclature for cardiac allograft vasculopathy-2010. J Heart Lung Transplant. 2010;29(7):717–27.
17. St Goar FG, Pinto FJ, Alderman EL, Valantine HA, Schroeder JS, Gao SZ, et al. Intracoronary ultrasound in cardiac transplant recipients. In vivo evidence of "angiographically silent" intimal thickening. Circulation. 1992;85(3):979–87.
18. Spes CH, Klauss V, Rieber J, Schnaack SD, Tammen AR, Uberfuhr P, et al. Functional and morphological findings in heart transplant recipients with a normal coronary angiogram: an analysis by dobutamine stress echocardiography, intracoronary Doppler and intravascular ultrasound. J Heart Lung Transplant. 1999;18(5):391–8.
19. Khandhar SJ, Yamamoto H, Teuteberg JJ, Shullo MA, Bezerra HG, Costa MA, et al. Optical coherence tomography for characterization of cardiac allograft vasculopathy after heart transplantation (OCTCAV study). J Heart Lung Transplant. 2013;32(6):596–602.
20. Hou J, Lv H, Jia H, Zhang S, Xing L, Liu H, et al. OCT assessment of allograft vasculopathy in heart transplant recipients. JACC Cardiovasc Imaging. 2012;5(6):662–3.
21. Johnson DE, Alderman EL, Schroeder JS, Gao SZ, Hunt S, DeCampli WM, et al. Transplant coronary artery disease: histopathologic correlations with angiographic morphology. J Am Coll Cardiol. 1991;17(2):449–57.
22. Rickenbacher PR, Pinto FJ, Chenzbraun A, Botas J, Lewis NP, Alderman EL, et al. Incidence and severity of transplant coronary artery disease early and up to 15 years after transplantation as detected by intravascular ultrasound. J Am Coll Cardiol. 1995;25(1):171–7.
23. Tsutsui H, Ziada KM, Schoenhagen P, Iyisoy A, Magyar WA, Crowe TD, et al. Lumen loss in transplant coronary artery disease is a biphasic process involving early intimal thickening and late constrictive remodeling: results from a 5-year serial intravascular ultrasound study. Circulation. 2001;104(6):653–7.
24. Shan P, Dong L, Maehara A, Nazif TM, Ali ZA, Rabbani LE, et al. Comparison between cardiac allograft vasculopathy and native coronary atherosclerosis by optical coherence tomography. Am J Cardiol. 2016;117(8):1361–8.
25. Cohn JM, Wilensky RL, O'Donnell JA, Bourdillon PD, Dillon JC, Feigenbaum H. Exercise echocardiography, angiography, and intracoronary ultrasound after cardiac transplantation. Am J Cardiol. 1996;77(14):1216–9.
26. Akosah KO, McDaniel S, Hanrahan JS, Mohanty PK. Dobutamine stress echocardiography early after heart transplantation predicts development of allograft coronary artery disease and outcome. J Am Coll Cardiol. 1998;31(7):1607–14.
27. Derumeaux G, Redonnet M, Soyer R, Cribier A, Letac B. Assessment of the progression of cardiac allograft vasculopathy by dobutamine stress echocardiography. J Heart Lung Transplant. 1998;17(3):259–67.
28. Spes CH, Klauss V, Mudra H, Schnaack SD, Tammen AR, Rieber J, et al. Diagnostic and prognostic value of serial dobutamine stress echocardiography for noninvasive assessment of cardiac allograft vasculopathy: a comparison with coronary angiography and intravascular ultrasound. Circulation. 1999;100(5):509–15.
29. Spes CH, Mudra H, Schnaack SD, Klauss V, Reichle FM, Uberfuhr P, et al. Dobutamine stress echocardiography for noninvasive diagnosis of cardiac allograft vasculopathy: a comparison with angiography and intravascular ultrasound. Am J Cardiol. 1996;78(2):168–74.
30. Mastrobuoni S, Bastarrika G, Ubilla M, Castano S, Azcarate P, Barrero EA, et al. Dual-source CT coronary angiogram in heart transplant recipients in comparison with dobutamine stress echocardiography for detection of cardiac allograft vasculopathy. Transplantation. 2009;87(4):587–90.
31. Ciliberto GR, Ruffini L, Mangiavacchi M, Parolini M, Sara R, Massa D, et al. Resting echocardiography and quantitative dipyridamole

technetium-99m sestamibi tomography in the identification of cardiac allograft vasculopathy and the prediction of long-term prognosis after heart transplantation. Eur Heart J. 2001;22(11):964–71.
32. Elhendy A, Sozzi FB, van Domburg RT, Vantrimpont P, Valkema R, Krenning EP, et al. Accuracy of dobutamine tetrofosmin myocardial perfusion imaging for the noninvasive diagnosis of transplant coronary artery stenosis. J Heart Lung Transplant. 2000;19(4):360–6.
33. Braggion-Santos MF, Lossnitzer D, Buss S, Lehrke S, Doesch A, Giannitsis E, et al. Late gadolinium enhancement assessed by cardiac magnetic resonance imaging in heart transplant recipients with different stages of cardiac allograft vasculopathy. Eur Heart J Cardiovasc Imaging. 2014;15(10):1125–32.
34. Pedrotti P, Bonacina E, Vittori C, Frigerio M, Roghi A. Pathologic correlates of late gadolinium enhancement cardiovascular magnetic resonance in a heart transplant patient. Cardiovasc Pathol. 2015;24(4):247–9.
35. Riesenkampff E, Chen CK, Kantor PF, Greenway S, Chaturvedi RR, Yoo SJ, et al. Diffuse myocardial fibrosis in children after heart transplantations: a magnetic resonance T1 mapping study. Transplantation. 2015;99(12):2656–62.
36. Ellims AH, Shaw JA, Stub D, Iles LM, Hare JL, Slavin GS, et al. Diffuse myocardial fibrosis evaluated by post-contrast t1 mapping correlates with left ventricular stiffness. J Am Coll Cardiol. 2014;63(11):1112–8.
37. Usman AA, Taimen K, Wasielewski M, McDonald J, Shah S, Giri S, et al. Cardiac magnetic resonance T2 mapping in the monitoring and follow-up of acute cardiac transplant rejection: a pilot study. Circ Cardiovasc Imaging. 2012;5(6):782–90.
38. Muehling OM, Wilke NM, Panse P, Jerosch-Herold M, Wilson BV, Wilson RF, et al. Reduced myocardial perfusion reserve and transmural perfusion gradient in heart transplant arteriopathy assessed by magnetic resonance imaging. J Am Coll Cardiol. 2003;42(6):1054–60.
39. Miller CA, Sarma J, Naish JH, Yonan N, Williams SG, Shaw SM, et al. Multiparametric cardiovascular magnetic resonance assessment of cardiac allograft vasculopathy. J Am Coll Cardiol. 2014;63(8):799–808.
40. Chih S, Ross HJ, Alba AC, Fan CS, Manlhiot C, Crean AM. Perfusion cardiac magnetic resonance imaging as a rule-out test for cardiac allograft vasculopathy. Am J Transplant. 2016;16(10):3007–15.
41. Ferencik M, Brady TJ, Hoffmann U. Computed tomography imaging of cardiac allograft vasculopathy. J Cardiovasc Comput Tomogr. 2012;6(4):223–31.
42. Bastarrika G, De Cecco CN, Arraiza M, Ubilla M, Mastrobuoni S, Pueyo JC, et al. Dual-source CT coronary imaging in heart transplant recipients: image quality and optimal reconstruction interval. Eur Radiol. 2008;18(9):1791–9.
43. Gregory SA, Ferencik M, Achenbach S, Yeh RW, Hoffmann U, Inglessis I, et al. Comparison of sixty-four-slice multidetector computed tomographic coronary angiography to coronary angiography with intravascular ultrasound for the detection of transplant vasculopathy. Am J Cardiol. 2006;98(7):877–84.
44. Romeo G, Houyel L, Angel CY, Brenot P, Riou JY, Paul JF. Coronary stenosis detection by 16-slice computed tomography in heart transplant patients: comparison with conventional angiography and impact on clinical management. J Am Coll Cardiol. 2005;45(11):1826–31.
45. Sigurdsson G, Carrascosa P, Yamani MH, Greenberg NL, Perrone S, Lev G, et al. Detection of transplant coronary artery disease using multidetector computed tomography with adaptative multisegment reconstruction. J Am Coll Cardiol. 2006;48(4):772–8.
46. Bastarrika G, Broncano J, Arraiza M, Azcarate PM, Simon-Yarza I, Levy Praschker BG, et al. Systolic prospectively ECG-triggered dual-source CT angiography for evaluation of the coronary arteries in heart transplant recipients. Eur Radiol. 2011;21(9):1887–94.
47. Bastarrika G, De Cecco CN, Arraiza M, Mastrobuoni S, Pueyo JC, Ubilla M, et al. Dual-source CT for visualization of the coronary arteries in heart transplant patients with high heart rates. AJR Am J Roentgenol. 2008;191(2):448–54.
48. Mittal TK, Panicker MG, Mitchell AG, Banner NR. Cardiac allograft vasculopathy after heart transplantation: electrocardiographically gated cardiac CT angiography for assessment. Radiology. 2013;268(2):374–81.
49. Shuman WP, Branch KR, May JM, Mitsumori LM, Lockhart DW, Dubinsky TJ, et al. Prospective versus retrospective ECG gating for 64-detector CT of the coronary arteries: comparison of image quality and patient radiation dose. Radiology. 2008;248(2):431–7.
50. Schepis T, Achenbach S, Weyand M, Raum P, Marwan M, Pflederer T, et al. Comparison of dual source computed tomography versus intravascular ultrasound for evaluation of coronary arteries at least one year after cardiac transplantation. Am J Cardiol. 2009;104(10):1351–6.
51. Adler G, Meille L, Rohnean A, Sigal-Cinqualbre A, Capderou A, Paul JF. Robustness of end-systolic reconstructions in coronary dual-source CT angiography for high heart rate patients. Eur Radiol. 2010;20(5):1118–23.
52. Taylor AJ, Cerqueira M, Hodgson JM, Mark D, Min J, O'Gara P, et al. ACCF/SCCT/ACR/AHA/ASE/ASNC/NASCI/SCAI/SCMR 2010 appropriate use criteria for cardiac computed tomography. A report of the American College of Cardiology Foundation Appropriate Use Criteria Task Force, the Society of Cardiovascular Computed Tomography, the American College of Radiology, the American Heart Association, the American Society of Echocardiography, the American Society of Nuclear Cardiology, the North American Society for Cardiovascular Imaging, the Society for Cardiovascular Angiography and Interventions, and the Society for Cardiovascular Magnetic Resonance. J Am Coll Cardiol. 2010;56(22):1864–94.
53. Ludman PF, Lazem F, Barbir M, Yacoub M. Incidence and clinical relevance of coronary calcification detected by electron beam computed tomography in heart transplant recipients. Eur Heart J. 1999;20(4):303–8.
54. von Ziegler F, Kaczmarek I, Knez A, Greif M, Rummler J, Meiser B, et al. Coronary calcifications detected by computed tomography are not markers of cardiac allograft vasculopathy. Transplantation. 2011;92(4):493–8.
55. Moro J, Almenar L, Igual B, Martinez-Dolz L, Sanchez E, Martin J, et al. Multislice CT in graft vascular disease. A pilot study. Transplant Proc. 2006;38(8):2563–5.
56. Pichler P, Loewe C, Roedler S, Syeda B, Stadler A, Aliabadi A, et al. Detection of high-grade stenoses with multislice computed tomography in heart transplant patients. J Heart Lung Transplant. 2008;27(3):310–6.
57. Iyengar S, Feldman DS, Cooke GE, Leier CV, Raman SV. Detection of coronary artery disease in orthotopic heart transplant recipients with 64-detector row computed tomography angiography. J Heart Lung Transplant. 2006;25(11):1363–6.
58. von Ziegler F, Leber AW, Becker A, Kaczmarek I, Schonermarck U, Raps C, et al. Detection of significant coronary artery stenosis with 64-slice computed tomography in heart transplant recipients: a comparative study with conventional coronary angiography. Int J Cardiovasc Imaging. 2009;25(1):91–100.
59. von Ziegler F, Rummler J, Kaczmarek I, Greif M, Schenzle J, Helbig S, et al. Detection of significant coronary artery stenosis with cardiac dual-source computed tomography angiography in heart transplant recipients. Transpl Int. 2012;25(10):1065–71.
60. Kepka C, Sobieszczansk-Malek M, Pregowski J, Kruk M, Bekta P, Opolski M, et al. Usefulness of dual-source computed tomography for the evaluation of coronary arteries in heart transplant recipients. Kardiol Pol. 2012;70(11):1111–9.
61. Khan R, Jang IK. Evaluation of coronary allograft vasculopathy using multi-detector row computed tomography: a systematic review. Eur J Cardiothorac Surg. 2012;41(2):415–22.

62. Wever-Pinzon O, Romero J, Kelesidis I, Wever-Pinzon J, Manrique C, Budge D, et al. Coronary computed tomography angiography for the detection of cardiac allograft vasculopathy: a meta-analysis of prospective trials. J Am Coll Cardiol. 2014;63(19):1992–2004.
63. Rohnean A, Houyel L, Sigal-Cinqualbre A, To NT, Elfassy E, Paul JF. Heart transplant patient outcomes: 5-year mean follow-up by coronary computed tomography angiography. Transplantation. 2011;91(5):583–8.
64. Globits S, De Marco T, Schwitter J, Sakuma H, O'Sullivan M, Rifkin C, et al. Assessment of early left ventricular remodeling in orthotopic heart transplant recipients with cine magnetic resonance imaging: potential mechanisms. J Heart Lung Transplant. 1997;16(5):504–10.
65. Bellenger NG, Marcus NJ, Davies C, Yacoub M, Banner NR, Pennell DJ. Left ventricular function and mass after orthotopic heart transplantation: a comparison of cardiovascular magnetic resonance with echocardiography. J Heart Lung Transplant. 2000;19(5):444–52.
66. Kronik G, Slany J, Mosslacher H. Comparative value of eight M-mode echocardiographic formulas for determining left ventricular stroke volume. A correlative study with thermodilution and left ventricular single-plane cineangiography. Circulation. 1979;60(6):1308–16.
67. Allison JD, Flickinger FW, Wright JC, Falls DG 3rd, Prisant LM, VonDohlen TW, et al. Measurement of left ventricular mass in hypertrophic cardiomyopathy using MRI: comparison with echocardiography. Magn Reson Imaging. 1993;11(3):329–34.
68. Pennell DJ, Sechtem UP, Higgins CB, Manning WJ, Pohost GM, Rademakers FE, et al. Clinical indications for cardiovascular magnetic resonance (CMR): Consensus Panel report. Eur Heart J. 2004;25(21):1940–65.
69. Sandstede J, Lipke C, Beer M, Hofmann S, Pabst T, Kenn W, et al. Age- and gender-specific differences in left and right ventricular cardiac function and mass determined by cine magnetic resonance imaging. Eur Radiol. 2000;10(3):438–42.
70. Natori S, Lai S, Finn JP, Gomes AS, Hundley WG, Jerosch-Herold M, et al. Cardiovascular function in multi-ethnic study of atherosclerosis: normal values by age, sex, and ethnicity. AJR Am J Roentgenol. 2006;186(6 Suppl 2):S357–65.
71. Myerson SG, Bellenger NG, Pennell DJ. Assessment of left ventricular mass by cardiovascular magnetic resonance. Hypertension. 2002;39(3):750–5.
72. Ferencik M, Gregory SA, Butler J, Achenbach S, Yeh RW, Hoffmann U, et al. Analysis of cardiac dimensions, mass and function in heart transplant recipients using 64-slice multi-detector computed tomography. J Heart Lung Transplant. 2007;26(5):478–84.
73. Bastarrika G, Arraiza M, De Cecco CN, Broncano J, Mastrobuoni S, Ubilla M, et al. Dual-source CT in heart transplant recipients: quantification of global left ventricular function and mass. J Thorac Imaging. 2009;24(2):103–9.
74. Bastarrika G, Arraiza M, De Cecco CN, Mastrobuoni S, Ubilla M, Rabago G. Quantification of left ventricular function and mass in heart transplant recipients using dual-source CT and MRI: initial clinical experience. Eur Radiol. 2008;18(9):1784–90.
75. Bastarrika G, Zudaire B, Ferreira M, Arraiza M, Saiz-Mendiguren R, Rabago G. Assessment of left atrial volumes and function in orthotopic heart transplant recipients by dual-source CT: comparison with MRI. Investig Radiol. 2010;45(2):72–6.
76. Cole WH. The increase in immunosuppression and its role in the development of malignant lesions. J Surg Oncol. 1985;30(3):139–44.
77. Roussel JC, Baron O, Perigaud C, Bizouarn P, Pattier S, Habash O, et al. Outcome of heart transplants 15 to 20 years ago: graft survival, post-transplant morbidity, and risk factors for mortality. J Heart Lung Transplant. 2008;27(5):486–93.
78. Budoff MJ, Gopal A. Incidental findings on cardiac computed tomography. Should we look? J Cardiovasc Comput Tomogr. 2007;1(2):97–105.
79. Earls JP. The pros and cons of searching for extracardiac findings at cardiac CT: studies should be reconstructed in the maximum field of view and adequately reviewed to detect pathologic findings. Radiology. 2011;261(2):342–6.
80. Hlatky MA, Iribarren C. The dilemma of incidental findings on cardiac computed tomography. J Am Coll Cardiol. 2009;54(16):1542–3.
81. Killeen RP, Dodd JD, Cury RC. Noncardiac findings on cardiac CT part I: pros and cons. J Cardiovasc Comput Tomogr. 2009;3(5):293–9.
82. White CS. The pros and cons of searching for extracardiac findings at cardiac CT: use of a restricted field of view is acceptable. Radiology. 2011;261(2):338–41.
83. Budoff MJ, Fischer H, Gopal A. Incidental findings with cardiac CT evaluation: should we read beyond the heart? Catheter Cardiovasc Interv. 2006;68(6):965–73.
84. Dewey M, Schnapauff D, Teige F, Hamm B. Non-cardiac findings on coronary computed tomography and magnetic resonance imaging. Eur Radiol. 2007;17(8):2038–43.
85. Kirsch J, Araoz PA, Steinberg FB, Fletcher JG, McCollough CH, Williamson EE. Prevalence and significance of incidental extracardiac findings at 64-multidetector coronary CTA. J Thorac Imaging. 2007;22(4):330–4.
86. Johnson KM. Extracardiac findings on cardiac computed tomography: a radiologist's perspective. J Am Coll Cardiol. 2010;55(15):1566–8.

Part VII

Where We Are: CT Assessment of Ventricular Function

CT of Cardiac Function and Wall Motion

35

Prabhakar Rajiah and Suhny Abbara

Functional evaluation is an important component of cardiovascular imaging, contributing to diagnosis, risk stratification, prognosis, determining optimal therapy, and follow-up after treatment. For example, left ventricular (LV) function is an important predictor of survival in patients following myocardial infarction [1] and CABG surgery [2] as well as other nonischemic cardiomyopathies. Right ventricular (RV) function is a prognostic determinant in conditions such as acute pulmonary embolism (PE), congenital heart disease (CHD), and arrhythmogenic right ventricular dysplasia (ARVD). Left atrial function is a predictor of recurrence of atrial fibrillation after pulmonary vein ablation. Although cardiac CT is primarily utilized in the evaluation of coronary arteries, it is also a valuable tool in the evaluation of cardiac function as well, particularly when echocardiography is not adequate and cardiovascular magnetic resonance (CMR) is contraindicated or associated with significant artifacts.

In this chapter, we review the role and technique of CT in the evaluation of ventricular and atrial function.

Imaging of Cardiac Function

There are several imaging modalities available for the evaluation of ventricular and atrial function, including echocardiography, magnetic resonance imaging (MRI), nuclear medicine, and angiography. *Echocardiography* is the most commonly used modality for the evaluation of cardiac function. It is widely available, inexpensive, portable, can be performed in hemodynamically unstable patients at bedside, does not have radiation, and there are no major contraindications. However, echocardiography is operator dependent and may be limited by acoustic windows, especially in patients with obesity, COPD, chest wall deformities, and surgeries, particularly in the evaluation of RV. It also relies on geometrical assumptions, which make evaluation of remodeled and complex hearts challenging. There is also poor contrast between blood and myocardium, as a result of which it has lower accuracy and reproducibility [3]. While LV volume is obtained by Simpson's rule, mass is evaluated in M-mode. Transesophageal echocardiography (TEE) has improved acoustic window, but there are associated complications of an invasive procedure and general anesthesia. New techniques such as 3D result in improved quantification, with higher accuracy and reproducibility [3], but add to the time and are prone to artifacts.

CMR has several advantages including good spatial and temporal resolutions, high contrast between blood and myocardium which allows accurate delineation of the endocardial contour, no radiation, and no geometrical assumptions. It can perform both qualitative and quantitative evaluation of global and regional systolic function, with possibilities of diastolic functional evaluation as well. CMR has been shown to be the gold standard in quantification of ventricular function, due to high accuracy and reproducibility [4]. Quantification is usually performed in short-axis view utilizing modified Simpson's method. Cine images in other planes including two, three, and four chamber are used to evaluate regional wall motion abnormalities. CMR also allows for anatomical evaluation and tissue characterization in the same study. However, CMR is contraindicated in patients with several intracardiac devices as well as claustrophobic patients. CMR is also not widely available, is expensive, requires higher technical expertise, takes longer time, and is challenging in patients with arrhythmia or those unable to lay flat. In children, intubation and anesthesia are often required.

Nuclear medicine techniques for quantification of LV function include gated radionuclide ventriculography (RVG), ECG-gated single-photon emission computed tomography (SPECT), and positron emission tomography (PET). With

P. Rajiah · S. Abbara (✉)
Department of Radiology, Cardiothoracic Imaging Division, UT Southwestern Medical Center, Dallas, TX, USA
Suhny.Abbara@utsouthwestern.edu

U. J. Schoepf (ed.), *CT of the Heart*, Contemporary Medical Imaging, https://doi.org/10.1007/978-1-60327-237-7_35

RVG or MUGA (multiple-gated acquisition), patient's RBCs are labelled, and ECG-gated cardiac scintigraphy is obtained over several heartbeats to generate a single composite cardiac cycle. This can quantify global and regional function and volumes, both at rest and stress. The advantage of this technique is that it does not rely on geometrical assumptions [5]. Disadvantages include lower temporal and spatial resolution and limited accuracy in arrhythmias. There are long preparation and examination times. Function can also be obtained from a gated SPECT utilized for myocardial perfusion imaging, by analyzing the ventricular contours [6], which correlates well with CMR [7]. Regional EF with handgrip has been shown to be highly sensitive and specific for coronary artery disease [8]. Disadvantages of SPECT include lower spatial resolution, inaccuracy in ischemia/infarct due to lower uptake in subendocardial region [9], and decreased accuracy in attenuation artifacts as well as patients with small or large hearts [3]. Variability has been noted with Tl-201 scans and between different software algorithms [3]. Repeated radionuclide injections and radiation dose are additional concerns. Similarly, function can be obtained from ECG-gated PET performed for myocardial perfusion and metabolism imaging, which correlates well with CMR [6]. PET has higher spatial resolution than SPECT but has lower temporal resolution than CMR, which results in underestimation of function. Due to inclusion of papillary muscles with myocardial wall, the volumes are lower than CMR [6]. Radiation is a concern with all the nuclear medicine techniques.

Cine ventriculography with catheter angiography is not routinely used for quantification of ventricular function. It is an invasive procedure, requires contrast, uses radiation, has geometric assumptions and restrictions from projection images. It is limited in evaluation of some regions, especially in complex, irregular shapes, and has significant variability in regional wall motion assessment due to variable cardiac rotation and lack of reliable landmarks [3].

Computed Tomography

Advantages and Disadvantages

CT scan has several advantages in the evaluation of ventricular function such as high isotropic spatial resolution, good temporal resolution, high contrast between ventricular lumen and myocardium, and multi-planar reconstruction capabilities. CT quantification does not rely on geometric assumptions. Additional information can be obtained on the morphology of the heart as well as coronary arteries and any adjacent structure. CT is not operator dependent, is widely available, and has rapid turnaround time, making it suitable for patients who cannot lay still for prolonged periods of time. For functional evaluation, CT is typically utilized when MRI is contraindicated or suboptimal due to artifacts or if echocardiography does not provide adequate information due to poor acoustic window, especially for right ventricle. Common contraindications for MRI include metallic objects in the eye, older versions of intracardiac devices (pacemakers, defibrillators), claustrophobia, and inability to lay flat for prolonged period. CT for functional evaluation has been considered an appropriate indication in the 2010 ACCF guidelines [10]. Disadvantages of CT include the use of ionizing radiation which is associated with several theoretical risks and the use of contrast media in patients with renal dysfunction which is associated with nephrotoxicity. Premedication is required for patients with history of contrast allergy. Image quality is compromised in patients with severe arrhythmias, with poor definition of borders, and with potential increases of radiation dose in some scanners due to the opening of image acquisition window.

Scan Mode

Cardiac cycle starts with isovolumetric contraction at the end of ventricular filling, followed sequentially by ventricular systole, isovolumic ventricular relaxation, and then diastole. To capture the cardiac volumes and function, ECG gating and high temporal resolution are required to essentially freeze the cardiac motion without any motion artifacts. Since multiple cardiac phases are required in the R-R interval, particularly end-systole (ES) and end-diastole (ED), retrospective ECG gating is required. The heart is scanned in the spiral mode, with the table continuously moving through the gantry, and images are acquired throughout the cardiac cycle, over multiple heartbeats. ECG tracing is also simultaneously acquired, and images are retrospectively reconstructed. A low pitch (<1.0), dependent on the heart rate, is utilized to image the heart throughout R-R interval with areas of oversampling. Due to this, there is an overlap of the same anatomy at different R-R intervals, which can be used for multisegment reconstruction. High spatial and temporal resolutions are required for accurate quantification. The highest possible spatial resolution should be selected to accurately delineate the endocardial borders and minimize partial volume averaging at the blood pool-myocardium interface which can be seen at the apex [3].

High temporal resolution is required to achieve artifact-free images of the myocardial contraction. A temporal resolution of 100–250 milliseconds (ms) is recommended for the evaluation of systole and diastole and higher if resolution of rapid ventricular filling and ejection phase is recommended. 80–90 milliseconds has been suggested for adequate evaluation of wall motion in CMR [3, 11], but 19.1 ms or less is necessary to avoid motion artifacts [12], especially in the posterior LV wall [11]. The temporal resolution of a scanner is determined primarily by the gantry rotation time. Since only a partial scan reconstruction algorithm is used, effective temporal resolution is the time taken to rotate the tube 180 plus fan angle. In the earlier scanners with few detectors, the gantry rotation time was long, with limited temporal resolution, as a result of which, the EDV can be underestimated and ESV can be overestimated since the position of ventricles at EDV and ESV is averaged over multiple heartbeats. However, improvements in scanner technology over the last decade have resulted in shorter gantry rotation times and improved temporal resolution. This is further improved in dual-source scanners, where the temporal resolution is one fourth of the gantry rotation time, resulting in effective temporal resolution of up to 75 milliseconds. Another option to improve temporal resolution in a spiral acquisition is to use multi-segment reconstruction, i.e., reconstruct data from same phase of cardiac cycle in consecutive heartbeats. The temporal resolution is equal to gantry rotation time divided by $2n$, with n being the number of segments. The higher the number of segments, the higher will be the temporal resolution. However, this requires a steady heart rate; otherwise there will be beat to beat variation of the position of the heart resulting in artifacts. Even with steady heartbeat, the heart may not be in the same location due to complex cardiac contraction. Multi-segment reconstruction may also require reduction of spiral pitch, which will increase scan time and thus radiation dose. Motion artifacts can be eliminated by using wide-array or volume scanners with z-coverage up to 16 cm or dual-source scanners with high pitch (up to 3.4), as a result of which the entire heart can be scanned in one heartbeat.

Medications and Contrast

Beta-blockers are routinely used in coronary CTA to reduce the heart rate and minimize coronary artery motion, but this is not required for evaluation of cardiac function. In addition, studies have shown there is a small but not negligible reduction in LV function after administration of propranolol in healthy subjects [13, 14] as well as those with heart disease [15, 16], due to negative inotropic action and increased ESV.

Contrast injection should be optimized depending on the chamber of interest. If both ventricles are being evaluated, a triphasic injection protocol is used to adequately opacify both the ventricles. With adequate contrast opacification of RV, i.e., >176 HU, the volume measurements are more comparable with CMR [17]. In the first phase, a full dose of contrast is administered at a rate of 4–7 ml/s to opacify the left ventricle. In the second phase, either a slower injection of contrast at 2–4 ml/s or a contrast saline admixture (50:50, 60:40, or 70:30) at the same rate of 4–7 ml/s is injected to opacify the right ventricle. In the final phase, saline flush is injected at 5–7 ml/s to eliminate the streak artifacts in SVC and the right atrium. Scan acquisition is triggered either by using a bolus tracking technique, with the ROI placed in the descending aorta, or a timing bolus technique following injection of a small bolus of contrast first, although this takes additional time and also wastes some amount of contrast [18]. Bolus tracking has been shown to provide more homogeneous enhancement [19]. Scanning is typically 4–6 s after peak aortic opacification [20].

Radiation Dose Reduction Strategies

With retrospective ECG gating, the radiation dose is significantly high since data is obtained throughout the cardiac cycle (Fig. 35.1), with values from 14.8 to 21.1 mSv [21]. However, the radiation dose can be reduced by using ECG-based tube current modulation, where the peak tube current is delivered only in specific cardiac phase(s), i.e., ED and ES, and ramped down to 4–20% of peak tube current for the rest of the R-R interval (Fig. 35.2). This technique has been shown to allow radiation dose savings of up to 60% [22, 23]. A prospective ECG-triggering mode, where data is acquired only in one portion of the cardiac cycle, is not useful for estimation of function. However, prospective ECG gating with wider padding can be utilized to evaluate cardiac function, although this does not provide any significant radiation dose savings compared to retrospective ECG gating [24]. Another technique is a prospectively ECG-triggered dual-step pulsing protocol in a dual-source scanner, in which a prospectively ECG-triggered window is obtained at low radiation dose (20% tube current) across a selected portion of cardiac cycle (10–90%), with a full tube current only in a selective portion of cardiac cycle (65–75% RR). X-ray tube is also turned off in between heartbeats. This provides both functional data at lower radiation dose as well as normal radiation dose data for detailed evaluation of coronary arteries. This provides accurate quantification compared to CMR with lower radiation dose (6.2 + 1.8 mSv) [21]. Other radiation dose reduction strategies can also be applied for functional evaluation, including lowering tube voltage, lowering tube current, automatic tube current modulation techniques, and iterative reconstruction algorithms.

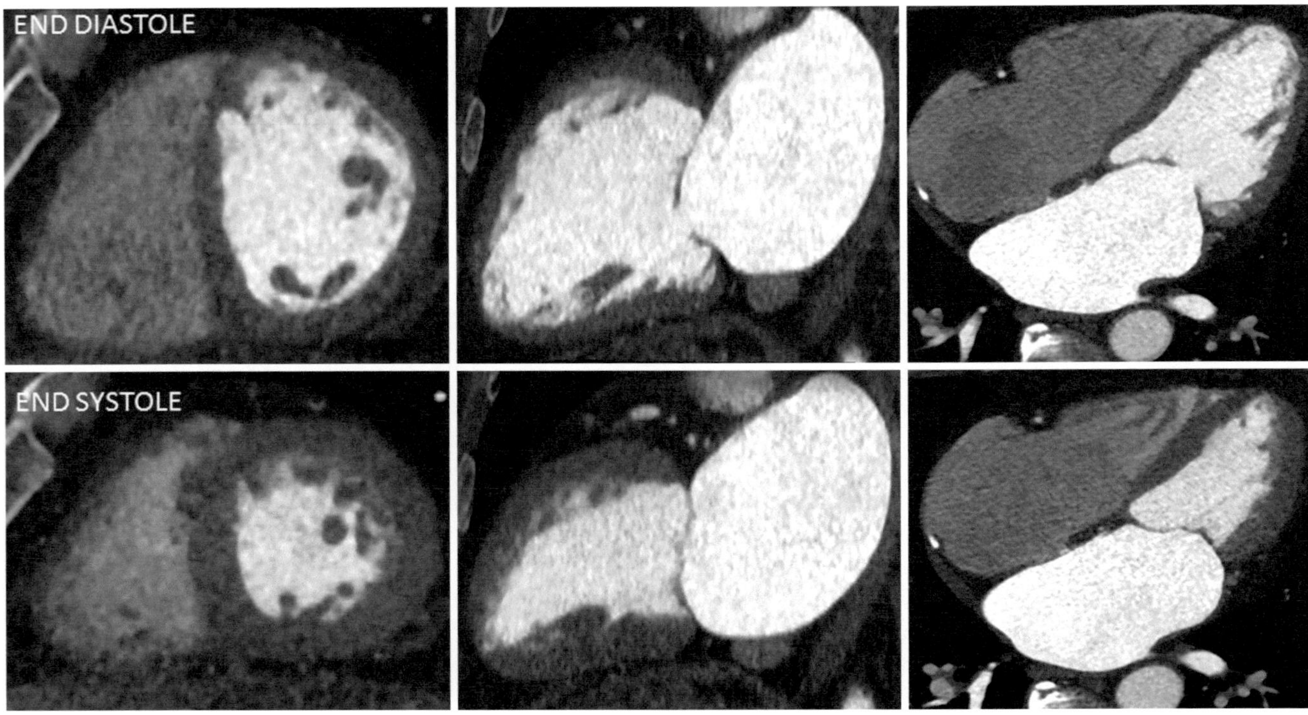

Fig. 35.1 Retrospective ECG gating without ECG-based tube current modulation. Short-axis (left), two-chamber (middle), and four-chamber (right) reconstructions of the heart at end-diastole (top row) and end-systole (bottom row). Since full tube current is delivered throughout the cardiac cycle, there is no significant difference in image quality between the two sets of images, albeit a high radiation dose

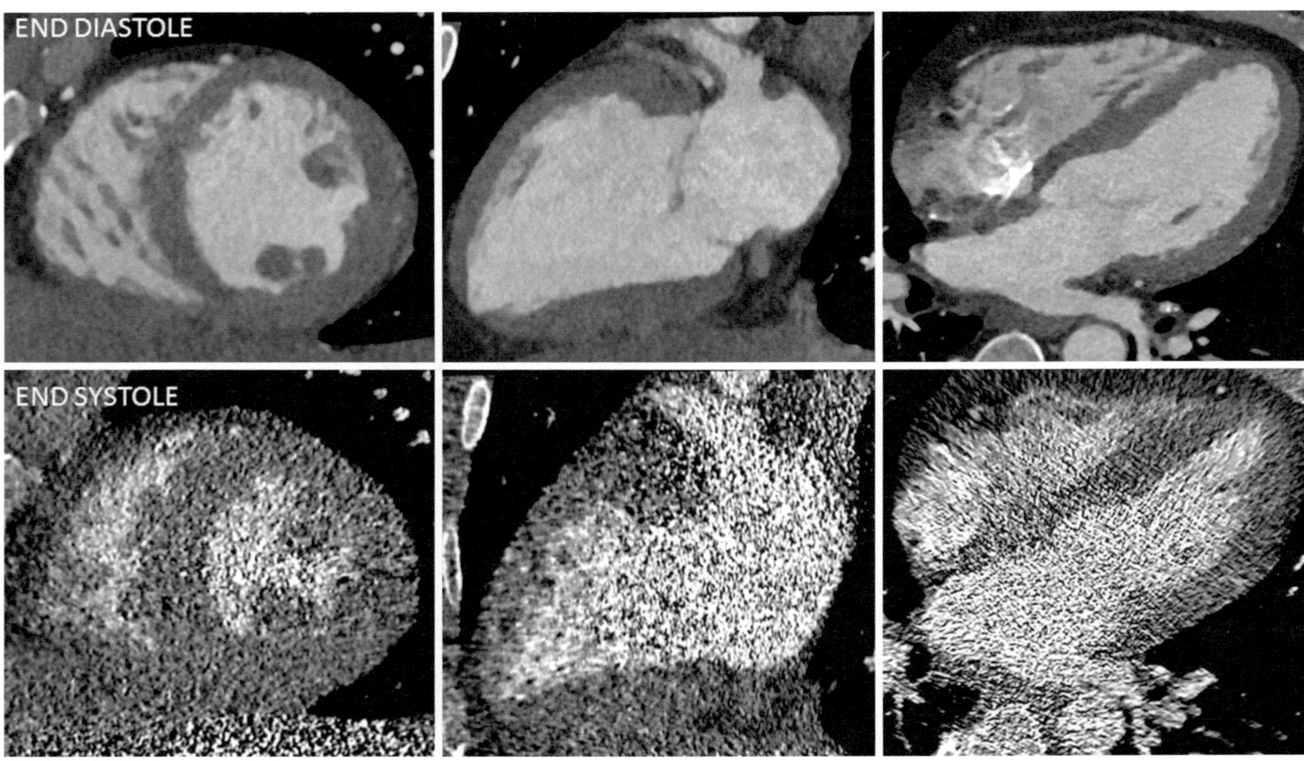

Fig. 35.2 Retrospective ECG gating with ECG-based tube current modulation. Short-axis (left), two-chamber (middle), and four-chamber (right) reconstructions of the heart at end-diastole (top row) and end-systole (bottom row). Note the higher noise seen in the end-systolic images since these images are obtained at 20% of maximum tube current. In spite of the higher noise at end-systole, these images are adequate for delineation of endocardial and epicardial contours for functional, volume, and mass measurements

Image Reconstruction

After acquisition of data, images are constructed at 5–10% increments throughout the R-R interval, generating either 10 or 20 cardiac phases. In a single-source scanner, no advantage is gained by using 20 instead of 10 phases, but there is an increase in reconstruction time and space taken for storing these images. In dual-source scanners with good temporal resolution, the full benefit of good temporal resolution may be gained by using 20 phases [20]. No significant difference in EF and volumes was noted between 10 and 20 phases, both for single-source [25] and dual-source scanners [26]. Images can be displayed as 2D cine loops, and most workstations allow manipulation of the planes in any direction. Typically short-axis, two-chamber, three-chamber, and four-chamber planes are used for qualitative global and regional functional evaluation. Thin slices are not mandatory for evaluation of function, with 1.5, 2.0, or 2.5 mm slices with no overlap of intervals of 1 or 1.5 mm commonly used. Noise reduction strategies, including iterative reconstruction, increase the CNR and hence improve the correlation of ventricular volumes, mass, and function with CMR [27].

Post Processing

Quantitation of the volumes and function can be performed using either manual, semiautomatic, or fully automatic techniques.

(a) *Area-length method.* In this technique, volume of the left ventricle (V) is calculated from the area (A) and length (L) of the left ventricle, using the formula $V = \frac{8}{3} \times \frac{A^2}{\pi L}$.
This is measured in one of the long-axis views (vertical or horizontal). The length is measured from mitral annulus to the apex, and the area is measured in the same plane. This technique uses geometrical assumptions to measure the volume, i.e., assuming an ellipsoid shape.

(b) *Biplane area-length method.* In this variation of the area-length product, both the vertical and horizontal long axes are used to calculate the volume. This method also relies on geometrical assumptions.

(c) *Simpson's method.* In Simpson's method, the volumes are determined by summing up areas of LV cavity at each short-axis slice and multiplying it with slice thickness, using the formula volume $\sum A_N \times S$, where A is the cross-sectional area and S is the section thickness. Multiple parallel short-axis slices are utilized. Endocardial contours are drawn, either manually, automatically, or semiautomatically, both at end-diastole and end-systole in all the slices along the entire length of ventricle (Fig. 35.3). Although the LV limits can be automatically determined using the software, determination of the most basal and apical slices can be challenging. The most basal slice is just forward to the atrioventricular ring and has myocardium in at least 50% of its perimeter. The most apical slice is the last image with contrast-opacified lumen. Determination of the correct ED and ES phase can also be done manually, semiautomatically, or automatically. End-diastole is defined as QRS onset, which corresponds to the phase with the largest cardiac dimension and following mitral valve closure. End-systole is the phase where the cardiac dimension is the smallest and precedes mitral valve opening. Papillary muscles are included in the ventricular lumen. For evaluation of myocardial volume, epicardial contours are drawn in end-diastolic phase, and the mass is calculated by using the formula $\sum A_N \times S$ x ṕ, where ṕ is the myocardial density (1.05 g/cm3). This three-dimensional technique is considered accurate since it does not rely on geometric assumptions. It has been shown superior to the area-length technique, which overestimates EDV, ESV, and SV [28] and agrees more with 2D echo, MRI, CVG, and gated SPECT. Sources of errors include inappropriate plane, selecting basal and apical slices, selecting ED and ES phases, and drawing endocardial and epicardial borders. Manual contouring, even with semiautomatic software, is time-consuming, subjective, and observer dependent. Semiautomatic and automatic techniques significantly shorten the processing time due to advanced software, automatic generation of cardiac views, automatic selection of ED and ES phases, and automatic segmentation. Automatic techniques also decrease interobserver variability without significant changes in volumes and function [29–31], although some studies showed differences in LVEDV [29].

Threshold-Based Segmentation

Threshold-based segmentation is an automatic technique that utilizes the differences in attenuation between the blood pool and myocardium. The mitral annular plane may have to be verified or defined manually since the contrast attenuation is similar in the atrium and ventricle, following which the contrast-filled LV is automatically segmented in all the phases. Ventricular volume is calculated by summing all the contiguous voxels whose attenuation is above that of a predefined threshold (Fig. 35.4). Although volumes are typically calculated from short-axis view in 2D, recent software also allow 3D volume quantification. Segmented pixels are displayed in color. If the segmentation does not look accurate, the attenuation threshold can be altered to make the color fit the cavity. In most softwares, the LV function automation works readily, while RV function requires some kind of manual correction. Time-volume curves can be generated since all the phases are segmented. This technique requires good opacification of the blood pool with contrast, with at least 150–200 HU attenuation difference between myocardium and blood pool. Errors will be seen if there is high attenuation material such as dense contrast in veins or right heart or pacemaker leads, which may lead to inclusion of RA or RV in LV blood pool. Similar errors can also emanate from unbroken column of contrast in VSD [30, 32]. In this technique, the papillary muscles are not included in the blood pool due to their different attenuation and hence do not contribute to the volume, as a result of which the EDV and ESV are smaller, with no change in EF [20]. Threshold-based technique has been shown to be accurate and reproducible with lower interobserver variability with shorter-processing time [3]. With manual contours, the papillary muscles are within the blood pool, and hence the volumes are larger, which correspond to MRI numbers due to similar measurement [33]. A study found differences of 5.6–30.1% for LV volumes, 5.8–9.4% for LV mass, and 4.3–6.0% for LV EF [34].

a

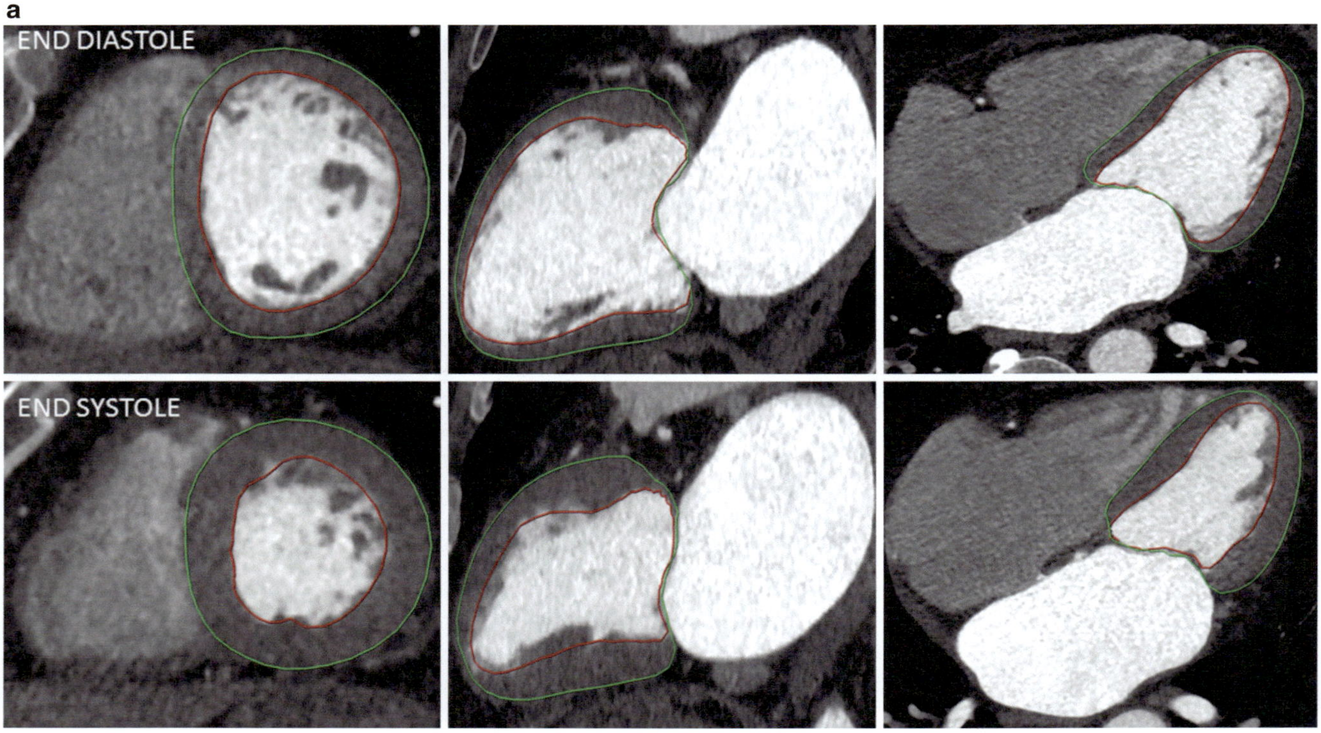

Fig. 35.3 Quantification of the left ventricle. (**a**) Values obtained from the above contours include ejection fraction, end-diastolic volume, end-systolic volume, stroke volume, cardiac output, and myocardial mass. All these can be indexed to the body surface area (BSA) (**b**) Short-axis (left), two-chamber (middle), and four-chamber (right) reconstructions of the heart at end-diastole (top row) and end-systole (bottom row). Endocardial (red) and epicardial (green) contours are drawn in the left ventricle, both in end-diastolic and end-systolic images.

b

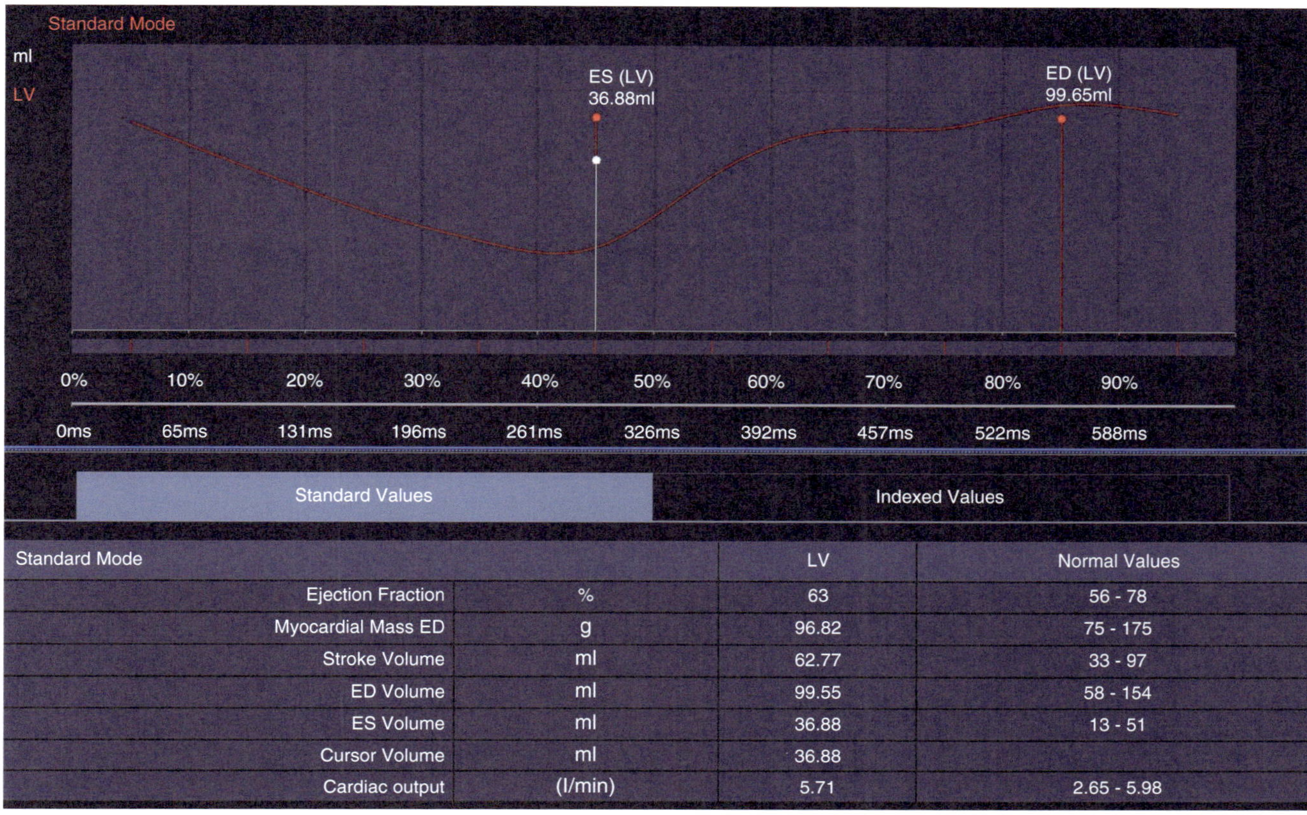

Standard Mode		LV	Normal Values
Ejection Fraction	%	63	56 - 78
Myocardial Mass ED	g	96.82	75 - 175
Stroke Volume	ml	62.77	33 - 97
ED Volume	ml	99.55	58 - 154
ES Volume	ml	36.88	13 - 51
Cursor Volume	ml	36.88	
Cardiac output	(l/min)	5.71	2.65 - 5.98

Fig. 35. 3 (continued)

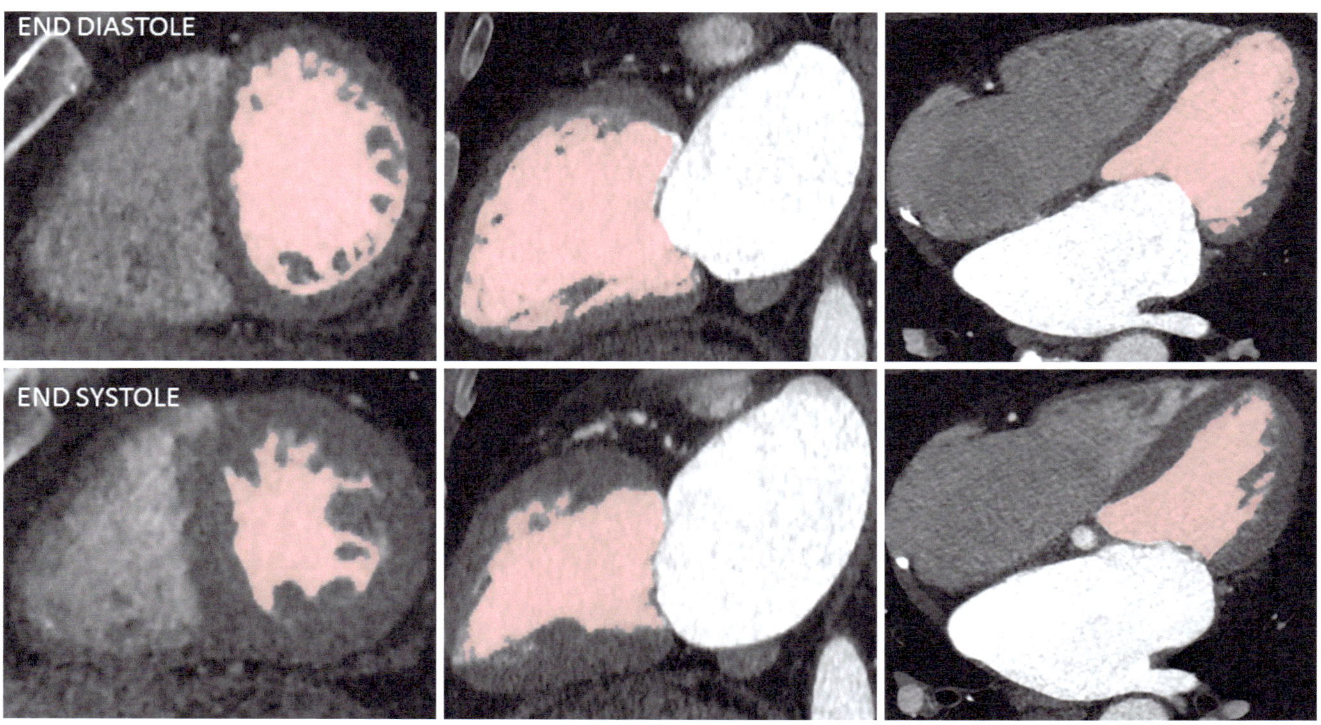

Fig. 35.4 Quantification using threshold segmentation. Short-axis (left), two-chamber (middle), and four-chamber (right) reconstructions of the heart at end-diastole (top row) and end-systole (bottom row). The threshold-based segmentation technique utilizes the differences in attenuation between contrast in the blood pool and the myocardium. All the contiguous voxels whose attenuation is above that of a predefined threshold are identified in pink. Ventricular volume is calculated by summing all these voxels

Interpretation of Results

Qualitative

Global function can be qualitatively evaluated in cine images at multiple planes. All the currently available softwares automatically generate the standard cardiac planes, typically a short-axis view and two long-axis views. Any other plane can also be generated by manual interaction. Global systolic function can be qualitatively classified as normal, reduced (mild, moderate, and severe), or hyperdynamic. Regional wall motion abnormalities can be evaluated using the 17-segment AHA model and multi-planar CT reconstructions, including short-axis, two-chamber, three-chamber, and four-chamber views. There are six basal, six mid, and four apical segments, accounting for 35%, 35%, and 30% of myocardial volume, respectively along with an apical cap. Regional wall motion can be classified as normal (inward motion in systole), hypokinesis (decreased wall motion), akinesis (no wall motion), and dyskinesis (paradoxical wall motion). Abnormalities have to be seen in two different views to be considered true positive.

Quantitative

Several quantitative parameters are derived from the post-processed images as above. Parameters of global systolic function include the *stroke volume*, which is the volume of blood ejected from the ventricle with each heartbeat, i.e., SV = EDV-ESV. This represents the blood ejected both forward and backward and hence includes regurgitant flow. The stroke volume of the right and left ventricles is the same, assuming there is no regurgitation or shunting. *Cardiac output (CO)*, the volume of blood pumped in 1 min, is SV × HR (ml/min). *Ejection fraction* is a percentage, which is SV/EDV × 100%. *Myocardial mass* is quantified as end-diastolic myocardial volume × density. Usually, a density of 1.05 g/cm3 is used. All these measurements can be indexed to the body surface area (BSA) to derive indexed values. If images are reconstructed in all cardiac phases, a time-volume curve can also be generated, which provides additional time-dependent variables such as peak ejection rate (PER), peak filling rate (PFR), time to PER, and time to PFR.

Regional wall motion can also be quantified using several indices if at least 8–10 cardiac phases are available. Normal LV ejection is a combination of radial wall thickening, circumferential shortening, and longitudinal shortening [11]. Parameters evaluated include *myocardial wall thickness*, which is calculated in orthogonal plane between endocardial and epicardial contour. Myocardium normally measures 6–8 mm in end-diastole and 10–14 mm in end-systole [35]. It is focally decreased in chronic ischemia or thickened in cardiomyopathy [36, 37]; *wall attenuation*, mean attenuation of the myocardial segment, which is decreased in infarction; and *systolic percentage wall thickening*, which represents regional percentage of wall thickening during systole (Ws-Wd/Wd × 100%). Normal wall thickening is 5 mm. Wall thickening is decreased in coronary artery stenosis, particularly with stress imaging due to regional hypoperfusion. In ischemic heart disease, wall motion may be difficult to evaluate, and wall thickening percentage is more accurate [11]: *wall motion* or *shortening*, displacement of points on the endocardial contour from ED to ES phase using displacement lines called chords, either in the longitudinal or circumferential plane. The length of each chord represents the amount of endocardial displacement; and *regional/segmental EF*, which represents the EF relative to a specific myocardial region/segment, is calculated by dividing ESV and EDV for a specific area beneath a myocardial segment or region [11]. Due to high variability of quantitative regional indices, qualitative or semiquantitative metrics are used, with graphics, color polar maps, and diagrams (Fig. 35.5).

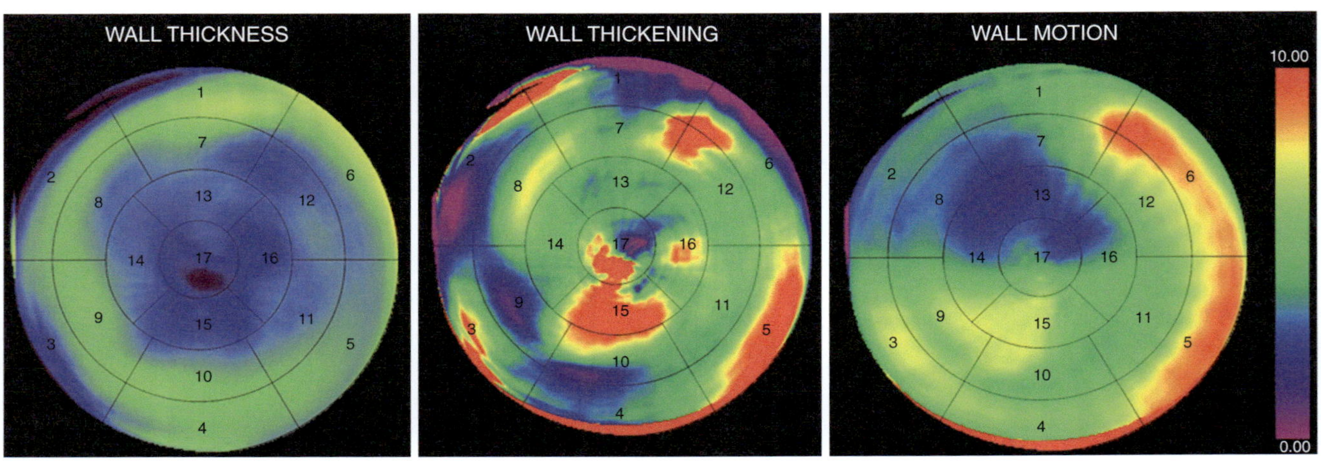

Fig. 35.5 Quantification of regional function. Polar maps showing values of myocardial wall thickness, myocardial wall thickening, and myocardial wall motion across the 17 myocardial segments as per AHA classification scheme

Diastolic Function

Diastolic dysfunction is an important factor providing diagnostic, therapeutic, and prognostic information in several disorders including CAD. This is typically performed with echocardiography. CT-derived transmitral velocity, mitral septal tissue velocity, and estimation of LV filling pressures have shown good correlation with echocardiogram [38] with comparable assessment of diastolic dysfunction; but this is not widely used clinically.

Left Ventricle

Normal functional values for the left ventricle are shown in Table 35.1 [36, 37, 39, 40]. Earlier studies showed overestimation of ESV and underestimation of EF in CT compared to CMR due to poorer temporal resolution of the earlier scanners [41, 42]. Several newer studies have shown excellent correlation between CT and CMR values, with single- and dual-source scanners of several detector widths, both at single- and multi-segment reconstruction [33, 43, 44]. Other studies have shown good correlation with and even superior accuracy than cineventriculography and transthoracic echocardiography [45, 46]. Interobserver variability of CT quantification ranges from 2% to 11% for LV EDV, 6% to 9% for ESV [11], and 2% to 8.5% for EF [3]. Most studies have also shown good sensitivity and accuracy of regional LV function assessment with CT compared to CMR, echocardiography, SPECT, and CVG [3].

Global systolic dysfunction is seen in several cardiomyopathies, both ischemic and nonischemic. Heart failure can present with either reduced or preserved ejection fractions. Hyperdynamic systolic function is seen in hypertrophic cardiomyopathies. LV function is important in the diagnosis, management, and prognosis of patients with ischemic heart disease, heart failure, malignant ventricular arrhythmia, chronic valvular regurgitation, type 2 diabetes mellitus, and congenital heart diseases [3].

Table 35.1 Normal regional LV functional parameters adapted from CMR data

	Men	Women
EDWT (mm)	7.6 ± 1.4	6.3 ± 1.0
ESWT (mm)	13.2 ± 1.8	12.2 ± 1.6
SWT (mm)	5.5 ± 0.8	5.8 ± 1.2
SWTH (%)	75 ± 16	96 ± 24

Data from Refs. [36, 37]

EDWT end-diastolic wall thickness, *ESWT* end-systolic wall thickness, *SWT* segmental wall thickening, *SWTH* segmental wall thickening percentage

Ischemic Heart Disease

LV dysfunction indicates CAD in symptomatic patients, although it is not highly sensitive. Contraction remains normal till a particular threshold for coronary blood flow is reached, below which there is an exponential fall in LV function. Dysfunction is also not specific and can happen in nonischemic cardiomyopathy, valvular heart disease, and other disorders. Wall motion abnormalities can be seen due to myocardial ischemia, hibernating myocardium, stunned myocardium, or infarct, with the last entity being irreversible. In myocardial ischemia, regional wall motion abnormalities are seen in the early stages of the disease. In acute myocardial infarction, akinesia is seen due to stunned myocardium, which may improve with revascularization [47]. Hibernating myocardium also shows functional abnormality, which improves with revascularization. CT has 89% sensitivity and 92% specificity in diagnosing abnormal segments using CMR as gold standard [48]. In patients with acute coronary syndrome (ACS) with negative troponin and EKG, coronary CTA alone has a 77% accuracy and 35% positive predictive value for detection of coronary stenosis, whereas adding functional CT improves accuracy to 87% and PPV to 80% [49] and also providing incremental value [50]. Wall motion abnormalities also highlight subtle coronary artery abnormalities that are not always evident on coronary CTA. In chronic infarct, regional wall motion abnormality such as akinesis or dyskinesis is seen with thinned myocardium in a vascular territory. Fat metaplasia, calcification, aneurysm, or pseudoaneurysm may be seen. Low EF predicts heart failure in patients with uncomplicated MI [51]. ESV is an additional independent prognostic factor in patients with previous MI and EF <40% [52]. Worsening LV EF and larger LV volumes predicted mortality in patients with CAD in the CONFIRM registry [53]. In the CASS registry, low EF was a better predictor of mortality than the number of vessels involved [2].

Heart Failure

Heart failure can be with preserved (HFpEF) or reduced ejection fraction (HFrEF). In restrictive cardiomyopathies such as amyloidosis, sarcoidosis, hemochromatosis, and glycogen storage disorders, the global systolic function is normal, but there is impaired diastolic relaxation. There is a direct correlation between LV EF and adverse outcomes including mortality. This relationship is not linear, but there is a cutoff, such as 45%, below which there is a linear relationship [2]. Nonischemic cardiomyopathies can be dilated, restrictive, hypertrophic cardiomyopathies, arrhythmogenic right ventricular dysplasia (ARVD), and unclassified disease. Most of these disorders have global systolic dysfunction, with regional wall motion abnormalities rarely seen, such as in myocarditis, sarcoidosis, and stress-induced cardiomyopathy. In dilated cardiomyopathy, the LV is dilated with global systolic dysfunction. Hypertrophic cardiomyopathy is characterized by LV thickening of several types and hyperdynamic global systolic function, with global systolic dysfunction seen in late phases of the disease. In stress-induced cardiomyopathy (Takotsubo cardiomyopathy), there is reversible global systolic dysfunction and hypokinesis/akinesis of the apical segments associated with normal contraction of the basal segments in a nonvascular distribution, which resembles a Japanese octopus pot. In reverse Takotsubo cardiomyopathy, there is hypokinesis/akinesis of the basal segments and normal contraction of apical segment. A common scenario is that in a patient with new onset heart failure and low to intermediate probability, CTA is used to exclude CAD, which can also provide functional information in the same study [10]. Similarly, in patients being evaluated for CRT, CT can provide functional information as well as venous anatomy in one study [20]. Intraventricular dysynchrony can also be evaluated to predict response to CRT [20]. Ventricular function is also accurately measured in CT in patients with cardiac transplants [54, 55] who are surviving longer, with 30% survival at 15 years [56]. In patients with left ventricular assist device (LVAD) for heart failure, CT provides accurate biventricular functional values, as well as comprehensive assessment of the device and its complications, such as location, angulation, thrombus, infection, fluid collections, pericardial effusion, and diaphragmatic hernia [57].

Right Ventricle

Right ventricle volumes and function can be qualitatively and quantitatively evaluated using retrospective ECG-gated data obtained from triphasic contrast injection protocol that opacifies both the ventricles simultaneously. Manual, automated, or semiautomated techniques can be used for quantifying volumes and function (Fig. 35.6), after determining the tricuspid annular plane. Normal values for the right ventricle in CT are shown in Table 35.2 [39]. Echocardiography is limited in the evaluation of RV due to its location behind the sternum which limits the acoustic window, complex shape which is exaggerated in abnormalities, heavy trabeculations, and thin wall [20]. CMR is considered the gold standard in the evaluation and quantification of RV [58]. However, CT is the ideal modality in the evaluation of patients who have contraindications to

a

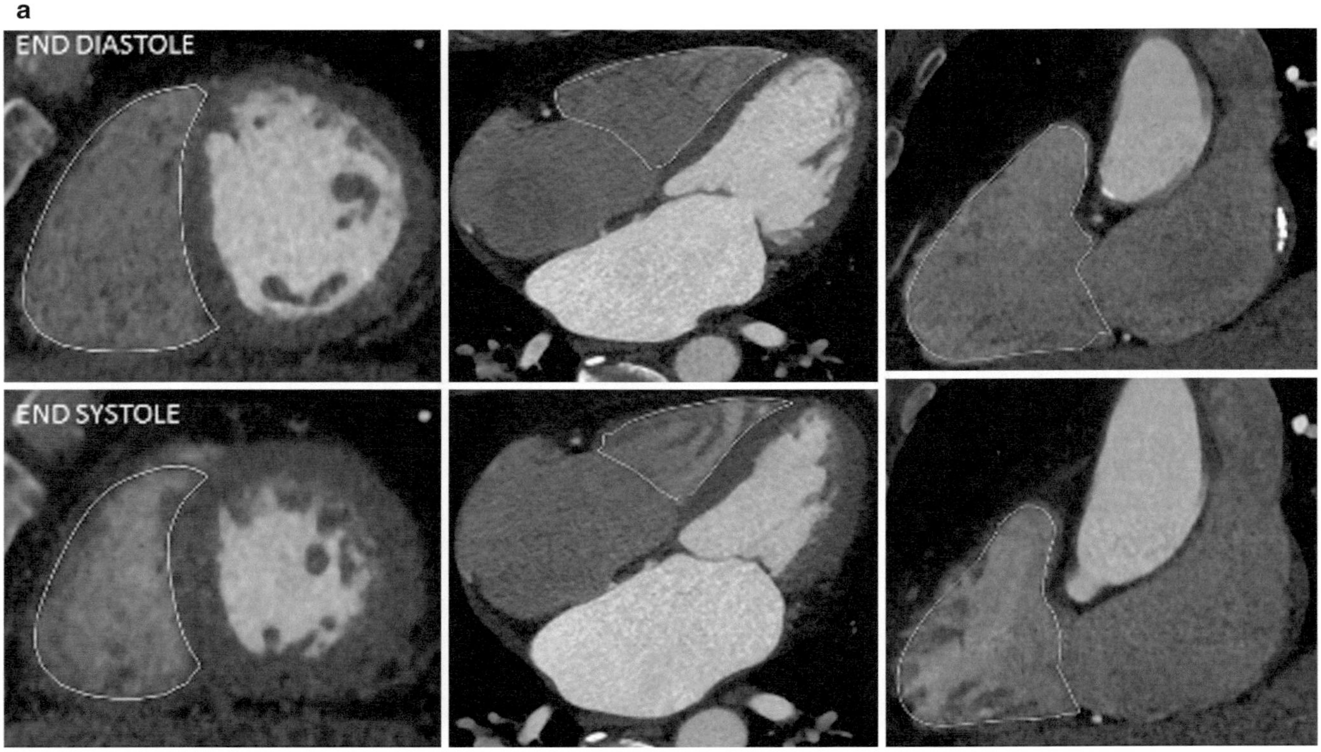

Fig. 35.6 Quantification of the right ventricle. (**a**) Short-axis (left), two-chamber (middle), and four-chamber (right) reconstructions of the heart at end-diastole (top row) and end-systole (bottom row). Endocardial (red) and epicardial (green) contours are drawn in the right ventricle both in end-diastolic and end-systolic images. (**b**) Values obtained from the above contours include ejection fraction, end-diastolic volume, end-systolic volume, stroke volume, cardiac output, and myocardial mass. All these can be indexed to the body surface area (BSA)

b

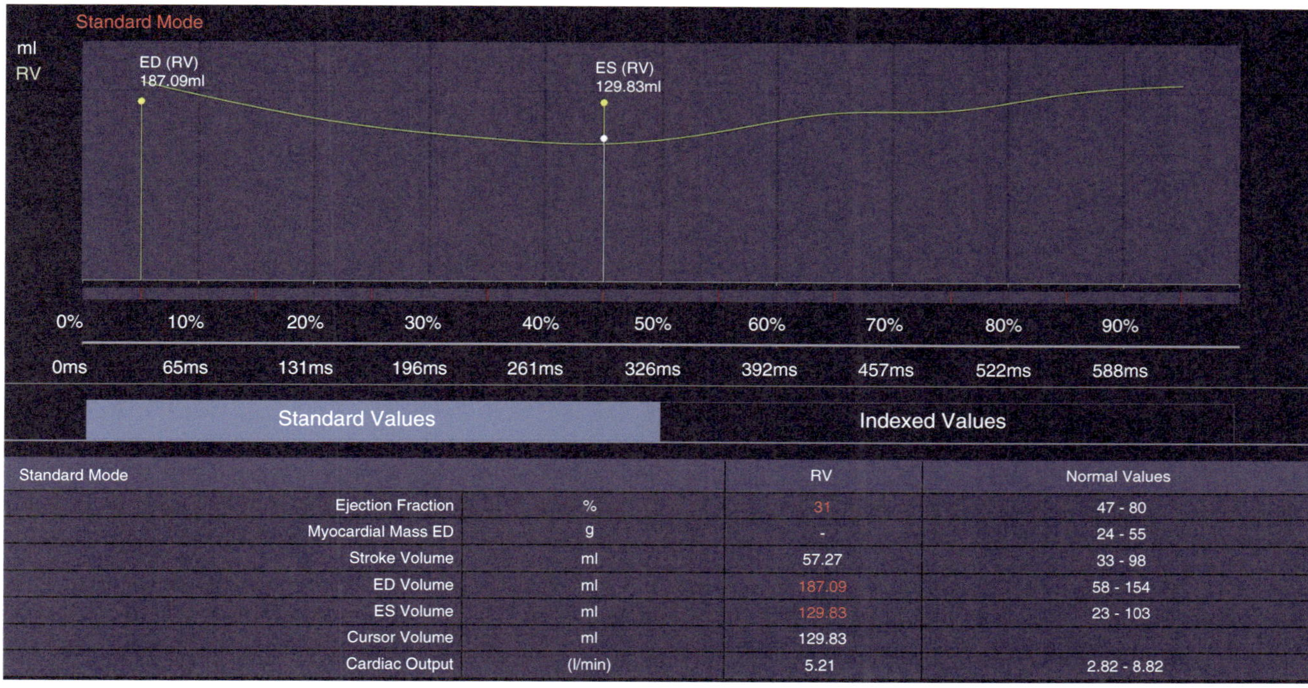

Fig. 35.6 (continued)

Table 35.2 Normal right ventricular values

ESD (mm)	29.6 ± 5.3
EDD (mm)	37.0 ± 5.7
EDV (ml)	174.9 ± 48.0
ESV (ml)	82.1 ± 29.2
EF (%)	57.9 ± 8.0

Adapted from Lin et al. [39], with permission

CMR or when artifacts are expected. Several studies have shown the high accuracy and reproducibility of CT compared to MRI in evaluation of RV function and volumes [59, 60].

RV function is an important parameter in the diagnosis, management, and prognosis of several disorders such as pulmonary embolism (PE), pulmonary hypertension, ARVD, and congenital heart disorders. In acute PE, RV dysfunction is seen when there is >30–40% of pulmonary arterial tree obstruction that has been shown to be an independent and powerful determinant of adverse prognosis [61], with higher ICU admission and death within 30 days [11]. Early identification of these high-risk patients will help in guiding them to catheter-directed thrombolysis or surgical embolectomy to reduce recurrence and death. Although ECG-gated CT is ideal for quantification of RV volumes, in the setting of acute PE, ECG gating is not always available and also not necessary. The regular axial plane or a four-chamber reconstruction can be used, and a RV/LV ratio >0.9 indicates elevated RV volume and RV strain [62] (Fig. 35.7a). Other secondary signs of RV strain include septal straightening or bowing (Fig. 35.7b), which is seen throughout cardiac cycle due to pressure overload and only in diastole for volume overload; dilated SVC (>25 mm), coronary sinus (>16 mm), and azygos vein (>25 mm); and reflux of contrast into IVC and hepatic veins [63] (Fig. 35.7c). CT can be utilized for serial changes in RV function and volumes, particularly with therapy and in those patients with contraindications for CMR (Fig. 35.8). RV dysfunction is an adverse prognostic determinant in other pulmonary disorders including cor pulmonale, interstitial lung diseases, obstructive sleep disorders, and pulmonary hypertension. For example, increased RVEDV and decreased EF have been associated with lower survival in cor pulmonale [64]. Higher RV volumes have been observed in liver diseases due to hepatopulmonary syndrome, portopulmonary hypertension, and TIPS therapy [65].

Congenital disorders including tetralogy of Fallot, transposition of great arteries, double outlet right ventricle, single ventricle physiologies, and shunt lesions (ASD, VSD, PDA, anomalous pulmonary venous return) may be associated with RV dilation and dysfunction [11]. For example, RV hypertrophy/dilation and dysfunction are seen in D-TGA following atrial switch procedure or in L-TGA due to inability of the morphologic right ventricle ("systemic ventricle")

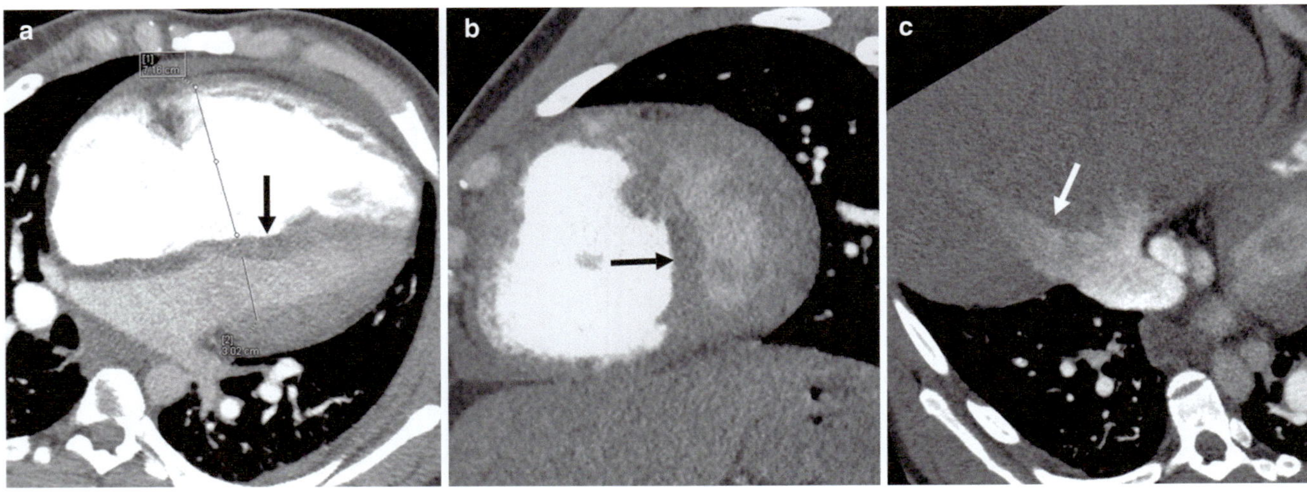

Fig. 35.7 Features of RV dysfunction in CT. (**a**) Axial CT scan shows RV/LV diameter ratio of 2.4. (**b**) Short-axis reconstruction of CT shows dilated RV and bowing of the interventricular septum (arrow) toward the LV. (**c**) Reflux of contrast in hepatic veins and IVC (arrow)

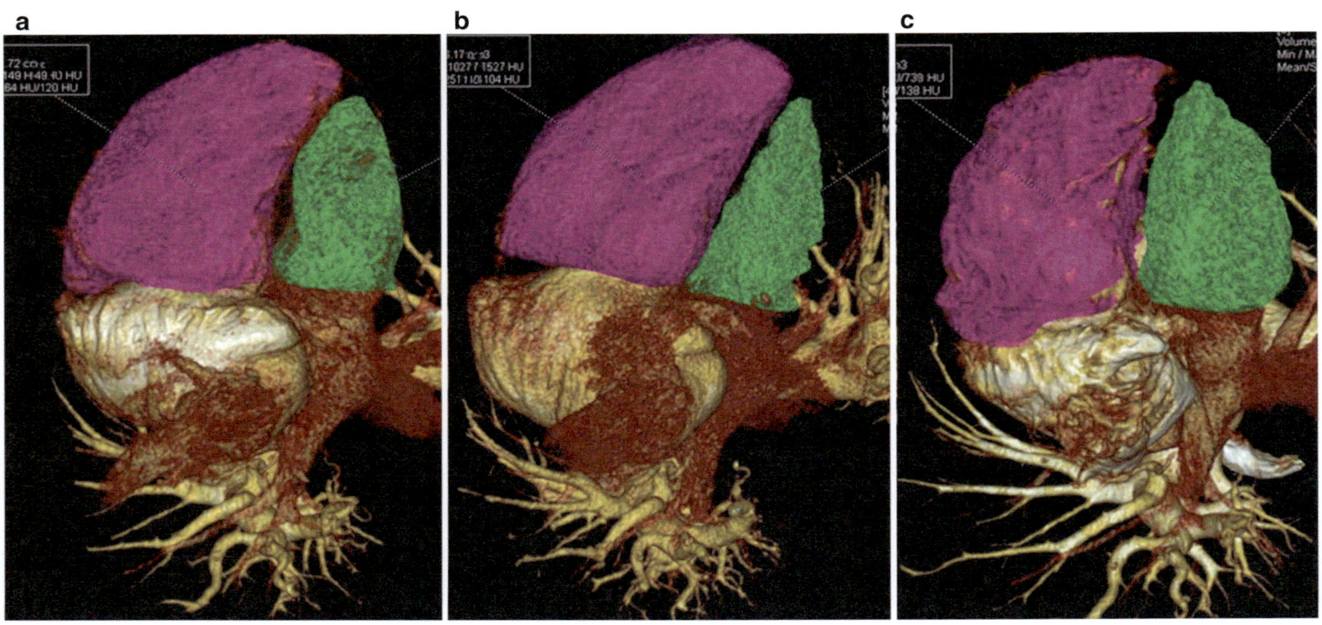

Fig. 35.8 Serial changes of RV volumes. 3D volume-rendered images in a patient with pulmonary hypertension show changes in RV volumes with time, with RVV/LVV values of 3.8 (**a**), 4.2 (**b**), and 2.6 (**c**) at 3 monthly intervals

to cope up with the systemic circulation. RV dysfunction and pulmonic regurgitation are common complications seen after surgical treatment of tetralogy of Fallot. RV function and volumes are important variables for repeat surgeries or interventional procedures such as percutaneous valve implantation. For example, pulmonary valve replacement is indicated in these patients when RVEDVI <170 ml/m^2 or RVDESVI <85 ml/m^2 [66] with lower cutoffs for chronic pulmonic regurgitation of 163 ml/m^2 and 80 ml/m^2, respectively [67].

Abnormal RV volumes and function are seen in several cardiomyopathies, particularly arrhythmogenic right ventricular dysplasia (ARVD). Recent task force criteria specify major criteria as a major wall motion abnormality (aneurysm, dyskinesis, dysynchrony, akinesia) along with RV dilation (EDVi >110 ml/m^2 in males, 100 ml/m^2 in females) or RV dysfunction (<40%). EDVi>100 ml/m^2 in males, 90 ml/m^2 in females, or RV dysfunction (40–45%) is considered as a minor criteria, although these criteria are derived from MRI [68]. ARVD is an appropriate indication for cardiac CT in 2010 ACCF guidelines [10]. Fatty tissue, bulging, and RV dilation help in distinguishing ARVD from tachyarrhythmia [69].

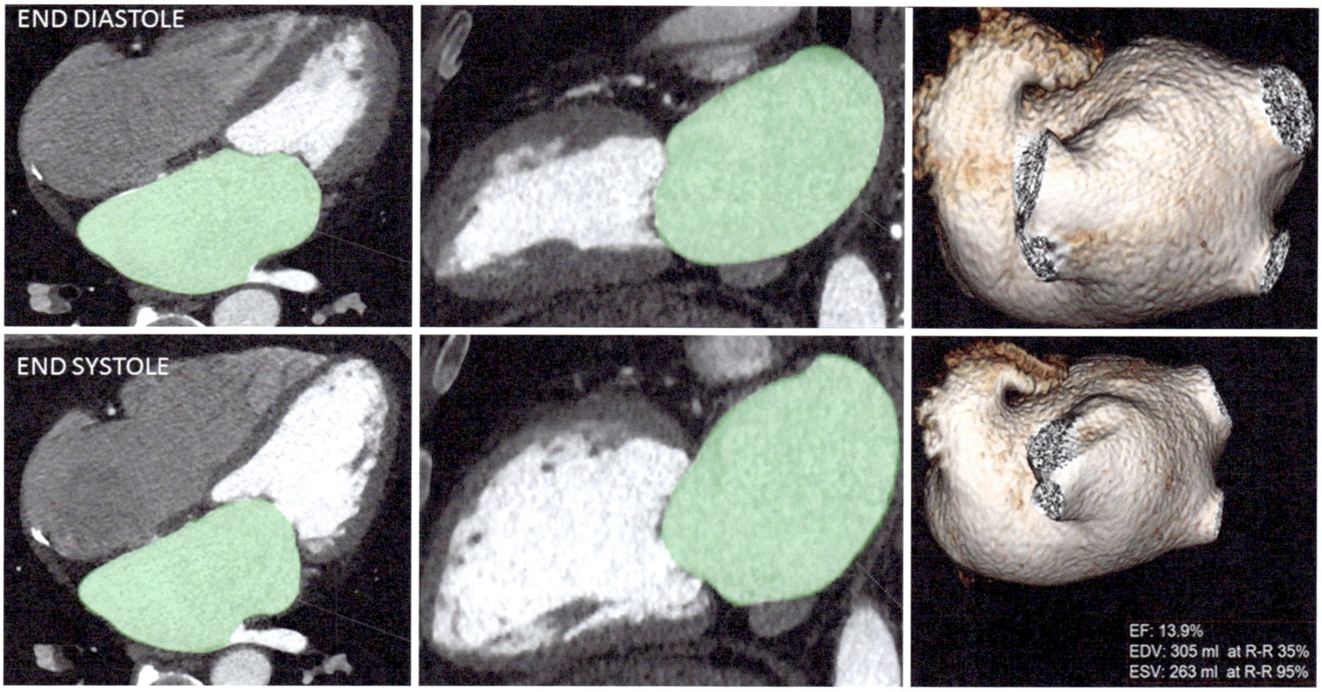

Fig. 35.9 Left atrial function. Short-axis (left), two-chamber (middle), and 3D volume-rendered (right) reconstructions of the heart at end-diastole (top row) and end-systole (bottom row). By segmenting (green) the left atrium both in end-diastole and end-systole, the left atrial volumes and function can be quantified. All these can be indexed to the body surface area (BSA)

Left Atrium

Left atrial volumes and function can be obtained from the same image data that is utilized for LV and RV quantification. Manual, semiautomated, or automated techniques are used to draw endocardial contours in the ED and ES phases with Simpson's method or used in threshold-based segmentation (Fig. 35.9).

Normal atrial filling has three phases, with an early rapid filling accounting for 75–80%, followed by diastasis accounting for 5%, and then an atrial systole accounting for 15–25% of LV blood volume [70]. Impaired relaxation of LV, with increased LA volume and lower LA EF, is seen in patients with restrictive cardiomyopathies (heart failure with preserved ejection fraction), and this can be used to distinguish it from other causes of LV hypertrophy including hypertension [71]. Although echocardiography is the most commonly used modality for evaluation of LA function, it has several limitations as discussed above. Body habitus and poor lateral resolution make it difficult to delineate the endocardium accurately in the posteriorly located left atrium, which results in lower atrial volumes and low accuracy and reproducibility [72–75]. CT values correlate with those of CMR, but usually, the LA volume is overestimated, and LA EF is underestimated [76].

Conclusion

CT provides accurate and reliable quantification of ventricular and atrial volumes and function, comparable to MRI and echocardiography. CT is used in specific circumstances where echocardiography is inadequate and MRI cannot be performed due to contraindications or artifacts. Retrospective ECG-gated spiral acquisitions are required for functional evaluation in CT, with the radiation dose minimized by using ECG-based tube current modulation.

References

1. Hammermeister KE, DeRouen TA, Dodge HT. Variables predictive of survival in patients with coronary disease. Selection by univariate and multivariate analyses from the clinical, electrocardiographic, exercise, arteriographic, and quantitative angiographic evaluations. Circulation. 1979;59(3):421–30.
2. Mock MB, Ringquist I, Fisher LD, et al. Survival of medically treated patients in the coronary artery surgery study (CASS) registry. Circulation. 1982;66:562–8.
3. Sayyed SH, Cassidy MM, Hadi MA. Use of multidetector computed tomography for evaluation of global and regional left ventricular function. J Cardiovasc Comput Tomogr. 2009;3(S1):S23–34.
4. Setser RM, Eischer SE, Lorenz CH. Quantification of left ventricular function with magnetic resonance images acquired in real time. J Magn Reson Imaging. 2000;12:430–8.

5. de Geus-Oei LF, Mavinkurve-Groothuis AM, Bellerson L, et al. Scintigraphic techniques for early detection of cancer treatment-induced cardiotoxicity. J Nucl Med. 2011;52(4):560–71.
6. Slart RH, Bax JJ, de Jong RM, et al. Comparison of gated PET with MRI for evaluation of left ventricular function in patients with coronary artery disease. J Nucl Med. 2004;45(2):176–82.
7. Bavelaar-Croon CD, Kayser HW, van der Wall EE, et al. Left ventricular function: correlation of quantitative gated SPECT and MR imaging over a wide range of values. Radiology. 2000;217(2):572–5.
8. Bodenheimer MMBV, Fooshee CM, Hermann GA, et al. Comparison of wall motion and regional ejection fraction at rest and during isometric exercise: concise communication. J Nucl Med. 1979;20:724–32.
9. Stollfuss JC, Haas F, Matsunari I, et al. Regional myocardial wall thickening and global ejection fraction in patients with low angiographic left ventricular ejection fraction assessed by visual and quantitative resting ECG-gated 99mTc-tetrofosmin single-photon emission tomography and magnetic resonance imaging. Eur J Nucl Med. 1998;25(5):522–30.
10. Taylor AJ, Cerqueira M, Hodgson JM, et al. ACCF/SCCT/ACR/AHA/ASE/ASNC/SCAI/SCMR 2010 appropriate use criteria for cardiac computed tomography. J Am Coll Cardiol. 2010;56(22):1864–94.
11. Savino G, Zwerner P, Herzog C, et al. CT of cardiac function. J Thorac Imaging. 2007;22:86–100.
12. Ritchie C, Godwin J, Crawford C, et al. Minimum scan speeds for suppression of motion artifacts in CT. Radiology. 1992;185:37–42.
13. Port S, Cobb FR, Jones RH. Effects of propranolol on left ventricular function in normal men. Circulation. 1989;61(12):358–66.
14. Mo YH, Jaw FS, Wang YC, et al. Effects of propranolol on the left ventricular volume of normal subjects during CT coronary angiography. Korean J Radiol. 2011;12(3):319.
15. Dell'Italia LJ, Walsh RA. Effect of intravenous metoprolol on left ventricular performance in Q-wave acute myocardial infarction. Am J Cardiol. 1989;63(3):166–71.
16. Jensen CJ, Jochims M, Hunold P, et al. Assessment of left ventricular function and mass in dual-source computed tomography coronary angiography: influence of beta-blockers on left ventricular function: comparison to magnetic resonance imaging. Eur J Radiol. 2010;74(3):484–91.
17. Lee H, Kim SY, Gebregziabher M, et al. Impact of ventricular contrast medium attenuation on the accuracy of left and right ventricular function analysis at cardiac multi detector-row CT compared with cardiac MRI. Acad Radiol. 2012;19(4):395–405.
18. Gao Y, Du X, Liang L, et al. Evaluation of right ventricular function by 64-row CT in patients with chronic obstructive pulmonary disease and cor pulmonale. Eur J Radiol. 2012;81(2):345–53.
19. Cademartiri F, Nieman K, van der Lugt A, et al. Intravenous contrast material administration at 16-detector row helical CT coronary angiography: test bolus versus bolus-tracking technique. Radiology. 2004;233(3):817–23.
20. Rizvi A, Deano RC, Bachman DP, et al. Analysis of ventricular function by computed tomography. J Cardiovasc Comput Tomogr. 2015;9(1):1–12.
21. Takx RAP, Moscariello A, Schoepf UJ, et al. Quantification of left and right ventricular function and myocardial mass: comparison of low-radiation dose 2nd generation dual-source CT and cardiac MRI. Eur J Radiol. 2012;81(4):e598–604.
22. Hausleiter J, Meyer T, Hadamitzky M, et al. Radiation dose estimates from cardiac multislice computed tomography in daily practice. Circulation. 2006;113:1305–10.
23. Hausleiter J, et al. A new algorithm for ECG-based tube current modulation ("MinDose") reduces radiation dose estimates in cardiac dual source CT angiography. Circulation. 2007;116(Suppl 16):II-575.
24. Feuchtner G, Goetti R, Plass A, et al. Dual-step prospective ECG-triggered 128-slice dual source CT for evaluation of coronary arteries and cardiac function without heart rate control a technical note. Eur Radiol. 2010;20:2092–9.
25. Ko YJ, Kim SS, Park WJ, et al. Comparison of global left ventricular function using 20 phases with 10-phase reconstructions in multidetector-row computed tomography. Int J Cardiovasc Imaging. 2012;28(3):603–11.
26. Puesken M, Fischbach R, Wenker M, et al. Global left-ventricular function assessment using dual-source multidetector CT: effect of improved temporal resolution on ventricular volume measurement. Eur Radiol. 2008;18(10):2087–94.
27. Wai B, Thai WE, Brown H, et al. Novel phase-based noise reduction strategy for quantification of left ventricular function and mass assessment by cardiac CT: comparison with cardiac magnetic resonance. Eur J Radiol. 2013;82:e337–41.
28. Lessick J, Ghersin E, Abadi S, Yalonetsky S. Accuracy of the long-axis area-length method for the measurement of left ventricular volumes and ejection fraction using multidetector computed tomograph. Can J Cardiol. 2008;24(9):685–9.
29. Greupner J, Zimmermann E, Hamm B, Dewey M. Automatic versus semiautomatic global cardiac function assessment using 64-row computed tomography. Br J Radiol. 2012;85(1015):e243–53.
30. Juergens KU, Seifarth H, Range F, et al. Automated threshold-based 3D segmentation versus short-axis planimetry for assessment of global left ventricular function with dual-source MDCT. Am J Roentgenol. 2008;190(2):308–14.
31. Plumhans C, Keil S, Ocklenburg C, et al. Comparison of manual, semi- and fully automated heart segmentation for assessing global left ventricular function in multidetector computed tomography. Investig Radiol. 2009;44(8):476–82.
32. van Ooijen PM, de Jonge GJ, Oudkerk M. Informatics in radiology: Postprocessing pitfalls in using CT for automatic and semiautomatic determination of global left ventricular function. Radiographics. 2012;32(2):589–99.
33. de Jonge GJ, can der Vleuten PA, Overbosch J, et al. Semiautomatic measurement of left ventricular function on dual source computed tomography using five different software tools in comparison with magnetic resonance imaging. Eur J Radiol. 2011;80(3):755–66.
34. Mao SS, Li D, Rosenthal DG, et al. Dual-standard reference values of left ventricular volumetric parameters by multidetector CT angiography. J Cardiovasc Comput Tomogr. 2013;7:234–40.
35. Juergens UK, Fischbach R. Left ventricular function studied with MDCT. Eur Radiol. 2006;16:342–57.
36. Alfakih K, Plein S, Thiele H, et al. Normal human left and right ventricular dimensions for MRI as assessed by turbo gradient echo and steady state free precession imaging sequences. J Magn Reson Imaging. 2003;17:323–9.
37. Sandstede J, Lipke C, Beer M, et al. Age and gender specific differences in left and right ventricular cardiac function and mass determined by cine magnetic resonance imaging. Eur Radiol. 2000;10:438–42.
38. Boogers MJ, van Werkhoven JM, Shuijf JD, et al. Feasibility of diastolic functional assessment with cardiac CT: feasibility study in comparison with tissue Doppler imaging. JACC Cardiovasc Imaging. 2011;4:246–56.
39. Lin FY, et al. Cardiac chamber volumes, function, and mass as determined by 64-multidetector row computed tomography: mean values among healthy adults free of hypertension and obesity. JACC Cardiovasc Imaging. 2008;1(6):782–6.
40. Nevsky G, Jacobs JE, Lim RP, et al. Sex-specific normalized reference values of heart and great vessel dimensions in cardiac CT angiography. Am J Roentgenol. 2011;196:788–94.
41. Juergens KU, Grude M, Maintz D, et al. Multi-detector row CT of left ventricular function with dedicated analysis software versus MR imaging: initial experience. Radiology. 2004;230:403–10.

42. Mahnken AH, Speuntrup E, Neithammer M, et al. Quantitative and qualitative assessment of left ventricular volume with ECG-gated multislice spiral CT: value of different image reconstruction algorithms in comparison to MRI. Acta Radiol. 2003;44(6):604–11.
43. van der Vleuten PA, Willems TP, Gotte MJ, et al. Quantification of global left ventricular function: comparison of multidetector computed tomography and magnetic resonance imaging. A meta-analysis and review of the current literature. Acta Radiol. 2006;47(10):1049–57.
44. Grude M, Juegens KU, Wichter T, et al. Evaluation of global left ventricular myocardial function with electrocardiogram gated multidetector computed tomography. Comparison with magnetic resonance imaging. Investig Radiol. 2003;38:653–61.
45. Asferg C, Usinger L, Kristensen TS, et al. Accuracy of multi-slice computed tomography for measurement of left ventricular ejection fraction compared with cardiac magnetic resonance imaging and two-dimensional transthoracic echocardiography: a systematic review and metaanalysis. Eur J Radiol. 2011;81:e756–62.
46. Dewey M, Muller M, Eddicks S, et al. Evaluation of global and regional left ventricular function with 16-slice computed tomography, biplane cineventriculography and two-dimensional transthoracic echocardiography: comparison with magnetic resonance imaging. J Am Coll Cardiol. 2006;48:2034.
47. Mahias-Narvarte AHKF, Willis PW. Evolution of regional left ventricular wall motion abnormalities in acute Q and non-Q wave myocardial infarction. American Heart Journal. 1987;113:1369–75.
48. Sarwar A, Shapiro MD, Nasir K, et al. Evaluating global and regional left ventricular function in patients with reperfused acute myocardial infarction by 64-slice multidetector CT: a comparison to magnetic resonance imaging. J Cardiovasc Comput Tomogr. 2009;3(3):170–7.
49. Seneviratne SK, Troung QA, Bamberg F, et al. Incremental diagnostic value of regional left ventricular function over coronary assessment by cardiac computed tomography for the detection of acute coronary syndrome in patients with acute chest pain: from the ROMICAT trial. Circ Cardiovasc Imaging. 2010;3(8):375–83.
50. Bezerra HG, Loureiro R, Irlbeck T, et al. Incremental value of myocardial perfusion over regional left ventricular function and coronary stenosis by cardiac CT for detection of acute coronary syndromes in high risk patients: a subgroup analysis of the ROMICAT trial. J Cardiovasc Comput Tomogr. 2011;5:382–91.
51. Candell-Riera JLJ, Santana C, Castell J, et al. Prognostic assessment of uncomplicated first myocardial infarction by exercise echocardiography and Tc-99m tetrofosmin gated SPECT. J Nucl Cardiol. 2001;81:122–8.
52. Antonini-Canterin FNG. Valutazione eoardiografica dei volume e della funzione sistolica globale del ventricolo sinistro. Ital Heart J. 2000;1:1261–72.
53. Arsanjani R, Berman DS, Gransar H, et al. Left ventricular function and volume with coronary CT angiography improves risk stratification and identification of patients at risk for incident mortality: results from 7758 patients in the prospective multinational CONFIRM observational cohort study. Radiology. 2014;273(1):70–7
54. Mastrobuoni S, Dell'aquila AM, Arraiza M, et al. Allograft morphology and function in heart transplant recipients surviving more than 15 years by magnetic resonance imaging and dual-source computed tomography. Eur J Cardiothorac Surg. 2011;40(1):e62–6.
55. Bastarrika G, Arraiza M, DeCecco CN, et al. Quantification of left ventricular function and mass in heart transplant recipients using dual-source CT and MRI: initial clinical experience. Eur Radiol. 2008;18(9):1784–90.
56. Taylor DO, Edwards LB, Aurora P, et al. Registry of the International Society for Heart and Lung Transplantation: twenty-fifth official adult heart transplant report—2008. J Heart Lung Transplant. 2008;27(9):943–56.
57. Acharya D, Singh S, Tallaj JA, et al. Use of gated cardiac computed tomography angiography in the assessment of left ventricular assist device dysfunction. ASAIO J. 2011;57:32–7.
58. Geva T. Is MRI the preferred method for evaluating right ventricular size and function in patients with congenital heart disease? Circ Cardiovasc Imaging. 2014;7:190–7.
59. Raman SV, Shah M, McCarthy B, et al. Multi-detector row cardiac computed tomography accurately quantifies right and left ventricular size and function compared with cardiac magnetic resonance. Am Heart J. 2006;151:736–44.
60. Guo YK, Gao HL, Zhang XC, et al. Accuracy and reproducibility of assessing right ventricular function with 64-section multidetector row CT: comparison with magnetic resonance imaging. Int J Cardiol. 2010;139:254–62.
61. Kang DK, Thilo C, Schoepf UJ, et al. CT signs of right ventricular dysfunction. J Am Coll Cardiol Img. 2011;4(8):841–9.
62. Quiroz R, Kucher N, Schoepf UJ, et al. Right ventricular enlargement on chest computed tomography: prognostic role in acute pulmonary embolism. Circulation. 2004;109(20):2401–4.
63. Staskiewicz G, Czekajska-Chehab E, Przegalinski J, et al. Widening of coronary sinus in CT pulmonary angiography indicates right ventricular dysfunction in patients with acute pulmonary embolism. Eur Radiol. 2010;20:1615–20.
64. Burgess MI, Mogulkoc N, Bright-Thomas RJ, et al. Comparison of echocardiographic markers of right ventricular function in determining prognosis in chronic pulmonary disease. J Am Soc Echocardiogr. 2002;15:633–9.
65. Dupont MVM, Dragean CA, Coche EE. Right ventricle function assessment by MDCT. Am J Roentgenol. 2011;196(1):77–86.
66. Therrien J, Provost Y, Merchant N, et al. Optimal timing for pulmonary valve replacement in adults after tetralogy of Fallot repair. Am J Cardiol. 2005;95:779–82.
67. Lee C, Kim YM, Lee CH, et al. Outcomes of pulmonary valve replacement in 170 patients with chronic pulmonary regurgitation after relief of right ventricular outflow tract obstruction: implications for optimal timing of pulmonary valve replacement. J Am Coll Cardiol. 2012;60:1005–14.
68. Marcus F, McKenna WJ, Sherrill D, et al. Diagnosis of arrhythmogenic right ventricular cardiomyopathy/dysplasia: proposed modification of the task force criteria. Eur Heart J. 2010;31(7):806–14.
69. Nakajima T, Kimura F, Kajimoto K, et al. Utility of ECG-gated MDCT to differentiate patients with ARVC/D from patients with ventricular tachyarrhythmias. J Cardiovasc Comput Tomogr. 2013;7:223–33.
70. Stojanovska J, Cronin P, Patel S, et al. Reference normal absolute and indexed values from ECG-gated MDCT: left atrial volume, function, and diameter. Am J Roentgenol. 2011;197(3):631–7.
71. Melenovsky V, Borlaug B, Rosen, et al. Cardiovascular features of heart failure with preserved ejection fraction versus non-failing hypertensive left ventricular hypertrophy in the urban Baltimore community. J Am Coll Cardiol. 2007;49:198.
72. Avelar E, Durst R, Rosito GA, et al. Comparison of the accuracy of multidetector computed tomography versus two-dimensional echocardiography to measure left atrial volume. Am J Cardiol. 2010;106(1):104–9.
73. Rodevan O, Bjornerheim R, Ljosland M, et al. Left atrial volumes assessed by three- and two-dimensional echocardiography compared to MRI estimates. Int J Card Imaging. 1999;15:397–410.
74. Christiaens L, Lequeux B, Ardilouze P, et al. A new method for measurement of LA volumes using 64-slice spiral CT: comparison with 2DE techniques. Int J Cardiol. 2009;131:217–24.
75. Kircher B, Abbott JA, Paul S, et al. Left atrial volume determination by biplane two-dimensional echocardiography: validation by cine CT. Am Heart J. 1991;121:864–71.
76. Wen Z, Zhang Z, Yu W, et al. Assessing the left atrial phase volume and function with dual-source CT: comparison with 3T MRI. Int J Cardiovasc Imaging. 2010;26:88–92.

Three-Chamber Function with Cardiac CT

36

Jongmin Lee

Basic Concepts

Congestive heart failure can be defined as the inability of the heart to pump blood forward at a sufficient rate to meet the metabolic demands of the body or the ability to do so only if the cardiac filling pressures are abnormally high. Congestive heart failure is regarded as the final and most severe manifestation of common forms of cardiac disease. To evaluate the progress or risk of heart failure, a comprehensive assessment of cardiac function is required.

The ability of the heart to pump blood is called the cardiac function. Traditionally, the mechanical function of heart has been described by the pressure, volume, and flow changes during a cardiac cycle [1]. The volumes, mass, and function of cardiac chambers provide important diagnostic and prognostic information for patients with ischemic or nonischemic cardiomyopathies [2].

Cardiac Output

A representative and comprehensive parameter of whole-heart function is cardiac output. Cardiac output is the sum of stroke volumes during 1 min, which can be expressed as "stroke volume x heart rate." Cardiac output is a parameter representing a ventricular pumping function normalized by the heart rate. Since theoretically the heart rate influences the ventricular ejection fraction and the stroke volume as a reverse correlation with the diastolic filling time, heart rate should be normalized for the objective comparison of a cardiac output function. The cardiac output is a relevant diagnostic and prognostic factor in various cardiovascular diseases and an important surrogate marker for a global cardiac function. In addition, cardiac output is a crucial factor for deciding whether a patient is a suitable candidate for cardiac transplant surgery.

Various methods to measure the cardiac output have been conceived and applied successfully. Direct measurement techniques for the cardiac output are accurate but invasive. Based on the Fick principle, which calculates the flow volume by the tissue consumption of a substance such as oxygen, the cardiac output can be acquired as a function of oxygen consumption, arterial and venous oxygen saturation, and blood hemoglobin concentration (Eq. 36.1).

$$Q = \frac{X_{tc}}{\left\{\left[[X]_a - [X]_v\right] \times [Hb] \times 1.36 \times 10\right\}} \quad (36.1)$$

Q, cardiac output; X_{tc}, tissue consumption of oxygen; $[x]_a$, arterial concentration of oxygen; $[x]_v$, venous concentration of oxygen; [Hb], concentration of hemoglobin [3]

Indicator dilution methods are other accurate options for measuring the cardiac output, but they are also invasive methods. Right heart catheterization-based thermodilution technique has been used as a gold standard method to determine cardiac output [4].

Indirect methods for the cardiac output measurement have been developed for a less invasive and simpler application. If the relationship between the pulse pressure and the stroke volume is assumed to be linear, the fractional change of the cardiac output can be acquired by the "fractional change of pulse pressure x fractional change of heart rate." For example, if both the pulse pressure and the heart rate increase up to 10%, the cardiac output increases 21% by the calculation as "1.1 * 1.1 = 1.21" [1]. A more simplified indirect solution is suggested by van Lieshout et al. [5]. Cardiac output is acquired based on an empirical assumption that each 1 mmHg pulse pressure is responsible for approximately 2 ml of stroke volume (CO = HR * PP * 2 ml). An additional empirical fact is that body surface area has a greater influence on cardiac output than body weight or body mass index. Therefore, patient-tailored cardiac output index based on body surface area is suggested as a useful marker [1].

J. Lee (✉)
Department of Radiology, Kyungpook National University, School of Medicine, Daegu, South Korea
e-mail: Jonglee@knu.ac.kr

U. J. Schoepf (ed.), *CT of the Heart*, Contemporary Medical Imaging, https://doi.org/10.1007/978-1-60327-237-7_36

Cardiac Function

The influencing factors of the cardiac pumping function can be classified as preload, afterload, and myocardial inotropic functions. Abnormal ventricular function can be classified as systolic and diastolic dysfunctions. The systolic dysfunction means an impaired myocardial contractility due to either a myocardial weakening or an increased afterload. Diastolic dysfunction typically refers to an impaired chamber filling with an increasing afterload of the chamber upstream.

Preload

The preload of cardiac ventricles can be evaluated using some morphometric markers such as end-diastolic volume (ventricular end-diastolic fiber length), stroke volume, ventricular dilatation, intrathoracic blood volume, and atrial ejection parameters. The atrial and ventricular preload may be influenced by the distribution of blood between the intrathoracic and extrathoracic compartments. The blood volume distribution is influenced by the body position, the intrathoracic pressure, the intrapericardial pressure, the venous tone, and the pumping action of skeletal muscle. Atrial contraction is a particularly important preload in the case of ventricular diastolic dysfunction.

How does the preload influence to a downstream function? The atrial stroke volume may control the downstream ventricular ejection function. The Frank-Starling law defined that the stroke volume of the cardiac chamber increases in response to the increase in the volume of blood filling the chamber (the end-diastolic volume) when all other factors remain constant. This reflective physiology is explained as a neurohormonal activation mechanism dominating myocardium. The Frank-Starling law explains how the preload can influence to the inotropic function (Fig. 36.1).

Afterload

The ventricular afterload can be estimated using markers such as end-systolic volume, stroke volume, ventricular mass, aortic distensibility (AD), aortic volume, and systemic vascular resistance or impedance. Since the arterial flow pattern is pulsatile with different heart rates, the resistance against the blood flow changes continuously and periodically. To explain the flow resistance in fluctuating arterial flow, a complex-valued generalization of resistance is used, which is the "impedance."

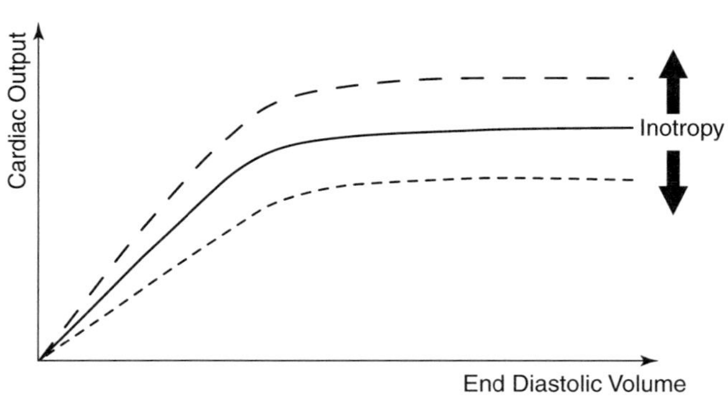

Fig. 36.1 The Frank-Starling law of the heart explains a positive provocation of end-diastolic volume (x-axis) to cardiac output (y-axis). By the ventricular inotropic function, the curve shifts to upward or downward

The ventricular afterload is influenced by the intraluminal pressure of great arteries, ventricular wall stress and tension, and end-diastolic volume and strain. An excessive ventricular dilatation state increases myocardial stress by Laplace law (i.e., tension = radius × pressure) and requires higher inotropic reflex by Frank-Starling law, which result in the excessive afterload of the ventricle. If the ventricular luminal volume increases, the perpendicular pressure to the myocardium increases due to the increased mass of contained blood. This pressure is a burden against the myocardial contraction and hence the afterload.

The aortic pressure is related to the peripheral vascular resistance (PVR), the arterial compliance, and the volume of blood. Based on the Ohm's law, the PVR can be simply acquired by the ratio of a pulse pressure (PP) and a stroke volume (i.e., PVR = PP/SV).

Inotropic State

The ventricular inotropic activity is influenced by the end-diastolic volume (preload), sympathetic nerve activity, circulating catecholamines, exogenously administered inotropic agents, physiologic depressants, pharmacologic depressants, loss of ventricular substance, and intrinsic myocardial depression. The sympathetic nerve activity is increased by norepinephrine released at sympathetic nerve endings and increases cardiac output. Therefore, the end-diastolic volume may not be changed because of the increased ventricular contractility and heart rate. The circulating catecholamines may be produced from adrenal gland and extracardiac sympathetic ganglia. The exogenous inotropic agents are cardiac glycosides, isoproterenol, sympathomimetic agents, calcium, caffeine, theophylline, etc. The physiologic depressants are myocardial hypoxia, hypercapnia, ischemia, and acidosis, and the pharmacologic depressants are guanidine, procainamide, barbiturates, anesthetics, and so on [6].

The in vivo ventricular contractility may be difficult to measure directly. Instead, the common markers representing myocardial inotropic function are stroke volume, ejection fraction, and their secondary derivatives. The ventricular ejection fraction is an extremely useful indirect clinical marker representing the myocardial contractility and is widely accepted for a routine clinical application. However, since the ejection fraction value may be confounded by the ventricular afterload, this cannot be an absolute myocardial contractility marker. In addition, a simple ratio between end-diastolic and end-systolic volumes doesn't reflect the size variability of ventricles, which influences to the stroke volume. For example, the athlete's heart can maintain the stroke volume and the left ventricle diastolic function in spite of the decreased ejection fraction in a resting state.

As an indirect but invasive method, the maximum pressure gradient rate (dP/dt_{max}) can be measured by the intraventricular catheterization. This value is usually acquired during isovolumetric contraction. The normal range of the left ventricular dP/dt_{max} has been suggested to be 1500–2000 mmHg/s [1]. Another potential indirect and noninvasive marker for the ventricular inotropic function is the strain. The myocardial strain imaging is available using echocardiography and cardiac MRI by tracking speckles and tagging matrix. However, it is limited to register speckles or matrix on CT images directly. Currently, based on the voxel tracking of a motion coherence algorithm, CT strain imaging was used to evaluate three-dimensional myocardial deformation during a cardiac cycle, and favorable results were reported to show myocardial inotropic function [7].

Cardiac CT

There has been uncertainty regarding the comprehensive evaluation of the left ventricular function using MDCT [8, 9]. However, from the beginning of MDCT, MDCT-derived cardiac function parameters have shown a significant correlation with reference values demonstrating its potency for routine clinical applications [10, 11]. A geometric chamber function evaluation by CT shows a significant accuracy and reproducibility compared with MRI [12]. In addition, a phantom study validated dual-source CT as the most accurate modality for the left ventricular function evaluation, which was better than 64-slice MDCT and MRI [13]. A large-scale prospective multinational observational cohort study using CONFIRM registry reported that an additional measurement of left ventricular function on CT coronary angiography could improve the risk stratification and identification of patients at risk for incident mortality. In this study, the LVEF, LVEDV, and LVESV demonstrated significant diversions of mortality curves [14]. Therefore, the cardiac CT function study, at least for left ventricle, should be in a consensus of clinical feasibility.

Due to the technical advances in MDCT, high-quality cine images can be acquired, and three-dimensional images of all cardiac chambers can be generated. In addition, many post-processing software applications supply an option to automatically evaluate three-chamber function. Since the automated segmentation of the right atrium has a limitation until now, the other three chambers are now candidates for automated segmentation (Fig. 36.2). The automated three-chamber function evaluation using MDCT has been extensively validated with cardiac MR data [2, 15].

	LV		RV		LA	
Parameter	Value	(Index)	Value	(Index)	Value	(Index)
Ejection Fraction%	69		60		33	
End Diastolic Volume(ml)	142	87	150	92	97	59
End Systolic Volume(ml)	45	27	61	37	65	39
Stroke Volume (ml)	97	59	90	55	32	20
Cardiac Output(L/min)	6.0	3.7	5.6	3.4		

	LV			LA	
Parameter	Value	(Index)	Parameter	Value	(Index)
Myocardial Mass (g)	107		Maximal Volume (ml)	123	75
Myocardial Volume (ml)	102		Cyclic Volume Change (ml)	58	36
LV/RV Regurgitation Fraction(%)	7.9		Reservoir Volume(ml)	27	

Heart Rate:	62 bpm
BSA:	1.6 m^2

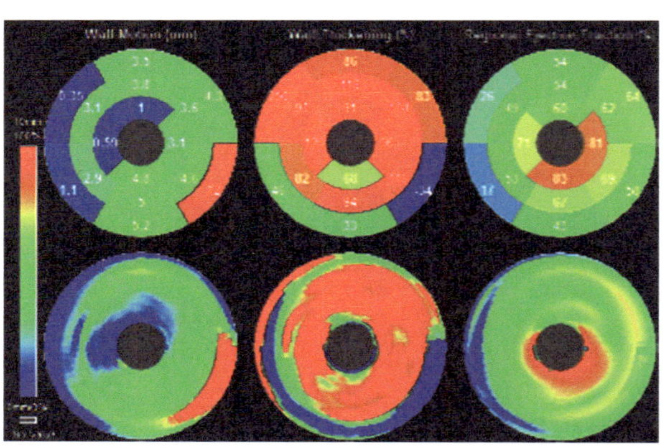

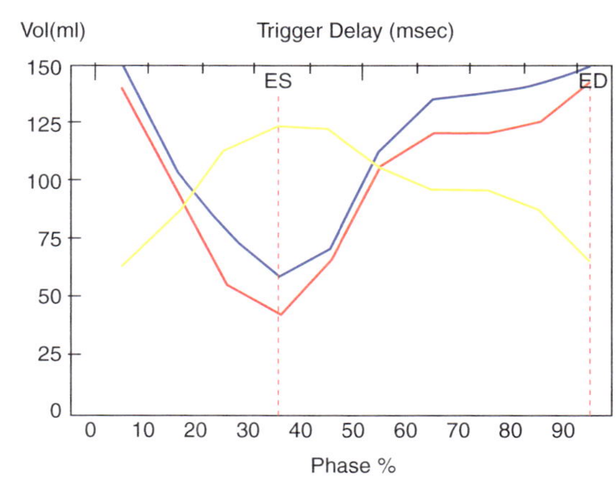

Fig. 36.2 The reports of the automated three-chamber function evaluation. The left atrial cyclic volume change (58 ml) is lower than left ventricular stroke volume (97 ml) due to the existence of conduit flow. In this software, the left atrial ejection fraction calculates the ejected volume fraction of active pumping

Although cardiac MR is the reference standard in determining left ventricular function, based on the clinical feasibility and high spatial resolution cardiac CT, CT-based function evaluation is becoming more feasible. In this chapter, the chamber function evaluation using MDCT will be discussed for each chamber. In addition, the comprehensive multichamber function evaluation will be discussed in viewpoints of hemodynamic ergonomics and morphometric markers.

Left Ventricular Function

The left ventricle is the most important chamber for the comprehensive cardiac pumping function, as the left ventricle is the final thrust for systemic arterial blood circulation against relatively high flow impedance. During one cardiac functional cycle, the left ventricular volume changes in a multimodal pattern. During systole, left ventricular functional phases comprise of isovolumic contraction and ejection. During diastole, isovolumic relaxation, rapid inflow, diastasis, and atrial systole phases are included. If CT images are reconstructed using ten phases for one cardiac cycle, the end-systolic phase and the diastasis phase match fourth and seventh to eighth phases, respectively (Fig. 36.3).

Morphometric markers representing left ventricular preload are the left ventricular end-diastolic volume index (LVEDVI) and the left atrial systolic volume index (LASVI). The markers for the left ventricular contractility includes left ventricular ejection fraction (LVEF), left ventricular stroke volume index (LVSVI), left ventricular cardiac output index (LVCI), myocardial strain, and adjusted left ventricular emptying fraction ($_{adj}$LVeFr). The markers for the afterload of left ventricle are LVESVI, left ventricular muscle mass index (LVMMI), PVR, aortic AD, and aortic blood volume and so on. The indices are normalized values by the body surface area in a unit of square meters.

Markers for Preload

To evaluate the preload of the left ventricle, the LVEDV can be used. In a retrospectively ECG-gated cardiac CT, all diastolic phases are included. When ten phase images are reconstructed during one cardiac cycle, the image with phase number 9 or 10 would be the end-diastolic image. Since images with phase number 7–10 show better image quality than systolic phases due to less motion, the LVEDV measurement is more accurate and reproducible in automated post-processing software. The LVEDV may be influenced by the left ventricular myocardial compliance or strain, the size of the subject or total blood volume, the left atrial stroke volume, and the intrathoracic blood volume.

Beta-adrenergic inhibitor such as propranolol has a negative inotropic action and is used for reducing heart rate during cardiac CT. However, there is a concern about its influence on other functional cardiac parameters. Since beta-blockers decrease heart rate, the left atrial volume may be increased as the preload for left ventricle. Subsequently, the left ventricular end-diastolic volume and the stroke volume will be increased by the Frank-Starling law. Several studies reported that a beta-blocker has no effect on the systolic and diastolic blood pressure; however it increases the end-systolic volume and decreases the ejection fraction. However, minor controversy exists regarding the effect of beta-blockers on the end-diastolic volume [16–19]. Recently, more papers suggested that the beta-blocker effect on end-diastolic volume is insignificant [20]. This means that the beta-blocker may not significantly influence the preload of the left ventricle.

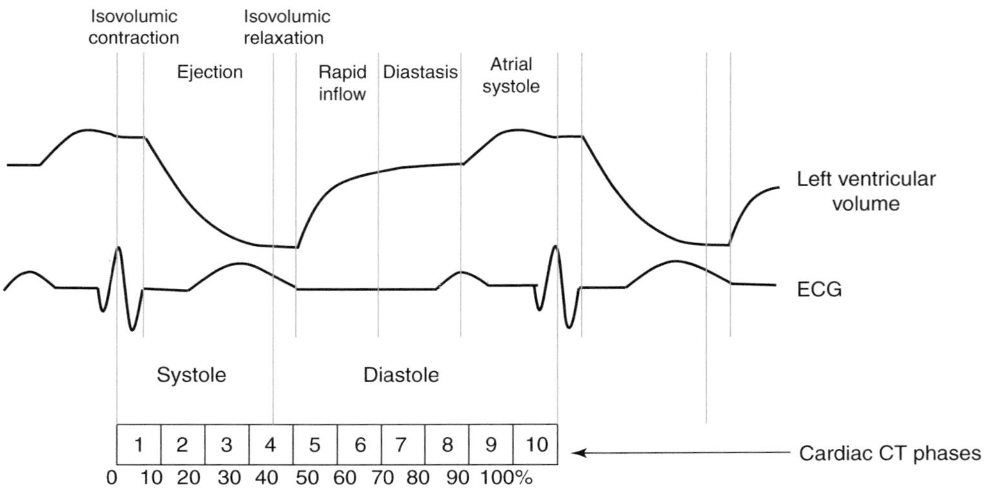

Fig. 36.3 Left ventricular time-volume curve during the cardiac cycle shows multimodal pattern. The usual cardiac phases for cardiac CT are diastasis and end-systolic phase, which match seventh to eighth and fourth series among reconstructed ten-phase cardiac CT image sets during a cardiac cycle

Markers for Inotropy

The ejection fraction, defined as the fraction of blood ejected from a ventricle with each heartbeat, is the most common parameter representing the left ventricular contractility and systolic function. The global ejection fraction of the left ventricle can be determined reliably by measuring the systolic and diastolic luminal volumes on the cardiac CT. In the cases of localized cardiomyopathy such as ischemic heart disease, due to compensatory hyperkinesia of normal myocardium, the global ejection fraction may be normal in spite of the regional wall motion abnormality [21].

Zeb et al. [22] evaluated the significance of the CT regional ejection fraction to depict the regional wall motion abnormality. By comparing CT results with SPECT myocardial perfusion and invasive coronary angiography, they suggested that the CT regional ejection fraction was comparable with SPECT perfusion imaging for depicting ischemic segments. In addition, they suggested that the CT regional ejection fraction showed a better performance than SPECT to determine significant coronary artery stenosis. Due to higher spatial resolution and image contrast, CT may detect a subtle change of regional wall motion. In addition, the regional wall motion abnormality detected on CT may be a sensitive presentation of myocardial ischemia.

As discussed in the basic concept section, the cardiac output is an important and common comprehensive marker for the cardiac pumping function. In cardiac CT, noninvasive measurement of the cardiac output has been attempted by adopting several complex mathematical and empirical formulae. Yee et al. [23] measured a left ventricular output using the bolus-timing scan for CT pulmonary angiography in a routine clinical setting. Using input variables including ascending and descending aortic radii, the geometric distance and the contrast media concentration between the ascending and descending aortas, a mathematically approximated left ventricular cardiac output was acquired. Although a clear validation of the method was not conducted, the feasibility on clinical practice is acceptable due to its simplicity without any additional risks to the patient.

From the preliminary bolus-timing scan data, a time-attenuation curve can be produced. Mahnken et al. [24] applied the Stewart-Hamilton equation to calculate a cardiac output using the area under the time-attenuation curve and the injected amount of contrast media as input variables. In addition, a conversion factor between the attenuation and real iodine concentration was included as an input constant (Eq. 36.2). To simulate the first pass flow without a recirculated contrast enhancement, a gamma variate function was additionally applied. As results, a significant correlation of the cardiac output and stroke volume data between a test-bolus technique and a geometric measurement was achieved.

$$\mathrm{CO} = \frac{Q^*}{\int_0^\infty c(t)\,dt} = \frac{K * f_{\mathrm{corr}} * Q}{A} \qquad (36.2)$$

Q the amount of indicator injected; $c(t)$ indicator concentration as a function of time; K the conversion factor between HU and Iodine concentration; A the area under the time-HU curve; $Q^*(=f_{\mathrm{corr}}{*}Q)$ the deconvolution correction factor

To avoid a complicated calculation for the cardiac output, a simple and indirect marker was recommended. A simple measurement of right-to-left cardiac transit time of contrast media during single-level bolus-timing scans presented a significant correlation with cardiac output index by MRI ($R^2 = 0.70$). A cut-off value of 20.5 s predicted cardiac dysfunction with 100% specificity and positive predictive value [25].

Strain is a concept of the continuum mechanics meaning "a deformation of a body without breakage from a reference configuration to a current configuration" [26]. In the case of the heart, a myocardial movement is driven by bimodal ergonomics, active systolic contraction, and passive diastolic relaxation. In addition, the myocardial movement is influenced by preload and its afterload. This complicated myocardial activity is expressed as the strain in cardiac imaging. In actuality, cardiac strain represents only the range of myocardial movement but cannot directly represent myocardial contractility or expansibility. However, the strain rate, which is the time derivative of the strain, may reflect active and passive motions of the myocardium. Currently, two-dimensional or three-dimensional myocardial strain is applied to evaluate the myocardial inotropic function.

Buss et al. [27] compared the endocardial strain and the strain rate between two-dimensional (2D) cardiac CT and echocardiography. Using a commercial tracking software, multidirectional endocardial strain was evaluated throughout one cardiac cycle. The results showed significant correlation with echocardiography and NT-pro-BNP level. Since the 2D cardiac CT strain imaging revealed significantly shorter processing time, high reproducibility, and lack of observation window limitation, non-inferiority to 2D echocardiography was disclosed.

In a recent study by Tanabe et al. [7] using cardiac CT and dedicated reconstruction software, 10-phase image sets are interpolated to 50 time frame image sets, and a three-dimensional left ventricular myocardial model is generated by image segmentation. From the mesh of the ventricular model, motion vectors and subsequent strain values can be acquired along longitudinal, radial, and circular directions. This strain evaluation presented an additional benefit of CT coronary angiography to detect an infarcted segment of myocardium.

Markers for Afterload

Just like typical fluid pumps, heart function may be influenced by the downstream flow impedance, referred to as afterload. Left ventricular afterload can be described as the aortic capacity to receive the left ventricular stroke volume. This aortic capacity may be related with intra-aortic blood mass, aortic wall stiffness or elasticity, and aortic morphology.

The aortic wall elasticity is a key factor for dampening the pulsatile energy of the entry flow and converting it to stabilized steady flow for the end organs. The aortic wall stiffness is an opposite concept to the dampening function and increases flow impedance throughout the aorta. Left ventricular output function is influenced by the aortic flow impedance, which is the afterload of left ventricular performance.

Ganten et al. [28] suggested the aortic AD as a marker for aortic wall stiffness (Eq. 36.3). Although the research was applied on abdominal aorta, the concept of the aortic AD may be applied on AAo and aortic arch for the left ventricular afterload evaluation.

$$D = \frac{\Delta A}{A_0 \cdot \Delta p} \qquad (36.3)$$

D, aortic distensibility; A, aortic cross-sectional area; A_0, minimum aortic cross sectional area during the cardiac cycle; p, blood pressure

Lee et al. [29] suggested the AWSI, which shows aortic wall stiffness consistently without any influence by different intraluminal pressures and aortic sizes. In ex vivo and in vivo experiments, AWSI showed a significantly higher accuracy than other stiffness factors including a classic compliance, Young's modulus of elasticity, beta-stiffness index, and aortic AD.

$$\text{AWSI} = \sqrt{\ln\left[\frac{\frac{-2b}{a^2}\cdot mBP}{\left\{1+\left(\frac{mBP}{a}\right)^2\right\}^2}\cdot\frac{1}{V_d}\right]} \qquad (36.4)$$

AWSI, aortic wall stiffness index; mBP, mean blood pressure; V_d, diastolic volume; a, b, model-specific constants

Left Atrial Function

Left Atrial Physiology

The left atrium comprises of three morphologically different compartments: anterior, venous, and appendage compartments. The left atrium modulates diastolic filling of the left ventricle through functional phases of reservoir, passive emptying and conduit, and active pumping (Fig. 36.4) [30]. The relative contribution to the left ventricular diastolic filling by left atrial phases comprises of 40%, 35%, and 25% of passive emptying (reservoir) volume, conduit volume, and active pumping volume, respectively [31]. At an early stage of left ventricular diastolic dysfunction, the relative contribution of active emptying increases with a reciprocally decreasing passive emptying. This change is noted as a decreased E/A ratio during the trans-mitral Doppler ultrasonography.

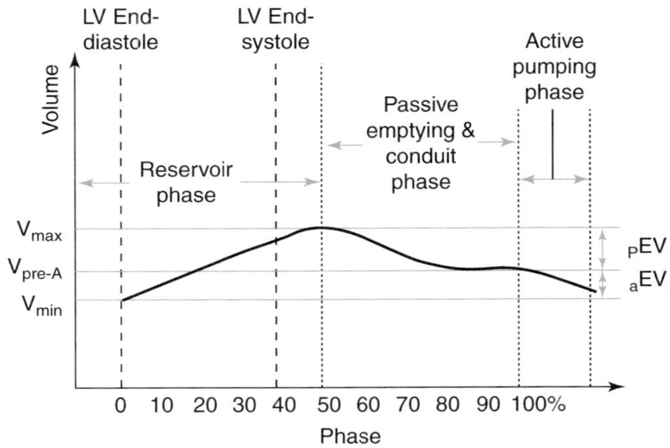

Fig. 36.4 Time-volume curve of left atrium shows bimodal pattern along functional phases. The reservoir phase is left atrial diastolic phase during left ventricular systole. The passive emptying and conduit and the active pumping phases generate weak bimodal curve during left atrial systole. The timing of the maximum volume can be beyond the left ventricular end-systole due to the isovolumic relaxation and superimposed conduit flow from pulmonary vein. $V_{pre\text{-}A}$ is the volume immediately before the late atrial contraction. $_p$EV is the passive emptying volume same as reservoir volume. aEV is the active emptying volume same as pumping volume

The reservoir phase of left atrium is during the left ventricular systolic phase. This phase may be influenced by the left atrial wall compliance, the descending motion of the left ventricular base during systole, and the LVESVI [32].

The passive emptying and conduit flow phase is shown during an early period of the left ventricular diastolic phase. In this phase, the left ventricular diastolic negative pressure allows left atrial blood to flow in. The passive decrease of the left atrial volume by a passive emptying can be described as the "reservoir volume." A direct inflow from pulmonary vein to left ventricle occurs through left atrium, which serves as a conduit role. The flow and its volume without left atrial volume change are called as a "conduit flow" and a "conduit volume," respectively [33].

During the conduit flow, the flow volume should not be related to the left atrial volume decrease. The sum of the passive emptying (reservoir) volume and the conduit volume is higher than the left atrial geometric volume decrease, because of the direct conduit flow through widely opened space from pulmonary vein to negatively loaded left ventricle [34]. The conduit flow is influenced by a paradoxical relationship between the left ventricular and left atrial relaxation capacities. The high left ventricular compliance will increase the conduit flow, whereas the high left atrial compliance will increase the reservoir volume with the relatively decreased conduit volume.

During the passive emptying of left atrium, both the conduit volume and the reservoir volume fill the relaxing left ventricle. The left atrial output volume should be the sum of the conduit volume, the reservoir volume, and the active ejection volume. However, the geometric volume measurement cannot present the total amount of the left atrial output volume due to the isovolumetric conduit phase. In this context, during the morphometric evaluation of a left atrial stroke volume, a simple subtraction of the end-diastolic volume by the end-systolic volume underestimates the left atrial output volume. The existence of the conduit flow is the reason why CT-based geometric left atrial stroke volume is shown to be lower than the left ventricular stroke volume (Fig. 36.5). The sane meaning of the morphometric "left atrial stroke volume" should be the sum of reservoir and pumping volumes, which equals to the cyclic volume change (Table 36.1).

The active pumping function of left atrium is during the late atrial contraction, which contributes up to 30% of the left ventricular stroke volume [35]. The left atrial active ejection may be governed by the Frank-Starling mechanism same as ventricles [36]. Therefore, the left atrial active emptying is influenced by the systemic venous return (preload) as well as the left ventricular end-diastolic pressure (afterload).

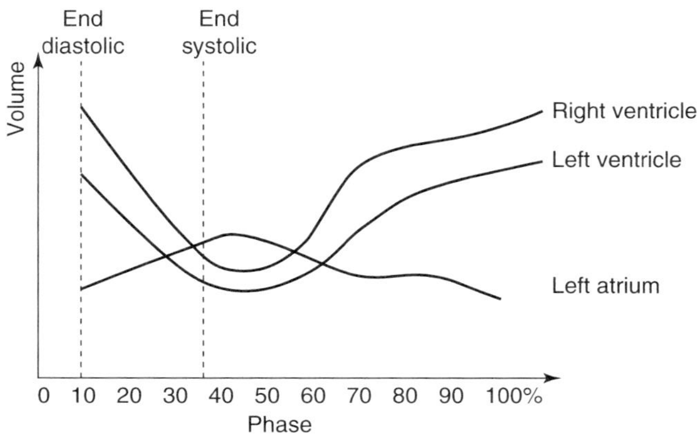

Fig. 36.5 The time-volume curves of three chambers. Along the cardiac phases, ventricles and left atrium reveal reciprocal change of their volumes. The right ventricular volume is usually higher than that of left ventricle. The left atrial curve height is shorter than that of left ventricle reflecting lower morphometric left atrial stroke volume than left ventricular stroke volume due to the conduit volume

Table 36.1 Nominations of fractional blood flow volumes from left atrium to left ventricle

Volumes	Synonyms	Definition
Reservoir volume	Passive emptying volume	Outflow in left atrial passive emptying phase
Conduit volume		Direct flow from pulmonary vein to left ventricle
Pumping volume	Active emptying volume, ejection volume	Outflow in left atrial active pumping phase
Stroke volume	Cyclic volume change	Reservoir volume + pumping volume
Output volume		Reservoir volume + conduit volume + pumping volume

Morphometric Markers for Left Atrial Function

The morphometric marker representing the preload of left atrium may be pulmonary vascular volume, $LAVI_{max}$, and left atrial expansion index. The markers for the left atrial systolic ability will be the left atrial ejection fraction (LAEF), LAaEF, and $_{adj}$LAeFr. The markers showing the afterload of left atrium are the minimum LAVI ($LAVI_{min}$), the left atrial passive ejection fraction (LApEF), LVESVI, LVMMI, LVSVI, and LVCI.

Reservoir Function

To evaluate the left atrial reservoir function, the measured left atrial volume can be utilized. The left atrial volume increase has been known as a strong predictor for adverse cardiovascular outcomes [37]. The left atrial volume change can be evaluated only with retrospective ECG gating since the pre-defined cardiac phase by prospective gaiting may miss the true maximum and minimum sizes of left atrium. Recently, Agner et al. [38] successfully validated CT-based left atrial volumetry with references by cardiac MR. They found that the cardiac CT overestimated the maximum and minimum left atrial volumes compared to cardiac MR (8% and 10%, respectively). This inter-modality discrepancy may be due to the difference between the spatial and temporal resolutions and image sharpness.

Since the venous compartment of left atrium possesses relatively less myocardial tissue and more venous wall attached to pericardium, the motion and contraction of the venous wall are weaker than the other compartments. Whereas, the venous compartment conducts a role of reservoir for the pulmonary venous return flow. The appendage compartment comprises of a thicker wall and pectinate muscles interconnecting the opposing walls. Due to the active contractile function and thick wall, the appendage is more resistant to overload than the other compartments; therefore, it is relatively insensitive to overloading. Paradoxically, if the appendage compartment shows dilatation with wall thinning, this feature may imply a long-standing volume overload of the left atrium, typically due to the left ventricular diastolic dysfunction with or without atrial fibrillation.

As another marker for left atrial volumetry, the $LAVI_{max}$ has been suggested. This index is a normalized maximum volume by the body surface area. According to the results of echocardiography, the $LAVI_{max}$ is the best parameter for cardiovascular outcome prediction and risk stratification [37]. Choi et al. [39] reported that $LAVI_{max}$ showed a significant predictability for the silent myocardial ischemia in a high-risk group. The $LAVI_{max}$ from echocardiography presented a higher adjusted odds ratio than LVEF, E/E' ratio, LVMI, and the diastolic left ventricular dysfunction.

The left atrial expansion index is another dynamic marker for the left atrial volumetry. The left atrial expansion capacity may reflect the reservoir function during left atrial diastole. To quantitate the expansion capacity, the left atrial expansion index was suggested by Hoit et al. [30]. The expansion index was calculated as the left atrial volume change per minimum left atrial volume $[(V_{max} - V_{min})/V_{min}]$.

Emptying Function

The three compartments of left atrium present different functional activities. The appendage shows the highest ejection fraction, whereas the venous compartment shows the lowest ejection fraction [40]. The LAA ejection fraction is not strongly related to the global and anterior compartmental function, whereas LAA function is reported to be more related to the left ventricular functional status [41]. The anterior compartment of left atrium has a smooth and movable wall and is not adhered by pericardium or venous structures. The anterior compartment presents a less compromised wall motion by surrounding structures and may properly reflect the left atrial performance. In the short-axis plane, the anterior compartment demonstrates a left atrial wall motion conveniently.

The LAEF may be calculated by a simple formula: $100 * (LAV_{max} - LAV_{min})/LAV_{max}$, where LAV is the left atrial volume. With some software, the LAEF shows the volume fraction by active pumping during systole (Fig. 36.2). The left atrial cyclic volume change implies the gap between the maximum and the minimum volumes. However, the maximum and the minimum volumes may not always match the left ventricular end-diastolic (100% of R-R interval) and the end-systolic (40% of R-R interval) phases. During the left ventricular early passive filling phase, left atrium can be more instantly dilated than the left atrial end-diastolic phase due to a superimposed conduit flow directly from pulmonary vein to the left ventricle (Fig. 36.4). Due to a concern about mismatching between cardiac phases and left atrial volumes, the gap between the maximum and the minimum volumes may be suitable for calculating the ejection fraction, in spite of a different concept from the ejection fraction by the left atrial active contraction.

To evaluate the passive emptying function of left atrium, the passive ejection fraction (pEF) can be used. The pEF is the passive emptying volume (pEV) per maximum left atrial volume $[(LAV_{max} - LAV_{pre\text{-}A})/LAV_{max}]$, where the $LAV_{pre\text{-}A}$ is the left atrial volume immediately before atrial contraction. For the active pumping function of left atrium, the active ejection fraction can be acquired as the active emptying volume ($LAV_{pre\text{-}A}$–LAV_{min}) over $LAV_{pre\text{-}A}$ (Fig. 36.4) [30].

Im et al. [42] suggested the $_{adj}$LAeFr as a marker for emptying function evaluation. The maximum and minimum left atrial volume indices were normalized by LAEF ($LAVI_{max}$/LAEF and $LAVI_{min}$/LAEF). The $_{adj}$LAEFr showed the best predictability for the recurrent atrial fibrillation as comparing with conventional markers including LVEF, LAV_{max}, LAV_{min}, LAEF, $LAVI_{max}$, and $LAVI_{min}$.

Afterload

The left atrial dilatation is a classical marker for left ventricular diastolic dysfunction, which is an increased afterload of left atrium. The left atrial volume increase can be either reversible by the instant volume overload or irreversible due to an eccentric wall remodeling. The aging, neurohumoral activation, and chronic atrial stretch may provoke the left atrial dilatation with histological changes including wall hypertrophy and fibrosis as eccentric left atrial remodeling [43]. In this background, eccentric remodeling may trigger episodes of atrial fibrillation.

The $LAVI_{min}$ is related to the afterload of left atrium. The $LAVI_{min}$ may be influenced by the left atrial elasticity and LVEDP and was reported as the best predictor for the major adverse cardiac events (MACE) in a study using 3D echocardiography [44].

With Doppler ultrasonography of the trans-mitral flow, the flow spectrum shows bimodal peaks due to the left atrial passive emptying flow (E velocity) and the active pumping flow (A velocity), whereas with cardiac CT with multiphase reconstruction during a cardiac cycle, the left ventricular time-volume curve and its time-differential curve can be acquired. The left ventricular volume gap between two adjacent phases shows the bimodal peaks in the time domain. If the volume gap is divided by the mitral valvular orifice area at the concordant phase, velocity values can be acquired. In the bimodal time-velocity curve, E and A velocities and E/A_{CT} can be measured on cardiac CT [45]. The E/A_{CT} represents the proportion of passive and active emptying volume during the left atrial systolic function. The E/A_{CT} is related with the left atrial afterload or the diastolic function of the left ventricle.

Global Function

The left atrial time-volume curve provides several potential markers to evaluate the atrial systolic and diastolic functions. However, since the volume is a three-dimensional scalar value, two-dimensional wall strain evaluation may be more sensitive to the geometric change of the left atrial wall. The total left atrial strain measured by echocardiography has been reported to be the best predictor of exercise capacity [46]. In light of the fact that the strain imaging of the left ventricular wall has been attempted using cardiac CT data, study results of CT-derived left atrial strain are expected in the literature soon.

Right Ventricular Function

Right Ventricular Physiology

The right ventricular function is different from the left ventricular function only by the magnitude of the peak systolic pressure due to the lower pulmonary vascular resistance (PLVR). The right ventricle comprises of thin myocardial wall that has a highly compliant nature. Due to this compliance, the right ventricle accommodates the changes of preload well. However the right ventricle is limited in overcoming the increased afterload due to its limited contractility. In this context, a common cause of the right ventricular failure is left ventricular failure. If right ventricular failure occurs due to the primary pulmonary process, it is called as the *cor pulmonale* [1].

Right ventricular failure has effects on right atrium and systemic venous return. The clinical presentation of the right ventricular failure contains systemic venous congestion noted as jugular vein dilatation, hepatomegaly, peripheral edema, IVC dilatation, and right atrial dilatation. The right ventricular dysfunction superimposed on left ventricular pathology is regarded as additional poor prognostic factor. Di Bella et al. [47] showed the combined right ventricular dysfunction after acute myocardial infarction significantly deteriorated patient prognosis. Right ventricular function may be additional information on left ventricular function during cardiac pathology evaluation using the cardiac CT.

In cases of acute pulmonary arterial hypertension such as acute massive pulmonary thromboembolism, a quick, simple, and noninvasive method for estimating right ventricular afterload may be indispensable to urgently inform therapeutic decision-making [48]. The morphometric markers representing the preload of right ventricle are RVEDVI and right atrial stroke volume index (RASVI). The markers for the right ventricular contractility evaluation may be the right ventricular ejection fraction (RVEF), right ventricular stroke volume index (RVSVI), and right ventricular output index (RVCI). The markers showing the afterload of right ventricle may comprise of RVESVI, right ventricular MMI (RVMMI), PLVR, pulmonary circulation volume, and pulmonary AD (AD).

Right Ventricular Contractility

The ejection fraction is a reliable marker for right ventricular systolic function. In patients with acute pulmonary thromboembolism combined by pulmonary arterial hypertension, RVEF and right ventricular end-systolic volume have been discovered to have significant implications [49]. With cardiac CT right ventricular volumetry requires more resources but may be less reliable than left ventricular volumetry due to prominent trabeculation, atypical morphology, indistinct basal boundary, and motion artifacts.

Sato et al. [50] suggested a simplified method to predict RVEF in patients with pulmonary hypertension. Using a retrospectively gated cardiac CT, the tricuspid annular plane systolic excursion (TAPSE) was measured during a cardiac cycle. Using a fitting equation between the TAPSE and ejection fraction values acquired by cardiac MRI, a simplified prediction equation for RVEF was suggested and sufficiently validated. The RVEF in the ml-equivalent unit was acquired as double value of TAPSE in millimeter. In pulmonary hypertension patients, 19.7 mm cut-off value of TAPSE was suggested to predict a reduced RVEF.

The right ventricular cardiac output or the cardiac index may be direct markers for the systolic function as left ventricle. In a study using a test-bolus scan data, the time-attenuation curves were drawn on main pulmonary arteries, and the right ventricular cardiac output was acquired using the modified Stewart-Hamilton equation (Eq. 36.2). Based on the reference standard data acquired during right heart catheterizations and thermodilution, the right ventricular cardiac output acquired from dynamic CT showed a significant correlation and clinical feasibility [51].

Afterload of the Right Ventricle

The pulmonary arterial pressure is an essential afterload of the right ventricle, and a pulmonary hypertension will increase the afterload of right ventricle. The pulmonary arterial hypertension escalates the right ventricular end-diastolic pressure, which relates to the dilatation of the right ventricle with a limited contractility.

The dilated right ventricle may shift interventricular septum to present an eccentric configuration of left ventricle in the short-axis plane. Yamasaki et al. [52] presented a simple predictor for pulmonary arterial hypertension among the patients with congenital heart diseases. The "eccentricity index" is acquired as a ratio between the orthogonal long and short diameters of left ventricular lumen in the short-axis plane. The eccentricity index values show a significant correlation with the right ventricular systolic pressure and the mean pulmonary arterial pressure from right heart catherization results. Also the eccentricity index correlates with cardiac MR functional parameters representing the right ventricular afterload such as RVESV and RVEF.

If the PLVR is measured, the evaluation of the right ventricular afterload should be more convenient. The pulmonary arterial flow impedance increases in patients with pulmonary thromboembolism, chronic obstructive pulmonary disease, and emphysema resulting in pulmonary arterial hypertension [53]. Müller et al. [53] measured the PLVR indirectly and noninvasively using the electron-beam CT data and Hagen-Poiseuille equation (Eq. 36.5). This study revealed a significant correlation between the noninvasively measured PLVR and catherization-based reference values ($r2$ = 073, regression coefficient = 1.001 after removing intercept).

$$\mathrm{PLVR}_{[\mathrm{Wood}]} = \frac{803 \cdot L_{B[m]}^{\;3}}{\mathrm{CO}^2_{[L/\min]} \cdot \left(\mathrm{PTT}_{M[s]} + 6.14\right)^2} \cdot \left[5 + 10 \cdot \left(\mathrm{HCT}_{L/L} - 0.52\right)\right] \tag{36.5}$$

L_B, patient's heights used for vascular length; HCT, hematocrit used for blood viscosity; PTT, pulmonary transit time; empirically acquired constants

Since this study is based on Hagen-Poiseuille law, inherent limitation by assumption such as a straight cylindrical tube, homogenous fluid (Newtonian fluid), laminar flow, steady non-pulsatile flow, and rigid wall without arterial compliance may not be overcome. However, the results demonstrate a feasibility of this technique in clinical practice.

Stiffening of pulmonary arterial wall attenuates its damping function against the pulsatile right ventricular outflow and subsequently increases the flow impedance as afterload. Using cardiac MDCT, Revel et al. [54] measured right ventricular and pulmonary arterial functional parameters to diagnose pulmonary hypertension. Image-based right pulmonary AD (area change/maximum area) has shown the best diagnostic value for pulmonary hypertension and has been useful for risk stratification.

Morphological alteration of pulmonary vasculature and the lungs on CT images may suggest increased right ventricular afterload. Pulmonary thromboembolism and extensive pulmonary parenchymal lesions including interstitial lung disease and chronic obstructive pulmonary disease may provoke pulmonary arterial hypertension.

Pulmonary arterial dilatation is a predictor for pulmonary hypertension. If the main pulmonary arterial diameter is greater than 29 mm at a distance of 2 cm from a pulmonary valve, pulmonary arterial hypertension could be predicted with 84% sensitivity and 75% specificity. If the main pulmonary artery shows the maximum transverse diameter larger than the adjacent AAo, pulmonary arterial hypertension could be suggested with 70% sensitivity and 92% specificity. The underline condition is that the AAo should not show the aneurysmal dilatation. In addition, the segmental pulmonary arterial enlargement greater than 1.25 times the caliber of the adjacent bronchus is another marker for pulmonary arterial hypertension [55].

A right ventricular deformation may suggest pulmonary arterial hypertension as well. Right ventricular enlargement, outflow tract dilatation and wall thickening, and flattening or leftward convexity of interventricular septum are classic image markers representing the elevated right ventricular end-diastolic pressure and pulmonary arterial hypertension. The right ventricular free wall thickness greater than 6 mm, RV/LV wall thickness ratio greater than 0.32, RV/LV luminal diameter ratio greater than 1.28, and MPA/AAo diameter ratio greater than 0.84 have been implicated with pulmonary arterial hypertension [56]. Lastly, the finding of bronchial artery hypertrophy greater than 1.5 mm was reported as a marker for pulmonary arterial hypertension [57].

Right Atrial Function

Theoretically, the morphometric markers representing the preload of right atrium are $\mathrm{RAVI}_{\max}$, vena cava size, intrathoracic pressure state, and intrapericardial pressure state. The markers for the right atrial contractility may be RAEF and RAaEF. The afterload of right atrium may be evaluated by $\mathrm{RAVI}_{\min}$, RA passive EF, RVESVI, RVMMI, RVSVI, and RVCI. In spite of these theoretically conceived markers, automated measurement of right atrial volume is limited to few commercial softwares due to the insufficient and nonhomogeneous enhancement, the irregular morphology, and motion artifacts.

Systemic venous congestion state is a type of increased preload of the right atrium. Although the exact volumetry is not feasible, a morphological change may reflect the increased preload. A vena caval enlargement used to be a sign for systemic venous congestion. However, this finding is related to many confounders such as the breath-holding capabilities, the strength of the Valsalva maneuver, and the original size of the venous structure. The retrograde vena caval or hepatic venous enhancement has been regarded as a sign representing the right heart dysfunction during a conventional slow-infusion contrast-enhanced CT [58]. However, dynamic contrast-enhanced CT with a high injection rate (>3 mL/s) could not maintain the feasibility of this systemic venous reflux sign

[59]. In cardiac CT, the sign of the retrograde opacification of inferior vena cava and hepatic vein may not be reliable for the prediction of the right cardiac dysfunction.

The TAPSE is known as a simple marker for the right ventricular function [50]. Sivak et al. [60] used the TAPSE for evaluating the right atrial function using cohorts of a normal and a pulmonary arterial hypertension. In echocardiography, the TAPSE is divided to two parts; $TAPSE_{RA}$ during the right atrial contraction and $TAPSE_{RV}$ before the right atrial contraction after tricuspid valve opening representing the right atrial passive emptying function. In a pulmonary arterial hypertension group, $TAPSE_{RV}$ shows a significant decrease, while the change of $TAPSE_{RA}$ is not significant. The late atrial contraction may be more preserved than the passive emptying function in the case of right atrial afterload increase.

The longitudinal strain of the right atrial wall evaluated by speckle-tracking echocardiography demonstrated its feasibility to predict increased afterload due to the right ventricular diastolic dysfunction [61]. Although no article about CT strain evaluation for right atrial function has been published, studies are expected in the near future.

Global Cardiac Function

The four cardiac chambers are working in a tight interrelated mode. Left ventricular diastolic dysfunction may increase the afterload of left atrium. An erroneous left atrial emptying function may provoke the right ventricular afterload increase. An increased left atrial emptying function will stimulate the left ventricular inotropic function, which is described as the Frank-Starling's law (Fig. 36.1). In this context, when evaluating global cardiac function, the function of the interrelated cardiac chambers is best when considered collectively.

To evaluate the function of the cardiac chambers simultaneously and comprehensively, the "three-chamber function" option can be used with commercially available post-processing software. By plotting the time-volume curves of left ventricle, left atrium, and right ventricle along cardiac phases (time domain), qualitative comparisons of the three-chamber function and the quantitative evaluation of the functional parameters are possible (Figs. 36.2 and 36.5).

For a quantitative evaluation of multichamber functional parameters, reference values are indispensable. However, the normal values of multichamber functional parameters show significant differences by the reports in the literature. These normal values show different ranges depending on the measuring techniques, ethnicity, age, sex, and cohort properties (Table 36.2); since the references may be different among cardiac CT centers, large-scale multicenter studies accounting for potential confounders are expected [62–65].

During the evaluation of the three-chamber function results, the major left ventricular functional parameters such as LVEDVI, LVESVI, LVEF, LVSVI, LVCI, and LVMMI are checked first. Subsequently the major left atrial functional parameters such as LAVImax, LAVImin, LASVI, and LAaEF are evaluated. Finally, the right ventricular functional parameters such as RVEF, Q_p/Q_s, RVEDVI, and RVSV are assessed (Figs. 36.6 and 36.7). In the scope of global cardiac function, the morphometric markers supporting the preload may be the vena cava size; however, its reliability is not accepted. The global inotropic

Table 36.2 An example of normal reference ranges for cardiac CT functional parameters in a single institute (Kyungpook National University Hospital)

	Left ventricle		Left atrium		Right ventricle	
	Male	Female	Male	Female	Male	Female
EDV(ml)	100–180	108–122			127–223	
ESV (ml)	28–66	28–52			53–111	
LVMM(mg)	129–205	100–158				
EF(%)	57–75	59–73			42–74	
SV(ml)	50–70				40–84	
CO(L/min)	4.0–8.0				3.2–9.6	
EDVI(ml/m^2)	57–88	47–74				
ESVI(ml/m^2)	16–33	11–24				
SVI(ml/m^2)	40–50		11–25	13–27	35–60	
CI(L/m^2)	2.5–4.5				2.0–5.4	
MMI(mg/m^2)	31–81					
$LAVI_{max}$			32–56	39–63		
$LAVI_{min}$			17–39	19–43		
EFI(%/m^2)			26–50	28–52		
LARsrV(ml)			16–28			
LACnV(ml)			18–25			
LAPmpV(ml)			13–18			

LARsrV left atrial reservoir volume, *LACnV* left atrial conduit volume, *LAPmpV* left atrial active pumping volume

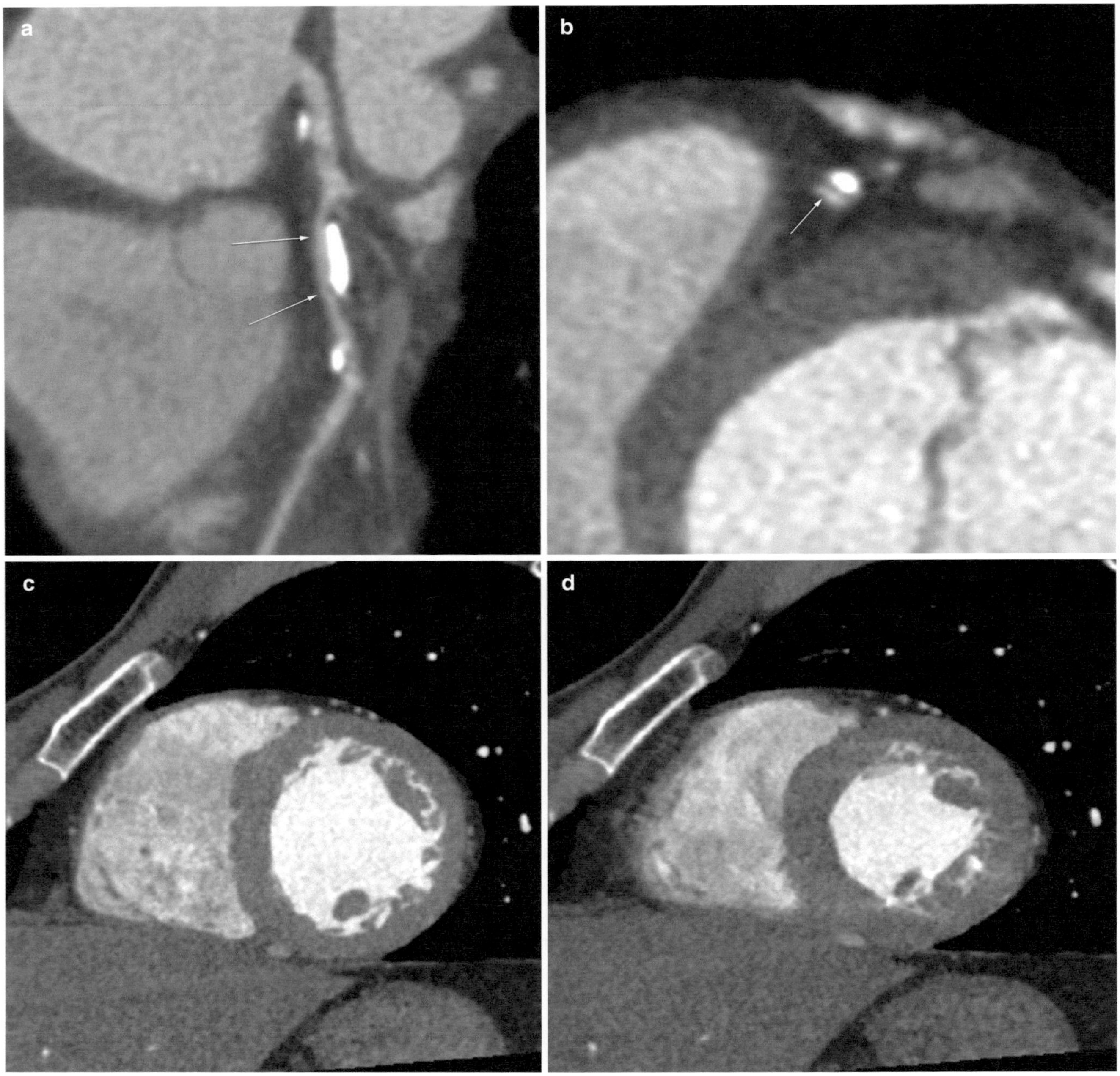

Fig. 36.6 A 64-year-old man presented atypical chest pain and was evaluated using cardiac CT. (**a**) Calcified atherosclerotic plaques (arrows) are noted in proximal and middle levels of left anterior descending artery (LAD) and left main coronary artery. (**b**) In en face view of LAD, significant luminal stenosis (arrow) is noted. (**c, d**) Short-axis cine images at mid-diastolic and end-systolic phases show left ventricular hypokinesia. (**e**) The three-chamber function report reveals upward shifting of ventricular time-volume curves. LVEDVI (89 mL/m^2) and LVESVI (48 mL/m^2) are increased. Global LVEF (46%) decreased slightly. Further calculated $LAVI_{max}$ (68 mL/m^2) and $LAVI_{min}$(41 mL/m^2) are increased. LAEFI (23 mL/m^2) is decreased. RVEF (40%) is slightly decreased. All the other parameters are in normal ranges. The conclusion is a significant coronary artery stenosis with LV systolic dysfunction accompanied by LA and RV systolic dysfunction

e

Parameter	LV Value	LV (Index)	RV Value	RV (Index)	LA Value	LA (Index)
Ejection Fraction%	46		40		14	
End Diastolic Volume(ml)	154	89	151	88	81	47
End Systolic Volume(ml)	82	48	91	53	70	41
Stroke Volume (ml)	71	41	60	35	11	6.4
Cardiac Output(L/min)	5.2	3.0	4.4	2.6		

LV Parameter	LV Value	LV (Index)	LA Parameter	LA Value	LA (Index)
Myocardial Mass (g)	107	1.8	Maximal Volume (ml)	115	67
Myocardial Volume (ml)	102		Cyclic Volume Change (ml)	45	26
LV/RV Regurgitation Fraction(%)	15		Reservoir Volume(ml)	0.0	

Heart Rate:	73 bpm
BSA:	1.7 m²

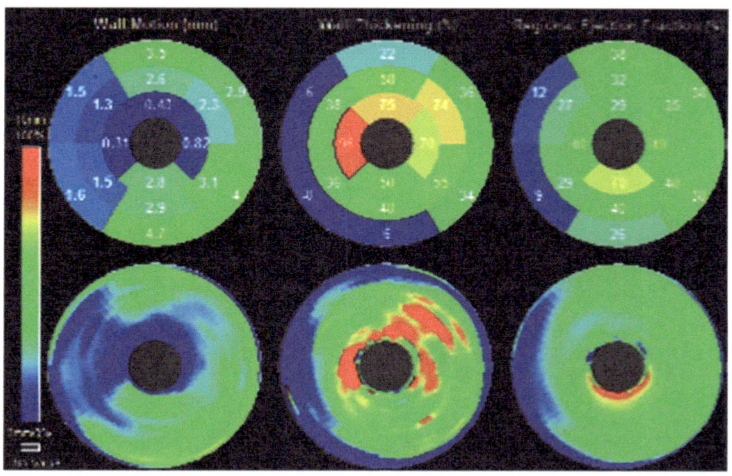

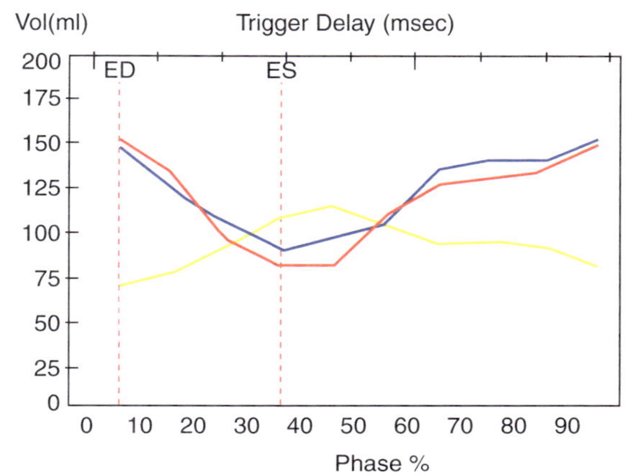

Fig. 36.6 (continued)

function can be evaluated by the markers such as LVEF, LVSVI, LVCI, and Q_p/Q_s. The markers for the afterload of whole heart may be LVESVI, PVR, AD, and aortic volume (Table 36.3).

As an integrated marker to show a comprehensive cardiac function, the Q_p/Q_s may be used to compare stroke volumes between right and left ventricles. In managing congenital heart diseases, the Q_p/Q_s is a reliable marker to diagnose and monitor a left-to-right shunt and to decide treatment strategy. The CT-based geometric measurement of the right and left ventricular stroke volumes can present the Q_p/Q_s values under the condition of an absent regurgitation in atrioventricular and ventriculoarterial valves. Recently, Yamasaki et al. [66] successfully validated Q_p/Q_s values, acquired using a 256-slice MDCT based on the right heart catheterization.

The myocardial strain of cardiac chambers may be a potential marker for a comprehensive multichamber function evaluation. Using the speckle-tracking echocardiography, four-chamber strain can be evaluated. When the mean and peak longitudinal strains are plotted in one graph, the relationship among four-chamber wall motions can be evaluated, and a comprehensive functional assessment of the heart may become possible. If the strain ratios between ventricles and between atria, the abnormal wall motion and its compensatory mechanism may be analyzed feasibly [67].

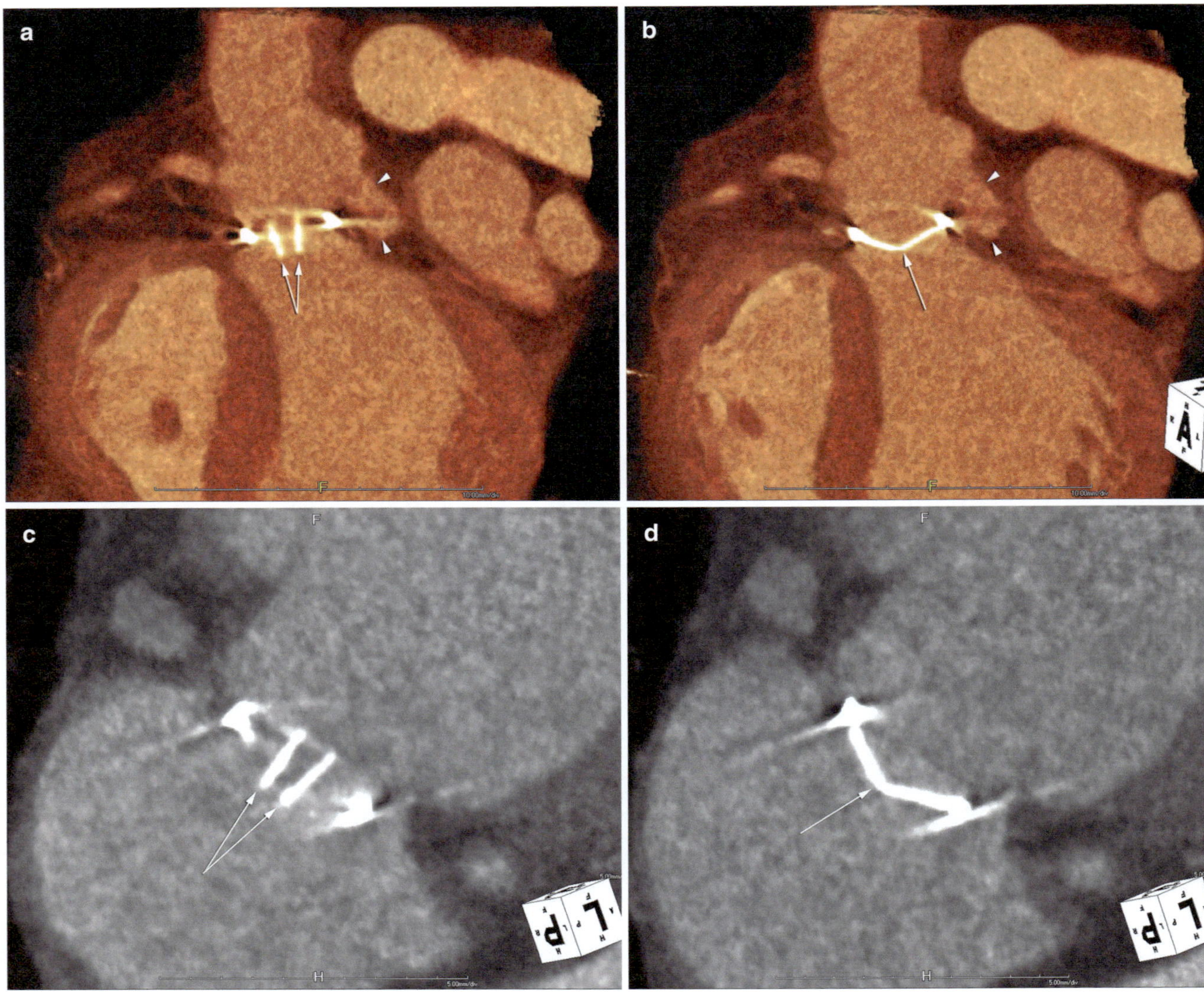

Fig. 36.7 A 47-year-old male complains resting dyspnea and chest discomfort. The patient has suffered from Behçet's disease, and valvuloplasties were performed 6 years ago. (**a**, **b**) Volume-rendered images along the left ventricular outflow tract reveal a well-functioning prosthetic aortic valve (arrows). Focal sinus of Valsalva aneurysm is noted (arrow heads) (**c**, **d**) Multiplanar longitudinal images show a well-functioning prosthetic mitral valve (arrows). (**e**, **f**) In four-chamber plane, left atrial dilatation and limited emptying are noted. Left ventricle (LV) shows dilatation. (**g**) The three-chamber function analysis report reveals upward shifting of all ventricular and left atrial time curves (right lower corner) suggesting chamber dilatation. LVEDVI(185), LVESVI(86), and LVMMI(95) are increased. LVEF [54] and PVR [5] are decreased. LVSVI and LVCI are not decreased. LAVImax(105) and LAVImin(84) are increased. The left atrial active pumping flow is not detected. The left atrial conduit flow volume seems to be increased with maintaining the fraction of reservoir volume. LAEFI [10] is decreased. The other functional parameters including right ventricle are within normal ranges. The prosthetic aortic and mitral valves are mechanically functioning well. However the left ventricle shows eccentric hypertrophy and dilatation with systolic dysfunction. Subsequently the left atrium dilates with systolic dysfunction. No left atrial active pumping function is detected suggesting the risk of atrial fibrillation. In conclusion, a functional aortic valvular stenosis should be considered if active Behçet's myocarditis can be excluded clinically

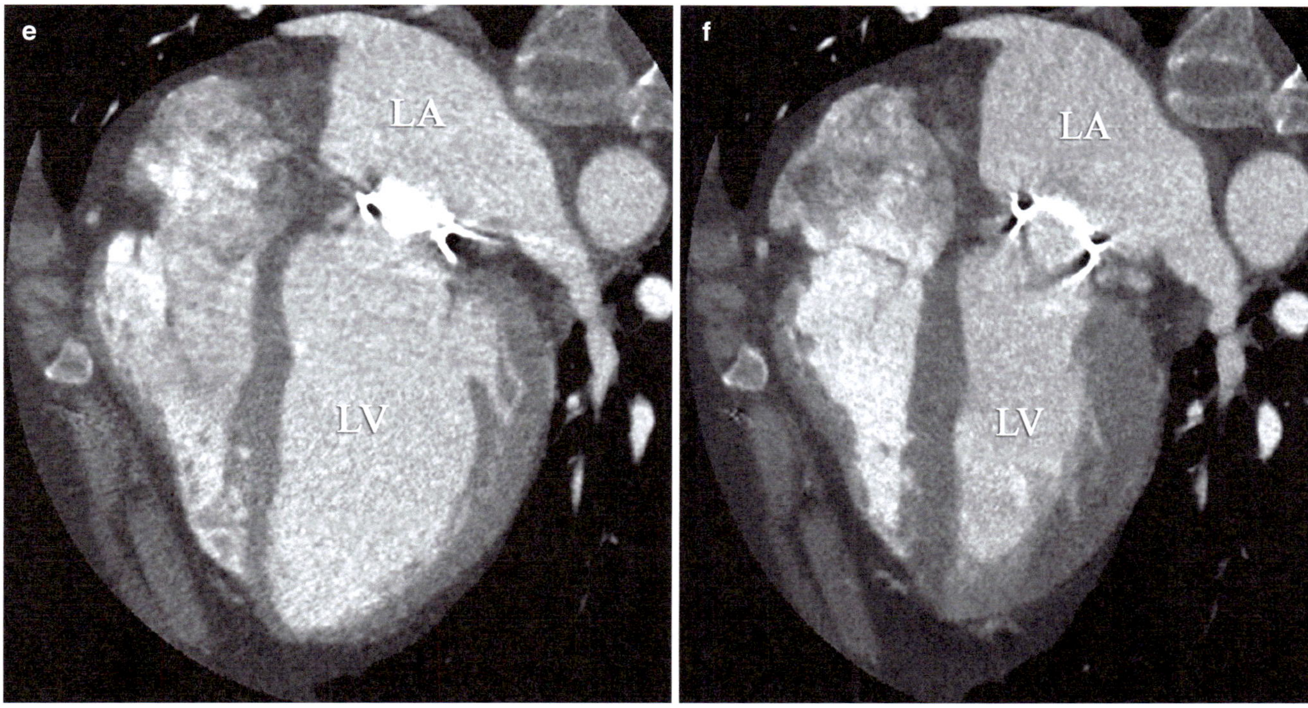

g

	LV		RV		LA	
Parameter	Value	(Index)	Value	(Index)	Value	(Index)
Ejection Fraction %	54		46		0.0	
End Diastolic Volume (ml)	370	186	257	130	167	84
End Systolic Volume (ml)	172	87	140	70	167	84
Stroke Volume (ml)	198	100	118	59	0.0	0.0
Cardiac Output (L/min)	14.5	7.3	8.6	4.3		

	LV			LA	
Parameter	Value	(Index)	Parameter	Value	(Index)
Myocardial Mass (g)	189	2.4	Maximal Volume (ml)	210	106
Myocardial Volume (ml)	179		Cyclic Volume Change (ml)	43	22
LV/RV Regurgitation Fraction (%)	41		Reservoir Volume (ml)	0.0	

Heart Rate:	73 bpm
BSA:	2.0 m^2

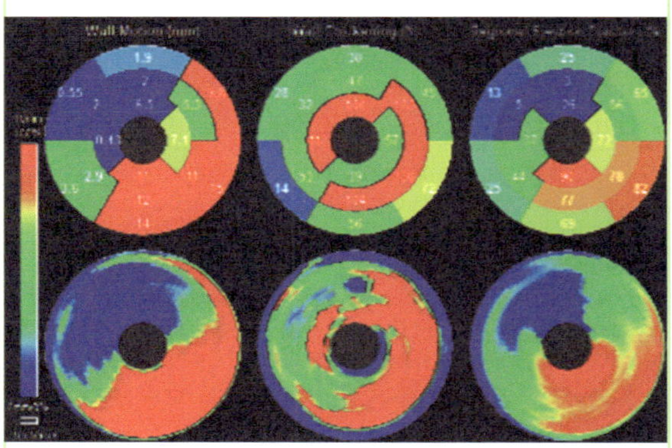

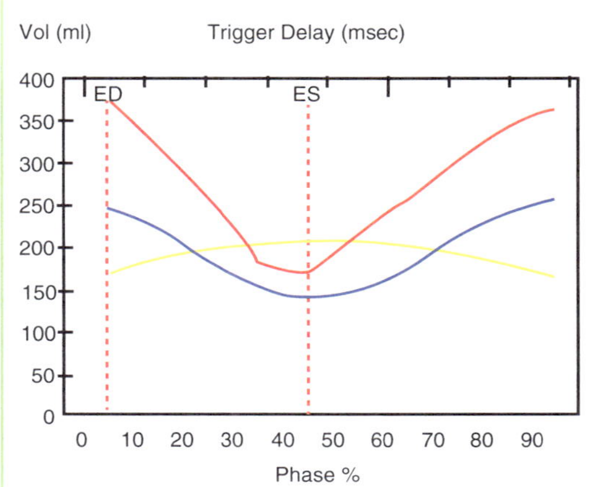

Fig. 36.7 (continued)

Table 36.3 Functional parameters of cardiac chambers

	Left ventricle	Left atrium	Right ventricle	Right atrium
Preload	LVEDVI, LASVI	$LAVI_{max}$, LAEI, pulmonary vessel size,	RVEDVI, RASVI	$RAVI_{max}$, VC size, intrathoracic pressure
Inotropy	LVEF, LVSVI, LVCI, strain, $_{adj}$LVeFr	LAEF, LAaEF, $_{adj}$LAeFr	RVEF, RVSVI, RVCI	RAEF, RAaEF
Afterload	LVESVI, LVMMI, PVR, AD, AWSI, aortic volume	$LAVI_{min}$, LApEF, LVESVI, LVMMI, LVSVI, LVCI, E/A_{CT}	RVESVI, RVMMI, PLVR, PTT, PAD, LAEI, RV, and pulmonary vascular deformation	$RAVI_{min}$, RApEF, RVESVI, RVMMI, RVSVI, RVCI, TAPSE

LAEpI left atrial expansibility index, *LVCI* left ventricular cardiac output index, *PTT* pulmonary transit time, *PAD* pulmonary arterial distensibility

Summary

Based on the high spatial resolution and acceptable temporal resolution, cardiac CT provides reliable information about the function of the cardiac chambers. Since the functions of four cardiac chambers are interrelated, the functional abnormality can be double checked by the adjacent chamber function. A functional compensatory mechanism among chambers can be evaluated. In addition, by analyzing the multiple chamber function simultaneously, a comprehensive global cardiac function can be evaluated.

The main expectation from current cardiac CT may comprise epicardial coronary arterial patency, the myocardial perfusion status, and the cardiac function as a circulation pump. The multichamber function evaluation will provide more valuable information about the cardiac performance in addition to CT coronary angiography. Based on the morphofunctional results, more reliable explanation about the patient's discomfort will be possible.

References

1. Mohrman DE, Heller LJ. Cardiovascular physiology, McGraw-Hill, New York; 2006. p. 47–70.
2. Fuchs A, Kuhl JT, Lonborg J, Engstrom T, Vejlstrup N, Kober L, et al. Automated assessment of heart chamber volumes and function in patients with previous myocardial infarction using multidetector computed tomography. J Cardiovasc Comput Tomogr. 2012;6(5):325–34.
3. Stouffer GA. Cardiovascular hemodynamics for the clinician, Wiley Blackwell, Oxford; 2008. p. 3-100.
4. Galie N, Hoeper MM, Humbert M, Torbicki A, Vachiery JL, Barbera JA, et al. Guidelines for the diagnosis and treatment of pulmonary hypertension: the task force for the diagnosis and treatment of pulmonary hypertension of the European Society of Cardiology (ESC) and the European Respiratory Society (ERS), endorsed by the International Society of Heart and Lung Transplantation (ISHLT). Eur Heart J. 2009;30(20):2493–537.
5. van Lieshout JJ, Wesseling KH. Continuous cardiac output by pulse contour analysis? Br J Anaesth. 2001;86(4):467–9.
6. Longo DL, Fauci AS, Kasper DL, Hauser SL, Jameson JL, Loscalzo J. Harrison's principles of internal medicine: McGraw-Hill; New York, 2012.
7. Tanabe Y, Kido T, Kurata A, Sawada S, Suekuni H, Kido T, et al. Three-dimensional maximum principal strain using cardiac computed tomography for identification of myocardial infarction. Eur Radiol. 2017;27(4):1667–75.
8. Mahnken AH, Katoh M, Bruners P, Spuentrup E, Wildberger JE, Gunther RW, et al. Acute myocardial infarction: assessment of left ventricular function with 16-detector row spiral CT versus MR imaging–study in pigs. Radiology. 2005;236(1):112–7.
9. Hundt W, Siebert K, Wintersperger BJ, Becker CR, Knez A, Reiser MF, et al. Assessment of global left ventricular function: comparison of cardiac multidetector-row computed tomography with angiocardiography. J Comput Assist Tomogr. 2005;29(3):373–81.
10. Raman SV, Shah M, McCarthy B, Garcia A, Ferketich AK. Multi-detector row cardiac computed tomography accurately quantifies right and left ventricular size and function compared with cardiac magnetic resonance. Am Heart J. 2006;151(3):736–44.
11. Yamamuro M, Tadamura E, Kubo S, Toyoda H, Nishina T, Ohba M, et al. Cardiac functional analysis with multi-detector row CT and segmental reconstruction algorithm: comparison with echocardiography, SPECT, and MR imaging. Radiology. 2005;234(2):381–90.
12. Maffei E, Messalli G, Martini C, Nieman K, Catalano O, Rossi A, et al. Left and right ventricle assessment with cardiac CT: validation study vs. cardiac MR. Eur Radiol. 2012;22(5):1041–9. Pubmed Central PMCID: 3321142.
13. Groen JM, van der Vleuten PA, Greuter MJ, Zijlstra F, Oudkerk M. Comparison of MRI, 64-slice MDCT and DSCT in assessing functional cardiac parameters of a moving heart phantom. Eur Radiol. 2009;19(3):577–83. Pubmed Central PMCID: 2816236.
14. Arsanjani R, Berman DS, Gransar H, Cheng VY, Dunning A, Lin FY, et al. Left ventricular function and volume with coronary CT angiography improves risk stratification and identification of patients at risk for incident mortality: results from 7758 patients in the prospective multinational CONFIRM observational cohort study. Radiology. 2014;273(1):70–7.
15. Mao SS, Li D, Vembar M, Gao Y, Luo Y, Lam F, et al. Model-based automatic segmentation algorithm accurately assesses the whole cardiac volumetric parameters in patients with cardiac CT angiography: a validation study for evaluating the accuracy of the workstation software and establishing the reference values. Acad Radiol. 2014;21(5):639–47.
16. Dell'Italia LJ, Walsh RA. Effect of intravenous metoprolol on left ventricular performance in Q-wave acute myocardial infarction. Am J Cardiol. 1989;63(3):166–71.
17. Port S, Cobb FR, Jones RH. Effects of propranolol on left ventricular function in normal men. Circulation. 1980;61(2):358–66.
18. Silke B, Verma SP, Frais MA, Reynolds G, Taylor SH. Comparative effects of metoprolol and celiprolol on cardiac hemodynamics and left ventricular volume at rest and during exercise-induced angina. Clin Pharmacol Ther. 1986;39(1):5–14.
19. Tsusaki H, Yonamine H, Tamai A, Shimomoto M, Kuwano K, Iwao H, et al. Left ventricular volume and function in cynomolgus monkeys using real-time three-dimensional echocardiography. J Med Primatol. 2007;36(1):39–46.

20. Mo YH, Jaw FS, Wang YC, Jeng CM, Peng SF. Effects of propranolol on the left ventricular volume of normal subjects during CT coronary angiography. Korean J Radiol. 2011;12(3):319–26. Pubmed Central PMCID: 3088849.
21. Martin GV, Sheehan FH, Stadius M, Maynard C, Davis KB, Ritchie JL, et al. Intravenous streptokinase for acute myocardial infarction. Effects on global and regional systolic function. Circulation. 1988;78(2):258–66.
22. Zeb I, Li D, Nasir K, Gupta M, Kadakia J, Gao Y, et al. Computerized left ventricular regional ejection fraction analysis for detection of ischemic coronary artery disease with multidetector CT angiography. Int J Cardiovasc Imaging. 2013;29(3):685–92. Pubmed Central PMCID: 4277887.
23. Yee S, Scalzetti EM. Measurement of cardiac output from dynamic pulmonary circulation time CT. Med Phys. 2014;41(6):061904.
24. Mahnken AH, Klotz E, Hennemuth A, Jung B, Koos R, Wildberger JE, et al. Measurement of cardiac output from a test-bolus injection in multislice computed tomography. Eur Radiol. 2003;13(11):2498–504.
25. Vanhoenacker PK, Van Hoe LR. A simple method to estimate cardiac function during routine multi-row detector CT exams. Eur Radiol. 2007;17(11):2845–51.
26. Truesdell C, Noll W, Antman SS. The non-linear field theories of mechanics. 3rd ed. Berlin, New York: Springer; 2004. xxix, 602 p. p.
27. Buss SJ, Schulz F, Mereles D, Hosch W, Galuschky C, Schummers G, et al. Quantitative analysis of left ventricular strain using cardiac computed tomography. Eur J Radiol. 2014;83(3):e123–30.
28. Ganten MK, Krautter U, von Tengg-Kobligk H, Bockler D, Schumacher H, Stiller W, et al. Quantification of aortic distensibility in abdominal aortic aneurysm using ECG-gated multi-detector computed tomography. Eur Radiol. 2008;18(5):966–73.
29. Seo J, Choi D, Rienmueller R, Lim JG, Chang Y, Lee J. Suggestion for a new image-based aortic wall stiffness evaluation technique: arterial wall stiffness index. Int J Cardiovasc Imaging. 2009;25(Suppl 1):83–94.
30. Hoit BD. Left atrial size and function: role in prognosis. J Am Coll Cardiol. 2014;63(6):493–505.
31. Prioli A, Marino P, Lanzoni L, Zardini P. Increasing degrees of left ventricular filling impairment modulate left atrial function in humans. Am J Cardiol. 1998;82(6):756–61.
32. Barbier P, Solomon SB, Schiller NB, Glantz SA. Left atrial relaxation and left ventricular systolic function determine left atrial reservoir function. Circulation. 1999;100(4):427–36.
33. Boudoulas KD, Paraskevaidis IA, Boudoulas H, Triposkiadis FK. The left atrium: from the research laboratory to the clinic. Cardiology. 2014;129(1):1–17.
34. Schweitzer A, Agmon Y, Aronson D, Abadi S, Mutlak D, Carasso S, et al. Assessment of left sided filling dynamics in diastolic dysfunction using cardiac computed tomography. Eur J Radiol. 2015;84(10):1930–7.
35. Rahimtoola SH, Ehsani A, Sinno MZ, Loeb HS, Rosen KM, Gunnar RM. Left atrial transport function in myocardial infarction. Importance of its booster pump function. Am J Med. 1975;59(5):686–94.
36. Hoit BD, Shao Y, Gabel M, Walsh RA. In vivo assessment of left atrial contractile performance in normal and pathological conditions using a time-varying elastance model. Circulation. 1994;89(4):1829–38.
37. Tsang TS, Abhayaratna WP, Barnes ME, Miyasaka Y, Gersh BJ, Bailey KR, et al. Prediction of cardiovascular outcomes with left atrial size: is volume superior to area or diameter? J Am Coll Cardiol. 2006;47(5):1018–23.
38. Agner BF, Kuhl JT, Linde JJ, Kofoed KF, Akeson P, Rasmussen BV, et al. Assessment of left atrial volume and function in patients with permanent atrial fibrillation: comparison of cardiac magnetic resonance imaging, 320-slice multi-detector computed tomography, and transthoracic echocardiography. Eur Heart J Cardiovasc Imaging. 2014;15(5):532–40.
39. Choi MJ, Kim JK, Kim SG, Yoon JW, Koo JR, Kim HJ, et al. Left atrial volume index is a predictor of silent myocardial ischemia in high-risk patients with end-stage renal disease. Int J Cardiovas Imag. 2013;29(7):1433–9. PubMed PMID: WOS:000325716000004. English.
40. Feuchtner GM, Dichtl W, Bonatti JO, Jodocy D, Muller S, Hintringer F, et al. Diagnostic accuracy of cardiac 64-slice computed tomography in detecting atrial thrombi. Comparative study with transesophageal echocardiography and cardiac surgery. Investig Radiol. 2008;43(11):794–801.
41. Christiaens L, Varroud-Vial N, Ardilouze P, Ragot S, Mergy J, Bonnet B, et al. Real three-dimensional assessment of left atrial and left atrial appendage volumes by 64-slice spiral computed tomography in individuals with or without cardiovascular disease. Int J Cardiol. 2010;140(2):189–96.
42. Im SI, Na JO, Kim SW, Choi CU, Kim JW, Yong HS, et al. Adjusted left atrial emptying fraction as a predictor of procedural outcome after catheter ablation for atrial fibrillation. Tex Heart Inst J. 2015;42(3):216–25. Pubmed Central PMCID: 4473613.
43. Nattel S, Burstein B, Dobrev D. Atrial remodeling and atrial fibrillation: mechanisms and implications. Circ Arrhythm Electrophysiol. 2008;1(1):62–73.
44. Caselli S, Canali E, Foschi ML, Santini D, Di Angelantonio E, Pandian NG, et al. Long-term prognostic significance of three-dimensional echocardiographic parameters of the left ventricle and left atrium. Eur J Echocardiogr. 2010;11(3):250–6.
45. Boogers MJ, van Werkhoven JM, Schuijf JD, Delgado V, El-Naggar HM, Boersma E, et al. Feasibility of diastolic function assessment with cardiac CT: feasibility study in comparison with tissue Doppler imaging. J Am Coll Cardiol Img. 2011;4(3):246–56.
46. Kusunose K, Motoki H, Popovic ZB, Thomas JD, Klein AL, Marwick TH. Independent association of left atrial function with exercise capacity in patients with preserved ejection fraction. Heart. 2012;98(17):1311–7.
47. Di Bella G, Siciliano V, Aquaro GD, De Marchi D, Rovai D, Carerj S, et al. Right ventricular dysfunction: an independent and incremental predictor of cardiac deaths late after acute myocardial infarction. Int J Cardiovasc Imaging. 2015;31(2):379–87.
48. Goldhaber SZ, Elliott CG. Acute pulmonary embolism: part II: risk stratification, treatment, and prevention. Circulation. 2003;108(23):2834–8.
49. Dogan H, Kroft LJ, Huisman MV, van der Geest RJ, de Roos A. Right ventricular function in patients with acute pulmonary embolism: analysis with electrocardiography-synchronized multi-detector row CT. Radiology. 2007;242(1):78–84.
50. Sato T, Tsujino I, Oyama-Manabe N, Ohira H, Ito YM, Sugimori H, et al. Simple prediction of right ventricular ejection fraction using tricuspid annular plane systolic excursion in pulmonary hypertension. Int J Cardiovasc Imaging. 2013;29(8):1799–805.
51. Pienn M, Kovacs G, Tscherner M, Johnson TR, Kullnig P, Stollberger R, et al. Determination of cardiac output with dynamic contrast-enhanced computed tomography. Int J Cardiovasc Imaging. 2013;29(8):1871–8.
52. Yamasaki Y, Nagao M, Kamitani T, Yamanouchi T, Kawanami S, Yamamura K, et al. Clinical impact of left ventricular eccentricity index using cardiac MRI in assessment of right ventricular hemodynamics and myocardial fibrosis in congenital heart disease. Eur Radiol. 2016;26(10):3617–25.
53. Muller HM, Tripolt MB, Rehak PH, Groell R, Rienmuller R, Tscheliessnigg KH. Noninvasive measurement of pulmonary vascular resistances by assessment of cardiac output and pulmonary transit time. Investig Radiol. 2000;35(12):727–31.

54. Revel MP, Faivre JB, Remy-Jardin M, Delannoy-Deken V, Duhamel A, Remy J. Pulmonary hypertension: ECG-gated 64-section CT angiographic evaluation of new functional parameters as diagnostic criteria. Radiology. 2009;250(2):558–66.
55. Tan RT, Kuzo R, Goodman LR, Siegel R, Haasler GB, Presberg KW. Utility of CT scan evaluation for predicting pulmonary hypertension in patients with parenchymal lung disease. Medical College of Wisconsin Lung Transplant Group. Chest. 1998;113(5):1250–6.
56. Chan AL, Juarez MM, Shelton DK, MacDonald T, Li CS, Lin TC, et al. Novel computed tomographic chest metrics to detect pulmonary hypertension. BMC Med Imaging. 2011;11:7. Pubmed Central PMCID: 3073886.
57. Remy-Jardin M, Duhamel A, Deken V, Bouaziz N, Dumont P, Remy J. Systemic collateral supply in patients with chronic thromboembolic and primary pulmonary hypertension: assessment with multi-detector row helical CT angiography. Radiology. 2005;235(1):274–81.
58. Collins MA, Pidgeon JW, Fitzgerald R. Computed tomography manifestations of tricuspid regurgitation. Br J Radiol. 1995;68(814):1058–60.
59. Yeh BM, Kurzman P, Foster E, Qayyum A, Joe B, Coakley F. Clinical relevance of retrograde inferior vena cava or hepatic vein opacification during contrast-enhanced CT. AJR Am J Roentgenol. 2004;183(5):1227–32.
60. Sivak JA, Raina A, Forfia PR. Assessment of the physiologic contribution of right atrial function to total right heart function in patients with and without pulmonary arterial hypertension. Pulm Circ. 2016;6(3):322–8.
61. Nourian S, Hosseinsabet A, Jalali A, Mohseni-Badalabadi R. Evaluation of right atrial function by two-dimensional speckle-tracking echocardiography in patients with right ventricular myocardial infarction. Int J Cardiovasc Imaging. 2017;33(1):47–56.
62. Lin FY, Devereux RB, Roman MJ, Meng J, Jow VM, Jacobs A, et al. Cardiac chamber volumes, function, and mass as determined by 64-multidetector row computed tomography: mean values among healthy adults free of hypertension and obesity. J Am Coll Cardiol Img. 2008;1(6):782–6.
63. Stojanovska J, Cronin P, Patel S, Gross BH, Oral H, Chughtai K, et al. Reference normal absolute and indexed values from ECG-gated MDCT: left atrial volume, function, and diameter. AJR Am J Roentgenol. 2011;197(3):631–7.
64. Stolzmann P, Scheffel H, Leschka S, Schertler T, Frauenfelder T, Kaufmann PA, et al. Reference values for quantitative left ventricular and left atrial measurements in cardiac computed tomography. Eur Radiol. 2008;18(8):1625–34.
65. Budoff MJ, Pagali SR, Hamirani YS, Chen A, Cheu G, Gao Y, et al. Sex-specific biatrial volumetric measurements obtained with use of multidetector computed tomography in subjects with and without coronary artery disease. Tex Heart Inst J. 2014;41(3):286–92. Pubmed Central PMCID: 4060347.
66. Yamasaki Y, Nagao M, Kawanami S, Kamitani T, Sagiyama K, Yamanouchi T, et al. One-stop shop assessment for atrial septal defect closure using 256-slice coronary CT angiography. Eur Radiol. 2017;27(2):697–704.
67. Addetia K, Takeuchi M, Maffessanti F, Nagata Y, Hamilton J, Mor-Avi V, et al. Simultaneous longitudinal strain in all 4 cardiac chambers: a novel method for comprehensive functional assessment of the heart. Circ Cardiovasc Imaging. 2016;9(3):e003895.

Part VIII

Where We Are: Cardiac Imaging Outside the Coronaries

Diseases of the Myocardium and Pericardium

37

Ana Paula S. Lima and Karen G. Ordovas

Computed tomography images of the heart can be used clinically for assessment of pericardial and myocardial diseases. Delineation of a normal pericardium and characterization of simple and complex pericardial collections can be performed with cardiac-gated CT. Several abnormalities of the myocardium can also be assessed with cardiac CT, particularly regarding cardiac morphology and perfusion, but also functional abnormalities. More commonly, myocardial diseases are identified as incidental findings on a chest CT for other clinical purposes and can aid to clinical management and risk stratification.

Pericardial Disease

Pericardial Anatomy

The pericardium is composed of an inner visceral layer, attached to the myocardium and epicardial fat, and an outer parietal layer containing serous fluid, normally up to 50 mL. On CT studies, the normal pericardium is usually less than 2 mm thick and if greater than 4 mm is considered abnormal (Fig. 37.1).

At the pericardial insertion points, reflections of pericardium are formed and may contain larger amount of serous fluid, the so-called sinuses and recesses. Two sinuses are formed by the pericardial reflections: the transvers sinus and the oblique sinus. The pericardial recesses are named the superior and inferior aortic recesses, left and right pulmonic recesses, posterior pericardial recess, left and right pulmonary vein recesses, and postcaval recess.

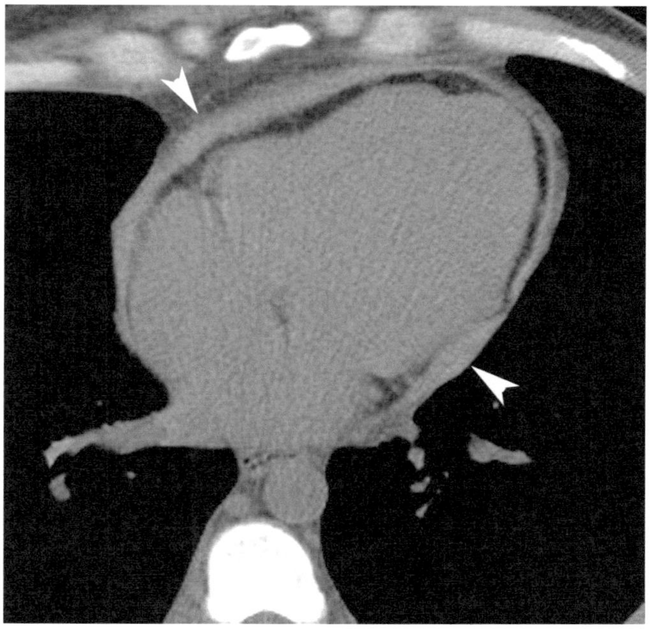

Fig. 37.1 Abnormally thick pericardium on cardiac CT

Pericardial sinuses and recesses can be confused for lymphadenopathy and masses, and therefore knowledge of its normal appearance on cross-sectional images is essential. The posterior extension of the superior pericardial recess (Fig. 37.2) often mimics right paratracheal adenopathy, whereas the anterior extension can be confused with aortic intramural hematoma, adenopathy, or mediastinal mass. Another common pitfall is the pulmonary vein recesses, particularly on the right, which can be mistaken for lymphadenopathy or pulmonary nodules (Fig. 37.3).

Pericardial Effusion

Accumulation of more than 50 ml of pericardial fluid is considered pericardial effusion. Pericardial effusions can rep-

A. P. S. Lima
Department of Radiology and Biomedical Imaging, University of California San Francisco, San Francisco, CA, USA

K. G. Ordovas (✉)
Department of Radiology, University of California San Francisco, San Francisco, CA, USA
e-mail: Karen.Ordovas@ucsf.edu

U. J. Schoepf (ed.), *CT of the Heart*, Contemporary Medical Imaging, https://doi.org/10.1007/978-1-60327-237-7_37

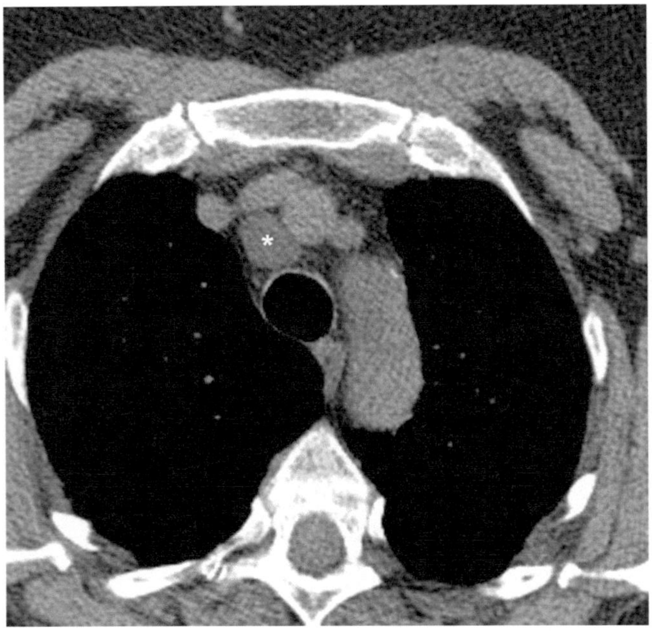

Fig. 37.2 Posterior aspect of the superior pericardial recess

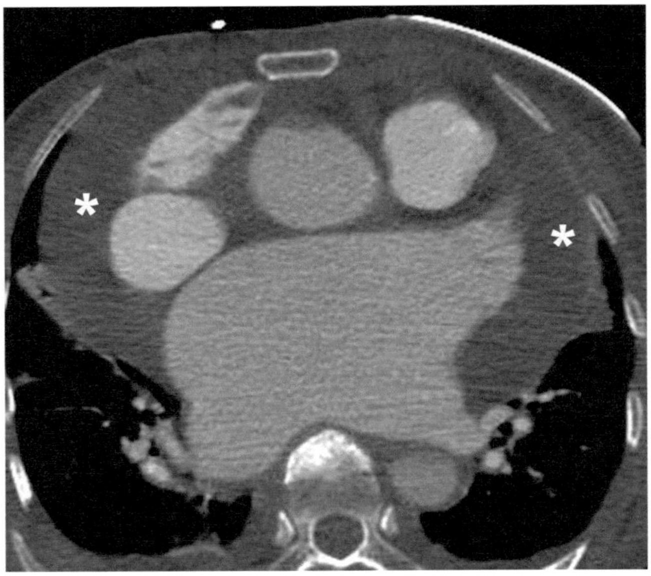

Fig. 37.4 Simple pericardial effusion

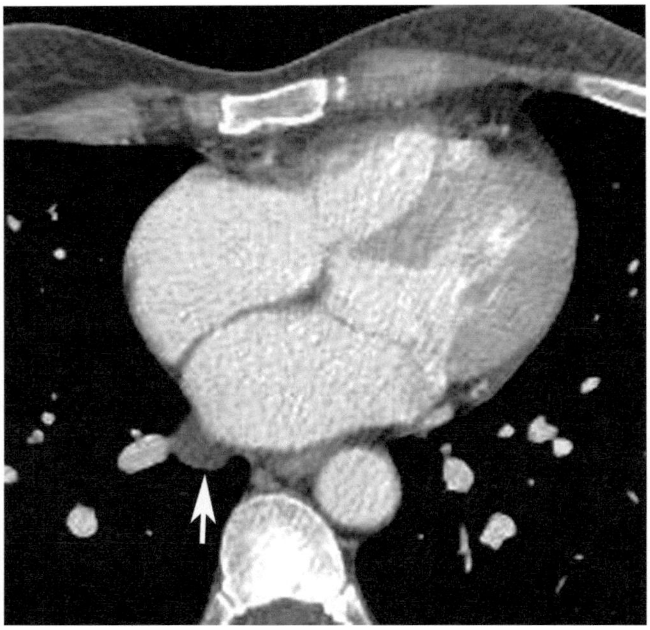

Fig. 37.3 Pulmonary vein recesses

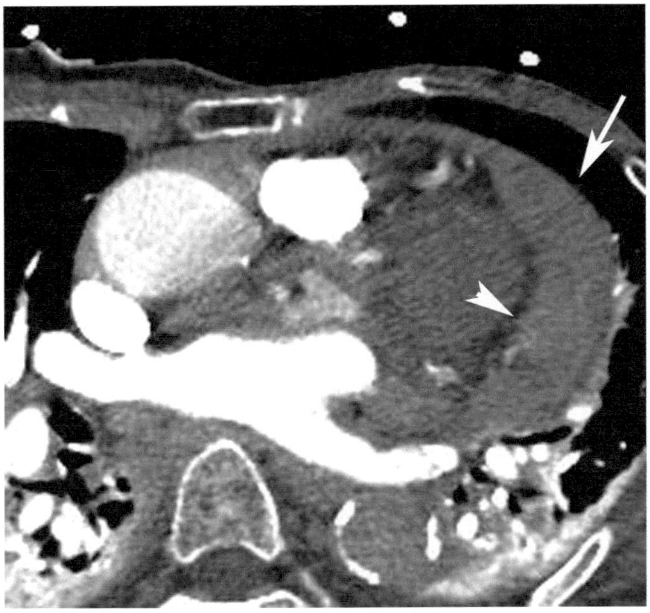

Fig. 37.5 Loculated pericardial effusion

resent transudate or exudate and have multiple mechanisms including inflammation, infection, trauma and iatrogenic insult.

The main role of cardiac CT in the assessment of pericardial effusion is to differentiate simple from complex collections, to delineate the distribution of loculated effusions, and to guide interventional procedures.

Simple pericardial effusion (transudate) has a density close to water on CT (Fig. 37.4). Differentiation of transudate from exudates is not always possible based on imaging appearance alone. However, increased and heterogeneous fluid density and areas of nondependent collections suggest exudates (Fig. 37.5).

The characterization of a hemorrhagic effusion, known as hemopericardium, may be very important for guiding clinical management. Hemopericardium can be seen in the setting of malignancy, trauma, or aortic rupture, and the CT

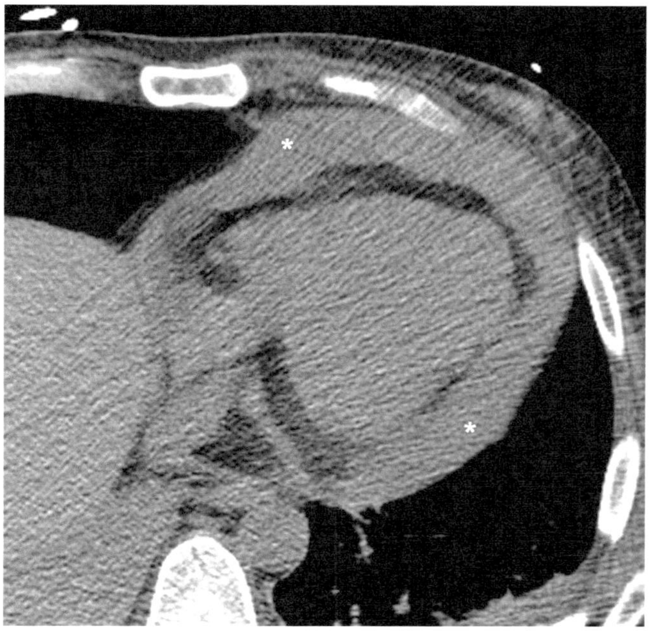

Fig. 37.6 Hemopericardium

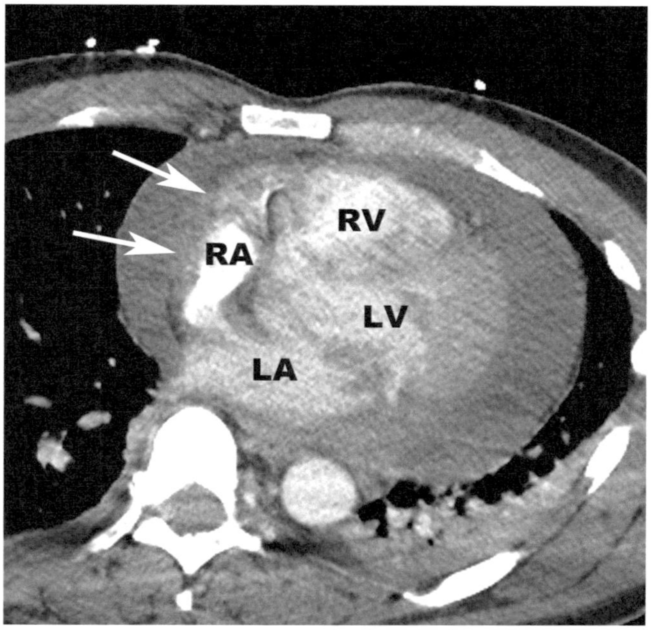

Fig. 37.7 Cardiac tamponade

appearance depends on the age of the bleeding. Acute hemopericardium has a high density on CT, whereas subacute hematomas present with a lower heterogeneous density (Fig. 37.6).

Pericardial Tamponade

Pericardial tamponade is characterized by impaired diastolic relaxation and ventricular filling due to accumulation of pericardial fluid that increases the intrapericardial pressure and causes an acute constrictive effect in the heart. Usually the hemodynamic effect is more pronounced on the lower pressure right atrium and ventricle and can compromise the venous return and cardiac output.

The volume and rapidity of fluid accumulation within the pericardium will determine patients' hemodynamic instability. In the acute setting, a volume as low as 150–200 ml can lead to tamponade, whereas a gradual accumulation in a chronic situation allows the pericardium to accumulate more than 1 L of fluid without hemodynamic instability.

The method of choice to interrogate the presence of cardiac tamponade is echocardiography. Cardiac CT showing a large effusion with compression of the right cardiac chambers can be diagnostic in the correct clinical scenario and can indeed be the first indication of a life-threatening diagnosis (Fig. 37.7). In addition, very commonly cardiac CT can identify the cause for the bleeding and expedite patient's clinical workup.

Pericarditis

Pericarditis is characterized by inflammation of the pericardial layers, usually without a definite etiology, but most commonly due to viral infections. Other conditions associated with pericarditis are thoracic radiation, collagen vascular diseases, uremia, myocardial infarction, and cardiac surgery. Tuberculosis is still a very common cause of pericarditis worldwide.

The classical clinical presentation of pericarditis is sharp and positional chest pain, often preceded by viral illness, diffuse ST segment elevation on ECG, and pericardial friction rub on physical examination.

The most common cardiac CT finding of pericarditis is pericardial thickening and enhancement, which is usually accompanied by effusion. Rarely, increased density of the epicardial and pericardial fat can be visualized. Pericardial enhancement is better appreciated in a late venous phase, usually more than 75 s after contrast injection (Fig. 37.8).

The presence of pericardial calcification and adhesions are suggestive of a chronic pericarditis and can be clearly delineate in a cardiac CT.

Constrictive Pericarditis

Patients with chronic pericarditis may develop pericardial fibrosis that impairs ventricular relaxation and leads to heart failure, a condition called constrictive pericarditis. Although many conditions can lead to constrictive pericarditis, the

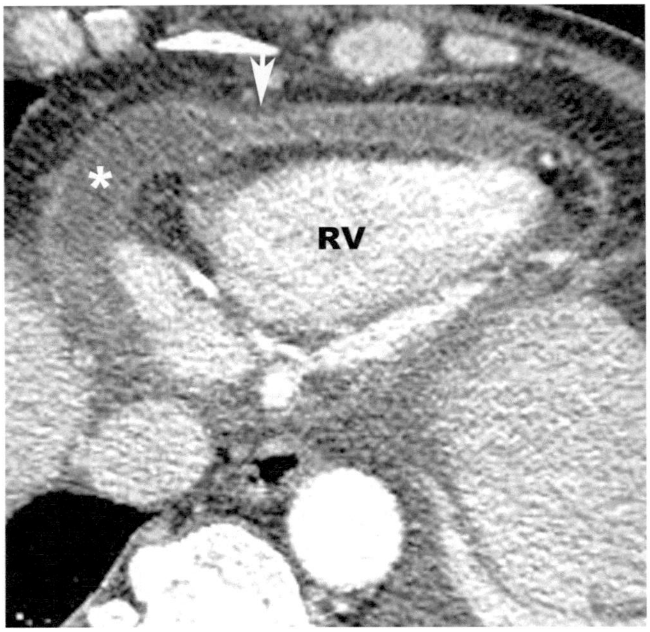

Fig. 37.8 Pericarditis with pericardial enhancement

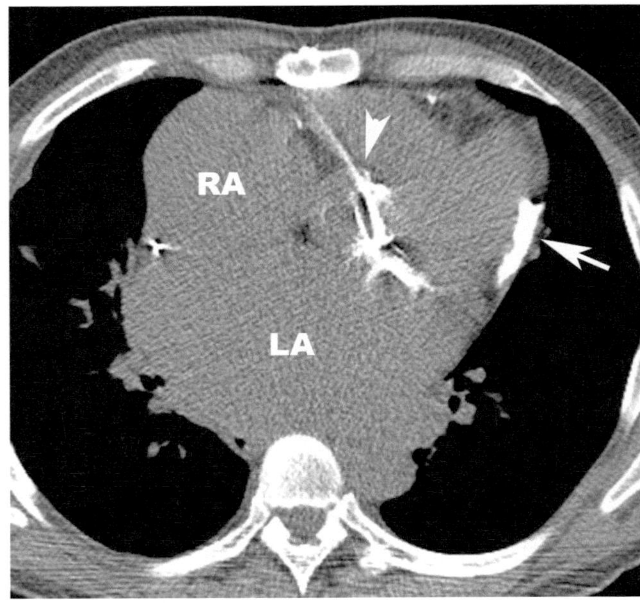

Fig. 37.9 Pericardial calcification and atrial enlargement in constrictive pericarditis

probability of this complication is related to the etiology and is high in bacterial pericarditis (20–30%), intermediate in immune-mediated and neoplastic pericarditis (2–5%), and low in viral pericarditis (<1%) [1].

Whereas in developing countries tuberculosis remains the main cause of constrictive pericarditis, the most common pericardial constriction insult in Europe and North America is cardiac surgery.

Constrictive pericarditis may have a subacute presentation or a more chronic and insidious clinical presentation with typical symptoms of dyspnea on exertion, fatigue, lower extremity swelling, and hepatic congestion. Occasionally, clinical presentation is atypical with symptoms resembling those of primary liver disease [2].

The most common type of constrictive pericarditis is the chronic fibrous type, characterized by thick fibrous pericardium, with calcifications in approximately 30% of the cases, which usually involve the atrioventricular grooves. Additional types of constrictive pericarditis include acute inflammatory, effusive-constrictive, and adhesive [3].

Echocardiography is often the first imaging test performed for evaluation of constrictive pericarditis, and classically demonstrates preserved left ventricular contractility, and signs of ventricular interdependence such as an early diastolic ventricular septal bounce. However, very rarely echocardiography is able to document the presence of pericardial thickening.

Cardiac CT is an excellent method to evaluate the pericardium in its entirety and to detect the presence of calcification (Fig. 37.9). Pericardial thickening of 4 mm or greater in a patient with constrictive/restrictive physiology is highly suggestive of constrictive pericarditis, and the specificity increases when thickness is greater than 6 mm. In approximately 20% of the cases, constrictive pericarditis is seen in the absence of a thick pericardium [3].

Additional morphologic abnormalities seen on cardiac CT are enlargement of the atria and, in advanced disease, narrowing and elongation of ventricles. Dilatation of the inferior vena cava and hepatic veins can also be seen. Contrast enhancement on late venous phases and large pericardial effusion suggests the inflammatory and effusive subtypes, respectively, whereas thick adhesions between the pericardial layers are characteristics of adhesive subtype of constrictive pericarditis. Although a retrospectively gated cardiac CT can demonstrate an early diastolic septal bounce, echocardiography and cardiac MRI are better methods to identify this abnormality.

Myocardium

CT as a Primary Tool for Myocardial Diseases

CT is rarely used as the primary technique for evaluation of myocardial diseases. However, evaluation of the myocardium is frequently performed in a comprehensive cardiac CT for ischemic heart disease assessment. Although coronary imaging is the most important application of CT in the assessment of cardiac diseases, modern scanners allow for visualization of perfusion defects and myocardial contraction abnormalities that can be used to characterize the hemo-

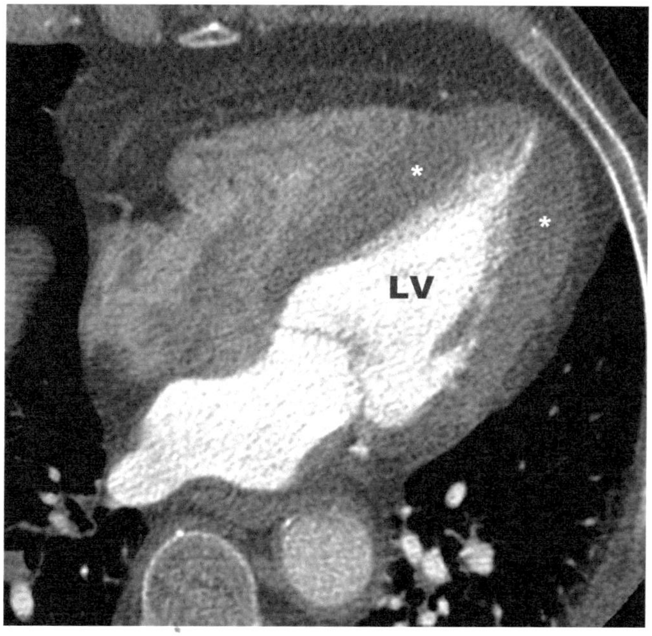

Fig. 37.10 Apical type of hypertrophic cardiomyopathy

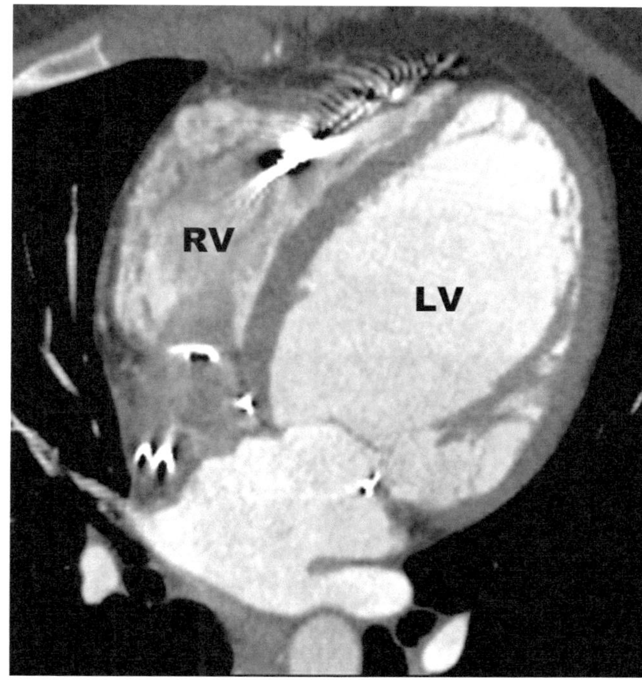

Fig. 37.11 Dilated cardiomyopathy on non-gated cardiac CT

dynamic significance of coronary lesions. In addition, delayed cardiac CT images can demonstrate areas of delayed myocardial enhancement that have been shown to correlate with the presence of myocardial scar and irreversible myocardial injury. Detailed discussion of the use of cardiac CT for myocardial perfusion and viability are discussed on a dedicated chapter of this book.

In patients with nonischemic myocardial disease, cardiac CT can provide additional information to echocardiography particularly in patients with hypertrophic cardiomyopathy. Cross-sectional imaging is commonly used in HCM patients to characterize the distribution and quantify the severity of myocardial hypertrophy, which could aid in risk stratification and guide therapy decisions (Fig. 37.10). It can also help differentiate between severe myocardial hypertrophy and myocardial mass. In patients with dilated cardiomyopathy, cardiac CT can provide precise quantification of ventricular volumes and function, which can be challenging for echocardiography when ventricular volumes are very large (Fig. 37.11). A common cardiac CT application in patients with dilated cardiomyopathy is assessment of ventricular thrombi suspected on echocardiography evaluation.

Incidental Cardiac CT Findings on Chest CT

Very commonly myocardial abnormalities are seen as incidental findings on chest CT or coronary CT studies and may in fact be important for establishing the diagnosis and informing patient management.

Calcifications

Myocardial calcifications can be easily identified on chest CT examinations and usually indicate sequela of a previous myocardial insult [4]. The most common type of myocardial calcification seen on CT are dystrophic calcifications within areas of necrotic scar due to an old myocardial infarction, which are usually subendocardial following a coronary territory (Fig. 37.12). Frequently, the presence of myocardial calcification is diagnostic of an old myocardial infarction which may be unknown to the patient and the medical team and would indicate the need for secondary prevention measures. Myocardial calcifications can also result from previous myocarditis, trauma, or iatrogenic injuries. Rarely, metastatic myocardial calcifications may occur in the setting of impaired calcium-phosphorus metabolism, usually in patients with chronic renal failure or hyperparathyroidism [5].

Wall Thinning and Aneurysm

Similar to myocardial calcifications, the presence of myocardial wall thinning reflects the presence of a previous insult to the cardiac muscle, which can be ischemic or nonischemic in etiology. Areas of wall thinning that match a coronary territory are classically due to sequel of a chronic myocardial infarction (Fig. 37.13). Diffuse myocardial wall thinning can be seen in the setting of dilated cardiomyopathy from several etiologies. Retrospectively cardiac-gated CT examinations can aid in functional characterization of areas of myocardial thinning. This functional assessment can be particularly useful in differentiating normal apical thinning, which should

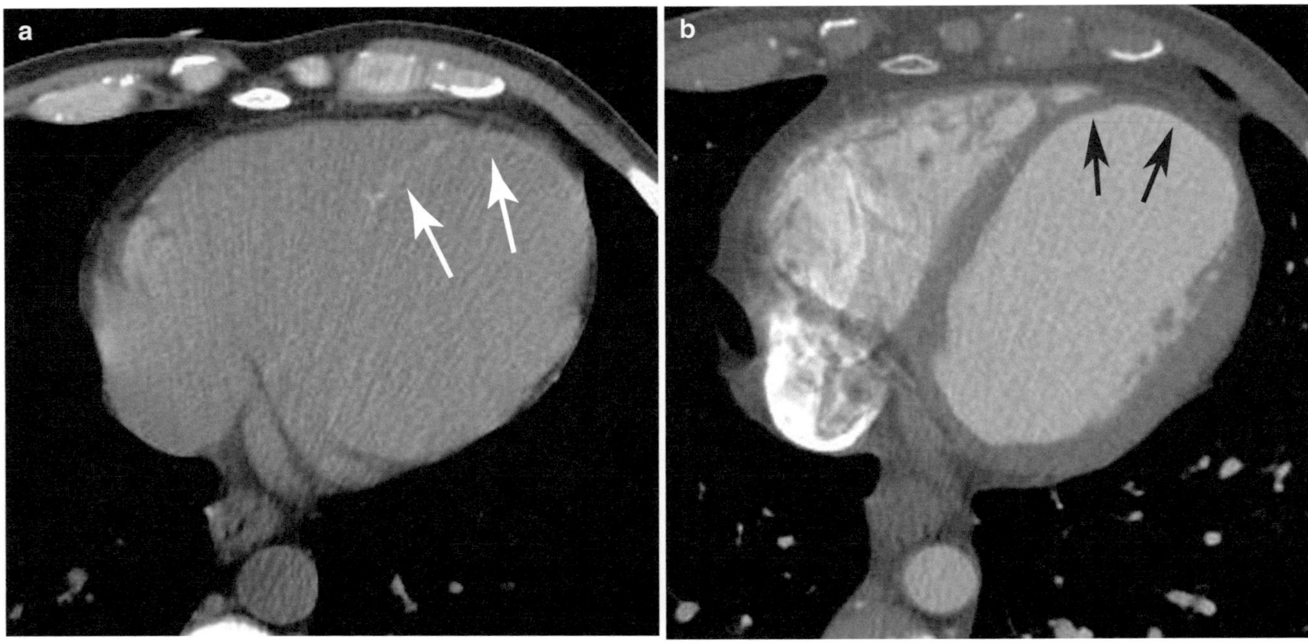

Fig. 37.12 (**a**, **b**) Myocardial calcification due to old myocardial infarction

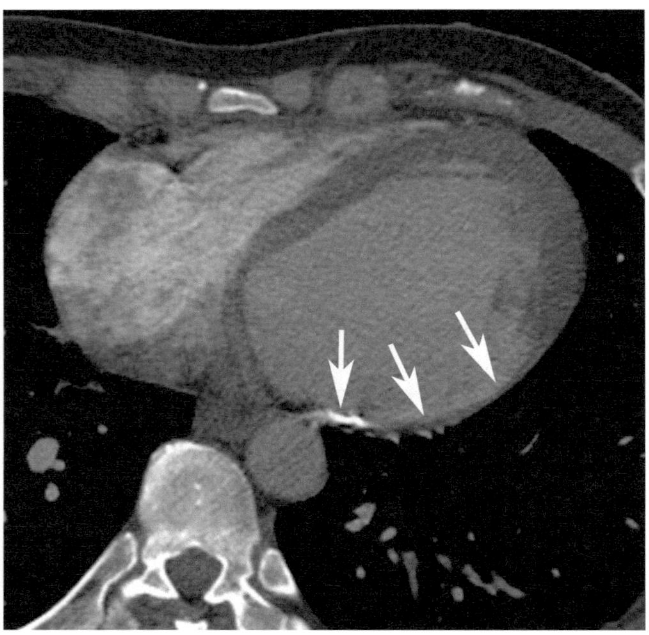

Fig. 37.13 Left ventricular wall thinning with associated calcification

show normal contractility, from an apical myocardial infarction [6].

When associated with outpouching of the ventricular walls in diastole, areas of wall thinning are characteristic of ventricular aneurysms. Detection of ventricular aneurysms may have a significant impact in clinical management as they are associated with increased risk of cardiovascular morbidity and mortality. True ventricular aneurysms usually involve the left apical and anterolateral walls and have a wide point of attachment with the chamber. These aneurysms increase the risk of thrombus formation and consequent embolic events. False ventricular aneurysms are most commonly seen in the diaphragmatic surface of the ventricle and impose a high risk of cardiac rupture, characterizing a cardiac urgency.

Hypoperfusion

In patients with an old myocardial infarction or myocardial ischemia at rest, areas of decreased subendocardial perfusion can be identified in cardiac CT and chest CT scans. This finding is particularly meaningful if matching the coronary territory of a vessel with evidence of atherosclerotic disease (Fig. 37.14). Although perfusion defects are easily identifiable in cardiac-gated CT for coronary artery disease evaluation, incidental areas of subendocardial perfusion abnormalities may be visualized on non-gate chest CT angiograms for pulmonary artery or aorta investigation. However, non-gated chest CT studies have a greater potential to be affected by motion and hard beaming artifact, which could limit the assessment of subendocardial perfusion defects [7].

Conclusion

Cardiac CT has great utility for evaluation of pericardia diseases, particularly as an aid to echocardiography in characterizing complex collections, loculation, and pericardial

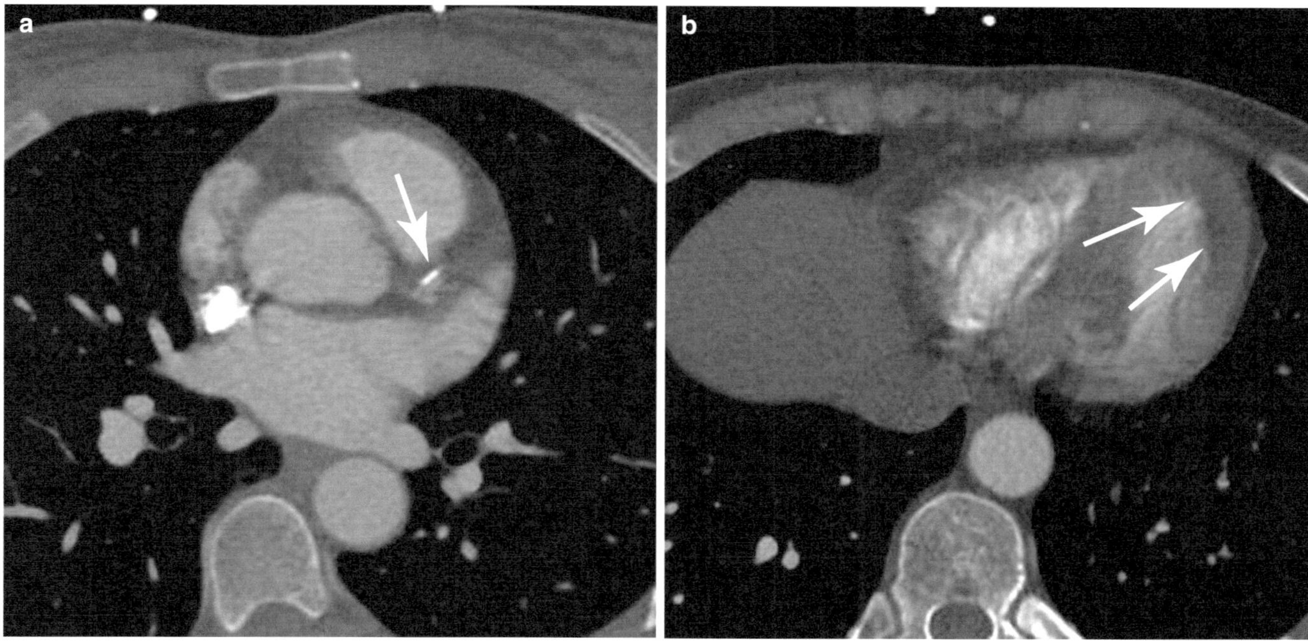

Fig. 37.14 (**a**, **b**) Subendocardial perfusion defect at rest in a patient with old myocardial infarction

constriction. Cardiac and chest CT can characterize ischemic myocardial injury as an area of wall thinning, aneurysm, abnormal contractility, impaired perfusion, and calcifications. More commonly, these myocardial abnormalities are incidental findings on a non-gated chest CT and could provide important insight for patients' diagnosis and management.

References

1. Fardman A, Charron P, Imazio M, et al. European guidelines on pericardial diseases: a focused review of novel aspects. Curr Cardiol Rep. 2016;18(5):46.
2. Garcia MJ. Constrictive pericarditis versus restrictive cardiomyopathy? J Am Coll Cardiol. 2016;67(17):2061–76.
3. Cummings KW, Green D, Johnson WR, et al. Imaging of pericardial diseases. Semin Ultrasound CT MR. 2016;37(3):238–54.
4. Austin CO, Kramer D, Canabal J, et al. A heart of stone: a case of acute development of cardiac calcification and hemodynamic collapse. J Cardiovasc Comput Tomogr. 2013;7(1):66–8.
5. Mana M, Sanguineti F, Unterseeh T, et al. Petrified myocardium: the age of stone? Circulation. 2013;126(9):1139–42.
6. Ferencik M, Abbara S, Hoffmann U, et al. Left ventricular thin-point detection using multidetector spiral computed tomography. Am J Cardiol. 2004;93(7):949–51.
7. Shriki JE, Shinbane J, Lee C, et al. Incidental myocardial infarct on conventional nongated CT: a review of spectrum of findings with gated CT and cardiac MRI correlation. AJR Am J Roentgenol. 2012;198(3):496–504.

CT of Cardiac and Paracardiac Masses

38

Harold Goerne and Prabhakar Rajiah

There is a broad spectrum of cardiac and paracardiac masses, which includes nonneoplastic as well as neoplastic lesions, both benign and malignant lesions. Paracardiac masses such as those involving the esophagus, tracheobronchial tree, lungs, pericardium, diaphragm, and lymph nodes are more common than the cardiac masses. The most common cardiac mass is a thrombus. The most common neoplastic lesion to involve the heart is metastasis, which is 20–40 times more common than primary neoplasms [1]. While the overall prevalence of cardiac metastasis is 1.23% [2], primary cardiac neoplasms have a prevalence of 0.001–0.056% [2, 3]. In adults, 75% of the primary cardiac neoplasms are benign, with myxoma being the most common (45–50%) type, followed by fibroelastoma (15%), lipoma (5–10%), and fibroma (2–4%). The most common primary cardiac malignancy is angiosarcoma (10%), followed by sarcomas with myoblastic or fibroblastic differentiation (5%) and rhabdomyosarcoma (2–5%) [4, 5]. Pediatric cardiac neoplasms are usually benign (90%) [6, 7], with rhabdomyoma (70%) being the most common neoplasm followed by fibroma (10%) [7, 8]. Malignant tumors are extremely rare in children, most of which are sarcomas, followed by lymphoma. The clinical manifestations of cardiac masses depend on the pathology and other features. Even benign cardiac neoplasms can be life-threatening depending on their location, size, and movement due to hemodynamic compromise, arrhythmia, or thromboembolism [9]. In addition, there are several normal variants that may mimic masses.

In this chapter, we review the role of computed tomography (CT) in the evaluation of cardiac masses, CT protocols, and the imaging appearances of common and uncommon cardiac and paracardiac masses.

H. Goerne
Department of Radiology, Cardiothoracic Imaging, UT Southwestern Medical Center, Dallas, TX, USA

P. Rajiah (✉)
Department of Radiology, Cardiothoracic Imaging Division, UT Southwestern Medical Center, Dallas, TX, USA

Imaging of Cardiac Masses

Imaging plays an important role in the evaluation of cardiac masses, since most of these are not amenable to biopsy due to their location and there is high risk of complications. Imaging is necessary to confirm the mass; determine the exact location, extension, and relationships; distinguish benign and malignant lesions, although a precise diagnosis is not always possible [4]; identify masses at risk of embolism and obstruction; and determine management options including biopsy, surgery, and serial follow-up. There are several imaging options available including echocardiography, magnetic resonance imaging (MRI), CT, and nuclear medicine. Transthoracic echocardiogram (TTE) is often the first imaging modality used in the evaluation of cardiac mass, with a mass often incidentally detected in this modality. It is widely available, inexpensive, and portable, has excellent temporal and good spatial resolutions, and can be performed in hemodynamically unstable patients, and there is no radiation exposure. However, it is operator-dependent, limited in patients with poor acoustic windows, and limited in imaging certain parts of the heart such as the right ventricle and apical regions, has limited field of view to image extracardiac structures, and does not have tissue characterization capabilities [10]. Transesophageal echocardiogram (TEE) can be used to overcome some of these limitations, particularly improving the spatial resolution, but is an invasive method [4]. MRI is an important modality in the evaluation of cardiac masses. It has excellent spatial and good temporal resolution, wide field of view, multiplanar imaging capabilities, and also tissue characterization capabilities, primarily due to inherent soft tissue contrast which can be augmented by several sequences and contrast administration, which help in distinguishing normal myocardium, fluid, edema, fat, fibrosis, and hemorrhage. Disadvantages of MRI include long acquisition times (30 min–1 h.), limited availability, need for higher technical expertise, inability to perform in hemodynamically unstable patients, and contraindications including claustrophobia, several cardiac

U. J. Schoepf (ed.), *CT of the Heart*, Contemporary Medical Imaging, https://doi.org/10.1007/978-1-60327-237-7_38

devices, and severe renal dysfunction [4]. Nuclear medicine techniques, primarily 18F-FDG-PET scan, are useful in assessing the metabolic activity of cardiac lesions, which helps in distinguishing benign from malignant lesions, staging of malignant lesions, and assessing response to therapy. Nuclear medicine techniques are associated with radiation and have lower spatial resolution.

CT in Cardiac Masses

CT has emerged as an important imaging modality in the evaluation of cardiac and paracardiac neoplasms. CT has several advantages including wide availability and rapid acquisition time. The excellent isotropic spatial resolution and multiplanar reconstruction capabilities of CT enable excellent, three-dimensional rendering of the masses, which is essential for surgical planning. The wide field of view of CT enables visualization of paracardiac and other extracardiac structures, which is essential for staging malignancies. CT is primarily used in the evaluation of cardiac masses in patients who cannot have MRI scan due to contraindications. It is also useful in specific situations where MRI or echocardiography cannot provide optimal information, for instance, the presence of calcification or evaluation of vascular supply of tumors. CT can also provide functional dynamic information. The principal disadvantages of CT are the use of ionizing radiation with its theoretical risks and iodinated contrast media which is associated with nephrotoxicity in patients with renal dysfunction.

CT Protocol

The cardiac CT protocol should be customized based on the specific clinical question, type, and location of the mass. All scans are performed with ECG gating to minimize cardiac motion. Prospective ECG triggering is the default mode due to lower radiation exposure, but retrospective ECG gating is recommended if ventricular functional estimation, mass mobility, and valvular motion need to be evaluated. It is also opted if coronary arteries are evaluated in patients with high or irregular heart rates. The radiation dose is higher for a retrospective gated mode, but it can be minimized by using ECG-based tube current modulation [4]. Usually, there is no need for beta-blocker and nitroglycerine predication for the evaluation of cardiac masses. The tube voltage and current are selected based on patient size. The scan range depends on the localization and extent of the mass. Occasionally the total extent of the mass may be seen only after the study, and hence a longer scan range may be necessary in such patients. For cardiac masses, it is advantageous to use a triphasic injection protocol which enables visualization of all the cardiac chambers as well as reduction of streak artifacts in the SVC and right atrium. This involves initial contrast injection at flow rate of 5–7 ml/s to opacify the left heart, followed by either a contrast injection at a slower rate of 2–4 ml/s or injection of a mixture of contrast and saline (50:50 or 60:40 ratio) at same flow rate of 5-7 ml/s to opacify the right heart and finally by saline bolus injection to minimize streak artifact. Additional non-contrast phase may be acquired if there is a concern of calcification, and a delayed phase may be acquired if there is a need for distinguishing thrombus from slow flow or for delayed enhancement. Images are reconstructed at submillimeter thickness (0.5–0.75 mm), with small field of view (200–250 mm) for the heart. In addition, full field-of-view 2 × 1 mm axial images, 2 × 2 mm coronal and sagittal multiplanar images, and 7 × 2 mm MIP axial images are reconstructed for the evaluation of lungs and other thoracic structures. With retrospective ECG-gated acquisitions, cine images of the heart can then be reconstructed in any desired plane.

Approach to Cardiac Masses

The first step in evaluation of a cardiac mass is to determine if it is a normal variant or a real mass. There are several normal variants discussed in detail below, which occur in characteristic locations with characteristic appearance. Awareness of these normal variants will prevent misdiagnosis as a cardiac mass. For masses, further determination includes if it is a nonneoplastic or neoplastic lesion, more particularly distinguishing benign from malignant lesion. Age, gender, symptoms, and other clinical history are important in helping to make this distinction. For instance, a mass adjacent to an akinetic segment in a patient with prior history of myocardial infarction is highly suggestive of a thrombus. A cardiac mass in a patient with known primary malignancy should alert the possibility of metastasis. There are several imaging features that help in distinguishing benign from malignant lesions. Some features of benign lesions are:

More common on the left; Smaller in size; Smooth, well-defined margins; Involvement of one compartment/chamber; No invasive features; May have a pedicle; No feeding artery; Calcification is rare; Pericardial effusion and metastasis are not seen.

Features of malignant lesions are; More common in the right, especially the atrium; Larger in size; Ill-defined, lobulated, invasive, and infiltrative margins; Involvement of multiple chambers or compartments (myocardium, pericardium, extracardiac); Broad base of attachment; Feeding artery may be present; Calcification may be seen in osteosarcoma; Pericardial effusion and metastasis may be seen.

Normal Variants

Prominent Crista Terminalis

Crista terminalis is a fibromuscular ridge located in the inner posterior aspect of the right atrium (RA), which divides this chamber into a trabeculated anterolateral wall and a smooth posterior wall [11]. Crista terminalis represents the junction of embryological primitive right atrium and sinus venosus and is caused by regression of the septum spurium, while the sinus venosus is incorporated into the right atrial wall. This regression shows a wide range of variations and can be prominent [12]. A prominent crista terminalis is one of the most common anatomical variants, which can mimic atrial neoplasm, thrombus, or vegetation [13]. On CT, it is seen as a linear and well-defined filling defect in the posterior wall of the right atrium (Fig. 38.1), which crosses the atrial wall from superior to inferior, with smooth borders and similar attenuation as that of the atrial wall with no contrast enhancement, which is well appreciated in four-chamber and axial planes.

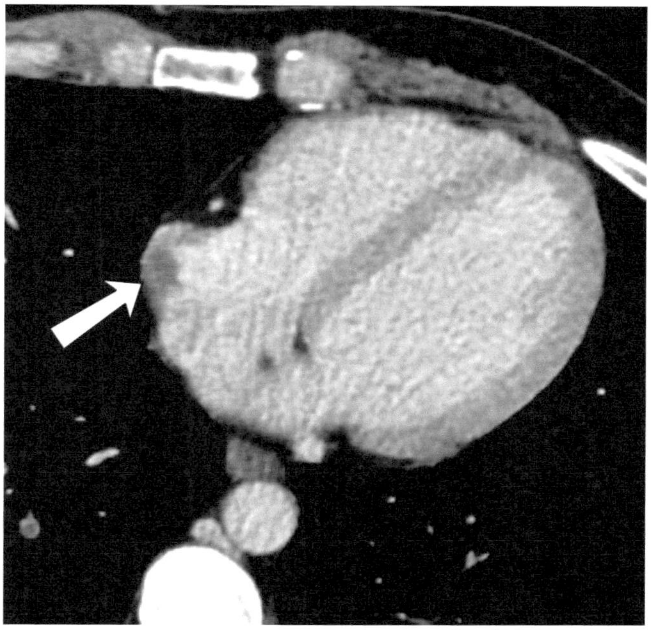

Fig. 38.1 Prominent crista terminalis. Axial CT scan shows a focal protrusion from the posterolateral aspect of the right atrium (arrow), characteristic of a prominent crista terminalis

Persistent Eustachian Valve

Eustachian valve is located at the junction between the inferior vena cava (IVC) and right atrium (RA) and directs oxygenated blood flow from the IVC toward the foramen ovale during fetal life [14]. After birth, with the closure of foramen ovale, the valve tends to regress as it has no specific function [15]. However, this valve can occasionally persist until adult life and when prominent, can be mistaken for mass on echocardiography. On CT, it is easy to recognize this variant, whose features depend on the size of the valve and can either be rigid and elongated or an undulating membrane [16]. Thebesian valve is located at the junction between the coronary sinus and RA.

Chiari Network

The Chiari network is a reticulum of fibers resembling a web located in the right atrium, between the Eustachian and Thebesian valves and the crista terminalis [17]. It is believed to be caused by incomplete resorption of the right side of the sinus venosus valve [17, 18]. The estimated prevalence is about 2% [17, 19] and is often detected incidentally in imaging, particularly echocardiogram. A patent foramen ovale is present in 83% of cases [17], with higher prevalence of atrial septal aneurysm and paradoxical embolism [18]. CT plays a role when echocardiogram is inconclusive and differential diagnosis such as thrombus or cor triatriatum dexter is considered. On CT, the network is hard to visualize when there is heterogeneous contrast in the right atrium.

Left Lateral Ridge

Left lateral ridge is located in the left atrium (LA) between the left superior pulmonary vein and left atrial appendage (LAA) [20]. This ridge is also called the Coumadin/warfarin ridge because it used to be often mistaken for thrombus and anticoagulation therapy was initiated. This is also called the ligament of Marshall and contains the oblique vein of Marshall, which is an embryological remnant of a left superior vena cava that drains into the coronary sinus

[21, 22]. On CT, it is easy to recognize this structure, since it usually has a rounded tip that gives a pedunculated appearance (Fig. 38.2).

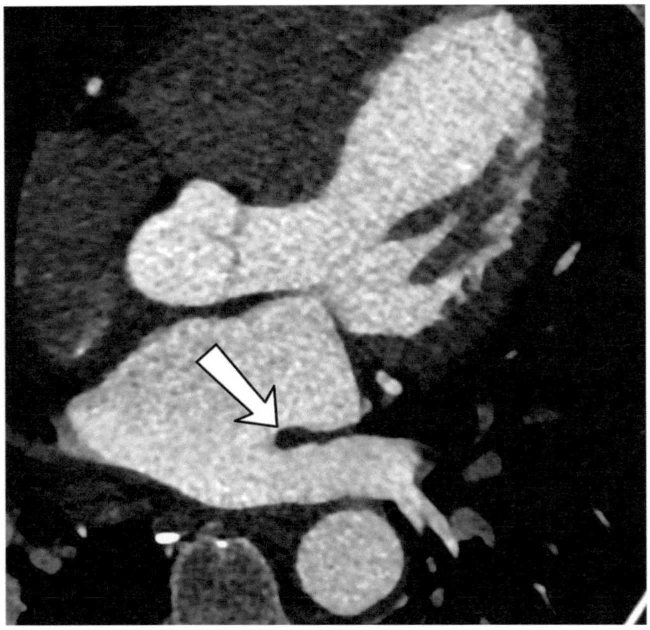

Fig. 38.2 Coumadin ridge. Axial CT scan shows a prominent ridge between the left superior pulmonary vein and the body of the left atrium, which is consistent with a Coumadin ridge (arrow)

Nonneoplastic Masses

Thrombus

Thrombus is the most common intracardiac mass [23]. Predisposing factors include wall motion abnormalities (myocardial infarction/dilated cardiomyopathy), atrial fibrillation, intracardiac devices, and hypercoagulable states [3]. Thrombus is most common in the left heart chambers. Left atrial thrombus is associated with atrial fibrillation and mitral valvular abnormalities and is most commonly seen in the posterior wall or the atrial appendage. On CT, thrombus is seen as a round or oval filling defect with low attenuation (Fig. 38.3). A left atrial appendage thrombus is often difficult to distinguish from contrast admixture. An attenuation threshold of 65 HU has sensitivity, specificity, and positive and negative predictive values of 94%, 97%, 94%, and 97%, respectively, in the diagnosis of thrombus [24]. Other studies have shown that there is no significant difference in the mean CT numbers of thrombus and slow flow (91.7 ± 11.6 HU vs. 85.2 ± 10.9 HU, respectively, $P = 0.241$), but the mean iodine concentration (mg/ml) as measured in a dual-energy CT is significantly different (3.53 ± 0.72 vs. 1.37 ± 0.31, respectively, $P < 0.001$) [25]. Ratio of left atrial appendage attenuation/ascending aorta of >0.75 has 100% negative predictive value in excluding thrombus [26]. A delayed phase (30 s from early phase) can distinguish slow flow from thrombus since a

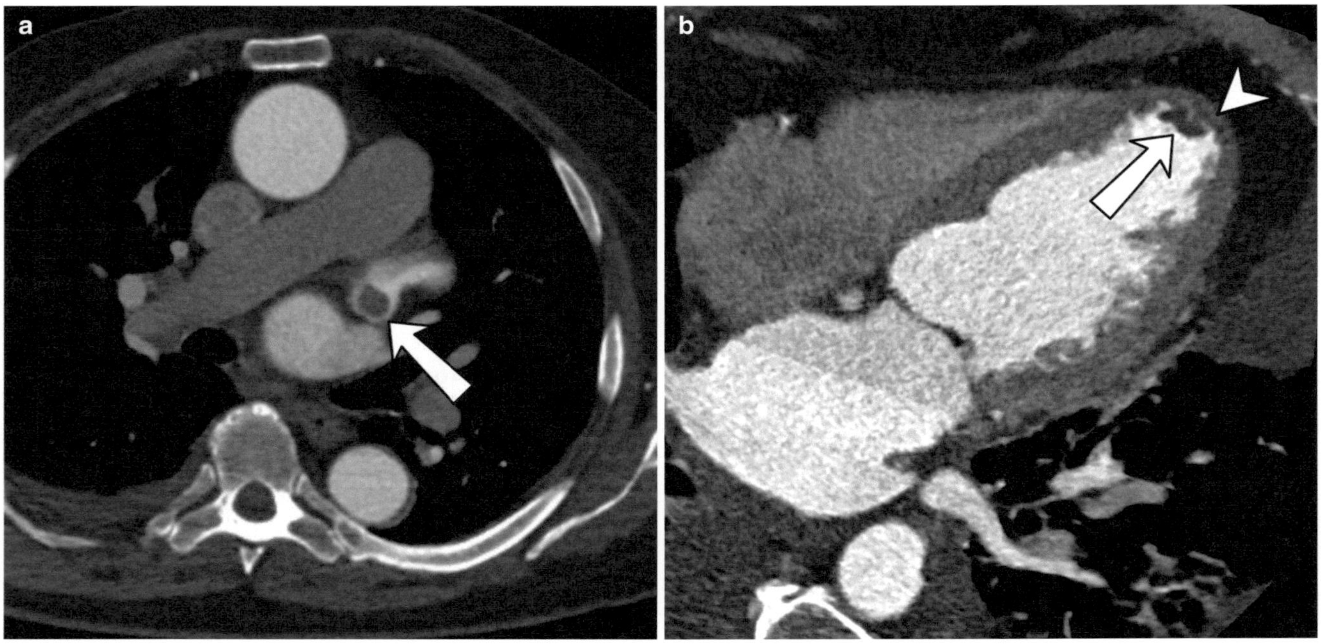

Fig. 38.3 Thrombus. (**a**) Axial CT shows a hypoattenuating filling defect in the left atrial appendage (arrow) consistent with a thrombus. (**b**) Four-chamber CT reconstruction shows a small hypoattenuating filling defect in the LV apex (arrow), consistent with a fresh thrombus. Note the subendocardial hypoattenuation in the apex related to hypoperfusion due to prior infarction (arrowhead)

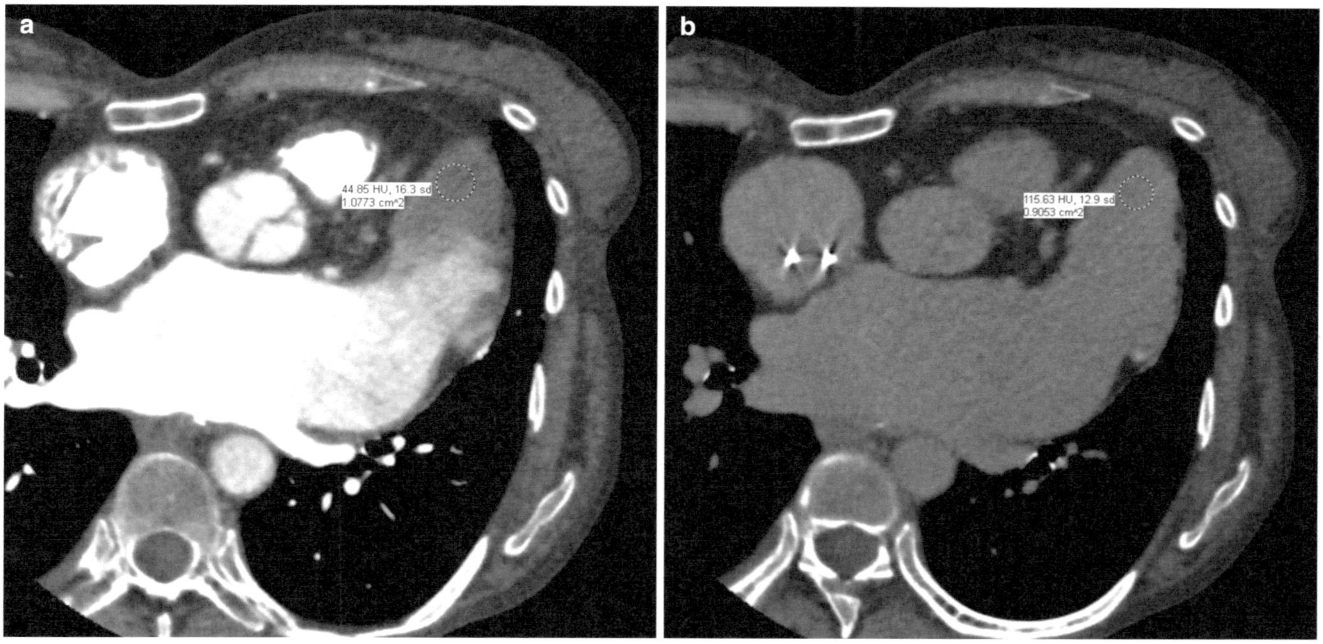

Fig. 38.4 Contrast admixture. (**a**) Axial CT scan shows a hypoattenuating filling defect in the left atrial appendage, which has an attenuation of 44.8 HU in the arterial phase (arrow). This could be either due to thrombus or contrast admixture. (**b**) Delayed phase axial CT scan in the same patient shows homogeneous opacification of the left atrial appendage with disappearance of the previously seen hypoattenuation. The mean attenuation in the delayed phase is 115 HU, and the left atrial appendage/ascending aorta ratio is 0.9. All these indicate that this is contrast admixture and not a thrombus

thrombus is present in both the phases with low attenuation, but contrast admixture is present only in the early phase (Fig. 38.4) [10]. Also, in the late phase, the left atrial appendage/ascending aorta attenuation ratio is lower in thrombus (0.29HU ± 0.12) than circulatory stasis (0.85 HU ± 0.12) [27]. Thrombus in the left ventricle has a crescentic shape with broad base and low attenuation but in some cases can be pedunculated [3]. It is closely associated with wall motion abnormalities. In the right chambers, thrombus is associated with central catheters or deep vein thrombosis and should be considered pulmonary emboli in transit [23]. Other causes include ARVD, Behcet's disease, metastases, and trauma. Chronic thrombus can be calcified and occasionally show some contrast enhancement due to vascularization (Fig. 38.5). Thrombus should also be distinguished from neoplasms such as myxoma. Features in favor of thrombus are - more common in ventricles than atria; common in left atrial appendage when located in the left atrium; smaller in size; rarely mobile or prolapsing; polypoidal; may be calcified; and no contrast enhancement. Features in favor of myxoma are - more common in the left atrium; particularly attached to the fossa ovalis, larger in size; villous or polypoid; usually pedunculated

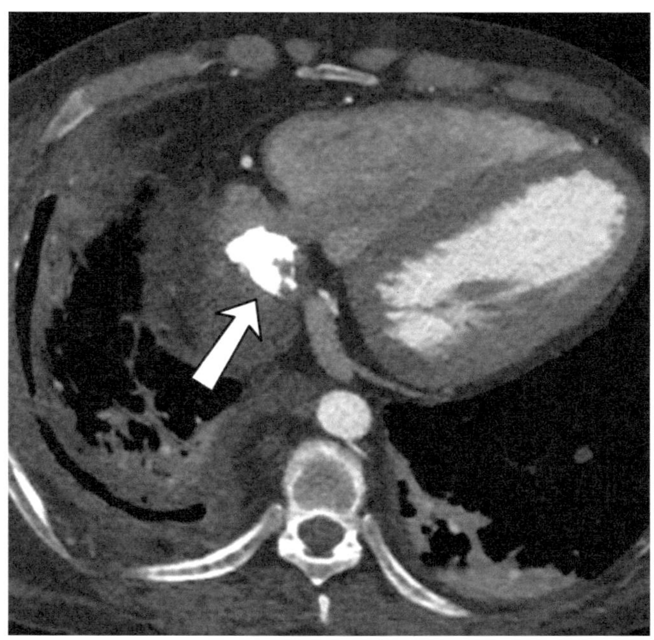

Fig. 38.5 Chronic thrombus. Axial CT scan shows a densely calcified chronic thrombus (arrow) in the right atrium

and mobile; may prolapse into AV valve; rarely calcified; and shows variable contrast enhancement [10, 27].

Lipomatous Hypertrophy of Interatrial Septum

Lipomatous hypertrophy of interatrial septum (LHIS) is a rare (1–8%) condition [28, 29] characterized by abnormal fatty deposition in the interatrial groove and inferior pyramidal space, which lies between the atrial walls surrounding the fossa ovalis (true septum) [30–32]. Although the exact etiology is not known, it is more common in obese patients with a high amount of epicardial fat and hence likely a metabolic condition. Histologically, there is increase in the number of adipocytes (hyperplasia) [33], both mature adipocytes and fetal fat cells (brown fat). Hypertrophy has also been shown [34, 35]. There is no capsule and hence this is not a true lipoma [29, 35]. On CT, there is increased thickness of interatrial septum >2 cm [32, 33, 35], with fat attenuation and the pathognomonic "dumbbell" shape that spares the fossa ovalis, which is devoid of fat (Fig. 38.6). The fat is contiguous with the epicardial fat, and the thickening is more extensive in cephalad than caudad region. There is no contrast enhancement, but this area shows uptake in FDG-PET scan, probably due to the presence of brown fat [29] or inflammation [32]. Occasionally, accumulation of fat can be extensive and may obstruct the right atrial inflow [32].

Caseous Mitral Annular Calcification

Caseous mitral annular calcification (CMAC) is a rare type of mitral annular calcification (MAC), with an estimated incidence of 2.7% of MAC [36], that is caused by degeneration and liquefaction necrosis, resulting in peripheral dense calcifications and central caseous admixture of liquid calcium, fatty acids, and cholesterol [37, 38]. It is more prevalent in elderly patients and in hypertension [39]. It can result in abnormal mitral flow, bradyarrhythmia, and AV blocks [39]. It is more common in the posterior mitral annulus and seen as a focal ovoid mass with a "shell" of peripheral calcification (>500 HU) with a slightly less hyperattenuating central component (350–500 HU) that represents the liquefied state [37, 39] (Fig. 38.7). There is no contrast enhancement, which distinguishes caseous MAC from neoplasm and abscess. Calcification also distinguishes it from abscess [40].

Pericardial Cyst

Pericardial cyst is a congenital abnormality caused by a pinched-off portion of the pericardium during development [41]. The wall of the cyst is composed of a thin layer of fibrous tissue and a single layer of mesothelial cells [42, 43]. It is most commonly (80%) seen in the right anterior cardiophrenic angle [44]. It is usually asymptomatic and

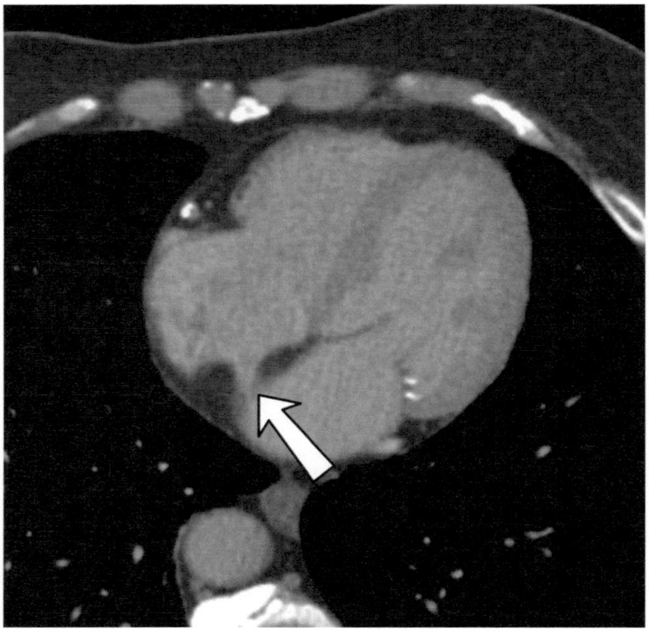

Fig. 38.6 Lipomatous hypertrophy of interatrial septum. Axial CT scan shows fatty infiltration of interatrial septum with sparing of the fossa ovalis (arrow), characteristic of lipomatous hypertrophy of the interatrial septum

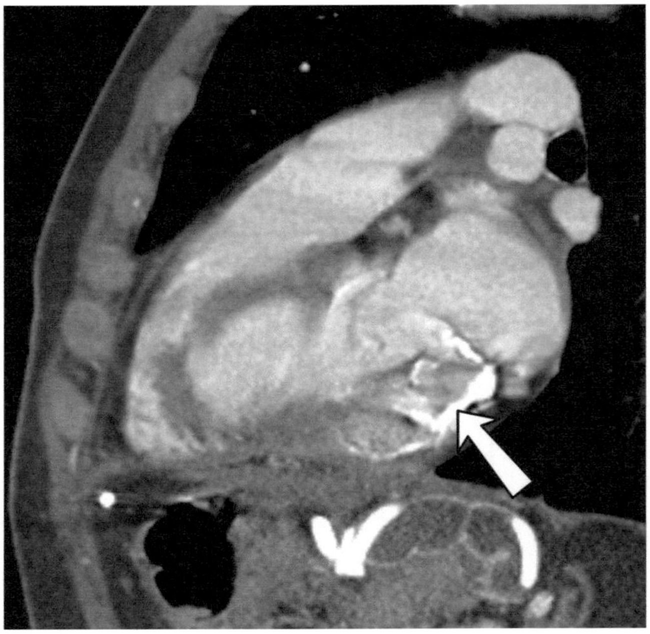

Fig. 38.7 Caseous MAC. Short-axis CT image shows coarse circumferential calcification of mitral annulus and heterogeneous lower-density central core with associated mass effect, consistent with caseous mitral annular calcification (arrow)

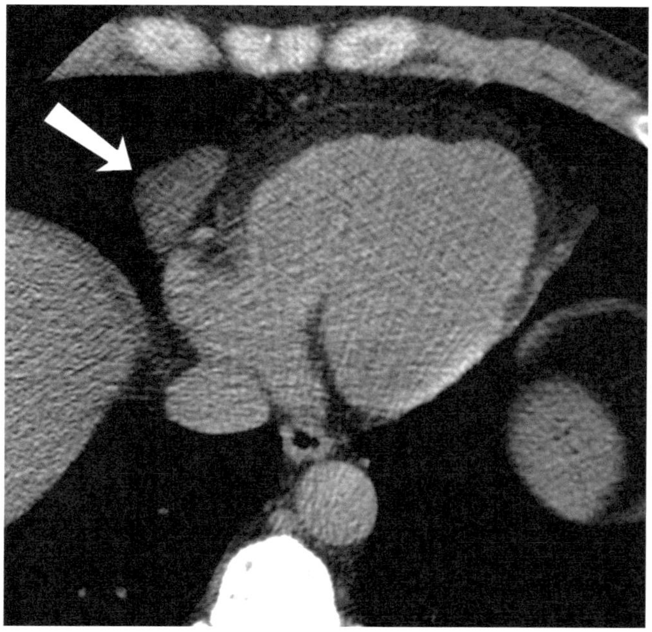

Fig. 38.8 Pericardial cyst. Axial CT scan shows a well-defined, unilocular, thin-walled, homogeneous cystic mass in the right cardiophrenic angle (arrow) in continuity with pericardium, consistent with a pericardial cyst

incidentally encountered in imaging but may occasionally present with chest pain or dyspnea. On CT, it is seen as a well-defined unilocular lesion with smooth border and homogenous density similar to water (−10 to 10 HU) (Fig. 38.8). Higher attenuation may be seen with infection or hemorrhage, and there is no contrast enhancement. Differential diagnosis includes other cystic mediastinal lesions, including bronchogenic cyst, esophageal duplication cyst, neurenteric cyst, thymic cyst, intrathoracic meningocele, mature cystic teratoma, and lymphangioma [43], which can be distinguished based on location. For example, duplication cyst is located adjacent to the esophagus, usually in a cervical location, and bronchogenic cyst is located around the carina, whereas a pericardial cyst is characteristically seen in the cardiophrenic angle. If the cyst communicates with the pericardial sac, it is then called a diverticulum.

Bronchogenic Cyst

Bronchogenic cyst is a congenital lesion resulting from abnormal budding of the embryonic ventral foregut [45].The wall of the cyst resembles the tracheobronchial epithelium, i.e., pseudostratified columnar respiratory epithelium, with variable amounts of smooth muscle, mucous glands, and cartilage [43]. It is most commonly seen in the mediastinum (85%) [45], usually adjacent to the carina or along the tracheobronchial tree. It can also be seen in lungs and rarely in other locations such as interatrial septum or in cardiac chambers [46–48]. On CT, it is seen as a well-defined thin-walled unilocular spherical lesion. The content is usually serous with attenuation similar to water, but occasionally it can be complex with soft tissue attenuation making it difficult to be distinguished from soft tissue mass. Air may be seen inside the cyst either due to infection or communication with tracheobronchial tree. There is no contrast enhancement of the cyst content, but the wall may enhance. It is usually asymptomatic but may produce symptoms when large due to compression of adjacent structures.

Hiatal Hernia

Hiatal hernia is a protrusion of the stomach into the thoracic cavity, with four reported types. Type I (sliding hernia) is the most common (85%), where the gastric cardia slides up into the posterior mediastinum [49]. Types II, III, and IV represent paraesophageal hernias, in which a part of the stomach lies anterior or lateral to the esophagus. In Type II, the GE junction remains in its normal position. Type III is a mixed hernia with features of Types I and II. Type IV is a giant paraesophageal hernia with one-third to one-half of the stomach protruding into the thoracic cavity [49]. It is common in patients >50 years. When large, hiatal hernia may produce posterior indentation of the left atrium and may be confused with a mass in echocardiogram. It is easy to identify in radiograph and barium swallow, but sometimes CT scan (Fig. 38.9) is required for establishing the diagnosis and distinguishing other sinister lesions in the posterior mediastinum. Gastric folds are seen within the hiatal hernia.

Other Nonneoplastic Masses

Coronary artery aneurysms and pseudoaneurysms can produce mass effect on the heart. *Coronary artery aneurysm* refers to a focal dilatation that is at least 1.5 times the normal diameter of the coronary artery and involves less than 50% of its length [50]. The most common cause of coronary aneurysm is atherosclerosis in adults and Kawasaki disease in childhood, with other causes including inflammatory disorders, connective tissue diseases, mycotic aneurysm, congenital (ALCAPA) or trauma/iatrogenic [50]. A giant coronary artery aneurysm can be seen with luminal thrombosis. CT is used in the diagnosis as well as establishment of relationship with adjacent structures (Fig. 38.10a). *Pseudoaneurysms* with or without luminal thrombus may also mimic a cardiac mass (Fig. 38.10b). *Coronary artery bypass graft aneurysm* can also produce mass effect on the heart. These are related to accelerated atherosclerosis, seen after 5 years of bypass surgery [51], whereas pseudoaneurysms may be present after 6 months, especially in the anastomotic sites [51]. Complications of CABG aneurysm include thrombosis, fistu-

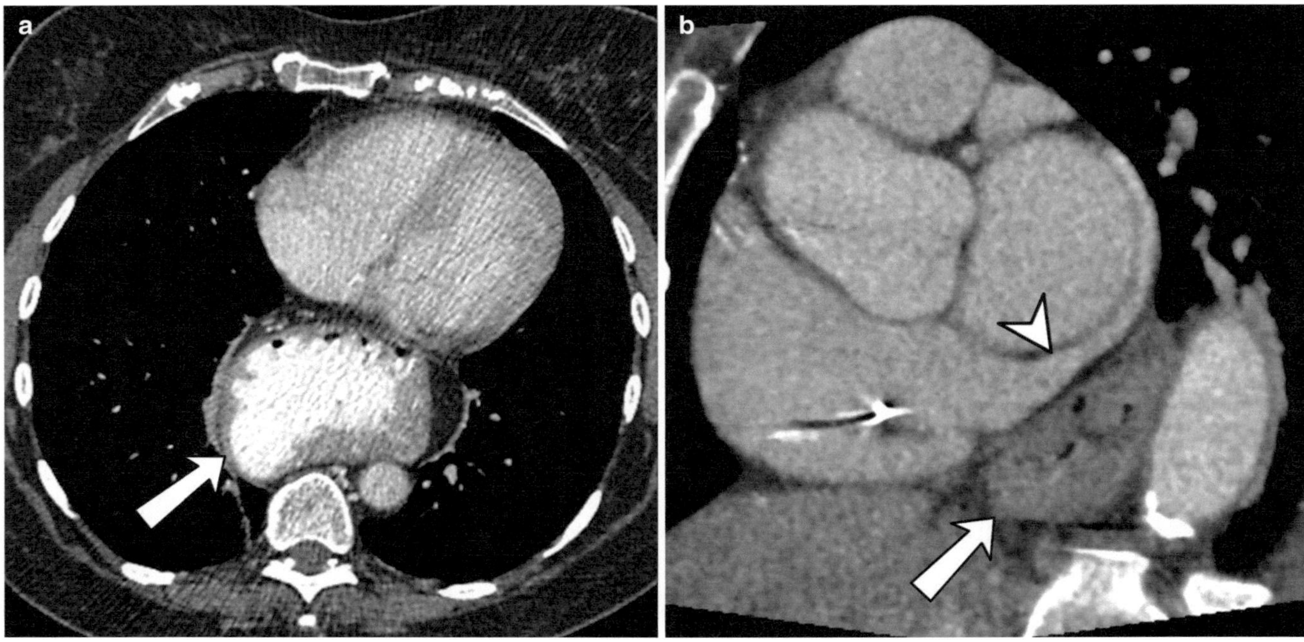

Fig. 38.9 Hiatal hernia. (**a**) Axial CT scan in a patient with suspected left atrial mass in echocardiogram shows indentation of posterior wall of the left atrium by a large hiatal hernia (arrow). (**b**) Short-axis CT reconstruction in another patient shows a paraesophageal hernia Type III (arrow) that displaces the left atrium and coronary sinus (arrowhead) cranially

las, and myocardial infarction. *Interatrial septal aneurysm* is a focal saccular deformity in the region of fossa ovalis caused by mobile interatrial tissue. It is diagnosed when the maximal septal excursion into either atrium is >1.5 cm. It is associated with a patent foramen ovale in 33% and ASD in 19%. Although increased risk of stroke has been reported in patients with atrial septal aneurysm and PFO, recent studies have shown no increased risk [52]. *Vegetations* of cardiac valves are seen in infective endocarditis. Predisposing factors include endocardial damage, prosthetic material, bacteremia, and congenital heart disease. The most common etiological agents are *Staphylococcus aureus* (31%) and Streptococcus viridans (17%) [53]. On CT, vegetation is seen as an irregular- or round-shaped hypoattenuating mass attached to a cardiac valve (Fig. 38.10c), usually in the low pressure side of the valve or in the subvalvular apparatus or in the ascending aorta. The motion of the vegetation and valvular dysfunction can be evaluated in retrospective gated cine images [54].

Benign Neoplasms

Myxoma

Myxoma is the most common primary cardiac neoplasm, accounting for 50% of these neoplasms. It is more common in women and those between 30 and 60 years [3]. The majority (60%) originate in the left atrium [55], typically from the fossa ovalis with a small pedicle or stalk. It can also be seen in the free wall of atrium, AV valve, or ventricle. Multiple myxomas are seen in 10% of cases, more common in younger men and those with familial syndromes. In Carney syndrome, myxomas often occur outside the left atrium and have higher recurrence rates [56]. Pathologically, myxoma is composed of myxoid stromal cells. There are two anatomical types, solid and papillary, with the former having firm and the latter having a friable gelatinous consistence [57]. The clinical manifestations depend on the type and size of the tumor, with the solid type producing obstruction of flow at AV valve and congestive cardiac failure, whereas the papillary type produces embolic/neurologic symptoms [57]. Fever, malaise, and weight loss may also be seen. Systemic emboli may be seen as a complication of left atrial myxomas, with most of them located in the central nervous system. Malignant behavior has been reported, characterized by recurrence, locally invasive features, extension outside heart and distal metastasis [58]. This has been shown to be faciliated by several cytokines and growth factors [58]. On CT, myxoma typically has round or ovoid shape and lobular or smooth borders with a narrow pedicle in 2/3 (Fig. 38.11a) and broad-based villous appearance in 1/3 [3] (Fig. 38.11b). Heterogeneous attenuation is seen. Calcifications are rare, more common in right atrial lesions. Heterogeneous contrast enhancement is seen in a small number of cases [55]. CT shows the motion and change in position of the mass, particularly prolapse of the mass into the ventricle (Fig. 38.11c), which is essential for surgical planning.

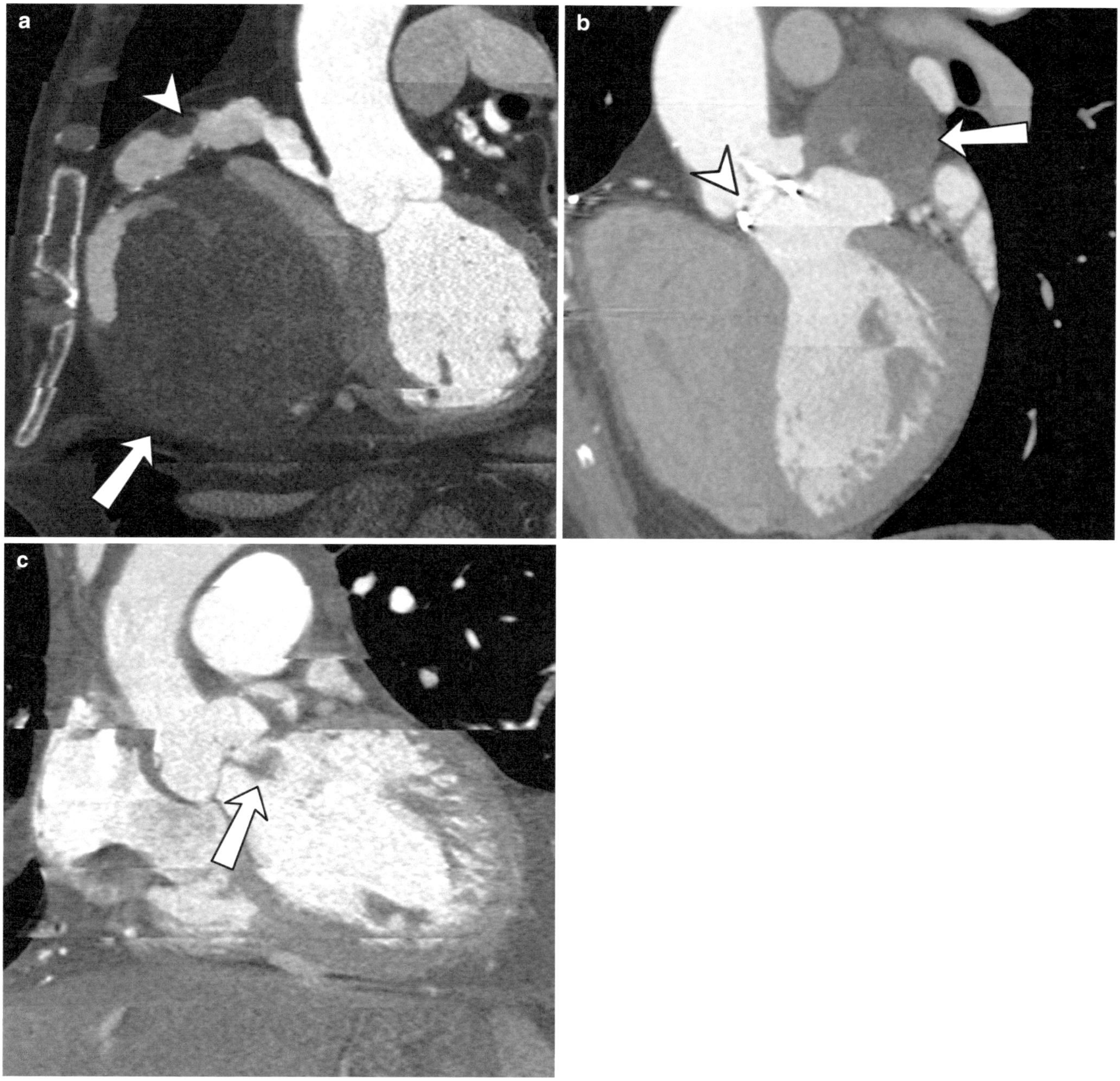

Fig. 38.10 Nonneoplastic masses. (**a**) Coronary aneurysm. Coronal CT reconstruction shows a giant right coronary aneurysm measuring up to 10 cm in diameter (arrow) that is producing extrinsic impression on the right ventricle. Note the diffuse and irregular dilatation in the proximal segment of RCA (arrowhead). (**b**) Pseudoaneurysm. Three-chamber CT reconstruction in another patient shows a partially thrombosed pseudoaneurysm (arrow) as a complication of endocarditis in prosthetic aortic valve (arrowhead). (**c**) Vegetation. Coronal CT reconstruction shows a linear and irregular mass related to a vegetation (arrow) in the ventricular aspect of the right leaflet of aortic valve in a patient with endocarditis

Fibroelastoma

Papillary fibroelastoma is the second most common primary neoplasm of the heart [4, 59, 60]. It can occur at any age but is more common in middle age and older adults with no sex predilection. The tumor usually is small in size (usually <2 cm) and has a cauliflower shape with a small stalk attached to the endocardial surface. Histologically, there is an avascular matrix of connective tissue composed of proteoglycans, collagen, and elastic fibers surrounded by a layer of hypertrophied endothelial cells [61]. Almost 80% of fibroelastomas are located in the surface of a valve [62], with predilection for aortic and mitral valves, usually in the non-ventricular surface, sparing the leaflet tips. However, it

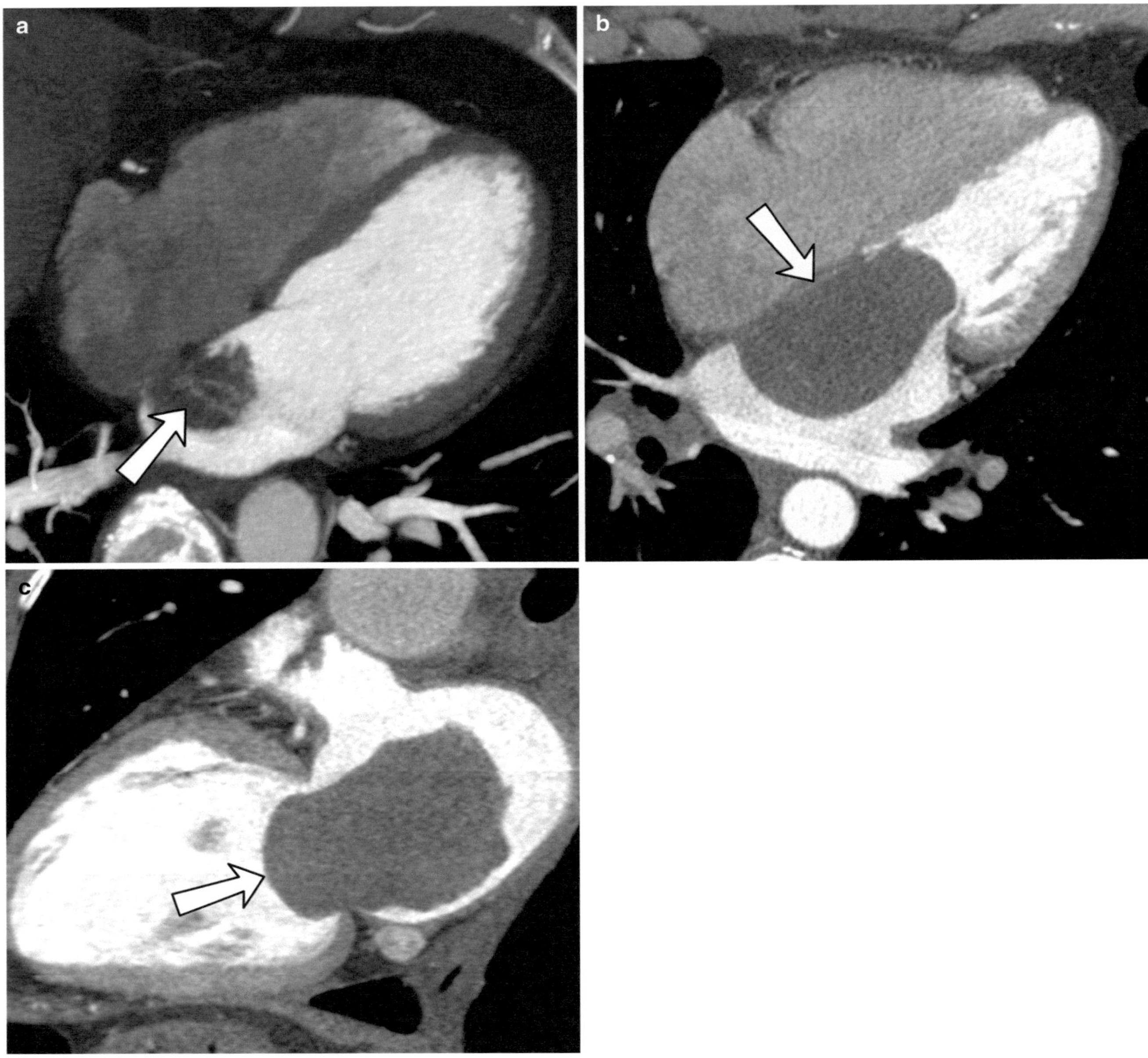

Fig. 38.11 Myxoma. (**a**) Four-chamber CT scan shows a characteristic polypoid left atrial mass (arrow) attached by a stalk to the fossa ovalis, consistent with a myxoma. (**b**) Four-chamber CT reconstruction in another patient shows a broad-based left atrial myxoma (arrow) that is attached to the interatrial septum. (**c**) Two-chamber view in the same patient as Fig. 38.11b shows the myxoma (arrow) prolapsing through the mitral valve into the left ventricle. There is near occlusion of the inlet of LV and mildly dilated left atrium

can occur in other locations such the chordae tendineae, LV apex, or LVOT. The friable composition of this tumor is a risk factor for rupture and embolic disease, and eventually it can obstruct one of the coronary ostia, resulting in angina [62]. Usually the diagnosis is made by echocardiogram, due to the small size and mobility. On CT, it appears as a small, homogeneous hypoattenuating mass with a thin stalk that is attached to the valve, sparing the free edges (Fig. 38.12). Lesions have been reported up to 70 mm [10]. Differential diagnosis includes vegetation, thrombus, Lambl's excrescences (fibrous strands at sites of valve closure), and hypertrophy of Arantius nodules (seen at free margin of aortic valve cusps). Vegetations are irregular with valvular destruction and systemic signs and symptoms. Usually fibroelastoma arises in the midportion of the leaflet, whereas the Lambl's excrescence arises from the line of closure [63]. Arantius nodules are small nodules in the tip of the ventricular side of the leaflets of semilunar valves, at exact point of coaptation. Fibroelastoma is surgically resected if it is symptomatic or mobile in the left heart.

Lipoma

Lipoma is a benign neoplasm consisting of mature adipose tissue surrounded by capsule. There is no gender predilection, and it is more common in middle and older ages. It can originate anywhere in the heart, either from the epicardial or subendocardial layers and rarely intramyocardial, and may extend into pericardial sac. Endocardial lipoma is seen in the LV or RA roof or along the septum. It can be asymptomatic but when larger can cause symptoms related to obstruction, compression, or arrhythmias [56]. It is usually solitary but may be multiple in tuberous sclerosis [56]. On CT, a lipoma is seen as a well-defined mass with homogeneous fat attenuation (<−50 UH) and broad base, with no contrast enhancement (Fig. 38.13). A lipoma of the interatrial septum can be distinguished from lipomatous hypertrophy by the involvement of the fossa ovalis and absence of dumbbell shape.

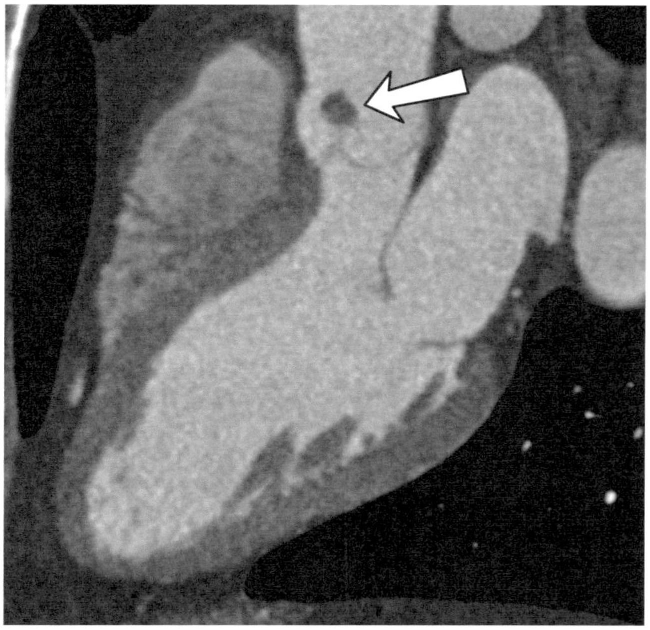

Fig. 38.12 Fibroelastoma. Three-chamber CT reconstruction shows a small round mass attached by a stalk to the edge of the right leaflet of aortic valve facing the aortic side, consistent with a fibroelastoma (arrow)

Hemangioma

Hemangioma is a benign vascular tumor and has three histologic types, capillary, cavernous, and arteriovenous [64], although some tumors have mix composition of the three types. It is usually a focal lesion, but diffuse angiomatosis may be occasionally seen [65]. Seventy-five percent of cardiac hemangiomas occur in adults [7, 66]. Seventy percent are seen in the ventricles, and 23% affect the right atrium, with left atrium rarely affected [64, 67]. Common locations are lateral wall of the LV and anterior wall of the RV. It can affect the endocardium, myocardium, or epicardium and can be intracavitary. On CT, it is seen as a well-defined round or

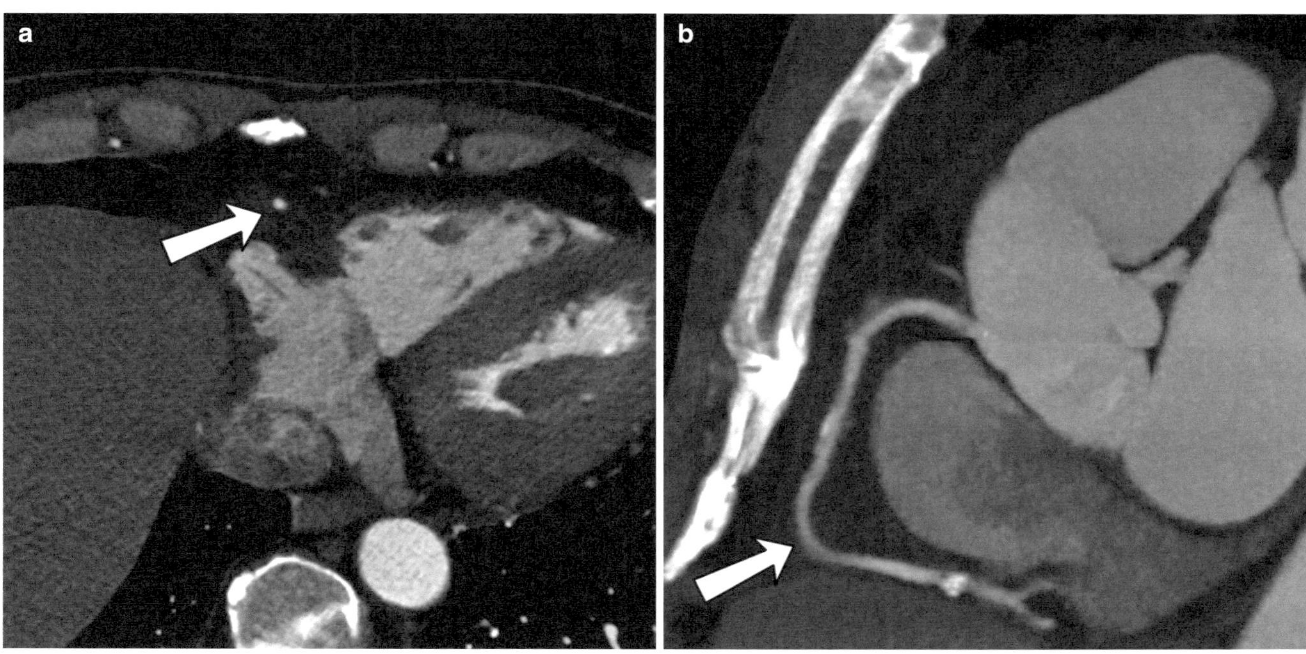

Fig. 38.13 Lipoma. (**a**) Axial CT scan shows a focal ill-defined fat attenuation mass in the right atrioventricular groove that displaces the right coronary artery laterally (arrow), consistent with a lipoma. (**b**) Sagittal reconstruction in the same patient shows the lipoma in the right atrioventricular groove displacing the acute angle of the right coronary artery laterally (arrow)

oval tumor when intracavitary but may mold the shape to adjacent structures when it is intramyocardial or epicardial. The attenuation is usually heterogeneous with some fat interspersed between the vascular components. Calcification may be present due to phleboliths. Contrast enhancement is intense (Fig. 38.14) and heterogenous in hemangioma, similar to other hypervascular tumors such as paragangliomas and sarcomas. Fat and calcium may help in distinguishing hemangioma from these lesions. Slow-flow hemangiomas may show little or no contrast enhancement. Although spontaneous regression has been reported, basically all hypervascular tumors require surgical excision.

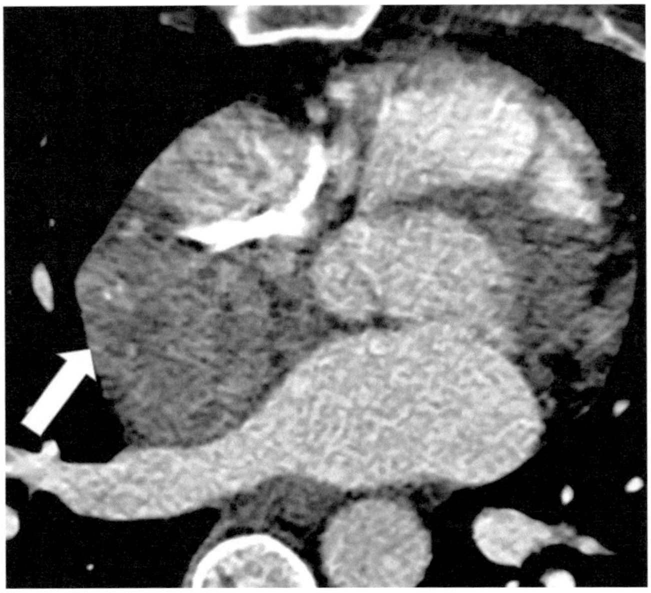

Fig. 38.14 Hemangioma. Axial CT scan shows an intensely enhancing mass in between the right and left atrium (arrow), which was proven to be a hemangioma

Paraganglioma

Paraganglioma is a rare tumor originating from chromaffin cells in sympathetic or parasympathetic chains, with only approximately 300 cases reported in the literature [68]. It can either be functioning (extra-adrenal pheochromocytoma) or nonfunctioning (chemodectoma) [56]. Ten percent of pheochromocytomas occur extra-adrenally. Paraganglioma is more common in young adults. It is usually encapsulated but can be infiltrative. It is more commonly seen in relation to great vessels than the heart and is commonly seen to originate from the paraganglia in posterior wall or roof of the left atrium, atrial septum, or the surrounding coronary arteries or aortic root. On CT, it is seen as a well-defined round or oval mass with heterogeneous attenuation and avid contrast enhancement (Fig. 38.15). Sometimes the contrast enhancement is heterogeneous due to central necrosis. Aggressive features with poor margins and extracardiac extension may also be seen. The use of nuclear medicine is helpful in localization of extra-adrenal

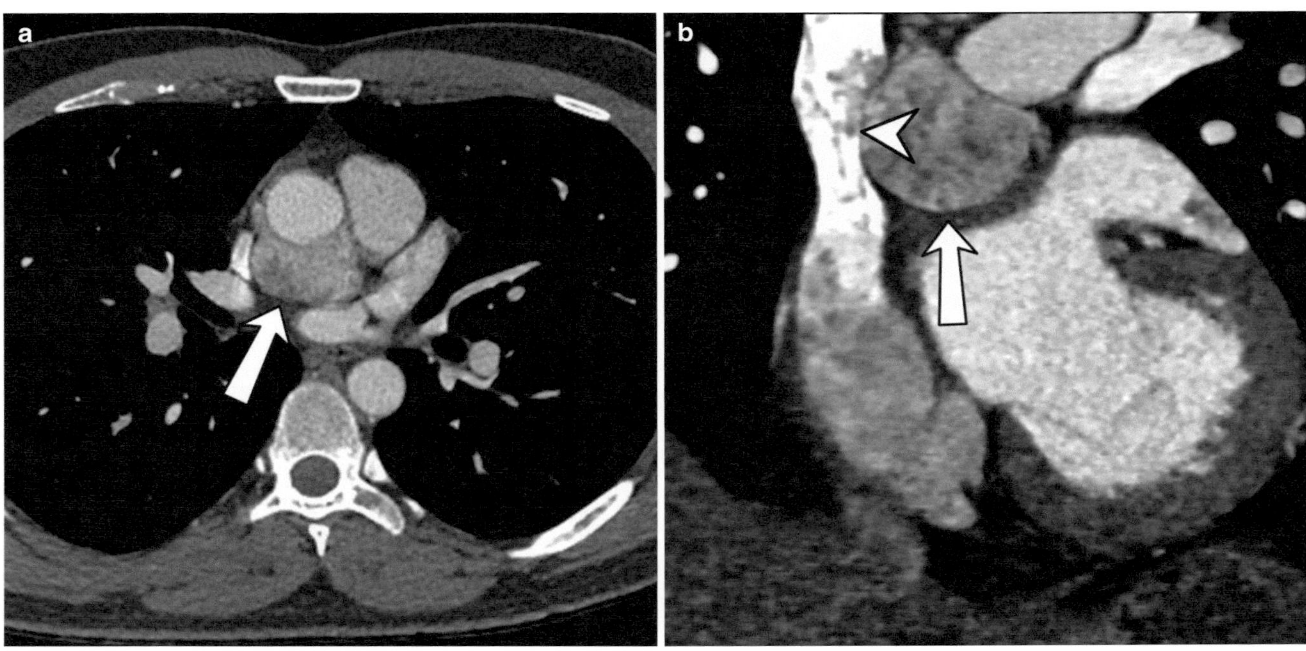

Fig. 38.15 Paraganglioma. (**a**) Axial CT scan shows an intensely enhancing mass in the posterior aspect of the ascending aorta (arrow). (**b**) Coronal CT reconstruction in the same patient shows an intensely enhancing intrapericardial mass (arrow) in the posterior aspect of the ascending aorta, which was biopsy proven to be a paraganglioma

paragangliomas with the use of I-131 or I-123 metaiodobenzylguanidine (MIGB), a norepinephrine analogue [56]. Surgical resection may be performed after embolization of feeding arteries to minimize bleeding.

Rhabdomyoma

Rhabdomyoma is the most common cardiac neoplasm (75%) in children. 60–90% of these tumors are multiple [7, 69]. There is a strong association with tuberous sclerosis complex (TSC), with 80% incidence of TSC in cardiac rhabdomyomas and 50% of patients with TSC having rhabdomyomas [7, 66]. Rhabdomyoma is considered a hamartoma and is well circumscribed but without a capsule and contains myocytes with disproportionate size and vacuoles that give the classic "spider cell" appearance [65]. Symptoms depend on the location and size of the tumor. It involves the ventricles and atria, equally on right and left. A common feature of this tumor is spontaneous regression [7], as a result of which surgery is not required, unless it is justified by clinical manifestations [65] such as arrhythmia or cardiac failure; otherwise serial imaging follow-up is recommended. For the same reason, this lesion is not seen in adults. On CT, the appearance is that of the normal myocardium, both in pre and post contrast. Hence, small lesions without mass effect can be difficult to visualize. Unlike fibroma, rhabdomyomas do not calcify.

Fibroma

Fibroma is the second most common tumor in infants and children. It has also been called cardiac fibromatosis or fibrous or fibroelastic hamartoma to suggest that it is not a true neoplasm [56, 65]. It is a solitary mass composed of collagen matrix, sometimes with elastic fibers [65]. In early ages, there is predominant cellularity (fibroblasts), but in adolescent and adults, it is predominantly acellular with only few layers of peripheral cells [66]. Calcification is common but hemorrhage, necrosis, and cysts are rare. It is often diagnosed in the first year of life with symptoms depending on the size and location, including obstruction, valvular dysfunction, or arrhythmias that can lead to syncope or sudden cardiac death [66]. It is more common in the left ventricle, commonly located in the LV free wall, ventricular septum, and RV wall [70], with the atrium rarely affected, particularly in patients with syndromes such as familial adenomatous polyposis, Gardner, and Gorlin syndromes. On CT, it is seen as an intramyocardial, homogeneous iso or hypoattenuating lesion with variable margins (Fig. 38.16). Central calcification may be seen in 25% of the cases [66]. Contrast enhancement is variable, ranging from no enhancement to heterogeneous enhancement, often delayed [10, 56]. Fibroma is distinguished from rhabdomyoma since it is usually solitary and has calcification, low attenuation, and delayed enhancement. Surgical resection is performed in symptomatic cases to prevent sud-

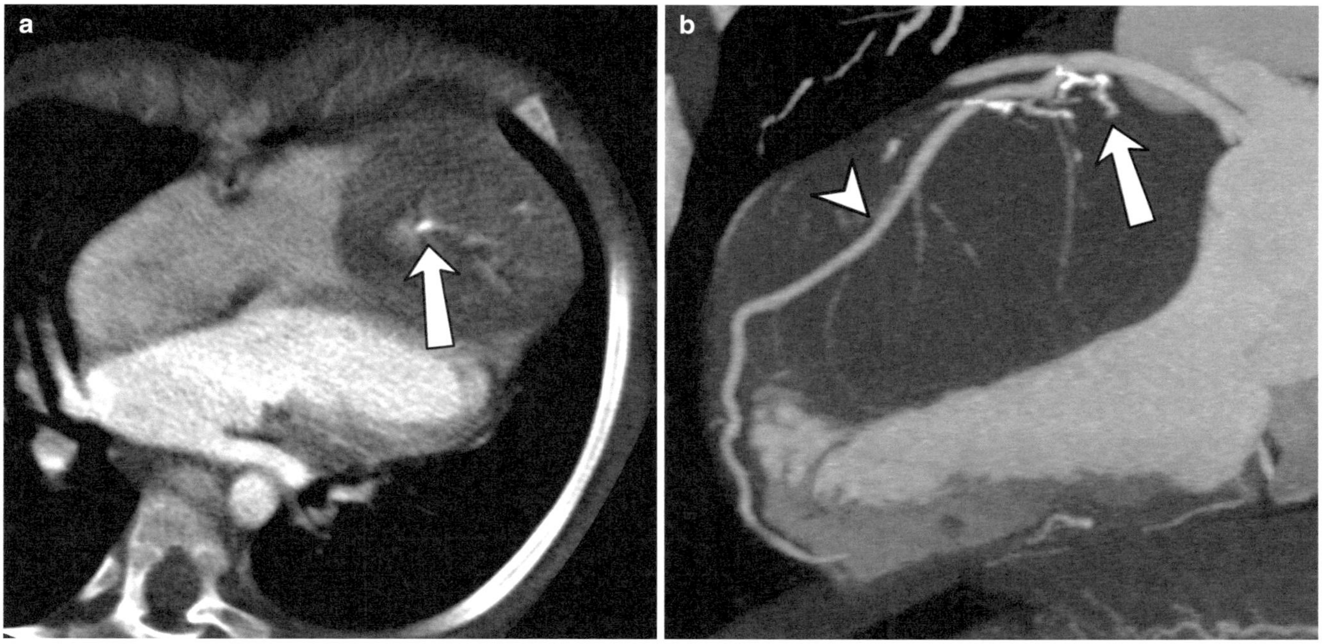

Fig. 38.16 Fibroma. (**a**) Four-chamber CT reconstruction shows a large hypoattenuating mass with central calcification in a child (arrow), consistent with a fibroma. (**b**) Sagittal reconstructed CT image in the same patient shows the large fibroma in the interventricular septum. Small calcifications are noted near the anterior surface of the tumor (arrow). The mid segment of LAD is surrounded by the tumor, showing the appearance of a myocardial bridge (arrowhead)

den cardiac death. There is no spontaneous regression and no reports of recurrence even after partial resection [65].

Less Common Benign Neoplasms

Less common benign tumors described in the literature include teratoma, lymphangioma, inflammatory myofibroblastic tumor, mesothelioma of the atrioventricular node, and Purkinje cell hamartoma (histiocytoid cardiomyopathy). Some of these neoplasms are less common in the heart but more common in the mediastinum, such as teratoma and lymphangioma. Cardiac teratoma is located in the pericardium (90%) [3] and has heterogeneous attenuation due to different components.

Malignant Neoplasms

Metastasis

Metastasis is more common than primary neoplasms of the heart. Cardiac metastasis is present in about 10–12% in autopsies with known malignancy [71]. Routes of spread to the heart include direct local spread and lymphatic, hematogenous, and transvenous routes. Lung cancer represents the most common primary neoplasm in patients with cardiac/pericardial metastasis, accounting for 37% of these patients [72], due to its proximity with the heart [73]. Other primary neoplasms to involve the heart are nonsolid malignancies (Kaposi's sarcoma, leukemia) (20%), breast (7%), esophagus, (6%) and skin (4.5%) [72]. Direct extension occurs from lung (Fig. 38.17a), esophageal, and other mediastinal neoplasms (Fig. 38.17b). Pericardium is the most frequent location of metastatic cardiac involvement due to rich lymphatics in visceral pericardium and manifests as pericardial effusion, thickening, irregularity, and nodules. Pericardial effusion is often the earliest finding, but it is difficult to diagnose a malignant effusion based on CT, and hence pericardiocentesis is often required [73]. Hematogenous extension through coronary arteries or veins often manifests with myocardial nodules or infiltration (Fig. 38.17c). This is usually associated with systemic metastases particularly lungs. Melanoma spreads to the heart in 64% of cases in an autopsy series [74]. Transvenous extension to the heart can occur either through the SVC (lung, lymphoma, thyroid cancers), IVC (renal (Fig. 38.17d), hepatic, adrenal cortex, or endometrial cancers; Wilms tumor; pheochromocytoma, endometrial, IVC leiomyosarcoma (Fig. 38.17e), invasive uterine leiomyoma (Fig. 38.17f)) or pulmonary vein (lung cancer). Renal cell carcinoma is the most common lesion in transvenous spread, often involving the right kidney [75], with 10% of the RCC with IVC extension reaching the right atrium [75]. The CT features of metastasis depend on the type of primary neoplasm and route of extension. CT not only provides evaluation of the heart and pericardium but also provides evaluation of the entire chest including assessment of lungs, mediastinum, bones, and soft tissue.

Sarcoma

Primary cardiac malignancies are rare and represent 25% of primary cardiac neoplasms, with most of them being sarcomas. Angiosarcoma is the most common subtype, with others being rhabdomyosarcoma, undifferentiated sarcoma (Fig. 38.18a), myxofibrosarcoma, osteosarcoma, leiomyosarcoma, and liposarcoma [10]. Rhabdomyosarcoma is the most common pediatric cardiac primary malignancy, usually the embryonic type. It is more common in adults, where it is of pleomorphic type, whereas in children, embryonic type is more common. Angiosarcoma typically arises in the right atrium, whereas osteosarcoma typically arises in the left atrium [76]. Sarcoma has infiltrative nature with lobulated borders, broad base, and heterogeneous enhancement with necrosis and hemorrhage. Calcifications/ossifications are often seen in osteosarcoma (Fig. 38.18b). Liposarcoma has fatty attenuation and soft tissue components. Extension of tumor and infiltration of adjacent structures are vital for surgical planning, which CT provides. Multiple lesions may be seen, and pulmonary metastasis is often present. Total resection is not possible in most of the cases, so surgery is just palliative.

Mesothelioma

Mesothelioma of the pericardium is a rare tumor of pericardial mesothelial cells, and its association with prior asbestos exposure is not clear, with only few cases with prior exposure [77]. There are three histological types: epithelial, spindle cell, and mixed [78]. The appearance of this tumor is very similar to pericardial metastasis with thickening/irregularity, diffuse plaque, solitary nodule (Fig. 38.19), or multiple masses. Calcifications may be seen. Contrast enhancement is usually present.

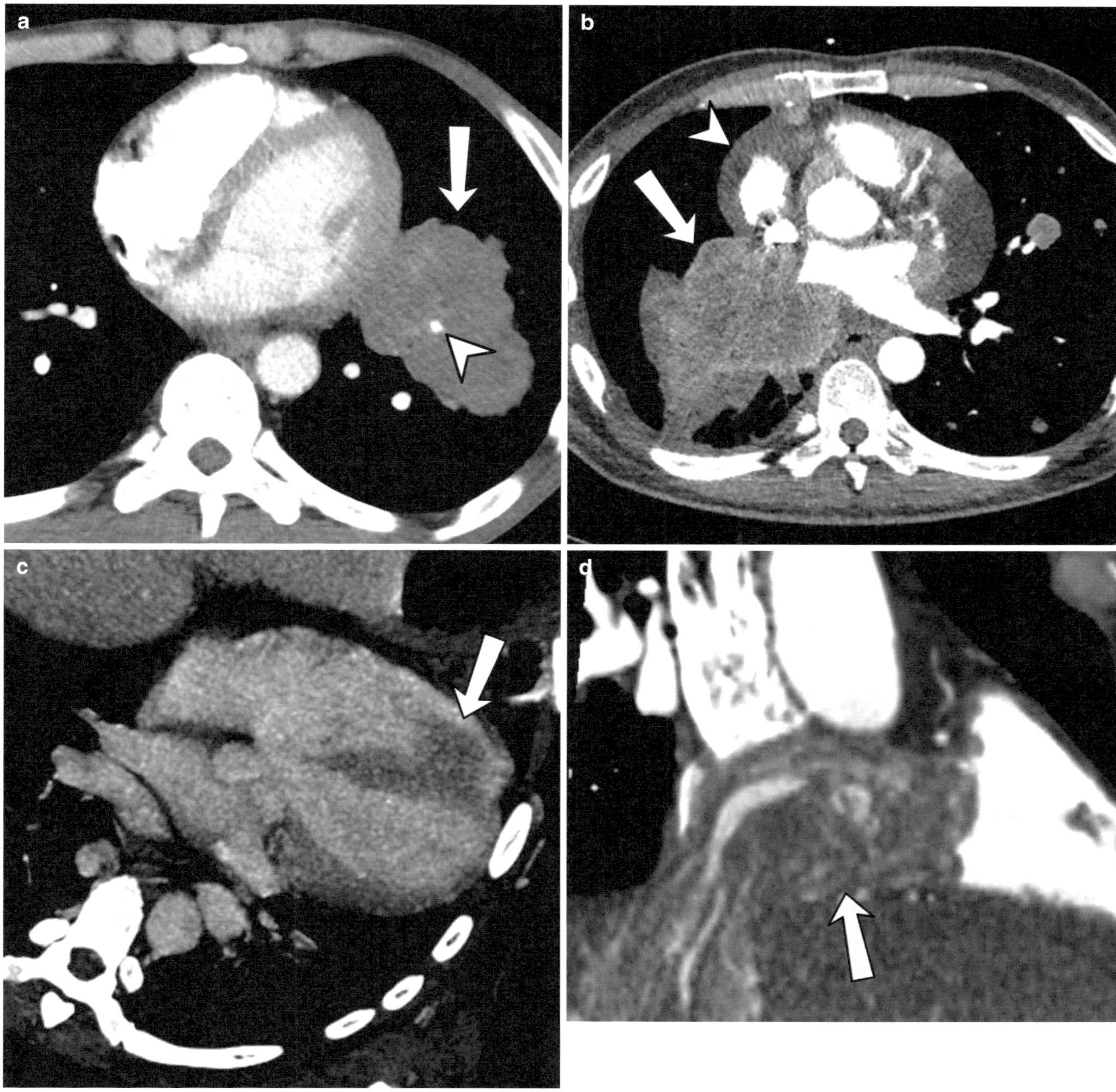

Fig. 38.17 Metastasis. (**a**) Axial CT image shows a bronchogenic neoplasm (arrow), which is encasing a pulmonary artery (arrowhead) and infiltrating the lateral wall of the left ventricle. (**b**) Axial CT scan in another patient with a metastatic clear cell sarcoma shows a large heterogeneous and lobulated mass (arrow) compressing the right superior pulmonary vein and right pulmonary artery, with infiltration of the pericardium and epicardial fat pad. Note the moderate pericardial effusion (arrowhead) and left lung nodules, which also represent metastases. (**c**) Four-chamber CT scan shows a well-defined intracavitary mass in the right ventricle (arrow), consistent with metastasis in a patient with known breast cancer. (**d**) Coronal CT reconstruction shows a large heterogeneous mass (arrow) in the inferior vena cava, which was an extension of renal cell carcinoma that invades the right atrium and the inlet of the right ventricle. (**e**) Coronal CT reconstruction in another patient shows a large invasive intravascular tumor in the infrarenal segment of IVC (arrow) that grows cranially until the IVC-right atrium junction. The mass shows heterogeneous enhancement. This is an intravascular leiomyosarcoma. (**f**) Coronal CT reconstruction shows a long tumor protruding into the right atrium from the inferior vena cava. Note the large and tortuous vessels (arrow) into the mass resembling an umbilical cord. This is a case of invasive leiomyoma from the uterus

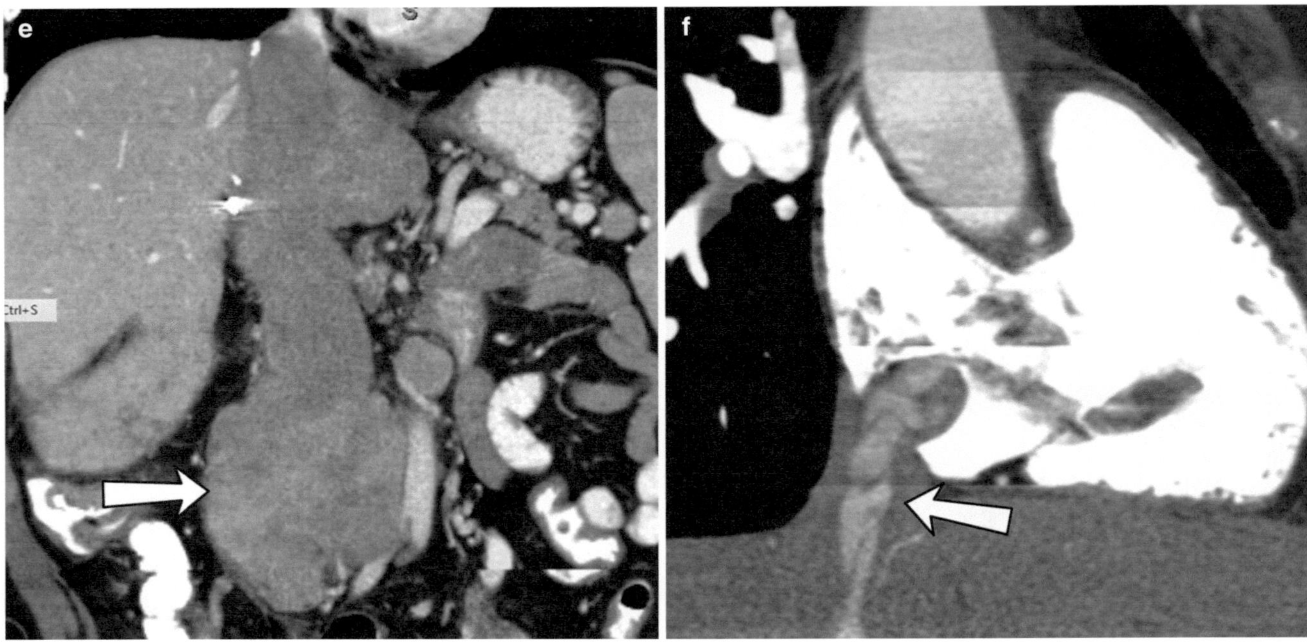

Fig. 38.17 (continued)

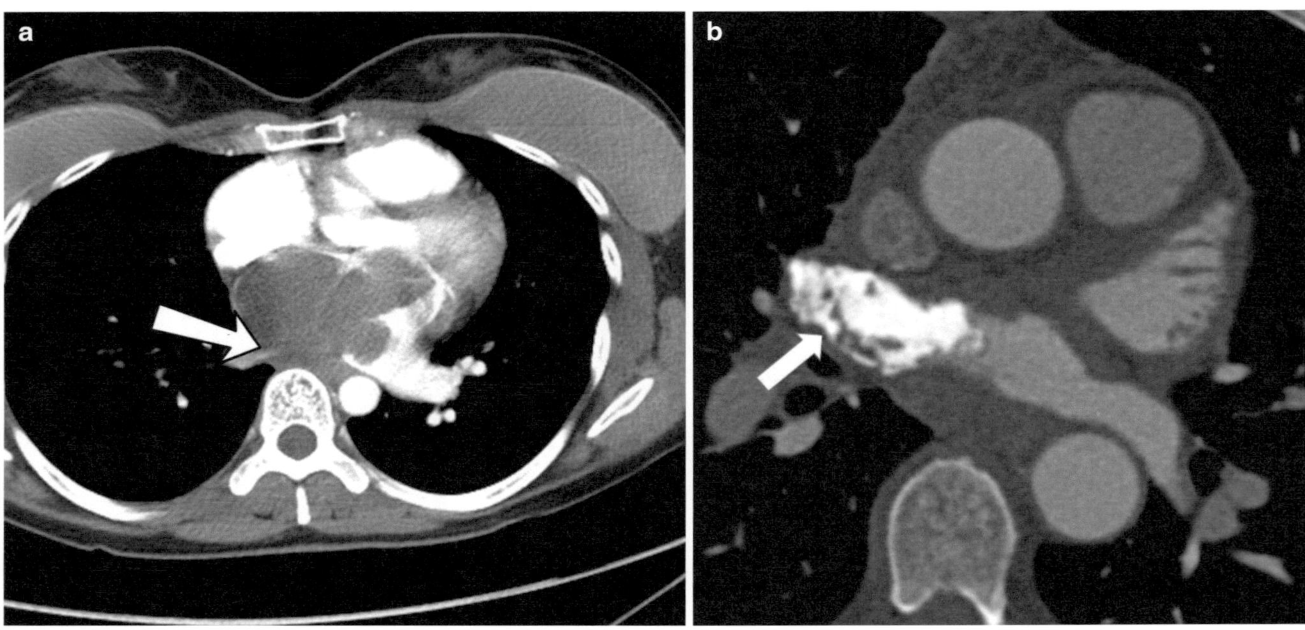

Fig. 38.18 Sarcoma. (**a**) Axial CT scan shows a large lobulated tumor in the left atrium with invasion of posterior wall (arrow), which was proven to be an intimal sarcoma. (**b**) Axial CT scan in another patient shows a densely ossified mass which is infiltrating into the right superior pulmonary vein (arrow), consistent with an osteosarcoma of the left atrium

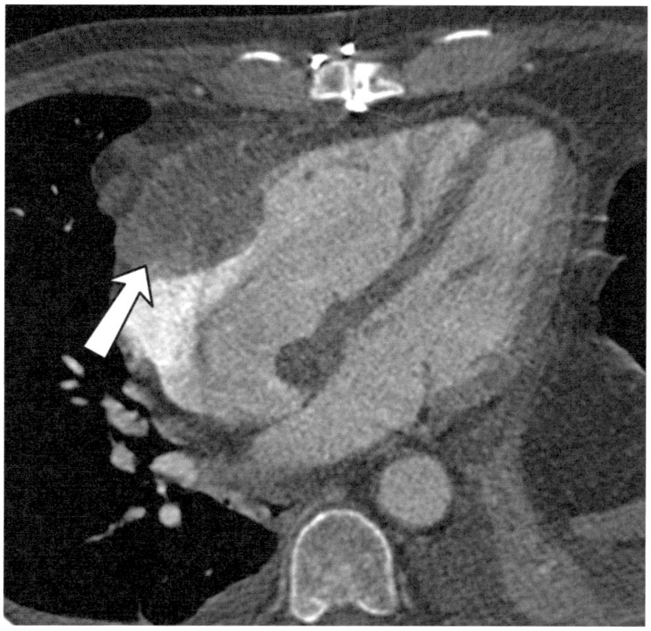

Fig. 38.19 Mesothelioma. Axial CT scan shows a large pericardial mass (arrow) adjacent to the right atrioventricular groove with mass effect and slight displacement of the right chambers consistent with pericardial mesothelioma

Lymphoma

Lymphomatous involvement of the heart is usually secondary to systemic disease. Primary lymphoma of the heart is extremely rare, accounting to 1.3% of primary cardiac neoplasms [10]. These primary lymphomas are usually non-Hodgkin B-cell type with aggressive behavior [10], usually associated with HIV/AIDS. Right atrium is the cavity that is most commonly involved. Pericardium, subepicardial fat, and atrioventricular groove are also affected. The tumor is ill-defined, diffuse, and infiltrative (Fig. 38.20a), and the spread is usually through the epicardial surface [79] or a large focal mass or multiple nodules with heterogeneous contrast enhancement. Pericardial effusion is a common feature. Although lymphoma can involve the coronary arteries, it typically encases the vessels without compression [80]. Leukemia is seen as diffuse infiltration (Fig. 38.20b).

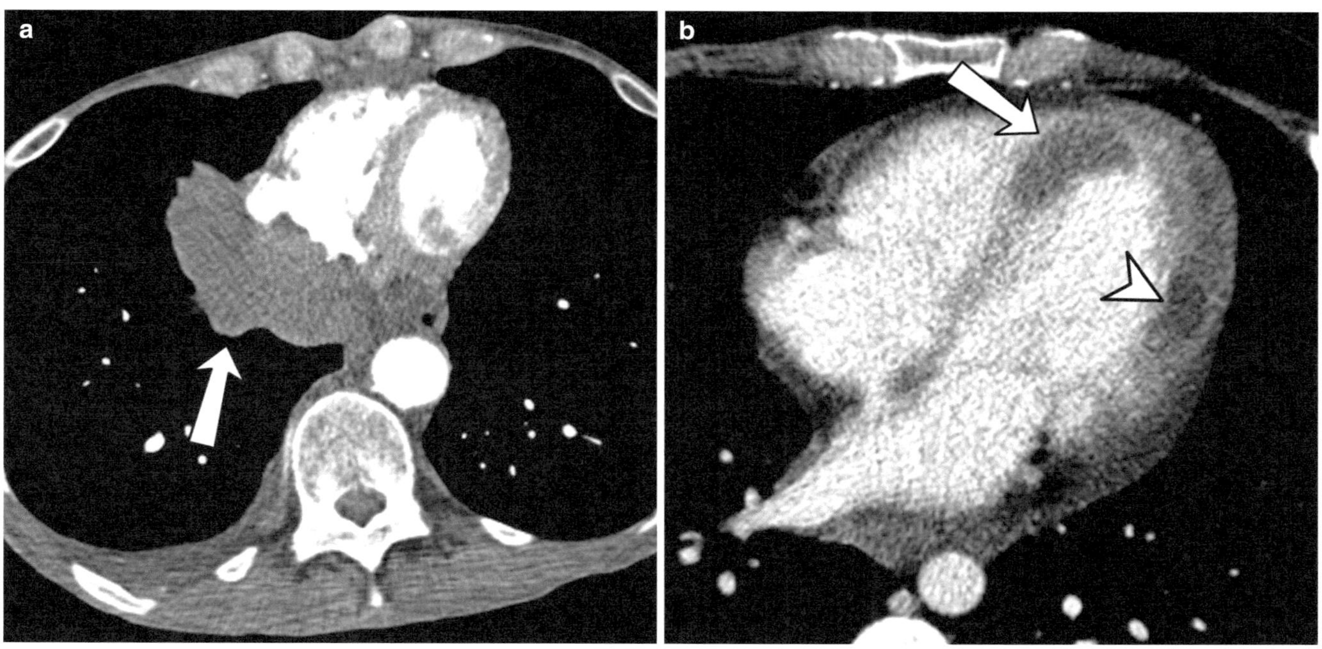

Fig. 38.20 Lymphoma. (a) Axial CT scan shows a large irregular paracardiac mass (arrow) that infiltrates the posterior wall of the right atrium, with minimal enhancement, which was proven to be a lymphoma. (b) Axial CT scan in another patient shows multiple hypoattenuating intramyocardial masses in the apical-septal (arrow) and mid-lateral (arrowhead) walls, related to cardiac involvement in a patient with known leukemia

Conclusion

CT is a valuable modality in the evaluation of cardiac masses and provides excellent information with regard to the location, extension, shape, size, attachment, and compromise of adjacent structures. CT is primarily used in the evaluation of cardiac masses in patients who cannot have MRI scan due to contraindications. It is also useful in specific situations where MRI or echocardiography cannot provide optimal information, for instance, the presence of calcification or evaluation of feeding arteries. CT can also provide functional dynamic information.

References

1. Burke A, Virmani R. Tumors of the heart and great vessels. Washington, DC: Amer Registry of Pathology; 1996.
2. Lam KY, Dickens P, Chan AC. Tumors of the heart. A 20-year experience with a review of 12,485 consecutive autopsies. Arch Pathol Lab Med. 1993;117(10):1027–31.
3. Kassop D, Donovan MS, Cheezum MK, et al. Cardiac masses on cardiac CT: a review. Curr Cardiovasc Imaging Rep [Internet]. 2014;7(8):9281. Available from: http://www.ncbi.nlm.nih.gov/pmc/articles/PMC4090749/pdf/12410_2014_Article_9281.pdf.
4. Hoey E, Ganeshan A, Nader K, Randhawa K, Watkin R. Cardiac neoplasms and pseudotumors: imaging findings on multidetector CT angiography. Diagn Interv Radiol. 2012;18(1):67–77.
5. Hoey ET, Mankad K, Puppala S, Gopalan D, Sivananthan MU. MRI and CT appearances of cardiac tumours in adults. Clin Radiol. 2009;64(12):1214–30.
6. Kumar N, Agarwal S, Ahuja A, Das P, Airon B, Ray R. Spectrum of cardiac tumors excluding myxoma: experience of a tertiary center with review of the literature. Pathol Res Pract. 2011;207(12):769–74.
7. Tao TY, Yahyavi-Firouz-Abadi N, Singh GK, Bhalla S. Pediatric cardiac tumors: clinical and imaging features. Radiographics. Radiological Society of North America. 2014;34(4):1031–46.
8. Beghetti M, Gow RM, Haney I, Mawson J, Williams WG, Freedom RM. Pediatric primary benign cardiac tumors: a 15-year review. Am Heart J. 1998;134(6):1107–14.
9. Motwani M, Kidambi A, Herzog BA, Uddin A, Greenwood JP, Plein S. MR imaging of cardiac tumors and masses: a review of methods and clinical applications. Radiology. 2013;268(1):26–43.
10. Rajiah P, Kanne JP, Kalahasti V, Schoenhagen P. Computed tomography of cardiac and pericardiac masses. J Cardiovasc Comput Tomogr. 2011;5(1):16–29.
11. Anavekar NS, Bonnichsen CR, Foley TA, et al. Computed tomography of cardiac pseudotumors and neoplasms. Radiol Clin N Am. 2010;48(4):799–816.
12. Akcay M, Bilen ES, Bilge M, Durmaz T, Kurt M. Prominent crista terminalis: as an anatomic structure leading to atrial arrhythmias and mimicking right atrial mass. J Am Soc Echocardiogr. 2007;20(2):197.e9–e10.
13. Salustri A, Bakir S, Sana A, Lange P, Mahmeed Al WA. Prominent crista terminalis mimicking a right atrial mass: case report. Cardiovasc Ultrasound. 6 ed. BioMed Central. 2010;8(1):47.
14. Gad A, Mannan J, Chhabra M, Zhang XXY, Narula P, Hoang D. Prominent Eustachian valve in newborns: a report of four cases. AJP Rep. 2016;6(1):e33–7.
15. Watson T, Kakar P, Srivastava S, Dhanjal TS. Eustachian valve remnant. Cardiol J. 2007;14(5):508–9.
16. Yavuz T, Nazli C, Kinay O, Kutsal A. Giant Eustachian valve with echocardiographic appearance of divided right atrium. Tex Heart Inst J. 2002;29(4):336–8.
17. Schneider B, Hofmann T, Justen MH, Meinertz T. Chiari's network: normal anatomic variant or risk factor for arterial embolic events? J Am Coll Cardiol. 1995;26(1):203–10.
18. Islam AKMM, Sayami LA, Zaman S. Chiari network: a case report and brief overview. J Saudi Heart Assoc. 2013;25(3):225–9.
19. Hightower JS, Taylor AG, Ursell PC, LaBerge JM. The Chiari network: a rare cause of intracardiac guide wire entrapment. J Vasc Interv Radiol. 2015;26(4):604–6.
20. Lodhi AM, Nguyen T, Bianco C, Movahed A. Coumadin ridge: an incidental finding of a left atrial pseudotumor on transthoracic echocardiography. World J Clin Cases. 2015;3(9):831–4.
21. Kim DT, Lai AC, Hwang C, et al. The ligament of Marshall: a structural analysis in human hearts with implications for atrial arrhythmias. J Am Coll Cardiol. 2000;36(4):1324–7.
22. Terpenning S, White CS. Imaging pitfalls, normal anatomy, and anatomical variants that can simulate disease on cardiac imaging as demonstrated on multidetector computed tomography. Acta Radiol Short Rep. 2015;4(1):1–15.
23. Kim DH, Choi SI, Choi J-A, et al. Various findings of cardiac thrombi on MDCT and MRI. J Comput Assist Tomogr. 2006;30(4):572–7.
24. Bittencourt MS, Achenbach S, Marwan M, et al. Left ventricular thrombus attenuation characterization in cardiac computed tomography angiography. J Cardiovasc Comput Tomogr. 2012;6(2):121–6.
25. Hong YJ, Hur J, Kim YJ, et al. Dual-energy cardiac computed tomography for differentiating cardiac myxoma from thrombus. Int J Cardiovasc Imaging. Springer Netherlands. 2014;30(Suppl 2(2)):121–8.
26. Patel A, Au E, Donegan K, et al. Multidetector row computed tomography for identification of left atrial appendage filling defects in patients undergoing pulmonary vein isolation for treatment of atrial fibrillation: comparison with transesophageal echocardiography. Heart Rhythm. 2008;5(2):253–60.
27. Hur J, Kim YJ, Lee H-J, et al. Left atrial appendage thrombi in stroke patients: detection with two-phase cardiac CT angiography versus transesophageal echocardiography 1. Radiology. 2009;251(3):683–90.
28. Czekajska-Chehab E, Tomaszewska M, Olchowik G, Tomaszewski M, Adamczyk P, Drop A. Lipomatous hypertrophy of the interatrial septum in ECG-gated multislice computed tomography of the heart. Med Sci Monit. 2012;18(7):MT54–9.
29. Fan C-M, Fischman AJ, Kwek BH, Abbara S, Aquino SL. Lipomatous hypertrophy of the interatrial septum: increased uptake on FDG PET. AJR Am J Roentgenol [Internet]. 2005;184(1):339–342. Available from: http://www.ajronline.org/doi/pdfplus/10.2214/ajr.184.1.01840339.
30. Anderson RH, Anderson RH, Webb S, Brown NA, Webb S, Brown NA. Clinical anatomy of the atrial septum with reference to its developmental components. Clin Anat. 1999;12(5):362–74.
31. Sánchez-Quintana D, Ho SY, Cabrera JA, Farré J, Anderson RH. Topographic anatomy of the inferior pyramidal space: relevance to radiofrequency catheter ablation. J Cardiovasc Electrophysiol. 2001;12(2):210–7.
32. Laura DM, Donnino R, Kim EE, Benenstein R, Freedberg RS, Saric M. Lipomatous atrial septal hypertrophy: a review of its anatomy, pathophysiology, multimodality imaging, and relevance to percutaneous interventions. J Am Soc Echocardiogr. 2016;29(8):717–23.
33. Heyer CM, Kagel T, Lemburg SP, Bauer TT, Nicolas V. Lipomatous hypertrophy of the interatrial septum: a prospective study of incidence, imaging findings, and clinical symptoms. Chest. 2003;124(6):2068–73.
34. O'Connor S, Recavarren R, Nichols LC, Parwani AV. Lipomatous hypertrophy of the interatrial septum: an overview. Arch Pathol Lab Med. 2006;130(3):397–9.
35. Xanthos T, Giannakopoulos N, Papadimitriou L. Lipomatous hypertrophy of the interatrial septum: a pathological and clinical approach. Int J Cardiol. 2007;121(1):4–8.

36. Pomerance A. Pathological and clinical study of calcification of the mitral valve ring. J Clin Pathol. 1970;23(4):354–61.
37. Shriki J, Rongey C, Ghosh B, et al. Caseous mitral annular calcifications: multimodality imaging characteristics. World J Radiol. 2010;2(4):143–7.
38. Harpaz D, Auerbach I, Vered Z, Motro M, Tobar A, Rosenblatt S. Caseous calcification of the mitral annulus: a neglected, unrecognized diagnosis. J Am Soc Echocardiogr. 2001;14(8):825–31.
39. Elgendy IY, Conti CR. Caseous calcification of the mitral annulus: a review. Clin Cardiol. Wiley Periodicals, Inc. 2013;36(10):E27–31.
40. Gilbert HM, Grodman R, Chung MH, Hartman G, Krieger KH, Hartman BJ. Sterile, Caseous mitral valve "abscess" mimicking infective endocarditis. Clin Infect Dis. 1997;24(5):1015–6.
41. Wang ZJ, Reddy GP, Gotway MB, Yeh BM, Hetts SW, Higgins CB. CT and MR imaging of pericardial disease. Radiographics. 2003;23(suppl_1):S167–80.
42. Kim JH, Goo JM, Lee HJ, et al. Cystic tumors in the anterior mediastinum. J Comput Assist Tomogr. 2003;27(5):714–23.
43. Jeung M-Y, Gasser B, Gangi A, et al. Imaging of cystic masses of the mediastinum. Radiographics. 2002;22(suppl_1):S79–93.
44. Rajiah P, Kanne JP. Computed tomography of the pericardium and pericardial disease. J Cardiovasc Comput Tomogr. 2010;4(1):3–18.
45. McAdams HP, Kirejczyk WM, Rosado-de-Christenson ML, Matsumoto S. Bronchogenic cyst: imaging features with clinical and histopathologic correlation. Radiology. 2000;217(2):441–6.
46. Seo N, Kang J-W, Lim C-H, Kim B, Lee HJ, Lim T-H. CT findings of an intracardiac bronchogenic cyst. Int J Cardiovasc Imaging. 2011;27(5):701–4.
47. Forcillo J, Dion D, Sauvageot C, Jeanmart H. Intraventricular bronchogenic cyst: a rare congenital anomaly. Ann Thorac Surg. 2015;100(3):1101–3.
48. Wang J, Zhu Q, Liang B, Shi H, Han P, Kong X. Left ventricular bronchogenic cyst. Ann Thorac Surg. 2016;101(2):744–6.
49. Dean C, Etienne D, Carpentier B, Gielecki J, Tubbs RS, Loukas M. Hiatal hernias. Surg Radiol Anat. 2012;34(4):291–9.
50. Díaz-Zamudio M, Bacilio-Pérez U, Herrera-Zarza MC, et al. Coronary artery aneurysms and ectasia: role of coronary CT angiography. Radiographics. 2009;29(7):1939–54.
51. Frazier AA, Qureshi F, Read KM, Gilkeson RC, Poston RS, White CS. Coronary artery bypass grafts: assessment with multidetector CT in the early and late postoperative settings. Radiographics. 2005;25(4):881–96.
52. Rajiah P, Kanne JP. Computed tomography of septal defects. J Cardiovasc Comput Tomogr. 2010;4(4):231–45.
53. Murdoch DR, Corey GR, Hoen B, et al. Clinical presentation, etiology, and outcome of infective endocarditis in the 21st century: the International Collaboration on Endocarditis-Prospective Cohort Study. Arch Intern Med. 2009;169(5):463–73.
54. Murillo H, Restrepo CS, Marmol-Velez JA, et al. Infectious diseases of the heart: pathophysiology, clinical and imaging overview. Radiographics [Internet]. 2016;36(4):963–983. Available from: http://pubs.rsna.org/doi/pdf/10.1148/rg.2016150225.
55. Grebenc ML, Rosado-de-Christenson ML, Burke AP, Green CE, Galvin JR. From the archives of the AFIP. Radiographics. 2002;22(3):673–89.
56. Araoz PA, Araoz PA, Mulvagh SL, et al. CT and MR imaging of benign primary cardiac neoplasms with echocardiographic correlation. Radiographics. 2000;20(5):1303–19.
57. Swartz MF, Lutz CJ, Chandan VS, Landas S, Fink GW. Atrial myxomas: pathologic types, tumor location, and presenting symptoms. J Card Surg. Blackwell Publishing Inc. 2006;21(4):435–40.
58. Amano J, Kono T, Wada Y, et al. Cardiac myxoma: its origin and tumor characteristics. Ann Thorac Cardiovasc Surg. 2003;9(4):215–21.
59. Auger D, Pressacco J, Marcotte F, Tremblay A, Dore A, Ducharme A. Cardiac masses: an integrative approach using echocardiography and other imaging modalities. Heart. BMJ Publishing Group Ltd and British Cardiovascular Society. 2011;97(13):1101–9.
60. Burke A, Jeudy J, Virmani R. Cardiac tumours: an update. Heart. 2008;94(1):117–23.
61. Barbier G, Vazquez Figueroa JG, Rinehart S, et al. Tissue characterization of a papillary fibroelastoma on the aortic valve by contrast-enhanced 320-detector row computed tomography. J Cardiovasc Comput Tomogr. 2010;4(5):345–7.
62. Mariscalco G, Bruno VD, Borsani P, Dominici C, Sala A. Papillary fibroelastoma: insight to a primary cardiac valve tumor. J Card Surg. 2010;25(2):198–205.
63. Daveron E, Jain N, Kelley GP, et al. Papillary fibroelastoma and Lambl's excrescences: echocardiographic diagnosis and differential diagnosis. Echocardiography. Blackwell Science Inc. 2005;22(5):461–3.
64. Hrabak-Paar M, Hübner M, Stern-Padovan R, Lušić M. Hemangioma of the interatrial septum: CT and MRI features. Cardiovasc Intervent Radiol. 2011;34(Suppl 2(S2)):S90–3.
65. Becker AE. Primary heart tumors in the pediatric age group: a review of salient pathologic features relevant for clinicians. Pediatr Cardiol. Springer-Verlag. 2000;21(4):317–23.
66. Burke A, Virmani R. Pediatric heart tumors. Cardiovasc Pathol. 2008;17(4):193–8.
67. Esmaeilzadeh M, Jalalian R, Maleki M, Givtaj N, Mozaffari K, Parsaee M. Cardiac cavernous hemangioma. Eur J Echocardiogr. The Oxford University Press. 2007;8(6):487–9.
68. Wang J-G, Han J, Jiang T, Li Y-J. Cardiac paragangliomas. J Card Surg. 2015;30(1):55–60.
69. Sparrow PJ, Kurian JB, Jones TR, Sivananthan MU. MR imaging of cardiac tumors. Radiographics. 2005;25(5):1255–76.
70. Beroukhim RS, Prakash A, Buechel ERV, et al. Characterization of cardiac tumors in children by cardiovascular magnetic resonance imaging: a multicenter experience. J Am Coll Cardiol. 2011;58(10):1044–54.
71. Abraham KP, Reddy V, Gattuso P. Neoplasms metastatic to the heart: review of 3314 consecutive autopsies. Am J Cardiovasc Pathol. 1990;3(3):195–8.
72. Klatt EC, Heitz DR. Cardiac metastases. Cancer. 1990;65(6):1456–9.
73. Chiles C, Woodard PK, Gutierrez FR, Link KM. Metastatic involvement of the heart and pericardium: CT and MR imaging. Radiographics. Radiological Society of North America. 2001;21(2):439–49.
74. Glancy DL, Roberts WC. The heart in malignant melanoma. A study of 70 autopsy cases. Am J Cardiol. 1968;21(4):555–71.
75. Oto A, Herts BR, Remer EM, Novick AC. Inferior vena cava tumor thrombus in renal cell carcinoma: staging by MR imaging and impact on surgical treatment. AJR Am J Roentgenol. 1998;171(6):1619–24.
76. Agaimy A, Rösch J, Weyand M, Strecker T. Primary and metastatic cardiac sarcomas: a 12-year experience at a German heart center. Int J Clin Exp Pathol. 2012;5(9):928–38.
77. Thomason R, Schlegel W, Lucca M, Cummings S, Lee S. Primary malignant mesothelioma of the pericardium. Case report and literature review. Tex Heart Inst J. Texas Heart Institute. 1994;21(2):170–4.
78. Suman S, Schofield P, Large S. Primary pericardial mesothelioma presenting as pericardial constriction: a case report. Heart. 2004;90(1):e4.
79. Jeudy J, Kirsch J, Tavora F, et al. From the radiologic pathology archives: cardiac lymphoma: radiologic-pathologic correlation. Radiographics. 2012;32(5):1369–80.
80. Shah RN, Simmons TW, Carr JJ, Entrikin DW. Primary cardiac lymphoma diagnosed by multiphase-gated cardiac CT and CT-guided percutaneous trans-sternal biopsy. J Cardiovasc Comput Tomogr. 2012;6(2):137–9.

39 Valvular Heart Disease and Prostheses

Gudrun M. Feuchtner

Valvular Imaging by Cardiac CTA: From Dream to Reality

Over decades, imaging of cardiac valves has been the domain of echocardiography [1], while the "shades-of-gray" obscured computed tomography (CT). From 2005 onward, multislice CT technology improved in terms of higher temporal and spatial resolution, along with the advent of ECG gating, which has made a dream come true: functional 4D cine imaging of cardiac valves. While the first steps with 16-slice CT in 2005 were limited to patients with low heart rates, nowadays, scanners with highest temporal resolution of >75 ms (in 2009, the second-generation 128-slice and in 2014 the third-generation 296-slice dual-source CT) have approached a temporal resolution to that of echocardiography and created new horizons in the dynamic assessment of cardiac valves and prosthetic heart valves (PHV), which are highlighted in this chapter.

Further, explanations of how to examine cardiac valves by computed tomography (CTA) and how to tailor a cardiac CT scan protocols to cardiac valves are provided. Based on current scientific evidence, the integration of CTA into the clinical work-up of patients in conjunction with other imaging modalities such as echocardiography or ^{18}flourdeoxyglucose (FDG) positron emission tomography (PET)/CT is discussed.

Technical CT Prerequisites

For the evaluation of cardiac valve function and anatomy, 64-slice CT or more advanced technology such as dual-source CT or volume CT scanners equipped with up to 296–320- slices is required. Furthermore, ECG gating including the acquisition of a multiphase CT dataset covering the entire cardiac cycle from R wave to R wave is fundamental for dynamic imaging. In order to obtain systolic and diastolic views of the valves and 4D cine loops of their function, image reconstruction of axial thin-slice source images (of 0.75–1 mm) at either 5 or 10% increments of the RR interval is recommended.

Retrospective ECG Gating

Retrospective ECG gating is the technique of first choice. Some vendors provide dedicated ECG-gating technology, such as for the "dual-source" CT (DSCT). Functional evaluation of valves [2] with prospective ECG triggering at a reduced mean radiation dose of 3.8 mSv is feasible. A DSCT scanner consists of two X-ray tubes operating at the same time. While one tube is turned "on" (full mAs, 100%), the second tube covers the entire cardiac cycle at 20% reduced tube mA, enabling the reconstruction of multiphase CT image datasets. The first tube (100% mAs) can be pulsed into any arbitrary phase of the cardiac cycle, either during the end-diastolic (70% of RR interval) in low heart rates <65 bpm or end-systolic phase (40% of RR interval) in patients with high heart rates >65 bpm), in order to ensure motion artifact-free visualization of coronary arteries. *More recently introduced CT systems are capable of "single-beat"* scans either "by using high-pitch" (pitch, 3.2–3.4) DSCT technology, or by "volume CT" approach: Equipped with a broad detector width of up to 16 cm, the entire volume of the heart is covered with one rotation during one heartbeat, enabling functional assessment of cardiac valves during one cardiac cycle.

Iodine Contrast Media Injection

For visualization of all four cardiac valves (right and left sided), a "biphasic split" contrast agent injection protocol is recommended [3]. A monophasic contrast agent bolus injection at a high flow rate of 4–6 mL/s, which is commonly

G. M. Feuchtner (✉)
Department of Radiology, Innsbruck Medical University, Innsbruck, Austria
e-mail: Gudrun.Feuchtner@i-med.ac.at

U. J. Schoepf (ed.), *CT of the Heart*, Contemporary Medical Imaging, https://doi.org/10.1007/978-1-60327-237-7_39

used for coronary CT angiography, typically results in lack of right chamber enhancement (due to significant "wash-out") without appropriate delineation of the tricuspid and pulmonary valve. In contrast, by using a "biphasic split protocol," homogenous right ventricular and atrial enhancement is feasible, due to a prolonged bolus transit time. The "biphasic split protocol" consists of a contrast agent bolus at high flow rate (5–6 cc/s), followed by a second bolus with a lower flow rate (3.0–4 cmL/s) [3] (volume 80% high flow versus 20% low flow). The second bolus may be mixed with saline solution or followed by a saline chaser.

The final administration of a saline solution optimizes bolus transit and geometry. A further advantage of a biphasic split protocol is the reduction of streak artifacts within the right chambers due to lower injection flow rate during the second phase [3].

Post-processing

Dedicated advanced 3D post-processing workstations equipped with multiplanar reformations (MPR) in three planes are required for the generation of valvular planes. Thin-slice MPR (1 mm slice width) are advantageous over thicker slices (>5 mm) and *maximum intensity projections* (MIP) as well are suitable, in order to ensure best display and highest resolution of thin structured such as valvular leaflets.

The following standardized planes for valves should be generated: *for the aortic valve*, left sagittal oblique, left coronal oblique, and orthogonal cross-sectional axial oblique views (see figures in following sections) through the valve and, for the mitral valve, four-chamber, three-chamber, and two-chamber views, as well as perpendicular short-axis mitral valve views.

3D Volume Rendering Technique, MIP, and 4D

Three-dimensional volume rendering technique (VRT) allows for the visualization of valvular leaflets, calcifications (Fig. 39.1), and heart valve prostheses. *Maximum intensity projections (MIP)* are less useful to fully visualize valves, since leaflets are thin. In such instances, the full spatial resolution of thin-slice MPR are advantageous. Finally, the generation of 4D cine imaging video loops during the entire cardiac cycle allows for evaluation of leaflet function and, in particular, prosthesis malfunction.

The Aortic Valve

Aortic Stenosis

Degenerative aortic stenosis (AS) is common in the elderly population with a prevalence of >2% and carries a poor prognosis with a 1- and 5-year survival of 60 and 32%, respectively. Its hallmark is severe aortic valve calcifications (Fig. 39.1). Open surgical aortic valve replacement (AVR) is the only effective treatment in cases of severe aortic stenosis. With up to 40% of patients being declined for conventional open-heart AVR due to an elevated risk profile, the new emerging transcatheter aortic valve implantation (TAVI) procedure provides an efficient minimally invasive treatment option with excellent long-term survival and outcome results.

Cardiac and aortoiliacal CTA is the modality of choice for planning of TAVI, in order to define the appropriate transcatheter access route (transaortal, transfermoral, transaxillary, or transapical) and to determine the optimal prosthesis size and in order to avoid complications such as coronary ostium overstenting or annulus rupture.

Beyond planning of TAVI, cardiac CTA allows for sizing of the aortic valve orifice area (AVA) and grading of aortic stenosis severity. For sizing of the AVA, the CTA images must be reconstructed during mid-systole (5–25% of RR interval), and the "best phase" with the smallest AVA should be selected (typically 25% of RR interval). Additionally, all short-axis views of the aortic valve from the tip of the leaflets caudally toward the annulus should be reviewed, in order to select the smallest AVA at the level of the orifice (Fig. 39.1).

Cardiac CTA has shown a good correlation with other modalities such as TTE or invasive catheterization for measuring the AVA [4–7], while a tendency towards AVA "overestimation" by CTA as compared to transthoracic echocardiography (TTE) has been observed. This can be explained by inter-modality differences: CTA provides direct anatomic AVA sizing, while TTE estimates the effective AVA based on transvalvular pressure gradient (VTI, velocity time integral) assuming left ventricular outflow tract (LVOT) circularity. However, LVOT is most commonly elliptic, thus explaining the inter-modality differences.

In practice, high-grade high-flow "classic" aortic stenosis (AS) is robustly diagnosed by TTE based on increased transvalvular flow and velocity. However, in patients with "low-flow-low-gradient" (paradoxical and classic, with preserved and impaired left ventricular ejection fraction) aortic stenosis, diagnosis by TTE is more difficult and typically requires stress echocardiography for affirmation. In those patients, anatomic sizing by AVA by cardiac CTA is a useful "true" anatomic parameter for estimation of the true severity of AS. Notably, in patients in whom TAVI is considered, CTA provides the advantage of concomitant aortic root and annulus sizing for TAVI planning and also provides an evaluation of coronary artery disease (CAD).

Furthermore, CTA allows for quantification of the aortic valve calcification (AVC) score (Agatston, volume, and mass score) on native ECG-gated unenhanced CT scan, as standardized performed for coronary artery calcium scores (CACS). The AVC score is a valuable prognostic marker, which predicts outcome in patients with severe asymptomatic AS [8] and assists decision-making in terms of whether to treat patients with surgical AVR or whether to postpone

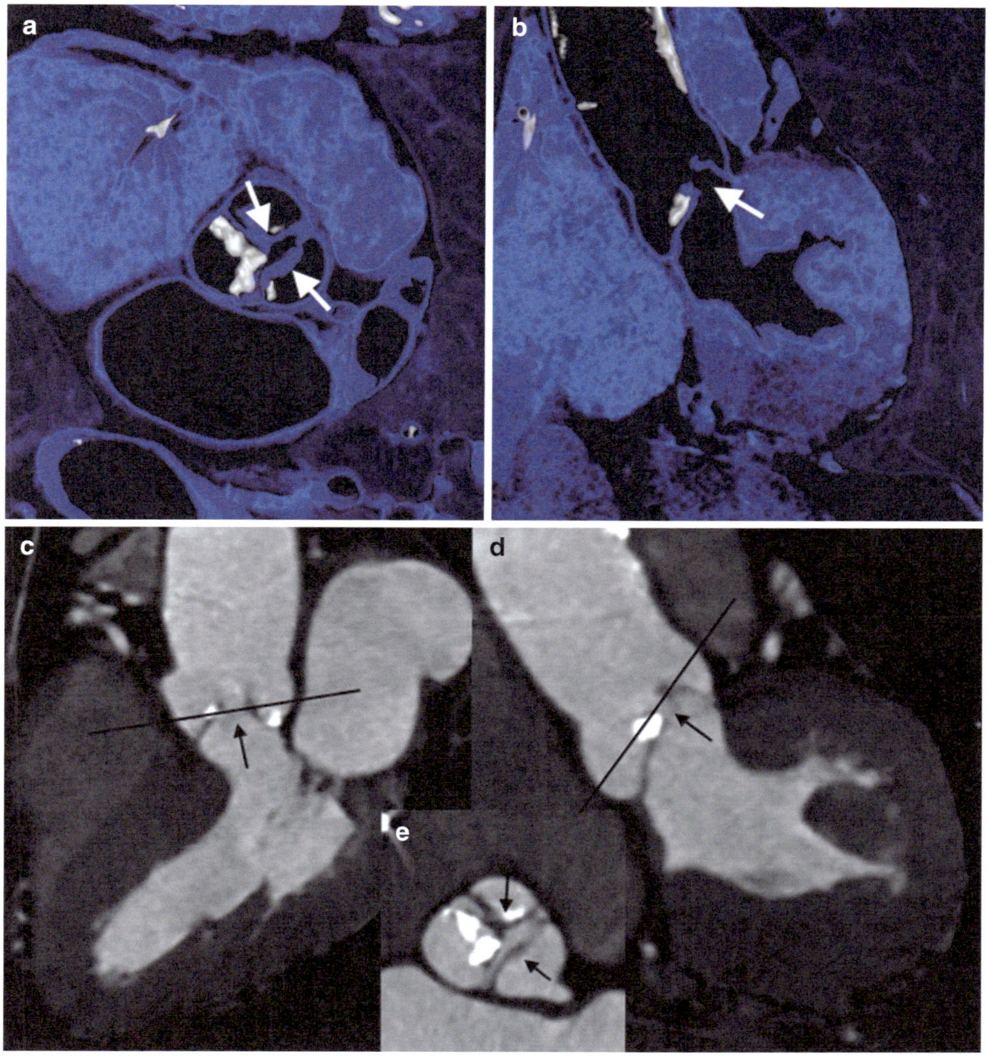

Fig. 39.1 Aortic stenosis (AS). An 82-year-old female with severe high grade AS III, severely calcified leaflets, and narrowing of the inner orifice area (**a**, **b**, *white arrows*) during mid-systolic phase, tricuspid aortic valve ("Mercedes-star-like") (**a**) with partial degenerative fusion of the left/right coronary cusp. Aortic valve by 3D volume rendering technique (VRT) (**a**, **b**). Multiplanar reformation (MPR) (**c**–**d**) of the aortic valve: C = left sagittal oblique (three-chamber view), D = axial oblique view of aortic valve, and E = left coronal oblique view. Image D allows for sizing of the inner aortic valve orifice area (AVA) (*black arrows denote severely stenosed AVA during mid-systole, 25% of the RR interval*). Black lines (**c**, **e**) indicate the level of cross-sectional view of aortic valve (**d**)

AVR and recommend optimal medical therapy. Both asymptomatic severe AS and low-flow-low-gradient AS [9] are considered as "Class IIA" indications for surgery [1]. Accordingly, the decision whether or not to perform conventional AVR or TAVI is usually influenced by a variety of prognostic markers, including the AVC score.

Aortic Valve Morphology

The normal aortic valve consists of three leaflets (*tricuspid*), the non-, left, and right coronary cusps, which symmetrically merge with a "Mercedes-star"-like appearance on axial slices by cardiac CTA during the diastolic phase.

The most common congenital abnormality is the "bicuspid" valve type (Fig. 39.2), where only two of the three leaflets are present. One of those leaflets may or may not show a "raphe," indicating the fusion site of two original leaflets. The "raphe" type is more common (80%). Due to the smaller orifice and a tendency toward degeneration, bicuspid valve malfunctions such as stenosis are more common than in normal tricuspid valves. During systolic phase, bicuspid valves are characterized by a "fish-mouth"-like opening of leaflets, with a round or oval shape (Fig. 39.2). Bicuspid valves are classified as either "type 0" (no raphe) or "type 1" (with raphe, 85%), with either fusion of left and right (L/R) (most common), right and non-coronary (R/N), or left and non-coronary (L/N) cusps. During diastole, the "linear sign" (Fig. 39.2) is pathognomonic for bicuspid valves, indicating a more-or-less symmetrical appearance, while minor deviations from absolute linearity are natural. A special designation is reserved for "type 2," the original tricuspid valve, which develops a "functional bicuspid" configuration of the leaflet opening due to secondary fusion of two leaflets of an originally tricuspid valve, due to degenerative aortic stenosis (most common) (Figs. 39.1a and 39.2a) or rheumatic disease (less common).

For an accurate diagnosis of a bicuspid valve, cardiac CTA yields a high sensitivity of 94% and a specificity of 100% [10], but functional CCTA datasets are required, including a systolic phase, to define whether leaflet fusion or raphe is present or not (type 1 and type 2). In contrast, the

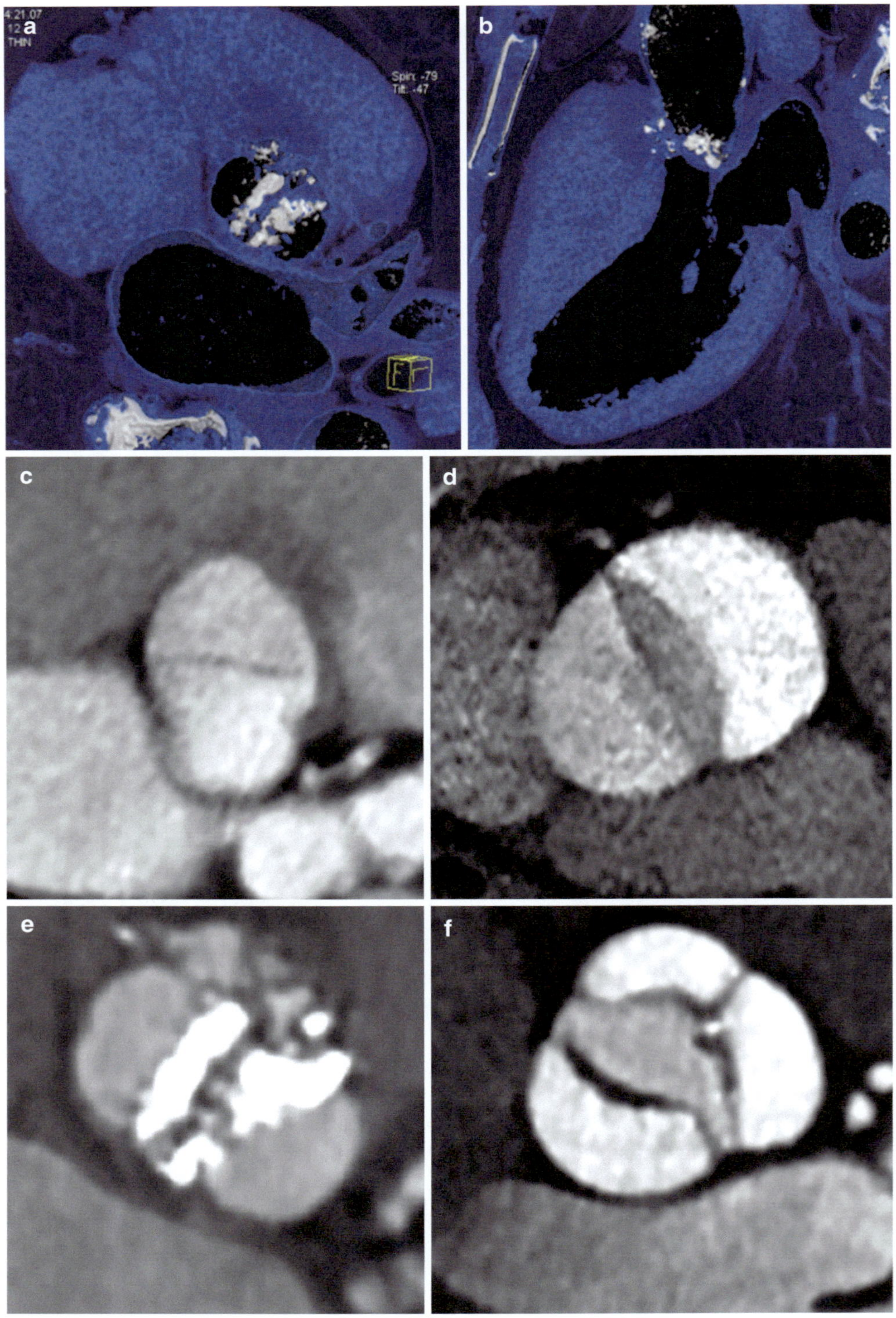

Fig. 39.2 Bicuspid valve types. (**a**) VRT with severe calcifications and degeneration "linear sign" during end-diastole, (**a**) axial and (**b**) three-chamber view, congenital type 0 (no raphe). (**c**) "*Linear sign*" during end-diastole (70% of RR interval) (type 0) and B "fish mouth" opening during mid-systole (25%RR interval) (type 0). Bicuspid valve congenital type 0 (without raphe, panel C/B/D/E) and type 1 (with raphe, **f**). (**d**) "Fish mouth" during mid-systole, mild degenerations, and fusion of left/right coronary cusp (R/L) during end-diastole (type 1 R/L). (**e**) "Linear sign" with severe calcification during end-diastole with fusion of non- (N) and right (R) coronary cusp (type 0 N/R)

bicuspid type 0 (no raphe) can be diagnosed during diastolic phase based on the "linear sign" [11].

In rare cases, a "quadricuspid" aortic valve may be present, consisting of four leaflets with an estimated incidence of 0.003–0.043% [12]. Another extremely rare congenital malformation is the "unicuspid valve," either the "acommissural" or "unicommissural type," consisting of one leaflet and a "hole-like" appearance, which often require surgery early after birth or in early adulthood due to a stenotic component.

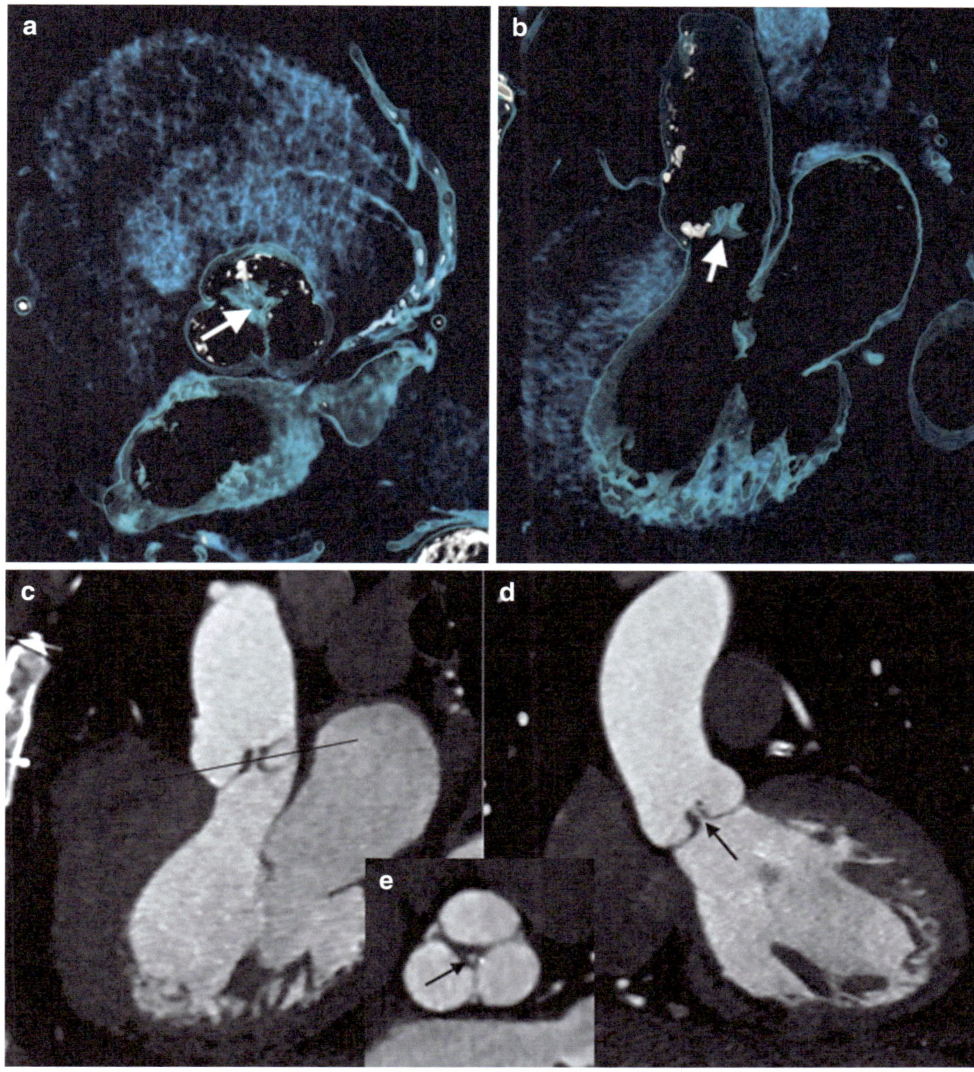

Fig. 39.3 Aortic regurgitation (AR). A 72-year-old male with moderate AR. During end-diastolic phase, small central incomplete leaflet adaption is shown ("poke hole"-like) (**a**) on 3D VRT (AB) and MPR (CDE). MPR in left sagittal oblique (three-chamber view) (**c**), axial oblique (**d**), and left coronal oblique (**e**) reconstructions. Note incomplete co-adaptation of leaflets (**c**, **e**, **d**). A central regurgitation orifice area (black arrow, **d**) can be visualized *during end-diastole (70% of RR interval)*. Black lines (**c**) indicate the level of cross-sectional oblique view of the aortic valve (**d**)

Aortic Regurgitation

Diagnosis of aortic regurgitation (AR) is primarily established by TTE in clinical practice based on Doppler regurgitant flow jet length and width and the pressure half-time (PHT) method. AR is further stratified into mild, moderate, and severe AR by TTE.

In patients with AR, cardiac CTA allows for direct visualization of incomplete leaflet margins adaption, and a "central regurgitant orifice area" (ROA) during the end-diastolic phase may be depicted (Fig. 39.3). Such findings should be included into a structured cardiac CTA reports. The anatomic ROA provides an estimate of the severity of AR; with <25 mm^2 ROA as cutoff for mild and >75 mm^2 ROA for severe AR [13]. CT image reconstruction is recommended between 60% and 80% of the RR interval; however, the cardiac phase with least cardiac motion and optimal image quality should be used when determining the ROA. Sizing of the ROA is recommended on oblique axial cross-sectional slices reformatted for aortic valve views. Mild and moderate AR [13] may create only tiny "poke hole"-like central leakages (Fig. 39.3) which may be difficult to visualize and limit the accuracy of CTA [14].

The most common request for cardiac CTA in clinical practice however is clarifying the etiology of AR such as aortic root aneurysm sizing, the characterization of cardiac masses such as vegetations causing AR, or the preoperative evaluation of CAD.

Furthermore, in patients with singular aortic valve disease and no other dysfunctional heart valves, the AR volume (mL) and fraction (%) can be calculated as the difference between left ventricular (LV) and right ventricular (RV) stroke volume. Notably, the absence of any other valvular dysfunction (mitral, pulmonary, or tricuspid) is an important prerequisite for the accurate quantification of the AR volume and fraction [15].

Mitral Valve

Mitral Stenosis

Mitral stenosis (MS) most commonly develops in the course of rheumatic disease on the valvular level due to nodular and/or diffuse thickening of the leaflets and chordae. Transthoracic echocardiography (TTE) enables an accurate functional diagnosis of MS and its severity (stratified into mild, MS I; moderate, MS II; and severe, MS III) depending on the increase in transvalvular flow velocity and pressure gradient. However, nodular and diffuse thickening and leaflet calcifications may be found incidentally on coronary CTA exams and should be reported (Fig. 39.4).

In addition, cardiac CT allows for sizing of the mitral orifice area (MOA) during the end-diastolic phase, which provides a reliable estimate of MS severity [16].

In patients with secondary MS due to orifice obstruction and atrial myxoma prolapse, CTA and MRI are the cross-sectional imaging modalities of choice to further characterize masses after an initial echocardiography screening. Atrial myxoma, which typically appears as round-shaped hypodense pedunculated masses arising from interatrial septum (e.g., fossa ovalis) with minor contrast uptake, may cause obstruction of the MOA during the diastolic phase. Prior to surgery, CTA allows for preoperative rule out of coronary artery disease and is able to accomplish two tasks with a single scan.

Mitral Regurgitation

Similar to aortic regurgitation, diagnosis of mitral regurgitation (MR) is firmly established by Doppler flow jet assessment during TTE, and cardiac CTA does not play a role in the primary diagnosis. Due to the saddle shape of mitral valve with irregular leaflet margins, the direct anatomic visualization of the mitral regurgitant orifice area (M-ROA) during end-systole is more difficult compared to the aortic valve, though technically feasible with a good correlation to TTE as shown in one study of 19 patients [17].

In patients with functional MR (FMR) due to heart failure and LV enlargement, the anatomy of the subvalvular apparatus and valve geometry is of interest for planning of novel minimally invasive or percutaneous mitral valve intervention techniques for annuloplasty. The subvalvular apparatus is highly variable due to anatomic variations in the posterior papillary muscle (PM) – both single and multiple heads – and insertions are often found. In patients with heart failure and FMR, increased tenting heights, mitral valve sphericity index, and more outward displacement of the PMs are found, which are indicators of FMR severity [18]. Beyond, CTA allows for 3D visualization of left circumflex artery (CX) course in relation to the mitral annulus. If the CX is located close to the annulus, patients may have an increased risk for fatal injury via perforation and bleeding while inserting mitral annuloplasty devices during open-heart surgery or during new investigative percutaneous techniques.

Mitral Valve Prolapse

During mid-end-systolic phase (25–40% of RR interval), direct visualization of mitral valve prolapse (MVP) by CTA [19] is feasible, and the exact measurement of leaflet excursion below the annulus is possible. A deviation of approximately >3 mm is usually regarded as "significant" MVP with functional relevance, causing mitral regurgitation. The recommended views for the sizing of prolapse excursion are two- and three-chamber views. Two different types of MVP are distinguished, the "bowing" ("billowing") type, which most commonly caused by primary myxomatous degenerative disease ("Barlow's disease") due to redundant leaflets forming round-shaped lesions and the "flail leaflet" type. A flail leaflet is characterized by free leaflet margin prolapse and usually occurs along with ruptured chordae, commonly due to rheumatic or inflammatory disease, or during acute myocardial infarct involving a papillary muscle. The exact anatomic assignment of the prolapse to the corresponding leaflet section (anterior A1, upper; A2, mid; and A3, caudal segment of the anterior leaflet or posterior P1, upper; P2, mid; and P3, caudal part of the posterior leaflet) is critical for planning surgical reconstruction. While 3D TEE usually provides this information, TTE typically does provide sufficient image quality. Beyond exact anatomic assignments, CTA also adds information about leaflet morphology such as whether calcifications are present or not (Fig. 39.5).

Degenerative Mitral Annular Calcification

CTA plays a major role in establishing diagnosis of degenerative mitral annular calcification (MAC) based on its clear detection of calcified masses. On TTE, large inhomogenous caseous/liquefaction necrosis type of MAC may mimic tumors due to their mass-like appearance, with potential invasion into periannular structures such as the myocardium. In such patients, cardiac CT (both unenhanced and contrast-enhanced CTA) is the modality of choice for ascertaining diagnosis, based on lack of contrast agent uptake and high CT densities (>130 HU) seen on unenhanced CT [20] (Fig. 39.6).

Pulmonary and Tricuspid Valve

The visualization of right-sided valves is a challenge, due to streak artifacts from contrast agent inflow. Such artifacts are minimized by using the biphasic contrast agent injection

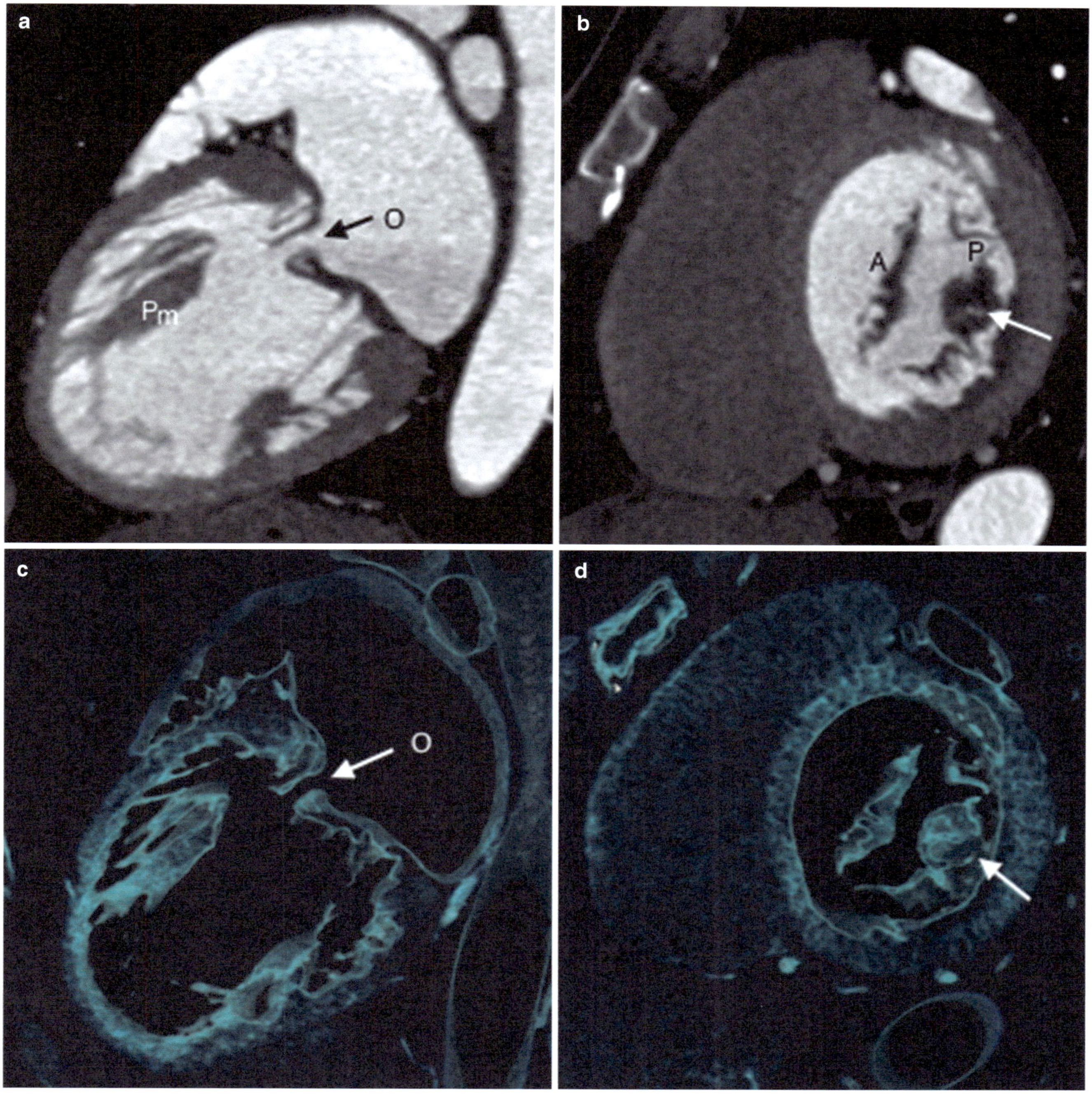

Fig. 39.4 Mitral stenosis/regurgitation, rheumatic disease. A 49-year-old female with rheumatic disease and combined MS/MR dysfunction. Diffuse A, anterior and nodular; P, posterior mitral leaflet thickening (involving P2/3 segment) (*arrows*) on two-chamber (**a**, **c**) and short-axis (**b**, **d**) views by MPR (**a**, **b**) and 3D VRT (**c**, **d**). *Arrows* (**a**, **c**) denote mitral valve orifice = O. Pm, papillary muscle thickening resulting in leaflet retraction and restricted leaflet motion

protocol described above [3] and designed to ensure homogenous attenuation of right cardiac chambers.

Infective Endocarditis

Diagnosis of infective endocarditis (IE) is made by applying major and minor Duke criteria, consisting of a combination of laboratory and imaging findings and either stratified as "definite," "possible," or "rejected." TTE and TEE are the primary imaging tools during initial patient triage. In patients with suspected paravalvular involvement and insufficient TTE/TEE imaging, cardiac CTA has been recently recognized as a "Class IIa" indication [1] by the American Heart Association (AHA) 2014 guidelines for the management of patients with valvular disease.

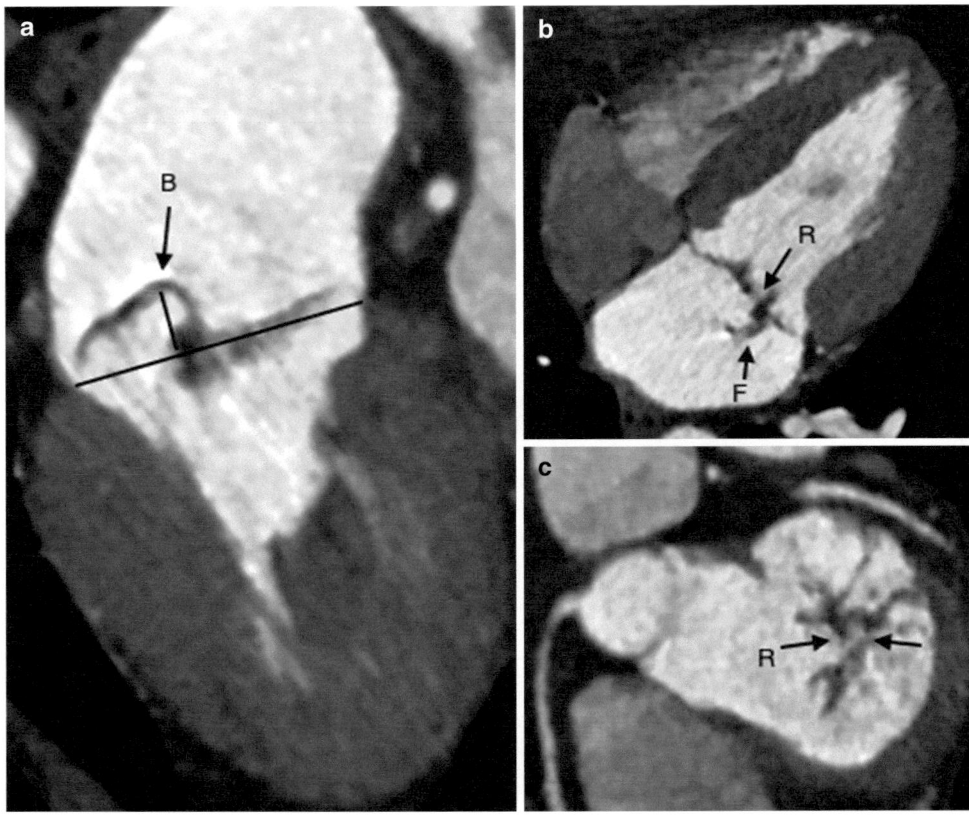

Fig. 39.5 Mitral regurgitation/prolapse. (**a**) A 66-year-old female with severe regurgitation (R) of the mitral valve caused by leaflet prolapse (B bowing and F flail leaflet), leading to central incomplete closure of leaflets (*arrow, right upper panel B*) prior to surgery. The regurgitant (R) orifice (*black arrows*) shows irregular borders (**c**). Three-chamber view (**a**), four-chamber view (**b**), and short axis through mitral valve plane (**c**). Black line indicates mitral annulus and orthogonal line the tenting height to maximal leaflet deviation below the annulus plane toward the LA (Bowing = B; A)

Similar to TTE and TEE, cardiac CTA allows for the visualization of specific lesions developing in the course of IE [21] with high accuracy. Specific lesions include (1) *vegetations*, defined as hypodense, round, irregular, or longitudinal masses attached to the valvular leaflets or the endocardium ("mural vegetations"). Consisting of inflammatory cells and granulomatous tissue, such lesions may uptake contrast at later stages, indicating the formation of organized connective tissue. Vegetations not treated by antibiotics or removed by surgical resection may calcify. The size of vegetations is varying from few millimeters up to >1 cm, with larger vegetations often having greater mobility. The size and mobility serve as a pivotal marker for a patients' individual risk for embolization into the systemic circulation, thus influencing the clinical decision management in terms of antibiotic conventional treatment versus surgical resection of large (>1 cm) and mobile vegetations.

Leaflet Perforations

During the course of inflammation, irregular or round-shaped lesions may occur within the cusp leading to a "torn" – aspect of leaflets typically causing severe valvular insufficiency (Fig. 39.7). A specific term is designated for the aneurysmal leaflet perforation type ("AR jet lesion") [22], occurring within the anterior mitral cusp, caused by an eccentric AR jet which create hole-like lesions in patients with chronic subacute.

Fistula

A communication between cardiac chambers and the aortic root may develop due to inflammatory arrosion, most commonly on atrioventricular valvular, annular, or the membranous ventricular septum level. Contrast agent continuity is revealed on cardiac CTA.

Paravalvular Abscess and Pseudoaneurysm

Paravalvular abscesses and pseudoaneurysm may be found in patients with severe IE. Such lesions, which more often occur after prosthetic heart valve endocarditis (PVE) than in native valvular IE, are described in greater detail in the next paragraph.

Prosthetic Heart Valves (PHV)

The imaging of prosthetic valves is a major challenge in clinical practice. The early and precise diagnosis of dysfunctional valves is pivotal in order to avoid fatal complications and adverse outcome. In prosthetic valve endocarditis (PVE), the 1-year mortality rate is high with 24.8–50% with improved survival for those undergoing early surgery [23]. Prosthetic heart valve (PHV) thrombosis carries an annual risk of thromboembolic events of 1–2% for mechanic and 1.46% [24] up to recently reported 13–40% for bioprosthesis detected by CCTA [25].

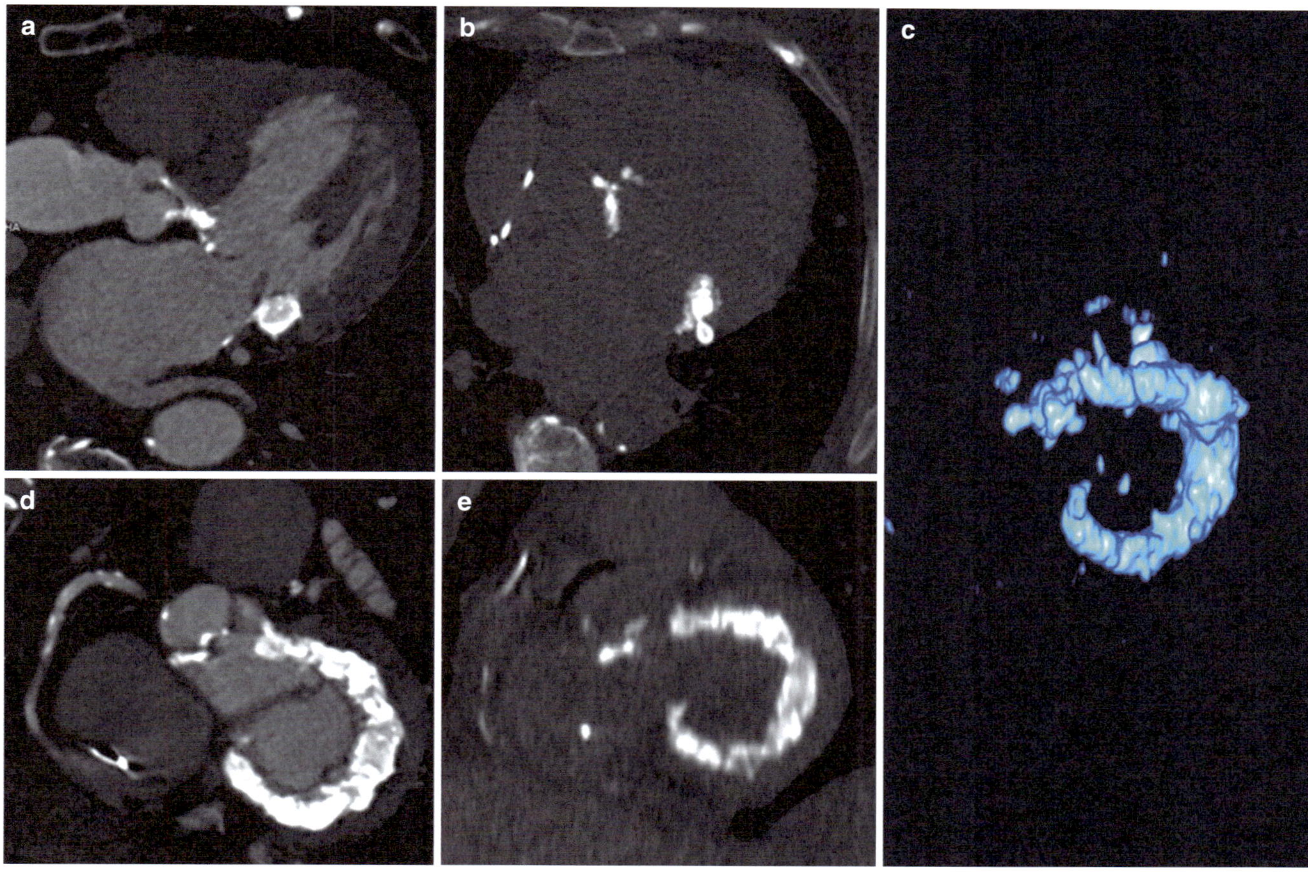

Fig. 39.6 Degenerative mitral annular calcification (MAC). An 80-year old female with 0-shape circumferential MAC (**e**) and an inner caseous/liquefaction necrosis (LN) aspect with lesser dense areas and a denser outer calcified shell. Mass-like aspect with myocardial invasion posterior (**c**). Contrast-enhanced (**a**, **b**) and non-contrast CT (**c**, **d**) and 3D VRT (**e**) reconstruction of MAC. Lack of contrast agent uptake within the mass (**a**, **c** versus **b**, **d**) allowed for a firm diagnosis of MAC. Oblique axial (**a**, **c**) and short-axis (**b**, **d**) views of the mitral valve

TTE and TEE are the primary imaging tools. However, reverberation artifacts from metal create individual device-related limitations in image quality of the paravalvular territory.

The advantage of CCTA is in the 3D visualization and 4D dynamics of leaflet motion, in addition to the complementary evaluation of coronary artery disease [26] or bypass graft patency prior to surgery.

Previous studies investigating CCTA in prosthetic valve dysfunction (PVD) reported good correlation [27–29] with up to 100% agreement in small sample-sized studies [27] involving surgery. In PHV endocarditis [30], the best diagnostic performance was observed for a combined CCTA/TEE approach. In contrast, for the evaluation of the paravalvular territory, CCTA performed superior to [30, 31] to TEE. Recent advances in CCTA technology in terms of temporal resolution further improved the visualization of small mobile masses attached to devices. Most recent data reveals improved performance of CCTA for mass detection [31] that may even outperform TEE, such as indicated in a study on transcatheter bioprosthetic valve thrombosis [25, 31].

Spectrum of CTA Findings in PHD

Masses are hypodense, round, longitudinal, or irregular-shaped lesions, representing either a "vegetation" in cases of infection and clinical signs of endocarditis, "thrombus/pannus," or "undermined areas requiring further work-up." CT attenuation is a valuable parameter to distinguish between thrombus and pannus, with increasing Hounsfield units (HU) indicating organization with neoangiogenesis and connective tissue proliferation of a thrombus [31–33]. A HU threshold of 145 provided high sensitivity (87.5%) and specificity (95.5%) in discriminating pannus from thrombus (Fig. 39.8). Furthermore, masses with a lower attenuation of HU <90 HU were associated with a higher success rate of complete thrombolysis, as compared to masses with attenuation >145 HU [32]. Similarly, the CT atten-

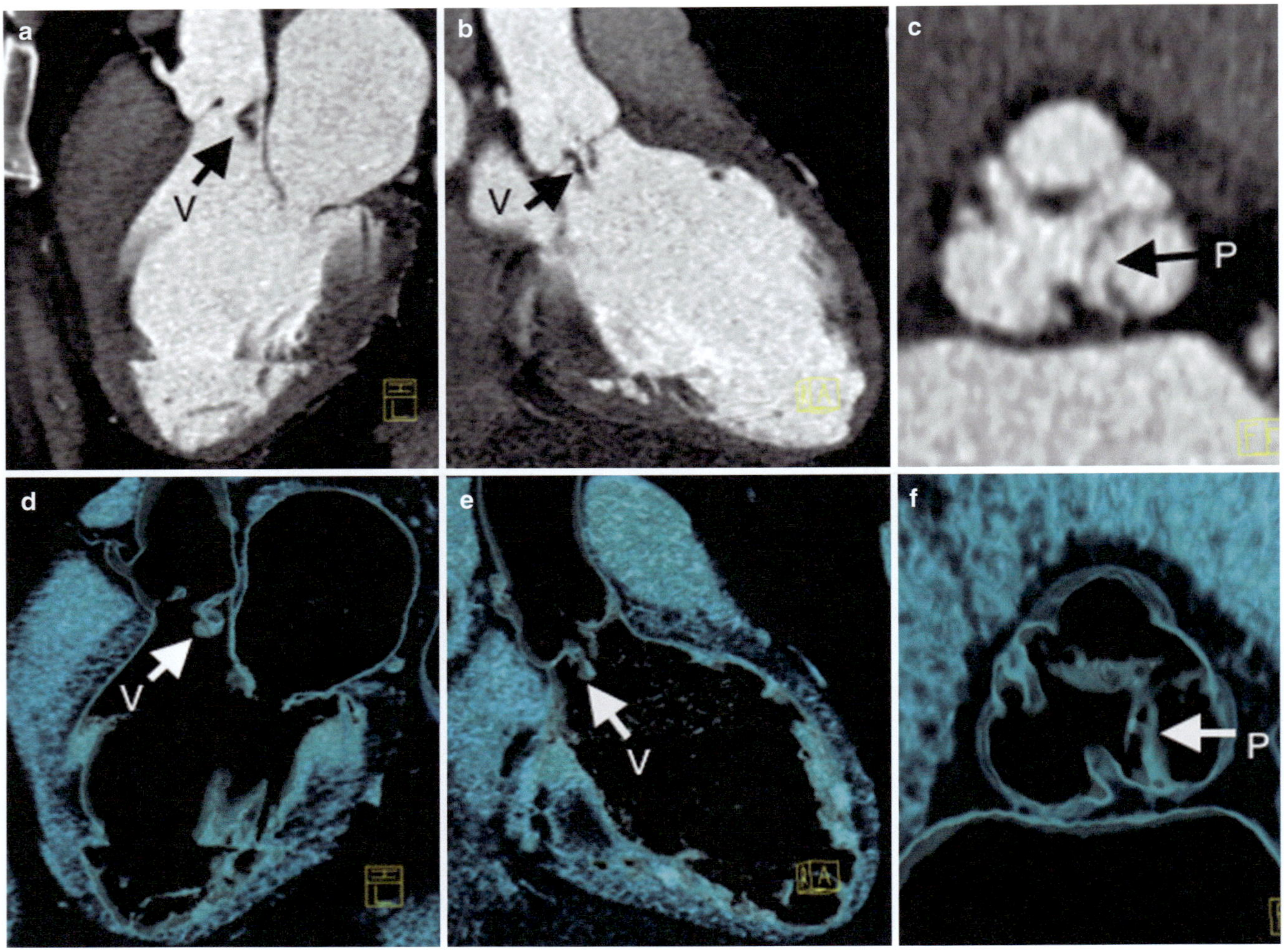

Fig. 39.7 Infective endocarditis. A 69-year-old man with septic shock and organ failure due to IE. V, vegetations, longitudinal hypodense masses, mobile, floating in the LVOT, and P, perforation of the left coronary cusp. Note small pseudodiverticula (2 mm) of ascending aorta at sino-tubular junction, indication infection uprising and periaortic fluid (abscess) confirmed by emergency surgery. Aortic valve was replaced. CTA was performed primarily for coronary artery evaluation prior to surgery. Three-chamber view (**a**, **c**), left sagittal oblique (**b**, **d**), and left coronal oblique and cross-sectional axial plane through aortic valve (**c**, **e**) with MPR (**a**–**c**) and 3D VRT (**d**–**e**)

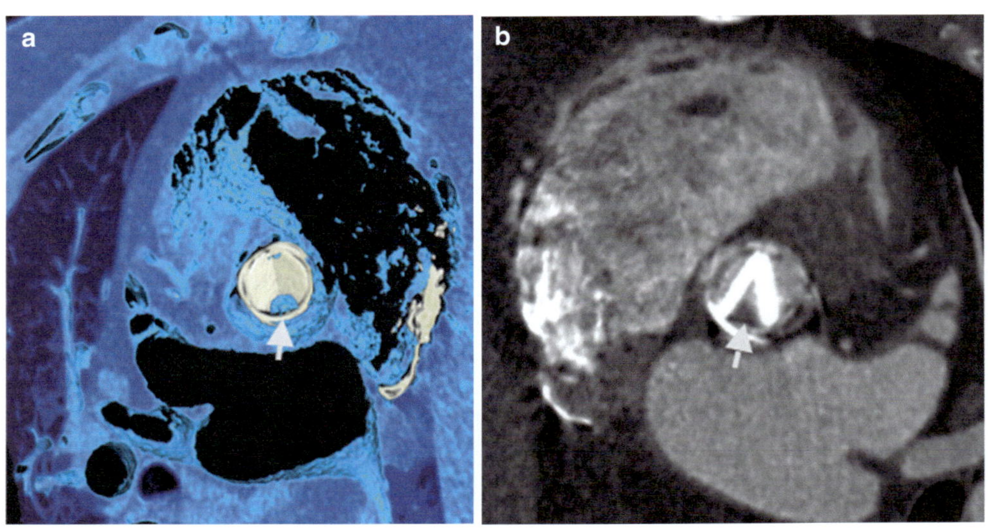

Fig. 39.8 (**a** and **b**) PHV 1. Thrombus/pannus at posterior circumference of mechanic bileaflet aortic prosthesis causing leaflet opening restriction with transvalvular pressure gradient increase corresponding to severe stenosis grade III. Hypodense mass was detected incidentally on CTA performed for coronary artery disease evaluation prior to surgery

uation of vegetations is variable depending on lesion age and degree of vascularization. Vegetations may or may not show minor uptake of contrast agent.

Special types of masses are lesions originating from the prosthetic valve apparatus, such as "degenerative lesions," which occur if biomaterial from a porcine or bovine bioprosthesis degenerates, which also appear "mass-like" with rather irregular or round contours. Degenerated bioprostheses are prone to develop infections, and the mass-like lesions are classified as "vegetations" when associated with symptoms of infection such as fever, C-reactive protein elevation, and/or positive blood cultures (Figs. 39.9 and 39.10).

Masses frequently cause functional PHV impairment such as stenosis or regurgitation. Patients with thrombi that do not respond to lysis and that cause PHV dysfunction are candidates for surgical resection.

A visual representation of a *pseudoaneurysm* on CT is defined as paravalvular cavity filled with contrast media. They mostly originate from a PHV annulus and grow large, often larger than 1 cm. On TTE, paravalvular flow jet is usually detected, while the exact size, extent, and anatomic position of a pseudoaneurysm often exceed the acoustic window on TTE. Therefore, CCTA is a valuable imaging tool to fully determine the size and paravalvular territory involved (Fig. 39.10) and is also beneficial for precise surgical planning.

Paravalvular leaks are often visualized on CT as contrast agent outflow at the annulus level, or flow from above to below, and seen in both infected and non-infected devices. Common causes are the undersizing of the PHV in relation to the annulus, which was observed in the early years (2008–2011) of transcatheter aortic valve implantation (TAVI) resulting in moderate up to severe paravalvular leakage with adverse prognosis.

Paravalvular abscess can be diagnosed by CTA based on the detection of a dense paravalvular infiltration with liquid-equivalent Hounsfield units (HU) of 0–30 HU and a surrounding layer of tissue with contrast uptake ("definite abscess"). Such a vascularized tissue layer may be present during arterial contrast injection or missing and appearing during the late phase (70 s after contrast agent injection). The formation of an outer vascularized layer with contrast uptake is often classified by cardiac surgeons as the "abscess cavity wall" and indicates connective fibrous tissue formation. In patients with an acute recent onset of infection, exclusively pure paravalvular liquid is seen on cardiac CTA. If the CT densities are not clearly related to liquid but reach above 30–40 HU, paravalvular abscesses may be difficult to discriminate from periprosthetic postsurgical fibrosis or material used to fix the device, such as the "fibroglue." Accordingly, in patients with an unclear focus of infection, an abscess should be suspected if a "dense" paravalvular infiltration with positive HU (loss of periaortic fatty tissue layer) is seen and ^{18}fluordeoxyglucose (FDG) positron emission tomography (PET) (^{18}FDG-PET/CT) [34] appended. ^{18}FDG-PET/CT increased the number of true positive cases diagnosed with PVE and improved the sensitivity from 70% to 97% ($p = 0.008$) if implemented as "major Duke" criterion into the diagnostic triage of patients with possible infective endocarditis. In such patients, the diagnosis of periprosthetic abscesses and dehiscence is of paramount importance, as surgical treatment is almost always required to ensure a favorable outcome.

Dehiscence, defined as the loosening of the prosthesis anchor within the annulus, is defined as rocking valve motion >10 degree above annulus and found in both infected and non-infected devices (e.g., due to suture loosening). Due to its ability to generate three-dimensional interactive oblique planes, CCTA is superior to TTE and TEE in showing the full circumferential extent of "dehiscence" and the degree of cranial or

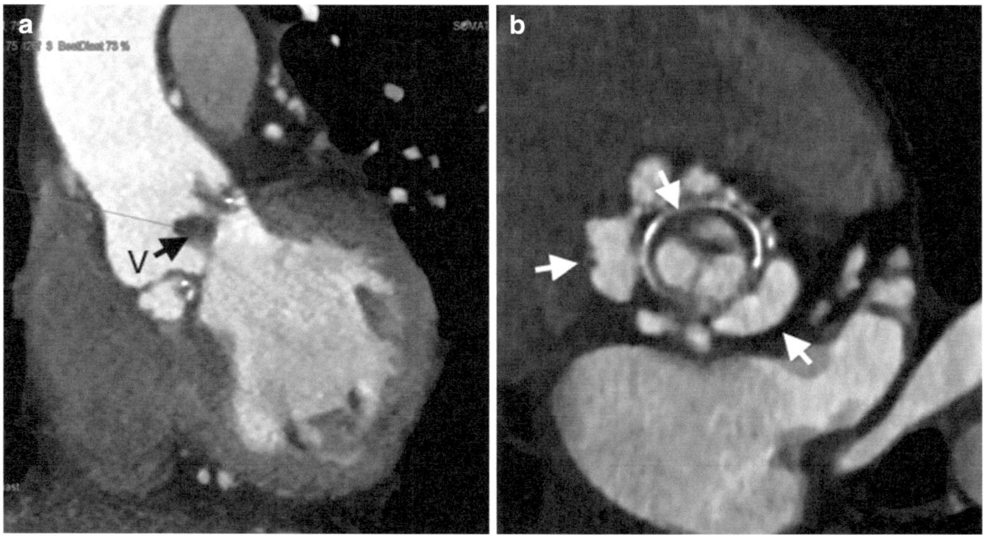

Fig. 39.9 PHV2. A 75-year-old male with structural bioprosthetic valve degeneration and infection. Mass-like vegetation (V), arrow, on left sagittal coronal planes (**a**) and corresponding cross-sectional axial oblique plaque through the aortic bioprosthesis (**b**). *Upper white arrow* denotes the stented prosthesis and attached diffuse thickening and pseudoaneurysm (*lateral white arrows*)

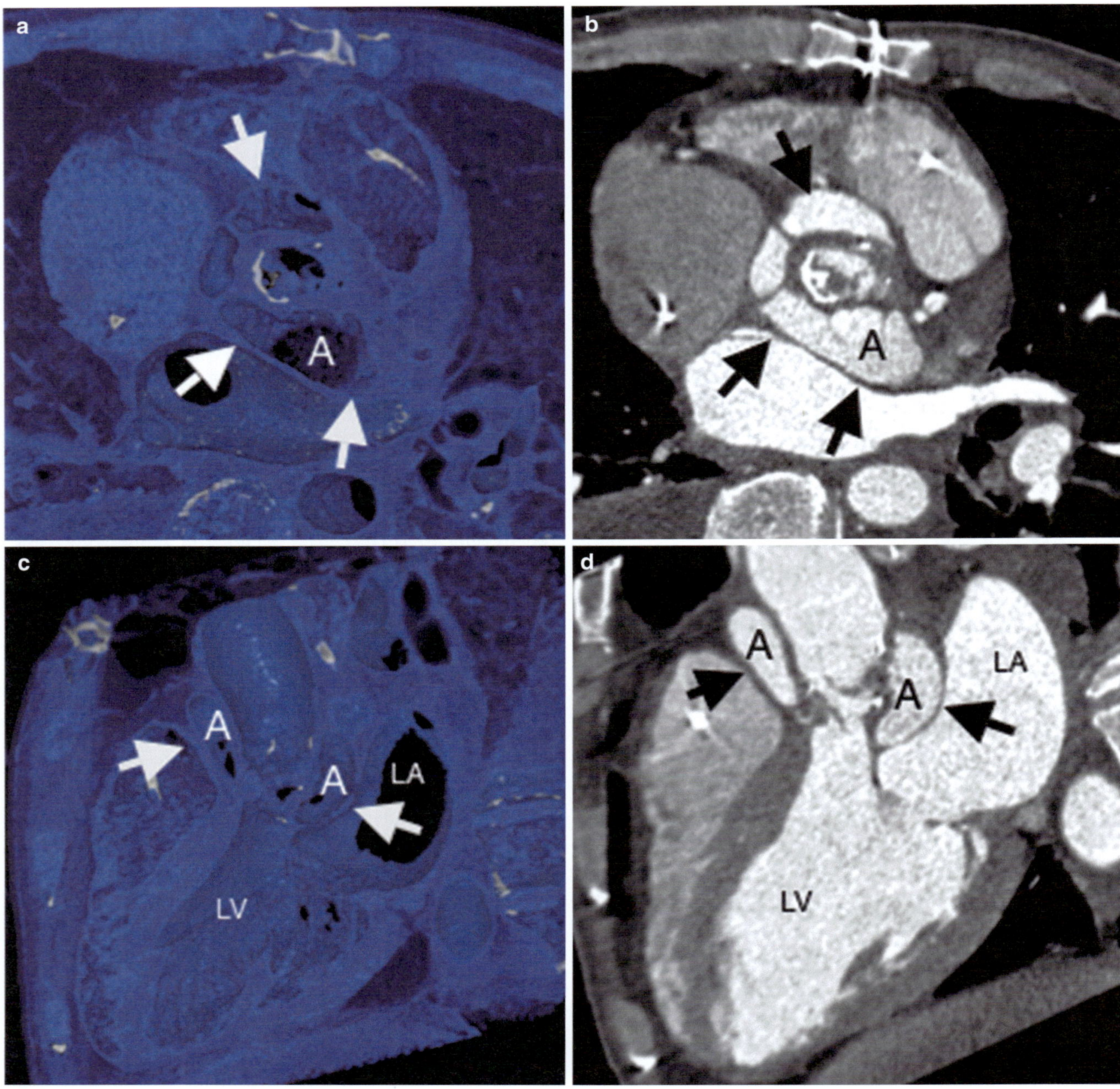

Fig. 39.10 PHV 3. Infected and degenerated bioprosthetic valve: large pseudoaneurysm (**a**) (white and black arrows) surrounding the aortic root and causing dehiscence and leaflet malfunction. Note thickened leaflets and calcified bioprosthetic valve due to inflammation and degeneration. (**a**, **c**) 3D VRT; (**b**, **d**) MPR; A, B, axial views; (**c**, **d**) three-chamber view; LA, left atrium; LV, left ventricle

caudal displacement of the device. Exact measurement of the "displacement angle" is feasible, and "rocking valve motion" can be visualized on 4D cine loops. Due to the risk of PHV device embolization, urgent surgery is necessary in "rocking valves" and with a high degree of annulus loosening, in order to avoid a fatal outcome.

Structural bioprosthetic valve degeneration (SVD) is due to degenerative processes of the porcine or bovine biomaterial on cellular level, affecting the leaflets (in stented PHV) and/or the PHV apparatus in fully biological devices such as aortic root grafts (e.g., the *Freestyle*™, *Medtronic*, or stentless valves); SVD is often seen as (1) thickening of the leaflets and/or (2) calcification and/or (3) "restricted leaflet motion" visualized on 4D cine images. The effective orifice area (EOA) can be sized [35] by CCTA, if image quality allows for measurement during early mid-systolic phase and serves as diagnostic parameter on CCTA with a good correlation to the EOA measured by TTE.

In fully biological aortic root grafts or new models of stent-less tissue valves, severe destruction may be found including paravalvular leak, aneurysmata, and dehiscence (Figs. 39.9 and 39.10).

"Stuck valve" (mechanical) is restricted leaflet motion with <70 degrees of opening angle during the systolic phase, measured in left coronal oblique and left sagittal oblique projections [36]. With mechanic valves, the opening angle depends on the individual device implanted, while less than 70° can be taken as a generalized valuable cutoff for restricted orifice opening. In one study, opening angles were found to be 64 vs 79 degrees in dysfunctional vs normal aortic valve prostheses ($P < 0.0001$) [36]. Common causes are patient-prosthesis mismatch (PPM) due to mal-sizing and the implantation of an oversized PHV or broken mechanic leaflets (Fig. 39.8).

One of the most common findings in PVD and PVE during TTE are increased transvalvular pressure gradients, or transvalvular or paravalvular regurgitation. Such functional abnormalities may be related to morphological findings such as thrombi, panni [31–33], or vegetation. In cases of unclear dysfunction, CCTA should be always requested to clarify the etiology of PVD. New data indicate a superior performance of CCTA over TTE for the detection of PHV masses [31].

Limitations of CCTA Artifacts

Among the variety of PHV models, artifacts depend on the specific material composition. Fortunately, most devices, in particular the most commonly implanted bileaflet type and the stent struts of bioprosthesis create only minor artifacts. However, hypodense beam hardening artifacts may mimic the presence of a pannus or thrombus apposition on the prosthesis rings. Only one mechanical monoleaflet tilting disc valve (Björk-Shiley, the "convexo-concave," composed of 51% cobalt, 20% chromium, 15% tungsten, and 15% nickel) causes severe artifacts, preventing the assessment of the paravalvular space and device. This type of PHV is rarely seen nowadays, as it was withdrawn from the market in 1986 due to outlet strut fractures (OSFs) with escape of the disc, resulting in embolization with fatal outcomes (0.7%). Notably, the average degree of opening angle was 60° for the first device (1979) and 70° for the second.

Furthermore, recent advances in CT technology (iterative reconstruction techniques [37] and prospective ECG triggering [38] allow for beam hardening artifact reduction. Prospective ECG triggering is recommended only in patients with regular heart rates. *Arrhythmia,* which is frequent in patients after PHV implantation, may result in misalignment artifacts hampering image quality due to RR interval variability.

Differentiation of Paravalvular Abscess and Periprosthetic Fibrosis

Dense tissue with CT attenuation values around 30–40 HU or above may create difficulties in distinguishing periprosthetic fibrosis from abscess. ^{18}FDG-PET/CT [34] has higher accuracy and recently showed an increase in sensitivity for diagnosis of PVE if a positive ^{18}FDG-PET/CT was recognized as "major Duke criterion."

Renal Dysfunction

A non-enhanced native CT scan in retrospective ECG-gated mode allows for the evaluation of the mechanic leaflet function and serves as valuable alternative imaging option for the assessment of mechanic leaflet function in patients with impaired renal function. However, unenhanced cardiac CTA does not permit the detection of masses such as thrombi or panni.

In conclusion, cardiac CTA is a valuable 3D imaging technique in the diagnostic work-up of patients with PHV dysfunction and should be systematically integrated after initial TTE/TEE screening. Specifically, the evaluation of the paravalvular territory such as the degree of the circumferential involvement in 3D views and to clarify etiology of PVD, such as the characterization of masses such as thrombi or panni, are indications for performing cardiac CTA. CTA offers the advantage of providing coronary artery disease evaluation prior to surgery.

Summary

Cardiac CTA has created new horizons in the evaluation of cardiac valves over the past 10 years. CTA offers an innovative 3D complementary imaging modality with added value in the clinical work-up algorithm in various specific settings.

References

1. Nishimura RA, Otto CM, Bonow RO, et al. 2014 AHA/ACC guideline for the management of patients with valvular heart disease: executive summary: a report of the ACC/AHA Task Force on Practice Guidelines. J Am Coll Cardiol. 2014;63(22):2438–88.
2. Feuchtner G, Göetti R, Plass A, Baumueller S, Stolzmann P, Scheffel H, Wieser M, Marincek B, Alkadhi H, Leschka S. Dual-step prospective ECG-triggered 128-slice dual-source CT for evaluation of coronary arteries and cardiac function without heart rate control: a technical note. Eur Radiol. 2010;20(9):2093–9.
3. Vrachliotis TG, Bis KG, Haidary A, Kosuri R, Balasubramaniam M, Gallagher M, Raff G, Ross M, O'neil B, O'neill W. Atypical chest pain: coronary, aortic, and pulmonary vasculature enhancement at

biphasic single-injection 64-section CT angiography. Radiology. 2007;243(2):368–76.
4. Feuchtner GM, Dichtl W, Friedrich GJ, et al. Multislice computed tomography for detection of patients with aortic valve stenosis and quantification of severity. J Am Coll Cardiol. 2006;47(7):1410–7.
5. Shah RG, Novaro GM, Blandon RJ, Whiteman MS, Asher CR, Kirsch J. Aortic valve area: meta-analysis of diagnostic performance of multi-detector computed tomography for aortic valve area measurements as compared to transthoracic echocardiography. Int J Cardiovasc Imaging. 2009;25(6):601–9.
6. Ropers D, Ropers U, Marwan M, Schepis T, Pflederer T, Wechsel M, Klinghammer L, Flachskampf FA, Daniel WG, Achenbach S. Comparison of dual-source computed tomography for the quantification of the aortic valve area in patients with aortic stenosis versus transthoracic echocardiography and invasive hemodynamic assessment. Am J Cardiol. 2009;104(11):1561–7.
7. Li X, Tang L, Zhou L, Duan Y, Yanhui S, Yang R, Wu Y, Kong X. Aortic valves stenosis and regurgitation: assessment with dual source computed tomography. Int J Cardiovasc Imaging. 2009;25(6):591–600.
8. Rosenhek R, Binder T, Porenta G, et al. Predictors of outcome in severe, asymptomatic aortic stenosis. N Engl J Med. 2000;343:611–61.
9. Pibarot P, Clavel MA. Management of paradoxical low-flow, low-gradient aortic stenosis: need for an integrated approach, including assessment of symptoms, hypertension, and stenosis severity. J Am Coll Cardiol. 2015;65(1):67–71.
10. Alkadhi H, Leschka S, Trindade PT, Feuchtner G, Stolzmann P, Plass A, Baumueller S. Cardiac CT for the differentiation of bicuspid and tricuspid aortic valves: comparison with echocardiography and surgery. AJR Am J Roentgenol. 2010;195(4):900.
11. Murphy DJ, McEvoy SH, Iyengar S, Feuchtner G, Cury RC, Roobottom C, Baumueller S, Alkadhi H, Dodd JD. Bicuspid aortic valves: diagnostic accuracy of standard axial 64-slice chest CT compared to aortic valve image plane ECG-gated cardiac CT. Eur J Radiol. 2014;83(8):1396–401.
12. Gouveia S, Martins JD, Costa G, Paramés F, Freitas I, Rebelo M, Trigo C, F Pinto F. Quadricuspid aortic valve - 10-year case series and literature review. Rev Port Cardiol. 2011;30(11):849–54.
13. Alkadhi H, Desbiolles L, Husmann L, Plass A, Leschka S, Scheffel H, Vachenauer R, Schepis T, Gaemperli O, Flohr TG, Genoni M, Marincek B, Jenni R, Kaufmann PA, Frauenfelder T. Aortic regurgitation: assessment with 64-section CT. Radiology. 2007;245(1):111–21.
14. Feuchtner GM, Dichtl W, Müller S, et al. 64-MDCT for diagnosis of aortic regurgitation in patients referred to CT coronary angiography. Am J Roentgenol. 2008;191:W1–7.
15. Feuchtner GM, Spoeck A, Lessick J, Dichtl W, Plass A, Leschka S, Mueller S, Klauser A, Scheffel H, Wolf F, Jaschke W, Alkadhi H. Quantification of aortic regurgitant fraction and volume with multi-detector computed tomography comparison with echocardiography. Acad Radiol. 2011;18(3):334–42.
16. Messika-Zeitoun D, Serfaty JM, Laissy JP, et al. Assessment of the mitral valve area in patients with mitral stenosis by multislice computed tomography. J Am Coll Cardiol. 2006;48:411–3.
17. Alkadhi H, Wildermuth S, Bettex DA. Mitral regurgitation: quantification with 16-detector row CT—initial experience. Radiology. 2006;238:454–63.
18. Delgado V, Tops L, Schujif JD, De Roos A, Brugada J, Schalij MJ, Thomas JD, Bax JJ. Assessment of mitral valve anatomy and geometry with multislice computed tomography. J Am Coll Cardiol Img. 2009;2(5):556–65.
19. Feuchtner G, Alkadhi H, Karlo C, et al. Cardiac CT angiography for the diagnosis of mitral valve prolapse: comparison with echocardiography. Radiology. 2010;254:374–83.
20. Srivatsa SS, Taylor MD, Hor K, Collins DA, King-Strunk M, Pelberg RA, Mazur W. Liquefaction necrosis of mitral annular calcification (LNMAC): review of pathology, prevalence, imaging and management: proposed diagnostic imaging criteria with detailed multi-modality and MRI image characterization. Int J Cardiovasc Imaging. 2012;28(5):1161–71. https://doi.org/10.1007/s10554-011-9935-x. Epub 24 Aug 2011.
21. Feuchtner GM, Stolzmann P, Dichtl W, et al. Multislice computed tomography in infective endocarditis: comparison with transesophageal echocardiography and intraoperative findings. J Am Coll Cardiol. 2009;53(5):436–44.
22. S M, Hangler H, Feuchtner G, Bartel T. Multimodality imaging reveals regurgitant jet lesion in aneurysmal anterior mitral leaflet: a severe complication of endocarditis. Eur Heart J. 2014;35(10):623.
23. Lalani T, Chu VH, Park LP, Cecchi E, Corey GR, Durante-Mangoni E, Fowler VG Jr, Gordon D, Grossi P, Hannan M, Hoen B, Muñoz P, Rizk H, Kanj SS, Selton-Suty C, Sexton DJ, Spelman D, Ravasio V, Tripodi MF, Wang A, International Collaboration on Endocarditis–Prospective Cohort Study Investigators. In-hospital and 1-year mortality in patients undergoing early surgery for prosthetic valve endocarditis. JAMA Intern Med. 2013;173(16):1495–504.
24. Egbe AC, Pislaru SV, Pellikka PA, et al. Bioprosthetic valve thrombosis versus structural failure: clinical and echocardiographic predictors. J Am Coll Cardiol. 2015;66(21):2285–94.
25. Makkar RR, Fontana G, Jilaihawi H, et al. Possible subclinical leaflet thrombosis in bioprosthetic aortic valves. N Engl J Med. 2015;373(21):2015–24.
26. Bettencourt N, Rocha J, Carvalho M, Leite D, Toschke AM, Melica B, Santos L, Rodrigues A, Gonçalves M, Braga P, Teixeira M, Simões L, Rajagopalan S, Gama V. Multislice computed tomography in the exclusion of coronary artery disease in patients with presurgical valve disease. Circ Cardiovasc Imaging. 2009;2(4):306–13.
27. Tsai IC, Lin YK, Chang Y, Fu YC, Wang CC, Hsieh SR, Wei HJ, Tsai HW, Jan SL, Wang KY, Chen MC, Chen CC. Correctness of multi-detector-row computed tomography for diagnosing mechanical prosthetic heart valve disorders using operative findings as a gold standard. Eur Radiol. 2009;19(4):857–67.
28. Symersky P, Budde RP, de Mol BA, Prokop M. Comparison of multidetector-row computed tomography to echocardiography and fluoroscopy for evaluation of patients with mechanical prosthetic valve obstruction. Am J Cardiol. 2009;104(8):1128–34.
29. Fagman E, Perrotta S, Bech-Hanssen O, Flinck A, Lamm C, Olaison L, Svensson G. ECG-gated computed tomography: a new role for patients with suspected aortic prosthetic valve endocarditis. Eur Radiol. 2012;22(11):2407–14.
30. Habets J, Tanis W, Reitsma JB, van den Brink RB, Mali WP, Chamuleau SA, Budde RP. Are novel non-invasive imaging techniques needed in patients with suspected prosthetic heart valve endocarditis? A systematic review and meta-analysis. Eur Radiol. 2015;25(7):2125–33.
31. Feuchtner G, Plank F, Mueller S, Schachner T, Bonaros N, Burghard P, Wolf F, Alhassan D, Blanke P, Leipsic J, Alkadhi H, Plass A, Spandorfer A, Felmly LM, De Cecco CN, Schoepf UJ. Cardiac computed tomography angiography for evaluation of prosthetic valve dysfunction. JACC Cardoivasc Imaging. 2017;10(1):91–3.
32. Gündüz S, Özkan M, Kalçik M, Gürsoy OM, Astarcioğlu MA, Karakoyun S, Aykan AÇ, Biteker M, Gökdeniz T, Kaya H, Yesin M, Duran NE, Sevinç D, Güneysu T. Sixty-four-section cardiac computed tomography in mechanical prosthetic heart valve dysfunction: thrombus or pannus. Circ Cardiovasc Imaging. 2015;8(12):e003246.
33. Tanis W, Habets J, van den Brink RB, Symersky P, Budde RP, Chamuleau SA. Differentiation of thrombus from pannus as the cause of acquired mechanical prosthetic heart valve obstruction by non-invasive imaging: a review of the literature. Eur Heart J Cardiovasc Imaging. 2014;15(2):119–29.

34. Saby L, Laas O, Habib G, Cammilleri S, Mancini J, Tessonnier L, Casalta JP, Gouriet F, Riberi A, Avierinos JF, Collart F, Mundler O, Raoult D, Thuny F. Positron emission tomography/computed tomography for diagnosis of prosthetic valve endocarditis: increased valvular (18)F-fluorodeoxyglucose uptake as a novel major criterion. J Am Coll Cardiol. 2013;61(23):2374–82.
35. Chenot F, Montant P, Goffinet C, Pasquet A, Vancraeynest D, Coche E, Vanoverschelde JL, Gerber BL. Evaluation of anatomic valve opening and leaflet morphology in aortic valve bioprosthesis by using multidetector CT: comparison with transthoracic echocardiography. Radiology. 2010;255(2):377–85.
36. Suchá D, Symersky P, Vonken EJ, Provoost E, Chamuleau SA, Budde RP. Multidetector-row computed tomography allows accurate measurement of mechanical prosthetic heart valve leaflet closing angles compared with fluoroscopy. J Comput Assist Tomogr. 2014;38(3):451–6.
37. Symersky P, Habets J, Westers P, de Mol BA, Prokop M, Budde RP. Prospective ECG triggering reduces prosthetic heart valve-induced artefacts compared with retrospective ECG gating on 256-slice CT. Eur Radiol. 2012;22(6):1271–7.
38. Suchá D, Willemink MJ, de Jong PA, Schilham AM, Leiner T, Symersky P, Budde RP. The impact of a new model-based iterative reconstruction algorithm on prosthetic heart valve related artifacts at reduced radiation dose MDCT. Int J Cardiovasc Imaging. 2014;30(4):785–93.

40 Cardiac Devices

Ian R. Drexler, Alan C. Legasto, Daniel B. Green, and Quynh A. Truong

Intracardiac devices and implants are commonly encountered in cardiac diagnostic imaging. These may range from prosthetic heart valves to ventricular assist devices. Familiarity by the interpreting physician with the normal and abnormal appearance of each device is essential for proper detection of device complications. While devices may be detected via computed tomography, beam hardening and streak artifacts may limit their full appearance, which is why it is important to know both the cross-sectional appearance and the scout or radiographic appearance of a device. This chapter reviews the normal appearance of common intracardiac devices as well as well as frequently seen artifacts.

Prosthetic Heart Valves and Valve Closure

Since the introduction of valve replacement surgery in the 1960s, approximately 90,000 valve substitutes have been implanted in the United States, and 280,000 have been implanted worldwide each year [1]. Currently, valves are classified as either mechanical, bioprosthetic, or percutaneous. The patient's age and surgical risk typically dictate what type of valve is placed.

Mechanical Heart Valves

Mechanical valves were the first type of prosthetic valve used clinically. They are designed to last many years, though require lifelong anticoagulation due to risk of clot formation [2]. Thus, in younger patients who will require a functioning valve for several decades, the mechanical heart valve is preferred. Mechanical heart valves may be either caged ball, single tilting disc, or bileaflet [3].

I. R. Drexler · A. C. Legasto · D. B. Green · Q. A. Truong (✉)
Department of Radiology, Weill Cornell Medicine,
New York, NY, USA
e-mail: qat9001@med.cornell.edu

Caged Ball Mechanical Heart Valve

The caged ball mechanical heart valve (Fig. 40.1) was the original type of prosthetic heart valve used. The Starr-Edwards valve was the first such valve, initially used as a prosthetic mitral valve. Although the caged ball valve is no longer used, thousands of patients still have them, so it is important to be familiar with their appearance [1]. In the closed position, the ball, or poppet, is at the base of the cage, creating a seal to prevent retrograde blood flow. Conversely, the ball is near the apex when it is open, allowing forward flow. The position of the poppet depends on the pressure differential between the two chambers the valve is traversing. A disadvantage of this design is that blood must be pumped around the ball, rather than centrally, which forces the left ventricle to work harder. It is important to note that the ball in the caged ball valve may be either radiolucent or radiopaque depending on the poppet material.

Single Tilting Disc and Bileaflet Mechanical Heart Valves

The single tilting disc valve offers advantages over the caged ball valve, including improved hemodynamics and structural stability. It consists of a metallic ring with a single circular disc connected via metal struts [4]. Like the caged ball valve, the disc opens when the pressure of one chamber exceeds that of the more distal chamber, such as when the left ventricular pressure exceeds aortic pressure during ventricular systole. However, risks of this type of valve include potential severe hemodynamic instability due to either pannus formation or valve thrombosis. For this reason, bileaflet valves are now the most commonly inserted mechanical valve [3].

Bileaflet Mechanical Valve

The bileaflet mechanical valve (Fig. 40.2) is composed of two semicircular discs that pivot about mechanical struts. This design provides improved hemodynamic flow compared to the tilting disc and caged ball valves, though it is susceptible to regurgitation.

U. J. Schoepf (ed.), *CT of the Heart*, Contemporary Medical Imaging, https://doi.org/10.1007/978-1-60327-237-7_40

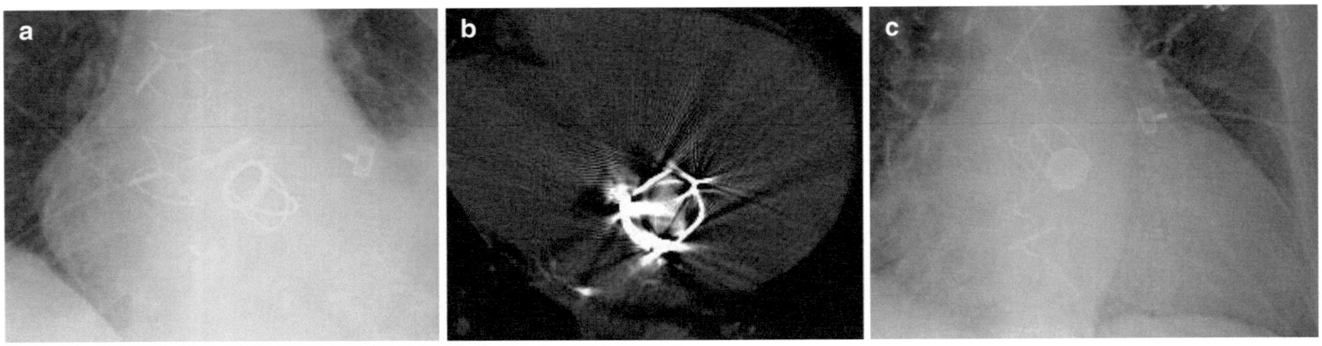

Fig. 40.1 Caged ball mechanical valve: Frontal radiograph (**a**) demonstrates the typical appearance of a caged ball mitral valve replacement. On CT transaxial imaging (**b**), the cage causes metallic beam hardening artifact, making evaluation limited. The caged ball device has also been used as an aortic valve replacement, as seen in a frontal chest radiograph (**c**)

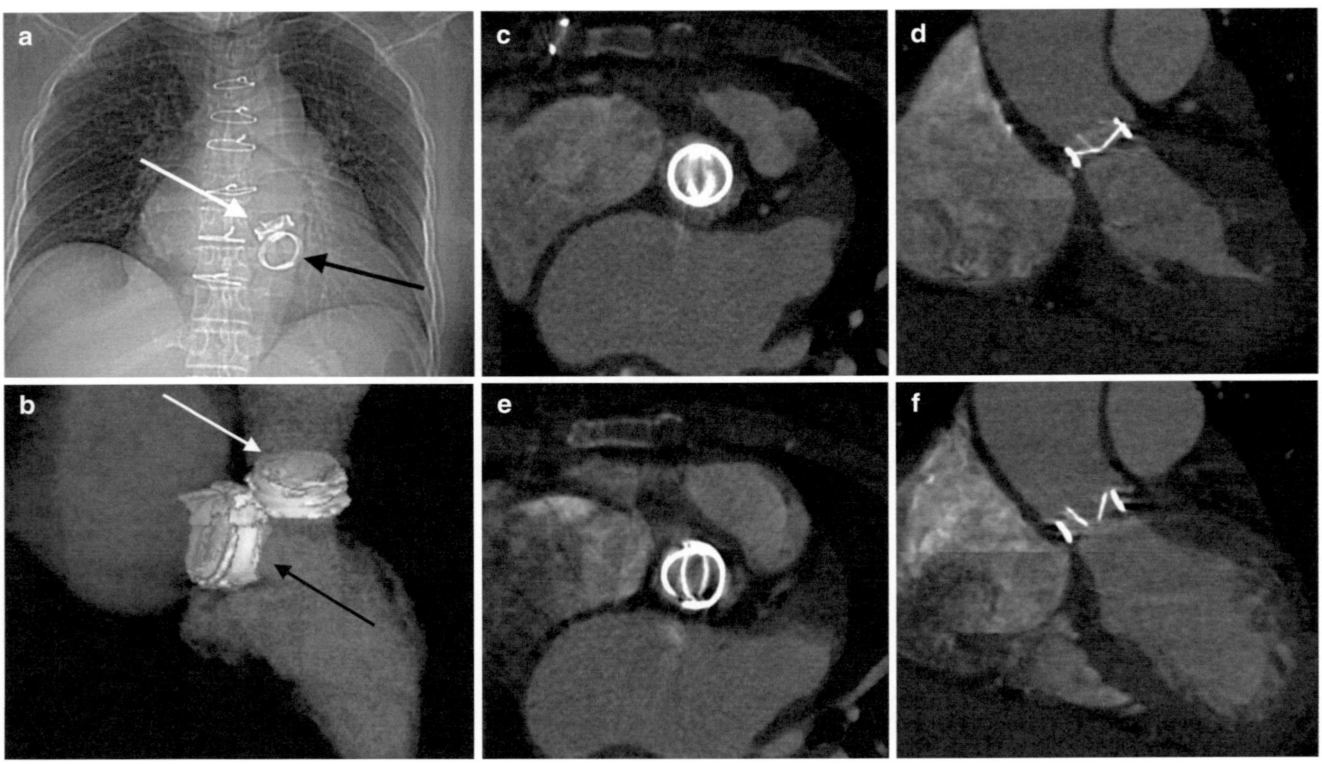

Fig. 40.2 Bileaflet mechanical valve: Scout image (**a**) and volume-rendered image (**b**) demonstrate mechanical valves in the aortic (*white arrow*) and mitral (*black arrow*) positions. Axial (**c**) and (**d**) coronal CT images show a bileaflet mechanical aortic valve in the closed position as during ventricular diastole and in the open position (**e**, **f**) as during ventricular systole

Bioprosthetic Valves

A major advantage of using bioprosthetic valves (Fig. 40.3) over mechanical valves is the lower incidence of antithromboembolic-related hemorrhages. Conversely, a disadvantage is the decreased longevity of the bioprosthetic valve due to a combination of tissue degeneration and calcification [5]. For these reasons, bioprosthetic valves can be used in elderly patients, who do not need their valves to last as long as younger patients' valves and who are at risk of falls, which can lead to major bleeding events if using anticoagulation.

Bovine pericardial prostheses, a type of bioprosthetic valve, have been used for aortic valve replacements (AVR) since the first-generation valves were introduced in the early 1970s. The second-generation valves, such as the Carpentier-

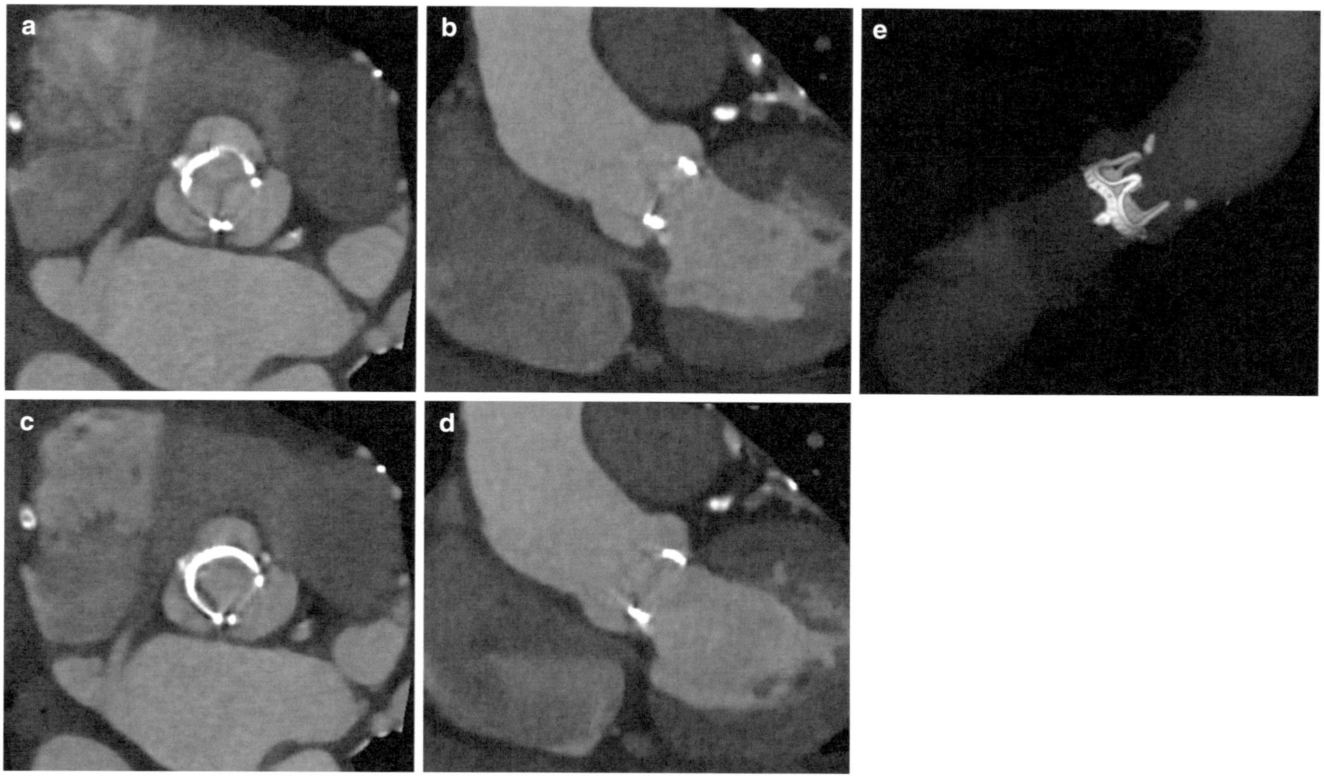

Fig. 40.3 Bioprosthetic aortic valve: CT images demonstrate en face and coronal views of a bioprosthetic aortic valve in the closed position (**a**, **b**) and in the open position (**c**, **d**). A volume-rendered image (**e**) demonstrates the bioprosthetic valve in place

Edwards pericardial bioprosthesis, allowed for a more advanced method of leaf mounting, resulting in more symmetrical opening of the valve compared to its first-generation predecessor [6].

Percutaneous Heart Valves

Most recent advancement in percutaneous interventions for structural heart disease includes transcatheter aortic valve replacement (TAVR) for severe aortic stenosis and percutaneous mitral clip for severe mitral regurgitation. Less commonly performed is transcatheter pulmonary valve implantation for congenital heart disease patients with right ventricular outflow tract (RVOT) dysfunction, either severe pulmonic stenosis or regurgitation, to minimize the number of open-heart surgeries over their lifetimes.

Transcatheter Aortic Valve Replacement [TAVR]

Aortic stenosis is the most common valvular heart disease. Patients with aortic stenosis develop increased left ventricular wall thickness and contractility, resulting in decreased diastolic compliance and myocardial fibrosis. In some cases, sudden cardiac death may result as a consequence of arrhythmias, low cardiac output, and ischemia. Transcatheter aortic valve replacement (TAVR) was developed as a treatment for those patients who are not surgical candidates for standard aortic valve replacements. The device is delivered arterially and is opened within the diseased aortic valve, displacing and replacing it [7].

Cardiac CT is typically obtained prior to TAVR placement for planning purposes. Important measurements to take include aortic annular size, the distance between the annulus and coronary ostia, and aortic valve area. The number of cusps and degree of cusp calcification should also be assessed. In addition to imaging of the heart, the aorta and iliofemoral arterial vessels are assessed for their dimensions and degree of atherosclerosis, which helps plan the interventional approach [8]. More recently, TAVRs have been used on patients who have had prior aortic valve replacements that have failed, creating a valve in valve. Post-TAVR CT (Fig. 40.4) may be obtained to evaluate for complications or causes of device failure (Fig. 40.5), which include periprosthetic aortic regurgitation, prosthetic endocarditis, valve migration, and valve injury [9, 10].

Mitral Valve Clip

Mitral regurgitation (MR) is the second most common valvular heart disease after aortic stenosis. If untreated, severe MR can lead to left ventricular failure, pulmonary hypertension, atrial fibrillation, and death. Nearly half of patients

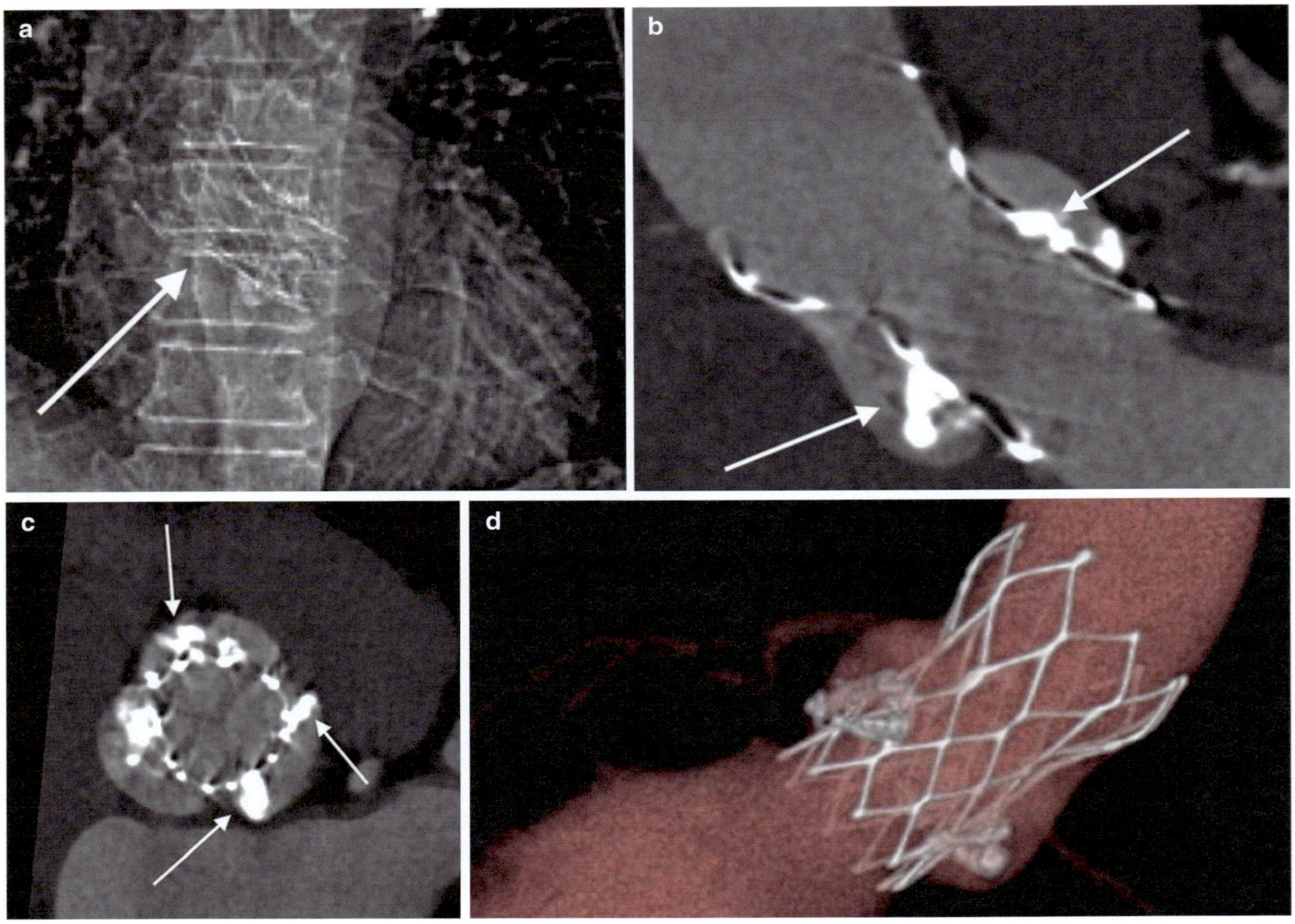

Fig. 40.4 Transcatheter aortic valve replacement (TAVR): Scout image (**a**) demonstrates the metallic TAVR overlying the spine (*white arrow*). En face (**b**) and sagittal (**c**) views demonstrate the TAVR on CT. Note the native aortic valve calcifications (*white arrows*) that have been peripherally displaced. Volume-rendered image (**d**) shows the valve in position

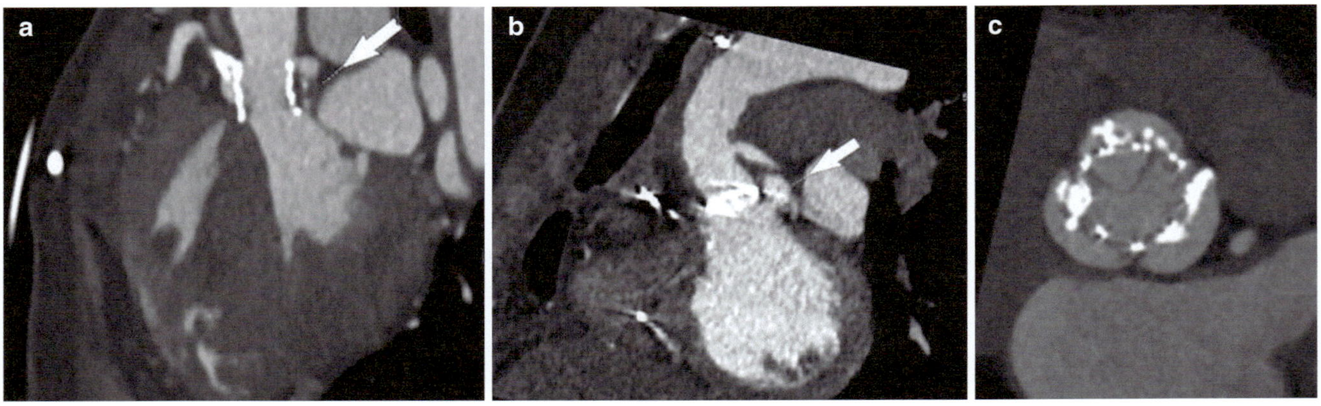

Fig. 40.5 TAVR complications: Multiplanar reformat CT images from three different patients demonstrate paravalvular leak (**a**), pseudoaneurysm formation (**b**), and restricted motion of the non-coronary cusp (**c**)

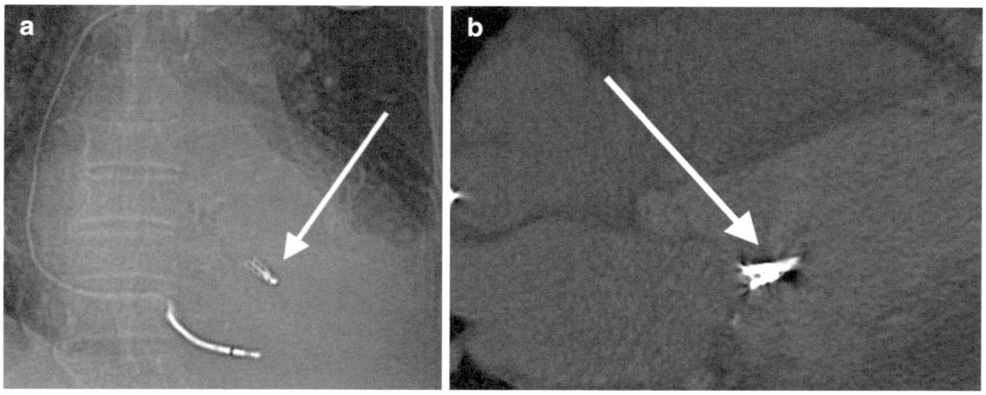

Fig. 40.6 Mitral Clip: Scout image (**a**) and four-chamber view CT slice (**b**) demonstrate a MitraClip device in place (*white arrows*)

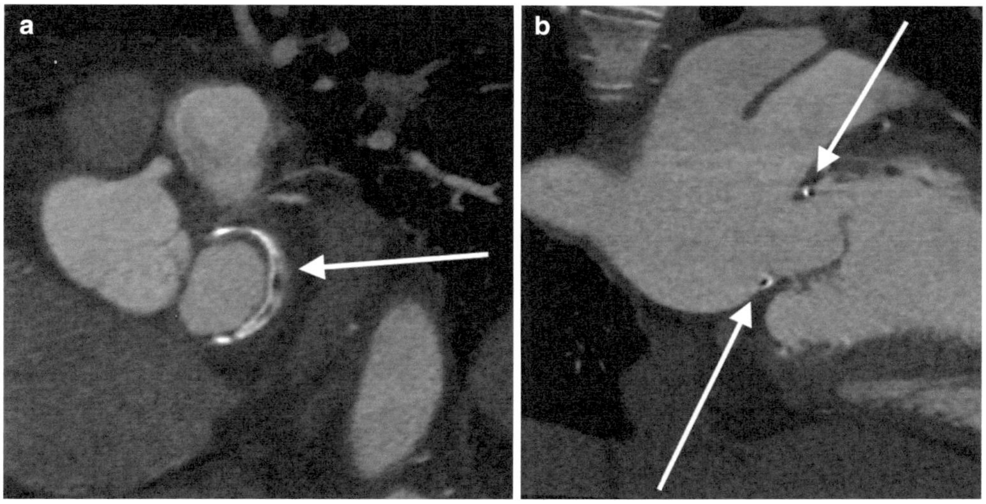

Fig. 40.7 Mitral valve annuloplasty: Multiplanar reformat CT images (**a**, **b**) show a mitral valve annuloplasty

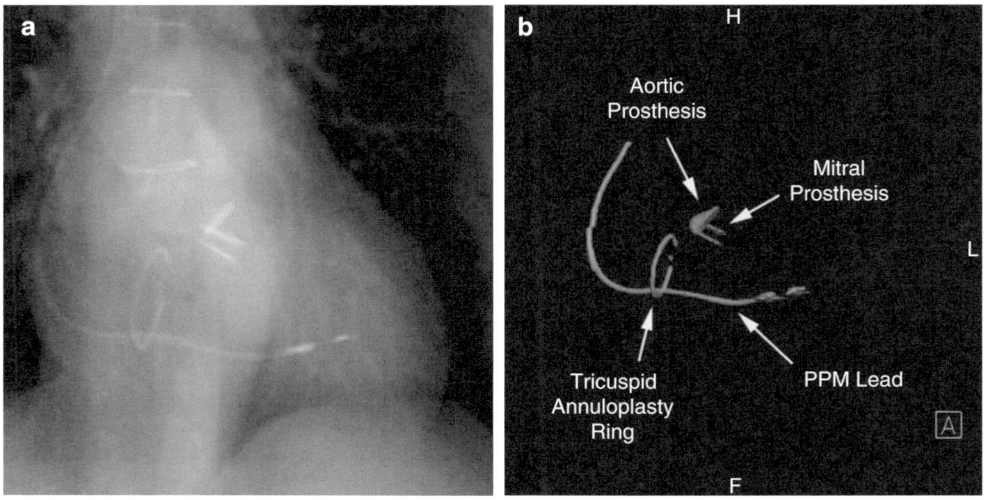

Fig. 40.8 Tricuspid annuloplasty: Chest radiograph (**a**) and volume-rendered image (**b**) demonstrate tricuspid annuloplasty as well as a pacemaker lead, mitral prosthesis, and aortic prosthesis

with MR in need of valve repair or replacement are considered high risk for surgical intervention. The MitraClip (Abbot Vascular, Abbot Park, IL) (Fig. 40.6) is a percutaneous method of repairing the mitral valve through mechanical coaptation of the mitral leaflets [11]. Potential risks include clip embolization and detachment from a single mitral leaflet [12].

Valvular Ring Annuloplasty

The concept of an annuloplasty (Figs. 40.7 and 40.8) first appeared in the 1950s. The idea that fixing the mitral annulus stems from the concept that functional mitral regurgitation is in part due to abnormal enlargement of the mitral annulus, which can lead to displacement of the normal coaptation between the anterior and posterior mitral leaflets [13]. Annuloplasty is commonly seen with repair of the tricuspid valve for severe tricuspid regurgitation. The annuloplasty ring is incomplete, to avoid interfering with the heart's sensitive conduction system. Complications of annuloplasty placement that can be assessed with CT include ring dehiscence and systolic anterior motion of the mitral valve [14].

Pacemakers, Implantable Cardioverter-Defibrillators, and Other EP Devices

Cardiac Rhythm Management Devices

Implantable pacemakers and implantable cardioverters-defibrillators are commonly seen on CT. It is often easier to assess the type of electrophysiologic device by looking at the scout view or, alternatively, a frontal radiograph, as metallic beam hardening artifact on cross-sectional images may cause confusion. The device's casing, or can, contains its software, hardware, and battery. The can, combined with the hardware, including the battery, capacitor, circuitry, and connector configuration, forms a fingerprint that is unique to each manufacturer, which facilitates identification on radiography [15]. There may be anywhere from one to three leads terminating in the heart, which defines single chamber, dual chamber, and biventricular devices. Risks of placement include infection, lead dislodgement, perforation, and clot formation.

Implantable Pacemakers

A single-chamber device (Fig. 40.9) is identified by the presence of a single lead terminating either within the right atrial appendage or right ventricle, whereas a dual-chamber device has two leads, typically terminating in the right atrium and right ventricle. Positioning of the right atrial and right ventricular leads are the same whether the device is a single- or dual-chamber system [16]. A biventricular device for cardiac resynchronization therapy (Figs. 40.10 and 40.11) has leads

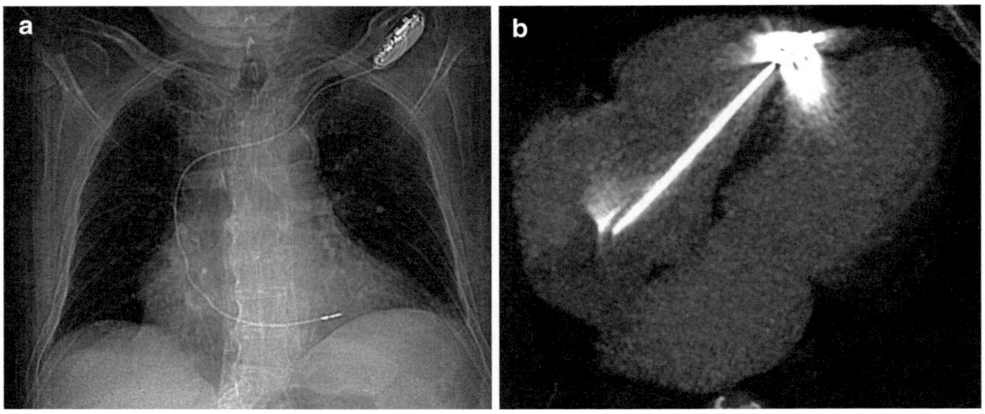

Fig. 40.9 Single-lead pacemaker: Scout frontal image (**a**) demonstrates a left chest wall single-lead pacemaker. A CT multiplanar reformat maximum intensity projection image (**b**) demonstrates the lead coursing from the right atrium and terminating in the right ventricular apex, where there is excessive metallic streak artifact

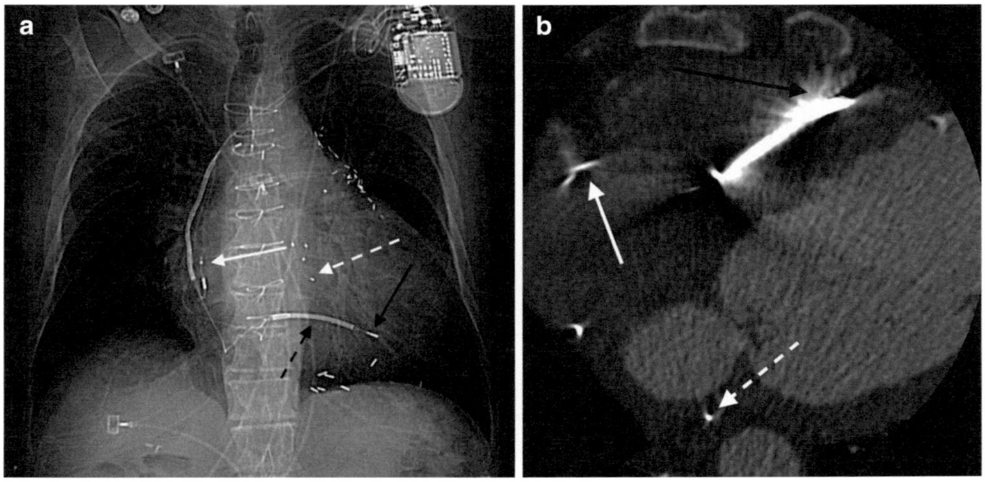

Fig. 40.10 Biventricular ICD/pacemaker: Scout image (**a**) demonstrates a biventricular ICD/pacemaker. The right ventricular lead terminates in the right ventricular apex (*solid black arrow*) and contains two shock coils (*dashed black arrow*). The left ventricular lead (*dashed white arrow*) enters the coronary sinus via the right atrium and terminates in one of its branches, such as the posterolateral branch. The right atrial lead (*solid white arrow*) terminates in the right atrial appendage. Axial CT image (**b**) demonstrates the same leads in the right ventricular apex (*solid black arrow*), right atrial appendage (*solid white arrow*), and the coronary sinus (*dashed white arrow*)

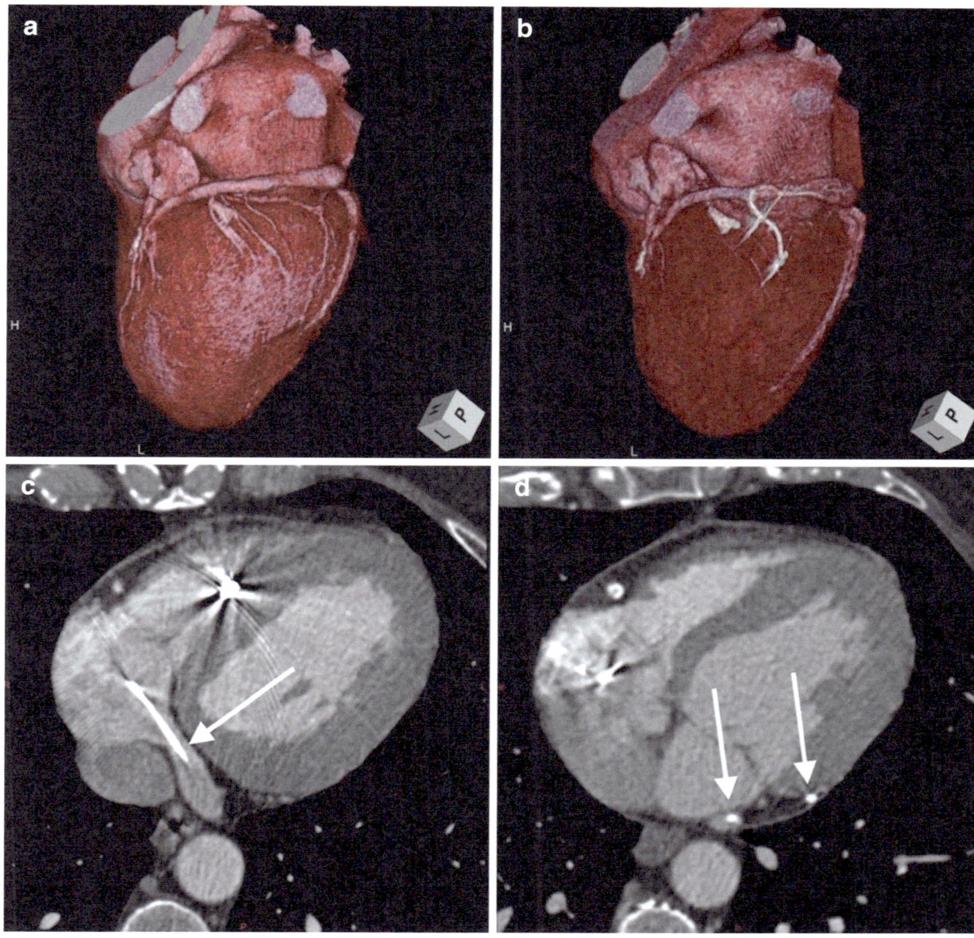

Fig. 40.11 Cardiac resynchronization therapy. Volume-rendered images before (**a**) and after (**b**) placement of a left ventricular lead into a branch of the coronary sinus. Axial cardiac CT images (**c**, **d**) showing the LV lead (*arrows*) course from the right atrium and into the coronary sinus

at the right atrial appendage, right ventricle, and a branch of the coronary sinus to pace the left ventricle.

Subcutaneous ICD

Patients who require an ICD over decades may require one or more lead extractions and replacements, each with a risk for morbidity. The presence of the lead itself in the vasculature imposes its own risks, including occlusion and infection. For these reasons, subcutaneous ICD (Fig. 40.12) insertion has become more commonplace [17].

Leadless Pacemaker

The risks of complication from conventional pacemakers, including pocket hematoma, pneumothoraces, and vascular obstruction, have led to the rise of leadless pacemakers (Fig. 40.13). Leadless pacemakers are endovascularly inserted into the right ventricle, where they are affixed to the myocardium [18]. While measuring less than 1 cm^3 in volume, they possess the same functionality as conventional pacemakers.

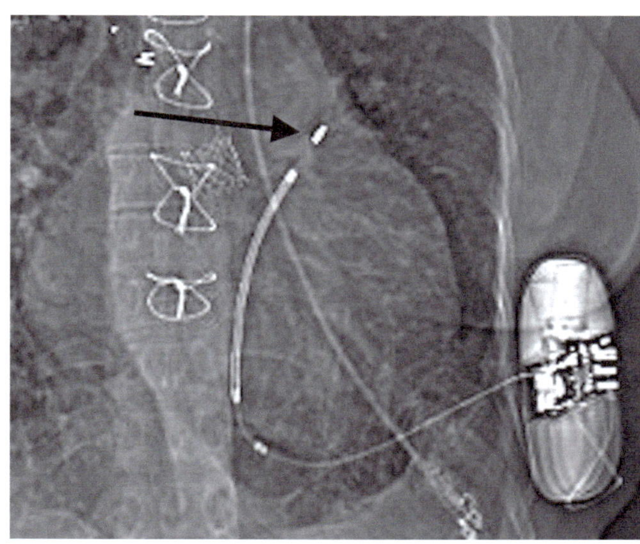

Fig. 40.12 Subcutaneous ICD: Scout image demonstrates a left chest wall subcutaneous ICD, with shock coil and lead tip (*arrow*) overlying the left heart shadow

Implantable Loop Recorder

The implantable loop recorder (ILR) (Fig. 40.14) is a single-lead ECG monitor that is subcutaneously inserted into the patient. The device stores ECG data either in response to patient activation or to a significant arrhythmia [19]. The battery lasts several years, and insertion is used for patients with unexplained syncope or with arrhythmias that may not be captured using shorter term ECG monitoring, such as with a Holter monitor [20]. The procedure is minimally invasive, with minimal risk of site infection and hematoma.

Atrial Septal and Ventricular Septal Closure Devices

Numerous devices have been used for closure of atrial and ventricular septal defects. The Amplatzer septal occluder (ASO) (St Jude Medical, St Paul, MN) is a percutaneously placed, self-expanding device that is used to close an ASD or, depending on the size, a VSD or PDA. The ASO (Figs. 40.15 and 40.16) is composed of a braided nitinol wire mesh and is shaped into two flat discs connected at a waist [21, 22]. The size of the occluder is dependent upon the size of the defect it is meant to close. With good positioning across an ASD, the left atrial disc will be in the left atrium, and the right atrial disc will be in the right atrium. An appropriately sized device should be disc-shaped, rather than mushroom-shaped [23]. An ASD or VSD may present with signs of left-to-right shunt, with symptoms typically worsening with larger defects and, in turn, larger pulmonary to systemic shunt fractions (Qp/Qs).

Additional occluders include the CardioSEAL septal occluder and the Gore Helex septal occluder. The CardioSEAL septal occluder was developed as an updated design of the double-umbrella device (Clamshell occluder) [24]. The Gore Helex septal occluder (HSO) is composed of polytetrafluorethylene membrane connected by a nitinol wire. Like the ASO, the Gore HSO has a double-disc shape [22].

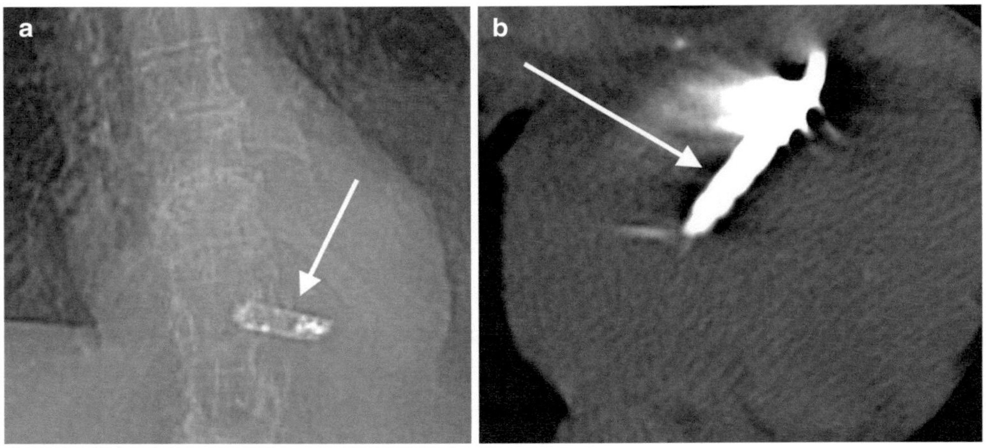

Fig. 40.13 Leadless pacemaker: Scout image (**a**) and axial CT (**b**) demonstrate the typical appearance and position of leadless pacemaker (*arrows*), which is inserted into the right ventricular apex. Extensive metallic beam hardening artifact on CT limits evaluation of the device itself, but its position and location are easily discernable

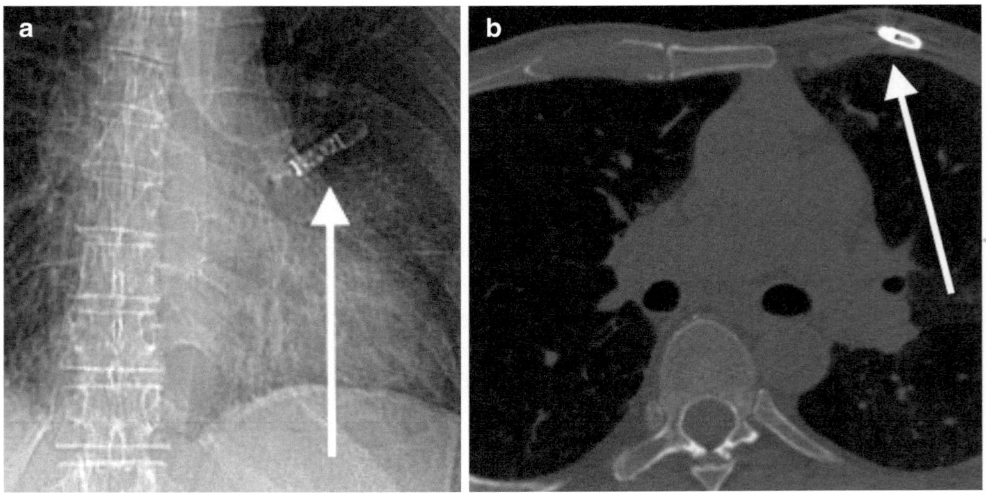

Fig. 40.14 Implantable loop recorder: Scout (**a**) and axial CT (**b**) images demonstrate implantable loop recorder (*arrows*), which is implanted in the subcutaneous tissues of the left anterior chest wall

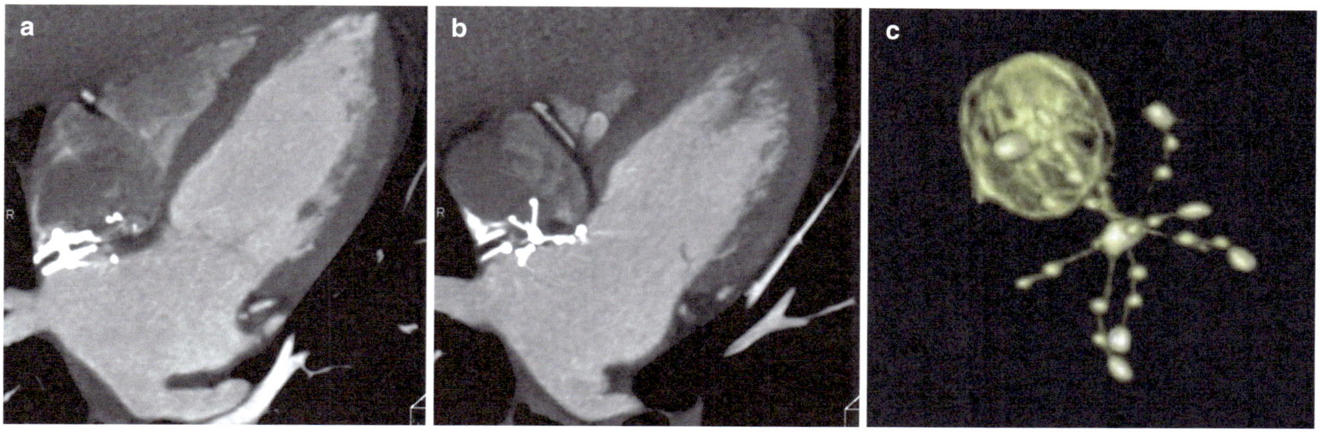

Fig. 40.15 Redo PFO closure: CT multiplanar reformat image (**a**) demonstrates an Amplatzer septal occluder that was placed to close off a patent foramen ovale after a CardioSEAL occluder (**b**) failed. A volume-rendered image (**c**) shows both devices together

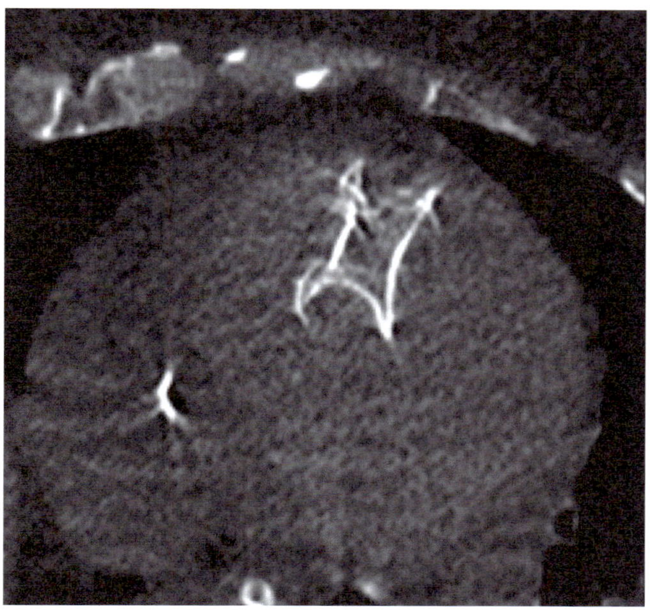

Fig. 40.16 Amplatzer septal occluder: Axial CT image demonstrates an Amplatzer septal occluder traversing the interatrial septum at the site of an atrial septal defect

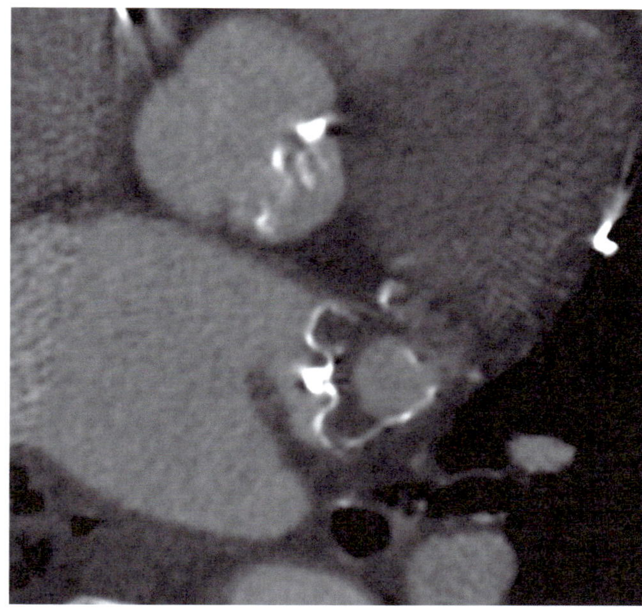

Fig. 40.17 WATCHMAN: A multiplanar reformat CT image demonstrates a WATCHMAN device in a patient's left atrial appendage. Note that there is thrombus contained within the WATCHMAN, which is preventing the thrombus from potentially embolizing into the systemic circulation, which could lead to cerebral infarction

Left Atrial Appendage Devices

Atrial fibrillation (AF) affects as many as 6 million people in the United States. Due to the increased risk of embolic stroke, which is thought to most often arise from thrombi in the left atrial appendage (LAA), patients are often kept on long-term anticoagulation therapy [25]. Prior to placing an atrial appending closure device, such as a WATCHMAN or LARIAT, a cardiac CT is performed to interrogate the left atrial appendage's anatomy, including its shape, size, and position relative to the pulmonary artery [26].

WATCHMAN Device

The WATCHMAN device (Boston Scientific, Natick, MA) (Fig. 40.17) is a self-expanding device designed for LAA closure. It is composed of a nitinol structure covered by a porous polyethylene terephthalate membrane. The device is introduced via a vascular sheath inserted into the femoral vein, and has the means to cross through the interatrial septum [26, 27]. Complications of the WATCHMAN device placement include device failure secondary to incomplete closure, infection, pericardial effusion, air embolism, thrombus formation during implantation, device embolization, and leak [28].

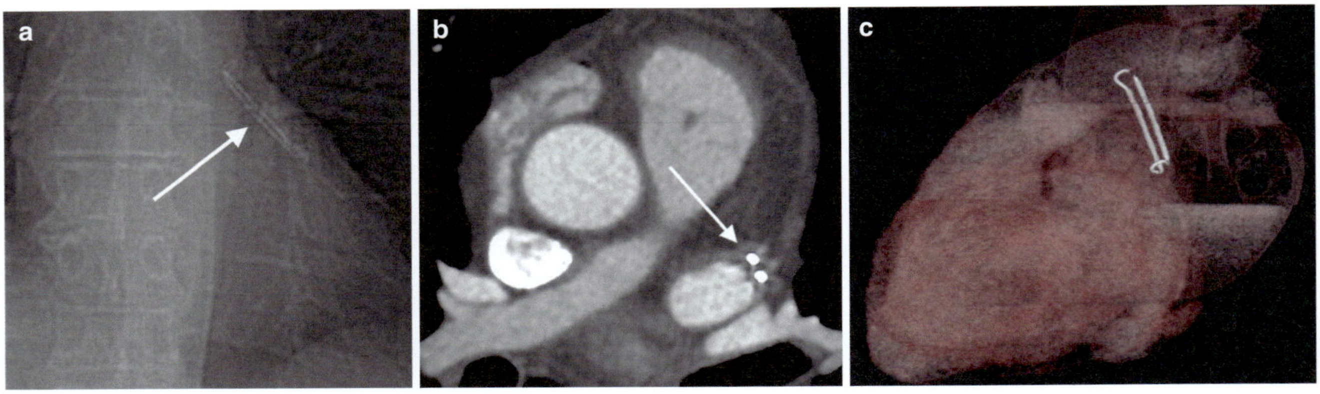

Fig. 40.18 AtriCure Clip: Scout image (**a**) demonstrates an AtriCure Clip (*arrow*), which is also seen on cross-sectional CT (**b**) and on volume-rendered imaging (**c**)

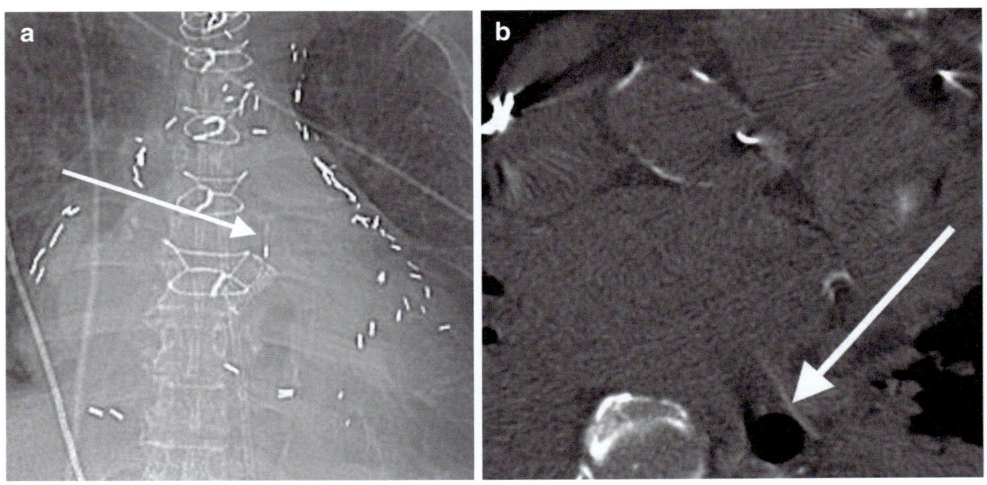

Fig. 40.19 Intra-aortic balloon pump: An intra-aortic balloon pump (IABP) tip is seen on a scout image (**a**). Note that it is the only radiopaque portion seen overlying the heart (*arrow*). Axial CT (**b**) demonstrates the balloon filled with air in the descending thoracic aorta (*arrow*)

AtriCure Clip

An AtriCure Clip (Fig. 40.18) is an atrial appendage excluder that is placed epicardially at the base of the appendage. It is composed of two parallel titanium tubes with elastic nitinol springs. Complications of placement include occlusion of the circumflex coronary artery and pulmonary arteries, bleeding, incomplete LAA closure, and device migration [29].

LARIAT Device

The LARIAT snare device (SentreHEART, Redwood City, CA) uses a transcatheter approach to exclude the LAA in patients with AF. The device utilizes magnetic-based guidewires in the LAA and pericardial space to capture and close off the LAA at its ostium, under fluoroscopic and echocardiographic guidance [30]. Contraindications to LARIAT placement include pericardial thickening, calcification, or adhesions which can interfere with pericardial access, a LAA width of >40 mm, a retro-pulmonary artery, pectus excavatum, and a posteriorly rotated heart [31].

Circulator Assist Devices

Short-Term

IABP

Since 1967, when the first intra-aortic balloon pump (IABP) was used, the IABP (Fig. 40.19) has become a ubiquitous circulatory support device in hospitals. During ventricular diastole, the balloon is inflated in the descending thoracic aorta, augmenting perfusion of the coronary arteries and cerebral circulation. Collapse during systole creates negative intra-aortic pressure, which decreases afterload and in turn reduces heart strain [32–34]. The distal tip of the IABP is radiopaque, allowing for its position to be easily detectible on radiography. If the balloon is too proximal within the aorta, it can occlude the great vessels, resulting in cerebral infarction or upper extremity ischemia. If the balloon is too distal, it can occlude the superior mesenteric arteries, resulting in bowel ischemia, or the renal arteries, resulting in renal failure. Thus, the ideal position of the balloon tip is 2–4 cm distal to the left subclavian artery.

Impella and TandemHeart

For years, the only mechanical circulatory device in use was the intra-aortic balloon pump. More recently, several devices have come to the market. The Impella (Abiomed, Danvers, MA) is a nonpulsatile axial flow pump used to move blood from the left ventricle into the ascending aorta. The Impella (Fig. 40.20) is typically placed into the femoral artery, either percutaneously or via surgical cutdown [35].

The TandemHeart (Cardiac Assist, Inc., Pittsburgh, PA) is a percutaneously placed mechanical circulatory assist device that creates a left atrium to femoral artery bypass. An inflow cannula is placed into the femoral artery and advanced into the left atrium via a transseptal puncture. Oxygenated blood is then pumped into the contralateral femoral artery. This results in reduced cardiac workload and oxygen demand [36].

Long-Term Assist Devices

Left ventricular assist devices (LVADs) have been used since the 1960s, initially to support patients who could not be weaned from cardiopulmonary bypass. Since that time, LVADs have evolved and today are on their third generation. The three situations LVADs are used today are as a bridge to heart transplantation, as destination therapy in patients who cannot undergo a heart transplant, and in patients who require myocardial recovery, such as after an episode of viral myocarditis [37]. First-generation LVADs utilized a pulsatile flow, while second-generation LVADs utilized continuous flow. The latter led to improved survival and decreased morbidity associated with first-generation LVADs, such as thromboembolism and ventricular arrhythmias [38]. Complications of LVADs are varied and include cannula obstruction, pericardial tamponade, thrombus formation, aortic stenosis and insufficiency, right-sided heart failure, and infection [39].

HeartWare Pump

The HeartWare (HeartWare Inc., Miami Lakes, FL) (Fig. 40.21) is a third-generation LVAD. Not only are the HeartWare and other third-generation LVADs smaller than their predecessors, but they also function better by utilizing

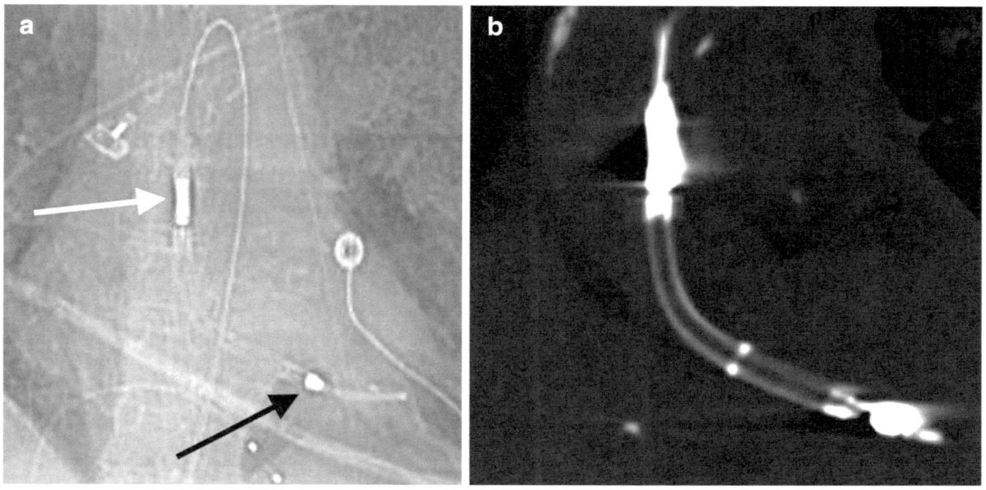

Fig. 40.20 Impella: Scout radiograph (**a**) demonstrates catheter in the aorta, attached to the Impella, which has radiopaque markers proximally (*white arrow*) and distally (*black arrow*). A multiplanar reformat CT image (**b**) shows what the Impella looks like in cross section

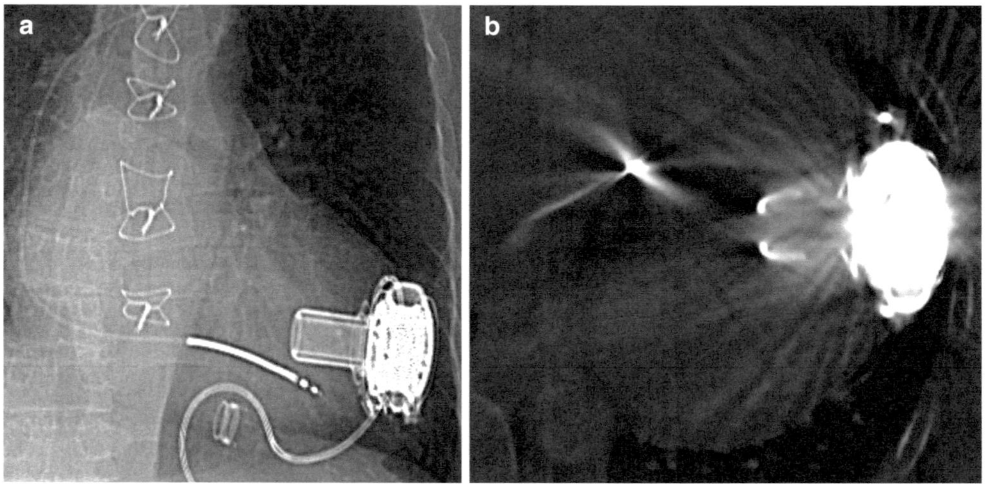

Fig. 40.21 HeartWare pump: Scout image (**a**) and axial CT image (**b**) demonstrate a normal appearance of the HeartWare pump in the LV apex

magnetic levitation [40]. The device consists of the pump, which is attached to a cuff at the left ventricular apex, and the outflow graft, which is attached to the ascending aorta.

HeartMate II

The HeartMate II (Thoratec Corp, Pleasanton, CA) (Fig. 40.22) is a second-generation, continuous flow LVAD [41]. The radiopaque inflow cannula, placed in the left ventricular apex, diverts blood from the left ventricle into the pump via the bend relief. The purpose of the bend relief is to allow the pump to be accommodated within the upper abdomen without kinking of the cannula. Note that the junction of the inflow cannula and bend relief is radiolucent. The blood exits the pump via the outflow cannula, which is anastomosed to the ascending aorta. The outflow cannula is often not visible on conventional radiography and scout CT images.

Other Devices

Swan-Ganz

The Swan-Ganz catheter (Fig. 40.23) is a pulmonary artery catheter that is used for hemodynamic monitoring [42]. The ideal position of the catheter tip is in either the left or right main pulmonary arteries. The tip should not go past the proximal interlobar pulmonary arteries, which extend approximately 2 cm from the hilum. Complications for placement of the catheter tip too distal include arterial occlusion leading to

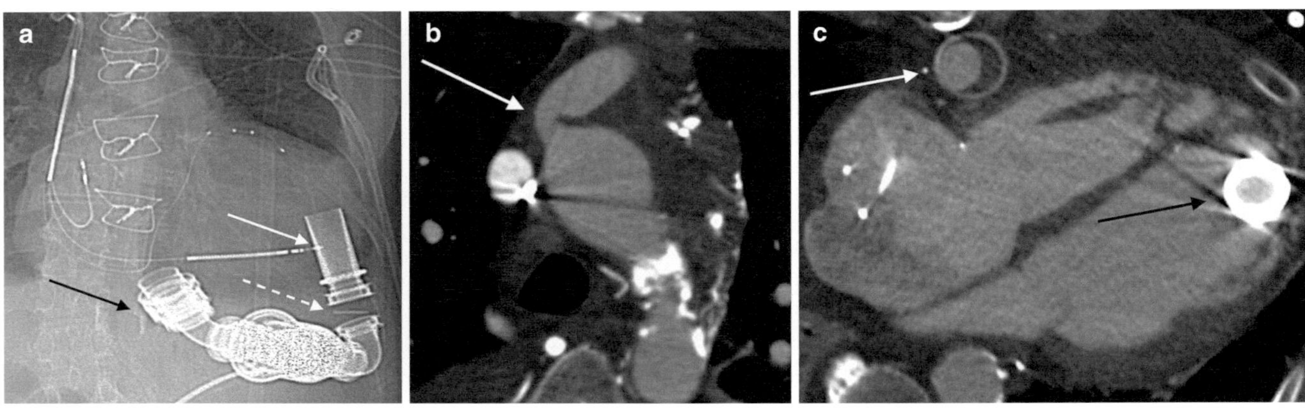

Fig. 40.22 HeartMate II: A scout image (**a**) shows the normal position of a HeartMate II LVAD. Notable structures include the inflow cannula (*white arrow*), bend relief (*white dashed arrow*), and outflow cannula (*black arrow*). Axial CT image (**b**) demonstrates the outflow cannula (*white arrow*) at the level of its anastomosis with the ascending aorta. An additional CT image (**c**) demonstrates the outflow cannula (*white arrow*) anterior the right atrioventricular groove and the inflow cannula (*black arrow*) in the left ventricular apex

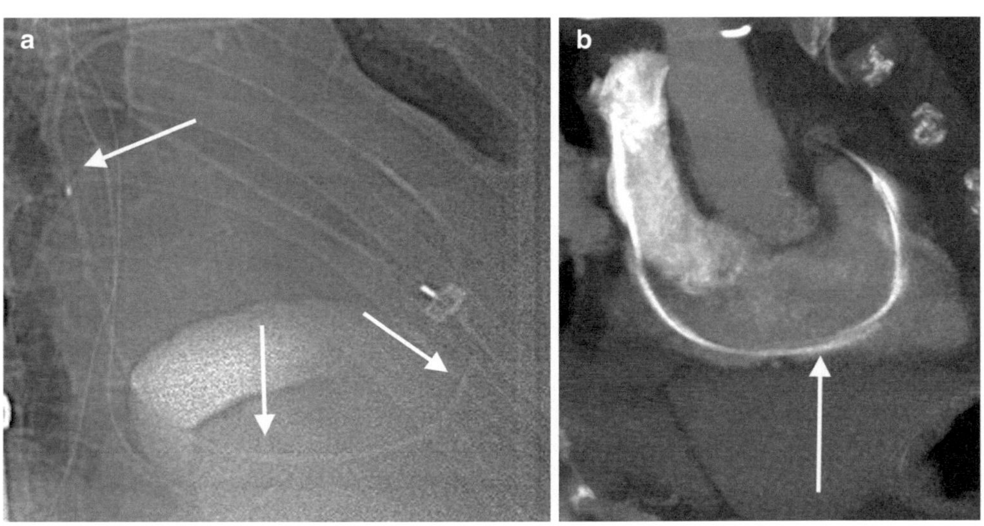

Fig. 40.23 Swan-Ganz catheter: Scout image (**a**) demonstrates a catheter (*white arrows*) overlying the left brachiocephalic vein and coursing into the superior vena cava, right atrium, right ventricle, and then right ventricular outflow tract. A CT maximum intensity projection multiplanar reformat image (**b**) demonstrates the same catheter in the SVC, right atrium, right ventricle, and right ventricular outflow tract

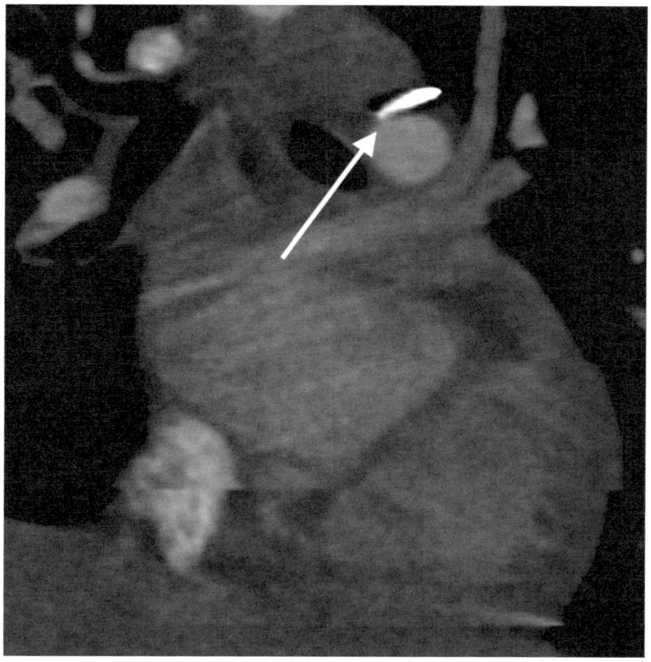

Fig. 40.24 PDA Clip: Multiplanar reformat CT image demonstrates a PDA clip (*arrow*) between the aortic arch and pulmonary artery

pulmonary infarction. Risks also include pulmonary artery rupture, pulmonary artery dissection, and pseudoaneurysm formation [43].

PDA Clip

A patent ductus arteriosus (PDA) (Fig. 40.24) is the persistent postnatal patency of an embryologic structure, the ductus arteriosus, which connects the pulmonary artery to the aorta, allowing for movement of oxygenated blood while in utero. Failure of the PDA to close after birth can lead to left-to-right shunting and, if untreated, can cause chronic strain on the heart, possibly resulting in Eisenmenger's syndrome. A PDA clip is a device that is surgically placed for permanent closure of the PDA [44], which can readily be seen in cardiac imaging.

Acknowledgments The authors would like to extend our gratitude to Benjamin W. Cobb for his assistance with imaging acquisition.

References

1. Pibarot P, Dumesnil JG. Prosthetic heart valves: selection of the optimal prosthesis and long-term management. Circulation. 2009;119:1034–48.
2. Habets J, Mali WPTM, Budde RPJ. Multidetector CT angiography in evaluation of prosthetic heart valve dysfunction. Radiographics. 2012;32:1893–905.
3. Tokunaga S, Tominaga R. Current status of the mechanical valve and bioprosthesis in Japan. J Artif Organs. 2008;11:53–9.
4. Pai GP, Ellison RG, Rubin JW, et al. Disc immobilization of Bjork-Shiley and Medtronic Hall valves during and immediately after valve replacement. Ann Thorac Surg. 1987;44:73–6.
5. Riess F-C, Bader R, Cramer E, et al. Hemodynamic performance of the Medtronic Mosaic porcine bioprosthesis up to ten years. Ann Thorac Surg. 2007;83:1310–8.
6. Puvimanasinghe J, Takkenberg J, Elijkemans M, et al. Comparison of Carpentier-Edwards pericardial and supraannular bioprostheses in aortic valve replacement. Eur J Cardio-thorac Surg. 2006;29:374–9.
7. Bonow RO, Leon MB, Doshi D, et al. Management strategies and future challenges for aortic valve disease. Lancet. 2016;387:1312–23.
8. Holmes DR, MacK MJ, Kaul S, et al. 2012 ACCF/AATS/SCAI/STS expert consensus document on transcatheter aortic valve replacement. J Am Coll Cardiol. 2012;59:1200–54.
9. Mylotte D, Piazza N. Transcatheter aortic valve replacement failure. Circ Cardiovasc Interv. 2015;8(4). pii: e002531.
10. Pislaru SV, Nkomo VT, Sandhu GS. Assessment of prosthetic valve function after TAVR. JACC Cardiovasc Imaging. 2016;9:193–206.
11. Wan B, Rahnavardi M, Tian DH, et al. A meta-analysis of MitraClip system versus surgery for treatment of severe mitral regurgitation. Ann Cardiothorac Surg. 2013;2:683–92.
12. Stewart MH, Jenkins JS. The evolving role of percutaneous mitral valve repair. Ochsner J. 2016;16:270–6.
13. Schwartz CF, Gulkarov I, Bohmann K, et al. The role of annuloplasty in mitral valve repair. J Cardiovasc Surg. 2004;45:419–25.
14. Maisano F, Skantharaja R, Denti P, et al. Mitral annuloplasty. Multimed Man Cardiothorac Surg. 2009;2009(918) MMCTS 2009:mmcts.2008.003640.
15. Jacob S, Shahzad MA, Maheshwari R, et al. Cardiac rhythm device identification algorithm using X-rays: CaRDIA-X. Heart Rhythm. 2011;8:915–22.
16. Costelloe CM, Murphy WA, Gladish GW, Rozner MA. Radiography of pacemakers and implantable cardioverter defibrillators. Am J Roentgenol. 2012;199:1252–8.
17. Aziz S, Leon AR, El-Chami MF. The subcutaneous defibrillator: a review of the literature. J Am Coll Cardiol. 2014;63:1473–9.
18. Reynolds D, Duray GZ, Omar R, et al. A leadless intracardiac transcatheter pacing system. N Engl J Med. 2016;374:533–41.
19. Paruchuri V, Adhaduk M, Garikipati NV, et al. Clinical utility of a novel wireless implantable loop recorder in the evaluation of patients with unexplained syncope. Heart Rhythm. 2011;8:858–63.
20. Shanmugam N, Liew R. The implantable loop recorder-an important addition to the armentarium in the management of unexplained syncope. Ann Acad Med Singap. 2012;41:115–24.
21. Bilkis AA, Alwi M, Hasri S, et al. The Amplatzer duct occluder: experience in 209 patients. J Am Coll Cardiol. 2001;37:258–61.
22. Tobis J, Shenoda M. Percutaneous treatment of patent foramen ovale and atrial septal defects. J Am Coll Cardiol. 2012;60:1722–32.
23. Lee T, Tsai I-C, Fu Y-C, et al. MDCT evaluation after closure of atrial septal defect with an Amplatzer septal occluder. Am J Roentgenol. 2007;188:W431–9.
24. Kaulitz R, Paul T, Hausdorf G. Extending the limits of transcatheter closure of atrial septal defects with the double umbrella device (CardioSEAL). Heart. 1998;80:54–9.
25. Chatterjee S, Herrmann HC, Wilensky RL, et al. Safety and procedural success of left atrial appendage exclusion with the lariat device. JAMA Intern Med. 2015;175:1104.
26. Wang Y, Di Biase L, Horton RP, et al. Left atrial appendage studied by computed tomography to help planning for appendage closure device placement. J Cardiovasc Electrophysiol. 2010;21:973–82.
27. Waksman R, Pendyala LK. Overview of the Food and Drug Administration circulatory system devices panel meetings on

WATCHMAN left atrial appendage closure therapy. Am J Cardiol. 2015;115:378–84.
28. Iskandar S, Vacek J, Lavu M, Lakkireddy D. Left atrial appendage closure for stroke prevention. Cardiol Clin. 2016;34:329–51.
29. Ailawadi G, Gerdisch MW, Harvey RL, et al. Exclusion of the left atrial appendage with a novel device: early results of a multicenter trial. J Thorac Cardiovasc Surg. 2011;142:1002–1009.e1.
30. Bartus K, Han FT, Bednarek J, et al. Percutaneous left atrial appendage suture ligation using the LARIAT device in patients with atrial fibrillation: initial clinical experience. J Am Coll Cardiol. 2013;62:108–18.
31. Ismail TF, Panikker S, Markides V, et al. CT imaging for left atrial appendage closure: a review and pictorial essay. J Cardiovasc Comput Tomogr. 2015;9:89–102.
32. Parissis H, Graham V, Lampridis S, et al. IABP: history-evolution-pathophysiology- indications: what we need to know. J Cardiothorac Surg. 2016;11:122.
33. Hurwitz LM, Goodman PC. Intraaortic balloon pump location and aortic dissection. AJR Am J Roentgenol. 2005;184:1245–6.
34. Ihdayhid AR, Chopra S, Rankin J. Intra-aortic balloon pump. Curr Opin Cardiol. 2014;29:285–92.
35. Rihal CS, Naidu SS, Givertz MM, et al. 2015 SCAI/ACC/HFSA/STS clinical expert consensus statement on the use of percutaneous mechanical circulatory support devices in cardiovascular care. J Am Coll Cardiol. 2015;65:e7–e26.
36. Brown JL, Estep JD. Temporary percutaneous mechanical circulatory support in advanced heart failure. Heart Fail Clin. 2016;12(3):385–98.
37. Kirklin JK, Naftel DC. Mechanical circulatory support: registering a therapy in evolution. Circ Heart Fail. 2008;1:200–5.
38. Lalonde SD, Alba AC, Rigobon A, et al. Clinical differences between continuous flow ventricular assist devices: a comparison between HeartMate II and HeartWare HVAD. J Card Surg. 2013;28:604–10.
39. Carr CM, Jacob J, Park SJ, et al. CT of left ventricular assist devices. Radiographics. 2010;30:429–44.
40. Sawa Y. Current status of third-generation implantable left ventricular assist devices in Japan, Duraheart and HeartWare. Surg Today. 2015;45:672–81.
41. Rodriguez LE, Suarez EE, Loebe M, Bruckner BA. Ventricular assist devices (VAD) therapy: new technology, new hope? Methodist Debakey Cardiovasc J. 2013;9:32–7.
42. Hunter TB, Taljanovic MS, Tsau PH, et al. Medical devices of the chest. Radiographics. 2004;24:1725–46.
43. Godoy MCB, Leitman BS, de Groot PM, et al. Chest radiography in the ICU: part 2, evaluation of cardiovascular lines and other devices. Am J Roentgenol. 2012;198:572–81.
44. Mandhan PL, Samarakkody U, Brown S, et al. Comparison of suture ligation and clip application for the treatment of patent ductus arteriosus in preterm neonates. J Thorac Cardiovasc Surg. 2006;132:672–4.

Part IX

Where We Are: Transcatheter Therapy Planning

CT in the Context of Transcatheter Aortic Valve Replacement

41

Eli Konen, Orly Goitein, and Arik Wolak

Aortic valve stenosis (aortic stenosis, AS) is the most common cause of left ventricular outflow obstruction in children and adults [1]. Severe AS is defined as maximum aortic valve velocity ≥4 m/s with an aortic valve area ≤1 cm^2, and/or the mean transvalvular gradient exceeds 40 mmHg [2]. Symptomatic AS includes a combination of the following: chest discomfort, heart failure, decreased exercise tolerance, effort dyspnea, and syncope. The main AS etiologies are calcific disease of a trileaflet valve or a congenitally abnormal valve (bicuspid or unicuspid) and rheumatic valve disease. In the Western world, calcific aortic disease of either a tricuspid or bicuspid valve is the most common cause. AS prevalence increases with age [3]. AS in younger patients is usually associated with congenitally abnormal valves, whereas trileaflet valve is more common in the elderly patients [4]. Usually, patients with AS and normal left ventricular systolic function remain asymptomatic until the stenosis is severe [5]. Once symptomatic, patients with severe AS who do not undergo valve replacement have a poor prognosis [6, 7]. Echocardiography is currently the main tool in the initial AS diagnosis and evaluation. Cardiac catheterization is recommended only if the noninvasive evaluation is nondiagnostic. The role of multidetector computed tomography (MDCT) in the initial evaluation of AS is minimal and limited to aortic valve calcification quantification [8], potentially beneficial in "paradoxical low-flow low-gradient" AS and in excluding pseudo-severe AS [9]. MDCT plays a key role in decision-making and procedure planning once procedure is indicated as will be discussed later. The poor prognosis of untreated symptomatic AS patients, together with enhanced survival rates following valve replacement, is the rational for the recommendation for early valve replacement. Percutaneous aortic balloon dilation is reserved for patients who are not eligible for surgical aortic valve replacement (SAVR) or serves as a bridge to valve replacement procedure [2].For more than 5 decades, SAVR, using either biological or mechanical valves, has been the gold standard treatment for severe symptomatic AS, severe AS with ejection fraction <50%, and severe asymptomatic AS in patients undergoing CABG [2, 10]. Although it offers an effective treatment option, it is still an extensive surgical procedure with an overall mortality rate ranging between 1.9% and 17% depending on the patient's risk group [11, 12]. As a rule, bioprosthetic valves tend to be less durable, while mechanical valves require lifelong anticoagulation treatment, both being prone to infections [13]. Due to high surgical risk or surgical contraindications, a significant portion of potential SAVR candidates will not benefit from the procedure. Therefore, during the last decade, percutaneous aortic valve replacement is becoming an increasingly growing alternative to SAVR, mainly for these high surgical risk patients [14–16]. Encouraging new data suggest that intermittent risk patients may also benefit from a percutaneous procedure [17]. Transcatheter aortic valve replacement (TAVR) is the replacement of the aortic valve without open heart surgery. The valve is delivered and positioned inside the diseased aortic valve through a blood vessel or through the apex of the heart using a delivery system, which is removed once the prosthetic valve is implanted. The catheter-based delivery system can be inserted using several approaches including transfemoral, transapical, axillary-subclavian, direct aortic (through the ascending aorta), and transcaval (through the femoral vein instead of the femoral artery and across from the inferior vena cava into the adjacent abdominal aorta) [18–20]. The transfemoral approach is performed under mild sedation while the delivery system is inserted into the femoral artery through a small incision in the groin and progressed along the artery to the correct position at the aortic valve. The transapical approach is performed under general anesthesia. A minimal surgical incision is made between the ribs followed by a small puncture of the cardiac apex where the

E. Konen · O. Goitein (✉)
Department of Diagnostic Imaging, Chaim Sheba Medical Center, Ramat Gan, Israel
e-mail: orly.goitein@sheba.health.gov.il

A. Wolak
Department of Cardiology, Shaare Zedek Medical Center, Jerusalem, Israel

U. J. Schoepf (ed.), *CT of the Heart*, Contemporary Medical Imaging, https://doi.org/10.1007/978-1-60327-237-7_41

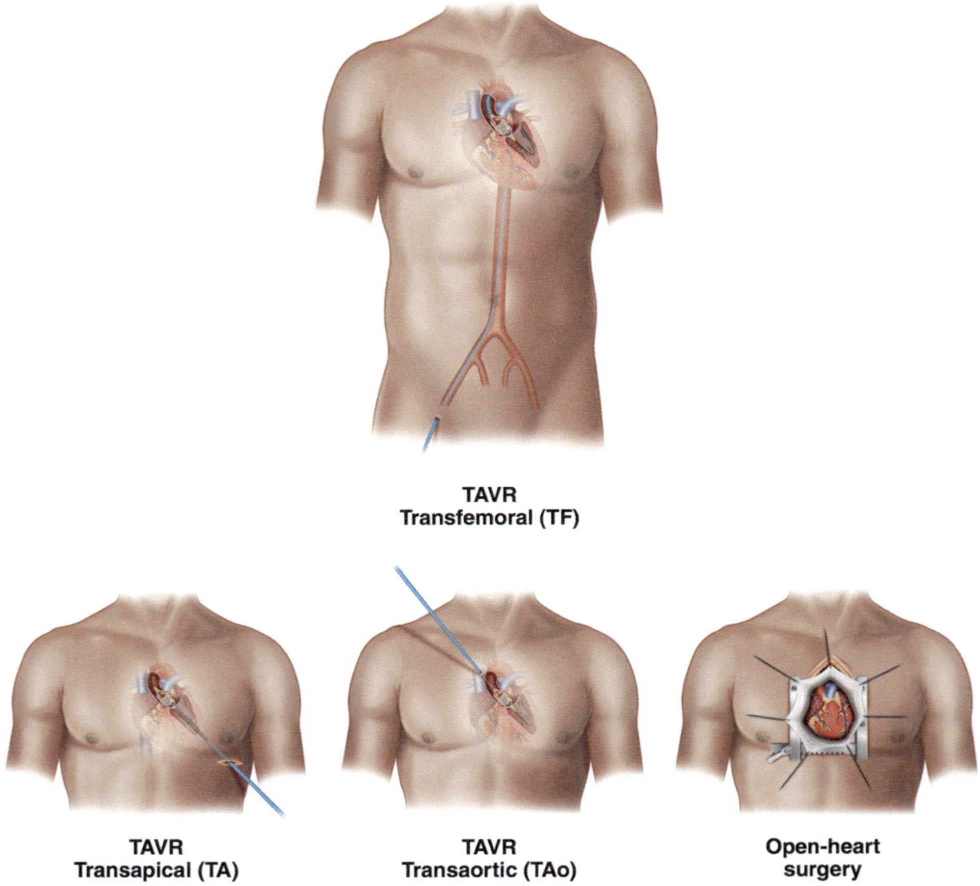

Fig. 41.1 Aortic valve replacement TAVR can be performed using several approaches: open heart surgery, transaortic, transapical, and transfemoral

delivery system is introduced into the left ventricle and through the left ventricular outflow tract to the correct position at the aortic valve (Fig. 41.1). Regardless of the approach, the procedure requires constant echocardiography guidance and pacemaker insertion for rapid pacing during the prosthetic valve final positioning and as backup if intra-procedural heart block occurs. Currently, there are several available TAVR systems (Fig. 41.2). The fundamental difference between these systems is in the aortic prostheses deployment method being either a self-expandable (SE) or balloon-expandable (BE) system [21].

Understanding the anatomy of the aortic valve components and surroundings – the aortic root, valvular leaflets, left ventricular outflow tract, origin of the coronary arteries, the mitral valve, and the conduction system – is essential for optimal patient selection and for achieving best TAVR result with minimal procedural complications. The aortic root is the anatomical location of TAVR procedure. It is located between the subpulmonary infundibulum anteriorly, the orifice of the mitral valve and the muscular ventricular septum posteriorly. It extends from the origin of the valvular leaflets at the left ventricle all the way distally to the sinotubular junction [22]. Four circumferential rings outline the aortic root. The first, the most basal one, is a virtual ring (the annulus) that is formed by joining the basal attachment of the valvar leaflets. The second is the anatomical ventriculoaortic junction (the "surgical" annulus). The third ring is the sinotubular junction. An additional fourth ring is seen in three dimensions, as the valve leaflets take the form of a three-pronged coronet, with the hinges from the supporting ventricular structures forming the "crown-like" ring (Fig. 41.3) [23]. The dimensions of the aortic root components vary in size and shape (circular vs. elliptic) between different individuals and change throughout the cardiac cycle by up to 20% [24]. The aortic valve is usually trileaflet, yet bicuspid aortic valve is a common abnormality and rarely unicuspid valve can be found. As for the aortic root, marked variations exist among individuals in the dimensions of all elements. Such disparities in the size of the leaflets can cause inaccurate measurements of the aortic annulus especially when acquiring measurements, using a two-dimensional modality. The left main and the right coronary arteries most often arise within the left and right sinuses of Valsalva just below the sinotubular junction, yet many times they can arise from a lower or higher position in the aortic root. Postmortem of normal hearts demonstrated an average distance of 12.6 and 13.2 mm from the orifice of the left main and right coronary arteries to the aortic annulus, respectively [23, 25] . The left

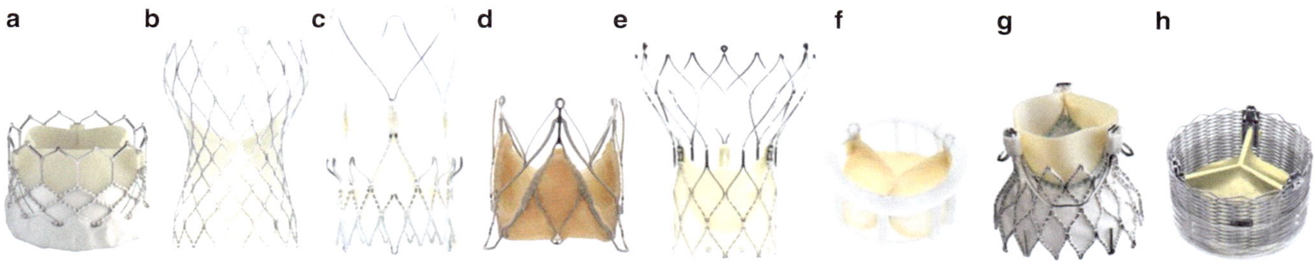

Fig. 41.2 Currently, eight transcatheter aortic valve replacement (TAVR) systems are commercially available in Europe (**a**–**h**), whereas two TAVR systems are approved by the US Food and Drug Administration in the United States (**a**, **b**). (**a**) Edwards Lifesciences Sapien 3 Valve (Edwards Lifesciences, Irvine, CA); (**b**) Medtronic CoreValve Evolut R (Medtronic, Minneapolis, MN); (**c**) Symetis Acurate neo Valve (Symetis, Ecublens VD, Switzerland); (**d**) JenaValve (JVT Research & Development Corp, Irvine, CA); (**e**) St. Jude Medical Portico Valve (St. Jude Medical, St. Paul, MN); (**f**) Direct Flow Medical Valve (Direct Flow Medical, Inc., Santa Rosa, CA); (**g**) Medtronic Engager Valve (Medtronic, Minneapolis, MN); and (**h**) Boston Scientific Lotus Valve (Boston Scientific, Marlborough, MA). (From Vahl et al. [27], with permission)

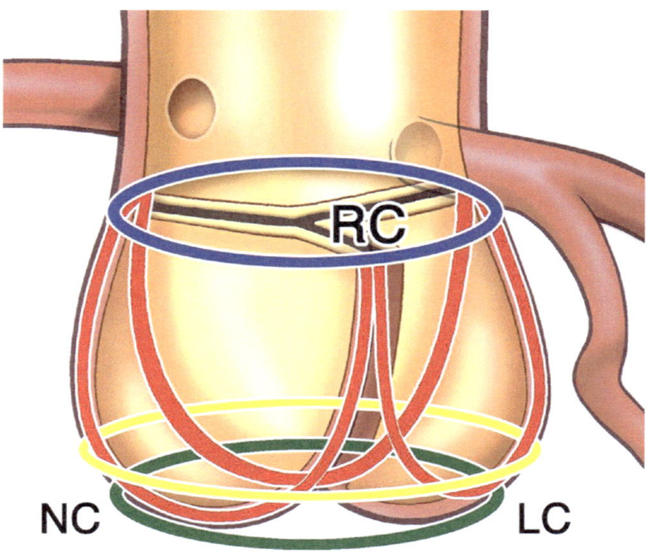

Fig. 41.3 Aortic root and anatomic location of aortic annulus. The three red rings represent the aortic valve cusps, with the green circle placed at the nadir of the aortic cusps denoting the annular plane. *LC* left coronary cusp, *NC* noncoronary cusp, *RC* right coronary cusp. (From Leipsic et al. [28], with permission)

ventricular outflow tract (LVOT) is a portion of the left ventricle through which blood passes to the aorta. LVOT characteristics which may hinder device positioning include changing angulation with age and the presence of subaortic asymmetrical septal hypertrophy [23].The aortic valve is located in proximity to all cardiac chambers including the conduction system. Therefore, it is only understandable why aortic valve procedures may cause heart block or intraventricular conduction abnormalities. The length of the membranous septum and the presence of basal septum calcifications were documented as associated with post-TAVR conduction abnormalities [26]. Patients with severe AS present with a wide variety of comorbidities that may impact their management strategy. Therefore, it is crucial that a multidisciplinary team will choose the best treatment approach on an individual basis, considering age, frailty, and anatomic and clinical features. The current general approach is to prefer SAVR for lower-risk young patients, TAVR for high-risk or inoperable patients, and medical palliative treatment to prohibitive-risk patients (Fig. 41.4) [27]. TAVR is currently evolving in three selected severe AS patients' groups: valve-in-valve for bioprosthetic valve failure, bicuspid aortic valve, and AS with concomitant valvular or coronary artery disease [27]. Per-patient TAVR procedure tailoring is the current standard of care. A dedicated "heart team" of collaborating physicians, which includes cardiologists, cardiac surgeons, and cardiac imaging experts (echocardiography, MDCT, and MRI), facilitates better communication and understanding of the complex anatomy at question [27–29].

MDCT offers comprehensive pre-procedural imaging and understanding of the aortic root structures relevant to the TAVR procedure, including the left ventricular outflow tract, aortic annulus, aortic sinuses, sinotubular junction, ascending aorta, coronary ostia height, procedure access route, and non-cardiac pathology which may affect the procedure (Table 41.1, Figs. 41.5, 41.6, 41.7, 41.8, and 41.9) [27, 28, 30–32]. Correct device sizing is key in preventing complications, including coronary occlusion, annular rupture, and paravalvular leak, severely affecting patient outcome [33, 34].

Acquisition Protocols

In order to evaluate the entire spectrum of aortic pathology and procedure access route, the scanning protocol should extend from the clavicles to the groin. A separate non-enhanced ECG-gated scan ("calcium score" scan) of the

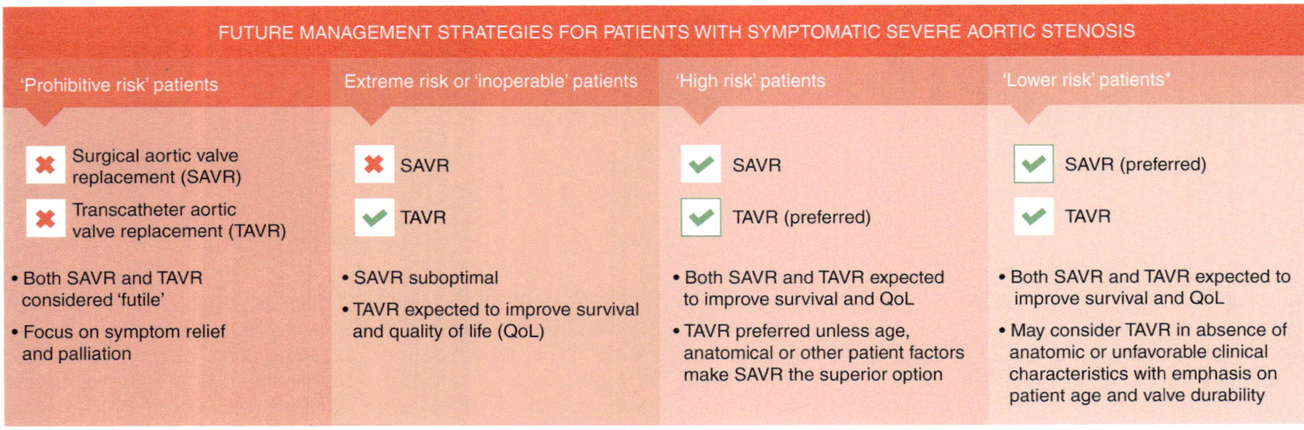

Fig. 41.4 TAVR, future expectations and barriers. Patients with severe aortic stenosis present with a spectrum of comorbidities that influence the treatment options available to them. The heart team will choose the optimal treatment strategy for individual patients based on their age, frailty, and anatomic and clinical characteristics. For patients undergoing transcatheter aortic valve replacement (TAVR), the bar for the performance standard is set by surgical aortic valve replacement (SAVR). TAVR has evolved as the preferred treatment for high-risk and inoperable patients. Because the durability of transcatheter heart valves and outcomes in lower-risk patients require further studies, SAVR remains the treatment of choice for such patients (From Vahl et al. [27], with permission)

Table 41.1 Pre-procedural TAVR CT report

Aortic annulus
Diameters (shortest, longest)
Annulus calcifications
Area and area-based diameters
Perimeter and perimeter-derived diameters
Aortic annulus plane for fluoroscopy
Left ventricular outflow tract calcifications
Aortic root
Sinotubular junction diameters
Sinus of Valsalva width and height
Coronary ostia to aortic annulus distance
Aorta
Ascending aorta, aortic arch, descending aorta width
Tortuosity, kinking, dissection, obstruction
Aortic valve
Aortic cusps length, calcifications
Cuspidity (bicuspid, tricuspid)
Vascular access
Iliofemoral arteries: minimal diameter
Tortuosity, angulation
Calcifications
Subclavian arteries – minimal diameter
Noncardiac findings
Findings that will affect procedure (change, postpone, cancel)

Modified from Achenbach et al. [30], with permission

heart with a limited field of view offers the ability to quantify the calcification burden in each of the aortic root components. It is imperative to scan the aortic root using ECG gating, which can be either retrospective or prospective or high-pitch mode. The ECG gating allows procurement of accurate, motion-free images. Retrospective gating may be helpful when high heart rates or atrial fibrillation is present. Due to the nature of severe aortic stenosis, administration of beta-blocker is not recommended, since it may result in further decrease of left ventricular function [35]. Isosorbide dinitrate spray is relatively contraindicated as well. Non-gated acquisition can be used for scanning the entire aorta and femoral vessels, thus decreasing both scan time and volume of administered contrast. Spatial resolution should be high with a reconstructed slice width ≤1.0 mm throughout the entire scan. Acquisition protocols vary and are determined by the specific scanner platform. Wide detector systems allow capture of the entire dataset with ECG gating. Spiral high-pitch ECG-gated scanning offers rapid cranio-caudal coverage, with a potential for further decrease in the contrast volume needed for adequate imaging [28, 30, 35–37].

Contrast Media and Radiation Exposure

Obtaining a satisfactory quality scan with a minimum contrast amount is of utmost importance in the elderly population of TAVR patients. It has been recently shown that contrast media volume can be substantially reduced, while maintaining adequate image quality, utilizing low-tube voltage acquisitions, and enhancing contrast conspicuity [36, 38–40].The risk for contrast-induced nephropathy following TAVR is non-negligible and is related to repeated contrast administration [41, 42]. In the TAVR patient population, it is associated with poor outcome and increased mortality [41, 43]. Radiation exposure is of less significance when the elderly TAVR population is considered, since the carcinogenic effects of radiation exposure require a lag time of at least 10 years [43]. When addressing TAVR procedures in younger

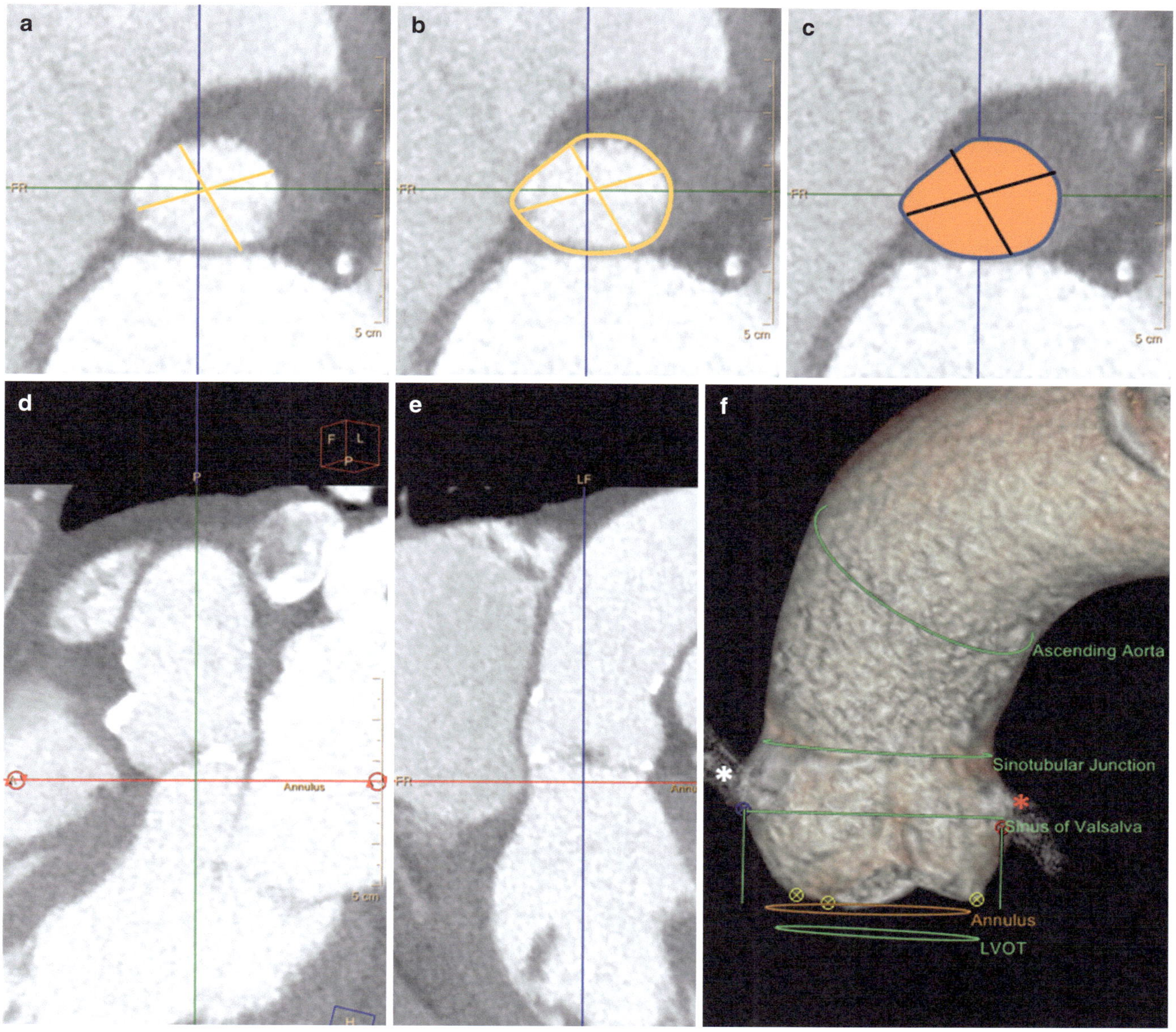

Fig. 41.5 Aortic annulus. (**a**) The aortic annulus obtained using two perpendicular pales through the nadir of the aortic cusps (**d**, **e**). Annulus diameters longest and shortest (in orange). (**b**) Aortic annulus perimeter and derived diameters (in orange). (**c**) Aortic annulus area and derived diameters (in orange). (**d**, **e**) Multiplanar reformats (MPR) serving for correct location at the annular plane at the nadir of the aortic valves (red). (**f**) Volume rendering of the aortic root demonstrating the aortic "rings": the left ventricular outflow tract (LVOT), the annulus (orange), the sinotubular junction, and the ascending aorta. The origin of the left main coronary artery (white asterisk), origin of the right coronary artery (red asterisk)

patients, radiation exposure issues cannot be overlooked and should be addressed appropriately.

Aortic Annulus Evaluation

The aortic annulus is a complex three-dimensional virtual ring at the base of the aortic cusps [23]. The annulus is oval in nature [23, 44, 45], and hence 3D imaging modalities including 3D transesophageal echocardiography (TEE) and MDCT are, by far, superior to 2D modalities such as 2D transthoracic echocardiography (TTE) or angiography [23, 24, 28, 30, 46–50]. Thus, MDCT is considered the gold standard for device sizing [27, 51, 52] . The anatomical structures at the aortic root change throughout the cardiac cycle. The annulus endures pulsatile changes as well as contour deformity caused by the adjacent structures such as the aortomitral tissue and left atrium [23, 53]. These annular cyclic changes need to be taken into consideration when choosing the device that needs to withstand them. Recently, some

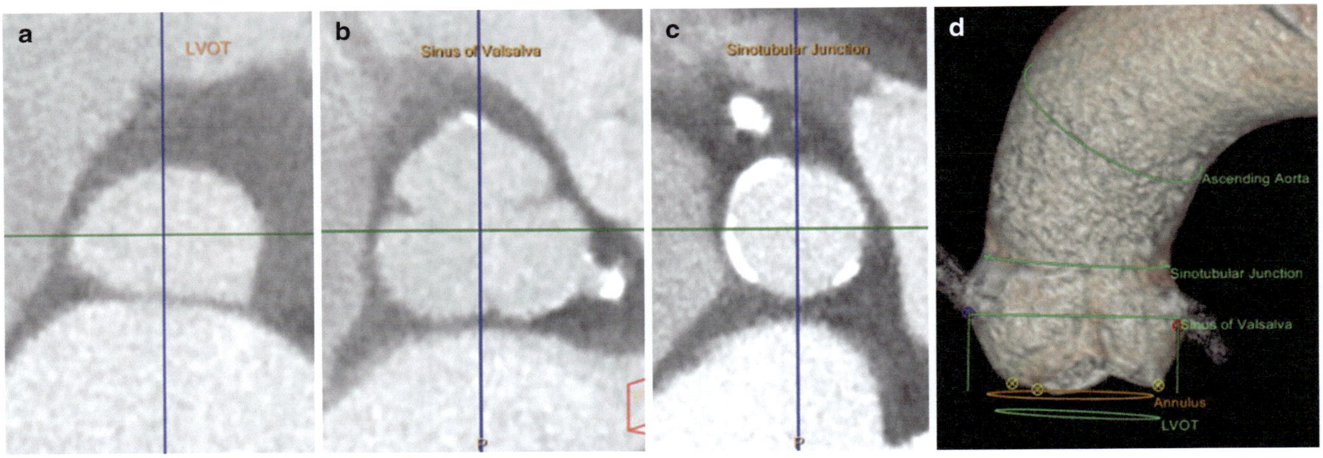

Fig. 41.6 (**a–c**) Cross section at the levels of the left ventricular outflow tract (LVOT) (**a**), sinuses of Valsalva (**b**), and the sinotubular junction (**c**). (**d**) Volume rendering of the aortic root demonstrating the corresponding aortic "rings" (**a–c**)

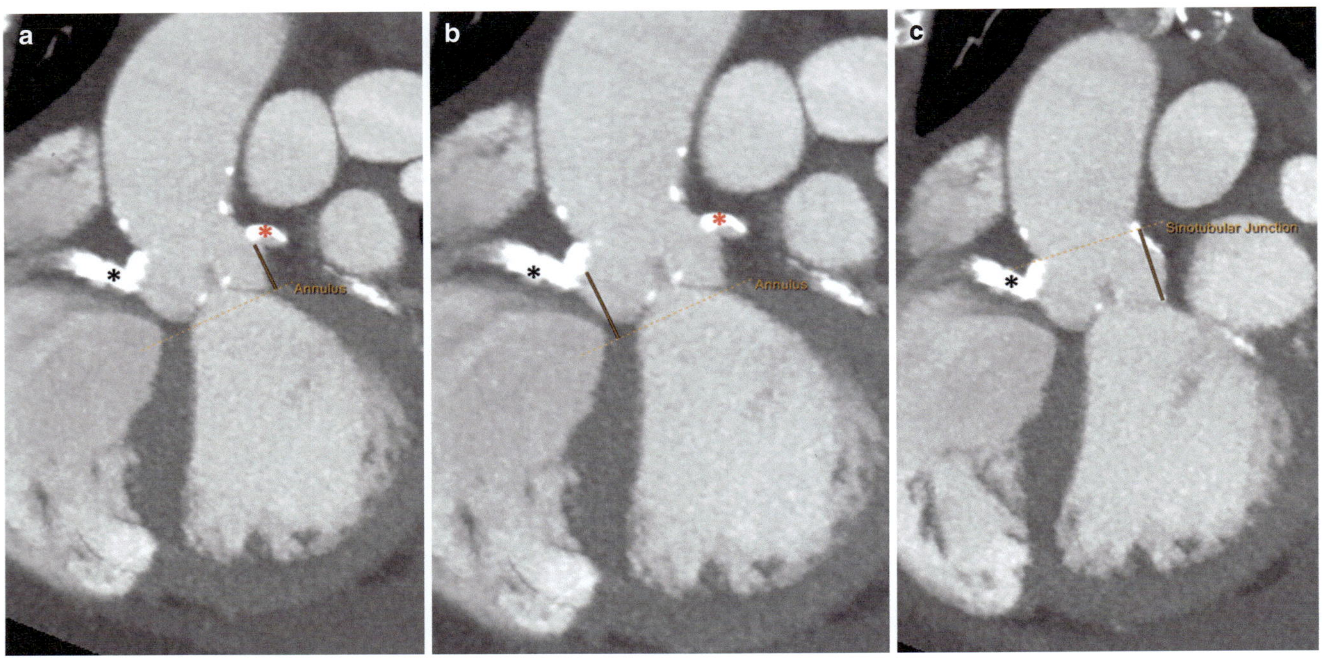

Fig. 41.7 Distance from the annulus to the origin of the coronary arteries. (**a**) Distance to the left main (LM) (red asterisk LM origin). (**b**) Distance to the right coronary artery (RCA) (black asterisk RCA origin). (**c**) Left coronary sinus height

authors have advocated the utilization of systolic phases in order to refrain from prosthesis under-sizing [24, 54]. However, if systolic phases are suboptimal, it is important to ensure adequate image quality using the best available phase. Current CT scanners offer isotropic data acquisition allowing precise, reproducible nonoperator-dependent measurements [46, 55, 56]. Accurate annular sizing should be performed using two orthogonal planes along the aortic root. The perpendicular plane immediately below the nadir of the aortic cusps represents the annulus. At this location, measurements should include diameters (shortest and longest), annular perimeter and area, and the calculated derived virtual diameters from both perimeter and area (Fig. 41.5) [28, 30, 32, 35, 46, 57]. MDCT perimeter- and area-derived virtual diameters have been shown to change the least during the cardiac cycle and are considered to be the most reliable diameter measurement [28, 30, 32, 35, 46, 57]. Dedicated application platforms for facilitating these measurements exist and are utilized in daily practice [54, 57–60]. Cases in which the annular size is borderline (for a certain device size) are particularly influenced by the geometric changes between systole and diastole. A comprehensive multimodal-

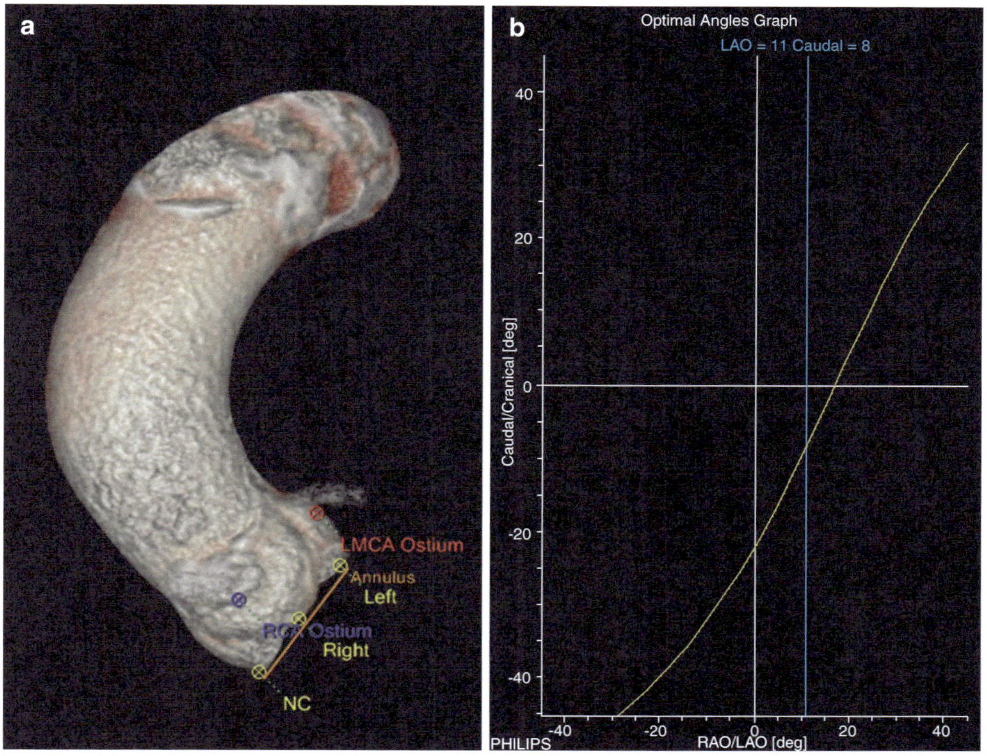

Fig. 41.8 Fluoroscopic projection angle predicted by MDCT. (**a**) Volume rendering of the aortic root aligning all three cusps in the same plane. (**b**) The "line of perpendicularity" demonstrating the preferred fluoroscopic angel for the procedure

ity approach incorporating MDCT, 3D TEE, and balloon sizing (during the procedure) is recommended when evaluating challenging cases [28, 54, 61]. Prosthesis sizing is undertaken using dedicated tables for each device. When sizing a device, one should consult with the most updated manufacturer instructions.

Aortic Root Evaluation

Other components of the aortic root should be addressed, including the distance of the coronary ostia location (Fig. 41.6), aortic cusp length and calcification, aortic sinuses width and degree of calcification, and sinotubular junction and ascending aorta size. These data are essential in fitting the appropriate device to the specific anatomy [30]. Prosthesis inappropriate sizing is associated with coronary occlusion, annular rupture, paravalvular regurgitation, and device embolization [62].

Aortic Annulus Plane for Fluoroscopy

The specific aortic root orientation is different for every patient with a general anterior right-sided angulation in most cases. The accurate position for each patient is easily depicted using MDCT data. Thus, providing a correct fluoroscopic (C-arm) angle in which all three coronary cusps are aligned in the same plane allows ease of utilization with the physical constraints of a catheterization suite (Fig. 41.9). This can be achieved both manually or using dedicated automated software. It is of high value for accurate device positioning and lowering the amount of aortograms and hence the contrast media volume needed for procedure completion [30, 46, 59, 63, 64].

Calcification Burden

The presence, quantity, and distribution of aortic root calcification are related to procedure outcome [65–69]. During a TAVR procedure, the native aortic valve leaflets are compressed by the inserted device rather than resected as in SAVR. TAVR prosthesis anchoring requires some degree of calcification; however, high calcification burdens in the aortic valve and LVOT are strong predictors for paravalvular aortic regurgitation (PAR) [65, 67–69]. Greater calcium burden in the left coronary cusp has been implicated as an independent predictor for the need for permanent pacemaker following the procedure [70]. LVOT calcification adjacent to the noncoronary cusp was demonstrated as a predictor for aortic root injury (Fig. 41.6) [71]. Other authors found a high total aortic calcification burden to be an integrative predictor for cardiac and all-cause mortality [66].

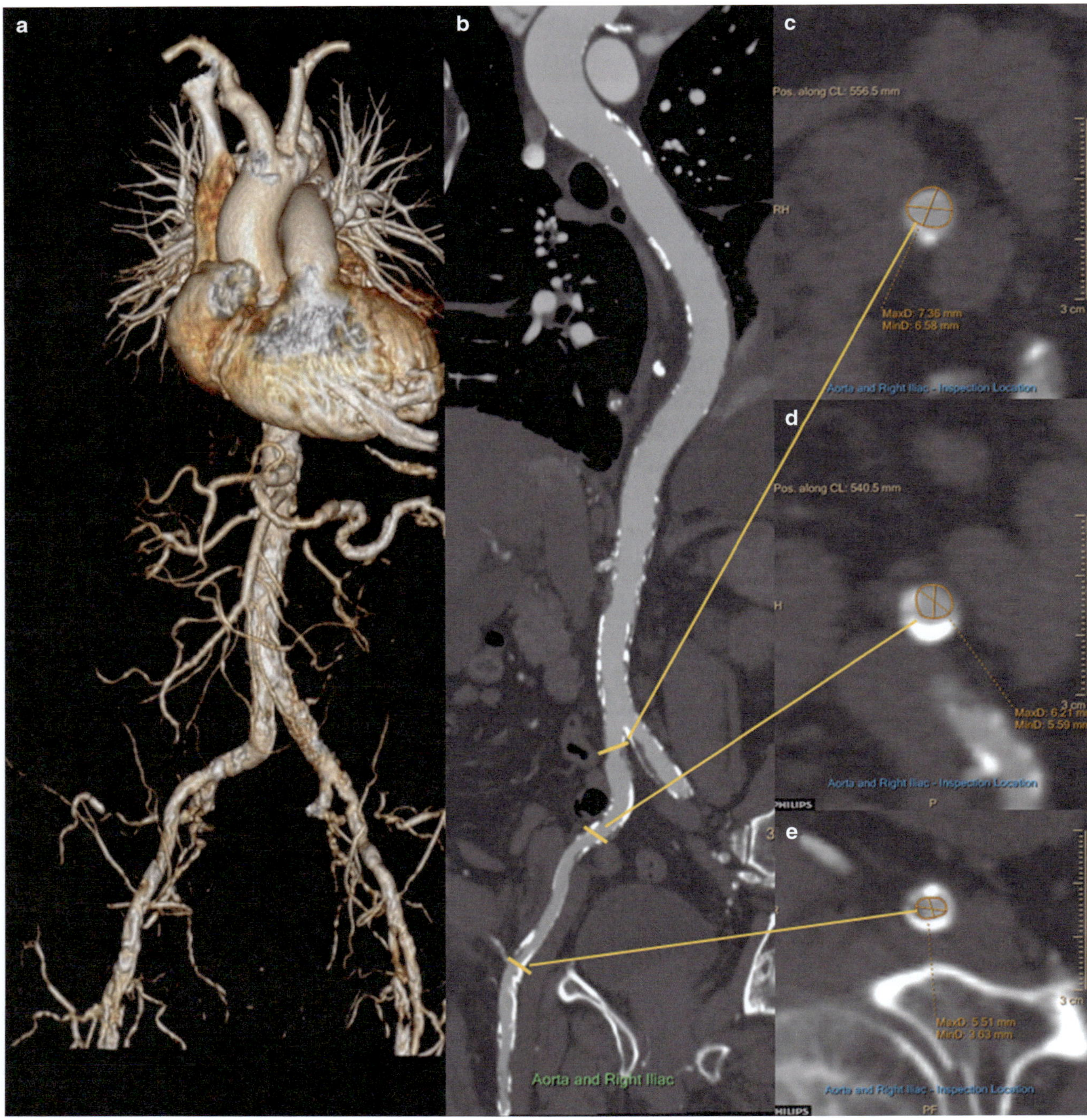

Fig. 41.9 Vascular access by MDCT (90-year-old TAVI patient). (**a**) Volume rendering (VR) of the entire aorta and femoral arteries demonstrating extensive atherosclerotic disease. (**b**) Curved multiplanar reformats (CMPR) of the aorta and the right iliac and femoral arteries demonstrating atherosclerotic disease. (**c–e**) Cross-sectional perpendicular slices for measurement of vascular diameters at the levels of right common iliac artery (**c**), right external iliac artery (**d**), and right common femoral artery (**e**). Note, the circumferential calcifications at this level, representing an unfavorable vascular access

Aortic Valve Cuspidity

Bicuspid aortic valve (BAV) is the most common congenital cardiac anomaly. Inherent abnormalities in the aortic valve are related to progressive calcification which leads to stenosis and dilatation of the proximal aorta segments [72]. Recently, a TAVR-oriented classification was suggested, dividing BAV into tri-commissural, bi-commissural raphe type and bi-commissural non-raphe type [73]. Short term outcome (within 30 days) of TAVR in patients with BAV was similar to that reported for those with normal, tricuspid valves although a higher rate of permanent pacemaker insertion was demonstrated for both BE and SE device types [73]. Some authors have reported a higher incidence of post-TAVR PAR in patients with BAV; however recent published data does not support this association [73, 74].

Procedure Access

Transfemoral arterial approach for TAVR was introduced in 2006 and is considered the preferred approach ever since [75]. Single-plane angiography is considered a minimal requirement for pre-TAVR vascular evaluation; however atherosclerotic burden assessment is considerably limited using this approach [76]. Major vascular complications are not uncommon and were described with a higher incidence especially in women [77–79]. Target vessel dimensions, tortuosity, and extent of calcifications are important factors when addressing procedure access (Fig. 41.9). Contrast-enhanced MDCT has been shown to have a greater predicative value for post-TAVR vascular complications as compared with angiography [18]. Potential contraindications for transfemoral approach include external sheath diameter exceeding the minimal arterial diameter, significant vessel tortuosity, and extensive peripheral vascular disease [75, 80]. Calcifications, in particular circumferential or near-circumferential, limit arterial expandability, thus increasing the potential risk for perforation or dissection [77, 80]. Routine implementation of pre-TAVR CT, along with ongoing decrease in the delivery system size requirements, holds promise for further lowering vascular complication rates [80].

Transfemoral approach is associated with lower mortality rate (30-day and 1-year) as compared with non-transfemoral approach [19, 20]. However, in the presence of prohibitive transfemoral access, alternative procedure routes exist, including transapical, transaortic, transcaval, and subclavian approaches.

Post-TAVR Outcomes

Successful device implantation is reported in more than 90% of patients [16, 33, 77, 81–83]. New-generation balloon-expandable devices have been introduced, significantly lowering mortality, with reported 1-year survival rates of 85.6% and 74.7% for the transfemoral and the transapical or transaortic approaches, respectively [78]. Post-TAVR complications include (in descending order of incidence) new conduction disorders requiring placement of a new permanent pacemaker (reported more in SE devices), major vascular and bleeding events, acute kidney injury, major stroke, and myocardial infarction [77] (Figs. 41.10 and 41.11). As cumulative experience increases and technical aspects of TAVR progress, a significant reduction in post-procedural complications is apparent, especially when comparing results between the earliest reports and the current literature [78, 82].The new-generation BE and SE devices incorporate several advanced technical alterations. Slimmer-profile systems (14–16F expandable sheaths) are related to less vascular injury and offer procedure availability for patients, who, previously, were not eligible for transfemoral approach. Ease of device manipulation is related to the decrease in adverse events such as device malpositioning, the need for a second valve-in-valve intervention, urgent surgery, or the need of cardiopulmonary support [78]. The current ability for device to repositioning or retrieval permits real-time procedure modifications. The wider range of valve sizes for both SE and BE devices allows better patient device adjustment. Paravalvular aortic regurgitation (PAR) is a much-discussed issue. Moderate (and greater) post-TAVR PAR is reported as associated with an increase in the overall mortality risk [78, 84, 85]. Some authors have found a higher incidence of PAR when comparing SE to BE valve; however this is not reported by all authors [21, 58, 82]. Adherence to MDCT sizing lowers the incidence of PAR [59, 86]. Reduced bioprosthesis leaflet motion was demonstrated utilizing four-dimensional MDCT but resolved following anticoagulation administration and was not associated with increased clinical events [87].

Catastrophic Procedure Complications

Coronary occlusion is rare and caused mainly by displacement of the calcified native valves over the coronary ostia. It was documented as more prevalent in women, heavily calcified cusps, balloon-expandable devices (twice as high), and "valve-in-valve" procedures [34]. A coronary height <12 mm, relatively small sinuses of Valsalva diameter (<30 mm), long aortic cusps, and narrow sinotubular junction were demonstrated in the majority of cases [30, 34, 88] (Fig. 41.7). Annular rupture is rare, described mostly as case reports, some of which suggest relation to prosthesis oversizing [62, 89, 90]. Other adverse outcomes include aortic dissection, device embolization, and tamponade. All of these are rare, acute complications requiring immediate intervention and are uniformly associated with poor outcome [88, 91, 92].

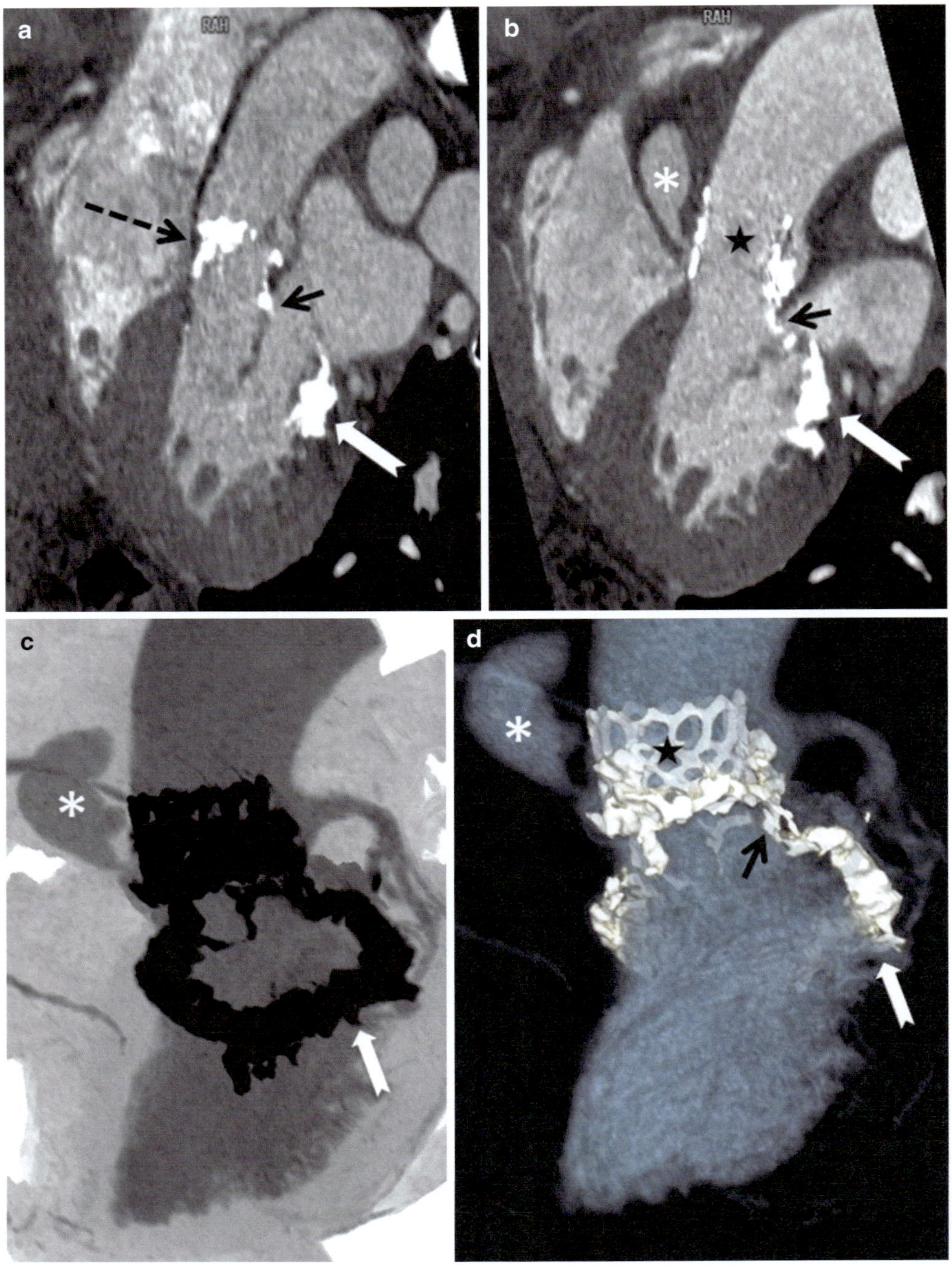

Fig. 41.10 Post-TAVI pseudoaneurysm. (**a**) Multiplanar reformats (MPR) of the left ventricular outflow tract (LVOT) before TAVI demonstrating heavy calcifications at the aortic annulus (dotted arrow), at the LVOT (black arrow), and at the mitral annulus (MAC) (white arrow). (**b**) MPR of the LVOT after TAVI demonstrating a pseudoaneurysm (white asterisk) originating at the aortic annulus. TAVI device is in place (black star). (**c**, **d**) MIP and volume rendering of the LVOT demonstrating the pseudoaneurysm (white asterisk), TAVI device (black star), MAC (white arrow), and LVOT calcifications (black arrow)

Valve-in-Valve: New Options for TAVR

In recent years, the utilization of aortic bioprosthetic valves is favored over mechanical valves due to their lower thrombogenicity [93]. However, bioprosthesis deterioration usually occurs by 10–15 years. TAVR valve-in-valve offers a noninvasive solution for failed bioprosthetic surgical valves. An overall 1-year survival of 83% was reported in a large international registry using both SE and BE devices [75, 94]. Smartphone platforms have been developed in order to guide accurate valve-in-valve proper sizing [95].

Evaluation of the Coronary Anatomy

Assessment of the coronary arteries using the data collected by TAVR study is feasible yet challenging. In the majority of these patients, it is recommended to avoid beta-blockers and nitrates prior to the acquisition; therefore, only limited rate control and

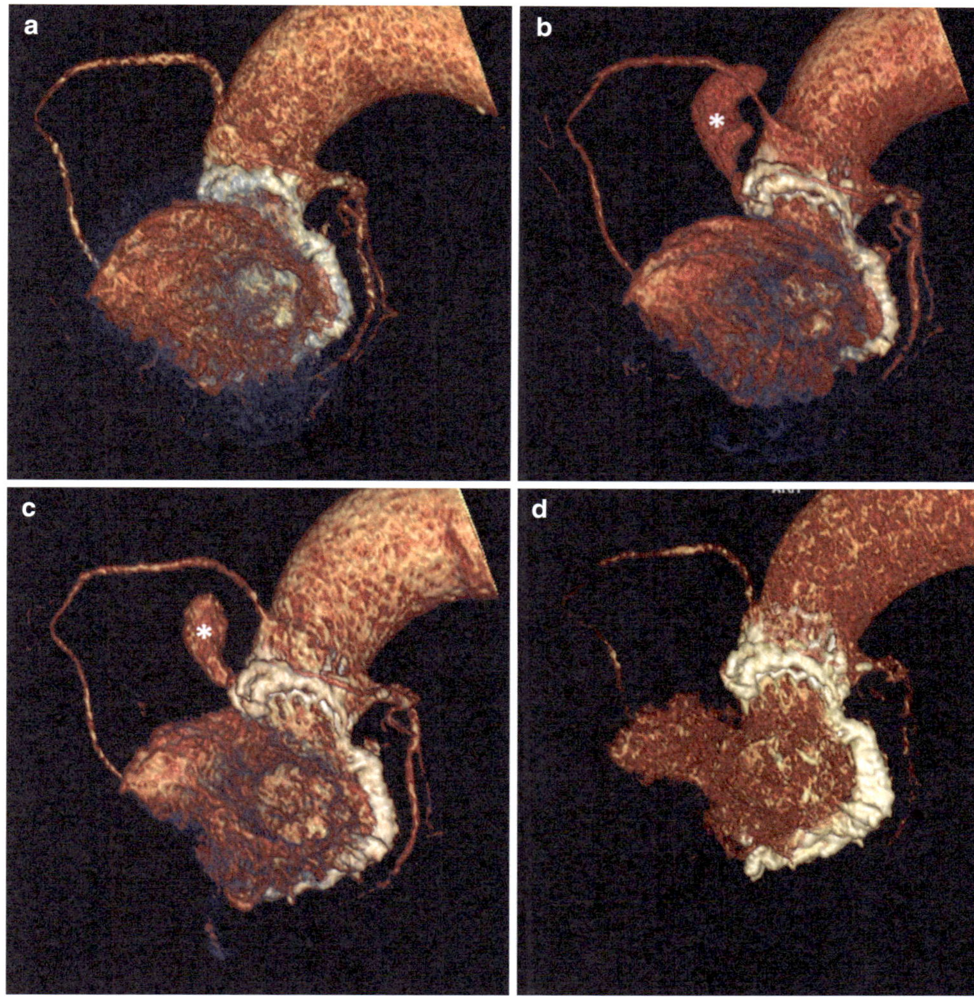

Fig. 41.11 Post-TAVI pseudoaneurysm follow-up (same patient as in Fig. 41.10). (**a**) Volume rendering (VR) pre-TAVI – normal study. (**b**) VR post-TAVI (2 days) demonstrating a pseudoaneurysm (white asterisk). (**c**) VR post-TAVI (2 months) demonstrating a decrease in size of the pseudoaneurysm (white asterisk). (**d**) VR post-TAVI (6 months) demonstrating resolution of the pseudoaneurysm with conservative treatment

coronary dilation are achieved during the scan. Additionaly owing to the nature of the TAVR target population (elderly and frail), it is usual to encounter breathing artifacts, blooming artifacts due to heavy calcification, and motion artifact due to arrhythmia (mostly atrial fibrillation and relative tachycardia). In one study of TAVR patients, sensitivity, specificity, and positive and negative predictive value of 96%, 73%, 72%, and 96%, respectively, were documented for the evaluation of only seven proximal segments (left main, proximal, and middle left anterior descending artery, proximal and middle right coronary artery, and proximal and middle circumflex artery) or bypass grafts [96]. Currently, it is a reasonable approach to perform an initial TAVR CTA study and to proceed to diagnostic invasive coronary angiography only if the data acquired is insufficient.

In conclusion, MDCT prior to TAVR provides imaging information which, when used properly, serves to reduce procedure-specific complications. It allows tailored, per-patient procedure planning including device type, size, procedure access route, procedure fluoroscopic angulation, and post-procedure follow-up. Multimodality imaging implementation prior to TAVR truly embodies the ideal of a comprehensive "heart team" incorporating imaging experts, cardiologists, and cardiac surgeons for optimal patient care.

References

1. American College of C, American Heart Association Task Force on Practice G, Society of Cardiovascular A, Bonow RO, Carabello BA, Chatterjee K, et al. ACC/AHA 2006 guidelines for the management of patients with valvular heart disease: a report of the American College of Cardiology/American Heart Association task force on practice guidelines (writing committee to revise the 1998 guidelines for the management of patients with valvular heart disease) developed in collaboration with the Society of Cardiovascular Anesthesiologists endorsed by the Society for Cardiovascular Angiography and Interventions and the Society of Thoracic Surgeons. J Am Coll Cardiol. 2006;48(3):e1–148.
2. Nishimura RA, Otto CM, Bonow RO, Carabello BA, Erwin JP 3rd, Guyton RA, et al. 2014 AHA/ACC guideline for the management of patients with valvular heart disease: a report of the American College of Cardiology/American Heart Association task force on practice guidelines. J Am Coll Cardiol. 2014;63(22):e57–185.

3. Eveborn GW, Schirmer H, Heggelund G, Lunde P, Rasmussen K. The evolving epidemiology of valvular aortic stenosis. The Tromso study. Heart. 2013;99(6):396–400.
4. Roberts WC, Ko JM. Frequency by decades of unicuspid, bicuspid, and tricuspid aortic valves in adults having isolated aortic valve replacement for aortic stenosis, with or without associated aortic regurgitation. Circulation. 2005;111(7):920–5.
5. Otto CM, Nishimura RA. New ACC/AHA valve guidelines: aligning definitions of aortic stenosis severity with treatment recommendations. Heart. 2014;100(12):902–4.
6. Kitai T, Honda S, Okada Y, Tani T, Kim K, Kaji S, et al. Clinical outcomes in non-surgically managed patients with very severe versus severe aortic stenosis. Heart. 2011;97(24):2029–32.
7. Leon MB, Smith CR, Mack M, Miller DC, Moses JW, Svensson LG, et al. Transcatheter aortic-valve implantation for aortic stenosis in patients who cannot undergo surgery. N Engl J Med. 2010;363(17):1597–607.
8. Messika-Zeitoun D, Aubry MC, Detaint D, Bielak LF, Peyser PA, Sheedy PF, et al. Evaluation and clinical implications of aortic valve calcification measured by electron-beam computed tomography. Circulation. 2004;110(3):356–62.
9. Cueff C, Serfaty JM, Cimadevilla C, Laissy JP, Himbert D, Tubach F, et al. Measurement of aortic valve calcification using multislice computed tomography: correlation with haemodynamic severity of aortic stenosis and clinical implication for patients with low ejection fraction. Heart. 2011;97(9):721–6.
10. Vahanian A, Alfieri O, Andreotti F, Antunes MJ, Baron-Esquivias G, Baumgartner H, et al. Guidelines on the management of valvular heart disease (version 2012): the joint task force on the management of Valvular heart disease of the European Society of Cardiology (ESC) and the European Association for Cardio-Thoracic Surgery (EACTS). Eur J Cardiothorac Surg. 2012;42(4):S1–44.
11. Mohr FW, Holzhey D, Mollmann H, Beckmann A, Veit C, Figulla HR, et al. The German aortic valve registry: 1-year results from 13,680 patients with aortic valve disease. Eur J Cardiothorac Surg. 2014;46(5):808–16.
12. Thourani VH, Suri RM, Gunter RL, Sheng S, O'Brien SM, Ailawadi G, et al. Contemporary real-world outcomes of surgical aortic valve replacement in 141,905 low-risk, intermediate-risk, and high-risk patients. Ann Thorac Surg. 2015;99(1):55–61.
13. Bach DS, Kon ND, Dumesnil JG, Sintek CF, Doty DB. Ten-year outcome after aortic valve replacement with the freestyle stentless bioprosthesis. Ann Thorac Surg. 2005;80(2):480–6. discussion 6-7.
14. Siemieniuk RA, Agoritsas T, Manja V, Devji T, Chang Y, Bala MM, et al. Transcatheter versus surgical aortic valve replacement in patients with severe aortic stenosis at low and intermediate risk: systematic review and meta-analysis. BMJ. 2016;354:i5130.
15. Indraratna P, Tian DH, Yan TD, Doyle MP, Cao C. Transcatheter aortic valve implantation versus surgical aortic valve replacement: a meta-analysis of randomized controlled trials. Int J Cardiol. 2016;224:382–7.
16. Siontis GC, Praz F, Pilgrim T, Mavridis D, Verma S, Salanti G, et al. Transcatheter aortic valve implantation vs. surgical aortic valve replacement for treatment of severe aortic stenosis: a meta-analysis of randomized trials. Eur Heart J. 2016;37(47):3503–12.
17. Leon MB, Smith CR, Mack MJ, Makkar RR, Svensson LG, Kodali SK, et al. Transcatheter or surgical aortic-valve replacement in intermediate-risk patients. N Engl J Med. 2016;374(17):1609–20.
18. Okuyama K, Jilaihawi H, Kashif M, Takahashi N, Chakravarty T, Pokhrel H, et al. Transfemoral access assessment for transcatheter aortic valve replacement: evidence-based application of computed tomography over invasive angiography. Circ Cardiovasc Imaging. 2014;8(1)
19. Chandrasekhar J, Hibbert B, Ruel M, Lam BK, Labinaz M, Glover C. Transfemoral vs non-transfemoral access for transcatheter aortic valve implantation: a systematic review and meta-analysis. Can J Cardiol. 2015;31(12):1427–38.
20. Thourani VH, Jensen HA, Babaliaros V, Suri R, Vemulapalli S, Dai D, et al. Transapical and transaortic transcatheter aortic valve replacement in the United States. Ann Thorac Surg. 2015;100(5):1718–26. discussion 26-7.
21. Abdel-Wahab M, Mehilli J, Frerker C, Neumann FJ, Kurz T, Tolg R, et al. Comparison of balloon-expandable vs self-expandable valves in patients undergoing transcatheter aortic valve replacement: the CHOICE randomized clinical trial. JAMA. 2014;311(15):1503–14.
22. Anderson RH. Clinical anatomy of the aortic root. Heart. 2000;84(6):670–3.
23. Piazza N, de Jaegere P, Schultz C, Becker AE, Serruys PW, Anderson RH. Anatomy of the aortic valvar complex and its implications for transcatheter implantation of the aortic valve. Circ Cardiovasc Interv. 2008;1(1):74–81.
24. Jurencak T, Turek J, Kietselaer BL, Mihl C, Kok M, van Ommen VG, et al. MDCT evaluation of aortic root and aortic valve prior to TAVI. What is the optimal imaging time point in the cardiac cycle? Eur Radiol. 2015;25(7):1975–83.
25. Cavalcanti JS, de Melo NC, de Vasconcelos RS. Morphometric and topographic study of coronary ostia. Arq Bras Cardiol. 2003;81(4):359–62, 5–8.
26. Hamdan A, Guetta V, Klempfner R, Konen E, Raanani E, Glikson M, et al. Inverse relationship between membranous septal length and the risk of atrioventricular block in patients undergoing transcatheter aortic valve implantation. JACC Cardiovasc Interv. 2015;8(9):1218–28.
27. Vahl TP, Kodali SK, Leon MB. Transcatheter aortic valve replacement 2016: a modern-day "through the looking-glass" adventure. J Am Coll Cardiol. 2016;67(12):1472–87.
28. Leipsic J, Gurvitch R, Labounty TM, Min JK, Wood D, Johnson M, et al. Multidetector computed tomography in transcatheter aortic valve implantation. JACC Cardiovasc Imaging. 2011;4(4):416–29.
29. Kappetein AP, Head SJ, Genereux P, Piazza N, van Mieghem NM, Blackstone EH, et al. Updated standardized endpoint definitions for transcatheter aortic valve implantation: the valve academic research Consortium-2 consensus document (VARC-2). Eur J Cardiothorac Surg. 2012;42(5):S45–60.
30. Achenbach S, Delgado V, Hausleiter J, Schoenhagen P, Min JK, Leipsic JA. SCCT expert consensus document on computed tomography imaging before transcatheter aortic valve implantation (TAVI)/transcatheter aortic valve replacement (TAVR). J Cardiovasc Comput Tomogr. 2012;6(6):366–80.
31. Wood DA, Tops LF, Mayo JR, Pasupati S, Schalij MJ, Humphries K, et al. Role of multislice computed tomography in transcatheter aortic valve replacement. Am J Cardiol. 2009;103(9):1295–301.
32. Apfaltrer P, Henzler T, Blanke P, Krazinski AW, Silverman JR, Schoepf UJ. Computed tomography for planning transcatheter aortic valve replacement. J Thorac Imaging. 2013;28(4):231–9.
33. Ludman PF, Moat N, de Belder MA, Blackman DJ, Duncan A, Banya W, et al. Transcatheter aortic valve implantation in the United Kingdom: temporal trends, predictors of outcome, and 6-year follow-up: a report from the UK Transcatheter aortic valve implantation (TAVI) registry, 2007 to 2012. Circulation. 2015;131(13):1181–90.
34. Ribeiro HB, Webb JG, Makkar RR, Cohen MG, Kapadia SR, Kodali S, et al. Predictive factors, management, and clinical outcomes of coronary obstruction following transcatheter aortic valve implantation: insights from a large multicenter registry. J Am Coll Cardiol. 2013;62(17):1552–62.
35. Blanke P, Schoepf UJ, Leipsic JA. CT in transcatheter aortic valve replacement. Radiology. 2013;269(3):650–69.
36. Matsumoto S, Yamada Y, Hashimoto M, Okamura T, Yamada M, Yashima F, et al. CT imaging before transcatheter aortic valve implantation (TAVI) using variable helical pitch scanning and its

diagnostic performance for coronary artery disease. Eur Radiol. 2017;27(5):1963–70.
37. Bittner DO, Arnold M, Klinghammer L, Schuhbaeck A, Hell MM, Muschiol G, et al. Contrast volume reduction using third generation dual source computed tomography for the evaluation of patients prior to transcatheter aortic valve implantation. Eur Radiol. 2016;26(12):4497–504.
38. Felmly LM, De Cecco CN, Schoepf UJ, Varga-Szemes A, Mangold S, McQuiston AD, et al. Low contrast medium-volume third-generation dual-source computed tomography angiography for transcatheter aortic valve replacement planning. Eur Radiol. 2017;27(5):1944–53.
39. Formosa A, Santos DM, Marcuzzi D, Common AA, Prabhudesai V. Low contrast dose catheter-directed CT angiography (CCTA). Cardiovasc Intervent Radiol. 2016;39(4):606–10.
40. Kok M, Turek J, Mihl C, Reinartz SD, Gohmann RF, Nijssen EC, et al. Low contrast media volume in pre-TAVI CT examinations. Eur Radiol. 2016;26(8):2426–35.
41. Abe M, Morimoto T, Akao M, Furukawa Y, Nakagawa Y, Shizuta S, et al. Relation of contrast-induced nephropathy to long-term mortality after percutaneous coronary intervention. Am J Cardiol. 2014;114(3):362–8.
42. Jochheim D, Schneider VS, Schwarz F, Kupatt C, Lange P, Reiser M, et al. Contrast-induced acute kidney injury after computed tomography prior to transcatheter aortic valve implantation. Clin Radiol. 2014;69(10):1034–8.
43. Hausleiter J. Reduced contrast media volumes for CT imaging of TAVI candidates. Eur Heart J Cardiovasc Imaging. 2016;17(1):11.
44. Al Ali AM, Altwegg L, Horlick EM, Feindel C, Thompson CR, Cheung A, et al. Prevention and management of transcatheter balloon-expandable aortic valve malposition. Catheter Cardiovasc Interv. 2008;72(4):573–8.
45. Messika-Zeitoun D, Serfaty JM, Brochet E, Ducrocq G, Lepage L, Detaint D, et al. Multimodal assessment of the aortic annulus diameter: implications for transcatheter aortic valve implantation. J Am Coll Cardiol. 2010;55(3):186–94.
46. Gurvitch R, Webb JG, Yuan R, Johnson M, Hague C, Willson AB, et al. Aortic annulus diameter determination by multidetector computed tomography: reproducibility, applicability, and implications for transcatheter aortic valve implantation. JACC Cardiovasc Interv. 2011;4(11):1235–45.
47. Hansson NC, Thuesen L, Hjortdal VE, Leipsic J, Andersen HR, Poulsen SH, et al. Three-dimensional multidetector computed tomography versus conventional 2-dimensional transesophageal echocardiography for annular sizing in transcatheter aortic valve replacement: influence on postprocedural paravalvular aortic regurgitation. Catheter Cardiovasc Interv. 2013;82(6):977–86.
48. Mylotte D, Dorfmeister M, Elhmidi Y, Mazzitelli D, Bleiziffer S, Wagner A, et al. Erroneous measurement of the aortic annular diameter using 2-dimensional echocardiography resulting in inappropriate CoreValve size selection: a retrospective comparison with multislice computed tomography. JACC Cardiovasc Interv. 2014;7(6):652–61.
49. Shibayama K, Mihara H, Jilaihawi H, Berdejo J, Harada K, Itabashi Y, et al. 3D assessment of features associated with transvalvular aortic regurgitation after TAVR: a real-time 3D TEE study. JACC Cardiovasc Imaging. 2016;9(2):114–23.
50. Wichmann JL, Varga-Szemes A, Suranyi P, Bayer RR, Litwin SE, De Cecco CN, et al. Transcatheter aortic valve replacement: imaging techniques for aortic root sizing. J Thorac Imaging. 2015;30(6):349–58.
51. Willson AB, Webb JG, Labounty TM, Achenbach S, Moss R, Wheeler M, et al. 3-dimensional aortic annular assessment by multidetector computed tomography predicts moderate or severe paravalvular regurgitation after transcatheter aortic valve replacement: a multicenter retrospective analysis. J Am Coll Cardiol. 2012;59(14):1287–94.
52. Yang TH, Webb JG, Blanke P, Dvir D, Hansson NC, Norgaard BL, et al. Incidence and severity of paravalvular aortic regurgitation with multidetector computed tomography nominal area oversizing or undersizing after transcatheter heart valve replacement with the Sapien 3: a comparison with the Sapien XT. JACC Cardiovasc Interv. 2015;8(3):462–71.
53. Hamdan A, Guetta V, Konen E, Goitein O, Segev A, Raanani E, et al. Deformation dynamics and mechanical properties of the aortic annulus by 4-dimensional computed tomography: insights into the functional anatomy of the aortic valve complex and implications for transcatheter aortic valve therapy. J Am Coll Cardiol. 2012;59(2):119–27.
54. Murphy DT, Blanke P, Alaamri S, Naoum C, Rubinshtein R, Pache G, et al. Dynamism of the aortic annulus: effect of diastolic versus systolic CT annular measurements on device selection in transcatheter aortic valve replacement (TAVR). J Cardiovasc Comput Tomogr. 2016;10(1):37–43.
55. Blanke P, Euringer W, Baumann T, Reinohl J, Schlensak C, Langer M, et al. Combined assessment of aortic root anatomy and aortoiliac vasculature with dual-source CT as a screening tool in patients evaluated for transcatheter aortic valve implantation. AJR Am J Roentgenol. 2010;195(4):872–81.
56. Schmidkonz C, Marwan M, Klinghammer L, Mitschke M, Schuhbaeck A, Arnold M, et al. Interobserver variability of CT angiography for evaluation of aortic annulus dimensions prior to transcatheter aortic valve implantation (TAVI). Eur J Radiol. 2014;83(9):1672–8.
57. Korosoglou G, Gitsioudis G, Waechter-Stehle I, Weese J, Krumsdorf U, Chorianopoulos E, et al. Objective quantification of aortic valvular structures by cardiac computed tomography angiography in patients considered for transcatheter aortic valve implantation. Catheter Cardiovasc Interv. 2013;81(1):148–59.
58. Athappan G, Patvardhan E, Tuzcu EM, Svensson LG, Lemos PA, Fraccaro C, et al. Incidence, predictors, and outcomes of aortic regurgitation after transcatheter aortic valve replacement: meta-analysis and systematic review of literature. J Am Coll Cardiol. 2013;61(15):1585–95.
59. Binder RK, Webb JG, Willson AB, Urena M, Hansson NC, Norgaard BL, et al. The impact of integration of a multidetector computed tomography annulus area sizing algorithm on outcomes of transcatheter aortic valve replacement: a prospective, multicenter, controlled trial. J Am Coll Cardiol. 2013;62(5):431–8.
60. Van Linden A, Kempfert J, Blumenstein J, Mollmann H, Kim WK, Alkaya S, et al. Manual versus automatic detection of aortic annulus plane in a computed tomography scan for transcatheter aortic valve implantation screening. Eur J Cardiothorac Surg. 2014;46(2):207–12. discussion 12.
61. Patsalis PC, Al-Rashid F, Neumann T, Plicht B, Hildebrandt HA, Wendt D, et al. Preparatory balloon aortic valvuloplasty during transcatheter aortic valve implantation for improved valve sizing. JACC Cardiovasc Interv. 2013;6(9):965–71.
62. Blanke P, Reinohl J, Schlensak C, Siepe M, Pache G, Euringer W, et al. Prosthesis oversizing in balloon-expandable transcatheter aortic valve implantation is associated with contained rupture of the aortic root. Circ Cardiovasc Interv. 2012;5(4):540–8.
63. Hell MM, Biburger L, Marwan M, Schuhbaeck A, Achenbach S, Lell M, et al. Prediction of fluoroscopic angulations for transcatheter aortic valve implantation by CT angiography: influence on procedural parameters. Eur Heart J Cardiovasc Imaging. 2017;18(8):906–14.
64. Holzamer A, Sitka E, Hengstenberg C, Schmid C, Debl K, Maier L, et al. Multislice computed tomography-based prediction of the implantation plane in transcatheter aortic valve implantation: deter-

mination of the line of perpendicularity and the implanter's views. Eur J Cardiothorac Surg. 2015;48(6):879–85. discussion 85-6.
65. Azzalini L, Ghoshhajra BB, Elmariah S, Passeri JJ, Inglessis I, Palacios IF, et al. The aortic valve calcium nodule score (AVCNS) independently predicts paravalvular regurgitation after transcatheter aortic valve replacement (TAVR). J Cardiovasc Comput Tomogr. 2014;8(2):131–40.
66. Harbaoui B, Montoy M, Charles P, Boussel L, Liebgott H, Girerd N, et al. Aorta calcification burden: towards an integrative predictor of cardiac outcome after transcatheter aortic valve implantation. Atherosclerosis. 2016;246:161–8.
67. Jilaihawi H, Makkar RR, Kashif M, Okuyama K, Chakravarty T, Shiota T, et al. A revised methodology for aortic-valvar complex calcium quantification for transcatheter aortic valve implantation. Eur Heart J Cardiovasc Imaging. 2014;15(12):1324–32.
68. Khalique OK, Hahn RT, Gada H, Nazif TM, Vahl TP, George I, et al. Quantity and location of aortic valve complex calcification predicts severity and location of paravalvular regurgitation and frequency of post-dilation after balloon-expandable transcatheter aortic valve replacement. JACC Cardiovasc Interv. 2014;7(8):885–94.
69. Koh EY, Lam KY, Bindraban NR, Cocchieri R, Planken RN, Koch KT, et al. Aortic valve calcification as a predictor of location and severity of paravalvular regurgitation after transcatheter aortic valve implantation. Interact Cardiovasc Thorac Surg. 2015;20(3):345–50.
70. Fujita B, Kutting M, Seiffert M, Scholtz S, Egron S, Prashovikj E, et al. Calcium distribution patterns of the aortic valve as a risk factor for the need of permanent pacemaker implantation after transcatheter aortic valve implantation. Eur Heart J Cardiovasc Imaging. 2016;17(12):1385–93.
71. Hansson NC, Norgaard BL, Barbanti M, Nielsen NE, Yang TH, Tamburino C, et al. The impact of calcium volume and distribution in aortic root injury related to balloon-expandable transcatheter aortic valve replacement. J Cardiovasc Comput Tomogr. 2015;9(5):382–92.
72. Sievers HH, Schmidtke C. A classification system for the bicuspid aortic valve from 304 surgical specimens. J Thorac Cardiovasc Surg. 2007;133(5):1226–33.
73. Jilaihawi H, Chen M, Webb J, Himbert D, Ruiz CE, Rodes-Cabau J, et al. A bicuspid aortic valve imaging classification for the TAVR era. JACC Cardiovasc Imaging. 2016;9(10):1145–58.
74. Mylotte D, Lefevre T, Sondergaard L, Watanabe Y, Modine T, Dvir D, et al. Transcatheter aortic valve replacement in bicuspid aortic valve disease. J Am Coll Cardiol. 2014;64(22):2330–9.
75. Webb JG, Chandavimol M, Thompson CR, Ricci DR, Carere RG, Munt BI, et al. Percutaneous aortic valve implantation retrograde from the femoral artery. Circulation. 2006;113(6):842–50.
76. Vahanian A, Alfieri O, Al-Attar N, Antunes M, Bax J, Cormier B, et al. Transcatheter valve implantation for patients with aortic stenosis: a position statement from the European Association of Cardio-Thoracic Surgery (EACTS) and the European Society of Cardiology (ESC), in collaboration with the European Association of Percutaneous Cardiovascular Interventions (EAPCI). Eur Heart J. 2008;29(11):1463–70.
77. Genereux P, Head SJ, Van Mieghem NM, Kodali S, Kirtane AJ, Xu K, et al. Clinical outcomes after transcatheter aortic valve replacement using valve academic research consortium definitions: a weighted meta-analysis of 3,519 patients from 16 studies. J Am Coll Cardiol. 2012;59(25):2317–26.
78. Herrmann HC, Thourani VH, Kodali SK, Makkar RR, Szeto WY, Anwaruddin S, et al. One-year clinical outcomes with SAPIEN 3 transcatheter aortic valve replacement in high-risk and inoperable patients with severe aortic stenosis. Circulation. 2016;134(2):130–40.
79. Kodali S, Williams MR, Doshi D, Hahn RT, Humphries KH, Nkomo VT, et al. Sex-specific differences at presentation and outcomes among patients undergoing transcatheter aortic valve replacement: a cohort study. Ann Intern Med. 2016;164(6):377–84.
80. Toggweiler S, Gurvitch R, Leipsic J, Wood DA, Willson AB, Binder RK, et al. Percutaneous aortic valve replacement: vascular outcomes with a fully percutaneous procedure. J Am Coll Cardiol. 2012;59(2):113–8.
81. Barbash IM, Finkelstein A, Barsheshet A, Segev A, Steinvil A, Assali A, et al. Outcomes of patients at estimated low, intermediate, and high risk undergoing transcatheter aortic valve implantation for aortic stenosis. Am J Cardiol. 2015;116(12):1916–22.
82. Chieffo A, Buchanan GL, Van Mieghem NM, Tchetche D, Dumonteil N, Latib A, et al. Transcatheter aortic valve implantation with the Edwards SAPIEN versus the Medtronic CoreValve Revalving system devices: a multicenter collaborative study: the PRAGMATIC plus initiative (pooled-RotterdAm-Milano-Toulouse in collaboration). J Am Coll Cardiol. 2013;61(8):830–6.
83. Kapadia SR, Svensson LG, Roselli E, Schoenhagen P, Popovic Z, Alfirevic A, et al. Single center TAVR experience with a focus on the prevention and management of catastrophic complications. Catheter Cardiovasc Interv. 2014;84(5):834–42.
84. Beohar N, Kirtane AJ, Blackstone E, Waksman R, Holmes D Jr, Minha S, et al. Trends in complications and outcomes of patients undergoing transfemoral transcatheter aortic valve replacement: experience from the PARTNER continued access registry. JACC Cardiovasc Interv. 2016;9(4):355–63.
85. Takagi H, Umemoto T, Group A. Impact of paravalvular aortic regurgitation after transcatheter aortic valve implantation on survival. Int J Cardiol. 2016;221:46–51.
86. Popma JJ, Gleason TG, Yakubov SJ, Harrison JK, Forrest JK, Maini B, et al. Relationship of annular sizing using multidetector computed tomographic imaging and clinical outcomes after self-expanding corevalve transcatheter aortic valve replacement. Circ Cardiovasc Interv. 2016;9(7)
87. Makkar RR, Fontana G, Jilaihawi H, Chakravarty T, Kofoed KF, de Backer O, et al. Possible subclinical leaflet thrombosis in bioprosthetic aortic valves. N Engl J Med. 2015;373(21):2015–24.
88. Holmes DR Jr, Mack MJ, Kaul S, Agnihotri A, Alexander KP, Bailey SR, et al. ACCF/AATS/SCAI/STS expert consensus document on transcatheter aortic valve replacement: developed in collabration with the American Heart Association, American Society of Echocardiography, European Association for Cardio-Thoracic Surgery, Heart Failure Society of America, mended hearts, Society of Cardiovascular Anesthesiologists, Society of Cardiovascular Computed Tomography, and Society for Cardiovascular Magnetic Resonance. J Thorac Cardiovasc Surg. 2012;144(3):e29–84.
89. Himbert D, Brochet E, Serfaty JM, Vahanian A. Contained aortic root rupture after transcatheter aortic valve implantation. Eur Heart J. 2010;31(24):2995.
90. Oda T, Okamura T, Miyazaki Y, Nakamura T, Mikamo A, Wada Y, et al. 1-year follow-up of contained aortic root rupture after transcatheter aortic valve replacement. JACC Cardiovasc Interv. 2016;9(3):295–6.
91. Eggebrecht H, Schmermund A, Kahlert P, Erbel R, Voigtlander T, Mehta RH. Emergent cardiac surgery during transcatheter aortic valve implantation (TAVI): a weighted meta-analysis of 9,251 patients from 46 studies. EuroIntervention. 2013;8(9):1072–80.
92. Rezq A, Basavarajaiah S, Latib A, Takagi K, Hasegawa T, Figini F, et al. Incidence, management, and outcomes of cardiac tampon-

ade during transcatheter aortic valve implantation: a single-center study. JACC Cardiovasc Interv. 2012;5(12):1264–72.
93. Brennan JM, Edwards FH, Zhao Y, O'Brien S, Booth ME, Dokholyan RS, et al. Long-term safety and effectiveness of mechanical versus biologic aortic valve prostheses in older patients: results from the Society of Thoracic Surgeons adult cardiac surgery National Database. Circulation. 2013;127(16):1647–55.
94. Dvir D, Webb JG, Bleiziffer S, Pasic M, Waksman R, Kodali S, et al. Transcatheter aortic valve implantation in failed bioprosthetic surgical valves. JAMA. 2014;312(2):162–70.
95. Bapat V. Valve-in-valve apps: why and how they were developed and how to use them. EuroIntervention. 2014;10(Suppl U):U44–51.
96. Hamdan A, Wellnhofer E, Konen E, Kelle S, Goitein O, Andrada B, et al. Coronary CT angiography for the detection of coronary artery stenosis in patients referred for transcatheter aortic valve replacement. J Cardiovasc Comput Tomogr. 2015;9(1):31–41.

CT for Minimally Invasive Repair of Mitral Valve and Other Structural Heart Diseases

42

John F. Mooney, Philipp Blanke, Shaw Hua Kueh, Stephanie Sellers, and Jonathon A. Leipsic

Minimally invasive procedures on the mitral valve and other cardiac structures offer a feasible alternative when the risk of surgery is unacceptably high. In particular, the success of transcatheter aortic valve replacement (TAVR) has led to the development of transcatheter mitral valve replacement (TMVR) implantation. With a high burden of mitral disease in an ageing population with significant comorbidities to contraindicate surgery, percutaneous repair or replacement is predicted to progressively expand.

The mitral valve poses a challenge to imaging and device implantation due to its complex shape and proximity to the left ventricular outflow tract (LVOT). CT offers excellent spatial and temporal resolution to define the anatomy of interest and relationship to surrounding structures. It can help determine accurate sizing for devices, provide images that correspond with fluoroscopy and screen for adverse risk and contraindication to procedures. Similar to the experience with TAVR, pre-procedural CT has the potential to accurately identify those at risk of complications and aid planning to minimize adverse outcomes. In addition to mitral procedures, CT is also used prior to structural procedures on atrial and septal defect, planning for pulmonary vein isolation and pulmonary valve replacement.

Minimally Invasive Repair or Replacement of the Mitral Valve

Procedural Overview

Mitral regurgitation is prevalent in over 10% of individuals aged greater than 75 years [1], with surgical repair or replacement the gold standard for treating significant mitral valve disorders [2]. However the risk of adverse peri- or post-operative morbidity and mortality may be unacceptably high in some patients. Risk categorization is commonly expressed with risk prediction tools like the Society of Thoracic Surgeons (STS) risk prediction model [3]. This includes pre-surgical morbidities like advanced age, underlying kidney failure, pre-existing heart failure as well as acute heart failure requiring active treatment with inotropes and balloon pump. In addition to the STS risk model, other risk factors that may preclude surgical intervention include patient frailty, highly calcified aorta, severe pulmonary hypertension and severe liver disease [4]. Patient characteristics also increase risk of morbidity and mortality, with older patients, those with low LVEF and those with an increased Charlson comorbidity index score more likely to be denied surgery [5].

Percutaneous repair or replacement of the mitral valve presents as a viable option for patients deemed too high a surgical risk. Current American College of Cardiology/American Heart Association (ACC/AHA) guidelines [4] list criteria for patients with mitral regurgitation that are potentially suitable for minimally invasive approach and include:

- Severely symptomatic heart failure (NYHA class III/IV) despite medical therapy.
- Chronic mitral regurgitation caused by leaflet degeneration (primary MR) as opposed to MR resulting from left ventricular remodelling (secondary MR).
- MR graded as moderate/severe to severe on echocardiography.
- The anatomy permits repair or replacement.
- The patient otherwise has a reasonable life expectancy.
- Comorbidities place the patient as an unacceptable surgical risk.

Transcutaneous mitral valve procedures have predominantly involved mitral repair rather than replacement. The MitraClip™ device (Abbott Vascular) has a widespread use, is the only FDA-approved device and has ongoing registry-based

J. F. Mooney · P. Blanke · S. H. Kueh · S. Sellers
Department of Radiology, University of British Columbia, Vancouver, BC, Canada

J. A. Leipsic (✉)
Department of Radiology, St. Paul's Hospital, Providence Healthcare, Vancouver, BC, Canada
e-mail: JLeipsic@providencehealth.bc.ca

U. J. Schoepf (ed.), *CT of the Heart*, Contemporary Medical Imaging, https://doi.org/10.1007/978-1-60327-237-7_42

evidence to its utility [6]. The concept of the MitraClip is derived from the Alfieri surgical repair of the mitral valve, where a double stitch between the anterior and posterior leaflets fixes the cusps where regurgitation is maximal. A double orifice is thereby created with two smaller inflow orifices. Access is gained by the femoral vein and transeptal puncture.

Experience with the MitraClip device has been presented in several registries and trials. The EVEREST I trial assessed feasibility and followed 24 patients with clips. Of these 13 had reduced MR sustained at 6 months [7]. The subsequent EVEREST II trial randomly assigned 279 patients to either surgical repair or percutaneous repair in a 2:1 ratio [8]. Outcomes were assessed at 30 days and 12 months with primary endpoints being survival, 30-day adverse outcomes, requirement for additional surgery and continued grade 3/4 MR. The overall findings were of greater efficacy in the surgical cohort (73% vs 55%), though with less adverse outcomes within the percutaneous repair group (15% vs 48%). The safety of percutaneous repair was confirmed in an analysis of high-risk candidates from the EVEREST II cohort. A total of 78 patients with estimated surgical mortality of 12% or greater were compared to a cohort that was screened but not enrolled [9]. The 12-month survival was 78% in the high-risk group receiving the device and 55% in the matched comparison group. In the treatment arm, there were improvements at 12 months in MR grade ≤2 (78%), left ventricular end-diastolic volume (172 ml to 140 ml, $p = 0.001$), NYHA class (89% III/IV at baseline, 74% I/II at 12 months, $p < 0.0001$) and rate of hospitalization (from 0.59 to 0.32, $p = 0.034$) [10]. Current guidelines recommend percutaneous mitral repair in patients with chronic primary MR, who are severely symptomatic despite optimal medical therapy and at prohibitive risk for surgery [4].

The safety and efficacy of the deployment of a transcatheter aortic valve for the relief of native mitral stenosis in the setting of severe mitral annular calcification (MAC) have been presented by a global registry to measure technique and outcomes [11]. A total of 64 patients with severe mitral annular calcification (NYHA III–IV) and an average Society of Thoracic Surgeons score of 14.4, from 32 centres, underwent compassionate deployment of a balloon-expandable transcatheter aortic device. The transapical (43.8%) followed by the transeptal (40.6%) and transatrial (15.6%) route was used. The device was deployed successfully in 72% of cases, with 11 requiring a second valve. A total of six patients had severe left ventricular outflow tract obstruction causing haemodynamic compromise, and of these two died. The 30-day all-cause mortality was 29.7% (12.5% cardiovascular cause, 17.2% non-cardiovascular cause), and of the survivors, 84% had improvement in symptoms (NYHA I–II). The frail state of many of the patients was observed as a significant contributor to mortality.

Devices specific for TMVR are currently undergoing feasibility trials. These include Tiara™ (Neovasc Inc. Richmond BC, Canada), CardiAQ™ (CardiAQ Valve Technologies, Irvine CA, USA), Tendyne™ (Tendyne Holdings, Roseville, MN, USA) and Twelve™ (Twelve Inc. Redwood City CA, USA). The devices incorporate distinct features to aid positioning. These include atrial skirts to aid apposition against the left atrial wall, tabs to engage the myocardium, anchors to engage the annulus and leaflets and paddles to engage the leaflets or apical tether. Transeptal implantation has not been successful, and the devices are designed for transapical delivery [10].

CT for Minimally Invasive Repair or Replacement of the Mitral Valve

Pre-procedural CT is commonly used to determine anatomical feasibility and to help with device sizing, deployment and vascular access for TAVR. It can also aid in defining adverse features such as subannular calcification, risk of coronary obstruction and excess annular dilation. Integration of CT imaging has led to improved outcomes after TAVR, with reduction in paravalvular leaks [12, 13] and vascular complications [14, 15]. The successful utility of CT in optimizing sizing for TAVR has led to its adoption for planning in TMVR.

Planning for mitral valve procedures using CT offers several advantages. It can accurately define annular dimensions in a reproducible fashion, calcification, and the anatomical landing zone and help with apical access and the detailed anatomy of the LVOT. It can also provide coplanar projection angles to assist implantation under fluoroscopy. Imaging considerations for a transcatheter mitral valve repair include a planimetric area >4.0 cm^2, minimal leaflet calcification where the device will grasp, limited flail width (<15 mm and flail gap <10 mm) and large central jet >6 cm^2 or >30% of the left atrial area (generally defined by echocardiogram) [8]. Mitral valve replacement requires determination of annular area and risk of LVOT obstruction. Oversizing can result in LVOT obstruction as well as potential rupture, and undersizing can result in valve embolization [11].

CT Acquisition

CT provides image quality of high-spatial and high-temporal resolution which is necessary for accurate sizing of the mitral valve. The constant motion of the mitral apparatus during the cardiac cycle requires rapid image acquisition with multidetector computed tomography (MDCT), typically with at least a 64-slice scanner. Image acquisition is synchronized to the ECG cycle and retrospective acquisition throughout the cardiac cycle performed. Contrast enhancement is required to enhance tissue boundaries. Retrospective acquisition allows the whole cardiac cycle to be imaged and any time point to be reconstructed. This allows assessment throughout the cardiac cycle albeit at higher radiation dose [16]. Image analysis is performed with multiplanar reformation (MPR) to provide thin two-dimensional planes through the three-dimensional data set allowing reconstruction in any plane [16].

Mitral Valve Anatomy

The mitral valve poses a challenge to both imaging and prosthetic implantation due to its complex anatomy, larger size and proximity to the left ventricular outflow tract. It is a complex three-dimensional structure composed of a saddle-shaped annulus, anterior and posterior leaflets, papillary muscles and chordae.

The annulus is a three-dimensional, nonplanar structure with two distinct peaks. It serves as the conduit between the left atrium and left ventricle and is incorporated in the left ventricle myocardium [17]. The posterior peak is at the insertion of the posterior leaflet and extends from the lateral to medial trigone. The anterior peak is defined by the intervalvular fibrosa (aka aorto-mitral curtain or aortic continuity) that lies between the mitral and aortic annulus. Between these peaks lies the nadir at the trigones. The intervalvular fibrosa lies between the mitral and aortic annulus and is anchored to the mitral annulus at the lateral and medial trigones [18].

The mitral valve is unique as it is the only cardiac valve to possess two leaflets – the anterior and posterior leaflets. The anterior leaflet is semi-circular in shape, whereas the posterior leaflet is rectangular. At each end are clefts, or commissures, which divide the leaflets. The posterior leaflet is divided further by clefts, creating three scallops labelled P1, P2 and P3 from lateral to medial. Though less distinct, by convention, the anterior leaflet is also categorized into corresponding scallops A1, A2 and A3.

Two papillary muscles (anterolateral and postero-medial) arise from the free wall of the left ventricle. Fibrous chordae run from each papillary muscle to the free edge of both leaflets. During systole, papillary muscle contraction brings the leaflets to coapt and prevent flow into the left atrium. In diastole, papillary muscle relaxation allows the leaflets to open.

Determining the Mitral Annular Area

MDCT also plays a critical role, owing to its exceptional spatial resolution, for the determination of the appropriateness of individual anatomy for TMVR. In particular, in the early days of TMVR, there are limited device sizes making accurate annular sizing and segmentation essential. Annular area can vary widely between patients, with estimates of annular area ranging from 7 to 10 cm^2 in healthy subjects [19] and between 11 and 20 cm^2 in patients with LV dilatation and functional MR. [19] This is reflected chiefly in an increased distance between the septal and lateral, also known as A2 to P2, distance compared to the intercommisural distance [20]. Accurately defining mitral dimensions has improved with 3D imaging techniques. Traditional 2D imaging techniques rely on accurate orientation to account for the nonplanar structure of the mitral apparatus, and estimated dimensions varied dependent on orientation [21]. A lack of consensus on defining the anterior boundary has also limited consistency in 2D measurement [22].

The use of 3D segmentation has improved accurate depiction of the mitral annulus [23] and is achieved by generating a cubic spline of manually placed points along the 3D contour. The LV long axis is identified, and seeding points are placed manually along the insertion of the posterior mitral leaflet and along the fibrous continuity with stepwise rotation at 22.5° to insert each point. Figure 42.1 illustrates the

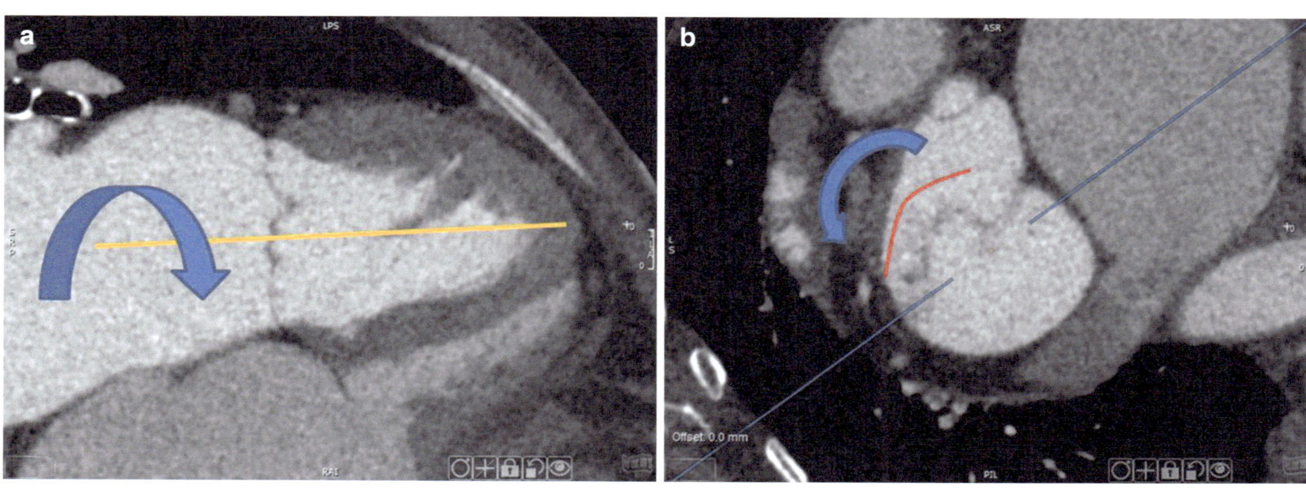

Fig. 42.1 Acquisition of the annular plane. (**a**) The long axis of the LV is identified and from this the short axis view obtained. (**b**) Rotation around the long axis allows positioning of seed points along the insertion of the posterior mitral leaflet and contour of the fibrous continuity, with rotation of the LV long axis by 22.5° in stepwise manner

acquisition of the long-axis and short-axis views, whereby rotation around the long axis allows planting of seed points in the short axis. In Fig. 42.2 the seed points have been set, and a method of least squares allows projection of the 3D image onto a 2D plane by defining the geometric plane.

The saddle-shaped annulus has long been shown to best define the geometry of the mitral annulus, but if one were to size a transcatheter device on the basis of this saddle-shaped annulus, the device would almost certainly result in LVOT obstruction. As a result, based on CT analyses, it has been proposed that the annulus be truncated anteriorly at the medical and lateral trigones to create a D-shaped annulus that excludes the annular apparatus [24]. This 'D'-shaped model uses CT to define the trigones and then the reconstructed 2D dimensions using a method of least squares plane. The initial step is to identify the trigones, where the anterior mitral valve leaflet separates from the atrioventricular junction to follow the fibrous continuity. Figure 42.3 demonstrates how the trigones are identified using the 3D saddle-shaped model reconstruction in short- and long-axis views.

With the trigones defined, the anterior and posterior segments can be demarcated and allow comparison between saddle-shaped and D-shaped models. The saddle-shaped model includes the anterior segment for the measurement of dimensions, and the D-shaped model excludes structure anterior to the trigone-to-trigone line, including the aorto-mitral continuity and anterior aortic peaks. The intercommisural distance is parallel to the trigone-to-trigone distance and perpendicular to the septal-to-lateral distance, transecting it through the virtual plane at the centroid [24].

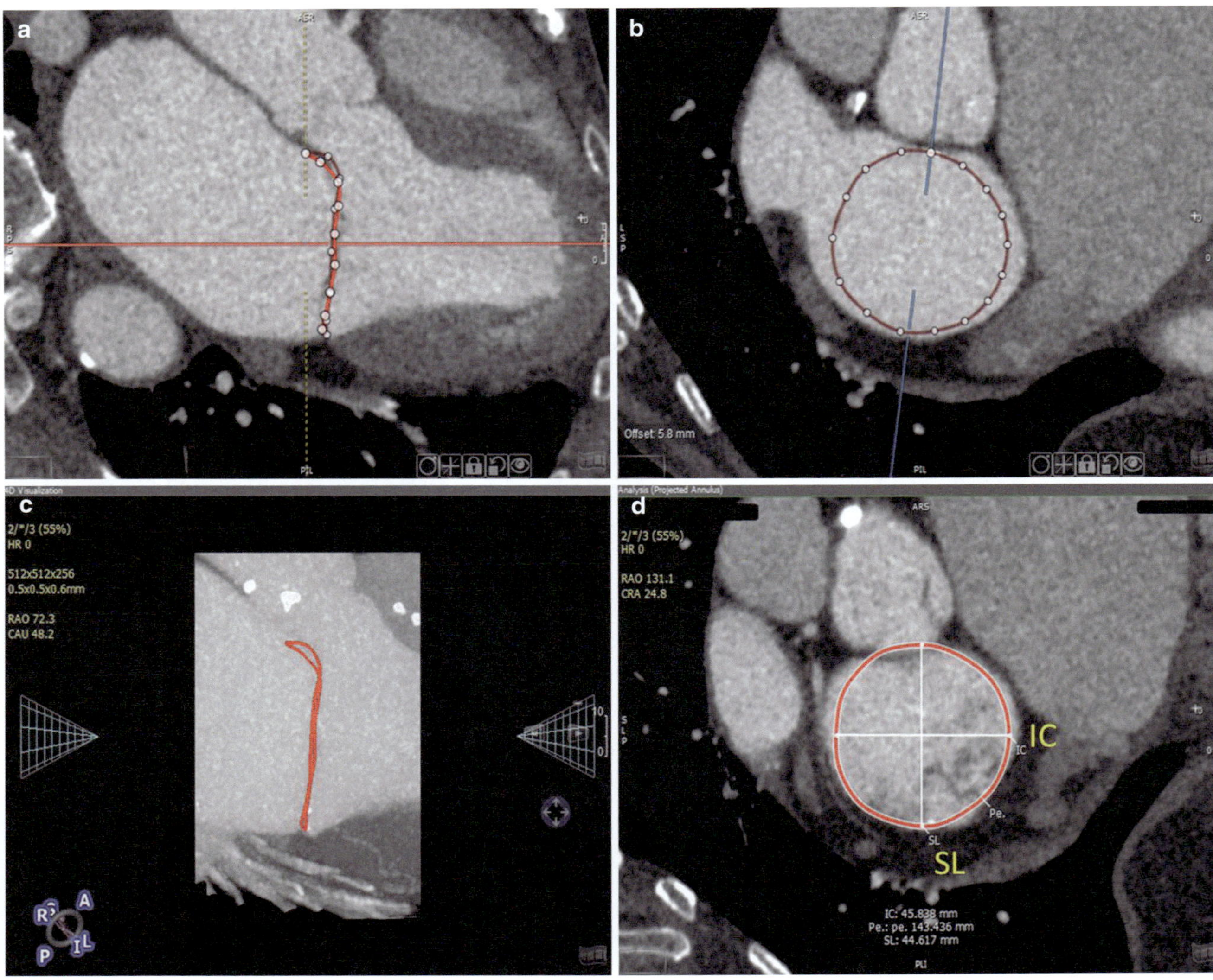

Fig. 42.2 Segmentation of the annulus. (**a**) Seeding points demonstrated in long axis. (**b**) The 16 seeding points in short axis. (**c**) 3-dimensional reconstruction of the saddle-shaped annulus superimposed on long-axis image. (**d**) Saddle-shaped annulus on short-axis view showing intercommisural (IC) and septa-lateral (SL) lines

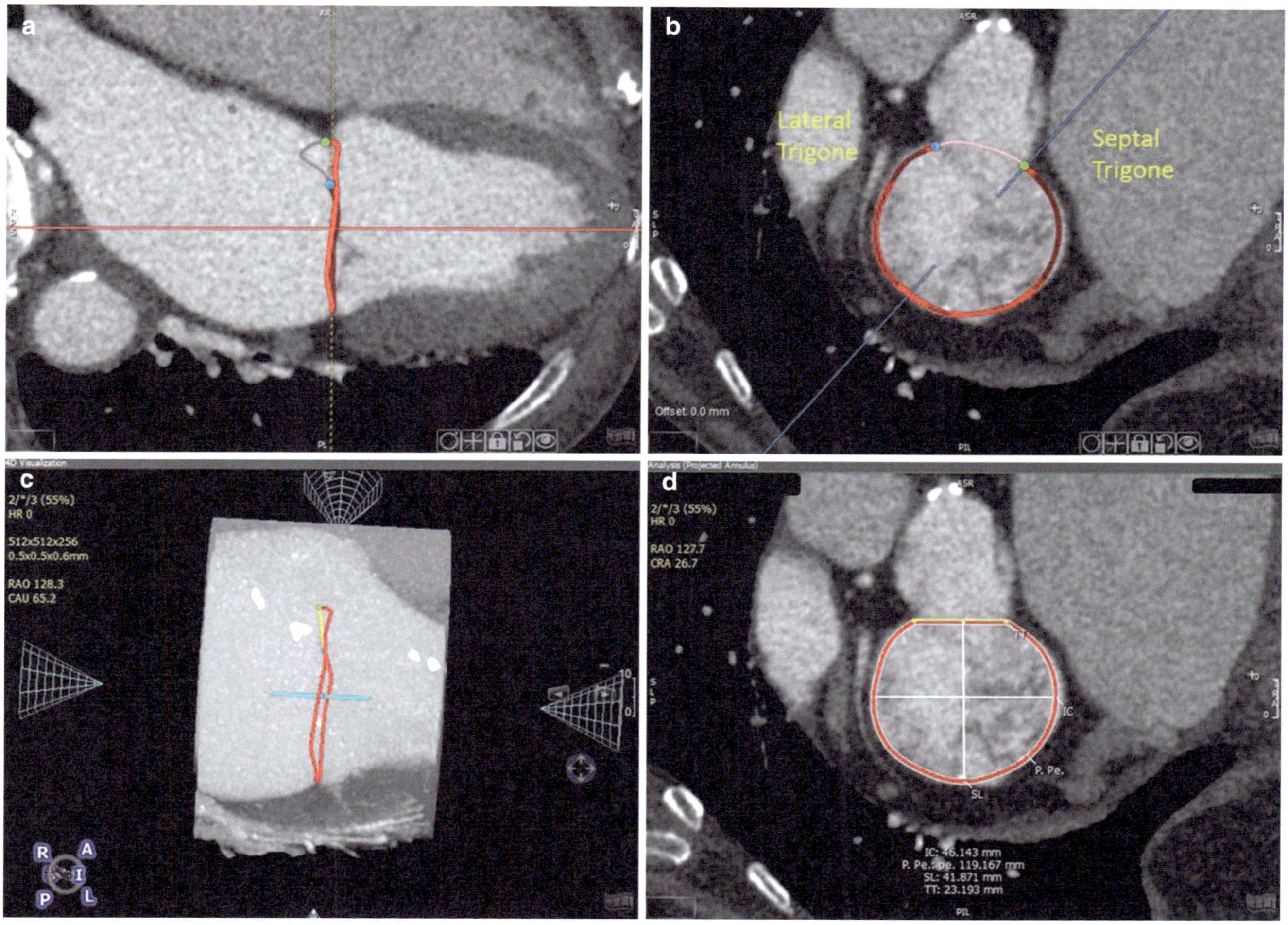

Fig. 42.3 Identification of trigones and definition of the D-shaped annulus. (**a**) Rotation on the long axis identifies trigones, where the mitral annulus separates from the intervalvular fibrosa. (**b**) Short-axis view with lateral (blue dot) and septal (green dot) trigones. (**c**, **d**) Construction of D-shaped annulus with omission of anterior segment in both long-axis (**c**) and short-axis (**d**) views

A D-shaped model is considered to have advantages over the saddle-shaped model. Firstly, it offers a standardized and reproducible method, with low interobserver variability, of estimating annular dimensions. Secondly, it resembles the cross-sectional area of TMVR devices which is of great relevance for correct sizing and implantation. This in turn reduces the risk of over- and undersizing, with the inherent risks of LVOT obstruction or paravalvular leak and device embolization, respectively. Thirdly, compared to the saddle-shaped model, there is less projection into the LVOT and the risks this poses [24].

The D-shaped method has identified variation in annular area between primary and secondary MR [20]. Primary causes relate to leaflet dysfunction and include leaflet prolapse, degeneration and destruction due to endocarditis or fibrosis. Secondary causes relate most commonly due to LV dilatation with or without prior infarction with tethering of the posterior leaflet with chordae rupture or annular dilatation due to dilated cardiomyopathy. Those with primary MR (in this case mitral valve prolapse) were found to have an absolute annular area 18% larger than those with secondary (functional) MR. Whether this in part relates to annular disjunction or frank septal-to-lateral enlargement is uncertain and will require further investigation. This is despite those patients with functional MR having overall larger LV volumes [20].

Landing Zone Characteristics

The surrounding anatomy of the annulus can be accurately defined with CT, including insertion at the atrioventricular junction, calcification and leaflets. The anatomy of the atrioventricular junction can vary between primary and secondary MR. Those with primary MR related to mitral valve prolapse may have mitral valvular disjunction, where the mitral leaflet insertion is displaced back into the atrium [25]. In secondary MR, changes in the surrounding myocardium can lead to leaflet tethering, reduced coaptation of leaflets and creation of a posterior myocardial shelf due to basal remodelling. Figure 42.4 demonstrates anatomical variation between valvular disjunction present in mitral valve prolapse (primary MR) and the presence of a prominent atrioventricular shelf in secondary mitral regurgitation [20].

CT can also readily demonstrate calcification and leaflet anatomy. Calcification on the mitral apparatus is a relatively common finding with advanced age. Extent of calcification can range from localized and mild to severe extending onto leaflets and rarely to caseous formation. The exact impact of annular calcification on self-expanding TMVR devices remains to be established, though significant calcification particularly when irregular is generally considered a contraindication to percutaneous valve implantation. Similarly, leaflet length, position and relationship to surrounding anatomy can be presented by CT. The length and anatomy of the leaflets can be determined in mid-diastole. The distance of the papillary muscles to the leaflets is also relevant, as closely tethered leaflets or direct papillary insertion to the leaflets may interfere with device anchoring [26].

Prediction of LVOT Obstruction

LVOT obstruction was a key cause of morbidity and mortality in the global registry for TMVR [11]. Proximity of the mitral annulus combined with unsuitable anatomy can lead to flow limitation or obstruction after implantation of prosthetic MV. Specific risk for LVOT obstruction relates to the anatomical relationship of the aorto-mitral angle, the LV size, the configuration of the interventricular septum and the device itself. Firstly, the angle between the mitral outflow and the LVOT long axis (aorto-mitral angle) poses risk where the angle is increased, and near-parallel angles pose minimal risk, whereas perpendicular angulation poses maximal risk. Secondly, a smaller overall left ventricular size may not be able to accommodate an implanted valve without threatening the LVOT. A third contribution to LVOT obstruction is hypertrophy at the basal septum that can accentuate the aorto-mitral angle and consequently diminish the LVOT area. Finally, the prosthetic device can protrude, or flare, into the LVOT and limit the cross-sectional area for systolic blood flow. Figure 42.5 compares a neo-LVOT with low risk of obstruction against one with very high risk of obstruction.

Determining the risk of LVOT obstruction is very important prior to TMVR. CT can provide insight by modelling device deployment and segmenting the residual LVOT with the virtual TMVR stent in place [27]. This predicted area of the neo-LVOT incorporates the influence of the aorto-mitral angle, LV size and basal hypertrophy and can indicate overall risk of obstruction. This approach is however limited as no discrete LVOT area has been established at which the risk of obstruction increases. It also will vary with loading conditions, residual LV function and the integrity of the choral apparatus. The stage of the cardiac cycle is also influential on obstruction, yet its role in determining LVOT remains unclear – minimal LVOT area occurs at end-systole – though this may have no influence on obstruction as maximal flow occurs early to mid-systole, proposing this stage may be more influential on risk on obstruction.

Fluoroscopic Angulation

CT can also assist valve implanters with coplanar views to assist coaxial device deployment, already utilized in TAVR

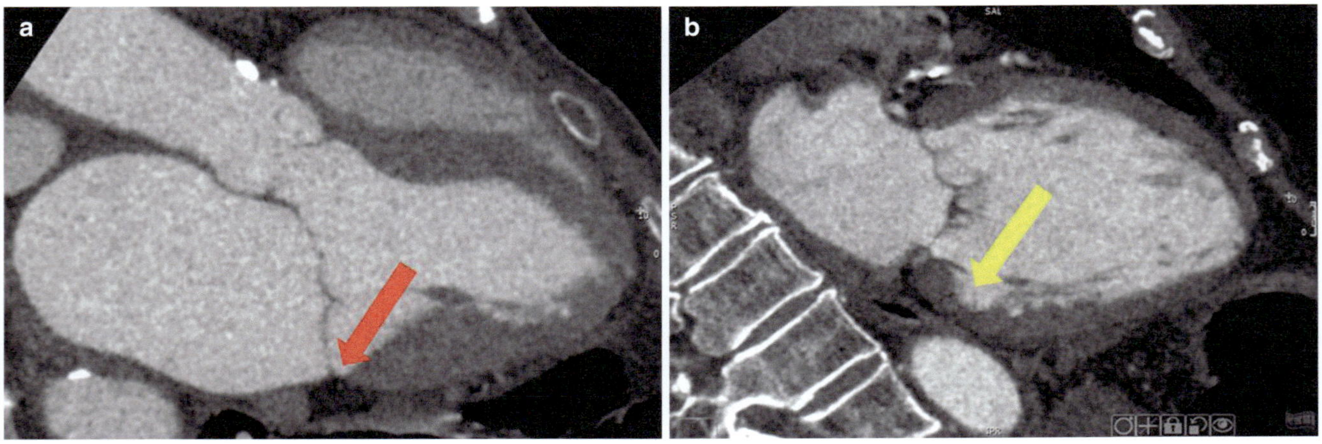

Fig. 42.4 The atrioventricular junction in (**a**) mitral valve prolapse with disjunction between MV insertion and atrioventricular junction (red arrow) and (**b**) functional mitral regurgitation with formation of an atrioventricular shelf adjacent to the MV insertion point (yellow arrow)

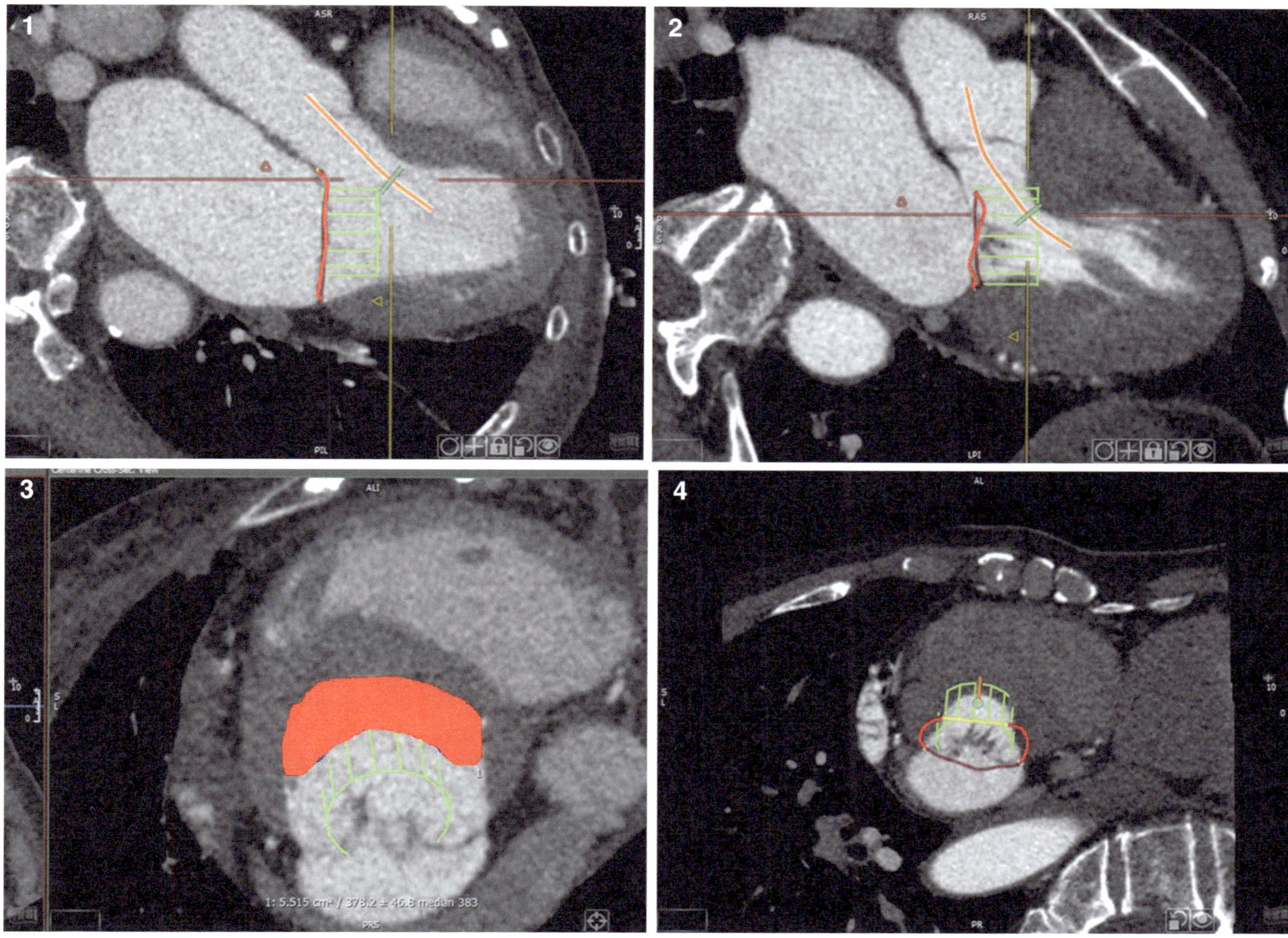

Fig. 42.5 CT data sets demonstrating prediction of neo-LVOT obstruction. Comparison between low- (1,3) and high-(2,4)risk cases for LVOT obstruction. The green cylinder simulates a 29 mm diameter device implant. The long-axis views demonstrate the neo-LVOT (shown by red bar), and the green bar represents the cross-sectional area. Image 1 shows an optimal LVOT tract and image 2 shows obstruction. In short-axis views, the cross-sectional area of the neo-LVOT is shown. Image 3 shows an optimal neo-LVOT area (highlighted in red) and image 4 shows complete obstruction

[28]. Plane segmentation on CT imaging can guide on the optimal angle (cranial or caudal) that corresponds to fluoroscopic projection, presenting implanters with an anatomical 'roadmap' prior to the procedure of what they can expect to see for coaxial deployment at corresponding C-arm angles [29]. The native annulus lies in an anterior-superior plane with angulation to the right. Projection angles have been assessed that correspond to the virtual lines that transect the annular plane – the septal-to-lateral line and trigone-to-trigone line. Figure 42.6 shows corresponding CT and fluoroscopic views with superimposed CT-derived annular geometry. Angulation of the arm to show the trigone-to-trigone line requires steep angulation (in this case RAO 77.3 CAU 51.8) that is not clinically practical.

In addition to the S curve of the mitral annulus, an en face angle is also commonly provided. This angle is meant to help guide the proceduralist as to how to position and direct his/her hands to allow for a perpendicular deployment. In Fig. 42.7, the 'en face' images and required C-arm projections are demonstrated, and Fig. 42.8 shows the projections required to emulate the septal-to-lateral line. It is worth noting that fluoroscopic angulation between the TT and SL views (as indicated along the red sigmoidal line in the figure); small changes in RAO angulation require corresponding larger changes in cranial or caudal angulation to maintain a coplanar angle.

The addition of a coronary sinus wire can aid in deployment, acting as a landmark by aligning with P1 along the floor of the coronary sinus and with P2. The guidewire path can also be represented in pre-procedural CT to help define the patient-specific relationship between the coronary sinus and P2 rather than relying on assumptions [29].

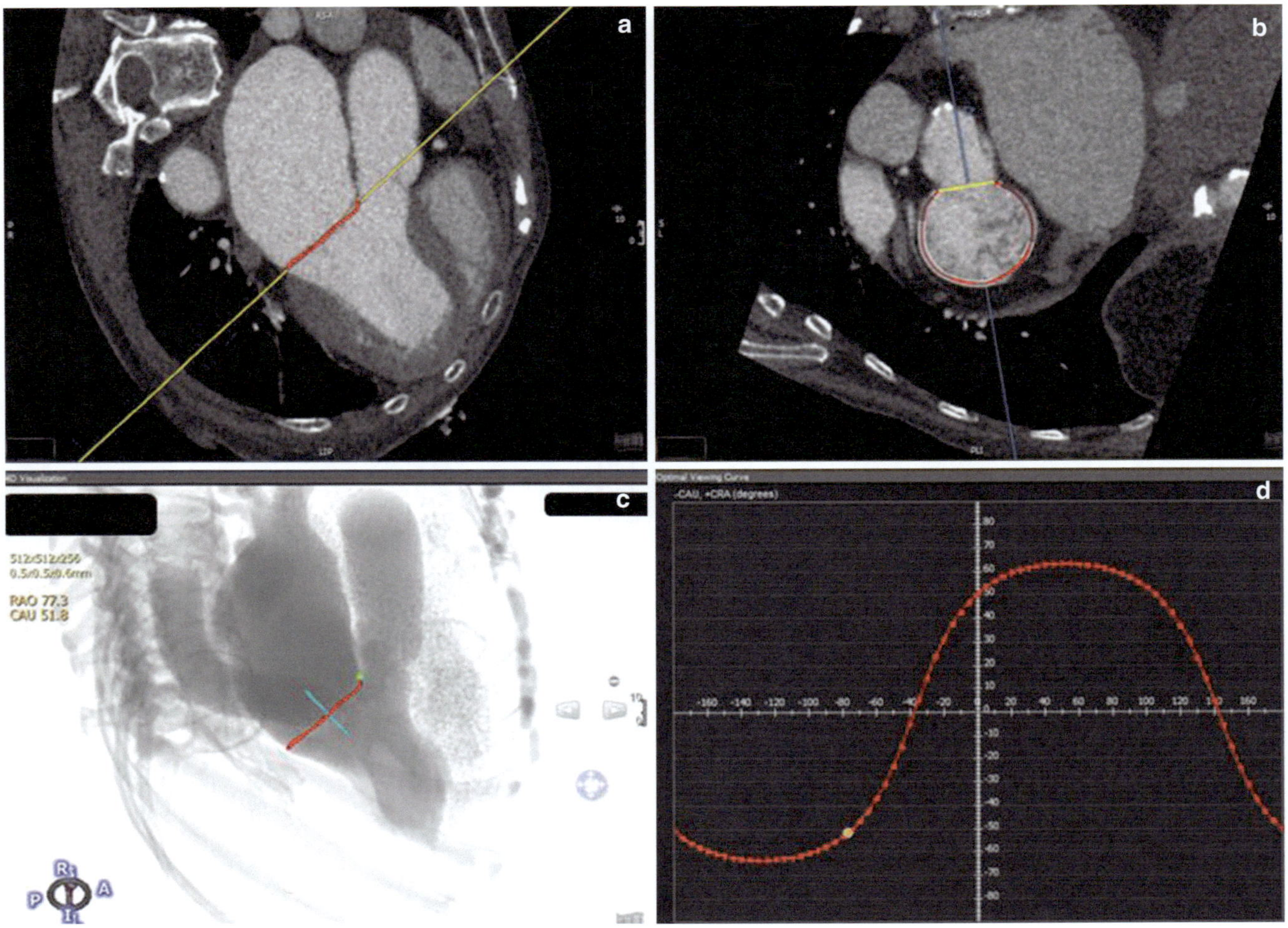

Fig. 42.6 Predicting fluoroscopic angulation along the trigone-to-trigone line. (**a**) shows transection of the annular plane at A2/P2. (**b**) demonstrates the en face view of the annular plane, with the D-shaped annulus shown. (**c**) superimposes the reconstructed annulus on corresponding fluoroscopy. (**d**) curve demonstrating optimal fluoroscopic projection angles as identified by yellow dot – note the T-T projection angles here are RAO 77.3, CAU 51.8 which can be clinically impractical to emulate

Defining Access Point

With current devices for TMVR often deployed transapically, pre-procedural CT can provide imaging of the anatomy required for catheter entry. A trajectory that is coaxial to the annular plan and bisects the centroid of the annulus can be provided that extends to the chest wall (Fig. 42.9) [10]. The relationship of this line to the corresponding line from the centroid to the 'true' apex can also be defined – this is often projected medial or inferior to the coaxial line. The trajectory line can then be assessed for proximity to papillary muscles, myocardial scar, the left anterior descending (LAD) coronary artery and any coronary grafts. The most appropriate intercostal space for chest wall access can also be determined.

Pulmonary Valve Implantation

Pulmonary valve replacement is generally required with worsening right function that can occur in patients with previous congenital heart surgery. It offers an alternative approach to redo surgery, angioplasty or stenting. The indications for replacement include severe pulmonary regurgitation, severe RV dilatation, severe RV dysfunction or worsening exercise function.

Pre-procedural imaging with CT can be used to assess the anatomy and aid with sizing [30]. Morphology of the RV outflow tract can be assessed for type and suitability for implant. Funnel-shaped outflow tracts (type 1) are high risk for valve embolization and not suitable, whereas tubular-shaped tracts offer better support. The conduit length from

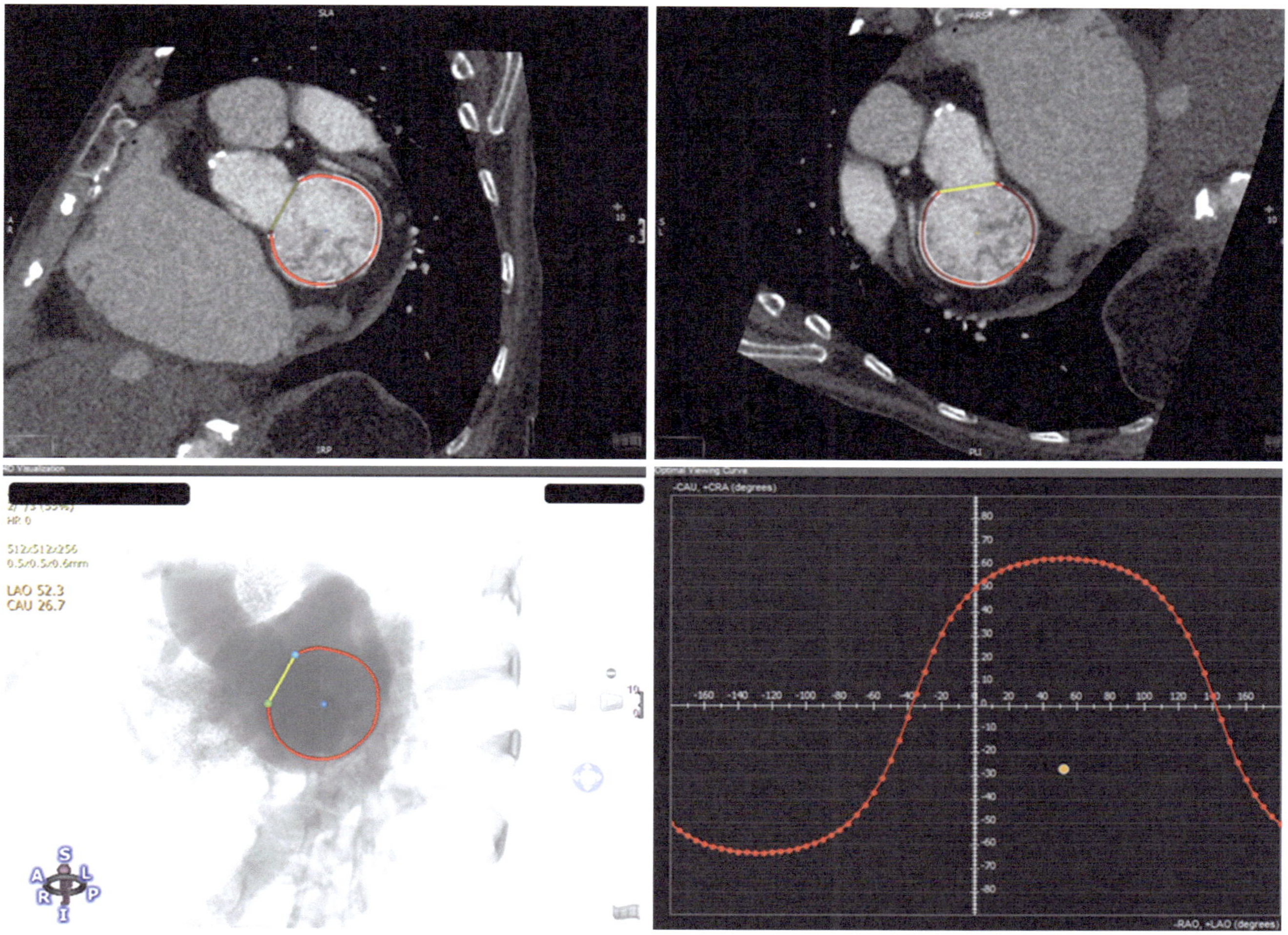

Fig. 42.7 Fluoroscopic angulation aimed to guide the positioning of the proceduralist's hands and the direction to proceed with the delivery catheter to achieve a perpendicular deployment (LAO 52.3, CAU 26.7)

the pulmonary bifurcation can also be determined, as can the internal diameter of the conduit.

Finally, proximity to the coronary vessels can be determined to avoid coronary compression with device deployment.

Percutaneous Closure of Atrial Septal Defects and Ventricular Septal Defects

CT can be used for planning of atrial septal defect (ASD) or patent foramen ovale (PFO) closure. Percutaneous devices employ a central waist with two umbrella-like discs at either end to fix the device to the atrial wall. With closure, transeptal flow and clot embolization can be disrupted.

Pre-procedural CT can determine defect size, rim distance, distorted or thinned septum and the presence of thrombus. Accurate sizing is required to determine device size, and coronal oblique images in end-systole are used. Rim measurement is also essential from the defect to surrounding anatomical structure. A rim of <3 mm is considered a contraindication for deployment, and for PFOs the minimum distance to the aorta or SVC should not exceed 9 mm [31].

CT can also be used for sizing prior to percutaneous ventricular septal defect (VSD) closure. The size and shape can be determined, measured in end-diastole. Proximity to the valves and the AV node can also be determined, which may contradict closure [32].

Pulmonary Vein Isolation

Radiofrequency ablation to isolate arrhythmogenic foci surrounding the pulmonary veins is an interventional procedure to treat atrial fibrillation. CT has a role in defining the pulmonary vein anatomy, presence of thrombus [33] and proximity to the oesophagus [34]. Additionally, CT imaging can be merged with electrical mapping systems to define the atrial border and vein location for the proceduralist [35].

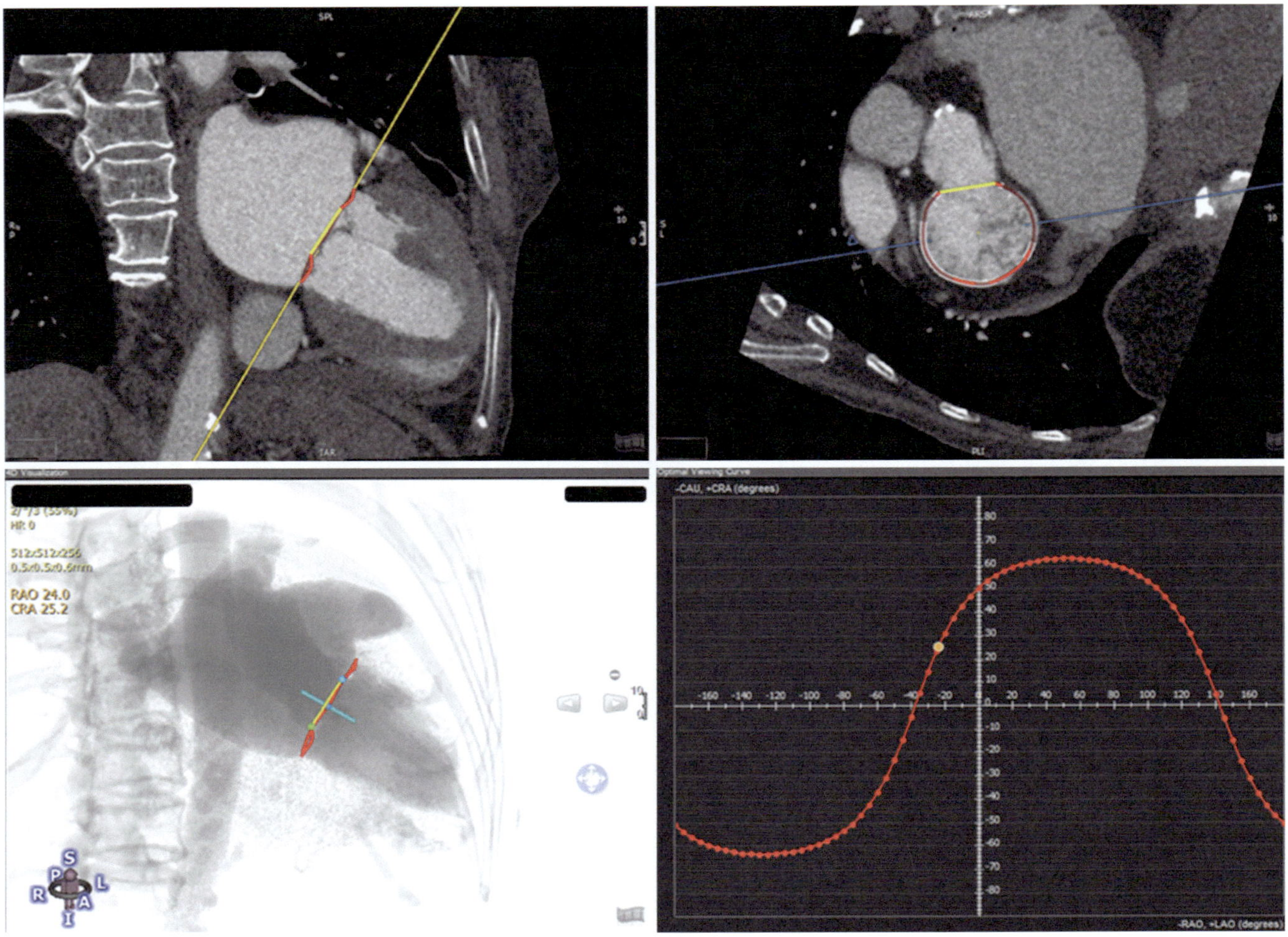

Fig. 42.8 Projection of the septal-to-lateral line. Note the predicted fluoroscopic angulation (RAO 24, CRA 25.2) is more clinically applicable

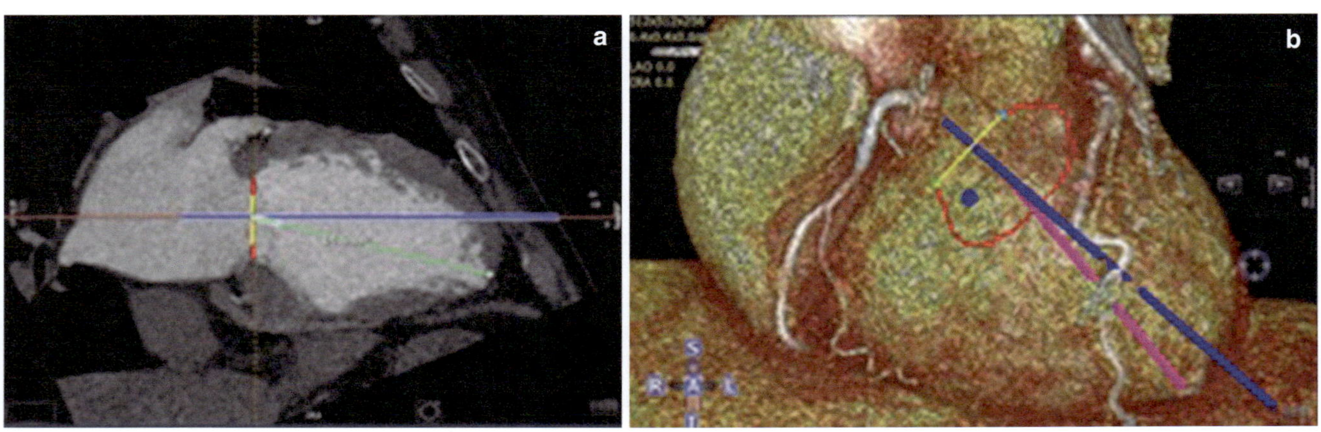

Fig. 42.9 Defining transapical access. (**a**) Two-chamber view demonstrating 'true axis' and coaxial trajectory. The green line represents the true long axis, and the blue line represents the trajectory that is coaxial to the annular plan and bisects the centroid of the reconstructed annulus. (**b**) Volume-rendered image depicting true axis (purple line) and coaxial trajectory (blue line). Proximity to the left anterior descending artery also demonstrated

The number, position and presence of accessory veins can be determined in pre-procedural CT. Most commonly there are four, two each side. Occasionally there can be a single ostium with the merger of the veins. Knowledge of vein anatomy is required to prevent injury and ensure all veins draining into the left atrium are isolated. Ostial size can also be determined, with smaller ostia more susceptible to stenosis.

The presence of thrombus in the left atrium or left atrial appendage can be shown on CT. Delayed phase imaging can discriminate filling defects due to thrombus from defects due to slow contrast filling as thrombus will persist in delayed phases. The presence of thrombus contraindicates proceeding with ablation.

Proximity to the oesophagus can be determined, with the left pulmonary veins commonly lying anterior. There is the potential risk of atrial-oesophageal fistula formation with ablation of ostia in close proximity to the oesophagus.

Conclusions

CT imaging prior to minimally invasive cardiac procedures is emerging as a vital tool. Excellent spatial and temporal resolution with wide-field views allows an understanding of the target and surrounding anatomy. Accurate sizing can determine appropriate device to minimize complications. Finally, higher-risk features can be identified to allow appropriate patient selection and minimization of morbidity and mortality.

References

1. Nkomo VT, Gardin JM, Skelton TN, Gottdiener JS, Scott CG, Enriquez-Sarano M. Burden of valvular heart diseases: a population-based study. Lancet. 2006;368:1005–11.
2. Maisano F, Alfieri O, Banai S, et al. The future of transcatheter mitral valve interventions: competitive or complementary role of repair vs. replacement? Eur Heart J. 2015;36:1651–9.
3. Shroyer AL, Coombs LP, Peterson ED, et al. The Society of Thoracic Surgeons: 30-day operative mortality and morbidity risk models. Ann Thorac Surg. 2003;75:1856–64. discussion 64-5.
4. Nishimura RA, Otto CM, Bonow RO, et al. 2014 AHA/ACC guideline for the management of patients with valvular heart disease: executive summary: a report of the American College of Cardiology/American Heart Association Task Force on Practice Guidelines. J Am Coll Cardiol. 2014;63:2438–88.
5. Mirabel M, Iung B, Baron G, et al. What are the characteristics of patients with severe, symptomatic, mitral regurgitation who are denied surgery? Eur Heart J. 2007;28:1358–65.
6. Nishimura RA, Vahanian A, Eleid MF, Mack MJ. Mitral valve disease--current management and future challenges. Lancet. 2016;387:1324–34.
7. Feldman T, Wasserman HS, Herrmann HC, et al. Percutaneous mitral valve repair using the edge-to-edge technique: six-month results of the EVEREST Phase I Clinical Trial. J Am Coll Cardiol. 2005;46:2134–40.
8. Feldman T, Foster E, Glower DD, et al. Percutaneous repair or surgery for mitral regurgitation. N Engl J Med. 2011;364:1395–406.
9. Whitlow PL, Feldman T, Pedersen WR, et al. Acute and 12-month results with catheter-based mitral valve leaflet repair: the EVEREST II (Endovascular valve edge-to-edge repair) high risk study. J Am Coll Cardiol. 2012;59:130–9.
10. Blanke P, Naoum C, Webb J, et al. Multimodality imaging in the context of Transcatheter mitral valve replacement: establishing consensus among modalities and disciplines. J Am Coll Cardiol Img. 2015;8:1191–208.
11. Guerrero M, Dvir D, Himbert D, et al. Transcatheter mitral valve replacement in native mitral valve disease with severe mitral annular calcification: results from the first multicenter global registry. JACC Cardiovasc Interv. 2016;9:1361–71.
12. Willson AB, Webb JG. Labounty TM, et al. 3-dimensional aortic annular assessment by multidetector computed tomography predicts moderate or severe paravalvular regurgitation after transcatheter aortic valve replacement: a multicenter retrospective analysis. J Am Coll Cardiol. 2012;59:1287–94.
13. Jilaihawi H, Kashif M, Fontana G, et al. Cross-sectional computed tomographic assessment improves accuracy of aortic annular sizing for transcatheter aortic valve replacement and reduces the incidence of paravalvular aortic regurgitation. J Am Coll Cardiol. 2012;59:1275–86.
14. Toggweiler S, Gurvitch R, Leipsic J, et al. Percutaneous aortic valve replacement: vascular outcomes with a fully percutaneous procedure. J Am Coll Cardiol. 2012;59:113–8.
15. Hayashida K, Lefevre T, Chevalier B, et al. Transfemoral aortic valve implantation new criteria to predict vascular complications. JACC Cardiovasc Interv. 2011;4:851–8.
16. Schoenhagen P, Numburi U, Halliburton SS, et al. Three-dimensional imaging in the context of minimally invasive and transcatheter cardiovascular interventions using multi-detector computed tomography: from pre-operative planning to intra-operative guidance. Eur Heart J. 2010;31:2727–40.
17. Levine RA, Triulzi MO, Harrigan P, Weyman AE. The relationship of mitral annular shape to the diagnosis of mitral valve prolapse. Circulation. 1987;75:756–67.
18. Berdajs D, Zund G, Camenisch C, Schurr U, Turina MI, Genoni M. Annulus fibrous of the mitral valve: reality or myth. J Card Surg. 2007;22:406–9.
19. Lee AP, Hsiung MC, Salgo IS, et al. Quantitative analysis of mitral valve morphology in mitral valve prolapse with real-time 3-dimensional echocardiography: importance of annular saddle shape in the pathogenesis of mitral regurgitation. Circulation. 2013;127:832–41.
20. Naoum C, Leipsic J, Cheung A, et al. Mitral annular dimensions and geometry in patients with functional mitral regurgitation and mitral valve prolapse: implications for transcatheter mitral valve implantation. J Am Coll Cardiol Img. 2016;9:269–80.
21. Hyodo E, Iwata S, Tugcu A, et al. Accurate measurement of mitral annular area by using single and biplane linear measurements: comparison of conventional methods with the three-dimensional planimetric method. Eur Heart J Cardiovasc Imaging. 2012;13:605–11.
22. Hahn RT, Abraham T, Adams MS, et al. Guidelines for performing a comprehensive transesophageal echocardiographic examination: recommendations from the American Society of Echocardiography and the Society of Cardiovascular Anesthesiologists. J Am Soc Echocardiogr. 2013;26:921–64.
23. Grewal J, Suri R, Mankad S, et al. Mitral annular dynamics in myxomatous valve disease: new insights with real-time 3-dimensional echocardiography. Circulation. 2010;121:1423–31.
24. Blanke P, Dvir D, Cheung A, et al. A simplified D-shaped model of the mitral annulus to facilitate CT-based sizing before transcatheter

mitral valve implantation. J Cardiovasc Comput Tomogr. 2014;8:459–67.
25. Hutchins GM, Moore GW, Skoog DK. The association of floppy mitral valve with disjunction of the mitral annulus fibrosus. N Engl J Med. 1986;314:535–40.
26. Cheung A, Webb J, Verheye S, et al. Short-term results of transapical transcatheter mitral valve implantation for mitral regurgitation. J Am Coll Cardiol. 2014;64:1814–9.
27. Blanke P, Naoum C, Dvir D, et al. Predicting LVOT obstruction in transcatheter mitral valve implantation: concept of the Neo-LVOT. J Am Coll Cardiol Img. 2017;10(4):482–5.
28. Gurvitch R, Wood DA, Leipsic J, et al. Multislice computed tomography for prediction of optimal angiographic deployment projections during transcatheter aortic valve implantation. JACC Cardiovasc Interv. 2010;3:1157–65.
29. Blanke P, Dvir D, Naoum C, et al. Prediction of fluoroscopic angulation and coronary sinus location by CT in the context of transcatheter mitral valve implantation. J Cardiovasc Comput Tomogr. 2015;9:183–92.
30. Ruiz CE, Kliger C, Perk G, et al. Transcatheter therapies for the treatment of valvular and paravalvular regurgitation in acquired and congenital valvular heart disease. J Am Coll Cardiol. 2015;66:169–83.
31. Webb G, Gatzoulis MA. Atrial septal defects in the adult: recent progress and overview. Circulation. 2006;114:1645–53.
32. Wahl A, Meier B. Patent foramen ovale and ventricular septal defect closure. Heart. 2009;95:70–82.
33. Romero J, Husain SA, Kelesidis I, Sanz J, Medina HM, Garcia MJ. Detection of left atrial appendage thrombus by cardiac computed tomography in patients with atrial fibrillation: a meta-analysis. Circ Cardiovasc Imaging. 2013;6:185–94.
34. Xu B, Gooley R, Seneviratne SK, Nasis A. Clinical utility of multidetector cardiac computed tomography in structural heart interventions. J Med Imaging Radiat Oncol. 2016;60:299–305.
35. Burke MC, Roberts MJ, Knight BP. Integration of cardiac imaging and electrophysiology during catheter ablation procedures for atrial fibrillation. J Electrocardiol. 2006;39:S188–92.

Cardiac CT: Electrophysiological Applications

43

Joan M. Lacomis, Iclal Ocak, Friedrich Knollmann, Andrew Voigt, and Raveen Bazaaz

Current electrophysiological applications of cardiac CT are primarily focused on evaluating patients with atrial fibrillation (AF) who are either a candidate for or who have been treated with pulmonary vein isolation (PVI) or left atrial appendage occlusion. In this chapter, we will review the importance of AF, describe methods of pulmonary vein isolation and LAA occlusion, and explore the role of CT imaging for these procedures.

Importance of Atrial Fibrillation

Atrial fibrillation is the most common sustained cardiac arrhythmia with a current prevalence of 6.1 million people affected in the USA and, with the incidence still increasing, an expected prevalence of 16 million people by 2050 [1, 2]. AF typically progresses from a syndrome of paroxysmal to persistent and thereon to permanent AF (Table 43.1).

AF is a significant cause of chronic left ventricular dysfunction and remains one of the leading causes of debilitating stroke imposing a tremendous burden on affected patients and the healthcare delivery system. Twenty-thirty percent of all strokes are due to AF [3–5].

J. M. Lacomis (✉) · I. Ocak
Department of Radiology, Thoracic Imaging Division, University of Pittsburgh Medical Center, University of Pittsburgh School of Medicine, Pittsburgh, PA, USA
e-mail: lacomisjm@upmc.edu

F. Knollmann
Department of Radiology, UCDavis Health, Sacramento, CA, USA

A. Voigt · R. Bazaaz
Heart and Vascular Institute, University of Pittsburgh Medical Center, Pittsburgh, PA, USA

Treatment of AF

Management of AF has long represented a significant clinical challenge. Since the publication of the AFFIRM trial in 2003 [6], it has been recognized that there is no clear clinical advantage to a rhythm control (vs a rate control) strategy among older patients who are minimally symptomatic. However, among symptomatic patients, AF can severely diminish quality of life. This has been used as an important justification for pursuing a sinus rhythm aggressively. For years, cardioversion and pharmacologic therapy were the mainstay treatments for AF and continue to play important roles in its management. AF is usually treated first with antiarrhythmic medications [7]. Recently, the association between AF, obesity, and obstructive sleep apnea (OSA) has been recognized. There is now emerging data suggesting that intensive lifestyle/weight loss intervention and therapy of OSA may reduce the symptomatic burden of AF [8, 9]. If a patient is hemodynamically compromised, electrical cardioversion is the treatment of choice [10]. However, AF is often refractory to or recurrent despite these treatments. The limited efficacy and known toxicity of antiarrhythmic drugs has led to the development of non-pharmacologic approaches.

The original Cox-Maze and its later modifications are surgical therapies for the treatment of AF. The newer catheter-based strategies for treating AF and/or preventing stroke in patients with AF represent nonsurgical options for patients who have failed traditional pharmacologic methods. The catheter-based strategies to treat AF include pulmonary vein isolation (PVI) with radiofrequency catheter ablation (RFCA) or cryoballoon ablation (CBA). More recently, LAA occluders have been deployed to reduce the risk of stroke in AF patients at risk for cardioembolic stroke who are also at high risk for bleeding as an alternative strategy to long-term oral anticoagulation [11].

Multidetector computed tomography (MDCT) is frequently used for preprocedural planning and identification of post-procedural complications. Imagers need to possess a thorough understanding of the procedures, including potential complications, the CT anatomy of the target

U. J. Schoepf (ed.), *CT of the Heart*, Contemporary Medical Imaging, https://doi.org/10.1007/978-1-60327-237-7_43

Table 43.1 Types of atrial fibrillation (AF)

AF category	Defining characteristic
Paroxysmal	Terminates spontaneously or with intervention within 7 days of onset
Persistent	Fails to self-terminate within 7 days and requires pharmacologic or electrical cardioversion to restore sinus rhythm
Permanent	Lasts longer than a year, and sinus rhythm is not possible
Lone	Occurs in adults <60 years of age without underlying cardiopulmonary disease
Isolated	Occurs without associated atrial tachycardia or aflutter

regions, the scanning and postprocessing techniques necessary to provide the needed anatomical information, and the pertinent report content for scans for these procedures.

Pulmonary Vein Isolation

Radiofrequency Catheter Ablation

In 1998, Haissaguerre and his colleagues identified the muscular sleeves of the distal PVs (adjacent to the left atrium (LA)) as an important source of ectopic beats initiating AF [12]. Over 90% of the ectopic beats initiating AF arise in the PVs with the culprit beats most often arising in the left superior pulmonary vein (LSPV) [12, 13]. The understanding of this relationship led to the development of the Cox-Maze-type surgeries followed by the interventional therapies of RFCA and CBA directed at causing anatomic scars to disrupt the electrical pathways between the initiating PVs and the substrate for propagation of AF, the posterior left atrium (PLA) [14]. RFCA was the first of these therapies and is still the most common. The technique itself has been modified over the years moving away from point ablation within the distal PVs to the current target of the pulmonary vein antral tissue in the PLA.

RFCA is a catheter-based procedure which is technically complex, time-consuming, and performed using general anesthesia at many centers. For the catheter-based procedures, the LA can only be accessed via a transfemoral approach, followed by trans-atrial septal puncture. RFCA is carried out by using an electrical current with alternating frequencies and results in hyperthermic cellular injury through a combination of coagulation and tissue necrosis [15]. The ablation catheter is navigated circumferentially around the bilateral PV inflow vestibules (i.e., PV antral regions) without entering any pulmonary venous ostia; using a point-by-point technique, multiple adjacent, approximately 4 millimeters in diameter, point ablation lesions are created. When complete, the discreet point lesions collectively form bilateral contiguous, linear, circumferential lesions to electrically isolate the bilateral antral PV tissue from the remainder of the PLA. Occasionally, another contiguous line of ablation lesions will be placed across the roof of the LA, extending between the vestibules [16–21], though the value of additional lines of ablation beyond PVI has been questioned by a more recent study [22].

Cryoballoon Ablation

CBA is currently the most widely used alternative to RFCA and was developed in part because of the often tedious and technically challenging nature of RFCA [23]. In addition, cryoablation may preserve the tissue architecture and be associated with less thrombus formation as compared to RFCA [24], though this has not been clearly established. Whereas RFCA is applied in a point-by-point mode and results in cellular necrosis by tissue heating, CBA is applied to the PV antral tissue with a balloon in a single-step mode and leads to cellular necrosis by freezing [25]. Like RFCA, the LA can only be accessed using a transfemoral approach followed by a trans-atrial septal puncture. Then, a balloon catheter is advanced over a guidewire into the ostium of a PV where it is inflated to completely occlude the ostium. Balloon occlusive pulmonary venography and electroanatomic mapping are often utilized to avoid positioning the cryoballoon within the PV during ablation. Balloon selections are based on PV ostial sizes on the preprocedural MDCT, though as experience with the technique has grown, in the vast majority of cases, the larger 28 mm cryoballoon is utilized. The CBA of each PV is performed in at least two 3–4 min freezing cycles. The operator monitors the temperature at the distal aspect of the balloon, with higher nadir (warmer) temperatures suggesting poor overall contact with antral tissue/inefficacy and lower nadir (colder) temperatures being worrisome for injury to collateral structures. The intracellular freezing is followed by injury during thawing due to a combination of ice crystals expanding and contracting in the intra- and extracellular spaces, thereby damaging cell walls and causing microvascular occlusions and ischemia. The combined local hemorrhagic and inflammatory responses lead to permanent cellular necrosis [25]. The balloon is deflated, and the single-step freezing process is repeated for each of the remaining PVs. Cryoballoon (CB) ostial ablation lesions form well-demarcated circumferential scars, electrically isolating the PVs from the LA [26].

In 2013, the STOP-AF trial, comparing CBA vs specific antiarrhythmic agents, demonstrated the safety and effectiveness of CBA for the treatment of PAF, with a 70% rate of freedom of AF recurrence at 1 year in the CBA group [23]. The more recent landmark "FIRE AND ICE" trial, comparing RFCA vs CBA, found that CBA was non-inferior to RFCA [25]. Single center trials and registry data showed freedom from AF of 45–72% for RFCA compared to 55–77% for CBA at follow-up ranging from 6 months to 2 years [27]. Two smaller single-center studies showed CBA in persistent AF patients has a 60–67% success rate at 1 year [25, 28].

The long-term outcomes for PV catheter ablation are not as good as initially hoped [29] with PV reconnection and repeat ablation procedures being common. This has prompted a search for additional targets for ablation and further investigation into the underlying LA substrate for AF. Although the majority of foci triggering AF have been mapped to the PVs, it has long been known that AF may also be triggered by arrhythmogenic foci originating from the right atrium (RA), LA, LAA, coronary sinus (CS), superior vena cava (SVC), or the vein of Marshall [12, 30–33]. The optimum treatment strategy including employing hybrid catheter-based and surgical techniques is an ongoing area of investigation.

CT Technique

Image Acquisition

The main goals of imaging are to delineate and display the PLA and its adjacent anatomy, typically in a combination of multiplanar reformats and 3D models, to identify any findings that may contraindicate or increase the complexity of the ablation, and to identify any significant incidental findings that warrant further investigation or intervention either pre- or post-ablation. Of note, it is increasingly common in recent years to perform pre-PVI anatomic mapping on patients who have had prior ablations and now have recurrent AF with a second ablation procedure planned. In such patients, it is also important to identify lasting complications from the prior ablation which may be unsuspected such as PV stenosis or occlusion.

Since AF patients who are candidates for RFCA or CBA typically have PAF or less commonly persistent AF, their rhythm may be AF or sinus at the time of CT which is typically obtained within 24 h pre-ablation [34–36]. Pre-ablation anatomic mapping of the PLA was initially described on four detector scanners without ECG gating [37]. As with other cardiac CT, modern scanning is now done on a minimum of 64 slice scanners. Since PLA anatomy can be accurately characterized with or without ECG gating, patients who are in AF can be successfully scanned without ECG gating, and retrospective gating is generally discouraged due to the higher radiation dose [36]. However, AF, especially if rate controlled, is less of a challenge for high-quality low-radiation ECG-gated acquisitions on the newest generation >64 slice MDCT scanners.

Regardless if an ECG-gated or a nongated acquisition is done, the z-axis coverage is increased from that of a coronary CTA to start the scan at the mid-aortic arch level to include the distal third of the superior pulmonary veins and the entire LAA. Although TEE is routinely done to exclude LAA thrombus, a limited repeat acquisition through the LAA can be done 60–90 s post-contrast injection if there is a question of pseudothrombus from mixing artifact from slow filling vs thrombus. Contrast dose and kvp are tailored for patient-specific weight, BMI, and renal function; the use of dual-barrel injectors with contrast timing, contrast/saline bolus profile, and injection rates can be the same as coronary CTA and can be done with a test bolus or automated bolus tracking [38–43].

Scans that are obtained post-PVI to evaluate for complications should image the entire chest as postop complications (or other pathologies accounting for patient's presentation) are not limited to the heart. ECG gating is dependent on a variety of factors including not only whether the scanner is sufficient for patient's rate and rhythm, but patient's clinical status which can range from minor symptoms to obtundation (see "Interpretation post-PVI") will also dictate the ability to ECG gate. The contrast volume is increased to cover the entire region, similar to an aortic CTA evaluation.

Postprocessing

Postprocessing includes multiplanar reformats (MPRs) and three-dimensional (3D) volume rendered models of the LA, LAA, and distal PVs. LA segmentation protocols for this purpose are available on all of the major vendor workstations. The 3D models are displayed from both epicardial (extra-atrial) and endocardial (intra-atrial) vantages; the esophagus can also be included on the epicardial views to show its location along the posterior atrial wall (Fig. 43.1a–c). Electrophysiologists reference these models for the ablation thus rendering the need for retrograde pulmonary venography obsolete. Typically, navigation of the catheter during ablation is performed using a combination of an electroanatomic mapping system, intracardiac echo, and fluoroscopy. At some centers, the epicardial 3D volume rendering is merged with the intraprocedural electroanatomic map so the progress of the ablation lines can be tracked in real time [44–47] (Fig. 43.2a, b).

PV ostial diameters are measured utilizing the MPRs to obtain true orthogonal obliques [42, 43]. Maximum PV ostial diameters occur during late atrial diastole (approximately 85% R-R), and minimum diameters occur during atrial systole (approximately 15% R-R) [44–48]. PV ostial diameters are needed to choose the appropriate size of the cryoballoon. Because of the dynamic nature of the PVs, measurements from ECG-gated studies should be obtained from the same phase on any subsequent post-ablation scans [48, 49].

Interpretation Pre-PVI

Interpretation of CT scans prior to PVI requires evaluation of axial source images, MPRs, and 3D models. Necessary anatomic information includes evaluation of the number and

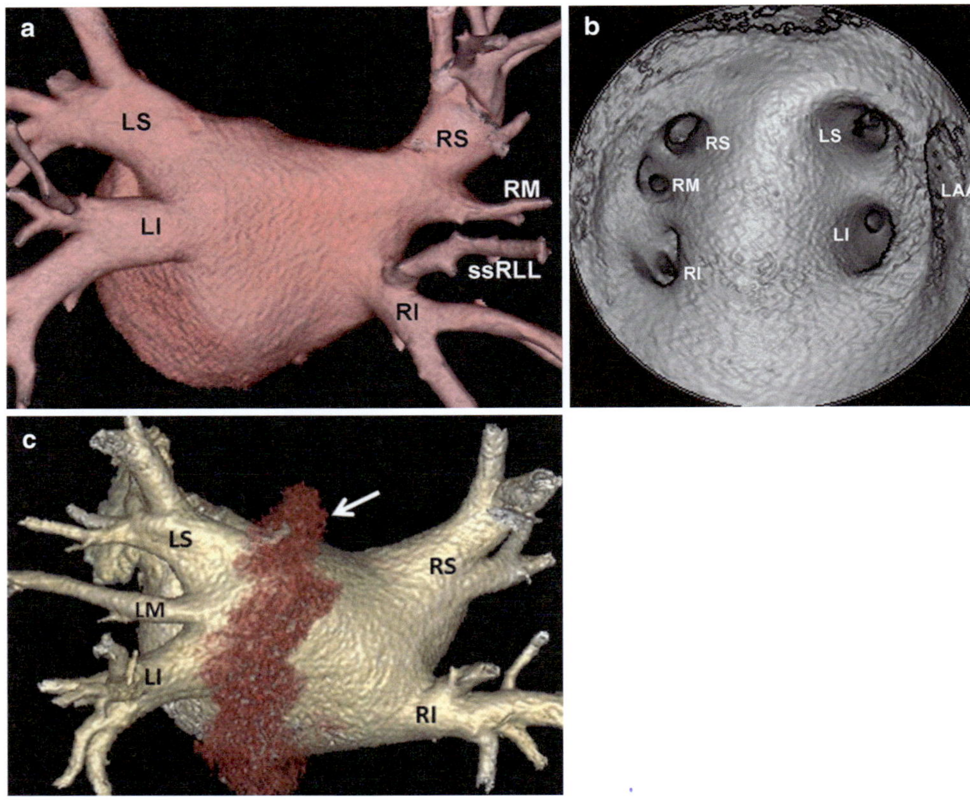

Fig. 43.1 (**a–c**): Standard 3D posterior left atrial models: Volume rendered PA epicardial view (**a**), endocardial view (**b**), and epicardial view including the esophagus (arrow) (**c**) of the posterior left atrium. (LS left superior pulmonary vein, LI left inferior pulmonary vein, RS right superior pulmonary vein, RI right inferior pulmonary vein, RM right middle lobe ostial branch, ssRLL superior segment RLL ostial branch, LM left middle pulmonary vein). In **2a**, ostial branches are labeled in white

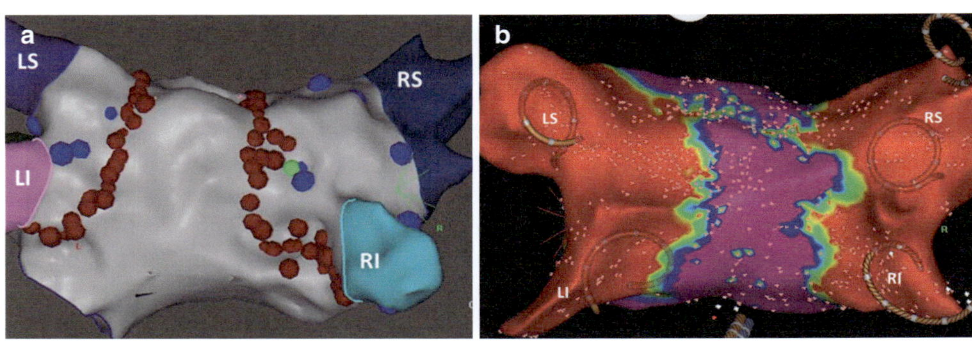

Fig. 43.2 (**a, b**): Electroanatomic mapping**:** In (**a**) a CARTO (BioSense, Diamond Bar, CA) electroanatomic map from a PA view of the PLA post-RFCA delineates the completed ablation lines. The red octagons represent the ablation points which collectively encircle the pulmonary vein antral tissue with the goal of electrical isolation. In (**b**) the corresponding CARTO endocardial voltage map, PA view post-RFCA, the red areas represent low voltage, and the purple areas represent normal voltage (viable tissue). Notice how wide the antral area is targeted for ablation surrounding the PVs. The overlying coiled objects are superimposed snapshots of the positions of the tip of the circular mapping catheter, used to validate electrical isolation of each of the veins

location of PVs, including the presence of conjoined or accessory veins, identification of ostial branches, the relative location of the esophagus along the posterior left atrial wall, and identification of any findings that may contraindicate or increase the complexity of the ablation.

Each PV can be divided into longitudinal segments between branch points in a retrograde manner extending from the LA, starting with the V_1 segment. The V_1 segment is between the PV ostium and the first branch point [35, 39] . If this length is within 5 mm of the ostium, the first branch is termed an ostial branch [35]. Ostial branches are important because they are at increased risk for stenosis. There is much variation between the different PVs in ostial diameters, angulations, and V_1 segment lengths [42, 43].The atrial wall between ipsilateral PVs is termed the intervenous saddle or carina [35]. There are two funnel-shaped, PV inflow vestibules or antral regions, right and left; each consists of all the PV ostia on the ipsilateral side and their intervenous saddles. The V_1 segments of the PVs, bilateral vestibules, and the interposed atrial wall comprise the PLA [35]. The remainder of the LA is divided into the roof, the appendage, the isthmus, and the septum [50]. The extensive electrical conduction system within the roof of the LA is termed Bachman's bundle; there is a complex network of interconnecting electrical pathways in the PLA. Of the more recently identified culprits in either the initiation or sustenance of AF, the identification of regions of functional reentry within the LA termed rotors is of most interest to imagers due to their association with underlying atrial fibrosis and the ability of cardiac magnetic resonance imaging to delineate fibrosis [51, 52].

Normally, all of the PVs drain into the LA; although variation in number and configuration of PVs entering the LA is common (Fig. 43.3), PVs which drain to structures other than the LA (i.e., the superior or inferior vena cavae, brachiocephalic vein, RA) are considered anomalous.

The classic description of four separate PVs with a superior and inferior ostium on the right and a superior and inferior on the left is the most common anatomic configuration and is referred to as conventional pulmonary venous anatomy (Fig. 43.1a). In several studies, some of which included only pre-RFCA AF patients, four PVs reportedly occur 60–82% of the time, but large population studies have not been done, and the true incidence is unknown [32, 34, 36, 37, 40, 43, 53]. Typically, the right superior pulmonary vein (RSPV) drains the right upper lobe (RUL) and usually the right middle lobe (RML); the right inferior (RIPV) drains the right lower lobe (RLL) and occasionally all or part of the RML; the left superior (LSPV) drains the left upper lobe (LUL) including the lingula; and the left inferior (LIPV) drains the left lower lobe (LLL) [32, 34, 36, 37, 40, 43, 53].

If variant PV anatomy is present, the right side tends to be more complex, often with accessory PVs, while the left side tends to be more simplified, as in the case of a conjoined vein. A conjoined or common vein occurs when the superior and inferior veins merge proximal to the LA and enter the LA as a single trunk of varying lengths [34, 40]. The resulting single pulmonary venous ostium is typically broad (Fig. 43.4a, e). Deciding if there is a short common trunk with large superior and inferior ostial branches versus two adjacent but separate left-sided veins with a small intervenous saddle can be difficult and may account for some of the variation in reported incidence of conjoined veins. While conjoined veins are usually on the left, they also rarely occur on the right, bilaterally or inferiorly (combined RIPV and LIPV) [34, 39, 40, 54]. The anatomic variant of a left common PV (LCPV) is often seen in clinical practice and has relevance for preprocedural planning for electrophysiologists. LCPV anatomy can be particularly challenging for operators contemplating a CBA approach, as the size of the common segment is sometimes larger than the diameter of the cryoballoon itself, forcing the operator to either switch to RFCA or to ablate using a more challenging segmental approach with multiple applications of cryothermal energy at the antral tissue surrounding the PV.

An accessory vein has its own independent atrio-pulmonary venous junction separate from the superior and inferior PVs on that side. Accessory veins are important as

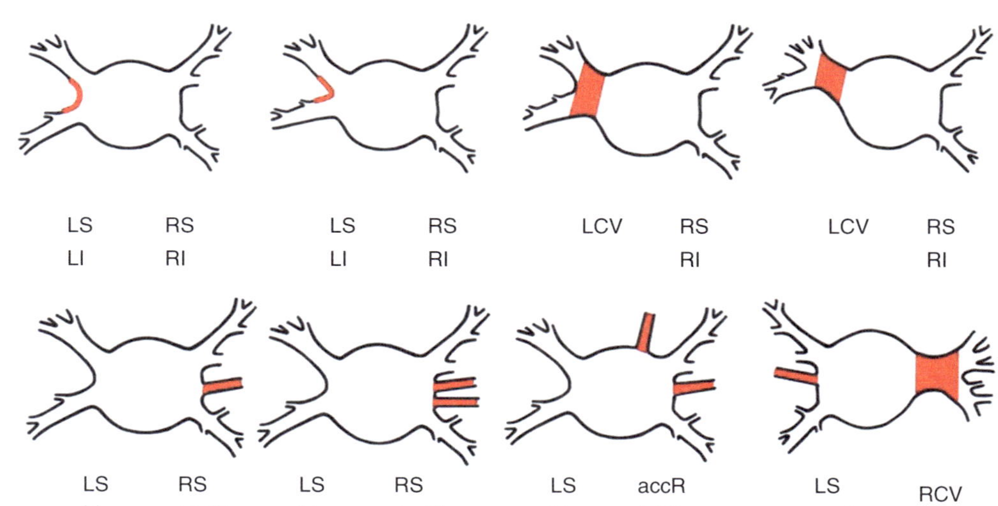

Fig. 43.3 Normal pulmonary vein variations: *Top row* (left to right): conventional anatomy with left superior (LS) and left inferior (LI) pulmonary veins widely separated, conventional anatomy with LS and LI immediately adjacent to each other, short left common vein (LCV), long LCV. *Bottom row* (left to right): accessory right middle vein (accR), two accessory right middle veins, top vein (TV) with or without a right middle vein, right common vein or left middle vein. Rarely, there can be bilateral common veins (not drawn)

their ostia may be smaller than those of the superior and inferior veins, exposing them to an increased risk of stenosis. It is important to know what segments or lobes of lung accessory veins are draining, because if complications such as hemodynamically significant pulmonary venous stenosis or thrombosis occur, the associated pulmonary parenchymal abnormalities will be reflected in the segment or lobe of lung drained by the affected vein.

There may be one or more accessory veins, typically on the right or toward the right posterior side of the roof of the LA. The frequency of accessory veins has been reported between 12% and 33% [39, 40, 43, 54]. The two most common accessory veins are the right middle lobe vein (which drains all or part of the right middle lobe (RML), accounting for 55–93% of accessory right-sided veins (Fig. 43.4b), and the superior segment right lower lobe (ssRLL) vein accounting for 28% of accessory right-sided veins (Fig. 43.4c). However, note that any third vein interposed between the RSPV and RIPV, regardless if it's draining the RML or ssRLL, has often been generically termed a "middle vein" [34, 37, 40, 53]. Rarely, accessory PVs can drain the basilar segments of the RLL. In addition, the occasional accessory vein on the left, which typically drains the lingula, is also commonly referred to as a "middle vein" (Fig. 43.4d) [32, 43, 44, 55–57].

The other interesting accessory vein is the "top vein" which enters the roof of the LA posteriorly, superomedial to the RSPV (Figs. 43.4c and 43.5b) [34, 44]. The top vein drains either the ssRLL or the posterior segment right upper lobe (psRUL) or a combination of the two. This should not be confused with another frequently seen normal structure, an accessory LAA. An accessory LAA is a small-sized, blind-ending, diverticula-like outpouching which contains a variable number of digitations [58]. The accessory LAA, which arises from the anterosuperior aspect of the LA roof, can be near the RSPV, more midline, or closer to the LSPV (Fig. 43.5a, b) [50].

In addition to evaluating PLA anatomy, scans are routinely evaluated for other significant findings. A well-opacified LAA can be assessed for thrombus, a contraindication to the procedure [15–21]. However, if the LAA is dilated and has slow flow, particularly if TEE shows spontaneous echo contrast indicating slow filling, it may be difficult to differentiate poor filling from thrombus. In fact, the two may look identical. There have been several proposed methods to differentiate pseudothrombus due to incomplete LAA opacification from LAA thrombus; the easiest is to obtain a second set of delayed images through the LAA at approximately 60–90 s post-contrast injection (Fig. 43.6a, b) [59].

While TEE is the standard of reference and the only approved imaging modality to assess for LAA thrombus, in a meta-analysis of 19 studies with 2955 patients, cardiac CT with the addition of delayed images was shown to be as

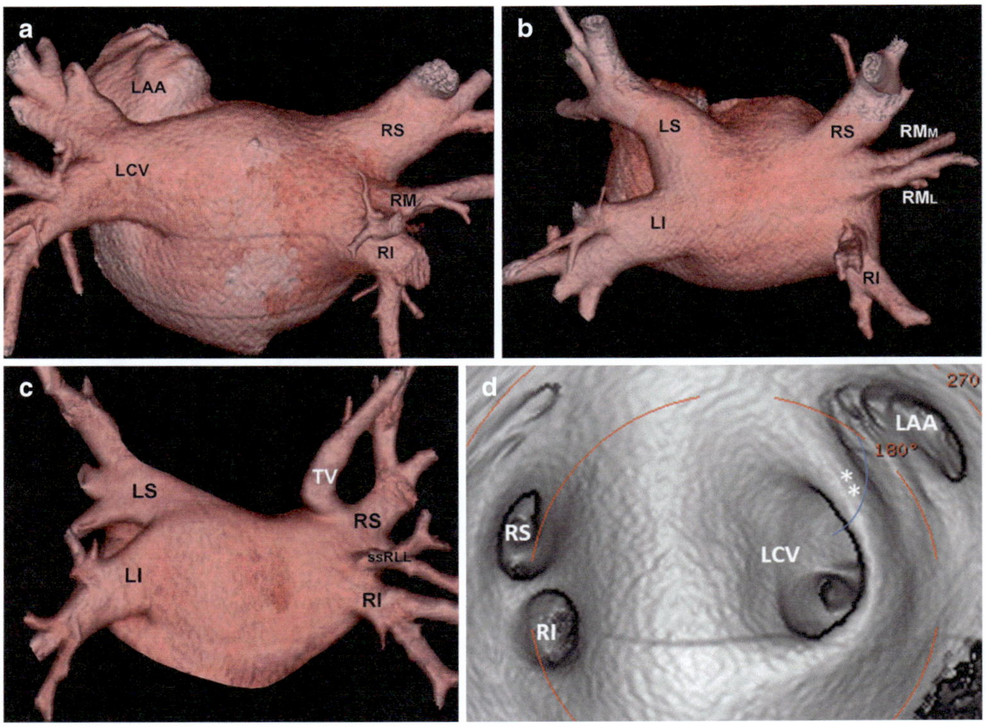

Fig. 43.4 (**a**–**d**): Normal pulmonary vein variations: (**a**) left common vein (LCV), accessory right middle pulmonary vein (RM) draining the entire right middle lobe; (**b**) two accessory "right middle" veins, separately draining the medial (RM_M) and lateral (RM_L) segments of the right middle lobe; (**c**) accessory superior segment right lower lobe pulmonary vein draining that lobe and accessory "top pulmonary vein" draining the posterior segment of the right upper lobe; (**d**) endocardial view showing the broad ostium of a LCV (LAA, left atrial appendage; RS, right superior pulmonary vein; RI, right inferior pulmonary vein; ** in 4d denotes the Ridge of Marshall)

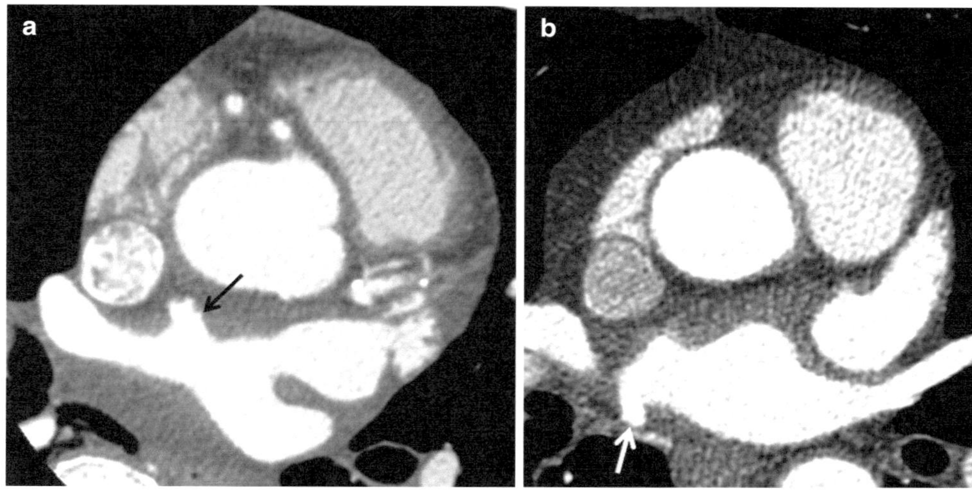

Fig. 43.5 (**a**, **b**): Accessory LAA: Both an accessory LAA and a top pulmonary vein (TV) typically arise in close proximity to the RSPV. In (**a**) the accessory LAA (black arrow) arises from the anterior aspect of the roof of the LA, whereas in (**b**), an accessory TV (white arrow) arises from the posterior aspect of the LA

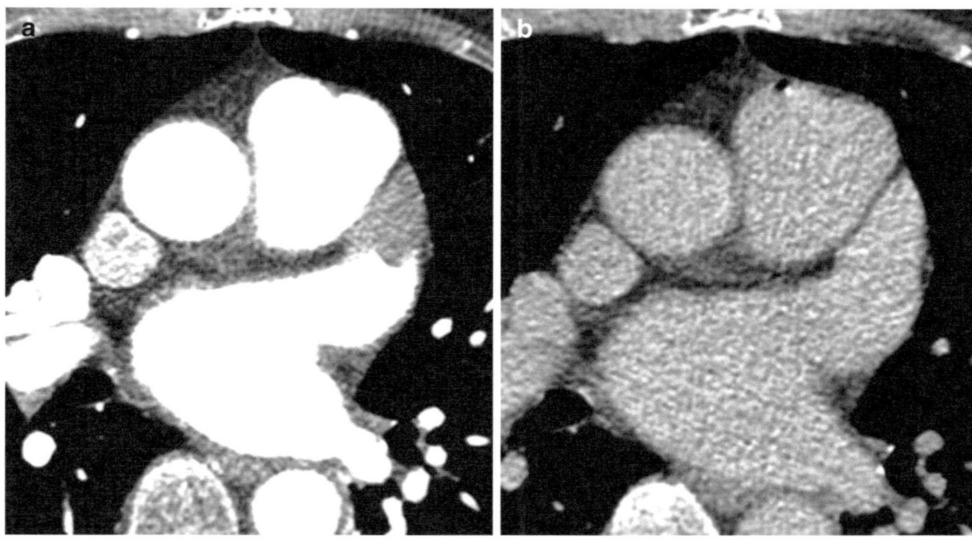

Fig. 43.6 (**a**, **b**): LAA pseudothrombus: Particularly as the LAA dilates, filling defects in the tip of the LAA are common on CTA (**a**) and could represent thrombus or pseudothrombus from slow LAA filling. Complete opacification of the LAA on delayed images (**b**) excludes the presence of true thrombus

accurate as TEE. In the meta-analysis, cardiac CT had an overall accuracy of 99% with a mean sensitivity of 100%, specificity of 99%, PPV of 92%, and NPV of 100% [59].

Any other abnormality of the LA, the RA, the atrial septum, or the azygous continuation of the IVC that may interfere with access to or ability to navigate a catheter within the PLA from a transfemoral approach should be reported [60]. Any abnormality of a structure in close proximity to the PLA, particularly if the abnormality exerts mass effect on the LA, such as a descending aortic aneurysm, esophageal dilatation, paraesophageal hernia, or mediastinal mass, should also be reported [42]. The esophagus warrants specific attention for RFCA cases as it is at risk for iatrogenic injury during the procedure due to its close proximity to the PLA. In addition to including the esophagus on the 3D epicardial volume rendering, specifying its location in the report in relation to the PLA is recommended. Anatomically, the esophagus is adjacent and posterior to the LA for approximately 5 cm of the length of the esophagus, either running midline, right or left para-midline, or obliquely from the LSPV to the RIPV.

Since catheter ablation for AF requires either general anesthesia or intravenous conscious sedation, incidental findings such as pneumonia, including aspiration after TEE, and coronary artery disease also need to be specifically addressed as their presence may warrant postponing or canceling the ablation. Similarly, findings such as a suspected lung carcinoma or other malignancies may affect the decision to proceed with an ablation until they are evaluated [25, 26, 38, 43].

Interpretation Post-PVI

The major role of CT post-PVI is to assess for complications. The overall major complication rate for PVI is estimated at 3.9–4.5% [24]. Both major and minor complications, listed in Table 43.2, can occur, most with either RFCA or CB ablation [21, 61–73]. Many are well-known complications that can occur with other interventional catheter-based cardiac procedures; there are also the risks associated with sedation and general anesthesia that are not included.

Of note, cardiac perforation and associated tamponade can occur during trans-atrial septal puncture, when manipulating the catheters in the LA and distal pulmonary veins or when performing the ablations, but are acutely apparent from clinical parameters and echocardiographic findings during these procedures and not reliant on MDCT for diagnosis. There are three complications noteworthy to PVI procedures: phrenic nerve injuries (PNI), atrio-esophageal fistula (AEF), and PV stenosis, the latter two of which are reliant on MDCT for diagnosis. Rapid and accurate interpretation of subtle CT findings of severe injury is paramount.

Atrio-esophageal Fistula

AEF is a rare but devastating complication only reported with RFCA. AEF occurs due to thermal injury to the esophagus through the LA wall. First described in 2004, there have only been a few published cases. The true incidence of unpublished occurrences is unknown, and many suspect the incidence is likely higher [57–61, 63, 64, 66]. In the published cases, patients presented from 2 days to 5 weeks post-ablation, and the incidence of mortality was over 50%.

The underlying problem is a thermal injury during the PLA ablation to the fragile anterior esophageal wall due to the anatomic close proximity of the esophagus and PLA. In some areas, the esophageal wall is in direct continuity with the posterior left atrial wall, and in other areas, there is a thin layer of fat interposed between the posterior wall of the LA and the anterior wall of the esophagus (Fig. 43.7a) [56, 74, 75]. If the thermal injury is severe enough, the esophagus can perforate. If the esophageal perforation goes undetected, the ensuing mediastinitis can extend to the LA wall which can also perforate, creating fistulous communication between the two [66–69, 72, 73, 76].

Early signs and symptoms of AEF are nonspecific and include chest pain, dysphagia, fever, and an elevated white blood cell count [61, 62, 69, 70, 77]. Patients may rapidly deteriorate as mediastinitis progresses over the span of hours to a few days. The diagnosis is easily missed in its early clinical stages. When the posterior left atrial wall is perforated, air from the esophagus may enter the LA, and signs of endocarditis, septic or air emboli, and overwhelming sepsis may develop. Patients are at risk for mental status changes, stroke, seizures, massive hematemesis, and rapid cardiovascular collapse with death. The mortality of >50% is in part attributed to significant delays in or missed diagnosis [61, 62, 71–75, 78].

Table 43.2 Reported complications of RFCA or CBA

Minor
Pleural effusion
Pericardial effusion
Hemodynamically insignificant pulmonary vein stenosis
Femoral vein catheterization complication: hematoma, arteriovenous fistula, pseudoaneurysm
Major
Pulmonary veins: dissection, perforation, severe stenosis, thrombosis, venous infarct, veno-occlusive disease with resultant PA hypertension
Cardiac perforation: hemopericardium, tamponade
LA intramural hematoma, dissection
Coronary arteries: spasm, ischemia, infarct
Cardiac dysrhythmias
Thromboembolic: stroke, transient ischemic attack (TIA), pulmonary or systemic emboli
Phrenic nerve palsy, paralysis
Atrio-esophageal fistula, esophageal perforation, mediastinitis

MDCT

MDCT is the primary imaging modality to assess for complications post-ablation [53, 66]. Early CT findings are those of mediastinitis such as fat stranding or a small mediastinal fluid collection and/or extraluminal gas locules in the region of the PLA or esophagus [14, 70, 72, 73] (Fig. 43.7b).

As the process progresses to a fistula, the posterior wall of the LA may become thickened and irregular or develop a pseudoaneurysm. Gas locules can occur within the pericardial space or within the wall or lumen of the PLA [14, 70, 72, 73]. Small pleural or pericardial effusions are relatively common minor complications post-RFCA; however, rapidly accumulating collections or pleural or pericardial enhancement should raise suspicion for AEF [14, 71] (Fig. 43.8a, b).

Confident MDCT diagnosis of an AEF is important to ensure adequate emergent treatment which requires surgical exploration with both esophageal and atrial repairs; TEE and esophagoscopy with CO_2 insufflation are contraindicated when AEF is suspected [21, 62, 77].

Pulmonary Vein Stenosis

Pulmonary vein stenosis (PVS) is a significant complication of catheter ablation for AF. There is significant variation in the reported incidence of severe, hemodynamically significant pulmonary vein stenosis, since post-PVI follow-up imaging is not always obtained. Also, the pulmonary veins undergo structural remodeling after ablation with a mean reduction in cross-sectional areas of roughly 5–10% [49]. A recent systematic review suggested that the incidence of PVS remains approximately 2% [49, 79]. Pathophysiology

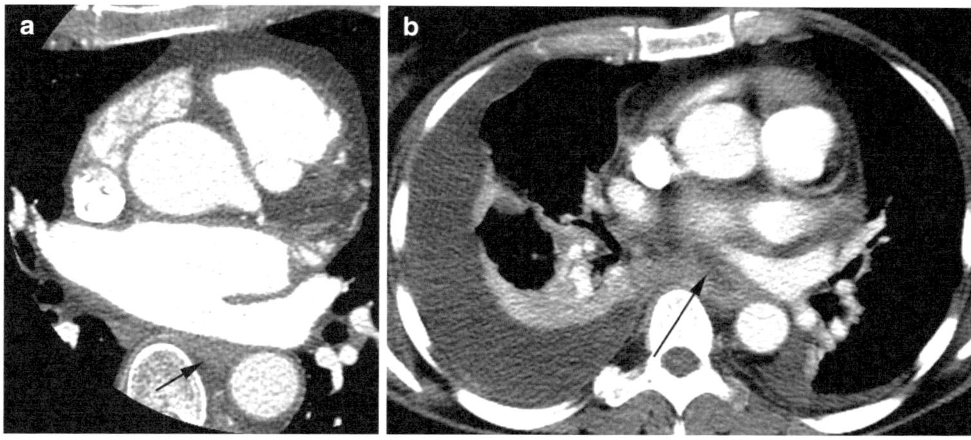

Fig. 43.7 (**a, b**): Atrio-esophageal fistula, early findings: The axial image from a CT obtained pre-ablation (**a**) shows the normal esophagus (arrow) toward the left side of the LA, immediately posterior and in direct continuity to the atrio-pulmonary venous junction of a long left common vein. Image (**b**) was obtained 5 days post-RFCA when the patient presented with chest pain. Note the signs of mediastinitis with a new, subtle fluid collection (arrow) in the mediastinum that is inseparable from the esophagus and abuts the posterior left atrial wall near the LSPV ostium with infiltration of the adjacent fat. There are also large right and small left pleural effusions; the former showed signs of loculation on more superior images (not shown). (From Lacomis et al. [14], with permission)

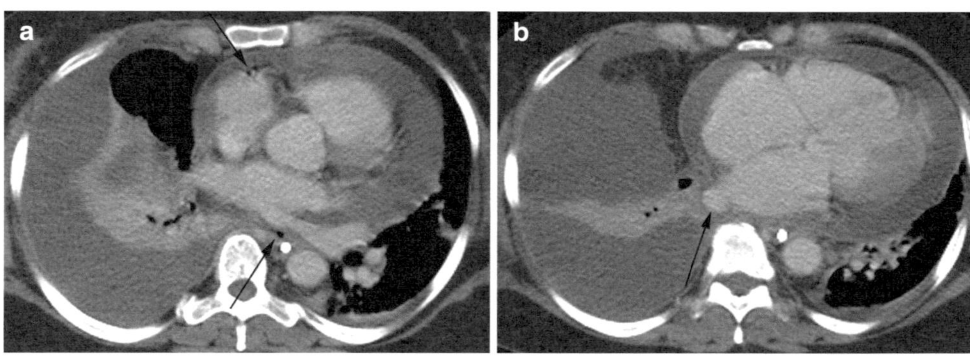

Fig. 43.8 (**a, b**): Atrio-esophageal fistula, late findings: The patient continued to clinically deteriorate with ongoing chest pain, new dyspnea, fever, and elevated white blood cell count and underwent CT of the chest, abdomen, and pelvis 48 h later which showed progression of findings and additional evidence of an atrio-esophageal fistula. There are new extraluminal gas locules adjacent to the esophagus and within the pericardial space (**a,** *arrows*)**.** A large pericardial effusion has developed, and the pericardium is enhancing (**a, b**). The right pleural effusion has markedly increased. In (**b**), there is a pseudoaneurysm (arrow) of the posterior left atrial wall, inferoposterior to the RIPV. A nasogastric tube is in the esophagus. (From Lacomis et al. [14], with permission)

of PVS after catheter ablation remains unclear but most likely due to irreversible progressive inflammation and collagen deposition in the PV wall adjacent to an ablation lesion [79]. PV stenosis is related to catheter position. The more distal positioning the catheter from the ostium, the higher the risk.

PV stenosis has been reported up to 2 years post-RFCA and, when severe, can result in PV thrombosis, venous infarct, pulmonary veno-occlusive disease, and pulmonary artery hypertension. Symptoms are often nonspecific and insidious in the onset such as vague chest pain, dyspnea, or cough, but patients can also present more acutely with sharp pleuritic chest pain and hemoptysis [19, 80].

MDCT

Acutely, an awareness of a recent history of PVI is necessary to avoid misdiagnosing the pulmonary findings of acute PV infarcts as pneumonia or pulmonary arterial infarcts (Fig. 43.9a–d) [19, 80–83]. CT can be more definitive, with direct assessment of the PVs, particularly when the pre-ablation CT is available for comparison. Obtaining the PV CT with ECG gating is recommended. This provides the best images for multiplanar reformatting and measurement of the ostial diameters. If ECG gating is not possible, non-ECG-gated CT images should be adequate for diagnosis of severe PV stenosis although diagnosis of mild or moderate areas of stenosis should be done more cautiously on non

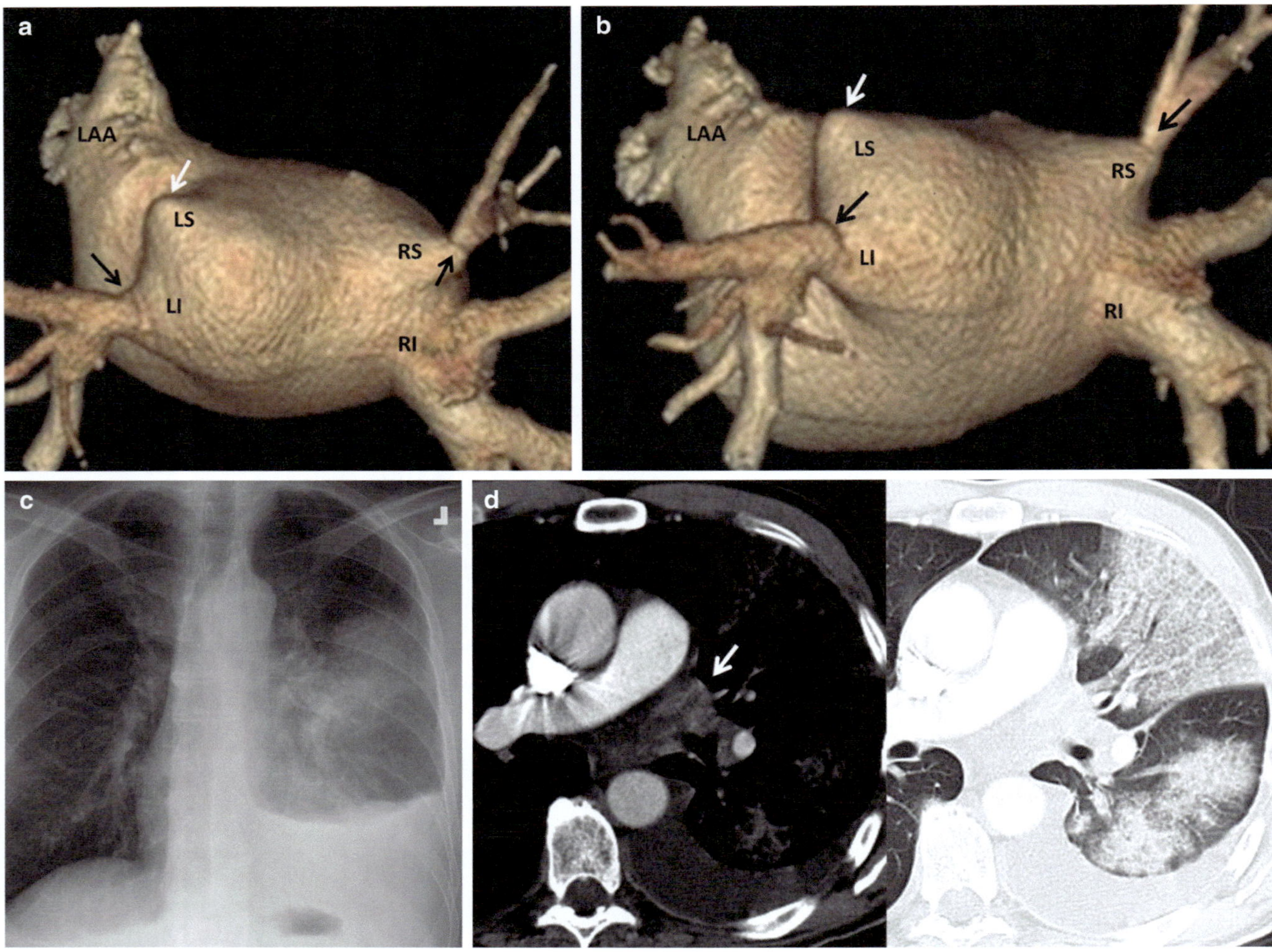

Fig. 43.9 (**a–d**): Pulmonary vein stenosis and occlusion: Epicardial (**a**, **b**) views of the PLA on a pre-ablation CT showing unexpected occlusion of the LSPV (white arrow) and stenoses of the RSPV and RIPV (black arrows). By history, the patient had an ablation 11 years earlier, followed 2 weeks later by a 6-week hospitalization for an "unusual pneumonia" with low-grade fevers and white count; all cultures and pleural fluid were negative. The initial PA radiograph from 11 years ago (**c**) shows large areas of airspace consolidation in the left mid- and lower lung zones with a moderate left pleural effusion. The initial chest CT (**d**) shows thrombus in the LSPV (white arrow) and large areas of ground glass opacity with intralobular septal thickening consistent with wedge-shaped venous infarcts in the lingula and left lower lobe with a left pleural effusion

ECG-gated CT images due to the variability of the PV diameters with different phases of the cardiac cycle [44, 48]. Both the minimum diameter and length of a stenosis should be assessed. Imaging criteria for the diagnosis of PVS include a reduction in PV long-axis diameter of >50% compared to pre-ablation study, corresponding to a reduction in PV cross-sectional area of >75%. Symptoms typically present when the severity of stenosis reaches 60% reduction in diameter [49]. A stenosis is likely more clinically significant if ancillary findings of fat infiltration in the adjacent mediastinum, enlarged reactive lymph nodes, peripheral lung opacities, and localized septal thickening due to veno-occlusive disease and localized pulmonary hypertension are found [19, 38, 80, 81, 84]. Noninvasive treatment of pulmonary vein stenosis following ablation with balloon angioplasty has been used as a treatment option for symptomatic patients although data suggest restenosis rates are relatively high ranging from 47% to 57% [19, 85].

Phrenic Nerve Injury

PNI during PVI is more common in CBA but can also occur in RFCA. It can result in either a palsy or paralysis and may be transient or permanent. A right-sided PNI is the most frequently observed complication with CBA. The risk of PNI due to CBA is reported between 6% and 24% [86]. The reported incidence of transient and persistent PNI resulting from ablation with the first-generation CB was 6% and 4%, respectively. The risk of PNI with the second-generation CB is even higher, with the reported incidence of transient and persistent PNI being 16–24% and 5–7%, respectively [87].

The underlying problem is a hypothermic (CBA) or thermal (RFCA) injury to the right phrenic nerve because of the proximity between the right phrenic nerve and the right PVs [87–89]. The right pericardiophrenic bundle, consisting of the right phrenic nerve, pericardiophrenic artery, and pericardiophrenic vein, courses along the lateral margin of the SVC passing close to the RSPV ostium [89–91]. Patients with unilateral PNI are typically asymptomatic, but dyspnea, particularly orthopnea, can occur.

MDCT

The right pericardiophrenic bundle is not consistently visualized on MDCT. New unilateral elevation of the right hemidiaphragm post-CBA is a sign of possible PNI and can be further evaluated with a fluoroscopic sniff test. In addition, Stroker et al. showed pre-CBA evaluation of the PVs with MDCT as a useful tool for predicting the risk of PNI. They found that large PV dimensions, ostial branches, and a short distance between the SVC and any of the right-sided PVs were associated with increased risk of PNI [86]. If the distance between the RSPV and right pericardiophrenic bundle is less than 10 mm, then there is a higher risk of PNI [89].

Injury to Pulmonary Parenchymal Tissue

CBA has recently been associated with acute injury involving the left mainstem bronchus which is often in close proximity to the ostium of the LSPV. Knight et al. demonstrated cryothermal injury to the left mainstem bronchus using a bronchoscope during CBA at the LSPV in three of ten patients [92]. The clinical relevance of this remains unclear, but it is postulated to be a cause for persistent dry cough seen in some patients post-CBA who do not have PNI. Case reports have also described hematomas adjacent to the RIPV, identified by CTA post-CBA in patients presenting with hemoptysis [93].

Left Atrial Appendage Occluder Procedures

Justification for LAA Occlusion

Many patients with AF face both symptoms resulting in diminution in quality of life (addressed by lifestyle interventions, anti-arrhythmic drugs, and catheter ablation) and an increased risk of stroke. Oral anticoagulation (AC) is the mainstay of prevention of stroke in AF patients. Currently, although there are several different risk scores that are used to identify patients with a high risk for stroke, patients with non-valvular AF are most commonly stratified for yearly stroke risk using the CHADS2 or the newer CHA2DS2-VASc score and are stratified for bleeding risk using the HAS-BLED score [94–97]. Patients with both a high risk of stroke (CHA2DS2-VASc score of at least 3) and elevated risks of bleeding on oral AC represent the target population for LAA occlusion procedures. However, because the CHA2Ds2-VASc score and other currently used risk scores have a poor predictive value with a C-statistic of 0.55–0.64, new thoughts of risk stratification for stroke are focused on the concept of assessing the LA for an underlying atrial myopathy including the presence of atrial fibrosis, dilatation, and loss of contractile function which leads to decreased LAA emptying velocities and blood stasis, thus increasing thrombogenicity [94, 98]. An interrelationship between complex LAA shapes, risk of thrombogenicity, and stroke has also been postulated [99–102]. Thus echocardiography (LA strain), cardiac MRI (LA and LAA flow, LAA morphology, fibrosis, LAA shape), and cardiac CT (LAA shape) have potential emerging roles in stroke risk stratification [103].

Although oral anticoagulation with a traditional vitamin K antagonist or a novel non-vitamin K antagonist drugs are effective therapies, they are not without risk. Only 65% of patients on oral warfarin are therapeutic on the agent, and there exists risk of a major hemorrhage in all patients on oral anticoagulation with an elevated HAS-BLED score [96].

The LAA is the primary source for thromboembolism in AF. In a review of 23 studies in patients with non-valvular AF, 91% of clots were localized to the LAA [104]. The role of occlusion of this structure to prevent thromboembolic complications from AF has been the subject of clinical investigation over the last decade. Increasing scientific evidence is leaning to a viable role for appendage occlusion in stroke prevention in non-valvular AF. In 2016, the US Centers for Medicare and Medicaid Services approved a device for endocardial LAA occlusion (LAAO) in patients considered suboptimal candidates for oral AC therapy. In Europe, per the 2016 European Society of Cardiology Management Guidelines for the management of AF, LAAO for stroke prevention in patients with AF and contraindications for long-term AC therapy has been given a class IIb recommendation [105]. The goal of LAA occlusion is to prevent thrombi formed in the LAA cavity from access to the LA and thus the systemic circulation.

Current LAA Occlusion Methods

There are three categories of LAA occlusion: surgical-based epicardial, catheter-based endocardial, and catheter-based endoepicardial. In addition, there are hybrid techniques combining surgical- and catheter-based techniques. Any of the techniques that include an epicardial component result in both electrical and mechanical exclusions of the LAA, so they have the added benefit of potential eventual elimination of LAA-initiated AF.

Surgical-Based Epicardial

Traditional open surgical techniques include stapling, suture ligation, and amputation done during other open heart surgical procedures. The main interest in the development of device-based LAA occluders is due to the low overall success rate of only 40% complete LAA exclusion by these traditional surgical methods (0% for staples, 23% for sutures, 73% for amputation) resulting in "incomplete exclusion" or recanalization and ongoing, even increased, risk of LAA source thromboemboli [106].

Multidetector CT is not routinely used in the preoperative assessment of the LAA for the traditional surgically based procedures; however, an incompletely surgically excluded LAA is occasionally encountered postoperatively even as an incidental finding when performing CT for other reasons (Fig. 43.10).

The AtriClip, or Gillinov-Cosgrove clip (Atricure, West Chester, OH), is a surgical device-based epicardial technique approved by the FDA in 2009 for LAA exclusion during other open cardiac surgeries in patients with a CHADS2 score of ≥2 and is now undergoing evaluation as a stand-alone minimally invasive thoracoscopic procedure in CHADS2 score of ≥2 patients who do not need other cardiac surgeries [107]. The AtriClip is a self-closing clip made of two parallel rigid titanium rods encasing elastic nitinol springs and wrapped in a braided polyester sheath that is placed epicardially around the base of the LAA and externally compresses to exclude the LAA cavity from the systemic circulation (Fig. 43.11).

Catheter-Based Endocardial

Catheter (percutaneous) endocardial device-based LAA occluders were originally described in 2001. This is a highly evolving field with discontinuation of some of the earlier devices, ongoing investigation of current utilized devices, and rapid introduction of new ones. Today, worldwide, the most widely used are the WATCHMAN device (Boston

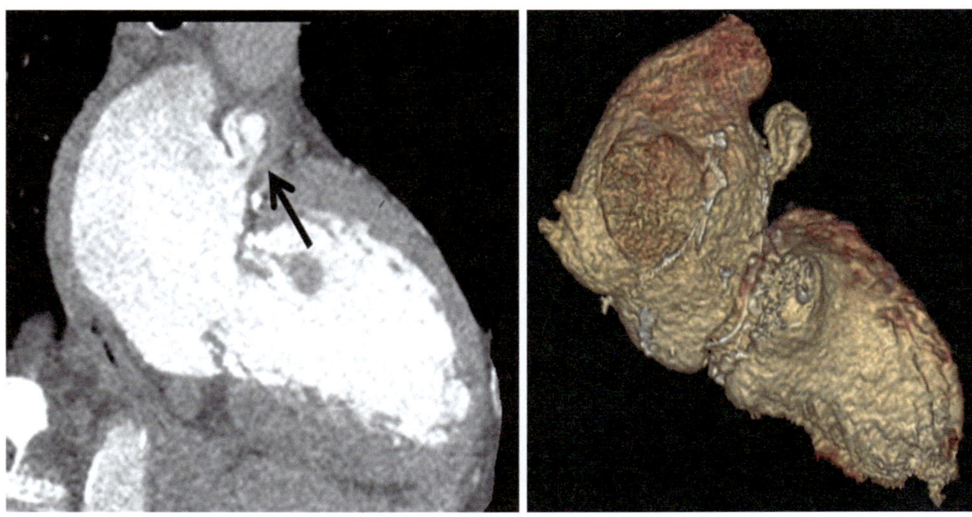

Fig. 43.10 Incomplete LAA exclusion: Multiplanar reformat in a two-chamber view of the heart and corresponding volume rendering showing an incompletely excluded LAA postsurgical epicardial LAA suturing (arrow) with focal central outpouching of contrast from the LA into the LA

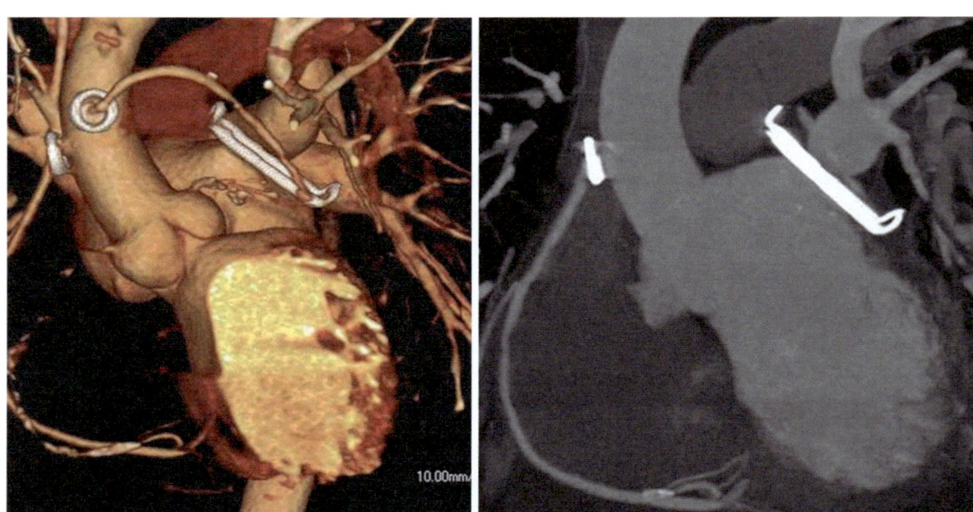

Fig. 43.11 AtriClip LAAO: Volume rendering and thick MIP reconstruction of the heart with a frontal cut showing the typical appearance of an AtriClip placed across the neck of the LAA during coronary artery bypass grafting; there is no residual LAA distal to the clip consistent with complete epicardial occlusion, thrombosis, and atrophy of the LAA. (Images courtesy of Pal Suranyi MD, PhD; Medical University of South Carolina, Charleston, SC, USA)

Scientific, Natick, MA), the original Amplatzer Cardiac Plug (ACP), and its newer version, the Amplatzer Amulet (Abbott Medical, Chicago, IL). The LAmbre (Lifetech Scientific Corp., Shenzhen, China) and the WaveCrest (J&J BWI Cardiovascular & Specialty Solutions Group, Diamond Bar, CA) are some examples of more recently developed devices and will be briefly mentioned. The access to the LAA for any of the endocardial occluders is done via transeptal LA access using fluoroscopic and TEE guidance.

The WATCHMAN device is CE mark approved and, in the USA as of July 2016, the only FDA-approved percutaneous method for LAA occlusion. The efficacy and safety of the WATCHMAN were evaluated in two prospective, randomized clinical trials, most notably the PROTECT-AF and the PREVAIL trials [11, 108]. The PROTECT-AF trial showed noninferiority of the WATCHMAN to warfarin and for the first time implicated the LAA in the pathogenesis of stroke in AF; however, there were periprocedural safety concerns including a 5% pericardial effusion rate. The PREVAIL trial failed to show noninferiority of the WATCHMAN to warfarin at preventing a combination of primary endpoints, met predefined procedural safety outcomes, and showed noninferiority to warfarin for the prevention of long-term ischemic events. FDA approval for the device was based on the combined data from the PROTECT, PREVAIL, and continued access protocols [11, 108, 109].

Clinical eligibility for a WATCHMAN requires that a patient has a demonstrable nonoptimal candidacy for anticoagulation, a CHADS score of ≥2/CHA2DS2-VASc score of ≥3, and the ability to tolerate short-term anticoagulation. The device consists of a radial, self-expanding nitinol frame with a 160 micron polyethylene terephthalate (PET) cap that blocks emboli from crossing it. Multiple fixation anchors around the perimeter of the frame attach the occluder to the LAA endothelium. The WATCHMAN is positioned by both intraprocedural TEE and fluoroscopy to accommodate the largest device that can optimally occlude the LAA orifice [109, 110] (Fig. 43.12).

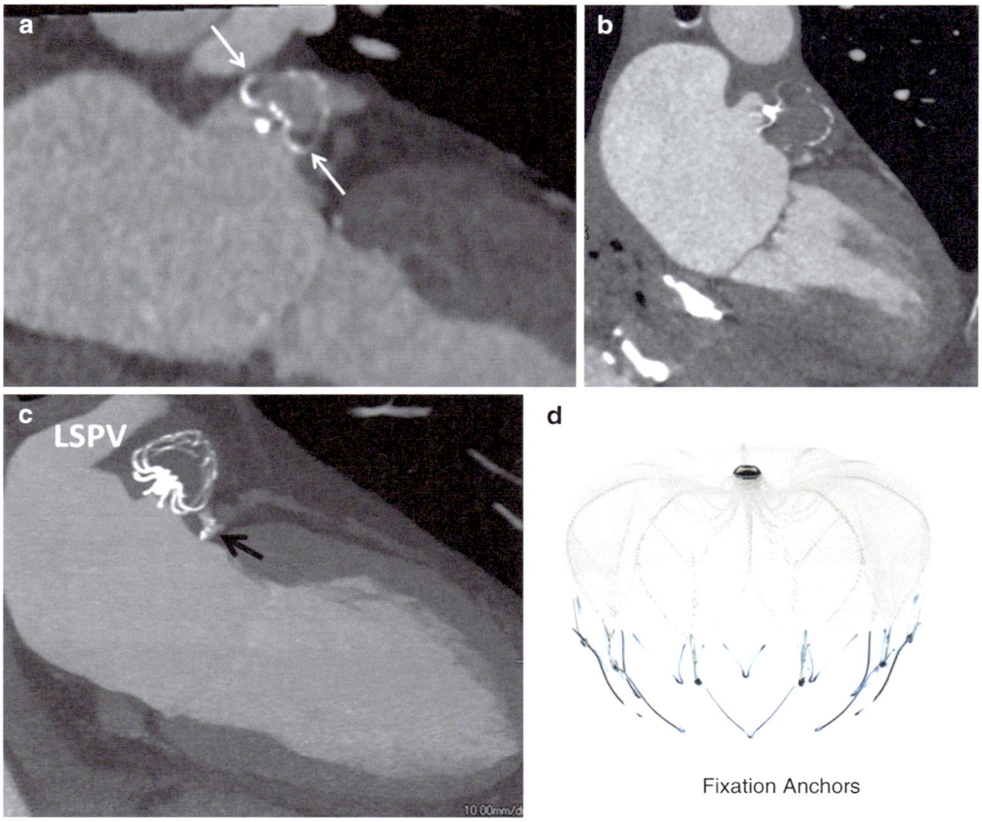

Fig. 43.12 (**a–d**): WATCHMAN LAAO: The WATCHMAN is an endocardial type of LAA occluder and is made of a self-expanding nitinol frame with a PET cap and ten fixation anchors around its periphery to attach to the LAA endothelium (**d**). The appropriate landing zone for the WATCHMAN is the neck of the LAA (**a**, **b**). Thrombus within or distal to the WATCHMAN in the lobar LAA is an expected finding and can fill the device (**b**) or be more laminar (**a**, *thin white arrows*); identification of thrombus on the outer surface (LAA side) of the PET cap or within the LA is abnormal and may warrant short-term anticoagulation (not shown). In (**c**), note the close proximity of the left main coronary artery (arrow) and the LSPV to the LAA. (A, B, courtesy of Orly Goitein, MD, Sheba Medical Center. C, Image c courtesy of Pal Suranyi, MD, PhD, University of South Carolina. D, image d courtesy of Boston Scientific.)

The ongoing Amulet IDE trial is a prospective, randomized, multicenter active control worldwide trial, designed to evaluate the safety and effectiveness of the Amulet LAAO. Subjects will be randomized in a 1:1 ratio between the Amulet (treatment) and a WATCHMAN (control). The trial will be conducted at up to 150 sites worldwide including US sites [111].

The first-generation ACP was CE mark approved and widely used in Europe [112]. The device design is based on the Amplatzer plugs that have a long-term success in atrial septal defect closure and other vascular procedures. The ACP has several components and is made of self-expanding nitinol mesh anchored by multiple fixation hooks on a polyester-covered lobe positioned in the neck of the LAA with a flexible connecting waist extending to a proximal polyester-covered disc which fits across to cover the LAA ostium on the LA side [113] (Fig. 43.13). The second-generation ACP, the Amulet, is similar in design with sizing and anchoring modifications made to accommodate larger LAA ostia and improve stability.

The LAmbre, CE mark approved and used in Europe, is another self-expanding LAA occluder made of a nitinol umbrella with hooks around its perimeter connected by a short central waist to a PET-filled disc-shaped cover. Similar to the ACP, the disc-shaped cover is positioned on the LA side of the LAA ostium; the umbrella-shaped portion is positioned approximately 5 mm distal to the LAA orifice within the LAA neck. The umbrella portion can be collapsed to facilitate repositioning during placement. The WaveCrest is CE mark approved and used in Europe. It is another umbrella-shaped device with a nitinol frame with anchors around the frame; an occlusive, polytetrafluoroethylene membrane covers the LA side of the device, and a polymer foam around the device faces the LAA side.

Catheter-Based Endoepicardial

The Lariat procedure is CE mark approved, currently only FDA approved for suture placement and knot tying in surgical procedures (i.e., soft tissue closure), but has not undergone any clinical trials for stroke prevention in AF patients. The Lariat procedure is used off-label when AF patients with a high risk of stroke have an absolute contraindication to even short-term oral anticoagulation. There is an ongoing FDA-approved clinical trial assessing the utility of LAA electrical isolation with the LARIAT device in conjunction with catheter-based pulmonary vein isolation in patients with persistent AF to see whether freedom from AF is improved over conventional techniques [111]. It is a percutaneous, catheter-based LAA epicardial suture ligation system that requires both endocardial (trans-atrial septal) and epicardial (subxiphoid pericardial) access with the assistance of both endo- and epicardial-based magnets to stabilize the LAA for placement.

CT Technique

During deployment, typically TEE and fluoroscopy are used for guidance. However, preprocedural planning relies on a combination of TEE and increasingly MDCT to assess the

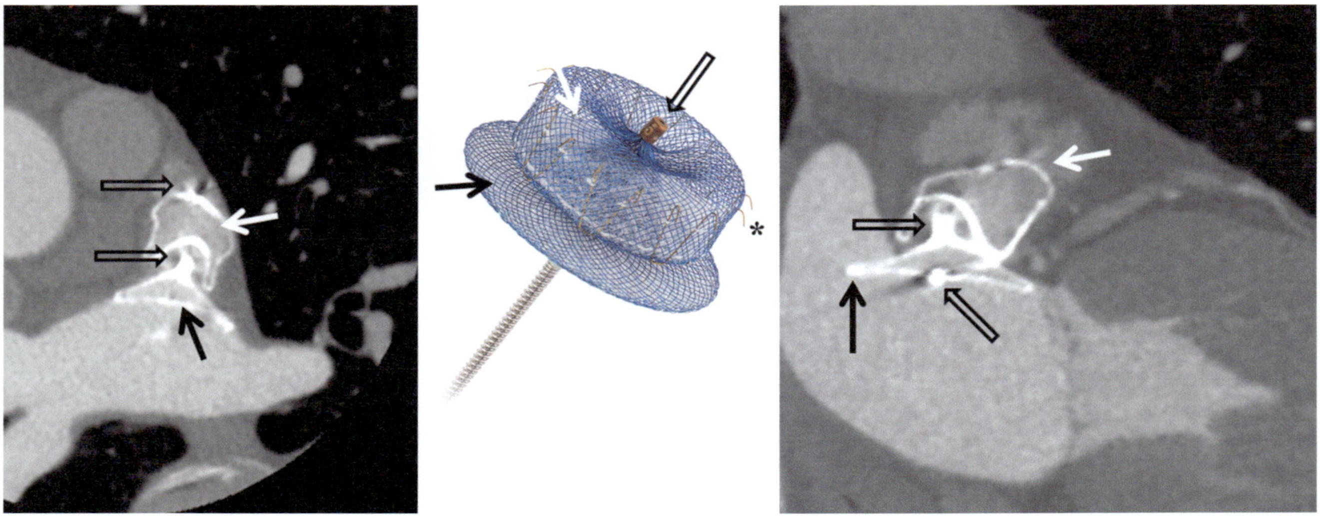

Fig. 43.13 Amplatzer Amulet LAAO: The Amulet is an endocardial type of LAA occluder made of a lobe (white arrow), with multiple fixation hooks (*) positioned in the neck of the LAA, a disc positioned on the LA side of the LAA ostium (black arrow), and a flexible rod waist (open black arrows) connecting the lobe and disc. (AMPLATZER, Amulet, and St. Jude Medical are trademarks of St. Jude Medical, LLC, or its related companies. Reproduced with permission of St. Jude Medical © 2017. All rights reserved; CT images of the Amulet courtesy of Orly Goitein, MD, Sheba Medical Center)

interatrial septal, LA and LAA anatomy, and the anatomic relationship of the LAA to adjacent anatomy and exclude LAA thrombus.

The CT scanner requirements (minimum of 64 slice MDCT scanners) and scan technique including the use of a second delayed acquisition through the LAA are the same as previously detailed for pre-PVI and post-PVI imaging with a few minor modifications.

As with pre-PVI patients, the z-axis of the scan starts at the mid-aortic arch, so the most cephalad extent of the LAA is imaged and covers the heart or the xiphoid process whichever is more distal (for Lariat evaluation). Similar to pre-PVI imaging, the decision to ECG gate or not gate the acquisition will be site dependent on the ability of the available scanner to obtain high-quality images of the LA and LAA in the setting of AF. Although, in normal sinus rhythm, maximum LAA dimensions occur during atrial diastole (ventricular systole), in persistent AF, the LAA dimensions change little over the course of the cardiac cycle. While a dedicated FOV for the heart is preferred, post-scan, reconstructing the data set with the FOV opened to include the anterior chest wall, is needed.

Postprocessing

Postprocessing for all occluders includes epicardial vantage 3D volume renderings of the LA and distal PVs with the LAA and of the LAA by itself. For potential Lariat patients, additional 3D volume renderings include the LA and distal PV model with addition of the MPA and with addition of the imaged sternum including the xiphoid and at least the anterior ribs.

LAA ostial sizing and additional LAA sizing parameters delineated below are most accurately measured on MDCT utilizing the MPRs to obtain true orthogonal obliques, although measurements have been required for some devices on the volume renderings [114]. It is important to be aware that measurements can vary with patient volume status. In addition, early experience with 3D printed models has shown their potential utility in preoperative planning for cardiovascular surgical procedures; others have suggested that, similarly, 3D printing of the LA and LAA may be helpful in pre-LAAO planning [115, 116].

Interpretation Pre-LAA Occluder

Left Atrial Appendage

The specific LAA measurements mentioned below are primarily obtained using TEE; however, MDCT measurements are increasingly being used as adjuncts so familiarity with these measurements is necessary.

The LAA is a complex and highly variable structure heterogeneously lined by fine pectinate muscles which should not be mistaken for intracardiac thrombus. The LAA wall is thin; between the pectinate muscles, it is often exceedingly paper thin, so it is at risk for perforation during the manipulation of catheters and device seating. The LAA is composed of three major components: an ostium, a neck (clinically referred to as the landing zone), and a lobar portion (Fig. 43.14).

The LAA Ostium

The LAA ostium is the well-defined junctional orifice between the LA and the LAA. LAA ostia can be ovoid, round, triangular, or waterdrop like or foot shaped [114]. The shape of the LAA ostium may influence device selection. The less round ostia are potentially greater risks for peridevice leaks [117]. Maximum ostial diameters and circumference are key components for occluder selection, since the occluders are available in fixed sizes (Fig. 43.14).

The LAA ostium is positioned above the left atrioventricular groove, typically at the level of the LSPV but can arise superiorly or inferiorly to the LSPV (Figs. 43.14 and 43.15). Inferior LAA ostia are also more posteriorly located and are notable because of their close proximity to the mitral valve [114].

The lateral ridge (i.e., Ridge of Marshall, "Coumadin," or "Warfarin" ridge) is the infolding of the LA wall that separates the LAA ostium from the adjacent PVs (Fig. 43.4b) [118]. The ridge is of variable widths, dependent on the amount of epicardial fat in its sulcus or groove on the extra-atrial side, so the distance between the LAA ostium and the left PVs varies between patients. The left PVs, particularly the LSPV, are at increased risk for compression by LAA occluders [118]. There are no current recommendations for providing CT measurements of the lateral ridge or measuring the distance between the left PVs and the LAA ostium.

Of note, other vascular structures can course between the LAA and LSPV on the epicardial side of the lateral ridge. These include a persistent left-sided SVC and the S-shaped sinoatrial nodal (SAN) artery [91, 119].

The LAA Neck

The neck of the LAA is the tubular junction between the ostium and the major lobar region and is the landing zone for anchoring the endocardial LAA occluders (Fig. 43.14). It is typically relatively smooth, but occasionally smaller secondary lobes can arise from the neck. Early branching of secondary lobes from the neck can interfere with device seating or, when proximal to the landing zone of the WATCHMAN (<10 mm from LAA ostium), may lead to peridevice leak.

The angle between the ostium, neck, and main lobe is reported on CT and TEE and influences the choice of delivery sheath; sharp angulation between the neck and main lobe

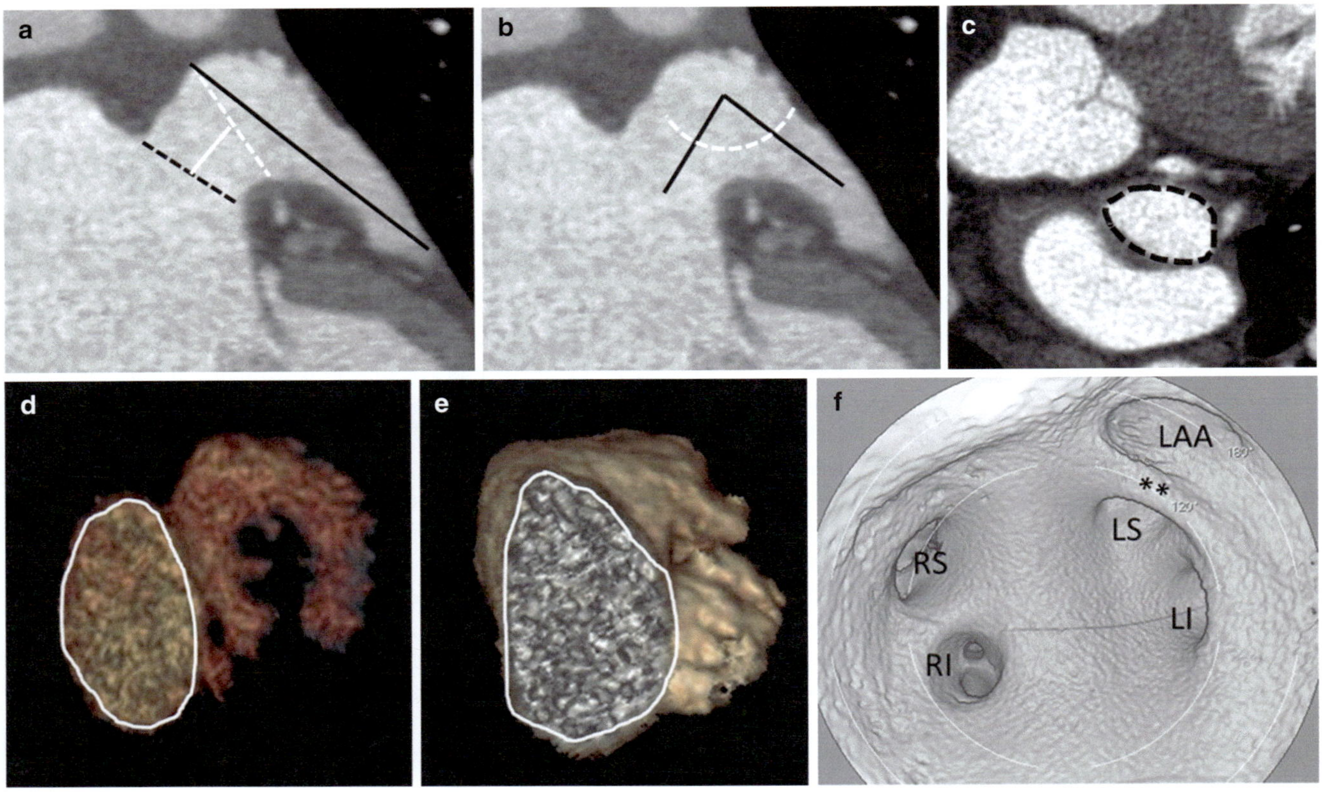

Fig. 43.14 (**a–f**): Left atrial appendage: This windsock shape LAA is divided into the ostium (**a**, dashed black line), interposing neck which is the landing zone for occluders (**a**, solid white line shows length of the neck; dashed white line denotes distal margin) and the lobar region (**a**, solid black line). Although standardly obtained on TEE, pre-LAAO measurements include the length of the largest lobe (**a**, solid black line) and angle between the ostium, neck, and dominant lobe (**b**); in (**c**) perimeter of the LAA ostium (black dashes) is obtained from a true orthogonal oblique perpendicular to the ostium; diameters are derived from the perimeter or can be measured directly. In (**a–c**), note all of the vascular structures in close proximity to the LAA neck and ostium. The LAA ostium comes in varying shapes, including oval and tear-dropped (**d**). The endocardial view (**e**) shows the superior location of this LAA ostium compared to the LSPV ostium, separated by the Ridge of Marshall (**)

can interfere with endocardial device manipulation to the landing zone.

The LAA Lobar Region

The lobar portion of the LAA is the longest part and can consist of single, double, or multiple lobes with varying degrees of trabeculation. In 2010, Wang et al. did an anatomical study of LAA morphology on MDCT and developed a classification system, based on the presence of absence of an obvious bend in the LAA [114].

An LAA with an obvious bend in the proximal or middle part of the dominant lobe is classified as a "chicken wing" shape. LAA without obvious bends in the main lobar region are classified as windsock (one dominant lobe), cauliflower (limited overall length with more complex internal structures), and cactus (dominant central lobe with secondary lobes extending outward both superiorly and inferiorly) shapes [114] (Fig. 43.15). There is an overlap in LAA morphological features among the different categories making some LAA difficult to categorize. Furthermore, as AF becomes persistent, the LAA undergoes structural remodeling, and some of the complexity of the lobulations is lost as the entire structure dilates and loses muscle mass and contractility.

Lobar anatomy, such as maximum available working depth for device deployment and potential prominent pectinate musculature, may affect suitability for a WATCMAN as the feet are situated within the lobar region. Conversely, devices such as the Amulet are positioned more ostially. As detailed earlier in this chapter, assessment of the LAA for thrombus vs pseudothrombus from underfilling and mixing artifacts requires scrutiny of both the early and late images. Pectinate muscles, fluid in adjacent pericardial recesses, and fat interposed between the LSPV and LAA should not be mistaken for thrombus.

Orientation of the LAA behind the main pulmonary artery and maximum transverse approach dimension of 45 mm or greater, which exceeds the size of the snare, are also relevant contraindications for the Lariat procedure (Fig. 43.16).

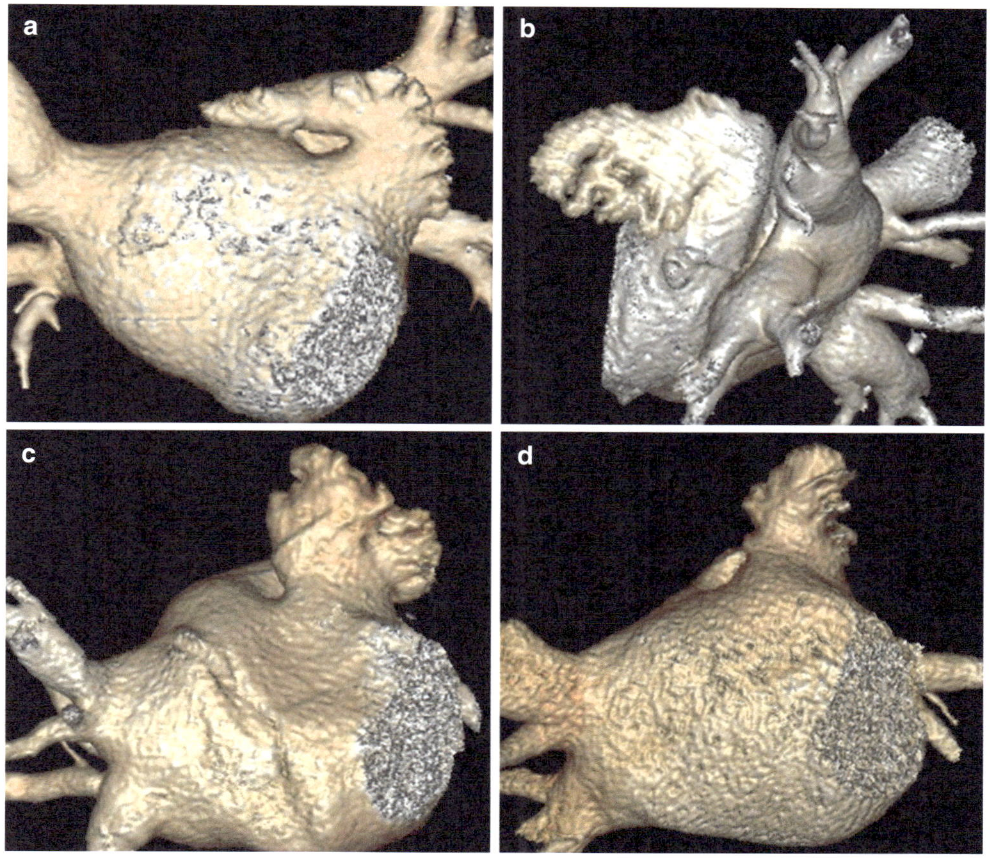

Fig. 43.15 Wings and things (**a–d**): LAA lobar morphology is classified into shapes depending on the presence or absence of an obvious bend within the main lobar region. LAA ostial shapes and position in relationship to the LSPV are variable. (**a**) Chicken wing (bend in the lobar region), (**b**) windsock (bend is at the junction of neck and lobar region), (**c**) cauliflower, (**d**) cactus. Note that in these examples, the LAA ostium is positioned inferior to the LSPV ostium, whereas in the earlier Fig. 43.1b, the LAA ostium is at the level of the PV's and in Figs. 43.4d and 43.14f, the LAA ostium is superior to the left common vein ostium

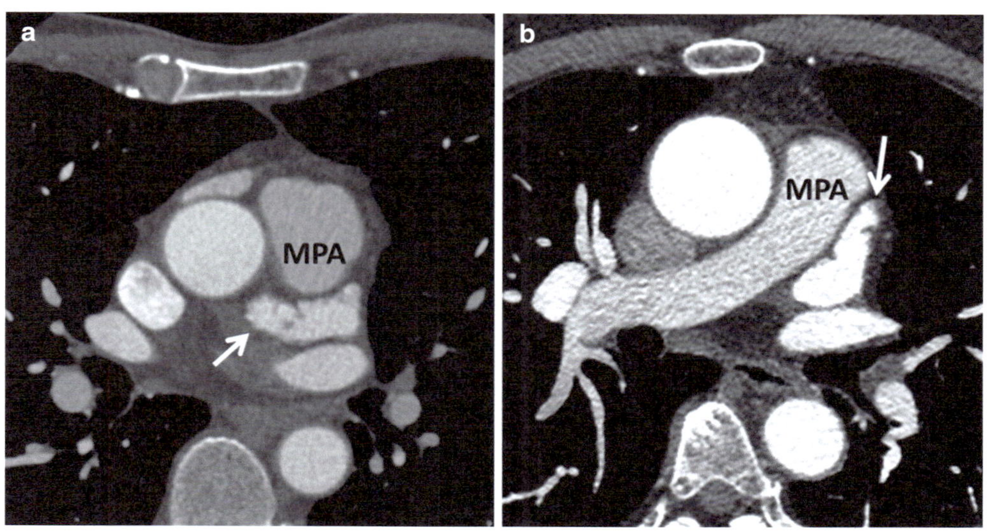

Fig. 43.16 Suitability for Lariat procedure: The position of the tip of the LAA (arrow) in relationship to the main pulmonary artery (MPA) is one of the anatomic factors determining suitability for a Lariat procedure. In (**a**) same patient as in Fig. 43.14a, the tip of the LAA is posterior to the MPA, so it is not reachable from a subxiphoid approach precluding candidacy for a Lariat, whereas in (**b**), same patient as in 43.14b, the LAA is directed anteriorly and to the left of the MPA which is a favorable LAA tip location for a Lariat

Extra-atrial Anatomy

Extra-atrial anatomy needs to be scrutinized for potential Lariat candidates, as there are additional exclusions for the Lariat system involving extra-atrial structures that can interfere with the pericardial puncture or the epicardial access route: a posteriorly oriented heart, any pericardial thickening or calcification, sternal-pericardial adhesions, and unfavorable sternal or chest wall anatomy such as pectus excavatum or severe scoliosis. Patients with a history of prior cardiac surgery or thoracic radiation with the exception of localized breast radiation are excluded prior to imaging.

Interpretation Post-LAA Occluder

Complications of the endocardial occluders include all of the same complications related to vascular and trans-atrial septal access as the catheter-based ablation procedures and some specific to the LAAO. Echocardiography is the primary imaging modality for the assessment of cardiac-related LAAO complications, but some are encountered on CT, so familiarity with possible complications is prudent.

Atrial Septal Defect

Similar to the ablation procedures, trans-atrial septal access can result in a persistent iatrogenic atrial septal defect, which can be seen on CT post-LAAO; the defect is usually small, <5 mm, usually being followed on echocardiography, and typically doesn't require treatment (Fig. 43.17) [120]. They may persist longer than a year but frequently eventually resolve spontaneously [120].

Cardiac Perforation and Pericardial Complications

The more serious complication of cardiac perforation presents during the LAAO procedure. Similar to the ablation procedures, incorrect location of the trans-atrial septal puncture, beyond the region of the fossa ovalis, is one of the causes of cardiac perforation and periprocedural significant pericardial effusion/hemopericardium and possible tamponade. Cardiac perforation, hemopericardium, and tamponade can also occur with perforation of the LA or LAA by the guidewires, catheters, or devices themselves and usually require emergency treatment [117, 121].

During the Lariat procedure, since the pericardium is directly punctured for access, pericarditis and pericardial effusion are common; a pericardial drain is typically placed for 24 h post-procedure, and short-term colchicine therapy is routinely administered [121, 122]. Postop CT should include evaluation of the pericardium for the accumulation of the pericardial effusion post-drain removal, hemopericardium, ongoing CT signs of pericarditis, or post-pericardiectomy syndrome as well as a search for other etiologies for chest pain and dyspnea.

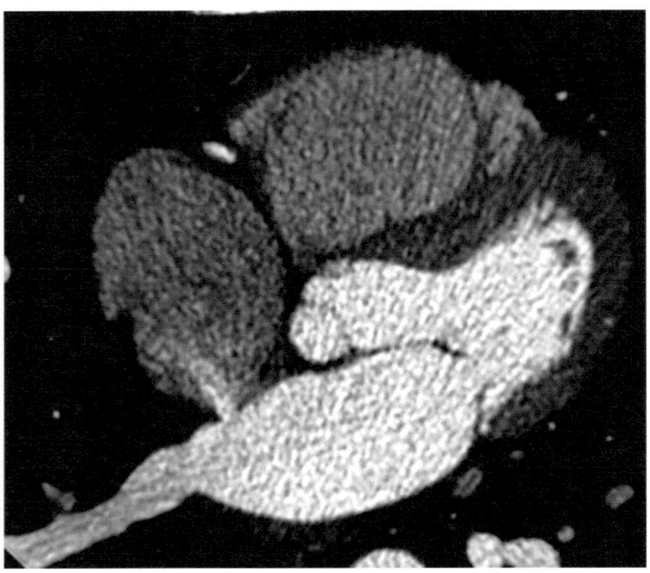

Fig. 43.17 Persistent atrial septal defect: A small, <5 mm ASD (arrow) and left to right shunt is persistent 6 months post-trans-atrial septal puncture for CBA; these small ASDs can occur with any of the procedures utilizing trans-atrial septal puncture including RFCA and LAAO

Device Embolization and Incomplete LAA Occlusion

Undersizing or inadequate seating of the endocardial devices can result in device migration or embolization requiring catheter or surgical retrieval; rates are low, reported between 0% and 3% [108, 117]. Similarly, peridevice leaks can result in residual flow into the LAA between the margin of the device and the wall of the LAA; if the peridevice leak is less than 5 mm wide, it is considered small and followed with echocardiography [117]. Peridevice leaks are common. A substudy of the PROTECT trial showed that 32% of the WATCHMAN patients had at least some degree of peridevice flow at 1 year [123]; multicenter experience in Europe reported 16% of ACP patients had a small peridevice leak at 6 months [124]. The Lariat suture may also incompletely occlude the LAA, but similar to other epicardial-based techniques, the leak is central. Malpositioned or oversized devices may also overlap the contiguous LSPV or the mitral valve leaflet.

Thrombus Formation

Over time, the endocardial devices endothelialize. CT identification of thrombus on the LAA side distal to an endocardial occluder or epicardial closure site is an expected finding. Thrombus on the LA side may indicate a need for short-term anticoagulation therapy. In the PROTECT trial, the incidence of some thrombus on the LA side of the WATCHMAN was approximately 4%. A higher incidence of thrombus on the flexible connecting waist of the ACP of approximately 14% was one of the reasons the device was redesigned.

Conclusion

The increasing disease burden caused by atrial fibrillation has led to new interventions aimed at restoring normal sinus rhythm and preventing embolic complications. Cardiac CT can help identify suitable candidates, plan the intervention, and diagnose complications. In some institutions, this application has become the most common indication for the clinical use of cardiac CT. Consequently, expertise in making the pertinent observations outlined in this chapter is of critical importance for the success of any cardiac CT program and offers a tremendous opportunity for interdisciplinary collaboration.

References

1. Go AS, et al. Prevalence of diagnosed atrial fibrillation in adults: national implications for rhythm management and stroke prevention: the AnTicoagulation and Risk Factors in Atrial Fibrillation (ATRIA) Study. JAMA. 2001;285(18):2370–5.
2. Miyasaka Y, et al. Secular trends in incidence of atrial fibrillation in Olmsted County, Minnesota, 1980 to 2000, and implications on the projections for future prevalence. Circulation. 2006;114(2):119–25.
3. Grond M, et al. Improved detection of silent atrial fibrillation using 72-hour Holter ECG in patients with ischemic stroke: a prospective multicenter cohort study. Stroke. 2013;44(12):3357–64.
4. Henriksson KM, et al. Comparison of cardiovascular risk factors and survival in patients with ischemic or hemorrhagic stroke. Int J Stroke. 2012;7(4):276–81.
5. Kishore A, et al. Detection of atrial fibrillation after ischemic stroke or transient ischemic attack: a systematic review and meta-analysis. Stroke. 2014;45(2):520–6.
6. Investigators, T.A.F.F.-u.I.o.R.M. A comparison of rate control and rhythm control in patients with atrial fibrillation. N Engl J Med. 2002;347(23):1825–33.
7. Fuster V, et al. ACC/AHA/ESC guidelines for the management of patients with atrial fibrillation: executive summary a report of the American College of Cardiology/American Heart Association Task Force on Practice Guidelines and the European Society of Cardiology Committee for Practice Guidelines and Policy Conferences (Committee to Develop Guidelines for the Management of Patients With Atrial Fibrillation) developed in collaboration with the North American society of pacing and electrophysiology. Circulation. 2001;104(17):2118–50.
8. Pathak RK, et al. Impact of CARDIOrespiratory FITness on arrhythmia recurrence in obese individuals with atrial fibrillation: the CARDIO-FIT study. J Am Coll Cardiol. 2015;66(9):985–96.
9. Pathak RK, et al. Long-term effect of goal-directed weight management in an atrial fibrillation cohort: a long-term follow-up study (LEGACY). J Am Coll Cardiol. 2015;65(20):2159–69.
10. Kim MH, et al. Clinical outcomes and costs associated with a first episode of uncomplicated atrial fibrillation presenting to the emergency room. Am J Cardiol. 2001;88(1):A7. 74-6.
11. Holmes DR Jr, et al. Prospective randomized evaluation of the Watchman Left Atrial Appendage Closure device in patients with atrial fibrillation versus long-term warfarin therapy: the PREVAIL trial. J Am Coll Cardiol. 2014;64(1):1–12.
12. Haissaguerre M, et al. Spontaneous initiation of atrial fibrillation by ectopic beats originating in the pulmonary veins. N Engl J Med. 1998;339(10):659–66.
13. Shah DC, et al. Electrophysiologically guided ablation of the pulmonary veins for the curative treatment of atrial fibrillation. Ann Med. 2000;32(6):408–16.
14. Lacomis JM, et al. CT of the pulmonary veins. J Thorac Imaging. 2007;22(1):63–76.
15. Oral H, et al. Catheter ablation for paroxysmal atrial fibrillation: segmental pulmonary vein ostial ablation versus left atrial ablation. Circulation. 2003;108(19):2355–60.
16. Pappone C, et al. Circumferential radiofrequency ablation of pulmonary vein ostia: a new anatomic approach for curing atrial fibrillation. Circulation. 2000;102(21):2619–28.
17. Lee R, et al. The closed heart MAZE: a nonbypass surgical technique. Ann Thorac Surg. 1999;67(6):1696–702.
18. Haissaguerre M, et al. Successful catheter ablation of atrial fibrillation. J Cardiovasc Electrophysiol. 1994;5(12):1045–52.
19. Packer DL, et al. Clinical presentation, investigation, and management of pulmonary vein stenosis complicating ablation for atrial fibrillation. Circulation. 2005;111(5):546–54.
20. Schwartzman D, Bazaz R, Nosbisch J. Catheter ablation to suppress atrial fibrillation: evolution of technique at a single center. J Interv Card Electrophysiol. 2003;9(2):295–300.
21. Pappone C, et al. Pulmonary vein denervation enhances long-term benefit after circumferential ablation for paroxysmal atrial fibrillation. Circulation. 2004;109(3):327–34.
22. Verma A, et al. Approaches to catheter ablation for persistent atrial fibrillation. N Engl J Med. 2015;372(19):1812–22.
23. Packer DL, et al. Cryoballoon ablation of pulmonary veins for paroxysmal atrial fibrillation: first results of the North American Arctic Front (STOP AF) pivotal trial. J Am Coll Cardiol. 2013;61(16):1713–23.
24. Lustgarten DL, Keane D, Ruskin J. Cryothermal ablation: mechanism of tissue injury and current experience in the treatment of tachyarrhythmias. Prog Cardiovasc Dis. 1999;41(6):481–98.
25. Kuck K-H, et al. Cryoballoon or radiofrequency ablation for paroxysmal atrial fibrillation. N Engl J Med. 2016;374(23):2235–45.
26. Khoueiry Z, et al. Outcomes after cryoablation vs. radiofrequency in patients with paroxysmal atrial fibrillation: impact of pulmonary veins anatomy. Europace. 2016;18(9):1343–51.
27. Ang R, et al. The hot and the cold: radiofrequency versus cryoballoon ablation for atrial fibrillation. Curr Cardiol Rep. 2015;17(9):631.
28. Guhl EN, et al. Efficacy of cryoballoon pulmonary vein isolation in patients with persistent atrial fibrillation. J Cardiovasc Electrophysiol. 2016;27(4):423–7.
29. Rillig A, et al. Six-year clinical outcomes after catheter ablation of atrial fibrillation in patients with impaired left ventricular function. J Cardiovasc Electrophysiol. 2015;26:1169.
30. Kholova I, Kautzner J. Morphology of atrial myocardial extensions into human caval veins: a postmortem study in patients with and without atrial fibrillation. Circulation. 2004;110(5):483–8.
31. Kurotobi T, et al. Marshall vein as arrhythmogenic source in patients with atrial fibrillation: correlation between its anatomy and electrophysiological findings. J Cardiovasc Electrophysiol. 2006;17(10):1062–7.
32. Scharf C, et al. Anatomy of the pulmonary veins in patients with atrial fibrillation and effects of segmental ostial ablation analyzed by computed tomography. J Cardiovasc Electrophysiol. 2003;14(2):150–5.
33. Dill T, et al. Pulmonary vein diameter reduction after radiofrequency catheter ablation for paroxysmal atrial fibrillation evaluated by contrast-enhanced three-dimensional magnetic resonance imaging. Circulation. 2003;107(6):845–50.
34. Lacomis JM, et al. Multi-detector row CT of the left atrium and pulmonary veins before radio-frequency catheter ablation for atrial fibrillation. Radiographics. 2003;**23 Spec No**:S35–48. discussion S48–50.
35. Lacomis J, et al. Direct comparison of CT & MRI for characterization of PLA morphology. J Interv Card Electrophysiol. 2006;16(1):7–13.
36. Kato R, et al. Pulmonary vein anatomy in patients undergoing catheter ablation of atrial fibrillation: lessons learned by use of magnetic resonance imaging. Circulation. 2003;107(15):2004–10.
37. Schwartzman D, Lacomis J, Wigginton WG. Characterization of left atrium and distal pulmonary vein morphology using

multidimensional computed tomography. J Am Coll Cardiol. 2003;41(8):1349–57.
38. Cronin P, et al. MDCT of the left atrium and pulmonary veins in planning radiofrequency ablation for atrial fibrillation: a how-to guide. AJR Am J Roentgenol. 2004;183(3):767–78.
39. Lacomis J, et al. 3D-Multidetector CT and variations in pulmonary venous and left atrial anatomy; implications in atrial fibrillation patients undergoing ablative therapy. Radiology. 2002;**S 225**:631.
40. Marom EM, et al. Variations in pulmonary venous drainage to the left atrium: implications for radiofrequency ablation. Radiology. 2004;230(3):824–9.
41. Cronin P. 2D or Not 2D that is the question, but 3D is the answer. Acad Radiol. 2007;14(7):769–71.
42. Cronin P, et al. Reliability of MDCT in characterizing pulmonary venous drainage, diameter and distance to first bifurcation: an interobserver study. Acad Radiol. 2007;14(4):437–44.
43. Cronin P, et al. Normative analysis of pulmonary vein drainage patterns on multidetector CT with measurements of pulmonary vein ostial diameter and distance to first bifurcation. Acad Radiol. 2007;14(2):178–88.
44. Lickfett L, et al. Changes of pulmonary vein orifice size and location throughout the cardiac cycle: dynamic analysis using magnetic resonance cine imaging. J Cardiovasc Electrophysiol. 2005;16(6):582–8.
45. Hsieh MH, et al. Double multielectrode mapping catheters facilitate radiofrequency catheter ablation of focal atrial fibrillation originating from pulmonary veins. J Cardiovasc Electrophysiol. 1999;10(2):136–44.
46. Zhong H, Lacomis JM, Schwartzman D. On the accuracy of CartoMerge for guiding posterior left atrial ablation in man. Heart Rhythm. 2007;4(5):595–602.
47. Bhakta D, Miller JM. Principles of electroanatomic mapping. Indian Pacing Electrophysiol J. 2008;8(1):32–50.
48. Choi SI, et al. Variation of the size of pulmonary venous ostia during the cardiac cycle: optimal reconstruction window at ECG-gated multi-detector row CT. Eur Radiol. 2005;15(7):1441–5.
49. Merchant FM, et al. Pulmonary vein remodeling following atrial fibrillation ablation: implications for the radiographic diagnosis of pulmonary vein stenosis. J Atr Fibrillation. 2016;9(2):1453.
50. Wongcharoen W, et al. Morphologic characteristics of the left atrial appendage, roof, and septum: implications for the ablation of atrial fibrillation. J Cardiovasc Electrophysiol. 2006;17(9):951–6.
51. Gal P, Marrouche NF. Magnetic resonance imaging of atrial fibrosis: redefining atrial fibrillation to a syndrome. Eur Heart J. 2017;38(1):14–9.
52. Calkins H, et al. HRS/EHRA/ECAS expert consensus statement on catheter and surgical ablation of atrial fibrillation: recommendations for personnel, policy, procedures and follow-up. A report of the Heart Rhythm Society (HRS) Task Force on catheter and surgical ablation of atrial fibrillation. Heart Rhythm. 2007;4(6):816–61.
53. Ghaye B, et al. Percutaneous ablation for atrial fibrillation: the role of cross-sectional imaging. Radiographics. 2003;**23 Spec No**:S19–33. discussion S48–50.
54. Lacomis J, et al. Ablation imaging of left atrial and pulmonary venous anatomy in atrial fibrillation patients: comparison of 3D-multidetector CT angiography and magnetic resonance angiography. Radiology. 2002;**S 225**:626.
55. Mangrum JM, et al. Intracardiac echocardiography-guided, anatomically based radiofrequency ablation of focal atrial fibrillation originating from pulmonary veins. J Am Coll Cardiol. 2002;39(12):1964–72.
56. Tsao HM, et al. Role of right middle pulmonary vein in patients with paroxysmal atrial fibrillation. J Cardiovasc Electrophysiol. 2001;12(12):1353–7.
57. Wittkampf FH, et al. Pulmonary vein ostium geometry: analysis by magnetic resonance angiography. Circulation. 2003;107(1):21–3.
58. Duerinckx AJ, Vanovermeire O. Accessory appendages of the left atrium as seen during 64-slice coronary CT angiography. Int J Cardiovasc Imaging. 2008;24(2):215–21.
59. Romero J, et al. Left atrial appendage closure devices. Clin Med Insights Cardiol. 2014;**8**(4251-CMC-Left-Atrial-Appendage-Closure-Devices.pdf):45–52.
60. Lazoura O, et al. Prevalence of left atrial anatomical abnormalities in patients with recurrent atrial fibrillation compared with patients in sinus rhythm using multi-slice CT. J Cardiovasc Comput Tomogr. 2012;6(4):268–73.
61. Sosa E, Scanavacca M. Left atrial-esophageal fistula complicating radiofrequency catheter ablation of atrial fibrillation. J Cardiovasc Electrophysiol. 2005;16(3):249–50.
62. Scanavacca MI, et al. Left atrial-esophageal fistula following radiofrequency catheter ablation of atrial fibrillation. J Cardiovasc Electrophysiol. 2004;15(8):960–2.
63. Kelly S, Bicknell SG, Sharma S. Left atrial wall hematoma after radiofrequency ablation for atrial fibrillation. AJR Am J Roentgenol. 2006;186(5):1317–9.
64. Ramakrishna G, et al. Endocardial flap of left atrial dissection following radiofrequency ablation. Pacing Clin Electrophysiol. 2003;26(8):1771–3.
65. Park HW, et al. Disseminated intravascular coagulation as a complication of radiofrequency catheter ablation of atrial fibrillation. J Cardiovasc Electrophysiol. 2005;16(9):1011–3.
66. Sonmez B, Demirsoy E, Yilmaz O. Atrioesophageal fistula: is it an unavoidable complication of radiofrequency ablation? J Thorac Cardiovasc Surg. 2003;126(5):1662–3. author reply 1663.
67. Gillinov AM, Pettersson G, Rice TW. Esophageal injury during radiofrequency ablation for atrial fibrillation. J Thorac Cardiovasc Surg. 2001;122(6):1239–40.
68. Doll N, et al. Esophageal perforation during left atrial radiofrequency ablation: is the risk too high? J Thorac Cardiovasc Surg. 2003;125(4):836–42.
69. Bunch TJ, et al. Temporary esophageal stenting allows healing of esophageal perforations following atrial fibrillation ablation procedures. J Cardiovasc Electrophysiol. 2006;17(4):435–9.
70. Schley P, Gulker H, Horlitz M. Atrio-oesophageal fistula following circumferential pulmonary vein ablation: verification of diagnosis with multislice computed tomography. Europace. 2006;8(3):189–90.
71. Pappone C, et al. Atrio-esophageal fistula as a complication of percutaneous transcatheter ablation of atrial fibrillation. Circulation. 2004;109(22):2724–6.
72. Malamis AP, Kirshenbaum KJ, Nadimpalli S. CT radiographic findings: atrio-esophageal fistula after transcatheter percutaneous ablation of atrial fibrillation. J Thorac Imaging. 2007;22(2):188–91.
73. Ripley KL, et al. Time course of esophageal lesions after catheter ablation with cryothermal and radiofrequency ablation: implication for atrio-esophageal fistula formation after catheter ablation for atrial fibrillation. J Cardiovasc Electrophysiol. 2007;18(6):642–6.
74. Lemola K, et al. Computed tomographic analysis of the anatomy of the left atrium and the esophagus: implications for left atrial catheter ablation. Circulation. 2004;110(24):3655–60.
75. Cury RC, et al. Relationship of the esophagus and aorta to the left atrium and pulmonary veins: implications for catheter ablation of atrial fibrillation. Heart Rhythm. 2005;2(12):1317–23.
76. Gillinov AM, et al. Esophageal perforation during left atrial radiofrequency ablation: is the risk too high? J Thorac Cardiovasc Surg. 2003;126(5):1661–2. author reply 1662.
77. Pappone C, et al. Atrial electroanatomic remodeling after circumferential radiofrequency pulmonary vein ablation: efficacy of an

anatomic approach in a large cohort of patients with atrial fibrillation. Circulation. 2001;104(21):2539–44.
78. Bunch TJ, et al. Outcomes after cardiac perforation during radiofrequency ablation of the atrium. J Cardiovasc Electrophysiol. 2005;16(11):1172–9.
79. Rostamian A, et al. The incidence, diagnosis, and management of pulmonary vein stenosis as a complication of atrial fibrillation ablation. J Interv Card Electrophysiol. 2014;40(1):63–74.
80. Ravenel JG, McAdams HP. Pulmonary venous infarction after radiofrequency ablation for atrial fibrillation. AJR Am J Roentgenol. 2002;178(3):664–6.
81. Saad EB, et al. Pulmonary vein stenosis after catheter ablation of atrial fibrillation: emergence of a new clinical syndrome. Ann Intern Med. 2003;138(8):634–8.
82. Burgstahler C, et al. Visualization of pulmonary vein stenosis after radio frequency ablation using multi-slice computed tomography: initial clinical experience in 33 patients. Int J Cardiol. 2005;102(2):287–91.
83. Yu WC, et al. Acquired pulmonary vein stenosis after radiofrequency catheter ablation of paroxysmal atrial fibrillation. J Cardiovasc Electrophysiol. 2001;12(8):887–92.
84. Saad EB, et al. Pulmonary vein stenosis after radiofrequency ablation of atrial fibrillation: functional characterization, evolution, and influence of the ablation strategy. Circulation. 2003;108(25):3102–7.
85. Mohr FW, et al. Curative treatment of atrial fibrillation with intraoperative radiofrequency ablation: short-term and midterm results. J Thorac Cardiovasc Surg. 2002;123(5):919–27.
86. Stroker E, et al. Anatomic predictors of phrenic nerve injury in the setting of pulmonary vein isolation using the 28-mm second-generation cryoballoon. Heart Rhythm. 2016;13(2):342–51.
87. Hai JJ, Tse HF. Phrenic nerve palsy in cryoballoon ablation: can it be prevented? Heart Rhythm. 2016;13(2):352–3.
88. Andrade JG, et al. The biophysics and biomechanics of cryoballoon ablation. Pacing Clin Electrophysiol. 2012;35(9):1162–8.
89. Horton R, et al. Locating the right phrenic nerve by imaging the right pericardiophrenic artery with computerized tomographic angiography: implications for balloon-based procedures. Heart Rhythm. 2010;7(7):937–41.
90. Matsumoto Y, et al. Detection of phrenic nerves and their relation to cardiac anatomy using 64-slice multidetector computed tomography. Am J Cardiol. 2007;100(1):133–7.
91. Cummings KW, et al. Cross-sectional imaging anatomy and pathologic conditions affecting thoracic nerves. Radiographics. 2017;37(1):73–92.
92. Verma N, et al. Bronchial effects of cryoballoon ablation for atrial fibrillation. Heart Rhythm. 2017;14(1):17–8.
93. Bessiere F, Chevalier P. Pulmonary vein hematoma after atrial fibrillation cryoablation: a new complication. Heart Rhythm. 2013;10(9):1359.
94. Lip GYH, et al. Refining clinical risk stratification for predicting stroke and thromboembolism in atrial fibrillation using a novel risk factor-based approach: The euro heart survey on atrial fibrillation. Chest. 2010;137(2):263–72.
95. Kosior DA. Risk stratification schemes for stroke in atrial fibrillation: the predictive factors still undefined. Pol Arch Med Wewn. 2015;125(12):889–90.
96. Pisters R, et al. A novel user-friendly score (HAS-BLED) to assess 1-year risk of major bleeding in patients with atrial fibrillation: the Euro Heart Survey. Chest. 2010;138(5):1093–100.
97. Steinberg BA, et al. Higher risk of death and stroke in patients with persistent vs. paroxysmal atrial fibrillation: results from the ROCKET-AF Trial. Eur Heart J. 2015;36(5):288–96.
98. Lee G, Sanders P, Kalman JM. Catheter ablation of atrial arrhythmias: state of the art. Lancet. 2012;380(9852):1509–19.
99. Burrell LD, et al. Usefulness of left atrial appendage volume as a predictor of embolic stroke in patients with atrial fibrillation. Am J Cardiol. 2013;112(8):1148–52.
100. Di Biase L, et al. Atrial fibrillation ablation strategies for paroxysmal patients: randomized comparison between different techniques. Circ Arrhythm Electrophysiol. 2009;2(2):113–9.
101. Anselmino M, et al. Left atrial appendage morphology and silent cerebral ischemia in patients with atrial fibrillation. Heart Rhythm. 2014;11(1):2–7.
102. Yamamoto M, et al. Complex left atrial appendage morphology and left atrial appendage thrombus formation in patients with atrial fibrillation. Circ Cardiovasc Imaging. 2014;7(2):337–43.
103. Fluckiger JU, et al. Left atrial flow velocity distribution and flow coherence using four-dimensional FLOW MRI: a pilot study investigating the impact of age and Pre- and Postintervention atrial fibrillation on atrial hemodynamics. J Magn Reson Imaging. 2013;38(3):580–7.
104. Blackshear JL, Odell JA. Appendage obliteration to reduce stroke in cardiac surgical patients with atrial fibrillation. Ann Thorac Surg. 1996;61(2):755–9.
105. Kirchhof P, et al. 2016 ESC Guidelines for the management of atrial fibrillation developed in collaboration with EACTS. Eur Heart J. 2016;37(38):2893–962.
106. Kanderian AS, et al. Success of surgical left atrial appendage closure: assessment by transesophageal echocardiography. J Am Coll Cardiol. 2008;52(11):924–9.
107. Ellis CR, Aznaurov SG. The left atrial appendage and thromboembolic stroke in atrial fibrillation: rationale for ligation by an epicardial approach: the AtriClip stroke trial. J Innov Card Rhythm Manag. 2015;6:2052–6.
108. Holmes DR, et al. Percutaneous closure of the left atrial appendage versus warfarin therapy for prevention of stroke in patients with atrial fibrillation: a randomised non-inferiority trial. Lancet. 2009;374(9689):534–42.
109. Reddy VY, et al. Percutaneous left atrial appendage closure for stroke prophylaxis in patients with atrial fibrillation: 2.3-Year Follow-up of the PROTECT AF (Watchman Left Atrial Appendage System for Embolic Protection in Patients with Atrial Fibrillation) Trial. Circulation. 2013;127(6):720–9.
110. Belgaid DR, et al. Prospective randomized evaluation of the watchman left atrial appendage closure device in patients with atrial fibrillation versus long-term warfarin therapy: the PREVAIL trial. Int J Cardiol. 2016;219:177–9.
111. Lee RJ, et al. Percutaneous alternative to the Maze procedure for the treatment of persistent or long-standing persistent atrial fibrillation (aMAZE trial): rationale and design. Am Heart J. 2015;170(6):1184–94.
112. Tzikas A, Sievert H, Holmes DR Jr. Percutaneous left atrial appendage occlusion in 2016. EuroIntervention. 2016;11(14):e1576–8.
113. Khattab AA, Meier B. Transcatheter left atrial appendage exclusion, gold or fool's gold? Eur Heart J Suppl. 2010;12(suppl_E):E35–40.
114. Wang Y, et al. Left atrial appendage studied by computed tomography to help planning for appendage closure device placement. J Cardiovasc Electrophysiol. 2010;21(9):973–82.
115. Pellegrino PL, et al. Left atrial appendage closure guided by 3D printed cardiac reconstruction: emerging directions and future trends. J Cardiovasc Electrophysiol. 2016;27(6):768–71.
116. Giannopoulos AA, et al. Cardiothoracic applications of 3-dimensional printing. J Thorac Imaging. 2016;31(5):253–72.
117. Wunderlich NC, et al. Percutaneous interventions for left atrial appendage exclusion: options, assessment, and imaging using 2D and 3D echocardiography. JACC Cardiovasc Imaging. 2015;8(4):472–88.

118. Cabrera JA, Saremi F, Sanchez-Quintana D. Left atrial appendage: anatomy and imaging landmarks pertinent to percutaneous transcatheter occlusion. Heart. 2014;100(20):1636–50.
119. Saremi F, et al. Arterial supply to sinuatrial and atrioventricular nodes: imaging with multidetector CT. Radiology. 2008;246(1):99–107; discussion 108-9.
120. Singh SM, Douglas PS, Reddy VY. The incidence and long-term clinical outcome of iatrogenic atrial septal defects secondary to transseptal catheterization with a 12F transseptal sheath. Circ Arrhythm Electrophysiol. 2011;4(2):166–71.
121. Price MJ, et al. Early safety and efficacy of percutaneous left atrial appendage suture ligation: results from the U.S. transcatheter LAA ligation consortium. J Am Coll Cardiol. 2014;64(6):565–72.
122. Stone D, Byrne T, Pershad A. Early results with the LARIAT device for left atrial appendage exclusion in patients with atrial fibrillation at high risk for stroke and anticoagulation. Catheter Cardiovasc Interv. 2015;86(1):121–7.
123. Viles-Gonzalez JF, et al. The clinical impact of incomplete left atrial appendage closure with the Watchman Device in patients with atrial fibrillation: a PROTECT AF (Percutaneous Closure of the Left Atrial Appendage Versus Warfarin Therapy for Prevention of Stroke in Patients With Atrial Fibrillation) substudy. J Am Coll Cardiol. 2012;59(10):923–9.
124. Tzikas A, et al. Left atrial appendage occlusion for stroke prevention in atrial fibrillation: multicentre experience with the AMPLATZER Cardiac Plug. EuroIntervention. 2016;11(10):1170–9.

Part X

Where We Are: Congenital Heart Disease

Special Technique Considerations for Congenital Heart Disease Imaging

44

Anthony M. Hlavacek

While the evaluation of patients with acquired coronary artery disease has been the major driving force behind many of the innovations in cardiac computed tomography (CT), this modality has proven to be a very useful imaging modality for patients with congenital heart disease as well. The high spatial resolution and isotropic nature of the resulting datasets allow viewing in multiple two-dimensional or curvilinear planes, along with the ability for excellent three-dimensional reconstructions. This inherent three-dimensional property of cardiac CT makes it useful for imaging tortuous vessels and defining complex anatomical relationships. With a scan time of only a few seconds or less, it is possible to image most children without sedation. Rapid image acquisition with current CT scanners results in minimal motion artifacts from breathing and poor cooperation. Unlike echocardiography, CT is window independent, has a large field of view, and provides excellent visualization of airway structures. In contrast to MRI, CT imaging is less likely to require sedation or anesthesia and is minimally affected by metallic devices, such as stents, coils, pacemakers, and defibrillators. For these reasons, cardiac CT is being increasingly utilized in patients with CHD [1], and recent expert census and guideline documents recommend its use for a variety of these patients [2, 3]. Given the varied imaging indications and complex anatomy and physiology in many of these patients, however, special techniques are often necessary to optimize the diagnostic information obtained [4]. This chapter assumes basic competence in cardiac CT imaging, including dose reduction strategies, but will provide recommendations regarding patient preparation, scan techniques, and reporting that can be utilized to optimize the diagnostic utility of cardiac CT in patients with CHD.

Patient Preparation

Imaging Environment

Most patients with CHD will be sent for cardiac CT with a known cardiac diagnosis, based on prior imaging and/or cardiac interventions. As a result, the CT is generally requested in order to address a specific clinical question to help guide medical or interventional management. In order to provide useful diagnostic information, each exam must be tailored for both a specific diagnosis and specific clinical question. This requires an in-depth knowledge of the patient's history, prior intervention(s), and common hemodynamic sequela of the patient's form of CHD. The acquisition protocol, technical parameters, and scan range will vary depending on the patient characteristics and clinical indication. For instance, a 2-year-old patient with a presumed vascular ring might be optimally scanned using a non-gated protocol with minimal or no sedation and aggressive dose reduction techniques, while a patient requiring optimal imaging of the coronary arteries will require a breath hold, slow heart rate, and the highest temporal and spatial resolution possible on the scanner platform. The imager should review the patient history and relevant clinical issues well before the patient arrives for the scan. He or she should be actively involved in guiding institutional imaging practices, patient preparation, image acquisition, and interpretation for each CT scan performed on patients with CHD. Ideally, the imager should be physically present during scan acquisition. Proficiency in cardiac CT for patients with CHD requires an expertise in both congenital cardiology and cardiac imaging; and the optimal imaging environment includes strong collaboration between radiologists, cardiologists, and cardiac surgeons.

Sedation Requirements

In patients with congenital heart disease, the risk of sedation must be weighed against the diagnostic information necessary. Depending on the available scanner platform and

A. M. Hlavacek (✉)
Department of Pediatrics, Division of Pediatric Cardiology, Medical University of South Carolina, Charleston, SC, USA
e-mail: hlavace@musc.edu

U. J. Schoepf (ed.), *CT of the Heart*, Contemporary Medical Imaging, https://doi.org/10.1007/978-1-60327-237-7_44

clinical indication, many patients can be scanned without sedation. Centers with newer-generation scanners utilizing ultrahigh pitch or volumetric scan modes can often achieve scan times of less than a second. With these techniques, it is usually possible to adequately visualize anatomy without sedation or a breath hold [5, 6]. Patients requiring detailed evaluation of the coronary arteries or evaluation of function will generally need to be able to cooperate with breathing instructions, however. The imager must take into account local resources, clinical indications, and patient age when determining the need for sedation.

Scans that do not require detailed coronary imaging or functional analysis are less susceptible to motion artifact. For these scans, infants <6 months of age can generally be swaddled and imaged without sedation (Fig. 44.1). The use of a pacifier and an oral dextrose solution can be helpful to keep the infant calm. Patients between 6 months and 3 years of age often require sedation to lie still in the scanner but can usually be imaged free breathing. Most children $\geq$3 years of age can cooperate with holding still in the scanner without sedation, unless they are developmentally delayed. The presence of a parent in the room or child life services may be helpful. Increasing experience with scanners utilizing volumetric acquisition or ultrahigh pitch scanning modes should result in a decrease in the need for sedation in children of all ages, due to the short acquisition time.

Scans that require coronary artery or functional analysis are more susceptible to motion artifact. Neonates that only require identification of the coronary artery origins prior to surgical repair can often be adequately imaged without sedation [6, 7]. However, when detailed coronary artery imaging (including detailed ostial anatomy) is indicated in a patient under 5–6 years of age, general anesthesia is frequently necessary to cooperate with breath holding (Table 44.1). Older children can often cooperate, particularly if breath holding is practiced with the patient prior to the scan. Practicing breath holds is also helpful to assess any respiratory variations in the heart rate, which is common in pediatric patients.

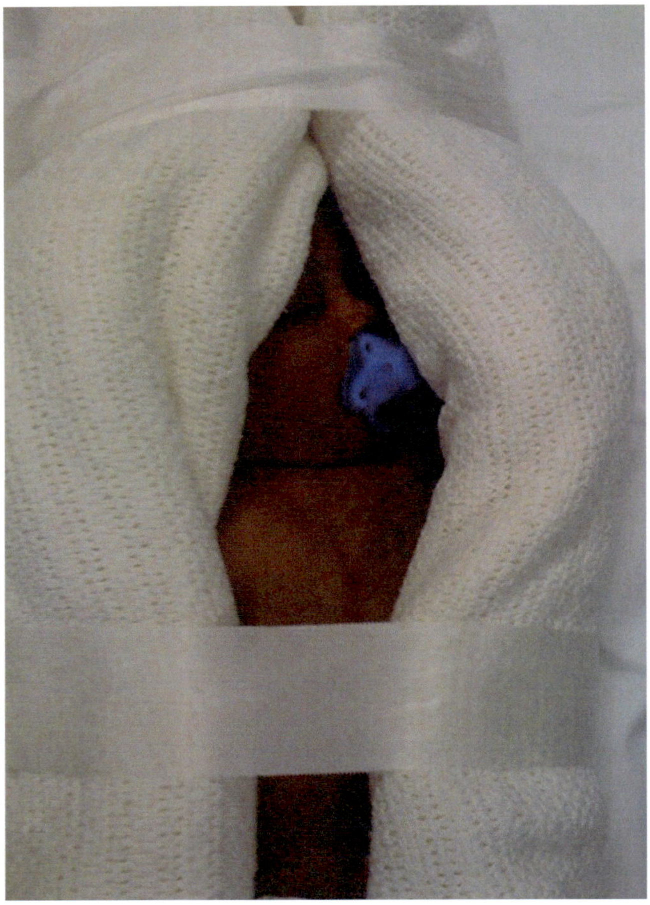

Fig. 44.1 This is an example of a method using blankets, tape, and a pacifier to swaddle and scan a 4-month-old infant without sedation

Intravenous Access

Peripheral IV access is most commonly utilized for contrast injection with congenital cardiac CT. Many central lines can be used as well, provided that manufacturer's recommended injection guidelines are utilized. Umbilical catheters should generally be avoided, however, given the frequently suboptimal and unpredictable contrast intensity caused by reflux of contrast into the liver (Fig. 44.2). Special precautions should be taken to avoid air bubbles in patients with CHD, since intracardiac shunting in patients with complex congenital heart disease can result in a systemic arterial embolus. In general, the largest gauge IV cannula feasible for the patient body size should be utilized.

The ideal location for contrast injection varies by cardiac defect and should be determined in advance. While the right antecubital vein is commonly utilized, an alternative location might be beneficial in certain diagnoses. Injections via the right upper extremity are generally preferred over the left arm, in order to avoid streak artifact in the arch vessels caused by residual high-density contrast in the left

Table 44.1 Sedation and anesthesia for cardiac scans in children

Sedation need	Detailed coronary/intracardiac anatomy or function indicated	Other indications
No sedation[a]	$\geq$ 5–6 years	<6 months or $\geq$ 3 yr
Sedation, free breathing	n/a	6 months – 3 years[b]
General anesthesia	$\leq$ 5–6 years	n/a

[a]Assuming normal developmental status
[b]Consider scanning without sedation if ultrahigh pitch or volumetric scan modes are available

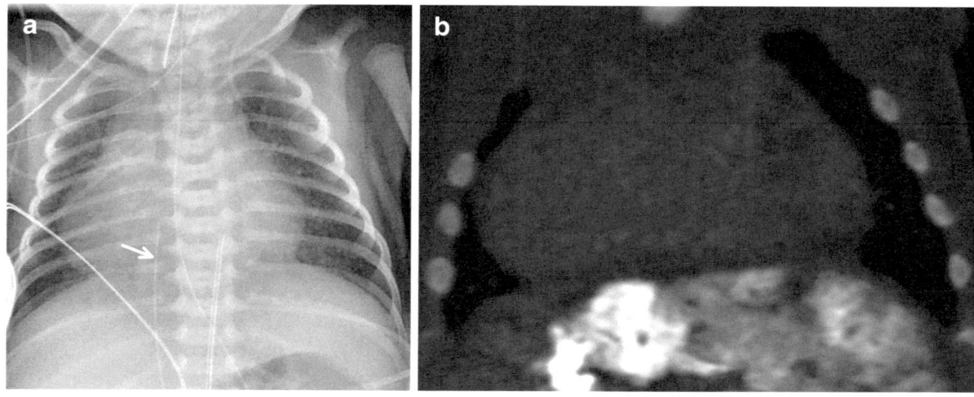

Fig. 44.2 Image (**a**) is a chest radiograph, in which an umbilical venous catheter (arrow) appears well placed within the atrium. Image (**b**) is a coronal reconstruction of a CT performed 3 h later. Contrast was injected via the catheter, but significant reflux of contrast into the liver resulted in a nondiagnostic study

brachiocephalic vein. Conversely, the left upper extremity would be preferable in a patient with situs inversus and might also be considered in someone with a persistent left superior vena cava (SVC). Injection via a lower extremity vein is often advantageous in neonates and infants, to avoid residual high-density contrast in the SVC, particularly when an abnormality in the vicinity of the SVC is suspected (right pulmonary artery/veins, right coronary, ascending aorta) [8]. Consideration of IV location can also be beneficial in patients with systemic venous abnormalities or occlusions, in order to optimize opacification of the structure of interest. For instance, injection via a lower extremity could definitively exclude a congenital interruption of the inferior vena cava, rather than relying on venous recirculation. On the other hand, the presence of an occlusive thrombus in the inferior vena cava might be better visualized with an upper extremity injection and acquisition during venous recirculation, due to the likelihood of incomplete mixing and beam-hardening artifact in the IVC resulting from a lower extremity injection.

Beta Blockade

It is well established that heart rate control improves image quality in the evaluation of coronary arteries and valve structures [9, 10]. The higher temporal resolution afforded by newer-generation scanners allows diagnostic images at higher rates, but the quality remains linked to heart rate [11]. Beta blockade can be safely used in most pediatric and adult patients [10, 12], although caution should be utilized in patients with potentially unstable hemodynamics. When newer-generation scanners are utilized, the coronary origins can usually be identified in infants without beta blockade [13]. Heart rate control should be considered in CHD patients when detailed coronary or valve imaging is needed but is unnecessary when extracardiac structures are the primary area of interest.

Acquisition Techniques

Injection Protocol

Adequate opacification of cardiac structures can be attained via manual or power injection, although the latter has been shown to provide superior image quality [14]. Although extravasation is a concern, power injection has been safely utilized in IV sizes as small as 24 gauge [15]. When attempting power injection via a small IV, however, a pressure-limited protocol and saline test injection are recommended. When injecting via a central line, manufacturer guidelines regarding flow rate and maximum pressure should be reviewed prior to use. When in doubt, hand injection should be considered.

A contrast volume of 1.5–2 ml/kg is generally used in pediatric patients, up to standard adult contrast volumes. When utilizing aggressive dose reduction strategies, particularly in small children and infants, contrast dilution with saline (2:1 contrast/saline ratio) can minimize beam-hardening artifacts. Contrast dilution also allows lengthening of the injection time, which creates a higher likelihood of optimal contrast enhancement of both venous and arterial structures in patients with complex anatomy or variable contrast transit times. Numerous injection protocols have been identified for patients with CHD. The most often utilized protocols are as follows:

- Dual-phase injection—with this protocol, contrast is injected at a consistent rate, followed by a saline flush. Due to its simplicity, it is the most frequently utilized protocol. It is ideal for patients with straightforward anatomy and a specific clinical question. Image acquisition is timed to the vessel of interest. For example, this protocol would be beneficial in a patient with an isolated coarctation of the aorta, in which only the aortic arch anatomy is required. In younger patients, utilizing a slow injection rate with this protocol often allows adequate opacification of most cardiovascular anatomy regardless of clinical indication.

- Triphasic injection—also known as a "biventricular protocol," this method consists of a two-phase contrast injection followed by a saline flush, ensuring simultaneous opacification of right and left heart structures. The two-phase contrast injection can be achieved by giving the second phase with diluted contrast or via a slower rate (e.g., 100% contrast followed by 30:70% contrast/saline ratio at constant rate vs. 100% contrast at 4 cc/sec followed by 2 cc/sec). The acquisition is timed for opacification of the aorta. This method is most useful in adult patients with repaired CHD, in whom evaluation of both coronary and right-sided cardiac structures is indicated.
- Venous two-phase injection protocol—with this method, a portion of the contrast is given (30–50%), followed by a 30–60 s pause and then injection of the remainder of the contrast via the dual-phase protocol above. This typically results in simultaneous opacification of systemic arterial and venous anatomy in a single acquisition, regardless of IV location. This method is useful in the initial evaluation of infants with heterotaxy syndromes, in whom complex arterial and venous connections are common.

Scan Triggering

The complex physiology that is present in patients with CHD often makes timing of the scan acquisition difficult. In adult CHD patients with significant ventricular dysfunction, valve regurgitation, or history of venous occlusion, a pre-scan timing bolus can be utilized to optimize the acquisition time. In most patients with congenital heart disease, however, automated bolus tracking is usually sufficient. Using this method, a region of interest (ROI) is selected, which will automatically initiate the scan upon reaching a pre-defined Hounsfield unit level within the relevant cardiac structure. The monitoring sequence should be set to initiate at least 2–3 s before completion of the contrast bolus. In patients with more complex anatomy, however, it can be challenging to identify the relevant cardiac structure on the pre-monitoring slice. In those patients, the ROI can be placed outside of the body. Instead of automatic triggering, the scan is manually initiated upon visualization of opacification during the monitoring sequence. This method, however, requires practice and a strong understanding of cardiac physiology. Each of the methods above requires a monitoring sequence to time scan acquisition, which increases the radiation exposure. For this reason, some advocate image acquisition at a fixed time from injection. This method can be useful in infants and small children, in whom a combination of higher heart rate and small IV size results in diffuse opacification of cardiovascular structures throughout the chest by the time the contrast bolus is complete. With this method, the contrast bolus should be lengthened to at least 10–15 s. The scan should then be timed to initiate once the contrast bolus is complete. The potential inability to detect IV malfunction prior to scan acquisition is a limitation to this method, however. Regardless of the triggering method, the imager should factor in the time required for scan initiation and acquisition time. This is particularly important in infants and small children, who have very fast circulation times. With these patients, it is frequently necessary to initiate the scan within a few seconds of completion of the contrast injection. If the acquisition time of the scanner mode is longer than average (>3–4 s), the injection time should be lengthened and consideration should be given to initiation of the scan before completion of the contrast bolus.

Sequence Selection

The discussion of scan selection below assumes a detailed understanding of available sequences, which is well described in the literature [16]. The first issue to consider when selecting a scan protocol for patients with congenital heart disease is whether ECG gating should be utilized. Functional assessment always requires cardiac gating. ECG gating is generally necessary to optimally evaluate structures that are prone to cardiac motion artifact (intracardiac anatomy, coronary arteries, and the aortic root), although newer ultrahigh pitch sequences are often able to accurately image these structures without cardiac gating [6, 17]. Most other patients can be scanned with a non-gated sequence, although image quality is often inferior to those obtained with ECG-gated sequences [18]. In addition to clinical indication, patient age and cooperation level should be considered. Aside from prospectively triggered high-pitch sequences, ECG-gated sequences are generally more prone to patient movement artifact. Therefore, one might choose a non-gated sequence to image poorly cooperative patients, rather than using sedation to perform an ECG-gated scan.

After deciding to use an ECG-gated sequence, one must choose whether to use a retrospectively gated helical sequence, prospectively triggered axial sequence, or a prospectively triggered ultrahigh pitch helical sequence. Retrospectively gated sequences are the most robust in patients with elevated heart rates or arrhythmias but also result in the highest radiation exposure [19]. Therefore, when other sequences are available, its use should be limited to those with significant arrhythmias or elevated heart rates. Radiation exposure is significantly decreased when a prospectively triggered axial sequence is utilized. This scan mode was initially limited to patients with a heart rate below 70, but it has been shown to generate diagnostic coronary imaging in children with heart rates as high as 140 using dual-source technology [20, 21]. More recently, prospectively gated volumetric scanning using a 320-slice scanner was shown to generate diagnostic coronary images in a group of patients ≤3 years of age (mean HR 111 ± 19), although diagnostic quality was compromised in patients ≤12.5 months or 5.6 kg [22]. Prospectively triggered ultrahigh pitch sequences offer the potential for further reduction in radiation dose but require a heart rate < 60–70 in order to consistently provide a detailed coronary evaluation [11, 23].

Lesion-Specific Recommendations

The general recommendations above should assist cardiac imaging specialists in obtaining highly diagnostic images on the majority of patients with CHD. Detailed, lesion-specific recommendations for all congenital heart defects are beyond the scope of this chapter but are available in a recent expert consensus document published by the Society of Cardiovascular CT [4]. Specific technical recommendations for selected lesions are listed below.

Thoracic Arterial Abnormalities

Straightforward pulmonary or aortic abnormalities should be scanned with the contrast bolus timed to the area of interest, using an injection lasting approximately 12–15 s. If abnormalities of both pulmonary and aortic anatomy are suspected, extending the contrast bolus to ~20 s, with the scan timed to the aorta, should allow simultaneous opacification of both circulations. One drawback of a lengthened contrast injection is that dense contrast entering the right atrium and ventricle at the time of image acquisition can obscure visualization of the right coronary artery, however. An alternative option in this scenario is to use the triphasic injection protocol described above.

Pulmonary Venous Anomalies

Optimal opacification of pulmonary venous anomalies is obtained by timing image acquisition to either the left atrium or ascending aorta. If the pulmonary venous return is obstructed, opacification may occur later than expected. In this scenario, a longer contrast injection with later image acquisition may be necessary. The scan range should be adjusted to include the suspected area of pulmonary venous return, which will often require including the majority of the thoracic cavity. If infradiaphragmatic TAPVR is suspected, the scan range should include the upper abdomen.

Systemic Venous Abnormalities

Venous imaging can be performed with a venous two-phase contrast bolus (described above), a longer contrast injection with late image acquisition, or with a delayed scan (venous phase). The timing of venous recirculation is dependent on the size of the patient, cardiac output, and intracardiac shunting. When needed, a delayed scan in the venous phase can be performed 30–60 s after the initial scan. If a patient has poor cardiac output, adequate venous opacification may take 120 s or longer. Superior central venous anatomy will be visualized earlier than the inferior vena cava. A higher contrast load (2.5–3 cc/kg) may be beneficial for optimal venous imaging, particularly in those requiring visualization of the inferior vena cava. These methods can also be helpful to evaluate the systemic venous baffles in patients who have undergone a Mustard or Senning procedure for transposition.

Cyanotic Heart Lesions

Before imaging patients with cyanotic congenital heart disease, one must consider the physiology present in the suspected lesion. Many patients with unrepaired cyanotic heart disease have right to left shunting within the heart, limiting pulmonary blood flow. In these patients, contrast injected into the heart will quickly enter the aortic circulation, with limited opacification of the pulmonary circulation. This physiology, for example, will be present in a patient with tetralogy of Fallot with significant pulmonary outflow obstruction (prior to repair). Patients with transposition physiology, on the other hand, usually have normal (or elevated) pulmonary blood flow. Rather, the presence of cyanosis in these patients is a result of poor mixing between the systemic and pulmonary circulations, which exist in parallel. In either scenario, the aorta will often opacify before the pulmonary arteries; and opacification of the pulmonary circulation will usually be proportional to the patient's oxygen saturation level. The contrast bolus should be lengthened in order to allow time for sufficient contrast to enter the pulmonary arteries. Timing of pulmonary arterial opacification will also depend on the source of pulmonary blood supply. In neonates/infants with pulmonary atresia or severe pulmonary stenosis, the pulmonary flow may originate from the ductus arteriosus or a systemic to pulmonary shunt (e.g., BT shunt), and contrast will reach the pulmonary arteries simultaneously with the aorta. In any patient with cyanotic heart disease, special precautions should be made to avoid air embolism during contrast injection.

Single Ventricle Physiology

Patients with single ventricle physiology generally follow a three-stage surgical palliation, which is described in Chap. 47. Many patients that follow this pathway require their first surgical intervention within the first 1–2 weeks of life. The first surgical procedure varies, dependent on the native anatomy, but often includes placement of a systemic to pulmonary shunt (e.g., Blalock-Taussig shunt). When imaging these patients before or after their first surgical procedure, one should note that the pulmonary arteries and aorta will opacify simultaneously.

The second procedure is called a Glenn (or Hemi-Fontan) procedure, and is generally performed at 4–6 months of age. With this, the superior vena caval flow is sent directly into the pulmonary arteries ("bilateral Glenn" if there are bilateral SVCs). In preparation for this procedure, CT is occasionally warranted to evaluate the upper systemic venous anatomy (right and/or left SVC) and pulmonary arteries. Therefore, the goal of CT imaging at this stage is simultaneous venous and arterial opacification. This is achieved by using a long injection (~15–18 s), with acquisition near the end of the injection. If there is high likelihood of upper central venous obstruction, consider injection in the foot to visualize the superior venous anatomy without streak artifact from dense contrast injection. Alternatively, one could perform a delayed image acquisition (venous phase) to ensure that the systemic veins are all opacified.

After the Glenn procedure, an injection in the upper extremity will directly opacify the pulmonary arteries through the anastomosis between the superior vena cava and pulmonary artery. Incomplete mixing of contrast, aortopulmonary collateral flow, and bilateral superior vena cavae will result in differential branch pulmonary artery opacification. This can result in a false-positive finding of pulmonary embolus (Fig. 44.3). Some patients develop collateral vessels from the upper systemic venous system to the pulmonary veins or lower systemic venous system. These are called "veno-venous collaterals," and their opacification is dependent on IV location. If the goal of the study is to evaluate the Glenn anastomosis or pulmonary arteries, injection in the lower extremity with bolus tracking in the superior vena cava is recommended, allowing opacification of the upper systemic veins via venous recirculation [24]. If the injection is lengthened, this method will simultaneously opacify the systemic arterial system and upper venous system (Fig. 44.4). If the injection is performed via an upper extremity, then a scan in the venous phase would be required to ensure homogeneous opacification of the pulmonary arteries, particularly in the presence of bilateral superior vena cavae.

The third surgical stage is called a Fontan procedure, which involves connection of the inferior vena caval flow into the pulmonary arteries. If the primary clinical question involves the aortic arch, intracardiac anatomy, or ventricular function,

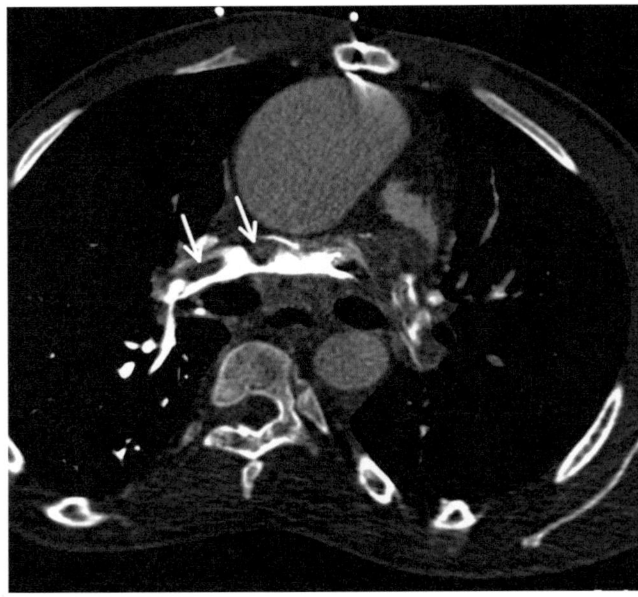

Fig. 44.3 Axial image from a cardiac CT performed on a patient with a history of a bilateral Glenn procedure. This is an example of how incomplete mixing of contrast within the pulmonary arteries in these patients can be mistaken for thrombus (arrows)

one can bolus track on the aorta using the appropriate acquisition protocol. Evaluation of the Fontan circuit is complex due to incomplete mixing within the circuit, differential streaming of into the pulmonary arteries, and variable timing of opacification of the superior and inferior venous system. These factors can result in nondiagnostic or false-positive evaluations for thrombus formation [25], which is common in this population. Numerous approaches have been recommended to address this issue. Regardless of strategy, one should consider using a larger amount of contrast (2.5–3 ml/kg, up to 150 mL). Traditionally, simultaneous injection in lower and upper extremity veins has been recommended in this patient group [26]. In order to get an adequate flow rate, this method usually requires placement of a femoral venous catheter. While this usually results in opacification of the entire Fontan circuit, most patients will still have incomplete mixing of contrast due to swirling and unopacified hepatic venous inflow. This is particularly a problem in patients with bilateral superior vena cavae. Some authors advocate a single acquisition in the venous phase, using a delay of 120–180 s after initiation of contrast injection [27]. This will result in homogenous opacification, allowing for identification of clots. However, the image quality will be inadequate for coronary imaging. A venous two-phase contrast protocol (as described in previous sections but using 50% of the contrast in the first phase) will allow opacification of the entire Fontan circuit while providing diagnostic imaging of the aorta and coronary arteries. However, since the opacification will not be homogeneous, a second scan in the venous phase will be necessary to more

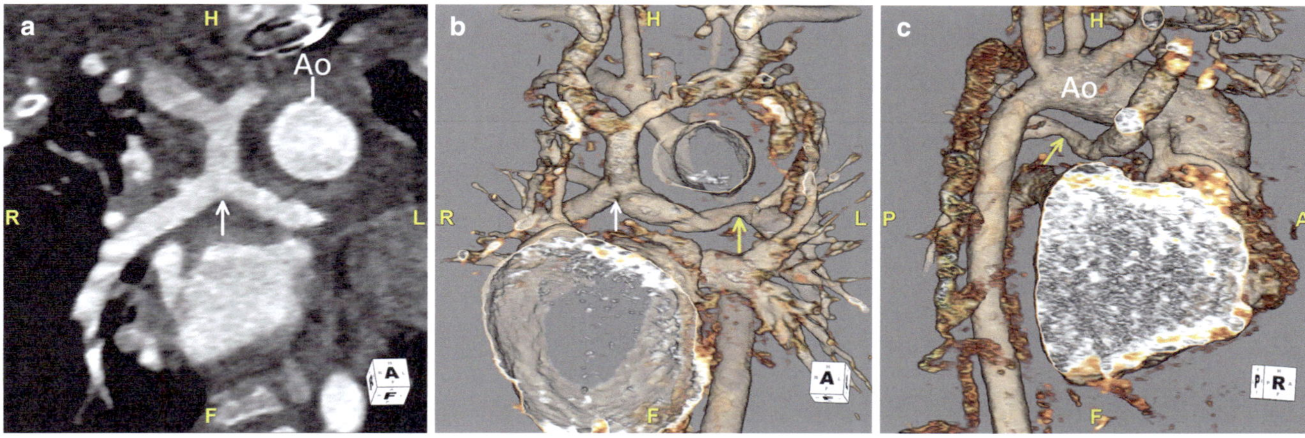

Fig. 44.4 In this patient with a history of Norwood and Glenn procedures for hypoplastic left heart syndrome, contrast was injected slowly via the foot, allowing opacification of the upper systemic veins and pulmonary arteries via venous recirculation, along with arterial opacification of the aorta in one acquisition (**a**) oblique coronal reconstruction; 3D volume-rendered images viewed from anterior (**b**) and rightward (**c**) perspectives). The connection between the superior vena cava and pulmonary arteries can be seen (white arrow), along with stenosis of the left pulmonary artery (yellow arrow). The reconstructed aorta can be visualized in detail as well (Ao)

definitively evaluate for a thrombus in the Fontan circuit. If an evaluation of function is needed, a multiphase acquisition will allow visualization of contrast streaming and can differentiate thrombus versus venous admixture better than a single cardiac phase acquisition. Dual-energy scanning has also been shown to be useful in this population when screening for thrombus formation [28].

Interpretation and Reporting

Given the complexity within the spectrum of native and repaired CHD, a collaborative approach between radiology and pediatric/adult congenital cardiology is recommended for interpretation of these studies. The use of multiplanar and 3D reconstruction software is also recommended when interpreting CT studies on patients with CHD, particularly when attempting to describe extracardiac abnormalities [29–31]. Furthermore, 3D reconstructions are often beneficial in communicating CT findings to cardiologists and surgeons that are less accustomed to visualizing axial CT images.

A segmental approach to interpretation and reporting has long been recognized as a fundamental concept in cardiac imaging for CHD [32–34]. A detailed description of segmental analysis can be found in Chap. 26 ("CT Spectrum of Congenital Heart Disease"). Briefly, the segmental approach involves a sequential evaluation of the three segments of the heart (atria, ventricles, and great arteries) and their connections (atrioventricular and ventriculo-arterial connections). This analysis should be utilized and applied in creating a structured report for each cardiac CT performed in patients with CHD. A recommended report template for cardiac findings with CHD is as follows:

- *Cardiac position*: [The heart is positioned leftward/midline/rightward, with apex pointing to the left, right, inferiorly.]
- *Segments*: [Atrial situs, ventricular looping, great arterial orientation, atrioventricular, and ventriculo-arterial connections.]
- *Systemic veins*: [Right superior vena cava, presence/absence of left superior vena cava. If left SVC, connections/bridging vein. Inferior vena cava is intact/interrupted.]
- *Pulmonary veins*: [Normal/abnormal pulmonary venous connection with _#_ pulmonary veins seen entering the left atrium. Anomalous pulmonary venous connections, if present.]
- *Atria*: [Size of right/left atrium. Interatrial septum is intact vs. atrial septal defect.]
- *AV valves*: [Appearance of tricuspid and mitral valves +/− motion.]
- *Ventricles*: [Size of right/left ventricle. Septum is intact vs. ventricular septal defect.]
- *Ventricular outflows*: [Description of subaortic and subpulmonic outflows.]
- *Semilunar valves*: [Appearance of pulmonary and aortic valves. +/− motion.]
- *Pulmonary arteries*: [Description main and branch pulmonary arteries/stenosis/embolus.]
- *Aorta*: [Aortic root and ascending aorta. Left/right arch with (normal/abnormal) branching pattern. Evidence of coarctation.]
- *Coronary arteries*: [Coronary origins and branching pattern, stenosis, filling defects.]
- *Ductus arteriosus*: [Patent/not patent, appearance.]
- *Collateral arteries*: [Aortopulmonary collaterals, venovenous collaterals.]
- *Pericardium*: [Normal, thickened, calcified, effusion.]

References

1. Han BK, Lesser AM, Vezmar M, Rosenthal K, Rutten-Ramos S, Lindberg J, Caye D, Lesser JR. Cardiovascular imaging trends in congenital heart disease: a single center experience. J Cardiovasc Comput Tomogr. 2013;7(6):361–6.
2. Cohen MS, Eidem BW, Cetta F, Fogel MA, Frommelt PC, Ganame J, Han BK, Kimball TR, Johnson RK, Mertens L, Paridon SM, Powell AJ, Lopez L. Multimodality imaging guidelines of patients with transposition of the great arteries: a report from the American Society of Echocardiography developed in collaboration with the Society for Cardiovascular Magnetic Resonance and the Society of Cardiovascular Computed Tomography. J Am Soc Echocardiogr. 2016;29(7):571–621.
3. Han BK, Rigsby CK, Hlavacek A, Leipsic J, Nicol ED, Siegel MJ, Bardo D, Abbara S, Ghoshhajra B, Lesser JR, Raman S, Crean AM. Computed tomography imaging in patients with congenital heart disease part I: rationale and utility. An expert consensus document of the Society of Cardiovascular Computed Tomography (SCCT): endorsed by the Society of Pediatric Radiology (SPR) and the North American Society of Cardiac Imaging (NASCI). J Cardiovasc Comput Tomogr. 2015;9(6):475–92.
4. Han BK, Rigsby CK, Leipsic J, Bardo D, Abbara S, Ghoshhajra B, Lesser JR, Raman SV, Crean AM, Nicol ED, Siegel MJ, Hlavacek A. Computed tomography imaging in patients with congenital heart disease, part 2: technical recommendations. An expert consensus document of the Society of Cardiovascular Computed Tomography (SCCT): endorsed by the Society of Pediatric Radiology (SPR) and the North American Society of Cardiac Imaging (NASCI). J Cardiovasc Comput Tomogr. 2015;9(6):493–513.
5. Han BK, Overman DM, Grant K, Rosenthal K, Rutten-Ramos S, Cook D, Lesser JR. Non-sedated, free breathing cardiac CT for evaluation of complex congenital heart disease in neonates. J Cardiovasc Comput Tomogr. 2013;7(6):354–60.
6. Bridoux A, Hutt A, Faivre JB, Flohr T, Duhamel A, Pagniez J, Remy J, Remy-Jardin M. Coronary artery visibility in free-breathing young children on non-gated chest CT: impact of temporal resolution. Pediatr Radiol. 2015;45(12):1761–70.
7. Vastel-Amzallag C, Le Bret E, Paul JF, Lambert V, Rohnean A, El Fassy E, Sigal-Cinqualbre A. Diagnostic accuracy of dual-source multislice computed tomographic analysis for the preoperative detection of coronary artery anomalies in 100 patients with tetralogy of Fallot. J Thorac Cardiovasc Surg. 2011;142(1):120–6.
8. Yang M, Mo XM, Jin JY, Zhang J, Liu B, Wu M, Teng GJ. Image quality and radiation exposure in pediatric cardiovascular CT angiography from different injection sites. AJR Am J Roentgenol. 2011;196(2):W117–22.
9. Dewey M, Vavere AL, Arbab-Zadeh A, Miller JM, Sara L, Cox C, Gottlieb I, Yoshioka K, Paul N, Hoe J, de Roos A, Lardo AC, Lima JA, Clouse ME. Patient characteristics as predictors of image quality and diagnostic accuracy of MDCT compared with conventional coronary angiography for detecting coronary artery stenoses: CORE-64 Multicenter International Trial. AJR Am J Roentgenol. 2010;194(1):93–102.
10. Mahabadi AA, Achenbach S, Burgstahler C, Dill T, Fischbach R, Knez A, Moshage W, Richartz BM, Ropers D, Schroder S, Silber S, Mohlenkamp S. Safety, efficacy, and indications of beta-adrenergic receptor blockade to reduce heart rate prior to coronary CT angiography. Radiology. 2010;257(3):614–23.
11. Gordic S, Husarik DB, Desbiolles L, Leschka S, Frauenfelder T, Alkadhi H. High-pitch coronary CT angiography with third generation dual-source CT: limits of heart rate. Int J Cardiovasc Imaging. 2014;30(6):1173–9.
12. Han BK, Lindberg J, Overman D, Schwartz RS, Grant K, Lesser JR. Safety and accuracy of dual-source coronary computed tomography angiography in the pediatric population. J Cardiovasc Comput Tomogr. 2012;6(4):252–9.
13. Cui Y, Huang M, Zheng J, Li J, Liu H, Liang C. Assessments of coronary artery visibility and radiation dose in infants with congenital heart disease on cardiac 128-slice CT and on cardiac 64-slice CT. Pediatr Cardiol. 2016;37(1):135–43.
14. Saake M, Lell MM, Rompel O, Gloeckler M, May M, Eller A, Achenbach S, Uder M, Wuest W. Contrast medium application in pediatric high-pitch cardiovascular CT angiography: manual or power injection? J Cardiovasc Comput Tomogr. 2014;8(4):315–22.
15. Amaral JG, Traubici J, BenDavid G, Reintamm G, Daneman A. Safety of power injector use in children as measured by incidence of extravasation. AJR Am J Roentgenol. 2006;187(2):580–3.
16. Halliburton S, Arbab-Zadeh A, Dey D, Einstein AJ, Gentry R, George RT, Gerber T, Mahesh M, Weigold WG. State-of-the-art in CT hardware and scan modes for cardiovascular CT. J Cardiovasc Comput Tomogr. 2012;6(3):154–63.
17. Beeres M, Schell B, Mastragelopoulos A, Herrmann E, Kerl JM, Gruber-Rouh T, Lee C, Siebenhandl P, Bodelle B, Zangos S, Vogl TJ, Jacobi V, Bauer RW. High-pitch dual-source CT angiography of the whole aorta without ECG synchronisation: initial experience. Eur Radiol. 2012;22(1):129–37.
18. Shuman WP, Leipsic JA, Busey JM, Green DE, Pipavath SN, Hague CJ, Koprowicz KM. Prospectively ECG gated CT pulmonary angiography versus helical ungated CT pulmonary angiography: impact on cardiac related motion artifacts and patient radiation dose. Eur J Radiol. 2012;81(9):2444–9.
19. Jin KN, Park EA, Shin CI, Lee W, Chung JW, Park JH. Retrospective versus prospective ECG-gated dual-source CT in pediatric patients with congenital heart diseases: comparison of image quality and radiation dose. Int J Cardiovasc Imaging. 2010;26(Suppl 1):63–73.
20. Duan Y, Wang X, Cheng Z, Wu D, Wu L. Application of prospective ECG-triggered dual-source CT coronary angiography for infants and children with coronary artery aneurysms due to Kawasaki disease. Br J Radiol. 2012;85(1020):e1190–7.
21. Paul JF, Rohnean A, Elfassy E, Sigal-Cinqualbre A. Radiation dose for thoracic and coronary step-and-shoot CT using a 128-slice dual-source machine in infants and small children with congenital heart disease. Pediatr Radiol. 2011;41(2):244–9.
22. Tada A, Sato S, Kanie Y, Tanaka T, Inai R, Akagi N, Morimitsu Y, Kanazawa S. Image quality of coronary computed tomography angiography with 320-row area detector computed tomography in children with congenital heart disease. Pediatr Cardiol. 2016;37(3):497–503.
23. Alkadhi H, Stolzmann P, Desbiolles L, Baumueller S, Goetti R, Plass A, Scheffel H, Feuchtner G, Falk V, Marincek B, Leschka S. Low-dose, 128-slice, dual-source CT coronary angiography: accuracy and radiation dose of the high-pitch and the step-and-shoot mode. Heart. 2010;96(12):933–8.
24. Ghadimi Mahani M, Agarwal PP, Rigsby CK, Lu JC, Fazeli Dehkordy S, Wright RA, Dorfman AL, Krishnamurthy R. CT for assessment of thrombosis and pulmonary embolism in multiple stages of single-ventricle palliation: challenges and suggested protocols. Radiographics. 2016;36(5):1273–84.
25. Prabhu SP, Mahmood S, Sena L, Lee EY. MDCT evaluation of pulmonary embolism in children and young adults following a lateral tunnel Fontan procedure: optimizing contrast-enhancement techniques. Pediatr Radiol. 2009;39(9):938–44.
26. Sandler KL, Markham LW, Mah ML, Byrum EP, Williams JR. Optimizing CT angiography in patients with Fontan physiology: single-center experience of dual-site power injection. Clin Radiol. 2014;69(12):e562–7.
27. Park EA, Lee W, Chung SY, Yin YH, Chung JW, Park JH. Optimal scan timing and intravenous route for contrast-enhanced computed tomography in patients after Fontan operation. J Comput Assist Tomogr. 2010;34(1):75–81.

28. Grewal J, Al Hussein M, Feldstein J, Kiess M, Ellis J, Human D, Leipsic J. Evaluation of silent thrombus after the Fontan operation. Congenit Heart Dis. 2013;8(1):40–7.
29. Di Sessa TG, Di Sessa P, Gregory B, Vranicar M. The use of 3D contrast-enhanced CT reconstructions to project images of vascular rings and coarctation of the aorta. Echocardiography. 2009;26(1):76–81.
30. Lee EY, Siegel MJ, Hildebolt CF, Gutierrez FR, Bhalla S, Fallah JH. MDCT evaluation of thoracic aortic anomalies in pediatric patients and young adults: comparison of axial, multiplanar, and 3D images. AJR Am J Roentgenol. 2004;182(3):777–84.
31. Lee EY, Tracy DA, Mahmood SA, Weldon CB, Zurakowski D, Boiselle PM. Preoperative MDCT evaluation of congenital lung anomalies in children: comparison of axial, multiplanar, and 3D images. AJR Am J Roentgenol. 2011;196(5):1040–6.
32. Brandt PW, Calder AL. Cardiac connections: the segmental approach to radiologic diagnosis in congenital heart disease. Curr Probl Diagn Radiol. 1977;7(3):1–35.
33. Lapierre C, Dery J, Guerin R, Viremouneix L, Dubois J, Garel L. Segmental approach to imaging of congenital heart disease. Radiographics. 2010;30(2):397–411.
34. Shinebourne EA, Macartney FJ, Anderson RH. Sequential chamber localization--logical approach to diagnosis in congenital heart disease. Br Heart J. 1976;38(4):327–40.

CT of Coronary Artery Anomalies

45

Long Jiang Zhang, Shahryar M. Chowdhury, and Guang Ming Lu

Coronary artery anomalies are defined as any coronary arterial pattern with a feature (e.g., origination, course, and termination) rarely encountered in the general population. Although coronary anomalies are rare, they are important to detect because they have been implicated in chest pain, syncope, myocardial infarctions, and even sudden death, especially in young adults [1–4]. Electrocardiogram-gated multi-detector row computed tomography (MDCT) of the heart allows the accurate and noninvasive depiction of congenital coronary anomalies in patients of all ages [5, 6]. MDCT has been shown to be superior to conventional coronary angiography in showing the origin and proximal path of anomalous coronary arteries [7]. This chapter briefly describes MDCT-reformatted techniques, normal coronary artery anatomy, MDCT coronary angiography findings in congenital coronary anomalies, and the clinical implications of these anomalies.

Special Considerations for Assessing Coronary Artery Anomalies

Important considerations should be taken when preparing and performing MDCT angiography for the assessment of coronary artery anomalies, which include the following: (1) Non-contrasted coronary artery calcium scans can suggest abnormal coronary origins in adults. However, delineating important details about the course, such as the presence of an intramural segment, is very difficult using non-contrasted scans alone. Thus, MDCT coronary angiography should be performed in these patients even if an abnormality is found on coronary artery calcium scoring scans. (2) CT scanning range should be properly adjusted to appropriately cover the potentially involved vascular structures. For example, in patients with the coronary to pulmonary artery fistula or other extracardiac termination, longer scanning range should be included. (3) Including systolic and diastolic cardiac phases into the acquisition, and the resultant reformatted CT images, can be very important to detect dynamic compression of abnormal coronary segments in coronaries that display myocardial bridging or abnormal origin of coronary artery from the opposite coronary sinus with an interarterial course. (4) Post-processing techniques such as multiplanar reformation (MPR) including curved planar reformation (CPR), maximal intensity projection (MIP), and volume rendering (VR) should be comprehensively used to show the anatomical relations between large vessels and heart chambers.

Normal Anatomic Features

Normally, myocardial blood flow is supplied by two main coronary arteries, the right coronary artery (RCA) and the left coronary artery (LCA) (Fig. 45.1) [8, 9].

Normal Coronary Artery Branches and Courses

The RCA originates from the right coronary sinus of Valsalva, descends in the anterior right atrioventricular groove, and usually gives off the conus branch (50–60%) as its first branch and then two or three large right ventricular wall branches. The acute marginal branch is the first large branch, which occasionally continues to the apex.

The LCA originates from the left coronary sinus of Valsalva, which bifurcates into the left circumflex (LCX) and left anterior descending (LAD) arteries or trifurcates with an additional intermediate ramus branch. The LAD usually descends in the anterior interventricular groove, giving off septal branches into the interventricular septum and diagonal branches descending toward the lateral margin of the left

L. J. Zhang (✉) · G. M. Lu
Department of Medical Imaging, Jinling Hospital, Medical School of Nanjing University, Nanjing, Jiangsu, China

S. M. Chowdhury
Division of Pediatric Cardiology, Department of Pediatrics, Medical University of South Carolina, Charleston, SC, USA

U. J. Schoepf (ed.), *CT of the Heart*, Contemporary Medical Imaging, https://doi.org/10.1007/978-1-60327-237-7_45

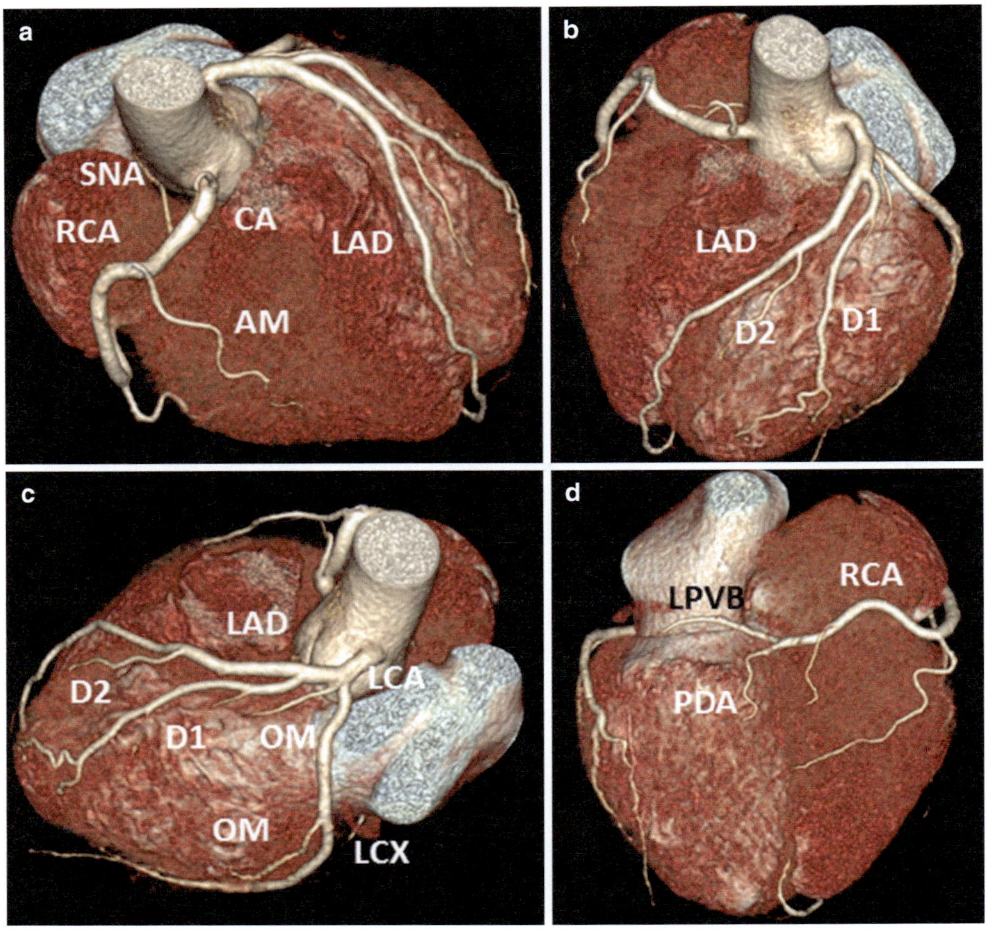

Fig. 45.1 Normal anatomy of the coronary arteries by MDCT coronary angiography. Volume-rendered CT angiogram with 3D reconstruction highlighting normal coronary anatomy. (**a**) Normal course of the RCA in the right interventricular groove shows an early CA branch. The second branch is the SNA. Afterwards AM branches supply the right ventricle. (**b**) The LAD runs in the interventricular sulcus with diagonal arteries supplying the lateral wall of the left ventricle. (**c**) The LCA splits into the LAD and LCX. The LCX runs in the left interventricular groove and gives off a number of OM branches. (**d**) In this right dominant system, the RCA gives rise to the PDA. The PDA appears somewhat small, likely associated with the LAD continuing around the apex of the heart to supply some of the inferior septum – also known as "wraparound" LAD, a normal variant. RCA = right coronary artery; CA = conus artery; AM = acute marginal artery; SNA = sinoatrial nodal artery; LCA = left coronary artery; LAD = left descending artery; D = diagonal; OM = obtuse marginal artery; LCX = left circumflex artery; PDA = posterior descending artery; LPVB = left ventricular posterior branch

ventricular wall. The LCX enters the left atrioventricular groove to supply obtuse marginal branches to the lateral and posterolateral walls of the left ventricle.

Coronary Dominance

In 70% of patients, the RCA gives off the posterior descending artery (PDA) and posterior left ventricular branches (right dominant supply). In the subjects with right coronary dominance, dysplasia or absence of the LCX can be often observed. In these cases, if the RCA supplies the typical LCX course, the RCA is referred to as "superdominant" (Fig. 45.1). In approximately 20% of patients, the PDA originates from the RCA, but branches from the LCX also supply this territory (codominant supply). In 10% of patients (left coronary dominant patients), the LCX supplies both the PDA and the posterior left ventricular branch [10]. In these patients, hypoplasia of the RCA is often found.

Sinoatrial Nodal Supply

Anatomic variations in the origin and course of the sinoatrial nodal artery (SNA) are important to recognize as it is occasionally misdiagnosed as a coronary artery fistula [11]. Sinoatrial nodal artery can be grouped into three types according to the origin, course, and termination [12]. (1) Right SNA (49.1%) originates from the RCA or right coronary sinus and courses between the right atrium and the root of aorta toward the ostium of the superior vena cava (SVC). (2) Left SNA (42.5%) originates from the proximal segment of the LCX and courses along the anterior wall of the left atrium, terminating at the ostium of the SVC. (3) Posterior SNA (8.4%) originates from the posterolateral segment of the LCX, LCA, or left ventricular posterior branch of the RCA. Entrance into the SVC can be classified as precaval (the SNA approaches the sinoatrial node anterior to the SVC), retrocaval (the SNA approaches the sinoatrial node posterior to the SVC), and pericaval (through multiple branches surrounding the SVC).

Classification, Prevalence, and Clinical Relevance of Coronary Anomalies

Coronary artery anomalies are found in 0.2–5.8% of individuals [2]. The majority of coronary artery anomalies are benign (anomalies that are usually not clinically significant). However, while having a low prevalence, malignant coronary artery anomalies can cause life-threatening sequelae such as cardiorespiratory arrest and sudden death. Various classification systems exist for coronary artery anomalies. No classification system is universally accepted. In this chapter, coronary anomalies are divided into the following three broad categories: anomalies of origin, anomalies of course, and anomalies of termination according to Kim et al.'s simplified classification of coronary artery anomalies (Table 45.1) [13–15]. Regardless of the classification system used, it is most important to delineate lesions that are benign versus those that are malignant especially when evaluating patients with concerning clinical symptoms such as angina, syncope, myocardial infarct, or sudden cardiac death [3, 14, 16].

Table 45.1 Classification of coronary artery anomalies

Anomalies of origin
High takeoff
Multiple ostia
Single coronary artery
Anomalous origin of coronary artery from the pulmonary artery[a]
Origin of coronary artery or branch from opposite or non-coronary sinus and an anomalous (retroaortic, interarterial[a], prepulmonic, septal [subpulmonic]) course
Anomalies of course
Myocardial bridging[a]
Duplication of arteries
Anomalies of termination
Coronary artery fistula[a]
Coronary arcade
Extracardiac termination

From Greenberg et al. [13], with permission
[a]Hemodynamically significant anomalies, which may contribute to myocardial perfusion abnormalities

Coronary Artery Anomalies of Origin

High Takeoff

High takeoff of a coronary artery is defined as origin of a coronary artery more than 1 cm above the sinotubular junction [10]. High takeoff of the RCA (Fig. 45.2a–c) is reported much more commonly than high takeoff of the LCA (Fig. 45.2d). This variant has no hemodynamic significance, but it may make selective invasive angiography more difficult [10, 15]. In addition, cardiac surgeons should be aware of this anomaly to avoid accidental cross-clamping or transection during surgery. In rare instances, high takeoff of a coronary artery may be associated with a malignant interarterial or intramural course – similar to those associated with origin of the coronary artery from the opposite sinus as described below (Fig. 45.2b–c).

Multiple Ostia

Multiple ostia have no significant clinical relevance. The LAD and LCX may arise separately with no LCA (Fig. 45.3a). This occurs in a small percentage (0.41%) of individuals, and invasive coronary angiography is technically difficult [14, 15, 17]. The RCA and the conus branch may arise separately from the right sinus (Fig. 45.3b). An aberrant conus artery arising separately from the RCA is particularly at risk for injury from ventriculostomy or other heart surgery.

Origin of Coronary Artery from the Posterior Sinus of Valsalva

An origin of the RCA or the LCA from the posterior sinus of Valsalva is rare. This anomaly has no clinical relevance (Fig. 45.4) unless accompanied by an interarterial or intramural course.

Single Coronary Artery

Single coronary artery is a rare congenital anomaly in which only one coronary artery arises from the aorta and supplies blood to the entire heart [18]. It is seen in only 0.002–0.04% of the population [2, 18, 19]. A single coronary artery may originate from either the right or left aortic sinus. In most cases, this single artery will give off two branches each with distributions of the typical RCA and LCA. Rarely, different distributions from that of the normal coronary artery tree may be observed, such as LCX from the RCA. In most cases this is a benign variant. However, patients with single

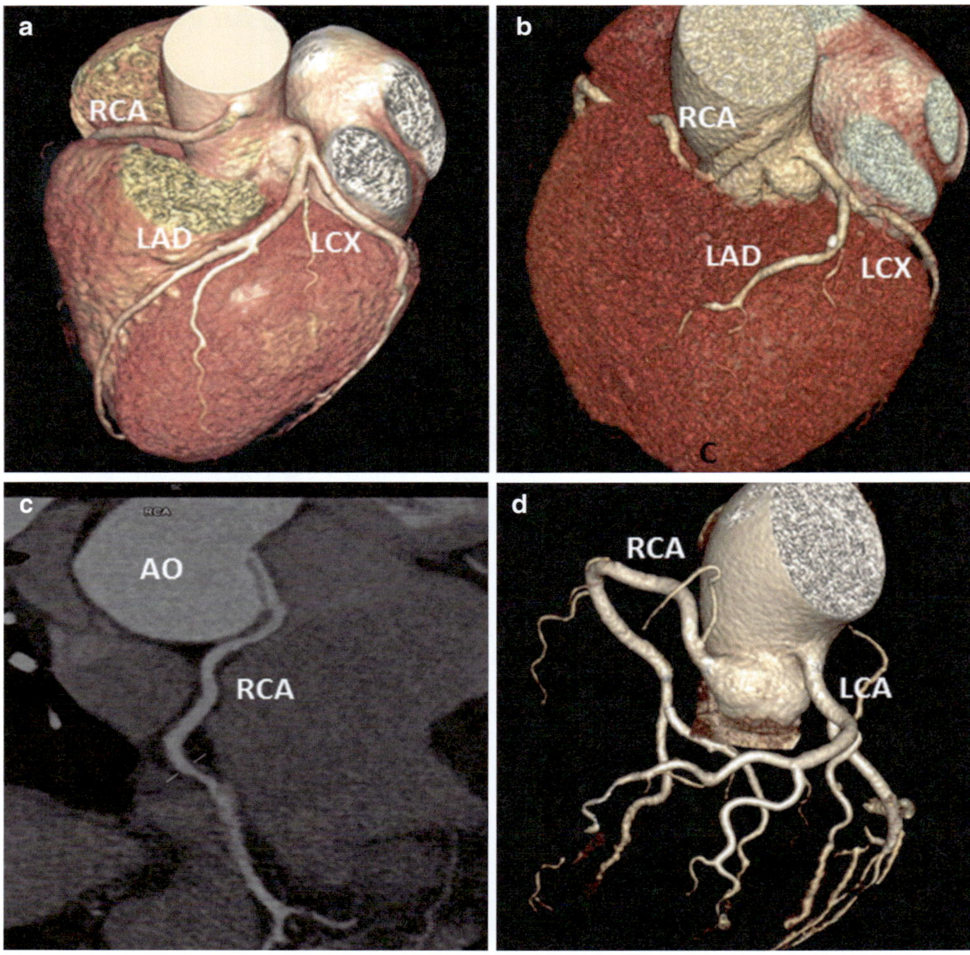

Fig. 45.2 High takeoff of the coronary arteries. (**a**) 3D volume reformatted CT angiogram showing the RCA arising from the ascending aorta above the sinotubular junction superior to the right sinus. (**b**) 3D volume reformatted CT angiogram showing the RCA arising from the ascending aorta above the sinotubular junction superior to the left sinus in close proximity to the left/right commissure. (**c**) Curved planar reformatted image showing the RCA arising from the ascending aorta coursing between the ascending aorta and pulmonary artery trunk, conferring increased risk for sudden cardiac death. Even if there is no interarterial course, these arteries may display an acute angle of takeoff and narrowed proximal course (such as in B) suggesting an intramural segment which is also a malignant finding. (**d**) A coronary artery tree image that shows the LCA arising from the ascending aorta above the sinotubular junction with a 90° angle from the aorta and widely patent proximal course – there is no evidence of an intermural course, and this is a benign finding. AO = aorta; LAD = left descending artery; LCA = left coronary artery; LCX = left circumflex artery; RCA = right coronary artery

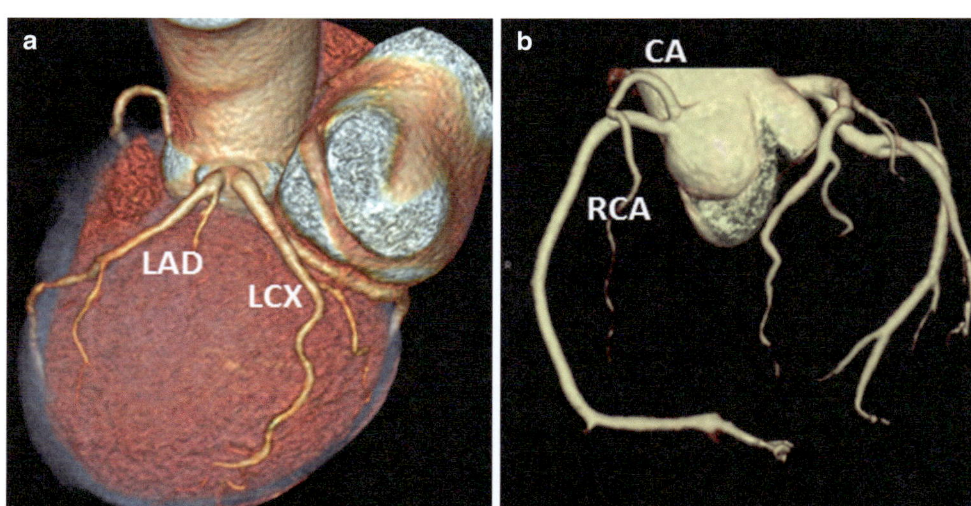

Fig. 45.3 Multiple ostia of the coronary arteries. (**a**) 3D volume reformatted CT angiogram shows the LAD and LCX originate separately from the left coronary sinus of Valsalva. (**b**) Coronary artery tree image shows the right coronary artery and conus artery separately originate from the right coronary sinus of Valsalva. CA = conus artery; LAD = left descending artery; RCA = right coronary artery; LCX = left circumflex artery

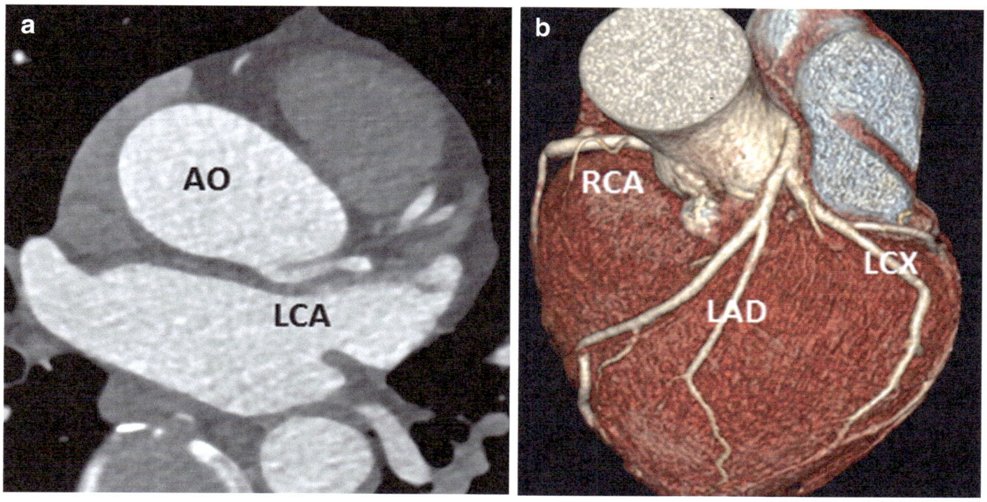

Fig. 45.4 Anomalous left coronary artery arising from posterior coronary sinus of Valsalva. (**a**) Axial contrast-enhanced CT angiography shows the left coronary artery arising from the non-coronary sinus of Valsalva. (**b**) 3D volume rendering reformatted CT image shows the left coronary artery arising from the non-coronary sinus of Valsalva with an otherwise unremarkable course. In the absence of an intramural or interarterial course, this is a benign lesion. AO = aorta; LAD = left descending artery; LCA = left coronary artery; LCX = left circumflex artery; RCA = right coronary artery

coronary artery are at increased risk for sudden death if a major coronary branch crosses between the pulmonary artery and the aorta.

Coronary Origin Stenosis and Atresia

Congenital coronary ostial atresia or hypoplasia is very rarely reported. It may be isolated or be associated with other congenital heart disease such as truncus arteriosus. Coronary ostial atresia or hypoplasia is usually associated with myocardial ischemia; the degree of severity is dependent upon the development of collaterals from the patent coronary system. The coronary ostium may also be occluded by a valve-like ridge [20]. This entity is often associated with congenital supra-aortic stenosis in patients with Williams syndrome and predisposes these patients to sudden cardiac death.

Origin of the Coronary Artery from the Opposite Sinus of Valsalva or Opposite Coronary Artery

Origin of the coronary artery from the contralateral sinus of Valsalva or contralateral coronary artery has multiple subtypes. Most commonly, the RCA may arise from the left coronary sinus of Valsalva or contralateral coronary artery in 0.03–0.17% of patients (Fig. 45.5) [3, 10, 15]. The LCA can arise from the right coronary sinus of Valsalva or opposite coronary artery (Fig. 45.6). In addition, the LCX or LAD may arise from the right coronary sinus of Valsalva or opposite coronary artery [15, 16]. An anomalous LCX most commonly arises from a separate ostium within the right sinus of Valsalva or as a proximal branch of the RCA (approximately 0.32–0.67% of the population) [2, 14, 21]. Anomalous LCX arteries most often take a retroaortic course, but more rarely it may take either an interarterial or a prepulmonic course. It may be an isolated anomaly with the LAD originating normally from the left coronary sinus or may be associated with other branch anomalies, such as origin of the LAD from the anomalous LCX. This anomaly has not been associated with sudden death. In all of these anomalies, the coronary ostium may be at the normal level, or the involved artery may have a high or low takeoff [20, 21].

A coronary artery arising from the contralateral sinus of Valsalva or opposite coronary artery can take any of four common courses, depending on the anatomic relationship of the anomalous vessel to the aorta and the pulmonary trunk: (a) interarterial (i.e., between the aorta and the pulmonary artery) (Figs. 45.5 and 45.6), (b) retroaortic, (c) prepulmonic, or (d) septal (subpulmonic) [2, 3, 10, 14, 15, 22]. It is of great clinical importance which course is taken. Retroaortic, prepulmonic, and septal (subpulmonic) courses are generally benign, while an interarterial course is malignant carrying a risk for sudden cardiac death. The mechanism behind sudden cardiac death in patients with an interarterial course is controversial. Some have argued that compression of the coronary artery between the aorta and pulmonary artery

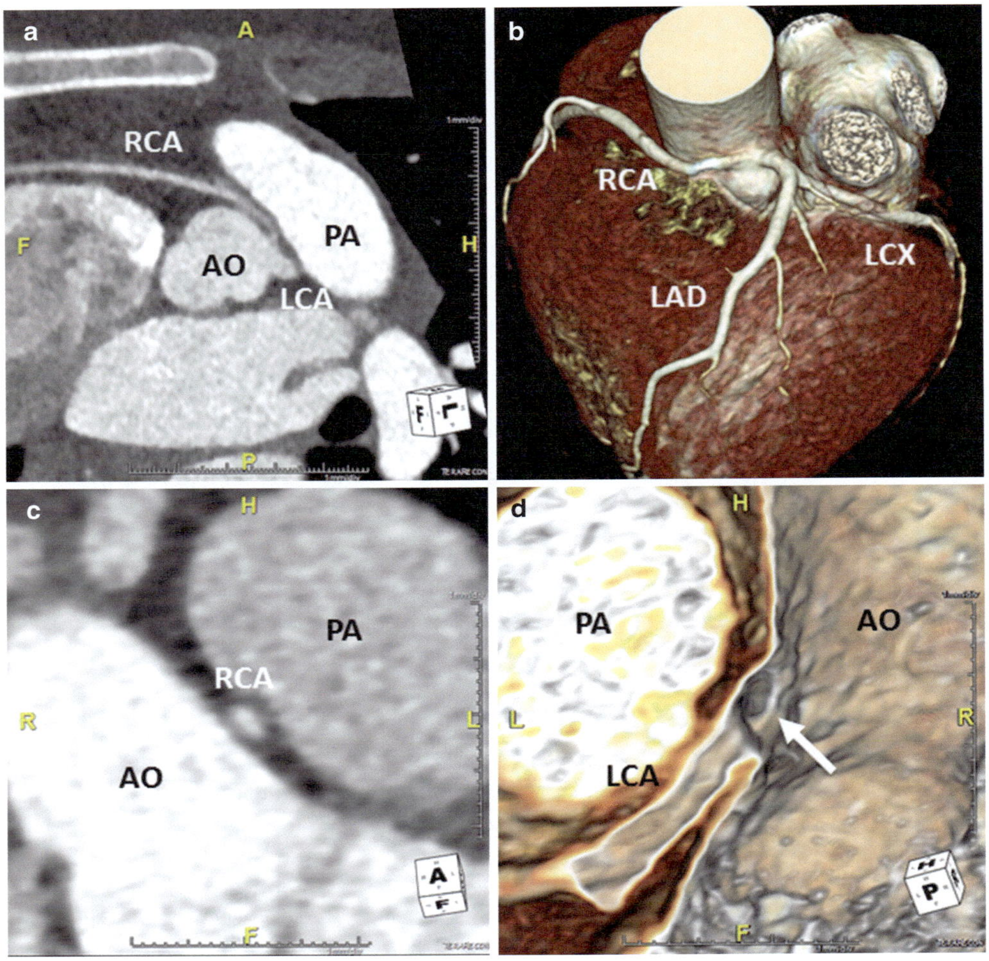

Fig. 45.5 Right coronary artery arising from the left coronary sinus of Valsalva (interarterial type). (**a**) Thin-slab maximum intensity projection CT image shows the right coronary artery arising from the left coronary sinus of Valsalva and coursing between the aortic root and pulmonary artery. (**b**) 3D volume-rendered reformatted CT reconstruction shows the separate origins of the LCA and RCA. (**c**) Multiplanar reformatted CT image shows the slit-like, eccentric shape of the proximal RCA. (**d**) 3D volume-rendered reformatted CT reconstruction can be used to visualize the eccentric RCA origin (arrow). In all images, note the acute angle of takeoff from the sinus, proximity to the left/right commissure, and slit-like orifice and proximal course, suggesting an intramural course. AO = aorta; PA = pulmonary artery; LAD = left descending artery; LCX = left circumflex artery; RCA = right coronary artery

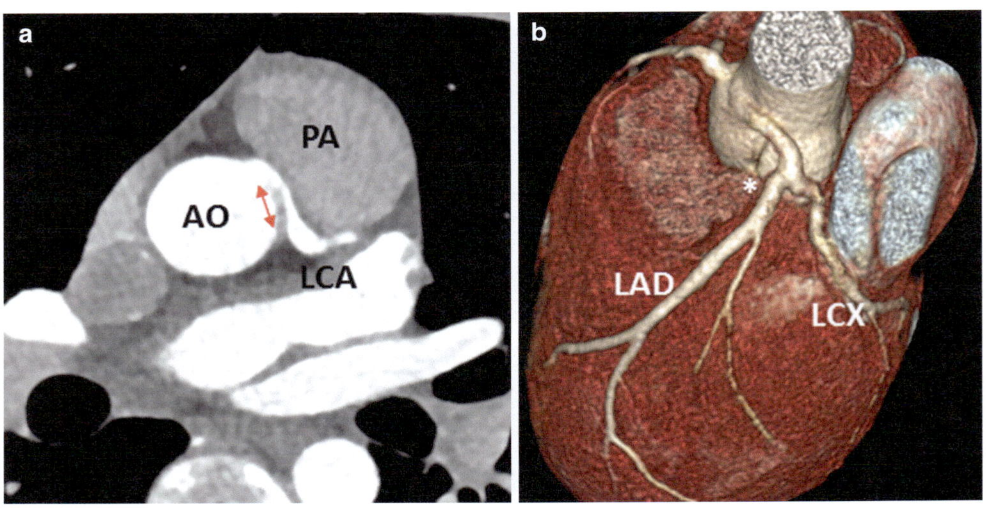

Fig. 45.6 Anomalous left coronary artery arising from right coronary sinus of Valsalva. (**a**) Axial contrast-enhanced CT angiography shows the left coronary artery arising from the right coronary sinus of Valsalva and coursing between the aortic root and pulmonary trunk. Note the acute angle of takeoff from the sinus, proximity to the left/right commissure, and slit-like orifice and proximal course, suggesting an intramural course. The intramural course ends when the LCA returns to normal size (arrow). (**b**) 3D volume rendering reformatted CT image shows the left coronary artery arising from the right coronary sinus of Valsalva near the intercoronary commissure (*)

during exercise contributes to ischemia and sudden death, while others have rejected that hypothesis [23–25].

Patients with an anomalous coronary origin are at risk for having an abnormal intramural proximal course – that is, the proximal coronary artery runs within the wall of the aorta. An intramural course is associated with increased risk for sudden death – higher in anomalous LCA versus RCA [2, 3, 21, 22, 26–32]. The vast majority of anomalous coronary arteries with an intramural course also display an interarterial course, though not all anomalous coronaries with an interarterial course have an intramural segment. A number of MDCT angiographic features are noted in patients with an intramural course: (1) The coronary origin and proximal course are narrow or slit-like, (2) the coronary originates eccentrically from the aortic sinus near the commissure, and (3) there is an acute angle of takeoff from the aortic sinus. One can determine where the intramural segment ends at the point when the distal coronary artery returns to a circular shape. Identifying the length of the intramural course by MDCT angiography can be important in guiding surgical "unroofing" procedure [33]. In addition, intramural coronaries are important to identify in patients who require coronary origin transfer procedures, such as the arterial switch procedure in patients with transposition of the great arteries or in patients undergoing the Ross procedure.

Origin of the Coronary Artery from the Pulmonary Trunk

Anomalous origin of the coronary artery from the pulmonary artery is one of the most clinically significant coronary artery anomalies. Anomalous origin of the LCA from the pulmonary artery (ALCAPA), also called Bland-White-Garland syndrome, is the most common type constituting 0.25–0.5% of all congenital heart disease (Fig. 45.7a, b) [15, 34–36]. Other types of this coronary artery anomaly include origin of the RCA from the pulmonary trunk (Fig. 45.7c, d), origin of

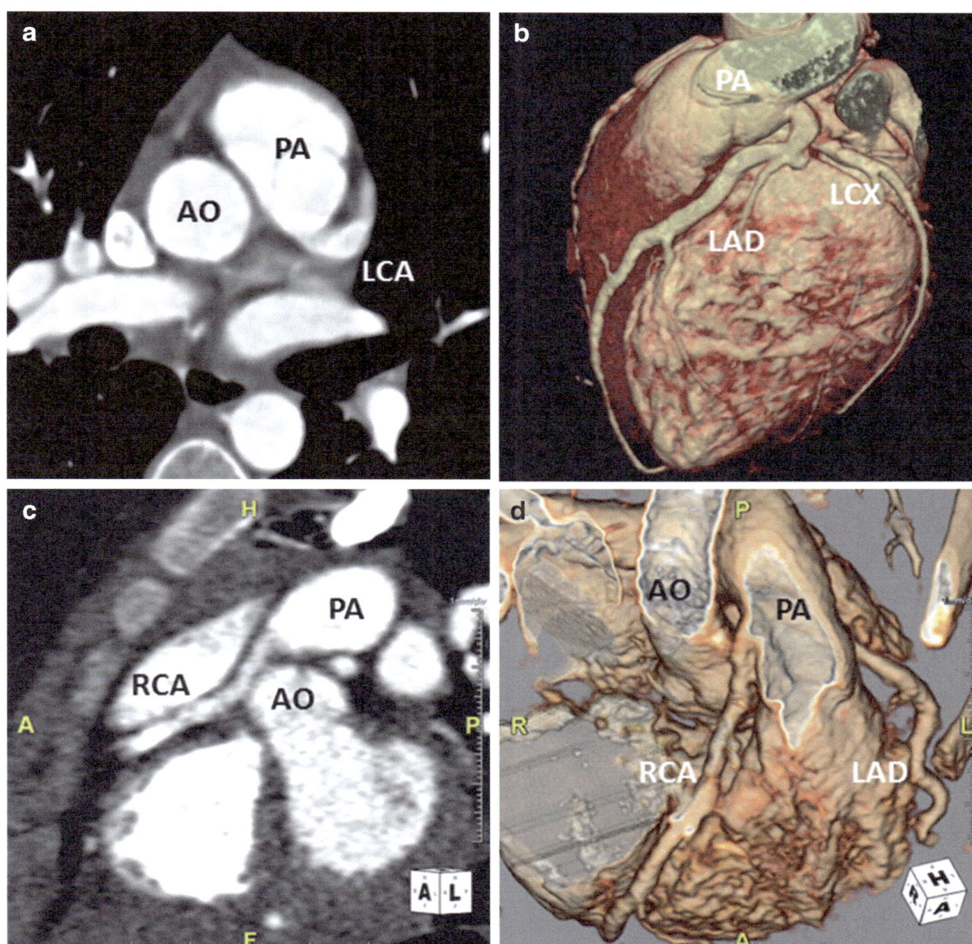

Fig. 45.7 Anomalous coronary artery arising from the pulmonary artery. (**a**) Axial contrast-enhanced CT image shows the LCA arising from the left-facing sinus of the pulmonary artery root. (**b**) 3D volume reformatted CT image shows the LCA arising from the pulmonary artery root. Note the coronary arteries appear dilated consistent with collateral development from the RCA system to the LCA. (**c**) Multiplanar reformatted CT image shows the RCA arising from the right-facing sinus of the pulmonary artery root. (**d**) 3D volume reformatted CT image shows the RCA arising from the pulmonary artery root. AO = aorta; LAD = left descending artery; LCX = left circumflex artery; PA = pulmonary artery; RCA = right coronary artery

LAD from pulmonary artery, and origin of LCX from pulmonary artery. There are rare reports of coronaries also originating from the branch pulmonary arteries.

ALCAPA can be classified into two types: infant and adult types. Clinical presentation is influenced by the development of collaterals from the RCA to the LCA system. In infants with poor collateralization, symptoms manifest in the first few months of life with symptoms due to myocardial ischemia – extreme fussiness with feeds, poor feeding, and poor growth. Without surgical repair, rapid death ensues in up to 90% of patients within weeks or months of birth [34]. In patients with greater collateralization, older infants and toddlers may present with symptoms of left-to-right shunting from the collateral retrograde through the LCA into the pulmonary artery. These patients display poor growth, tachypnea, and left heart enlargement. These patients often have poor ventricular function and atrioventricular valve regurgitation. In adult type with significant collateralization, ALCAPA syndrome may be asymptomatic. Alternatively, adults with ALCAPA may develop myocardial infarction, left ventricular dysfunction, mitral valve regurgitation, or silent myocardial ischemia, leading to sudden cardiac death.

MDCT coronary angiography can directly visualize the LCA arising from the main pulmonary artery, which is the diagnostic hallmark of ALCAPA syndrome (Fig. 45.7a, b). Most often, the LCA originates from the left-facing pulmonary sinus. Less often, the LCA originates from the non-facing pulmonary sinus. Other indirect signs, such as the dilated and tortuous RCA and LCA, dilated intercoronary collateral vessels, left ventricular hypertrophy and dilatation, and dilated bronchial arteries, can also be found in this entity [35].

Surgical correction is the standard treatment for the patients with ALCAPA syndrome. The aim of surgery is to restore a two-coronary-artery circulation system. In neonates with poor collateralization, early correction is required. In asymptomatic adults with adequate collateralization, surgery should be considered when extensive delayed subendocardial enhancement caused by myocardial infarction is seen on magnetic resonance imaging [35]. The preferred surgery includes a coronary button transfer, the Takeuchi procedure, as it is the most anatomic correction and has excellent long-term results. In adult patients with adequate collateralization, alternative approaches include placement of a coronary artery bypass graft (CABG) or ligation of the origin of the LCA to stop competitive flow. A combined approach in adults may be preferred. After surgery, MDCT angiography is often used to ensure there is no kinking of the LCA after button transfer and to assess the patency of bypass grafts if symptoms recur.

Coronary Artery Anomalies of Course

Myocardial Bridging

Coronary arteries generally course epicardially. Myocardial bridging is a congenital anomaly characterized by muscular encasement of a coronary artery segment that has dipped into the myocardium [15, 36, 37]. It is reported the prevalence of myocardial bridging ranges from 15% to 85% in autopsy studies; however, it is only seen in 0.5–2.5% of invasive angiographic studies [36]. MDCT coronary angiography displays better sensitivity than invasive angiography with a reported incidence of 3.5–30% [36–38]. Myocardial bridging is most commonly localized in the middle segment of the LAD; but it can be found in other coronary arteries. Multiple myocardial bridges can be observed in the same or different coronary arteries and their branches. Additionally, segments of the coronary artery proximal to the myocardial bridge are more vulnerable to atherosclerotic plaques due to abnormal blood flow profiles, increasing the risk of myocardial ischemia [36, 37].

Myocardial bridges can be divided into two types: superficial bridges (75%) (Fig. 45.8) and deep bridges (25%) (Fig. 45.9) although no uniform depth criteria have been set to classify myocardial bridges [38]. Deep myocardial bridge often denotes the completely encased coronary artery, which often results in compression of involved coronary segment during the systolic phase. Superficial myocardial bridges are encased incompletely by myocardium; however, long superficial MB can result in severe stenosis during the cardiac cycle (Fig. 45.7).

Myocardial bridging is asymptomatic in the vast majority of patients [8]. However, there is evidence that myocardial bridging can be responsible for angina pectoris, myocardial infarction, life-threatening arrhythmias, or even death in certain patients, especially those with deep myocardial bridge or long superficial bridging [39, 40].

The MDCT coronary angiogram can clearly show the presence, course, and anatomical features of intramuscular coronary arteries [36, 41]. When myocardial bridging is suspected, systolic and diastolic phase reformation is recommended to assess the luminal narrowing during the systolic phase. Other indirect findings include a "milking" effect which can be found during the systolic and diastolic phase reformatted CT images or 4D cine and a "step-down-step-up" phenomenon induced by systolic compression of the tunneled segment in sagittal MPR or VR reformatted images.

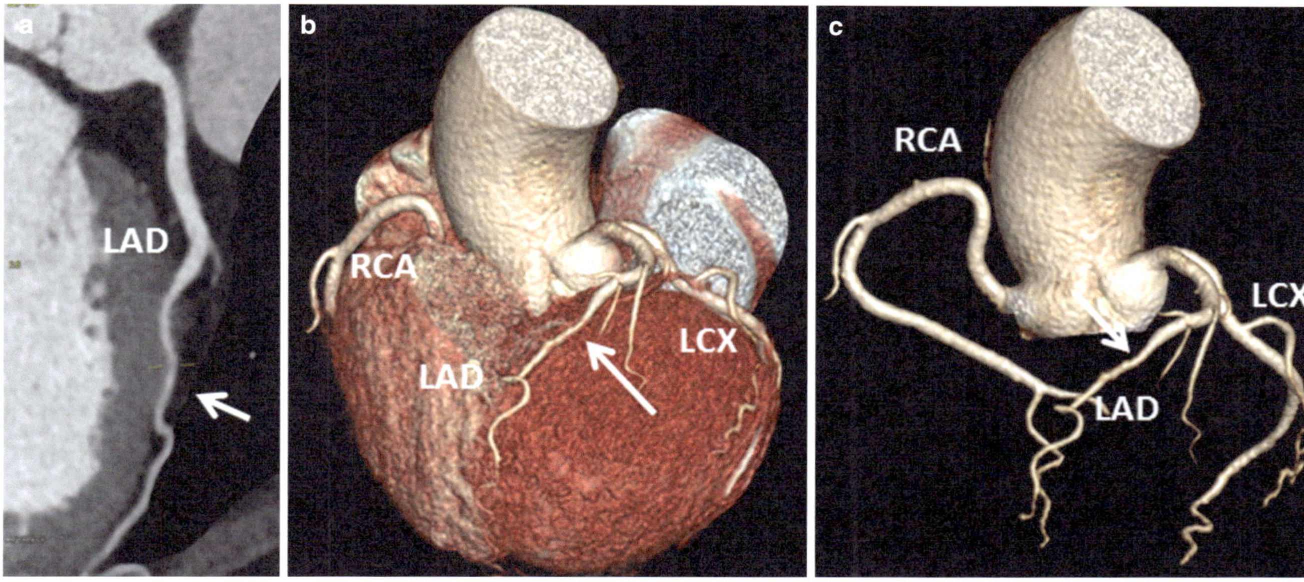

Fig. 45.8 Superficial myocardial bridging of the left anterior descending artery. (**a**) Curved planar reformatted image shows the superficial intramural course (arrow) of the mid-segment of the left anterior descending artery. Note the LAD is not entirely encased in myocardium consistent with a superficial myocardial bridge. (**b**) 3D volume reformatted CT image and (**c**) coronary artery tree image show moderate stenosis of intramyocardial segment of the LAD artery (arrow). LAD = left descending artery; LCX = left circumflex artery; RCA = right coronary artery

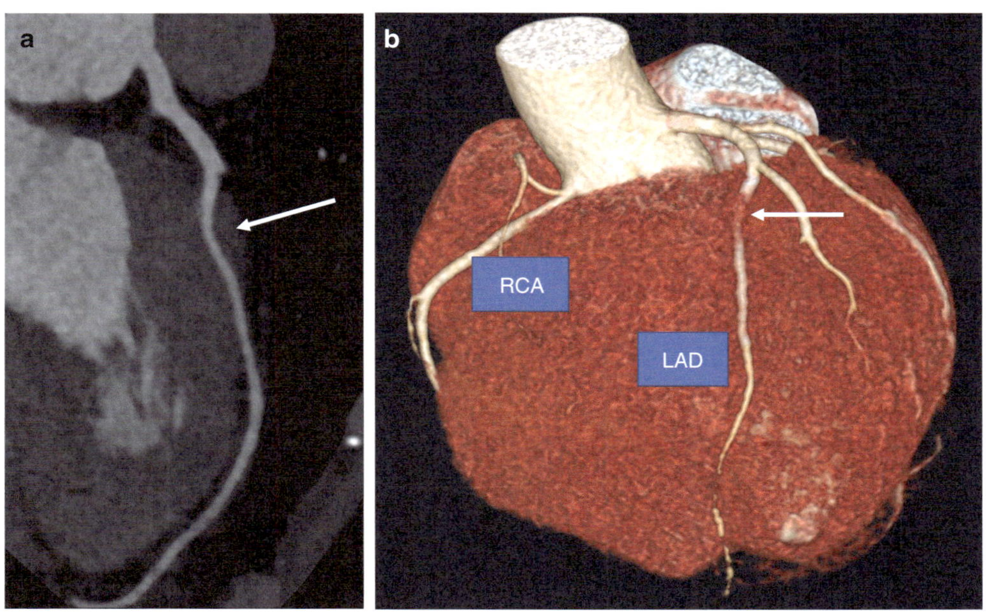

Fig. 45.9 Deep myocardial bridging of the left anterior descending artery. (**a**) Curved planar reformatted image shows deep intramural course with 4 mm covering myocardium (arrow) of the mid-segment of the left anterior descending artery. Note 2 mm is the cutoff value for determining the superficial and deep myocardial bridging. (**b**) 3D volume reformatted CT image shows the covering myocardium in the mid-segment of the left anterior descending artery (arrow). RCA = right coronary artery; LAD = the left anterior descending artery

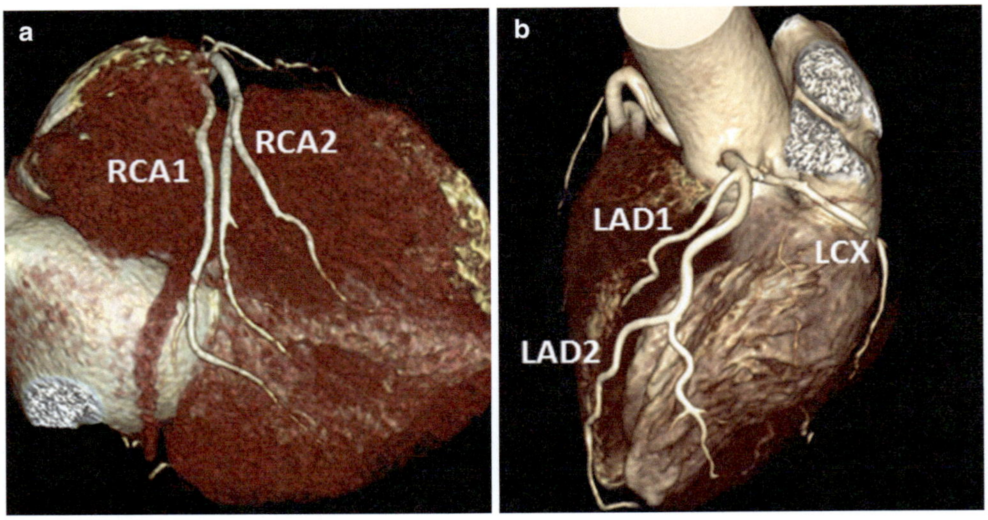

Fig. 45.10 Coronary artery duplication. (**a**) 3D volume reformatted CT image showing a duplicated right coronary artery. (**b**) 3D volume reformatted CT angiogram showing a short LAD (LAD1) coursing and terminating in the anterior interventricular sulcus without reaching the apex and a long LAD (LAD2) reaching the apex. CA = conus artery; LAD = left descending artery; LCX = left circumflex artery; RCA = right coronary artery

Coronary Artery Duplication

Coronary artery duplication can occur in both the RCA and LCA. Duplication of the RCA is rare; few cases are reported in the literature (Fig. 45.10a) [15]. LAD duplication is more common occurring in 0.13–1% of the general population [15, 42]. LAD duplication consists of a short LAD coursing and terminating in the proximal interventricular sulcus without reaching the apex and a secondary LAD originating from the LCA (Fig. 45.10b) or RCA and entering the distal anterior interventricular sulcus and coursing to the apex [15, 42]. LAD duplication should not be confused with an LAD and a diagonal branch running parallel to each other. Such a parallel diagonal branch does not reenter the anterior interventricular sulcus and take over the course of the distal LAD. Coronary artery duplication is a benign anomaly, but it may complicate surgical intervention when aortocoronary bypass or other coronary artery surgeries are performed. It is also important to identify in congenital heart diseases where transection of the right ventricular outflow tract would be considered (i.e., tetralogy of Fallot) as an LAD off the RCA would be disrupted in such a case.

Coronary Artery Anomalies of Termination

Coronary Artery Fistula

Coronary artery fistula is a condition in which a communication exists between a coronary artery and a cardiac chamber and a great vessel or other vascular structure [15]. Coronary artery fistulae are rare, with the reported prevalence of 0.002% in the general population and approximately 0.1–0.2% of all patients undergoing selective coronary angiography [43–45]. Although most patients have no symptoms, some patients may have exertional dyspnea and fatigue. Symptom severity depends on the degree of shunt and left- or right-heart overload, i.e., the size of the origin of the fistula and the drainage sites. Large coronary artery fistulae can cause myocardial ischemia, congestive heart failure, endocarditis, thrombosis, pulmonary hypertension, and/or embolic events. These symptoms may not develop until late adulthood.

Coronary fistulae more commonly involve the RCA (60% of cases) than the LCA (40%) [15]. In less than 5% of cases, fistulae originate from both the LCA and the RCA. The most common site of drainage is the pulmonary artery (Fig. 45.11a, b), followed by the right ventricle (Fig. 45.11c, d) and the right atrium (Fig. 45.12a, b). Drainage into the left atrium (Fig. 45.12c, d) or left ventricle occurs in less than 10% of cases [45–47].

On MDCT coronary angiography, the involved coronary artery is often dilated or tortuous, and the site of drainage can be clearly visualized. In coronary artery fistula to pulmonary artery, the contrast ejection sign can be found in pulmonary artery trunk.

Coronary Arcade

Coronary arcade is a direct communication between the RCA and the LCA, which is large enough to visualize by invasive coronary angiography or MDCT coronary angiography but without significant coronary artery stenosis. Coronary arcade should be differentiated from collateral vessels on the basis of the prominent straight connection between the two unobstructed major arteries, often at or near the level of the crux, which is different from the tortuous

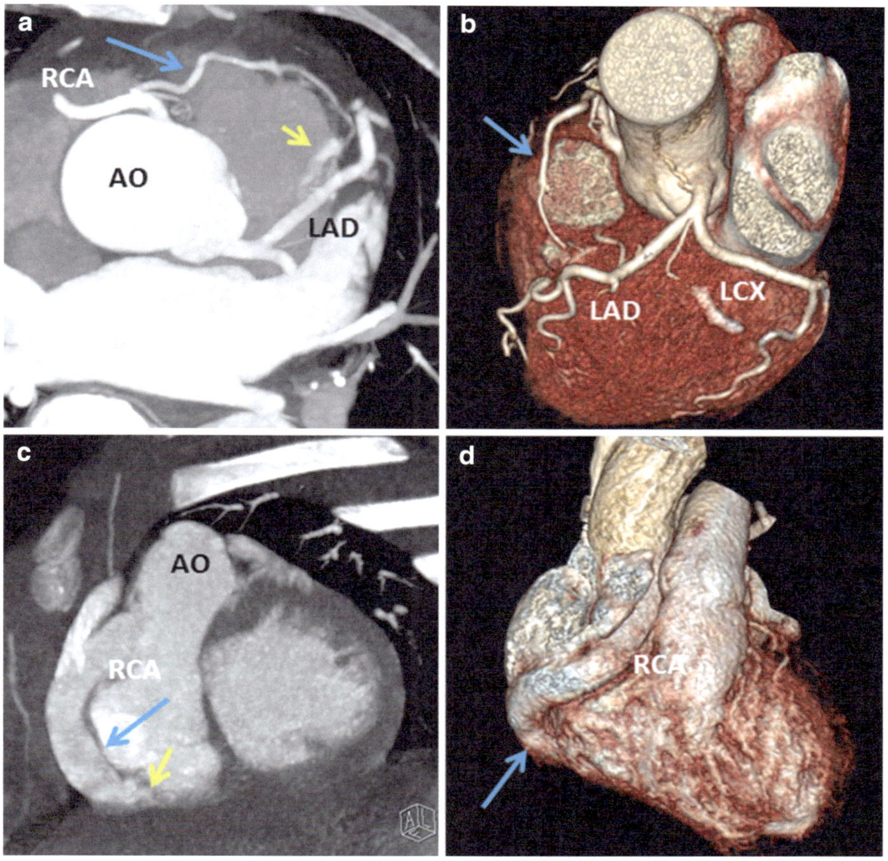

Fig. 45.11 Right coronary artery fistulae. (**a**) Thin-slab maximum-intensity projection image shows tortuous vessels (blue arrow) in the vicinity of the pulmonary artery trunk. The fistula orifice displays the typical ejection sign into the pulmonary artery (yellow arrow). (**b**) 3D volume reformatted CT angiogram shows the tortuous vessels (blue arrow) near the excluded pulmonary artery. (**c**) Thin-slab maximum-intensity projection image shows the dilated proximal RCA and large fistula (blue arrow) terminating into the right ventricle (yellow arrow). (**d**) 3D volume reformatted CT angiogram shows the dilated proximal RCA and large fistula (blue arrow) terminating into the right ventricle. AO = aorta; LAD = left descending artery; LCX = left circumflex artery; RCA = right coronary artery

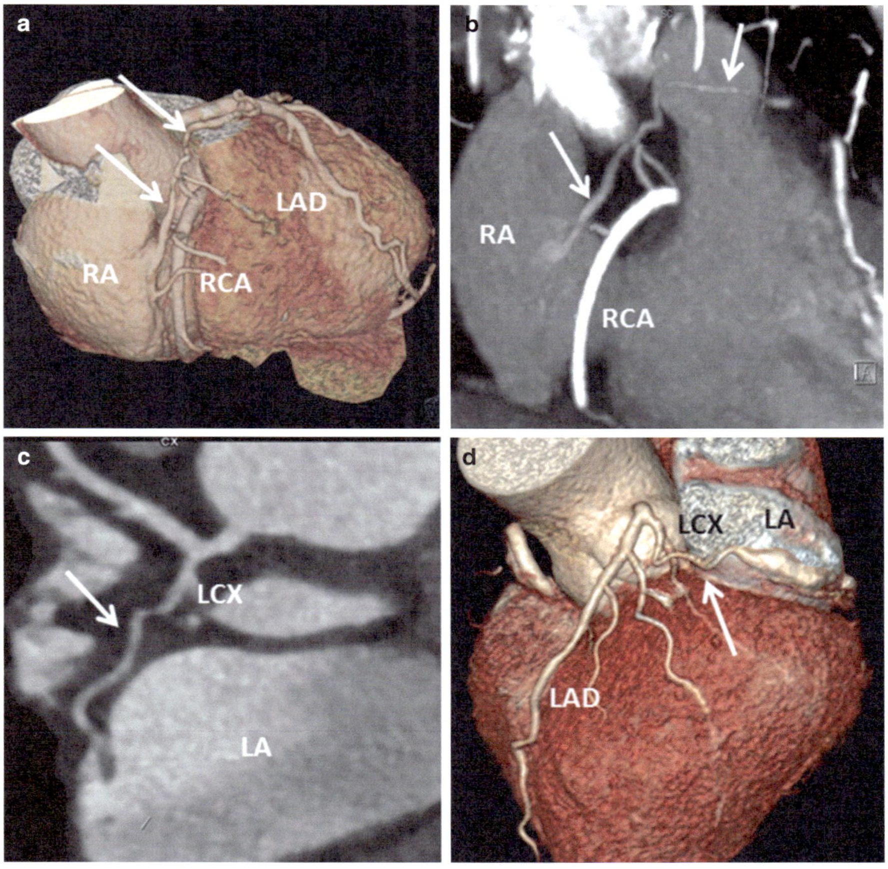

Fig. 45.12 Left coronary artery fistulae. (**a**) 3D volume reformatted CT angiogram shows a tortuous vessel (arrows) traveling from the LAD to the RA. (**b**) Thin-slab maximum-intensity projection image shows the tortuous vessel (arrows) displaying the typical ejection sign into the right atrium. (**c**) Thin-slab maximum-intensity projection image shows a tortuous vessel (arrow) traversing from the LCX to the LA. (**d**) 3D volume reformatted CT angiogram shows a tortuous vessel (arrows) traveling from the LCX to the LA. LA = left atrium; LAD = left descending artery; LCX = left circumflex artery; RA = right atrium; RCA = right coronary artery

collateral vessels [15]. In addition, coronary arcade should be differentiated from coronary to pulmonary artery fistula; the former has no direct communication between the coronary artery and pulmonary artery.

Extracardiac Termination

Systemic arterial termination of a coronary artery is uncommon. Connections may exist between the coronary arteries and extracardiac vessels such as the bronchial, internal mammary, pericardial, anterior mediastinal, superior and inferior phrenic, and intercostal arteries and the esophageal branch of the aorta. This entity can be distinguished from coronary artery fistula in that the coronary artery is not usually enlarged and tortuous. Most coronary-systemic arterial communications are not significant, except for the presence of atherosclerosis in the native coronary artery originating from systemic arterial communication [15].

It may be difficult to identify a coronary artery terminating into extracardiac artery by MDCT coronary angiography due to the small caliber of the vessels involved. Therefore, ensuring adequate scanning range and careful slice by slice observation in thin-slice axial contrast-enhanced CT images is key for diagnosing these coronary-systemic arterial communications.

Summary

In conclusion, coronary artery anomalies include anomalies of origin, course, and termination. These anomalies can clearly and accurately be visualized by state-of-the-art MDCT coronary angiography owing to high spatial resolution and three-dimensional imaging capability. It is important to identify and report those anomalies that are malignant, such as interarterial or intramural course in patients with an anomalous coronary origin. Due to its superior ability to depict coronary artery anomalies than conventional invasive coronary angiography, MDCT coronary angiography is the first-line choice for imaging coronary artery anomalies.

References

1. Angelini P. Coronary artery anomalies: an entity in search of an identity. Circulation. 2007;115(10):1296–305.
2. Perez-Pomares JM, de la Pompa JL, Franco D, Henderson D, Ho SY, Houyel L, Kelly RG, Sedmera D, Sheppard M, Sperling S, Thiene G, van den Hoff M, Basso C. Congenital coronary artery anomalies: a bridge from embryology to anatomy and pathophysiology--a position statement of the development, anatomy, and pathology ESC Working Group. Cardiovasc Res. 2016;109(2):204–16.
3. Sundaram B, Kreml R, Patel S. Imaging of coronary artery anomalies. Radiol Clin N Am. 2010;48(4):711–27.
4. Angelini P. Novel imaging of coronary artery anomalies to assess their prevalence, the causes of clinical symptoms, and the risk of sudden cardiac death. Circ Cardiovasc Imaging. 2014;7(4):747–54.
5. van Ooijen PM, Dorgelo J, Zijlstra F, Oudkerk M. Detection, visualization and evaluation of anomalous coronary anatomy on 16-slice multidetector-row CT. Eur Radiol. 2004;14(12):2163–71.
6. Datta J, White CS, Gilkeson RC, Meyer CA, Kansal S, Jani ML, Arildsen RC, Read K. Anomalous coronary arteries in adults: depiction at multi-detector row CT angiography. Radiology. 2005;235(3):812–8.
7. Shi H, Aschoff AJ, Brambs HJ, Hoffmann MH. Multislice CT imaging of anomalous coronary arteries. Eur Radiol. 2004;14(12):2172–81.
8. Young PM, Gerber TC, Williamson EE, Julsrud PR, Herfkens RJ. Cardiac imaging: Part 2, normal, variant, and anomalous configurations of the coronary vasculature. AJR Am J Roentgenol. 2011;197(4):816–26.
9. Dodd JD, Ferencik M, Liberthson RR, Cury RC, Hoffmann U, Brady TJ, Abbara S. Congenital anomalies of coronary artery origin in adults: 64-MDCT appearance. AJR Am J Roentgenol. 2007;188(2):W138–46.
10. Shriki JE, Shinbane JS, Rashid MA, Hindoyan A, Withey JG, DeFrance A, Cunningham M, Oliveira GR, Warren BH, Wilcox A. Identifying, characterizing, and classifying congenital anomalies of the coronary arteries. Radiographics. 2012;32(2):453–68.
11. Schoepf UJ. CT of the heart: principles and applications. In: Contemporary cardiology. Totowa: Humana Press; 2005.
12. Zhang LJ, Wang YZ, Huang W, Chen P, Zhou CS, Lu GM. Anatomical investigation of the sinus node artery using dual-source computed tomography. Circ J. 2008;72(10):1615–20.
13. Greenberg MA, Fish BG, Spindola-Franco H. Congenital anomalies of coronary artery: classification and significance. Radiol Clin North Am. 1989;27:1127–46.
14. Kang JW, Seo JB, Chae EJ, Jang YM, Do KH, Lee JS, Song JW, Lim TH. Coronary artery anomalies: classification and electrocardiogram-gated multidetector computed tomographic findings. Semin Ultrasound CT MR. 2008;29(3):182–94.
15. Kim SY, Seo JB, Do KH, Heo JN, Lee JS, Song JW, Choe YH, Kim TH, Yong HS, Choi SI, Song KS, Lim TH. Coronary artery anomalies: classification and ECG-gated multi-detector row CT findings with angiographic correlation. Radiographics. 2006;26(2):317–33. discussion 333-314
16. Raimondi F, Bonnet D. Imaging of congenital anomalies of the coronary arteries. Diagn Interv Imaging. 2016;97(5):561–9.
17. Danias PG, Stuber M, McConnell MV, Manning WJ. The diagnosis of congenital coronary anomalies with magnetic resonance imaging. Coron Artery Dis. 2001;12(8):621–6.
18. Aldana-Sepulveda N, Restrepo CS, Kimura-Hayama E. Single coronary artery: spectrum of imaging findings with multidetector CT. J Cardiovasc Comput Tomogr. 2013;7(6):391–9.
19. Desmet W, Vanhaecke J, Vrolix M, Van de Werf F, Piessens J, Willems J, de Geest H. Isolated single coronary artery: a review of 50,000 consecutive coronary angiographies. Eur Heart J. 1992;13(12):1637–40.
20. Frescura C, Basso C, Thiene G, Corrado D, Pennelli T, Angelini A, Daliento L. Anomalous origin of coronary arteries and risk of sudden death: a study based on an autopsy population of congenital heart disease. Hum Pathol. 1998;29(7):689–95.
21. Bunce NH, Lorenz CH, Keegan J, Lesser J, Reyes EM, Firmin DN, Pennell DJ. Coronary artery anomalies: assessment with free-breathing three-dimensional coronary MR angiography. Radiology. 2003;227(1):201–8.
22. Lim JC, Beale A, Ramcharitar S, Medscape. Anomalous origination of a coronary artery from the opposite sinus. Nat Rev Cardiol. 2011;8(12):706–19.

23. Barth CW 3rd, Roberts WC. Left main coronary artery originating from the right sinus of Valsalva and coursing between the aorta and pulmonary trunk. J Am Coll Cardiol. 1986;7(2):366–73.
24. Lorenz EC, Mookadam F, Mookadam M, Moustafa S, Zehr KJ. A systematic overview of anomalous coronary anatomy and an examination of the association with sudden cardiac death. Rev Cardiovasc Med. 2006;7(4):205–13.
25. Angelini P, Walmsley RP, Libreros A, Ott DA. Symptomatic anomalous origination of the left coronary artery from the opposite sinus of valsalva. Clinical presentations, diagnosis, and surgical repair. Tex Heart Inst J. 2006;33(2):171–9.
26. Ashrafpoor G, Danchin N, Houyel L, Ramadan R, Belli E, Paul JF. Anatomical criteria of malignancy by computed tomography angiography in patients with anomalous coronary arteries with an interarterial course. Eur Radiol. 2015;25(3):760–6.
27. Krupinski M, Urbanczyk-Zawadzka M, Laskowicz B, Irzyk M, Banys R, Klimeczek P, Gruszczynska K, Baron J. Anomalous origin of the coronary artery from the wrong coronary sinus evaluated with computed tomography: "high-risk" anatomy and its clinical relevance. Eur Radiol. 2014;24(10):2353–9.
28. Zhang LJ, Wu SY, Huang W, Zhou CS, Lu GM. Anomalous origin of the right coronary artery originating from the left coronary sinus of valsalva with an interarterial course: diagnosis and dynamic evaluation using dual-source computed tomography. J Comput Assist Tomogr. 2009;33(3):348–53.
29. Zhang LJ, Yang GF, Huang W, Zhou CS, Chen P, Lu GM. Incidence of anomalous origin of coronary artery in 1879 Chinese adults on dual-source CT angiography. Neth Hear J. 2010;18(10):466–70.
30. Cheezum MK, Ghoshhajra B, Bittencourt MS, Hulten EA, Bhatt A, Mousavi N, Shah NR, Valente AM, Rybicki FJ, Steigner M, Hainer J, MacGillivray T, Hoffmann U, Abbara S, Di Carli MF, DeFaria Yeh D, Landzberg M, Liberthson R, Blankstein R. Anomalous origin of the coronary artery arising from the opposite sinus: prevalence and outcomes in patients undergoing coronary CTA. Eur Heart J Cardiovasc Imaging. 2017;18(2):224–35.
31. Lee HJ, Hong YJ, Kim HY, Lee J, Hur J, Choi BW, Chang HJ, Nam JE, Choe KO, Kim YJ. Anomalous origin of the right coronary artery from the left coronary sinus with an interarterial course: subtypes and clinical importance. Radiology. 2012;262(1):101–8.
32. Chaitman BR, Lesperance J, Saltiel J, Bourassa MG. Clinical, angiographic, and hemodynamic findings in patients with anomalous origin of the coronary arteries. Circulation. 1976;53(1):122–31.
33. Gulati R, Reddy VM, Culbertson C, Helton G, Suleman S, Reinhartz O, Silverman N, Hanley FL. Surgical management of coronary artery arising from the wrong coronary sinus, using standard and novel approaches. J Thorac Cardiovasc Surg. 2007;134(5):1171–8.
34. Schwartz ML, Jonas RA, Colan SD. Anomalous origin of left coronary artery from pulmonary artery: recovery of left ventricular function after dual coronary repair. J Am Coll Cardiol. 1997;30(2):547–53.
35. Pena E, Nguyen ET, Merchant N, Dennie C. ALCAPA syndrome: not just a pediatric disease. Radiographics. 2009;29(2):553–65.
36. Hazirolan T, Canyigit M, Karcaaltincaba M, Dagoglu MG, Akata D, Aytemir K, Besim A. Myocardial bridging on MDCT. AJR Am J Roentgenol. 2007;188(4):1074–80.
37. Corban MT, Hung OY, Eshtehardi P, Rasoul-Arzrumly E, McDaniel M, Mekonnen G, Timmins LH, Lutz J, Guyton RA, Samady H. Myocardial bridging: contemporary understanding of pathophysiology with implications for diagnostic and therapeutic strategies. J Am Coll Cardiol. 2014;63(22):2346–55.
38. Konen E, Goitein O, Sternik L, Eshet Y, Shemesh J, Di Segni E. The prevalence and anatomical patterns of intramuscular coronary arteries: a coronary computed tomography angiographic study. J Am Coll Cardiol. 2007;49(5):587–93.
39. Morales AR, Romanelli R, Tate LG, Boucek RJ, de Marchena E. Intramural left anterior descending coronary artery: significance of the depth of the muscular tunnel. Hum Pathol. 1993;24(7):693–701.
40. Ferreira AG Jr, Trotter SE, Konig B Jr, Decourt LV, Fox K, Olsen EG. Myocardial bridges: morphological and functional aspects. Br Heart J. 1991;66(5):364–7.
41. Lu GM, Zhang LJ, Guo H, Huang W, Merges RD. Comparison of myocardial bridging by dual-source CT with conventional coronary angiography. Circ J. 2008;72(7):1079–85.
42. Bozlar U, Ugurel MS, Sari S, Akgun V, Ors F, Tasar M. Prevalence of dual left anterior descending artery variations in CT angiography. Diagn Interv Radiol. 2015;21(1):34–41.
43. Saboo SS, Juan YH, Khandelwal A, George E, Steigner ML, Landzberg M, Rybicki FJ. MDCT of congenital coronary artery fistulas. AJR Am J Roentgenol. 2014;203(3):W244–52.
44. Said SA, el Gamal MI, van der Werf T. Coronary arteriovenous fistulas: collective review and management of six new cases--changing etiology, presentation, and treatment strategy. Clin Cardiol. 1997;20(9):748–52.
45. Zhang LJ, Zhou CS, Wang Y, Jin Z, Yu W, Zhang Z, Zhang B, Fang X, Cui X, Li K, Huang W, Zheng L, Ji XM, Hoffman C, Schoepf UJ, Lu GM. Prevalence and types of coronary to pulmonary artery fistula in a Chinese population at dual-source CT coronary angiography. Acta Radiol. 2014;55(9):1031–9.
46. Zhou CS, Zhang LJ, Wang YN, Yu W, Huang W, Zhang B, Zhao YE, Chen X, Zheng L, Zhang ZQ, Jin ZY, Lu GM. Incidence and classification diagnosis of coronary artery fistula at dual-source CT coronary angiography. Zhonghua Yi Xue Za Zhi. 2012;92(47):3336–40.
47. Lim JJ, Jung JI, Lee BY, Lee HG. Prevalence and types of coronary artery fistulas detected with coronary CT angiography. AJR Am J Roentgenol. 2014;203(3):W237–43.

CT Spectrum of Congenital Heart Disease

46

David Steflik and Anthony M. Hlavacek

Congenital heart disease (CHD) is a relatively common problem, affecting approximately 0.8% of newborn infants [1]. An understanding of the CT findings of congenital heart diseases and their postoperative complications is important for the radiologist, since patients with palliated or repaired congenital heart disease are living longer and many of them will require lifelong care and imaging.

Imaging Algorithms

The initial imaging algorithm for patients with suspected CHD usually includes an echocardiogram and possible chest radiograph [2]. However, echocardiography is limited by acoustic windows, relatively small field of view, and inability to image airway structures. Magnetic resonance imaging (MRI) also has been added to the imaging armamentarium. MRI provides excellent anatomic and functional information and is particularly valuable in the evaluation of valvular and myocardial function, but it is time-consuming, and it is contraindicated in many patients with pacemakers and in some with implantable cardioverter-defibrillators [3–6].

Cardiac CT is being increasingly used in the evaluation of patients with congenital heart disease and has several advantages over MRI [7–9]. It is more available and less time-consuming than MRI [10, 11]. Fast scan protocols limit the need for sedation, which is a significant risk in patients with congenital heart disease [12]. Current scanners provide high spatial resolution, enabling visualization of small structures; high temporal resolution, which can minimize respiratory and cardiac motion artifacts; and isotropic voxels, allowing for reconstructions with excellent resolution. CT allows a more complete evaluation of lung parenchyma than MRI. CT, unlike MRI, is not hampered by postoperative metal artifacts. Limitations of CT include the lack of the functional capabilities of MRI, the radiation exposure, and the necessity for intravenous administration of contrast material. Nevertheless, CT is enjoying broader use because of its ease of use and widespread availability, and thus, an understanding of the CT features of CHD is essential to ensure a correct diagnosis.

After acquisition of the image set, the data should be reviewed in a segmental fashion, as discussed below. This chapter reviews the native CT appearances of common congenital heart malformations. The CT spectrum of postoperative congenital heart disease is covered in Chap. 46. The CT techniques for evaluating congenital heart disease in children are discussed in Chap. 43.

Sequential Segmental Analysis

Sequential segmental analysis forms the basis of morphologic assessment of the heart. There are three segments within the heart: atria, ventricles, and great arteries. Each segment is defined by the morphology of its structures, rather than their relative location within the chest or connections to other structures. The connections of these different anatomic segments must also be described, which will then correlate with the physiology seen by the clinician at the bedside.

The first structures that must be objectively evaluated are the atria. The most reliable ways to assess the atria are its appendages, which are easily seen on cardiac CT [13]. The right atrial appendage is broad and triangular, with pectinate muscles extending into the body of the atrium (Fig. 46.1a). The left atrial appendage is narrow and "fingerlike," with pectinate muscles confined to the appendage (Fig 46.1b). The right atrium usually receives the inferior vena cava, unless the intrahepatic portion is interrupted. In the traditional classification system, the usual relationship of the atria is termed "situs solitus." The mirror-image relationship, with the morphologic right atrium leftward of the morphologic right atrium, is termed "situs inversus." When there are two right or left atrial appendages, which is found in atrial isomerism, or heterotaxy, the arrangement is classically

D. Steflik · A. M. Hlavacek (✉)
Department of Pediatrics, Division of Pediatric Cardiology, Medical University of South Carolina, Charleston, SC, USA
e-mail: hlavace@musc.edu

U. J. Schoepf (ed.), *CT of the Heart*, Contemporary Medical Imaging, https://doi.org/10.1007/978-1-60327-237-7_46

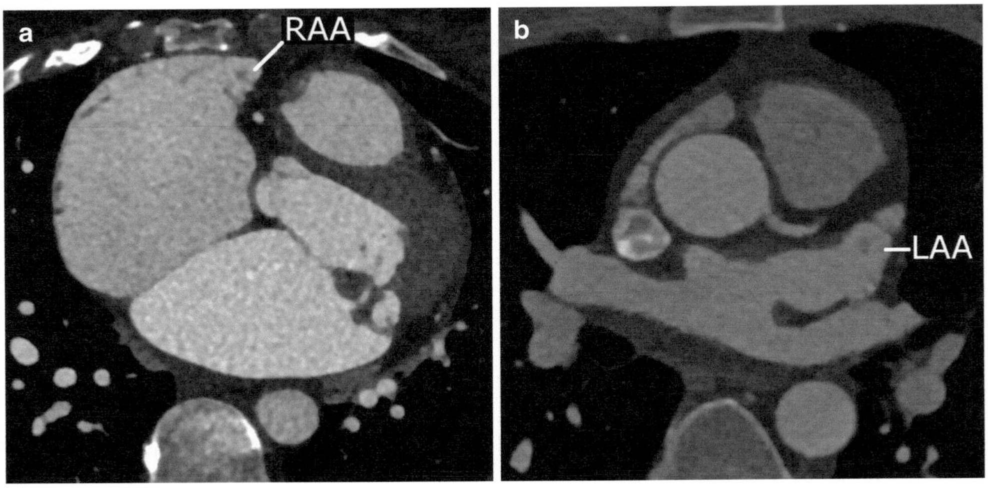

Fig. 46.1 Axial images displaying the typical characteristics of right and left atrial appendages. Note that the right atrial appendage (**a**) has a broad base with pectinate muscles extending into the body of the atrium, while the left atrial appendage (**b**) is generally narrow with pectinate muscles confined to the body of the appendage (*RAA* right atrial appendage, *LAA* left atrial appendage)

called "situs ambiguous," although defining the atrial arrangement as "right" or "left atrial isomerism" is more descriptive [14].

The next structures that must be systematically assessed are the ventricles. The right ventricle is most readily identified by coarse apical trabeculations and a moderator band, while the left ventricle has relatively fine apical trabeculations. When the respective atrioventricular valves are patent, the morphologic right ventricle is noted to have a muscular infundibulum separating the tricuspid valve from the semilunar valve, while the left ventricle has fibrous continuity between the mitral valve and semilunar valve (if present). The usual relationship between the ventricles is termed "D-looped," while the mirror-image arrangement is termed "L-looped." In the rare instance that the ventricles cannot be described in a right-left relationship, the arrangement is often termed "X-looped."

Once the atrial and ventricular orientations are defined, the atrioventricular connections can be described. If the right atrium (RA) is connected to the right ventricle (RV) and the left atrium (LA) is connected with the left ventricle (LV), the atrioventricular connections are termed "concordant." "Discordant" atrioventricular connections exist when the RA connects to the LV and the LA connects with the RV. When atrial isomerism is present, the connections are termed "mixed." A "univentricular" connection exits when there is double inlet to one ventricle (generally left) or there is the absence of one atrioventricular connection (as in classical tricuspid atresia).

Finally, the connections and orientation of the great arteries must be assessed. A concordant ventriculoarterial connection exists when the morphologic RV connects to the pulmonary artery and the morphologic LV connects with the aorta. A discordant ventriculoarterial connection (or "transposition") exists when the morphologic RV connects to the aorta and the morphologic LV connects with the pulmonary artery. The ventriculoarterial connection can also be described as "double outlet" (usually from the RV) or "common," as is found with truncus arteriosus. The orientation of the great arteries is generally defined by the location of the aortic valve relative to the pulmonary valve. In a normal heart, the aortic valve is oriented posterior and rightward to the pulmonary valve. With usual transposition ("D-transposition"), the aortic valve is generally anterior and rightward of the pulmonic valve, but is usually anterior and leftward in congenitally corrected transposition ("L-transposition").

Atrial Septal Defects

Atrial septal defects represent 8–10% of congenital heart defects [15]. Secundum, primum, and sinus venosus defects constitute the three most common types of ASD. Secundum defects are the most common type of atrial septal defect, constituting 75% of defects [16]. A secundum ASD is a defect in the central portion of the atrial septum, or the area containing the fossa ovalis (Fig. 46.2). These defects can be large, and are usually solitary, but can also consist of multiple smaller communications. Primum defects reside in the apical (inferior) portion of the atrial septum and are contiguous with the atrioventricular valves. These defects are generally considered to fall within the spectrum of atrioventricular septal defects and are generally accompanied by a "cleft" mitral valve. Sinus venosus defects involve a deficiency of the wall that separates the right pulmonary veins from the superior vena cava (or infrequently inferior vena cava) and thus the right atrium, creating an interatrial communication (Fig. 46.3). All sinus venosus defects are associated with anomalous drainage of at least one of the right pulmonary veins, usually with connection of the right superior pulmonary vein to the superior vena cava [17]. The least common

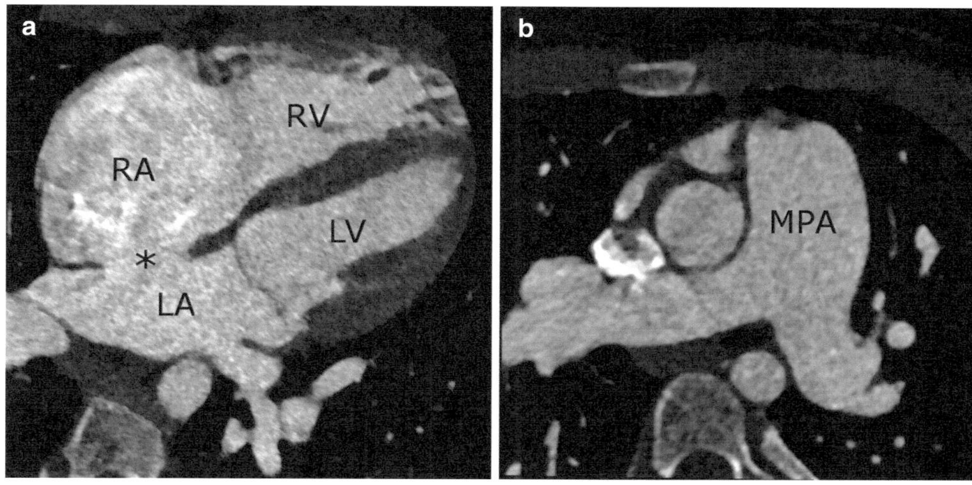

Fig. 46.2 (**a**) "Four-chamber view" displaying a secundum atrial septal defect (*). The right atrium and ventricle are dilated. (**b**) Axial image revealing dilation of the main pulmonary artery, which is common in atrial septal defects (*RA* right atrium, *RV* right ventricle, *LA* left atrium, *LV* left ventricle, *MPA* main pulmonary artery)

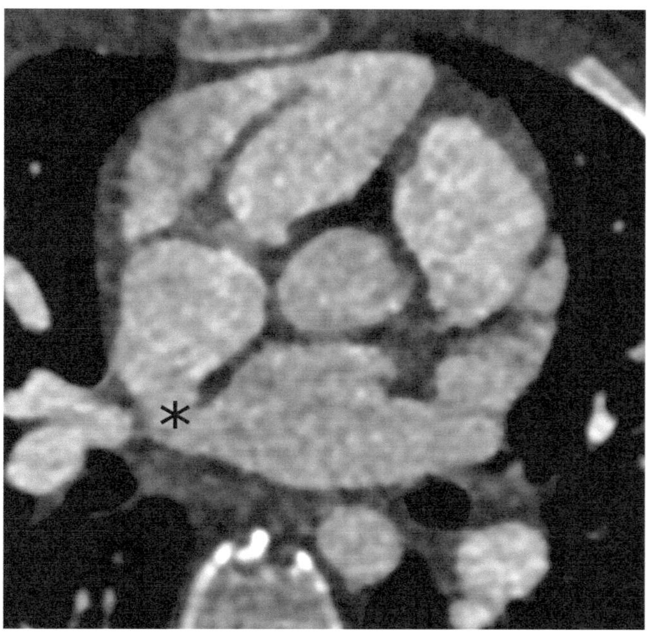

Fig. 46.3 Axial image revealing the typical location of a superior sinus venosus defect (*)

form of ASD is the coronary sinus defect, in which the coronary sinus is at least partially "unroofed," resulting in a communication from the LA to RA. Comprising <1% of ASD, it is usually seen in association with heterotaxy syndromes with bilateral superior vena cavae, although it can also occur in isolation. The major determinant of the magnitude and direction of any atrial-level shunt is the relative compliance of the ventricles. Significant left to right shunts can lead to right atrial and ventricular enlargement and flow-related elevations in pulmonary arterial pressures but rarely result in irreversible pulmonary hypertension.

The CT features of atrial septal defects are discontinuity of a portion of the interatrial septum with contrast-enhanced blood seen in the defect. Cardiac CT can reliably define the location and size of atrial septal defects in larger children and adults [18], particularly when cardiac gating is applied, but will occasionally be inaccurate in non-gated studies or with smaller children and infants. When compared to transthoracic and transesophageal echocardiography in adult patients, cardiac CT has been shown to be superior in determining candidacy for device closure in the catheterization laboratory [19] and can define device protrusion or malposition after closure [20, 21]. It can also be helpful for preoperative assessment of pulmonary venous drainage in patients with sinus venosus defects [22, 23]. Patients with a hemodynamically significant defect will display dilation of the right ventricle and main pulmonary artery on cardiac CT. Ventricular volume measurements can be utilized to quantify the degree of left to right shunt [18, 24].

The differential diagnostic consideration for secundum ASD is a patent foramen ovale, in which there is incomplete fusion between the septum primum and septum secundum which creates a flap-like opening at the foramen ovale. There is no structural deficiency of septal tissue. The patent foramen is small and stays closed as long as left atrial pressure is greater than right atrial pressure, but it can reopen when right atrial pressure increases, such as with a Valsalva maneuver, coughing, or sneezing. In this case, the blood can flow from the right to left atrium.

Ventricular Septal Defects

Ventricular septal defects (VSD) are the most common congenital heart lesions identified during childhood, making up 20–30% of congenital heart defects [25]. There are multiple classification schemes for ventricular septal defects, but the most straightforward method is to define the defect as muscular, perimembranous, or subarterial. Muscular defects are

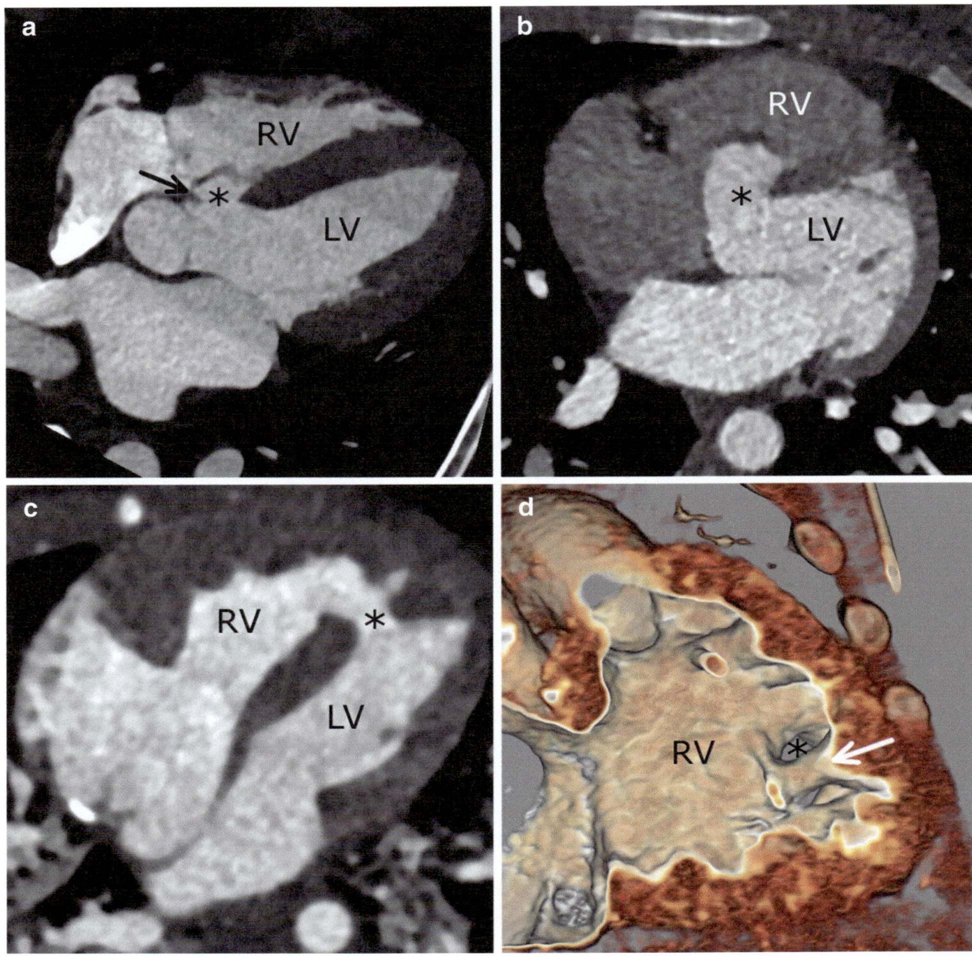

Fig. 46.4 (**a**) "Four-chamber view" in a patient with a perimembranous ventricular septal defect. Note that the defect (*) is in fibrous continuity with the tricuspid and aortic valve (black arrow). (**b**) Axial image in a patient whose perimembranous defect has been closed spontaneously by aneurysmal tricuspid valve tissue (*). (**c**) "Four-chamber view" in an infant with an apical muscular ventricular septal defect (*). (**d**) 3D volume-rendered image from the same patient in which the free wall of the right ventricle has been cropped, providing an "en-face" view of the ventricular septum. The defect is inferior to the moderator band (white arrow) (*RV* right ventricle, *LV* left ventricle)

completely surrounded by muscular septum (Fig. 46.4). Based on the location on the right ventricular aspect of the septum, muscular defects may be further described as inlet, mid-muscular, apical, or outlet. Perimembranous defects (also known as membranous, conoventricular, or infracristal defects) border the membranous septum, usually resulting in fibrous continuity between the tricuspid and aortic valves (Fig. 46.4). These defects are the most common type of VSD, accounting for up to 80% of defects identified at surgery or autopsy [26]. Subarterial defects (also known as supracristal, conal, infundibular, subpulmonary, or doubly committed) result in fibrous continuity between the pulmonary and aortic valves, due to an absence of a subpulmonary infundibulum. Perimembranous and subarterial defects can be accompanied by aortic valve prolapse into the VSD, resulting in insufficiency. Subaortic membranes and muscular subpulmonary stenosis are also more frequent in patients with a perimembranous defect.

The degree of left to right shunt through a ventricular septal defect is dependent upon the size of the defect and the relative pulmonary and systemic vascular resistances. Small defects are generally well tolerated and often close spontaneously. Significant pulmonary overcirculation from a large ventricular-level shunt results in left atrial and ventricular dilation, poor growth, and tachypnea. If left unrepaired, large defects will result in irreversible pulmonary hypertension.

Patent Ductus Arteriosus

A patent ductus arteriosus is a normal finding in nearly every fetus, with usual functional closure within 24 h after full-term birth [27]. Excluding premature infants, the ductus remains patent in about 1 in 2000 live births, accounting for about 7% of congenital heart disease [28]. With decreasing gestation or other congenital abnormalities, the incidence increases dramatically [29].

With CT, an isolated ductus is usually visualized as a tubular structure extending from the underside of the aortic arch just below the origin of the left subclavian artery to the

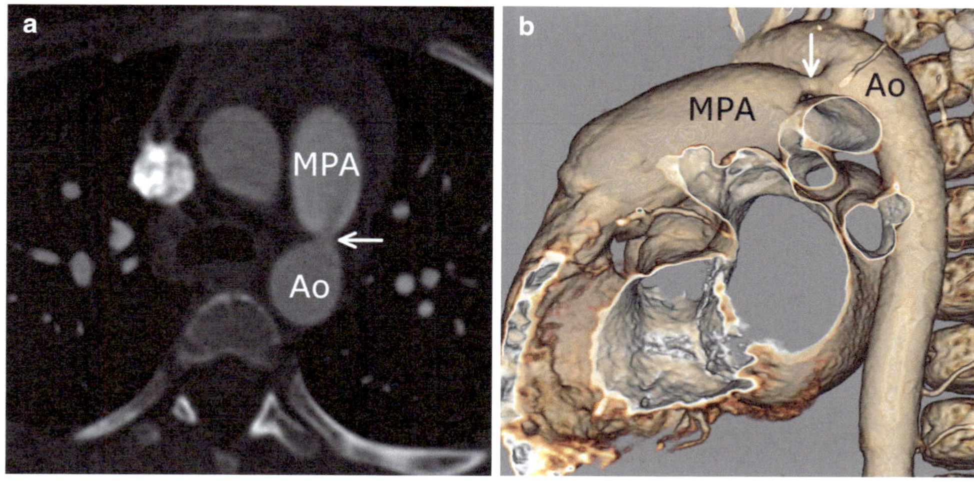

Fig. 46.5 Axial (**a**) and 3D volume-rendered (**b**) images in an infant with a patent ductus arteriosus (arrow) connecting the main pulmonary artery to the descending aorta (*MPA* main pulmonary artery, *Ao* aorta)

left pulmonary artery (Fig. 46.5). The communication between the pulmonary arteries is best seen on sagittal or oblique reformations. After birth, it usually begins constricting at the pulmonary artery end, resulting in a conical shape. However, numerous ductal shapes have been described [30]. The ductus arteriosus may become aneurysmal and calcified, which may lead to rupture [30, 31]. The degree of left to right shunt through a patent ductus is dependent upon its diameter and length. The shunt is also dependent on the difference between the pulmonary and systemic vascular resistances [16]. The physiology is similar to VSD, with large shunts resulting in left atrial and ventricular dilation, poor growth, and tachypnea.

Atrioventricular Septal Defects

Atrioventricular septal defects (AVSD), also known as atrioventricular canal or endocardial cushion defects, account for 5% of congenial heart disease. Atrioventricular septal defects include a wide array of anatomical variants that all have a defect of the atrioventricular septum and abnormalities of the atrioventricular (AV) valves. Many of these patients will have a common AV valve, with shunting at both the atrial and ventricular levels (Fig. 46.6). Others will have separate AV valves, with shunting at the atrial level, ventricular level, both, or neither. The defect in the atrioventricular septum results in an aortic valve that is displaced anteriorly, creating a "gooseneck deformity" that predisposes these patients to subaortic stenosis. The physiology and clinical manifestations of atrioventricular septal defects are determined by the location and amount of left to right shunting that occurs through the corresponding septal defects, along with the degree of AV valve regurgitation. Patients with primarily atrial-level shunting will have physiology similar to a secundum ASD, while patients with significant ventricular-level shunting will have physiology similar to a VSD (see above). The presence of significant AV valve regurgitation will worsen any heart failure symptoms present. CT findings include atrial enlargement, ventricular dilation (right, left, or biventricular), and dilation of the pulmonary arteries.

Pulmonary Stenosis

Pulmonary stenosis most commonly occurs at the level of the valve but can also be intracavitary (within the body of the RV), subvalvar (in the pulmonary infundibulum), supravalvar (at the sinotubular junction), or more distal in the main or branch pulmonary arteries. It is imperative to determine the level(s) of obstruction, as treatment differs accordingly. Typical pulmonary valve stenosis results in doming of the pulmonary valve in systole, but the valve can also be dysplastic with markedly thickened leaflets. Subvalvar obstruction can occur in isolation but is usually found in the presence of other abnormalities. "Double-chambered right ventricle" is a specific form of pulmonary obstruction resulting from hypertrophied muscle bundles that septate the RV into a high-pressure proximal chamber and a low-pressure distal chamber. It is mostly associated with ventricular septal defects of the perimembranous variety. Peripheral pulmonic stenosis occurs mainly with other cardiac defects but can be an isolated lesion. Diffuse pulmonary artery hypoplasia/stenosis is found in both Alagille and Williams syndromes. In addition to visualization of the level of pulmonary outflow obstruction (Fig. 46.7), cardiac CT will reveal right ventricular hypertrophy.

Tetralogy of Fallot

Tetralogy of Fallot (TOF) is the most common form of cyanotic congenital heart disease. The multiple anatomic features of Tetralogy of Fallot result from a single anatomic

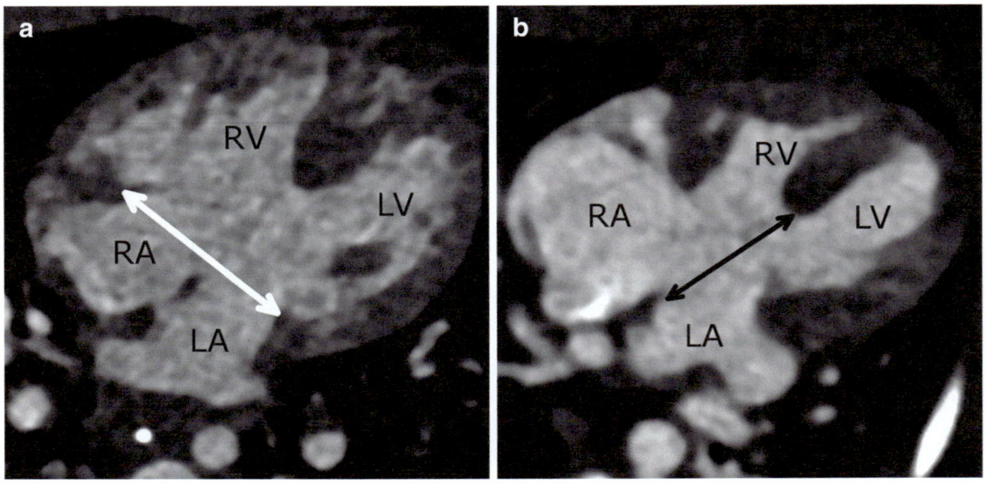

Fig. 46.6 Axial (**a**) and "four-chamber view" (**b**) in two infants with an atrioventricular septal defect. In the "complete" form, there is a common atrioventricular valve (white arrow) along with a large septal defect (black arrow), allowing shunting at the atrial and ventricular levels (*RA* right atrium, *RV* right ventricle, *LA* left atrium, *LV* left ventricle)

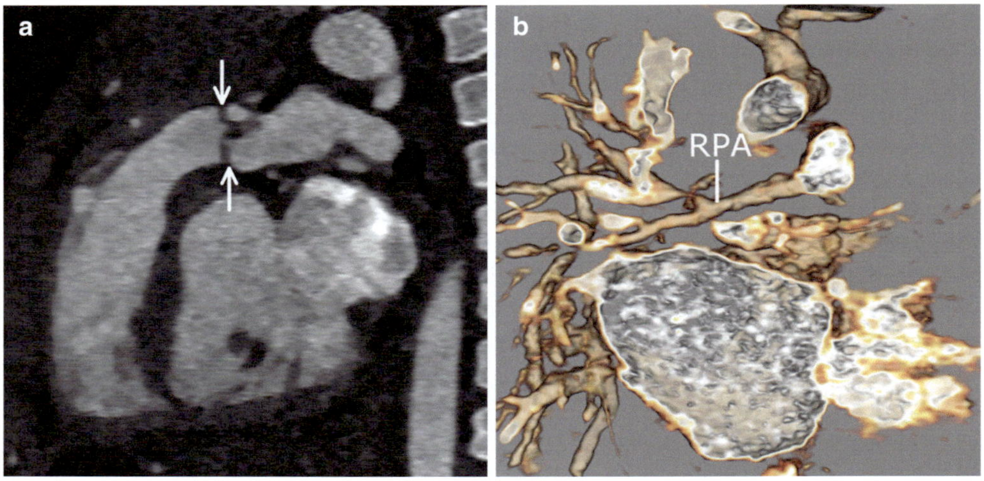

Fig. 46.7 (**a**) Oblique sagittal image in a child with valvar pulmonary stenosis. Note the thickened valve (arrows). (**b**) 3D volume-rendered image views from an anterior perspective, revealing diffuse hypoplasia of the right pulmonary artery, along with multiple focal stenoses, in a child with Williams syndrome (*RPA* right pulmonary artery)

abnormality: the anterior displacement of the outlet septum. This anterior displacement results in subvalvar pulmonary stenosis, an anterior malalignment VSD, "over-riding" aorta, and right ventricular hypertrophy (Fig. 46.8). The pulmonary valve is often hypoplastic or stenotic. The most extreme form of this abnormality is TOF with pulmonary atresia (also known as pulmonary atresia with VSD), in which the pulmonary circulation is supplied by a patent ductus arteriosus or aortopulmonary collateral arteries (Fig. 46.8d). CT has been shown to be highly accurate in the identification of pulmonary arterial supply in these patients [32, 33]. In 3–5% of patients with TOF, the pulmonary valve is absent, resulting in massive dilation of the main and branch pulmonary arteries during fetal development. The physiology and clinical manifestations of TOF are primarily influenced by the degree of pulmonary outflow obstruction. In those with no or little obstruction to pulmonary blood flow, the oxygen saturations may be normal, and the physiology is similar to a large VSD, with pulmonary overcirculation and heart failure symptoms. As the degree of pulmonary obstruction increases, cyanosis becomes more apparent as a result of increased right to left shunting through the VSD.

Aortic Stenosis

The precise incidence of aortic stenosis is unknown, given that minor malformations such as bicuspid aortic valve are common and generally asymptomatic in childhood. The incidence of congenital bicuspid valve is 1.3% of the population, making it the most common congenital heart defect. Approximately 60–75% of patients with congenital aortic stenosis are at the valve level [16]. Among those with congenital aortic stenosis, about 20% will have some other form of congenital heart disease, most commonly VSD, coarctation, or PDA [34]. Bicuspid aortic valve is common in patients with Turner's syndrome, while patients with supravalvar stenosis often have Williams syndrome. Similar to pulmonary stenosis, aortic stenosis can occur in the subvalvar, valvar, or supravalvar region

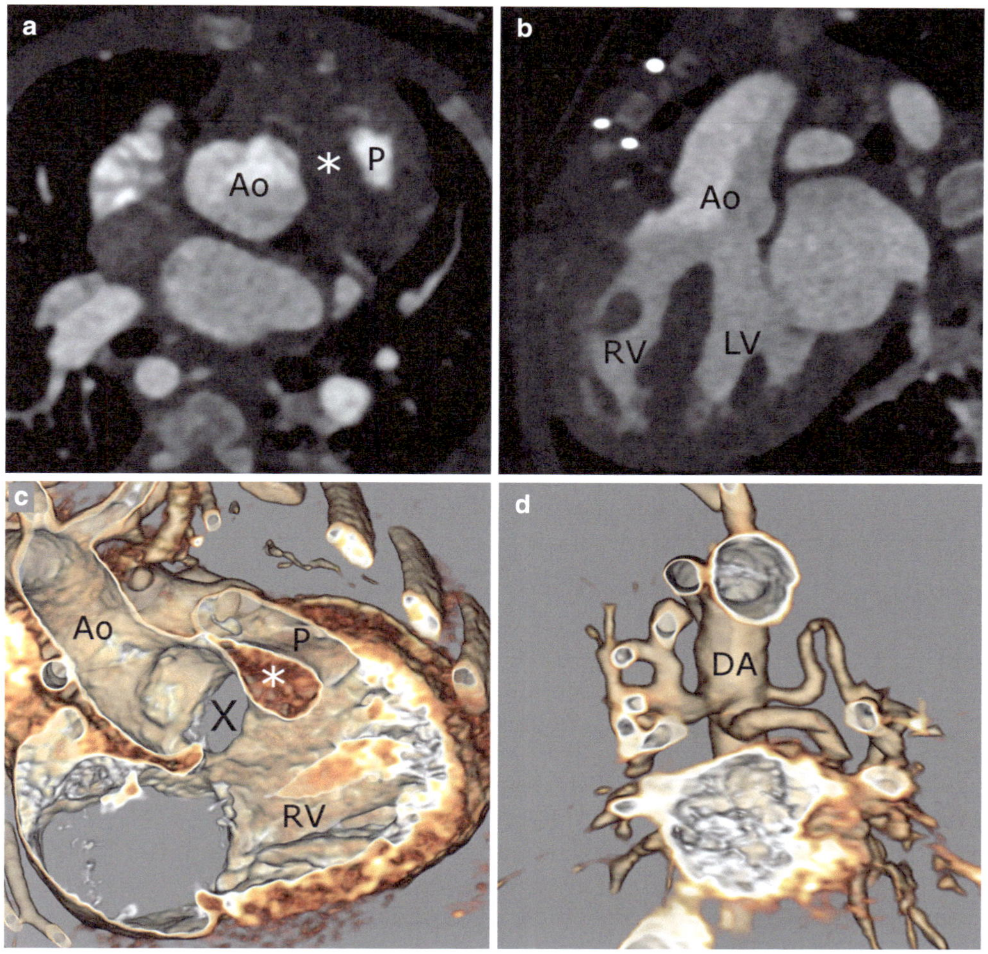

Fig. 46.8 (**a**) Axial image in an infant with tetralogy of Fallot. Anterior deviation of the outlet septum (*) results in narrowing of the pulmonary outflow. (**b**) Oblique sagittal slice in the same infant, displaying an aorta that "overrides" the ventricular septum. (**c**) 3D volume-rendered image from the same patient in which the free wall of the right ventricle has been cropped, providing an "en-face" view of the ventricular septum. The anteriorly deviated outlet septum (*) is seen, resulting in pulmonary outflow obstruction and a ventricular septal defect (X). (**d**) 3D volume-rendered reconstruction viewed from an anterior perspective in an infant with tetralogy of Fallot with pulmonary atresia and multiple AP collaterals. Three collateral vessels are seen originating from the descending aorta, with one vessel supplying the right lung and two collateral vessels supplying the left lung (*Ao* aorta, *P* pulmonary outflow, *RV* right ventricle, *LV* left ventricle, *DA* descending aorta)

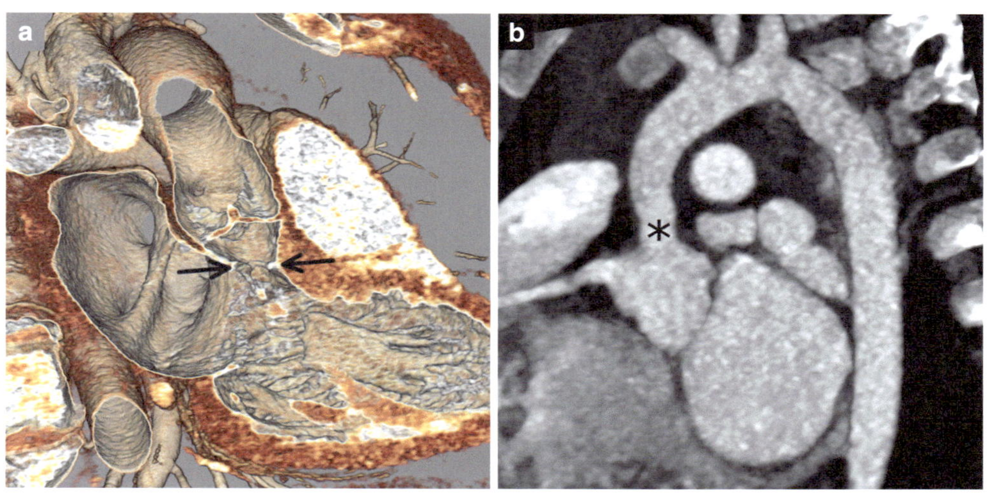

Fig. 46.9 (**a**) 3D volume-rendered reconstruction in a "three-chamber view" demonstrating a discrete subaortic membrane (arrows). (**b**) Maximum intensity projection image in an oblique sagittal plane revealing supravalvar aortic stenosis consisting of tubular hypoplasia of the ascending aorta (*)

(Fig. 46.9). Abnormal septal tissue growth, as in hypertrophic cardiomyopathy, and subaortic membranes can cause obstruction below the level of the valve. Valvar aortic stenosis is most commonly due to abnormal fusion of valve commissures, resulting in a bicuspid or, rarely, unicuspid aortic valve. Older patients with aortic stenosis often have thickened, dysplastic valves. The most common form of a bicuspid aortic valve results from fusion of the right and left leaflets. Supravalvar stenosis is the least common form and commonly occurs at the level of the sinotubular junction, although diffuse hypoplasia of the ascending aorta can occur as well. In addition to visualization of the level of obstruction, cardiac CT will reveal left ventricular hypertrophy.

Coarctation of the Aorta

Coarctation of the aorta makes up 6–8% of congenital heart disease [16]. Genetically, it is associated with Turner's syndrome. There is also a strong association between coarctation and bicuspid aortic valve. Coarctation of the aorta typically occurs in the region distal to the left subclavian artery (also known as the aortic isthmus), near the insertion of the ductus arteriosus. CT will often reveal a discrete narrowing with a prominent posterior "shelf" (Fig. 46.10). This type is classically called the "juxtaductal" or "adult" form, although it is often seen in infants as well. Older children and adults will often display aortic dilatation proximal and distal to the coarctation and collateral vessel formation on CT. Collateral circulation is usually via the internal mammary arteries and the intercostal arteries. Increased collateral flow through intercostal vessels can cause notching of the posterior third through eighth ribs. The "infantile" or "preductal" form results in long-segment hypoplasia of the aortic isthmus (Fig. 46.10). Neonates with severe coarctation of the aorta can present in cardiogenic shock once the ductus arteriosus closes. CT has been shown to be highly accurate in describing the anatomy prior to surgical repair [35, 36].

Interrupted Aortic Arch

Interrupted aortic arch (IAA) is defined as the lack of luminal continuity between the ascending and descending aortas. [37]. The type of interrupted arch is classified by the location of the discontinuity. Type A interruptions are located distal to the left subclavian artery and are associated with aortopulmonary window defects [38]. If the interruption occurs between the left carotid and subclavian arteries, it is called a type B interruption. Type B interruptions frequently have a ventricular septal defect with posterior malalignment of the outlet septum and are the most common form of IAA. An interruption between the brachiocephalic and left carotid arteries (or between the carotid arteries) is called a type C interruption, which is the rarest form of IAA. Like other critical left-sided obstructive lesions (critical aortic stenosis, coarctation, hypoplastic left heart syndrome, etc.), neonates with IAA are dependent on ductal patency for systemic blood flow (Fig. 46.11). Those that are not identified and treated after birth present with cardiogenic shock as the ductus arteriosus closes. Management is thus aimed at maintaining patency of the ductus arteriosus until ultimate surgical intervention. CT has been shown to be useful in this diagnosis and often plays an important role in the preoperative evaluation [39].

Ebstein's Anomaly

Ebstein's anomaly is a rare disorder, making up <1% of congenital heart defects. It has been associated with maternal

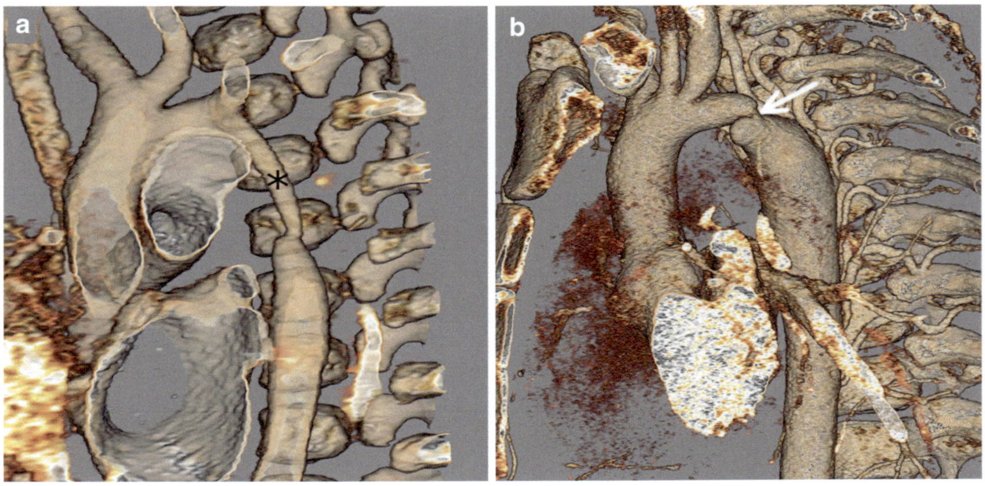

Fig. 46.10 Both images are 3D volume-rendered reconstructions in an oblique sagittal "candy cane view." Image (**a**) displays the "infantile form" of coarctation, with tubular hypoplasia of the aortic isthmus (*). Image (**b**) reveals the "adult form" of coarctation, with discrete narrowing (arrow) and numerous engorged spinal and intercostal arteries due to collateral flow

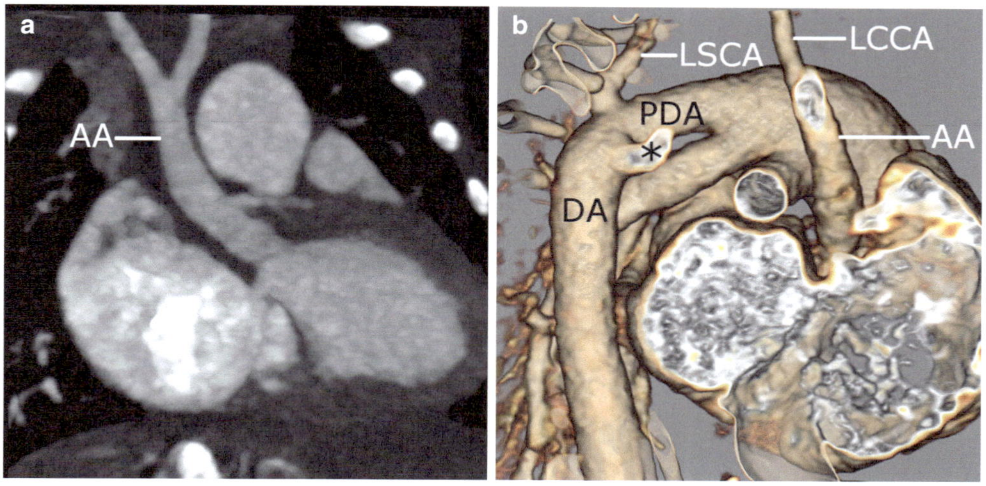

Fig. 46.11 These images are from a neonate with a type B interrupted aortic arch and aberrant right subclavian artery. (**a**) Maximum intensity projection image in a coronal plane displaying a hypoplastic ascending aorta that supplies only the right and left common carotid arteries. (**b**) 3D volume-rendered reconstruction viewed from a rightward perspective, revealing the interruption between the left common carotid and left subclavian arteries. A patent ductus arteriosus provides blood flow to the descending aorta, which supplies an aberrant right subclavian artery (*) (*AA* ascending aorta, *DA* descending aorta, *LCCA* left common carotid artery, *LSCA* left subclavian artery, *PDA* patent ductus arteriosus)

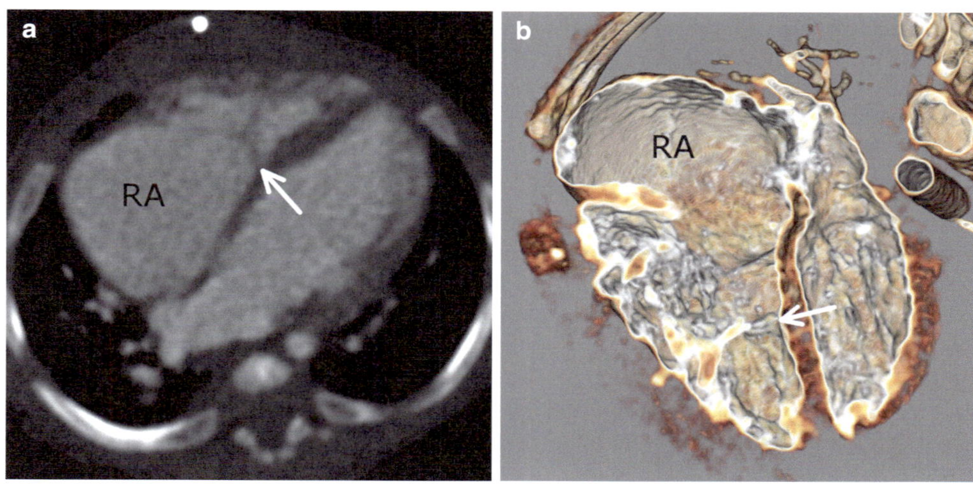

Fig. 46.12 Axial image (**a**) and 3D volume-rendered reconstruction in a "four-chamber view" (**b**) in two patients with Ebstein's anomaly. Note the apical displacement of the septal leaflet of the tricuspid valve (arrow) and dilation of the right atrium (RA)

lithium use, but most cases are idiopathic. The typical CT finding of Ebstein's anomaly consists of apical and rotational displacement of the tricuspid valve toward the right ventricular outflow tract, resulting in an "atrialization" of the right ventricle proximal to the displaced tricuspid valve [40] (Fig. 46.12). There is also a tethering and fenestration of the TV anterior leaflet with significant TV annular dilation. As a result of tricuspid regurgitation during fetal life, neonates with severe Ebstein's anomaly often display massive dilation of the right atrium and atrialized right ventricle.

The physiology and clinical presentation in Ebstein's anomaly depend on the degree of tricuspid regurgitation and atrialization of the right ventricle. Neonates with severe tricuspid regurgitation and atrialization lack the ability to generate adequate flow across the pulmonary valve, resulting in right to left shunting at the atrial level and cyanosis. Those with the most extreme forms are ductal dependent at birth, requiring single-ventricle palliation strategies [41]. Those with the mildest disease experience minimal symptoms. Other patients with greater severity require surgical intervention later in childhood or early adulthood due to progressive exercise intolerance.

Transposition of the Great Arteries (D-TGA)

This anomaly is characterized by concordant atrioventricular connections with discordant ventriculoarterial connec-

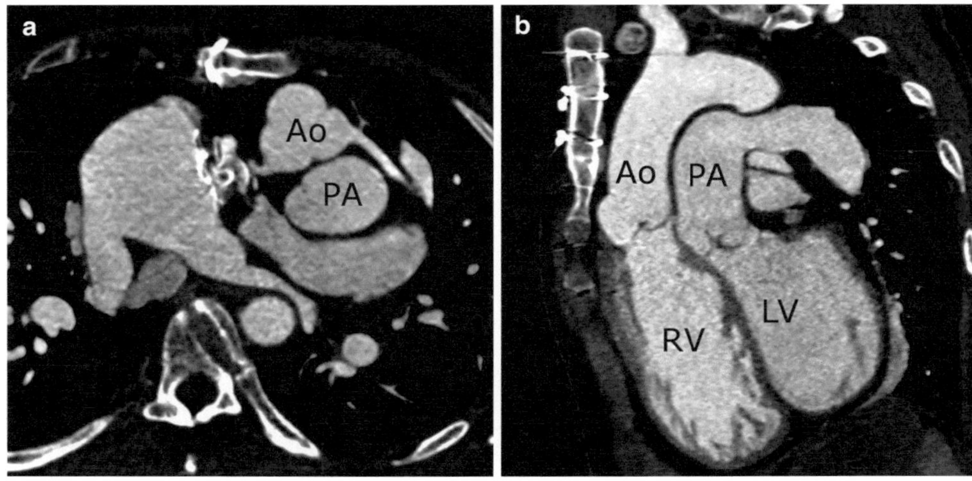

Fig. 46.13 Images (**a**) (axial) and (**b**) (oblique sagittal) are from an adult with transposition of the great arteries (D-TGA). The aorta and main pulmonary artery leave the heart in a parallel fashion, with the aortic valve residing anterior and rightward of the pulmonary valve (*Ao* aorta, *PA* main pulmonary artery, *RV* right ventricle, *LV* left ventricle)

tions. The aorta arises from the morphologic right ventricle and is anterior and to the right of the pulmonary artery, which arises from the morphologic left ventricle (Fig. 46.13). Many patients with TGA also have an ASD and/or VSD as well. In transposition physiology, the systemic and pulmonary circulations are in parallel, whereas in the usual circulation, these circulations are in series. As a result, pulmonary venous blood (oxygenated) is pumped back into the pulmonary circulation, while systemic venous return (deoxygenated) is pumped back into the systemic circulation. In order to be compatible with life, there must be mixing of these two circulations to allow oxygenated blood to reach the systemic circulation and deoxygenated blood to reach the lungs. Mixing is most effective at the atrial level, but shunting at the ventricular level or patent ductus arteriosus can contribute as well. Neonates with inadequate mixing of the two circulations are born with severe hypoxemia, which can result in metabolic acidosis due to inadequate oxygen delivery. These patients are usually taken for emergent balloon septostomy in the catheterization laboratory to create a larger atrial communication, allowing increased mixing. Coronary abnormalities are common and must be defined prior to surgical repair. Neonatal repair is the standard approach, with rare exceptions.

Congenitally Corrected Transposition (L-TGA)

Congenitally corrected transposition of the great arteries (CCTGA) results when the atrioventricular and ventriculoarterial connections are both discordant. Hence, CCTGA is occasionally called "double discordance." This results in systemic venous return emptying normally into the morphologic RA and then passing through a mitral valve into the morphologic LV and then to the lungs via the pulmonary artery. This pulmonary venous return then empties normally into a morphologic LA, then through a tricuspid valve and a morphologic RV, and then to the body via the aorta (Fig. 46.14). The vast majority of these patients will have associated lesions, including VSD, pulmonary stenosis, and/or tricuspid valve abnormalities [42]. In the context of usual atrial arrangement ("situs solitus"), the morphologic right ventricle will be left sided ("L-looped") causing the aortic valve to be positioned anterior and leftward to the pulmonary valve (Fig. 46.14). Hence, this defect is occasionally called "L-TGA." However, approximately 5% of these patients have a mirror-image atrial arrangement ("situs inversus"), which would cause the aortic valve to be positioned anterior and rightward. For this reason, CCTGA is the preferred terminology.

Viewed in simplistic terms, the physiology in CCTGA is normal, given that systemic venous return is sent to the lungs and pulmonary venous return is sent to the body. This is supported by the fact that some patients are not identified until their teenage years or adulthood. However, the right ventricle is not morphologically designed to pump against systemic afterload, and many patients will eventually develop heart failure symptoms due to right ventricular systolic dysfunction. Presentation and symptomology during childhood are largely dependent on associated abnormalities (VSD, pulmonary stenosis, or complete heart block).

Double Outlet Right Ventricle

In double outlet right ventricle, both great arteries arise from the right ventricle (≥50% of the circumference of both arterial valves). Usually, both arterial valves are separated from the mitral valve by a muscular infundibulum. The orientation of the great arteries is variable. There is always a VSD, which is conventionally described in relation to the nearest arterial valve: subaortic, subpulmonary, doubly committed (equally close to both arterial valves), or noncommitted (distant from both arterial valves). Often, the arterial valve that is furthest from the VSD has subvalvar or valvar stenosis, but there is great variability with this lesion. The most common variant of DORV has a subaortic VSD and pulmonary stenosis

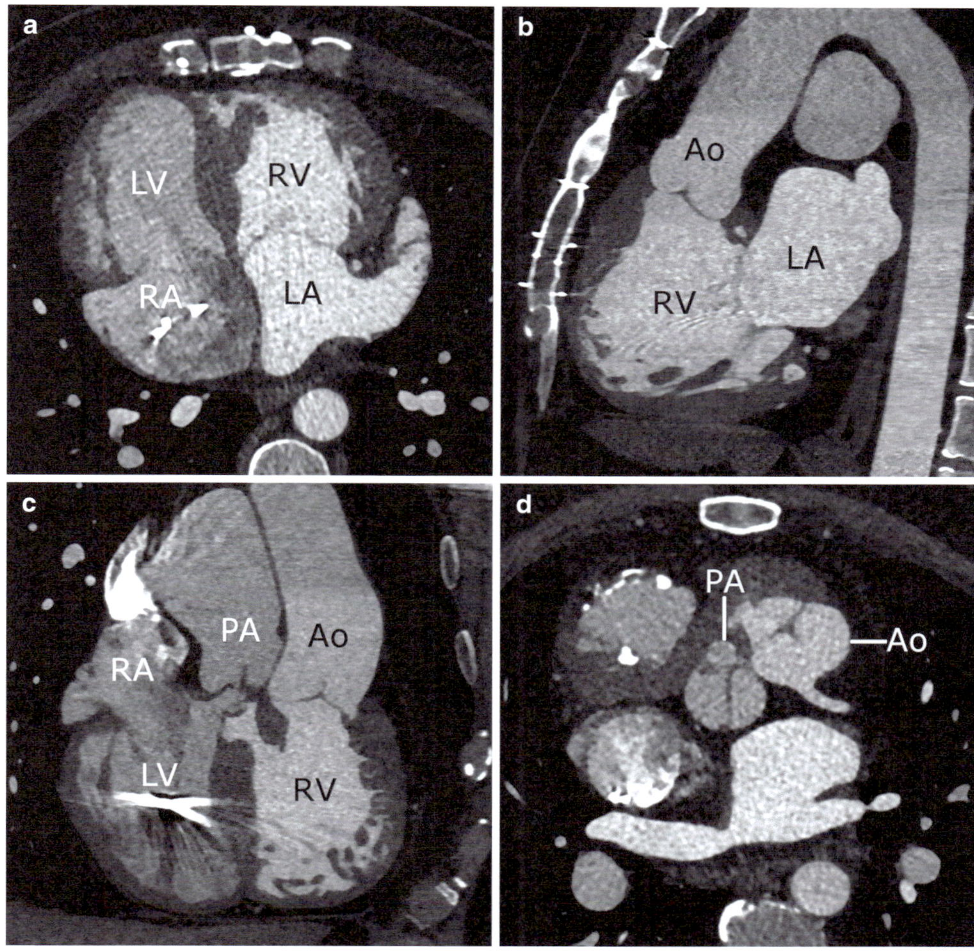

Fig. 46.14 These images are from a patient with congenitally corrected transposition (L-TGA). (**a**) In this axial image, the discordant atrioventricular connections can be seen. (**b**) Oblique sagittal image revealing "double discordance," with the left atrium supplying the right ventricle, which is connected to the aorta. (**c**) Oblique coronal image, also displaying "double discordance" (right atrium→left ventricle→pulmonary artery). As is common with this defect, one can identify a repaired ventricular septal defect, subpulmonary obstruction, parallel great arteries, and a pacemaker lead in the left ventricle due to complete heart block. (**d**) This axial image reveals that the aortic valve is anterior and leftward to the pulmonary valve (*RA* right atrium, *RV* right ventricle, *LA* left atrium, *LV* left ventricle, *MPA* main pulmonary artery, *Ao* aorta)

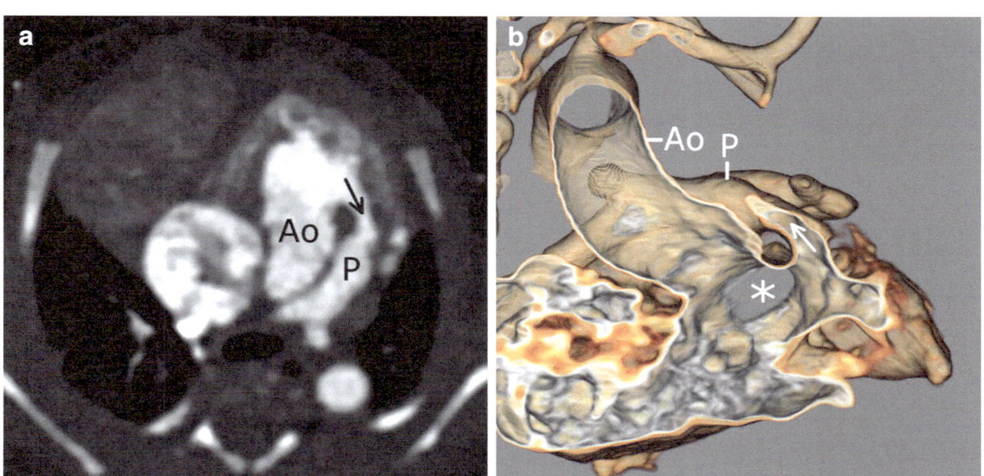

Fig. 46.15 (**a**) Axial image in an infant with double outlet right ventricle and a subaortic ventricular septal defect. The pulmonary outflow (arrow) reveals both subvalvar stenosis and valvar hypoplasia. (**b**) 3D volume-rendered image from the same patient in which the free wall of the right ventricle has been cropped, providing an "en-face" view of the ventricular septum. Note the subaortic ventricular septal defect (*) and pulmonary outflow obstruction (arrow). (*Ao* aorta, *P* pulmonary artery)

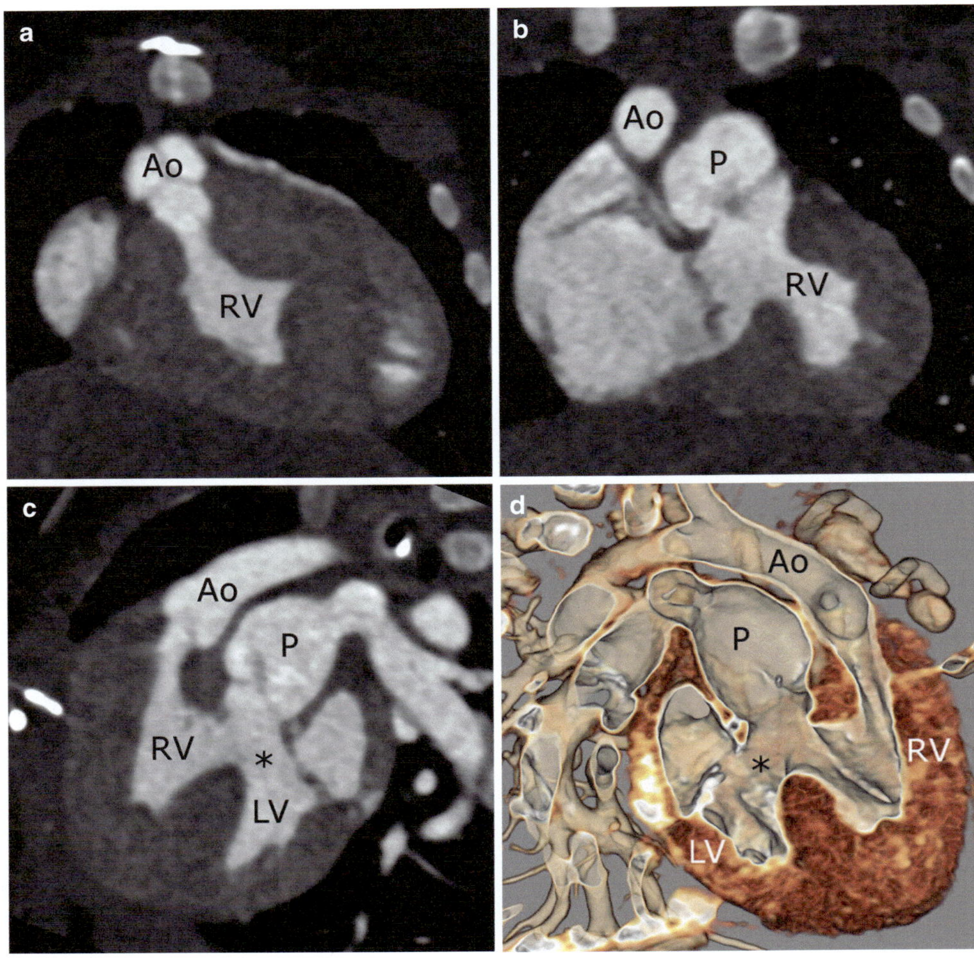

Fig. 46.16 These images are from an infant with double outlet right ventricle and subpulmonary ventricular septal defect. Images (**a**, **b**) are coronal slices (**a** is anterior to **b**), revealing a hypoplastic aortic outflow and widely patent pulmonary outflow from the right ventricle. The aorta is seen diving posteriorly to the right of the pulmonary artery. Images (**c**, **d**) (oblique sagittal plane and 3D volume-rendered reconstruction), showing both great arteries originating from the right ventricle. The only egress from the left ventricle is via a ventricular septal defect (*). Note the narrow aortic outflow and hypoplastic aortic arch (*Ao* aorta, *P* pulmonary, *RV* right ventricle, *LV* left ventricle)

(Fig. 46.15), providing physiology similar to TOF (see above), depending on the degree of pulmonary outflow obstruction. The type with a subpulmonary VSD is commonly called a "Taussig-Bing anomaly" and is associated with aortic hypoplasia and/or coarctation (Fig. 46.16). A biventricular repair is feasible in most cases, with baffling of the VSD patch to one of the arterial valves.

Truncus Arteriosus

Truncus arteriosus is a rare cardiac anomaly, accounting for <1% of congenital heart disease. It is frequently associated with DiGeorge syndrome, especially when it is paired with an interrupted aortic arch. With truncus arteriosus (also known as "common arterial trunk"), there is a single artery supplying blood flow to the pulmonary, systemic, and coronary circulations (Fig. 46.17). A subarterial-type ventricular septal defect is always present, although there may be additional septal defects. The single semilunar valve, often called the "truncal valve," can be comprised of one to five leaflets, although it is most often tricuspid [43]. Truncal valve stenosis and/or regurgitation is common. Truncus arteriosus is classified into three major types. Type 1 is the most common, with a short main pulmonary artery segment giving rise to both branch pulmonary arteries. Type II is the next most common, with both branch pulmonary arteries arising separately from the posterior wall of the common trunk. In type III, both pulmonary arteries separate from the lateral walls of the common trunk. A type IV was described in the original classification scheme, but is no longer felt to represent a form of truncus arteriosus [44]. Aortic arch abnormalities are a common associated finding, with 21–36% of patients having a right aortic arch and approximately 11% displaying an interrupted arch [45]. Truncus arteriosus is one of the few congenital heart defects in which a ductus arteriosus is not present during fetal life, unless there is an interrupted aortic arch.

Vascular Rings

Vascular rings represent approximately 1–2% of congenital heart defects, although this is likely an underestimate, since

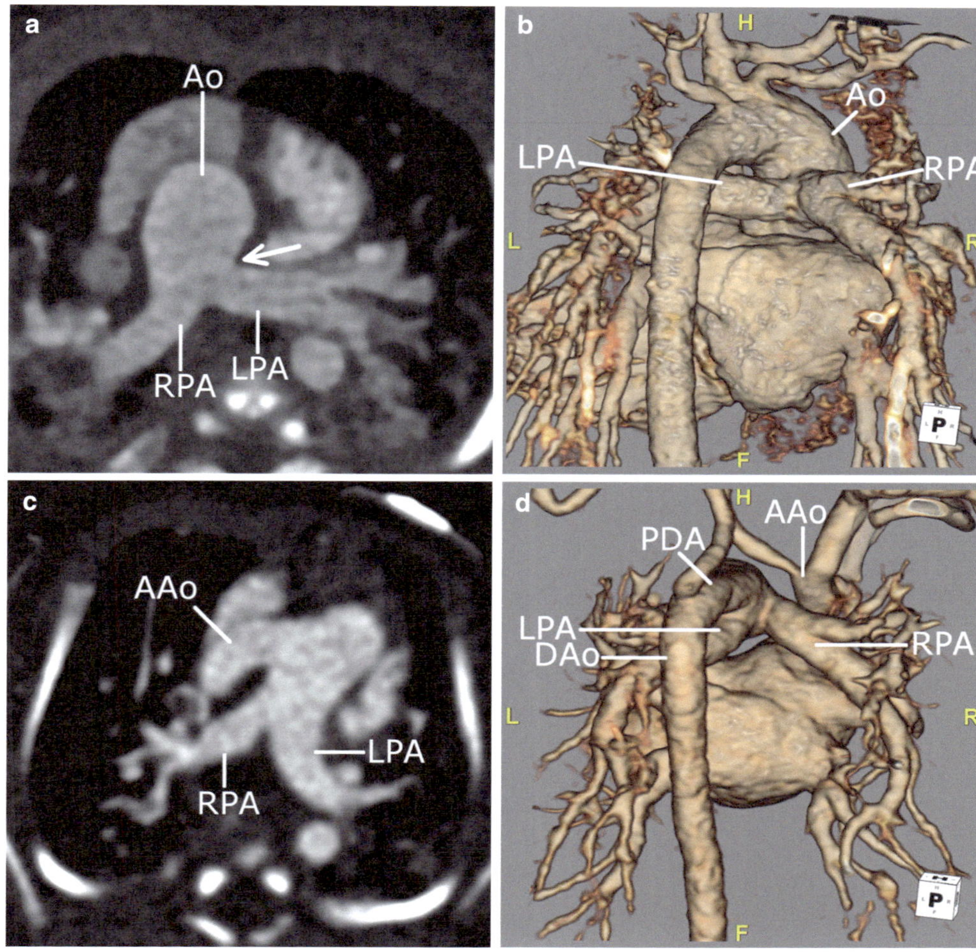

Fig. 46.17 Images (**a**, **b**) (axial slice, 3D volume-rendered reconstruction viewed from posterior perspective) are from an infant with truncus arteriosus type I. Aortic and pulmonary blood flow originate from a common trunk. A short main pulmonary artery (arrow) supplies a right and left pulmonary artery, with the aorta continuing superiorly to provide systemic blood flow. Images (**c**, **d**) are from an infant with truncus arteriosus and an interrupted aortic arch (axial slice, 3D volume-rendered reconstruction viewed from posterior perspective). A common trunk supplies the pulmonary arteries and a hypoplastic ascending aorta. The descending aorta is supplied by a patent ductus arteriosus (*Ao* aorta, *RPA* right pulmonary artery, *LPA* left pulmonary artery, *AAo* ascending aorta, *PDA* patent ductus arteriosus, *DAo* descending aorta)

many patients are asymptomatic [46]. Vascular rings are defined as an arch anomaly in which the trachea and esophagus are completely encircled by vascular structures (or ligamentous structures with a vascular origin). There is insufficient space to cover all forms of vascular rings, but the two most common types are double aortic arch and right aortic arch with an aberrant left subclavian and diverticulum of Kommerell. A more detailed coverage of vascular rings can be found in a review by Ramos-Duran [47].

A double aortic arch results from persistence of both the right and left aortic arches, each providing ipsilateral carotid and subclavian arteries (Fig. 46.18). In 80% of cases, the right arch is dominant, with the left arch being smaller and more caudal [47]. Occasionally a segment of either arch is atretic (usually left), persisting only as a ligamentous structure.

A right aortic arch with an aberrant left subclavian and diverticulum of Kommerell is the second most commonly identified vascular ring. In this lesion, after coursing to the right of the trachea, an outpouching (Kommerell's diverticulum) can be seen originating from the leftward aspect of the descending aorta behind the trachea and esophagus, continuing as the left subclavian (Fig. 46.19). Also originating from this diverticulum, a ductus arteriosus or ligamentum connects anteriorly to the main pulmonary artery to complete the ring.

With any type of confirmed or suspected vascular ring, CT can accurately define the aortic arch anatomy and branching pattern [48]. In addition, evidence of airway compression can also be identified [49]. The caliber and course of vascular structures can help identify ligamentous structures, such as the ligamentum arteriosum or an atretic arch segment [47].

Anomalous Pulmonary Venous Connections

By definition, a pulmonary venous connection is anomalous whenever it connects to a structure other than another pulmonary vein or the left atrium. Totally anomalous pulmonary venous connection (TAPVC) occurs when the entire lung drains anomalously. When at least one pulmo-

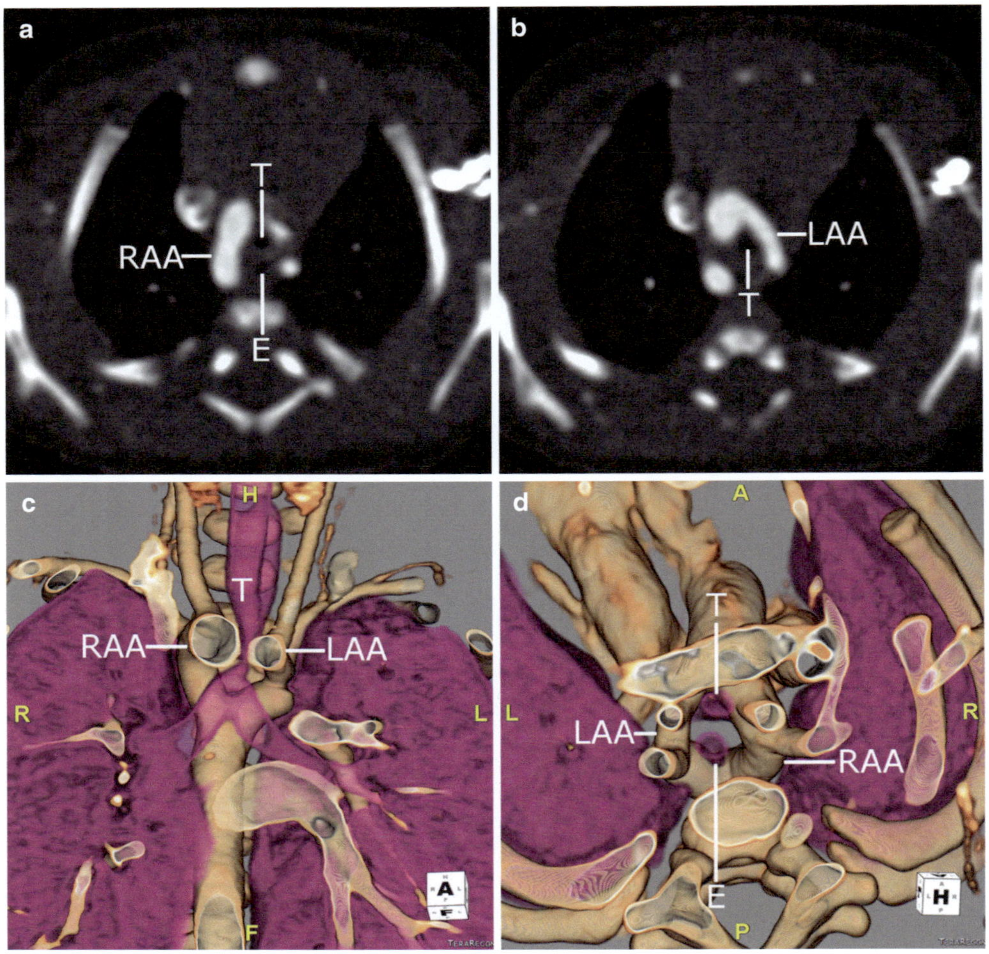

Fig. 46.18 Infant with a double aortic arch. (**a**) Axial slice, showing a dominant right aortic arch. (**b**) Axial slice, displaying a smaller left aortic arch. (**c**, **d**) 3D volume-rendered reconstructions viewed from anterior (**c**) and superior (**d**) perspectives, revealing both aortic arches encircling the trachea and esophagus. Note that the right arch is superior to the left arch, which is typical. The double arch results in significant compression of the trachea in this patient (*RAA* right aortic arch, *LAA* left aortic arch, *T* trachea, *E* esophagus)

nary vein connects normally to the left atrium, the condition is considered partially anomalous pulmonary venous connection (PAPVC). CT performs particularly well in the visualization of anomalous pulmonary venous connections and is being increasingly used in patients with these lesions [50, 51].

The most widely accepted classification system of TAPVC splits the types into supracardiac, cardiac, infracardiac (or infradiaphragmatic), and mixed [46] (Fig. 46.20). With exception of the mixed type, all of the pulmonary veins usually connect to a confluence posterior to the left atrium prior to reaching the ultimate location of drainage. In the supracardiac type, this confluence drains superiorly via a vertical vein into either the innominate vein, the azygous vein, or the superior vena cava. In the cardiac type, the pulmonary venous system drains directly into the coronary sinus or the right atrium. With the infracardiac type, the confluence drains inferiorly via a vertical vein, through the diaphragm and into the portal venous system, hepatic veins, or the inferior vena cava. The mixed type contains a combination of any of the above, without any pulmonary veins draining normally to the left atrium. In order to be compatible with life, there must be an atrial-level communication with right to left shunting. The clinical sequelae are primarily determined by the presence/absence of obstruction to pulmonary venous return. Obstruction generally occurs within the pulmonary venous drainage itself (e.g., within the vertical vein) but can also occur at the atrial septum. The presence of obstruction results in profound cyanosis and decreased cardiac output. Obstruction is most commonly seen in patients with infracardiac TAPVC and is rarely seen with the cardiac type, with the supracardiac type falling somewhere between the two [52]. Although TAPVC is considered a "cyanotic heart defect," with right to left shunting at the atrial level, the anomalous pulmonary venous connection itself also results in a left to right shunt, with oxygenated blood directed back into the pulmonary circulation. Therefore, patients with unobstructed TAPVC

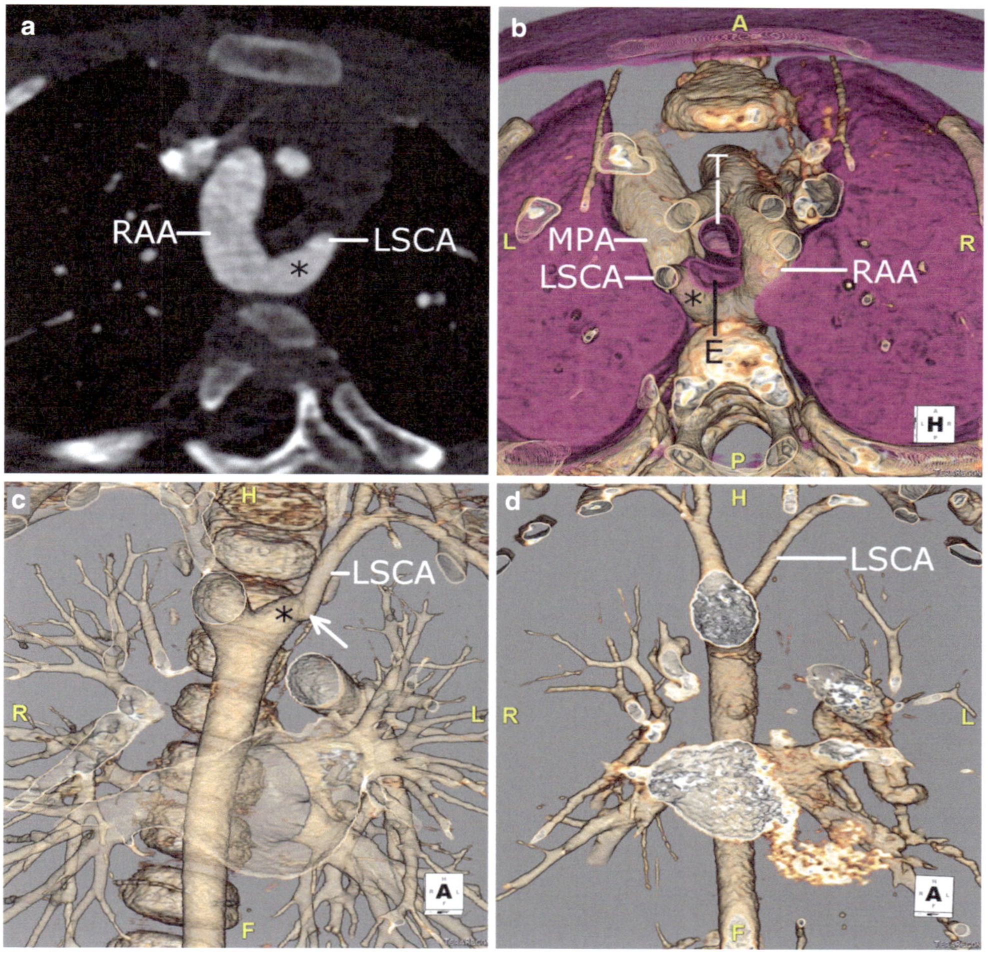

Fig. 46.19 Images (**a**–**c**) are from a child with a right aortic arch with an aberrant left subclavian artery and diverticulum of Kommerell. (**a**) Axial image showing an aortic arch to the right of the trachea, supplying an aberrant left subclavian artery. Note the diverticulum (*), which has a similar caliber to the aortic arch. (**b**) 3D volume-rendered reconstruction viewed from a superior perspective, revealing the right aortic arch and aberrant left subclavian partially encircling the trachea and esophagus. A ligamentum (not seen) will connect the diverticulum (*) and main pulmonary artery, completing the vascular ring. (**c**) 3D volume-rendered reconstruction viewed from an anterior perspective. The arrow highlights that there is an "elbow" and distinct change in caliber as the diverticulum transitions to the left subclavian artery, created by the presence of a ligamentum tethering this area to the main pulmonary artery. Image (**d**) is taken from a patient that also has a right aortic arch with an aberrant left subclavian. This patient did not have a vascular ring. In contrast to image (**c**), note the absence of a diverticulum of Kommerell, resulting in a left subclavian artery with a uniform caliber and course. This appearance of the left subclavian confirms the absence of a ligamentum in this area and, therefore, the absence of a vascular ring (*RAA* right aortic arch, *LSCA* left subclavian artery, *MPA* main pulmonary artery, *T* trachea, *E* esophagus)

display a net physiology of a large left to right shunt, with right ventricular enlargement, tachypnea, and poor weight gain.

There are numerous forms of PAPVC, with descriptions encompassing pulmonary venous connections to nearly any systemic vein in the thorax. The most common types of PAPVC are drainage of the left upper pulmonary vein to the innominate vein, right upper pulmonary vein to the superior vena cava, and right pulmonary veins draining into the inferior vena cava (Fig. 46.21). The last type is the typical drainage seen with the entity called "Scimitar syndrome." The physiology of PAPVC is similar to an atrial septal defect, with dilation of the right ventricle and pulmonary arteries noted on CT. The degree of left to right shunting is determined by the proportion of the lung draining anomalously. Patients with anomalous drainage of a single segment of the lung are often asymptomatic, while patients with numerous lung segments draining anomalously will have symptoms similar to unobstructed TAPVC. Obstruction is rare with PAPVC.

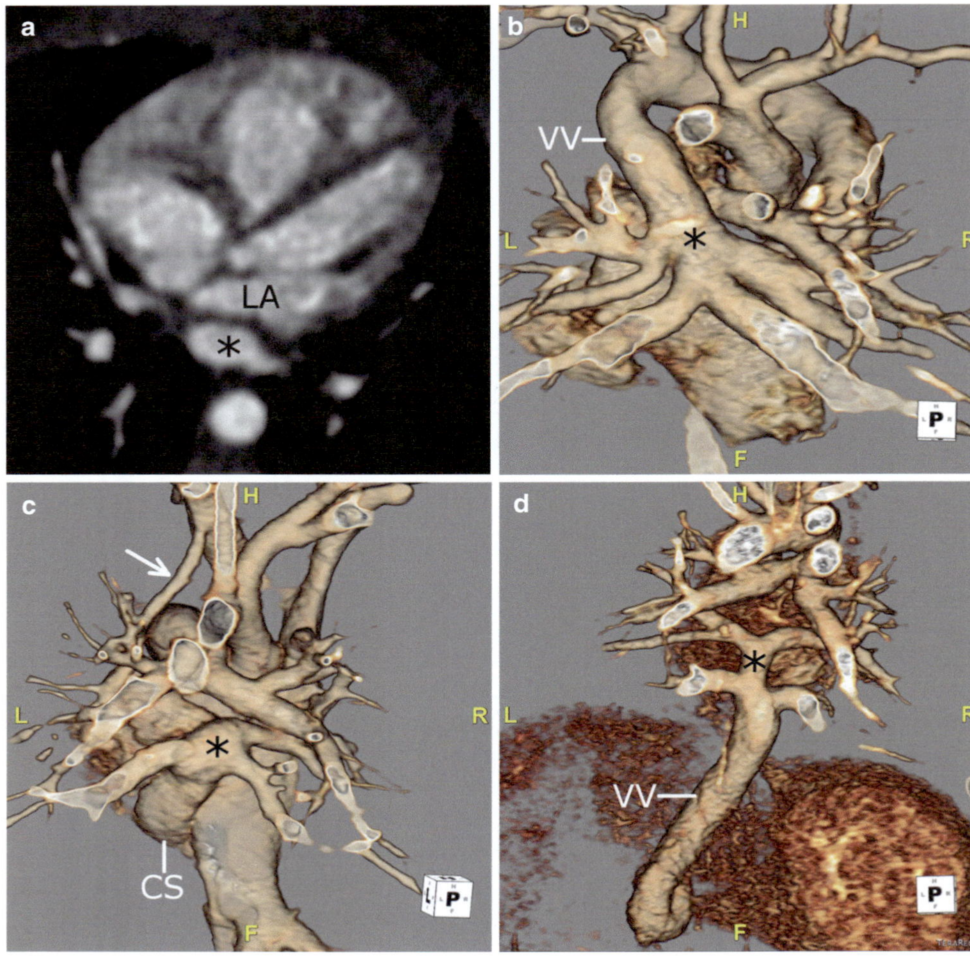

Fig. 46.20 These images are all from infants with totally anomalous pulmonary venous connections. (**a**) Axial image displaying a confluence (*) posterior to the left atrium, which should alert the imager to the presence of totally anomalous pulmonary venous connection. Images (**b–d**) are 3D volume-rendered reconstructions viewed from a posterior perspective. (**b**) Supracardiac connection, with a vertical vein connecting the pulmonary venous confluence (*) to the brachiocephalic vein. (**c**) Cardiac connection, with the confluence (*) draining into the coronary sinus. This patient has mixed connections, as the left upper pulmonary vein drains into the brachiocephalic vein. (**d**) Infracardiac connection, with a vertical vein connecting the pulmonary venous confluence (*) to the portal vein (*LA* left atrium, *VV* vertical vein, *CS* coronary sinus)

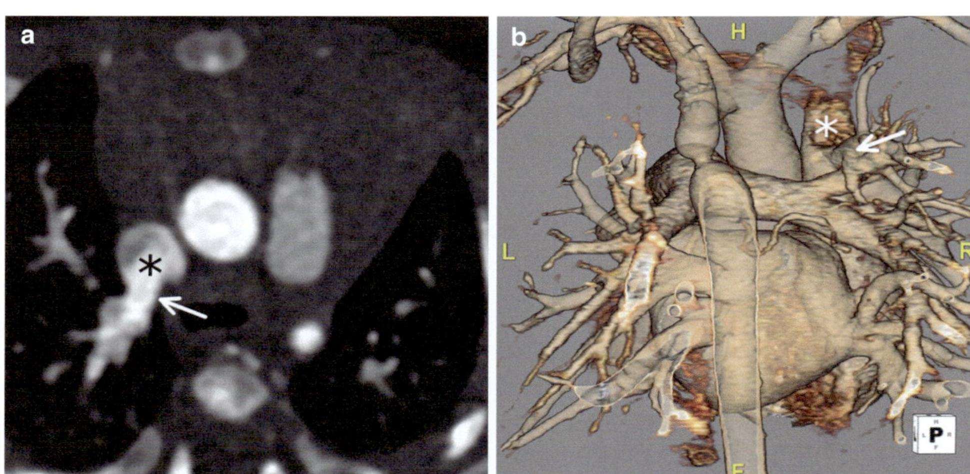

Fig. 46.21 (**a**) Axial image, showing an anomalous connection of the right upper pulmonary vein (arrow) to the superior vena cava (*). (**b**) 3D volume-rendered reconstruction in the same patient viewed from a posterior perspective, displaying the right upper pulmonary vein (arrow) connecting to the superior vena cava (*) superior to the right pulmonary artery. The other pulmonary veins can be seen draining normally into the left atrium. A discrete coarctation of the aorta can be seen as well, which was the primary indication for the scan

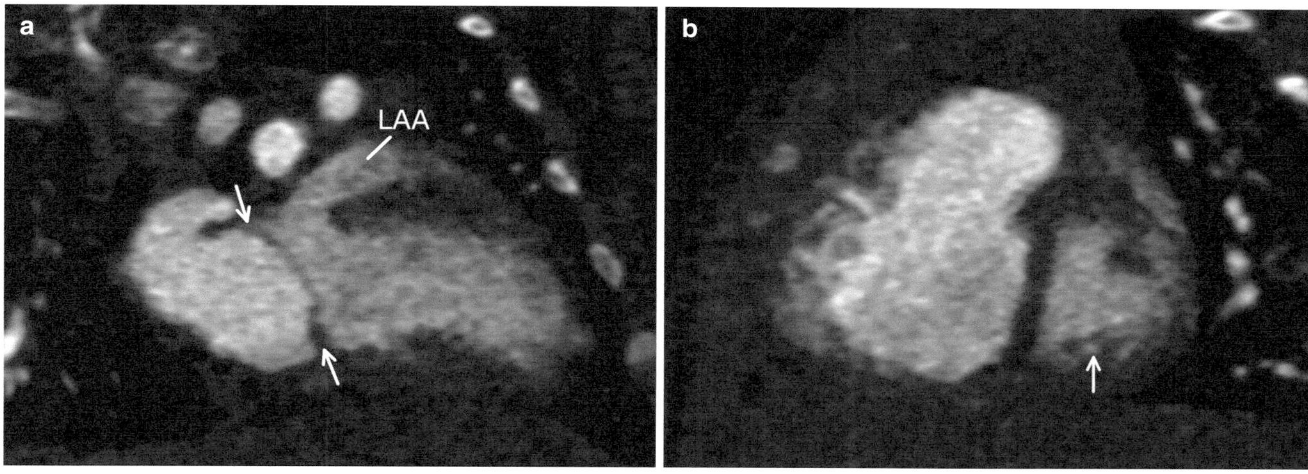

Fig. 46.22 (**a**) "Two-chamber view" in a patient with cor triatriatum. A membrane (arrows) can be seen above the left atrial appendage, distinguishing it from a supramitral ring. (**b**) "Short axis" image, showing the small orifice in the membrane (arrow), through which all pulmonary venous return must flow (*LAA* left atrial appendage)

Cor Triatriatum

Cor triatriatum is a rare defect, making up less than 0.5% of all congenital heart disease [53]. In the classic form, there is a discrete membrane within the left atrium separating the pulmonary venous return from the remainder of the left atrium. In these patients, the only route of egress for pulmonary venous blood toward the mitral valve is an opening within the membrane. This membrane is always located in the area between the pulmonary venous ostia and left atrial appendage (Fig. 46.22). This location differentiates it from a supramitral ring, which is located between the left atrial appendage and mitral valve. A variant from classical cor triatriatum is called "partial cor triatriatum," in which some, but not all, of the pulmonary veins are separated from the left atrium by the membrane.

Hypoplastic Left Heart Syndrome

Hypoplastic left heart syndrome (HLHS) includes a spectrum of left ventricular hypoplasia that results in a small left ventricle that is unable to support a full cardiac output. The most common type is a combination of mitral atresia and aortic atresia, followed by mitral and aortic stenosis [54]. In patients with aortic atresia, there remains a small ascending aorta which must remain patent in order for retrograde filling of the coronary arteries (Fig. 46.23). While diffuse aortic hypoplasia is very common in patients with HLHS, a discrete coarctation is present in 80% of patients [55]. Special attention should be given in evaluating the atrial septum, tricuspid valve, pulmonary veins, and coronary arteries, as HLHS is associated with abnormalities in each.

After birth, ductal patency is required for systemic perfusion in patients with HLHS, with aortic arch and coronary flow occurring in a retrograde fashion. An unrestrictive atrial communication is essential as well, particularly in patients with mitral atresia. Pulmonary venous return is thus diverted to the right ventricle, which must then supply both systemic and pulmonary flows. There are no curative surgical options for HLHS, but there is a staged single-ventricle palliative approach that is discussed in Chap. 47 ("The Use of Cardiovascular CT in Repaired CHD").

Pulmonary Atresia with Intact Ventricular Septum

The variable anatomy in pulmonary atresia with an intact ventricular septum includes the size of the right ventricular cavity, tricuspid valve, and coronary arteries. The right ventricular size correlates with the tricuspid valve annular size. The tricuspid valve is frequently abnormal, varying from small and stenotic to large and Ebstein's-like. The tricuspid annulus size also correlates with the presence of coronary fistulae connecting to the right ventricle [56] (Fig. 46.24). These fistulae can often be identified on CT and are a major prognostic factor in survival [57]. Some patients have a condition termed "right ventricular-dependent coronary circulation," in which stenosis or atresia in the proximal coronary arteries results in coronary flow that is dependent on flow from these fistulae. The pulmonary atresia is often complete muscular atresia of the right ventricular outflow tract, but a third of patients have a patent right ventricular outflow tract with membranous atresia of the pulmonary valve leaflets [56]. Regardless of the type of pulmonary atresia, there is usually an intact main pulmonary artery segment.

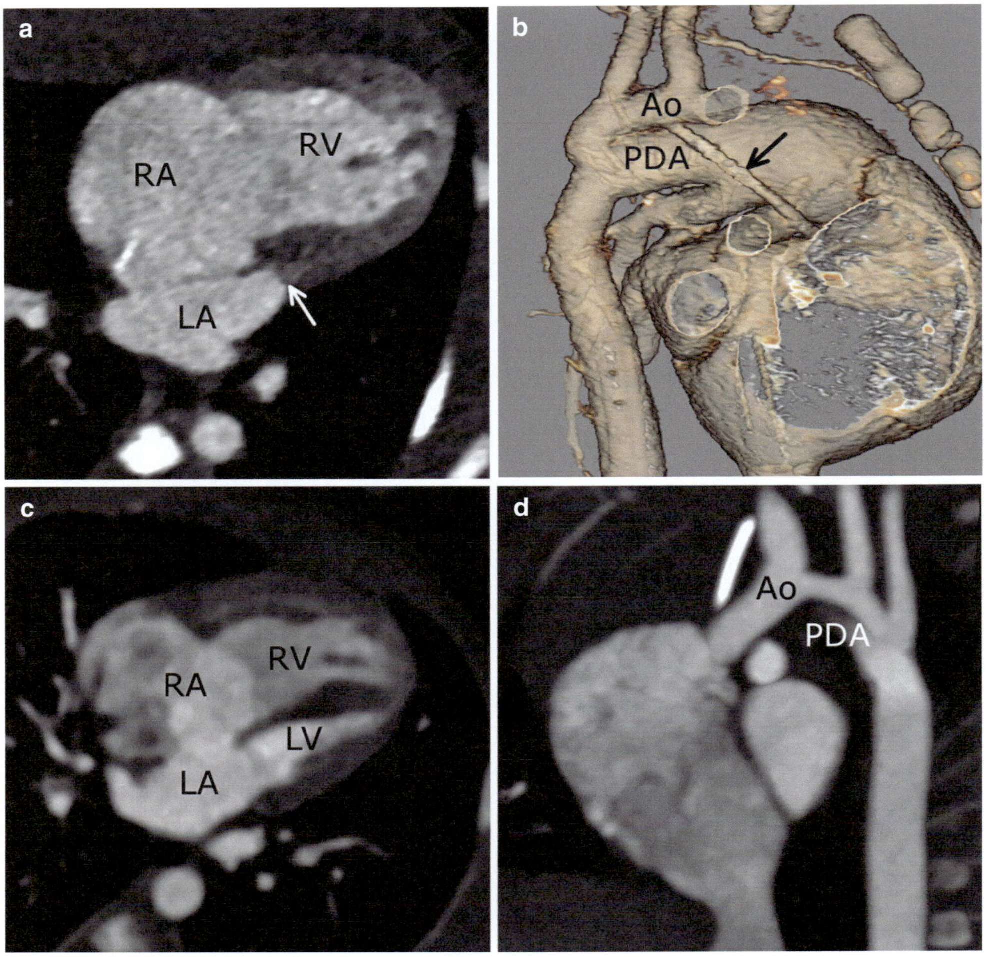

Fig. 46.23 (**a**) "Four-chamber view" in an infant with mitral and aortic atresia, resulting in hypoplasic left heart syndrome. The atretic mitral valve is seen (white arrow), with severe hypoplasia of the left ventricle. An atrial septal defect is seen, which is the only route of egress from the left atrium. The right atrium and ventricle are dilated. (**b**) 3D volume-rendered reconstruction in the same patient viewed from a rightward perspective. Aortic blood flow is supplied via a patent ductus arteriosus. Note the severely hypoplastic ascending aorta (black arrow), which is filled retrograde to supply blood flow to the coronary arteries. (**c**) "Four-chamber view" in another infant with a less severe form of hypoplastic left heart, with mitral and aortic stenosis. The mitral valve is patent, resulting in a mildly hypoplastic left ventricle. Contrast can be seen streaming left to right through an atrial septal defect. (**d**) Maximum intensity projection in a "candy cane" view from the same patient, displaying a hypoplastic aortic arch with a coarctation. There is a patent ductus arteriosus, augmenting flow to the descending aorta (*RA* right atrium, *RV* right ventricle, *LA* left atrium, *LV* left ventricle, *Ao* aorta, *PDA* patent ductus arteriosus)

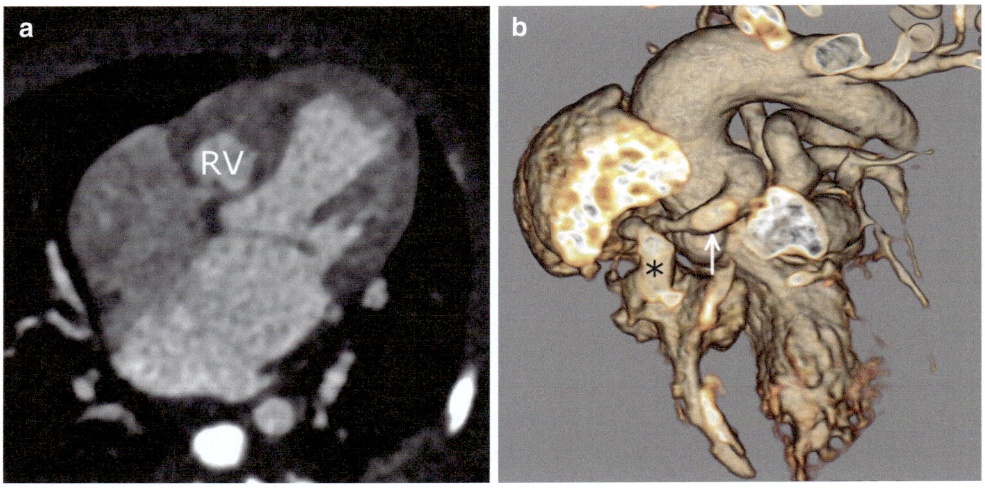

Fig. 46.24 (**a**) "Four-chamber view" in an infant with pulmonary atresia with intact ventricular septum. The tricuspid valve is patent, but the lack of egress results in the typical appearance of a severely hypoplastic and hypertensive right ventricle (RV). (**b**) 3D volume-rendered reconstruction in another patient with this diagnosis, revealing a dilated single coronary artery (arrow) with a large fistulous connection to the right ventricle (*), which is common in this entity

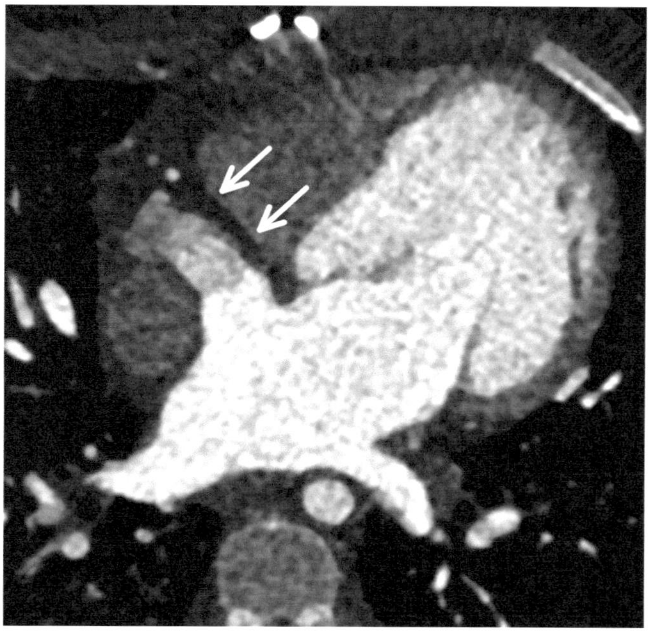

Fig. 46.25 "Four-chamber view" in a patient with tricuspid atresia. Note the plate-like atresia (arrows), which is the typical appearance in this lesion and represents the absence of a connection between the right atrium and ventricle. This patient has an intact ventricular septum, so no contrast is seen in the right ventricle

Tricuspid Atresia

In patients with tricuspid atresia, there is no connection between the right atrium and right ventricle, with no identifiable tricuspid valve tissue (Fig. 46.25). This contrasts with the mitral atresia that is seen with HLHS, in which there is a connection between the left atrium and left ventricle, but an atretic valve can generally be identified. The right ventricle is generally hypoplastic, dependent on the presence and size of a ventricular septal defect. If the ventricular septum is intact, there is usually pulmonary atresia [16]. If a VSD is present, the right ventricular outflow is generally patent. Tricuspid atresia is accompanied by concordant ventriculoarterial connections in 80% of patients, but transposed and double outlet ventricular connections have been described [58]. Patients with tricuspid atresia who have transposed great arteries will often have aortic arch hypoplasia or coarctation. All patients with tricuspid atresia are ultimately managed with staged single-ventricle palliation (see Chap. 45).

Double Inlet Left Ventricle

Double inlet left ventricle (DILV) is comprised of both AV valves emptying into the morphologic left ventricle (Fig. 46.26). A diminutive right ventricle is always present but exists as simply an outlet chamber. The size of the right ventricle is dependent upon the size of the VSD, which is its only source of inflow. There is variability in the orientation of the ventricles and arterial arrangement. The most common form of DILV has transposition of the great arteries with L-looped ventricles (morphologic right ventricle on the left) and a leftward and anterior aorta. The second most common form has transposition of the great arteries with D-looped ventricles (morphologic right ventricle on the right) and a rightward and anterior aorta. Only 15% of patients with DILV have normally related great arteries, an anomaly also known as "Holmes heart." Those with transposition are prone to also have aortic arch hypoplasia, while those with normally related great arteries generally display pulmonary stenosis [16]. All patients with DILV are ultimately managed with staged single-ventricle palliation (see Chap. 45).

Systemic Venous Abnormalities

The two most common systemic venous abnormalities are persistent left superior vena cava (LSVC) and interrupted inferior vena cava. Neither abnormality results in symptoms, but their identification is important prior to interventional catheterizations or surgical procedures requiring cardiopulmonary bypass.

The incidence of LSVC is approximately 0.3% and is much greater in those with congenital heart disease [59]. It can be identified on CT, starting at the confluence of the left jugular and subclavian veins. It is variable in size and often empties into an enlarged coronary sinus (Fig. 46.27). Occasionally, the coronary sinus is "unroofed," and the LSVC is seen emptying directly into the left atrium. There is occasionally an innominate vein that serves as a communication between the LSVC and RSVC.

An interrupted IVC carries an incidence of about 0.2% and has a strong association with left atrial isomerism [60]. It results from an absence of a hepatic segment of the IVC. The infra-hepatic segment of the IVC is routed via a dilated azygous system, which then empties into the atrium by way of the superior vena cava. While identification of the hepatic portion of the IVC by CT is dependent upon the site of contrast injection, scan delay, and length of scan field, a dilated azygous can often be identified lateral to the descending aorta regardless of the scan protocol (Fig. 46.28).

Heterotaxy Syndromes

Heterotaxy syndromes highlight the importance of the segmental approach to describing cardiac and extracardiac structures. Heterotaxy is generally described as an abnor-

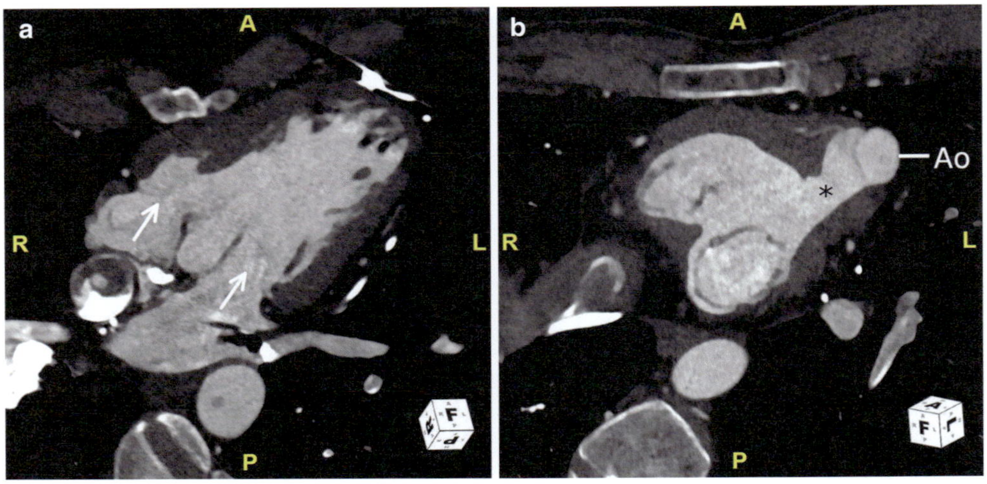

Fig. 46.26 (**a**) "Four-chamber view" in a patient with double inlet left ventricle. Both atrioventricular valves (arrows) empty into a morphologic left ventricle. (**b**) "Short axis view" in the same patient, showing a ventricular septal defect (*) leading to a left-sided morphologic right ventricle that supplies the aorta (Ao). This segmental arrangement is common with this entity, and the size of the ventricular septal defect must be described in order to determine the adequacy for providing systemic blood flow

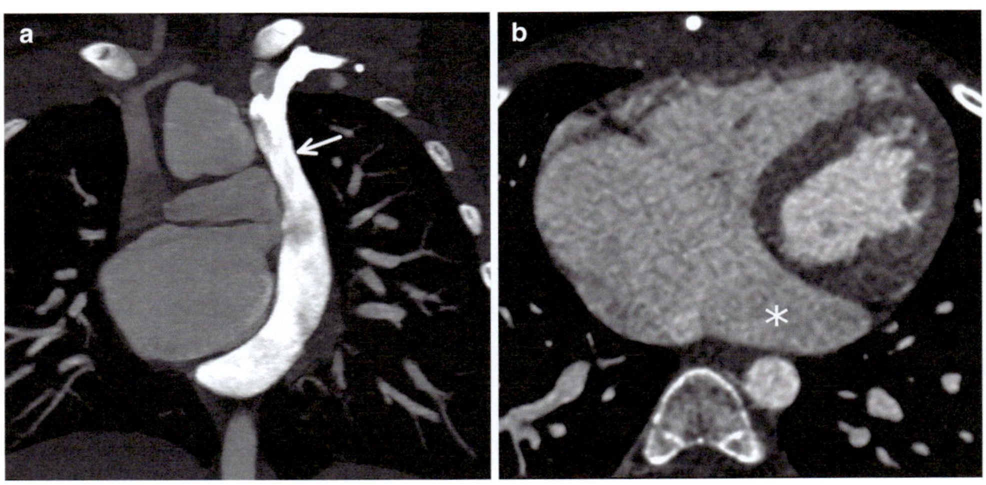

Fig. 46.27 (**a**) Maximum intensity projection in a coronal plane. Contrast has been injected in the left arm, displaying a persistent left superior vena cava (arrow) with connection to the coronary sinus. A bridging innominate vein is absent. (**b**) Axial image in another patient with a persistent left superior vena cava. Dilation of the coronary sinus (*) provides a clue to investigate for this entity

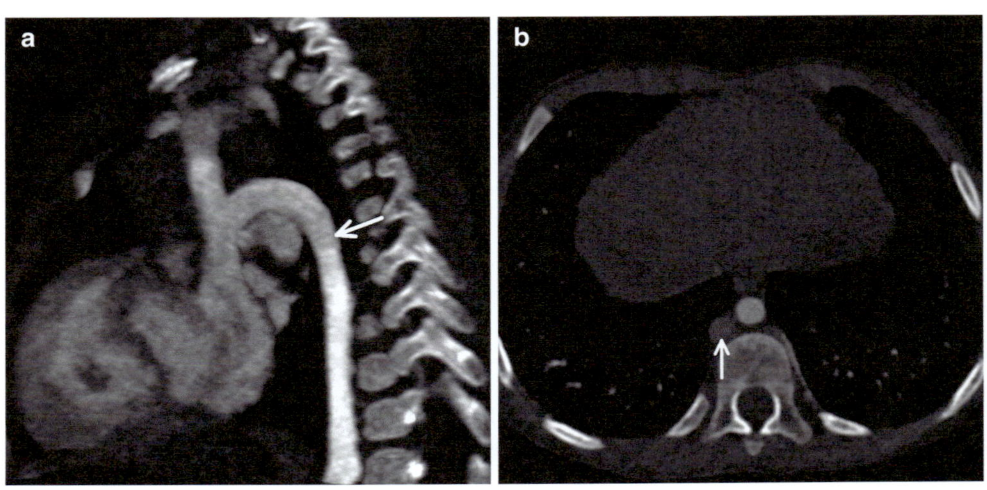

Fig. 46.28 (**a**) Maximum intensity projection in a sagittal plane. In this patient with interruption of the inferior vena cava, contrast was injected in the foot, opacifying a dilated azygous vein (arrow). (**b**) Axial image. Although contrast was injected via an upper extremity, this entity can be identified by visualizing the dilated azygous vein lateral to the descending aorta (arrow)

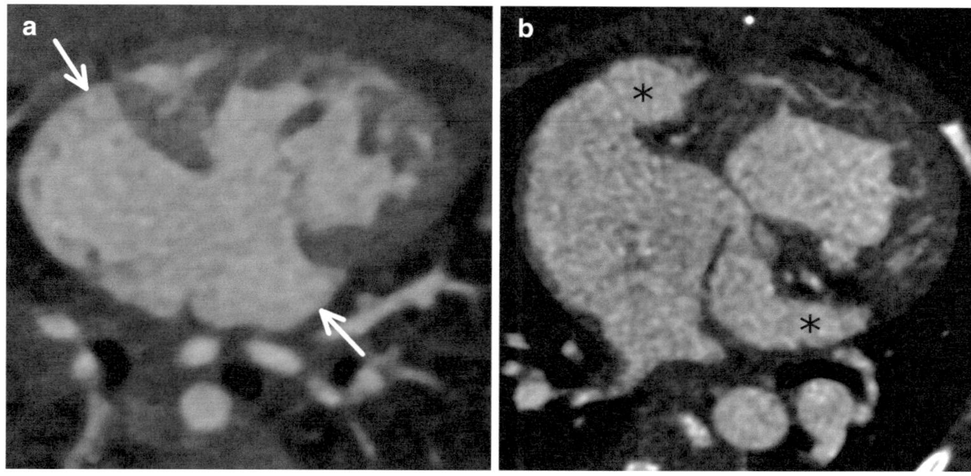

Fig. 46.29 (**a**) "Four-chamber view" in a patient with visceral heterotaxy and an unbalanced atrioventricular septal defect. Two broad-based atrial appendages are seen (arrows), consistent with right atrial isomerism. (**b**) "Four-chamber view" in another patient with visceral heterotaxy and an unbalanced atrioventricular septal defect. In this patient, there are two narrow atrial appendages (*), consistent with left atrial isomerism

mal arrangement of thoracic and abdominal viscera that is neither situs solitus (normal) nor situs inversus (mirror image). The complex of anomalies can be grouped into two categories, right atrial isomerism and left atrial isomerism, based on the appearance of the atrial appendages (Fig. 46.29). The former is also known as "asplenia syndrome" and the latter known as "polysplenia syndrome," although there is poor correlation between splenic anatomy and cardiac findings.

Right atrial isomerism is associated with TAPVC, absent coronary sinus, common atrium, pulmonary atresia, DORV, and single-ventricle physiology [61]. Left atrial isomerism is associated with an interrupted IVC, congenital heart block, and LVOT obstruction. Bilateral superior vena cavae and AVSD are common in both types of isomerism. The physiology is dictated by the constellation of findings.

References

1. Gatzoulis MA, Webb GD. Adults with congenital heart diseases: a growing population. Edinburgh: Churchill Livingstone; 2003.
2. Kaemmerer H, Stern H, Fratz S, Prokop M, Schwaiger M, Hess J. Imaging in adults with congenital cardiac disease (ACCD). Thorac Cardiovasc Surg. 2000;48(6):328–35. https://doi.org/10.1055/s-2000-8344.
3. Boxt LM. Magnetic resonance and computed tomographic evaluation of congenital heart disease. J Magn Reson Imaging. 2004;19(6):827–47. https://doi.org/10.1002/jmri.20077.
4. de Roos A, Roest AA. Evaluation of congenital heart disease by magnetic resonance imaging. Eur Radiol. 2000;10(1):2–6. https://doi.org/10.1007/s003300050002.
5. Gutierrez FR, Siegel MJ, Fallah JH, Poustchi-Amin M. Magnetic resonance imaging of cyanotic and noncyanotic congenital heart disease. Magn Reson Imaging Clin N Am. 2002;10(2):209–35.
6. Haramati LB, Glickstein JS, Issenberg HJ, Haramati N, Crooke GA. MR imaging and CT of vascular anomalies and connections in patients with congenital heart disease: significance in surgical planning. Radiographics. 2002;22(2):337–47; discussion 348–339. https://doi.org/10.1148/radiographics.22.2.g02mr09337.
7. Kulkarni A, Hsu HH, Ou P, Kutty S. Computed tomography in congenital heart disease: clinical applications and technical considerations. Echocardiography. 2016;33(4):629–40. https://doi.org/10.1111/echo.13147.
8. Han BK, Rigsby CK, Hlavacek A, Leipsic J, Nicol ED, Siegel MJ, Bardo D, Abbara S, Ghoshhajra B, Lesser JR, Raman S, Crean AM. Computed tomography imaging in patients with congenital heart disease part I: rationale and utility. An expert consensus document of the Society of Cardiovascular Computed Tomography (SCCT): endorsed by the Society of Pediatric Radiology (SPR) and the North American Society of Cardiac Imaging (NASCI). J Cardiovasc Comput Tomogr. 2015;9(6):475–92. https://doi.org/10.1016/j.jcct.2015.07.004.
9. Han BK, Lesser AM, Vezmar M, Rosenthal K, Rutten-Ramos S, Lindberg J, Caye D, Lesser JR. Cardiovascular imaging trends in congenital heart disease: a single center experience. J Cardiovasc Comput Tomogr. 2013;7(6):361–6. https://doi.org/10.1016/j.jcct.2013.11.002.
10. Goo HW, Park IS, Ko JK, Kim YH, Seo DM, Park JJ. Computed tomography for the diagnosis of congenital heart disease in pediatric and adult patients. Int J Cardiovasc Imaging. 2005;21(2–3):347–65; discussion 367. https://doi.org/10.1007/s10554-004-4015-0.
11. Leschka S, Oechslin E, Husmann L, Desbiolles L, Marincek B, Genoni M, Pretre R, Jenni R, Wildermuth S, Alkadhi H. Pre- and postoperative evaluation of congenital heart disease in children and adults with 64-section CT. Radiographics. 2007;27(3):829–46. https://doi.org/10.1148/rg.273065713.
12. Girshin M, Shapiro V, Rhee A, Ginsberg S, Inchiosa MA Jr. Increased risk of general anesthesia for high-risk patients undergoing magnetic resonance imaging. J Comput Assist Tomogr. 2009;33(2):312–5. https://doi.org/10.1097/RCT.0b013e31818474b8.
13. Wolla CD, Hlavacek AM, Schoepf UJ, Bucher AM, Chowdhury S. Cardiovascular manifestations of heterotaxy and related situs abnormalities assessed with CT angiography. J Cardiovasc Comput Tomogr. 2013;7(6):408–16. https://doi.org/10.1016/j.jcct.2013.11.008.
14. Loomba RS, Hlavacek AM, Spicer DE, Anderson RH. Isomerism or heterotaxy: which term leads to better understanding? Cardiol Young. 2015;25(6):1037–43. https://doi.org/10.1017/s1047951115001122.
15. Hoffman JI, Kaplan S. The incidence of congenital heart disease. J Am Coll Cardiol. 2002;39(12):1890–900.
16. Allen HD, Driscoll DJ, Shaddy RE, Feltes TF. Moss and Adams' heart disease in infants, children, and adolescents: including the fetus and young adult, vol. 1. 8th ed. Philadelphia: Lippincott Williams & Wilkins; 2013.

17. Anderson RH, Spicer DE, Hlavacek AM, Cook AC, Backer CL. Wilcox's surgical anatomy of the heart. 4th ed. Cambridge, UK: Cambridge University Press; 2013.
18. Osawa K, Miyoshi T, Morimitsu Y, Akagi T, Oe H, Nakagawa K, Takaya Y, Kijima Y, Sato S, Kanazawa S, Ito H. Comprehensive assessment of morphology and severity of atrial septal defects in adults by CT. J Cardiovasc Comput Tomogr. 2015;9(4):354–61. https://doi.org/10.1016/j.jcct.2015.04.007.
19. Ko SF, Liang CD, Yip HK, Huang CC, Ng SH, Huang CF, Chen MC. Amplatzer septal occluder closure of atrial septal defect: evaluation of transthoracic echocardiography, cardiac CT, and transesophageal echocardiography. AJR Am J Roentgenol. 2009;193(6):1522–9. https://doi.org/10.2214/AJR.09.2854.
20. Lee T, Tsai IC, Fu YC, Jan SL, Wang CC, Chang Y, Chen MC. MDCT evaluation after closure of atrial septal defect with an Amplatzer septal occluder. AJR Am J Roentgenol. 2007;188(5):W431–9. https://doi.org/10.2214/ajr.06.0709.
21. Marini D, Ou P, Boudjemline Y, Kenny D, Bonnet D, Agnoletti G. Midterm results of percutaneous closure of very large atrial septal defects in children: role of multislice computed tomography. EuroIntervention. 2012;7(12):1428–34. https://doi.org/10.4244/eijv7i12a223.
22. Amat F, Le Bret E, Sigal-Cinqualbre A, Coblence M, Lambert V, Rohnean A, Paul JF. Diagnostic accuracy of multidetector spiral computed tomography for preoperative assessment of sinus venosus atrial septal defects in children. Interact Cardiovasc Thorac Surg. 2011;12(2):179–82. https://doi.org/10.1510/icvts.2010.251298.
23. Lembcke A, Razek V, Kivelitz D, Rogalla N, Rogalla P. Sinus venosus atrial septal defect with partial anomalous pulmonary venous return: diagnosis with 64-slice spiral computed tomography at low radiation dose. J Pediatr Surg. 2008;43(2):410–1.
24. Yamasaki Y, Nagao M, Kawanami S, Kamitani T, Sagiyama K, Yamanouchi T, Sakamoto I, Yamamura K, Yabuuchi H, Honda H. One-stop shop assessment for atrial septal defect closure using 256-slice coronary CT angiography. Eur Radiol. 2017;27:697. https://doi.org/10.1007/s00330-016-4407-2.
25. Reller MD, Strickland MJ, Riehle-Colarusso T, Mahle WT, Correa A. Prevalence of congenital heart defects in metropolitan Atlanta, 1998–2005. J Pediatr. 2008;153(6):807–13. https://doi.org/10.1016/j.jpeds.2008.05.059.
26. Jacobs JP, Burke RP, Quintessenza JA, Mavroudis C. Congenital Heart Surgery Nomenclature and Database Project: ventricular septal defect. Ann Thorac Surg. 2000;69(4 Suppl):S25–35.
27. Rudolph AM, Drorbaugh JE, Auld PA, Rudolph AJ, Nadas AS, Smith CA, Hubbell JP. Studies on the circulation in the neonatal period. The circulation in the respiratory distress syndrome. Pediatrics. 1961;27:551–66.
28. Mitchell SC, Korones SB, Berendes HW. Congenital heart disease in 56,109 births. Incidence and natural history. Circulation. 1971;43(3):323–32.
29. Kitterman JA, Edmunds LH Jr, Gregory GA, Heymann MA, Tooley WH, Rudolph AM. Patent ducts arteriosus in premature infants. Incidence, relation to pulmonary disease and management. N Engl J Med. 1972;287(10):473–7. https://doi.org/10.1056/nejm197209072871001.
30. Schneider DJ, Moore JW. Patent ductus arteriosus. Circulation. 2006;114(17):1873–82. https://doi.org/10.1161/circulationaha.105.592063.
31. Sardesai SH, Marshall RJ, Farrow R, Mourant AJ. Dissecting aneurysm of the pulmonary artery in a case of unoperated patent ductus arteriosus. Eur Heart J. 1990;11(7):670–3.
32. Lin MT, Wang JK, Chen YS, Lee WJ, Chiu HH, Chen CA, Chiu SN, Wu ET, Lu CW, Huang SC, Chen SJ, Chiu IS, Chang CI, Wu MH. Detection of pulmonary arterial morphology in tetralogy of Fallot with pulmonary atresia by computed tomography: 12 years of experience. Eur J Pediatr. 2012;171(3):579–86. https://doi.org/10.1007/s00431-011-1621-4.
33. Meinel FG, Huda W, Schoepf UJ, Rao AG, Cho YJ, Baker GH, Hlavacek AM. Diagnostic accuracy of CT angiography in infants with tetralogy of Fallot with pulmonary atresia and major aortopulmonary collateral arteries. J Cardiovasc Comput Tomogr. 2013;7(6):367–75. https://doi.org/10.1016/j.jcct.2013.11.001.
34. Braunwald E, Goldblatt A, Aygen MM, Rockoff SD, Morrow AG. Congenital aortic stenosis. I. Clinical and hemodynamic findings in 100 patients. II. Surgical treatment and the results of operation. Circulation. 1963;27:426–62.
35. Xu J, Zhao H, Wang X, Bai Y, Liu L, Liu Y, Wei M, Li J, Zheng M. Accuracy, image quality, and radiation dose of prospectively ECG-triggered high-pitch dual-source CT angiography in infants and children with complex coarctation of the aorta. Acad Radiol. 2014;21(10):1248–54. https://doi.org/10.1016/j.acra.2014.04.019.
36. Budoff MJ, Shittu A, Roy S. Use of cardiovascular computed tomography in the diagnosis and management of coarctation of the aorta. J Thorac Cardiovasc Surg. 2013;146(1):229–32. https://doi.org/10.1016/j.jtcvs.2013.01.024.
37. Backer CL, Mavroudis C. Congenital Heart Surgery Nomenclature and Database Project: patent ductus arteriosus, coarctation of the aorta, interrupted aortic arch. Ann Thorac Surg. 2000;69(4 Suppl):S298–307.
38. Braunlin E, Peoples WM, Freedom RM, Fyler DC, Goldblatt A, Edwards JE. Interruption of the aortic arch with aorticopulmonary septal defect. An anatomic review. Pediatr Cardiol. 1982;3(4):329–35. https://doi.org/10.1007/bf02427036.
39. Yang DH, Goo HW, Seo DM, Yun TJ, Park JJ, Park IS, Ko JK, Kim YH. Multislice CT angiography of interrupted aortic arch. Pediatr Radiol. 2008;38(1):89–100. https://doi.org/10.1007/s00247-007-0662-3.
40. Schreiber C, Cook A, Ho SY, Augustin N, Anderson RH. Morphologic spectrum of Ebstein's malformation: revisitation relative to surgical repair. J Thorac Cardiovasc Surg. 1999;117(1):148–55.
41. Attenhofer Jost CH, Connolly HM, Dearani JA, Edwards WD, Danielson GK. Ebstein's anomaly. Circulation. 2007;115(2):277–85. https://doi.org/10.1161/circulationaha.106.619338.
42. Allwork SP, Bentall HH, Becker AE, Cameron H, Gerlis LM, Wilkinson JL, Anderson RH. Congenitally corrected transposition of the great arteries: morphologic study of 32 cases. Am J Cardiol. 1976;38(7):910–23.
43. Van Praagh R, Van Praagh S. The anatomy of common aorticopulmonary trunk (truncus arteriosus communis) and its embryologic implications. A study of 57 necropsy cases. Am J Cardiol. 1965;16(3):406–25.
44. Collett RW, Edwards JE. Persistent truncus arteriosus; a classification according to anatomic types. Surg Clin North Am. 1949;29(4):1245–70.
45. Konstantinov IE, Karamlou T, Blackstone EH, Mosca RS, Lofland GK, Caldarone CA, Williams WG, Mackie AS, McCrindle BW. Truncus arteriosus associated with interrupted aortic arch in 50 neonates: a Congenital Heart Surgeons Society study. Ann Thorac Surg. 2006;81(1):214–22. https://doi.org/10.1016/j.athoracsur.2005.06.072.
46. Keane JF, Lock JE, Fyler DC. Nadas' pediatric cardiology. 2nd ed. Philadelphia: Saunders; 2006.
47. Ramos-Duran L, Nance JW Jr, Schoepf UJ, Henzler T, Apfaltrer P, Hlavacek AM. Developmental aortic arch anomalies in infants and children assessed with CT angiography. AJR Am J Roentgenol. 2012;198(5):W466–74. https://doi.org/10.2214/AJR.11.6982.
48. Leonardi B, Secinaro A, Cutrera R, Albanese S, Trozzi M, Franceschini A, Silvestri V, Toma P, Carotti A, Pongiglione G. Imaging modalities in children with vascular ring and pulmo-

nary artery sling. Pediatr Pulmonol. 2015;50(8):781–8. https://doi.org/10.1002/ppul.23075.

49. Lee EY, Zurakowski D, Waltz DA, Mason KP, Riaz F, Ralph A, Boiselle PM. MDCT evaluation of the prevalence of tracheomalacia in children with mediastinal aortic vascular anomalies. J Thorac Imaging. 2008;23(4):258–65. https://doi.org/10.1097/RTI.0b013e31817fbdf7.
50. Dyer KT, Hlavacek AM, Meinel FG, De Cecco CN, McQuiston AD, Schoepf UJ, Pietris NP. Imaging in congenital pulmonary vein anomalies: the role of computed tomography. Pediatr Radiol. 2014;44(9):1158–68; quiz 1155–7. https://doi.org/10.1007/s00247-014-3044-7.
51. Bonelli-Sica JM, de la Mora-Cervantes R, Diaz-Zamudio M, Castillo-Castellon F, Ramirez-Carmona R, Velazquez-Moreno J, Kimura-Hayama E. Dual-source 256-MDCT for diagnosis of anomalous pulmonary venous drainage in pediatric population. AJR Am J Roentgenol. 2013;200(2):W163–9. https://doi.org/10.2214/ajr.11.8348.
52. Jonas RA, Smolinsky A, Mayer JE, Castaneda AR. Obstructed pulmonary venous drainage with total anomalous pulmonary venous connection to the coronary sinus. Am J Cardiol. 1987;59(5):431–5.
53. Krasemann Z, Scheld HH, Tjan TD, Krasemann T. Cor triatriatum: short review of the literature upon ten new cases. Herz. 2007;32(6):506–10. https://doi.org/10.1007/s00059-007-2882-6.
54. Tweddell JS, Hoffman GM, Mussatto KA, Fedderly RT, Berger S, Jaquiss RD, Ghanayem NS, Frisbee SJ, Litwin SB. Improved survival of patients undergoing palliation of hypoplastic left heart syndrome: lessons learned from 115 consecutive patients. Circulation. 2002;106(12 Suppl 1):I82–9.
55. Hawkins JA, Doty DB. Aortic atresia: morphologic characteristics affecting survival and operative palliation. J Thorac Cardiovasc Surg. 1984;88(4):620–6.
56. Hanley FL, Sade RM, Blackstone EH, Kirklin JW, Freedom RM, Nanda NC. Outcomes in neonatal pulmonary atresia with intact ventricular septum. A multiinstitutional study. J Thorac Cardiovasc Surg. 1993;105(3):406–23, 424–407; discussion 423–404.
57. Seguela PE, Houyel L, Loget P, Piot JD, Paul JF. Critical stenosis of a right ventricle to coronary artery fistula seen at dual-source CT in a newborn with pulmonary atresia and intact ventricular septum. Pediatr Radiol. 2011;41(8):1069–72. https://doi.org/10.1007/s00247-011-2068-5.
58. Tandon R, Edwards JE. Tricuspid atresia. A re-evaluation and classification. J Thorac Cardiovasc Surg. 1974;67(4):530–42.
59. Sanders JM. Bilateral superior vena cavae. Anat Rec. 1946;94:657–62.
60. Mayo J, Gray R, St Louis E, Grosman H, McLoughlin M, Wise D. Anomalies of the inferior vena cava. AJR Am J Roentgenol. 1983;140(2):339–45. https://doi.org/10.2214/ajr.140.2.339.
61. Rubino M, Van Praagh S, Kadoba K, Pessotto R, Van Praagh R. Systemic and pulmonary venous connections in visceral heterotaxy with asplenia. Diagnostic and surgical considerations based on seventy-two autopsied cases. J Thorac Cardiovasc Surg. 1995;110(3):641–50. https://doi.org/10.1016/s0022-5223(95)70095-1.

The Use of Cardiovascular CT in Repaired CHD

47

B. Kelly Han, Andrew Crean, and John R. Lesser

Advances in medical and surgical care of patients with congenital heart disease (CHD) have resulted in expected survival for even the most complex lesions [1]. There is an increasing prevalence of CHD in all age groups, the majority of patients with CHD are now adults, and the number reaching older adulthood is rapidly rising [2–4]. Patients with repaired or palliated CHD require serial diagnostic evaluations throughout their lives [5]. The improved spatial and temporal resolution, rapid image acquisition, and radiation dose reduction of newer generation scanners have dramatically increased the applicability of computed tomography (CT) to patients with congenital heart disease of all ages [6]. Cardiovascular CT is increasingly used in patients with CHD when echocardiography is not sufficient and cardiac magnetic resonance imaging (CMR) is contraindicated, unlikely to provide adequate image quality due to artifact, or considered high risk due to scan time or anesthesia when needed [7, 8]. Cardiovascular CT in congenital heart disease will be optimally used in settings where all advanced diagnostic modalities are available so that the test with the best information and least risk can be chosen for each individual patient and clinical indication.

CT is an important diagnostic modality for select patients with CHD after intervention, from the neonate to the adult patient. Evaluation of CHD is considered an appropriate indication on the most recent consensus document on the use of cardiovascular CT [9]. Table 47.1 lists consensus recommendations for the use CT in CHD [8].

B. K. Han (✉)
Department of Advanced Congenital Cardiac Imaging, Minneapolis Heart Institute and the Children's Hospitals and Clinics of Minnesota, Minneapolis, MN, USA
e-mail: khan@chc-pa.org

A. Crean
Department of Cardiology, Ottawa Heart Institute, University of Ottawa, Ottawa, ON, Canada

J. R. Lesser
Minneapolis Heart Institute Foundation, Minneapolis, MN, USA

Risk of Cardiovascular CT in Repaired and Palliated CHD

The risks of cardiovascular CT include peripheral IV access, exposure to iodinated contrast in almost all patients, limited anesthesia in patients for whom a breath hold is required when unable to cooperate due to hemodynamic or developmental status, and radiation exposure. Anesthesia risk includes both the procedural risk of adverse event and the risk for long-term adverse neurodevelopmental outcome for repeated exposure at young ages [10–14]. Children with congenital heart disease, particularly hospitalized patients or those with unrepaired cyanotic heart disease, are at the highest risk for an adverse event with anesthesia [15]. When anesthesia is needed for breath holding, it is usually limited to a single imaging sequence (high heart rate coronary imaging or functional imaging acquired over several heartbeats) and is of short duration.

Cumulative radiation exposure is of particular concern for congenital heart disease patients requiring repeated diagnostic testing and intervention. These CHD patients may have a relatively high cumulative radiation exposure, where approximately 75% is catheterization based in the current era [16]. Studies have shown that cardiovascular CT has lower radiation exposure than catheterization when modern CT scanner technology is available [17]. The reported radiation dose from cardiac CT in patients with CHD varies from less than 1 millisievert to 18 mSv [18–22]. Recent trends show many CHD scans can be performed at a dose of approximately 1 mSv including anatomic evaluation and ECG-triggered exams for coronary evaluation [20, 21, 23]. The image quality required for high-resolution coronary imaging is rarely needed for CHD CT studies. CT in CHD is optimally performed in centers with the appropriate attention to CT dose reduction and modern CT equipment. The scan planning is individualized and includes decisions about aggressive radiation dose reduction with direct physician input concerning patient preparation, data acquisition as well as interpretation of each scan [22, 24].

U. J. Schoepf (ed.), *CT of the Heart*, Contemporary Medical Imaging, https://doi.org/10.1007/978-1-60327-237-7_47

Table 47.1 Situations in which cardiovascular CT may be appropriate in repaired CHD

Presence of CMR unsafe implant or foreign body (retained pacing leads, non-MR compatible pacemaker/defibrillator, neurostimulator)
Poor CMR image quality (known or expected) due to metallic artifact
Unable to fit in MRI scanner due to obesity or severe claustrophobia
Neonate or young patient requiring evaluation of postoperative complex anatomy, particularly if considered higher risk for adverse event with sedation or anesthesia required for CMR, and the CT scan can be performed with no or limited sedation
Critically ill patient with repaired CHD of any age that may not tolerate breath holding or length of CMR scan
Evaluation of ventricular assist device or ECMO cannula positioning
Patient requiring CT for evaluation of extracardiac anatomy in addition to palliated or repaired CHD (e.g., lung parenchyma, airway, skeletal abnormality)
Preoperative patients with prior sternotomy considered high risk for vascular injury with sternal reentry due to an anterior coronary artery, conduit, or sternal adhesions
Evaluation of prosthetic valve function or structural integrity (calcification, stenosis, coaptation defect, leaflet immobility, paravalvular leak, endocarditis, or clot)
Evaluation of calcification within vessels and surgical conduits prior to catheter-based intervention (e.g., balloon angioplasty, transcatheter valve replacement, stent placement)
Coronary artery imaging in CHD (a) Patient needing detailed preoperative coronary artery evaluation in addition to assessment of complex cardiac anatomy (b) Patient with symptoms and signs suggestive of atherosclerotic coronary artery disease and a history of CHD, prior coronary intervention, or high-risk Kawasaki disease (c) Young symptomatic patients with known or suspected coronary anomaly, particularly if CMR is unlikely to provide complete assessment or more likely to require anesthesia (d) Delineation of coronary anatomy prior to surgical or percutaneous pulmonary valve implantation (e) Evaluation of coronary artery after any surgery requiring coronary artery manipulation or reimplantation

Modified from Han et al. [8]

The Use of Cardiovascular CT in Repaired and Palliated CHD

Patients with repaired or palliated CHD referred for cardiovascular CT will have prior diagnostic studies and interventions. The cardiac imager must know the underlying CHD diagnosis, prior interventions and diagnostic studies, and the clinical question so that a targeted exam may be performed. Optimal CT imaging in CHD requires close collaboration between CT imagers, cardiologists, and surgeons.

The most common indications for cardiovascular CT after intervention in CHD are:

- Coronary artery evaluation after surgical manipulation or reimplantation
- Aortic arch evaluation after surgical or catheter-based intervention
- Transposition of the great arteries, s/p atrial and arterial switch
- Tetralogy of Fallot, s/p palliation or complete repair
- Univentricular heart disease through all stages of palliation

Diagnosis-Specific Preparation and CT Scan Protocols

Coronary Artery Imaging After Intervention in CHD

Coronary imaging in patients with repaired CHD is recommended for definition of coronary artery anatomy after surgical manipulation, prior to repeat intervention on the RVOT, to assess the relationship to the RVOT and sternum, and for assessment of coronary lesions in symptomatic patients and in certain adult patient undergoing repeat cardiac intervention to determine the need for concurrent coronary intervention [5] (Figs. 47.1 and 47.2). Coronary imaging is often one aspect of a complete evaluation of congenital heart disease, and the scan preparation will include consideration of all aspects of the patients CHD anatomy requiring evaluation for clinical management.

Definition of Coronary Artery Subsequent to Coronary Intervention

Patients who have undergone surgical coronary intervention/manipulation in repair of a congenital heart defect include patients who have undergone an arterial switch operation, the Nikaidoh or Ross procedure, and unroofing or reimplantation of an anomalous origin of the coronary artery from the pulmonary artery or aortic root (ALCAPA or AAOCA). (See section on TGA for coronary evaluation after intervention).

Definition of Coronary Artery Anatomy Prior to Right Ventricular Outflow Tract (RVOT) Intervention

Coronary imaging is required prior to repeat RVOT intervention for definition of the coronary artery relationship to both the sternum and the right ventricular outflow tract. RVOT replacement is one of the most common repeat surgical procedures performed in patients of all ages with congenital heart disease, required in certain forms of tetralogy of Fallot, truncus arteriosus, the Rastelli procedure, Ross procedure, and in some patients after the arterial switch procedure [5, 25]. Coronary location can determine the optimal sternal reentry and location of pulmonary conduit in the setting of a coronary artery proximal to the RVOT or existing conduit. Transcatheter valves are currently used in existing conduits primarily for conduit stenosis, with prestenting in many cases to create a circumferential landing

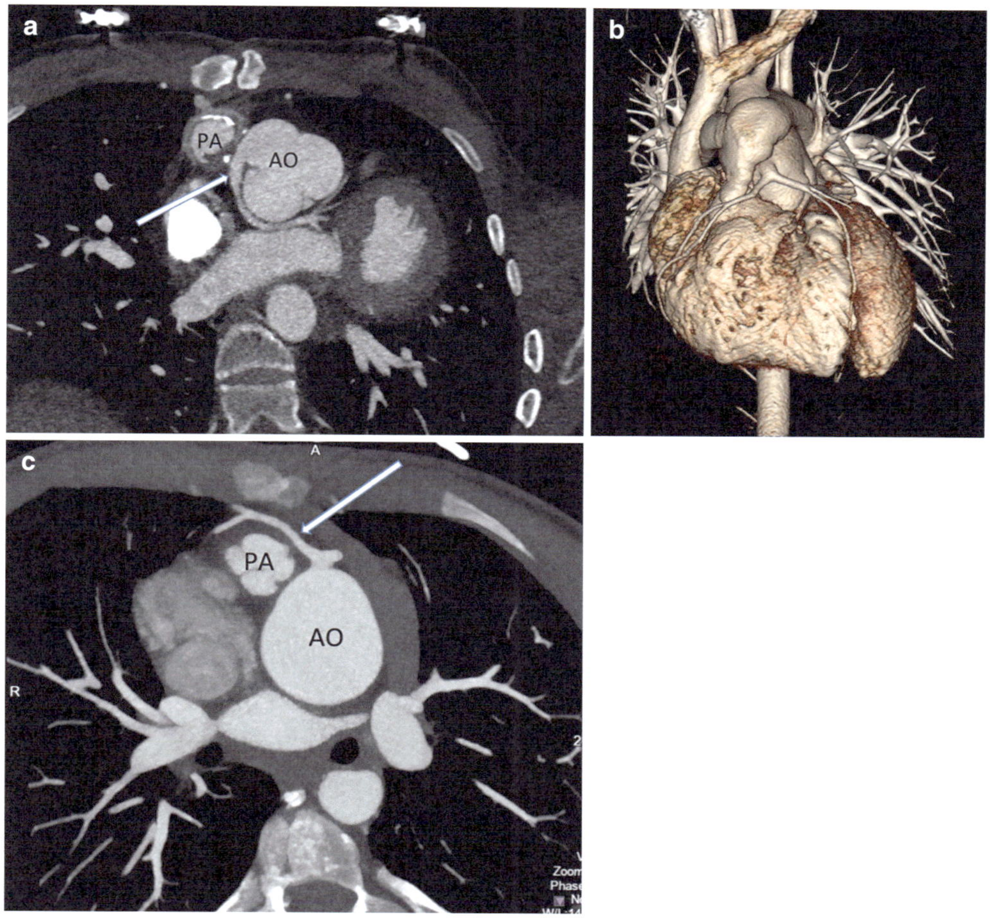

Fig. 47.1 Coronary relationship to the sternum and RVOT after arterial switch or Rastelli procedure. (**a**) Axial 2D image of the left coronary artery as it arises from the right-facing sinus in this patient after Rastelli procedure. The coronary artery (arrow) runs between the neo-aorta and the calcified pulmonary homograft, concerning for potential coronary compression with transcatheter valve placement. (**b** and **c**) This coronal 3D reconstruction (**b**) shows a single coronary artery arising from the right coronary sinus of the neo-aortic root after arterial switch procedure, coursing anterior to the RVOT after LeCompte maneuver. The 2D image (**c**) from the same patient shows the right coronary artery coursing anterior to the RVOT and directly posterior to the sternum (arrow). Note the dilated neo-aortic root additionally

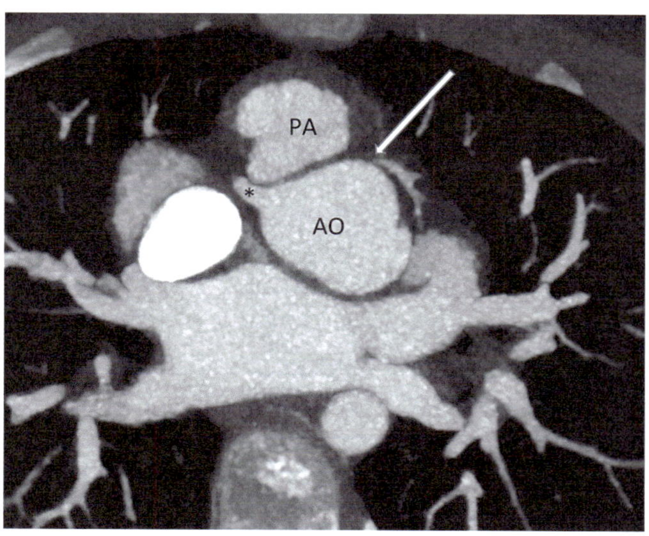

Fig. 47.2 Left main ostial coronary artery stenosis after the arterial switch operation. 2D image showing the left main coronary artery is severely narrowed at the ostium after arterial switch procedure (arrow). The right coronary ostium is widely patent (*)

zone for the valve. In a multi-institution study, 17% of patients undergoing transcatheter pulmonary valve placement were found to have abnormal coronary artery pattern, and 5% of patients had coronary compromise on test balloon prior to valve insertion [26, 27]. Transcatheter valves within a stent cause significant artifact in MRI, and CT angiography can visualize valvular detail or endocarditis/thrombus if suspected [28–30].

High-Resolution Coronary Imaging in Patients with CHD

As patients with CHD enter middle and late adulthood, they may acquire coronary artery disease and require coronary intervention [31]. High-resolution coronary imaging should be pursued in patients with repaired or palliated CHD and symptoms suggestive of ischemia. It is also recommended that male patients over the age of 35 and postmenopausal women undergo coronary evaluation prior to planned cardiac intervention to determine the need for concurrent coronary intervention [5, 32].

Potential anatomic findings after coronary artery intervention:

- Ostial or proximal coronary artery narrowing after arterial switch operation or the Ross procedure
- Right coronary artery lesion after Nikaidoh (due to leftward translocation of the aorta)
- Anomalous coronary artery may run adjacent or over the RVOT in patient requiring re-intervention
- Atherosclerotic coronary lesions in adult CHD patients

Pediatric and Adult Congenital Coronary CT Scan Recommendations

- The coronary artery detail needed for clinical management in CHD will vary by indication:
  - For course and location of the coronary arteries prior to RVOT intervention, minimal acquisition window and aggressive dose reduction should be used. On highest pitch or volumetric scanners, coronary course can often be determined with a younger patient quietly breathing.
  - For symptomatic patients and those requiring detailed coronary imaging to rule out a coronary lesion, optimal image quality is necessary and may require medication to reduce heart rate. Small children may need intubation for a breath hold.
- Contrast injection should be modified so that coronary artery anatomy and congenital anatomy may be evaluated in the same scan acquisition whenever possible. This may require a prolonged or dual-contrast-phase injection technique. If a shunt lesion is suspected, then a contrast density gradient is required across the heart and is achieved through judicious manipulation of contrast: saline ratio in each phase of a dual-phase injection [7].

Aortic Arch

Aortic arch imaging is one of the most frequent indications for CT imaging in patients with congenital heart disease who have previously undergone intervention (Figs. 47.3 and 47.4). The most common prior interventions are repair of aortic coarctation and repair of interrupted aortic arch. Advanced imaging is recommended every 5 years according to the current ACHD clinical guidelines [5]. Long-term survival for patients with repaired aortic coarctation is decreased compared to the general population, and many patients require re-intervention [33]. Younger age at repair results in better long-term survival but a higher rate of re-intervention. Preoperative hypertension and age over 20 years at the time of repair are independent risk factors for mortality [34]. Aortic coarctation is repaired utilizing end-to-end anastomosis, left subclavian flap repair, interposition graft, or catheter-based balloon angioplasty and stenting [35]. Patients with aortic coarctation may also have a bicuspid aortic valve or abnormal mitral valve and other left-sided obstructive lesions. CT imaging is particularly relevant to patients who have previously undergone stent placement in the aorta [36]. Aortic coarctation is one of the lesions that may present in adulthood in a patient imaged for other reasons.

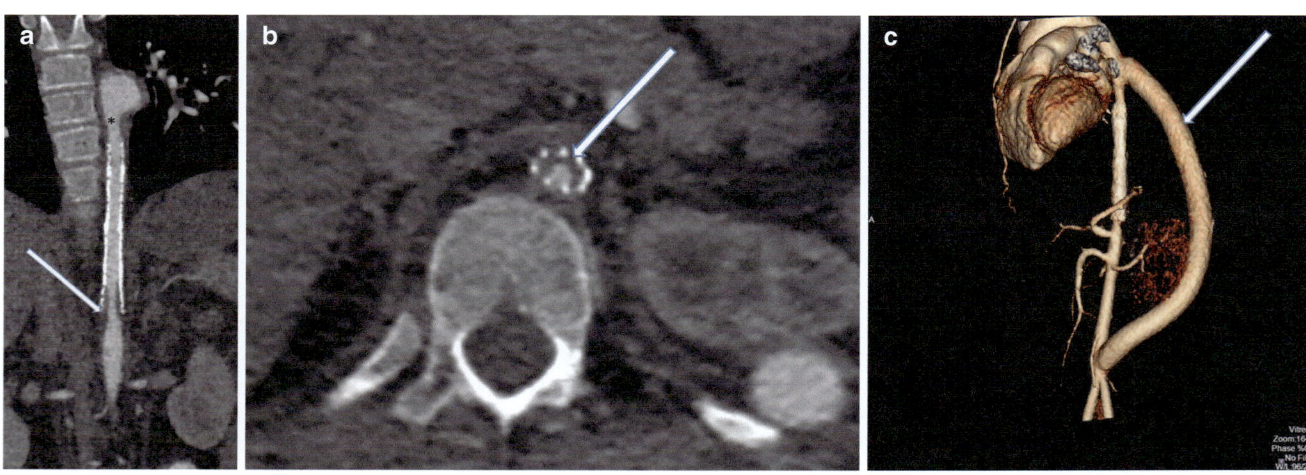

Fig. 47.3 Recurrent coarctation after stenting for thoracic aortic coarctation (mid-aortic syndrome). (**a** and **b**) There is recurrent aortic coarctation (*) in the mid thoracic aorta proximal to multiple stents placed to treat coarctation/mid-aortic syndrome. There is intimal proliferation causing obstruction at the distal end of the stents. Image B shows a 2D cross section of the distal stent in the same area. (**c**) 3D reconstruction of an interposition graft (arrow) from the proximal descending thoracic aorta to the abdominal aorta to bypass the obstruction in the same patient

Common Anatomic Findings After Aortic Arch Intervention

- Recurrent aortic arch obstruction (in stent stenosis, homograft stenosis, or arch obstruction adjacent to the site or prior repair)
- Aortic aneurysm or pseudoaneurysm
- Aortic dissection

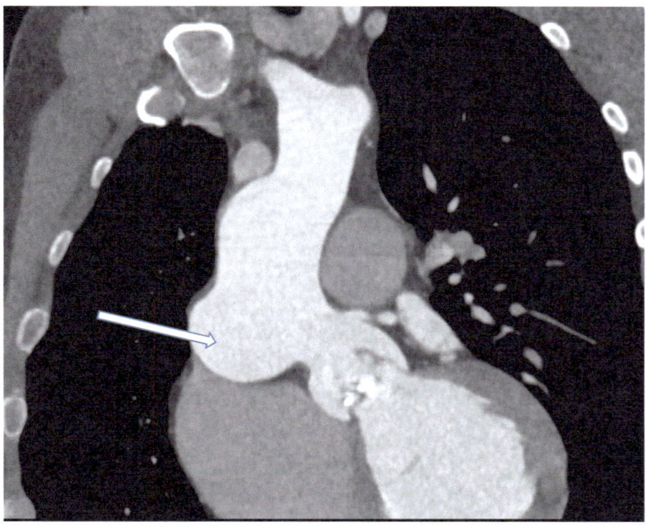

Fig. 47.4 Ascending aorta pseudoaneurysm after prior aortic valvotomy. Unexpected severe dilation of the ascending aorta (arrow, 6.5 cm) at the site of aortic entry for prior aortic valvotomy to treat aortic stenosis. Note calcified aortic valve leaflets. Scan was performed to evaluate the proximal descending aorta in the area of prior coarctation repair, which was unremarkable

Scan Modifications

- Standard IV placement and timing of contrast to the aorta unless other lesions require evaluation.
- Extend cranial scan range slightly; anomalous coronary arteries may arise from the proximal ascending aorta.
- Aggressive dose reduction may be used in most cases. Heart rate-lowering medications are only needed if coronary imaging is required.
- If a bicuspid valve needs evaluation in addition to the aorta, systolic image acquisition is best (Sievers classification).

Transposition Complexes

Transposition complexes include a wide variety of anatomic and hemodynamic lesions requiring different surgical approaches for repair or palliation. For isolated ventricular-arterial discordance, surgical pathway is determined by the relationship of the great arteries to the ventricular chambers and the ability of the valves to be used in the alternate circulation, particularly the pulmonary valve suitability for the aortic position. For patients with both atrioventricular and ventricular-arterial discordance, the surgical approach is determined by associated lesions, function of the right ventricle and tricuspid valve in the systemic circulation, and concerns regarding long-term outcomes for a systemic right ventricle. Some centers consider primary transplant as an option when indicated rather than a double switch (atrial and arterial switch) procedure (Figs. 47.5 and 47.6).

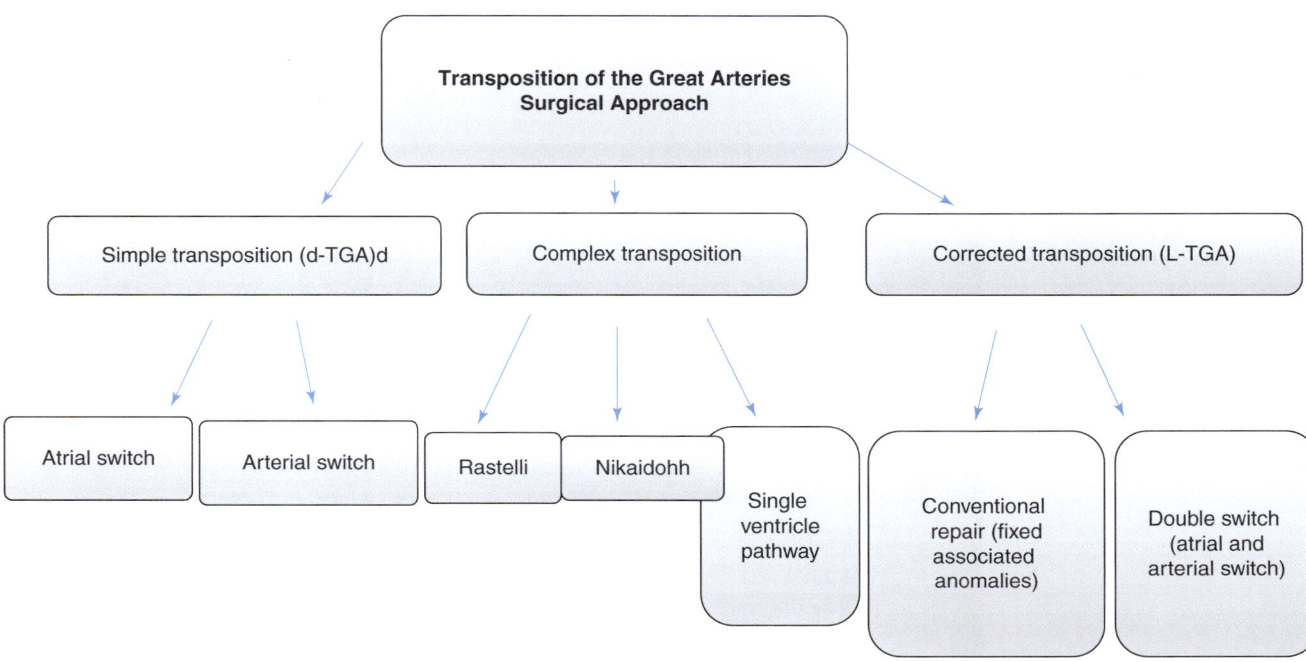

Fig. 47.5 Surgical treatment approaches to transposition of the great arteries

d-TGA s/p Atrial Switch

Until the 1980s most patients with isolated ventricular-arterial discordance (most commonly d-TGA) underwent an atrial switch operation with the systemic and pulmonary venous return baffled to the opposite atrium, essentially creating physiologically corrected transposition with a systemic right ventricle and a subpulmonary left ventricle (Figs. 47.7, 47.8, 47.9, and 47.10). Predictors of mortality include associated cardiac defects, RV dysfunction, and tricuspid regurgitation [37]. These patients have a high rate of sinus node dysfunction requiring pacemaker placement. An implantable defibrillator is considered for patients with low systemic ejection fraction [38].

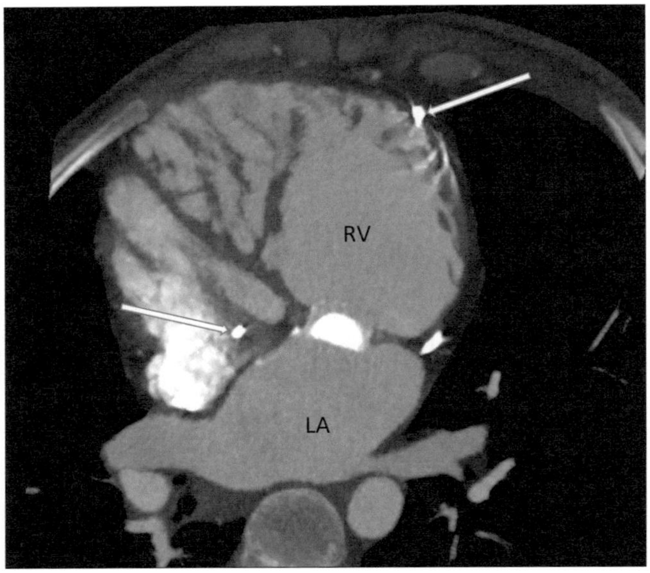

Fig. 47.6 Systemic RV failure in L-TGA. This image shows an enlarged and hypertrophied systemic right ventricle in a patient with L-TGA (also called physiologically corrected transposition). Heart block is common, and both epicardial and transvenous pacer leads are seen (arrows). Severe systemic tricuspid regurgitation required prosthetic valve replacement

Common Lesions After the Atrial Switch Operation

- Systemic and pulmonary venous baffle obstruction (most common in the superior vena cava baffle to the left atrium)
- Systemic RV dysfunction
- Tricuspid (systemic AV valve) regurgitation
- Subpulmonary obstruction due to septal displacement into the LVOT

Scan Modifications

- Biventricular injection protocol (triphasic, two-phase contrast and saline) (Fig. 47.11).
- Lengthen monitoring sequence if high suspicion for baffle obstruction and the heart will fill via collaterals.
- ECG-gated functional scan if quantification of function is needed (use aggressive dose reduction since function analysis performed in 6–8 mm slices).
- May quantify regurgitation by stroke volume differences if closely correlated to echocardiography.

d-TGA s/p Arterial Switch

The earliest patients who underwent arterial switch are now in young adulthood. In most cases the coronary arteries are transferred to the neo-aortic root (Figs. 47.12 and 47.13). An exception is in a patient after an Aubert procedure or the Nikaidoh procedure. In the Aubert procedure, the coronary is

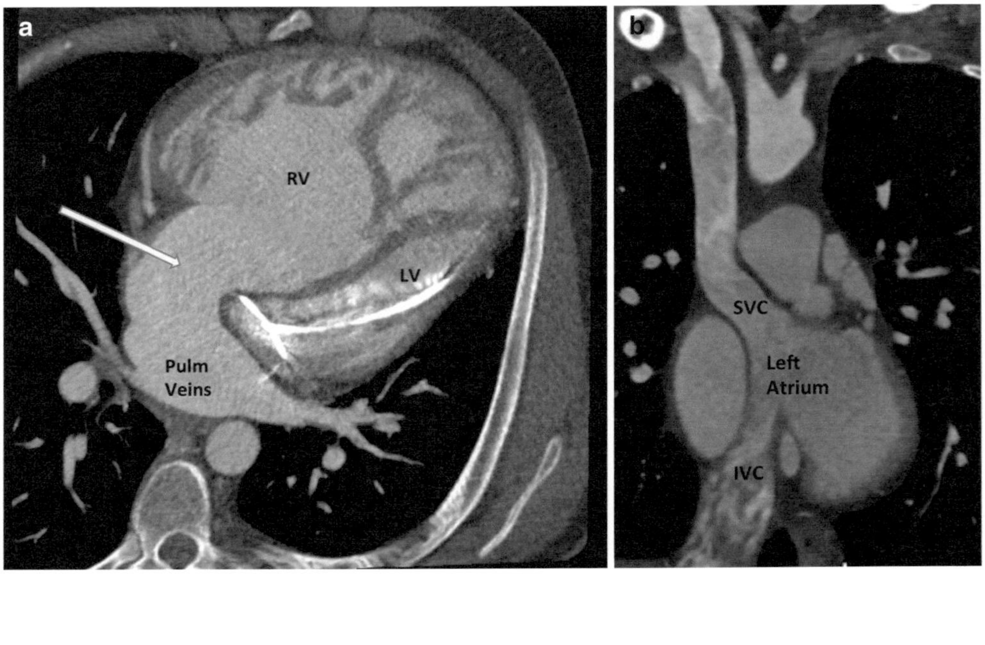

Fig. 47.7 d-TGA after atrial switch operation (Senning). (**a**) A patent pulmonary venous baffle (arrow) to the hypertrophied and enlarged systemic right ventricle in a patient after the atrial switch operation. (**b**) Note the pacer lead into the apex of the thin-walled subpulmonary left ventricle

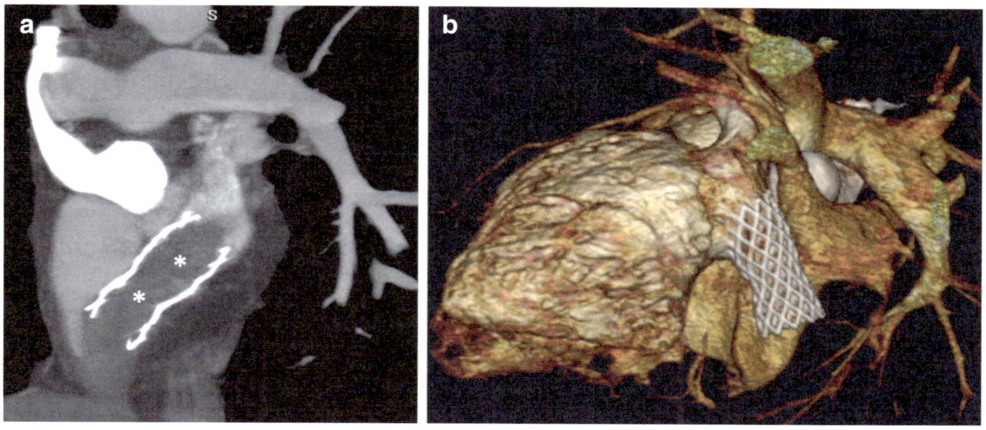

Fig. 47.8 *d*-TGA with Mustard palliation, systemic venous baffle stenting. (**a**) Coronal view to show the inferior limb of the systemic venous baffle (asterisk) which has been stented open. Note that the relatively low attenuation inside the stent does *not* imply thrombosis but simply early time point of imaging post contrast injection before recirculation of opacified blood through the IVC. (**b**) Volume-rendered image of the same patient to demonstrate the clarity with which cardiac CT can assess and depict stented structures

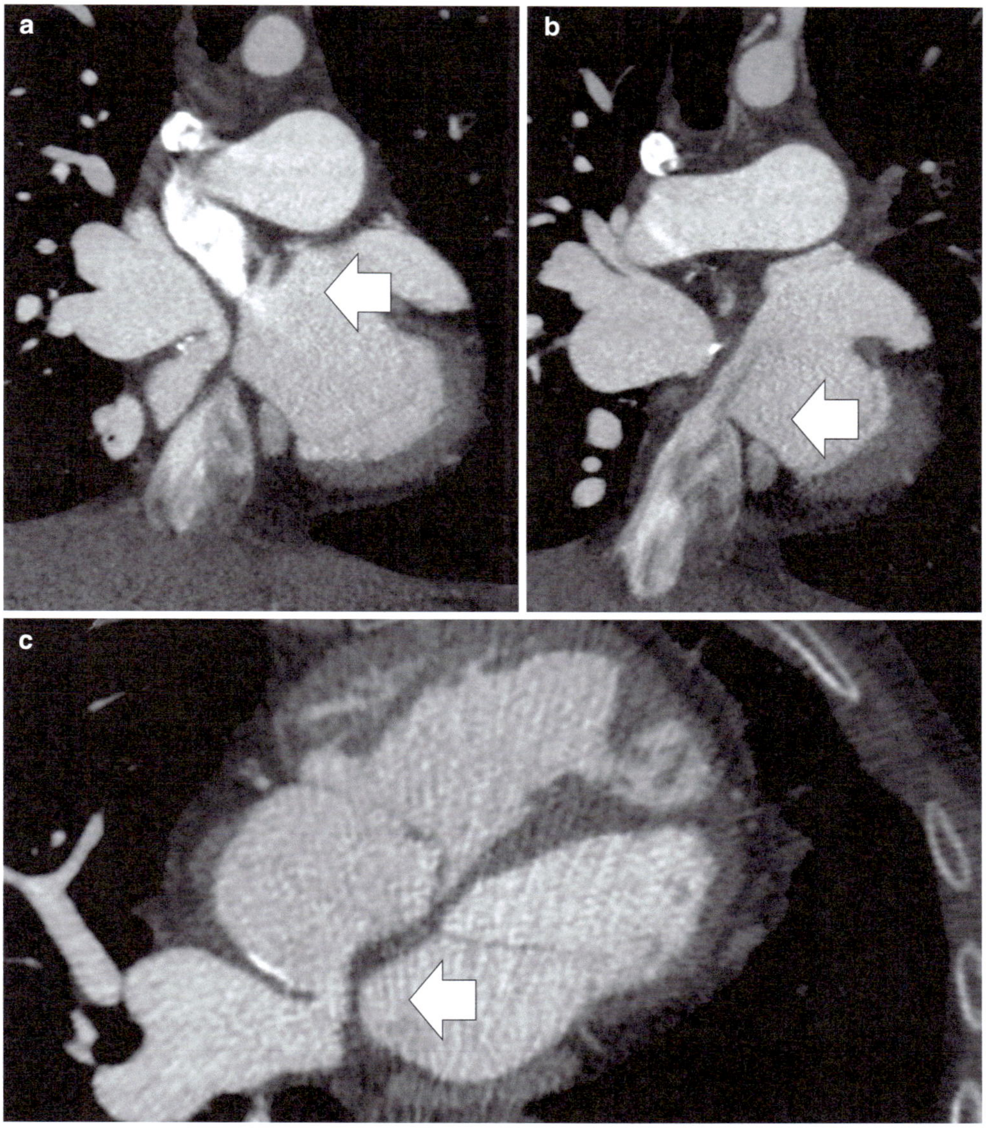

Fig. 47.9 Multilevel baffle obstruction in an adult with Mustard palliation of *d*-transposition of the great arteries. (**a**) Coronal view demonstrating focal narrowing at the distal end of the superior limb of the systemic venous baffle (arrow). (**b**) Coronal view demonstrating similar narrowing of the distal inferior limb of the systemic venous baffle (arrow). (**c**) Axial view in the same patient. The left-sided pulmonary veins are occluded (not shown); the right-sided veins (asterisk) drain through a stenosed baffle (arrow) into the left atrium

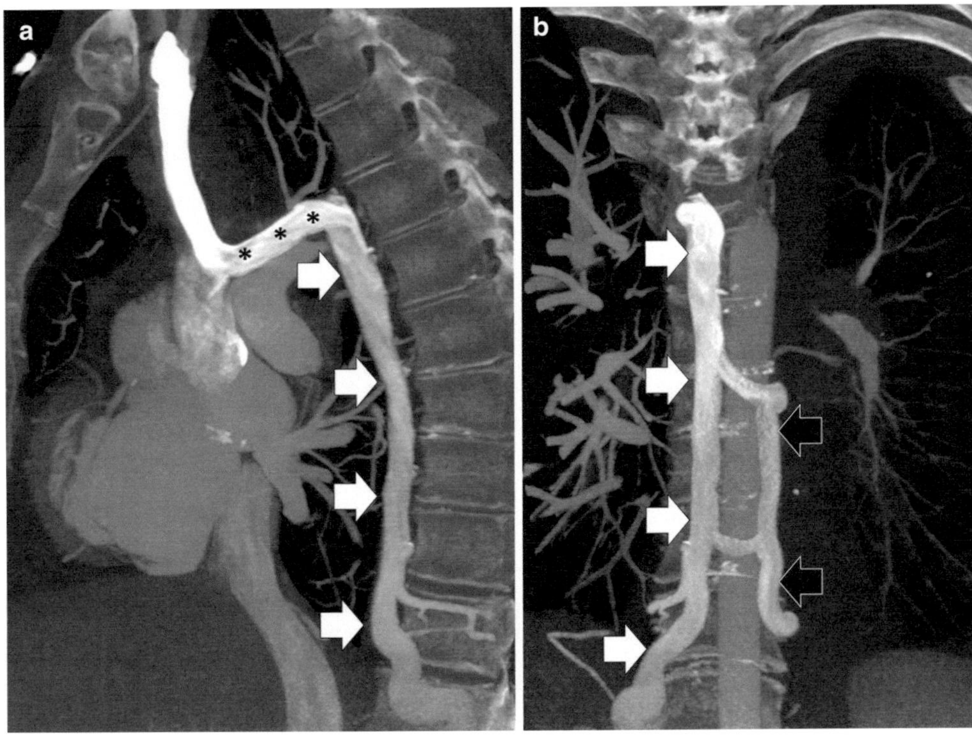

Fig. 47.10 Baffle obstruction with azygous system off-loading. (**a**) Sagittal and (**b**) coronal maximum intensity projection reconstructions from the same patient as the preceding image (Fig. 47.9). The azygous (white arrows) and hemiazygous (black arrows) systems are significantly dilated. In a patient with Mustard palliation of *d*-TGA, this implies obstruction of the superior venous limb. Blood from the head and neck passes down the SVC but – upon meeting resistance to forward flow through the baffle – passes retrograde along the azygous arch (black asterisks) and down into the azygous system. This collateral pathway allows blood from the upper body to enter the inferior limb of the systemic venous baffle via the IVC instead

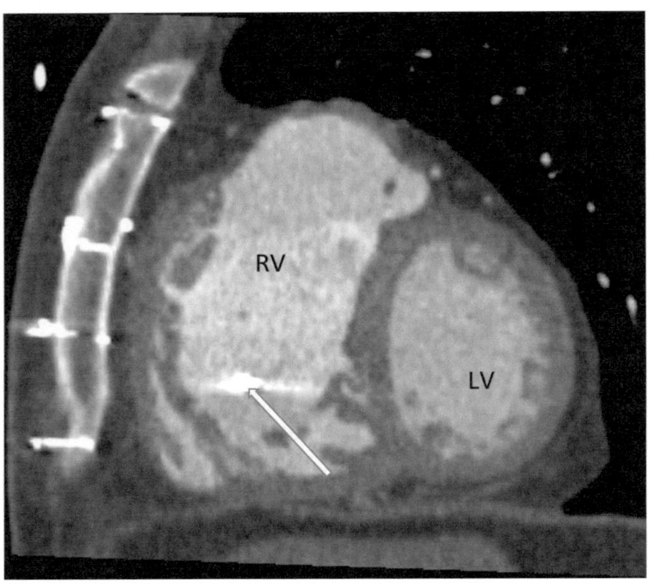

Fig. 47.11 Ventricular function assessment by cardiovascular CT: This ECG-gated and pulse-modulated CT dataset is reconstructed in a diastolic interval in the short axis plane for quantification of biventricular size and systolic function. Note the enlarged RV and the pacer lead artifact (arrow). A biventricular (triphasic, two-phase contrast and saline) injection protocol was used to opacify both the right and left ventricle at the time of image acquisition

baffled through the neo-pulmonary valve, and in the Nikaidoh procedure, the aorta is translocated leftward and closer to the VSD. After the Nikaidoh the right coronary artery is at risk for mid-vessel narrowing. Overall, the hemodynamic results and quality of life after the arterial switch operation have been excellent [39]. The risks for coronary lesions include a stormy postoperative course, single or intramural coronary artery, or two coronary ostia arising close to each other. There is a bimodal risk of coronary events, in the early post-operative era and then again around 10 years postoperatively. Eight to 10% of patients will have coronary stenosis or occlusion after the arterial switch operation [39, 40]. Cardiovascular CT has complete agreement with invasive angiography for assessment of coronary artery anatomy after the arterial switch procedure. Lesions are ostial or in the proximal coronary artery course [41]. Some consider coronary CT preferable for this indication since the catheter can alter the coronary course and mask ostial narrowing during selective coronary angiography.

Valvular and supravalvular PS are common in d-TGA post arterial switch, as the branch pulmonary arteries are stretched anteriorly over the neo-aortic root to the neo-pulmonary valve. Repeat intervention on the RVOT is the most common intervention after the arterial switch procedure.

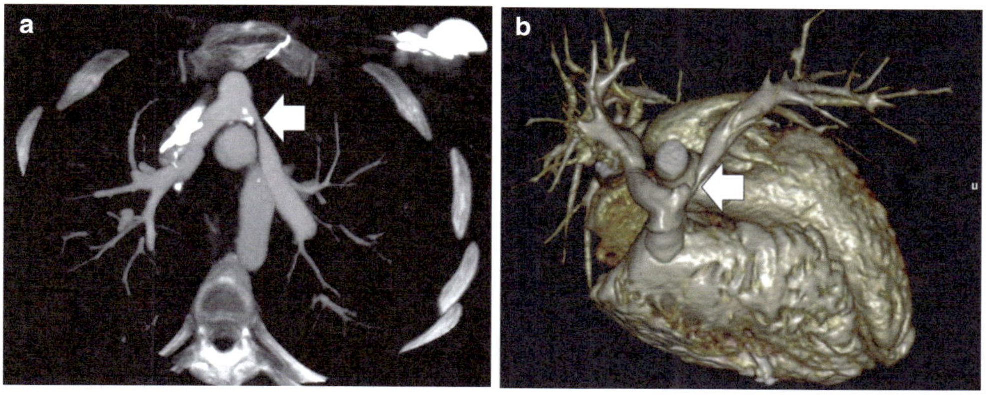

Fig. 47.12 d-TGA following arterial switch procedure. (**a**) Axial MIP and (**b**) volume render of CT dataset in a patient who has had the arterial switch procedure for a diagnosis of *d*-TGA. Focal areas of narrowing in the pulmonary arteries are not uncommon following the LeCompte maneuver; in this instance there is a focal stenosis on the proximal left pulmonary artery (arrows). Stenoses of this severity usually impact flow and will generally be stented – subsequent stent surveillance is then almost always carried out by CT rather than CMR

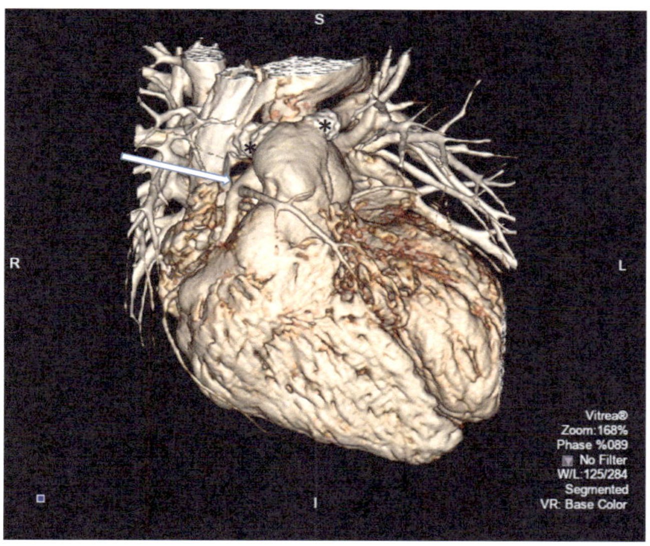

Fig. 47.13 3D volume-rendered image of a single right coronary artery with the left anterior descending coronary artery coursing anterior to the RVOT (arrow) after LeCompte maneuver. Note the stents in the proximal branch pulmonary arteries bilaterally (*)

The relationship of the coronary artery to the RVOT is critical for catheter-based intervention, and the relationship to both the RVOT and the sternum is critical for those undergoing surgical RVOT placement.

Most Common Residual Hemodynamic Lesions

- RVOT obstruction at the level of the neo-pulmonary valve or branch pulmonary arteries
- Neo-aortic stenosis or insufficiency
- Narrowing of the ascending aorta at the neo-aortic root anastomosis
- Neo-aortic root dilation
- Ostial coronary artery lesions after arterial switch procedure
- Mid RCA lesions after the Nikaidoh procedure

Scan Modification

- Consider medication to control heart rate if high-resolution coronary artery imaging needed (at least once in adulthood and patients with symptoms of ischemia).
- Biventricular (triphasic) contrast injection protocol to opacify both the right and left side of the heart.
- Extend scan range to include the proximal ascending aorta and branch pulmonary arteries.

Tetralogy of Fallot

Tetralogy of Fallot includes the most common form with pulmonary stenosis and the less common forms of absent pulmonary valve and pulmonary artery atresia with aortopulmonary collaterals. Repair of all forms of tetralogy involves closure of the VSD with establishment of unobstructed pulmonary blood flow. Relief of pulmonary obstruction is achieved with pulmonary valvotomy, transannular patch, and RV-PA conduit. Patients with absent pulmonary valve require pulmonary artery plication, and those with aortopulmonary collaterals will have aortopulmonary collaterals ligated or closed via catheter intervention. Tetralogy with absent pulmonary valve may also have issues with compression of surrounding structures by the very enlarged pulmonary arteries. Cardiac CT is ideal for identification of complications including both airway and coronary artery compression.

All patients require interval postoperative evaluation to monitor right ventricular size and function, residual/recurrent pulmonary artery or conduit stenosis and/or insufficiency, left ventricular dysfunction, and aortic root dilation. Risk of sudden death increases significantly approximately 25 years postoperatively. Risk factors include prior ventriculotomy, increased RVEDV and RVESV, decreased RV EF, and ventricular ectopy. As patients enter adulthood, they are more likely to have EP devices and to be referred for CT imaging [42, 43].

Pulmonary valve placement is the most commonly performed procedure in adult congenital heart disease and is commonly performed in patients with prior repair of TOF [44, 45]. An RVOT conduit is also required for certain forms of transposition with pulmonary stenosis and insufficiency and truncus arteriosus and for neo-pulmonary root stenosis not amenable to transcatheter therapy. Transcatheter valves are placed in existing conduits. Research into placement in the native RVOT is underway but not widely performed. Coronary compression with transcatheter valve placement has been reported to result in death, and pre-intervention coronary evaluation is required. Coronary arteries running anterior to the RVOT or immediately adjacent to the RVOT are most problematic. Percutaneous valve endocarditis may become a significant problem in follow-up. CT is uniquely suited to assess this complication given that all echo modalities have difficulty imaging the anterior location of the pulmonary valve, particularly if the RVOT was stented prior to valve placement. (Figures 47.14 and 47.15 show vegetation on the pulmonary valve and hematoma in the RVOT).

Most Common Residual Lesions

- Main pulmonary artery or conduit stenosis and branch pulmonary artery stenosis
- Pulmonary insufficiency
- Right ventricular dilation and dysfunction
- Tricuspid regurgitation
- Aortic root dilation [46, 47]
- Left ventricular dysfunction

Scan Modifications

- Biventricular (triphasic) injection protocol to opacify right and left side of the heart.
- Extend scan range to include proximal ascending aorta and branch pulmonary arteries.
- Use aggressive dose reduction for coronary evaluation if lesions are not suspected.
- ECG-gated scan using aggressive dose reduction if ventricular volumes and function are needed for clinical management.

Single Ventricle Heart Disease

Single ventricle heart disease includes a variety of lesions where either ventricle is inadequate to support a separate pulmonary and systemic circulation. Surgical palliation creates separation of the venous and arterial circulation by allowing passive flow of systemic venous flood to the lungs, with the single ventricle pumping pulmonary venous blood to the body. Survival through all stages of palliation has improved in the last decades and is now 60–80% at 10 years, with most mortality in the first year of life [48, 49]. Advanced diagnostics are required in single ventricle (SV) heart disease between stages of palliation and for serial lifelong assessment. Echocardiography alone is inadequate for evaluation of thoracic vasculature [50]. At most centers, the current standard is invasive catheterization before both stage 2 (Glenn) and stage 3 (Fontan) procedure. Catheterization and anesthesia have a relatively high rate of procedural adverse events in palliated single ventricle heart disease [15, 51]. Noninvasive evaluation with both cardiovascular magnetic resonance (CMR) and cardiovascular CT has been shown to be diagnostically equivalent to invasive evaluation prior to stage 2 SV palliation, with fewer procedural adverse events, less sedation/anesthesia use, and peripheral rather than

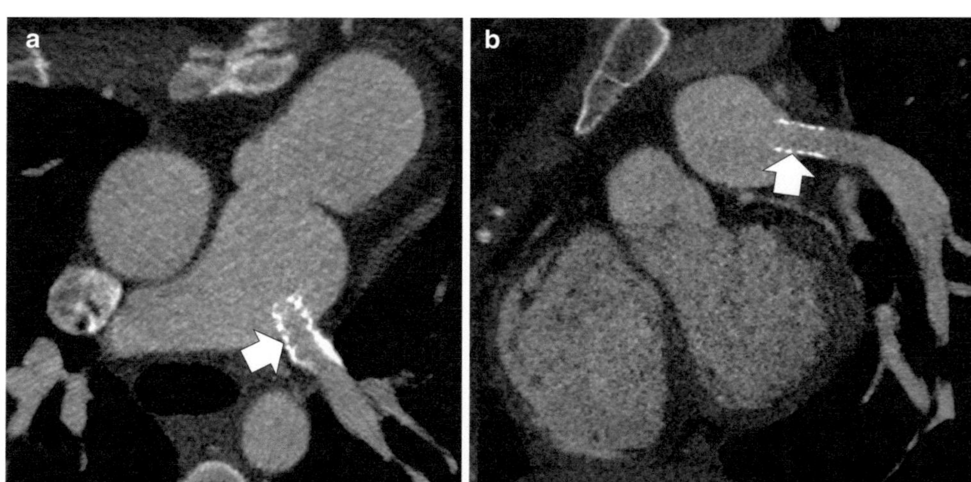

Fig. 47.14 Pulmonary artery hypoplasia in tetralogy of Fallot. (**a**) Axial and (**b**) sagittal reconstructions which show a normal-sized right pulmonary artery but a diffusely small left pulmonary artery. Note that the LPA had an origin stenosis at birth which has subsequently been stented (arrow)

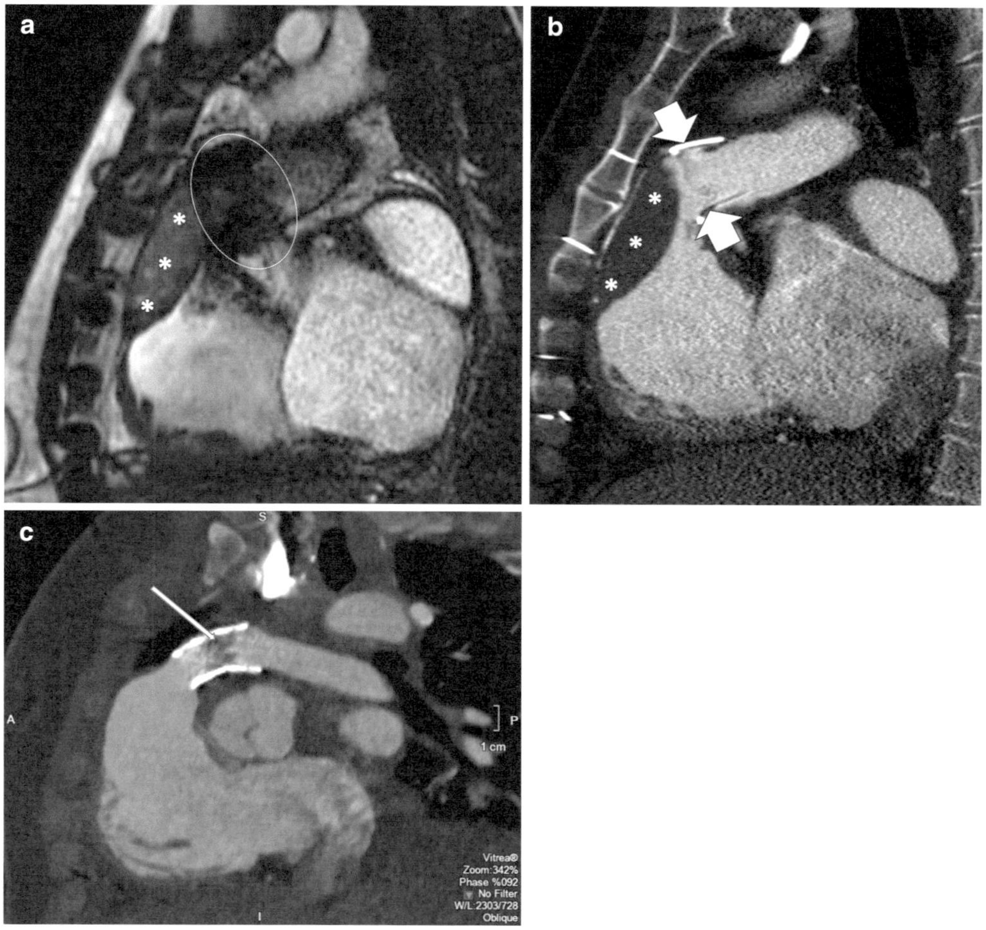

Fig. 47.15 (**a** and **b**) RVOT obstruction clarified by cardiac CT. (**a**) Sagittal oblique view of the right ventricular outflow tract by cine CMR – there is a convex lesion (asterisks) bulging into, and narrowing, the RVOTO. Beyond this is an area of signal dephasing (white oval), where the underlying anatomy is unclear. (**b**) CT reconstruction of the same area demonstrates the convex lesion, which from attenuation values can be inferred to be hematoma and demonstrates that the poorly visualized area on CMR is in fact a pulmonary valve replacement (arrows) – although the valve itself is tissue, the metallic valve struts can cause significant artifact in a magnetic field. (**c**) Transcatheter pulmonary valve endocarditis visualized by CT: This 2D sagittal image is from a patient with a clinical diagnosis of endocarditis in the setting of a rapidly increasing RVOT gradient after transcatheter pulmonary valve placement. Vegetations are visualized as low attenuation material within the stent (arrow), confirmed at the time of surgical valve replacement

central IV access [52, 53]. Diagnostic accuracy compared to surgical findings is excellent, and outcomes through the next stage of palliation and up to 8 years after the Fontan are similar [54]. A retrospective evaluation of pre-Fontan cardiac catheterizations determined that over 50% did not add information [55], and future diagnostic algorithms will include cardiovascular CT when patients face MRI contraindications due to the high rate of pacemaker placement and interventions such as pulmonary artery stenting and coil embolization of aortopulmonary and veno-veno collateral vessels.

Common Anatomic Findings Between Stages 1 and 2

- Aortopulmonary or Sano (RV-PA) shunt stenosis
- Branch pulmonary artery stenosis
- Aortic coarctation
- Central venous occlusion
- Aortopulmonary and veno-veno collateral vessels

Scan Recommendations [7]

Complete assessment of both systemic venous and arterial vasculature is needed for second-stage surgical planning (Figs. 47.16 and 47.17). Central venous obstruction from previous surgical lines is common and may affect choice of IV site.

- Consider lower extremity or right arm IV to avoid scatter artifact from dense contrast in the innominate vein.
- Consider late image acquisition so arterial and venous vasculature can be obtained in a single dataset or a routine delayed venous scan.

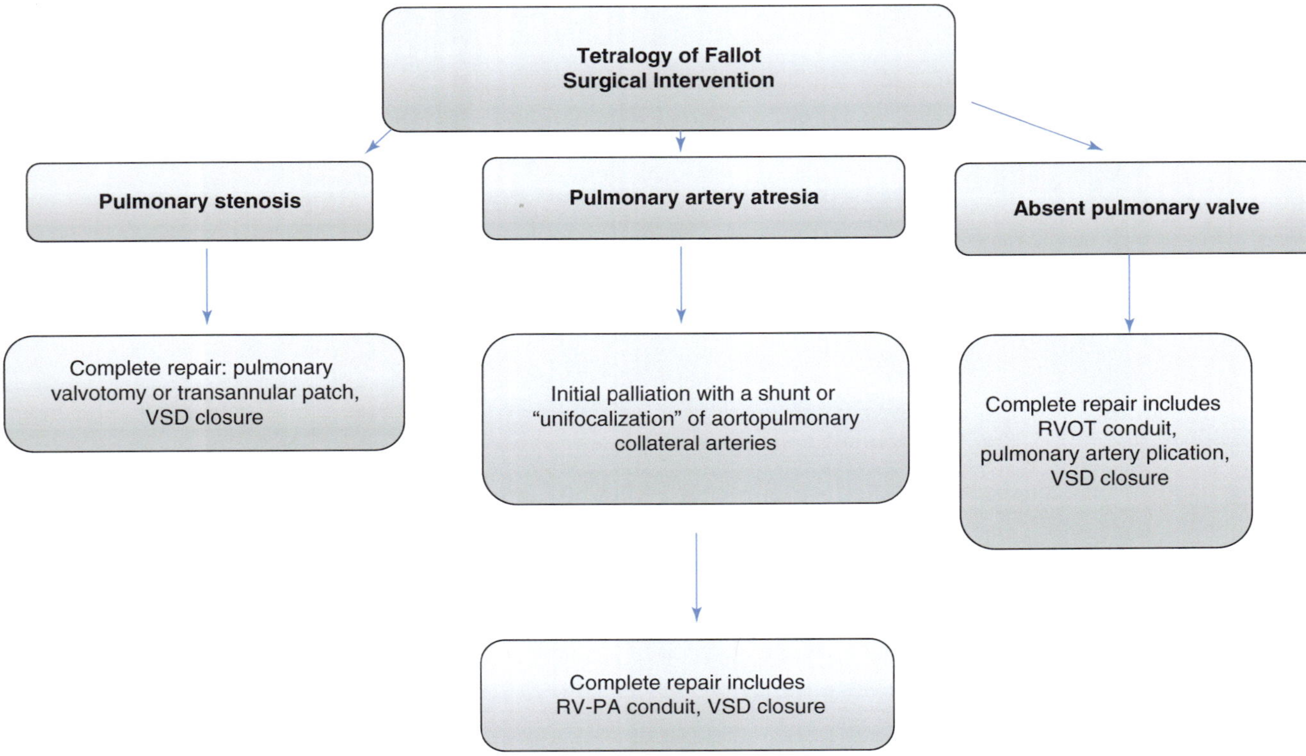

Fig. 47.16 Surgical intervention for tetralogy of Fallot

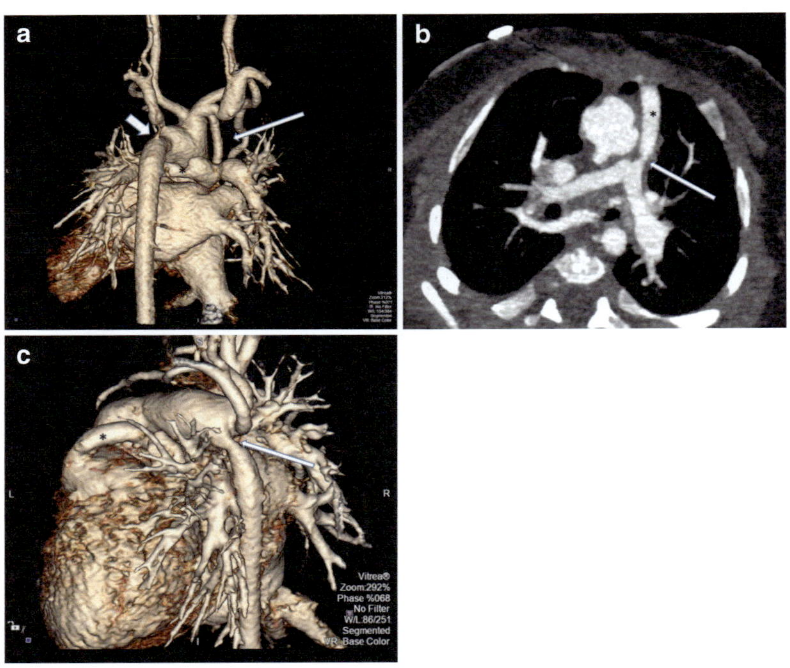

Fig. 47.17 Common findings after first-stage palliation of single ventricle heart disease. (**a**) This 3D volume-rendered dataset is a posterior view of an aortopulmonary shunt to the main pulmonary artery (arrow), with proximal stenosis of the left pulmonary artery (*). Note the size discrepancy between the reconstructed aorta and the proximal descending aorta at the distal Norwood anastomosis (short arrow). (**b**) This axial 2D image shows narrowing (arrow) at the distal RV-PA conduit (*) at the insertion to the branch pulmonary arteries. The RV-PA conduit is also called a Sano shunt and is placed from the anterior right ventricle to the branch pulmonary arteries as part of the first-stage single ventricle palliation, an alternative to an aortopulmonary shunt (see Figure a). (**c**) This 3D volume-rendered image shows aortic coarctation at the distal Norwood anastomosis as the reconstructed aorta inserts into the proximal descending aorta (arrow). The Sano shunt from the anterior surface of the right ventricle is also visualized (*)

Common Anatomic Findings Between Stages 2 and 3

- SVC to PA narrowing and branch pulmonary artery stenosis
- Aortic coarctation,
- Central venous occlusion
- Aortopulmonary and veno-veno collateral vessels

Scan Recommendations

- Consider lower extremity IV to avoid scatter artifact from dense contrast in the superior vena cava to pulmonary artery connection (Fig. 47.18).
- Consider late image acquisition so SVC to PA connection is visualized in the venous phase. Since the head is larger relative to body surface area in an infant, there is robust opacification of the superior central venous system prior to inferior vena cava opacification. If detailed inferior vena cava anatomy is needed (interrupted IVC), a lower extremity IV or a routine delayed venous scan should be considered.

Common Anatomic Findings After Third-Stage Palliation

- Narrowing along the Fontan pathway (SVC, IVC, or branch pulmonary arteries)
- Fenestration patency or occlusion
- Aortic coarctation
- Clot within the Fontan pathway, pulmonary arteries, or rudimentary ventricle
- Aortopulmonary and veno-veno collaterals
- Assessment of ventricular function
- Plastic bronchitis

Scan Acquisition Considerations and Recommendations After Third-Stage Palliation (Fontan)

Streaming of contrast primarily into one pulmonary artery is relatively common after the Fontan and can complicate assessment of the contralateral pulmonary artery (Figs. 47.19, 47.20, 47.21, and 47.22). Opacification of the inferior portion

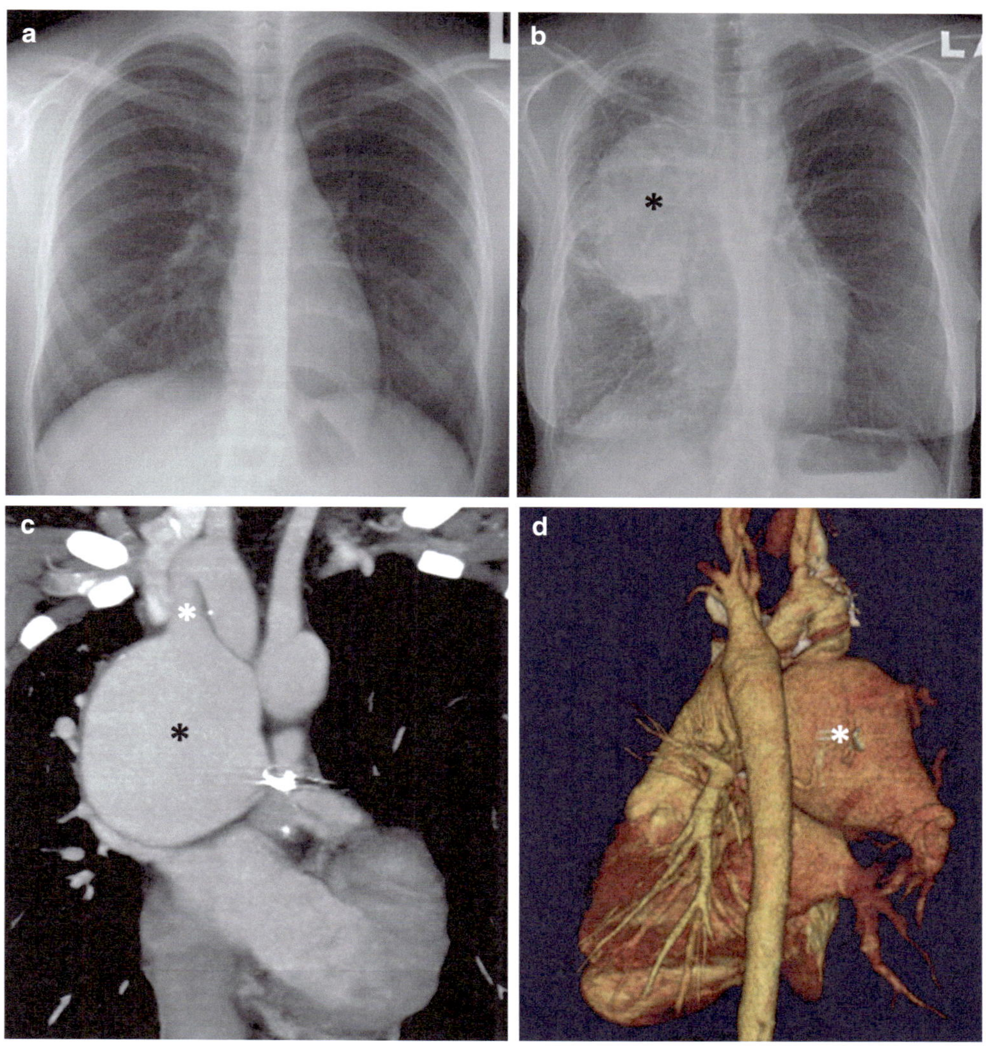

Fig. 47.18 Pulmonary artery aneurysm following BT shunt. (**a**) CXR with normal cardiopulmonary silhouette. (**b**) CXR of same patient 10 years later, now showing an abnormal configuration to the right para-mediastinal border. (**c**) Massive aneurysmal dilatation of the right main pulmonary artery (black asterisk) at the insertion of the BT shunt (white asterisk). (**d**) Volume-rendered image to show the size of the PA aneurysm (asterisk) relative to surrounding structures

of the Fontan pathway is also difficult and variable, depending on the type of Fontan connection and hemodynamics. Older style atrio-pulmonary artery connections and dilated lateral tunnel Fontan pathways will fill much later than extracardiac or non-dilated lateral tunnel Fontan connections. Filling is also delayed in the presence of high pulmonary artery pressures, ventricular dysfunction, and venous occlusion with extensive veno-veno collateralization. Chest CT performed acutely for chest pain or breathlessness may result in radiologists unfamiliar with this kind of circulation reporting large central "thrombi," which in reality are streaming artifacts due to incomplete mixing of opacified and unopacified blood.

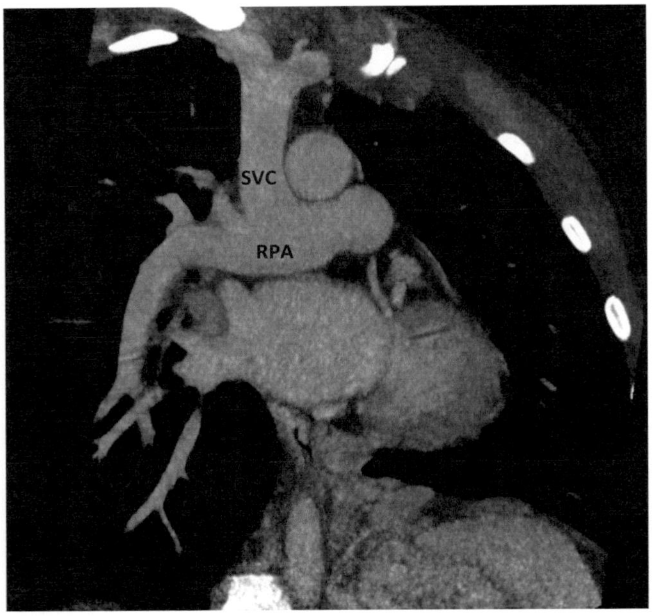

Fig. 47.19 Glenn superior vena cava to pulmonary artery anastomosis: This 2D MIP of a venous phase angiogram shows the superior vena cava connection to the right pulmonary artery after second-stage single ventricle palliation. The aortopulmonary shunt or Sano RV-PA conduit is taken down as part of this procedure

Scan Modifications

- Consider a two-phase contrast bolus with a 30–60 s pause between phases. This will allow opacification of the venous structures during image acquisition.
- A low-dose (70 or 80 kVp) ECG-triggered functional scan with a narrow acquisition window can be used to assess contrast flow in the superior vena cava to Fontan pathway.
- Delayed scan is useful for evaluation of the Fontan pathway, anywhere from 60 to 90 s after the initial contrast injection depending on risk factors.
- The huge right atrium which can be seen in adult patients with a classic RA-PA Fontan may rarely take over 5 min for full mixing of iodine and blood to occur due to the extremely slow swirling flow (referred to by echo as "smoke") that occurs.

Functional Cardiovascular CT Imaging in CHD

Quantification of ventricular volumes and function is used in clinical management for many indications in CHD. Examples include the timing of RVOT conduit placement in patients with pulmonary stenosis and insufficiency and the placement of defibrillators in patients with failing systemic and single right ventricles. On newer generation scanners with acceptable temporal resolution, cardiovascular CT is equivalent to

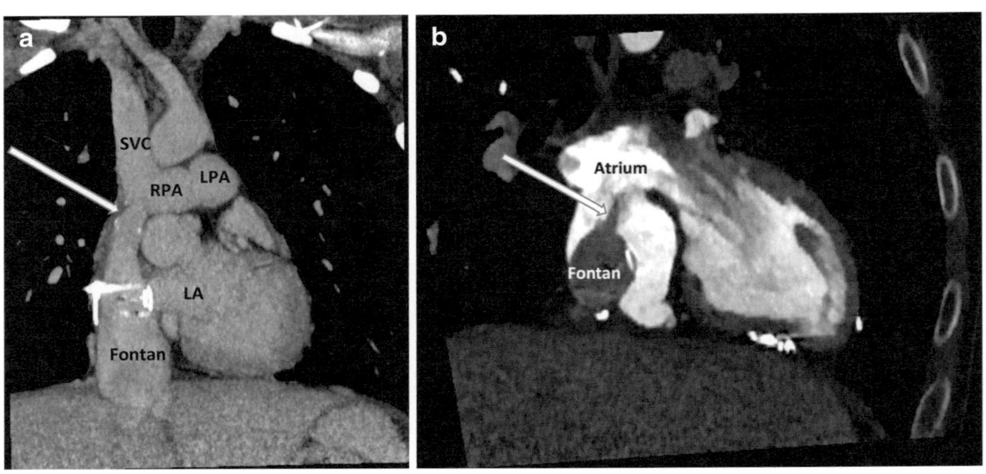

Fig. 47.20 CT imaging after the Fontan procedure: (**a**) A venous phase angiogram that shows narrowing of the lateral tunnel Fontan as it inserts into the undersurface of the RPA (arrow). The superior vena cava portion of the pathway is widely patent. Note the pacer lead artifact and the fenestration closure device between the Fontan and the atrium. (**b**) This image is a single phase of a functional dataset obtained to evaluate the Fontan pathway and fenestration status and quantify ventricular function. The arrow points to unopacified blood passing from the lateral tunnel Fontan pathway, through a fenestration and into the atrium which is opacified with contrast returning from the lungs. Note pacer lead on the epicardial surface of the heart

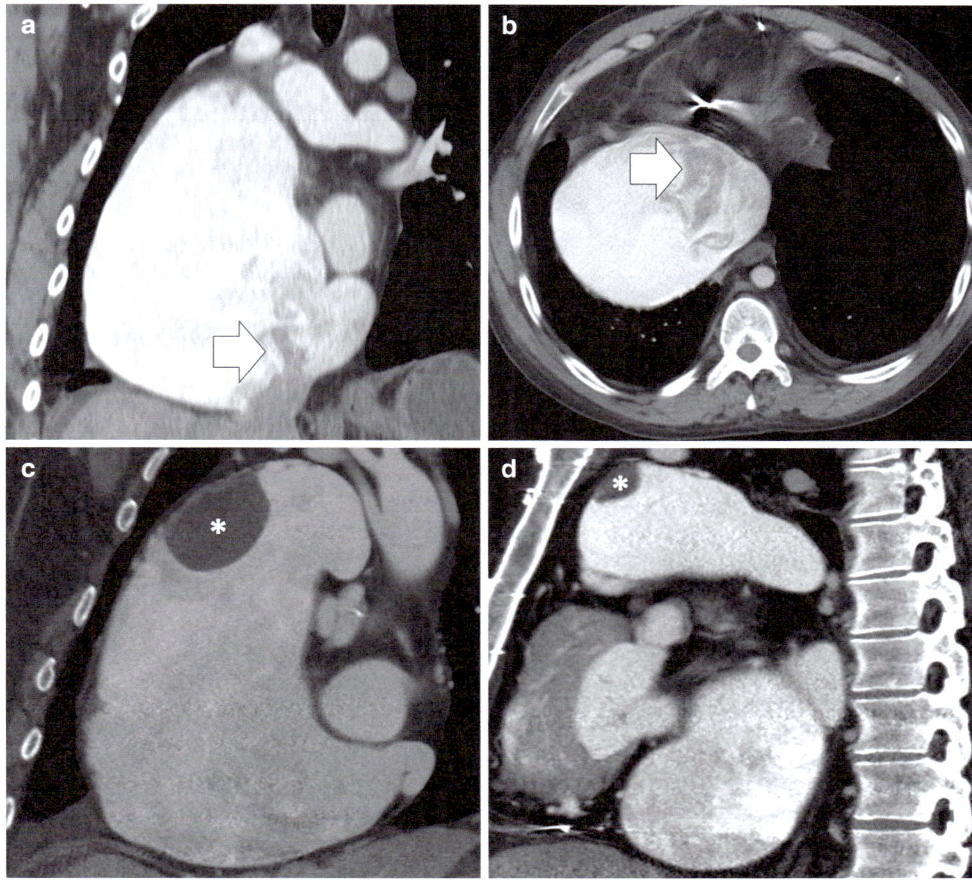

Fig. 47.21 Thrombus and pseudo-thrombus in a Fontan circuit. (**a**) Sagittal and (**b**) axial images demonstrating swirling unopacified blood from the IVC entering the right atrium (arrows). On echo this may be mistaken for thrombus on occasion. The same error may be avoided on CT by acquiring a delayed phase several minutes after injection of a sufficient volume of contrast. (**c**, **d**) Sagittal images in another patient with an RA-PA Fontan demonstrating thrombus in the RA and proximal main PA (asterisks)

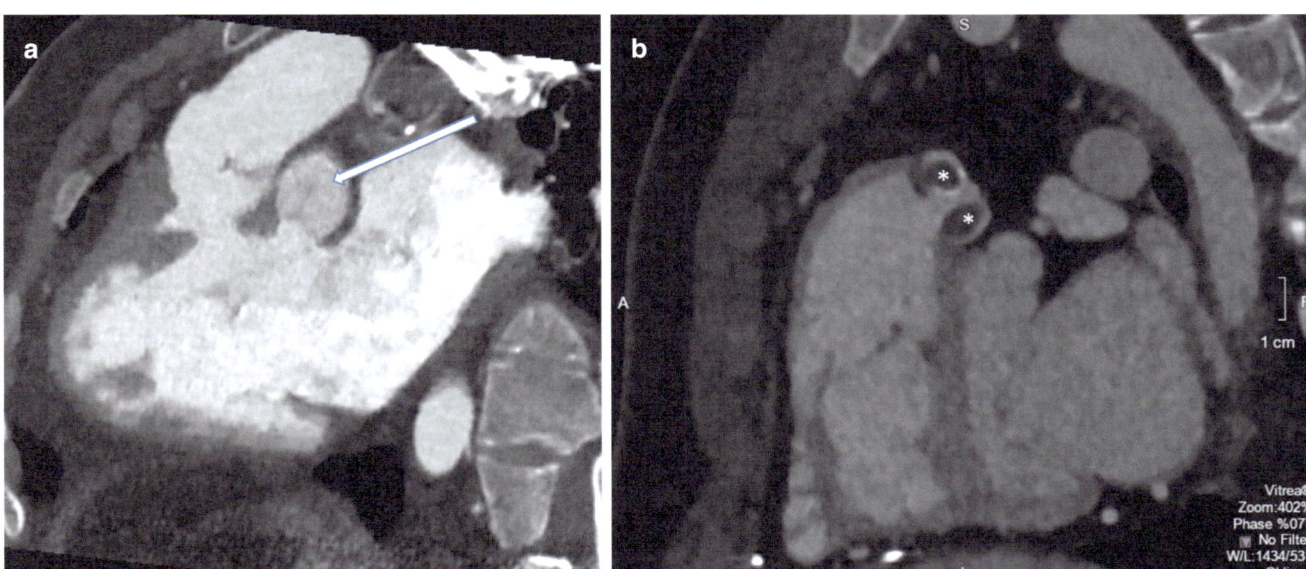

Fig. 47.22 (**a**) This figure shows retained pulmonary valve leaflets in a patient who had ligation of the pulmonary valve as part of Fontan completion. The retained valve leaflets in the systemic circulation predisposes to clots (**b**), which are seen in another patient. Newer palliative procedures oversew the pulmonary valve at the level of the valve leaflets to avoid this complication

CMR for right and left ventricular volumes and function as long as contrast opacification is adequate for the chamber being evaluated [56–58]. Functional datasets are reconstructed in a short axis stack with 6–8 mm slices, and a higher noise level is tolerated without loss of diagnostic accuracy. 70 and 80 kVp can be used for functional imaging in most patients with an estimated dose of 1–2.5 mSv [59].

Common Indications for Functional Analysis in CHD

- Quantification of right ventricular volumes and ejection fraction to determine the optimal timing of surgical or transcatheter pulmonary valve placement in patients with pulmonary stenosis or insufficiency and echocardiographic evidence of right ventricular enlargement or dysfunction (s/p TOF or any surgery requiring placement of a pulmonary artery conduit).
- Calculation of ejection fraction for patients with echocardiographic evidence of systemic ventricular systolic dysfunction (single ventricle, systemic right or left ventricle) to guide medical management of heart failure, placement of EP devices, and advanced heart therapies (VAD, transplant).
- Evaluation of ejection fraction and ventricular dyssynchrony in pacemaker-dependent patients to determine need for biventricular pacing and to guide optimal lead placement (concomitant coronary sinus imaging is important for these cases) [60].
- Evaluation of prosthetic valve function in patients with unexplained systolic gradient, for evaluation of paravalvular leak or for possible mass/vegetation (clot/endocarditis)
- Evaluation of complex AV valve attachments in subarterial obstruction, after AV canal defect, corrected transposition, s/p Rastelli.
- Calculation of stroke volume difference to estimate regurgitation (only possible in biventricular circulation). If more than one regurgitant lesion or shunt is present on the echocardiogram, only the total stroke volume difference can be reported, and echocardiography must be used to determine severity of individual lesions.

References

1. Khairy P, Ionescu-Ittu R, Mackie AS, Abrahamowicz M, Pilote L, Marelli AJ. Changing mortality in congenital heart disease. J Am Coll Cardiol. 2010;56(14):1149–57.
2. Marelli AJ, Ionescu-Ittu R, Mackie AS, Guo L, Dendukuri N, Kaouache M. Lifetime prevalence of congenital heart disease in the general population from 2000 to 2010. Circulation. 2014;130(9):749–56.
3. Tutarel O, Kempny A, Alonso-Gonzalez R, Jabbour R, Li W, Uebing A, et al. Congenital heart disease beyond the age of 60: emergence of a new population with high resource utilization, high morbidity, and high mortality. Eur Heart J. 2014;35(11):725–32.
4. Baumgartner H. Geriatric congenital heart disease: a new challenge in the care of adults with congenital heart disease? Eur Heart J. 2014;35(11):683–5.
5. Warnes CA, Williams RG, Bashore TM, Child JS, Connolly HM, Dearani JA, et al. ACC/AHA 2008 guidelines for the management of adults with congenital heart disease: a report of the American College of Cardiology/American Heart Association task force on practice guidelines (writing committee to develop guidelines on the management of adults with congenital heart disease). Developed in collaboration with the American Society of Echocardiography, Heart Rhythm Society, International Society for Adult Congenital Heart Disease, Society for Cardiovascular Angiography and Interventions, and Society of Thoracic Surgeons. J Am Coll Cardiol. 2008;52(23):e143–263.
6. Han BK, Lesser AM, Vezmar M, Rosenthal K, Rutten-Ramos S, Lindberg J, et al. Cardiovascular imaging trends in congenital heart disease: a single center experience. J Cardiovasc Comput Tomogr. 2013;7(6):361–6.
7. Han BK, Rigsby CK, Leipsic J, Bardo D, Abbara S, Ghoshhajra B, et al. Computed tomography imaging in patients with congenital heart disease, part 2: technical recommendations. An expert consensus document of the Society of Cardiovascular Computed Tomography (SCCT): endorsed by the Society of Pediatric Radiology (SPR) and the North American Society of Cardiac Imaging (NASCI). J Cardiovasc Comput Tomogr. 2015;9(6):493–513.
8. Han BK, Rigsby CK, Hlavacek A, Leipsic J, Nicol ED, Siegel MJ, et al. Computed tomography imaging in patients with congenital heart disease part I: rationale and utility. An expert consensus document of the Society of Cardiovascular Computed Tomography (SCCT): endorsed by the Society of Pediatric Radiology (SPR) and the North American Society of Cardiac Imaging (NASCI). J Cardiovasc Comput Tomogr. 2015;9(6):475–92.
9. Taylor AJ, Cerqueira M, Hodgson JM, Mark D, Min J, O'Gara P, et al. ACCF/SCCT/ACR/AHA/ASE/ASNC/NASCI/SCAI/SCMR 2010 appropriate use criteria for cardiac computed tomography. A report of the American College of Cardiology foundation appropriate use criteria task force, the Society of Cardiovascular Computed Tomography, the American College of Radiology, the American Heart Association, the American Society of Echocardiography, the American Society of Nuclear Cardiology, the North American Society for Cardiovascular Imaging, the Society for Cardiovascular Angiography and Interventions, and the Society for Cardiovascular Magnetic Resonance. J Cardiovasc Comput Tomogr. 2010;4(6):407 e1–33.
10. Gottlieb EA, Andropoulos DB. Anesthesia for the patient with congenital heart disease presenting for noncardiac surgery. Curr Opin Anaesthesiol. 2013;26(3):318–26.
11. Ing C, DiMaggio C, Whitehouse A, Hegarty MK, Brady J, von Ungern-Sternberg BS, et al. Long-term differences in language and cognitive function after childhood exposure to anesthesia. Pediatrics. 2012;130(3):e476–85.
12. Flick RP, Katusic SK, Colligan RC, Wilder RT, Voigt RG, Olson MD, et al. Cognitive and behavioral outcomes after early exposure to anesthesia and surgery. Pediatrics. 2011;128(5):e1053–61.
13. Ing CH, DiMaggio CJ, Whitehouse AJ, Hegarty MK, Sun M, von Ungern-Sternberg BS, et al. Neurodevelopmental outcomes after initial childhood anesthetic exposure between ages 3 and 10 years. J Neurosurg Anesthesiol. 2014;26(4):377–86.
14. DiMaggio C, Sun LS, Ing C, Li G. Pediatric anesthesia and neurodevelopmental impairments: a Bayesian meta-analysis. J Neurosurg Anesthesiol. 2012;24(4):376–81.

15. Ramamoorthy C, Haberkern CM, Bhananker SM, Domino KB, Posner KL, Campos JS, et al. Anesthesia-related cardiac arrest in children with heart disease: data from the Pediatric Perioperative Cardiac Arrest (POCA) registry. Anesth Analg. 2010;110(5):1376–82.
16. Downing TE, McDonnell A, Zhu X, Dori Y, Gillespie MJ, Rome JJ, et al. Cumulative medical radiation exposure throughout staged palliation of single ventricle congenital heart disease. Pediatr Cardiol. 2015;36(1):190–5.
17. Watson TG, Mah E, Joseph Schoepf U, King L, Huda W, Hlavacek AM. Effective radiation dose in computed tomographic angiography of the chest and diagnostic cardiac catheterization in pediatric patients. Pediatr Cardiol. 2013;34(3):518–24.
18. Johnson JN, Hornik CP, Li JS, Benjamin DK Jr, Yoshizumi TT, Reiman RE, et al. Cumulative radiation exposure and cancer risk estimation in children with heart disease. Circulation. 2014;130(2):161–7.
19. Podberesky DJ, Angel E, Yoshizumi TT, Toncheva G, Salisbury SR, Alsip C, et al. Radiation dose estimation for prospective and retrospective ECG-gated cardiac CT angiography in infants and small children using a 320-MDCT volume scanner. AJR Am J Roentgenol. 2012;199(5):1129–35.
20. Vastel-Amzallag C, Le Bret E, Paul JF, Lambert V, Rohnean A, El Fassy E, et al. Diagnostic accuracy of dual-source multislice computed tomographic analysis for the preoperative detection of coronary artery anomalies in 100 patients with tetralogy of Fallot. J Thorac Cardiovasc Surg. 2011;142(1):120–6.
21. Han BK, Lindberg J, Overman D, Schwartz RS, Grant K, Lesser JR. Safety and accuracy of dual-source coronary computed tomography angiography in the pediatric population. J Cardiovasc Comput Tomogr. 2012;6(4):252–9.
22. Young C, Taylor AM, Owens CM. Paediatric cardiac computed tomography: a review of imaging techniques and radiation dose consideration. Eur Radiol. 2011;21(3):518–29.
23. Meinel FG, Henzler T, Schoepf UJ, Park PW, Huda W, Spearman JV, et al. ECG-synchronized CT angiography in 324 consecutive pediatric patients: spectrum of indications and trends in radiation dose. Pediatr Cardiol. 2015;36(3):569–78.
24. Halliburton SS, Abbara S, Chen MY, Gentry R, Mahesh M, Raff GL, et al. SCCT guidelines on radiation dose and dose-optimization strategies in cardiovascular CT. J Cardiovasc Comput Tomogr. 2011;5(4):198–224.
25. Khairy P, Van Hare GF, Balaji S, Berul CI, Cecchin F, Cohen MI, et al. PACES/HRS expert consensus statement on the recognition and management of arrhythmias in adult congenital heart disease. Heart Rhythm. 2014;11(10):e102–65.
26. Morray BH, McElhinney DB, Cheatham JP, Zahn EM, Berman DP, Sullivan PM, et al. Risk of coronary artery compression among patients referred for transcatheter pulmonary valve implantation: a multicenter experience. Circ Cardiovasc Interv. 2013;6(5):535–42.
27. McElhinney DB, Hellenbrand WE, Zahn EM, Jones TK, Cheatham JP, Lock JE, et al. Short- and medium-term outcomes after transcatheter pulmonary valve placement in the expanded multicenter US melody valve trial. Circulation. 2010;122(5):507–16.
28. Han BK, Moga FX, Overman D, Carter C, Lesser JR. Diagnostic value of contrast-enhanced multiphase computed tomography for assessment of percutaneous pulmonary valve obstruction. Ann Thorac Surg. 2016;101(4):e115–6.
29. Habets J, Tanis W, van Herwerden LA, van den Brink RB, Mali WP, de Mol BA, et al. Cardiac computed tomography angiography results in diagnostic and therapeutic change in prosthetic heart valve endocarditis. Int J Cardiovasc Imaging. 2014;30(2):377–87.
30. Wijesekera H, Seneviratne S, Woolley I. Cardiac computed tomography in endocarditis. Heart. 2010;96(19):1604.
31. Stulak JM, Dearani JA, Burkhart HM, Ammash NM, Phillips SD, Schaff HV. Coronary artery disease in adult congenital heart disease: outcome after coronary artery bypass grafting. Ann Thorac Surg. 2012;93(1):116–22; discussion 22–3.
32. Bhatt AB, Foster E, Kuehl K, Alpert J, Brabeck S, Crumb S, et al. Congenital heart disease in the older adult: a scientific statement from the american heart association. Circulation. 2015;131(21):1884–931.
33. Pedersen TA. Late morbidity after repair of aortic coarctation. Dan Med J. 2012;59(4):B4436.
34. Brown ML, Burkhart HM, Connolly HM, Dearani JA, Cetta F, Li Z, et al. Coarctation of the aorta: lifelong surveillance is mandatory following surgical repair. J Am Coll Cardiol. 2013;62(11):1020–5.
35. Egan M, Holzer RJ. Comparing balloon angioplasty, stenting and surgery in the treatment of aortic coarctation. Expert Rev Cardiovasc Ther. 2009;7(11):1401–12.
36. Holzer R, Qureshi S, Ghasemi A, Vincent J, Sievert H, Gruenstein D, et al. Stenting of aortic coarctation: acute, intermediate, and long-term results of a prospective multi-institutional registry--Congenital Cardiovascular Interventional Study Consortium (CCISC). Catheter Cardiovasc Interv. 2010;76(4):553–63.
37. Khairy P, Landzberg MJ, Lambert J, O'Donnell CP. Long-term outcomes after the atrial switch for surgical correction of transposition: a meta-analysis comparing the Mustard and Senning procedures. Cardiol Young. 2004;14(3):284–92.
38. Khairy P, Van Hare GF, Balaji S, Berul CI, Cecchin F, Cohen MI, et al. PACES/HRS expert consensus statement on the recognition and management of arrhythmias in adult congenital heart disease: executive summary. Heart Rhythm. 2014;11(10):e102–65.
39. Villafane J, Lantin-Hermoso MR, Bhatt AB, Tweddell JS, Geva T, Nathan M, et al. D-transposition of the great arteries: the current era of the arterial switch operation. J Am Coll Cardiol. 2014;64(5):498–511.
40. Ou P, Khraiche D, Celermajer DS, Agnoletti G, Le Quan Sang KH, Thalabard JC, et al. Mechanisms of coronary complications after the arterial switch for transposition of the great arteries. J Thorac Cardiovasc Surg. 2013;145(5):1263–9.
41. Ou P, Celermajer DS, Marini D, Agnoletti G, Vouhe P, Brunelle F, et al. Safety and accuracy of 64-slice computed tomography coronary angiography in children after the arterial switch operation for transposition of the great arteries. J Am Coll Cardiol Img. 2008;1(3):331–9.
42. Khairy P, Aboulhosn J, Gurvitz MZ, Opotowsky AR, Mongeon FP, Kay J, et al. Arrhythmia burden in adults with surgically repaired tetralogy of Fallot: a multi-institutional study. Circulation. 2010;122(9):868–75.
43. Khairy P, Dore A, Poirier N, Marcotte F, Ibrahim R, Mongeon FP, et al. Risk stratification in surgically repaired tetralogy of Fallot. Expert Rev Cardiovasc Ther. 2009;7(7):755–62.
44. Geva T. Indications for pulmonary valve replacement in repaired tetralogy of fallot: the quest continues. Circulation. 2013;128(17):1855–7.
45. Ferraz Cavalcanti PE, Sa MP, Santos CA, Esmeraldo IM, de Escobar RR, de Menezes AM, et al. Pulmonary valve replacement after operative repair of tetralogy of Fallot: meta-analysis and meta-regression of 3,118 patients from 48 studies. J Am Coll Cardiol. 2013;62(23):2227–43.
46. Le Gloan L, Mongeon FP, Mercier LA, Dore A, Marcotte F, Ibrahim R, et al. Tetralogy of Fallot and aortic root disease. Expert Rev Cardiovasc Ther. 2013;11(2):233–8.
47. Warnes CA, Child JS. Aortic root dilatation after repair of tetralogy of Fallot: pathology from the past? Circulation. 2002;106(11):1310–1.
48. d'Udekem Y, Xu MY, Galati JC, Lu S, Iyengar AJ, Konstantinov IE, et al. Predictors of survival after single-ventricle palliation: the impact of right ventricular dominance. J Am Coll Cardiol. 2012;59(13):1178–85.

49. DiBardino DJ. Long-term progression and survival following Norwood Single Ventricle Reconstruction. Curr Opin Cardiol. 2015;30(1):95–9.
50. Stern KW, McElhinney DB, Gauvreau K, Geva T, Brown DW. Echocardiographic evaluation before bidirectional Glenn operation in functional single-ventricle heart disease: comparison to catheter angiography. Circ Cardiovasc Imaging. 2011;4(5):498–505.
51. Rabbitts JA, Groenewald CB, Mauermann WJ, Barbara DW, Burkhart HM, Warnes CA, et al. Outcomes of general anesthesia for noncardiac surgery in a series of patients with Fontan palliation. Paediatr Anaesth. 2013;23(2):180–7.
52. Brown DW, Gauvreau K, Powell AJ, Lang P, Colan SD, Del Nido PJ, et al. Cardiac magnetic resonance versus routine cardiac catheterization before bidirectional glenn anastomosis in infants with functional single ventricle: a prospective randomized trial. Circulation. 2007;116(23):2718–25.
53. Han BK, Vezmar M, Lesser JR, Michalak G, Grant K, Dassenko D, et al. Selective use of cardiac computed tomography angiography: an alternative diagnostic modality before second-stage single ventricle palliation. J Thorac Cardiovasc Surg. 2014;148(4):1548–54.
54. Brown DW, Gauvreau K, Powell AJ, Lang P, del Nido PJ, Odegard KC, et al. Cardiac magnetic resonance versus routine cardiac catheterization before bidirectional Glenn anastomosis: long-term follow-up of a prospective randomized trial. J Thorac Cardiovasc Surg. 2013;146(5):1172–8.
55. Banka P, McElhinney DB, Bacha EA, Mayer JE Jr, Gauvreau K, Geva T, et al. What is the clinical utility of routine cardiac catheterization before a Fontan operation? Pediatr Cardiol. 2010;31(7):977–85.
56. Aho MR, Gebregziabher M, Schoepf UJ, Suranyi P, Lee H, Gregg D, et al. Impact of right ventricular contrast attenuation on the accuracy of right ventricular function analysis at cardiac multi-detector-row CT. Eur J Radiol. 2010;73(3):560–5.
57. Greupner J, Zimmermann E, Grohmann A, Dubel HP, Althoff TF, Borges AC, et al. Head-to-head comparison of left ventricular function assessment with 64-row computed tomography, biplane left cineventriculography, and both 2- and 3-dimensional transthoracic echocardiography: comparison with magnetic resonance imaging as the reference standard. J Am Coll Cardiol. 2012;59(21):1897–907.
58. Rizvi A, Deano RC, Bachman DP, Xiong G, Min JK, Truong QA. Analysis of ventricular function by CT. J Cardiovasc Comput Tomogr. 2015;9(1):1–12.
59. Lesser AM, Newell MC, Samara MA, Gornick C, Grant K, Garberich R, et al. Radiation dose and image quality of 70 kVp functional cardiovascular computed tomography imaging in congenital heart disease. J Cardiovasc Comput Tomogr. 2016;10(2):173–8.
60. Niazi I, Dhala A, Choudhuri I, Sra J, Akhtar M, Tajik AJ. Cardiac resynchronization therapy in patients with challenging anatomy due to venous anomalies or adult congenital heart disease. Pacing Clin Electrophysiol: PACE. 2014;37(9):1181–8.

Part XI

Where We Are: The Heart and Beyond

CT Imaging of the Heart-Lung Axis

48

Michelle C. Williams and Edwin J. R. van Beek

The heart and lungs are intimately related in terms of both anatomy and physiology. Their close proximity in the thorax means that CT imaging of one organ also visualises at least part of the other. The shared physiology of respiration and circulation has implications in both health and disease. Diseases that affect one of these organs have secondary implications for the other. In addition shared aetiologies, such as smoking, or similar mechanistic pathways, such as systemic inflammation, can lead to the coexistence of both respiratory and cardiovascular diseases. Thus, CT imaging of the heart-lung axis is frequently encountered in clinical practice and a holistic approach to cardiothoracic imaging is therefore required.

This chapter will discuss some of the key imaging relationships between the heart and the lungs, including pulmonary hypertension, thromboembolic disease, chronic lung diseases and atherosclerosis.

CT Imaging Methods to Assess The Heart-Lung Axis

Cardiovascular disease may be identified on CT imaging performed to assess the lungs, such as CT pulmonary angiography (CTPA) or high-resolution CT of the chest (HRCT, Fig. 48.1). As a rule, electrocardiogram (ECG) gating is not used for these types of studies, and therefore motion artefact will impact the ability to assess the coronary arteries. Nevertheless, coronary artery calcification can be identified, and a qualitative or semiquantitative assessment is usually feasible.

Coronary artery calcium can be assessed on CT images which are not optimised for traditional calcium scoring [1]. This includes images performed without ECG gating, contrast-enhanced images and images where cardiac-optimised reconstruction algorithms or slice thickness/interval have not been used. It may be possible to perform quantitative calcium scoring on these images, by application of the Agatston or other calcium scoring methods. However differences in the acquisition and reconstruction of these images will mean that the resulting calcium score may be overestimated [1, 2]. Nevertheless, these techniques have been shown to correlate with traditional Agatston scores [1]. Ordinal calcium scores can also be used to assess coronary artery calcification on these non-optimised CT images [3, 4]. This method assesses the presence and quantity of calcification in the major epicardial vessels (none, mild, moderate, severe) and provides a summed score. Vascular calcification is influenced by age and gender as well as cardiovascular risk; therefore, these results should be communicated in the context of the patient's age and gender [5].

CT scans performed to assess respiratory disease can also provide information on the heart structure and function. These cardiovascular findings may be incidental or related to the presenting complaint. This includes identification of dilated cardiac chambers, dilated great vessels and valvular calcification [6, 7]. Valvular calcification may indicate the presence of incidental aortic stenosis, particularly in elderly populations [8]. A combination of cardiovascular CT findings and traditional risk factors can be used to stratify patients at risk, and this is associated with prognosis [9]. Evidence of congenital cardiovascular disease and malignancy can also be diagnosed and may lead to further dedicated imaging examinations.

Respiratory disease is frequently identified on CT imaging performed to assess the heart [10]. It is now widely accepted that for cardiac CT, a wide field of view to assess the imaged lungs and other extra-cardiac findings within the scanned volume should be reconstructed and assessed [11, 12]. For some patients the respiratory findings may be the cause of their symptoms, such as patients with chest pain and a pulmonary embolism. For others the respiratory findings will require further assessment and follow-up, such as the identification of lung nodules (Fig. 48.2).

M. C. Williams (✉) · E. J. R. van Beek
Edinburgh Imaging Facility QMRI, University of Edinburgh, Edinburgh, UK
e-mail: michelle.williams@ed.ac.uk

U. J. Schoepf (ed.), *CT of the Heart*, Contemporary Medical Imaging, https://doi.org/10.1007/978-1-60327-237-7_48

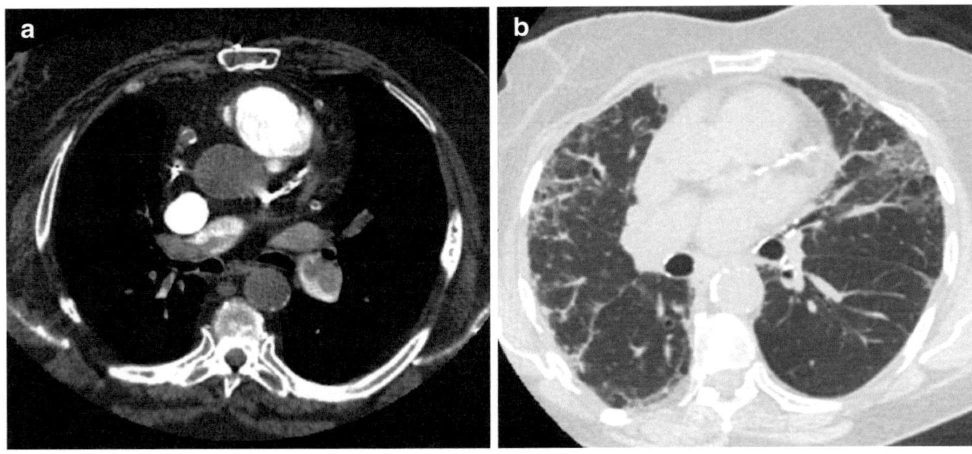

Fig. 48.1 Cardiovascular disease identified as coronary artery calcification on (**a**) CTPA in a patient with pulmonary embolism (**b**) high-resolution CT of the chest in a patient with idiopathic pulmonary fibrosis

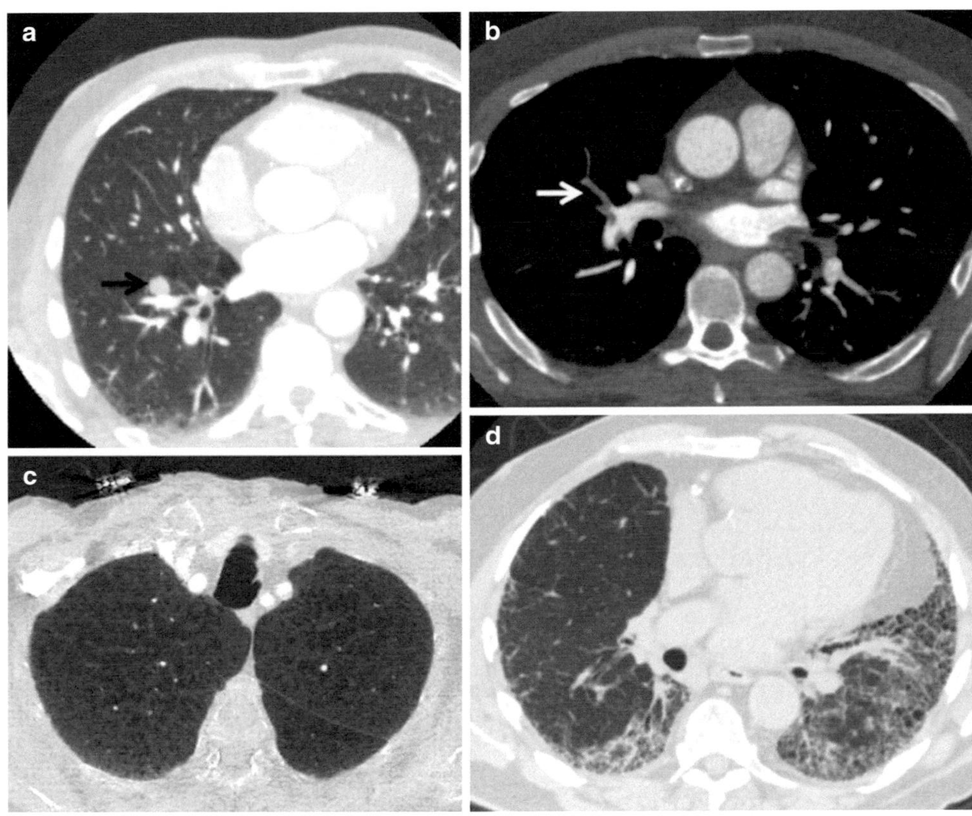

Fig. 48.2 Extra-cardiac findings identified in the lungs on CT coronary angiography with (**a**) lung malignancy, (**b**) pulmonary embolism, (**c**) emphysema and (**d**) pulmonary fibrosis

In addition to visual assessment of the lungs, a variety of automated software tools can be applied. The extent of emphysema can be quantified based on attenuation density [13, 14]. Interstitial lung disease can be identified based on attenuation density and texture analysis [14, 15]. Automated software can also be used to identify lung nodules and track their dimensions and volume on follow-up imaging. Modern CT techniques can also be used to assess lung function. Dual-energy imaging can be used to create pulmonary blood volume images, which can be used to assess pulmonary perfusion in areas of infarction or in lung tumours [16]. Dynamic contrast-enhanced CT of the lungs can be used to quantify pulmonary perfusion [17].

A direct simultaneous assessment of the cardiovascular and respiratory system can be planned, for instance, in patients referred for lung transplantation [18]. Patients presenting with acute chest pain may benefit from a combined "triple-rule-out" scan in selected cases [19, 20]. This technique allows for simultaneous assessment of the coronary arteries for coronary artery disease, the pulmonary arteries for the presence of pulmonary embolism and the aorta for aortic dissection. However, this is a highly challenging technique due to the requirement of contrast opacification in three separate time intervals, resulting in a high frequency of non-diagnostic examinations, as well as exposing the patient to an increased radiation dose and volume of contrast [19, 20]. Therefore, the routine use of triple-rule-out CT for all patients attending to the emergency department is not recommended.

Shared Aetiology and Pathogenesis

Respiratory and cardiovascular diseases share a number of factors in their aetiology and pathogenesis. The most important shared risk factor for cardiovascular and respiratory diseases is smoking. Globally over 6 million deaths per year can be linked to the effects of tobacco [21]. The proportion of deaths attributable to tobacco is 71% for lung cancer, 42% for chronic obstructive pulmonary disease (COPD) and 10% for cardiovascular disease [21]. In addition, smokers have an excess of mortality not accounted for by these known associations [22].

In addition to smoking, there is overlap between other traditional cardiovascular risk factors and the risk of respiratory disease. A recent meta-analysis identified an increased prevalence of risk factors for cardiovascular disease amongst patients with COPD [23]. In particular there was an increased prevalence of hypertension (meta-odds ratio (OR) 1.33, 95% confidence interval (CI) 1.13–1.56, $p = 0.0007$), diabetes (1.36, 95% CI 1.21–1.53, $p < 0.0001$) and a history of ever having smoked (4.25, 95% CI 3.23–5.60, $p < 0.0001$) [23]. Interestingly, no association between the presence of COPD and the prevalence of obesity or dyslipidaemia was demonstrated [23]. Occupational exposure to asbestos is linked to an increased risk of both respiratory and cardiovascular disease [24]. Exposure to airborne pollution or particulate matter is associated with increased respiratory and cardiovascular morbidity and mortality [25–27].

Inflammation plays an important role in the development of both cardiovascular and respiratory diseases [28]. Biomarkers of systemic inflammation are increased in patients with reduced lung function [29] and in patients with symptomatic and asymptomatic cardiovascular disease [30, 31]. Smoking is associated with an increase in inflammatory biomarkers, even after smoking cessation [30]. Blood-borne inflammatory cells make up an important part of the atherosclerotic plaque, and inflammatory cytokines are involved in the progression of atherosclerosis [32].

Lung inflammation is central to the development of COPD, and low-grade systemic inflammation has been linked to an increase in complications, more rapid decline in lung function and increased hospitalisation [29]. Systemic inflammation in patients with COPD is associated with poorer clinical outcomes and increased prevalence of comorbidities such as heart disease, diabetes and hypertension [33]. Secondary markers of inflammation such as elastin degradation products are also increased in patients with COPD [34]. Inflammation is central to a number of other respiratory diseases such as pulmonary fibrosis, bronchiectasis and cystic fibrosis. In addition, inflammation has an important role in the development of lung cancer, through complex and incompletely understood mechanisms [35]. Thus, inflammation is a shared pathogenesis between a variety of respiratory and cardiovascular diseases and may represent a potential therapeutic target [36].

However, a recent population study of 1154 patients identified that, although airflow limitation was an independent predictor of atherosclerosis, systemic inflammation was not [37]. In addition, air flow limitation and endothelial dysfunction appear to be unrelated, independent predictors of the presence of atherosclerosis [38]. Thus, the links between respiratory and cardiovascular diseases and inflammation are complex and remain incompletely understood.

Overall, there is overwhelming evidence that there is a combined effect of cardiovascular disease and COPD, affecting outcomes. The COPDGene study demonstrated comorbidities had a major impact on clinical outcomes [39], while cardiovascular disease was directly associated with COPD severity, reduced functional status and quality of life [40]. In a different cohort, the ECLIPSE study, it was also demonstrated that patients with COPD had increased coronary artery risk with adverse outcomes in terms of morbidity and mortality [39–41].

Pulmonary Hypertension and The Heart

Pulmonary hypertension is defined as a mean pulmonary artery pressure of 25 mmHg or above on catheterisation of the right side of the heart [42]. There are multiple causes of pulmonary hypertension, which the widely used clinical classification divides into five groups (pulmonary arterial hypertension, Group 1; pulmonary hypertension due to left heart disease, Group 2; pulmonary hypertension due to chronic lung disease and/or hypoxia, Group 3; chronic thromboembolic pulmonary hypertension, Group 4; and pulmonary hypertension due to unclear multifactorial mechanisms, Group 5) [43]. Thus, there is significant overlap in the requirement for imaging both the heart and the lungs in patients with suspected or known pulmonary hypertension.

Acute Pulmonary Embolism

Acute pulmonary embolism can lead to changes in the heart and lungs that can be identified by echocardiography, CT and perfusion scintigraphy (Fig. 48.3). Right heart strain on

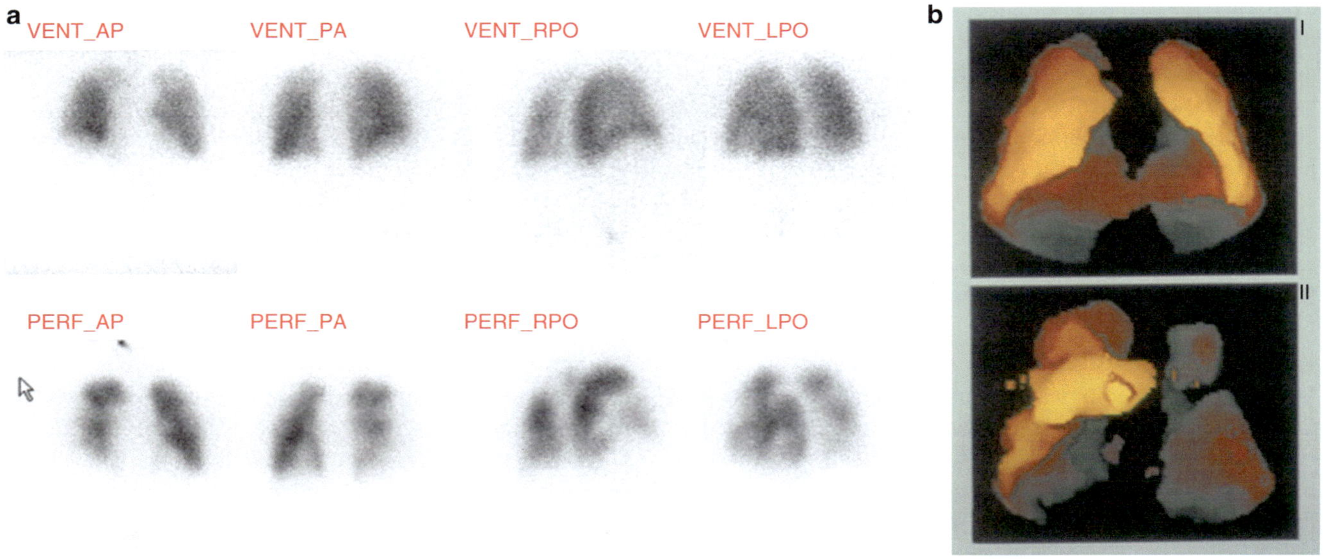

Fig. 48.3 Examples of SPECT images of the lungs. Planar SPECT images (**a**) with normal ventilation images and multiple perfusion defects, indicating a high probability of PE. Reconstructed SPECT images (**b**) in a separate patient showing normal ventilation on the superior image and multiple perfusion defects on the inferior image

CTPA is indicated by the presence of dilation of the right ventricle, dilation of the right atrium, an increase in the right ventricle to left ventricle ratio (RV/LV), bowing of the interventricular septum, dilation of the main and branch pulmonary arteries and regurgitation of contrast into the inferior vena cava or azygos vein (Fig. 48.4). An increased RV/LV ratio is associated with an increased severity if pulmonary embolism [44]. Increased mortality has been identified in patients with an increased RV/LV ratio, with bowing of the interventricular septum, regurgitation of contrast into the inferior vena cava and increased volume of the right ventricle [45]. Hence, these CT findings in the heart on CTPA may identify patients who require more aggressive treatment with fibrinolytic agents or follow-up.

Chronic Thromboembolic Pulmonary Hypertension

After treatment of an acute pulmonary embolism, these cardiac features can resolve following normalisation of the pulmonary artery pressures. However, in a small proportion of patients, chronic thromboembolic pulmonary hypertension may develop [46]. After an acute embolic event, the cumulative incidence of developing chronic thromboembolic pulmonary hypertension is between 0.1 and 9.1% at 2 years [47]. However, routine imaging follow-up after acute pulmonary embolism is not currently recommended [47, 48]. CT features of chronic thromboembolic pulmonary hypertension include endothelialised thrombus or webs, pulmonary artery stenosis or occlusion and features of right heart strain and ventricular remodelling (Fig. 48.5). In addition changes in the lung parenchyma can be identified by CT including infarction and mosaic perfusion [49]. Finally, initial studies have shown that CT perfusion may be useful in assessing patients after large pulmonary embolism, as incomplete peripheral resolution may lead to persistent perfusion abnormalities and increased risk of pulmonary hypertension [17].

Pulmonary Hypertension Secondary to Lung Disease

A variety of mechanisms lead to the development of pulmonary hypertension in patients with respiratory diseases such as COPD or idiopathic pulmonary fibrosis (Fig. 48.6). COPD causes obliteration of the pulmonary vascular bed through parenchymal destruction, and the cross-sectional area of small pulmonary vessels correlates with the severity of pulmonary artery hypertension [50]. The vascular responses to cigarette smoke include vasoconstriction, vascular remodelling, intima hyperplasia and muscular changes of the vessel wall [51]. Hypoxia leads to vasoconstriction and inhomogeneous perfusion [52]. In addition hyperinflation in COPD can impair right and left ventricular filling [53].

These changes in the pulmonary vasculature lead to subsequent alterations in the right ventricle. Patients with COPD are five times more likely to have disease of the pulmonary circulation compared to matched controls or the general public and two times more likely to develop heart failure [23]. Enlargement of the pulmonary artery diameter compared to the diameter of the aorta in patients with COPD is associated

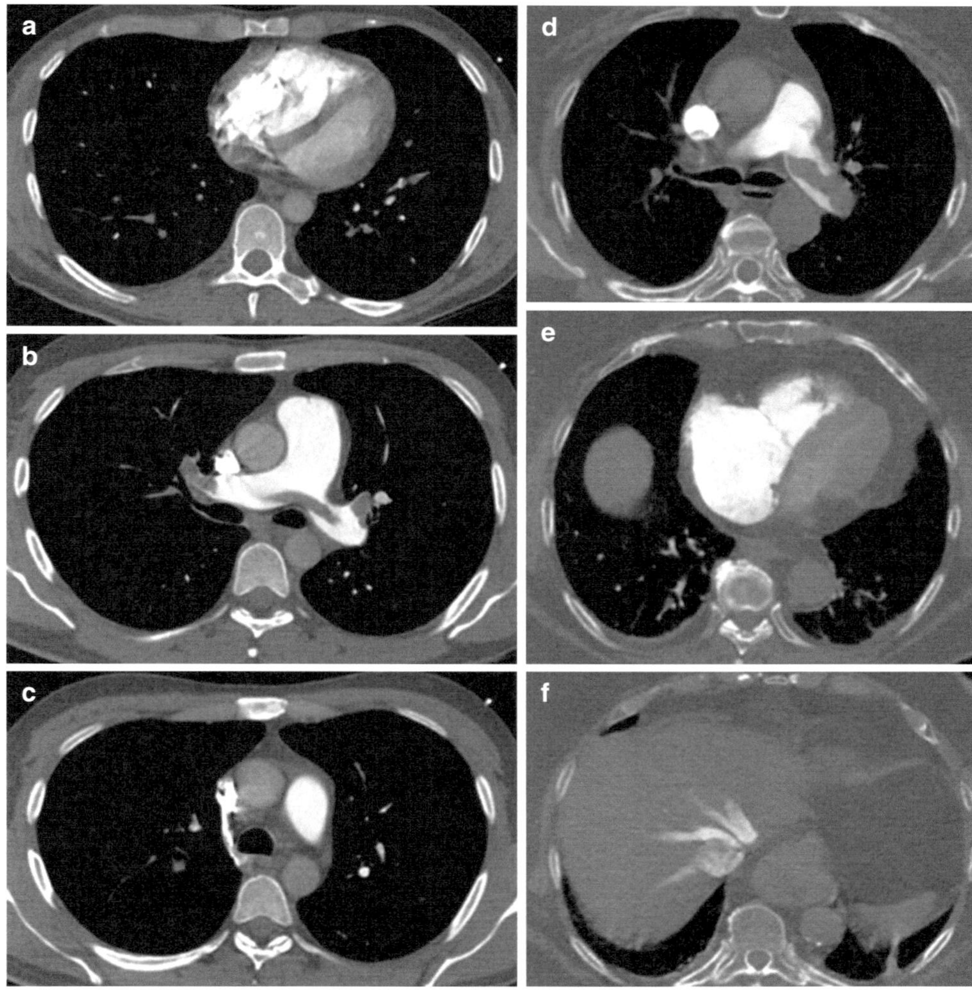

Fig. 48.4 CTPA images from two patients showing evidence of right heart strain. In the first patient with a saddle pulmonary embolism CT shows (**a**) a dilated right ventricle, an increased right ventricle to left ventricle ratio and bowing of the interventricular septum, (**b**) dilation of the main pulmonary artery and (**c**) and reflux of contrast into the azygos vein. The second patient has pulmonary embolism in (**d**) the left and right pulmonary arteries, (**e**) dilation of the right ventricle and right atrium and (**f**) regurgitation of contrast into the inferior vena cava

with the development of pulmonary hypertension and increased mortality [54]. Furthermore, patients with features of pulmonary hypertension are more likely to suffer repeated and more severe exacerbations of COPD [55]. However, there is significant capacity within the lungs and heart to compensate for these changes, and only 5–10% of patients with severe COPD develop pulmonary hypertension [56].

Other Causes of Pulmonary Hypertension

Other causes of pulmonary hypertension include hereditary causes and drug-induced and connective tissue diseases (Fig. 48.7). Pulmonary hypertension can occur in patients with congenital heart disease [57] (Fig. 48.8). In addition idiopathic pulmonary hypertension may be diagnosed after exclusion of other causes. The combined endpoint of all causes of chronic pulmonary hypertension is morphological and functional changes in the right ventricle (Fig. 48.9). This includes thinning, dilation and hypertrophy of the right ventricle, septal bowing of the left ventricle, tricuspid regurgitation and changes in cardiac output [58]. Eventually this will result in right heart failure and secondary changes within the lung parenchyma.

Atherosclerosis and Respiratory Disease

The coexistence of coronary artery disease and respiratory disease can be identified on CT. The link between cardiovascular disease and COPD (chronic obstructive pulmonary disease) has been extensively studied. Patients with COPD have an increased frequency of cardiovascular disease, and cardiovascular disease is associated with more severe disease, hospitalisation, morbidity and mortality. In addition there is a higher frequency of coronary artery disease in other respiratory diseases including bronchiectasis and interstitial lung disease. With the advancing use of low-dose CT to screen

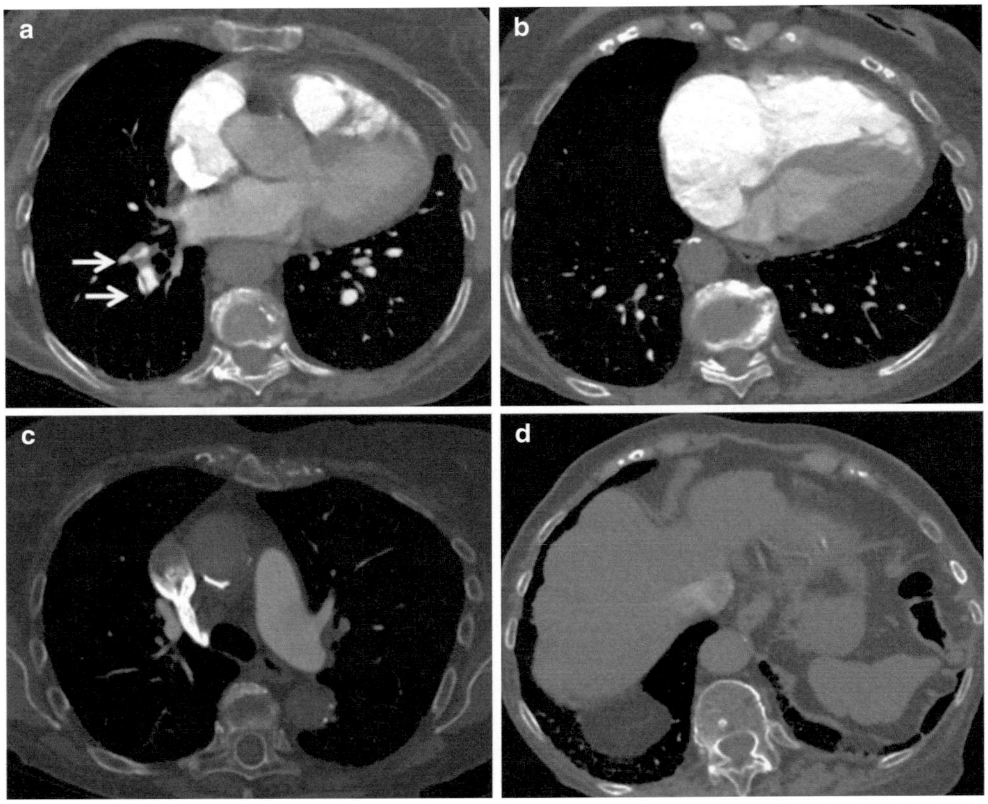

Fig. 48.5 Chronic thromboembolic pulmonary hypertension with (**a**) mural thrombus and web in the right pulmonary artery branches (arrows), (**b**) dilation of the right ventricle, dilation of the right atrium and an increased right ventricle to left ventricle ratio, (**c**) regurgitation of contrast into the azygos vein and (**d**) regurgitation of contrast into the inferior vena cava

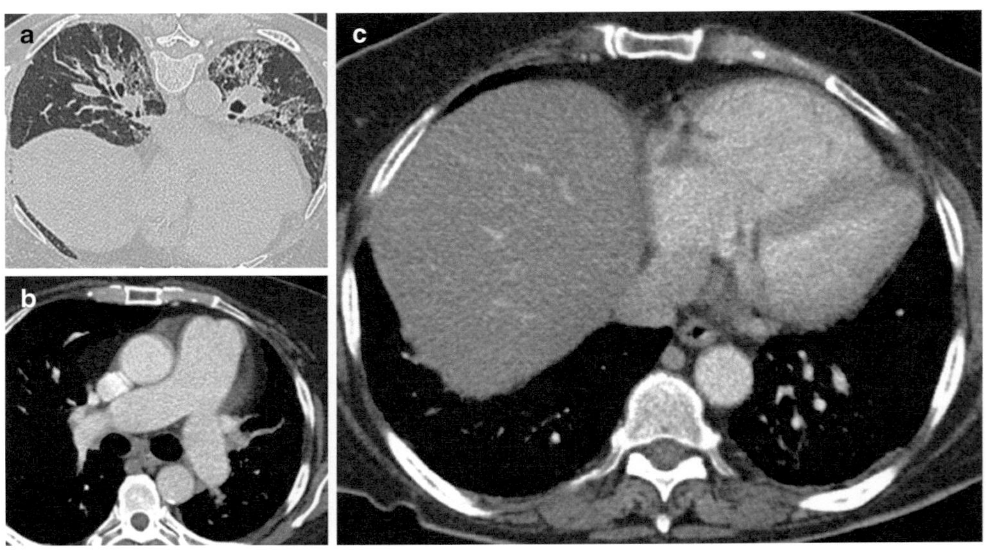

Fig. 48.6 Pulmonary hypertension in a patient with idiopathic pulmonary fibrosis (**a**), dilation of the main pulmonary artery (**b**) and dilation of the right ventricle (**c**)

patients at risk of lung cancer, there will also be an opportunity to identify asymptomatic or undiagnosed coronary artery disease in these patients.

Cardiovascular Disease and COPD

Several cohort studies in patients with COPD have shown a correlation between cardiovascular disease and COPD [59–61]. A recent meta-analysis identified a 2.5-fold higher risk of cardiovascular disease in patients with COPD [23]. Subgroup analysis showed similar rates of coronary heart disease (meta-OR 1·86, 95% CI 1.51–2.30; $p < 0.0001$) and myocardial infarction (2.71, 95% CI 1.69–4.35; $p < 0.0001$) but increased rates of angina pectoris (8.16, 95% CI 3.08–21.59; $p < 0.0001$) [23]. Interestingly there was no increase in cerebrovascular disease in patients with COPD (1.32; 95% CI 0.99–1.76; $p = 0.06$) [23].

However, studies relying on patient-reported frequency of cardiovascular disease are potentially limited by referral or

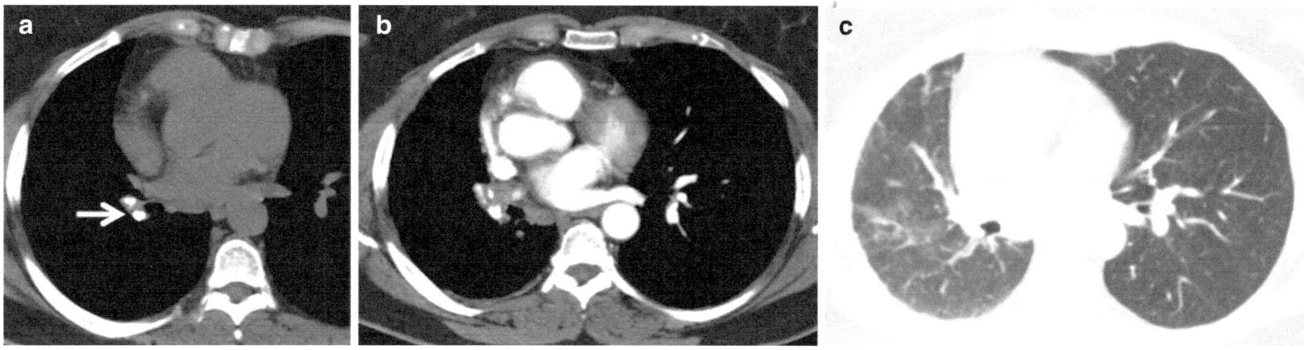

Fig. 48.7 Right pulmonary artery occlusion due to histoplasmosis (arrow) with (**a**) non-contrast CT, (**b**) contrast-enhanced CT and (**c**) lung windows

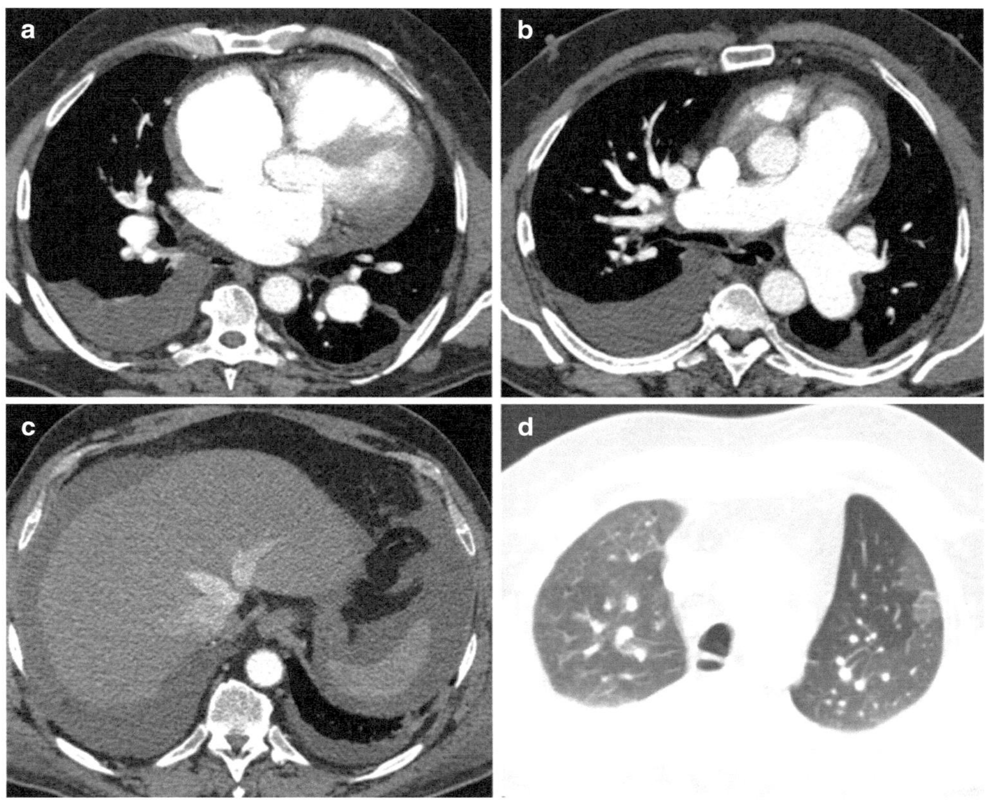

Fig. 48.8 CT imaging in a patient with an atrial septal defect with (**a**) hypertrophy of the right ventricle and right atrium, (**b**) dilation of the pulmonary arteries and pleural effusion, (**c**) regurgitation of contrast into the inferior vena cava (**d**) and interstitial lung changes

recollection bias. The assessment of coronary artery calcification on CT can provide a more robust assessment of cardiovascular risk. Coronary artery calcification is a marker of atherosclerosis, and patients with an increased volume of coronary artery calcification have a higher risk of myocardial infarction and mortality [62]. Several studies have shown that patients with emphysema on CT or airflow limitation by spirometry have more coronary artery calcification than those with normal lungs [37, 63]. However, in the Multi-Ethnic Study of Atherosclerosis (MESA) where 3642 asymptomatic patients underwent cardiac CT, lung function assessed with spirometry and emphysema assessed on CT were not independently associated with coronary artery calcification [63]. However, these investigators did find an association between spirometry and carotid intima-media thickness amongst smokers and percent emphysema and ankle brachial index amongst smokers and non-smokers [63]. Both COPD and cardiovascular diseases are a heterogeneous mix of pathologies, potentially leading to these differences in the assessment of coronary artery calcification.

Cardiovascular disease is linked with morbidity in patients with COPD. In the COPDGene cohort, physician diagnosed self-reported cardiovascular disease was associated with reduced functional status and poorer quality of life [40].

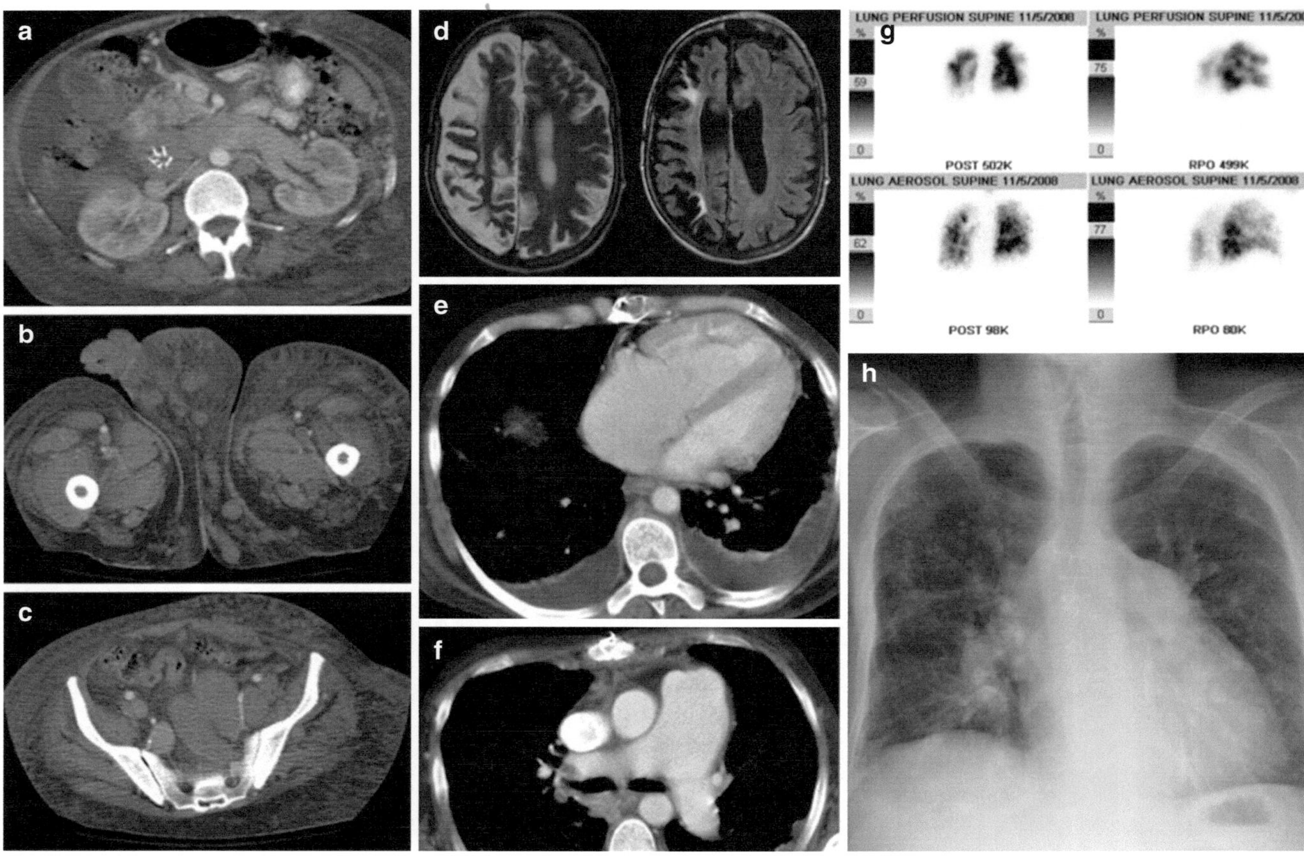

Fig. 48.9 Pulmonary hypertension and right heart failure in a patient with Klippel-Trenaunay-Weber syndrome with (**a**) mega vena cava containing an inferior vena cava filter, (**b**) multiple enlarged cutaneous veins, (**c**) enlarged iliac veins, (**d**) MRI of the brain showing hemi-hypertrophy, (**e**) dilation of the right ventricle, right atrium and pleural effusions, (**f**) dilation of the main pulmonary artery, (**g**) perfusion defects in the lungs identified on SPECT and (**h**) chest x-ray showing cardiomegaly and enlarged pulmonary arteries

Patients with COPD have an increased risk of hospitalisation for cardiovascular disease compared to age- and sex-matched controls [60, 64]. Coronary artery calcification in patients with COPD is linked with an elevated risk of myocardial infarction [4]. Patients with COPD have a higher incidence of major adverse cardiovascular events compared to patients without COPD who have similar levels of coronary artery calcification [65]. Patients with COPD also have an increased frequency of atrial and ventricular arrhythmias [23, 66]. In addition the presence of coronary artery calcification is associated with increased disease severity in patients with COPD [4].

Cardiovascular disease is linked with increased mortality in patients with COPD [64]. Compared to age- and sex-matched controls, patients with COPD had an increased risk of cardiovascular mortality (risk ratio 2.07, 95% CI 1.82–2.36) and all-cause mortality (risk ratio 2.82, 95% CI 2.61–3.05) [60]. In a cohort of patients with COPD, Romme et al. identified that coronary artery calcification and thoracic aortic calcification were associated with arterial stiffness and mortality [67]. In a study of 942 patients from the ECLIPSE study cohort (672 with COPD, 199 smokers with normal spirometry and 71 non-smokers), coronary artery calcification was associated with reduced exercise capacity and increased mortality [41]. After adjusting for age, gender and pack years, a calcium score percentile above 90% was associated with a hazard ratio for mortality of 1.77 (95% CI 1.04–3.01) [41].

Nevertheless, subclinical cardiovascular disease is under diagnosed in patients with COPD [68, 69]. The overlapping symptoms can make the diagnosis difficult. Therefore a high index of suspicion is required in the assessment of patients with COPD in order not to miss this important secondary diagnosis. The radiologist plays a vital role in bridging the gap between pulmonary medicine and cardiology in this respect.

Cardiovascular Disease and Other Respiratory Diseases

In addition to COPD, an increased prevalence of cardiovascular disease has been identified in patients with a variety of other respiratory diseases. In a study of 42 patients with fibrosing idiopathic interstitial pneumonias, the prevalence of asymptomatic coronary artery disease diagnosed with CT and myocardial perfusion scintigraphy was between 12% and 26% [70]. Invasive coronary angiography performed prior to lung transplantation for patients with advanced COPD or interstitial lung disease identified occult coronary artery disease in half of the patients [69]. The risk of cardiovascular disease and stroke is also higher for patients with bronchiectasis [71].

Cardiovascular Disease and Lung Cancer Screening

Low-dose non-contrast CT imaging is now widely used for lung cancer screening [72]. It is possible to identify coronary artery calcification on these CT scans, and the presence of coronary artery calcification correlates with cardiovascular and all-cause mortality [3, 73–75]. Traditional Agatston scoring would be time consuming in these screening studies. However, an ordinal visual calcium score can be performed which correlates with traditional Agatston score and with mortality [3, 73, 74].

Extra-cardiac Findings in the Lungs on Cardiac CT

Extra-cardiac incidental findings can be identified in the lungs on cardiac CT [76–81]. This includes findings that may explain the patient's symptoms of chest pain (such as pulmonary embolism) or breathlessness (such as emphysema or pulmonary fibrosis). In addition, clinically occult diagnoses may be made such as the presence of previously unknown lung cancer. Occasionally malignancy may be the cause of chest pain, such as when a lung cancer extends into the pericardium or with metastases in the heart.

Incidental findings were identified in more than a third of cardiac CT scans in a large Scottish population study [82]. However, significant findings that require further investigation or treatment are much less common, representing only 16% [83]. Half of clinically significant extra-cardiac findings occur in the lungs [83]. A meta-analysis identified that previously unknown malignancy was identified in 0.7% of cardiac CT scans, with 70% of these being lung cancer [84]. Such incidental findings can have important clinical and economic implications, particularly if further follow-up imaging is required [85, 86].

Lung nodules represent a quarter of clinically significant extra-cardiac findings identified on CT coronary angiography [83]. These may require follow-up with repeat CT scans, positron emission tomography or referral to a respiratory multidisciplinary team. Guidelines from the Fleischner Society and the British Thoracic Society can be used to stratify management based on nodule size and risk factors [87].

Conclusion

Computed tomography imaging can assess both the heart and the lungs in a single, rapid diagnostic test. There is an important overlap between cardiovascular and respiratory diseases, which may be mediated through shared aetiologies, such as smoking, or shared pathological mechanisms, such as inflammation. Cardiovascular disease may be identified on imaging performed to assess respiratory disease and vice versa. Abnormalities of the right heart can be a common endpoint of a variety of causes of pulmonary hypertension including thromboembolic, respiratory and cardiac diseases. Coronary artery calcification can be used as a marker of the presence of coronary artery disease in patients being assessed with CT for respiratory disease. Incidental extra-cardiac findings in the lungs are frequently identified on cardiac CT and may have important clinical and economic implications. Thus imaging of the heart-lung axis is an important feature of CT imaging of the heart, where the radiologist plays a key role in providing insight and helps triage the patient to appropriate care pathways.

References

1. Budoff MJ, NASIR K, Kinney GL, Hokanson JE. Coronary artery and thoracic calcium on noncontrast thoracic CT scans: comparison of ungated and gated examinations in patients from the COPD gene cohort. J Cardiovasc Comput Tomogr. 2011;5(2):113–8.
2. Steiner RM, Budoff MJ, Khurram N, Kinney GL, Hokanson JE, Barr RG, Nath H, Lopez-Garcia C, Black-Shinn J, and Casaburi R. Coronary artery calcium on non-contrast thoracic CT scans; comparison of ECG gated and non-gated examinations in patients from the COPD gene cohort. In A2616–16. American Thoracic Society. 2011. doi:https://doi.org/10.1164/ajrccm-conference.2011.183.1_MeetingAbstracts.A2616.
3. Shemesh J, Henschke CI, Shaham D, Yip R, Farooqi AO, Cham MD, McCauley DI, et al. Ordinal scoring of coronary artery calcifications on low-dose CT scans of the chest is predictive of death from cardiovascular disease. Radiology. 2010;257(2):541–8.
4. O'Hare PE, Ayres JF, O'Rourke RL, Slaughter RE, Marshall HM, Bowman RV, Fong KM, Yang IA. Coronary artery calcification on computed tomography correlates with mortality in chronic obstructive pulmonary disease. J Comput Assist Tomogr. 2014;38(5):753–9.
5. McClelland RL, Chung H, Detrano R, Post W, Kronmal RA. Distribution of coronary artery calcium by race, gender, and age: results from the Multi-ethnic Study of Atherosclerosis (MESA). Circulation. 2006;113(1):30–7.
6. Foley PWX, Hamaad A, El-Gendi H, Leyva F. Incidental cardiac findings on computed tomography imaging of the thorax. BMC Res Notes. 2010;3(1):326; BioMed Central Ltd.
7. McKie SJ, Hardwick DJ, Reid JH, Murchison JT. Features of cardiac disease demonstrated on CT pulmonary angiography. Clin Radiol. 2005;60(1):31–8.

8. Liu F, Coursey CA, Grahame-Clarke C, Sciacca RR, Rozenshtein A, Homma S, Austin JHM. Aortic valve calcification as an incidental finding at CT of the elderly: severity and location as predictors of aortic stenosis. AJR Am J Roentgenol. 2006;186(2):342–9.
9. Jairam PM, Gondrie MJA, Grobbee DE, Mali WPTM, Jacobs PCA, van der Graaf Y, PROVIDI Study Group. Incidental imaging findings from routine chest CT used to identify subjects at high risk of future cardiovascular events. Radiology. 2014;272(3):700–8.
10. Kim JW, Kang E-Y, Yong HS, Kim YK, Ok HW, Yu-Whan O, Ki YL, Han H. Incidental extracardiac findings at cardiac CT angiography: comparison of prevalence and clinical significance between precontrast low-dose whole thoracic scan and postcontrast retrospective ECG-gated cardiac scan. Int J Cardiovasc Imaging. 2009;25(1):75–81; Springer Netherlands.
11. van Beek EJR, Thompson B. Should we include full field of view in assessment of cardiac CT? J Cardiovasc Comput Tomogr. 2008;2(1):64; author reply 64–5.
12. Mirsadraee S, van Beek EJR. Cross-sectional cardiac imaging: prevalence and significance of extracardiac findings. J Thorac Imaging. 2014;29(2):92–7.
13. Galbán CJ, Han MLK, Boes JL, Chughtai KA, Meyer CR, Johnson TD, Galbán S, et al. Computed tomography-based biomarker provides unique signature for diagnosis of COPD phenotypes and disease progression. Nat Med. 2012;18(11):1711–5.
14. Balbinot F, da Costa Batista Guedes Á, Nascimento DZ, Zampieri JF, Alves GRT, Marchiori E, Rubin AS, Hochhegger B. Advances in imaging and automated quantification of pulmonary diseases in non-neoplastic diseases. Lung. 2016;194(6):871–9.
15. Xu Y, van Beek EJR, Hwanjo Y, Guo J, McLennan G, Hoffman EA. Computer-aided classification of interstitial lung diseases via MDCT: 3D adaptive multiple feature method (3D AMFM). Acad Radiol. 2006;13(8):969–78; Elsevier.
16. Otrakji A, Digumarthy SR, Lo Gullo R, Flores EJ, Shepard J-AO, Kalra MK. Dual-energy CT: spectrum of thoracic abnormalities. Radiographics. 2016;36(1):38–52.
17. Mirsadraee S, Reid JH, Connell M, MacNee W, Hirani N, Murchison JT, van Beek EJ. Dynamic (4D) CT perfusion offers simultaneous functional and anatomical insights into pulmonary embolism resolution. Eur J Radiol. 2016;85(10):1883–90.
18. Wild J, Arrigo M, Isenring BD, Buergi U, Kurowski T, Schuurmans MM, Huber LC, Benden C. Coronary artery disease in lung transplant candidates: role of routine invasive assessment. Respiration/Int Rev Thorac Dis. 2015;89(2):107–11.
19. Burris AC, Boura JA, Raff GL, Chinnaiyan KM. Triple rule out versus coronary CT angiography in patients with acute chest pain: results from the ACIC consortium. JACC Cardiovasc Imaging. 2015;8(7):817–25.
20. Ayaram D, Bellolio MF, Murad MH, Laack TA, Sadosty AT, Erwin PJ, Hollander JE, Montori VM, Stiell IG, Hess EP. Triple rule-out computed tomographic angiography for chest pain: a diagnostic systematic review and meta-analysis. Edited by Alan E Jones. Acad Emerg Med. 2013;20(9):861–71.
21. WHO. 2012. Mortality attributable to tobacco. http://www.who.int/tobacco/publications/surveillance/rep_mortality_attributable/en/.
22. Carter BD, Abnet CC, Feskanich D, Freedman ND, Hartge P, Lewis CE, Ockene JK, et al. Smoking and mortality--beyond established causes. N Engl J Med. 2015;372(7):631–40.
23. Chen W, Thomas J, Sadatsafavi M, FitzGerald JM. Risk of cardiovascular comorbidity in patients with chronic obstructive pulmonary disease: a systematic review and Meta-analysis. Lancet Respir Med. 2015;3(8):631–9.
24. Rong Y, Luo X, Zhang Z, Cui X, Liu Y, Chen W. Occupational exposure to asbestos and cardiovascular related diseases: a meta-analysis. Prev Med Rep. 2015;2:920–6.
25. Samoli E, Atkinson RW, Analitis A, Fuller GW, Green DC, Mudway I, Anderson HR, Kelly FJ. Associations of short-term exposure to traffic-related air pollution with cardiovascular and respiratory hospital admissions in London, UK. Occup Environ Med. 2016;73(5):300–7.
26. Langrish JP, Bosson J, Unosson J, Muala A, David E, Newby NL, Mills AB, Sandström T. Cardiovascular effects of particulate air pollution exposure: time course and underlying mechanisms. J Intern Med. 2012;272(3):224–39.
27. Hoek G, Krishnan RM, Beelen R, Peters A, Ostro B, Brunekreef B, Kaufman JD. Long-term air pollution exposure and cardio- respiratory mortality: a review. Environ Health. 2013;12(1):43.
28. Van Eeden S, Leipsic J, Paul Man SF, Sin DD. The relationship between lung inflammation and cardiovascular disease. Am J Respir Crit Care Med. 2012;186(1):11–6.
29. Gan WQ, Man SFP, Senthilselvan A, Sin DD. Association between chronic obstructive pulmonary disease and systemic inflammation: a systematic review and a meta-analysis. Thorax. 2004;59(7):574–80.
30. McEvoy JW, Nasir K, DeFilippis AP, Lima JA, Bluemke DA, Hundley WG, Barr RG, et al. Relationship of cigarette smoking with inflammation and subclinical vascular disease: the multi-ethnic study of atherosclerosis. Arterioscler Thromb Vasc Biol. 2015;35(4):1002–10.
31. Seifarth H, Schlett CL, Lehman SJ, Bamberg F, Donnelly P, Januzzi JL, Koenig W, Truong QA, Hoffmann U. Correlation of concentrations of high-sensitivity troponin T and high-sensitivity C-reactive protein with plaque progression as measured by CT coronary angiography. J Cardiovasc Comput Tomogr. 2014;8(6):452–8.
32. Falk E. Pathogenesis of atherosclerosis. J Am Coll Cardiol. 2006;47(8 Suppl):C7–C12.
33. Miller J, Edwards LD, Agustí A, Bakke P, Calverley PMA, Celli B, Coxson HO, et al. Comorbidity, systemic inflammation and outcomes in the ECLIPSE cohort. Respir Med. 2013;107(9):1376–84.
34. Maclay JD, McAllister DA, Rabinovich R, Haq I, Maxwell S, Hartland S, Connell M, et al. Systemic elastin degradation in chronic obstructive pulmonary disease. Thorax. 2012;67(7):606–12.
35. Conway EM, Pikor LA, Kung SHY, Hamilton MJ, Lam S, Lam WL, Bennewith KL. Macrophages, inflammation, and lung cancer. Am J Respir Crit Care Med. 2016;193(2):116–30.
36. King PT. Inflammation in chronic obstructive pulmonary disease and its role in cardiovascular disease and lung cancer. Clin Transl Med. 2015;4(1):68.
37. Gudmundsson G, Margretardottir OB, Sigurdsson MI, Harris TB, Launer LJ, Sigurdsson S, Olafsson O, Aspelund T, Gudnason V. Airflow obstruction, atherosclerosis and cardiovascular risk factors in the AGES Reykjavik study. Atherosclerosis. 2016;252(September):122–7.
38. Chandra D, Gupta A, Strollo PJ, Fuhrman CR, Leader JK, Bon J, Slivka WA, et al. Airflow limitation and endothelial dysfunction. Unrelated and independent predictors of atherosclerosis. Am J Respir Crit Care Med. 2016;194(1):38–47; American Thoracic Society.
39. Putcha N, Han MLK, Martinez CH, Foreman MG, Anzueto AR, Casaburi R, Cho MH, et al. Comorbidities of COPD have a major impact on clinical outcomes, particularly in African Americans. Chronic Obstr Pulm Dis. 2014;1(1):105–14.
40. Black-Shinn JL, Kinney GL, Wise AL, Regan EA, Make B, Krantz MJ, Graham Barr R, et al. Cardiovascular disease is associated with COPD severity and reduced functional status and quality of life. COPD. 2014;11(5):546–51; Taylor & Francis.
41. Williams MC, Murchison JT, Edwards LD, Agustí A, Bakke P, Calverley PMA, Celli B, et al. Coronary artery calcification is increased in patients with COPD and associated with increased morbidity and mortality. Thorax. 2014;69(8):718–23.
42. Hoeper MM, Bogaard HJ, Condliffe R, Frantz R, Khanna D, Kurzyna M, Langleben D, et al. Definitions and diagnosis of pulmonary hypertension. J Am Coll Cardiol. 2013;62(25 Suppl):D42–50.

43. Simonneau G, Gatzoulis MA, Adatia I, Celermajer D, Denton C, Ghofrani A, Gomez Sanchez MA, et al. Updated clinical classification of pulmonary hypertension. J Am Coll Cardiol. 2013;62(25 Suppl):D34–41.
44. Reid JH, Murchison JT. Acute right ventricular dilatation: a new helical CT sign of massive pulmonary embolism. Clin Radiol. 1998;53(9):694–8.
45. Becattini C, Agnelli G, Germini F, Vedovati MC. Computed tomography to assess risk of death in acute pulmonary embolism: a meta-analysis. Eur Respir J. 2014;43(6):1678–90; European Respiratory Society.
46. Pengo V, Lensing AWA, Prins MH. Incidence of chronic thromboembolic pulmonary hypertension after pulmonary embolism. N Engl J Med. 2004;350(22):2257–64.
47. Konstantinides S, Torbicki A, Agnelli G. 2014 ESC guidelines on the diagnosis and management of acute pulmonary embolism. Eur Heart J. 2014;35(45):3145–6.
48. Exter d, Paul L, van Es J, Kroft LJM, Erkens PMG, Douma RA, Mos ICM, Jonkers G, et al. Thromboembolic resolution assessed by CT pulmonary angiography after treatment for acute pulmonary embolism. Thromb Haemost. 2015;114(1):26–34.
49. Ley S, Ley-Zaporozhan J, Pitton MB, Schneider J, Wirth GM, Mayer E, Düber C, Kreitner K-F. Diagnostic performance of state-of-the-art imaging techniques for morphological assessment of vascular abnormalities in patients with chronic thromboembolic pulmonary hypertension (CTEPH). Eur Radiol. 2012;22(3):607–16.
50. Matsuoka S, Washko GR, Dransfield MT, Yamashiro T, San Jose Estepar R, Diaz A, Silverman EK, Patz S, Hatabu H. Quantitative CT measurement of cross-sectional area of small pulmonary vessel in COPD: correlations with emphysema and airflow limitation. Acad Radiol. 2010;17(1):93–9.
51. Barberà JA. Mechanisms of development of chronic obstructive pulmonary disease-associated pulmonary hypertension. Pulm Circ. 2013;3(1):160–4.
52. Kent BD, Mitchell PD, McNicholas WT. Hypoxemia in patients with COPD: cause, effects, and disease progression. Int J Chron Obstruct Pulmon Dis. 2011;6:199–208.
53. O'Donnell DE, K A W. Lung hyperinflation in COPD: applying physiology to clinical practice. COPD Res Pract. 2015;1:4.
54. Shin S, King CS, Whitney Brown A, Albano MC, Atkins M, Sheridan MJ, Ahmad S, et al. Pulmonary artery size as a predictor of pulmonary hypertension and outcomes in patients with chronic obstructive pulmonary disease. Respir Med. 2014;108(11):1626–32.
55. Wells JM, Morrison JB, Bhatt SP, Nath H, Dransfield MT. Pulmonary artery enlargement is associated with cardiac injury during severe exacerbations of COPD. Chest J. 2016;149(5):1197–204.
56. Naeije R. Pulmonary hypertension and right heart failure in chronic obstructive pulmonary disease. Proc Am Thorac Soc. 2005;2(1):20–2.
57. Dimopoulos K, Wort SJ, Gatzoulis MA. Pulmonary hypertension related to congenital heart disease: a call for action. Eur Heart J. 2014;35(11):691–700; The Oxford University Press.
58. Peña E, Dennie C, Veinot J, Muñiz SH. Pulmonary hypertension: how the radiologist can help. Radiographics. 2012;32(1):9–32.
59. Eriksson B, Lindberg A, Müllerova H, Rönmark E, Lundbäck B. Association of heart diseases with COPD and restrictive lung function--results from a population survey. Respir Med. 2013;107(1):98–106.
60. Curkendall SM, deLuise C, Jones JK, Lanes S, Stang MR, Goehring E, She D. Cardiovascular disease in patients with chronic obstructive pulmonary disease, Saskatchewan Canada cardiovascular disease in COPD patients. Ann Epidemiol. 2006;16(1):63–70.
61. Huiart L, Ernst P, Suissa S. Cardiovascular morbidity and mortality in COPD. Chest J. 2005;128(4):2640–6.
62. Budoff MJ, J E Hokanson KNASIR, Shaw LJ, Kinney GL, Chow D, DeMoss D, et al. Progression of coronary artery calcium predicts all-cause mortality. JACC Cardiovasc Imaging. 2010;3(12):1229–36; Elsevier.
63. Barr RG, Ahmed FS, Carr JJ, Hoffman EA, Jiang R, Kawut SM, Watson K. Subclinical atherosclerosis, airflow obstruction and emphysema: the MESA lung study. Eur Respir J. 2012;39(4):846–54; Alhaj EK, Alhaj NE, Bergmann SR, Hecht H, Matarazzo TJ, Smith S, Alhaj N, Alhaj M, Nelson S. Coronary artery calcification and emphysema. Can J Cardiol. 2008;24(5):369–72.
64. Sidney S, Sorel M, Charles P, Quesenberry C dL, Lanes S, Eisner MD. COPD and incident cardiovascular disease hospitalizations and mortality: Kaiser Permanente medical care program. Chest J. 2005;128(4):2068–75.
65. Gaisl T, Schlatzer C, Schwarz EI, Possner M, Stehli J, Sievi NA, Clarenbach CF, et al. Coronary artery calcification, epicardial fat burden, and cardiovascular events in chronic obstructive pulmonary disease. Edited by James D Chalmers. PLoS One. 2015;10(5): e0126613; Public Library of Science.
66. Konecny T, Park JY, Somers KR, Konecny D, Orban M, Soucek F, Parker KO, et al. Relation of chronic obstructive pulmonary disease to atrial and ventricular arrhythmias. Am J Cardiol. 2014;114(2):272–7.
67. Romme EAPM, McAllister DA, Murchison JT, van Beek EJR, Petrides GS, Price COS, Rutten EPA, Smeenk FWJM, Wouters EFM, MacNee W. Associations between COPD related manifestations: a cross-sectional study. Respir Res. 2013;14(1):129.
68. Ye C, Younus A, Malik R, Roberson L, Shaharyar S, Veledar E, Ahmad R, et al. Subclinical cardiovascular disease in patients with chronic obstructive pulmonary disease: a systematic review. QJM. 2016; https://doi.org/10.1093/qjmed/hcw135.
69. Reed RM, Eberlein M, Girgis RE, Hashmi S, Iacono A, Jones S, Netzer G, Scharf S. Coronary artery disease is under-diagnosed and under-treated in advanced lung disease. Am J Med. 2012;125(12):1228.e13–22.
70. Cassagnes L, Gaillard V, Monge E, Faivre J-B, Delhaye C, Molinari F, Petyt G, et al. Prevalence of asymptomatic coronary disease in fibrosing idiopathic interstitial pneumonias. Eur J Radiol. 2015;84(1):163–71.
71. Navaratnam V, Millett ERC, Hurst JR, Thomas SL, Smeeth L, Hubbard RB, Brown J, and Quint JK. 2016. Bronchiectasis and the risk of cardiovascular disease: a population-based study. Thorax, BMJ Publishing Group Ltd and British Thoracic Society, 72:thoraxjnl-2015-208188.
72. National Lung Screening Trial Research Team, Church TR, Black WC, Aberle DR, Berg CD, Clingan KL, Duan F, et al. Results of initial low-dose computed tomographic screening for lung Cancer. N Engl J Med. 2013;368(21):1980–91.
73. Chiles C, Duan F, Gladish GW, Ravenel JG, Baginski SG, Snyder BS, DeMello S, Desjardins SS, Munden RF, NLST Study Team. Association of coronary artery calcification and mortality in the national lung screening trial: a comparison of three scoring methods. Radiology. 2015;276(1):82–90.
74. Sverzellati N, Cademartiri F, Bravi F, Martini C, Gira FA, Maffei E, Marchianò A, et al. Relationship and prognostic value of modified coronary artery calcium score, FEV1, and emphysema in lung cancer screening population: the MILD trial. Radiology. 2012;262(2):460–7. https://doi.org/10.1148/radiol.11110364.
75. Jacobs PC, Gondrie MJA, van der Graaf Y, de Koning HJ, Isgum I, van Ginneken B, Mali WPTM. Coronary artery calcium can predict all-cause mortality and cardiovascular events on low-dose CT screening for lung cancer. Am J Roentgenol. 2012;198(3):505–11; American Roentgen Ray Society.
76. Koonce J, Schoepf JU, Nguyen SA, Northam MC, Ravenel JG. Extra-cardiac findings at cardiac CT: experience with 1,764 patients. Eur Radiol. 2009;19(3):570–6; Springer-Verlag.
77. Kirsch J, Araoz PA, Steinberg FB, Fletcher JG, McCollough CH, Williamson EE. Prevalence and significance of incidental

extracardiac findings at 64-multidetector coronary CTA. J Thorac Imaging. 2007;22(4):330–4.
78. Lehman SJ, Abbara S, Cury RC, Nagurney JT, Hsu J, Goela A, Schlett CL, et al. Significance of cardiac computed tomography incidental findings in acute chest pain. Am J Med. 2009;122(6):543–9; Elsevier.
79. Schietinger BJ, Bozlar U, Hagspiel KD, Norton PT, Greenbaum HR, Wang H, Isbell DC, et al. The prevalence of extracardiac findings by multidetector computed tomography before atrial fibrillation ablation. Am Heart J. 2008;155(2):254–9; Elsevier.
80. Kawano Y, Tamura A, Goto Y, Shinozaki K, Zaizen H, Kadota J. Incidental detection of cancers and other non-cardiac abnormalities on coronary multislice computed tomography. Am J Cardiol. 2007;99(11):1608–9; Elsevier.
81. Burt JR, Iribarren C, Fair JM, Norton LC, Mahbouba M, Rubin GD, Hlatky MA, Go AS, Fortmann SP, Atherosclerotic Disease, Vascular Function, Genetic Epidemiology (ADVANCE) Study. Incidental findings on cardiac multidetector row computed tomography among healthy older adults: prevalence and clinical correlates. Arch Intern Med. 2008;168(7):756–61; American Medical Association.
82. Scot-Heart Investigators. CT coronary angiography in patients with suspected angina due to coronary heart disease (SCOT-HEART): an open-label, parallel-group, multicentre trial. Lancet. 2015;385(9985):2383–91.
83. Karius P, Schuetz GM, Schlattmann P, Dewey M. Extracardiac findings on coronary CT angiography: a systematic review. J Cardiovasc Comput Tomogr. 2014;8(3):174–82. e1–6.
84. Flor N, Di Leo G, Squarza SA, Tresoldi S, Rulli E, Cornalba G, Sardanelli F. Malignant incidental extracardiac findings on cardiac CT: systematic review and meta-analysis. Am J Roentgenol. 2013;201(3):555–64; American Roentgen Ray Society.
85. Showkathali R, Sen A, Brickham B, Dworakowski R, Wendler O, MacCarthy P. 'Incidental findings' during TAVI work-up: more than just an inconvenience. EuroIntervention. 2015;11(4):465–9.
86. Goehler A, McMahon PM, Lumish HS, Carol CW, Munshi V, Gilmore M, Chung JH, et al. Cost-effectiveness of follow-up of pulmonary nodules incidentally detected on cardiac computed tomographic angiography in patients with suspected coronary artery disease. Circulation. 2014;130(8):668–75.
87. MacMahon H, Austin JHM, Gamsu G, Herold CJ, Jett JR, Naidich DP, Patz EF, Swensen SJ. Guidelines for management of small pulmonary nodules detected on CT scans: a statement from the Fleischner Society. Radiology. 2005;237(2):395–400.

49 Ischemic Stroke: The Role of Cardiac CT

Jin Hur and Byoung Wook Choi

Stroke is a leading cause of mortality and long-term disability worldwide [1, 2]. While the etiology of ischemic stroke is often found in the cervicocranial vasculature, approximately 20% results from high-risk cardiac abnormalities [3, 4]. Because cardiac embolism has a treatable source, identification of cardioembolic sources in stroke patients is important for appropriate therapeutic management. Currently, echocardiography is frequently used in the workup of patients with ischemic stroke to identify potential cardiac embolic sources [5–7]. Transesophageal echocardiography (TEE) is highly accurate in the detection of left atrial thrombus, patent foramen ovale (PFO), atrial septal aneurysm (ASA), and aortic atheroma [8–12].

Cardiac computed tomography (CT) can be used to evaluate not only the coronary arteries but also other cardiac structures such as the left atrial appendage (LAA), myocardium, valves, and septa [13–16]. Recent advances in multidetector computed tomography (MDCT) allow quick and accurate evaluation of cardiac anatomy and thoracic aorta by cardiac CT. Because the cause of embolic stroke is commonly either from carotid atherosclerosis or from the heart, these potential sources of emboli need to be investigated to accurately prescribe secondary stroke prevention.

Given the clinical importance of ischemic stroke arising from the heart and aorta, we discussed the potential clinical application cardiac CT in an ischemic stroke population, detailing on the diagnosis of cardioembolic sources based on the latest available evidence and published guidelines.

Cardioembolic Stroke

Cardioembolic stroke is estimated to be the causative factor in 20 to 40% of all stroke cases [1]. Because cardiac embolism has a treatable source, identification of cardioembolic sources in stroke patients is important for appropriate therapeutic management. Cardioembolic sources can be divided into two categories, major sources or minor sources (Table 49.1) [17, 18]. Major sources of embolism have an established causal relationship with stroke, and their identification is therefore usually clinically relevant. Minor sources of embolism, on the other hand, have an ill-described or weak causal relationship with stroke, and their relevance in a given situation is much less certain. Therefore, in terms of therapeutic management, detection of major sources is more important.

Echocardiography is indicated in patients in whom cardioembolism is suspected but unproven. Transthoracic echocardiography (TTE) should be used as a screening test; although, in the absence of clinical or simple test evidence of cardiac disease, the likelihood of discovering a major embolic source is low [19]. TEE provides superior anatomical information in relation to the aortic arch, left atrium, and the mitral and aortic valves. In patients in whom the mechanism of stroke remains uncertain after initial workup, recent reports suggest that TEE, performed soon after symptom onset, may identify a source of embolism in 30–45% of cases [9–12]. However, TEE is a semi-invasive procedure that required special skills for proper performance and interpretation.

Cardiac CT is a well-established but not widely used technique for imaging cardioembolic sources. Cardiac CT provides high-quality noninvasive images of the heart, great vessels, and coronary vasculature [13–16]. Therefore, cardiac CT has the ability to provide high-quality noninvasive images of uniform sections of the heart, thus allowing the possible detection of potential cardiac embolic sources. However, CT imaging has fundamental disadvantages including radiation dose and use of iodine contrast medium [20–22].

J. Hur (✉) · B. W. Choi
Department of Radiology, Yonsei University School of Medicine, Severance Hospital, Seoul, South Korea
e-mail: khuhz@yuhs.ac

U. J. Schoepf (ed.), *CT of the Heart*, Contemporary Medical Imaging, https://doi.org/10.1007/978-1-60327-237-7_49

Table 49.1 Proximal sources of embolism

Major sources	Minor sources
Atrial dysrhythmias	Interatrial septal abnormalities
Atrial fibrillation Atrial flutter	Patent foramen ovale Atrial septal defect Atrial septal aneurysm
Left atrial thrombus	Spontaneous echo contrast (blood stasis)
Left ventricular thrombus	Pulmonary atriovenous malformation
Cardiac tumors	Mitral valve prolapse
Vegetation Infective Noninfective (marantic)	Valvular calcification Mitral annular calcification Aortic valve stenosis
Prosthetic cardiac valve	
Complex aortic atheroma	

Cardioembolic Sources

Investigation of potential embolic sources is an important diagnostic step in managing patients with acute ischemic stroke or transient ischemic attack, especially when the mechanism is considered to be embolic.

Cardiac Thrombus

The left atrium (LA) or LAA is an important location of thrombus formation and subsequent cardioembolic events, especially in association with dysrhythmias, such as atrial fibrillation (AF) [23, 24]. Currently, TEE has emerged as the most sensitive technique for the detection of intracardiac thrombi and is believed to be the single best modality for patients with suspected intracardiac thrombi [6–9]. Although TEE is widely available, it is a semi-invasive test, usually performed under conscious sedation.

A noninvasive method with high reliability and accuracy comparable to TEE for the identification of LA or LAA thrombus would be of significant clinical value. Cardiac CT is a sensitive tool for detecting intracardiac thrombi. In several studies, investigators have reported that intracardiac thrombi can be detected with CT (Figs. 49.1 and 49.2) [25–30]. The diagnostic accuracy of cardiac CT has been extensively studied indicating a high negative predictive value (NPV). Nonetheless, there have been major discrepancies between reported positive predictive values (PPV) and accuracy estimates. A recent meta-analysis study demonstrated overall high accuracy of cardiac CT compared with TEE for the detection of LA or LAA thrombus in patients with AF. The investigators included 19 studies with a total of 2955 patients, and the weighted mean sensitivity and specificity were 96% (95% CI, 92–100%) and 92% (95% CI, 91–93%), whereas PPV and NPV were 41% (95% CI, 37–44%) and 99% (95% CI, 99–100%), respectively [28].

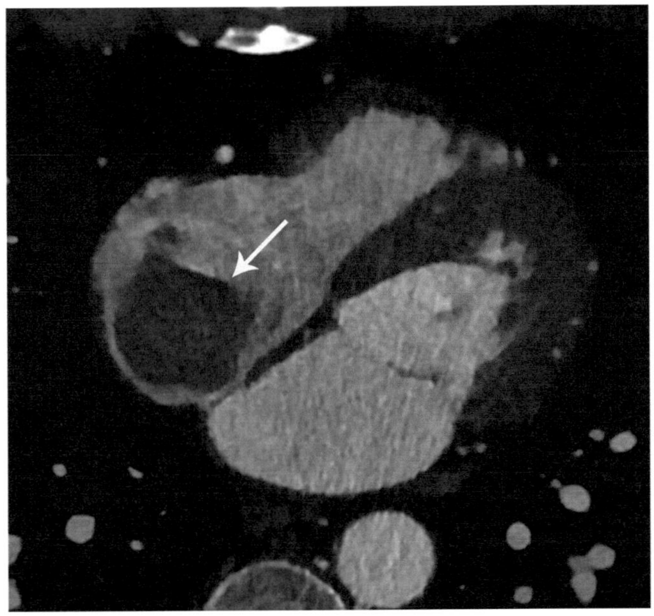

Fig. 49.1 Image in a 48-year-old man with stroke. Axial cardiac CT image shows a large oval-shaped filling defect (arrow) in RA. The mass was confirmed as a thrombus which was resolved on follow-up transthoracic echocardiography after anticoagulation therapy. RA right atrium

This is because pseudo-filling defect such as blood stasis can also cause an apparent filling defect on CT images, thereby mimicking a thrombus.

Left ventricular (LV) thrombus formation is frequently associated with ischemic heart disease or dilated cardiomyopathy, which is a potential source of embolic stroke [31]. Contrast-enhanced magnetic resonance imaging (MRI) has a higher sensitivity and specificity than TEE for LV thrombus detection, especially for apical thrombi, because echocardiography cannot clearly show the myocardium-thrombus interface at the apex [32]. Delayed-enhancement CMR (DE-CMR) imaging has been validated as a sensitive method for LV thrombus detection [33]. Because DE-CMR identifies a thrombus based on tissue characteristics rather than anatomic appearance, it enables a thrombus to be delineated from the myocardium and chamber cavity irrespective of location or morphology (Fig. 49.3). A previous study reported that DE-CMR detected thrombi in 7% of subjects (55 patients), while cine-CMR identified thrombi in only 4.7% (37 patients). Among the 55 patients with LV thrombi identified using DE-CMR, 44% (24 of 55) had cine-CMR analyses negative for thrombi [33]. Cardiac CT can also clearly depict the endocardial border with high resolution and can easily detect a LV thrombus. On CT, left ventricular thrombus shows a significantly lower CT attenuation than normally perfused myocardial wall (Fig. 49.4) [34].

Recently, left atrial occlusion devices have been recognized as a treatment option for preventing embolic stroke

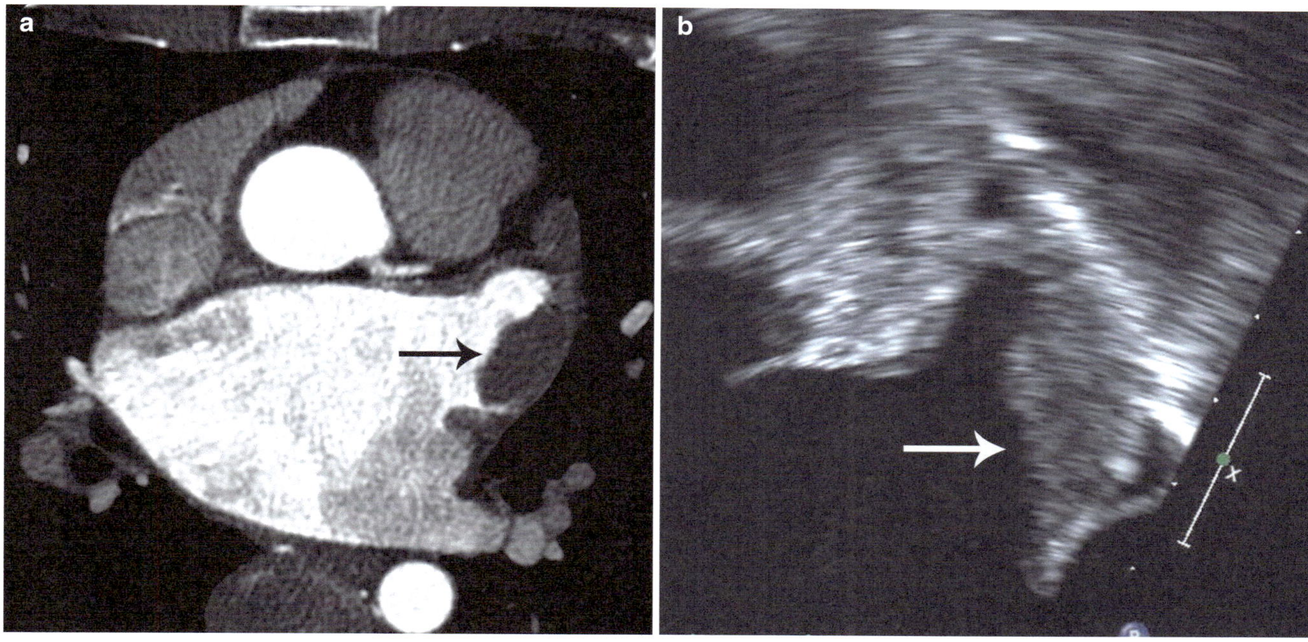

Fig. 49.2 Images in a 41-year-old man with stroke and atrial fibrillation. (**a**) Axial cardiac CT image shows an oval filling defect (arrow) in the LAA. The left atrium was enlarged due to atrial fibrillation. (**b**) TEE image shows an oval-shaped echogenic thrombus (arrow) in the LAA. LAA, left atrial appendage; TEE, transesophageal echocardiography

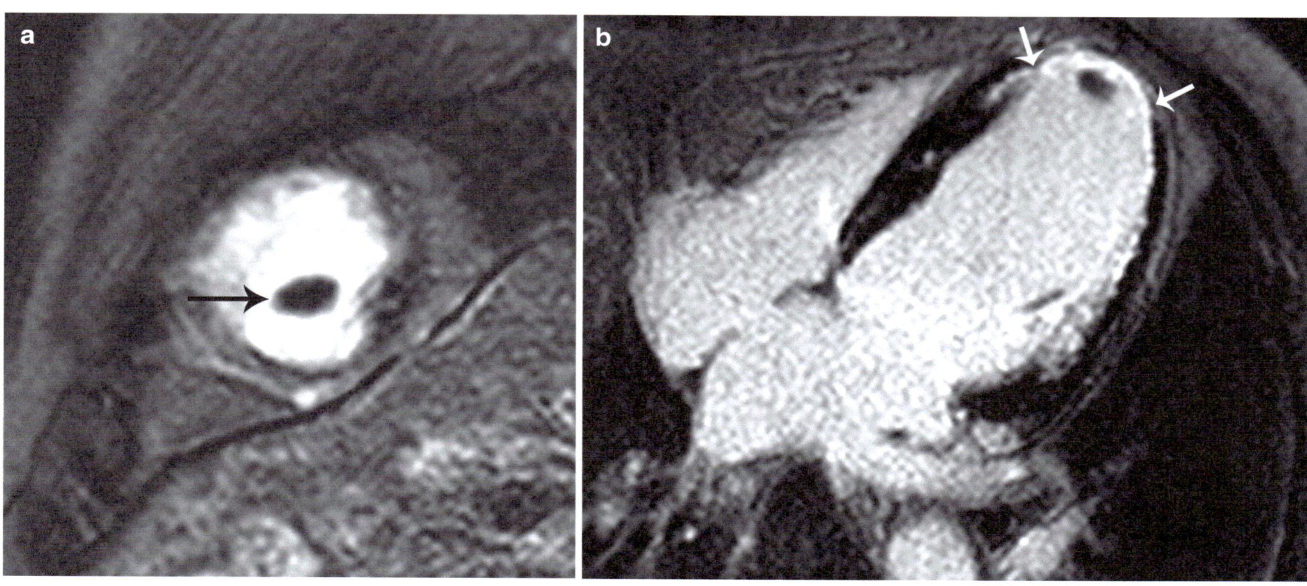

Fig. 49.3 Images in a 70-year-old man with stroke and myocardial infarction. (**a**) On short-axis DE-CMR, the mass shows black signal intensity without delayed enhancement (arrow) in LV apex. The mass was confirmed as a thrombus which was resolved on follow-up transthoracic echocardiography after anticoagulation therapy. (**b**) On four-chamber DE-CMR, the LV myocardium shows diffuse delayed contrast enhancement in the apical wall (arrows) from myocardial infarction. LV, left ventricle

in patients with AF who are intolerant to warfarin therapy [35]. With excellent NPV, cardiac CT has the ability to potentially exclude thrombus in LAA and may obviate the need for pre-procedural TEE in some cases. Cardiac CT can also be used to measure the size of the LAA, which is typically used before procedure for LAA occlusion, a procedure that can reduce the risk of stroke in patients with AF [36].

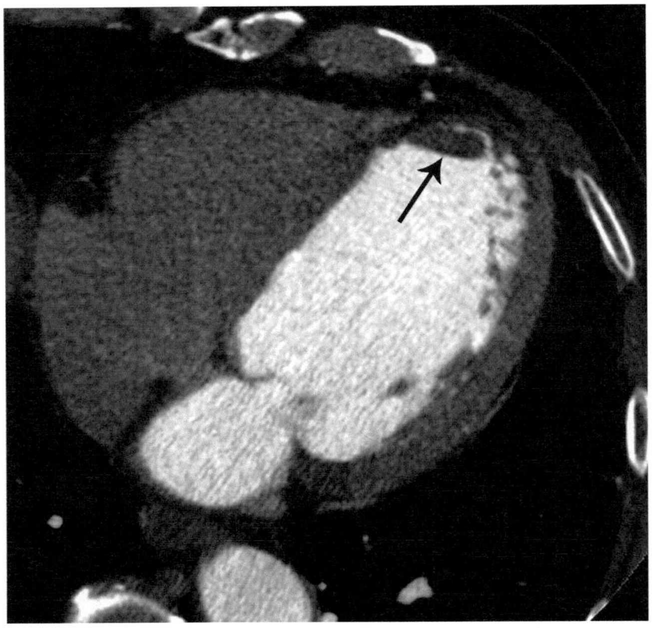

Fig. 49.4 Image in a 62-year-old man with stroke and myocardial infarction. Axial cardiac CT shows an oval-shaped filling defect (arrow) in the LV apex, which was confirmed as a thrombus. LV, left ventricle

Spontaneous Echo Contrast (Blood Stasis)

Spontaneous echo contrast (SEC) is a smoke-like echo phenomenon with a swirling pattern of blood flow that can be observed on echocardiography, most often within the LAA. The reduced atrial contraction associated with atrial fibrillation leads to blood stasis, which facilitates thrombus formation in the LAA.

Spontaneous echo contrast (SEC) caused by slow blood flow during atrial fibrillation, as seen at ultrasonography, also can cause an apparent filling defect on CT images and thereby mimic a thrombus (Fig. 49.5). These pseudo-filling defects seen on CT images represent incomplete mixing of CT contrast material and blood. Therefore, it may be difficult to differentiate between a thrombus and a pseudo-filling defect caused by blood stasis with a single-phase CT scanning. The blood stasis phenomenon appears when LA dysfunction causes an incomplete mixing of contrast agent and blood. Therefore, the delayed phase scanning will allow for the complete mixing of contrast agent and blood (Fig. 49.6) [37–39]. In sub-analysis of 753 patients from recent meta-analysis study, in which delayed images were obtained, sensitivity and specificity were 100% (95% CI, 96–100%) and 99% (95% CI, 98–100%), respectively. Likewise, the PPV significantly increased to 92% while maintaining a high NPV of 100% and an overall diagnostic accuracy of 99% (95% CI, 98–100%) [28]. This result suggested that cardiac CT using delayed imaging is a reasonable alternative to TEE for evaluating LAA or LA thrombus and differentiating from blood stasis.

Although delayed imaging with cardiac CT has excellent sensitivity and specificity for thrombus, it requires rescanning within 1 min. This would require preknowledge of thrombus or high suspicion of LA or LAA thrombus as this could double radiation exposure by requiring a second scan. One concern regarding the use of cardiac CT for LAA evaluation is radiation. However, CT has most recently undergone technical and acquisition changes that substantially reduce the dose of radiation [40].

Cardiac Tumor

Although cardiac tumors are rare, diagnosis and refined characterization of these masses are important due to the high morbidity and mortality associated with the functional consequences of such tumors and the potential for arrhythmia or emboli [41]. It is clinically important to differentiate cardiac tumors from cardiac tumor-like lesions, such as thrombi, because of the different therapeutic strategies used to treat these lesions.

Myxomas are the most common cardiac tumor, and they are associated with a high rate of embolic events (30–40%) [42]. Imaging plays a key role in establishing the diagnosis of patients with cardiac myxomas and thrombi because the clinical presentation is often diverse and nonspecific. Magnetic resonance imaging (MRI) is presently the modality of choice to evaluate cardiac tumors (Fig. 49.7). Optimal tumor characterization may be achieved with cardiac MRI, which provides an unrestricted field of view and superior soft-tissue depiction without ionizing radiation [43, 44]. Cardiac CT can be used to detect cardiac tumors. Several useful imaging characteristics can be found based on CT for differentiating cardiac myxomas from thrombi. Cardiac myxomas tend to be larger than thrombi and originate in the fossa ovalis or interatrial septum, whereas thrombi are smaller than myxomas and are usually seen in the LAA (Fig. 49.8) [45]. However, CT lacks the superior soft-tissue contrast abilities of MRI and is therefore not suitable for differentiating between cardiac myxomas and thrombi. Therefore, it may be challenging to differentiate a cardiac myxoma from an atrial thrombus based on CT imaging features because both can be localized at the left atrial septum and be irregular in shape. A recent study of dual-energy cardiac CT demonstrated that iodine concentration obtained from the dual-energy CT data is a feasible quantitative parameter in differentiating cardiac myxomas from thrombi [46]. This result suggested that dual-energy cardiac CT can be a helpful complementary tool to differentiate a myxoma from a thrombus in cases in which echocardiography or conventional contrast CT is inconclusive.

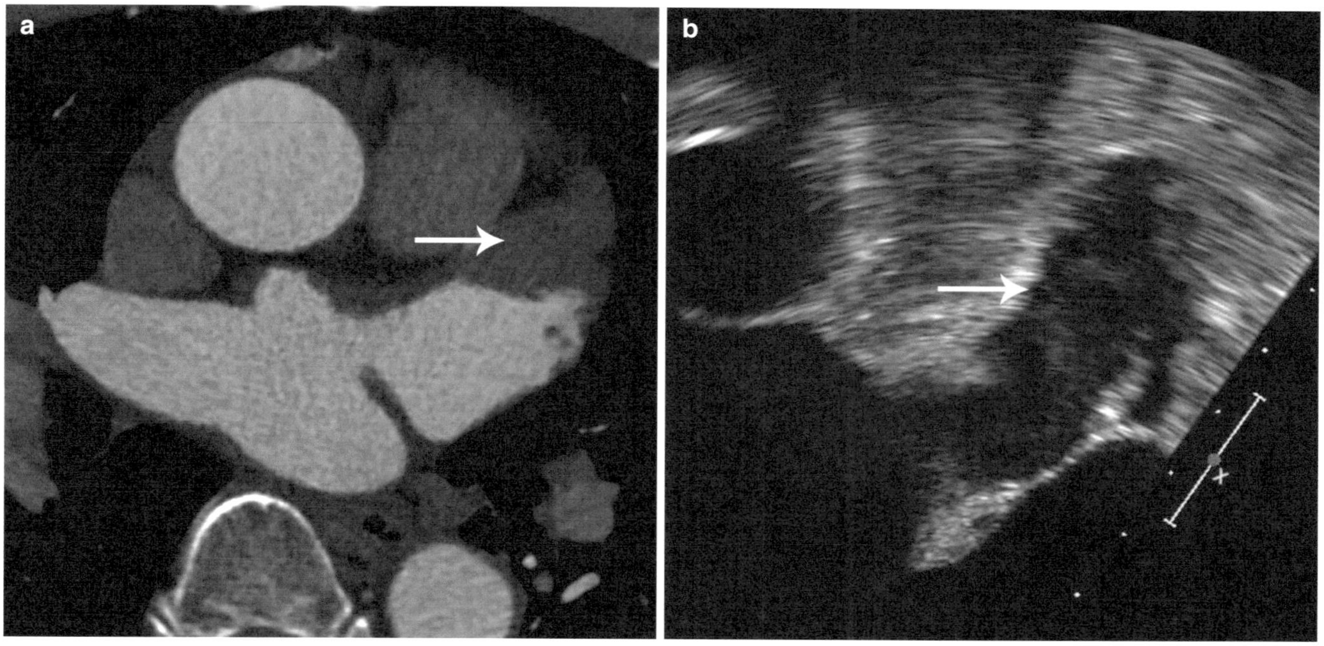

Fig. 49.5 Images in a 62-year-old woman with stroke and atrial fibrillation. (**a**) Axial cardiac CT image shows triangular filling defect (arrow) in the LAA. (**b**) TEE image obtained on the same day after CT image acquisition shows moderate spontaneous echo contrast (arrow) with no thrombus in the LAA. LAA, left atrial appendage; TEE, transesophageal echocardiography

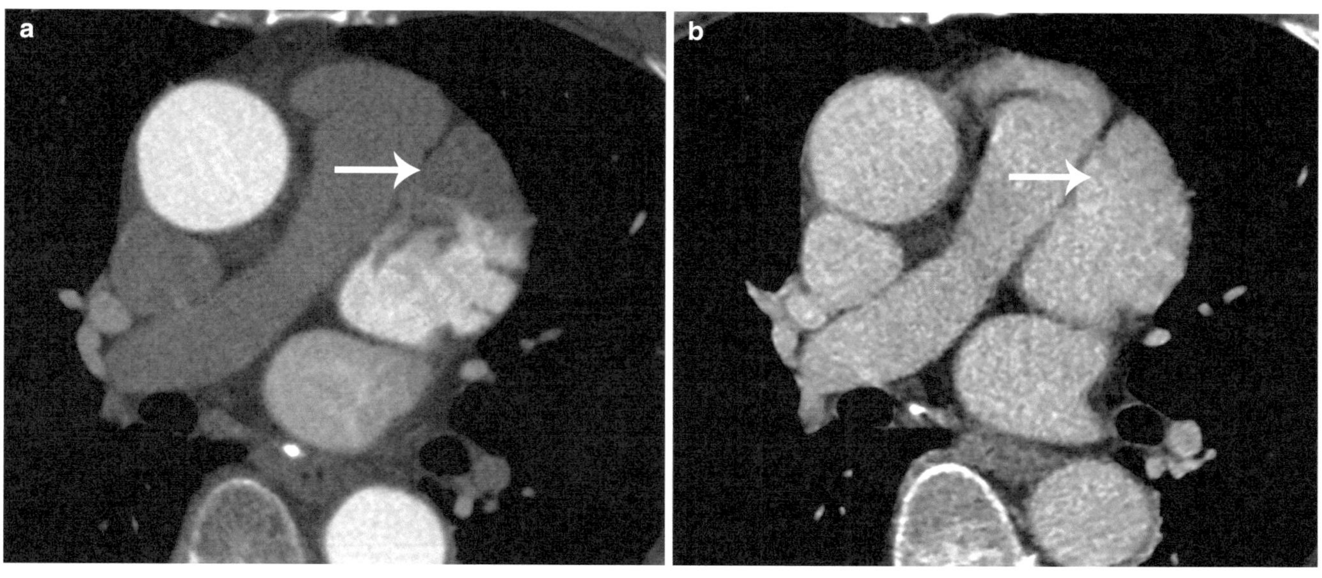

Fig. 49.6 Images in a 68-year-old man with stroke. (**a**) Axial early-phase cardiac CT image shows triangular filling defect (arrow) in LAA. (**b**) Axial late-phase cardiac CT image shows no filling defect (arrow) in LAA. The defect caused by blood stasis disappeared at late-phase imaging. LAA, left atrial appendage

Interarterial Septal Abnormalities

A paradoxical embolism is a type of stroke or arterial thrombosis caused by a thrombus of venous origin through a defect in the heart, such as a patent foramen ovale (PFO) or an atrial septal defect (ASD), that creates the potential for right-to-left shunting of blood.

A patent foramen ovale constitutes a potential conduit for right-to-left shunting and has a high frequency of occurrence in young adults with cryptogenic ischemic stroke [47]. TEE with agitated saline injection and Valsalva maneuver is the accepted reference standard modality for the diagnosis of PFO [48, 49]. A previous study demonstrated that CT has lower sensitivity compared to TEE in

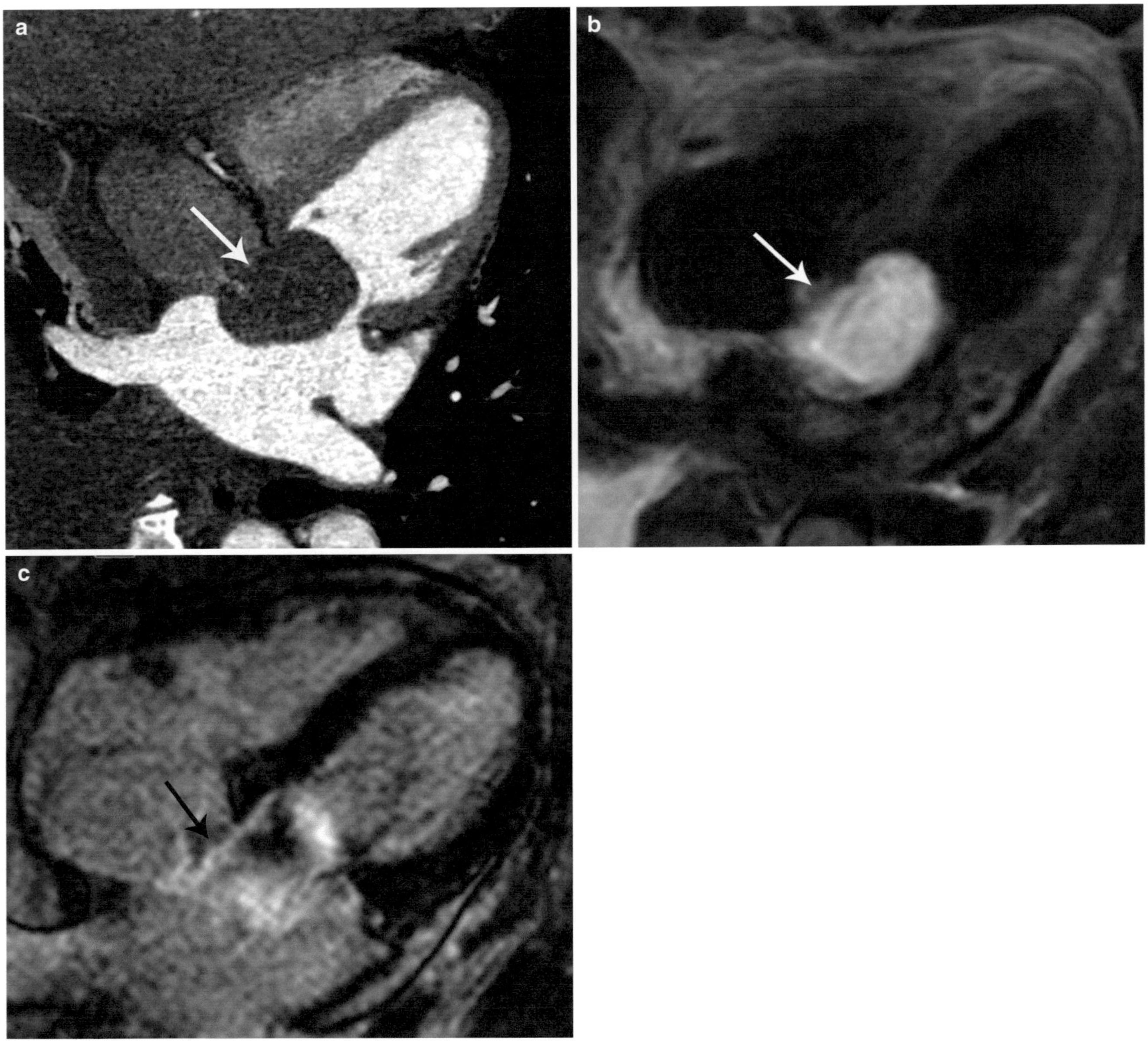

Fig. 49.7 Images in a 56-year-old man with stroke. (**a**) Axial cardiac CT shows a large filling detect (arrow) in LA. (**b**) A four-chamber T2-weighted black blood double inversion spin echo CMR image shows a high signal intensity mass (arrow) in LA. (**c**) On four-chamber DE-CMR, the mass shows strong contrast enhancement, suggestive of tumor (arrow). The mass was pathologically confirmed after surgical resection as a myxoma

the detection of PFO [50]. This is because PFO requires a provocative maneuver for diagnosis, which is impossible to do with CT. However, an interatrial septal channel with a contrast jet from the left atrium to the right atrium on CT is very confirmative finding of a PFO (Fig. 49.9) [50]. A channel-like appearance of the interatrial septum and the characteristic direction of the contrast jet toward the inferior vena cava help differentiate a PFO from an ASD [51]. An atrial septal aneurysm (ASA) is defined as exaggerated excursion of the septum into the arterial chamber, characterized by redundant and excessively mobile tissue in the region of the fossa ovalis. A previous study showed that a PFO with concomitant ASA is associated with a high risk of paradoxical embolism [52].

An ASD is the most common congenital heart lesion found in adults. Patients with an ASD and a right-to-left shunt are at risk for a stroke due to paradoxical embolization. The typical feature of an ASD on cardiac CT studies is a sharply defined defect in the septum with a contrast jet perpendicular to the atrial septum (Fig. 49.10) [51].

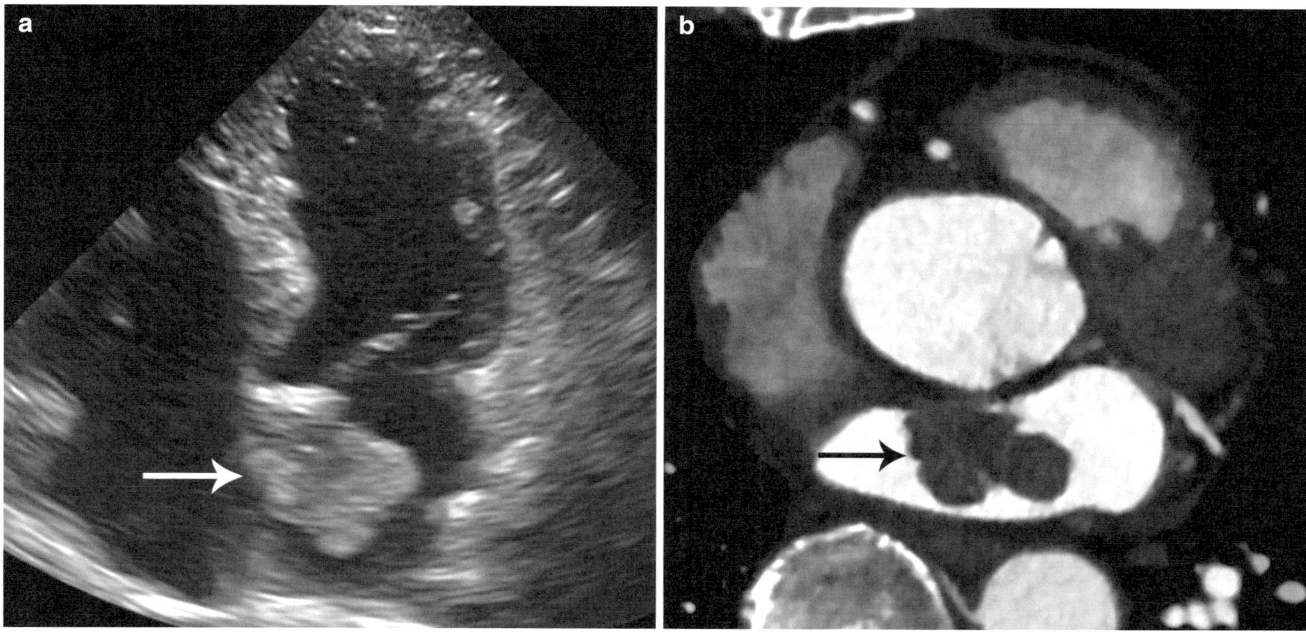

Fig. 49.8 Images in a 58-year-old man with stroke. (**a**) TTE image shows an oval-shaped echogenic mass in the LA. (**b**) Axial cardiac CT shows a lobulated filling detect (arrow) in LA. The mass was pathologically confirmed after surgical resection as a myxoma. LA, left atrium; TTE, transthoracic echocardiography

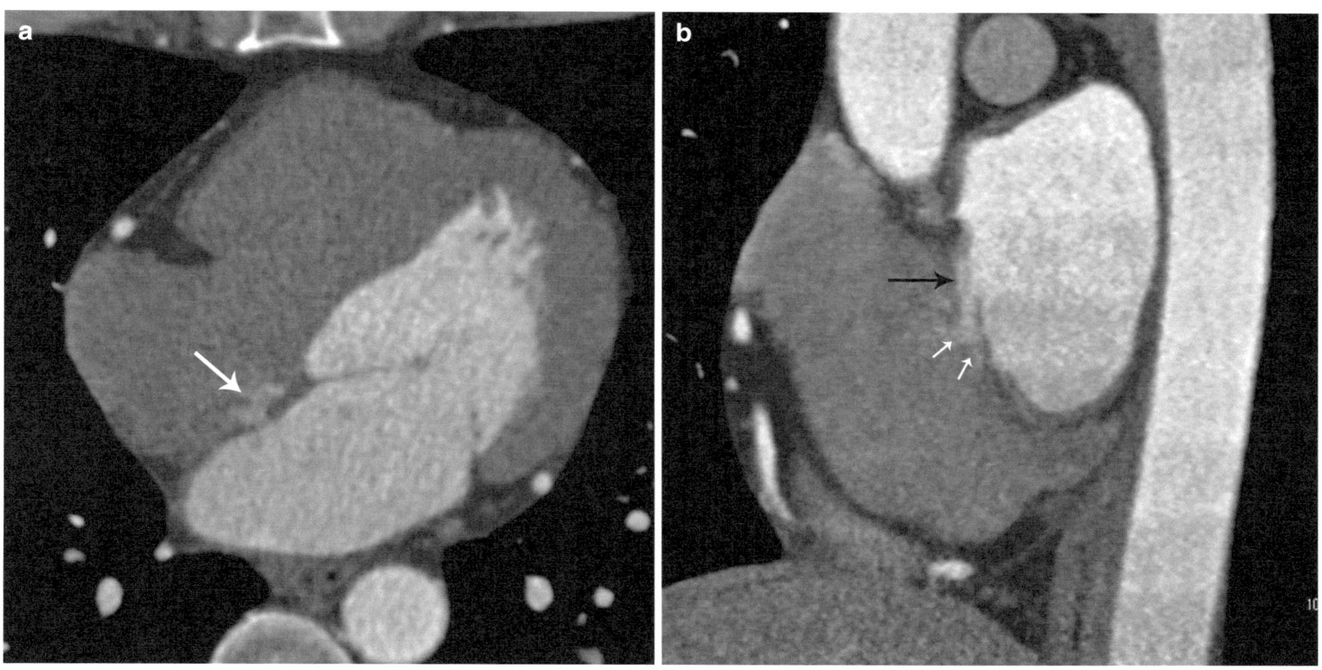

Fig. 49.9 Images in a 43-year-old man with stroke. (**a**) Axial cardiac CT image shows contrast agent jet (arrow) from LA to RA. (**b**) Oblique sagittal reformatted CT image shows the flap-like appearance of the interatrial septum (arrow) and contrast agent jets from LA to RA toward inferior vena cava (small arrows) consistent with patent foramen ovale

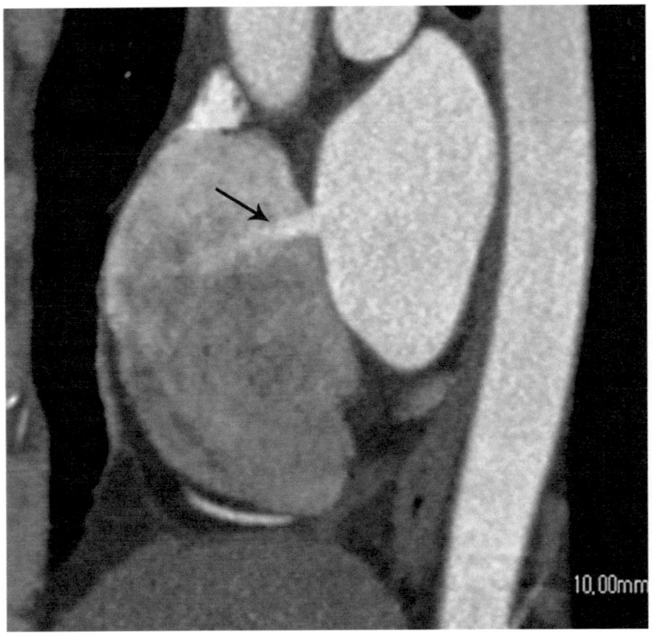

Fig. 49.10 Image in a 55-year-old woman with stroke. Oblique sagittal reformatted CT image shows a contrast jet from LA and RA (arrow) through the ASD. The direction of the jet is perpendicular to the interatrial septum. ASD atrial septal defect

Valvular Vegetation

The incidence of ischemic stroke associated with infective endocarditis is 15–20% [53]. Mitral valve involvement carries greater stroke risk than aortic valve involvement [54]. Embolic risk is also increased by mobility, consistency, extent, and size [54, 55]. Currently, echocardiography is the first-line imaging tool for the detection of valvular vegetation [56]. CT can be used to evaluate suspected vegetation or periannular complications such as abscesses or mycotic aneurysms (Fig. 49.11). A recent meta-analysis data proved that the addition of cardiac CT to TEE can improve the detection of periannular complications and vegetations, in patients with prosthetic heart valve endocarditis [57].

Valvular Calcification

Mitral annular calcification is a risk factor of stroke. A previous study of population-based cohort of 1159 subjects in an elderly demonstrated that mitral annular calcification was associated with twice the risk of stroke, independent of traditional risk factors for stroke [58]. Cardiac CT is useful modality in the evaluation of the extent and location of mitral annular calcification [59]. On CT, mitral annulus calcifications are often found around the posterior annulus of the mitral valve on CT and may cause systemic embolism in association with infective endocarditis or liquefaction of calcifications (Fig. 49.12).

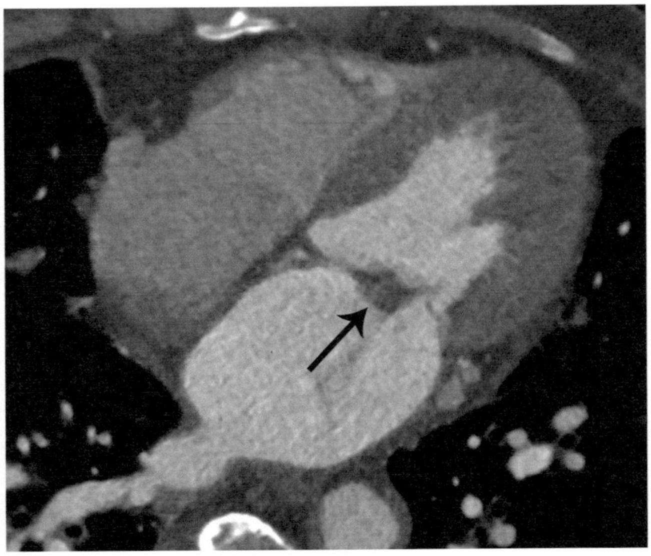

Fig. 49.11 Image in a 56-year-old man with stroke. Axial cardiac CT image shows an oval-shaped filling defect in the mitral valve (arrow). The mass was pathologically confirmed as vegetation

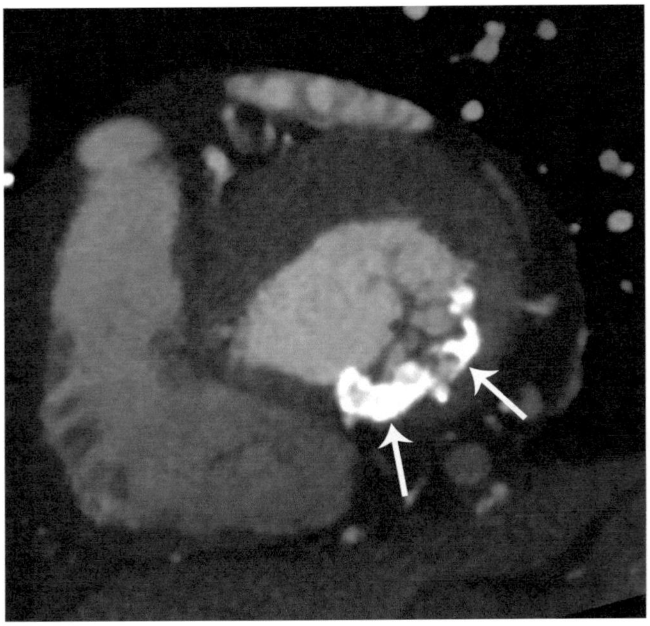

Fig. 49.12 Image in a 74-year-old man with stroke. A short-axis reformatted cardiac CT image shows severe calcifications in the mitral annulus (arrows)

The common causes of aortic stenosis are congenital, calcific degenerative, and rheumatic. Even in the absence of hemodynamically significant left ventricular outflow obstruction, there is a significant increase in the risk of death from cardiovascular events, including stroke, which may be the result of embolic fragments detaching from the thickened valve leaflets. CT is sensitive modality to evaluate the presence and extent of aortic valvular calcifications. Previous study demonstrated that cardiac CT enables quantification of aortic valvular calcifications through a calcium-scoring method and grading of the stenosis degree by measuring the valve area on mid-systolic images [60].

Aortic Atheroma

Aortic atheroma of the proximal aortic arch is important source of embolism in patients with ischemic stroke [61, 62]. Complex morphological features of the plaque, such as ulcerations or superimposed thrombi, have been shown to increase the risk of stroke [62, 63]. Echocardiography, CT, and MRI are the principal means of imaging atherosclerotic plaques in the aorta. TEE has been the primary echocardiographic method for visualizing atherosclerotic plaques in the thoracic aorta and remains the imaging standard for this indication [64, 65]. Compared with TEE, CT is much more useful for measuring plaque thickness, discovering ulceration, and examining its components (Fig. 49.13). CT has some advantages in the evaluation of aortic plaque because of the ability to reconstruct high-quality multidimensional images and enable a retrospective review with the same quality of reproducibility [66]. Radiation dose exposure and contrast medium are the most serious obstacles when using CT for patients with possible embolic stroke. CT is also a static imaging modality that cannot be used to evaluate plaque mobility, an important factor in risk stratification.

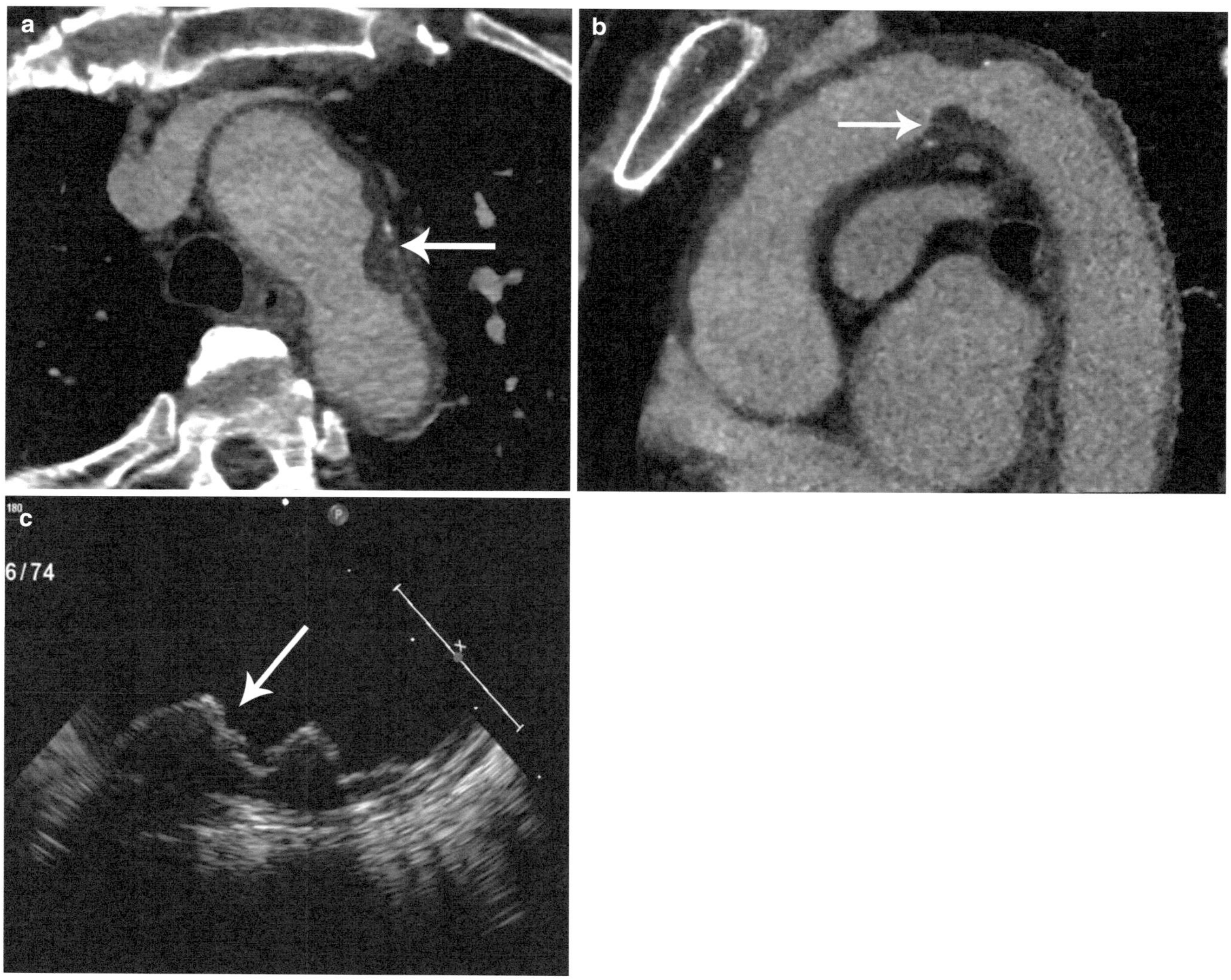

Fig. 49.13 Images in a 71-year-old man with recurrent stroke. (**a**) Axial and (**b**) coronal reformatted cardiac CT images show an aortic plaque (arrows) on the aortic arch. (**c**) TEE image shows an echogenic aortic plaque (arrow) on the aortic arch

Conclusion

Investigation of potential embolic sources is an important diagnostic step in managing patients with acute ischemic stroke or transient ischemic attack, especially when the mechanism is considered to be embolic. During the past decade, cardiac CT has been tested and compared with TEE for the diagnosis of cardioembolic sources. Many studies showed that cardiac CT is a very useful and powerful modality for the detection of cardioembolic sources in stroke patients. However, based on current evidence, cardiac CT is not recommended for the use in the initial evaluation of intracardiac structures in stroke patients [67]. In addition, cardiac CT imaging has fundamental disadvantages including radiation dose and use of iodine contrast media. Continued technological advances requiring less contrast and ionizing radiation could increase the importance of cardiac CT in this field in the near future.

References

1. Bonita R. Epidemiology of stroke. Lancet. 1992;339:342–4.
2. Sacco RL, Adams R, Albers G, et al. Guidelines for prevention stroke in patients with ischemic stroke or transient ischemic attack. Stroke. 2006;37:577–617.
3. Albers GW, Amarenco P, Easton JD, Sacco RL, Teal P. Antithrombotic and thrombolytic therapy for ischemic stroke. Chest. 2004;126:483S–512S.
4. Kistler JP. Cerebral embolism. Compr Ther. 1996;22:515–30.
5. McNamara RL, Lima JA, Whelton PK, Powe NR. Echocardiographic identification of cardiovascular sources of emboli to guide clinical management of stroke: a cost-effectiveness analysis. Ann Intern Med. 1997;127:775–87.
6. Pearson AC, Labovitz AJ, Tatineni S, Gomez CR. Superiority of transesophageal echocardiography in detecting cardiac source of embolism in patients with cerebral ischemia of uncertain etiology. J Am Coll Cardiol. 1991;17:66–72.
7. Leung DY, Black IW, Cranney GB, et al. Selection of patients for transesophageal echocardiography after stroke and systemic embolic events: role of transthoracic echocardiography. Stroke. 1995;26:1820–4.
8. Daniel WG, Mugge A. Transesophageal echocardiography. N Engl J Med. 1995;332:1268–79.
9. de Bruijn SF, Agema WR, Lammers GJ, et al. Transesophageal echocardiography is superior to transthoracic echocardiography in management of patients of any age with transient ischemic attack or stroke. Stroke. 2006;37:2531–44.
10. Harloff A, Handke M, Reinhard M, et al. Therapeutic strategies after examination by transesophageal echocardiography in 503 patients with ischemic stroke. Stroke. 2006;37:859–64.
11. Rauh R, Fischereder M, Spengel FA. Transesophageal echocardiography in patients with focal cerebral ischemia of unknown cause. Stroke. 1996;27:691–4.
12. Strandberg M, Marttila RJ, Helenius H, Hartiala J. Transoesophageal echocardiography in selecting patients for anticoagulation after ischaemic stroke or transient ischaemic attack. J Neurol Neurosurg Psychiatry. 2002;73:29–33.
13. Nikolaou K, Flohr T, Knez A, et al. Advances in cardiac CT imaging: 64-slice scanner. Int J Cardiovasc Imaging. 2004;20:535–40.
14. Raff GL, Gallagher MJ, O'Neill WW, Goldstein JA. Diagnostic accuracy of noninvasive coronary angiography using 64-slice spiral computed tomography. J Am Coll Cardiol. 2005;46:552–7.
15. Mollet NR, Cademartiri F, van Mieghem CA, et al. High-resolution spiral computed tomography coronary angiography in patients referred for diagnostic conventional coronary angiography. Circulation. 2005;112:2318–23.
16. Boxt LM, Lipton MJ, Kwong RY, Rybicki F, Clouse ME. Computed tomography for assessment of cardiac chambers, valves, myocardium and pericardium. Cardiol Clin. 2003;21:561–85.
17. Adams HP Jr, Bendixen BH, Kappelle LJ, et al. Classification of subtype of acute ischemic stroke: definitions for use in a multicenter clinical trial. Stroke. 1993;24:35–41.
18. Doufekias E, Segal AZ, Kizer JR. Cardiogenic and aortogenic brain embolism. J Am Coll Cardiol. 2008;51:1049–59.
19. Wolber T, Maeder M, Atefy R, et al. Should routine echocardiography be performed in all patients with stroke? J Stroke Cerebrovasc Dis. 2007;16:1–7.
20. Hausleiter J, Meyer T, Hermann F, et al. Estimated radiation dose associated with cardiac CT angiography. JAMA. 2009;301:500–7.
21. Heinrich MC, Häberle L, Müller V, Bautz W, Uder M. Nephrotoxicity of iso-osmolar iodixanol compared with nonionic low-osmolar contrast media: meta-analysis of randomized controlled trials. Radiology. 2009;250:68–86.
22. Honoris L, Zhong Y, Chu E, et al. Comparison of contrast enhancement, image quality and tolerability in coronary CT angiography using 4 contrast agents: a prospective randomized trial. Int J Cardiol. 2015;186:126–8.
23. Agmon Y, Khandheria BK, Gentile F, Seward JB. Echocardiographic assessment of the left atrial appendage. J Am Coll Cardiol. 1999;34:1867–77.
24. Al-Saady NM, Obel OA, Camm AJ. Left atrial appendage: structure, function and role in thromboembolism. Heart. 1999;82:547–55.
25. Achenbach S, Sacher D, Ropers D, et al. Electron beam computed tomography for the detection of left atrial thrombi in patients with atrial fibrillation. Heart. 2004;90:1477–8.
26. Shapiro MD, Neilan TG, Jassal DS, et al. Multidetector computed tomography for the detection of left atrial appendage thrombus: a comparative study with transesophageal echocardiography. J Comput Assist Tomogr. 2007;31:905–9.
27. Singh NK, Nallamothu N, Zuck VP, Issa ZF. Left atrial appendage filling defects on 64-slice multidetector computed tomography in patients undergoing pulmonary vein isolation: predictors and comparison to transesophageal echocardiography. J Comput Assist Tomogr. 2009;33:946–51.
28. Romero J, Husain SA, Kelesidis I, Sanz J, Medina HM, Garcia MJ. Detection of left atrial appendage thrombus by cardiac computed tomography in patients with atrial fibrillation: a meta-analysis. Circ Cardiovasc Imaging. 2013;6:185–94.
29. Kim YY, Klein AL, Halliburton SS, et al. Left atrial appendage filling defects identified by multidetector computed tomography in patients undergoing radiofrequency pulmonary vein antral isolation: a comparison with transesophageal echocardiography. Am Heart J. 2007;154:1199–205.
30. Hur J, Kim YJ, Nam JE, et al. Thrombus in the left atrial appendage in stroke patients: detection with cardiac CT angiography: a preliminary report. Radiology. 2008;249:81–7.
31. Vaitkus PT, Barnathan ES. Embolic potential, prevention and management of mural thrombus complicating anterior myocardial infarction: a meta-analysis. J Am Coll Cardiol. 1993;22:1004–9.
32. Srichai MB, Junor C, Rodriguez LL, et al. Clinical, imaging, and pathological characteristics of left ventricular thrombus: a comparison of contrast-enhanced magnetic resonance imaging, transthoracic echocardiography, and transesophageal echocardiography with surgical or pathological validation. Am Heart J. 2006;152:75–84.

33. Weinsaft JW, Kim HW, Shah DJ, et al. Detection of left ventricular thrombus by delayed-enhancement cardiovascular magnetic resonance prevalence and markers in patients with systolic dysfunction. J Am Coll Cardiol. 2008;52:148–57.
34. Bittencourt MS, Achenbach S, Marwan M, et al. Left ventricular thrombus attenuation characterization in cardiac computed tomography angiography. J Cardiovasc Comput Tomogr. 2012;6:121–6.
35. Holmes DR, Reddy VY, Turi ZG, et al. PROTECT AF Investigators. Percutaneous closure of the left atrial appendage versus warfarin therapy for prevention of stroke in patients with atrial fibrillation: a randomized non-inferiority trial. Lancet. 2009;374:534–42.
36. Garcia-Fernandez MA, Perez-David E, Quiles J, et al. Role of left atrial appendage obliteration in stroke reduction in patients with mitral valve prosthesis: a transesophageal echocardiographic study. J Am Coll Cardiol. 2003;42:1253–8.
37. Hur J, Kim YJ, Lee HJ, et al. Left atrial appendage thrombi in stroke patients: detection with two-phase cardiac CT angiography versus transesophageal echocardiography. Radiology. 2009;251:683–90.
38. Kim SC, Chun EJ, Choi SI, et al. Differentiation between spontaneous echocardiographic contrast and left atrial appendage thrombus in patients with suspected embolic stroke using two-phase multidetector computed tomography. Am J Cardiol. 2010;106:1174–81.
39. Hur J, Kim YJ, Lee HJ, et al. Dual-enhanced cardiac CT for detection of left atrial appendage thrombus in patients with stroke: a prospective comparison study with transesophageal echocardiography. Stroke. 2011;42:2471–7.
40. Budoff MJ. Maximizing dose reductions with cardiac CT. Int J Cardiovasc Imaging. 2009;25:279–87.
41. Castillo JG, Silvay G. Characterization and management of cardiac tumors. Semin Cardiothorac Vasc Anesth. 2010;14:6–20.
42. Bjessmo S, Ivert T. Cardiac myxoma: 40 years' experience in 63 patients. Ann Thorac Surg. 1997;63:697–700.
43. Sparrow PJ, Kurian JB, Jones TR, Sivananthan MU. MR imaging of cardiac tumors. Radiographics. 2005;25:1255–76.
44. Kim EY, Choe YH, Sung K, Park SW, Kim JH, Ko YH. Multidetector CT and MR imaging of cardiac tumors. Korean J Radiol. 2009;10:164–75.
45. Scheffel H, Baumueller S, Stolzmann P, et al. Atrial myxomas and thrombi: comparison of imaging features on CT. AJR Am J Roentgenol. 2009;192:639–45.
46. Hong YJ, Hur J, Kim YJ, et al. Dual-energy cardiac computed tomography for differentiating cardiac myxoma from thrombus. Int J Card Imaging. 2014;30:121–8.
47. Kerut EK, Norfleet WT, Plotnick GD, et al. Patent foramen ovale: a review of associated conditions and the impact of physiological size. J Am Coll Cardiol. 2001;38:613–23.
48. Woods TD, Patel A. A critical review of patent foramen ovale detection using saline contrast echocardiography: when bubbles lie. J Am Soc Echocardiogr. 2006;19:215–22.
49. Pinto FJ. When and how to diagnose patent foramen ovale. Heart. 2005;91:438–40.
50. Kim YJ, Hur J, Shim CY, et al. Patent foramen ovale: diagnosis with multidetector CT: comparison with transesophageal echocardiography. Radiology. 2009;250:61–7.
51. Kim YJ, Hur J, Choe KO, et al. Interatrial shunt detected in coronary computed tomography angiography: differential features of a patent foramen ovale and an atrial septal defect. J Comput Assist Tomogr. 2008;32:663–7.
52. Mas JL, Arquizan C, Lamy C, et al. Recurrent cerebrovascular events associated with patent foramen ovale, atrial septal aneurysm, or both. N Engl J Med. 2001;345:1740–6.
53. Mylonakis E, Calderwood SB. Infective endocarditis in adults. N Engl J Med. 2001;345:1318–30.
54. Cabell CH, Pond KK, Peterson GE, et al. The risk of stroke and death in patients with aortic and mitral valve endocarditis. Am Heart J. 2001;142:75–80.
55. Di Salvo G, Habib G, Pergola V, et al. Echocardiography predicts embolic events in infective endocarditis. J Am Coll Cardiol. 2001;37:1069–76.
56. Daniel WG, Mugge A, Martin RP, et al. Improvement in the diagnosis of abscesses associated with endocarditis by transesophageal echocardiography. N Engl J Med. 1991;324:795–800.
57. Habets J, Tanis W, Reitsma JB, et al. Are novel non-invasive imaging techniques needed in patients with suspected prosthetic heart valve endocarditis? A systematic review and meta-analysis. Eur Radiol. 2015;25:2125–33.
58. Benjamin EJ, Plehn JF, D'Agostino RB, et al. Mitral annular calcification and the risk of stroke in an elderly cohort. N Engl J Med. 1992;327:374–9.
59. Higgins J, Mayo J, Skarsgard P. Cardiac computed tomography facilitates operative planning in patients with mitral calcification. Ann Thorac Surg. 2013;95:e9–11.
60. Budoff MJ, Takasu J, Katz R, et al. Reproducibility of CT measurements of aortic valve calcification, mitral annulus calcification, and aortic wall calcification in the multi-ethnic study of atherosclerosis. Acad Radiol. 2006;13:166–72.
61. Amarenco P, Cohen A, Tzourio C, et al. Atherosclerotic disease of the aortic arch and the risk of ischemic stroke. N Engl J Med. 1994;331:1474–9.
62. The French Study of Aortic Plaques in Stroke Group. Atherosclerotic disease of the aortic arch as a risk factor for recurrent ischemic stroke. N Engl J Med. 1996;334:1121–221.
63. Tunick PA, Rosenzweig BP, Katz ES, Freedberg RS, Perez JL, Kronzon I. High risk for vascular events in patients with protruding aortic atheromas: a prospective study. J Am Coll Cardiol. 1994;23:1085–90.
64. Rana BS, Monaghan MJ, Ring L, Shapiro LS, Nihoyannopoulos P. The pivotal role of echocardiography in cardiac sources of embolism. Eur J Echocardiogr. 2011;12:25–31.
65. Pepi M, Evangelista A, Nihoyannopoulos P, et al. European Association of Echocardiography. Recommendations for echocardiography use in the diagnosis and management of cardiac sources of embolism: European Association of Echocardiography. Eur J Echocardiogr. 2010;11:461–76.
66. Ko Y, Park JH, Yang MH, et al. Significance of aortic atherosclerotic disease in possibly embolic stroke: 64-multidetector row computed tomography study. J Neurol. 2010;257:699–705.
67. Taylor AJ, Cerqueira M, Hodgson JM, Mark D, Min J, O'Gara P, et al. ACCF/SCCTA/ACR/AHA/ASE/ASNC/NASCI/SCAI/SCMR 2010 appropriate use criteria for cardiac computed tomography. A report of the American college of cardiology foundation appropriate use criteria task force, the society of cardiovascular computed tomography, the American college of radiology, the American heart association, the American society of echocardiography, the American society of nuclear cardiology, the north American society for cardiovascular imaging, the society for cardiovascular angiography and interventions, and the society for cardiovascular magnetic resonance. J Am Coll Cardiol. 2010;56:1864–94.

Incidental Findings on CT Angiography and How to Manage Them

50

Seung Min Yoo, Hwa Yeon Lee, and Charles S. White

Because of recent technologic advances, coronary CT angiography (CTA) has become a potent imaging tool in the evaluation of patients with atypical chest pain (i.e., low to intermediate risk for both stable angina and acute coronary syndrome) [1]. Coronary CTA is expected to be increasingly used in clinical practice due to its high sensitivity and a negative predictive value that approaches 100% [2]. A major reason for performing coronary CTA is to evaluate coronary artery disease, and it is vital for interpreting physicians to focus on identifying abnormalities in the coronary arteries. However, neighboring organs such as central portions of the lungs, mediastinum, aorta, esophagus, upper abdominal organs, and thoracic skeleton are typically included in the examination, regardless of whether a restricted field of view (Fig. 50.1) or a full field of view is used for the evaluation of coronary arteries. Thus, it is critical that all interpreting physicians be careful not to overlook extracardiac incidental findings (Fig. 50.2). This chapter will discuss the most important incidental findings and an approach to their follow-up and management.

Use of a Small Versus Wide Field of View on Coronary CT Angiography

A discussion of the concept of the small and wide fields of view is a prerequisite to understand the ongoing debate regarding appropriate field of view in interpreting coronary CTA. The "small or restricted field of view" is a primary tool for analysis of coronary arteries using 16–25 cm^2 of coverage and thin collimation <1 mm. In contrast, "wide or full field of view" provides full coverage (35–40 cm^2) with thicker collimation of 2–5 mm encompassing the entire transverse extent of the chest. The latter is an additional reconstruction that may be obtained in order to provide and overread for extracardiac incidental findings [3, 4]. Because of the small size of the coronary arteries, reconstruction with a small field of view is required to maximize spatial resolution by reducing pixel size, facilitating precise analysis of the degree of stenosis and characterize plaque in these small structures. However, because all structures within a given CT slice have already been exposed to radiation, wide field of view images can be obtained without additional radiation dose.

The prevalence of incidental extracardiac findings (Tables 50.1 and 50.2) demonstrated on coronary CTA is fairly high ranging up to 67.0% on the wide field of view image with considerable variation in frequency due to study design and definition [3–17]. Of these, the prevalence of clinically important findings needing further work-up or management is less common and ranges from 1.2% to 22.7% [18]. It is certainly true that more malignant lesions (Fig. 50.3) will be found in wide field of view because a substantial number of lung cancers occur in the peripheral portion of the lungs, and most of breast tissue is excluded from a small field of view on coronary CTA. Earlier detection of lung or breast cancer may lead to curable surgical resection and favorable outcomes. In spite of this potential benefit, several reports [14, 19–22] have advocated exclusive use of small of view, although a larger group has favored the additional use of a wide field of view in interpreting coronary CTA [3, 4, 9, 11, 12, 15–18, 23–28]. There are differing opinions even within specialties [4, 14, 18–22, 27, 29]. The main reason for the controversy is the high prevalence of false-positive findings (i.e., low prevalence of malignancy less than 0.4%) on the larger field of view and lack of proven benefit of CT screening of lung cancer prior to the publication of the National Lung Screening Trial (NLST) [19, 20]. Work-up of numerous indeterminate lung nodules that ultimately prove to be benign may lead to extra cost, morbidity related to downstream testing and intervention, a low but potential risk of

S. M. Yoo
Department of Radiology, CHA University Bundang Medical Center, Bundang, South Korea

H. Y. Lee
Smile Radiologic Clinic, Seoul, South Korea

C. S. White (✉)
Department of Diagnostic Radiology, University of Maryland Medical Center, Baltimore, MD, USA
e-mail: cwhite@umm.edu

U. J. Schoepf (ed.), *CT of the Heart*, Contemporary Medical Imaging, https://doi.org/10.1007/978-1-60327-237-7_50

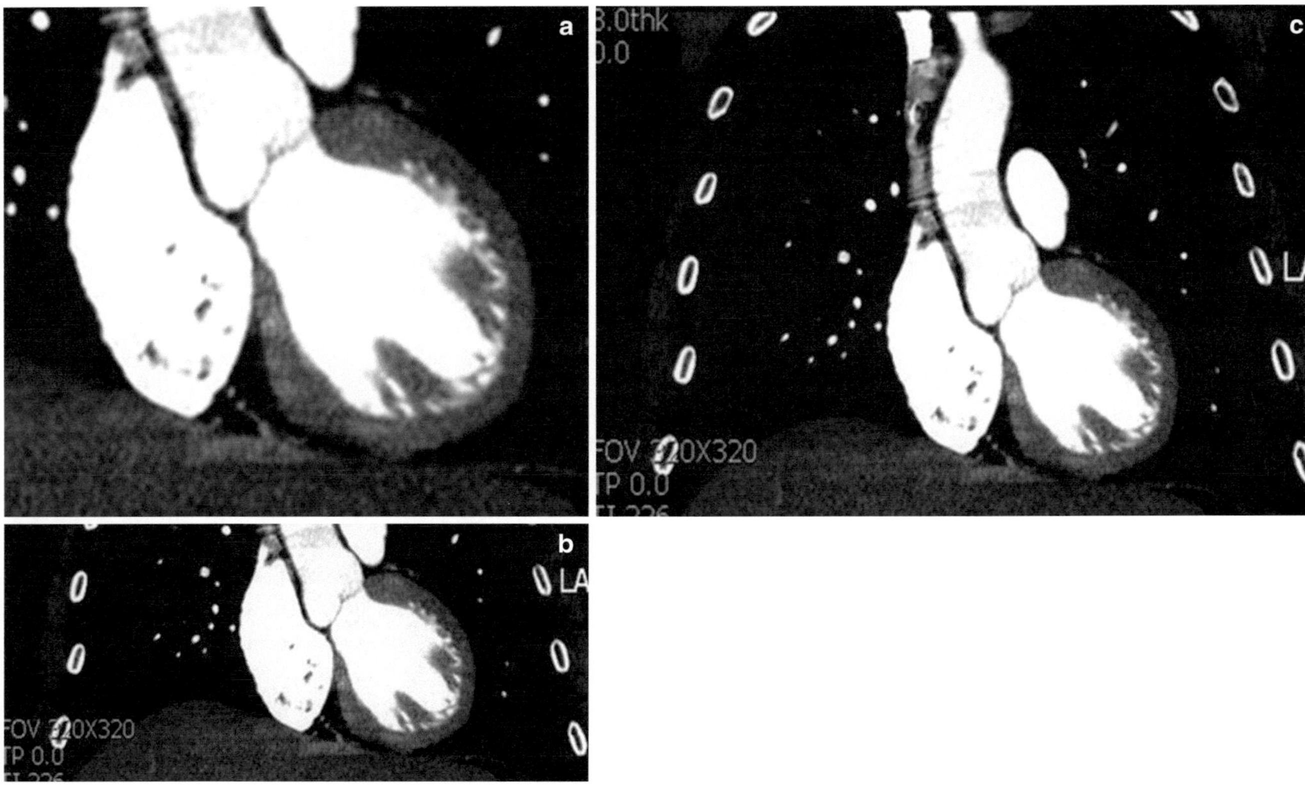

Fig. 50.1 Representative small (**a**) and wide (**b**) field of views on dedicated coronary CTA compared with the wide field of view (**c**) of triple rule-out protocol. The small field of view on dedicated coronary CTA includes the central lung parenchyma, aorta, mediastinum, bony structures, and abdominal organs. The wide field of view on dedicated coronary CTA includes about two-thirds of total lung volume

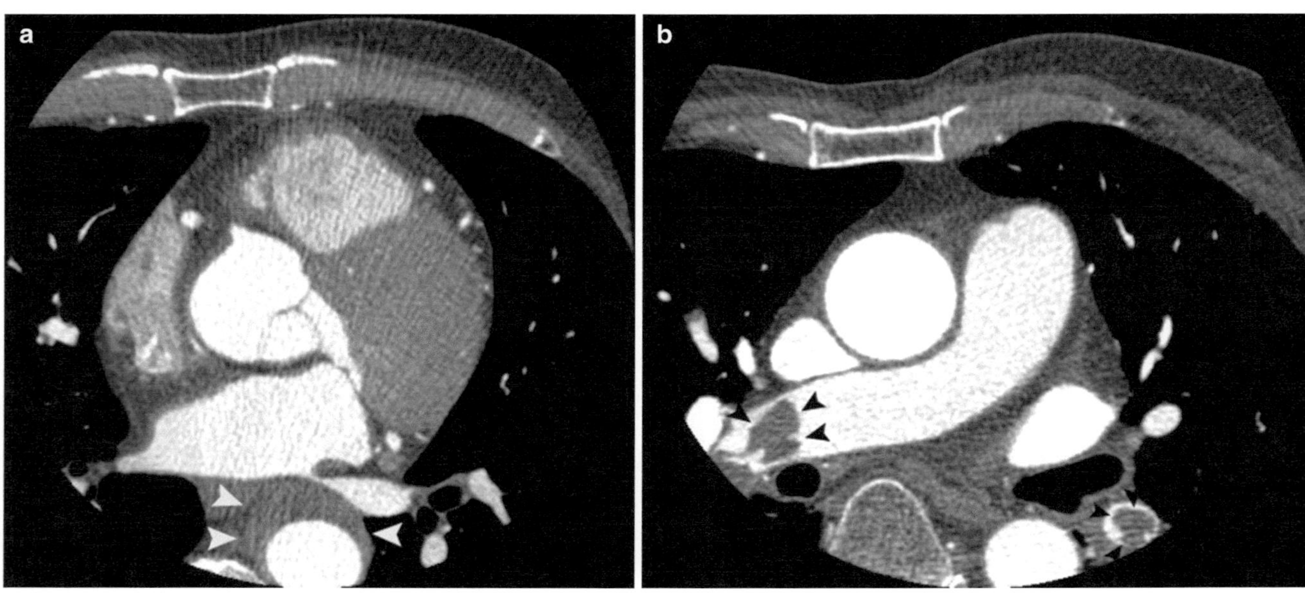

Fig. 50.2 Various important extracardiac findings demonstrated on small field of view coronary CTA image. Stanford type B intramural hematoma (arrowheads in **a**), central pulmonary emboli (arrowheads in **b**), esophageal wall thickening in a patient with gastroesophageal reflux disease (arrowheads in **c**), anterior mediastinal mass (arrowheads in **d**), and central lung cancer (arrows in **e**) are demonstrated even using a small coronary CTA field of view. Thus, all interpreters should be familiar with important extracardiac findings

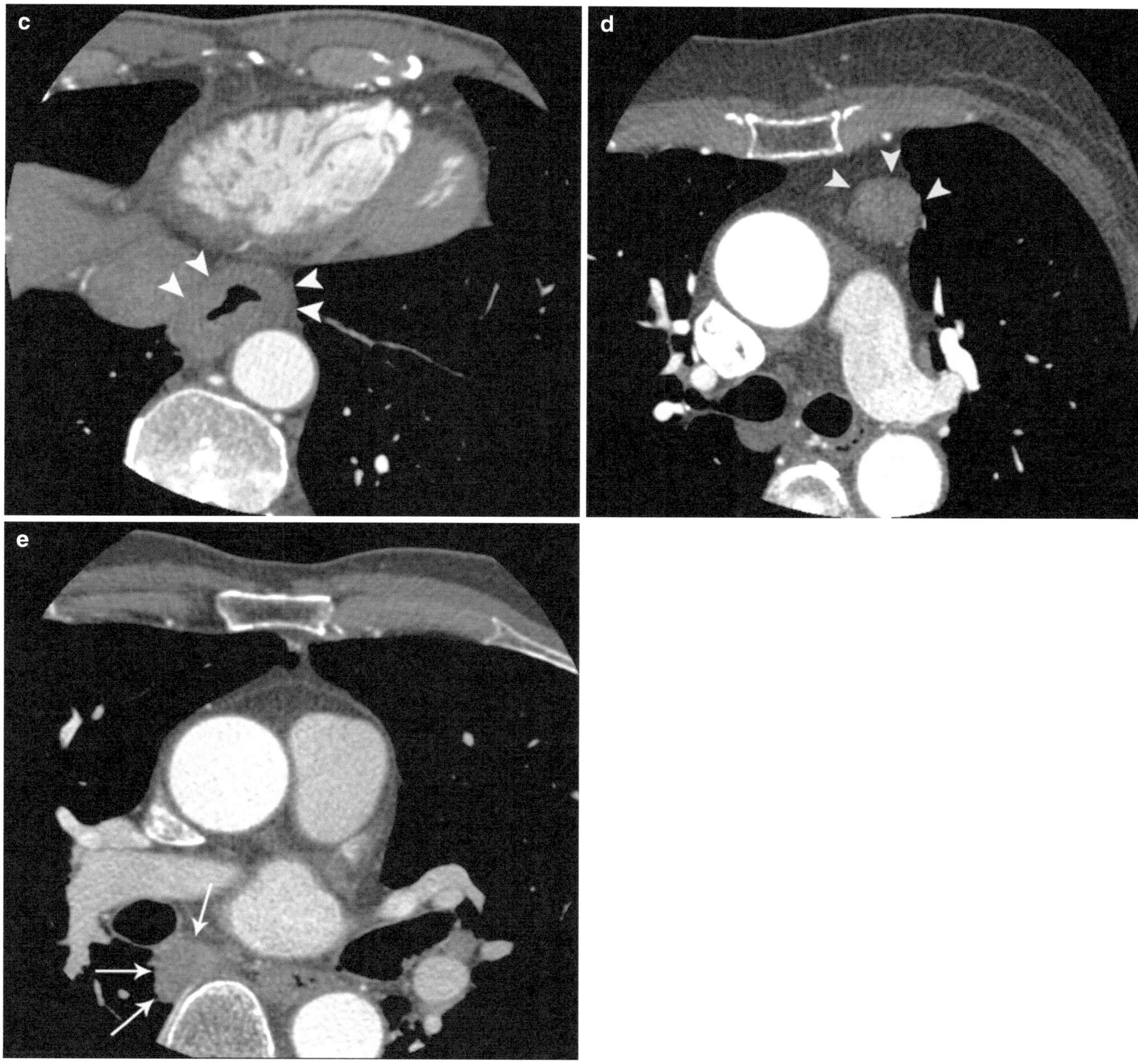

Fig. 50.2 (continued)

radiation-induced cancer, and anxiety on the part of both physicians and patients.

Results from the NLST indicated a lung cancer and overall mortality benefit for low-dose chest CT screening compared with screening with chest radiography. The randomized trial of more than 53,000 asymptomatic subjects who had a smoking history of more than 30 pack-years and were 55–74 years of age showed a 20.3% reduction of lung cancer mortality in the CT arm compared with chest radiography arm [30]. Based on the result of NLST, it seems reasonable to suggest that a wide field of view of coronary CTA be reconstructed and evaluated in the subset of patients who fit the entry criteria of the NLST.

However, even this suggestion should be viewed with caution because of differences in the patient selection. The individuals who enrolled in the NLST were entirely asymptomatic, whereas nearly all patients who undergo coronary CTA are referred for chest pain. Such a distinct referral pattern may affect the prevalence and characteristics of incidental extracardiac findings. In addition, the specifics of imaging protocols are different between low-dose chest CT and coronary CTA. The former is a nonenhanced CT with low radiation exposure, whereas the latter is obtained with intravenous contrast media and a higher radiation exposure due to ECG gating, potentially permitting lung nodules and certain other incidental findings to be more easily identified. For example, aortic dissection would be directly visible on coronary CTA but would be unlikely to be detected on a lung cancer screening study.

Table 50.1 Potentially clinically significant incidental extracardiac findings

Incidental finding	Prevalence (%)
Pulmonary nodule ≥4 mm	0.4–16.5%
Pulmonary consolidation	0.4–6.2%
Marked mediastinal lymphadenopathy	0.1–2.3%
Hiatal hernia	0.2–6.4%
Aortic dissection	0.0–0.3%
Aortic aneurysm	0.3–1.6%
Pulmonary embolism	0.0–1.9%
Breast nodule	0.0–0.6%
Fracture	0.0–0.3%
Metastatic bone destruction	Frequency not available
Pleural effusion	0.1–4.0%
Adrenal nodule	0.0–0.8%
Indeterminate hepatic nodule	0.0–2.3%
Cholelithiasis	0.1–3.6%

Moreover, there is inconsistency in the use of wide field of view in the radiologic practices depending on body part. Only small field of view images are typically reconstructed in other parts of body such as the orbits, inner ear, sinuses, and thoracic spine CT, even though radiation is received through the entire transverse CT section [29]. Lastly, it should be remembered that the typical *z*-axis coverage of dedicated coronary CTA does not include the upper one-third of the entire chest volume (i.e., tracheal carina to lung apices) [15]. This may lead to the false assumption that the entirety of both lungs is normal among patients undergoing a normal dedicated coronary CTA and their treating clinicians. Therefore, until a randomized trial is available to provide an overview about cost-effectiveness and outcome benefits, reconstruction of only a small field of view may be acceptable in patients undergoing dedicated coronary CTA, particularly in those of different age and smoking habits as compared with enrollees in NLST [29].

Table 50.2 Benign incidental extracardiac findings

Incidental finding	Prevalence (%)
Pulmonary nodule <4 mm	1.7–9.3%
Benign hepatic cyst	1.1–6.6%
Simple renal cyst	0.1–0.3%
Benign adrenal adenoma	0.1–0.6%

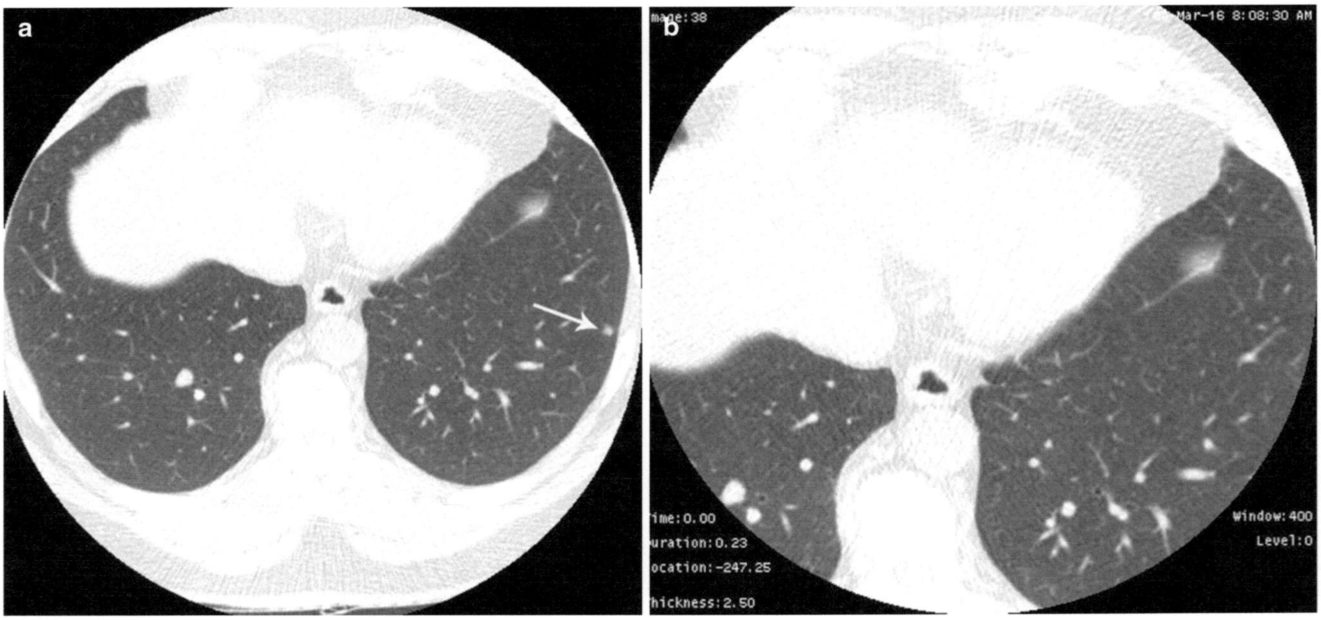

Fig. 50.3 Various important extracardiac findings identified only on a wide field of view coronary CTA image. (**a**, **b**) Solid pulmonary nodule 5 mm in diameter (arrow in **a**) is demonstrated in the left lower lobe on wide field of view image at the level of inferior cardiac margin in a 42-year-old male smoker. Note that the nodule is not visible on a small field of view image (**b**). (**c**) Enhancing 8 mm nodule (arrows in **c**) is demonstrated in the lateral portion of the left breast on a wide field of view coronary CTA image at the level of pulmonary artery bifurcation in a 42-year-old female patient. This nodule was not visible on a small field of view image. Breast ultrasonography was recommended in the patient for further evaluation. D. Right seventh rib destruction (arrowheads on **d**) is noted on a wide field of view bone setting image at the level of the right main pulmonary artery in an 81-year-old man. However, this lesion is not demonstrated on a small field of view image (**e**). The patient ultimately proved to have a rectal cancer

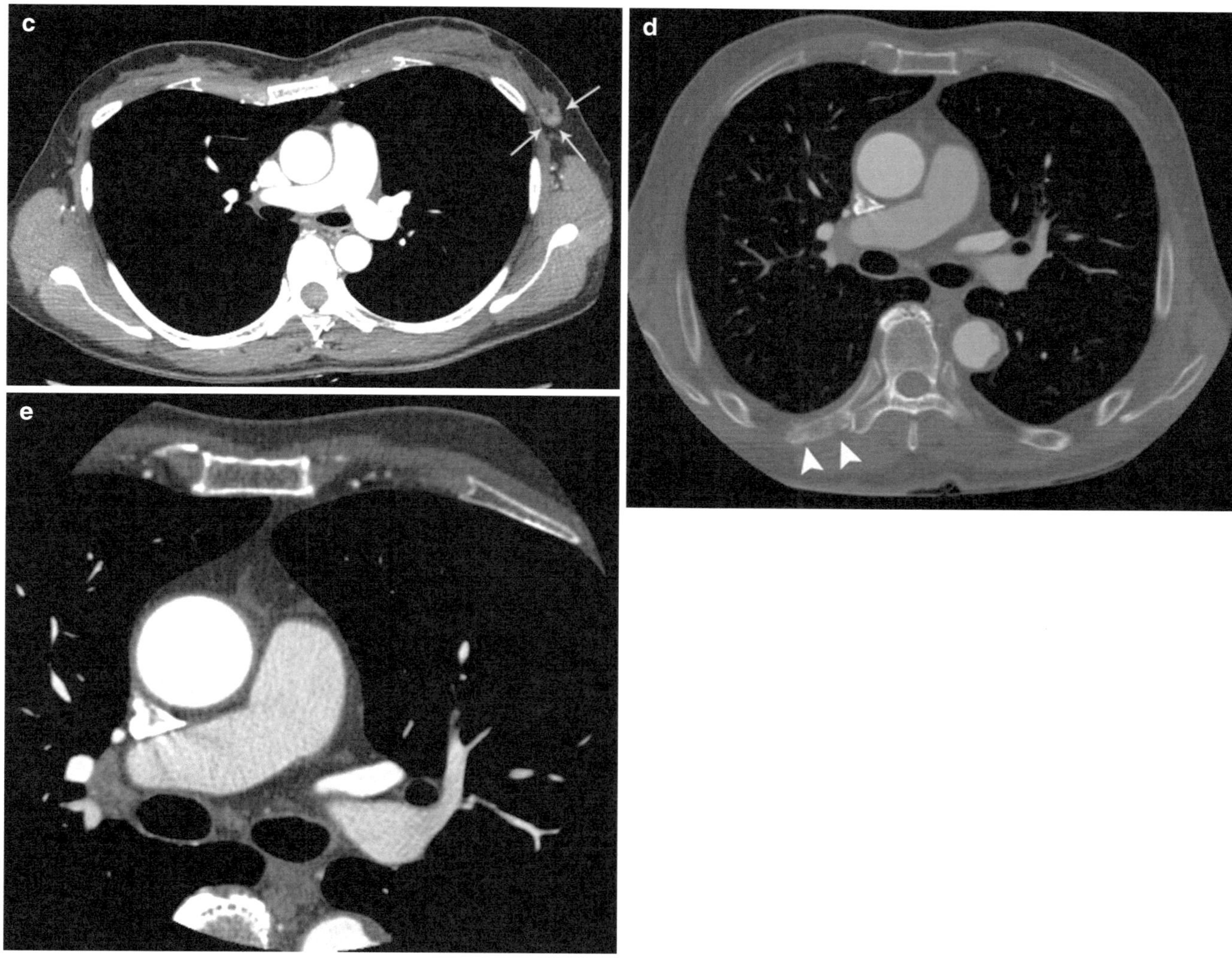

Fig. 50.3 (continued)

In the setting of acute chest pain, there is less debate than in stable angina regarding the use of a wide field of view (either dedicated coronary CTA or triple rule-out protocol) because an alternative cause of acute chest pain such as peripheral pulmonary embolism (Fig. 50.4), pneumonia, pneumothorax, rib fracture, cholecystitis, or pancreatitis can be identified when the coronary artery component is negative [13, 27]. According to one study, clinically important extracardiac findings that potentially changed patient management were identified up to 5% of patients presenting with acute chest pain. Thus, a stronger case can be made for a large field of view reconstruction in these patients [13, 31].

Practical Tips to Avoid Overlooking Important Incidental Findings

Because at least 8–22% (mean, 14%) of lung parenchyma, mediastinum, bone, chest wall, aorta, pulmonary arteries, and upper abdominal organs are included even in a small field of view [32], interpreters should be careful not to miss important extracardiac findings. Dedicated analysis of the coronary arteries with submillimeter collimation should be performed with a small field of view, and interpretation with three major image settings (mediastinal, lung, and bone window settings) should be routinely performed to analyze all organs visualized within the field of view beyond the coronary arteries, even if only a small field of view image is used [23, 33]. In contrast, if wide field of view images are available, the coronary arteries should be interpreted with small field of view image using submillimeter collimation, whereas extracardiac findings should be separately analyzed on wide field of view images with the three different window settings using 2–5 mm collimation. The typical Hounsfield unit (HU) levels and widths for mediastinal, lung, and bone window settings are 50 and 350, −500 and 1800, and 500 and 2000, respectively [33]. As a rule axial images are the best option to identify extracardiac findings. Although it is not routinely used in clinical practice, additional reconstruction of coronal or sagittal views may provide additional information to

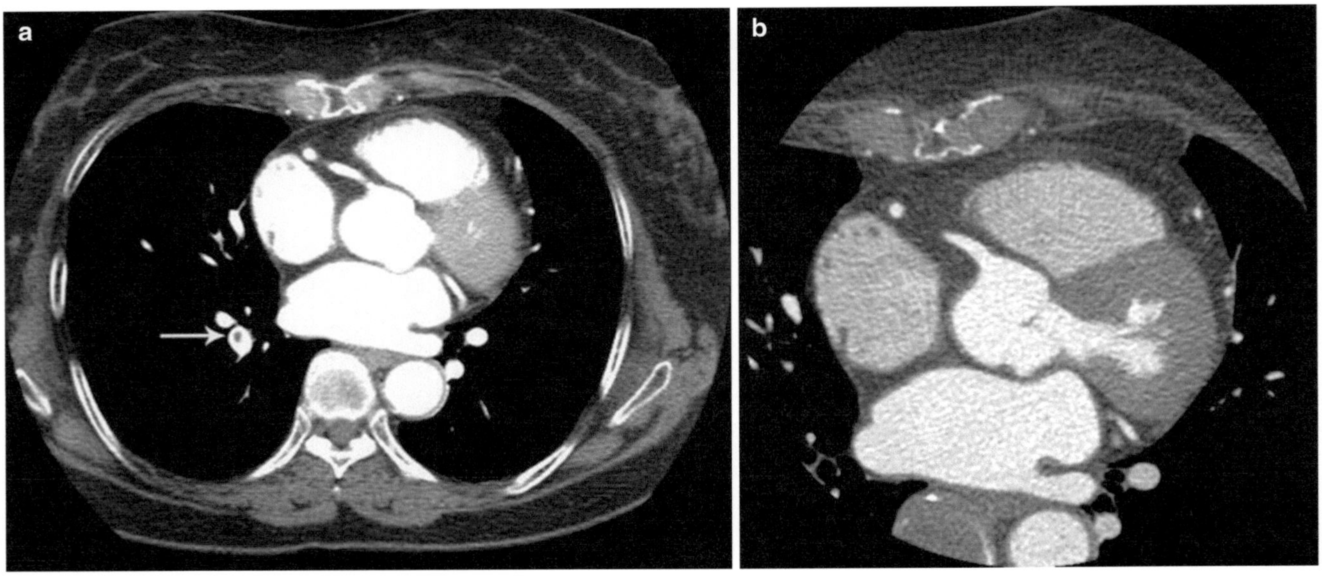

Fig. 50.4 Peripheral pulmonary embolism in a segmental pulmonary artery in the right lower lobe is identified only on a wide field of view image at the level of the left atrium in a 71-year-old woman. The patient presented with acute chest pain and the primary concern was acute coronary syndrome. Dedicated coronary CTA showed normal coronary arteries. Segmental pulmonary embolus is demonstrated on the wide field of view image (arrow on **a**), but not the small field of view image (**b**), thus showing the potential benefits of wide field of view imaging to provide an alternative cause of chest pain. Although most central pulmonary emboli are visible on a small field of view image, this may not be the case for more peripheral emboli

determine the precise location of a pulmonary nodule near a fissure or to identify vertebral pathology such as a compression fracture [33]. If an extracardiac finding is encountered, a multidisciplinary approach can be made used to select the next appropriate step. Importantly, those who interpret cardiac CTA should keep in mind that incidental extracardiac findings should always be compared on any previous studies to avoid unnecessary and potentially costly follow-up examinations.

Incidental Findings and How to Manage Them

Lung

An incidental pulmonary nodule is the most frequent finding in the evaluation of wide field of view on coronary CTA. The prevalence of all incidental pulmonary nodules and indeterminate pulmonary nodules needing further work-up is 0.9–36.2% and 0.4–16.5%, respectively [18]. A pulmonary nodule is defined as a relatively well-defined area of increased attenuation less than 3 cm in diameter. Certain characteristics can lead to a specific diagnosis. The presence of fat (HU of less than −10) in the pulmonary nodule on nonenhanced CT is diagnostic of benign hamartoma (Fig. 50.5). Central, diffuse, lamellated, or popcorn shape calcification in a smoothly marginated nodule is a typical CT finding of benign pulmonary nodule. In contrast, eccentric calcification in a pulmonary nodule does not necessarily indicate a benign etiology.

If an indeterminate nodule is found on coronary CTA, the nodule can be followed by the Fleischner Society recommendations. The recommendations classify lung nodules based on size and the presence or absence of risk factors such as smoking history or known primary cancer. Follow-up CT is not recommended in small (<4 mm) pulmonary nodules in a nonsmoker. In contrast, indeterminate pulmonary nodule more than 4 mm irrespective of risk factors should be followed by low-dose chest CT for up to 2 years to confirm resolution or stability. Stability over 2 years typically indicates that a solid pulmonary nodule is benign. However, an indeterminate pulmonary nodule with ground-glass attenuation should be followed more than 2 years because ground-glass or part-solid nodules that prove to be malignant typically have a longer doubling time [34].

Mediastinum

The most frequent significantly abnormal finding in the mediastinum is lymph node enlargement. Lymph node size less than 10 mm in short diameter is usually benign. If there is lymph node enlargement ≥10 mm in short diameter (Fig. 50.6) on coronary CTA, it should be further characterized by its shape and as well as any history of malignancy. The presence of a central fatty hilum or calcification in an enlarged lymph node or the concomitant presence of pneumonia may indicate

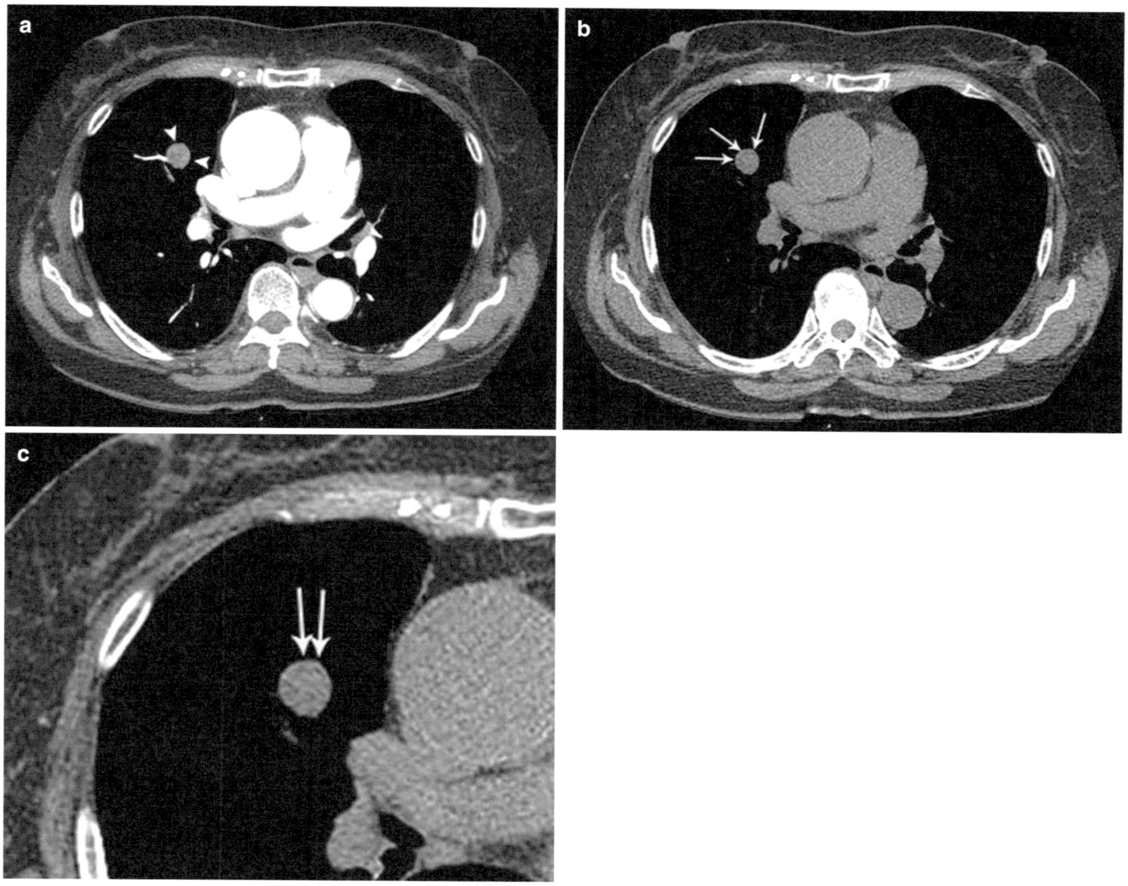

Fig. 50.5 Incidental pulmonary hamartoma in a 60-year-old female patient. Pulmonary nodule is demonstrated in the right middle lobe in enhanced (arrowheads in **a**), nonenhanced (arrows in **b**) wide field of view, and magnified (arrows in **c**) images at the level of the main pulmonary artery. Note fat attenuation (arrows in **c**) indicative of pulmonary hamartoma

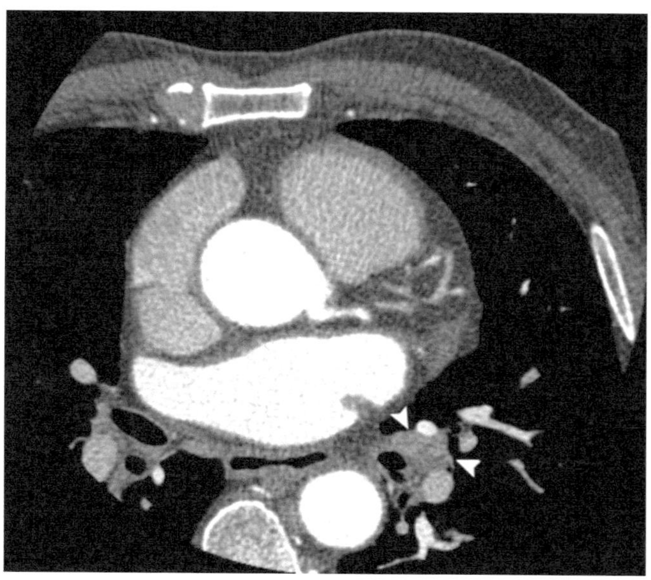

Fig. 50.6 Indeterminate left hilar lymph node enlargement on a small field of view image in a 66-year-old male. Left hilar lymph node enlargement (arrowheads) measuring about 12 mm in short diameter is demonstrated on a small field of view image of coronary CTA at the level of the left atrium. Follow-up chest CT was recommended

a benign etiology. In contrast, lymph node enlargement that lacks benign features should be followed by CT or further evaluated [23, 33]. Conglomerate lymph node enlargement with peripheral rim or diffuse enhancement can be a finding in tuberculous or malignant lymph node enlargement. Another frequent mediastinal finding is an esophageal abnormality such as hiatal hernia or esophageal wall thickening. The gastroesophageal junction is located above the diaphragmatic hiatus on CT in patients with a hiatal hernia. This finding may explain symptoms of chest pain due to gastroesophageal reflux disease. If gastroesophageal reflux disease is suspected, endoscopic evaluation can be performed.

Aorta

The clinical presentation of aortic dissection and acute coronary syndrome can be quite similar. Thus, the aorta should be evaluated carefully on coronary CTA even when using a small field of view. Aortic dilatation or aneurysm is a frequent incidental finding on coronary CTA. An aortic aneurysm (Fig. 50.7) is defined as aortic dilatation more than 150%

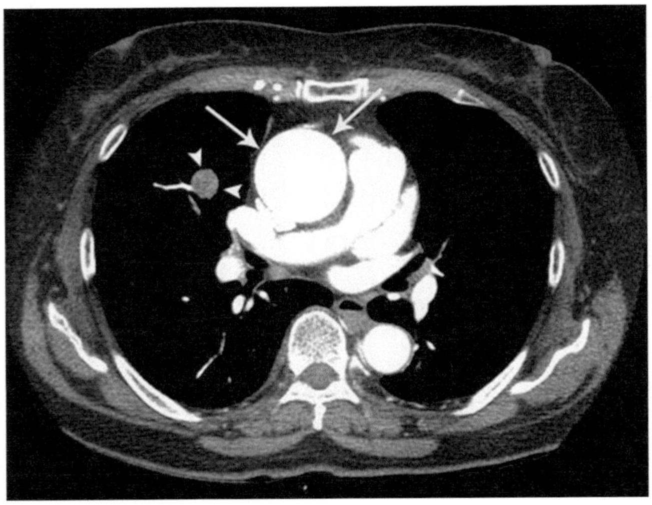

Fig. 50.7 Ascending aortic aneurysm on a small field of view image in a 60-year-old female patient. This is the same patient with Fig. 50.5 who has hamartoma (arrowheads) in the right middle lobe. Note ascending aortic aneurysm (arrows) measuring approximately 50 mm in diameter

(often 5 cm in diameter) compared with size of a normal aorta. Six months to 1 year CT follow-up is recommended to evaluate changes in the aortic diameter. If there is greater than 1 cm aortic dilatation over the course of a year, surgical intervention should be considered.

Pulmonary Artery

Most central pulmonary emboli may be visible even in a small field of view image on coronary CTA. However, it should be stressed that dedicated coronary CTA targets the left circulation but not the right. Thus, the visibility of central pulmonary emboli depends on the degree of enhancement in the pulmonary arteries. In contrast, peripheral pulmonary embolism in segmental or subsegmental pulmonary arteries may only be noted on a wide field of view. In patients with pulmonary embolism demonstrated on CTA, lower extremity Doppler ultrasonography can be recommended to evaluate for deep vein thrombosis.

Breast

The prevalence of breast nodules found on coronary CTA is up to 0.6% [3, 4, 14, 26, 32]. If a breast nodule (Fig. 50.3c) is identified on a wide field of view coronary CTA image, ultrasonography and mammography should be performed to exclude early breast cancer.

Thoracic Skeleton and Pleura

It is important to identify the presence of acute rib fractures because they may be an alternative cause of chest pain [33]. It is of value to remember that rib fractures can occur without a history of blunt trauma, for example, due to chronic cough or stress-related injury. It is also important to identify any metastatic rib lesion (Fig. 50.3d) or vertebral destruction to avoid unnecessary additional examinations to confirm the diagnosis. Pleural effusion is another common incidental finding. Pleural effusion in the dependent portion of the chest with low density (<20 HU) and no enhancement usually indicates a transudate. Although the presence of pleural linear or nodular enhancement, loculation, or high attenuation of content (HU >20) may suggest exudative or complicated effusion, the absence of such findings does not completely exclude an exudative or malignant pleural effusion [33].

Upper Abdominal Organs

Frequent abdominal incidental findings are cysts (Fig. 50.8), hemangiomas, adrenal nodules (Fig. 50.9), and gallbladder or renal stones. Most hepatic nodules less than 10 mm in diameter are benign in asymptomatic patients. Standard recommendations such as the Fleischner guidelines for indeterminate lung nodule do not exist for follow-up of incidental hepatic nodules in low-risk patients [23]. Peripheral nodular enhancement on the arterial phase of CT is typical for a hemangioma. Occasionally, hepatocellular carcinoma or hypervascular metastasis such as melanoma may be a cause of hepatic nodule with high attenuation on coronary CTA. Thus, the possibility of malignant hepatic nodule should be considered in patients with CT features of liver cirrhosis or history or a primary focus of cancer. According to the recently published Liver Imaging-Reporting and Data System (LI-RADS), a nodule demonstrated on CT in patients at high risk for hepatocellular carcinoma (e.g., liver cirrhosis) should be considered at least as an indeterminate nodule (≥LR-3), irrespective of size. In this scenario, dynamic abdomen CT is recommended [35]. It should be kept in mind that coronary CTA is not the optimal examination to identify hepatic nodules because it is not obtained in a parenchymal venous phase.

An incidental adrenal nodule is another common abdominal finding within the field of view of coronary CTA. Hounsfield units less than 10 on nonenhanced CT images often indicate a benign adenoma because most adenomas contain a fatty component. However, adrenal adenomas with scanty fat often have a higher CT attenuation on nonenhanced CT. In such cases, a dedicated abdominal CT study showing a characteristic washout pattern is helpful to discriminate an adenoma from a malignant lesion. Greater than 40% washout on a 15 min delayed CT image indicates an adenoma [23].

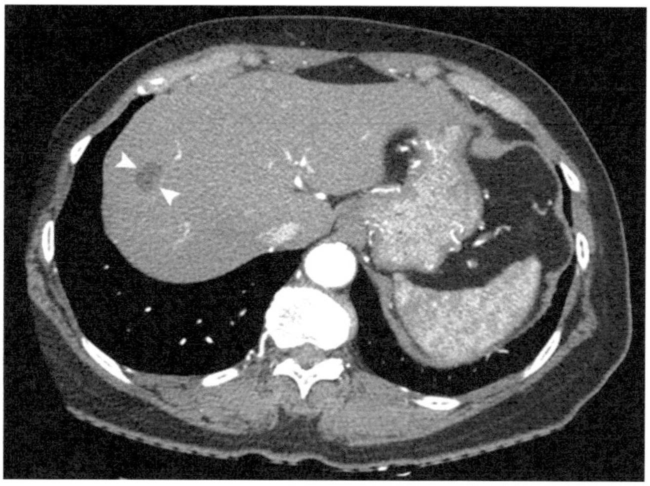

Fig. 50.8 Hepatic cyst in a 50-year-old male patient. Hepatic cyst with typical low attenuation (i.e., HU near zero) (arrowheads) is noted on a wide field of view image at the level of dome of liver

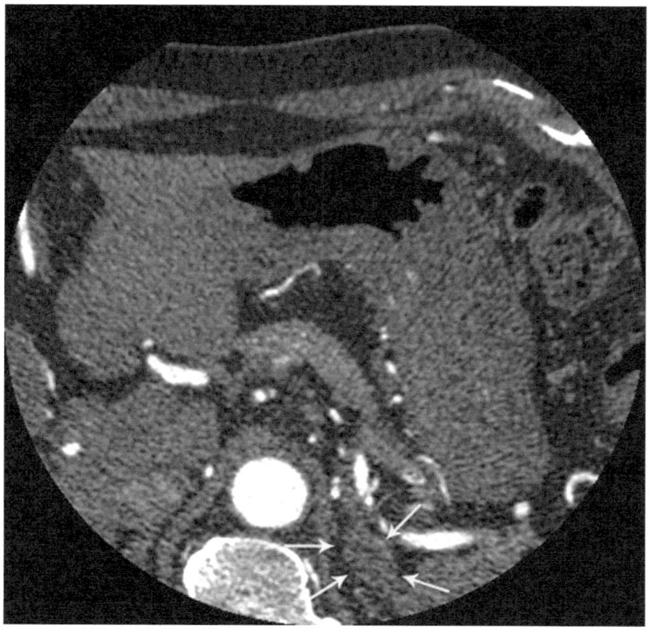

Fig. 50.9 Nonspecific left adrenal nodule in a 50-year-old male patient. Nonspecific left adrenal nodule (arrows) measuring approximately 10 mm is noted on a small field of view image at the level of adrenal gland. In this instance, the characteristic washout pattern is helpful to discriminate an adenoma from malignant lesion. Greater than 40% washout on a 15 min delayed CT image indicates an adenoma

Conclusion

Many important extracardiac findings are demonstrated even on the small field of view image of coronary CTA. Thus, interpreting physicians irrespective of specialty should be familiar with various important extracardiac findings. In the acute chest pain setting, additional reconstructions and analysis with a wide field of view may be valuable to identify an alternative cause of chest pain. For patients with stable angina, a small field of view image on coronary CTA may be acceptable to evaluate extracardiac findings.

References

1. Taylor AJ, Cerqueira M, Hodgson JM, Mark D, Min J, O'Gara P, Rubin GD, American College of Cardiology Foundation Appropriate Use Criteria Task Force; Society of Cardiovascular Computed Tomography; American College of Radiology; American Heart Association; American Society of Echocardiography; American Society of Nuclear Cardiology; North American Society for Cardiovascular Imaging; Society for Cardiovascular Angiography and Interventions; Society for Cardiovascular Magnetic Resonance, Kramer CM, Berman D, Brown A, Chaudhry FA, Cury RC, Desai MY, Einstein AJ, Gomes AS, Harrington R, Hoffmann U, Khare R, Lesser J, McGann C, Rosenberg A, Schwartz R, Shelton M, Smetana GW, Smith SC Jr. ACCF/SCCT/ACR/AHA/ASE/ASNC/NASCI/SCAI/SCMR 2010 appropriate use criteria for cardiac computed tomography. A report of the American college of cardiology foundation appropriate use criteria task force, the society of cardiovascular computed tomography, the American college of radiology, the American heart association, the American society of echocardiography, the American society of nuclear cardiology, the north American society for cardiovascular imaging, the society for cardiovascular angiography and interventions, and the society for cardiovascular magnetic resonance. J Am Coll Cardiol. 2010;56(22):1864–94.
2. Kim HR, Yoo SM, Rho JY, Lee HY, White CS. MDCT evaluation of atherosclerotic coronary artery disease: what should radiologists know? Int J Cardiovasc Imaging. 2014;30(Suppl 1):1–11.
3. Johnson KM, Dennis JM, Dowe DA. Extracardiac findings on coronary CT angiograms: Limited versus complete image review. AJR Am J Roentgenol. 2010;195(1):143–8.
4. Onuma Y, Tanabe K, Nakazawa G, Aoki J, Nakajima H, Ibukuro K, Hara K. Noncardiac findings in cardiac imaging with multidetector computed tomography. J Am Coll Cardiol. 2006;48:402–6.
5. Hunold P, Schmermund A, Seibel RM, Grönemeyer DH, Erbel R. Prevalence and clinical significance of accidental findings in electron-beam tomographic scans for coronary artery calcification. Eur Heart J. 2001;22(18):1748–58.
6. Horton KM, Post WS, Blumenthal RS, Fishman EK. Prevalence of significant noncardiac findings on electron-beam computed tomography coronary artery calcium screening examinations. Circulation. 2002;106(5):532–4.
7. Schragin JG, Weissfeld JL, Edmundowicz D, Strollo DC, Fuhrman CR. Non-cardiac findings on coronary electron beam computed tomography scanning. J Thorac Imaging. 2004;19(2):82–6.
8. Dewey M, Schnapauff D, Teige F, Hamm B. Non-cardiac findings on coronary computed tomography and magnetic resonance imaging. Eur Radiol. 2007;17(8):2038–43.
9. Kirsch J, Araoz PA, Steinberg FB, Fletcher JG, McCollough CH, Williamson EE. Prevalence and significance of incidental extracardiac findings at 64-multidetector coronary CTA. J Thorac Imaging. 2007;22(4):330–4.
10. Kawano Y, Tamura A, Goto Y, Shinozaki K, Zaizen H, Kadota J. Incidental detection of cancers and other non-cardiac abnormalities on coronary multislice computed tomography. Am J Cardiol. 2007;99(11):1608–9.
11. Northam M, Koonce J, Ravenel JG. Pulmonary nodules detected at cardiac CT: comparison of images in limited and full fields of view. AJR Am J Roentgenol. 2008;191(3):878–81.

12. Kim JW, Kang EY, Yong HS, Kim YK, Woo OH, Oh YW, Lee KY, Han H. Incidental extracardiac findings at cardiac CT angiography: comparison of prevalence and clinical significance between precontrast low-dose whole thoracic scan and postcontrast retrospective ECG-gated cardiac scan. Int J Cardiovasc Imaging. 2009;25(Suppl 1):75–81.
13. Lehman SJ, Abbara S, Cury RC, Nagurney JT, Hsu J, Goela A, Schlett CL, Dodd JD, Brady TJ, Bamberg F, Hoffmann U. Significance of cardiac computed tomography incidental findings in acute chest pain. Am J Med. 2009;122(6):543–9.
14. Machaalany J, Yam Y, Ruddy TD, Abraham A, Chen L, Beanlands RS, Chow BJ. Potential clinical and economic consequences of noncardiac incidental findings on cardiac computed tomography. J Am Coll Cardiol. 2009;54(16):1533–41.
15. Haller S, Kaiser C, Buser P, Bongartz G, Bremerich J. Coronary artery imaging with contrast-enhanced MDCT: extracardiac findings. AJR Am J Roentgenol. 2006;187(1):105–10.
16. Lee CI, Tsai EB, Sigal BM, Plevritis SK, Garber AM, Rubin GD. Incidental extracardiac findings at coronary CT: clinical and economic impact. AJR Am J Roentgenol. 2010;194(6):1531–8.
17. Kim TJ, Han DH, Jin KN, Won Lee K. Lung cancer detected at cardiac CT: prevalence, clinicoradiologic features, and importance of full-field-of-view images. Radiology. 2010;255(2):369–76.
18. Earls JP. The pros and cons of searching for extracardiac findings at cardiac CT: studies should be reconstructed in the maximum field of view and adequately reviewed to detect pathologic findings. Radiology. 2011;261(2):342–6.
19. Budoff MJ, Fischer H, Gopal A. Incidental findings with cardiac CT evaluation: should we read beyond the heart? Catheter Cardiovasc Interv. 2006;68(6):965–73.
20. Budoff MJ, Gopal A. Incidental findings on cardiac computed tomography. Should we look? J Cardiovasc Comput Tomogr. 2007;1(2):97–105.
21. Iribarren C, Hlatky MA, Chandra M, Fair JM, Rubin GD, Go AS, Burt JR, Fortmann SP. Incidental pulmonary nodules on cardiac computed tomography: prognosis and use. Am J Med. 2008;121(11):989–96.
22. Hlatky MA, Iribarren C. The dilemma of incidental findings on cardiac computed tomography. J Am Coll Cardiol. 2009;54(16):1542–3.
23. Sosnouski D, Bonsall RP, Mayer FB, Ravenel JG. Extracardiac findings at cardiac CT: a practical approach. J Thorac Imaging. 2007;22(1):77–85.
24. Douglas PS, Cerqueria M, Rubin GD, Chin AS. Extracardiac findings: what is a cardiologist to do? JACC Cardiovasc Imaging. 2008;1(5):682–7.
25. Greenberg-Wolff I, Uliel L, Goitein O, Shemesh J, Rozenman J, Di Segni E, Konen E. Extra-cardiac findings on coronary computed tomography scanning. Isr Med Assoc J. 2008;10(11):806–8.
26. Yiginer O, Bas S, Pocan S, Yildiz A, Alibek S. Incidental findings of cardiac MSCT: who might benefit from scanning the entire thorax on Ca score imaging? Int J Cardiol. 2010;140(2):239–41.
27. Rumberger JA. Noncardiac abnormalities in diagnostic cardiac computed tomography: within normal limits or we never looked! J Am Coll Cardiol. 2006;48(2):407–8.
28. Colletti PM. Incidental findings on cardiac imaging. AJR Am J Roentgenol. 2008;191(3):882–4.
29. White CS. The pros and cons of searching for extracardiac findings at cardiac CT: use of a restricted field of view is acceptable. Radiology. 2011;261(2):338–41.
30. National Lung Screening Trial Research Team, Aberle DR, Berg CD, Black WC, Church TR, Fagerstrom RM, Galen B, Gareen IF, Gatsonis C, Goldin J, Gohagan JK, Hillman B, Jaffe C, Kramer BS, Lynch D, Marcus PM, Schnall M, Sullivan DC, Sullivan D, Zylak CJ. The national lung screening trial: overview and study design. Radiology. 2011;258(1):243–53.
31. Takakuwa KM, Halpern EJ. Evaluation of a "triple rule-out" coronary CT angiography protocol: use of 64-Section CT in low-to-moderate risk emergency department patients suspected of having acute coronary syndrome. Radiology. 2008;248(2):438–46.
32. Fantauzzi J, MacArthur A, Lu M, Jeudy J, White CS. Quantitative assessment of percentage of lung parenchyma visualized on cardiac computed tomographic angiography. J Comput Assist Tomogr. 2010;34(3):385–7.
33. Teague SD, Rissing S, Mahenthiran J, Achenbach S. Learning to interpret the extracardiac findings on coronary CT angiography examinations. J Cardiovasc Comput Tomogr. 2012;6(4):232–45.
34. Naidich DP, Bankier AA, MacMahon H, Schaefer-Prokop CM, Pistolesi M, Goo JM, Macchiarini P, Crapo JD, Herold CJ, Austin JH, Travis WD. Recommendations for the management of subsolid pulmonary nodules detected at CT: a statement from the Fleischner society. Radiology. 2013;266(1):304–17.
35. Mitchell DG, Bruix J, Sherman M, Sirlin CB. LI-RADS (Liver Imaging Reporting and Data System): summary, discussion, and consensus of the LI-RADS management working group and future directions. Hepatology. 2015;61(3):1056–65.

Part XII

Where We Are: The Bigger Picture

Prognosis and Outcome: State of the Evidence

51

Asim Rizvi, Hadi Mirhedayati Roudsari, James K. Min, and Fay Y. Lin

Coronary artery disease (CAD) remains the leading cause of mortality in the developed world despite improvements in diagnostic modalities and therapies targeted at reducing disease burden. The recent advent of coronary computed tomography angiography (CCTA) has gained interest as a promising noninvasive anatomic alternative to stress imaging techniques for diagnosis of anatomically obstructive CAD. CCTA has demonstrated high diagnostic accuracy for obstructive CAD, with a sensitivity, specificity, positive predictive value (PPV), and negative predictive value (NPV) of 95%, 83%, 64%, and 99%, respectively, compared to invasive coronary angiography (ICA) for >50% stenosis in the ACCURACY (Assessment by Coronary Computed Tomographic Angiography of Individuals Undergoing Invasive Coronary Angiography) study and of 99%, 89%, 93%, and 100%, respectively, in the meta-analyses [1, 2]. More recently, the PROMISE (PROspective Multicenter Imaging Study for Evaluation of chest pain) study showed that CCTA is a safe strategy for initial evaluation of CAD and demonstrated similar downstream major adverse cardiovascular events (MACE) with reduced risk of myocardial infarction (MI) or all-cause mortality (ACM) in comparison to stress imaging techniques (hazard ratio [HR], 0.66; 95% CI 0.44–1.00; $p = 0.049$) [3].

Currently, scientific guidelines recommend the appropriate use of CCTA for diagnosis of CAD in different patient populations [4–6]. However, the prognostic value of CCTA and the impact of CCTA on downstream outcomes are important for patient risk stratification and management. The purpose of this chapter is to discuss the current literature using CCTA as a prognostic tool.

A. Rizvi (✉)
Department of Radiology, Dalio Institute of Cardiovascular Imaging, NewYork-Presbyterian Hospital and the Weill Cornell Medical College, New York, NY, USA

Department of Radiology, Mayo Clinic, Rochester, MN, USA
e-mail: drasimrizvi@gmail.com; rizvi.asim@mayo.edu

H. M. Roudsari · J. K. Min · F. Y. Lin
Department of Radiology, NewYork-Presbyterian Hospital and the Weill Cornell Medical College, New York, NY, USA

Prognostic Significance of CCTA for All-Cause Mortality

CCTA-evaluated CAD has demonstrated incremental prognostic value in chronic stable outpatients for ACM (Table 51.1). The earliest data from Min et al. determined the prognostic value of 16-detector row CCTA for ACM in 1127 patients without known CAD [7]. After a 15-month follow-up, the number of vessels affected by moderate or severe stenosis as well as proximal left anterior descending artery stenosis demonstrated independent predictive value above and beyond clinical risk factors (all $p < 0.001$). Survival decreased with higher Duke scores, with 96% survival for 2 moderate stenoses or 1 severe stenosis ($p < 0.013$) and 85% survival for moderate left main coronary artery stenosis ($p < 0.001$), respectively (Fig. 51.1). Notably, authors concluded that a negative CCTA for CAD confers significantly decreased risk of ACM compared to the remainder of the population (0.3% vs. 4.8%; HR 0.12, 95% confidence interval [CI] 0.02–0.89) [7]. This study was followed up with a large ($n = 5330$), multicenter cohort utilizing 64-detector row CCTA in patients without known CAD [8]. Over a period of 2.3 years, the HR for ACM in patients with obstructive CAD (≥70% stenosis) was 2.44 (95% CI 1.61–3.72, $p < 0.001$). Risk increased with each additional diseased vessel, with an HR of 2.23, 3.29, and 7.35 for 1-, 2-, and 3-vessel diseases, respectively (all $p < 0.001$). Additionally, CCTA evaluation of left ventricular ejection fraction (LVEF) improved prediction of ACM above and beyond CCTA measures of obstructive CAD, with worse outcomes for LVEF ≤50% (adjusted HR [aHR] 1.56, 95% CI 1.04–2.36, $p = 0.03$) [8].

CCTA also demonstrates high diagnostic accuracy for nonobstructive plaque, which has prognostic significance as well [9, 10]. Ostrom et al. examined ACM after 64-detector row CCTA in 2538 symptomatic patients without known CAD over 78 ± 12 months [11]. The survival rates for patients with 1-, 2-, and 3-vessel nonobstructive (<50% stenosis) CAD versus obstructive (≥50% stenosis) CAD were reported as 97.3%, 95%, and 93.1% versus 92.9%, 89.7%, and 80%, respectively (Fig. 51.2). The risk-adjusted HR for

U. J. Schoepf (ed.), *CT of the Heart*, Contemporary Medical Imaging, https://doi.org/10.1007/978-1-60327-237-7_51

Table 51.1 Studies evaluating the prognostic significance of coronary computed tomographic angiography for predicting all-cause mortality and major adverse cardiovascular events

Author	Year	Patients (*n*)	Follow-up	Study design	Outcomes	Population
Min et al. [7]	2007	1127	15 ± 4 months	Retrospective	ACM	Patients with chest pain syndrome
Pundziute et al. [13]	2007	100	16 months	Prospective	Cardiac death, nonfatal MI, UA, revascularization	Patients with known or suspected CAD
Ostrom et al. [11]	2008	5538	78 ± 12 months	Retrospective	ACM	Patients with chest pain syndrome
Gaemperli et al. [14]	2008	220	14 ± 4 months	Retrospective	ACM, MI, UA, revascularization	Patients without known CAD
Carrigan et al. [16]	2009	227	2 ± 1 years	Retrospective	Cardiac death, nonfatal MI, revascularization	Patients with suspected CAD
Hadamitzky et al. [73]	2009	1150	18 months	–	Cardiac death, MI, UA, revascularization	Patients with suspected CAD
Gopal et al. [18]	2009	454	40 ± 9 months	Prospective	Cardiac death, MI	Patients with suspected CAD
Abidov et al. [19]	2009	199	2 years	Prospective	Cardiac death, MI, UA, revascularization.	Patients with suspected CAD and inconclusive stress tests
Rubinshtein et al. [17]	2009	545	18 ± 6 months	Prospective	Cardiac death, MI, revascularization	Patients with suspected CAD
Motoyama et al. [67]	2009	1059	27 ± 10 months	–	Acute coronary syndrome	Patients with suspected or known CAD
Aldrovandi et al. [15]	2009	187	24 months	Prospective	Cardiac death, nonfatal MI, UA, revascularization	Patients with suspected MI
Chow et al. [21]	2010	2076	16 ± 8 months	Prospective	Cardiac death, MI	Patients with known or suspected CAD
Min et al. [20]	2010	172	22 ± 5 months	Prospective	Cardiac death, MI, UA, revascularization	Patients with known or suspected CAD
Min et al. [8]	2010	5330	2 ± 1 years	Retrospective	ACM	Patients without known CAD
Lin et al. [12]	2011	2583	3 ± 1 years	Prospective	ACM	Patients without known CAD
Kristensen et al. [22]	2011	312	16 months	Prospective	Cardiac death, MI, UA, revascularization	Patients with NSTEMI
Beigel et al. [74]	2013	959	27 months	Prospective	ACM, UA, revascularization	Patients with chest pain syndrome
Dougoud et al. [28]	2014	218	6.9 years	Prospective	Cardiac death, nonfatal MI, UA, revascularization	Patients with suspected CAD

Abbreviations: *ACM* all-cause mortality, *MI* myocardial infarction, *UA* unstable angina, *CAD* coronary artery disease

3-vessel nonobstructive CAD was elevated at 1.7 (95% CI 1.49–2.05), as were those for 1-, 2-, and 3-vessel obstructive CAD at 1.8 (95% CI 1.4–2.51), 2.3 (95% CI 1.91–2.93), and 2.6 (95% CI 2–3.37), respectively ($p < 0.001$ for all). These findings revealed that CCTA-diagnosed CAD was able to predict ACM in symptomatic patients irrespective of age, sex, and conventional risk factors [11]. Lin et al. also evaluated the independent predictive value of nonobstructive CAD diagnosed by 64-detector row CCTA in a multicenter cohort of 2583 patients without prior CAD over 3.1 ± 0.5 years [12]. An adjusted HR of 1.98 (95% CI 1.06–3.69, $p = 0.03$) was observed for the presence of nonobstructive CAD overall, with the highest risk seen among patients with 3-vessel nonobstructive CAD (HR 4.75, 95% CI 2.10–10.75, $p < 0.001$) or those with nonobstructive CAD affecting ≥5 segments (HR 5.12, 95% CI 2.16–12.10, $p < 0.001$). Moreover, the presence of nonobstructive plaque was associated with higher risk of mortality even among patients with <10% Framingham-estimated 10-year risk (3.4% over 3 years, log-rank $p < 0.001$) and among patients with no medically treatable CAD risk factors, including diabetes, dyslipidemia, and hypertension (6.7% over 3 years, log-rank $p < 0.001$), with annualized mortality rates that would reclassify these supposedly low-risk patients [12]. Thus, the identification of nonobstructive and obstructive CAD by CCTA both portend elevated mortality above and beyond CAD risk factors and traditional risk scores.

Prognostic Significance of CCTA for Major Adverse Cardiovascular Events

CCTA risk stratification for MACE is also well demonstrated by study investigators (Table 51.1) [13–22]. The earliest data on MACE was reported by Pundziute and colleagues [13]. Over a mean follow-up of 16 months, 100

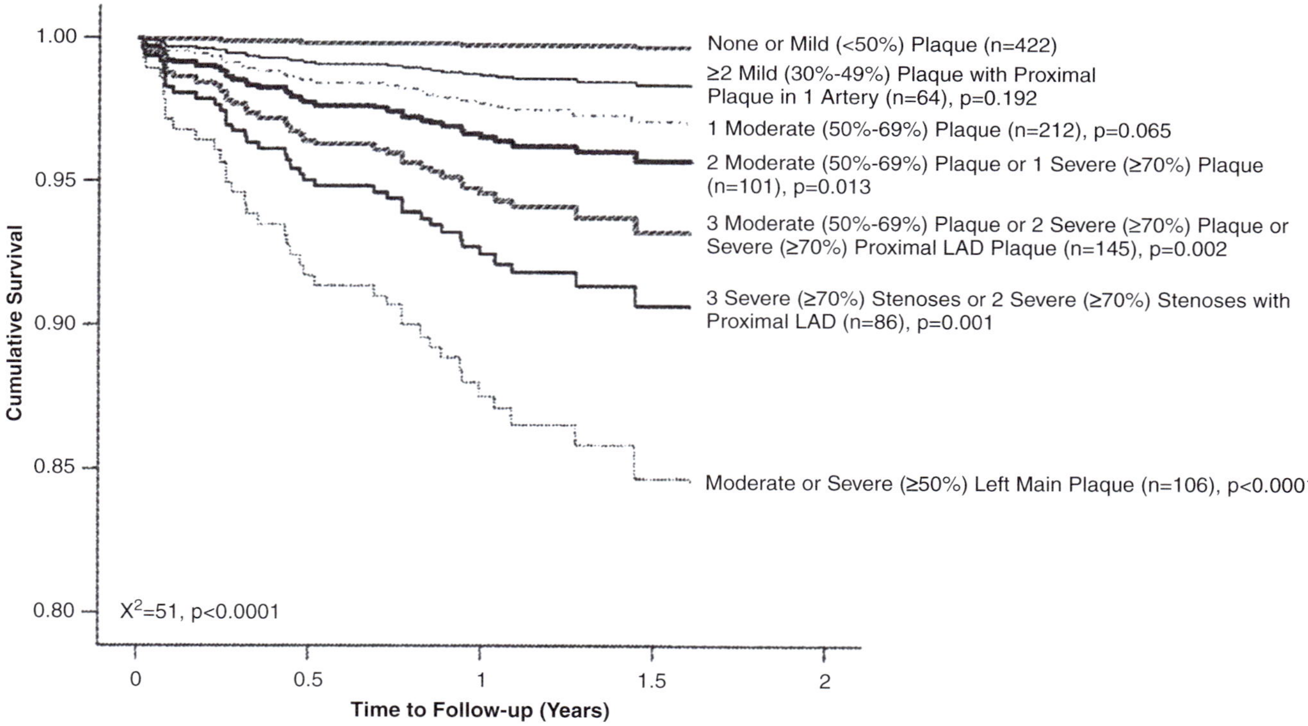

Fig. 51.1 Cumulative survival in patients exhibiting coronary plaque by the Duke prognostic coronary artery disease index. Risk-adjusted $p < 0.001$ (adjusted for age, family history, and dyslipidemia). *LAD* left anterior descending artery. (From Min et al. [7], with permission)

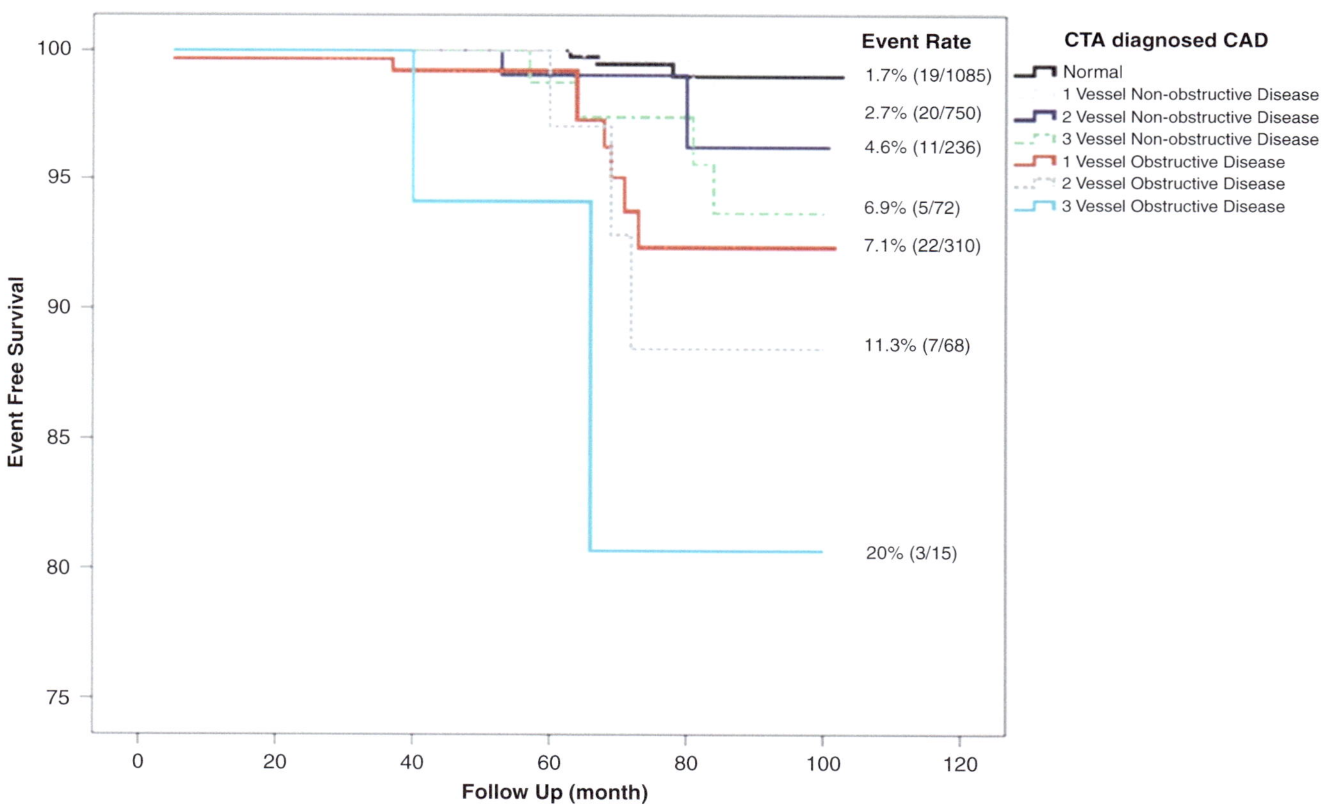

Fig. 51.2 Risk-adjusted event-free survival by CCTA-diagnosed CAD stratified by severity of disease and number of diseased coronary arteries. Risk adjustment for age, gender, hypercholesterolemia, diabetes mellitus, smoking, hypertension, family history of premature CAD, and coronary artery calcium score. All-cause mortality increased significantly by increasing severity of CCTA-diagnosed CAD and number of diseased coronary arteries. *CCTA* coronary computed tomographic angiography, *CAD* coronary artery disease. (From Ostrom et al. [11], with permission)

symptomatic patients with known or suspected CAD were observed for MACE defined as cardiac death, unstable angina, nonfatal MI, and revascularization. Patients without CAD had an excellent prognosis compared to patients with any evidence of CAD, with reported first-year event rates of 0% and 30%, respectively (log-rank $p < 0.005$). The greatest risk of MACE was seen in patients with any coronary plaque (aHR 8.8; 95% CI 1.1–70), obstructive CAD (aHR 28; 95% CI 3.3–239), and left main or left coronary artery disease (aHR 35; 95% CI 4.3–288) ($p < 0.05$ for all). In aggregate, a CCTA showing no evidence of CAD could assure a high negative predictive value for MACE, with a dose effect evident for increasing extent and severity of CCTA-visualized CAD [13].

Most notably, the CONFIRM (The Coronary CT Angiography EvaluatioN For clinical Outcomes: An InterRnational Multicenter) registry has provided important data regarding the incremental prognostic significance of CCTA [23]. Using CONFIRM data, Leipsic and colleagues evaluated the risk of MACE in 5262 patients with suspected CAD but without medically modifiable CAD risk factors [24]. Over a mean follow-up of 2.3 ± 1.2 years, increased risk of MACE was observed in patients with obstructive CAD (risk-adjusted HR 6.64; 95% CI 3.68–12.00; $p \leq 0.001$). Furthermore, there was a dose-response relationship between the number of obstructed vessels and the risk of MACE, with the greatest hazard seen in patients with 3-vessel obstructive CAD or left main CAD (HR 11.69; 95% CI 5.38, 25.4; $p \leq 0.001$). Notably, an extremely low incidence of MACE was reported in patients without any evidence of CAD on CCTA as compared with those with obstructive CAD (0.31% versus 2.06%) [24]. Further still, the CONFIRM investigators demonstrated the prognostic value of CCTA findings with long-term follow-up. Cheruvu et al. followed 1884 patients without CAD for the outcomes of ACM and MACE [25]. Over a mean follow-up of 5.6 ± 1.3 years, the risk of ACM increased with the severity of CAD and the number of diseased vessels, with the highest risk seen in those with 3-vessel or left main obstructive (>50% stenosis) CAD (HR: 2.87; 95% CI 1.57–5.23; $p = 0.001$). During the same follow-up duration, an increased risk of MACE was observed in patients with obstructive CAD (HR 6.63; 95% CI 3.91–11.26; $p < 0.001$) as compared to those with nonobstructive CAD (HR: 2.20; 95% CI 1.31–3.67; $p = 0.003$). The incidence of MACE in patients with no CAD was reported as 5.6% as compared to 13.24% and 36.28% in patients with nonobstructive and obstructive CAD, respectively ($p < 0.001$) [25].

In addition, the prognostic value of CCTA for MACE has been confirmed in meta-analyses [26, 27]. One meta-analysis of 28 studies by Habib et al. comprised of 41,690 individuals with an average of 1.96 years of follow-up for a composite outcome of ACM, cardiac death, MI, unstable angina, or revascularization [27]. Patients with obstructive CAD and nonobstructive CAD had increased odds of cardiac death or MI with demonstrated odds ratios (OR) of 14.92 (95% CI 6.78–32.85) and 6.41 (95% CI 2.44–16.8), respectively, when compared with those with no CAD [27].

In a recent small study ($n = 218$) with a longer follow-up duration of 6.9 years, Dougoud et al. found annual event rates for composite MACE (mortality, nonfatal MI, and late revascularization) in patients with obstructive CAD (≥50%), nonobstructive CAD (<50%), and normal coronary arteries on CCTA to be 6.0%, 2.7%, and 0.3%, respectively (log-rank $p = 0.001$) [28]. Thus, the prognostic value of the presence or absence of CAD detected by CCTA is durable and incremental to clinical risk factors alone.

The Confirm Registry

The CONFIRM registry is a large, prospective, dynamic observational study and represents 27,125 consecutive patients who have undergone ≥64-detector row CCTA [23]. The study design and methods have been described elsewhere [23]. The primary objective of this study is to assess the prognostic significance of CCTA for the prediction of future adverse CAD events including ACM, MI, unstable angina (UA), target vessel revascularization, and CAD-related hospitalization [23]. The scale of the CONFIRM registry has allowed detailed examination of the prognostic value of CCTA in multiple patient subgroups.

Prognostic Significance of CCTA by Age and Gender

The ability of CCTA to risk stratify younger and older men and women is fundamental to guide the appropriate application of CCTA across diverse populations. To that end, Min and colleagues examined 24,775 patients without known CAD for age- and sex-specific outcomes utilizing the CONFIRM registry [29]. Over 2.3 years of follow-up, the risk of ACM was significantly higher in younger patients with CAD (<65 years) compared to older patients with CAD (≥65 years), with an adjusted HR of 4.00 versus 2.46 for 2-vessel CAD and 6.19 versus 3.10 for 3-vessel CAD ($p < 0.001$ for both) (Fig. 51.3). Moreover, gender-specific risk stratification revealed that women had increased risk of ACM compared to men for 3-vessel CAD, with an adjusted HR of 4.21 versus 3.27 ($p < 0.001$ for all) (Figure 51.4) [29].

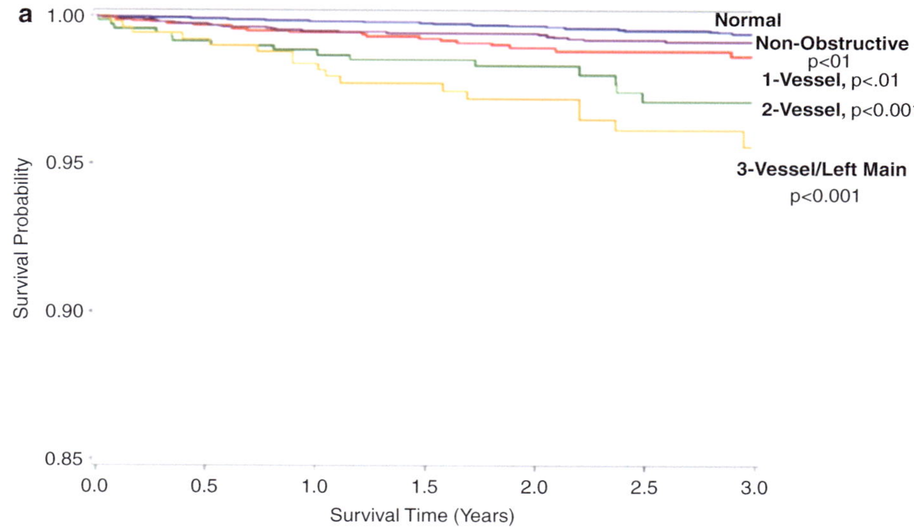

At Risk	Year 0	Year 1	Year 2	Year 3
Normal	8646	8010	4693	2474
Non-Obstructive	5103	4717	2606	1287
1-Vessel	1807	1693	1049	481
2-Vessel	692	640	419	180
3-Vessel/Left Main	501	466	306	151

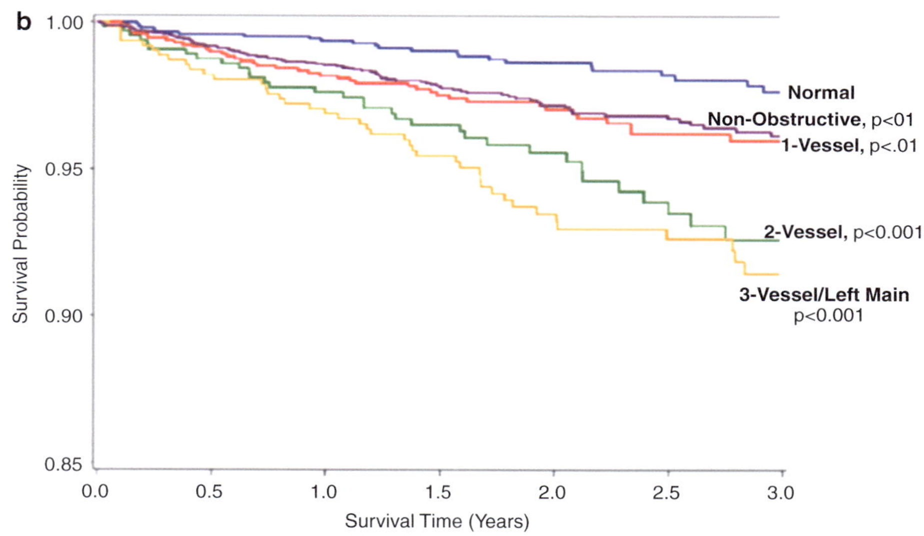

At Risk	Year 0	Year 1	Year 2	Year 3
Normal	1500	1347	837	433
Non-Obstructive	3011	2720	1475	643
1-Vessel	1311	1180	698	301
2-Vessel	654	588	323	144
3-Vessel/Left Main	629	568	358	173

Fig. 51.3 Unadjusted all-cause 3-year Kaplan-Meier survival by presence, extent, and severity of CAD by CCTA as stratified by age <65 or ≥65 years. Although rates of mortality in relationship to CAD extent are lower in patients age <65 years (**a**), patients age <65 years with 2- and 3-vessel CAD experience a higher relative rate of mortality referenced to patients age <65 years with no CAD in comparison with patients age ≥65 years with 2- and 3-vessel CAD referenced to patients age ≥65 years with no CAD (**b**). *CAD* coronary artery disease, *CCTA* coronary computed tomographic angiography. (From Min et al. [29], with permission)

Prognostic Significance of CCTA Based on Ethnic Differences

Prior studies have reported that the epidemiology, pathology, and prognosis of CAD may vary across different ethnicities [30–34]. Using data from CONFIRM registry, Hulten and colleagues evaluated the prognostic significance of CCTA in a total of 16,451 patients among three subgroups of Caucasian, East Asian, and African ethnicities [35]. When comparing patients with obstructive CAD and those with nonobstructive CAD, the annual incidence of death or MI was 2.2% versus 0.7% among Caucasians (aHR 2.77, 95%

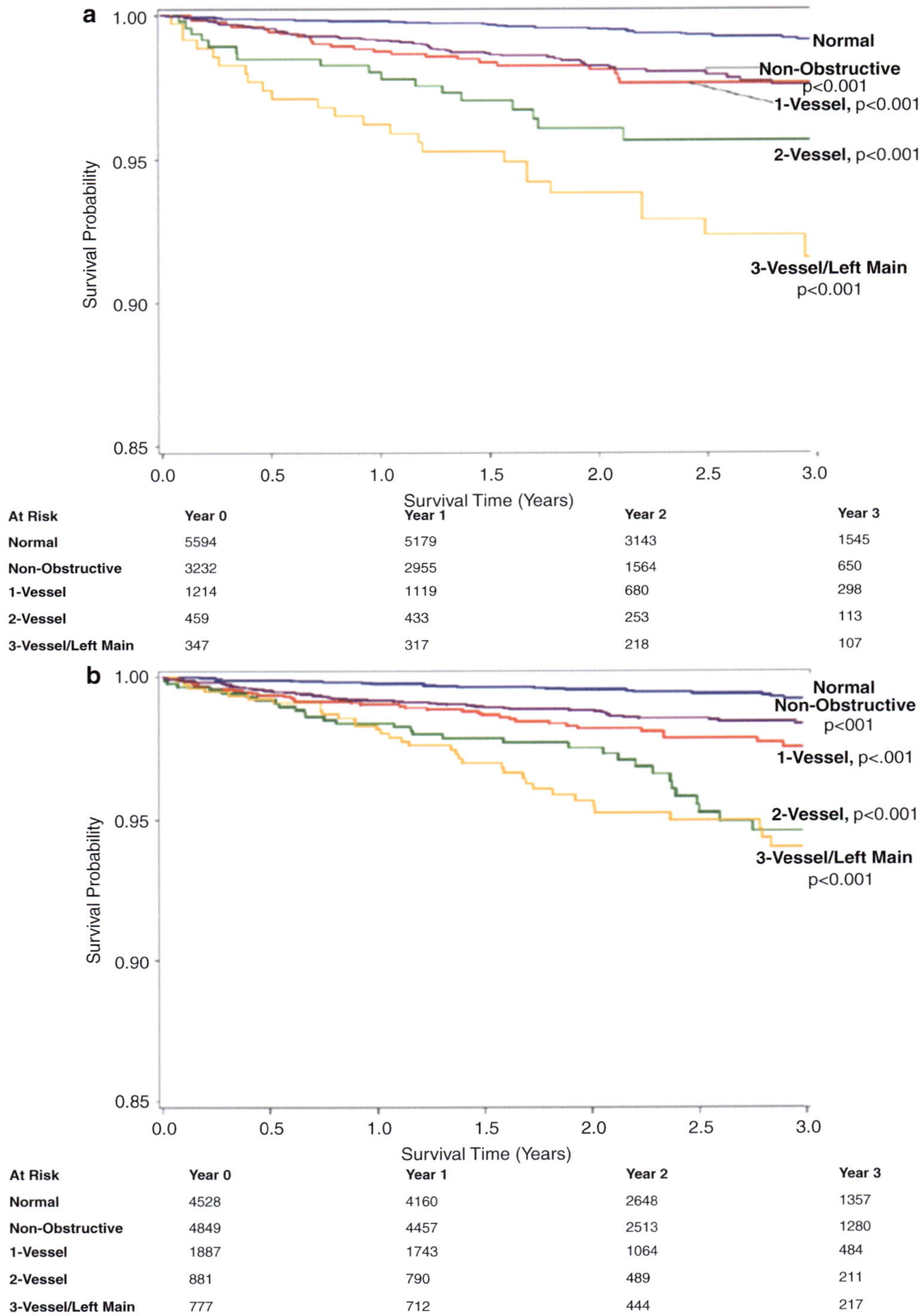

Fig. 51.4 Unadjusted all-cause 3-year Kaplan-Meier Survival by presence, extent, and severity of CAD by CCTA as stratified by Sex. Although rates of mortality in relationship to CAD extent are lower in women, women with 3-vessel CAD experience a higher relative rate of mortality referenced to women with no CAD (**a**) in comparison with men with 3-vessel CAD referenced to men with no CAD (**b**). *CAD* coronary artery disease, *CCTA* coronary computed tomographic angiography. (From Min et al. [29], with permission)

CI 1.73–4.43, $p < 0.001$), 4.8% versus 1.1% among Africans (aHR 6.25, 95% CI 1.12–34.97, $p = 0.037$), and 0.8% versus 0.1% among East Asians (aHR 4.84, 95% CI 2.24–10.9, $p < 0.001$). Interestingly, East Asians had a lower risk of events (aHR 0.25, 95% CI 0.16–0.38, $p < 0.001$) when compared to Caucasians and Africans [35].

Prognostic Significance of CCTA Above and Beyond Coronary Artery Calcium Scoring

Coronary artery calcium (CAC) scoring derived from non-contrast CT has been shown to be a useful test for identifying atherosclerotic plaque burden. In patients without chest pain symptoms, the absence of CAC has been associated with a lower risk of future cardiovascular adverse events. However, the relationship between CAC scoring and CCTA for prognostication was uncertain prior to investigations within the CONFIRM cohort. First, Villines and the CONFIRM investigators evaluated the prognostic value of CCTA in 10,037 symptomatic patients without coronary artery calcium without known CAD [36]. Over a median follow-up of 2.1 years, no difference was noted in the rate of ACM in patients with CAC scores of 0, despite the presence of obstructive CAD ($p = 0.7$). MACE occurred in 3.9% of patients with CAC scores of 0 and obstructive CAD (HR 5.7, 95% CI 2.5–13.1, $p < 0.001$) compared to 0.8% of patients with CAC scores of 0 and nonobstructive CAD. Further, CAC scoring in symptomatic patients did not provide incremental prognostic benefit for predicting MACE compared to clinical risk factors and CCTA alone ($p = 0.84$) [36]. Al-Mallah et al. examined the incremental prognostic value of CAC scoring and CCTA over clinical risk stratification in 8627 symptomatic patients without known CAD who were observed for MACE for a median follow-up duration of 25 months [37]. After adjusting for clinical risks, a CAC score >400 and detection of obstructive CAD by CCTA were found to be significant predictors of MACE (HR 4.8, 95% CI 2.9–8.1 versus HR 3.9; 95% CI 2.7–5.5, respectively, $p < 0.05$ for both). Furthermore, obstructive CAD detection by CCTA showed incremental prognostic value over clinical risk stratification and CAC scoring (C-statistics 0.82 vs. 0.79, $p = 0.002$) [37].

Cho et al. examined CCTA and CAC scoring in asymptomatic patients [38]. During a median follow-up of 2.5 years, patients with obstructive 2- and 3-vessel CAD or left main CAD had increased risk of ACM and MACE ($p < 0.05$ for both) compared to those without CAD. Both CAC scoring and CAD detection by CCTA improved performance over standard risk factors for predicting ACM and MACE (likelihood ratio $p < 0.05$ for all). However, incremental discriminatory ability was only shown for MACE. Net reclassification improvement (NRI) was not observed when CCTA was added to the risk factors plus CAC scoring model. Thus, among asymptomatic patients, CCTA is not useful for risk stratification beyond combined assessment by risk factors with CACS [38].

Prognostic Significance of CCTA in Diabetic Patients

People with diabetes mellitus (DM) demonstrate increased risk of CAD and display adverse outcomes after surviving a CAD event [39]. The study investigators therefore assessed the prevalence, extent, severity, and prognosis of CAD in DM and non-DM patients without known CAD who underwent CCTA [40].

In a recent investigation utilizing CONFIRM data, Blanke et al. evaluated the long-term prognostic value of CCTA among DM patients compared with non-DM individuals [41]. A total of 1823 DM patients were identified and propensity-matched to 1823 non-DM patients with 5-year follow-up. The presence of CAD on CCTA was graded as none (0%), nonobstructive (1–49%), or obstructive (≥50%) stenosis. The study reported that DM patients did not display increased risk of mortality compared with non-DM patients in the absence of CAD (aHR of DM 1.32, 95% CI 0.78–2.24, $p = 0.30$). However, DM patients did display heightened risk of mortality compared with non-DM patients when they had nonobstructive CAD (HR 2.10, 95% CI 1.43–3.09, $p < 0.001$). Notably, the mortality risk in this population was even higher than non-DM patients with obstructive disease ($p < 0.001$). The authors concluded that among DM patients, CCTA-assessed nonobstructive and obstructive CAD was associated with significantly increased risk of ACM and MACE at 5-year follow-up, when compared with non-DM patients [41].

Prognostic Significance of CCTA Based on CAD Severity and Left Ventricular Ejection Fraction

CCTA acquisition protocols that span systole can evaluate LVEF in addition to CAD severity. Utilizing data from the CONFIRM registry, Arsanjani and colleagues assessed the gradations of LVEF and volumes measured with CCTA among 7758 patients [42]. During a follow-up of 2.2 years, worse LVEF was independently associated with mortality for moderately reduced (<45% but ≥35%) and severely reduced (<35%) LVEF, with a demonstrated HR of 3.14 and 5.19, respectively ($p < 0.001$). Moreover, LVEF demonstrated improved discrimination for mortality [area under the receiver operating characteristic curve (AUC) = 0.816] when compared with CAD risk factors alone (AUC = 0.781) or CAD risk factors combined with CAD extent and severity (AUC = 0.799) ($p < 0.001$). The study concluded that left ventricular dysfunction improves risk prediction and discrimination for ACM [42].

Prognostic Significance of CCTA in Patients with Acute Chest Pain

Acute-onset chest pain is one of the most common presentations for patient visits to the emergency department (ED). Given the high sensitivity and NPV for the detection of coronary stenosis, CCTA may allow for timely diagnosis, improved risk stratification, and appropriate triage of patients, especially those with low to intermediate risk. Accordingly, numerous studies have evaluated the long-term outcome of patients with negative CCTAs who were discharged from the ED [43].

The CT-STAT (Coronary Computed Tomographic Angiography for Systematic Triage of Acute Chest Pain Patients to Treatment) was a multicenter trial that included 699 low-risk ED patients [44]. These prospectively enrolled patients were either randomly allocated to CCTA (n = 361) or to myocardial perfusion scintigraphy (MPS) (n = 338). The study investigators compared the efficiency, cost, and safety of CCTA in the evaluation of patients with acute chest pain and low risk of ACS. The primary outcome was time to diagnosis. The investigators also showed a cost reduction in patients randomized to CCTA. The study found that patients in the CCTA arm had a 54% reduction in time to diagnosis and 38% reduction in costs. Notably, there was no difference in MACE between the two study groups [44]. Further, the ACRIN-PA (American College of Radiology Imaging Network-Pennsylvania) study evaluated the safety (defined as the absence of MI or cardiac death during 30-day follow-up) of this CCTA strategy in low- to intermediate-risk patients who presented to the ED [45]. Of the 640 patients with negative CCTA, none of them died or had a MI within 30 days of presentation. In addition, early CCTA led to a shorter mean hospital stay (18 h versus 24.8 h) and an increased rate of ED discharge when compared to standard of care (50% versus 23%) [45].

ROMICAT (Rule Out Myocardial Infarction/Ischemia Using Computer Assisted Tomography) was a double-blind, prospective, observational study that demonstrated excellent sensitivity and NPV of CCTA to rule out ACS in 368 patients with inconclusive clinical evaluation of acute chest pain in the ED [46]. The subsequent ROMICAT II study followed 368 ED patients who presented with acute chest pain, negative initial troponin, and ECG findings for 2 years [47]. The investigators found that the cumulative probability of 2-year MACE significantly increased with CCTA-stratified CAD categories, with 0%, 5%, and 30% for no CAD, nonobstructive CAD, and obstructive CAD, respectively (log-rank $p < 0.001$). Adding evaluation of regional wall motion abnormalities (RWMA) improved risk stratification, with 2-year MACE events of 0.9%, 15%, 10%, and 62% for no stenosis or RWMA, RWMA but no stenosis, stenosis but no RWMA, and both stenosis and RWMA, respectively (log-rank $p < 0.001$). The addition of CT stenosis beyond the clinical Thrombolysis In Myocardial Infarction (TIMI) risk score improved discrimination for predicting MACE (0.84 vs. 0.61, $p < 0.001$), and addition of RWMA further improved the prediction (0.91, $p < 0.001$) compared to combined TIMI risk score and CT stenosis alone [47].

In aggregate, these studies support the use of CCTA as an efficient, safe, and cost-effective alternative to the traditional triage methods for low- and low-to-intermediate-risk ED patients to exclude obstructive CAD as the etiology of chest pain while allowing for a faster ED discharge. Thus, the Society of Cardiovascular Computed Tomography (SCCT) recently published guidelines for the appropriate use of CCTA in the diagnosis of acute chest pain in patients with suspicion of ACS in the ED [48]. Utilizing CCTA in these patients may lead to increased downstream invasive coronary angiography (ICA) and coronary revascularization.

The ACCF/SCCT/ACR/AHA/ASE/ASNC/NASCI/SCAI/SCMR 2010 Appropriate Use Criteria for Cardiac Computed Tomography lists the use of CCTA as appropriate for "detection of CAD in symptomatic patients without known heart disease—acute symptoms with suspicion of ACS (urgent presentation) (Appropriate, score 7)" in patients with the following [49]:

- Normal ECG and cardiac biomarkers and low-intermediate pretest probability of CAD
- ECG uninterpretable and low-intermediate pretest probability of CAD
- Nondiagnostic ECG or equivocal cardiac biomarkers and low-intermediate pretest probability of CAD

In theory, a triple rule-out (TRO)-CT protocol is attractive for ED evaluation of chest pain because it may allow for exclusion of ACS, aortic dissection (AD), and pulmonary embolus (PE) in a single scan [50]. However, TRO-CT has potential disadvantages of increased radiation and contrast dose, higher imaging costs, and decreased image quality. Burris and colleagues compared the diagnostic yield of TRO-CT with CCTA for assessment of obstructive (>50% stenosis) CAD, AD, and PE in 12,834 patients with acute chest pain in the multicenter ACIC (Advanced Cardiovascular Imaging Consortium) registry [51, 52]. The overall diagnostic yield was similar for TRO-CT and CCTA (18.3% versus 17.4%, $p = 0.37$). TRO-CT demonstrated no additional yield for CAD detection as compared to CCTA (15.5% versus 17.2%, $p = 0.093$). TRO-CT exhibited slightly higher diagnostic yield compared to CCTA in the detection of AD (1.7 vs. 1.1%, $p = 0.046$) and PE (1.1 vs. 0.4%, $p = 0.004$), but the clinical magnitude was very small. Therefore, they concluded that there is no clear clinical benefit from routine use of TRO-CT in patients with acute chest pain [52].

Prognostic Significance of CCTA in Patients with Known CAD

Prior data have reported risk stratification of coronary artery bypass (CABG) patients utilizing ICA [53]. However, CCTA can risk stratify CABG patients noninvasively on the basis of native vessel anatomy and graft patency [54–57]. To date, limited data is available to assess the prognostic utility of CCTA in CABG patients.

In an investigation by Small et al., the authors evaluated ACM in 657 CABG patients from a multicenter registry of

10,628 patients who underwent CCTA, over 20 months of follow-up [58]. CAD severity was categorized by two models: unprotected coronary territories (UCT) representing the number of vessels with CAD and coronary artery protection score (CAPS) defined as a summary of native vessel disease and graft patency. In multivariate analysis, the UCT (HR 1.35, 95% CI 0.98–1.84, $p = 0.004$) and CAPS (HR 1.35, 95% CI 1.17–1.56, $p < 0.001$) were both independent predictors of ACM. Furthermore, CAPS improved discrimination and reclassification compared with clinical risk factors alone (C-statistics, 0.75 vs. 0.64, $p < 0.001$; NRI, 27.2%, $p = 0.003$), although UCT did not [58].

Prognostic Significance of CCTA Plaque Characteristics

Previous studies have shown that approximately 60% of high-risk plaques are not associated with anatomically significant stenosis [59, 60]. CCTA assessment of plaque characteristics may permit early identification of vulnerable plaque that would be missed by luminal evaluation alone [61–65]. Study investigators examined atherosclerotic plaque characteristics by CCTA in patients with ACS and stable angina, analyzing positive remodeling (PR), spotty calcification (SC), and consistency of non-calcified plaque (NCP <30 HU or 30 HU < NCP <150 HU) [66]. The study found that among CCTA assessment of culprit lesions in patients with ACS and stable angina, PR (87% vs. 12%), SC (63% vs. 21%), and NCP <30 HU (79% vs. 9%) were significantly more prevalent in ACS patients ($p < 0.001$ for all) [66]. In a subsequent investigation, Motoyama et al. evaluated two atherosclerotic plaque characteristics, PR and low attenuation plaque (LAP) detected by CCTA, for predicting acute coronary events in >1000 patients with established or suspected CAD who were followed for 27 ± 10 months [67]. Both features were found to be independent predictors of acute coronary events (HR 23, 95% CI 7–75, $p < 0.001$]. The authors reported that the likelihood of ACS in patients with 1- or 2-feature positive plaques was significantly higher compared to patients without these plaque features or patients with no plaques (22.2% vs. 3.7% vs. 0.5%, log-rank $p < 0.001$) (Fig. 51.5). Importantly, the plaques associated with early ACS had larger LAP volume when compared with those associated with late ACS [67]. In addition, Imazeki and colleagues demonstrated that remodeling detected on CCTA closely correlated with IVUS, and the remodeling index (RI) was significantly larger in patients with ACS (1.19 ± 0.18) than in those with stable angina (0.89 ± 0.10, $P < 0.001$) [68]. Further, in a ROMICAT II subanalysis, the presence of high-risk plaque (HRP) characteristics (PR, LAP, SC, and napkin-ring sign) was evaluated for prognosis of ACS in patients with acute chest pain [69]. The study findings

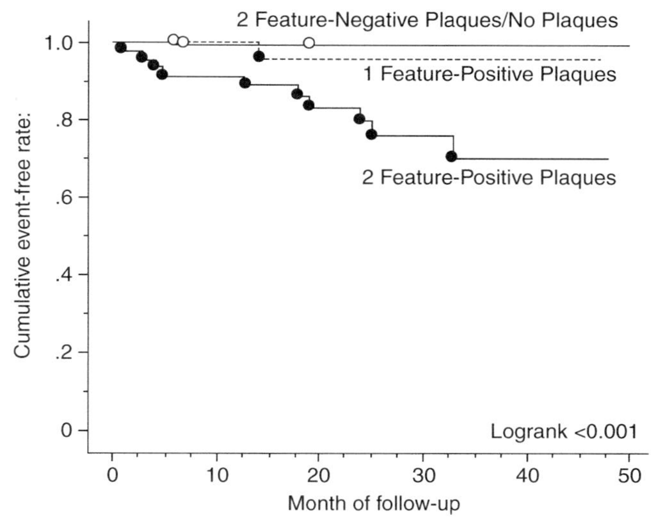

Fig. 51.5 Kaplan-Meier Curve for development of ACS on the basis of plaque characteristics. Patient stratification according to the presence of 2- and 1-feature positive and 2-feature negative plaques/no plaques. The y-axis represents cumulative event-free rate (log-rank $p < 0.001$). *ACS* acute coronary syndrome. (From Motoyama et al. [67], with permission)

showed that presence of HRP on CCTA was a significant predictor of ACS (OR 8.9, 95% CI 1.8–43.3, $p = 0.006$) after adjusting for a ≥50% coronary artery stenosis (OR 38.6, 95% CI 14.2–104.7, $p < 0.001$) [69].

These findings shed light on the prognostic power of CCTA beyond the detection of stenosis severity and highlight the importance of assessing non-stenotic coronary artery morphology and atherosclerotic plaque characteristics, which are difficult to evaluate through stress testing and ICA luminology alone.

Prognostic Significance of CCTA as Compared to Myocardial Perfusion Scintigraphy

As the prognostic value of myocardial perfusion scintigraphy (MPS) has been supported by a large body of literature, CCTA has often been compared to MPS for predictive value. In this regard, Shaw et al. propensity-matched 693 patients who underwent CCTA with 3067 patients who underwent MPS for evaluation of new-onset chest pain. The study found similar risk stratification by Duke prognostic CAD index by CCTA and by percentage of ischemic myocardium by MPS [70]. Van Werkhoven and colleagues evaluated the incremental prognostic significance of CCTA and MPS in 541 patients over a median of 672 days [71]. CCTA and MPS were found to be complementary, with an incremental predictive value of obstructive CAD by CCTA above and beyond MPS and baseline risk factors. The annualized event rate was 1.0% in patients with a normal CCTA and MPS, 3.7–3.8% in those with an abnormal CCTA or MPS, and 9.0% in those with both an abnormal CCTA and an abnormal MPS (log-rank $p < 0.005$) [71].

Downstream Outcomes After CCTA

PROMISE and SCOT-HEART (Scottish COmputed Tomography of the HEART) are two large trials that provide insight into the diagnosis, management, and outcomes in patients with stable angina [3, 72]. The PROMISE study compared the outcomes of CCTA and functional stress testing in 10,003 symptomatic patients without diagnosed CAD [3]. At a median follow-up of 25 months, there was no significant difference in the incidence of MACE for CCTA (3.3%) and functional-testing (3.0%) groups (aHR 1.04, 95% CI 0.83–1.29, $p = 0.75$). In addition, the CCTA group showed a reduced risk of death or nonfatal MI (HR 0.66, 95% CI 0.44–1.00, $p = 0.049$) compared to the functional-testing group. Despite an increased rate of ICA in the CCTA group compared with the functional-testing group (12.2% vs. 8.1%), there was a lower rate of ICA that showed no obstructive CAD within 90 days in the CCTA group (3.4% vs. 4.3%, $p = 0.02$). The study findings therefore revealed that CCTA was not associated with better clinical outcomes than functional testing in symptomatic patients with suspected CAD [3]. The SCOT-HEART trial assessed 4146 patients with stable angina by CCTA plus standard care or standard care alone [72]. In the CCTA group, an increased certainty of diagnosis of angina due to CAD was observed at 6 weeks (relative risk [RR] 1.79, 95% CI 1.62–1.96, $p < 0.001$). Furthermore, the CCTA group had a strong trend toward 38% reduction in cardiac death or nonfatal MI related to CAD at a median follow-up of 1.7 years (aHR 0.62, 95% CI 0.38–1.01, $p = 0.053$) [72].

Conclusion

CCTA provides vital prognostic information beyond its high diagnostic performance for CAD evaluation. A CCTA that detects no coronary plaque accurately predicts a very low rate of major adverse cardiovascular events. Major studies including the CONFIRM registry, the ROMICAT trial, the PROMISE study, and the SCOT-HEART study have provided a robust evidence base for risk prediction with CCTA in diverse populations for broad application to patient care.

References

1. Budoff MJ, Dowe D, Jollis JG, Gitter M, Sutherland J, Halamert E, Scherer M, Bellinger R, Martin A, Benton R, Delago A, Min JK. Diagnostic performance of 64-multidetector row coronary computed tomographic angiography for evaluation of coronary artery stenosis in individuals without known coronary artery disease: results from the prospective multicenter ACCURACY (Assessment by Coronary Computed Tomographic Angiography of Individuals Undergoing Invasive Coronary Angiography) trial. J Am Coll Cardiol. 2008;52:1724–32.
2. Mowatt G, Cook JA, Hillis GS, Walker S, Fraser C, Jia X, Waugh N. 64-slice computed tomography angiography in the diagnosis and assessment of coronary artery disease: systematic review and meta-analysis. Heart. 2008;94:1386–93.
3. Douglas PS, Hoffmann U, Patel MR, Mark DB, Al-Khalidi HR, Cavanaugh B, Cole J, Dolor RJ, Fordyce CB, Huang M, Khan MA, Kosinski AS, Krucoff MW, Malhotra V, Picard MH, Udelson JE, Velazquez EJ, Yow E, Cooper LS, Lee KL, Investigators P. Outcomes of anatomical versus functional testing for coronary artery disease. N Engl J Med. 2015;372:1291–300.
4. Taylor AJ, Cerqueira M, Hodgson JM, Mark D, Min J, O'Gara P, Rubin GD, American College of Cardiology Foundation Appropriate Use Criteria Task F, Society of Cardiovascular Computed T, American College of R, American Heart A, American Society of E, American Society of Nuclear C, North American Society for Cardiovascular I, Society for Cardiovascular A, Interventions, Society for Cardiovascular Magnetic R, Kramer CM, Berman D, Brown A, Chaudhry FA, Cury RC, Desai MY, Einstein AJ, Gomes AS, Harrington R, Hoffmann U, Khare R, Lesser J, McGann C, Rosenberg A, Schwartz R, Shelton M, Smetana GW, Smith SC Jr. ACCF/SCCT/ACR/AHA/ASE/ASNC/NASCI/SCAI/SCMR 2010 appropriate use criteria for cardiac computed tomography. A report of the American college of cardiology foundation appropriate use criteria task force, the society of cardiovascular computed tomography, the American college of radiology, the American heart association, the American society of echocardiography, the American society of nuclear cardiology, the north American society for cardiovascular imaging, the society for cardiovascular angiography and interventions, and the society for cardiovascular magnetic resonance. J Am Coll Cardiol. 2010;56:1864–94.
5. Abbara S, Arbab-Zadeh A, Callister TQ, Desai MY, Mamuya W, Thomson L, Weigold WG. SCCT guidelines for performance of coronary computed tomographic angiography: a report of the Society of Cardiovascular Computed Tomography Guidelines Committee. J Cardiovasc Comput Tomogr. 2009;3:190–204.
6. Raff GL, Abidov A, Achenbach S, Berman DS, Boxt LM, Budoff MJ, Cheng V, DeFrance T, Hellinger JC, Karlsberg RP, Society of Cardiovascular Computed T. SCCT guidelines for the interpretation and reporting of coronary computed tomographic angiography. J Cardiovasc Comput Tomogr. 2009;3:122–36.
7. Min JK, Shaw LJ, Devereux RB, Okin PM, Weinsaft JW, Russo DJ, Lippolis NJ, Berman DS, Callister TQ. Prognostic value of multidetector coronary computed tomographic angiography for prediction of all-cause mortality. J Am Coll Cardiol. 2007;50:1161–70.
8. Min JK, Lin FY, Dunning AM, Delago A, Egan J, Shaw LJ, Berman DS, Callister TQ. Incremental prognostic significance of left ventricular dysfunction to coronary artery disease detection by 64-detector row coronary computed tomographic angiography for the prediction of all-cause mortality: results from a two-centre study of 5330 patients. Eur Heart J. 2010;31:1212–9.
9. Pundziute G, Schuijf JD, Jukema JW, Decramer I, Sarno G, Vanhoenacker PK, Boersma E, Reiber JH, Schalij MJ, Wijns W, Bax JJ. Evaluation of plaque characteristics in acute coronary syndromes: non-invasive assessment with multi-slice computed tomography and invasive evaluation with intravascular ultrasound radiofrequency data analysis. Eur Heart J. 2008;29:2373–81.
10. Voros S, Rinehart S, Qian Z, Joshi P, Vazquez G, Fischer C, Belur P, Hulten E, Villines TC. Coronary atherosclerosis imaging by coronary CT angiography: current status, correlation with intravas-

cular interrogation and meta-analysis. JACC Cardiovasc Imaging. 2011;4:537–48.
11. Ostrom MP, Gopal A, Ahmadi N, Nasir K, Yang E, Kakadiaris I, Flores F, Mao SS, Budoff MJ. Mortality incidence and the severity of coronary atherosclerosis assessed by computed tomography angiography. J Am Coll Cardiol. 2008;52:1335–43.
12. Lin FY, Shaw LJ, Dunning AM, Labounty TM, Choi JH, Weinsaft JW, Koduru S, Gomez MJ, Delago AJ, Callister TQ, Berman DS, Min JK. Mortality risk in symptomatic patients with nonobstructive coronary artery disease: a prospective 2-center study of 2,583 patients undergoing 64-detector row coronary computed tomographic angiography. J Am Coll Cardiol. 2011;58:510–9.
13. Pundziute G, Schuijf JD, Jukema JW, Boersma E, de Roos A, van der Wall EE, Bax JJ. Prognostic value of multislice computed tomography coronary angiography in patients with known or suspected coronary artery disease. J Am Coll Cardiol. 2007;49:62–70.
14. Gaemperli O, Valenta I, Schepis T, Husmann L, Scheffel H, Desbiolles L, Leschka S, Alkadhi H, Kaufmann PA. Coronary 64-slice CT angiography predicts outcome in patients with known or suspected coronary artery disease. Eur Radiol. 2008;18:1162–73.
15. Aldrovandi A, Maffei E, Palumbo A, Seitun S, Martini C, Brambilla V, Zuccarelli A, Tarantini G, Weustink AC, Mollet NR, Ruffini L, Crisi G, Ardissino D, de Feyter PJ, Krestin GP, Cademartiri F. Prognostic value of computed tomography coronary angiography in patients with suspected coronary artery disease: a 24-month follow-up study. Eur Radiol. 2009;19:1653–60.
16. Carrigan TP, Nair D, Schoenhagen P, Curtin RJ, Popovic ZB, Halliburton S, Kuzmiak S, White RD, Flamm SD, Desai MY. Prognostic utility of 64-slice computed tomography in patients with suspected but no documented coronary artery disease. Eur Heart J. 2009;30:362–71.
17. Rubinshtein R, Halon DA, Gaspar T, Peled N, Lewis BS. Cardiac computed tomographic angiography for risk stratification and prediction of late cardiovascular outcome events in patients with a chest pain syndrome. Int J Cardiol. 2009;137:108–15.
18. Gopal A, Nasir K, Ahmadi N, Gul K, Tiano J, Flores M, Young E, Witteman AM, Holland TC, Flores F, Mao SS, Budoff MJ. Cardiac computed tomographic angiography in an outpatient setting: an analysis of clinical outcomes over a 40-month period. J Cardiovasc Comput Tomogr. 2009;3:90–5.
19. Abidov A, Gallagher MJ, Chinnaiyan KM, Mehta LS, Wegner JH, Raff GL. Clinical effectiveness of coronary computed tomographic angiography in the triage of patients to cardiac catheterization and revascularization after inconclusive stress testing: results of a 2-year prospective trial. J Nucl Cardiol. 2009;16:701–13.
20. Min JK, Feignoux J, Treutenaere J, Laperche T, Sablayrolles J. The prognostic value of multidetector coronary CT angiography for the prediction of major adverse cardiovascular events: a multicenter observational cohort study. Int J Cardiovasc Imaging. 2010;26:721–8.
21. Chow BJ, Wells GA, Chen L, Yam Y, Galiwango P, Abraham A, Sheth T, Dennie C, Beanlands RS, Ruddy TD. Prognostic value of 64-slice cardiac computed tomography severity of coronary artery disease, coronary atherosclerosis, and left ventricular ejection fraction. J Am Coll Cardiol. 2010;55:1017–28.
22. Kristensen TS, Kofoed KF, Kuhl JT, Nielsen WB, Nielsen MB, Kelbaek H. Prognostic implications of nonobstructive coronary plaques in patients with non-ST-segment elevation myocardial infarction: a multidetector computed tomography study. J Am Coll Cardiol. 2011;58:502–9.
23. Min JK, Dunning A, Lin FY, et al. Rationale and design of the CONFIRM (Coronary CT angiography evaluation for clinical outcomes: an international multicenter) registry. J Cardiovasc Comput Tomogr. 2011;5:84–92.
24. Leipsic J, Taylor CM, Grunau G, et al. Cardiovascular risk among stable individuals suspected of having coronary artery disease with no modifiable risk factors: results from an international multicenter study of 5262 patients. Radiology. 2013;267:718–26.
25. Cheruvu C, Precious B, Naoum C, et al. Long term prognostic utility of coronary CT angiography in patients with no modifiable coronary artery disease risk factors: results from the 5 year follow-up of the CONFIRM international multicenter registry. J Cardiovasc Comput Tomogr. 2016;10:22–7.
26. Abdulla J, Asferg C, Kofoed KF. Prognostic value of absence or presence of coronary artery disease determined by 64-slice computed tomography coronary angiography a systematic review and meta-analysis. Int J Cardiovasc Imaging. 2011;27:413–20.
27. Habib PJ, Green J, Butterfield RC, Kuntz GM, Murthy R, Kraemer DF, Percy RF, Miller AB, Strom JA. Association of cardiac events with coronary artery disease detected by 64-slice or greater coronary CT angiography: a systematic review and meta-analysis. Int J Cardiol. 2013;169:112–20.
28. Dougoud S, Fuchs TA, Stehli J, Clerc OF, Buechel RR, Herzog BA, Leschka S, Alkadhi H, Kaufmann PA, Gaemperli O. Prognostic value of coronary CT angiography on long-term follow-up of 6.9 years. Int J Cardiovasc Imaging. 2014;30:969–76.
29. Min JK, Dunning A, Lin FY, et al. Age- and sex-related differences in all-cause mortality risk based on coronary computed tomography angiography findings results from the international multicenter CONFIRM (coronary CT angiography evaluation for clinical outcomes: an international multicenter registry) of 23,854 patients without known coronary artery disease. J Am Coll Cardiol. 2011;58:849–60.
30. Budoff MJ, Yang TP, Shavelle RM, Lamont DH, Brundage BH. Ethnic differences in coronary atherosclerosis. J Am Coll Cardiol. 2002;39:408–12.
31. Shaw LJ, Shaw RE, Merz CN, et al., and American College of Cardiology-National Cardiovascular Data Registry I. Impact of ethnicity and gender differences on angiographic coronary artery disease prevalence and in-hospital mortality in the American college of cardiology-national cardiovascular data registry. Circulation. 2008;117:1787–801.
32. Detrano R, Guerci AD, Carr JJ, et al. Coronary calcium as a predictor of coronary events in four racial or ethnic groups. N Engl J Med. 2008;358:1336–45.
33. Ferdinand KC. Coronary artery disease in minority racial and ethnic groups in the United States. Am J Cardiol. 2006;97:12A–9A.
34. McClelland RL, Chung H, Detrano R, Post W, Kronmal RA. Distribution of coronary artery calcium by race, gender, and age: results from the multi-ethnic study of atherosclerosis (MESA). Circulation. 2006;113:30–7.
35. Hulten E, Villines TC, Cheezum MK, et al., and Investigators C. Usefulness of coronary computed tomography angiography to predict mortality and myocardial infarction among Caucasian, African and east Asian ethnicities (from the CONFIRM [coronary CT angiography evaluation for clinical outcomes: an international multicenter] registry). Am J Cardiol. 2013;111:479–85.
36. Villines TC, Hulten EA, Shaw LJ, et al., and Investigators CR. Prevalence and severity of coronary artery disease and adverse events among symptomatic patients with coronary artery calcification scores of zero undergoing coronary computed tomography angiography: results from the CONFIRM (coronary CT angiography evaluation for clinical outcomes: an international multicenter) registry. J Am Coll Cardiol. 2011;58:2533–40.
37. Al-Mallah MH, Qureshi W, Lin FY, et al. Does coronary CT angiography improve risk stratification over coronary calcium scoring in symptomatic patients with suspected coronary artery disease? Results from the prospective multicenter international CONFIRM registry. Eur Heart J Cardiovasc Imaging. 2014;15:267–74.
38. Cho I, Chang HJ, Sung JM, et al., and Investigators C. Coronary computed tomographic angiography and risk of all-cause mortality and nonfatal myocardial infarction in subjects without chest pain

syndrome from the CONFIRM Registry (coronary CT angiography evaluation for clinical outcomes: an international multicenter registry). Circulation. 2012;126:304–13.

39. Buse JB, Ginsberg HN, Bakris GL, et al., American Heart A and American Diabetes A. Primary prevention of cardiovascular diseases in people with diabetes mellitus: a scientific statement from the American Heart Association and the American Diabetes Association. Circulation. 2007;115:114–26.
40. Rana JS, Dunning A, Achenbach S, et al. Differences in prevalence, extent, severity, and prognosis of coronary artery disease among patients with and without diabetes undergoing coronary computed tomography angiography: results from 10,110 individuals from the CONFIRM (COronary CT angiography evaluation for clinical outcomes): an international multicenter registry. Diabetes Care. 2012;35:1787–94.
41. Blanke P, Naoum C, Ahmadi A, et al. Long-term prognostic utility of coronary CT angiography in stable patients with diabetes mellitus. JACC Cardiovasc Imaging. 2016;9(11):1280–8.
42. Arsanjani R, Berman DS, Gransar H, et al., and Investigators C. Left ventricular function and volume with coronary CT angiography improves risk stratification and identification of patients at risk for incident mortality: results from 7758 patients in the prospective multinational CONFIRM observational cohort study. Radiology. 2014;273:70–7.
43. Samad Z, Hakeem A, Mahmood SS, Pieper K, Patel MR, Simel DL, Douglas PS. A meta-analysis and systematic review of computed tomography angiography as a diagnostic triage tool for patients with chest pain presenting to the emergency department. J Nucl Cardiol. 2012;19:364–76.
44. Goldstein JA, Chinnaiyan KM, Abidov A, et al., and Investigators C-S. The CT-STAT (coronary computed tomographic angiography for systematic triage of acute chest pain patients to treatment) trial. J Am Coll Cardiol. 2011;58:1414–22.
45. Litt HI, Gatsonis C, Snyder B, et al. CT angiography for safe discharge of patients with possible acute coronary syndromes. N Engl J Med. 2012;366:1393–403.
46. Hoffmann U, Bamberg F, Chae CU, et al. Coronary computed tomography angiography for early triage of patients with acute chest pain: the ROMICAT (rule out myocardial infarction using computer assisted tomography) trial. J Am Coll Cardiol. 2009;53:1642–50.
47. Schlett CL, Banerji D, Siegel E, et al. Prognostic value of CT angiography for major adverse cardiac events in patients with acute chest pain from the emergency department: 2-year outcomes of the ROMICAT trial. JACC Cardiovasc Imaging. 2011;4:481–91.
48. Raff GL, Chinnaiyan KM, Cury RC, et al. SCCT guidelines on the use of coronary computed tomographic angiography for patients presenting with acute chest pain to the emergency department: a report of the Society of Cardiovascular Computed Tomography Guidelines Committee. J Cardiovasc Comput Tomogr. 2014;8:254–71.
49. Taylor AJ, Cerqueira M, Hodgson JM, Mark D, Min J, O'Gara P, Rubin GD, American College of Cardiology Foundation Appropriate Use Criteria Task F, Society of Cardiovascular Computed T, American College of R, American Heart A, American Society of E, American Society of Nuclear C, North American Society for Cardiovascular I, Society for Cardiovascular A, Interventions and Society for Cardiovascular Magnetic R. ACCF/SCCT/ACR/AHA/ASE/ASNC/NASCI/SCAI/SCMR 2010 Appropriate use criteria for cardiac computed tomography. A report of the American college of cardiology foundation appropriate use criteria task force, the society of cardiovascular computed tomography, the American college of radiology, the American heart association, the American society of echocardiography, the American society of nuclear cardiology, the north American society for cardiovascular imaging, the society for cardiovascular angiography and interventions, and the society for cardiovascular magnetic resonance. J Cardiovasc Comput Tomogr. 2010;4:407 e1–33.
50. Halpern EJ. Triple-rule-out CT angiography for evaluation of acute chest pain and possible acute coronary syndrome. Radiology. 2009;252:332–45.
51. Chinnaiyan KM, Depetris AM, Al-Mallah M, et al. Rationale, design, and goals of the advanced cardiovascular imaging consortium (ACIC): a blue cross blue shield of Michigan collaborative quality improvement project. Am Heart J. 2012;163:346–53.
52. Burris AC 2nd, Boura JA, Raff GL, Chinnaiyan KM. Triple rule out versus coronary CT angiography in patients with acute chest pain: results from the ACIC consortium. JACC Cardiovasc Imaging. 2015;8:817–25.
53. Liao L, Kong DF, Shaw LK, Sketch MH Jr, Milano CA, Lee KL, Mark DB. A new anatomic score for prognosis after cardiac catheterization in patients with previous bypass surgery. J Am Coll Cardiol. 2005;46:1684–92.
54. Weustink AC, Nieman K, Pugliese F, Mollet NR, Meijboom WB, van Mieghem C, ten Kate GJ, Cademartiri F, Krestin GP, de Feyter PJ. Diagnostic accuracy of computed tomography angiography in patients after bypass grafting: comparison with invasive coronary angiography. JACC Cardiovasc Imaging. 2009;2:816–24.
55. Bassri H, Salari F, Noohi F, Motevali M, Abdi S, Givtaj N, Raissi K, Haghjoo M. Evaluation of early coronary graft patency after coronary artery bypass graft surgery using multislice computed tomography angiography. BMC Cardiovasc Disord. 2009;9:53.
56. Lee R, Lim J, Kaw G, Wan G, Ng K, Ho KT. Comprehensive noninvasive evaluation of bypass grafts and native coronary arteries in patients after coronary bypass surgery: accuracy of 64-slice multidetector computed tomography compared to invasive coronary angiography. J Cardiovasc Med (Hagerstown). 2010;11:81–90.
57. Hamon M, Lepage O, Malagutti P, Riddell JW, Morello R, Agostini D, Hamon M. Diagnostic performance of 16- and 64-section spiral CT for coronary artery bypass graft assessment: meta-analysis. Radiology. 2008;247:679–86.
58. Small GR, Yam Y, Chen L, et al. Prognostic assessment of coronary artery bypass patients with 64-slice computed tomography angiography: anatomical information is incremental to clinical risk prediction. J Am Coll Cardiol. 2011;58:2389–95.
59. Falk E, Shah PK, Fuster V. Coronary plaque disruption. Circulation. 1995;92:657–71.
60. Virmani R, Burke AP, Kolodgie FD, Farb A. Vulnerable plaque: the pathology of unstable coronary lesions. J Interv Cardiol. 2002;15:439–46.
61. Hoffmann MH, Shi H, Schmitz BL, et al. Noninvasive coronary angiography with multislice computed tomography. JAMA. 2005;293:2471–8.
62. Motoyama S, Anno H, Sarai M, et al. Noninvasive coronary angiography with a prototype 256-row area detector computed tomography system: comparison with conventional invasive coronary angiography. J Am Coll Cardiol. 2008;51:773–5.
63. Hoffmann U, Moselewski F, Nieman K, et al. Noninvasive assessment of plaque morphology and composition in culprit and stable lesions in acute coronary syndrome and stable lesions in stable angina by multidetector computed tomography. J Am Coll Cardiol. 2006;47:1655–62.
64. Motoyama S, Kondo T, Anno H, Sugiura A, Ito Y, Mori K, Ishii J, Sato T, Inoue K, Sarai M, Hishida H, Narula J. Atherosclerotic plaque characterization by 0.5-mm-slice multislice computed tomographic imaging. Circ J. 2007;71:363–6.
65. Achenbach S, Moselewski F, Ropers D, et al. Detection of calcified and noncalcified coronary atherosclerotic plaque by contrast-enhanced, submillimeter multidetector spiral computed tomography: a segment-based comparison with intravascular ultrasound. Circulation. 2004;109:14–7.

66. Motoyama S, Kondo T, Sarai M, et al. Multislice computed tomographic characteristics of coronary lesions in acute coronary syndromes. J Am Coll Cardiol. 2007;50:319–26.
67. Motoyama S, Sarai M, Harigaya H, et al. Computed tomographic angiography characteristics of atherosclerotic plaques subsequently resulting in acute coronary syndrome. J Am Coll Cardiol. 2009;54:49–57.
68. Imazeki T, Sato Y, Inoue F, Anazawa T, Tani S, Matsumoto N, Takayama T, Uchiyama T, Saito S. Evaluation of coronary artery remodeling in patients with acute coronary syndrome and stable angina by multislice computed tomography. Circ J. 2004;68:1045–50.
69. Puchner SB, Liu T, Mayrhofer T, et al. High-risk plaque detected on coronary CT angiography predicts acute coronary syndromes independent of significant stenosis in acute chest pain: results from the ROMICAT-II trial. J Am Coll Cardiol. 2014;64:684–92.
70. Shaw LJ, Berman DS, Hendel RC, Borges Neto S, Min JK, Callister TQ. Prognosis by coronary computed tomographic angiography: matched comparison with myocardial perfusion single-photon emission computed tomography. J Cardiovasc Comput Tomogr. 2008;2:93–101.
71. van Werkhoven JM, Schuijf JD, Gaemperli O, et al. Prognostic value of multislice computed tomography and gated single-photon emission computed tomography in patients with suspected coronary artery disease. J Am Coll Cardiol. 2009;53:623–32.
72. Investigators S-H. CT coronary angiography in patients with suspected angina due to coronary heart disease (SCOT-HEART): an open-label, parallel-group, multicentre trial. Lancet. 2015;385:2383–91.
73. Hadamitzky M, Freissmuth B, Meyer T, et al. Prognostic value of coronary computed tomographic angiography for prediction of cardiac events in patients with suspected coronary artery disease. JACC Cardiovasc Imaging. 2009;2:404–11.
74. Beigel R, Brosh S, Goitein O, et al. Prognostic implications of non-obstructive coronary artery disease in patients undergoing coronary computed tomographic angiography for acute chest pain. Am J Cardiol. 2013;111:941–5.

Cardiac CT: Comparative Cost-Effectiveness

52

Christopher L. Schlett

The Need for Comparative Cost-Effectiveness

Across the world, but particularly in developed countries, we are facing the problem of rising health-care costs in the era of limited resources. Between 2005 and 2015, the health-care expenditure as portion of the gross domestic product increased by 12% within the OECD countries while the USA remains the country with the highest expenditure (2015: $3.2 trillion, 16.9% of the gross domestic product) [1, 2]. Since the increase in spending is limited at some point, we have to make decisions on different levels. Unlike most daily decision, many health-care decisions have significant consequences and involve essential uncertainties and trade-offs. However, high health-care expenditures are not necessarily inappropriate, and any level of spending might be considered "appropriate," depending on the value gained by that investment.

The aim of comparative effectiveness research (CER) in general is to compare alternative approaches to patient care. Using randomized controlled trials (RCTs) – one of the three important types of CER – broadly accepted evidence can be generated to support one or the other strategy; however, RCTs also have their limitations, e.g., measuring long-term effects. Cost-effectiveness analysis (CEA) is another method in the broader CER framework although comparative cost data are currently not routinely evaluated in most countries, including the USA [3]. CEA is one of the five major cost analysis types (cost minimization, cost-benefit, cost-consequence, cost-effectiveness, cost-utility) and the most common type published in medical literature beside cost-utility analysis. In general, CEA evaluates the difference in health outcomes for two or more interventions or diagnostic strategies in relation to their cost difference.

The need for CER, and particularly CEA, usually arises when the value of a new intervention or diagnostic test is unclear compared to the existing, standard-of-care practice, like it was for cardiac CT. Comparisons can become complex when more than one outcome is being considered; for example, a new diagnostic test is more effective but has substantially higher severe side effects and associated costs. Today, CEA is one of the multiple considerations that form reimbursement decisions by different institutions across the world including, e.g., the National Institute for Health and Care Excellence (NICE) in the UK and the Institute for Quality and Efficiency in Health Care in Germany. However, from an industry point of view, it can be argued that CEA is a form of price control, which leads to reduced returns to industry and to lower research and development expenditure and stifles future innovations. Nevertheless, CER and CEA became a popular and important tool in medicine including the evaluation of novel diagnostic test strategies like cardiac CT.

A Primer for Cost-Effectiveness Analysis

A few basic elements should briefly be reviewed for a better understanding of the results derived from CEA regarding cardiac CT. While costs seem to be a more simple measure, the quantification of health outcomes is complex – a typically used metric is quality-adjusted life-year (QALY). It takes into account both, the quality and the quantity of life lived, using the following equation: "QALY = time * utility." The utility itself covers multiple health metrics which are combined into a single overall measure and ranges from 0 (equals to "dead") to 1 (equals to "perfect health"). For all other health states in-between, there is a deduction [4]; for example, for major cardiac events, commonly used utility weights range from 0.70 to 0.85 [5], but utility weights vary by many factors (e.g., gender) and must be carefully chosen.

Another challenge is to derive accurate cost estimates, and both measuring and modeling of this parameter can be complex, too. The costs of a cardiac CT exam include the fees associated with performing the scan as well as

C. L. Schlett (✉)
Department of Diagnostic and Interventional Radiology, University Medical Center Freiburg, Freiburg, Germany
e-mail: Christopher.Schlett@post.harvard.edu

U. J. Schoepf (ed.), *CT of the Heart*, Contemporary Medical Imaging, https://doi.org/10.1007/978-1-60327-237-7_52

downstream costs associated with the imaging test (including additional diagnostic tests, therapeutic procedures, etc.). Even the actual cost just for the CT scan is difficult to determine since it is often a fraction of the charged price and varies among hospitals, states, and countries. This inherent lack of consistency in costs can be a stumbling block for accurate CEA. In the USA, many CEAs use cost estimates typically derived from the US Centers for Medicare and Medicaid Services (CMS) average payments.

A frequently used tool in CEA is the incremental cost-effectiveness ratio (ICER). It was initially described in 1977 by Drs. Weinstein and Stason and serves as a summary measure in the comparison of two different interventions or diagnostic strategies (e.g., A vs. B) while it is defined as "ICER = [cost-A - cost-B] / [outcome-A - outcome-B]" [6]. The ICER can be used as a decision rule in resource allocation if a willingness-to-pay value can be determined; e.g., in the UK, NICE has formally acknowledged a range from £20,000 to £30,000 per QALY, but higher thresholds can be argued for special circumstances such as treatments for rare conditions; in other European countries, a threshold of €80,000 per QALY and in the USA a threshold of $50,000 per QALY are often considered as appropriate. However, these thresholds may not necessarily reflect a society's willingness to pay, and alternative methods have been suggested, including thresholds based on per capita incomes or benchmark interventions [7].

Also, the chosen time horizon can impact the results significantly. CEA assessing cardiac CT for stable chest pain patients are more likely to choose a lifetime horizon given the chronic disease character, while CT for acute chest pain would focus more on short-term costs/effects. Similarly, the chosen perspective has great impact on the CEA results. Each stakeholder within the health-care system (e.g., governments, insurance companies, hospitals, physicians, employers, patients) has a different perspective with regard to cost and effect; thus, what could be considered cost-effective from a societal standpoint is not necessarily cost-effective from the perspective of an individual hospital. Nevertheless, most CEA studies apply the societal perspective in the academic environment [8].

Before deriving the CEA results, the therapeutic and diagnostic strategies must be formulated. One way are decision trees, which are a schematic representation of all of the clinically and policy relevant features of the decision problem. They include "Decision Nodes" (a choice between alternatives strategies), "Chance Nodes" (possible events determined by probability), and "Terminal Nodes" (outcomes associated with a given pathway) as illustrated in Fig. 52.1. Another approach are Markov models, which represent a mathematical modeling technique derived from matrix algebra. Those are recursive decision trees that are used for modeling conditions that have events which may occur repeatedly over time (e.g., nonfatal myocardial infarcts) and/or for modeling predictable events that occur over time (e.g., developing coronary stenosis). Central elements of all Markov models are mutually exclusive health states and the transition between states, which reflect events (Fig. 52.2). The time spent in each health state determines overall expected outcome. Analyzing the model often includes sensitivity analysis and/or Monte Carlo simulations to model the given uncertainty.

Comparative Cost-Effectiveness of Cardiac CT for Acute Chest Pain Patients

Two major RCTs have been conducted assessing comparative effectiveness and cost of cardiac CT in patients with suspicion of acute coronary syndrome – ACRIN-PA (American College of Radiology Imaging Network, Pennsylvania) and ROMICAT II (Rule Out Myocardial Infarction using Computer Assisted Computed Tomography) [9, 10]. Optimally, a strategy including early CCTA would reduce costs and provide more cost-effective care in the triage of patients with suspicion of acute coronary syndrome. Both studies found a significant reduction in length of stay and a higher rate of direct discharge from the emergency department with no alteration in safety [9, 10]. In ROMICAT II, no reduction in overall costs was observed [9]; costs in the emergency department decreased ($2101 vs. $2566 in CCTA vs. standard of care), while in contrast, the costs during hospitalization slightly increased using CCTA ($4026 vs. $3874), potentially due to the higher number of revascularizations [9]. Cost data for ACRIN-PA have not yet been released.

Only a few CEA studies, limited to the USA, are available comparing different triage strategies in patients with suspicion of acute coronary syndrome. In a study by Khare et al. [11], the authors found that a triage strategy including CCTA would dominate other strategies, such as stress echocardiography or stress ECG, regarding its cost-effectiveness (ICER, $29,738/QALY for CCTA, if compared with stress echocardiography, and $7332/QALY, if compared with the stress ECG).

In another study by Ladapo et al. using first-order Monte Carlo microsimulations for 55-year-old men and women, a triage strategy including early CCTA resulted in an ICER of $6400/QALY for men, and it was actually cost-saving for women ($6630 for CCTA and $7010 for standard of care) [12]. This finding was driven by their observation that the CCTA strategy was cheaper in women than in men ($6630 vs. $10,190). These findings were sensitive to several parameters, including correctly classifying a patient as healthy by CCTA or the time horizon over which patients could return to the emergency department, but the authors found that CCTA remained in the range of what is typically considered cost-effective in most sensitivity analyses [12].

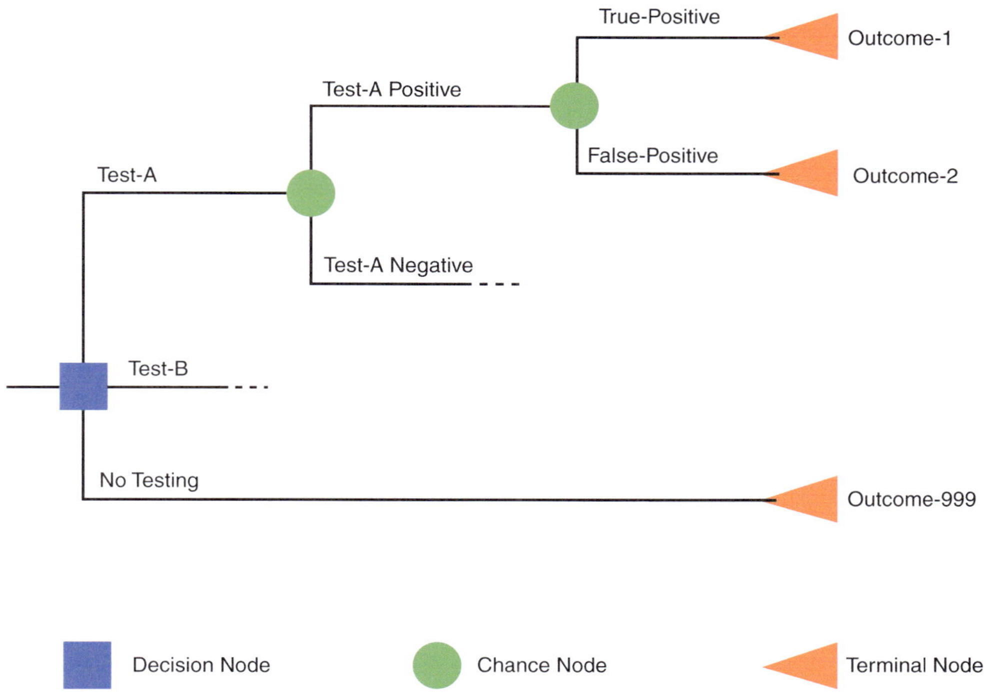

Fig. 52.1 Decision Tree. A simplified version of a decision tree comparing different diagnostic tests vs. no testing. The decision tree consists typically of three node types: "Decision Nodes," representing a choice between alternatives strategies; "Chance Nodes," possible events determined by a probability; and "Terminal Nodes," outcomes associated with a given pathway. By "Rolling Back" the decision tree, costs and health outcome can be determined for each test strategy

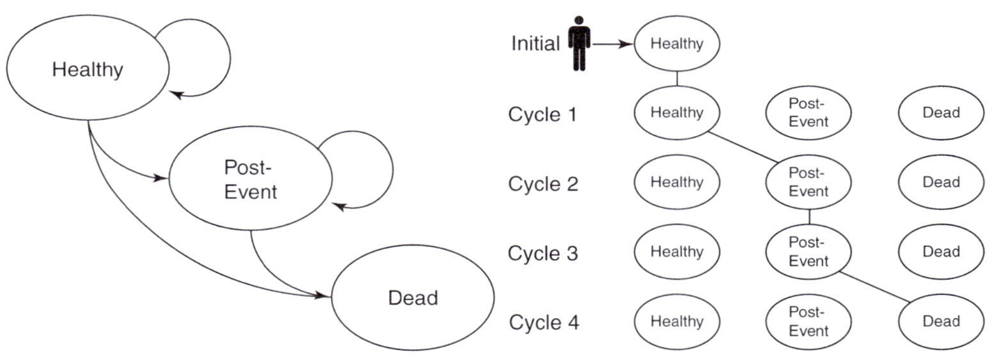

Fig. 52.2 Example of a Markov model and Monte Carlo simulation. The Markov model (left part) consists of different health states with one starting state (e.g., "Healthy") and one absorbing state (e.g., "Dead"), which is a state that, once entered, cannot be left. A patient is always in one of a finite number of discrete health states. All events are represented as transitions from one state to another. Monte Carlo simulation (right part) can be used to evaluate a Markov model. The simulation determines the prognoses of a large number of individual patients. Each patient begins in the starting state, and at the end of each cycle, the transition to another health state is based on a probability. The patient is given credit for each cycle spent in a non-absorbing state, and each state may be adjusted for quality of life. The simulation is stopped when the patient enters the absorbing state

Thus, CCTA may have the potential to be a cost-effective alternative compared to a traditional triage of patients with suspicion of acute coronary syndrome; however, it has to hold up against other, newer strategies such as using high-sensitivity troponin in future research.

Comparative Cost-Effectiveness Analysis of Cardiac CT for Stable Chest Pain

Comparative effectiveness and cost of cardiac CT to other testing strategies for patients with stable chest pain have been evaluated in several randomized controlled trials, including the two large trials PROMISE and SCOT-HEART [13, 14]. Regarding the effectiveness determined as occurrence of major cardiac events, PROMISE revealed low event rates, which showed no difference between the two strategies at 2.1 years (3.3% vs. 3.0% for cardiac CTA vs. functional testing, $p = 0.75$). In SCOT-HEART, event rate (overall death or MI) was about twofold higher than for the PROMISE trial and showed a reduction of nearby 40% by cardiac CT vs. standard of care (HR, 0.62; 95% CI, 0.38–1.01; $p = 0.053$). In general, the use of diagnostic testing improves angina and quality of life; however, this improvement does not vary significantly between the randomized testing strategy, which was also observed in other, smaller studies assessing health status by, e.g., the Seattle Angina Questionnaire (SAQ) [15].

Assessing the comparative costs for the diagnostic testing strategies, SCOT-HEART trial showed slightly higher costs in the CCTA arm at 6 months (difference, \$462, $p < 0.0001$), which mainly reflects the difference in upfront procedural cost. There were neither differences in cost associated with outpatient and inpatient services nor medication use (all $p \geq 0.16$). Similarly, in the PROMISE trial, the costs were not different through 3 years of follow-up (difference: \$627, p = NS) [16].

Although 3 years is a relative long follow-up for a randomized controlled trial, it cannot reflect a lifelong horizon, which is relevant for decision-making. More importantly, stable chest pain must be often considered as a chronic disease, and therefore a lifelong horizon becomes even more relevant.

Several CEAs have been conducted, including long-term outcome modeling such as Markov cohort simulation and state-transition microsimulation [17]. These studies demonstrate a high heterogeneity; the most relevant studies have been listed in Table 52.1. One of the most comprehensive CEAs was published in 2015 by Genders et al. which considered most but not all possible imaging tests as well as several national perspectives, including the USA, the UK, and the Netherlands [18]. They found that a strategy that began with CCTA, continued with cardiac stress imaging if CCTA found at least coronary stenosis, and that ended with invasive coronary angiography (ICA) if stress imaging induced any ischemia, maximized QALYs and was cost-effective in the USA (ICER, \$22,000/QALY for men and \$21,000/QALY for women) and the Netherlands (ICER, €38,000/QALY for men and €18,000/QALY for women). For the UK, the results were more divergent. For men, the preferred strategy with an ICER of £7000/QALY began with CCTA and continued with optimal medical therapy without ICA, if CCTA found only moderate CAD, or if stress imaging induced only mild ischemia. In women, the preferred strategy was stress echocardiography followed by ICA if echocardiography induced mild or moderate ischemia (ICER £7000/QALY).

A comparable study using gender-stratified analysis by Ladapo et al. [19] using a typical case of a 55-year-old female or male patient with stable chest pain found that CCTA with stress testing was the performed strategy with an ICER ranging from \$26,200/QALY in men to \$35,000/QALY in women; however, differences in health outcomes were small, and CCTA raised overall costs, partly through the follow-up of incidental findings. Although results from Medicare data showed a decrease of overall CAD-related costs after 9 months if patients underwent CCTA rather than imaging stress test [20], a higher rate of invasive downstream testing after CCTA has been reported, for example, in the SPARC registry and the PROMISE trial [13, 21]. The long-term value regarding costs and, more importantly, regarding health outcome of this is quite controversial and only partially included in the CEA studies [17].

Nevertheless, many CEA studies suggested that strategies which began with CCTA and were followed by cardiac stress imaging were cost-effective for patients with stable chest pain [22–24]. However, in sensitivity analyses, the optimal diagnostic imaging strategy depends strongly on the pretest CAD probability (Fig. 52.3). For CCTA, cost-effectiveness was often reached in cohorts with low-intermediate pretest probability of CAD; in contrast, ICA becomes a cost-effective strategy in patients with a high pretest CAD probability (≥70%). But sensitivity analysis revealed also other influencing factors, such as test characteristics and costs of a test.

In summary, results from different CERs suggest that CCTA may serve as an initial gatekeeper test resulting in cost-effectiveness under varying assumptions in patients presenting with stable chest pain with a low to intermediate pretest probability of CAD. Similarly, the 2016 updated NICE guidelines, which considered already the results of the PROMISE and SCOT-HEART trial, recommend CCTA as a first-line modality for patients presenting with new-onset chest pain due to suspected CAD in the UK [25].

Cost-Effectiveness Analysis Regarding Reporting Incidental Findings on Cardiac CT

While most CEAs regarding cardiac CT mainly focus whether CCTA is a cost-effective diagnosis strategy for chest pain patients, other questions remain open and can be addressed with similar statistical techniques. One example is a CEA study by Goehler et al. [26]. Their objective was to assess from a society perspective and lifelong horizon – whether reporting pulmonary nodules, incidentally detected in CCTA, would be cost-effective. Using a validated lung cancer simulation model, they found for a typical chest pain cohort that reporting and following up pulmonary nodules according to the guidelines of the international societies led to a reduction in cumulative lung cancer mortality (4.6% relative reduction) and consecutively to higher QALY; however, also downstream testing increased. Thus, the ICER for the overall cohort was \$154,700/QALY, which is significantly above the normally assumed willingness-to-pay threshold. One reason for this observation is the phenomenon of competing risks where the majority of patients undergoing cardiac CT die of CAD and other causes, rather than of lung cancer [26, 27]. Even if restricting the cohort to smokers, an ICER of \$129,800/QALY remained above the assumed willingness-to-pay threshold.

Although these CEA data do not support reporting pulmonary nodules incidentally detected on cardiac CT, the international guidelines still recommend to report incidental

Table 52.1 Cost-effectiveness analysis of cardiac CT for stable chest pain

Year of publication, first author, Reference	Time frame	Perspective	Country of analysis	Imaging algorithms compared	Threshold willingness to pay ($ or € /QALY)	Reference case analysis	Suggested initial imaging test for low-intermediate pretest probability	Optimal strategy depends on
2009, Ladapo [19]	Lifetime	Health-care system	USA	CCTA + xECG/ICA, xECG + CCTA/ICA, TCA ± ICA, xECG ± ICA, xECHO ± ICA, SPECT ± ICA, ICA, vs. no testing	US$50,000/ QALY	55-year-old men and women with pretest probability of 70% and 30%, respectively	CCTA	Pretest probability, (risks of) radiation exposure, and sensitivity of CCTA
2009, Genders [23]	Lifetime	Patient, physician, hospital, health-care system, society	Netherlands, USA	CCTA ± ICA vs. ICA	€80,000/QALY	60-year-old men and women (men pretest probability of 79%; women pretest probability of 65%)	CCTA	Optimization criterion (i.e., outcomes), pretest probability, sensitivity/specificity of CCTA
2009, Kreisz [28]	Short term (10 years)	Health-care system	Australia	CCTA ± ICA vs. ICA	AUS$50,000 / QALY	Patients referred for ICA with pretest probability of 10–90%	CCTA	Pretest probability
2010, Min [29]	Short term and lifetime	Health-care payer	USA	CCTA ± ICA, CCTA ± SPECT/ICA, SPECT ± ICA, SPECT ± CCTA/ICA, vs. ICA	US$50,000 / QALY	55-year-old men with pretest probability of 30%	CCTA	CCTA sensitivity, SPECT sensitivity, pretest probability, cost tests
2012, Meyer [30]	Short term	Health-care payer	USA	CCTA (dual energy) vs. SPECT	n/a	51- to 71-year-old men and women with pretest probability of 80%	CCTA	Sensitivity, age, cost tests, pretest probability
2013, Genders [31]	Short term and lifetime	Health-care system	Netherlands	CCTA vs. xECG	€80,000/QALY	46- to 66-year-old men and women with pretest probability of 70%	CCTA	Pretest probability
2015, Genders [18]	Lifetime	Health-care system, society	USA, UK, Netherlands	CCTA, Stress Test (CMR, SPECT, xECHO), CCTA ± Stress Test (CMR , SPECT, xECHO), vs. ICA	For USA: $50,000/QALY For UK: £25,000/ QALY For Netherlands: €80,000/QALY	60-year-old men and women with low to intermediate probability for CAD	CCTA (for USA, Netherlands, UK men)xECHO (for UK women)	Pretest probability, False-positive rate
2016, Agus [32]	Short term (1 year)	Health-care system	UK	CCTA vs. Stress Test	£20,000/QALY	57.8 ± 10.0 years, 56% male; 42/22/36% of low-/ intermediate-/high- pretest probability of CAD	CCTA	Pretest probability
2016, Bertoldi [33]	Lifelong	Health-care system	Brazilian	CCTA, Stress Test (xECG, xECHO, CMR) vs. ICA	I$11,909-35,727/ QALY	60 years, intermediate (50%) pretest probability of CAD	CCTA	Cost tests, pretest probability

Abbreviations used: *CMR* cardiac magnetic resonance imaging, *ICA* invasive angiography, *CCTA* coronary CT angiography, *QALY* quality-adjusted life-year, *ICER* incremental cost-effectiveness ratio, *xECG* stress electrocardiography, *xECHO* stress echocardiography

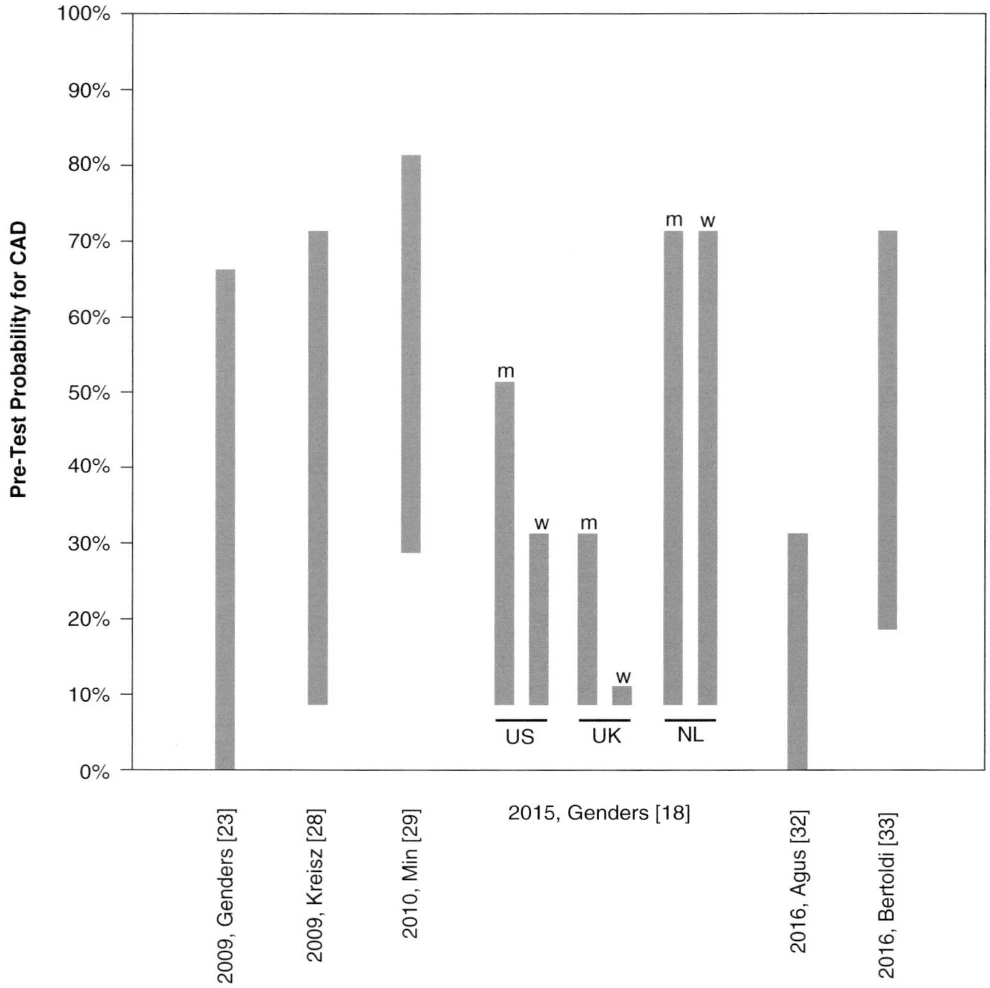

Fig. 52.3 Sensitivity analysis regarding pretest probability for CAD. The bar graphs demonstrate under which assumed pretest probabilities for CAD CCTA remain the preferred strategy. USA denotes the United States, UK the United Kingdom, NL the Netherlands, m male patients, w female patients

findings, and most radiologists follow these recommendations across the word, illustrating that decision-making is not only a process of economic evaluation.

References

1. OECD.Stat, Health expenditure and financing. Joint OECD, EUROSTAT and WHO Health Accounts SHA Questionnaires (JHAQ). https://stats.oecd.org/index.aspx?DataSetCode=SHA
2. US Centers for Medicare & Medicaid Services National Health Expenditures 2015 Highlights. https://ccf.georgetown.edu/wp-content/uploads/pdfs/highlights.pdf
3. Goehler A, Gazelle GS. Examining the use of comparative and cost-effectiveness analyses in radiology. AJR Am J Roentgenol. 2014;203(5):939–44.
4. Torrance GW. Measurement of health state utilities for economic appraisal. J Health Econ. 1986;5(1):1–30.
5. Hanmer J, et al. Report of nationally representative values for the noninstitutionalized US adult population for 7 health-related quality-of-life scores. Med Decis Mak. 2006;26(4):391–400.
6. Weinstein MC, Stason WB. Foundations of cost-effectiveness analysis for health and medical practices. N Engl J Med. 1977;296(13):716–21.
7. Marseille E, et al. Thresholds for the cost-effectiveness of interventions: alternative approaches. Bull World Health Organ. 2015;93:118–24.
8. Russell LB, et al. The role of cost-effectiveness analysis in health and medicine. Panel on cost-effectiveness in health and medicine. JAMA. 1996;276(14):1172–7.
9. Hoffmann U, et al. Coronary CT angiography versus standard evaluation in acute chest pain. N Engl J Med. 2012;367(4):299–308.
10. Litt HI, et al. CT angiography for safe discharge of patients with possible acute coronary syndromes. N Engl J Med. 2012;366(15):1393–403.
11. Khare RK, et al. Sixty-four-slice computed tomography of the coronary arteries: cost-effectiveness analysis of patients presenting to the emergency department with low-risk chest pain. Acad Emerg Med. 2008;15(7):623–32.
12. Ladapo JA, et al. Cost-effectiveness of coronary MDCT in the triage of patients with acute chest pain. AJR Am J Roentgenol. 2008;191(2):455–63.
13. Douglas PS, et al. Outcomes of anatomical versus functional testing for coronary artery disease. N Engl J Med. 2015;372(14): 1291–300.
14. Investigators, S-H. CT coronary angiography in patients with suspected angina due to coronary heart disease (SCOT-HEART): an open-label, parallel-group, multicentre trial. Lancet. 2015;385(9985):2383–91.

15. Min JK, et al. Coronary CT angiography versus myocardial perfusion imaging for near-term quality of life, cost and radiation exposure: a prospective multicenter randomized pilot trial. J Cardiovasc Comput Tomogr. 2012;6(4):274–83.
16. Fordyce CB, Newby DE, Douglas PS. Diagnostic strategies for the evaluation of chest pain: clinical implications from SCOT-HEART and PROMISE. J Am Coll Cardiol. 2016;67(7):843–52.
17. van Waardhuizen CN, et al. Diagnostic performance and comparative cost-effectiveness of non-invasive imaging tests in patients presenting with chronic stable chest pain with suspected coronary artery disease: a systematic overview. Curr Cardiol Rep. 2014;16(10):537.
18. Genders TS, et al. The optimal imaging strategy for patients with stable chest pain: a cost-effectiveness analysis. Ann Intern Med. 2015;162(7):474–84.
19. Ladapo JA, et al. Clinical outcomes and cost-effectiveness of coronary computed tomography angiography in the evaluation of patients with chest pain. J Am Coll Cardiol. 2009;54(25):2409–22.
20. Min JK, et al. Costs and clinical outcomes in individuals without known coronary artery disease undergoing coronary computed tomographic angiography from an analysis of Medicare category III transaction codes. Am J Cardiol. 2008;102(6):672–8.
21. Hachamovitch R, et al. Patient management after noninvasive cardiac imaging results from SPARC (study of myocardial perfusion and coronary anatomy imaging roles in coronary artery disease). J Am Coll Cardiol. 2012;59(5):462–74.
22. Genders TS, et al. Coronary computed tomography versus exercise testing in patients with stable chest pain: comparative effectiveness and costs. Int J Cardiol. 2013;167(4):1268–75.
23. Genders TS, et al. CT coronary angiography in patients suspected of having coronary artery disease: decision making from various perspectives in the face of uncertainty. Radiology. 2009;253(3):734–44.
24. Dorenkamp M, et al. Direct costs and cost-effectiveness of dual-source computed tomography and invasive coronary angiography in patients with an intermediate pretest likelihood for coronary artery disease. Heart. 2012;98(6):460–7.
25. Moss AJ, et al. The updated NICE guidelines: cardiac CT as the first-line test for coronary artery disease. Curr Cardiovasc Imaging Rep. 2017;10(5):15.
26. Goehler A, et al. Cost-effectiveness of follow-up of pulmonary nodules incidentally detected on cardiac computed tomographic angiography in patients with suspected coronary artery disease. Circulation. 2014;130(8):668–75.
27. Lu MT, et al. Lung cancer screening eligibility in the community: cardiovascular risk factors, coronary artery calcification, and cardiovascular events. Circulation. 2016;134(12):897–9.
28. Kreisz FP, et al. The pre-test risk stratified cost-effectiveness of 64-slice computed tomography coronary angiography in the detection of significant obstructive coronary artery disease in patients otherwise referred to invasive coronary angiography. Heart Lung Circ. 2009;18(3):200–7.
29. Min JK, et al. Cost-effectiveness of coronary CT angiography versus myocardial perfusion SPECT for evaluation of patients with chest pain and no known coronary artery disease. Radiology. 2010;254(3):801–8.
30. Meyer M, et al. Cost-effectiveness of substituting dual-energy CT for SPECT in the assessment of myocardial perfusion for the workup of coronary artery disease. Eur J Radiol. 2012;81(12):3719–25.
31. Genders TS, et al. Coronary computed tomography versus exercise testing in patients with stable chest pain: comparative effectiveness and costs. Int J Cardiol. 2013;167(4):1268–75.
32. Agus AM, et al. The cost-effectiveness of cardiac computed tomography for patients with stable chest pain. Heart. 2016;102(5):356–62.
33. Bertoldi EG, et al. Long-term cost-effectiveness of diagnostic tests for assessing stable chest pain: modeled analysis of anatomical and functional strategies. Clin Cardiol. 2016;39(5):249–56.

Barriers to Greater Clinical Implementation

53

David C. Levin

Coronary artery disease (CAD) is a ubiquitous and dangerous disease. It was estimated that in the United States in 2010, almost 1.5 million individuals either died of CAD or experienced a new nonfatal myocardial infarction (MI), a recurrent MI, or a new silent MI [1]. Other than in patients who present with an acute MI and can be diagnosed by an ECG and/or enzyme measurements, the way to definitively establish the presence of CAD is through the use of noninvasive imaging – principally radionuclide myocardial perfusion imaging (MPI), stress echocardiography (SE), or coronary CT angiography (CCTA). None of the federal or commercial payers have yet agreed to cover the use of these techniques for screening asymptomatic individuals, but given the nature of CAD, clinicians should have a low threshold for ordering these tests in patients with suggestive symptoms and risk factors. The question is, which test to use first? In the author's opinion, the answer in most patients is CCTA.

Our research group (the Center for Research on Utilization of Imaging Services – CRUISE – in the Department of Radiology at Thomas Jefferson University Hospital) has studied utilization patterns of these three tests in the US Medicare fee-for-service population from 2001 through 2014. We use the nationwide Medicare Part B databases, covering over 37 million fee-for-service enrollees, but not including over 15 million people in managed Medicare Advantage plans. The results are surprising and in some ways disturbing. The data are presented as utilization rates per 1000 Medicare fee-for-service enrollees. Total rates are shown, as well as those by cardiologists and radiologists – the two specialties most heavily involved in cardiac imaging. Although the data come from the Medicare population (mostly over age 65), there is no reason to believe that the trends are different in the younger, commercially insured population. It should be noted that the trend lines reflect just the primary codes for MPI and SE and are not affected by code bundling that occurred in echocardiography in 2009 or MPI in 2010.

Figure 53.1 shows the trends in MPI. The total rate per 1000 rose sharply from 63.4 in 2001 to peak at 88.0 in 2006, an increase of 39% in only 5 years. The next 3 years saw a gradual progressive decline. Beginning in 2010, the decline accelerated, and by 2014 the rate had dropped to 58.7, i.e., below what it had been 13 years earlier. Most MPI exams are performed by cardiologists. Their utilization rate trend generally parallels the trend for total MPI exams and shows a sharp increase through 2006, followed by a relatively flat period for the next 3 years and then followed in turn by a prolonged decline starting in 2010. The role of radiologists is much less and never showed the same sort of increase in the early 2000s. Beginning in 2006, the radiologists' rate trend demonstrated a gradual progressive decline.

One can speculate about why participation by cardiologists rose so sharply between 2001 and 2006 and then dropped so sharply in more recent years. Most of the use by cardiologists occurred in private offices. In the early 2000s, it was the best noninvasive test available for suspected CAD (CCTA was in its infancy). The literature to that point had generally supported its efficacy, and cardiologists were enthusiastic about it. It was a well-reimbursed procedure that did not require much image post-processing and was not difficult to read. In addition to the primary CPT-4 code for the MPI exam itself, there were "add-on" codes almost always used for determination of left ventricular wall motion and ejection fraction (EF). These made the procedure even more lucrative, since a claim for services then included three separate codes. However, beginning in 2010, the Centers for Medicare and Medicaid Services (CMS) made an important change by bundling the add-on codes for wall motion and EF together with the primary MPI code. From then on, when an MPI exam was performed along with wall motion and EF studies, only the new single-bundled code could be used when the claim was filed. The global reimbursement for the single-bundled code was 36% lower than the sum of the

D. C. Levin (✉)
Department of Radiology, Thomas Jefferson University Hospital, Philadelphia, PA, USA
e-mail: david.levin@jefferson.edu

U. J. Schoepf (ed.), *CT of the Heart*, Contemporary Medical Imaging, https://doi.org/10.1007/978-1-60327-237-7_53

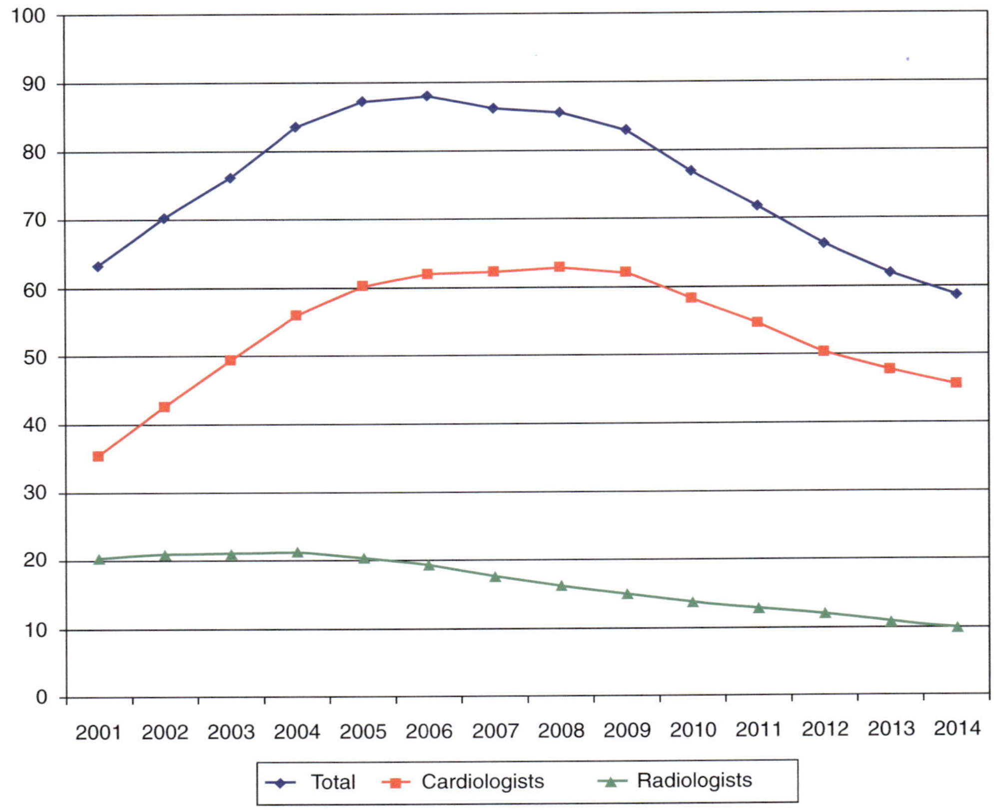

Fig. 53.1 Utilization rates of radionuclide myocardial perfusion imaging (MPI) in the Medicare fee-for-service population, 2001 through 2014. Vertical axis shows examinations per 1000 beneficiaries. In addition to the total rates, data are shown for cardiologists and radiologists, who together provide the vast majority of MPI studies. The small proportions of examinations performed by other specialists are not shown. (Adapted from Levin et al. [24], with permission)

reimbursements for the three codes prior to 2010. Since SPECT cameras are expensive to purchase and maintain, and technologists must be hired to operate them, the new lower payment levels posed financial difficulties for office practices. It appears that many cardiologists closed their offices or sold them to hospitals and became hospital employees. Another factor was the rise of the radiology benefits management companies (RBMs). These companies and the commercial insurers who were their clients imposed preauthorization requirements for expensive high-tech procedures like MPI. No longer could a cardiologist simply order an MPI exam and get it done. Now, he/she had to go through the process of obtaining preauthorization, a process that was often time-consuming and inconvenient and could result in a denial. With the "double whammy" of a drop in reimbursement and the hassle of the preauthorization process, it isn't surprising that enthusiasm for MPI diminished.

The trends for SE are shown in Fig. 53.2. SE is generally not included in preauthorization programs – i.e., it can be ordered and performed without preauthorization. The total utilization rate stayed relatively unchanged from 2001 through 2010 but then began a 4-year period of decline. The rate had been 12.6 in 2010 but declined to 10.2 by 2014. Cardiologists perform the vast majority of SEs, and their trend again closely parallels the total trend. Radiologists have essentially no role in SE, and therefore no trend line is shown.

The CCTA trends are shown in Fig. 53.3. Note that the scale is far lower than that for MPI (Fig. 53.1). The year 2006 is the first year shown because that was the first year in which specific codes for CCTA were available. In that first year, the total CCTA utilization rate was 0.99 per 1000. In 2007, the rate more than doubled to 2.1. Indeed, it seemed as if this new and exciting procedure was poised for a rapid rise in use. But to the surprise and disappointment of many in the field, nothing of the sort happened. Instead, a sharp decline was seen, reaching a nadir of 1.07 in 2012 and 2013. A small increase to 1.11 occurred in 2014, but it is too early to tell if this represents the start of a more favorable trend. Utilization rates among both cardiologists and radiologists peaked in 2007 (at 1.26 and 0.67, respectively) but then declined in subsequent years. The decline was steeper among cardiologists, and their rate had dropped to only 0.47 by 2014. Among radiologists, the utilization rate reached its nadir in 2010 but then began to increase slowly, reaching 0.59 in 2014. Comparing the overall data for MPI and CCTA reveals that in 2014, there were 53 times as many MPI studies performed as CCTAs in this population.

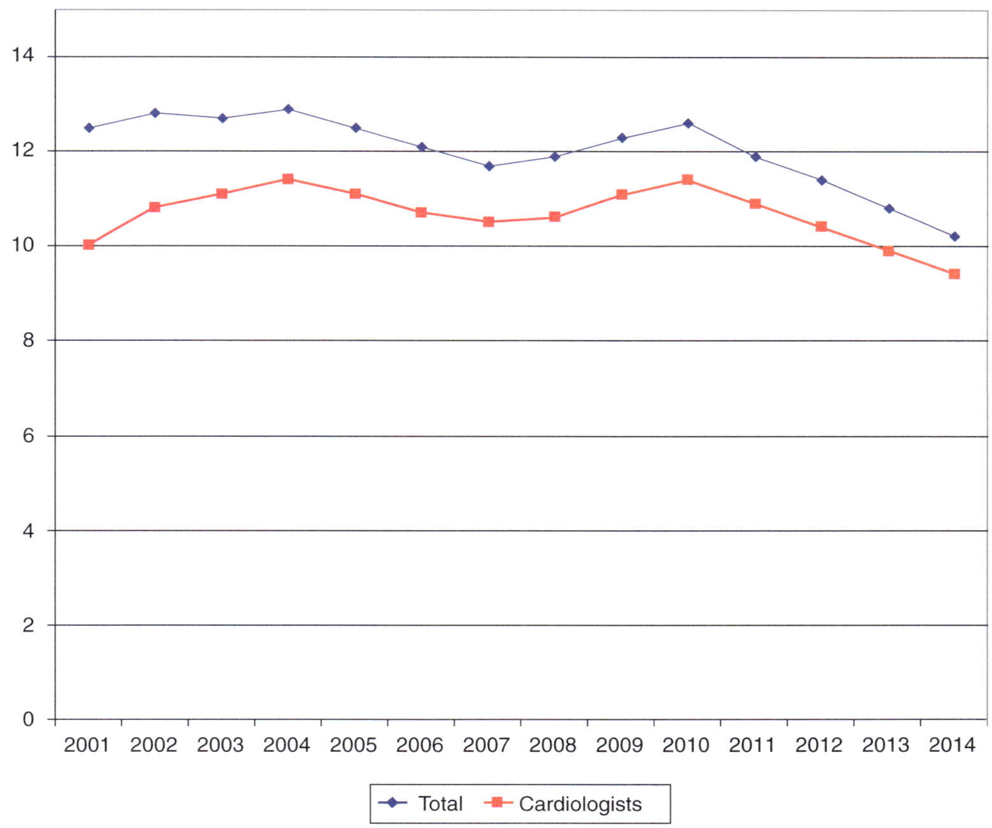

Fig. 53.2 Utilization rates of stress echocardiograms (SEs) in the Medicare fee-for-service population, 2001 through 2014. Vertical axis shows examinations per 1000 beneficiaries. Total rates and rates for cardiologists are shown. Radiologists have essentially no role in SE. The differences between the total rates and those for cardiologists are attributable to SEs performed by a variety of other specialists, particularly primary care physicians and internists. (Adapted from Levin et al. [24], with permission)

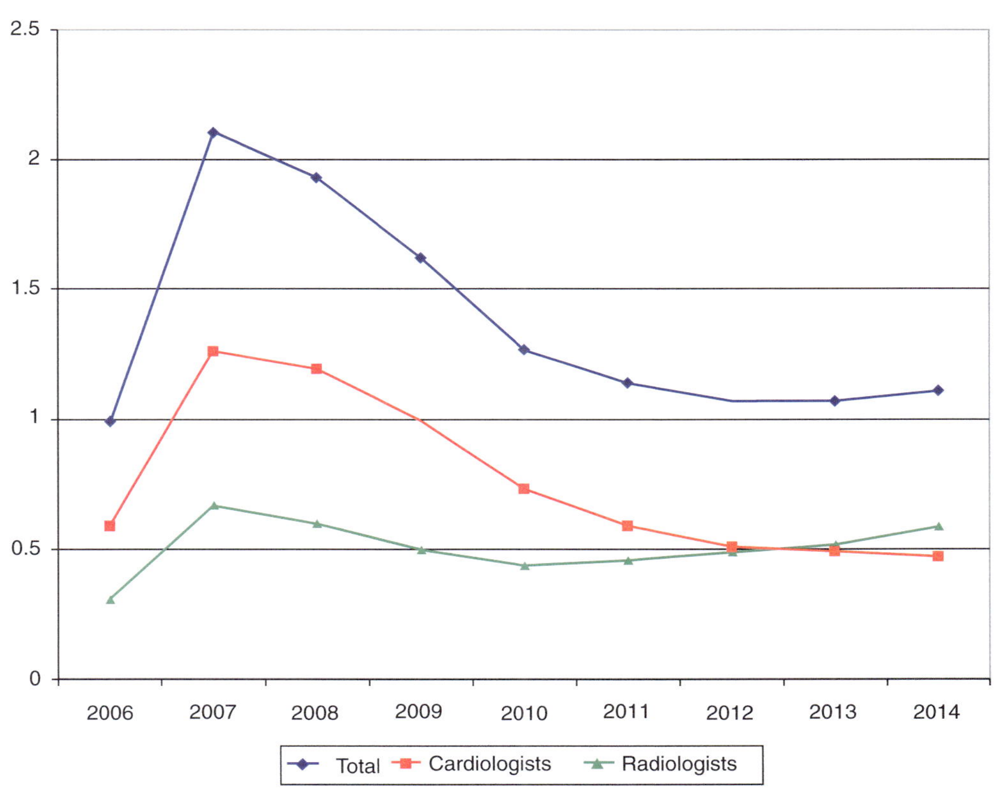

Fig. 53.3 Utilization rates of coronary CT angiography (CCTA) in the Medicare fee-for-service population, 2006 through 2014. 2006 was the first year in which specific codes for CCTA were available. Vertical axis shows examinations per 1000 beneficiaries. In addition to total rates, data are shown for radiologists and cardiologists, who together provide the vast majority of CCTAs. The small proportions of examinations provided by other specialists are not shown. (Adapted from Levin et al. [24], with permission)

Why Has CCTA Failed to Grow More Rapidly?

The answer to this question is not clear-cut and is probably multifactorial. Here are some of the reasons: (1) Multidetector row CT scanners are expensive, particularly those of the latest generations. (2) CCTA can take up considerable scanner time and may slow throughput of other patients undergoing noncardiac scans. Busy hospital radiology departments may have difficulty allocating the necessary time for cardiac exams. (3) The procedure is often labor-intensive for the interpreting physician. Formatting and post-processing take time, and often multiple phases must be examined to get a complete exam. (4) Some patients are difficult to image, particularly those with heavily calcified plaques; those who are obese, have rapid heart rates, or arrhythmias; or those who are unable to hold their breath or remain still. (5) Preauthorization requests are sometimes denied by the RBMs, and the hassle the ordering physician must endure can be discouraging. RBMs and payers are more likely to deny recently developed tests like CCTA than older ones. (6) The procedure is not well reimbursed, given the time it takes and its labor-intensive nature. For example, Medicare's national professional component reimbursement for CCTA is $121, compared with $80 for a SPECT MPI. The physician time required for the former may be 3–4× that for the latter. (7) Cardiologists may be reluctant to interpret CCTAs because it would require them to report any abnormalities in the lungs or mediastinum, areas in which they may not feel comfortable. (8) Old habits sometimes die hard; cardiologists who have become accustomed to doing MPI or SE on their patients may be unwilling to give up those procedures.

Is CCTA Being Used Appropriately?

In this author's opinion, the answer to the question is no, CCTA is not being used appropriately. It should be used far more often than it is. In many instances, it should replace MPI as the first imaging test to be used in patients with suspected CAD. There are number of reasons for this, as we discuss below.

The Inadequacy of the Clinical Workup of Suspected CAD when It Relies on More Traditional Noninvasive Imaging

In 2008, three major multicenter trials of CCTA were reported – the ACCURACY trial, the CORE 64 trial, and the Dutch university hospital trial of Meijboom et al. [2–4]. These studies reported on the accuracy of CCTA, using invasive coronary angiography (ICA) as the gold standard in 230, 291, and 360 patients, respectively. All these patients had been worked up by experienced cardiologists and referred for ICA because of high clinical concern for CAD. Many of the workups had included MPI. One of the most striking findings of the three studies was the high percentage of patients who proved to have normal coronary arteries or nonobstructive disease on ICA. In the ACCURACY trial, 75% of the patients had either normal vessels or nonobstructive disease (≤50% stenosis) [2]. In the CORE 64 trial, 44% had either normal vessels or nonobstructive disease [3]. In the Dutch trial [4], there were 151 patients who were diagnosed clinically with typical angina pectoris, yet 30% were found to have normal coronary arteries or nonobstructive disease on ICA. There were 77 sicker patients who were thought clinically to have unstable angina, yet 25% of them had normal vessels or nonobstructive disease. The sickest group of all was 50 patients thought to have non-ST-elevation myocardial infarction, but even in this group, 16% had normal coronary arteries or nonobstructive disease. What these striking data from the three trials show is that the clinical workup of individuals with suspected CAD, which generally includes the use of more traditional imaging techniques like MPI or SE, is not reliable. Too many patients who do not need to go to the cardiac catheterization lab are being sent there for ICA.

Even more striking data comes from the study of Patel et al. [5] which reported on almost 400,000 patients in the National Cardiovascular Data Registry of the American College of Cardiology. All received elective ICA, and 84% had undergone prior noninvasive testing (primarily with MPI) before ICA. Among patients with positive noninvasive tests, 59% had either no disease or nonobstructive CAD. Conversely, among those with negative noninvasive test results, 28% actually did have obstructive CAD on ICA. In other words, the clinical workups of these patients, most of which included noninvasive testing, yielded many false negatives and even more false positives. Here again is further evidence that too many patients are being sent for ICA who do not need it.

The Inability of MPI to Rule Out CAD

A number of studies have shown that negative results on an MPI exam do not exclude the presence of significant CAD [6–12]. Patients with multiple nonobstructive coronary plaques may have normal MPI studies because such plaques do not restrict coronary blood flow, even during exercise. But plaques of this sort can usually be detected on CCTA. This will allow the treating physician to begin aggressive medical therapy, in an effort to avert future disease progression. False-negative MPI results can also occur when obstructing stenoses are present in all three major coronary arteries, as this can lead to balanced ischemia. In addition, in patients with dominant left coronary arteries, left main coronary stenosis can lead to uniform reduction of perfusion of the entire left ventricle and a false-negative MPI exam.

By contrast, the negative predictive value of CCTA is close to 100% [2, 4, 10, 12]. This means it will be a better gatekeeper to the catheterization lab than MPI. If a patient with suspected CAD has an adequate CCTA with a negative result, the treating physician can be assured the patient does not need to undergo ICA.

Direct Comparison of CCTA and MPI

A recent study by Arbab-Zadeh et al. directly compared CCTA with MPI [13]. Patients in the study all underwent the two noninvasive imaging tests and then proceeded to have ICA as the gold standard. Among 245 patients without a previous history of CAD, the per-patient results for CCTA and MPI, respectively, were as follows: sensitivity 0.91 vs 0.55, specificity 0.80 vs 0.70, PPV 0.81 vs 0.63, and NPV 0.91 vs 0.63. The authors concluded that CCTA was more accurate than MPI for the diagnosis of CAD. Another important study was that of Moscariello et al. [14]. They evaluated 185 consecutive patients with chest pain and a positive MPI exam. All patients also underwent CCTA and ICA. Of the 185, ICA revealed that, despite the positive MPI, 110 of them (59%) had either normal coronary arteries or mild nonobstructive plaques. MPI obviously had a high rate of false positives. But in comparison, on a per-patient basis, CCTA had a sensitivity of 100%, specificity of 93.6%, PPV of 91.5%, and NPV of 100%. The better performance of CCTA, and particularly its high NPV, suggests that it ought to be the first imaging test performed in patients with suspected CAD, in preference to MPI or SE.

The Value of CCTA as a Prognostic Examination

MPI is not able to accurately detect nonobstructing coronary artery plaques but CCTA can. Several CCTA studies have compared Kaplan-Meier survival in three groups of patients – those with completely normal coronary arteries, those with nonobstructive CAD, and those with obstructive lesions (≥50% stenosis). Lin et al. [15] found that among 2583 patients who underwent CCTA and were followed for over 3 years, the presence of any nonobstructive plaque was associated with higher mortality (hazard ratio [HR] 1.98) compared with individuals with completely normal coronary arteries. Mortality was progressively greater in patients with nonobstructive CAD in 1, 2, and 3 vessels. Thus, even in patients with mild, low-risk atherosclerotic disease, CCTA can provide valuable prognostic information. Chow et al. [16] followed 2076 patients after CCTA for a mean of 16 months for the occurrence of major adverse cardiac events (MACE). The annual MACE rate was 0.13% in patients whose CCTA exam had demonstrated normal coronary arteries, 0.52% in those with only nonobstructing plaques, 1.44% in those with single-vessel obstructive CAD, 4.3% in those with two-vessel obstructive CAD, and 9.79% in those with three-vessel obstructive CAD.

The results of the large CONFIRM registry, reported by Min et al. [17], provided more evidence of the prognostic value of CCTA. They studied over 24,000 patients without known CAD who underwent CCTA and were followed for all-cause mortality for a mean of 2.3 years. Compared with patients having normal coronary arteries by CCTA, those with nonobstructive disease had a higher risk of mortality (HR 1.62). Additional mortality risk was associated with single-vessel obstructive CAD (HR 2.00), two-vessel obstructive CAD (HR 2.92), and three-vessel or left main obstructive CAD (HR 3.70). Similar findings have been demonstrated by others as well [18–20]. Taken together, these studies point to another great strength of CCTA – its ability to stratify risk and enhance the decision-making process of clinical cardiologists. The studies have shown that while patients with nonobstructive CAD by CCTA may not need PCI or CABG, they are at higher risk than patients with completely normal coronary arteries. They need to be given aggressive medical therapy and, if necessary, counseled about lifestyle modification to prevent disease progression. CCTA also noninvasively allows assessment of risk of one-, two-, and three-vessel obstructive disease, so decisions can be made about whether to send the patient for ICA and possible percutaneous or surgical intervention.

The Advantages of CCTA as the First Imaging Test in Patients with Acute Chest Pain Presenting to the Emergency Department

Approximately 8 million patients present to EDs each year complaining of acute chest pain [21, 22]. It is the second most common chief complaint in ED patients. As much as $8 billion is spent on those patients for subsequent hospitalizations and evaluations that turn out to be negative. Conversely, 2–8% of these cases have acute coronary syndromes that are missed on the initial evaluations. This is obviously a significant public health problem, and it is important to improve efficiency and accuracy of the workup of these ED cases. Recent studies have shown that such improvement is possible through greater use of CCTA.

Goldstein et al. [23, 24] randomized 699 acute chest pain patients to CCTA or MPI as part of their workup in the ED. They found that in the CCTA group, time to diagnosis was reduced by 54%, and cost of ED care was reduced by 38%. In the patients whose index ED imaging test was normal, there was no difference between the two groups in the 6-month incidence of MACE. In another ED study, Litt et al. [24, 25] randomized 908 acute chest pain patients to CCTA and another 462 to traditional care, in which the patient's physicians determined which tests to order. Patients in the CCTA cohort were more frequently discharged directly from the ED (50% vs 23%), had shorter length of stay in the ED (18 h vs 25 h), and had a higher rate of detection of CAD (9.0 vs 3.5%). Of the patients undergoing CCTA, 640 had normal results, and none of them died or experienced an MI within 30 days. Hoffmann et al. [26] studied 1000 ED patients with acute chest pain but no ECG or troponin abnormalities. The patients were randomized to early CCTA or standard evaluation. Mean length of stay was shorter by 7.6 h in the CCTA group. More patients were discharged directly from the ED (47% vs 12%). There was no significant difference between the two groups in incidence of MACE at 28 days. Poon et al. [27] randomized 894 ED patients each to CCTA or standard evaluation (serial ECGs and troponins). The CCTA cohort had a 14% rate of admission to the hospital, compared with 40% among the standard evaluation cohort. Mean length of stay in the ED was 7.7 h among the CCTA group, compared with 11.5 h among the standard evaluation group. Symptoms requiring return to the hospital within 30 days occurred in 1.3% in the CCTA group, compared with 3.6% in the standard evaluation group. The latter group was more than seven times as likely to subsequently undergo ICA without revascularization. There were no cardiac deaths in either group during 30 days of follow-up. Three acute MIs occurred in the CCTA group, compared with six in the standard evaluation group. It seems quite apparent from these four studies of patients presenting to EDs with acute chest pain that early CCTA is the preferred pathway to expeditious diagnosis and disposition.

Advantages of CCTA

Although ICA is still considered the gold standard in diagnosing CAD because of its higher spatial resolution, it is important to recognize that CCTA offers some substantial advantages. It is noninvasive, has less risk and cost, and can be done on an outpatient basis. Reconstructed CCTA images of the coronary arteries can be rotated and viewed from an infinite number of angles, whereas ICA images can only be viewed from the six or seven angles at which the image intensifier was positioned during the contrast injections. On CCTA, the coronary arteries can be viewed in cross section, whereas that is not possible with ICA. Lastly, small calcified plaques are usually not visualized on ICA because the X-ray beam is not sensitive in detecting small calcific deposits, whereas CT is highly sensitive in doing so. Since these small calcified plaques rarely narrow the lumen, their presence will often be missed on ICA when in fact they may be the early harbingers of nonobstructive CAD in what otherwise would appear to be "normal" coronary arteries. Thus ICA may underestimate a patient's atherosclerotic disease burden [28].

Conclusions

The cardiac imaging community is facing a peculiar paradox. There is abundant evidence showing that CCTA is the most appropriate initial imaging test in patients with suspected CAD. The evidence has been presented at length here and elsewhere in this textbook. Yet CCTA is far less commonly utilized than older, less effective tests like MPI and SE (recall that in the Medicare population, MPI is used 53 times as often as CCTA). Possible reasons for this have been discussed earlier. Hopefully some of the obstacles preventing greater use of CCTA will be resolved as time goes on. The imaging equipment will undoubtedly become faster, more efficient, and more automated, thus allowing radiologic technologists to do most of the work without requiring the presence of a physician. Advances in software and machine learning are already occurring and will allow for computer-aided identification of exams that are normal. We must do a better job at educating our primary care colleagues and the nurse practitioners and physician assistants who work for them about the advantages accruing to early use of CCTA in their chest pain patients. Cardiologists and other cardiac imagers who have become overly accustomed to using MPI (perhaps because they own the equipment) should be encouraged to change their approach. As Arbab-Zadeh has pointed out [28], CCTA has come a long way and is ready for prime time. Cardiologists and radiologists must work together to make it happen.

References

1. Go AS, Mozaffarian D, Roger VL, et al. Executive summary: heart disease and stroke statistics – 2014 update. A report from the American Heart Association. Circulation. 2014;129:399–410.
2. Budoff MJ, Dowe D, Jollis JG, et al. Diagnostic performance of 64-multidetector row coronary computed tomographic angiography for evaluation of coronary artery stenosis in individuals without known coronary artery disease. J Am Coll Cardiol. 2008;52:1724–32.
3. Miller JM, Rochitte CE, Dewey M, et al. Diagnostic performance of coronary angiography by 64-row CT. N Engl J Med. 2008;359:2324–36.
4. MeijboomWB MMFL, Schuijf JD, et al. Diagnostic accuracy of 64-slice computed tomography coronary angiography. J Am Coll Cardiol. 2008;52:2135–44.
5. Patel MR, Peterson ED, Dai D, et al. Low diagnostic yield of elective coronary angiography. N Engl J Med. 2010;362:886–95.

6. Schuijf JD, Wijns W, Jukema JW, et al. Relationship between noninvasive coronary angiography with multi-slice computed tomography and myocardial perfusion imaging. J Am Coll Cardiol. 2006;48:2508–14.
7. Weustink AC, Moller NR, Neefjes LA, et al. Diagnostic accuracy and clinical utility of noninvasive testing for coronary artery disease. Ann Intern Med. 2010;152:630–9.
8. Mark DB, Berman DS, Budoff MJ, et al. ACCF/ACR/AHA/NASCI/SAIP/SCAI/SCCT expert consensus document on coronary computed tomographic angiography. Circulation. 2010;121:2509–43.
9. Dorbala S, Hachamovitch R, Carli MF, et al. Myocardial perfusion imaging and multidetector computed tomographic coronary angiography. J Am Coll Cardiol. 2006;48:2515–7.
10. Marwick TH, Cho I, Hartaigh B, Min JK. Finding the gatekeeper to the cardiac catheterization laboratory: coronary CT angiography or stress testing? J Am Coll Cardiol. 2015;65:2747–56.
11. Dilsizian V, Taillefer R. Journey in evolution of nuclear cardiology. Will there be another quantum leap with the F-18 labeled myocardial perfusion tracers? J Am Coll Cardiol Cardiovasc Imaging. 2012;5:1269–84.
12. Chinnaiyan KM, Raff GL, Goraya T, et al. Coronary computed tomography angiography after stress testing. Results from a multicenter statewide registry, ACIC (Advanced Cardiovascular Imaging Consortium). J Am Coll Cardiol. 2012;59:688–95.
13. Arbab-Zadeh A, Di Carli MF, Cerci R, et al. Accuracy of computed tomographic angiography and single-photon emission computed tomography-acquired myocardial perfusion imaging for the diagnosis of coronary artery disease. Circ Cardiovasc Imaging. 2015;8:e003533.
14. Moscariello A, Vliegenthart R, Schoepf UJ, et al. Coronary CT angiography versus conventional cardiac angiography for therapeutic decision making in patients with high likelihood of coronary artery disease. Radiology. 2012;265:385–92.
15. Lin FY, Shaw LJ, Dunning AM, et al. Mortality risk in symptomatic patients with nonobstructive coronary artery disease. J Am Coll Cardiol. 2011;58:510–9.
16. Chow BJW, Wells GA, Chen L, et al. Prognostic value of 64-slice cardiac computed tomography. J Am Coll Cardiol. 2010;55:1017–102817.
17. Min JK, Dunning A, Lin FY, et al. Age- and sex-related differences in all-cause mortality risk based on coronary computed tomography angiography findings. J Am Coll Cardiol. 2011;58:849–60.
18. Russo V, Zavalloni A, Reggiani MLB, et al. Incremental prognostic value of coronary CT angiography in patients with suspected coronary artery disease. Circulation Cardiovasc Imaging. 2010;3:351–9.
19. Van Werkhoven JM, Cademartiri F, Seitun S, et al. Diabetes: prognostic value of CT coronary angiography – comparison with a nondiabetic population. Radiology. 2010;256:83–92.
20. Naisis A, Meridith IT, Sud PS, Cameron JD, Troupis JM, Seneviratne SK. Long-term outcome after CT angiography in patients with possible acute coronary syndrome. Radiology. 2014;272:674–82.
21. Galperin-Aizenberg M, Cooke TS, Hollander JE, Litt HI. Cardiac CT angiography in the emergency department. AJR Am J Roentgenol. 2015;204:463–74.
22. Levin DC, Parker L, Halpern EJ, Julsrud PR, Rao VM. The lack of growth in use of coronary CT angiography: is it being appropriately used? AJR Am J Roentgenol. 2011;196:862–7.
23. Goldstein JA, Chinnaiyan KM, Abidov A, et al. The CT-STAT (coronary computed tomographic angiography for systematic triage of acute chest pain patients to treatment) trial. J Am Coll Cardiol. 2011;58:1414–22.
24. Levin DC, Parker L, Halpern EJ, Rao VM. Recent trends in imaging for suspected coronary artery disease: what is the best approach? J Am Coll Radiol. 2016;13:381–6.
25. Litt HI, Gatsonis C, Snyder B, et al. CT angiography for safe discharge of patients with possible acute coronary syndromes. N Engl J Med. 2012;366:1393–403.
26. Hoffmann U, Truong QA, Schoenfeld DA, et al. (ROMICAT-II) coronary CT angiography versus standard evaluation in acute chest pain. N Engl J Med. 2012;367:299–308.
27. Poon M, Cortegiano M, Abramowicz AJ, et al. Associations between routine coronary computed tomographic angiography and reduced unnecessary hospital admissions, length of stay, recidivism rates, and invasive coronary angiography in the emergency department triage of chest pain. J Am Coll Cardiol. 2013;62:543–52.
28. Arbab-Zadeh A. What will it take to retire invasive coronary angiography? J Am Coll Cardiol Img. 2016;9:565–7.

A Test on the Move: Cardiac CT in China as a Case Study

54

Bin Lu, Weihua Yin, Xinshuang Ren, and Siyu Chen

Cardiovascular Diseases in China

With the rapid economic growth and increased life expectancy, China's population is experiencing rapid transitions; the leading health problems and the challenges imposed on the health system by epidemiological and demographic factors have also changed in recent years. An epidemic of cardiovascular diseases (CVD) in China is emerging as a result of lifestyle changes, urbanization, and the accelerated process of aging. The incidence of CVD is continuously increasing and will remain as an upward trend in the next decades.

In 2014, cardiovascular disease was the leading cause of death in China among both urban and rural areas. Cardiovascular mortality was higher in rural areas than urban areas since 2009. Among rural areas in 2014, cardiovascular mortality was 2.96‰, while cardiac mortality was 1.44‰, and cerebrovascular mortality was 1.52‰ (cerebral hemorrhage 0.75‰, cerebral infarction 0.45‰). Cardiovascular mortality in urban areas was 2.62‰, while cardiac mortality was 1.36‰, and cerebrovascular mortality was 1.26‰ (cerebral hemorrhage 0.52‰, cerebral infarction 0.42‰) [1, 2]. Figure 54.1 shows major disease mortality changes from 1990 to 2014 in rural and urban areas throughout China [3]. The causes of mortality in different provinces of China were systemically analyzed from 1990 to 2013 [3]. Lower respiratory infarction was the primary cause of death in 16 provinces, and another 15 provinces had cerebrovascular disease as the main cause in 1990. Furthermore, in 2013, cerebrovascular disease had been the primary cause of death in 27 provinces and ischemic heart disease in another 5 provinces. Chronic noninfectious diseases including ischemic heart disease, stroke, chronic obstructive pulmonary disease, and neoplasm have a major impact on the human lifespan. The age-adjusted mortality rate of cardiovascular disease decreased from 3.89‰ in 1990 to 3.07‰ in 2013, but the cardiovascular mortality number increased by 46% as a result of the increase in the elder population.

B. Lu (✉) · W. Yin · X. Ren · S. Chen
Department of Radiologic Imaging, Fuwai Hospital, Chinese Academy of Medical Sciences and Peking Union Medical College, National Center of Cardiovascular Diseases, Beijing, China

Cardiovascular Risk Factors in China

Hypertension

According to the 2015 Chinese residents' nutrition and chronic disease status report, incidence of hypertension had increased to 25.2% in residents older than 18 years old, totaling about 270 million people who suffered from hypertension [4]. In 2010, 2043 patients died of hypertension in China, accounting for 24.6% of all-cause death. In the past 50 years, four nationwide hypertension sampling surveys have been done in China; the incidence of hypertension increased among the population of individuals over 15 years old, with rates of 5.1%, 7.7%, 13.6%, and 17.6% in 1959, 1979, 1991, and 2002, respectively [5]. Although many studies have suggested the control of hypertension is an effective strategy to prevent cardiovascular events, systemic analysis of serial cross-sectional health survey data showed that only a small percentage of hypertensive patients achieved the goal of blood pressure control. In 1991, the awareness rate, treatment rate, and control rate of hypertension in China were only 22.4%, 12.0%, and 3.0%, respectively [6]. With the increase of government expenditure on health and improvement of residential health awareness, these same rates increased to 26.1%, 22.8%, and 6.1% in 2009 (Fig. 54.2) [6].

Prior studies showed anxiety, alcohol, salt intake, and obesity were important risk factors of hypertension. A meta-analysis, including eight prospective studies, showed the odds ratio of hypertension in people with anxiety compared to those without was 1.55 (95%CI 1.24–1.94) [7]. Salt intake is higher in Chinese residents in comparison to people from western countries. A study in Shanghai including 19,519 residents, aged 35–91 years old, showed the odds ratio to be 1.117 (95%CI 1.102–1.223) comparing hypertension in people who intake

U. J. Schoepf (ed.), *CT of the Heart*, Contemporary Medical Imaging, https://doi.org/10.1007/978-1-60327-237-7_54

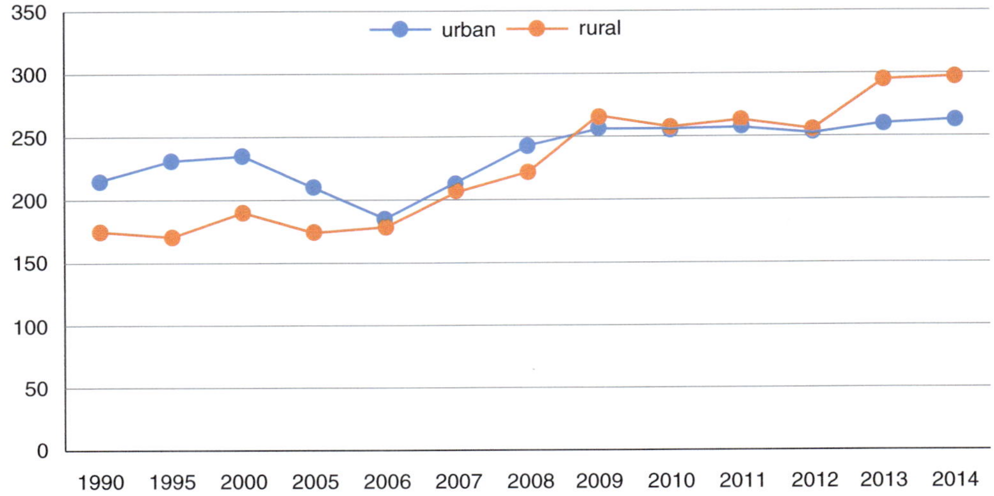

Fig. 54.1 Mortality rates of CVD in urban and rural Chinese populations (China: 1990–2013). (Courtesy of National Center of Cardiovascular Disease of China.)

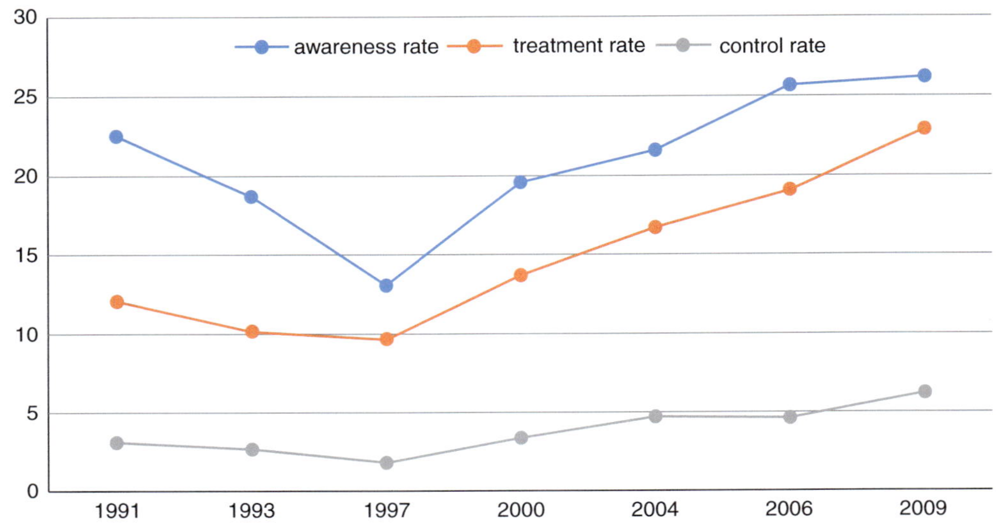

Fig. 54.2 Awareness rate, treatment rate, and control rate of hypertension from 1991 to 2009. (Courtesy of National Center of Cardiovascular Disease of China.)

more than 12 g salt per day and a control group that intakes 6–12 g salt per day [8].

It is important to emphasize secondary hypertension as well, considering more than 10% of hypertension results from renal disease, endocrine dysfunction, and obstructive sleep apnea syndrome [9]. A study in the Xinjiang province showed that 14.76% of hypertensive patients were diagnosed with secondary hypertension; the proportion increased to 21.9% in young patients, and it decreased to 9.85% in elder patients [10]. Renal hypertension was the most common type of secondary hypertension.

Smoking

China is known to have one of the highest smoking rates for adult men since 1984 among countries worldwide. In 2010, a global survey covering 28 provinces in China showed that the smoking rate of Chinese males over 15 years old was 52.9%, while the rate was 2.4% in females [11, 12]. Smoking rates in male doctors and teachers were 40% and 36.5%, respectively, which were higher than the rates in most other countries. A 2012 survey collecting information on a particular population (18–59 years old) in China showed the smoking rate was 55.3% in males and 1.4% in females. Males in the construction industry had the highest smoking rate (58.6%), with the average amount smoked was 15.6 cigarettes per day (15.7% in male, 10.3 in female) [13]. Smoking in adolescents is a serious problem in China. A meta-analysis summarized the smoking prevalence state in adolescents aged 12–17 years old from 1981 to 2010. The smoking rate among male students fluctuated between 39.04% and 46.03%, while the smoking rate among female students, increasing rapidly in recent years, was between 2.47% and 19.44% [14]. Current smoking rate in 2010 was 17.4% in male students and 3.26% in female students.

Tendency of smoking at young age warrants attention. In 2010, GATS survey showed the proportion of students who smoked a whole cigarette before 13 years old in relation to those who were currently smoking was 55.9% in males and 57.0% in females; furthermore, 52.7% of current smokers aged 20–34 years old became daily smokers before 20 years old. Given the high smoking rate in China, secondhand smoke exposure (SHS) reached up to 74.1% in males and 71.6% in females in 2010. About 738 million people suffered from SHS [15]. A prospective study in China showed smoking to be important risk factor of mortality in adults. The relative risk (RR) and population attribute risk (PAR) of all smokers were 1.23 (95%CI 1.18–1.27) and 7.9%. RR and PAR were 1.18 (95%CI 1.13–1.23) and 10.0% in male smokers and 1.27 (95%CI 1.19–1.34) and 3.5% in female smokers [16]. Respiratory disease, cardiovascular disease, and cancer were common causes of death in smokers; 24.1% of male smokers and 4.0% of female smokers died from cardiovascular disease.

The smoking cessation rate increased from 9.42% in 1996 to 16.9% in 2010, and about 16.1% of smokers intended to quit in the next 12 months [15]. The smoking cessation rate for rural areas within Midwest China was very low (1.9%). Though smoking cessation rate increased, there was no change in relapse rate, which was 32.5% in 2002 and 33.1% in 2010 [11, 15]. In order to reduce potential damage caused by SHS, regulations on cigarette control took effect in Beijing on June 1, 2015. Per these regulations, smoking was banned in enclosed public locations, and the advertisement, sales promotion, and sponsorship of cigarettes were prohibited; violators will be fined up to 10,000 yuan.

Hyperlipidemia

Multiple prospective cohort studies certified that serum total cholesterol (TC) and low-density lipoprotein (LDL) are important risk factors associated with cardiovascular events. Total triglyceride (TG) was also shown to be predictive of cardiovascular disease.

According to several international studies, total cholesterol and low-density lipoprotein (LDL) are lower in the Chinese population compared to those in western countries. In 2001, a cross-sectional survey of a nationally representative sample of 15,540 Chinese adults, ages 35–74, showed that the prevalence of hypercholesterolemia was relatively high (24.8%), especially among citizens in developed areas, as well as in middle-aged and elderly individuals [17, 18]. The percentage of adults with controlled blood cholesterol was low in China; only 3.5% of men and 1.5% of women were under control [17]. Chronic disease monitoring in China reported the average levels of serum total cholesterol (TC) and total glyceride (TG) in people older than the age of 18 from 31 provinces. The average level of TC and TG was 4.06 mmol/l and 1.45 mmol/l in men and 4.03 mmol/l and 1.21 mmol/l in women, respectively [19]. Incidence of hyperlipidemia (TC >6.22 mmol/l) was highest in men aged 45–59 years old and in women older than 60 years. The distribution of hyperlipidemia was in accordance to the area. Incidence of hyperlipidemia was higher in urban and eastern areas compared to rural, middle, and western areas [19].

Dyslipidemia in teenagers is a major health problem in China. China's 2002 Nutrition and Health Survey showed that the incidence of hypercholesterolemia (TC >220 mg/dl or 5.72 mmol/l) in children and teenagers (3–18 years old) was 0.8% (1.4% in urban areas, 0.6% in rural areas). The incidence rate of hypertriglyceridemia among this population (TG >150 mg/dl or 1.70 mmol/l) was 2.8% (2.5% in urban areas, 2.9% in rural areas) [20]. A meta-analysis including data from 2001 to 2011 showed incidence of hyperlipidemia in teenagers increased with time. Obese teenagers were more likely to have hyperlipidemia, especially those with family history of hyperlipidemia [21].

Diabetes

China's chronic disease monitor report, published in 2013, reflects the prevalence of diabetes in recent years. Based on 98,658 samples from 162 monitor centers in 31 provinces, the incidence of diabetes in China was 9.7% [22]. Incidence increased with age, and it was higher in urban areas than in rural areas regardless of gender. Regarding people younger than 60 years old, incidence was higher in males; however, incidence was higher in females among people older than 60 years.

In order to investigate the effect of diabetes on mortality in the Chinese population, 690 individuals with newly diagnosed diabetes and 519 nondiabetic individuals were enrolled and monitored for 23 years [23]. In total, 338 (56.5%) diabetic patients and 100 (20.3%) nondiabetic patients died during the follow-up. Cardiovascular disease was the major cause of death for patients with diabetes; collectively, 47.5% of males and 49.7% of females died of cardiovascular disease, with nearly half of them passing due to stroke (52.3% of males, 42.3% of females). Incidence of all-cause mortality per year in patients with diabetes was 3 times that of the incidence in nondiabetic individuals (male, 36.9‰ vs 13.3‰; female, 27.1‰ vs 9.2‰). Diabetic females had higher risk of cardiovascular mortality than diabetic males (HR 6.9 vs 3.5).

The Daqing Diabetes Prevention Study was the first and longest-running lifestyle intervention research study for diabetes worldwide. Individuals in the experimental group were under positive lifestyle intervention for 6 years. After 20 years of follow-up, the results showed that lifestyle intervention reduces the risk of diabetes by 51%. The cumulative incidence rate of diabetes in people with lifestyle intervention was 80% and a rate of 93% in the control group. Adjusted to age and grouping random factors, incidence of diabetes in the experimental group was still lower than that in control group, and the odds ratio for lifestyle intervention was 0.57 (95%CI 0.41–0.81). The onset of diabetes in the experimental group was 3.6 years later than that in control group [24]. In addition, lifestyle intervention decreases the risk of severe retinopathy (laser treatment or blindness) by 47% [25]. For patients with impaired glucose tolerance in the Daqing Diabetes Prevention Study, lifestyle intervention decreased the all-cause mortality by 29% and cardiovascular mortality by 41% [26].

The 3B study approach investigated risk factors for cardiovascular disease among type 2 diabetics [27]. In total, 25,817 diabetic patients from 104 hospitals were included. The average age was 62.6 years old, and 47% of the enrolled patients were male. In all, 72% of these patients had hypertension or hyperlipidemia. Incidence of cardiovascular events in diabetic patients with combined hypertension or hyperlipidemia was six times that of patients with isolated diabetes. Independent predictors of cardiovascular events included the following: low BMI (<24 kg/m^2), no smoking or drinking, high-level education, and course of, diabetes for less than 5 years.

Overweight and Obesity

Incidence of individuals who are overweight (BMI 24.0–27.9 kg/m^2) or obese (BMI >28.0 kg/m^2) increased in recent years with changes in lifestyle and development of economy. China's 2002 Nutrition and Health Survey showed the overweight rate was 17.6%, and the obesity rate was 5.6% [28]. Nutrition and health status surveillance of nine provinces showed overweight and obesity rates increased rapidly over the past 20 years, reaching 44% in 2011 [29]. The Chronic Disease Monitor Program in China reports that in 2010, the overweight rate, obesity rate, and central obesity rate were 30.6%, 12.0%, and 40.7%, respectively. These rates were much higher than the rates reported in 2002 [30]. Sample surveys in the Guangdong province showed central obesity rate increased from 12.9% in 2002 to 23.7% in 2010, which implied a change of obesity type [31]. The prevalence of obesity in adolescents was not optimistic. Data from the National Survey on Chinese Students' Physical Fitness and Health between 1985 and 2010 showed an obvious increase of overweight and obesity rate in students aged 7–18 years old. The overweight and obesity rates in 2010 were 8.7 times and 38.1 times those in 1985 (overweight, 9.6% vs 1.1%; obesity, 5.0% vs 0.1%) [32].

Obesity, especially central obesity, was an important cardiovascular risk factor. A prospective study including 270,000 participants, aged 35–74 years old, showed positive correlation between waistline and new-onset diabetes. Waistline/height ratio (WHtR) is a simple indicator evaluating the extent of central obesity. Several Chinese studies showed individuals with central obesity (WHtR >0.50) had increased risk of cardiovascular disease.

Lack of Physical Activity

A cross-sectional study including 460,000 adults, aged 35–74 years old, showed that the average physical activity level was 21.7 MET-h/d, mainly attributed to occupational activity (62%) and housework (26%) [33]. China's Nutrition and Health Survey reported citizen physical activity decreased from 1991 to 2011, especially occupational activity. Male occupational activity decreased from 382 MET-h/w to 264 MET-h/w in 2011, while female occupational activity decreased from 420 MET-h/w to 243 MET-h/w [34]. The percentage of exercise remains low with less than 7 MET--h/w in males and less than 7 MET-h/w in females. A 2011 survey of students aged 11–18 years old showed that the rate of reaching standard physical activity was only 19.9%, 25.1% in boys and 14.6% in girls [35].

Results from an additional study showed that physical activity negatively relates to incidence of diabetes. This Chinese multicenter study showed morbidity of diabetes decreased with increased physical activity. Mortality risk of ischemic heart disease (HR 1.20–1.71), ischemic stroke (HR 1.05–1.53), and diabetes (HR1.11–1.45) was higher in people with lack of physical activity than those with sufficient physical activity [36].

Unreasonable Diet

Dietary structure in China has changed in recent years [37]. Characteristics of the new dietary structure that are against the prevention of cardiovascular disease include the following: decrease in cereal intake, obvious increase in fat intake, low intake of vegetables and fruits, and high intake of salt (15.9 g/d). The Chinese Nutrition and Health Survey showed that the percentage of people getting more than 30% energy from fat increased from 35.8% in 1989 to 55.0% in 2009. Sodium intake decreased in recent years but remains at a high level (4.7 g/d). Potassium intake increased in recent years, yet it is still below recommended dose (2 g/d). A nationwide disease survey of 970,000 people showed that more than 60% of citizens are aware of the negative effects of salt on health and 40% of citizens had taken measures to decrease salt intake.

A prospective research study conducted in Shanghai showed that compliance score to diet recommendation negatively relates to all-cause mortality and cardiovascular mortality [38]. The amount of vegetable and fruits consumed in the diet negatively relates to coronary artery disease. Cardiovascular risk decreased by 38% in the females with a high intake of vegetables and fruits (medium 814 g/d) compared with those with a low intake (medium 274 g/d) [39]. There was no significant difference found among male citizens. In addition, the amount of salt intake positively relates with onset hypertension; however, potassium intake negatively relates with this condition. A meta-analysis showed that low-sodium intake can remarkably decrease systolic blood pressure by 4.9 mmHg and diastolic blood pressure by 1.5 mmHg [40].

Air Pollution

A great number of studies show that particulate matter (PM) in the air, especially PM2.5, presents as an independent risk factor of cardiovascular disease [41]. Recent studies evaluated the relationship between exposure duration and onset of cardiovascular disease, as well as cardiovascular mortality. Particular matters such as PM2.5, SO_2, and NOx prove to relate with cardiovascular disease. The following chart summarizes studies that evaluated the effect of PM2.5 (Table 54.1) [42–48]. From 2010 to 2012, a study was conducted in Beijing to monitor air condition and showed that ischemic heart disease onset and mortality increased by 0.27% (95%CI 0.21–0.33%) and 0.25% (95%CI 0.10–0.40%), respectively, with every 10 ug/m^3 increase in PM2.5. PM2.5 had a hysteresis effect on the onset of ischemic heart disease as the onset rate increased at the first, second, and third day after exposure of PM2.5. Also, the results showed that people older than 65 years were more sensitive to PM2.5; the correlation between onset ischemic heart disease and the concentration of PM2.5 in people older than 65 was stronger than those younger than 65.

Studies showed long-term exposure to outdoor air pollution had a greater impact on cardiovascular disease. In a cohort study, researchers retrieved air condition data from an air condition monitoring station and analyzed the relationship between particulate matter exposure and cardiovascular mortality according to the results of a 10-year (1991–2000) follow-up [50]. Baseline PM exposure dose was correlated with cardiovascular mortality: every 10 ug/m^3 increase in concentration of total PM, SO_2, and NOx leads to an increase of cardiovascular mortality risk by 0.9% (95%CI 0.3–1.5%), 3.2% (95%CI 2.3–4.0%), and 2.3% (95%CI 0.6–4.1%), respectively. A cohort study in Shenyang including 24,845 people showed that every 20 ug/m^3 increase in SO_2 leads to a 19% (OR 1.19, 95%CI 1.05–1.34) increase in hypertension among males. No correlation was found in female participants. Moreover, a cohort study conducted in Hong Kong evaluated the relationship between PM exposure and cardiovascular disease mortality in older participants (>65 years old) during 10–13-year follow-up. The results showed that cardiovascular mortality increased by 22% (HR 1.22, 95%CI 1.08–1.39), ischemic heart disease mortality by 42% (HR 1.42, 95%CI 1.16–1.73), and cerebrovascular mortality by 24% (HR 1.24, 95%CI 1.00–1.53) with every 10 ug/m^3

Table 54.1 Relationship between PM2.5 concentrations and CVD mortality

Monitoring time	Region	PM2.5 concentrations (mean)	Outcome indicator/No.	CVD risk (95% CI)
2004–2005	Shanghai [42]	56.4 μg/m^3	Total mortality/79,530	Every 10 μg/m^3 increase, mortality of CVD increases 0.41% (0.01–0.82%)
2004–2008	Xian [43]	176.7 μg/m^3	——	Every 10 μg/m^3 increase, mortality of CVD increases 0.27% (0.08–0.46%), mortality of coronary heart diseases increases 0.39% (0.14%, 0.65%)
2004–2008	Xian [44]	Median 2004 184.9 μg/m^3 2005 194.9 μg/m^3 2006 206.8 μg/m^3 2007 193.7 μg/m^3 2008 179.1 μg/m^3	Mortality of CVD/22,051	Every 100 μg/m^3 increases, mortality of CVD, coronary heart diseases, and stroke increases 6.18%, 8.23%, and 5.13%, respectively
2006–2008	Shenyang [45]	75 μg/m^3	Total mortality/60,938	Every 10 μg/m^3 increases, mortality of CVD increases 0.53% (0.09–0.97%); mortality of CVD in population aged ≥75 years old increases 0.64% (0.02–1.24%)
2007–2008	Guangzhou [46]	70.1 μg/m^3	Total mortality/58,400	Every 10 μg/m^3 increases, mortality of CVD increases 1.22% (0.63–1.68%)
2006–2011	Shanghai [47]	55 μg/m^3	Mortality of out-of-hospital coronary heart diseases/18,202	Every 10 μg/m^3 increases, mortality of out-of-hospital coronary heart diseases increases 0.68% (0.14–1.21%)
2010–2012	Beijing [48]	96.2 μg/m^3	Mortality of ischemic heart diseases/53,247	Every 10 μg/m^3 increases, mortality of ischemic heart diseases increases 0.25% (0.10–0.40%)

From National Health and Family Planning Commission of the People's Republic of China [49], with permission increase in PM2.5. A large amount of epidemiologic evidence proves the correlation between air pollution and cardiovascular disease; but, as most of the studies were observational, more experimental studies were needed for further evaluation.

Cardiovascular Disease

Cerebrovascular Disease

The Department of Health in China has organized a nationwide health survey every 5 years since 1993. According to the reports, incidence of cerebrovascular disease in China increased in recent years, and the incidence in urban areas was higher than that in rural areas. China Health Statistics Yearbook 2015 reported cerebrovascular mortality in urban areas was 1.26‰, cerebral hemorrhage mortality was 0.52‰, and cerebral infarction mortality was 0.42‰ for the year 2014. For that same year, cerebrovascular mortality in rural areas was 1.52‰, while cerebral hemorrhage mortality was 0.75‰, and cerebral infarction mortality was 0.45‰. The related figures suggest a higher mortality rate in rural areas than in urban areas. Cerebrovascular mortality rate increased with age, and the rate was higher in men than in women after adjusted to age, regardless of the region (Fig. 54.3).

China's 2010 Chronic Disease and Risk Factor Surveillance investigated 98,658 adults to figure out the incidence of transient ischemic attack adjusted to age was 2.27%. Transient ischemic attack (TIA) was common in older female with low education, smoking history, hypertension, myocardial infarction, or diabetes. Only 3.08% of adults were aware of the disease, and only 4.07% of TIA patients received recommended therapy [51].

Coronary Artery Disease

According to the nationwide health survey, incidence of ischemic heart disease in 2008 was 15.9‰ in urban areas and 4.8‰ in rural areas, which was much higher than incidence rates in 2003 (12.4‰ in urban areas, 4.6‰ in rural areas) [52].

Coronary artery mortality was 1.08‰ in urban areas and 1.05‰ in rural areas for the year 2014; furthermore, mortality rate in men was higher than that in women. Coronary artery disease mortality rate increased in recent years. Mortality rate in rural areas increased rapidly since 2012 and closely approached the rate in urban areas in 2014 (Fig. 54.4). Rate of acute myocardial infarction had an upward trend from 2002 to 2014. The mortality rate rose fast since 2005, and mortality rate in rural areas went over the rate in urban areas since 2007 (Fig. 54.5) [52].

Heart Failure

In 2000, the prevalence of chronic heart failure among the Chinese population aged 35–74 years was 0.9%: 0.7% in men and 1.0% in women. Prevalence was higher in the north than the south and higher in urban areas. The prevalence of heart failure increased significantly with age. During the past two to three decades, the main cause for heart failure has shifted from rheumatic valvular heart disease to coronary heart disease [53].

The preliminary results from the China Heart Failure Registry Study (China-HF) showed that currently the average age of patients with heart failure is 66 ± 15 years old and has been rising. From this population, 54.5% of HF patients are male, and 84.7% of the patients were at III–IV levels according to the NYHA functional classification criteria. The main comorbidities with heart failure have changed significantly: the proportion with valvular diseases

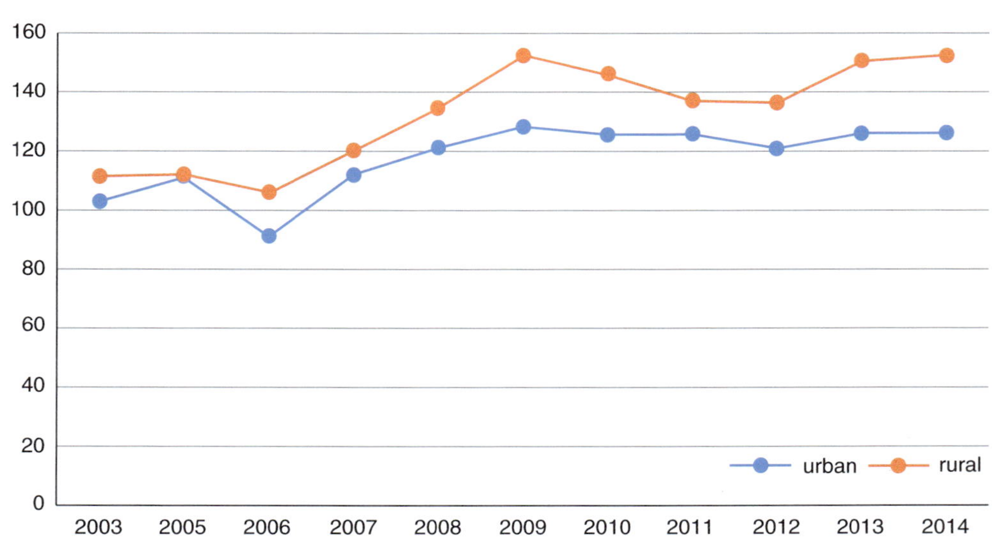

Fig. 54.3 Trends in stroke mortality (China: 2003–2014). (Courtesy of National Center of Cardiovascular Disease of China.)

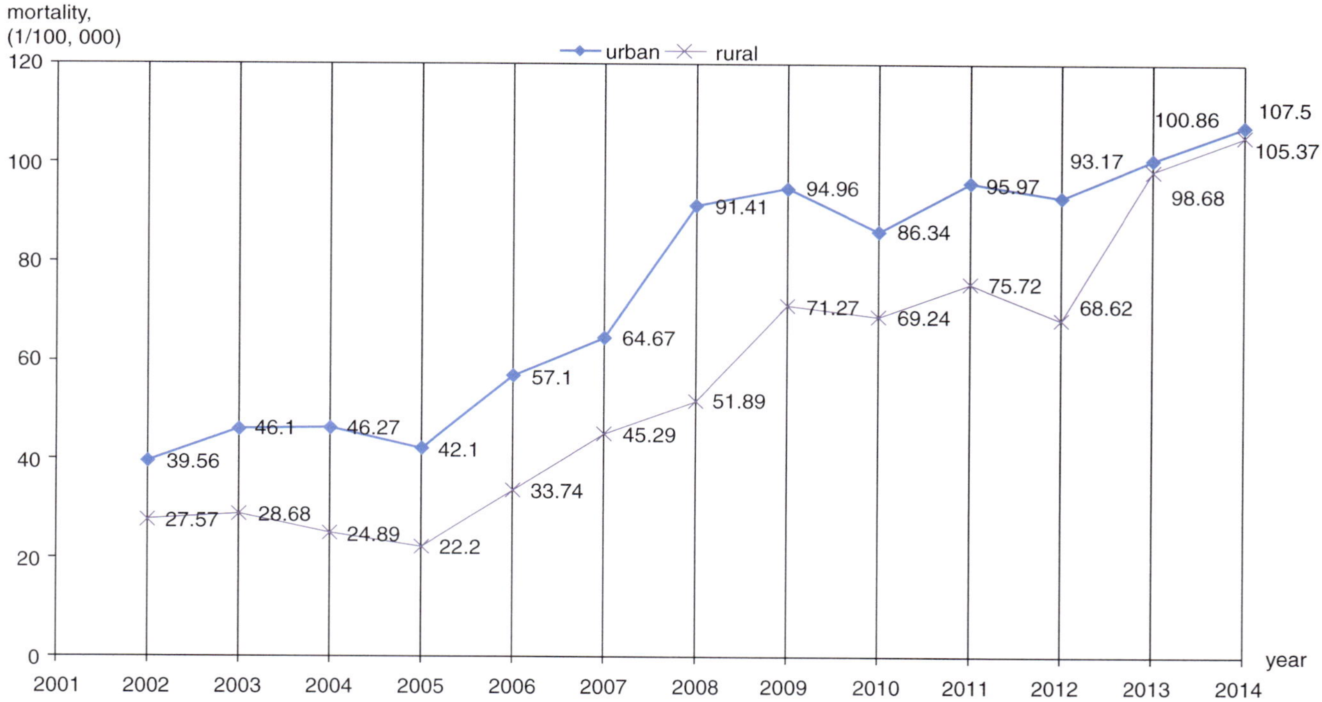

Fig. 54.4 Coronary heart disease mortality trends in urban and rural areas between 2002 and 2014. (Courtesy of National Center of Cardiovascular Disease of China.)

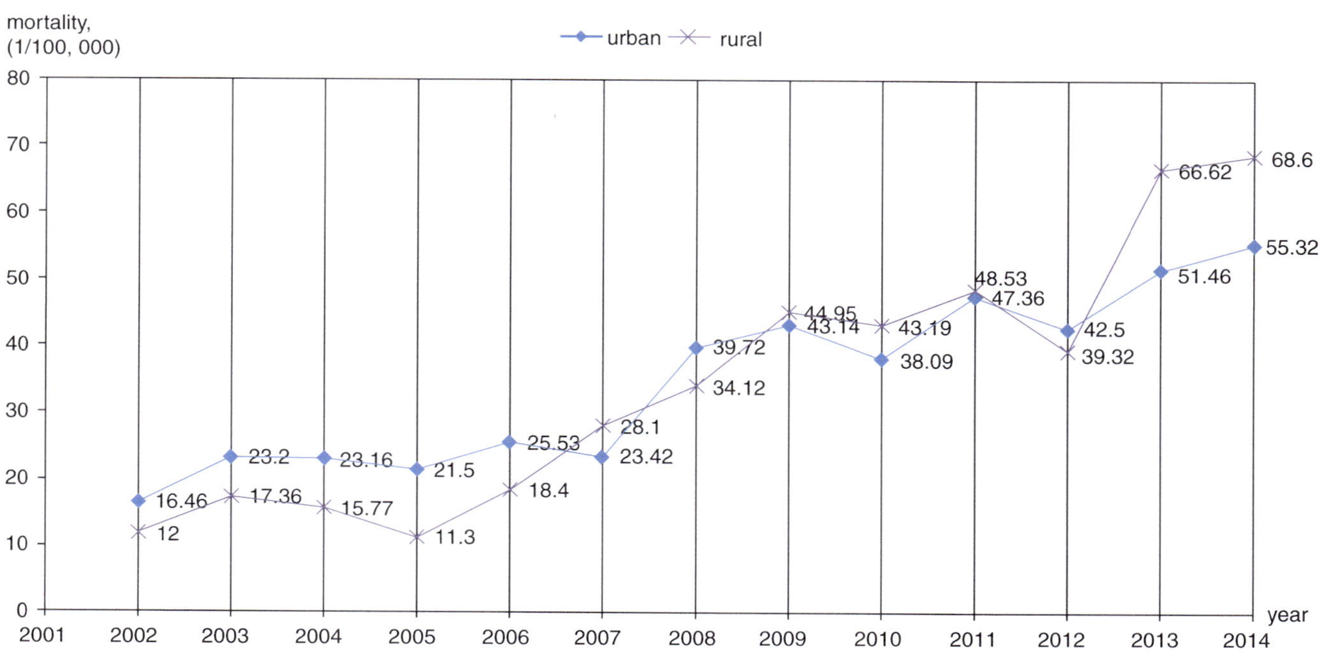

Fig. 54.5 Acute myocardial infarction mortality trends in urban and rural areas between 2002 and 2014. (From National Health and Family Planning Commission of the People's Republic of China [49], with permission.)

has gradually decreased; coronary artery disease (49.4%), hypertension (54.6%), and chronic kidney disease (29.7%) have become the most common comorbidities. Infection (45.9%) continues to be the primary reason for the onset of heart failure, followed by fatigue or stress (26.0%) and then myocardial ischemia (23.1%). The usage of diuretics in patients during hospitalization has not changed significantly. The usage of digoxin showed a downward trend due to the effects of international clinical trials. The use of angiotensin II receptor antagonist (24.6%), aldosterone receptor antagonist (55.4%), and beta-receptor blocker (50.6%) has increased significantly [54].

Medical Care Expenditure [55–57]

Since 1980, the amount of inpatients increased and amplified rapidly after 2000. The medical cost of cardiovascular disease increased correspondingly. The growth rate of medical costs was even higher than the rate of GDP, which resulted from the increasing need for inpatient services and high proportion of unreasonable medicine use.

The number of discharged patients diagnosed with cardiovascular disease was 17,938,600 in 2014, accounting for 12.75% of total inpatients. From this inpatient total, 6.63% were patients with heart disease, and 6.12% were patients with cerebrovascular disease. Ischemic heart disease (6,553,700 per year), acute myocardial infarction (541,400 per year), and cerebral infarction (5,319,900 per year) were the main diagnoses among the patients; the others were hypertension (2,526,100 per year), intracranial hemorrhage (1,299,900 per year), and rheumatic heart disease (250,100 per year).

The growth rate of inpatients diagnosed with cardiovascular disease was 10.10% per year, faster than average inpatient growth rate (6.33%). The growth rate rank in patients with cardiovascular disease included the following: cerebral infarction (12.3%), ischemic heart disease (11.74%), intracranial hemorrhage (9.76%), acute myocardial infarction (8.12%), hypertension (8.06%), hypertensive cardiomyopathy and nephropathy (5.82%), and rheumatic heart disease (1.43%).

Hospitalization costs for acute myocardial infarction in 2014 totaled $1.34 billion, while intracranial hemorrhage was $2.08 billion and cerebral infarction $4.70 billion. The growth rates of these conditions were 32.02%, 18.90%, and 24.96% per year, respectively, since 2004. Single hospitalization cost of acute myocardial infarction, intracranial hemorrhage, and cerebral infarction was 24,706 yuan, 15,929.7 yuan, and 8,841.4 yuan, respectively. The growth rates were 8.72%, 6.63%, and 2.81% per year.

Drug expenses for cardiovascular disease in hospitals with more than 100 beds were 65.6 billion yuan. The top five expenses were drugs improving cardiovascular circulation, myocardial nutrition and drugs improving coronary flow, lipid-lowering drugs, calcium channel blockers, and angiotensin receptor blockers.

Current Practice of Cardiac Imaging (CT) in China

High-Technology Medical Equipment

Many researchers have reported on inequities in health status, healthcare, health insurance, and healthcare workforce in China; yet, only a small number of studies have focused on equity in distribution of high-technology medical equipment, such as computed tomography (CT). He et al. examined the issue using panel data from multiple provinces in 2006 and 2009, providing information not only about the numbers of CTs and magnetic resonance imaging (MRI) but also detailed characteristics about these types of equipment such as machine model, price, and government subsidies for purchasing the machine. To inform China policymaking on allocation of CTs and MRIs, He et al. compare the growth of the high-technology equipment between the study provinces and a group of selected industrialized countries [58].

Examining equity in distribution of CTs and MRIs in China is particularly important for several reasons. First, unnecessary allocation and overuse of these two types of high-technology medical equipment have been a known part of the medical arms race in industrialized countries. Given the rapid economic growth in China, with the world's second largest economy, some experts were concerned that a similar phenomenon of medical race might occur in China, although they have not conducted empirical analyses to quantify their concerns. Second, availability of healthcare resources, including CT and other types of high-technology medical equipment, is important in defining the healthcare system's performance. One analysis of all 30 Organization for Economic Cooperation and Development (OECD) countries concluded that distributions of CTs positively correlate with total health expenditure per capita and economic incentives to hospitals [59]. Researchers from developing countries have also paid attention to CT disseminations. Third, there is a huge gap in socioeconomic development among eastern, middle, and western regions of China. Because the eastern region has more healthcare resources, an arms race among hospitals may exacerbate the equity problem in China's allocation of healthcare resources across regions. Fourth, one study reported that the number of CTs in China increased 55.4% and the number of MRIs increased 90.2% from 2002 to 2005 [60]. While the newer versions of the equipment quickly provide higher-quality images at greater prices, they also raise issues of equity regarding which hospitals purchased them and whether the government subsidized the purchase [61].

Finally, in response to the heavy investment in high-technology medical equipment by hospitals, China's central government implemented a policy in 2005 called the Chinese Certificate of Need (CON), which aims to improve "appropriate allocation and efficient use of large medical equipment" through regional health planning and quota control. Nevertheless, it remains an unsettled question whether implementation of the policy results in reasonable growth and more equitable distributions of CT and MRI.

As shown in Table 54.2, there are substantial geographic, demographic, and economic differences among the study sites analyzed by He et al. [58]. Shanghai has the highest population density and lowest rural population percentage, and it was ranked first in GDP per capita among the four cities in 2009.

Table 54.3 shows CT distributions in the selected OECD countries. Among the selected countries, Japan had the highest number of CTs in 2009 (97.3%), while the UK had the lowest level (7.4%). In comparison, the study sample in China is lower than that of the UK.

Most of the selected OECD countries had a growing number of CTs between 2006 and 2009 except Australia and the UK, both of which had negative growth of CTs. In comparison, all the study sites in China had a positive growth rate of CTs from 2006 to 2009, and the growth rate was higher than most of the selected OECD countries.

He et al. found that China had lower numbers of CTs per million people in 2009 than most of the selected OECD countries, despite the increases in its CT numbers from 2006 to 2009 being higher than most of the OECD countries. These findings suggest that China is the largest developing country but still lags behind the developed countries in high-technology medical equipment, such as CTs. On the other hand, with the rapid economic development and large population, the number of CTs in China increased substantially in these years [58].

Table 54.2 Description of the study sites in 2009

Study site	Shanghai	Zhejiang	Shanxi	Hunan
Location	Eastern China	Eastern China	Northwest China	Central China
Number of cities within site	/	14	13	17
Area (10,000 km^2)	0.63	10.18	20.58	21.18
Population	19	47	38	69
Population density (person/km^2)	3049	463	183	326
Percentage of rural population (%)	11.4	42.1	56.5	56.8
GDP per capita (CNY)	78,326	48,196	21,659	19,479
Rank of GDP per capita	1	5	16	20

Table 54.3 Number of CTs in the study sites and the selected OECD countries

Study sites in China	2009	Change from 2006 to 2009 (%)
Shanghai	7.6	62.7
Zhejiang	8.3	31.0
Shanxi	8.5	63.8
Hunan	6.0	42.2
OECD countries		
Australia	38.8	−30.7
Austria	29.9	1.0
Canada	13.9	15.8
Denmark	23.7	50.0
Finland	20.5	38.5
Greece	33.9	28.4
Ireland	15.8	23.4
Israel	7.7	42.6
Iceland	34.5	42.6
Japan	97.3	5.1
New Zealand	14.6	18.7
R.O. Korea	37.1	10.1
UK	7.4	−1.3
USA	34.3	6.5
Entire sample	41.8	1.04

Despite the improvement in equity status of CTs in some of the study sites, He et al. found that the distributions of CTs positively correlated with economic development level across all cities in the four study sites in either 2006 or 2009. He et al. also found that the vast majority of CTs were imported and only a small percentage were made by domestic Chinese firms, indicating that China is still at a low level of high-technology medical equipment development [58].

Cardiac CT Imaging

Cardiac CT and its main application, coronary CT angiography (CTA), remain a challenge because of rapid cardiac motion in combination with small dimensions and complex anatomy. It requires a dedicated CT system, ECG-synchronized data acquisition or image reconstruction, as well as advanced post-processing and interpretation. Nationwide surveys describing cardiac CT utilization have been performed in the USA and Germany, but there is a lack of data from China. While the use of coronary CTA has increased sharply, there are inadequate data describing the number, indications, and acquisition techniques of coronary CTA examinations. Also, there may be significant regional imbalance regarding utilization of cardiac CT, data acquisition, contrast injection protocols, radiation exposure, and diagnostic analytic skills across China.

Fuwai Hospital launched a national survey to investigate the utilization of cardiac CT in China and to develop a national coronary CTA information database, allowing comparisons between our findings and those from other countries. A 25-item questionnaire was designed. Initial questions were used for the following: to identify a contact person at each hospital; to confirm the availability of at least one advanced, dedicated CT scanner; and to confirm that the volume of coronary CTA procedures exceeded 100 in the last 12 months. Only hospitals fulfilling these criteria were included in the subsequent analysis. This survey was conducted from December 2014 to February 2015. The remaining questions pertained to the type of facility, the indications for cardiac CT, patient preparation, and technical aspects of the acquisition protocols. Additional questions referred to storage and interpretation of cardiac CT data sets and future needs for cardiac CT.

Hospitals in China are organized according to a three-tier system. They are designated as primary, secondary, or tertiary institutions that are recognized by the hospital's ability to provide different levels of medical care and medical education and conduct medical research. Based on the level of service, size, medical technology, and available medical equipment, the three tiers are further subdivided into three subsidiary levels A, B, and C, resulting in a total of nine levels. Our survey focused on tertiary hospitals, because primary and secondary hospitals in China typically do not perform cardiac CT. The final minimal sample size was 240, to include a buffer of 5%. Finally, after the removal of hospitals that refused participation, there were 152 hospitals that participated in this study with at least 1 dedicated CT (64 rows or above) performing more than 100 CTA in the last year (Fig. 54.6). The median annual number of coronary CTA procedures performed at these institutions was 1037 (range, 150–8072).

Common clinical indications for coronary CTA included the following: exclusion of coronary artery disease in patients with low to intermediate likelihood of disease in 100% of centers (152/152); screening to rule out coronary artery disease in asymptomatic individuals in 95% (145/152); exclusion of coronary anomalies in 64% (98/152); evaluation for pericardial disease in 39% (59/152); follow-up of patients with coronary stents in 28% (43/152); diagnosis of coronary artery disease in patients with a high pretest likelihood in 21% (32/152); and triple rule-out in 18% (28/152). Maurer listed coronary CTA indications in Germany and other countries, which were different from our findings (Table 54.4).

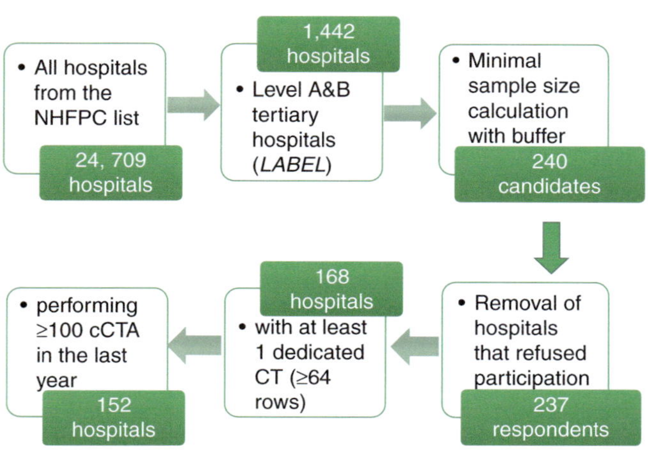

Fig. 54.6 A total of 152 tertiary hospitals in China were randomized enrolled for the nationwide survey of cardiac CT imaging

Beta-blockers were routinely used by 30.3% (46/152) of hospitals regardless of the heart rates before coronary CTA and administered based on heart rate limits in the remaining sites. The respective thresholds were 65–74 beats/minute at 57 of 152 sites (38%), 75–84 beats/minute at 34 (22%) sites, and 85–100 beats/minute at 15 (10%) hospitals. Routine administration of sublingual nitroglycerin prior to cardiac CT was reported by 131/152 respondents (86%). In all hospitals (100%), patient breath-hold capacity was tested before the scan. The majority (96/152, 63%) of respondents stated that they did not perform cardiac CT in patients with atrial fibrillation, 35 (23%) did so occasionally and depending on circumstances, and 21 (14%) stated they did routinely.

Tube current was adjusted to the patient's body weight or body mass index by 90/152 sites (59%), and 123 sites (81%) used lead aprons to shield the thyroid gland and/or genitals. Prospectively ECG-triggered image acquisition was used in more than 90% of cases by 20/152 hospitals (13%), between 50% and 89% of all cases by 47 hospitals (31%), between

Table 54.4 Coronary CTA indications in China and in other countries

Indications	Frequency% in China [62]	Frequency% in Germany (Maurer [63])	Frequency% in worldwide countries)
Exclusion of CAD in patients with low-intermediate pretest likelihood	100 (152/152)	91 (41/45)	97 (164/169)
Exclusion of CAD in healthy people	95 (145/152)	20 (9/45)	34 (58/169)
Follow-up of coronary bypass	66 (101/152)	78 (35/45)	76 (128/169)
Exclusion of coronary anomaly	64 (98/152)	80 (36/45)	92 (156/169)
Evaluation of pericardial disease	39 (59/152)	4 (2/45)	Not applicable
Follow-up of patients' coronary stents	28 (43/152)	36 (16/45)	33 (56/169)
Diagnosis of CAD in patients with a high pretest likelihood	21 (32/152)	22 (10/45)	33 (55/169)
Triple rule-out	18 (28/152)	53 (24/45)	44 (75/169)

11% and 49% by 70 hospitals (46.0%), and in 10% or less by 15 sites (10%). In addition, 57 hospitals (38%) had experience with the use of novel coronary CTA acquisition techniques, including single-shot snap, high-pitch, or prospective acquisition. Iterative reconstruction algorithms were used by 125 hospitals (82%). In our survey, 24 of 152 hospitals (16%) identified >15 mSv as the modal value of radiation dose, 64/152 (42%) stated 10–15 mSv, 48 (32%) cited a range of 6–9 mSv, 16 hospitals (11%) quoted 3–5 mSv, and no hospitals stated <3 mSv (Fig. 54.7). The median dose among all hospitals was 10–15 mSv, but after adjustment by coronary CTA volume, the median dose among all patients was between 6 and 9 mSv.

Regarding contrast media suppliers, we investigated the market shares of domestic and foreign vendors and found that 43/152 hospitals (28%) used foreign products for almost all patients (≥90%), 44 (29%) used foreign products in most of their patients (50–89%), 32 hospitals (21%) used foreign contrast agents in less than half of their studies (11–49%), and 33 hospitals (22%) used foreign products in few or no cases (≤10%). Only 24/152 sites (16%) adjusted the contrast injection rate based on patient body weight or body mass index. Over 97% used biphasic or triphasic injection protocols for contrast injection (biphasic, 74%; triphasic, 23%; and monophasic, 3%).

The vast majority of respondents (145/152; 95%) stored image data in PACS, and the remaining 7 sites stored them on compact disks. The average duration of a coronary CTA examination was estimated to be 14.2 min (median 15 min; range 5–30 min, Fig. 54.8), the average estimated post-processing time was 13.6 min (median 15 min; range 5–25 min), and the estimated time required for interpretation and reporting was 18.0 min (median 20 min; range 8–30 min).

Only 46/152 centers (30%) reported that they also evaluated pulmonary and other non-cardiac structures. In most hospitals (123/152, 81%), coronary artery calcium scores (Agatston scores) were not calculated. Instead, a qualitative degree of calcification (i.e., mild, moderate, and severe) was reported.

To our knowledge, this is the first nationwide survey describing cardiac CT, and especially coronary CTA utilization, in mainland China. We used random sampling of hospitals in all Chinese provinces in order to reflect geographic differences in population and economic status. Routine components of cardiac CT including scanner technology, clinical indications, image acquisition techniques, contrast media injections protocols, image reconstruction and interpretation, and clinical challenges are described. This study provides a comprehensive picture of current cardiac CT utilization in China.

It was initiated and conducted by the Chinese International Regional Committee of the Society of Cardiovascular Computed Tomography (SCCT IRC China). In order to limit expenses, questionnaires were collected by either the marketing team of GE Healthcare China or the authors themselves. However, random verification of questionnaires provided by GE addressed concerns regarding commercial bias.

Together with other professional organizations, SCCT released appropriate use criteria for cardiac CT in 2010 and two guidelines for the interpretation and reporting of coronary CTA in 2009 and 2014 [62]. The authors of this report, as members of the cardiothoracic group of Chinese Society of Radiology, published a Chinese coronary CTA guideline in January 2011 in the form of an expert consensus document. These documents played a significant role in promoting the development of cardiac CT in China. Nevertheless,

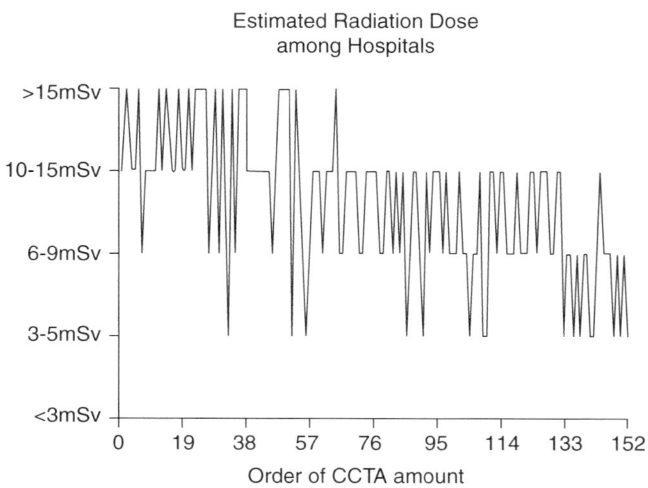

Fig. 54.7 Estimated radiation dose among hospitals were 6–9 mSv in median

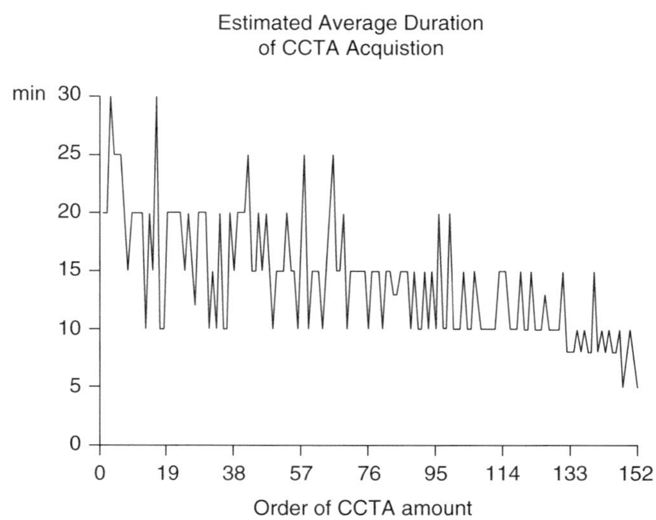

Fig. 54.8 The average duration of a coronary CTA examination was estimated to be 15 min (range 5–30 min)

the survey results suggest that the utilization of cardiac CT in mainland China is still limited by several factors. First, high-end cardiac CT scanners are not uniformly available. Although the hospitals targeted by our survey were of the highest level in China, one third of candidate hospitals did not have a dedicated, high-end cardiac CT scanner available. Participating hospitals were all public; thus obtaining such an expensive scanner (64+ CT) via government procurement is difficult. Furthermore, a percentage of the participating hospitals are centers specialized on cancer care, pediatric hospitals, maternity hospitals, mental hospitals, and traditional Chinese medicine hospitals, and as such, cardiovascular diseases are not their major concern. Second, several of the clinical scenarios which were considered appropriate and frequent indications for coronary CTA by the hospitals in this survey are actually inappropriate by current clinical guidelines. For example, 95% of respondents stated that they performed coronary CTA in clinically healthy individuals, which is rated as inappropriate in current guidelines [65]. While a few experts recommend the use of coronary CTA as a screening test, these so-called "health check-up" indications may reflect an undesirable trend of aggressive marketing of cardiac CT [66]. Chinese physicians may not always refuse a patients' "unreasonable" request, especially in areas of rapidly evolving healthcare and in certain socioeconomic environments [67]. Third, the estimated radiation dose was relatively high, reflecting choices of acquisition parameters. In a seminal paper, Hausleiter et al. reported dose data from the PROTECTION I study and demonstrated that the estimated radiation dose of coronary CTA on a global scale in 2007 was 12 mSv, as compared to 15 mSv in East Asia [68]. In the past 8 years, several effective strategies to reduce radiation dose have become available, with submillisievert coronary CTA feasible in selected patients [69]. Nevertheless, estimated doses differed significantly among sites. Some of the most effective strategies for dose reduction, including prospectively ECG-triggered acquisition, tube current adjustment, particularly in combination with iterative reconstruction algorithms, were not frequently used [70]. These approaches for dose reduction are largely dependent on CT hardware and software. Even if available on the scanner platform, technicians may require a more user-friendly operating interface, supporting "point-of-care" decisions to use low-dose techniques, rather than uniform use of "one-size-fits-all" protocols ordered by supervisors.

Fourth, we found significant variability in all aspects of cardiac CT performance, including the number of annual coronary CTA procedures, which varied from 150 to over 8000 per year; radiation dose, which varied from 3–5 mSv to >15 mSv; as well as cumulative time required for scanning, processing, and reporting, which varied from 18 min to 85 min. Many factors may cause these inequalities, including whether a site was a teaching versus non-teaching hospital, the local economic level, and the interest of hospital leaders and radiology directors. We believe that the best approach to alleviate this diversity is continuing education [69]. The Chinese Society of Radiology and SCCT should promote education and training programs similar to those of other academic societies [72].

We believe that our data provides an overview of the current practice of cardiac CT in mainland China and provides interesting insights into the different practical aspects of its routine use. The results of our survey show that cardiac CT with modern CT systems has become an established radiological modality in China after nearly 10 years of evolution, but at the same time, the method would benefit from more sophisticated and uniform application and performance. Education is most likely the key to achieve further improvement. Being the first study of its kind, the study will serve as a baseline for future studies to judge changes in coronary CTA as well as other related procedures in China.

Current Scientific Research of Cardiovascular CT in China

As cardiovascular disease is widely distributed in China, the scientific research of cardiovascular CT is also increasing. Here we investigated the different types of cardiovascular CT research from July 2015 to June 2016 (Table 54.5).

Table 54.5 Published papers on cardiovascular CT in China from July 2015 to June 2016

Research topics	Radiology journal	Cardiology journal	Other journals	In total
Dose and image quality	21	2	5	28
CAD diagnosis	4	2		6
CT-guided PCI	3	2	1	6
CT plaque imaging	2		1	3
Functional CT imaging		2	2	4
Congenital heart diseases	3		1	4
Pulmonary vessel diseases	2		3	5
Valvular diseases	1	2		3
Adipose tissue volume of pericardium	1	1	2	4
Biomarkers and CCTA		6	6	12
Other rare diseases	2		1	3
In total	39	17	22	78

Information Sources

SCI-EXPANDED was searched electronically from July 1, 2015 to June 31, 2016, utilizing the keywords and word variant of CT, cardiac CT, and coronary heart disease. The search criteria was as follows: (TS=(((computed tomography) OR ((multi-slice spiral CT) OR (multi-slice CT) OR (multi-row spiral CT))) AND ((heart OR cardiac OR (heart disease) OR cardiovascular) OR ((coronary artery) OR (coronary artery disease) OR (coronary heart disease)))) AND CU=(CHINA)) AND type: (Article). The article number was 167. Exclusion criteria include case reports, reviews, meta-analysis, comments, and letters. We also excluded research for cardiovascular US, MRI, SPECT, and PET-CT of other diseases and research not done in China. Finally, 78 articles were included.

Published Papers on Cardiovascular CT by Chinese Researchers in 2016

The research field can be concluded to radiation dose and image quality, coronary artery disease, congenital heart disease, pulmonary disease, valvular disease, epicardial and pericoronary adipose tissue, biomarkers, and other rare diseases. For the departments of the author, 39 authors came from radiology, 17 came from cardiology, and 22 came from other departments. The 22 authors from other departments are distributed in surgery, ICU, fundamental school, CT companies, etc.

Radiation Dose and Image Quality

In the last year, articles about radiation dose and image quality of cardiovascular CT were 28 in total, including the contrast medium dose, image processing and three-dimensional reconstruction, and image quality control. The prospective ECG-triggered high-pitch coronary CT angiography at 70 kVp in a clinical setting was investigated.

Coronary Artery Disease

There were 19 articles focused on the diagnosis of coronary artery disease. Among them, six studies were about CAD diagnosis, six about CT-guided PCI, three about plaque imaging, and four about cardiac functional CT (myocardial CT perfusion, FFR-CT).

Congenital Heart Disease

The congenital heart disease is a constant topic in China due to the huge population. Four articles were focused on congenital heart disease last year, including the tetralogy of Fallot, the vascular ring, the aortic arch branching variation, and the variation of the left atrial appendage.

Pulmonary Disease

Five articles of pulmonary disease on cardiovascular CT were published last year, mostly focused on risk factors of acute and chronic pulmonary embolism.

Valvular Disease

On evaluation of valvular disease, computed tomography had become one of the standard imaging modalities for preprocedural annular sizing prior to transcatheter aortic valve replacement (TAVR) and mitral annulus repair. Three articles were published on the cardiac CT evaluation of valvular disease last year. They might be used for choosing valve device and complication treatment.

Epicardial and Pericoronary Adipose Tissue

Epicardial and pericoronary adipose tissue was found to correlate with coronary heart disease. Thus, an increasing interest of relationship between adipose tissue and coronary heart disease was studied. In the last year, four articles were published on this region.

Biomarkers

Biomarkers of coronary artery calcification were also studied. Instead of radiologists, most studies were done by cardiologists and fundamental researchers. There were 12 articles on this topic. The biomarkers for coronary artery calcification were associated with cystatin C, big endothelin-1, and osteocalcin-positive endothelial progenitor cells. The coronary artery calcification was associated with low serum testosterone in elderly men with stable CAD and serum gamma-glutamyltransferase in type 2 diabetes mellitus. Hyperphosphatemia, angiotensin-converting enzyme 2, and FGF-23 were correlated with coronary artery calcification in

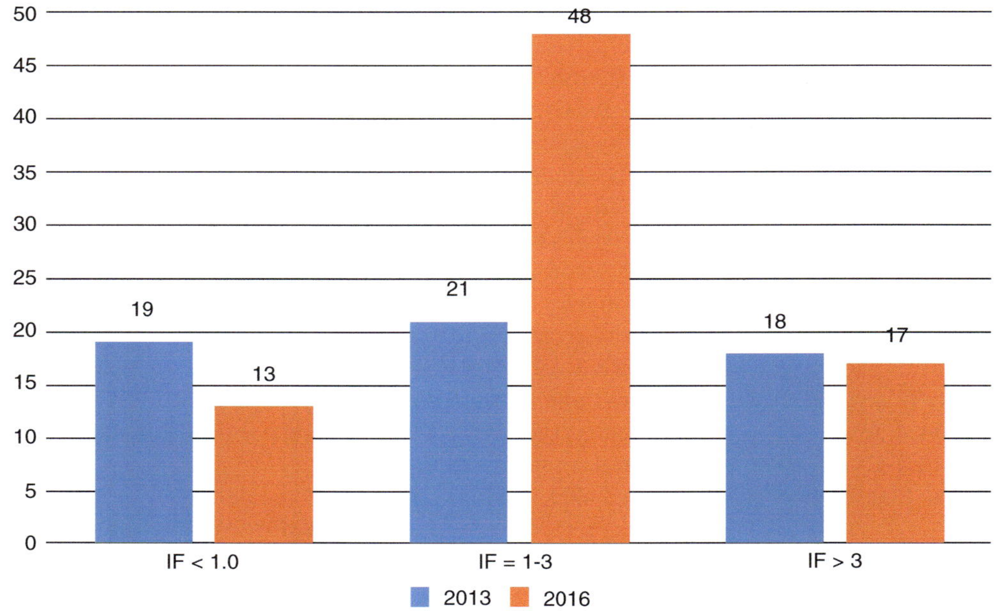

Fig. 54.9 Comparisons of different impact factors and paper volumes of published papers between 2013 and 2016 on cardiovascular CT in China

peritoneal dialysis patients. Genetic circulating microRNAs miR-134, miR-3135b, and miR-2861 were correlated with coronary artery calcification in symptomatic patients. SNPs that are associated with CAD may also increase the risk of calcification with aortic arch. This might suggest utilization of radiomics in the future, which combines the radiology feature with their clinical features, gene information, and pathology information.

Other Rare Diseases

Three other studies include detection of aortic rupture using postmortem computed tomography, detection of coronary artery dissection, and detection of cardiac tumor.

Impact Factors of Published Papers on Cardiovascular CT

For published papers on cardiovascular CT in China last year, there were 13 original papers for SCI-IF <1.0, 48 papers for SCI-IF 1.0–3.0, and 19 papers for SCI-IF >3.0. Compared with 2013, although the quality of papers was not obviously increased, the number of SCI-IF 1.0–3.0 papers increased from 21 to 48. This suggested that much more research had been done on cardiovascular CT in China. We also hope that the high-quality research will come soon, which will be mentioned in the articles below (Fig. 54.9).

References

1. Ministry of Health of the People's Republic of China. Statistics Year Book of Health of the People's Republic of China. Beijing: Pecking Union Medical College Press; 2009–2012.
2. National Health and Family Planning Commission of the People's Republic of China. Year Book of Health and Family Planning in the People's Republic of China. Beijing: Pecking Union Medical College Press; 2015.
3. Zhou MG, Wang HD, Zhu J, et al. Cause-specific mortality for 240 causes in China during 1990–2013: a systematic subnational analysis for the Global Burden of Disease Study 2013. Lancet. 2016;387:251–72.
4. Report of Nutrition and Chronic Diseases in China. 2015. http://www.labagd.com/Item/14257.aspx.
5. Li LM, Rao KQ, Kong LZ, et al. A description on the Chinese national nutrition and health survey in 2002. Chin J Epidemiol. 2005;07:478–84.
6. Xi B, Liang Y, Reilly KH, et al. Trends in prevalence, awareness, treatment, and control of hypertension among Chinese adults 1991-2009. Int J Cardiol. 2012;158(2):326–9.
7. Pan Y, Cai W, Cheng Q, et al. Association between anxiety and hypertension: a systematic review and meta-analysis of epidemiological studies. Neuropsychiatr Dis Treat. 2015;11:1121–30.
8. Survey on prevalence and risk factors for primary hypertension among communities in Changing District, Shanghai. Geriatr Health Care. 2012;18(1):19–22.
9. Wang JG, Li LH. Hypertension series: the differential diagnosis and treatment for secondary hypertension- continued. Chin Circ J. 2012;27(2):85–6.
10. Li NF, Wang L, Zhou KM, et al. Analysis of etiology of the patients with hypertension from the People's Hospital of Xinjiang Uygur Autonomous Region. Chin J Cardiol. 2007;35(9):865–8.
11. Yang GH, Fan LX, Tan J, et al. Smoking in China: Findings of the 1996 National Prevalence Survey. JAMA. 1999;282(13):1247–53.
12. Yang GH, Li Q, Hsia J. Prevalence of smoking in China in 2010. N Engl J Med. 2011;364(25):2469–70.

13. Huang ZJ, Wang LM, Zhang M, et al. Smoking behavior among the Chinese employed floating population aged 18-59 in 2012. Chin J Epidemiol. 2014;35(11):1192–7.
14. Han J, Che XG. A meta-analysis of cigarette smoking prevalence among adolescents in China: 1981-2010. Int J Environ Res Public Health. 2015;12:4617–30.
15. Yang GH. Global Adult Tobacco Survey (GATS)-China Report. Beijing: Three-Gorgas Press; 2010, 2011.11.
16. Gu D, Kelly TN, Wu X, et al. Mortality attributable to smoking in China. N Engl J Med. 2009;360(2):150–9.
17. He J, Gu D, Reynolds K, et al. Serum total and lipoprotein cholesterol levels and awareness, treatment, and control of hypercholesterolemia in China. Circulation. 2004;110(4):405–11.
18. Yang WY, Xiao JZ, Yang ZJ, et al. Serum lipids and lipoproteins in Chinese men and women. Circulation. 2012;125:2212–21.
19. Li JH, Mi SQ, Li YC, et al. The levels and distribution of serum lipids in Chinese adults, 2010. Chin J Prev Med. 2012;46(7):607–12.
20. Zhao WH, Zhang J, Li Y. Report of Chinese nutrition and health status: blood lipid 2002 [J]. People's Medical Publishing House. 2002.
21. Ding WQ, Dong HB, Mi J, et al. Prevalence of dyslipidemia in Chinese children and adolescents: a Meta-analysis. Chin J Epidemiol. 2015;36(1):71–7.
22. Xu Y, Wang L, He J, et al. Prevalence and control of diabetes in Chinese adults. JAMA. 2013;310(9):948–58.
23. An YL, Zhang P, Wang JP, et al. Cardiovascular and all-cause mortality over a 23-year period among Chinese with newly diagnosed diabetes in the Da Qing IGT and Diabetes Study. Diabetes Care. 2015;38(7):1365–71.
24. Li GW, Zhang P, Wang J, et al. Long-term effect of lifestyle interventions to prevent diabetes in the China Da Qing Diabetes Prevention Study: a 20-year follow-up study. Lancet. 2008;371:1783–9.
25. Gong Q, Gregg EW, Wang J, et al. Long-term effects of a randomised trial of a 6-year lifestyle intervention in impaired glucose tolerance on diabetes-related microvascular complications: the China Da Qing Diabetes Prevention Outcome Study. Diabetologia. 2011;54(2):300–7.
26. Li GW, Zhang P, Wang JP, et al. Cardiovascular mortality, all-cause mortality, and diabetes incidence after lifestyle intervention for people with impaired glucose tolerance in the Da Qing Diabetes Prevention Study: a 23-year follow-up study. Lancet Diabetes Endocrinol. 2014;2(6):474–80.
27. Ji L, Hu D, Pan C, et al. Primacy of the 3B approach to control risk factors for cardiovascular disease among type 2 diabetes. Am J Med. 2013;126(10):925e11–22.
28. Ma GS, Li YP, Wu YF, et al. The prevalence of body weight and obesity and its change among Chinese people during 1992 to 2002. Chin J Prev Med. 2005;39(5):311–5.
29. Gordon Larsen P, Wang H, Popkin BM. Overweight dynamics in Chinese children and adults. Obes Rev. 2014;15(S1):37–48.
30. Li XY, Jiang Y, Hu N, et al. Prevalence and characteristic of overweight and obesity among adults in China, 2010. Chin J Prev Med. 2012;46(8):683–6.
31. Lao XQ, Ma WJ, Sobko T, et al. Overall obesity is leveling-off while abdominal obesity continues to rise in a Chinese population experiencing rapid economic development: analysis of serial cross-sectional health survey data 2002–2010. Int J Obes. 2015;39(2):288–94.
32. Ma J, Cai XH, Wang HJ, et al. The trend analysis of overweight and obesity in Chinese students during 1985-2010. Chin J Prev Med. 2012;46(9):776–80.
33. Du HD Li LM, Whitlock G, et al. Patterns and socio-demographic correlates of domain-specific physical activities and their associations with adiposity in the China Kadoorie Biobank Study. BMC Public Health. 2014;14:826.
34. Ng SW, Howard AG, Wang HJ, et al. The physical activity transition among adults in China: 1991–2011. Obes Rev. 2014;15(S1):27–36.
35. Chen Y, Zheng Z, Yi J, et al. Associations between physical inactivity and sedentary behaviors among adolescents in 10 cities in China. BMC Public Health. 2014;14(1):744.
36. Fan S, Chen J, Huang J, et al. Physical activity level and incident type 2 diabetes among Chinese adults. Med Sci Sports Exerc. 2015;47(4):751–6.
37. Zhai FY, Yan XG. Survey Report on the Status of Nutrition and Health of the Chinese People in 2002: Series Two, Status of Diet and Nutrients consumption, vol. 7. Beijing: People's Medical Publishing House; 2006.
38. Yu D, Zhang X, Xiang YB, et al. Adherence to dietary guidelines and mortality: a report from prospective cohort studies of 134,000 Chinese adults in urban Shanghai. Am J Clin Nutr. 2014;100(2):693–700.
39. Yu D, Zhang X, Gao YT, et al. Fruit and vegetable intake and risk of CHD: results from prospective cohort studies of Chinese adults in Shanghai. Br J Nutr. 2014;111(2):353–62.
40. Du S, Neiman A, Batis C, et al. Understanding the patterns and trends of sodium intake, potassium intake, and sodium to potassium ratio and their effect on hypertension in China. Am J Clin Nutr. 2014;99(2):334–43.
41. Brook RD, Rajagopalan S, Pope CA 3rd, et al. Particulate matter air matter air pollution and cardiovascular disease: an update to the scientific statement from the American Heart Association. Circulation. 2010;121(21):2331–78.
42. Kan H, London SJ, Chen G, et al. Differentiating the effects of fine and coarse particles on daily mortality in Shanghai, China. Environ Int. 2007;33:376–84.
43. Huang W, Cao J, Tao Y, et al. Seasonal variation of chemical species associated with short-term mortality effects of PM(2.5) in Xi'an, a Central City in China. Am J Epidemiol. 2012;175(6):556–66.
44. Zhao K, Cao JY, Wen XM. Correlation between PM2.5 pollution in air and mortality of residents in urban area, Xi'an. [Chinese]. J Prev Med Inf. 2011;27(4):257–62.
45. Ma Y, Chen R, Pan G, et al. Fine particulate air pollution and daily mortality in Shenyang, China. Sci Total Environ. 2011;409:2473–7.
46. Yang C, Peng X, Huang W, et al. A time-stratified case-crossover study of fine particulate matter air pollution and mortality in Guangzhou, China. Int Arch Occup Environ Health. 2012;85(5):579–85.
47. Dai J, Chen R, Meng X, et al. Ambient air pollution, temperature and out-of-hospital coronary deaths in Shanghai, China. Environ Pollut. 2015;203:116–21.
48. Xie W, Li G, Zhao D, et al. Relationship between fine particulate air pollution and ischaemic heart disease morbidity and mortality. Heart. 2015;101:257–63.
49. National Health and Family Planning Commission of the People's Republic of China. China Health and Family Planning Statistics Yearbook. Beijing: Peking Union Medical College Press; 2015.
50. Cao J, Yang C, Li J, et al. Association between long-term exposure to outdoor air pollution and mortality in China: a cohort study. J Hazard Mater. 2011;186:1594–600.
51. Wang Y, Zhao X, Jiang Y, et al. Prevalence, knowledge, and treatment of transient ischemic attacks in China. Neurology. 2015;84(23):2354–61.
52. Ministry of Health Statistics Center. 2008 China health services survey – 4th Family health survey. China Statistics Press. 2009.
53. Gu DF, Huang GY, He J, et al. Investigation of prevalence and distributing feature of chronic heart failure in Chinese adult population. Chin J Cardiol. 2003;31(1):3–6.
54. Zhang J, Zhang YH, et al. China heart failure registry study–a multicenter, prospective investigation for preliminary analysis on etiology, clinical features and treatment in heart failure patients. Chin Circ J. 2015;30(5):413–6.
55. Ministry of Health of People's Republic of China. National health statistics annual report 1980–2001 [J], vol. 01: China Statistics Press; 1985. p. 56.

56. Ministry of Health of People's Republic of China. China health statistics yearbook [J]. China Statistics Press. 2002–2012.
57. National Health and Family Planning Commission of the People's Republic of China. China statistical yearbook of health and family planning [J]. Beijing: People's Medical Publishing House; 2013–2015.
58. He D, Yu H, Chen Y. Equity in the distribution of CT and MRI in China: a panel analysis. Int J Equity Health. 2013;12:39.
59. Oh E-H, Imanaka Y, Evans E. Determinants of the diffusion of computed tomography and magnetic resonance imaging. Int J Technol Assess Health Care. 2005;21:73–80.
60. Ma J, Lu M, Quan H. From a national, centrally planned health system to a system based on the market: lessons from China. Health Aff (Millwood). 2008;27:937–48.
61. X-ray computed tomography. Wikipedia 2012. http://en.Wikipedia.org/wik/x-ray_computed_tomography.
62. Liu K, Hsieh C, Zhuang N, Gao Y, Li ZN, Ren XS, Yang L, Zhang JY, Budoff MJ, Lu B. Current utilization of cardiac computed tomography in mainland China: a national survey. J Cardiovasc Comput Tomogr. 2016;10(1):76–81. https://doi.org/10.1016/j.jcct.2015.11.004. PMID26699712.
63. Maurer MH, Hamm B, Dewey M. Survey regarding the clinical practice of cardiac CT in Germany: indications, scanning technique and reporting. RöFo. 2009;181:1135e1143.
64. Leipsic J, Abbara S, Achenbach S, et al. SCCT guidelines for the interpretation and reporting of coronary CT angiography: a report of the Society of Cardiovascular Computed Tomography Guidelines Committee. J Cardiovasc Comput Tomogr. 2014;8:342–58.
65. Kim YJ, Yong HS, Kim SM, Kim JA, Yang DH, Hong YJ. Korean guidelines for the appropriate use of cardiac CT. Korean J Radiol. 2015;16:251–85.
66. Muhlestein JB, Lappe DL, Lima JA, et al. Effect of screening for coronary artery disease using CT angiography on mortality and cardiac events in high-risk patients with diabetes: the FACTOR-64 randomized clinical trial. JAMA. 2014;312:2234–43.
67. Blumenthal D, Hsiao W. Lessons from the East—China's rapidly evolving health care system. N Engl J Med. 2015;372:1281–5.
68. Hausleiter J, Meyer T, Hermann F, et al. Estimated radiation dose associated with cardiac CT angiography. JAMA. 2009;301:500–7.
69. Stehli J, Fuchs TA, Bull S, et al. Accuracy of coronary CT angiography using a submillisievert fraction of radiation exposure: comparison with invasive coronary angiography. J Am Coll Cardiol. 2014;64:772–80.
70. Zhao L, Plank F, Kummann M, et al. Improved non-calcified plaque delineation on coronary CT angiography by sonogram-affirmed iterative reconstruction with different filter strength and relationship with BMI. Cardiovasc Diagn Ther. 2015;5:104–12.
71. Schindera ST, Treier R, von Allmen G, et al. An education and training programme for radiological institutes: impact on the reduction of the CT radiation dose. Eur Radiol. 2011;21:2039–45.
72. Garcia MJ, Blankstein R, Budoff MJ, et al. COCATS 4 Task Force 7: Training in Cardiovascular Computed Tomographic Imaging. J Am Coll Cardiol. 2015;65:1810–21.

Part XIII

Where We Are Going: The Genes and the Heart

55 Differences and Disparities in Cardiovascular Medicine Related to Gender, Race, and Ethnicity: The Role of Cardiac CT

John W. Nance

Knowledge of demographic *differences* in physiology, pathology, and therapeutic response is necessary for optimal patient diagnosis and treatment. However, there are demographic, socioeconomic, and geographic differences in healthcare access, disease occurrence, and resultant morbidity/mortality that transcend biology; these differences constitute healthcare and health status *disparities*. Some differences in healthcare quality are due to clinical appropriateness/need and patient preferences, which may be appropriate, but there is also well-established discrimination as well as differences in the operation of healthcare systems leading to unnecessary, unjust, and avoidable inequities. An understanding of both unavoidable biological differences and avoidable disparities in cardiovascular health and care is necessary to appropriately select patients for cardiac CT, interpret the findings, and guide further management. Differences and disparities, as defined above, will be discussed concurrently.

A brief note is warranted on the categorizations discussed throughout this chapter. *Race* is a sociopolitical construct, rather than a biological or genotypic construct, and conclusions regarding racial differences in pathophysiology should be interpreted accordingly. Likewise, *ethnicity* (in this chapter, Hispanic or not Hispanic) is a cultural distinction with tremendous intra-ethnic heterogeneity. Shifts in the definitions of race and ethnicity can change faster than shifts in disease burden or pathophysiology, necessitating constant surveillance to identify relevant differences and eliminate disparities. *Sex* will be used to denote biological (i.e., chromosomal) differences, whereas *gender* differences are sociocultural. Finally, the volume and quality of data on cardiovascular health for different populations are variable, leading to unfortunate but unavoidable gaps in the following discussion. Rectifying the disparities in both healthcare quality and healthcare knowledge should remain a high priority.

J. W. Nance (✉)
Department of Radiology, Medical University of South Carolina, Charleston, SC, USA
e-mail: nancej@musc.edu

History

There have been significant changes in the global burden of cardiovascular disease over the past several decades, which are beyond the scope of this chapter. Interestingly, however, there is a dramatic and ongoing reevaluation of heart disease burden in varied populations. Some of this shift is due to changing risk profiles, treatment strategies, and actual disease prevalence; however, there is likely also a component of prior and ongoing information bias. For example, hypertension and hypertensive heart disease were reported as twice as frequent in American blacks compared to whites in the 1920s, but coronary heart disease (CHD) was considered uncommon in blacks, possibly due to missed cases [1]. This generally accepted medical "fact" was relatively slow to change, until the increased focus on disparities in minority health over the past three decades. The US Department of Health and Human Services Secretary's Task Force on Black and Minority Health was published in 1985 and provided one of the earlier comprehensive surveys of heart health in various populations, showing higher average annual age-adjusted death rates for heart disease in blacks versus whites, particularly in the younger and female subsets. While a significant portion of this difference can be attributed to differences in hypertension, the study also found that CHD mortality rates were in fact similar in black and white men and higher in black than white women [2]. These differences were attributed to disparities in care in the pivotal release of the Institute of Medicine's report, *Unequal Treatment: Confronting Racial and Ethnic Disparities in Health Care*, in 2002 [3]. Disparities specific to cardiovascular care were likewise highlighted in the Henry J. Kaiser Family Foundation's report, *Racial/Ethnic Differences in Cardiac Care: The Weight of the Evidence*, also released in 2002.

The history of cardiovascular disease in women suffers from similar flaws: While past data suggested that cardiovascular disease, and CHD in particular, were predominantly diseases of men, there was likely a component of information bias given historic gender disparities in clinical trial

U. J. Schoepf (ed.), *CT of the Heart*, Contemporary Medical Imaging, https://doi.org/10.1007/978-1-60327-237-7_55

inclusions and the more common atypical presentation of acute coronary syndromes in women. Indeed, CHD has killed more American women than men on an annual basis since 1984 [4]. Furthermore, there are gender differences in anatomic burden of disease that do not correlate linearly with clinical outcome (discussed below), further obfuscating interpretations of historic studies on disease prevalence and extent. While management recommendations are similar in men and women, some of these long-standing biases apparently persist, and there are continued disparities in time to diagnosis and implementation of recommended medical and surgical treatment [5].

Race and Ethnicity

The burden of cardiovascular disease spares no race or ethnicity, but significant heterogeneity exists between and even within different subpopulations (Table 55.1). Outcome disparities can be attributed to patient-, provider-, and system-level problems. On a patient level, there are differences in the rates and prognostic implications of cardiovascular disease risk factors, but there are also differences in disease prevalence and expression that are independent of risk factors, implying more complex underlying pathophysiologic mechanisms. On a provider level, different races and ethnicities are subject to varying types and levels of risk factor modulation, diagnostic strategies, and therapeutic interventions. Access to care, infrastructure, and insurance coverage constitutes the major system-level disparities currently encountered.

Table 55.1 Racial and ethnic differences in cardiovascular disease[a]

	African origin	Asian origin	Hispanic origin
Risk factors	Much higher rates and lower control of hypertension Twice as likely to have diabetes	More nontraditional risk factors and smoking in certain subpopulations	Nearly twice the rate of diabetes and metabolic syndrome, particularly among Mexican-Americans
Disease burden	Approximately 30% higher mortality rate from cardiovascular disease Worse outcomes in the presence of cardiovascular disease	Approximately 50% lower mortality rate from cardiovascular disease	Approximately 30% lower mortality rate from cardiovascular disease Higher rates of heart failure Worse outcomes in the presence of cardiovascular disease
Imaging findings	Less coronary artery calcium and angiographically obstructive disease Greater left ventricular mass Relatively more noncalcified plaque	Less coronary artery calcium Lower left ventricular mass Less nonobstructive and obstructive CAD	Less coronary artery calcium Less nonobstructive and obstructive CAD

[a]Figures are relative to non-Hispanic whites

Patients of African Descent

Black patients overall have worse risk factor profiles than whites, particularly hypertension, diabetes, and obesity (the latter most pronounced in women). The predictive value of some risk factors (e.g., hypertension and diabetes) is greater than whites, while the value of others (such as lipoprotein [a]) is lower [1]. The consequent burden of cardiovascular disease, particularly hypertensive heart disease, is dramatic, with three to five times higher cardiovascular mortality associated with hypertension in blacks compared to whites.

The spectrum and burden of CHD in blacks are more nuanced. For example, the prevalence of myocardial infarction is higher in white males, but incidence is higher in black males (prevalence and incidence are higher in black females compared to white counterparts). Blacks are more likely to present with atypical symptoms, seek care later than whites, and are subject to greater delays prior to receiving medical or surgical treatments. Perhaps most unsettling, the outcomes of CHD are significantly worse in blacks, with higher mortality at younger ages [1].

Surprisingly, black patients have less angiographically significant coronary artery disease (CAD) than white counterparts, despite worse risk factor profiles and outcomes [6]. The reasons for this apparent paradox are unclear; one of the leading theories is that the overall worse risk factor profile and relatively increased rates of hypertensive heart disease and left ventricular hypertrophy provide a more malignant substrate for adverse events. Cardiac CT, both coronary calcium scoring and coronary CT angiography (cCTA), has provided another possible mechanism: blacks tend to have overall decreased coronary artery calcium and calcified plaques, while having relatively more noncalcified disease [7, 8], possibly reflecting pathophysiologic differences in the stability of underlying atherosclerosis (Fig. 55.1). There is conflicting data on the prognostic implications of these findings, with some studies reporting differing outcomes associated with coronary artery calcium burden (as measured by unenhanced CT calcium scoring) in blacks and others showing no significant difference [9, 10]. The overall prognostic patterns in cCTA seem to hold across populations, with very low risk of future events in patients without any atherosclerotic disease and progressively worse outcomes in patients with nonobstructive and obstructive CAD. Interestingly, data from the large CONFIRM registry also showed that patients with African ethnicity had the highest relative increase in adverse events (specifically, all-cause mortality and myocardial infarction) when obstructive versus nonobstructive disease was present, again arguing for an increased clinical susceptibility to disease in blacks [11].

How do we apply this information to daily cardiac CT practice? While there are clearly differences in risk factor profiles, there is no evidence to suggest that these differences should be exploited in cardiac CT ordering patterns. However, the relatively lower amounts of calcified plaque and greater amounts of noncalcified plaque in blacks, combined with worse outcomes in the presence of any disease,

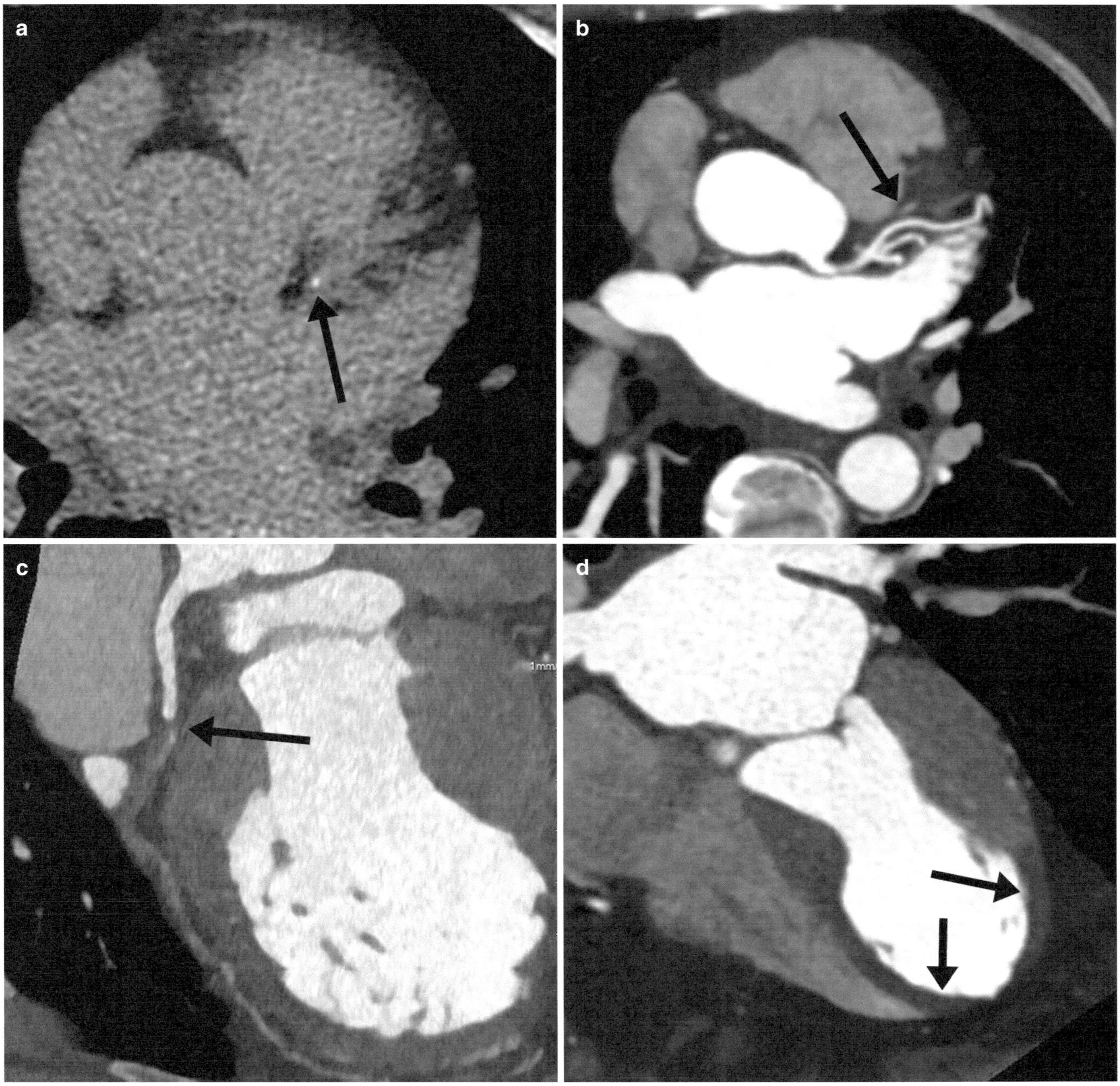

Fig. 55.1 A 59-year-old black woman presented to the emergency department with atypical chest pain. Calcium scoring revealed a single punctate focus of calcium (arrow in **a**), corresponding to an Agatston score of 1. Despite the low Agatston score, cCTA revealed occlusion of the proximal LAD at the level of the takeoff of the first diagonal branch (arrows in **b** and **c**). The corresponding LAD territory was thinned and severely hypokinetic on functional images (arrows in **d**). The patient was subsequently taken to catheterization, where angioplasty and stenting of the LAD occlusion (arrow in **e**) were performed

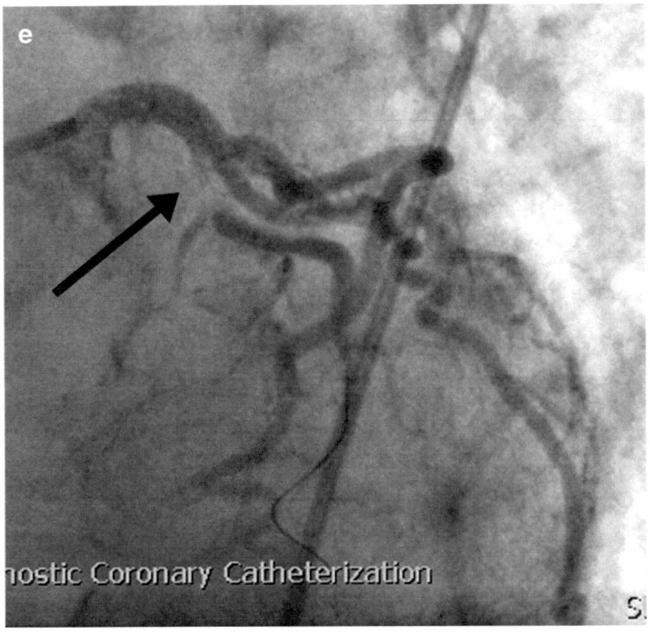

Fig. 55.1 (continued)

might warrant more heavy weighting for cCTA over simple coronary artery calcium scoring in clinical situations in which both would be appropriate. Noncalcified and nonobstructive disease also warrant specific mention in cCTA reports. Finally, the optimal clinical management of black patients who have undergone cardiac CT is likely a high-yield area for future research, particularly in the blooming era of personalized medicine. For example, do black patients with noncalcified nonobstructive disease but increased myocardial mass require more aggressive follow-up or medical management? Future studies should help validate personalized treatment algorithms.

Hispanics

Among the well-studied racial and ethnic minorities, Hispanics show the greatest underlying heterogeneity, with varying regions of origin, acculturation levels, and contributions of European, African, and Native American ancestry. As a group Hispanics have an overall worse risk profile than non-Hispanic whites, with particularly high levels of diabetes and metabolic syndrome. Despite this increased risk, Hispanics suffer lower levels of subclinical cardiovascular disease on imaging (coronary artery calcium and left ventricular mass) [7, 12] and have lower rates of total cardiovascular disease and CHD; this phenomenon is sometimes termed the "Hispanic paradox." As in patients of African descent, Hispanic patients presenting with acute coronary syndrome and myocardial infarction experience longer delays before treatment and suffer worse outcomes compared to non-Hispanic whites [13]. Similar to other immigrant populations, Hispanics in the United States suffer increasing levels of cardiovascular disease as acculturation increases. Interestingly, Hispanics with low acculturation have been shown to demonstrate a paradoxical relationship between socioeconomic status and endpoints of cardiovascular disease relative to other Western populations, i.e., worse outcomes with higher socioeconomic status. This relationship reverts back to the expected, inverse relationship between socioeconomic status and outcomes as acculturation increases [14].

Imaging studies have shown that cCTA has good sensitivity and specificity for the detection of coronary artery stenosis [15] and that coronary artery calcium scoring and cCTA findings independently predict death or myocardial infarction in Hispanics [11]. There is no available evidence to suggest that cardiac CT should be ordered, acquired, or interpreted differently in Hispanic compared to non-Hispanic white patients.

Patients of Asian Descent

Comparative racial and ethnic research involving Asian populations is less studied. Asians, particularly East Asians, tend to have better risk profiles than whites and other racial/ethnic minorities, with correspondingly less subclinical and clinical cardiovascular disease. East Asians are unique among racial and ethnic minorities in having similar outcomes compared to whites following adverse cardiac events. Calcium scoring and cCTA demonstrate good sensitivity and specificity and hold independent prognostic value in Asians; however, East Asians have been shown to have less than expected mortality and nonfatal myocardial infarction in the presence of atherosclerosis on cCTA [11]. Nevertheless, there is no evidence to suggest that race-specific ordering, acquisition, or interpretation should be applied to Asian populations.

Gender

Cardiovascular disease is the leading killer of women in the United States, and while overall mortality from heart disease has decreased since 2001, mortality in women under 45 years old has increased. CHD prevalence is lower in all women compared to all men, but this differential decreases with advancing age, and in absolute numbers, more women than men die of cardiovascular disease annually [4]. Global epidemiological figures are similar – heart disease is the leading cause of death in women in all major high-income economies and the majority of middle- and low-income economies [16].

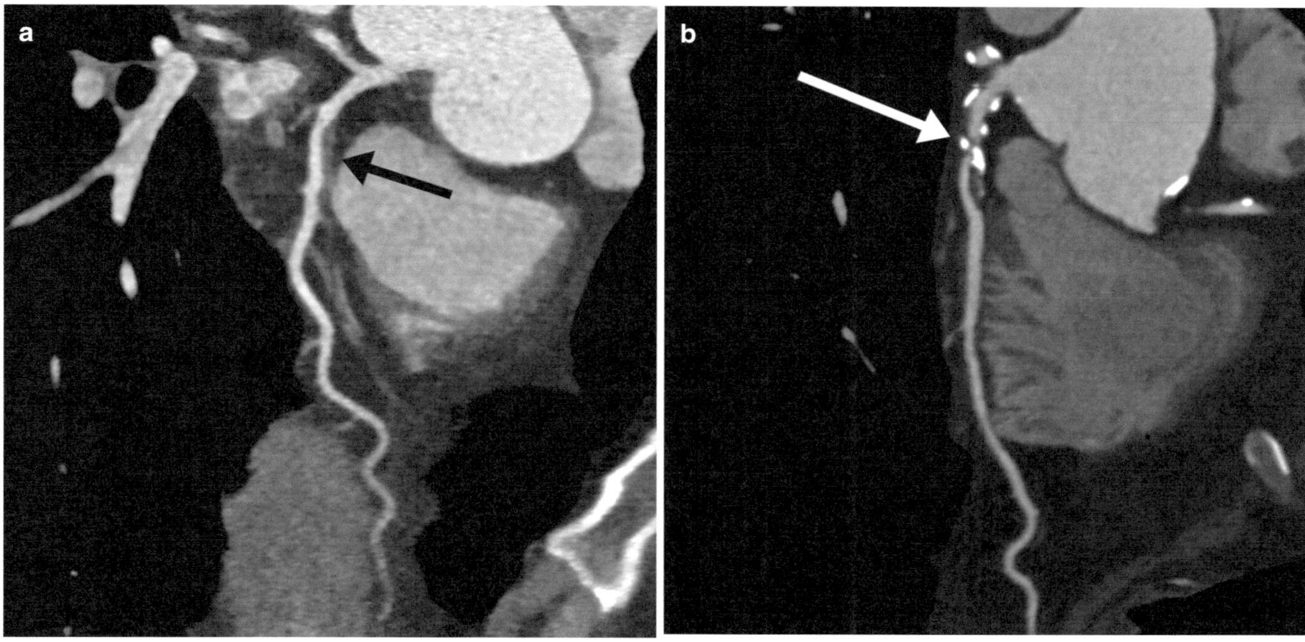

Fig. 55.2 A 54-year-old white woman presented to the emergency department with chest pain. There was no detectable coronary calcium. cCTA revealed nonobstructive noncalcified plaque in the proximal to mid-LAD (arrow in **a**). Contrast with the obstructive mixed calcified and noncalcified plaque in this 57-year-old white man presenting with chest pain (arrow in **b**)

Unfortunately, awareness of heart disease in women lags behind the actual burden, both among patients and providers, which can lead to suboptimal management or delays in presentation and diagnosis. Despite similar guidelines for the prevention and management of cardiovascular disease in men and women, there is disparity in their implementation. Symptomatic women are less likely to be referred for noninvasive imaging, angiography, or revascularization (Fig. 55.2). Women with angiographic evidence of CHD are less likely to receive optimal primary and secondary therapy. Women have poorer outcomes following acute coronary syndrome and higher risks of intracranial bleeding following thrombolytics. They are less likely to receive and wait longer for diagnostic and invasive procedures while admitted and less likely to receive recommended pharmacotherapy upon discharge. Finally, adverse outcomes are more common in women following revascularization [5].

Differences in pathophysiology, risk factor profile and relative risks, and presentation of cardiovascular disease between women and men can help explain some, but not all, of the variations in management and outcomes. Estrogen is thought to play a protective role in premenopausal women, helping to explain the gap in CHD prevalence in younger women compared to younger men; recall that the gap narrows in older women and men. Indeed, postmenopausal changes in atherosclerotic plaque composition have been identified, with higher rates of lipid-laden plaques with necrotic cores, more inflammatory changes, and a greater propensity for plaque rupture in women >50 years old. Women under 50 years old have significantly higher rates of plaque erosion (versus rupture) compared to older counterparts. In women of all ages, there is less obstructive CAD compared to men, both in an asymptomatic population and in those presenting with acute coronary syndrome. Up to 20% of women presenting with acute coronary syndrome have angiographically normal coronary arteries, with ischemia caused by microvascular disease. For this reason, the term "ischemic heart disease" (IHD), which includes obstructive CAD, nonobstructive CAD, and microvascular disease, is preferred over "CAD."

Traditional, emerging, and sex-specific risk factors play a role in comprehensive risk stratification in women. Application of global risk scores (such as the Framingham Risk Score) is a class I indication in asymptomatic adults without a clinical history. The American Heart Association's (AHA) women-specific guidelines further specifies that asymptomatic women should be classified into three different risk categories – high risk, at risk, and ideal cardiovascular health – with the reasoning that traditional scoring (e.g., Framingham Risk Score) is relevant in identifying high-risk women but suboptimal to ensure low risk given the high lifetime burden of cardiovascular disease in women (nearly one in two) [17]. Symptomatic women should also be classified into low, intermediate, and high risk of IHD. Because of the higher prevalence of atypical symptoms in women, risk stratification is more heavily weighted toward age and risk factors rather than clinical presentation. In general, women are considered low risk if premenopausal (e.g., 50s or younger), intermediate risk in their 60s, and high risk in their 70s. Women with multiple cardiac risk factors, functional disability, and extensive comorbidities should be elevated one risk category, and women with peripheral arterial disease or long-standing, poorly controlled diabetes are considered high-risk equivalents [18].

Current consensus statements are mixed on the appropriate use of cCTA in varied populations. For example, the AHA consensus statement on the role of noninvasive testing in women with suspected IHD states that imaging evaluation of women with low risk for IHD (in the acute or stable settings) is inappropriate and that cCTA is only appropriate in women with intermediate to high risk with an abnormal 12-lead rest ECG [18]. In contrast, the ACCF/AHA/ACP/AATS/PCNA/SCAI/STS guidelines for the diagnosis and management of patients with stable IHD states that cCTA may be appropriate in patients with intermediate pretest probability of IHD who are able to exercise and in patients with low to intermediate probability who are not able to exercise [19]. ACCF/SCCT/ACR/AHA/ASE/ASNX/NASCI/SCAI/SCMR appropriate use criteria for cCTA state that cCTA is also acceptable in low to intermediate probability patients presenting with acute chest pain, low probability asymptomatic patients with family history of premature CAD, and intermediate probability asymptomatic patients without known CAD [20]. Clearly, further work needs to be done to improve the quality of evidence, including sex-specific evidence, and refine optimal diagnostic strategies.

The diagnostic accuracy of cCTA is comparable in women and men, with >90% sensitivity and specificity in the 70–90% range for obstructive CAD [18]. As a general rule, calcified and obstructive CAD prevalence and extent in women lag behind men by approximately 10 years; accordingly, women undergoing cCTA tend to be older, with higher risk according to traditional risk stratification methods. Notably, over twice as many women (60–70%) as men (~30%) with suspected IHD undergoing invasive coronary angiography have nonobstructive CAD [21].

Several studies have demonstrated sex-specific differences in the prognostic value of various cCTA parameters. While women and men have similar outcomes with regard to extent and severity of obstructive CAD, only women show elevated risk-adjusted mortality for the presence and extent of nonobstructive CAD [18] and may therefore benefit from more aggressive risk factor modification and medical therapy. Accordingly, nonobstructive CAD (particularly when >2 major epicardial vessels are involved) should be highlighted in cCTA reports. Importantly, the absence of CAD (obstructive or nonobstructive) portends a very favorable prognosis in both men and women [22].

To date, routine clinical practice has underexploited the unique ability of cCTA to noninvasively identify nonobstructive CAD in women. There are no societal guidelines on recommended therapy for patients with signs and symptoms of IHD and nonobstructive CAD. Ischemia on stress testing is often dismissed as "false positive" due to lack of obstructive disease on anatomic imaging, and secondary preventative strategies are rarely implemented [23]. cCTA may have a more prominent role with evolving diagnostic and treatment paradigms for IHD other than obstructive CAD, which tends to disproportionately affect women.

References

1. Clark LT. Issues in minority health: atherosclerosis and coronary heart disease in African Americans. Med Clin North Am. 2005;89(5):977–1001, 994.
2. Savage DD. Highlights from the Department of Health and Human Services Task Force on Black and Minority Health. J Natl Black Nurses Assoc. 1986;1(2):16–23.
3. Institute of Medicine (US) Committee on Understanding and Eliminating Racial and Ethnic Disparities in Health Care. Ethnic disparities in health. In: Smedley BD, Stith AY, Nelson AR, editors. Unequal treatment: confronting racial and ethnic disparities in health care. Washington, DC: National Academies Press (US); 2003.
4. Mozaffarian D, et al. Executive summary: heart disease and stroke statistics--2016 update: a report from the American Heart Association. Circulation. 2016;133(4):447–54.
5. Shah T, Palaskas N, Ahmed A. An update on gender disparities in coronary heart disease care. Curr Atheroscler Rep. 2016;18(5):28.
6. Liao Y, et al. The relative effects of left ventricular hypertrophy, coronary artery disease, and ventricular dysfunction on survival among black adults. JAMA. 1995;273(20):1592–7.
7. Bild DE, et al. Ethnic differences in coronary calcification: the Multi-Ethnic Study of Atherosclerosis (MESA). Circulation. 2005;111(10):1313–20.
8. Nance JW Jr, et al. Coronary atherosclerosis in African American and white patients with acute chest pain: characterization with coronary CT angiography. Radiology. 2011;260(2):373–80.
9. Detrano R, et al. Coronary calcium as a predictor of coronary events in four racial or ethnic groups. N Engl J Med. 2008;358(13):1336–45.
10. Doherty TM, Tang W, Detrano RC. Racial differences in the significance of coronary calcium in asymptomatic black and white subjects with coronary risk factors. J Am Coll Cardiol. 1999;34(3):787–94.
11. Hulten E, et al. Usefulness of coronary computed tomography angiography to predict mortality and myocardial infarction among Caucasian, African and East Asian ethnicities (from the CONFIRM [Coronary CT Angiography Evaluation for Clinical Outcomes: an International Multicenter] Registry). Am J Cardiol. 2013;111(4):479–85.
12. Gardin JM, et al. Do differences in subclinical cardiovascular disease in Mexican Americans versus European Americans help explain the Hispanic paradox? Am J Cardiol. 2010;105(2):205–9.
13. Graham G. Racial and ethnic differences in acute coronary syndrome and myocardial infarction within the United States: from demographics to outcomes. Clin Cardiol. 2016;39(5):299–306.
14. Gallo LC, et al. Do socioeconomic gradients in subclinical atherosclerosis vary according to acculturation level? Analyses of

Mexican-Americans in the multi-ethnic study of atherosclerosis. Psychosom Med. 2009;71(7):756–62.
15. Jug B, et al. Influence of race and ethnicity on diagnostic performance of 64-slice multidetector coronary computed tomographic angiography. Int J Cardiol. 2013;168(2):1521–3.
16. Gholizadeh L, Davidson P. More similarities than differences: an international comparison of CVD mortality and risk factors in women. Health Care Women Int. 2008;29(1):3–22.
17. Mosca L, et al. Effectiveness-based guidelines for the prevention of cardiovascular disease in women--2011 update: a guideline from the American Heart Association. J Am Coll Cardiol. 2011;57(12):1404–23.
18. Mieres JH, et al. Role of noninvasive testing in the clinical evaluation of women with suspected ischemic heart disease: a consensus statement from the American Heart Association. Circulation. 2014;130(4):350–79.
19. Fihn SD, et al. 2012 ACCF/AHA/ACP/AATS/PCNA/SCAI/STS Guideline for the diagnosis and management of patients with stable ischemic heart disease: a report of the American College of Cardiology Foundation/American Heart Association Task Force on Practice Guidelines, and the American College of Physicians, American Association for Thoracic Surgery, Preventive Cardiovascular Nurses Association, Society for Cardiovascular Angiography and Interventions, and Society of Thoracic Surgeons. J Am Coll Cardiol. 2012;60(24):e44–e164.
20. Taylor AJ, et al. ACCF/SCCT/ACR/AHA/ASE/ASNC/NASCI/SCAI/SCMR 2010 appropriate use criteria for cardiac computed tomography. A report of the American College of Cardiology Foundation Appropriate Use Criteria Task Force, the Society of Cardiovascular Computed Tomography, the American College of Radiology, the American Heart Association, the American Society of Echocardiography, the American Society of Nuclear Cardiology, the North American Society for Cardiovascular Imaging, the Society for Cardiovascular Angiography and Interventions, and the Society for Cardiovascular Magnetic Resonance. J Am Coll Cardiol. 2010;56(22):1864–94.
21. Jespersen L, et al. Stable angina pectoris with no obstructive coronary artery disease is associated with increased risks of major adverse cardiovascular events. Eur Heart J. 2012;33(6):734–44.
22. Min JK, et al. Age- and sex-related differences in all-cause mortality risk based on coronary computed tomography angiography findings results from the International Multicenter CONFIRM (Coronary CT Angiography Evaluation for Clinical Outcomes: an International Multicenter Registry) of 23,854 patients without known coronary artery disease. J Am Coll Cardiol. 2011;58(8):849–60.
23. Pepine CJ, et al. Emergence of nonobstructive coronary artery disease: a woman's problem and need for change in definition on angiography. J Am Coll Cardiol. 2015;66(17):1918–33.

56 Cardiac CT Radiomics

Márton Kolossváry and Pál Maurovich-Horvat

Medical imaging modalities have undergone great improvements in the past decades. State-of-the-art scanners can depict anatomical structures at previously unimaginable detail, while also providing functional information regarding pathologies. No matter how sophisticated our imaging techniques might be, our interpretation of results is still based predominantly on visual inspection. Qualitative assessment of radiological images discards vast amount of information, while relying on greatly subjective and hard to reproduce expert opinions [1, 2]. In the era of personalized medicine where subtle differences in the genome are seen as opportunities for new personalized therapies [3], superficial visual assessment of pathologies seems outdated.

Radiomics is the process of extracting numerous quantitative image-based features from radiological examinations, to create large datasets where each abnormality is characterized by hundreds of different parameters [4, 5]. These parameters are used to create "big data" datasets, which can be analyzed using machine learning techniques to find new meaningful patterns and relationships in the data (Fig. 56.1).

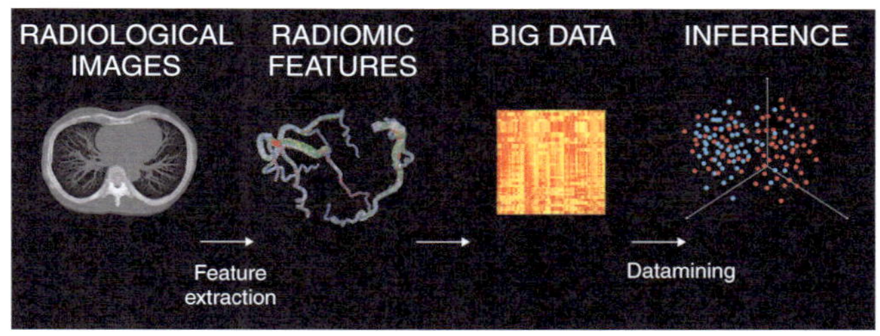

Fig. 56.1 Pipeline of radiomics-based patient analysis. After image acquisition, new novel radiomics-based image characteristics are extracted to quantify different lesion properties. The hundreds of variables are joined together to create "big data" databases. Machine learning is used to find new meaningful connections between the parameters and the clinical outcome data. Based on the results, new imaging biomarkers can be identified which have the potential to increase the diagnostic accuracy of radiological examinations

Concept of Radiomics

In radiological images, each voxel represents a separate measurement of some physical characteristic in that given area or volume. Basically, radiological examinations are a vast number of physical measurements done in a spatial coordinate system. In CT, the amount of radiation absorption in the given voxel is utilized to create the image (for details see Chap. 2). Different tissue components all absorb radiation to a different extent; thus the Hounsfield units (HU) mirror the underlying tissue structure of a given voxel. Therefore, it is reasonable to assume that spatial heterogeneity of a coronary atherosclerotic lesion on CT might correlate with known histological morphologies and thus could give additional prognostic information above stenosis severity.

Several qualitative imaging markers representing coronary plaque heterogeneity have been identified on coronary CT angiography (CTA). These have been shown to correlate with histological abnormalities and major adverse cardiac events (MACE) to some degree [6, 7]. Being qualitative markers, they are prone to interobserver variations and require much experience. Furthermore, there are aspects of heterogeneity which are difficult to comprehend by visual inspection. Subtle differences in HU values are undetectable by eye sight, while they might hold valuable information of underlying tissue architecture. Much of radiomics is about mathematically quantifying these fine textural properties, shape of the lesion, and the spatial distribution of HU values on radiological images.

M. Kolossváry (✉) · P. Maurovich-Horvat
Cardiovascular Imaging Research Group, Heart and Vascular Center, Semmelweis University, Budapest, Hungary
e-mail: p.maurovich-horvat@cirg.hu

U. J. Schoepf (ed.), *CT of the Heart*, Contemporary Medical Imaging, https://doi.org/10.1007/978-1-60327-237-7_56

Classification of Radiomic Techniques

Radiomic techniques can be divided into four major groups: (1) intensity-based metrics, which measure different properties of the distribution of HU values; (2) texture-based analysis, which quantifies the spatial heterogeneity of the lesion; (3) shape-based measures, which quantify the three-dimensional geometry of an abnormality; and (4) transform-based metrics, which transform the image from the spatial domain to the frequency or scale domain. Summary of radiomic techniques can be found in Fig. 56.2.

Radiomic Features

Intensity-Based Metrics

Intensity-based metrics are often also called *first-order statistics*, meaning that statistics are derived from individual voxels themselves, discarding all spatial and relational information. These metrics can easily be calculated by segmenting out the given voxels and then calculating the statistics on the array of voxel values. This is also referred to as *histogram analysis*, since the calculated statistics resemble some property of the distribution of the voxel values.

Parameters Representing the Average and Spread of the Data

The following statistics are the most common metrics used in practice: *mean* which is the closest point to all other points, *median* which is the middle element of an ordered array of values, *minimum* and *maximum* which reflect the most extreme points in the distribution, *percentiles* which are cutoff points for a given proportion of the distribution, and *interquartile range*, which are two distinguished data points, that define the 25th and the 75th percentile, which indicate the spread of middle 50% of the data points. While previous statistics represent information regarding the values and the range of the distribution, they do not express any information regarding the shape of the distribution. There are an infinite number of different distributions which have the same mean or interquartile range but have very different shapes (Fig. 56.3).

Parameters Representing the Shape of the Distribution

The concept of distribution shape is grasped using so-called moments. Moments are defined as the average of the values (x_i) minus a given value (c) raised to a given power (q). If $c = 0$ and $q = 1$, the moment equals the *mean*. If c = *the mean* (μ), we call our moments *central moments*. If $c = \mu$ and $q = 2$, then we obtain the *variance*, which informs us about how spread-out our data is from the mean. The square root of the variance is the *standard deviation (SD)*, which also quantifies the spread of the data, and in cases of normally distributed data, it gives information where approximately 68% of the data is situated around the mean. If we divide our central moments with the SD on the *qth* power, then we obtain *standardized* or *normalized central moments*. If $c = \mu$ and $q = 3$ and we standardize by SD^3, then we define *skewness*, which quantifies the asymmetry of the distribution. Negative skew means the left tail is longer and a considerable proportion of the distribution is shifted to the right, while positive skew indicates just the opposite. If $c = \mu$ and $q = 4$ and we normalize by SD^4, we come to the *kurtosis*, which basically quantifies the number of outliers in the data. The smaller the value, the more data points are in the proximity of the mean, while higher values indicate that a larger proportion of the data points are located beyond one SD distance of the mean, as compared to the normal distribution. Higher degree moments can also be defined but are seldom used due to exhaustive calculations and difficult interpretation.

Parameters Representing the Diversity of Values

While previous statistics quantified the spread and the shape of the distribution, they do not give any information regarding the diversity of the data, meaning how dissimilar the data points are. Voxel values can also be viewed as signals with different intensities. Concepts from signal processing—a subfield of information theory—can be implemented to quantify heterogeneity of voxel values. *Energy* is the sum of all squared elements and quantifies the overall magnitude of voxel intensities in the image. *Uniformity* is the sum of squared probabilities of each given voxel value. If there is only one value present, then uniformity is 1; the more different values there are, the smaller the probabilities of each value; thus the squared sum will be closer

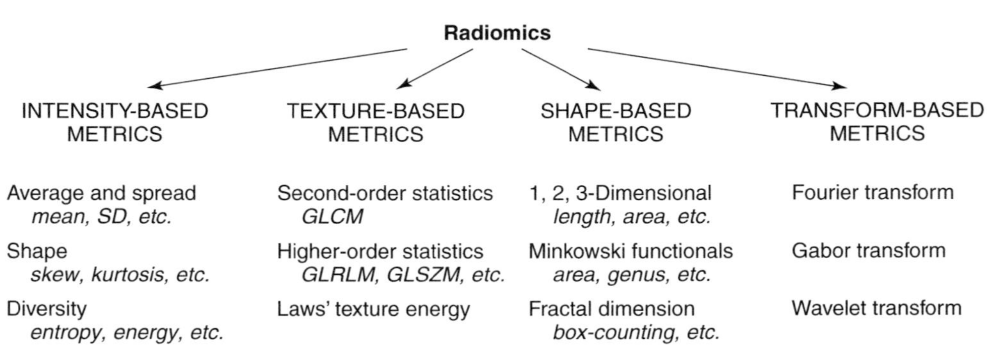

Fig. 56.2 Classification of different radiomic techniques. (From Kolossvary et al. [5], with permission)

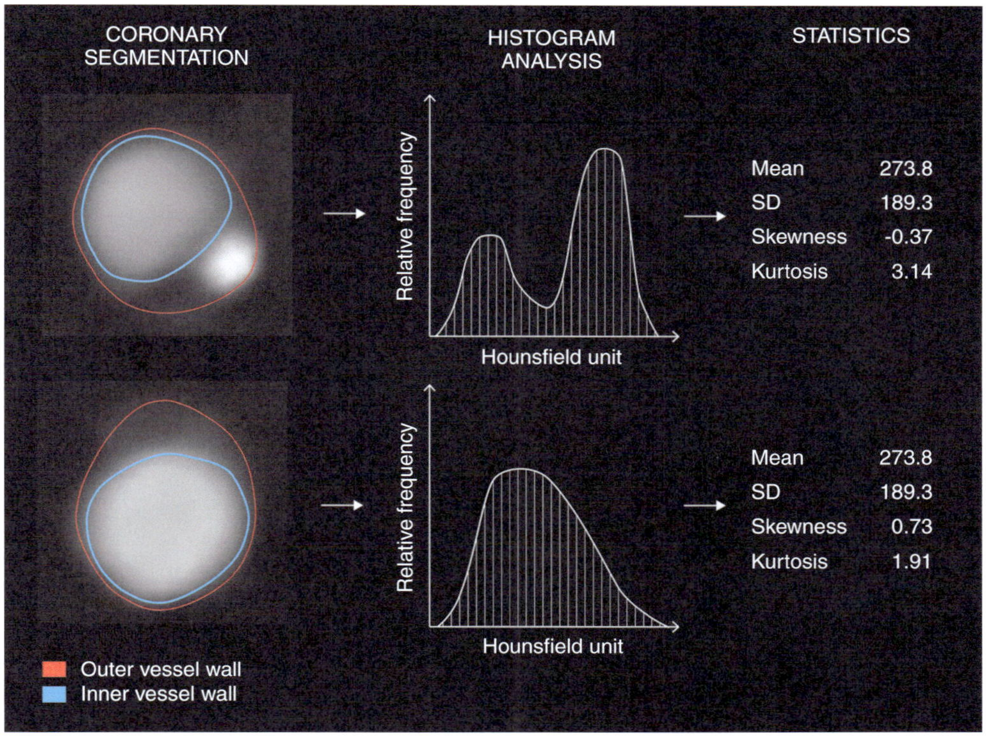

Fig. 56.3 Pipeline for calculating first-order statistics on two representative examples of coronary lesions. First the coronary arteries need to be segmented. Then histograms need to be created showing the relative frequency of given HU values. From these different statistics can be calculated. The image also justifies the use of several different parameters to reflect a lesion, since the average attenuation values and the standard deviations are the same, while only higher moments can differentiate between these two plaques. (From Kolossvary et al. [5], with permission)

to 0. *Shannon entropy* is a measure to quantify the amount of information contained in the data [8]. In cases where there are two outcomes and both are equally probable (e.g., a coin toss), then we are at maximum uncertainty about the outcome of a toss, since both occur with the same probability; thus the unpredictability is at maximum. However, if one outcome is more probable than the other (biased coin), then we have some assumption about what the outcome might be, since one of the events is more probable; thus our uncertainty is smaller. This shows that higher probability (p) events carry less information, because we could have guessed what might happen, while rare events carry more information, since their occurrence is scarce and highlights only a few instances. Entropy quantifies this uncertainty or randomness, by weighting the information content of an event (which is defined as $\log_2 p$) with its relative frequency in the dataset and then adding up all these values for all the events and multiplying it by minus one. The result is called the commonly used term: *bits*. It quantifies the minimum number of required binary elements to describe all possible entries in the data. Higher values indicate that more bits are required to describe the data suggesting higher uncertainty meaning greater heterogeneity, while smaller values indicate just the opposite. Overall, high SD and entropy and low uniformity all represent increased heterogeneity.

Utilization and Potential Pitfalls of Intensity-Based Metrics

Several of the abovementioned metrics have been used to quantify coronary lesions. One of the first attempts to utilize quantitative information from cardiac CT scans was the Agatston score [9]. The calcium score of a lesion is computed by calculating the area of voxels with attenuation values greater than 130 HU and multiplying it by a weighting factor based on the maximum attenuation value of the given lesion (for details see Chap. 2). This simple idea of taking the area of calcium in a lesion and multiplying it by a number is one of the best cardiovascular risk stratification methods we have to date [10, 11]. It is also feasible to quantify volumetric quantities of plaque components using coronary CTA [12]. Unfortunately, there is only limited information regarding the prognostic value of different quantitative plaque components on MACE. Versteylen et al. have shown total plaque volume, total noncalcified volume, per-plaque maximal volume, noncalcified percentage, and plaque burden to be all significantly larger in acute coronary syndrome patients, as compared to non-acute coronary syndrome controls [13]. Furthermore, adding quantitative plaque characteristics to the Framingham risk score (FRS) and qualitative CTA reading results significantly improves the diagnostic performance of the model, as compared to FRS and qualitative information (area under the curve: 0.64 vs. 0.79, $p < 0.05$, respectively).

As attractive it may seem to measure quantitative metrics regarding coronary plaques, there are major potential pitfalls that we must not forget. These metrics are all based on absolute HU values. It has been shown in ex vivo studies that using a different CT scanner for the measurements changed the observed median Agatston score significantly (Philips, 353; Toshiba, 410; GE, 469; Siemens, 332; $p < 0.05$). Furthermore, the limited inter-platform reproducibility resulted in up to 6.5% of the intermediate-risk patients reclassified into either low- or high-risk groups [14]. Moreover, using different image reconstruction algorithms on the same examination also had a significant effect on observed values and risk prediction [15]. Same tendencies can be observed for coronary CTA scans as well. It seems there is also a considerable amount of inter-vendor variation [16], and higher levels of iteration during image reconstruction may also have an effect on observed values [17, 18]. Furthermore, there is no consensus on the cutoff values for identifying different tissue components, which is mainly due to the aforementioned reasons, and because of different plaque components, HU ranges overlap significantly, due to the similar molecular composition and limited spatial- and low-contrast resolution of current CT scanners [19, 20]. Therefore, several different cutoff values have been proposed [12, 21]. In addition, these are all population-based results; thus individual variations can be significantly larger. Furthermore, most of these statistics are related to the mean, which is a very robust statistic since it is calculated using each voxel value. Therefore, if such alterations can be observed averaging hundreds of thousands of voxel values, then individual voxel values show considerably larger variations, which would have a great effect on personalized patient management based on these metrics.

Overall, intensity-based metrics can quantify the distribution and heterogeneity of our data. However, there are major concerns, due to the lack of quantification standards, the concerns of reproducibility, the effects of noise, etc. Finally, these metrics all discard spatial information; therefore measures of diversity only reflect properties of the distribution, which has nothing to do with spatial heterogeneity.

Texture-Based Metrics

Earlier metrics discarded the spatial relation of the voxels to each other. This seems conceptually flawed since we know plaque composition has a significant effect on plaque vulnerability, and plaque composition is expressed by the spatial interrelationship of the voxels on coronary CTA. Even so, it is very hard to conceptualize this spatial interaction between the image points. This problem first emerged from the analysis of satellite imagery in the 1970s and is referred to as texture analysis. *Texture* is a broad concept, which tries to describe patterns in an image. Patterns are basically repetitions of different characteristics, such as shape, color, intensity, etc. Texture analysis tries to mathematically define these ideas by calculating different statistics which are based on the spatial relationship of two or more image points and not simply on the voxel values themselves.

Second-Order Statistics

Haralick et al. proposed the idea of *gray-level co-occurrence matrix (GLCM)* [22]. GLCMs or *gray-tone spatial dependencies matrix (GTSDM)* is a *second-order statistics* meaning that the statistics calculated from these values are based on the relationship of two voxels. The main idea is not to look at intensity values themselves, but to examine how many times similar intensity values occur next to each other at a given distance and direction. To achieve this, first our image values must be discretized, meaning that they need to be partitioned into n non-overlapping groups. Next raw GLCMs are created. For simplicity, we will continue assuming we have a 2D image, for example, a cross section of a lesion, not a 3D dataset. To derive a GLCM, two parameters need to be given: distance and direction. Distance refers to how far away we look from our reference voxel, for example, the voxels next to a reference voxel are at a distance of 1. Direction is usually an angle, where the voxels to the east of a reference voxel are at an angle of 0°, ones to the northeast are at 45°, ones to the north are at 90°, and ones to the northwest are at 135°. As we will see, there is no need to define the remaining four directions, since they can be derived from one of the earlier defined directions.

In a GLCM there are as many rows as there are column, which is equal to the number of intensity groups (n) to which we discretized our image. The rows are labeled as i, and the columns as j. A value in the *ith* row and *jth* column (location defined as $[i, j]$) in the raw GLCM enumerates how many times in our image a voxel of value j is located at a given distance and in a certain direction with respect to any one of the voxels in the image that have a value of i. For example, in a raw GLCM where distance is 1 and the angle is 0°, the value in the 3rd column and the 2nd row is equal to the number of times a value of 3 occurs to the right of a value of 2 in the whole image. As stated earlier, one needs to only calculate these GLCMs in four directions since the other four can be derived from the opposite GLCM by transposing the matrix, which means we simply mirror the values on the main diagonal, which goes through the matrix from the top-left to the bottom-right. For example, the value in the *ith* row and *jth* column in a GLCM of distance 1 and angle 0° is equal to the value in the *jth* row and *ith* column in the GLCM of distance 1 and an of angle 180°. This is because it is equivalent to ask how many times a value j occurs to the right of value i and to ask how many times does value i occur to the left of j. Therefore, we can simply add up these corresponding GLCMs to receive four symmetrical (value in *ith* row and *jth* column equals the value in *jth* row and *ith* column) matrices. Since the absolute number of occurrences is not very informative, because we do not know whether, for example, 42 is a large value or not, we change the values in the raw GLCM to relative frequencies, which we get by simply dividing each entry by the sum of the entries.

These matrices already tell us a lot of information. The values on the main diagonal represent the probability of two voxels having the same value at a given direction and angle. The further away we go from the diagonal, the greater the difference between the two voxels. Two extremes would be a matrix with only elements on the diagonals, which means that there are only identical intensity values in the given direction in our image. On the other extreme, if each entry in the GLCM is the same, then our intensity values occur at random in our picture in the given direction.

Haralick originally proposed 14 different metrics that can be derived from the GLCMs, but many more are used [23]. Basically, all parameters are derived by weighting the entries of the matrix based on some objective and then summing them up. These values are the following, but not limited to: *angular second moment/uniformity/energy* is calculated just as is the first-order case, by squaring the elements of the GLCM and then summing them up. Values close to 1 indicate few highly probable values in the GLCM, which means that the same two values occur usually next to each other, while a uniformity close to 0 would mean that different valued voxels occur next to each other at random. *Contrast* is calculated by multiplying the elements of the GLCM by a weight and then summing all the values. The weight for a value in the *ith* row and *jth* column of the GLCM equals the difference between the intensity *i* and *j* squared. This emphasizes values where there is a large difference in the intensities of neighboring voxels, because elements on the diagonal (which means the two pixels have the same intensity) receive a weight of 0, while the further away we move from the main diagonal (where there are bigger differences between the two voxels), the higher the weights, which increases exponentially. Therefore, higher values of contrast indicate bigger differences between the voxels at a given direction and distance, while smaller values indicate uniformity between the voxel values. *Homogeneity/inverse difference moment* is just the opposite of contrast. We want to express the amount of uniformity in the image; thus we want to give bigger weights to elements close to the main diagonal of the GLCM and smaller weights to values farther away from it. To achieve this, we take the same weight as before and multiply the values by the reciprocal of this weight. Since the denominator would be 0 for elements on the diagonal, we add 1 to it for all weights. Pipeline for deriving GLCMs is shown in Fig. 56.4.

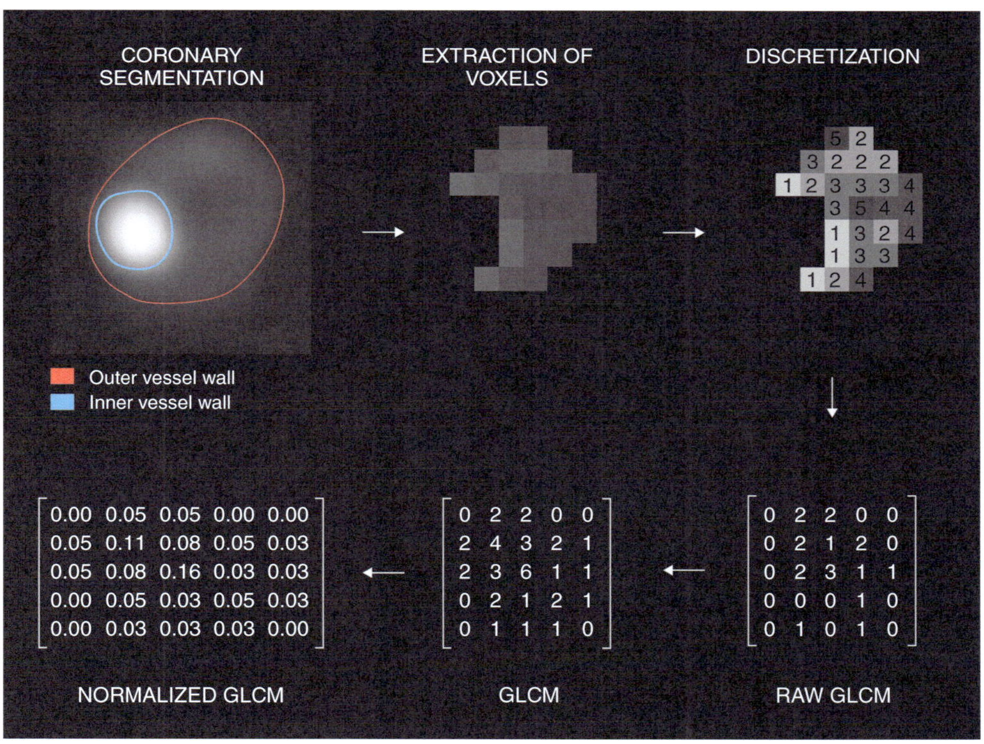

Fig. 56.4 Pipeline for calculating gray-level co-occurrence matrices (GLCM). First the coronary arteries need to be segmented. Then the voxels need to be extracted from the images. Next the images need to be discretized into *n* different value groups. Then a given direction and distance is determined to calculate the GLCM (distance 1, angle 0°). Raw GLCMs are created by calculating the number of times a value *j* occurs to the right of value *i*. This value is then inserted into the *ith* row and *jth* column of the raw GLCM. To achieve symmetry, the transpose is added to the raw GLCM. Next, the matrix is normalized by substituting each value by its frequency; this results in the normalized GLCM. Afterward, different statistics can be calculated from the GLCMs. To get rotationally invariant results, statistics are calculated in all four directions and then averaged. (From Kolossvary et al. [5], with permission)

These and several other measures can be calculated from the GLCMs. The values are a function of the angle at which we examined neighboring voxels. It is rational to suppose that texture is rotationally invariant. If we rotate our image by 90°, we should still get the same value for contrast or homogeneity. Texture is an intrinsic property of the image; it cannot have high and low contrast at the same time. To solve this discrepancy, the statistics calculated in all four directions are averaged.

Higher-Order Statistics

While second-order statistics looked at the relationship of two voxels, *higher-order statistics* assess the relationship of three or more voxels. Galloway proposed the idea of *gray-level run length matrix (GLRLM)*, which not only looks at pairs of voxels, but rather assesses how many identical-value voxels occur in a given direction next to each other [24]. Similarly, we can create such matrices in four different directions in 2D. The rows of the GLRLM represent again the given attenuation values, while the columns represent the given run lengths. Thus, an entry x in the *ith* row and *jth* column would mean that in the image it occurs x times that i intensity voxels are next to each other j times in the given direction.

Galloway proposed five easy statistics that can be calculated from these matrices, but many more exist [23]. *Short runs emphasis* takes each value in the matrix and divides it by its run length squared and then adds up all the values; thus short runs are emphasized, while long run lengths are diminished. *Long runs emphasis* does just the opposite; it multiplies each value of the matrix by its run length squared instead of dividing it and then sums all the values, thus emphasizing long runs. *Gray-level nonuniformity* highlights the dissimilarity of the voxels in the picture. It is calculated by adding up the number of different run lengths for a given intensity value and then squaring and summing them. If the runs are equally distributed throughout the HU values, then the value is minimal, while unevenly distributed gray-level intensities create large values. *Run length nonuniformity* adds up the number of times the given run length occurred for all gray values and then squares and adds them up. Instead of measuring intensity nonuniformity, this measures run length nonuniformity. These metrics are usually divided by the total number of runs to normalize it. The last statistics, *run percentage* is the ratio of the total number of runs to the number of voxels. It has the lowest value in cases of linear structures, where we have few long runs. Pipeline for deriving GLRLMs can be found in Fig. 56.5.

Several other concepts have also been introduced, such as the *gray level gap length matrix (GLGLM)*, which is similar to GLRLMs, but instead of quantifying how long same value voxels occur, it calculates how many voxels we need to travel in a direction to find a voxel with the same value [25]. The *gray-level size zone matrix (GLSZM)* is also similar to GLRLM but quantifies how many voxels of the same value are connected to each other, irrespective of direction [26]. The *neighborhood gray-tone difference matrix (NGTDM)* tries to mimic human perception mechanisms by including a whole neighborhood of voxels for calculating statistics [27]. Methods to eliminate the problem of image discretization have also been proposed, such as the *multiple gray-level size zone matrix (MGLSZM)*, which calculates the metrics for several different gray-level quantizations, which are summed using a weighted average [28].

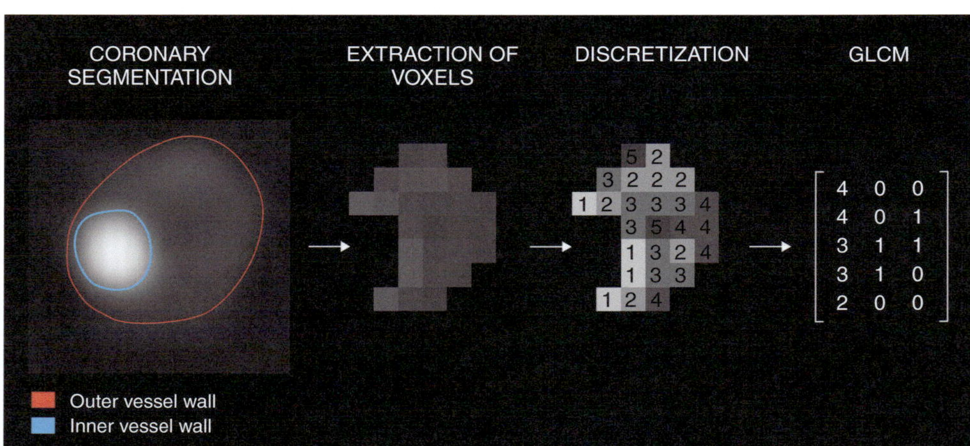

Fig. 56.5 Pipeline for calculating gray-level run length matrices (GLRLMs). First the coronary arteries need to be segmented. Next the voxels need to be extracted from the images. Then the images need to be discretized into n different value groups. Next a given direction (angle 0°) is determined. GLRLMs are created by calculating the number of times a i value voxels occur next to each other in the given direction. The *ith* row and *jth* column of the GLRLM represent how many times it occurs in the image and that i value voxels are next to each other j times. To get rotationally invariant results, the statistics calculated in different directions are averaged. (From Kolossvary [5], with permission)

Laws' Texture Energy Measures

Laws proposed a different method for quantifying different texture properties [29]. Instead of calculating metrics based on the relationship of neighboring voxels, he suggested filtering the image for specific structures. This is done by *convolution*, which simply means that we replace each pixel in the image with a weighted value of its neighbors. The values that we use as weights for filtering are stored in the *kernel* matrix. The convolution technique is used in daily practice to reconstruct images with sharper or smoother kernels. The sharp kernel improves spatial resolution, enhances edges, and reduces metallic or blooming artifacts (e.g., stents, heavy calcification). A sharper kernel generates images with higher spatial resolution but increases the image noise, whereas a smoother kernel generates images with lower noise but with reduced spatial resolution.

If we choose our kernel values carefully, we can emphasize different textures, such as edges or ripples, while canceling out other effects. Laws proposed five one-dimensional filters which can be combined to achieve two- or three-dimensional complex filters. Through convolution of our original image and the kernel, we receive a new image, which we can then analyze, usually calculating the energy as proposed earlier in the chapter.

Utilization and Potential Pitfalls of Texture-Based Metrics

Texture-based methods have been implemented to classify tumor heterogeneity [30], but cardiac implementations are scares. This is mainly due to several difficulties specific to cardiac imaging that are less prominent in tumors. Atherosclerotic lesions are very small; therefore only a limited number of voxels depict the abnormality. These statistics are robust in cases when there are a sufficient number of data points. While the submillimeter resolution of high-tech scanners is adequate for clinical decision-making and even volumetric analysis, it might not be enough for texture analysis. Furthermore, while anatomical planes are suitable for heterogeneity analysis of tumors, since they are directionally invariant, coronary arteries are complex 3D structures which have a specific direction; thus simple anatomical slices are inadequate for analysis. Finally, while a 2D plane can resemble the heterogeneity of a tumor, it may not be sufficient for atherosclerotic lesions, since they are complex 3D structures, where heterogeneity needs to be assessed in 3D, on the course of the coronary artery. Despite these potential limitations, there are promissing results of appling radiomics to identify vulnerable plaques from coronary CTA images. Kolossvary et al showed that texture-based radiomic statistics significantly outperformed conventional volumetric quantitative parameters to identify napkin-ring sign plaques from coronary CTA images [23].

Shape-Based Metrics

Coronary lesions are complex 3D objects. As the ratio and the spatial distribution of different plaque components change, also does the *shape* of the lesion. Shape is an abstract concept trying to quantify different geometrical properties of objects. Shape-based metrics can be grouped based on the dimension in which we do our measurements.

One-Dimensional (1D) Metrics

1D metrics are basically based on the diameters of the lesion. The diameter can be measured on the longest axes or the shortest axes or in any arbitrary direction. They can also be compared to other entities, as in the case of *diameter stenosis*, where the diameter of the lesion is divided by the vessel diameter on cross-sectional images to assess stenosis severity on coronary CTA. Furthermore, from these values many different metrics can be calculated, such as the ratio of longest diameter to the shortest diameter, which is close to 1 in case of cylindrical objects and gets bigger as the abnormality becomes elliptic, or the difference between the longest and the shortest diameter which also quantifies roundness.

Two-Dimensional (2D) Metrics

2D metrics are based on cross sections of the lesion. From these images several different parameters can be calculated. These are mainly based on different areas or on different border lengths. In most cases these 2D metrics are used to approximate more complex 3D metrics, since they are simpler to calculate. For example, *lesion area* is a measure used to describe the size of a lesion. Most common in case of coronary CTA is the *area stenosis*, which is the ratio of the vessel wall area to the vessel area. This metric is commonly used to assess positive remodeling.

Three-Dimensional (3D) Metrics

3D metrics aim to quantify different geometrical properties of the lesion. Many of these concepts originate from rigid body mechanics. All 3D objects have three so-called principal axes or eigenvectors, which are mutually perpendicular to each other and intersect at the center of mass. Torque applied around these principal axes acts independently, meaning that if we push or rotate our object along one principal axis, it will not rotate in any other direction. These eigenvectors also have corresponding *eigenvalues*, which can be interpreted as weights proportional to the amount of mass or HU intensities located in that direction.

Several different parameters can be derived from the eigenvectors, such as: *asymmetry* is defined as 1 minus the square root of the ratio of the smallest and the largest eigenvalues. In cases where HU values are distributed equally in all directions of the principal axes, then asymmetry is 0, while in cases where the distribution is imbalanced in the three directions, then it is close to 1. *Compactness* is a scaled product of the three eigenvalues divided by the volume of the lesion. The less spread-out our lesion is, the higher the compactness. *Roundness* is the difference of the biggest eigenvalue of the smallest enclosing and the largest enclosed ellipse. It describes how closely similar the lesion is to an ellipse. Small values indicate similarity to an ellipse, while larger values indicate more rounded shape.

Minkowski Functionals

Minkowski functionals originate from the area of integral geometry [31] and quantify different properties of complex geometrical structures. They can be implemented to calculate characteristics on 2D and 3D images from the number of connected and non-connected voxels, edges, and vertices. The results of some functionals are commonly known parameters such as *area* and *circumference* in 2D or *volume* and *surface area* in 3D [32]. Furthermore, the *Euler characteristic* or *genus* can be calculated which can be seen as a connectivity parameter representing the number of separate voxel groups containing a signal minus the number of completely enclosed regions where there is no signal. These values can be calculated on several images derived from the original image using different thresholds to receive an array of different values which can be statistically analyzed.

Fractal Dimension

Fractal geometry examines the self-similarity of objects. Fractals exhibit expanding symmetry by repeating patterns that are present at each scale. Conventional objects showing no fractal geometry scale their characteristics by a scalar on the power of the dimension meaning: if we scale a 1D object, for example, a line by two, then the length of the line will increase by 2^1. If we double the edge length of a 2D polygon, for example, a square, then the area will increase by 2^2. If we scale the radius of a 3D object such as a sphere, then its volume will increase by 2^3. For such geometrical objects, the fractal dimension is equal to the topological dimension and it is an integer. However, fractals behave differently. For example, a line whose topological dimension is 1 can have a fractal dimension anywhere between 1 and 2. If we were to scale this line by 2, then its length would not be twice as long. Actually, its length is undefined, since if we were to enlarge our image, then we would see more and more detail which affects the length of the line, but this continues infinitely as we magnify our image.

Fractal dimension is a measure for quantifying the spatial complexity of an object and is proportional to how the detail of the image changes as we alter the scale [33]. *Rényi dimensions* generalize the concept of fractal dimensions from which several different definitions can be gained. The *box-counting dimension* or *Minkowski-Bouligand dimension* is the easiest, we simply calculate how many voxels contain the image, and then we repeat this many times with a finer grid. We then plot the number of occupied voxels versus the reciprocal of the scale on a log-log plot. The box-counting dimension will be equal to the slope of the regression line that connects the points. The *information* and the *correlation* dimension can also be calculated from Rényi dimensions [34, 35].

Utilization and Potential Pitfalls of Shape-Based Metrics

To date, mainly the effect of 1D parameters on later MACE rates has been investigated. Conventionally, stenosis severity is expressed by diameter stenosis in the daily routine. Several studies have shown the prognostic value of diameter stenosis on later MACE rates, but long-term effects still remain a question [36]. Furthermore, lesion length has also been shown to effect later outcomes in patients undergoing percutaneous coronary intervention [37]. Most commonly used 2D shape-based metric is the cross-sectional area, which is used to calculate *positive remodeling*, which has been shown to be a vulnerability feature of rupture-prone plaques [38].

The main concern with shape-based metrics trying to quantify some geometrical aspect of a coronary lesion is that plaques grow along the coronary arteries, which have complex 3D shapes. The difficulty is that the length of a lesion is not equal to the distance measured between the origin and the end of lesion on the image, but instead equal to the distance along the coronary artery between the two points. Therefore, if we measure shape-based metrics not accounting for coronary geometry, then we are also including geometrical information regarding the arteries themselves. This might not be a problem, since coronary geometry and shape-based metrics can be very much interrelated, but little is known how they might affect each other. Finally, complex shape-based radiomic features require complex computational algorithms which are currently not implemented in clinical software.

Transform-Based Metrics

Images are two- or three-dimensional datasets where the pixels are positioned in the *spatial domain*. Transform-based metrics convert these images from the spatial domain to a different coordinate system, for example, the *frequency domain*, which uses information taken from the rate at which image intensity values change to describe the image, instead of using spatial coordinates for this purpose.

Fourier and Gabor Transforms

Fourier and *Gabor transforms* originate from signal processing. Fourier transform takes a 1D signal and decomposes it to a series of sinusoidal waves. Applying 1D Fourier transforms in both the x and the y imaging planes, we can transform our image to a 2D frequency domain. Gabor transform is similar to the Fourier transform but first filters the image by applying a Gaussian filter. This can be useful for image analysis, since the image can be filtered from specific frequencies such as noise, or different characteristics can be emphasized on the picture, for instance, edges. Using the *inverse Fourier transform*, the original image can be reconstructed from these sine and cosine frequencies. After transforming back our images, we can extract different statistics from our filtered images, such as texture-based metrics mentioned earlier.

Wavelet Transforms

While Fourier transform can be used to analyze the frequency component of a signal or an image, we lose all our spatial information. *Wavelet transform* on the other hand not only contains frequency information but also includes spatial information as well [39]. Basically we can sacrifice frequency precision to gain spatial information. By setting the values of two parameters, we can weight frequency over temporal information or vice versa. Therefore, a family of transformed pictures can be obtained from which statistical parameters can be calculated.

Utilization and Potential Pitfalls of Transform-Based Metrics

Fourier and Gabor transforms are extensively used for image filtering to increase quality. Their main application is not to produce quantitative parameters for image classification; thus their utilization as a classifier is scarce. Wavelet transforms are becoming increasingly popular since they incorporate spatial and frequency information as well. With the tuning of the parameters, infinite number of statistics can be derived from them. This poses a potential problem, since the selection of high accuracy classifiers from numerous potential parameters is prone to overfitting.

Conclusions

Radiology has undergone unprecedented developments over the past years. While medical images were only seen as rough representations of underlying pathologies in the past, the improvement of spatial and temporal resolution all leads to increased image quality allowing us to view radiologists as in vivo pathologists. This also means that radiologists are subjected to vast amounts of information, to the point that might not be comprehensible by humans. Radiomics has the potential to vastly increase our knowledge of the underlying pathological processes, but this requires new specialists who are familiar with new concepts which incorporate scientific fields such as computer vision and data science. Radiomics together with genetics, proteomics, and metabolomics has the potential to change our understanding of human diseases. We are at the dawn of a new era, where illnesses are no longer represented by a single value, but by a myriad of parameters. Thus, medical professionals need to get comfortable with relying more and more on quantitative data, rather than our medical assumptions. If we are unwilling to join this transition, we might be left behind.

References

1. Jones BK, Buckwalter AJ, McCarthy FE, DeYoung RB, El-Khoury YG, Dolan L, Gannon HF, Inwards YC, Klein JM, Kyriakos M, McCarthy FE, Rosenberg EA, Siegal PG, Unni KK, Fayad L, Kransdorf JM, Murphey DM, Panicek MD, Rubin AD, Sundaram M, Vanel D. Reliability of histopathologic and radiologic grading of cartilaginous neoplasms in long bones. J Bone Joint Surg Am. 2007;89(10):2113–23. https://doi.org/10.2106/JBJS.F.01530.
2. Rutkow IM. Surgical decision making. The reproducibility of clinical judgement. Arch Surg. 1982;117(3):337–40.
3. Barabasi AL, Gulbahce N, Loscalzo J. Network medicine: a network-based approach to human disease. Nat Rev Genet. 2011;12(1):56–68. https://doi.org/10.1038/nrg2918.
4. Gillies RJ, Kinahan PE, Hricak H. Radiomics: Images Are More than Pictures, They Are Data. Radiology. 2016;278(2):563–77. https://doi.org/10.1148/radiol.2015151169.
5. Kolossvary M, Kellermayer M, Merkely B, Maurovich-Horvat P. Cardiac computed tomography radiomics: a comprehensive review on radiomic techniques. J Thorac Imaging. 2017;33(1):26–34. https://doi.org/10.1097/RTI.0000000000000268.
6. Feuchtner G, Kerber J, Burghard P, Dichtl W, Friedrich G, Bonaros N, Plank F. The high-risk criteria low-attenuation plaque <60 HU and the napkin-ring sign are the most powerful predictors of MACE: a long-term follow-up study. Eur Heart J Cardiovasc Imaging. 2016. https://doi.org/10.1093/ehjci/jew167.
7. Otsuka K, Fukuda S, Tanaka A, Nakanishi K, Taguchi H, Yoshikawa J, Shimada K, Yoshiyama M. Napkin-ring sign on coronary CT angiography for the prediction of acute coronary syndrome. JACC Cardiovasc Imaging. 2013;6(4):448–57. https://doi.org/10.1016/j.jcmg.2012.09.016.
8. Shannon CE. A mathematical theory of communication. Bell Syst Tech J. 1948;27(3):379–423. https://doi.org/10.1002/j.1538-7305.1948.tb01338.x.
9. Agatston AS, Janowitz WR, Hildner FJ, Zusmer NR, Viamonte M Jr, Detrano R. Quantification of coronary artery calcium using ultrafast computed tomography. J Am Coll Cardiol. 1990;15(4):827–32.
10. McClelland RL, Jorgensen NW, Budoff M, Blaha MJ, Post WS, Kronmal RA, Bild DE, Shea S, Liu K, Watson KE, Folsom AR, Khera A, Ayers C, Mahabadi AA, Lehmann N, Jockel KH, Moebus S, Carr JJ, Erbel R, Burke GL. 10-Year coronary heart disease risk prediction using coronary artery calcium and traditional risk factors: derivation in the MESA (Multi-Ethnic Study of Atherosclerosis) with validation in the HNR (Heinz Nixdorf Recall) study and the DHS (Dallas Heart Study). J Am Coll Cardiol. 2015;66(15):1643–53. https://doi.org/10.1016/j.jacc.2015.08.035.
11. Polonsky TS, McClelland RL, Jorgensen NW, Bild DE, Burke GL, Guerci AD, Greenland P. Coronary artery calcium score and risk classification for coronary heart disease prediction. JAMA. 2010;303(16):1610–6. https://doi.org/10.1001/jama.2010.461.
12. Brodoefel H, Reimann A, Heuschmid M, Tsiflikas I, Kopp AF, Schroeder S, Claussen CD, Clouse ME, Burgstahler

C. Characterization of coronary atherosclerosis by dual-source computed tomography and HU-based color mapping: a pilot study. Eur Radiol. 2008;18(11):2466–74. https://doi.org/10.1007/s00330-008-1019-5.
13. Versteylen MO, Kietselaer BL, Dagnelie PC, Joosen IA, Dedic A, Raaijmakers RH, Wildberger JE, Nieman K, Crijns HJ, Niessen WJ, Daemen MJ, Hofstra L. Additive value of semiautomated quantification of coronary artery disease using cardiac computed tomographic angiography to predict future acute coronary syndrome. J Am Coll Cardiol. 2013;61(22):2296–305. https://doi.org/10.1016/j.jacc.2013.02.065.
14. Willemink MJ, Vliegenthart R, Takx RA, Leiner T, Budde RP, Bleys RL, Das M, Wildberger JE, Prokop M, Buls N, de Mey J, Schilham AM, de Jong PA. Coronary artery calcification scoring with state-of-the-art CT scanners from different vendors has substantial effect on risk classification. Radiology. 2014;273(3):695–702. https://doi.org/10.1148/radiol.14140066.
15. Szilveszter B, Elzomor H, Karolyi M, Kolossvary M, Raaijmakers R, Benke K, Celeng C, Bartykowszki A, Bagyura Z, Lux A, Merkely B, Maurovich-Horvat P. The effect of iterative model reconstruction on coronary artery calcium quantification. Int J Cardiovasc Imaging. 2016;32(1):153–60. https://doi.org/10.1007/s10554-015-0740-9.
16. Symons R, Morris JZ, Wu CO, Pourmorteza A, Ahlman MA, Lima JA, Chen MY, Mallek M, Sandfort V, Bluemke DA. Coronary CT angiography: variability of CT scanners and readers in measurement of plaque volume. Radiology. 2016:161670. https://doi.org/10.1148/radiol.2016161670.
17. Precht H, Kitslaar PH, Broersen A, Dijkstra J, Gerke O, Thygesen J, Egstrup K, Lambrechtsen J. Influence of adaptive statistical iterative reconstruction on coronary plaque analysis in coronary computed tomography angiography. J Cardiovasc Comput Tomogr. 2016. https://doi.org/10.1016/j.jcct.2016.09.006.
18. Fuchs TA, Fiechter M, Gebhard C, Stehli J, Ghadri JR, Kazakauskaite E, Herzog BA, Husmann L, Gaemperli O, Kaufmann PA. CT coronary angiography: impact of adapted statistical iterative reconstruction (ASIR) on coronary stenosis and plaque composition analysis. Int J Cardiovasc Imaging. 2013;29(3):719–24. https://doi.org/10.1007/s10554-012-0134-1.
19. Pohle K, Achenbach S, Macneill B, Ropers D, Ferencik M, Moselewski F, Hoffmann U, Brady TJ, Jang IK, Daniel WG. Characterization of non-calcified coronary atherosclerotic plaque by multi-detector row CT: comparison to IVUS. Atherosclerosis. 2007;190(1):174–80. https://doi.org/10.1016/j.atherosclerosis.2006.01.013.
20. Sun J, Zhang Z, Lu B, Yu W, Yang Y, Zhou Y, Wang Y, Fan Z. Identification and quantification of coronary atherosclerotic plaques: a comparison of 64-MDCT and intravascular ultrasound. AJR Am J Roentgenol. 2008;190(3):748–54. https://doi.org/10.2214/AJR.07.2763.
21. Takahashi S, Kawasaki M, Miyata S, Suzuki K, Yamaura M, Ido T, Aoyama T, Fujiwara H, Minatoguchi S. Feasibility of tissue characterization of coronary plaques using 320-detector row computed tomography: comparison with integrated backscatter intravascular ultrasound. Heart Vessel. 2016;31(1):29–37. https://doi.org/10.1007/s00380-014-0577-5.
22. Haralick RM, Shanmugam K, Dinstein I. Textural features for image classification. IEEE Trans Syst Man Cybern. 1973;SMC-3(6):610–21. https://doi.org/10.1109/TSMC.1973.4309314.
23. Kolossváry M, Karády J, Szilveszter B, Kitslaar P, Hoffmann U, Merkely B, Maurovich-Horvat P. Radiomic features are superior to conventional quantitative computed tomographic metrics to identify coronary plaques with napkin-ring sign. Circ Cardiovasc Imaging. 2017;10(12):e006843.
24. Galloway MM. Texture analysis using gray level run lengths. Comput Graphics Image Process. 1975;4(2):172–9. https://doi.org/10.1016/S0146-664X(75)80008-6.
25. Xinli W, Albregtsen F, Foyn B. Texture analysis using gray level gap length matrix. Paper presented at the Selected papers from the 9th Scandinavian conference on Image analysis: theory and applications of image analysis II: theory and applications of image analysis II, Uppsala, Sweden; 1995.
26. Thibault G, Fertil B, Navarro C, Pereira S, Cau P, Levy N, Sequeira J, Mari J-L. Shape and texture indexes application to cell nuclei classification. Int J Pattern Recognit Artif Intell. 2013;27(01):1357002. https://doi.org/10.1142/s0218001413570024.
27. Amadasun M, King R. Textural features corresponding to textural properties. IEEE Trans Syst Man Cybern. 1989;19(5):1264–74. https://doi.org/10.1109/21.44046.
28. Thibault G, Angulo J, Meyer F. Advanced statistical matrices for texture characterization: application to cell classification. IEEE Trans Biomed Eng. 2014;61(3):630–7. https://doi.org/10.1109/TBME.2013.2284600.
29. Laws KI. Textured image segmentation. A Dissertation Presented to the Faculty of the Graduate School. University of Southern California; 1980.
30. O'Connor JP, Rose CJ, Waterton JC, Carano RA, Parker GJ, Jackson A. Imaging intratumor heterogeneity: role in therapy response, resistance, and clinical outcome. Clin Cancer Res. 2015;21(2):249–57. https://doi.org/10.1158/1078-0432.CCR-14-0990.
31. Minkowski H. Volumen und Oberfläche. Math Ann. 1903;57:447.
32. Larkin TJ, Canuto HC, Kettunen MI, Booth TC, Hu DE, Krishnan AS, Bohndiek SE, Neves AA, McLachlan C, Hobson MP, Brindle KM. Analysis of image heterogeneity using 2D Minkowski functionals detects tumor responses to treatment. Magn Reson Med. 2014;71(1):402–10. https://doi.org/10.1002/mrm.24644.
33. Mandelbrot B. How long is the coast of Britain? statistical self-similarity and fractional dimension. Science. 1967;156:636–8.
34. Rose CJ, Mills SJ, O'Connor JP, Buonaccorsi GA, Roberts C, Watson Y, Cheung S, Zhao S, Whitcher B, Jackson A, Parker GJ. Quantifying spatial heterogeneity in dynamic contrast-enhanced MRI parameter maps. Magn Reson Med. 2009;62(2):488–99. https://doi.org/10.1002/mrm.22003.
35. Lopes R, Betrouni N. Fractal and multifractal analysis: a review. Med Image Anal. 2009;13(4):634–49. https://doi.org/10.1016/j.media.2009.05.003.
36. Kolossváry M, Szilveszter B, Merkely B, Maurovich-Horvat P. Plaque imaging with CT – a comprehensive review on coronary CT angiography based risk assessment. Cardiovasc Diagn Ther. 2017. https://doi.org/10.21037/cdt.2016.11.06.
37. Claessen BE, Smits PC, Kereiakes DJ, Parise H, Fahy M, Kedhi E, Serruys PW, Lansky AJ, Cristea E, Sudhir K, Sood P, Simonton CA, Stone GW. Impact of lesion length and vessel size on clinical outcomes after percutaneous coronary intervention with everolimus- versus paclitaxel-eluting stents pooled analysis from the SPIRIT (Clinical Evaluation of the XIENCE V Everolimus Eluting Coronary Stent System) and COMPARE (Second-generation everolimus-eluting and paclitaxel-eluting stents in real-life practice) Randomized Trials. JACC Cardiovasc Interv. 2011;4(11):1209–15. https://doi.org/10.1016/j.jcin.2011.07.016.
38. Motoyama S, Kondo T, Sarai M, Sugiura A, Harigaya H, Sato T, Inoue K, Okumura M, Ishii J, Anno H, Virmani R, Ozaki Y, Hishida H, Narula J. Multislice computed tomographic characteristics of coronary lesions in acute coronary syndromes. J Am Coll Cardiol. 2007;50(4):319–26. https://doi.org/10.1016/j.jacc.2007.03.044.
39. Dettori L, Semler L. A comparison of wavelet, ridgelet, and curvelet-based texture classification algorithms in computed tomography. Comput Biol Med. 2007;37(4):486–98. https://doi.org/10.1016/j.compbiomed.2006.08.002.

57 Advanced Methods for Coronary Artery Plaque Analysis

Pál Maurovich-Horvat and Udo Hoffmann

The quest to identify vulnerable patients and perhaps even individual atherosclerotic coronary plaques that will cause future acute coronary events remains to be one of the greatest challenges of modern cardiovascular medicine [1–3]. Current guidelines on diagnostic strategies of patients with stable coronary artery disease (CAD) focus on the detection of significant coronary artery stenosis or myocardial ischemia [4]. Needless to say that such a strategy will not identify the patients who die suddenly due to acute coronary events without prior clinical manifestations of CAD [5]. It has been demonstrated by postmortem investigations that majority of acute coronary syndromes are caused by plaque rupture and subsequent sudden luminal thrombosis [6–8]. Rupture-prone atherosclerotic lesions have been termed as vulnerable plaques, which have distinct characteristics from stable lesions. The differences in morphology and functional and metabolic characteristics provide a unique opportunity for non-invasive cardiac imaging to identify these lesions before they cause acute events (Fig. 57.1) [9–11]. Moreover, it has been demonstrated that on a patient level, the total quantity of plaques (i.e., plaque burden) has a strong predictive value for myocardial infarction [12, 13]. Therefore, it appears that the assessment of coronary plaque morphology and plaque burden is potentially very important for prediction of future cardiovascular events [7, 14, 15]. Coronary computed tomography angiography (CTA) is a unique imaging technique that allows for the non-invasive depiction of the global coronary plaque burden, not just the individual plaques and luminal stenosis [16].

P. Maurovich-Horvat (✉)
Cardiovascular Imaging Research Group, Heart and Vascular Center, Semmelweis University, Budapest, Hungary
e-mail: p.maurovich-horvat@cirg.hu

U. Hoffmann
Department of Cardiovascular Imaging, Massachusetts General Hospital, Boston, MA, USA

Plaque Characterization

It has been demonstrated that vulnerable plaques harbor the same morphologic characteristics as ruptured plaques, with the only difference lying in the intact thin fibrous cap [8]. Vulnerable plaques are generally large and contain a large necrotic core covered by markedly attenuated and inflamed fibrous caps; therefore these plaques are identified as thin-cap fibroatheromas (TCFA) in histology [9, 17]. Thin fibrotic cap is defined as a cap thickness of <65 μm, which is beyond the spatial resolution limit of the state-of-the-art CT scanners (≈0.4 mm); therefore the non-invasive morphometric assessment of the fibrotic cap is currently not feasible [8]. However, histopathologic investigations have revealed that vulnerable plaques prone to rupture need to grow in a sizeable extent in all three spatial dimensions [17, 18]. Furthermore, it has been shown that the necrotic core length of vulnerable plaques ranges between 2 and 17 mm (mean 8 mm) and the area of the necrotic core in 80% of vulnerable plaques is larger than 1.0 mm^2 [17]. These spatial dimensions are above the plaque detection threshold of coronary CTA (>1 mm plaque thickness) [19]. In addition, 95% of vulnerable plaques are confined to the proximal coronary segments, where coronary CTA has the best accuracy due to the large vessel diameter and less frequent motion artifacts [17, 20]. Therefore, the non-invasive assessment of coronary plaques and the identification of high-risk lesions with coronary CTA might be feasible. The conventional coronary CTA plaque classification scheme is based on the presence and quantity of calcific plaque components; thus the following plaque categories can be differentiated: calcified, partially calcified (mixed), and non-calcified plaque (NCP). Partially calcified lesions can be further divided into predominant calcified and predominant non-calcified plaques (Fig. 57.2). In clinical reports, the description of plaques as "non-calcified" is preferable to "soft" or "lipid rich" as low CT density (HU) levels do not necessarily correlate closely with pathology or biochemistry [21].

U. J. Schoepf (ed.), *CT of the Heart*, Contemporary Medical Imaging, https://doi.org/10.1007/978-1-60327-237-7_57

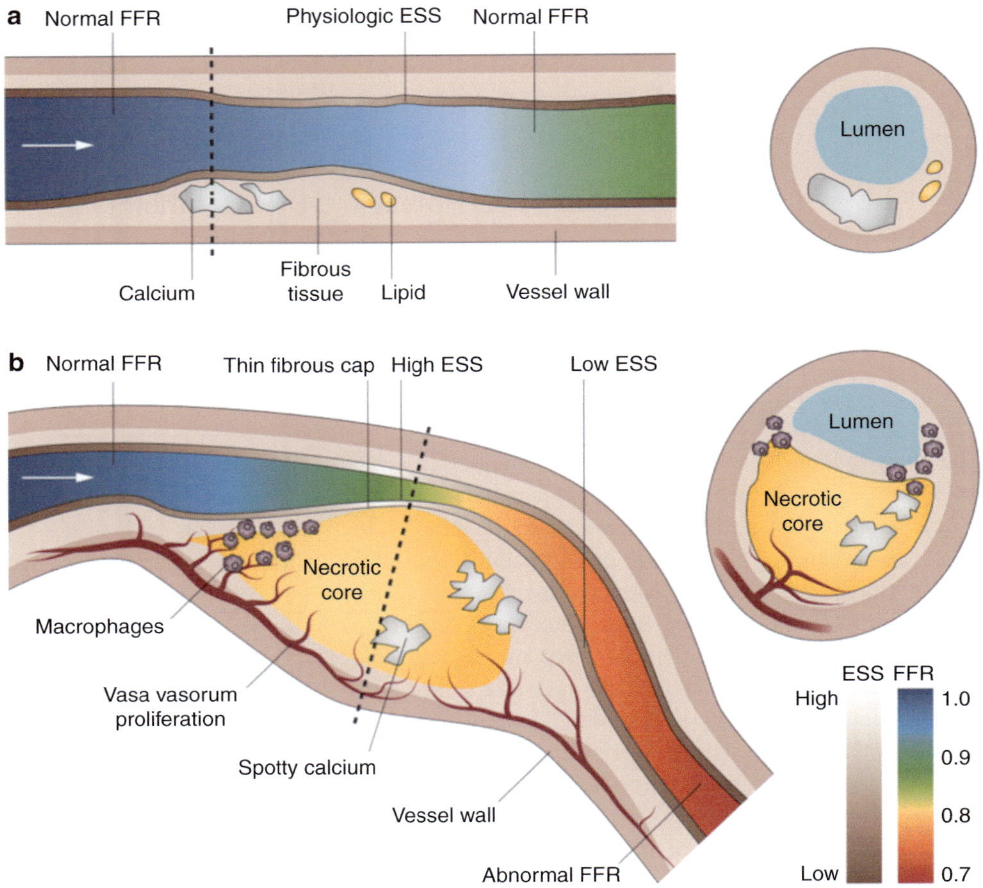

Fig. 57.1 The morphologic and functional characteristics of stable and vulnerable plaques. (**a**) Fibrocalcific lesion with calcification and small lipid pools considered to be a stable plaque. The plaque causes mild luminal narrowing without ischemia (FFR >0.8; green color). The ESS in the vicinity of the plaque is in the normal range. (**b**) A thin-cap fibroatheroma with a large lipid-rich necrotic core, thin fibrous cap, neovascularization, spotty calcium, and presence of inflammatory cells is a vulnerable plaque. Despite the positively remodeled vessel wall at the site of the plaque, the lesion causes luminal narrowing and ischemia (FFR <0.8; red color). The downstream plaque region with low ESS promotes plaque growth, whereas the high ESS at the most stenotic part can trigger plaque rupture. Abbreviations: ESS, endothelial shear stress; FFR, fractional flow reserve. (From Maurovich-Horvat et al. [11], with permission)

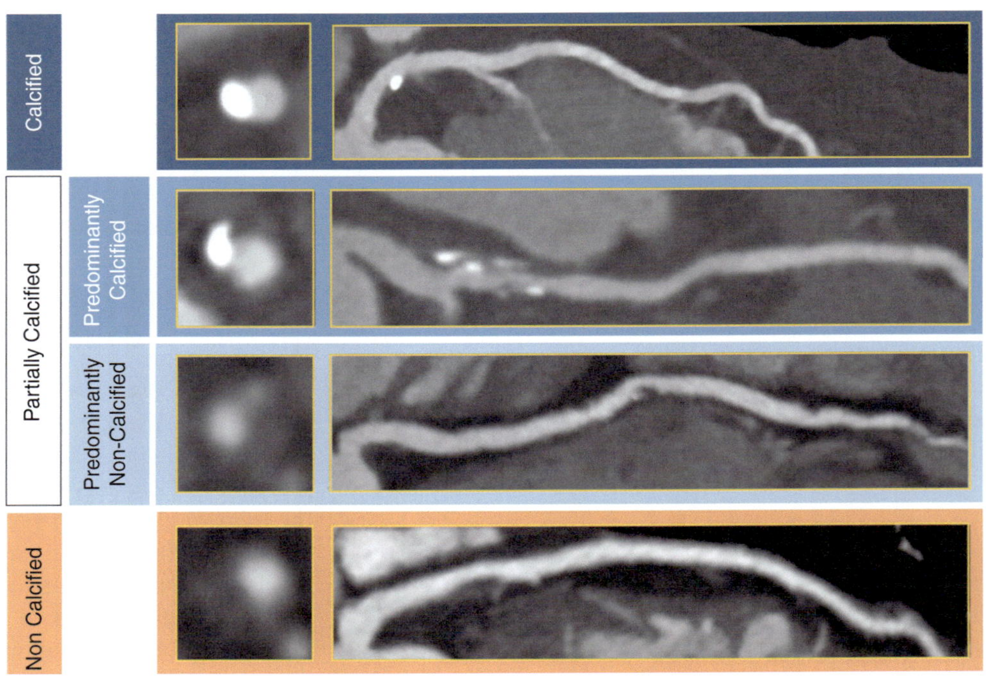

Fig. 57.2 The conventional coronary CTA plaque classification scheme is based on the presence and quantity of calcium. The following plaque categories can be differentiated: calcified, partially calcified (mixed), and non-calcified plaque. Partially calcified lesions can be further divided into predominantly calcified and predominantly non-calcified plaques. The figure shows cross-sectional images and curved multiplanar reconstructions of various plaque types

Low-Attenuation Plaque

Despite the challenges associated with CT density-based plaque assessment, several investigators have attempted to correlate HU measurements with plaque lipid content using intravascular ultrasound (IVUS) or histology as reference standard. NCPs with high CT attenuation correlated with fibrous tissue, and those with low densities correlated with necrotic core and fibro-fatty tissue [22]. In general, plaques with a mean attenuation of <30 HU are considered low-attenuation plaques and have been associated to increased risk of acute coronary events [23]. However, almost all investigators reported a substantial overlap of CT densities between fibrous and lipid-rich plaques, which precludes the reliable identification of high-risk lesions based solely on HU measurements [22, 24]. Furthermore, it is important to note that the measurement of plaque attenuation is affected by several technical factors, such as the adjacent intraluminal iodinated contrast attenuation, tube voltage, slice thickness, and reconstruction filter [25–28]. Despite of these limitations associated to HU measurements, low CT attenuation is a well-established high-risk coronary plaque feature.

Positive Remodeling

The seminal work of Glagov demonstrated that the growth of the lipid-rich atherosclerotic plaques initially manifests with outward plaque expansion (i.e., positive vessel remodeling) to preserve the coronary lumen and flow [29]. Therefore, it should be noted that positively remodeled plaques might be missed if assessed solely by luminal narrowing measurements, such as invasive coronary angiography. Positive remodeling is associated with plaque vulnerability, abundance of macrophages, and increased necrotic core [30]. Coronary CTA can visualize the vessel wall; therefore it is well suited to measure cross-sectional diameter and area. The remodeling index is calculated as the vessel cross-sectional area at the site of stenosis divided by the average of proximal and distal reference areas [31, 32]. A ≥1.1 remodeling index was suggested for the definition of positive remodeling in coronary CTA, which corresponds to a 10% increase in cross-sectional area at the site of the stenosis relative to the reference sites [32, 33]. The pioneering work of Motoyama and colleagues demonstrated a strong association between ACS and the presence of positively remodeled plaques as assessed by coronary CTA [23]. Furthermore, positive remodeling had the best diagnostic performance among other high-risk plaque features (low attenuation, spotty calcification) to identify the culprit lesions in ACS patients (sensitivity 87%, specificity 88%, PPV 89%, NPV 85%) [23]. The same group demonstrated in a follow-up study using serial coronary CTA that the high-risk plaques only resulted in an acute coronary event if they were associated with plaque progression and suggested that among plaques with features of vulnerability, those with a higher degree of progression have much greater likelihood to result in ACS [34, 35].

Napkin-Ring Sign

A histopathologic study demonstrated that among plaque features that are potentially accessible by non-invasive imaging techniques, the size of necrotic core (>3.5 mm^2) is one of the best discriminators between vulnerable plaques and stable lesions [10, 14]. Therefore, the detection of large necrotic core might be a promising target for coronary CTA to risk-stratify individual coronary plaques. Since lipid-rich tissue is associated with low attenuation in coronary CTA, plaque cross section with centrally located area of low attenuation might be indicative of the presence of large lipid-rich necrotic core. In an ex vivo coronary CTA investigation, the authors demonstrated that plaques with a large necrotic core have a distinct attenuation pattern, which was termed as the napkin-ring sign (NRS) [36]. The NRS is a qualitative plaque feature, and it can be defined in a non-calcified plaque cross section by the presence of two features: (1) a central area of low CT attenuation that is apparently in contact with the lumen, (2) which is surrounded by a ring-like higher attenuation plaque tissue (Fig. 57.3) [11, 36]. A histopathologic investigation showed that the area of necrotic core was more than twice as large in NRS plaques than in non-NRS plaques (median 1.10 mm^2 vs. 0.46 mm^2, $p = 0.05$) [37]. Furthermore the specificity of NRS to identify TCFA was excellent (94.1%) [38]. Two large prospective studies demonstrated that the presence of NRS is an independent predictor of future acute coronary events (independent of the presence of positive remodeling and low attenuation) [39, 40]. The NRS appears to be a signature of plaques with large necrotic core; furthermore longitudinal investigations show strong prognostic value of this plaque feature to predict future coronary events.

Spotty Calcium

Calcification is a *condicio sine qua non* of advanced atherosclerosis [41]. However, the effect of calcification on plaque instability is not fully understood [42–44]. Histopathology studies have demonstrated that most plaque ruptures contain some calcification; however, approximately two-thirds of these are microcalcifications that are not detectable by coronary CTA [45]. In coronary CTA, spotty calcification is defined as a small (less than 3 mm), hyperdense plaque component surrounded by non-calcified plaque tissue [23]. Spotty calcifications can be classified as small (<1 mm), intermediate (1–3 mm), and large (>3 mm) calcifications, and it seems

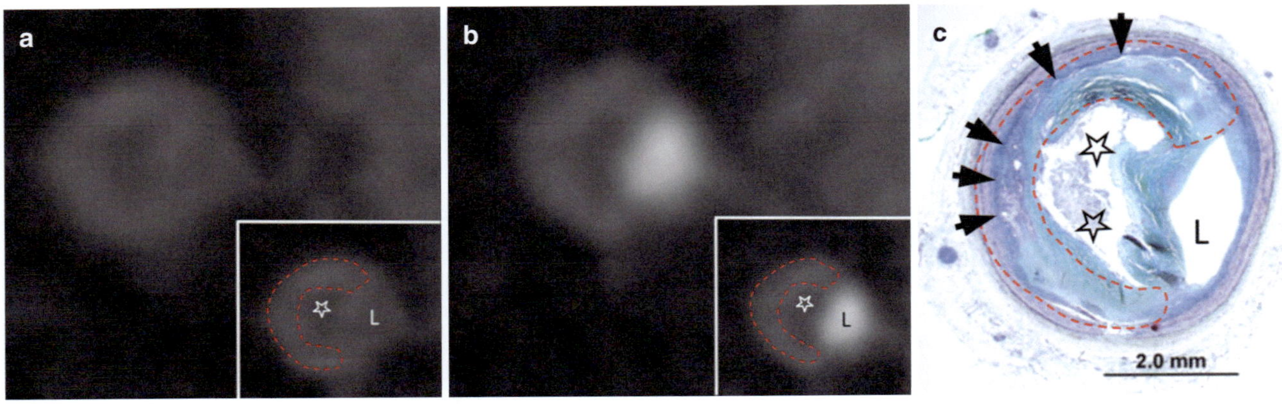

Fig. 57.3 Cross sections of a non-calcified coronary plaque with napkin-ring sign. The circumferential outer rim of the plaque (red dashed line) has a higher CT attenuation in both the non-contrast (panel A) and contrast-enhanced (panel B) images as compared to the attenuation within the central part of the plaque. The corresponding histopathological section (panel C) demonstrates a high-risk plaque with large necrotic core. The stars indicate the necrotic core, which correlates with the low-attenuation plaque core on the CT images, whereas the outer portion of the plaque contains fibrous plaque tissue correlating to the high-attenuation CT rim. Notably, the low-attenuation central part of the plaque is apparently in contact with the lumen (panel B). L: lumen (From Maurovich-Horvat et al. [36], with permission)

that small spotty calcium shows the strongest association with vulnerable plaques [46]. Several large studies demonstrated that spotty calcium is a sensitive but not very specific marker of high-risk coronary plaques [23, 47–50].

Plaque Quantification

Rapture-prone plaques and culprit lesions in patients who suffered ACS tend to have large size; therefore it is reasonable to hypothesize that coronary CTA plaque quantification might have an incremental value in risk stratification over traditional CTA plaque assessment [9, 11]. In line with this notion, coronary CTA studies of ACS and stable angina pectoris (SAP) patients demonstrated that the culprit plaques in patients with ACS have larger plaque volume than stable lesions in patients with SAP [50]. In addition, patients with unstable angina quantitative coronary CTA analysis revealed that plaques with morphological features of plaque disruption (e.g., intraplaque contrast dye penetration) had larger volume and contained more low CT attenuation plaque components as compared to plaques with no signs of disruption [51].

Invasive and non-invasive imaging studies have demonstrated that coronary atherosclerosis is a dynamic process. Plaques change size, morphology, and composition over few months, gaining or losing high-risk features [52–54]. The probability that a plaque remains unstable and eventually causes a clinical event increases with the number of plaques. Several longitudinal studies have demonstrated that a larger plaque burden is associated with adverse outcome [12, 13]. A sub-study of the COURAGE trial (Clinical Outcomes Utilizing Revascularization and Aggressive Drug Evaluation) showed that plaque burden is a stronger predictor of future major adverse cardiovascular events than ischemic myocardium burden [13]. In line with these observations, a recent study showed that patients with five or more than five coronary segments with non-obstructive atherosclerotic plaque have a similar risk of developing adverse coronary event as patients with obstructive CAD with less than five coronary segments involved [12]. Segment stenosis score (SSS) and segment involvement score (SIS) are semiquantitative metrics to quantify plaque burden [55]. The SSS is calculated by grading all coronary segments as 0, no stenosis/no plaque; 1, <50% stenosis; 2, 50–69% stenosis; and 3, ≥70% stenosis, whereas SIS is the number of segments that contain any plaque. Both SSS and SIS are independent predictors of coronary events [56–59]. Similarly, results from the CONFIRM (Coronary CT Angiography Evaluation for Clinical Outcomes: an International Multicenter) registry also showed SIS to be an independent predictor of major adverse events (hazard ratio, 1.22; CI, 1.03–1.44) [60]. The CONFIRM risk score is a combination of clinical cardiovascular risk, the number of proximal coronary segments with stenosis greater than 50%, and the number of proximal segments with partially calcified or calcified plaques. The combined risk score outperforms all clinical risk prediction scores and significantly improves prediction of all-cause mortality [60]. Automated software tools are now available for plaque quantification and characterization and have the potential to improve the reproducibility, accuracy, and efficiency of coronary CTA-based plaque burden assessment (Fig. 57.4). A recent study demonstrated that patients who developed ACS had a higher total plaque volume and total NCP volume at the baseline; therefore it seems that semiautomatic plaque quantification provides additional prognostic value for ACS over both clinical risk factors and traditional CT reading (including calcium score, segment stenosis score, lesion severity, and number of segments with NCP) [61]. The accuracy of automated quantification of coronary plaque by coronary CTA

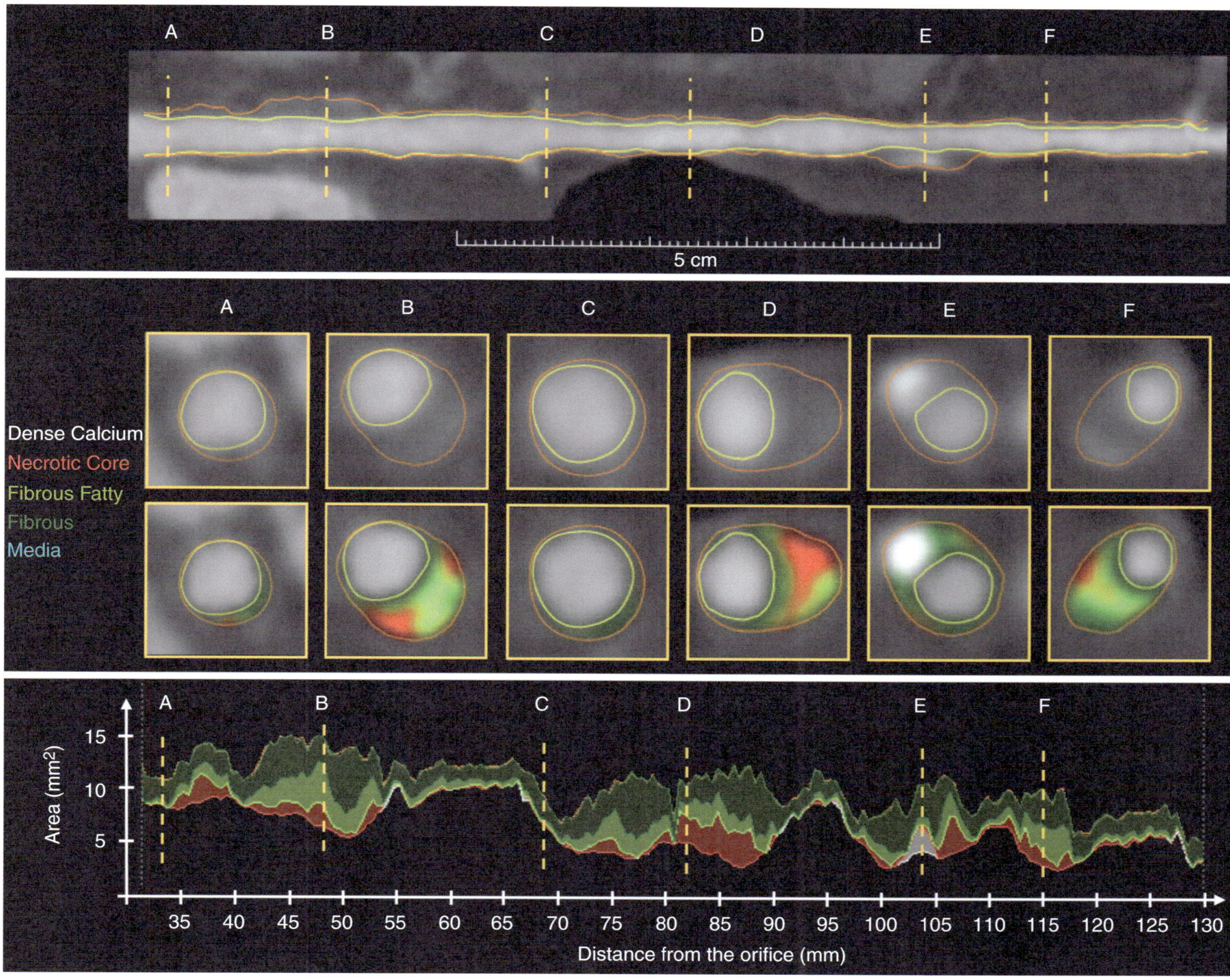

Fig. 57.4 Semiautomated plaque characterization and quantification using a dedicated software tool. The upper panel represents a stretched view of a segmented left anterior descending coronary artery. The orange line indicates the outer vessel wall, whereas the yellow line indicates the lumen. The middle panel shows plaque cross sections along the vessel without and with color overlay. The lower panel illustrates the areas of different plaque components. The letters from A to F represent the location of the cross-sectional images

was successfully validated against gray-scale intravascular ultrasound (IVUS) and virtual histology IVUS [22, 62, 63]. It is important to note that automated plaque quantification software tools provide a good intra-platform reproducibility but poor inter-platform reproducibility; therefore it is recommended to use the same software for serial or comparative assessments [64].

Functional Plaque Assessment FFR_{CT} and ESS_{CT}

Fractional flow reserve (FFR) derived from coronary CTA (FFR_{CT}) is a promising non-invasive marker of coronary physiology [65]. The diagnostic performance of FFR_{CT} is superior to anatomical coronary stenosis assessment alone when compared with the reference standard invasive FFR measurement [66, 67]. Importantly, FFR_{CT} can be derived from coronary CTA dataset acquired in a standard fashion, without the need for additional imaging, extra radiation, or any medication (Fig. 57.5). It has been demonstrated that FFR identifies hemodynamically significant lesions likely to produce ischemia-related symptoms; however, it is less clear why FFR might predict the subsequent risk for ACS resulting from plaque rupture and coronary thrombosis [68]. The presence of a large plaque volume, large low-attenuation plaque volume, and higher positive remodeling index was found to be strongly predictive of reduced FFR regardless of the degree of stenosis on multivariable analysis [69]. It is proposed that the presence of plaques with large necrotic cores may be associated with the inability of the vessel to dilate and may predispose to ischemia and abnormal FFR

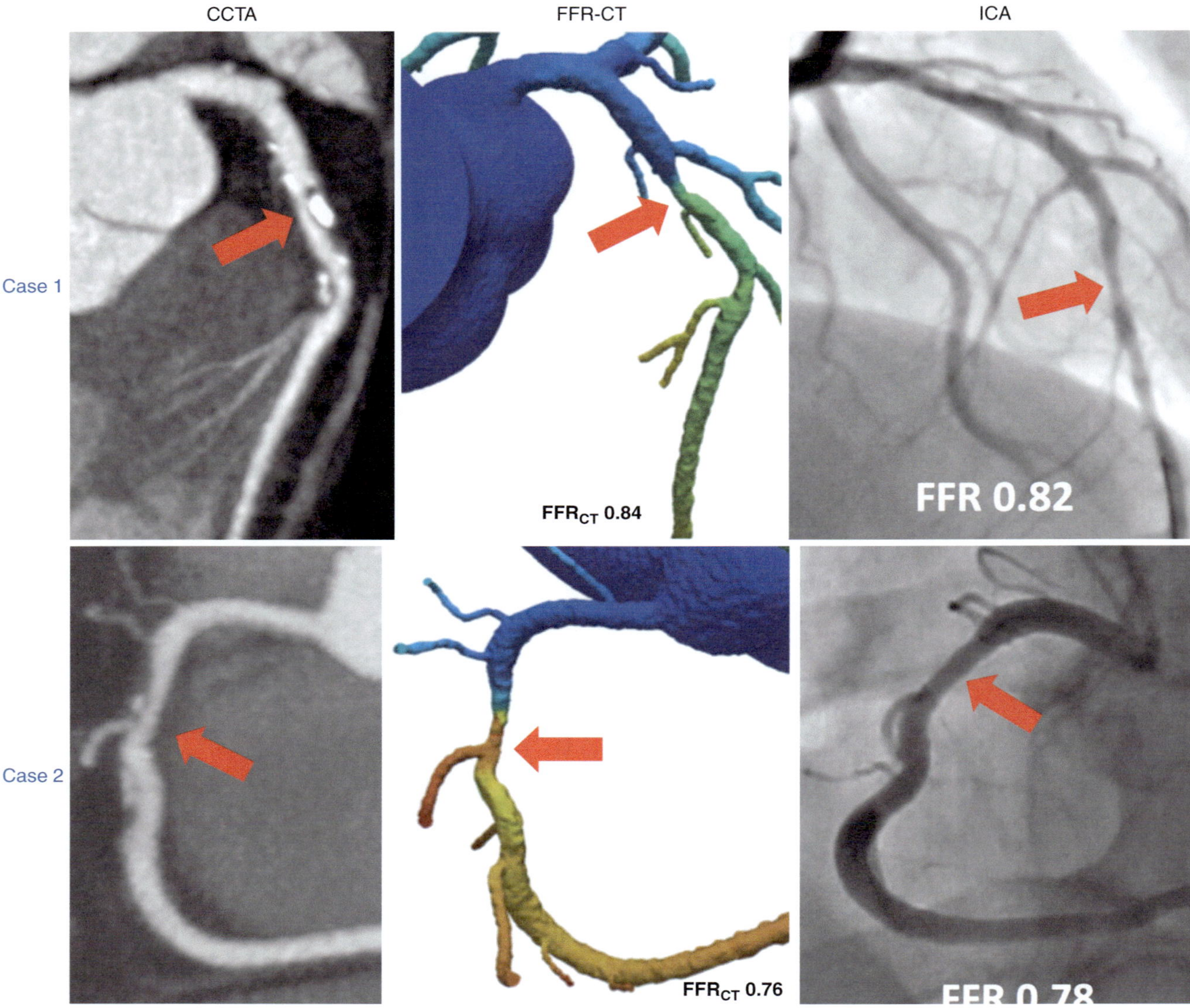

Fig. 57.5 Both cases (upper and lower panels) represent severe stenosis (approximately 70%) as depicted by coronary CTA. FFR-CT demonstrates no lesion-specific ischemia (0.86) in the first case, whereas the FFR-CT shows ischemia (0.70) in the second case. Both coronary CTA stenosis severities and the FFR-CT values were confirmed by ICA. The arrows indicate severe luminal narrowing both in coronary CTA and ICA. Abbreviations: CTA, computed tomography angiography; FFR, fractional flow reserve; ICA, invasive coronary angiography (Courtesy of HeartFlow Inc., Redwood City, CA, USA)

[68]. Therefore, FFR seems to be an important determinant of lesion vulnerability.

Plaques develop at specific areas of coronary arteries where flow is disturbed, such as the outer walls of bifurcations, in side branches, and in the inner curve of the arteries. These predilection sites are characterized by low and oscillatory endothelial shear stress [70, 71]. On the other hand, it seems that high endothelial shear stress (ESS) is a key component in atherosclerotic plaque destabilization, arterial wall remodeling, and atherosclerosis progression [72]. ESS is the tangential force generated by the friction of flowing blood on the endothelial surface of the arterial wall [73].

Abnormal FFR, the flow perturbations, the altered ESS, and lesion strain might be responsible for the development of rupture-prone lesion [74, 75]. Furthermore, patients with an obstructive coronary plaque may in fact develop an ACS due to the high ESS-induced thrombus formation [76]. Therefore the determination of blood flow-related functional parameters might improve the atherosclerotic lesion characterization [77]. The three-dimensional dataset acquired by coronary CTA allows for computational fluid dynamics and the simulation of patient-specific hemodynamic parameters including FFR_{CT} and ESS_{CT}, which highly likely will improve the accuracy of coronary CTA to detect vulnerable plaques.

Spectral Plaque Assessment

Conventional single-energy coronary CTA faces a significant challenge in differentiating components of non-calcified plaques (e.g., lipid-rich vs. fibrous) [78]. Several studies have shown considerable overlap in Hounsfield units between lipid-rich and fibrous non-calcified plaques inherent to the limited spatial and soft-tissue resolution of CT [79]. Spectral or multi-energy CT imaging has a great potential to improve morphological plaque assessment. Spectral CT allows for both monochromatic energy imaging and material basis decomposition. Materials and tissues can be distinguished by evaluating material density images [80]. The tissue characterization capabilities of spectral CT may improve the identification of lipid-rich components of non-calcified plaque tissue [81]. Furthermore, density and atomic number histograms of materials can be derived within regions of interests. It has been demonstrated that this histogram analysis is able to differentiate between components of renal stones and may also be applied to evaluate components of coronary calcifications such as calcium oxalate and hydroxyapatite [82]. In addition, spectral CT imaging of gold-labeled high-density lipoprotein (Au-HDL) nanoparticles designed to target activated macrophages showed promising results in atherosclerotic mice model [83]. The results in animal studies are encouraging and might open new avenues in multi-contrast spectral imaging. The capabilities of spectral CT imaging are promising; however, further studies are warranted to determine the proper methods for plaque assessment by this emerging technology.

Coronary CTA Radiomics

For long, radiological images have been regarded as pictures of the inner body. However, radiological images are in fact multidimensional datasets consisting of voxels, and each voxel value represents a specific measurement based on physical tissue characteristics. *Radiomics* is the process of obtaining quantitative parameters from these spatial datasets, in order to create "big data" databases, where each lesion is characterized by hundreds of different parameters (Fig. 57.6) [84, 85]. These features aim to

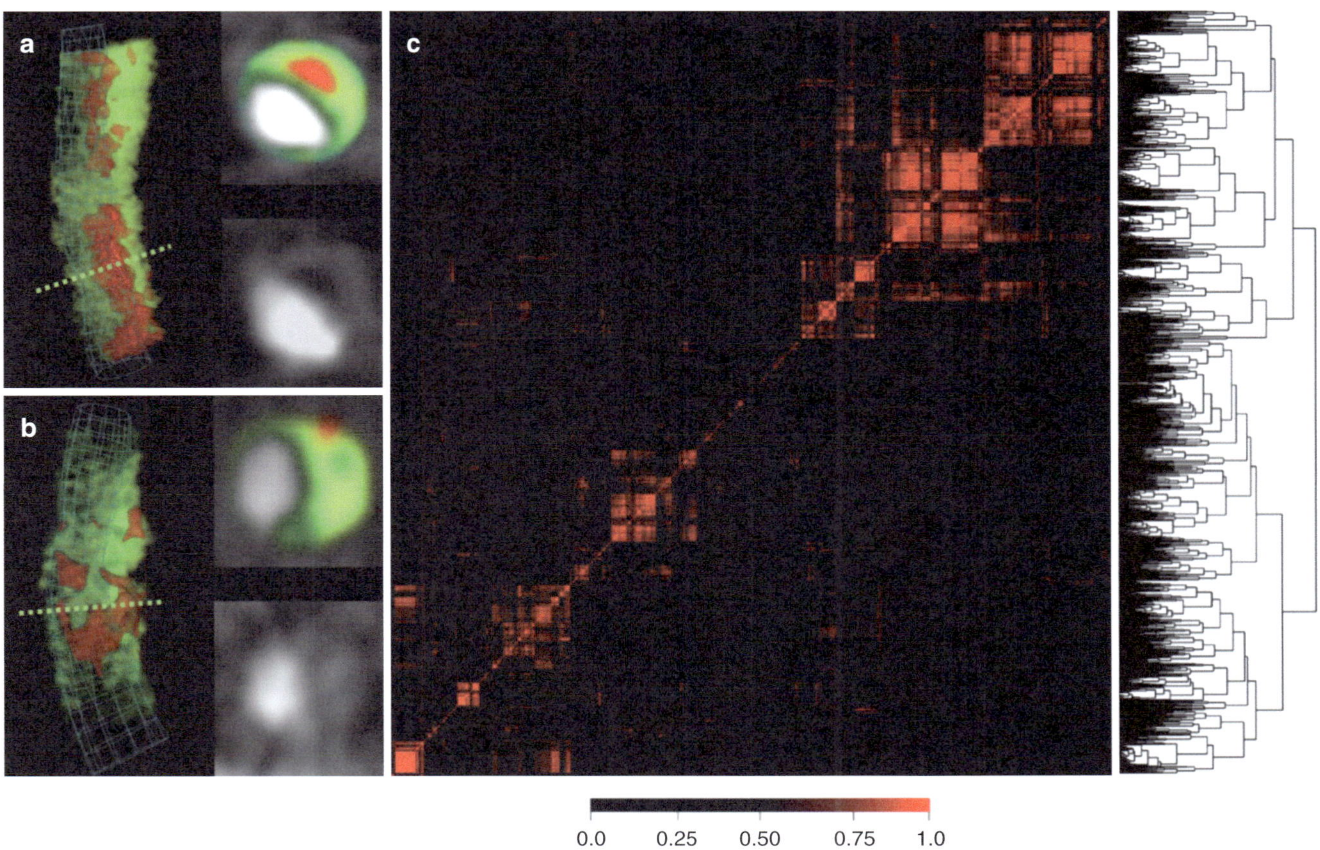

Fig. 57.6 Panel A shows volume rendered and cross-sectional images of a plaque with napkin-ring sign (NRS). Panel B represents a plaque with no NRS. Green dashed lines indicate the location of cross-sectional planes. Colors indicate different CT attenuation values. NCP, non-calcified plaque; NRS, napkin-ring sign. Panel C: heatmap of a covariance matrix of more than 7000 radiomic features. A dendrogram of the corresponding hierarchical clustering can be seen on the right side of the image [89]

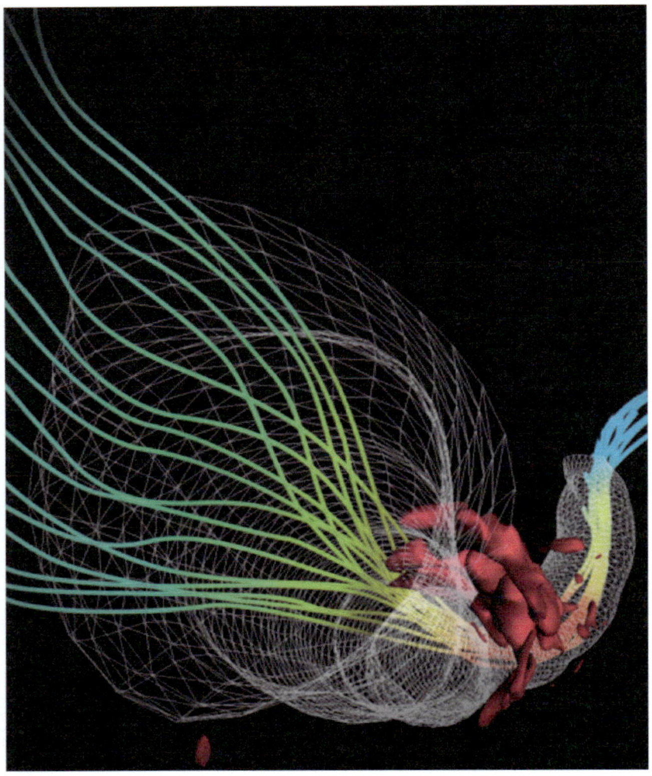

Fig. 57.7 Combined image of functional and anatomical plaque features represented in a three-dimensional artistic illustration

quantify morphological characteristics difficult or impossible to comprehend by visual assessment [86]. As the number of examinations grows, the limitations of human visual perception influence the overall diagnostic accuracy of radiological examinations [87]. This results in increased inter- and intra-reader variability [88]. The quantitative nature of radiomics has the potential to greatly decrease this variability and therefore increase the diagnostic accuracy of radiological examinations. Therefore, one of the main advantages of radiomics in coronary CTA imaging might be to decrease the reader dependency of determining high-risk plaque features [89]. Furthermore, radiomics has the potential to identify new imaging biomarkers and improve risk stratification and early disease detection based on coronary CTA datasets. Please see for more details section 56 on Cardiac CT radiomics.

A holistic approach of combining functional and morphological parameters with clinical and genetic information is a promising technique to change our understanding and treatment of cardiovascular diseases and can facilitate personalized risk assessment to identify vulnerable patients and vulnerable plaques (Fig. 57.7).

References

1. Braunwald E. Epilogue: what do clinicians expect from imagers? J Am Coll Cardiol. 2006;47(8 Suppl):C101–3. doi:S0735-1097(06)00163-X [pii]. https://doi.org/10.1016/j.jacc.2005.2.072.
2. Heidenreich PA, Trogdon JG, Khavjou OA, Butler J, Dracup K, Ezekowitz MD, Finkelstein EA, Hong Y, Johnston SC, Khera A, Lloyd-Jones DM, Nelson SA, Nichol G, Orenstein D, Wilson PW, Woo YJ, American Heart Association Advocacy Coordinating Committee; Stroke Council; Council on Cardiovascular Radiology and Intervention; Council on Clinical Cardiology; Council on Epidemiology and Prevention; Council on Arteriosclerosis; Thrombosis and Vascular Biology; Council on Cardiopulmonary; Critical Care; Perioperative and Resuscitation; Council on Cardiovascular Nursing; Council on the Kidney in Cardiovascular Disease; Council on Cardiovascular Surgery and Anesthesia, and Interdisciplinary Council on Quality of Care and Outcomes Research. Forecasting the future of cardiovascular disease in the United States: a policy statement from the American Heart Association. Circulation. 2011;123(8):933–44. https://doi.org/10.1161/CIR.0b013e31820a55f5.
3. Waxman S, Ishibashi F, Muller JE. Detection and treatment of vulnerable plaques and vulnerable patients: novel approaches to prevention of coronary events. Circulation. 2006;114(22):2390–411.
4. Libby P. Mechanisms of acute coronary syndromes and their implications for therapy. N Engl J Med. 2013;368(21):2004–13.
5. Writing Group Members, Mozaffarian D, Benjamin EJ, Go AS, Arnett DK, Blaha MJ, Cushman M, Das SR, de Ferranti S, Despres JP, Fullerton HJ, Howard VJ, Huffman MD, Isasi CR, Jimenez MC, Judd SE, Kissela BM, Lichtman JH, Lisabeth LD, Liu S, Mackey RH, Magid DJ, DK MG, Mohler ER 3rd, Moy CS, Muntner P, Mussolino ME, Nasir K, Neumar RW, Nichol G, Palaniappan L, Pandey DK, Reeves MJ, Rodriguez CJ, Rosamond W, Sorlie PD, Stein J, Towfighi A, Turan TN, Virani SS, Woo D, Yeh RW, Turner MB, American Heart Association Statistics Committee; Stroke Statistics Subcommittee. Heart disease and stroke statistics-2016 update: a report from the American Heart Association. Circulation. 2016;133(4):e38–360.
6. Burke AP, Farb A, Malcom GT, Liang YH, Smialek J, Virmani R. Coronary risk factors and plaque morphology in men with coronary disease who died suddenly. N Engl J Med. 1997;336(18):1276–82.
7. Falk E, Nakano M, Bentzon JF, Finn AV, Virmani R. Update on acute coronary syndromes: the pathologists' view. Eur Heart J. 2013;34(10):719–28.
8. Virmani R, Kolodgie FD, Burke AP, Farb A, Schwartz SM. Lessons from sudden coronary death: a comprehensive morphological classification scheme for atherosclerotic lesions. Arterioscler Thromb Vasc Biol. 2000;20(5):1262–75.
9. Narula J, Garg P, Achenbach S, Motoyama S, Virmani R, Strauss HW. Arithmetic of vulnerable plaques for noninvasive imaging. Nat Clin Pract Cardiovasc Med. 2008;5(Suppl 2):S2–10. https://doi.org/10.1038/ncpcardio1247.
10. Finn AV, Nakano M, Narula J, Kolodgie FD, Virmani R. Concept of vulnerable/unstable plaque. Arterioscler Thromb Vasc Biol. 2010;30(7):1282–92.
11. Maurovich-Horvat P, Ferencik M, Voros S, Merkely B, Hoffmann U. Comprehensive plaque assessment by coronary CT angiography. Nat Rev Cardiol. 2014;11(7):390–402.

12. Bittencourt MS, Hulten E, Ghoshhajra B, O'Leary D, Christman MP, Montana P, Truong QA, Steigner M, Murthy VL, Rybicki FJ, Nasir K, Gowdak LH, Hainer J, Brady TJ, Di Carli MF, Hoffmann U, Abbara S, Blankstein R. Prognostic value of nonobstructive and obstructive coronary artery disease detected by coronary computed tomography angiography to identify cardiovascular events. Circ Cardiovasc Imaging. 2014;7(2):282–91.
13. Mancini GB, Hartigan PM, Shaw LJ, Berman DS, Hayes SW, Bates ER, Maron DJ, Teo K, Sedlis SP, Chaitman BR, Weintraub WS, Spertus JA, Kostuk WJ, Dada M, Booth DC, Boden WE. Predicting outcome in the COURAGE trial (clinical outcomes utilizing revascularization and aggressive drug evaluation): coronary anatomy versus ischemia. JACC Cardiovasc Interv. 2014;7(2):195–201.
14. Narula J, Nakano M, Virmani R, Kolodgie FD, Petersen R, Newcomb R, Malik S, Fuster V, Finn AV. Histopathologic characteristics of atherosclerotic coronary disease and implications of the findings for the invasive and noninvasive detection of vulnerable plaques. J Am Coll Cardiol. 2013;61(10):1041–51.
15. Ferencik M, Schlett CL, Ghoshhajra BB, Kriegel MF, Joshi SB, Maurovich-Horvat P, Rogers IS, Banerji D, Bamberg F, Truong QA, Brady TJ, Nagurney JT, Hoffmann U. A computed tomography-based coronary lesion score to predict acute coronary syndrome among patients with acute chest pain and significant coronary stenosis on coronary computed tomographic angiogram. Am J Cardiol. 2012;110(2):183–9.
16. Achenbach S, Friedrich MG, Nagel E, Kramer CM, Kaufmann PA, Farkhooy A, Dilsizian V, Flachskampf FA. CV imaging: what was new in 2012? J Am Coll Cardiol Img. 2013;6(6):714–34.
17. Virmani R, Burke AP, Farb A, Kolodgie FD. Pathology of the vulnerable plaque. J Am Coll Cardiol. 2006;47(8 Suppl):C13–8.
18. Kolodgie FD, Burke AP, Farb A, Gold HK, Yuan J, Narula J, Finn AV, Virmani R. The thin-cap fibroatheroma: a type of vulnerable plaque: the major precursor lesion to acute coronary syndromes. Curr Opin Cardiol. 2001;16(5):285–92.
19. van der Giessen AG, Toepker MH, Donelly PM, Bamberg F, Schlett CL, Raffle C, Irlbeck T, Lee H, van Walsum T, Maurovich-Horvat P, Gijsen FJ, Wentzel JJ, Hoffmann U. Reproducibility, accuracy, and predictors of accuracy for the detection of coronary atherosclerotic plaque composition by computed tomography: an ex vivo comparison to intravascular ultrasound. Investig Radiol. 2010;45(11):693–701.
20. Hoffmann U, Ferencik M, Cury RC, Pena AJ. Coronary CT angiography. J Nucl Med. 2006;47(5):797–806.
21. Leipsic J, Abbara S, Achenbach S, Cury R, Earls JP, Mancini GJ, Nieman K, Pontone G, Raff GL. SCCT guidelines for the interpretation and reporting of coronary CT angiography: a report of the Society of Cardiovascular Computed Tomography Guidelines Committee. J Cardiovasc Comput Tomogr. 2014;8(5):342–58.
22. Voros S, Rinehart S, Qian Z, Vazquez G, Anderson H, Murrieta L, Wilmer C, Carlson H, Taylor K, Ballard W, Karmpaliotis D, Kalynych A, Brown C 3rd. Prospective validation of standardized, 3-dimensional, quantitative coronary computed tomographic plaque measurements using radiofrequency backscatter intravascular ultrasound as reference standard in intermediate coronary arterial lesions: results from the ATLANTA (assessment of tissue characteristics, lesion morphology, and hemodynamics by angiography with fractional flow reserve, intravascular ultrasound and virtual histology, and noninvasive computed tomography in atherosclerotic plaques) I study. JACC Cardiovasc Interv. 2011;4(2):198–208.
23. Motoyama S, Kondo T, Sarai M, Sugiura A, Harigaya H, Sato T, Inoue K, Okumura M, Ishii J, Anno H, Virmani R, Ozaki Y, Hishida H, Narula J. Multislice computed tomographic characteristics of coronary lesions in acute coronary syndromes. J Am Coll Cardiol. 2007;50(4):319–26. https://doi.org/10.1016/j.jacc.2007.03.044.
24. Pohle K, Achenbach S, Macneill B, Ropers D, Ferencik M, Moselewski F, Hoffmann U, Brady TJ, Jang IK, Daniel WG. Characterization of non-calcified coronary atherosclerotic plaque by multi-detector row CT: comparison to IVUS. Atherosclerosis. 2007;190(1):174–80.
25. Achenbach S, Boehmer K, Pflederer T, Ropers D, Seltmann M, Lell M, Anders K, Kuettner A, Uder M, Daniel WG, Marwan M. Influence of slice thickness and reconstruction kernel on the computed tomographic attenuation of coronary atherosclerotic plaque. J Cardiovasc Comput Tomogr. 2010;4(2):110–5.
26. Cademartiri F, Mollet NR, Runza G, Bruining N, Hamers R, Somers P, Knaapen M, Verheye S, Midiri M, Krestin GP, de Feyter PJ. Influence of intracoronary attenuation on coronary plaque measurements using multislice computed tomography: observations in an ex vivo model of coronary computed tomography angiography. Eur Radiol. 2005;15(7):1426–31.
27. Ferencik M, Chan RC, Achenbach S, Lisauskas JB, Houser SL, Hoffmann U, Abbara S, Cury RC, Bouma BE, Tearney GJ, Brady TJ. Arterial wall imaging: evaluation with 16-section multidetector CT in blood vessel phantoms and ex vivo coronary arteries. Radiology. 2006;240(3):708–16.
28. Suzuki S, Furui S, Kuwahara S, Kaminaga T, Yamauchi T, Konno K, Yokoyama N, Isshiki T. Accuracy of attenuation measurement of vascular wall in vitro on computed tomography angiography: effect of wall thickness, density of contrast medium, and measurement point. Investig Radiol. 2006;41(6):510–5. https://doi.org/10.1097/01.rli.0000209662.24569.c7.
29. Glagov S, Weisenberg E, Zarins CK, Stankunavicius R, Kolettis GJ. Compensatory enlargement of human atherosclerotic coronary arteries. N Engl J Med. 1987;316(22):1371–5. https://doi.org/10.1056/NEJM198705283162204.
30. Varnava AM, Mills PG, Davies MJ. Relationship between coronary artery remodeling and plaque vulnerability. Circulation. 2002;105(8):939–43.
31. Achenbach S, Ropers D, Hoffmann U, MacNeill B, Baum U, Pohle K, Brady TJ, Pomerantsev E, Ludwig J, Flachskampf FA, Wicky S, Jang IK, Daniel WG. Assessment of coronary remodeling in stenotic and nonstenotic coronary atherosclerotic lesions by multidetector spiral computed tomography. J Am Coll Cardiol. 2004;43(5):842–7.
32. Mintz GS, Nissen SE, Anderson WD, Bailey SR, Erbel R, Fitzgerald PJ, Pinto FJ, Rosenfield K, Siegel RJ, Tuzcu EM, Yock PG. American College of Cardiology Clinical Expert Consensus Document on Standards for Acquisition, Measurement and Reporting of Intravascular Ultrasound Studies (IVUS). A report of the American College of Cardiology Task Force on Clinical Expert Consensus Documents. J Am Coll Cardiol. 2001;37(5):1478–92.
33. Gauss S, Achenbach S, Pflederer T, Schuhback A, Daniel WG, Marwan M. Assessment of coronary artery remodelling by dual-source CT: a head-to-head comparison with intravascular ultrasound. Heart. 2011;97(12):991–7.
34. Motoyama S, Ito H, Sarai M, Kondo T, Kawai H, Nagahara Y, Harigaya H, Kan S, Anno H, Takahashi H, Naruse H, Ishii J, Hecht H, Shaw LJ, Ozaki Y, Narula J. Plaque characterization by coronary computed tomography angiography and the likelihood of acute coronary events in mid-term follow-up. J Am Coll Cardiol. 2015;66(4):337–46.
35. Ahmadi A, Leipsic J, Blankstein R, Taylor C, Hecht H, Stone GW, Narula J. Do plaques rapidly progress prior to myocardial

infarction? The interplay between plaque vulnerability and progression. Circ Res. 2015;117(1):99–104.
36. Maurovich-Horvat P, Hoffmann U, Vorpahl M, Nakano M, Virmani R, Alkadhi H. The napkin-ring sign: CT signature of high risk coronary plaques? JACC Cardiovasc Imaging. 2010;3(4):440–05.
37. Seifarth H, Schlett CL, Nakano M, Otsuka F, Karolyi M, Liew G, Maurovich-Horvat P, Alkadhi H, Virmani R, Hoffmann U. Histopathological correlates of the napkin-ring sign plaque in coronary CT angiography. Atherosclerosis. 2012;224(1):90–6.
38. Maurovich-Horvat P, Schlett CL, Alkadhi H, Nakano M, Otsuka F, Stolzmann P, Scheffel H, Ferencik M, Kriegel MF, Seifarth H, Virmani R, Hoffmann U. The napkin-ring sign indicates advanced atherosclerotic lesions in coronary CT angiography. J Am Coll Cardiol Img. 2012;5(12):1243–52.
39. Otsuka K, Fukuda S, Tanaka A, Nakanishi K, Taguchi H, Yoshikawa J, Shimada K, Yoshiyama M. Napkin-ring sign on coronary CT angiography for the prediction of acute coronary syndrome. J Am Coll Cardiol Img. 2013;6(4):448–57.
40. Feuchtner G, Kerber J, Burghard P, Dichtl W, Friedrich G, Bonaros N, Plank F. The high-risk criteria low-attenuation plaque <60 HU and the napkin-ring sign are the most powerful predictors of MACE: a long-term follow-up study. Eur Heart J Cardiovasc Imaging. 2016;18:772. https://doi.org/10.1093/ehjci/jew167.
41. Otsuka F, Finn AV, Virmani R. Do vulnerable and ruptured plaques hide in heavily calcified arteries? Atherosclerosis. 2013;229(1):34–7.
42. Huang H, Virmani R, Younis H, Burke AP, Kamm RD, Lee RT. The impact of calcification on the biomechanical stability of atherosclerotic plaques. Circulation. 2001;103(8):1051–6.
43. Maldonado N, Kelly-Arnold A, Vengrenyuk Y, Laudier D, Fallon JT, Virmani R, Cardoso L, Weinbaum S. A mechanistic analysis of the role of microcalcifications in atherosclerotic plaque stability: potential implications for plaque rupture. Am J Phys Heart Circ Phys. 2012;303(5):H619–28.
44. Mauriello A, Servadei F, Zoccai GB, Giacobbi E, Anemona L, Bonanno E, Casella S. Coronary calcification identifies the vulnerable patient rather than the vulnerable plaque. Atherosclerosis. 2013;229(1):124–9. https://doi.org/10.1016/j.atherosclerosis.2013.03.010.
45. Burke AP, Weber DK, Kolodgie FD, Farb A, Taylor AJ, Virmani R. Pathophysiology of calcium deposition in coronary arteries. Herz. 2001;26(4):239–44.
46. van Velzen JE, de Graaf FR, de Graaf MA, Schuijf JD, Kroft LJ, de Roos A, Reiber JH, Bax JJ, Jukema JW, Boersma E, Schalij MJ, van der Wall EE. Comprehensive assessment of spotty calcifications on computed tomography angiography: comparison to plaque characteristics on intravascular ultrasound with radiofrequency backscatter analysis. J Nucl Cardiol. 2011;18(5):893–903.
47. Kim SY, Kim KS, Seung MJ, Chung JW, Kim JH, Mun SH, Lee YS, Lee JB, Ryu JK, Choi JY, Chang SG. The culprit lesion score on multi-detector computed tomography can detect vulnerable coronary artery plaque. Int J Cardiovasc Imaging. 2010;26(Suppl 2):245–52.
48. Kitagawa T, Yamamoto H, Horiguchi J, Ohhashi N, Tadehara F, Shokawa T, Dohi Y, Kunita E, Utsunomiya H, Kohno N, Kihara Y. Characterization of noncalcified coronary plaques and identification of culprit lesions in patients with acute coronary syndrome by 64-slice computed tomography. JACC Cardiovasc Imaging. 2009;2(2):153–60.
49. Ozaki Y, Okumura M, Ismail TF, Motoyama S, Naruse H, Hattori K, Kawai H, Sarai M, Takagi Y, Ishii J, Anno H, Virmani R, Serruys PW, Narula J. Coronary CT angiographic characteristics of culprit lesions in acute coronary syndromes not related to plaque rupture as defined by optical coherence tomography and angioscopy. Eur Heart J. 2011;32(22):2814–23. https://doi.org/10.1093/eurheartj/ehr189.
50. Pflederer T, Marwan M, Schepis T, Ropers D, Seltmann M, Muschiol G, Daniel WG, Achenbach S. Characterization of culprit lesions in acute coronary syndromes using coronary dual-source CT angiography. Atherosclerosis. 2010;211(2):437–44.
51. Madder RD, Chinnaiyan KM, Marandici AM, Goldstein JA. Features of disrupted plaques by coronary computed tomographic angiography: correlates with invasively proven complex lesions. Circ Cardiovasc Imaging. 2011;4(2):105–13.
52. Arbab-Zadeh A, Fuster V. The myth of the "vulnerable plaque": transitioning from a focus on individual lesions to atherosclerotic disease burden for coronary artery disease risk assessment. J Am Coll Cardiol. 2015;65(8):846–55.
53. Kubo T, Maehara A, Mintz GS, Doi H, Tsujita K, Choi SY, Katoh O, Nasu K, Koenig A, Pieper M, Rogers JH, Wijns W, Bose D, Margolis MP, Moses JW, Stone GW, Leon MB. The dynamic nature of coronary artery lesion morphology assessed by serial virtual histology intravascular ultrasound tissue characterization. J Am Coll Cardiol. 2010;55(15):1590–7.
54. Iwasaki K, Matsumoto T. Dynamic change of high-risk plaque detected by coronary computed tomographic angiography in patients with subclinical coronary artery disease. Int J Cardiovasc Imaging. 2016;32:1667. https://doi.org/10.1007/s10554-016-0957-2.
55. Min JK, Shaw LJ, Devereux RB, Okin PM, Weinsaft JW, Russo DJ, Lippolis NJ, Berman DS, Callister TQ. Prognostic value of multidetector coronary computed tomographic angiography for prediction of all-cause mortality. J Am Coll Cardiol. 2007;50(12):1161–70.
56. Andreini D, Pontone G, Mushtaq S, Bartorelli AL, Bertella E, Antonioli L, Formenti A, Cortinovis S, Veglia F, Annoni A, Agostoni P, Montorsi P, Ballerini G, Fiorentini C, Pepi M. A long-term prognostic value of coronary CT angiography in suspected coronary artery disease. JACC Cardiovasc Imaging. 2012;5(7):690–701.
57. Dougoud S, Fuchs TA, Stehli J, Clerc OF, Buechel RR, Herzog BA, Leschka S, Alkadhi H, Kaufmann PA, Gaemperli O. Prognostic value of coronary CT angiography on long-term follow-up of 6.9 years. Int J Cardiovasc Imaging. 2014;30(5):969–76.
58. Hadamitzky M, Taubert S, Deseive S, Byrne RA, Martinoff S, Schomig A, Hausleiter J. Prognostic value of coronary computed tomography angiography during 5 years of follow-up in patients with suspected coronary artery disease. Eur Heart J. 2013;34(42):3277–85.
59. Al-Mallah MH. Does coronary CT angiography improve risk stratification over coronary artery calcium scoring in symptomatic patients with a low pre-test probability of coronary artery disease and a CAC of zero? Reply. Eur Heart J Cardiovasc Imaging. 2014;15(2):232–3.
60. Hadamitzky M, Achenbach S, Al-Mallah M, Berman D, Budoff M, Cademartiri F, Callister T, Chang HJ, Cheng V, Chinnaiyan K, Chow BJ, Cury R, Delago A, Dunning A, Feuchtner G, Gomez M, Kaufmann P, Kim YJ, Leipsic J, Lin FY, Maffei E, Min JK, Raff G, Shaw LJ, Villines TC, Hausleiter J, Investigators C. Optimized prognostic score for coronary computed tomographic angiography: results from the CONFIRM registry (COronary CT Angiography EvaluatioN For Clinical Outcomes: An InteRnational Multicenter Registry). J Am Coll Cardiol. 2013;62(5):468–76.
61. Versteylen MO, Kietselaer BL, Dagnelie PC, Joosen IA, Dedic A, Raaijmakers RH, Wildberger JE, Nieman K, Crijns HJ, Niessen WJ, Daemen MJ, Hofstra L. Additive value of semiautomated quantification of coronary artery disease using cardiac computed tomographic angiography to predict future acute coronary syndrome. J Am Coll Cardiol. 2013;61(22):2296–305.
62. Voros S, Rinehart S, Qian Z, Joshi P, Vazquez G, Fischer C, Belur P, Hulten E, Villines TC. Coronary atherosclerosis imaging by coronary CT angiography: current status, correlation with intravascular interrogation and meta-analysis. JACC Cardiovasc Imaging. 2011;4(5):537–48.

63. Boogers MJ, Broersen A, van Velzen JE, de Graaf FR, El-Naggar HM, Kitslaar PH, Dijkstra J, Delgado V, Boersma E, de Roos A, Schuijf JD, Schalij MJ, Reiber JH, Bax JJ, Jukema JW. Automated quantification of coronary plaque with computed tomography: comparison with intravascular ultrasound using a dedicated registration algorithm for fusion-based quantification. Eur Heart J. 2012;33(8):1007–16.
64. Oberoi S, Meinel FG, Schoepf UJ, Nance JW, De Cecco CN, Gebregziabher M, Costello P, Weininger M. Reproducibility of noncalcified coronary artery plaque burden quantification from coronary CT angiography across different image analysis platforms. AJR Am J Roentgenol. 2014;202(1):W43–9.
65. Taylor CA, Fonte TA, Min JK. Computational fluid dynamics applied to cardiac computed tomography for noninvasive quantification of fractional flow reserve: scientific basis. J Am Coll Cardiol. 2013;61(22):2233–41.
66. Min JK, Leipsic J, Pencina MJ, Berman DS, Koo BK, van Mieghem C, Erglis A, Lin FY, Dunning AM, Apruzzese P, Budoff MJ, Cole JH, Jaffer FA, Leon MB, Malpeso J, Mancini GB, Park SJ, Schwartz RS, Shaw LJ, Mauri L. Diagnostic accuracy of fractional flow reserve from anatomic CT angiography. JAMA. 2012;308(12):1237–45.
67. Norgaard BL, Leipsic J, Gaur S, Seneviratne S, Ko BS, Ito H, Jensen JM, Mauri L, De Bruyne B, Bezerra H, Osawa K, Marwan M, Naber C, Erglis A, Park SJ, Christiansen EH, Kaltoft A, Lassen JF, Botker HE, Achenbach S, Group NXTTS. Diagnostic performance of noninvasive fractional flow reserve derived from coronary computed tomography angiography in suspected coronary artery disease: the NXT trial (analysis of coronary blood flow using CT angiography: next steps). J Am Coll Cardiol. 2014;63(12):1145–55.
68. Ahmadi A, Stone GW, Leipsic J, Serruys PW, Shaw L, Hecht H, Wong G, Norgaard BL, O'Gara PT, Chandrashekhar Y, Narula J. Association of coronary stenosis and plaque morphology with fractional flow reserve and outcomes. JAMA Cardiol. 2016;1(3):350–7.
69. Park HB, Heo R, Ó Hartaigh B, Cho I, Gransar H, Nakazato R, Leipsic J, Mancini GB, Koo BK, Otake H, Budoff MJ, Berman DS, Erglis A, Chang HJ, Min JK. Atherosclerotic plaque characteristics by CT angiography identify coronary lesions that cause ischemia: a direct comparison to fractional flow reserve. JACC Cardiovasc Imaging. 2015;8(1):1–10.
70. Stary HC, Blankenhorn DH, Chandler AB, Glagov S, Insull W Jr, Richardson M, Rosenfeld ME, Schaffer SA, Schwartz CJ, Wagner WD, et al. A definition of the intima of human arteries and of its atherosclerosis-prone regions. A report from the Committee on Vascular Lesions of the Council on Arteriosclerosis, American Heart Association. Circulation. 1992;85(1):391–405.
71. Chatzizisis YS, Coskun AU, Jonas M, Edelman ER, Feldman CL, Stone PH. Role of endothelial shear stress in the natural history of coronary atherosclerosis and vascular remodeling: molecular, cellular, and vascular behavior. J Am Coll Cardiol. 2007;49(25):2379–93.
72. Samady H, Eshtehardi P, McDaniel MC, Suo J, Dhawan SS, Maynard C, Timmins LH, Quyyumi AA, Giddens DP. Coronary artery wall shear stress is associated with progression and transformation of atherosclerotic plaque and arterial remodeling in patients with coronary artery disease. Circulation. 2011;124(7):779–88.
73. Slager CJ, Wentzel JJ, Gijsen FJ, Schuurbiers JC, van der Wal AC, van der Steen AF, Serruys PW. The role of shear stress in the generation of rupture-prone vulnerable plaques. Nat Clin Pract Cardiovasc Med. 2005;2(8):401–7.
74. Fearon WF. Is a myocardial infarction more likely to result from a mild coronary lesion or an ischemia-producing one? Circ Cardiovasc Interv. 2011;4(6):539–41.
75. Gijsen FJ, Wentzel JJ, Thury A, Mastik F, Schaar JA, Schuurbiers JC, Slager CJ, van der Giessen WJ, de Feyter PJ, van der Steen AF, Serruys PW. Strain distribution over plaques in human coronary arteries relates to shear stress. Am J Phys Heart Circ Phys. 2008;295(4):H1608–14.
76. Yong AS, Pennings GJ, Chang M, Hamzah A, Chung T, Qi M, Brieger D, Behnia M, Krilis SA, Ng MK, Lowe HC, Kritharides L. Intracoronary shear-related up-regulation of platelet P-selectin and platelet-monocyte aggregation despite the use of aspirin and clopidogrel. Blood. 2011;117(1):11–20.
77. Han D, Starikov A, Ó Hartaigh B, Gransar H, Kolli KK, Lee JH, Rizvi A, Baskaran L, Schulman-Marcus J, Lin FY, Min JK. Relationship between endothelial wall shear stress and high-risk atherosclerotic plaque characteristics for identification of coronary lesions that cause ischemia: a direct comparison with fractional flow reserve. J Am Heart Assoc. 2016;5(12) https://doi.org/10.1161/JAHA.116.004186.
78. Danad I, Fayad ZA, Willemink MJ, Min JK. New applications of cardiac computed tomography: dual-energy, spectral, and molecular CT imaging. JACC Cardiovasc Imaging. 2015;8(6):710–23.
79. Leber AW, Knez A, Becker A, Becker C, von Ziegler F, Nikolaou K, Rist C, Reiser M, White C, Steinbeck G, Boekstegers P. Accuracy of multidetector spiral computed tomography in identifying and differentiating the composition of coronary atherosclerotic plaques: a comparative study with intracoronary ultrasound. J Am Coll Cardiol. 2004;43(7):1241–7.
80. Willemink MJ, Leiner T, Maurovich-Horvat P. Cardiac CT imaging of plaque vulnerability: hype or Hope? Curr Cardiol Rep. 2016;18(4):37. https://doi.org/10.1007/s11886-016-0714-0.
81. Machida H, Tanaka I, Fukui R, Shen Y, Ishikawa T, Tate E, Ueno E. Current and novel imaging techniques in coronary CT. Radiographics. 2015;35(4):991–1010.
82. Kulkarni NM, Eisner BH, Pinho DF, Joshi MC, Kambadakone AR, Sahani DV. Determination of renal stone composition in phantom and patients using single-source dual-energy computed tomography. J Comput Assist Tomogr. 2013;37(1):37–45.
83. Cormode DP, Roessl E, Thran A, Skajaa T, Gordon RE, Schlomka JP, Fuster V, Fisher EA, Mulder WJ, Proksa R, Fayad ZA. Atherosclerotic plaque composition: analysis with multicolor CT and targeted gold nanoparticles. Radiology. 2010;256(3):774–82.
84. Gillies RJ, Kinahan PE, Hricak H. Radiomics: images are more than pictures, they are data. Radiology. 2016;278(2):563–77.
85. Kolossvary M, Kellermayer M, Merkely B, Maurovich-Horvat P. Cardiac computed tomography radiomics: a comprehensive review on radiomic techniques. J Thorac Imaging. 2017;33:26. https://doi.org/10.1097/RTI.0000000000000268.
86. Davnall F, Yip CS, Ljungqvist G, Selmi M, Ng F, Sanghera B, Ganeshan B, Miles KA, Cook GJ, Goh V. Assessment of tumor heterogeneity: an emerging imaging tool for clinical practice? Insights Imaging. 2012;3(6):573–89.
87. Krupinski EA, Berbaum KS, Caldwell RT, Schartz KM, Kim J. Long radiology workdays reduce detection and accommodation accuracy. J Am Coll Radiol. 2010;7(9):698–704.
88. Puchner SB, Liu T, Mayrhofer T, Truong QA, Lee H, Fleg JL, Nagurney JT, Udelson JE, Hoffmann U, Ferencik M. High-risk plaque detected on coronary CT angiography predicts acute coronary syndromes independent of significant stenosis in acute chest pain: results from the ROMICAT-II trial. J Am Coll Cardiol. 2014;64(7):684–92.
89. Kolossváry M, Karády J, Szilveszter B, Kitslaar P, Hoffmann U, Merkely B, Maurovich-Horvat P. Radiomic features are superior to conventional quantitative computed tomographic metrics to identify coronary plaques with napkin-ring sign. Circ Cardiovasc Imaging. 2017;10(12).

Part XIV

Where We Are Going: Risk Prediction and Management: The Next Wave

Coronary CT Angiography for Screening, Risk Stratification, and Management of Asymptomatic Patients: State of the Evidence

58

Felix G. Meinel and Matthias Renker

Unlike coronary artery calcium scoring, coronary CTA is generally not established as a tool for screening and risk stratification of asymptomatic individuals. The most recent multi-society appropriate use guidelines rate coronary CTA as "rarely appropriate" in asymptomatic patients with low to intermediate risk for CAD [1]. They suggest that coronary CTA "may be appropriate" in asymptomatic patients with a high risk for CAD (>20% ten-year CAD risk or CAD equivalent such as diabetes or peripheral artery disease) [1]. Compared to coronary artery calcium scoring, coronary CTA is associated with a higher radiation dose and the risks of contrast material administration. These risks are small but real [2, 3] and need to be carefully weighed when considering coronary CTA as a screening test in large populations of individuals with no signs or symptoms of CAD.

Commissioned by the World Health Organization, Wilson and Jungner in 1968 published ten criteria for diseases that may be amenable to successful screening programs [4]. They are now considered the "classic" WHO criteria, also known as Wilson's criteria (Table 58.1). Criteria 1–7 on this list clearly apply to CAD and indeed make it seem like an obvious candidate for screening. Item 8 is a challenge: There is far-reaching consensus whom to treat in *symptomatic* patients with CAD, but this is not so clear for *asymptomatic* patients. The paragraph "Role for Management" in this chapter discusses the practical consequences of finding evidence of CAD in an asymptomatic individual. Even more challenging are the requirements for a successful screening program that were formulated in the "modified" WHO criteria published in 2008 [5] (Table 58.2). The key items on that list are 4 and 10. For screening to be justified, there should be evidence (in the form of randomized controlled trials) that the program is effective and that the overall benefits of screening outweigh the harm. As will be discussed in the paragraph "Impact" below, such evidence does not currently exist with regard to coronary CTA screening for CAD.

Table 58.1 Wilson and Jungner classic screening criteria

The condition should be an important health problem
There should be a treatment for the condition
Facilities for diagnosis and treatment should be available
There should be a latent stage of the disease
There should be a test or examination for the condition
The test should be acceptable to the population
The natural history of the disease should be adequately understood
There should be an agreed policy on whom to treat
The total cost of finding a case should be economically balanced in relation to medical expenditure as a whole
Case finding should be a continuous process, not just a "once and for all" project

From Wilson and Jungner[4], with permission

Table 58.2 Synthesis of emerging screening criteria proposed over the past 40 years

The screening program should respond to a recognized need
The objectives of screening should be defined at the outset
There should be a defined target population
There should be scientific evidence of screening program effectiveness
The program should integrate education, testing, clinical services, and program management
There should be quality assurance, with mechanisms to minimize potential risks of screening
The program should ensure informed choice, confidentiality, and respect for autonomy
The program should promote equity and access to screening for the entire target population
Program evaluation should be planned from the outset
The overall benefits of screening should outweigh the harm

From Andermann et al.[5], with permission

F. G. Meinel (✉)
Department of Diagnostic and Interventional Radiology, Rostock University Medical Center, Rostock, Germany
e-mail: felix.meinel@med.uni-rostock.de

M. Renker
Department of Cardiology, Kerckhoff Heart and Thorax Center, Bad Nauheim, Germany

U. J. Schoepf (ed.), *CT of the Heart*, Contemporary Medical Imaging, https://doi.org/10.1007/978-1-60327-237-7_58

Utilization

Although the benefit/risk profile of coronary CTA in asymptomatic individuals remains controversial, it is not infrequently performed. The CONFIRM registry enrolled 27,125 patients who underwent coronary CTA in six countries between 2003 and 2009; at least 7590 (28%) of these individuals were asymptomatic for coronary artery disease [6]. In a 2009 survey of 169 institutions providing cardiac CT in 38 countries, 34% reported performing cardiac CT "for the exclusion of CAD in clinically healthy patients" [7]. A more recent survey (conducted 2014–2015) analyzed the patterns of coronary CTA utilization in 152 tertiary care hospitals with advanced CT systems across China [8]. As many as 95% of these hospitals listed "screening to rule out coronary artery disease in asymptomatic individuals" as one of their clinical indications for performing coronary CTA studies. The use of coronary CTA in asymptomatic patients as part of self-referred health "checkup" examinations has indeed become a growing trend, particularly in Asia. But also in Western countries, it is not uncommon to see radiology or cardiology practices advertising coronary CT angiography to the public for "checkup" examinations.

Diagnostic Yield

Asymptomatic Individuals with Low Cardiovascular Risk

Table 58.3 provides an overview of published cohorts of low-risk, asymptomatic patients who underwent coronary CTA. In individuals with a calcium score of zero, a prevalence of nonobstructive plaque on the order of 6% and a prevalence of obstructive CAD from non-calcified plaque of <1% have been reported (Table 58.3). Similar prevalence rates were found in a cohort of young adults under the age of 45 (mean age 40, Table 58.3). Others have reported a prevalence of 33–58% for nonobstructive CAD and 4–5% for obstructive CAD even in such relatively low-risk groups as normal-weight individuals and middle-aged sportsmen (Table 58.3).

Association with Coronary Artery Calcium Score

The amount of coronary artery calcium as determined by CT calcium scoring is predictive of coronary CTA findings in asymptomatic individuals. In a 2015 analysis of the CONFIRM registry, the prevalence of obstructive CAD was 42% in patients with a CACS of >100 compared to 9% in patients with a CACS of ≤100 [16].

Association with Clinical Risk Factors

Not surprisingly, the diagnostic yield of coronary CTA increases in cohorts with cardiovascular risk factors. This has been shown for smoking, diabetes, hypertension, and chronic kidney disease (Table 58.4). The prevalence of subclinical CAD in asymptomatic patients is also associated with less well-established cardiovascular risk factors such as the inflammatory marker C-reactive protein and subclinical hypothyroidism (Table 58.4). Thus, larger cohorts of coronary CTA performed in asymptomatic individuals provide an opportunity to investigate the effect of established cardiovascular risk factors on subclinical coronary atherosclerosis and identify novel risk factors for CAD.

Table 58.4 Coronary CTA findings in asymptomatic individuals: correlation with cardiovascular risk factors

Risk factor	Correlation with coronary CTA findings	References
Chronic kidney disease	Yes	[17]
Arterial stiffness	Yes	[18]
Smoking	Yes	[19, 20]
Hypertension	Yes	[21]
Diabetes	Yes	[22]
Metabolic syndrome	Yes	[23]
C-reactive protein	Yes	[24]
Subclinical hypothyroidism	Yes	[25]

Table 58.3 Major publications on the diagnostic yield of coronary CTA in asymptomatic low-risk patients

Author	Year	Target population	*n*	Age (years[a])	No CAD(%)	Nonobstructive CAD(%)	Obstructive CAD (%)	Reference
Braber TL	2016	Middle-aged sportsmen	318	54.7	36.8	57.9	5.3	[9]
Kim S	2015	Normal weight	2078	53.4	63.1	33.2	3.7	[10]
Lee MS	2013	Zero calcium score	6531	49.8	93.2	6.1	0.7	[11]
Cho I	2013	Zero calcium score	4491	48	93.0	6.2	0.8	[12]
Kim KJ	2013	Low risk	2133	48.7	87.3	11.4	1.3	[13]
Jin KN	2012	Young adults (<45 years)	914	40.4	90.6	8.4	1.0	[14]
Yoo DH	2011	Zero calcium score	6040	50.1	93.1	6.1	0.8	[15]

Publications with $n \geq 200$ are listed
[a]Mean or median

Specific High-Risk Groups

Studies on coronary CTA screening for asymptomatic CAD have been performed in a number of specific high-risk groups (Table 58.5) with the largest number of publications focusing on patients with diabetes mellitus. In patients with diabetes without symptoms of CAD, only 20–31% have normal coronary arteries on coronary CTA, while 36–48% show nonobstructive CAD and 23–44% obstructive CAD (Table 58.6). Patients with familial hypercholesterolemia represent another specific high-risk group with an exceptionally high expected diagnostic yield of coronary CTA. In a cohort of 101 statin-treated asymptomatic patients with familial hypercholesterolemia, coronary CTA demonstrated nonobstructive CAD in 59% of patients and obstructive CAD in 26% [34]. HIV infection has been recognized as a major risk factor for accelerated atherosclerosis. Indeed, in one cohort of 55 HIV-infected individuals with low cardiovascular risk (as determined by traditional risk factors), coronary CTA revealed a 29% prevalence of obstructive CAD [44].

Prognostic Value

General Asymptomatic Population

Does coronary CTA have incremental value over CACS in asymptomatic subjects? In one publication from the CONFIRM registry, a population of 7590 subjects without chest pain and without a history of coronary artery disease was followed for a median period of 24 months [6]. This was a mixed population of patients with Framingham risk scores ranging from low to high. All-cause mortality as well as a composite of all-cause mortality and nonfatal myocardial infarction served as endpoints in this analysis. While both CACS and coronary CTA improved risk stratification beyond standard clinical risk factors, the incremental benefit of adding coronary CTA to clinical risk factors and CACS was minimal and not considered clinically meaningful [6].

Table 58.5 Publications on coronary CTA in asymptomatic individuals from specific high-risk groups

Risk group	References
Diabetes mellitus	[26–33]
Familial hypercholesterolemia	[34–36]
Peripheral or cerebral artery disease	[37–40]
Status post mediastinal radiotherapy for Hodgkin's lymphoma	[41, 42]
Morbid obesity	[43]
HIV positive	[44–46]
Smokers	[19, 20]
Family history of early-onset coronary artery disease	[47]

Association with Coronary Artery Calcium Score

The CONFIRM registry investigators also analyzed the prognostic value of coronary CTA findings in relationship to the calcium score [16]. In their analysis of 3217 asymptomatic patients, coronary CTA had incremental prognostic value over clinical risk factors (Framingham risk score) for patients with a CACS of >100 but not for those with a CACS of ≤100 [16]. In the group of asymptomatic individuals with a CACS of >100, the incremental benefit of coronary CTA for risk prediction was greatest in patients with an intermediate CACS (101–400) and declined in patients with higher CACS (>400). The primary conclusion of this study was that coronary CTA for risk stratification in asymptomatic patients may be appropriate in patients with an intermediate CACS (101–400) but is probably not useful in patients with lower or higher CACS.

Association with Clinical Risk Factors

Other authors looked at more selected groups of patients with cardiovascular risk factors. One published cohort consisted of 711 asymptomatic patients with a "high a priori risk of CAD", which was defined as either a high estimated cardiovascular lifetime risk or a borderline or mildly abnormal ECG-treadmill stress test result [48]. The primary endpoint was a

Table 58.6 Major publications on the diagnostic yield of coronary CTA in asymptomatic patients with diabetes

Author	Year	*n*	Age (years[a])	Diabetes duration(years[a])	No CAD(%)	Nonobstructive CAD(%)	Obstructive CAD (%)	Reference
Kang SH	2016	591	62.2	12.5	28.4	39.9	31.6	[27]
Halon DA	2016	630	63.5	10.1	20.6	48.3	31.1	[28]
Kim JJ	2015	933	63.4	11.7	20.7	39.1	40.1	[29]
Kim JJ	2015	284	64.9	13.1	20.1	36.3	43.7	[30]
Dedic A	2015	378	56	Not stated	22.8	44.4	32.8	[31]
Idilman IS	2015	273	58.6	4.7	24.2	40.6	35.2	[32]
Min JK	2014	400	60.4	Not stated	30.0	42.2	27.8	[33]
Muhlestein JB	2014	336	61.5	12.3	31.3	46.1	22.6	[26]

Publications with $n \geq 200$ are listed
[a]Mean or median

composite of cardiac death and nonfatal myocardial infarction. Findings at coronary CTA were significant predictors of events during a mean follow-up of 2.7 years. In particular, a segment involvement score of ≥5 was significantly associated with adverse events. However, this analysis did not adjust for CACS and therefore does not demonstrate an incremental prognostic value of coronary CTA over CACS.

Specific High-Risk Groups

Six relatively large cohorts have investigated the prognostic value of coronary CTA in asymptomatic patients with diabetes (Table 58.7). All found a substantially increased hazard for adverse events in asymptomatic patients with obstructive CAD at CTA (Table 58.7), and all but one also reported a (smaller) risk increase in patients with nonobstructive CAD compared to those with no CAD. Three of these cohorts adjusted the prognostic value of coronary CTA for results of CACS and found an incremental prognostic value of coronary CTA findings over CACS in asymptomatic individuals with diabetes. One cohort study investigated the prognostic value of coronary CTA in 70 asymptomatic patients on hemodialysis [49]. In this relatively small cohort, cumulative event rates of 36% vs. 0% in patients with vs. without obstructive CAD at CTA were reported.

Role for Management

Primary Prevention in Individuals at Risk for Coronary Artery Disease

Implementing current state of knowledge, national and European guidelines advocate primary prevention in terms of cardiovascular risk factor reduction as the most important strategy in any individual being at risk for CAD. These guidelines therefore pertain to potential candidates of screening as well, so that aggressive risk factor reduction appears to be the most important management approach in high-risk individuals. Beyond lifestyle changes (e.g., dietary measures, physical activity, weight reduction, and avoidance of any tobacco exposure), optimal medical treatment is recommended to meet specific treatment targets that are adjusted to proposed risk categories. For low-density lipoprotein cholesterol (LDL-C, the primary lipid analysis with respect to management), the treatment target approach is presently a consensus recommendation comprised in the 2016 European guidelines on the management of dyslipidemias for applicability and compliance reasons, while its benefit is not conclusively proven [50]. Explicit LDL-C target levels were discontinued in the 2013 US national guidelines [51]. The rationale and details for non-lipid treatment strategies and goals for cardiovascular disease prevention are covered in recent national guidelines such as those on the assessment of cardiovascular risk [52], lifestyle, diet and exercise [53], and management of obesity [54].

Treatment Implications by Coronary Calcium Scoring

As indicated above, CAC testing has been validated by multiple studies and has been shown to be a very robust predictor of adverse cardiovascular events in the general population, as well as in specific risk groups such as the elderly and diabetics. Importantly, CAC has been shown to help guide medical therapy. A CAC score ≥75th percentile (for age and gender) or ≥300 Agatston units is considered high risk by means of the 2013 ACC/AHA guideline on the treatment of blood cholesterol to reduce atherosclerotic cardiovascular risk in adults and warrant high-dose statins [52]. In the randomized St. Francis Heart study, atorvastatin reduced cardiovascular events by 42% in those with a CAC score >400 Agatston units (number needed to treat for the reduction of 1 myocardial infarction or death, 17) [55].

Table 58.7 Major publications on the prognostic value of coronary CTA in asymptomatic patients with diabetes

Author	Year	*n*	Age (years[a])	Diabetes duration(years[a])	Obstructive CAD (%)	HR for obstructive CAD(most adjusted)	95%-CI	Reference
Kang SH	2016	591	62.2	12.5	31.6	14.4	1.6–134.7	[27]
Halon DA	2016	630	63.5	10.1	31.1	6.6	3.3–13.1	[28]
Kim JJ	2015	933	63.4	11.7	40.1	2.0	1.2–3.3	[29]
Dedic A	2015	378	56	Not stated	32.8	9.5	0.9–104.2	[31]
Min JK	2014	400	60.4	Not stated	27.8	1.8[b]	1.2–2.8[2]	[33]
Muhlestein JB	2014	336	61.5	12.3	22.6	5.4	1.0–27.7	[26]

Publications with $n \geq 200$ are listed
[a]Mean or median
[b]The HR in the paper by Min et al. refers to each grade increment in maximum stenosis severity (0%, 1–49%, 50–69%, >70%)

Management recommendations based on current guidelines are as follows [52]:

- CAC score ≥75th percentile or ≥300 Agatston units should be treated with high-dose statins.
- CAC score <75th percentile and<300 Agatston units should be treated with low−/moderate-dose statins.
- CAC score = 0 should be considered for lifestyle modification.

In the multiethnic study of atherosclerosis (MESA), individuals with a CAC score ≥100 Agatston units showed an estimated benefit for acetylsalicylic acid regardless of risk factors (number needed to treat = 92, estimated 5-year number needed to harm = 442 for major bleeding) [56]. Reversely, a benefit for acetylsalicylic acid in individuals with CAC of 0 Agatston units was very unlikely (5-year number needed to treat = 2036 for individuals with low cardiovascular risk and 808 for elevated traditional risk status; 5-year number needed to harm = 442 for major bleeding). Comparable data exist for angiotensin-converting enzyme inhibitors.

Treatment Implications by Coronary CT Angiography

Through optimized downstream prescription of preventive therapies and altered use of myocardial revascularization procedures, the SCOT-HEART trial has demonstrated outcome modification by coronary CTA in patients presenting with suspected angina due to CAD [57]. Altogether, coronary CTA was associated with a reduction of fatal/nonfatal myocardial infarction of approximately 50% in this symptomatic population.

For asymptomatic patients, there is currently no conclusive evidence that coronary CTA-directed medical management or revascularization reduces morbidity or mortality (see paragraph "Impact" below). Likewise, there are no guidelines available on how coronary CTA findings should guide the management of asymptomatic patients. If coronary CTA is performed in asymptomatic patients at risk for CAD, it appears reasonable to manage these patients similar to patients with stable chest pain. Patients with moderate (50–69%) stenosis should be recommended to receive stress cardiac imaging (stress MRI or nuclear stress test) to detect myocardial ischemia, and patients with severe (≥70%) stenosis should be recommended to undergo diagnostic coronary angiography. Additionally, aggressive risk factor modification and low-dose acetylsalicylic acid should be considered in all patients with more than minimal CAD at coronary CTA.

Impact

Only one randomized controlled trial has evaluated the effectiveness of coronary CTA screening to reduce cardiovascular morbidity and mortality in asymptomatic individuals. In the FACTOR-64 trial, 900 asymptomatic individuals with diabetes were randomized to CAD screening with coronary CTA or optimal diabetes care according to established standards [26]. In the coronary CTA arm, the CT results were used for clinical decision-making. Individuals with normal coronary arteries were recommended to continue standard diabetes mellitus care. Participants with evidence of CAD by coronary CTA or a coronary artery calcium score >10 were recommended to begin a more aggressive risk factor modification including tighter control of LDL-C, triglycerides, HbA_{1C}, and blood pressure. Additionally, patients with moderate (50–69%) stenosis were recommended to receive stress cardiac imaging, and patients with severe (≥70%) stenosis were recommended to undergo diagnostic coronary angiography. Patients were followed for a mean of 4 years. The trial's primary outcome was a composite endpoint of all-cause mortality, nonfatal myocardial infarction, and unstable angina requiring hospitalization.

The trial's main result was that coronary CTA screening and CTA-directed management did not significantly reduce event rates compared to the control group (6.2% vs. 7.6%; hazard ratio, 0.80 [95% confidence interval, 0.49–1.32]; $P = 0.38$). Although discouraging, this result should not be regarded as refuting the idea of screening coronary CTA in high-risk asymptomatic individuals once and for all. The event rate in the FACTOR-64 trial was low, much lower than the estimation that was used for sample size calculations. Hence, the trial was not powered to detect a moderate risk reduction. The rate of coronary CTA-driven revascularizations was also low (5.8%). These observations suggest that the trial participants had a relatively low-risk profile and/or that the standard care was unusually stringent and effective. Therefore, further randomized trials with larger sample sizes and higher-risk inclusion criteria (e.g., longer-standing diabetes) are warranted. There was also some "contamination" in the trial as only 395 (87.4%) of the 452 participants in the CTA arm actually received a CT scan. In an as-treated analysis, the event rates for the primary endpoint were 5.6% vs. 7.9% (HR, 0.69 [95% CI, 0.41–1.16]; $P = 0.16$) indicating a trend toward a benefit of CTA screening.

Conclusions

Screening for CAD in asymptomatic individuals is generally not considered an appropriate application of coronary CTA by existing guidelines. Nevertheless, the practice is not uncommon. The diagnostic yield of coronary CTA in low-risk asymptomatic patients is low with obstructive coronary artery disease found in approximately 1% of low-risk individuals in most studies. The prevalence of asymptomatic CAD increases with the presence of established cardiovascular risk factors such as smoking, hypertension, diabetes, and chronic kidney disease. Coronary CTA has a particularly high diagnostic yield in specific high-risk subgroups of asymptomatic individuals such as patients with diabetes or familial hypercholesterolemia. In asymptomatic patients with diabetes, only 20–31% have normal coronary arteries on coronary CTA with 36–48% showing nonobstructive CAD and 23–44% showing obstructive CAD. Findings at coronary CTA have incremental prognostic value over coronary artery calcium scoring in high-risk groups (in particular, patients with diabetes), while the incremental prognostic value is probably not meaningful in a more mixed population. The only randomized controlled trial on the impact of coronary CTA screening in asymptomatic diabetic patients did not show a significant reduction in cardiovascular events. However, screening for CAD in asymptomatic high-risk individuals – in particular, patients with diabetes – remains a possible future application of coronary CTA. More randomized trials are needed to assess whether coronary CTA screening can decrease morbidity and mortality in these patients.

References

1. Wolk MJ, et al. ACCF/AHA/ASE/ASNC/HFSA/HRS/SCAI/SCCT/SCMR/STS 2013 multimodality appropriate use criteria for the detection and risk assessment of stable ischemic heart disease: a report of the American College of Cardiology Foundation Appropriate Use Criteria Task Force, American Heart Association, American Society of Echocardiography, American Society of Nuclear Cardiology, Heart Failure Society of America, Heart Rhythm Society, Society for Cardiovascular Angiography and Interventions, Society of Cardiovascular Computed Tomography, Society for Cardiovascular Magnetic Resonance, and Society of Thoracic Surgeons. J Am Coll Cardiol. 2014;63(4):380–406.
2. Meinel FG, et al. Radiation risks from cardiovascular imaging tests. Circulation. 2014;130(5):442–5.
3. Meinel FG, et al. Contrast-induced acute kidney injury: definition, epidemiology, and outcome. Biomed Res Int. 2014;2014:859328.
4. Wilson JMG, Jungner G. Principles and practice of screening for disease. Public Health Paper Number 34. 1968 [cited 18 Oct 2016]; Available from: http://www.who.int/iris/handle/10665/37650.
5. Andermann A, et al. Revisiting Wilson and Jungner in the genomic age: a review of screening criteria over the past 40 years. Bull World Health Organ. 2008;86(4):317–9.
6. Cho I, et al. Coronary computed tomographic angiography and risk of all-cause mortality and nonfatal myocardial infarction in subjects without chest pain syndrome from the CONFIRM registry (coronary CT angiography evaluation for clinical outcomes: an international multicenter registry). Circulation. 2012;126(3):304–13.
7. Maurer MH, et al. Indications, imaging technique, and reading of cardiac computed tomography: survey of clinical practice. Eur Radiol. 2012;22(1):59–72.
8. Liu K, et al. Current utilization of cardiac computed tomography in mainland China: a national survey. J Cardiovasc Comput Tomogr. 2016;10(1):76–81.
9. Braber TL, et al. Occult coronary artery disease in middle-aged sportsmen with a low cardiovascular risk score: the Measuring Athlete's Risk of Cardiovascular Events (MARC) study. Eur J Prev Cardiol. 2016;23(15):1677–84.
10. Kim S, et al. Normal-weight obesity is associated with increased risk of subclinical atherosclerosis. Cardiovasc Diabetol. 2015;14:58.
11. Lee MS, et al. Asymptomatic subjects with zero coronary calcium score: coronary CT angiographic features of plaques in event-prone patients. Int J Cardiovasc Imaging. 2013;29(Suppl 1):29–36.
12. Cho I, et al. Prevalence and prognostic implication of non-calcified plaque in asymptomatic population with coronary artery calcium score of zero. Korean Circ J. 2013;43(3):154–60.
13. Kim KJ, et al. The prevalence and characteristics of coronary atherosclerosis in asymptomatic subjects classified as low risk based on traditional risk stratification algorithm: assessment with coronary CT angiography. Heart. 2013;99(15):1113–7.
14. Jin KN, et al. Subclinical coronary atherosclerosis in young adults: prevalence, characteristics, predictors with coronary computed tomography angiography. Int J Cardiovasc Imaging. 2012;28(Suppl 2):93–100.
15. Yoo DH, et al. Significance of noncalcified coronary plaque in asymptomatic subjects with low coronary artery calcium score: assessment with coronary computed tomography angiography. Int J Cardiovasc Imaging. 2011;27(Suppl 1):27–35.
16. Cho I, et al. Incremental prognostic utility of coronary CT angiography for asymptomatic patients based upon extent and severity of coronary artery calcium: results from the COronary CT Angiography EvaluatioN For Clinical Outcomes InteRnational Multicenter (CONFIRM) study. Eur Heart J. 2015;36(8):501–8.
17. Cho I, et al. Coronary atherosclerosis detected by coronary CT angiography in asymptomatic subjects with early chronic kidney disease. Atherosclerosis. 2010;208(2):406–11.
18. Nam HJ, et al. Association between brachial-ankle pulse wave velocity and occult coronary artery disease detected by multi-detector computed tomography. Int J Cardiol. 2012;157(2):227–32.
19. Yi M, et al. Coronary CT angiography findings based on smoking status: do ex-smokers and never-smokers share a low probability of developing coronary atherosclerosis? Int J Cardiovasc Imaging. 2015;31(Suppl 2):169–76.
20. Kim JA, et al. Relationship between amount of cigarette smoking and coronary atherosclerosis on coronary CTA in asymptomatic individuals. Int J Cardiovasc Imaging. 2013;29(Suppl 1):21–8.
21. Im TS, et al. Grade-response relationship between blood pressure and severity of coronary atherosclerosis in asymptomatic adults: assessment with coronary CT angiography. Int J Cardiovasc Imaging. 2014;30(Suppl 2):105–12.
22. Gurudevan S, et al. Impaired fasting glucose is associated with increased severity of subclinical coronary artery disease compared to patients with diabetes and normal fasting glucose: evaluation by coronary computed tomographic angiography. BMJ Open. 2016;6(8):e005148.
23. Ryu J, et al. Relation of coronary atherosclerosis and metabolic syndrome in asymptomatic subjects: evaluation with coronary CT angiography. Int J Cardiovasc Imaging. 2013;29(Suppl 2):101–7.
24. Yang DH, et al. Association between C-reactive protein and type of coronary arterial plaque in asymptomatic patients: assessment with coronary CT angiography. Radiology. 2014;272(3):665–73.
25. Park YJ, et al. Impact of subclinical hypothyroidism on the coronary artery disease in apparently healthy subjects. Eur J Endocrinol. 2011;165(1):115–21.
26. Muhlestein JB, et al. Effect of screening for coronary artery disease using CT angiography on mortality and cardiac events in high-risk

patients with diabetes: the FACTOR-64 randomized clinical trial. JAMA. 2014;312(21):2234–43.
27. Kang SH, et al. Long-term prognostic value of coronary CT angiography in asymptomatic type 2 diabetes mellitus. JACC Cardiovasc Imaging. 2016;9(11):1292–300.
28. Halon DA, et al. Coronary computed tomography (CT) angiography as a predictor of cardiac and noncardiac vascular events in asymptomatic type 2 diabetics: a 7-year population-based cohort study. J Am Heart Assoc. 2016;5(6):e003226.
29. Kim JJ, et al. Impact of diabetes duration on the extent and severity of coronary atheroma burden and long-term clinical outcome in asymptomatic type 2 diabetic patients: evaluation by coronary CT angiography. Eur Heart J Cardiovasc Imaging. 2015;16(10):1065–73.
30. Kim JJ, et al. A prospective two-center study on the associations between microalbuminuria, coronary atherosclerosis and long-term clinical outcome in asymptomatic patients with type 2 diabetes mellitus: evaluation by coronary CT angiography. Int J Cardiovasc Imaging. 2015;31(1):193–203.
31. Dedic A, et al. Prognostic value of coronary computed tomography imaging in patients at high risk without symptoms of coronary artery disease. Am J Cardiol. 2016;117(5):768–74.
32. Idilman IS, et al. Nonalcoholic fatty liver disease is associated with significant coronary artery disease in type 2 diabetic patients: a computed tomography angiography study 2. J Diabetes. 2015;7(2):279–86.
33. Min JK, et al. Incremental prognostic value of coronary computed tomographic angiography over coronary artery calcium score for risk prediction of major adverse cardiac events in asymptomatic diabetic individuals. Atherosclerosis. 2014;232(2):298–304.
34. Neefjes LA, et al. CT coronary plaque burden in asymptomatic patients with familial hypercholesterolaemia. Heart. 2011;97(14):1151–7.
35. Ten Kate GJ, et al. The effect of LDLR-negative genotype on CT coronary atherosclerosis in asymptomatic statin treated patients with heterozygous familial hypercholesterolemia. Atherosclerosis. 2013;227(2):334–41.
36. Neefjes LA, et al. Accelerated subclinical coronary atherosclerosis in patients with familial hypercholesterolemia. Atherosclerosis. 2011;219(2):721–7.
37. Hromadka M, et al. Incidence of severe coronary stenosis in asymptomatic patients with peripheral arterial disease scheduled for major vascular surgery. Int Angiol. 2016;35(4):411–7.
38. Calvet D, et al. Predicting asymptomatic coronary artery disease in patients with ischemic stroke and transient ischemic attack: the PRECORIS score. Stroke. 2014;45(1):82–6.
39. den Dekker MA, et al. Prevalence of severe subclinical coronary artery disease on cardiac CT and MRI in patients with extra-cardiac arterial disease. Eur J Vasc Endovasc Surg. 2013;46(6): 680–9.
40. Yoon YE, et al. Incidence of subclinical coronary atherosclerosis in patients with suspected embolic stroke using cardiac computed tomography. Int J Cardiovasc Imaging. 2011;27(7):1035–44.
41. Daniels LA, et al. Screening for coronary artery disease after mediastinal irradiation in Hodgkin lymphoma survivors: phase II study of indication and acceptancedagger. Ann Oncol. 2014;25(6):1198–203.
42. Girinsky T, et al. Prospective coronary heart disease screening in asymptomatic Hodgkin lymphoma patients using coronary computed tomography angiography: results and risk factor analysis. Int J Radiat Oncol Biol Phys. 2014;89(1):59–66.
43. Lubanski MS, et al. Subclinical coronary atherosclerosis identified by coronary computed tomographic angiography in asymptomatic morbidly obese patients. Heart Int. 2010;5(2):e15.
44. d'Ettorre G, et al. Significant coronary stenosis detected by coronary computed angiography in asymptomatic HIV infected subjects. J Infect. 2012;64(1):82–8.
45. Fitch KV, et al. Subclinical myocyte injury, fibrosis and strain in relationship to coronary plaque in asymptomatic HIV-infected individuals. AIDS. 2016;30(14):2205–14.
46. Ketlogetswe KS, et al. Lower adiponectin is associated with subclinical cardiovascular disease among HIV-infected men. AIDS. 2014;28(6):901–9.
47. Kral BG, et al. Noncalcified coronary plaque volumes in healthy people with a family history of early onset coronary artery disease. Circ Cardiovasc Imaging. 2014;7(3):446–53.
48. Plank F, et al. The diagnostic and prognostic value of coronary CT angiography in asymptomatic high-risk patients: a cohort study. Open Heart. 2014;1(1):e000096.
49. de Bie MK, et al. CT coronary angiography is feasible for the assessment of coronary artery disease in chronic dialysis patients, despite high average calcium scores. PLoS One. 2013;8(7):e67936.
50. Catapano AL, et al. 2016 ESC/EAS Guidelines for the Management of Dyslipidaemias: The Task Force for the Management of Dyslipidaemias of the European Society of Cardiology (ESC) and European Atherosclerosis Society (EAS)Developed with the special contribution of the European Association for Cardiovascular Prevention & Rehabilitation (EACPR). Eur Heart J. 2016;37(39):2999–3058.
51. Stone NJ, et al. 2013 ACC/AHA guideline on the treatment of blood cholesterol to reduce atherosclerotic cardiovascular risk in adults: a report of the American College of Cardiology/American Heart Association Task Force on Practice Guidelines. J Am Coll Cardiol. 2014;63(25 Pt B):2889–934.
52. Goff DC Jr, et al. 2013 ACC/AHA guideline on the assessment of cardiovascular risk: a report of the American College of Cardiology/ American Heart Association Task Force on Practice Guidelines. Circulation. 2014;129(25 Suppl 2):S49–73.
53. Eckel RH, et al. 2013 AHA/ACC guideline on lifestyle management to reduce cardiovascular risk: a report of the American College of Cardiology/American Heart Association Task Force on Practice Guidelines. J Am Coll Cardiol. 2014;63(25 Pt B):2960–84.
54. Jensen MD, et al. 2013 AHA/ACC/TOS guideline for the management of overweight and obesity in adults: a report of the American College of Cardiology/American Heart Association Task Force on Practice Guidelines and The Obesity Society. J Am Coll Cardiol. 2014;63(25 Pt B):2985–3023.
55. Arad Y, et al. Coronary calcification, coronary disease risk factors, C-reactive protein, and atherosclerotic cardiovascular disease events: the St. Francis heart study. J Am Coll Cardiol. 2005;46(1):158–65.
56. Miedema MD, et al. Use of coronary artery calcium testing to guide aspirin utilization for primary prevention: estimates from the multi-ethnic study of atherosclerosis. Circ Cardiovasc Qual Outcomes. 2014;7(3):453–60.
57. Williams MC, et al. Use of coronary computed tomographic angiography to guide management of Patients with coronary disease. J Am Coll Cardiol. 2016;67(15):1759–68.

Part XV

Where We Are Going: Lesion-specific Ischemia, Infarction, and Viability

Transluminal Attenuation Gradient and Other CT Techniques for Gauging Lesion Significance

59

Yeon Hyeon Choe, Jin-Ho Choi, and Sung Mok Kim

Coronary CT angiography (CCTA) has emerged as the noninvasive modality of choice for imaging of the coronary arteries and serves as a gatekeeper to interventional treatment of coronary artery disease (CAD) [1, 2]. However, severe motion and blooming artifacts are associated with elevated heart rates, calcifications, and stents, respectively, and can often times hinder the evaluation of image sets. Despite the high diagnostic performance of CCTA for the detection of stenosis, not all lesions are hemodynamically significant. Current CT technology does not allow for clear vessel wall-lumen delineation due to limited spatial resolution; however, the use of commercialized software tools can help radiologists detect stenotic lesions semiautomatically [3, 4]. Notably, even with the use of software, manual interaction is necessary to define the luminal contour. Thus, efforts have been made to enhance the diagnostic capability of CCTA through the use of CT fractional flow reserve (CT-FFR), vasodilator stress myocardial CT perfusion (CTP), and transluminal attenuation gradients (TAG) [5–7].

Y. H. Choe (✉)
Department of Radiology, HVSI Imaging Center, Heart Vascular Stroke Institute, Samsung Medical Center, Sungkyunkwan University School of Medicine, Seoul, South Korea
e-mail: yhchoe@skku.edu

J.-H. Choi
Division of Cardiology, Department of Medicine (J-H C), Samsung Medical Center, Sungkyunkwan University School of Medicine, Seoul, South Korea

S. M. Kim
Department of Radiology, HVSI Imaging Center, Heart Vascular Stroke Institute, Seoul, South Korea

Theoretical Background of TAG

Enhancement in the vessel lumen depends on various factors including contrast volume and concentration, injection speed, CT scan protocols including tube voltage (kVp), as well as patient body habitus and sex [8]. Contrast attenuation-time curves in a certain anatomical region can depict upslope, peak, and downslope (Fig. 59.1). Blood in the coronary artery propagates from the proximal segment to distal segments as time lapses. The normal mean flow velocity in the coronary arteries is 40 ± 19 cm/s (peak diastolic velocity, 64 ± 26 cm/s; peak systolic velocity, 34 ± 22 cm/s) using Doppler guidewire technique [9]. The peak diastolic velocity in the distal left anterior descending coronary artery (LAD) is 21.2 ± 7.9 cm/s using transthoracic Doppler echocardiography [10].

On CCTA image sets, small decreases in contrast opacification were observed going from proximal to distal segments of the coronary arteries [11]. The attenuation gradients were steeper in patients with obstructive coronary artery diseases [11–13]. According to Steigner et al. [11], three distinct coronary contrast opacification gradients (gradients according to distance from the coronary ostium [G(d)], lumen cross-sectional area [G(a)], and lumen short-axis diameter [G(s)]) could be measured within a single heartbeat using a 320-slice CT scanner. Notably, gradient variations between cardiac phases, heart rates, body habitus, and readers were low. Gradients in patients with lesions were significantly different ($p < 0.021$) than in patients considered normal at CCTA. For all patients, the gradients defined with respect to the coronary lumen cross-sectional area and short-axis diameters were highly linear, not significantly influenced by the coronary artery (left anterior descending artery [LAD] versus left circumflex [LCX] versus right coronary artery [RCA]), and only have minute variations with respect to individual patient parameters. While 64-slice CT results also showed abnormalities in

U. J. Schoepf (ed.), *CT of the Heart*, Contemporary Medical Imaging, https://doi.org/10.1007/978-1-60327-237-7_59

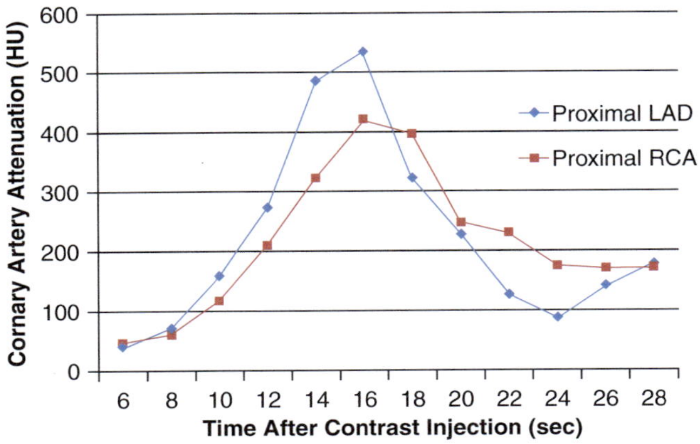

Fig. 59.1 Time-attenuation curves of the coronary arteries. The graph shows time-attenuation curves of the coronary arteries (left anterior descending branch, LAD; right coronary artery, RCA) obtained from two different patients, respectively. Dynamic CT was performed under adenosine stress after a 50 mL bolus of contrast material (400 Ig/mL) was administered at 5 mL/s

TAG values in patients with obstructive CAD [12], Park et al. claimed that a decrease in TAG is associated with a decrease in coronary luminal diameter (transluminal diameter gradient [TDG]) [14].

Techniques for TAG

Theoretically, whole-heart coverage at a single gantry rotation in a single heartbeat using 256-slice or 320-slice CT is advantageous for TAG measurement. Attenuation along a vessel does not reflect contrast density at a single time point using a 64-slice CT [12] (Fig. 59.2).

Contrast enhancement should be strong enough to allow automatic detection of vessel luminal contour using dedicated software. TAG can be affected by scan timing [15], rendering scans optimal before the peak enhancement of the coronary artery [15, 16]. Additionally, it is desirable to obtain CT images during the upslope period (ascending leg) of the time-attenuation curve of CCTA [15], as dynamic scanning shows increasing TAG at time points after peak attenuation in the coronary arteries (Fig. 59.3) [14]. TAG may fluctuate along the course of the coronary tree due to CT technical causes, for example, motion artifacts and variations in photon flux. Chow et al. [17] used corrected coronary opacification (CCO) within coronary lumen normalized to the aorta.

Current CT software analysis techniques allow for easy analysis of TAG assuming vessel centerlines are drawn correctly. Automated gradient calculation software shows no difference between manual and automated methods despite varying body mass index categories, presence and severity of coronary artery disease, plaque composition, or reconstruction algorithms [18].

Notably, the LAD coronary artery is different from the RCA in TAG, as the LAD has more bifurcations such as septal and diagonal branches [14, 17]. Therefore, TAG may vary according to coronary anatomy. For example, the LAD and LCX coronary arteries taper more rapidly along the vessel length than the RCA. TAG may be associated with branching of coronary arteries and is relatively constant in the segments between the branches, while TAGs of larger and smaller vessels may be different.

Coronary Flow Measurement with CT

Lackner et al. [19] suggested that the CT data in an experimental model simultaneously acquired for the coronary and aorta time-density curves enables qualitative and semiquantitative assessment of stenotic changes in flow. In a study by Bovenschulte et al., the ratio of upslopes of the coronary artery and aorta, derived from the time-density curve data using a 64-slice CT, was used as a measure of the difference in the slope of density increase in the coronary artery and aorta [20]. All examinations of hemodynamically relevant stenosis ($\geq$70%) and insignificant stenoses produced ratios of $\leq$0.55 and $\geq$0.77, respectively.

Lardo et al. [21] proposed a new method for noninvasive measurement of absolute coronary blood flow (CBF) termed transluminal attenuation flow encoding (TAFE). They applied TAFE to calculate absolute CBF using four vessel input parameters including TAG, cross-sectional area, length, and the contrast bolus duration derived from the arterial input function in animal studies (Fig. 59.4). TAFE-derived CBF divided by myocardial mass strongly correlated with microsphere myocardial blood flow ($R^2 = 0.90$, $p < 0.001$). In human studies, TAFE-derived CBF in the LAD, LCX, and RCA was 26.4 ± 10.7 mL/min, 20.1 ± 13.0 mL/min, and 43.2 ± 40.9 mL/min, respectively. CBF per unit mass was 0.93 ± 0.48 mL/g/min. Interobserver variability was minimal with excellent correlation ($R = 0.96$, $p < 0.0001$) and agreement (mean difference, 4.2 mL/min).

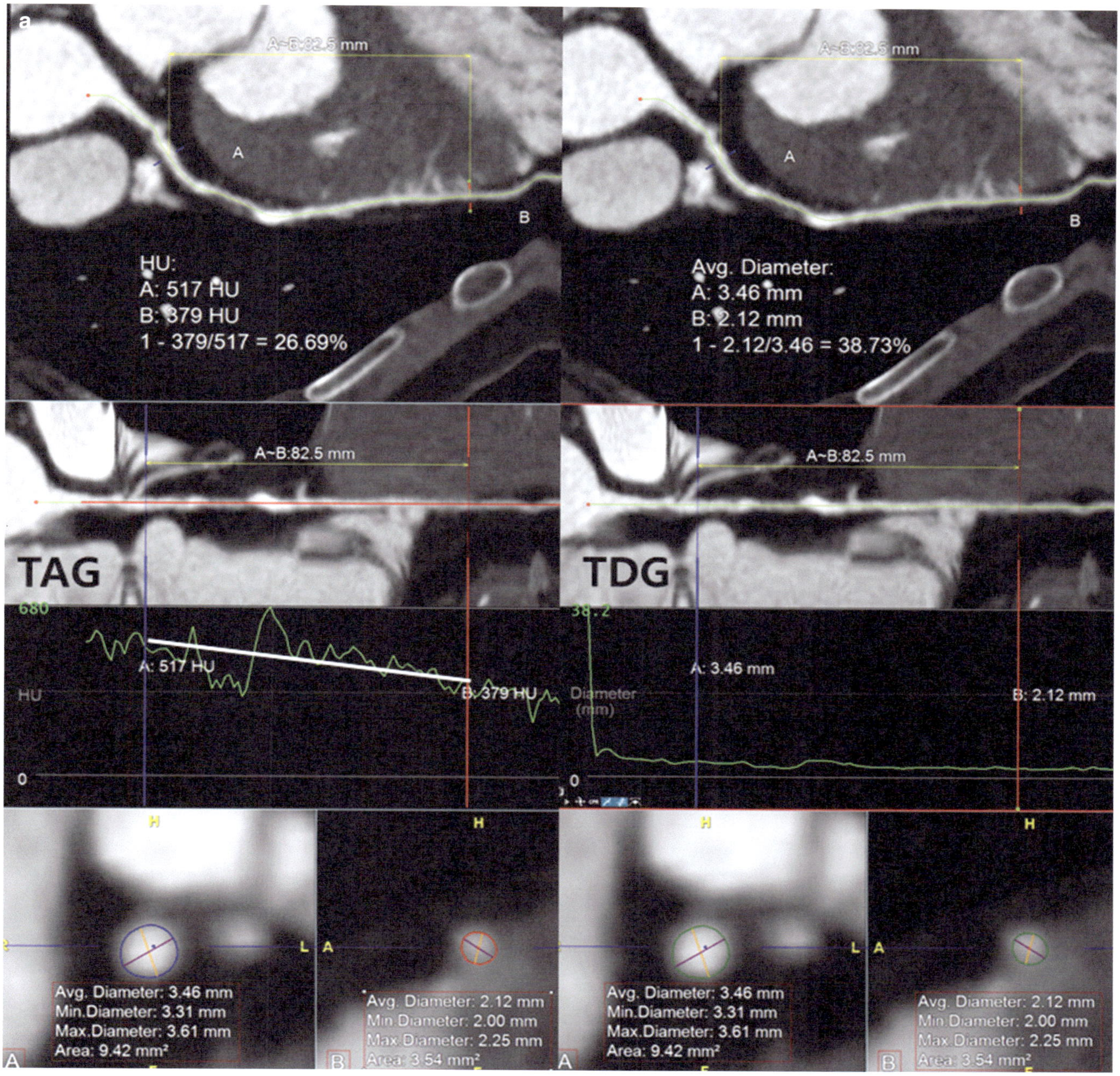

Fig. 59.2 TAG and TDG measurement. (**a**) Transluminal attenuation gradient (TAG) and transluminal diameter gradient (TDG) were calculated in the left anterior descending branch (LAD) using a single-heartbeat acquisition with a 320-slice CT. TAG was −16.7 HU/cm and TDG was 0.162 mm/cm. (**b**) LAD segmental lesion measured 60% stenosis (arrow) by quantitative coronary angiography, and fractional flow reserve with adenosine-induced hyperemia was 0.64

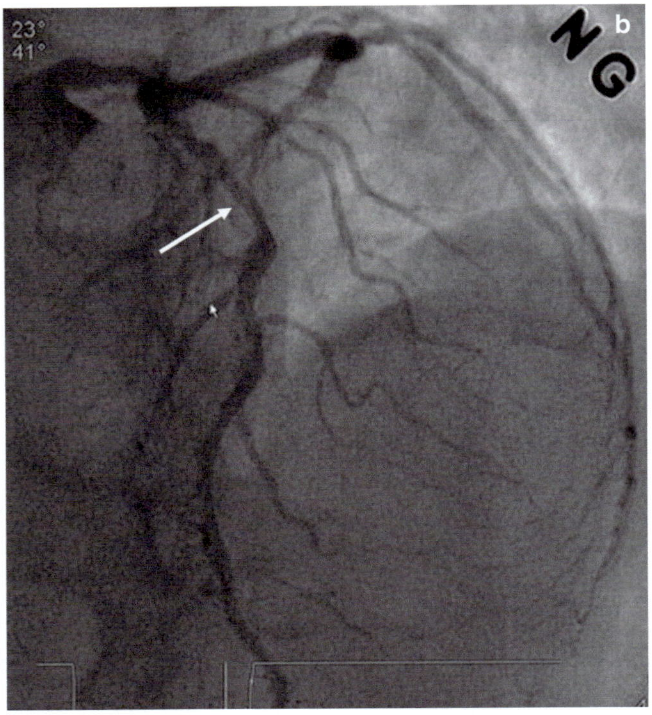

Fig. 59.2 (continued)

Contrast Density Difference

Contrast density difference (CDD) is defined as the decline in luminal contrast attenuation over a coronary lesion (Fig. 59.5) [22]. CDD was significantly greater in hemodynamically relevant lesions, as defined by invasive fractional flow reserve (FFR), compared to nonsignificant lesions (26.0 ± 20.2% vs. 16.6 ± 10.9%; $p = 0.013$). At a threshold of ≥24%, CDD predicted hemodynamically significant lesions with a specificity of 75%, sensitivity of 33%, PPV of 35%, and NPV of 73% [22]. TAG showed no significant difference between hemodynamically significant and nonsignificant lesions (−14.2 ± 14.2 HU/cm vs. −11.0 ± 12.8 HU/cm; $p = 0.45$). In the receiver operating characteristic (ROC) curve analysis, AUCs for CDD, TAG (threshold, −6.5 HU/cm), and visual assessment of CCTA were 0.67 (95% CI, 0.54–0.8), 0.56 (95% CI, 0.41–0.71), and 0.61 (95% CI, 0.48–0.74), respectively. The AUC for CDD was not significantly higher compared to TAG and visual stenosis assessment.

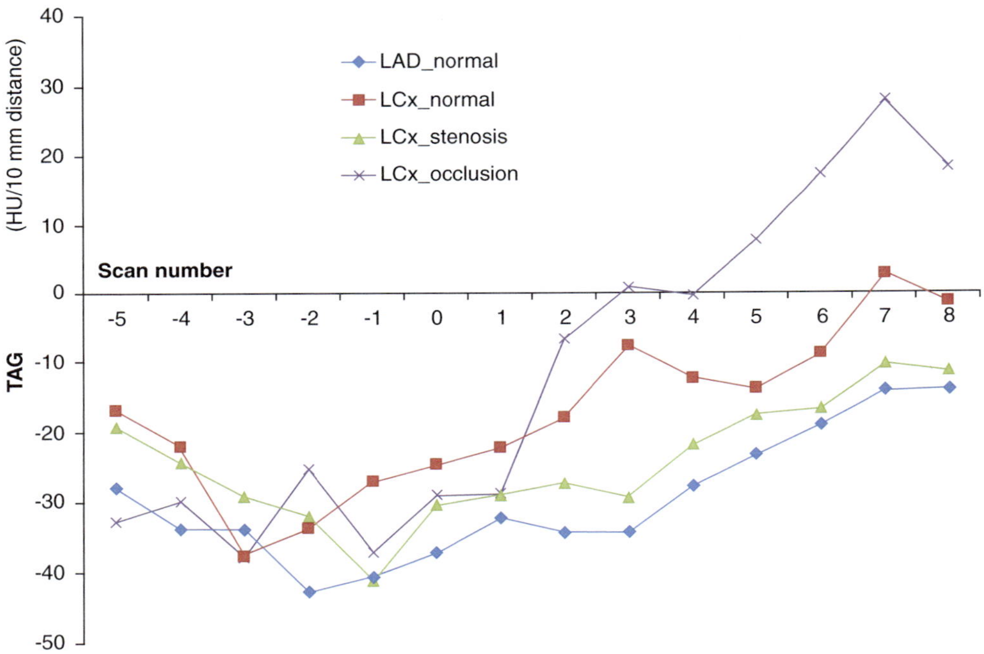

Fig. 59.3 Changes in TAG over time in each coronary artery with dynamic scanning in an animal model. Scan number was coded as zero when attenuation of the ascending aorta reached its peak. There were no significant differences in transluminal attenuation gradient (TAG) values between stenotic and normal left circumflex coronary artery (LCX) or between stenotic LCX and normal left anterior descending coronary artery (LAD) at each time point (all, $p > 0.05$). Significant difference in TAG values was only found between normal LAD and occluded LCX in the fifth to eighth repeated scans and between stenotic LCX and occluded LCX in the third to eighth repeated scans (all, $p < 0.05$). (From Park et al. [14], with permission)

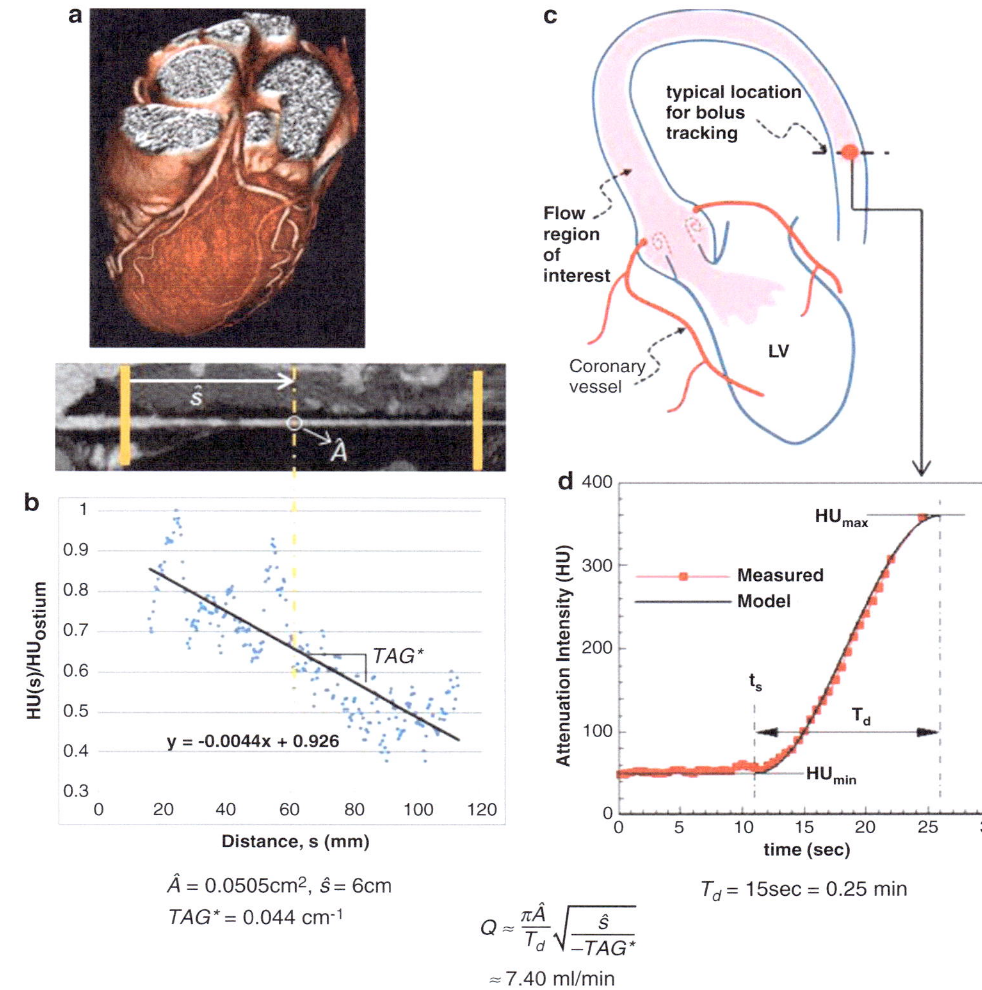

Fig. 59.4 Implementation of transluminal attenuation flow encoding (TAFE). After 3D isotemporal acquisition of the whole heart (**a**), multiplanar reformations of the three primary coronary vessels are generated (**b**). TAG is computed (**b**, lower panel) between two user-defined proximal and distal boundary locations. The average distance between the user-defined point(s) and the average cross-sectional area (**a**) over the user-defined length is automatically calculated. The contrast bolus duration (Td) is the temporal element of contrast dispersion and is derived from AIF measured in the descending aorta (**c**, **d**). Once these four CT-based parameters have been isolated, an equation (bottom) can be used to calculate coronary flow in mL/min. AIF arterial input function, TAG transluminal attenuation gradient. (From Lardo et al. [21], with permission)

Corrected Coronary Attenuation

Coronary attenuation variability after contrast material injection may occur due to the lack of temporal uniformity on 64-slice CT systems. The corrected coronary attenuation (CCO) is calculated as the quotient of the attenuation in the coronary artery and aorta (CCO, coronary artery attenuation/aorta attenuation) (Fig. 59.6) [17]. According to Chow et al., in normal arteries, the mean CCO was 0.979 ± 0.070 (median, 0.965; interquartile range [IQR], 0.940–1.005) [17]. Normal CCO variability (difference between highest CCO and lowest CCO) was measured as 0.100 ± 0.042 (median, 0.099; IQR, 0.073–0.128). Changes in CCO across coronary stenoses seem to predict abnormal resting coronary blood flow (Thrombolysis in Myocardial Infarction [TIMI] flow grade < 3) [17]. Compared with the CCO variability in nonobstructive arteries, the CCO difference was significantly greater in arteries with obstructive CAD (diameter stenoses ≥50%) (0.191 ± 0.214; median, 0.106; interquartile range [IQR], 0.042–0.296) (p = 0.004), and the proportion of abnormal CCO differences increased with worsening diameter stenosis ($p < 0.001$). Similarly, CCO differences were greater in arteries with TIMI flow grade < 3 (0.406 ± 0.226) compared to coronaries with normal flow (0.078 ± 0.078, $p < 0.001$). With CCO differences (threshold, >0.184 [mean CCO difference + 2 standard deviations]), abnormal coronary flow (TIMI flow grade < 3) was identified with a sensitivity, specificity, positive predictive value, and negative predictive value of 83.3% (95% confidence interval [CI], 57.7–95.6%), 91.2% (95% CI, 75.2–97.7%), 83.3% (95% CI, 57.7–95.6%), and 91.2% (95% CI, 75.2–97.7%), respectively. Notably, the accuracy of this method was 88.5% with very good agreement (kappa = 0.75; 95% CI, 0.55–0.94).

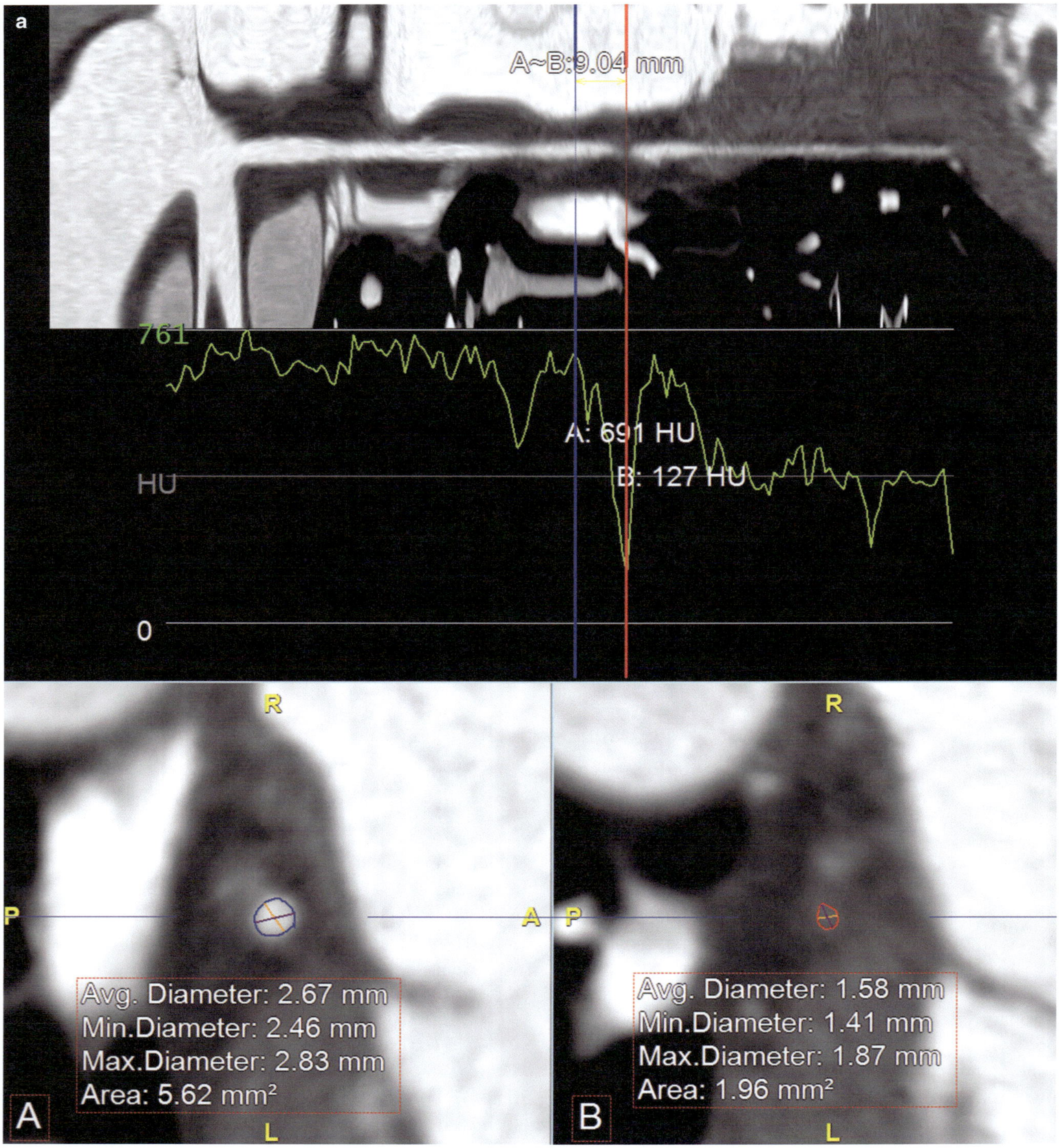

Fig. 59.5 Coronary density difference. (**a**) Coronary density difference measures 82% for the focal severe stenosis with soft plaques in left circumflex artery. (**b**) Invasive coronary angiography reveals severe stenosis (arrow) in distal vessel with FFR = 0.4

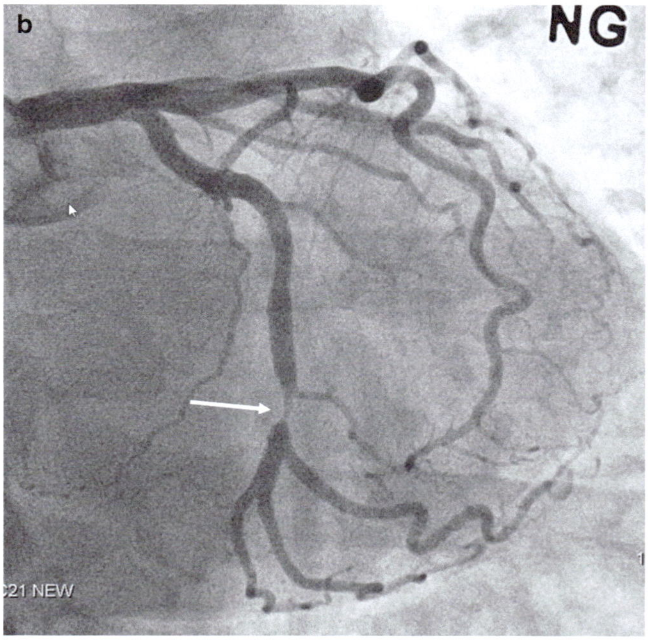

Fig. 59.5 (continued)

Transluminal Diameter Gradient

Coronary artery intraluminal attenuation was shown to decrease with diminution of vessel diameters (Fig. 59.7) [14]. In a study by Park et al., a moderate correlation was found between TAG and transluminal diameter gradient (TDG) ($r = 0.580$; $p < 0.0001$) in 152 coronary arteries of 62 patients [14]. Separate analysis of significant and nonsignificant stenosis groups also showed a significant correlation between TAG and TDG ($r = 0.610$ [$p < 0.0001$] for nonsignificant stenosis; $r = 0.565$ [$p = 0.0001$] for significant stenosis) (Fig. 59.8). In addition, TAG-positive arteries exhibited significantly greater TDG values in groups with ($p < 0.0001$) and without significant stenosis ($p < 0.0001$). There were no significant differences in TAG values between groups with significant stenosis (diameter stenosis ≥50%) and without significant stenosis ($p = 0.884$), whereas a significant difference was found in TDG values (−0.379 [IQR, 0.377] versus −0.273 [IQR, 0.191], $p = 0.021$). However, it should be noted that coronary artery attenuation also depends on the coronary flow physiology and CT technical factors.

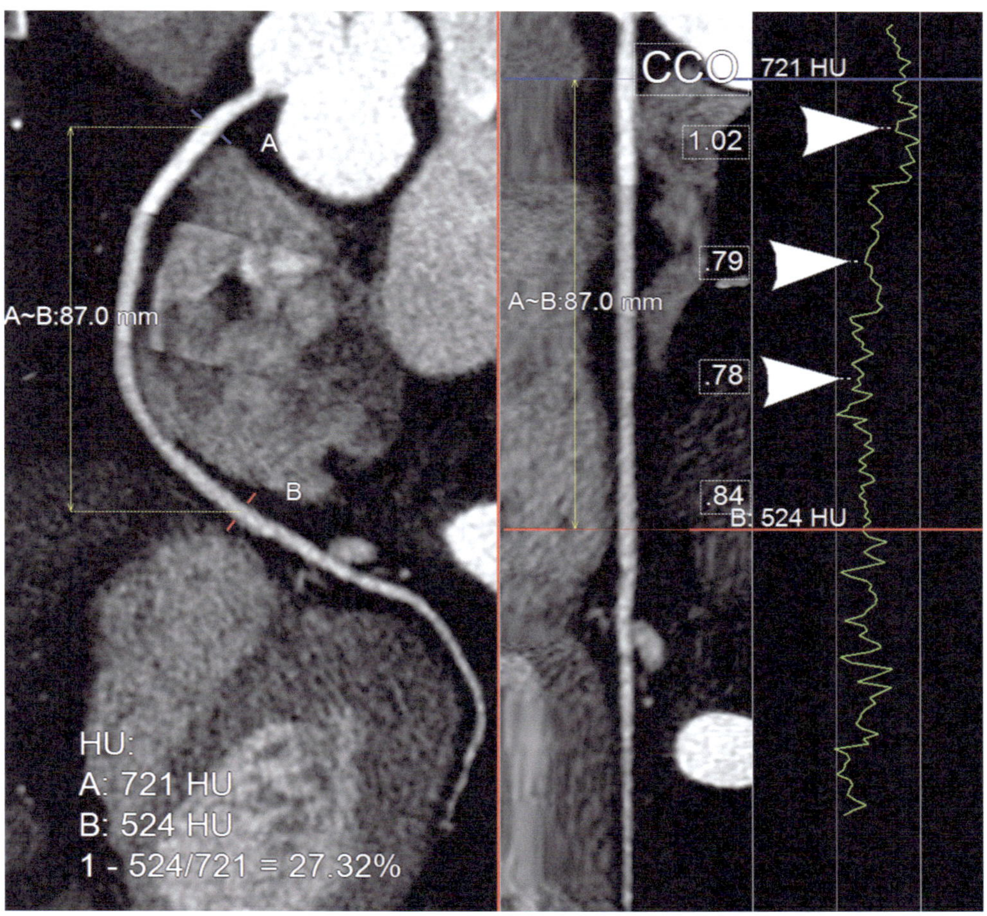

Fig. 59.6 Corrected coronary attenuation (CCO). CCO was calculated as 1.02, 0.79, 0.78, and 0.84, respectively, in four sequential segments of right coronary artery on images obtained from a 64-slice CT system. Note the stepwise changes (arrows) in the attenuation curve according to each imaging slab

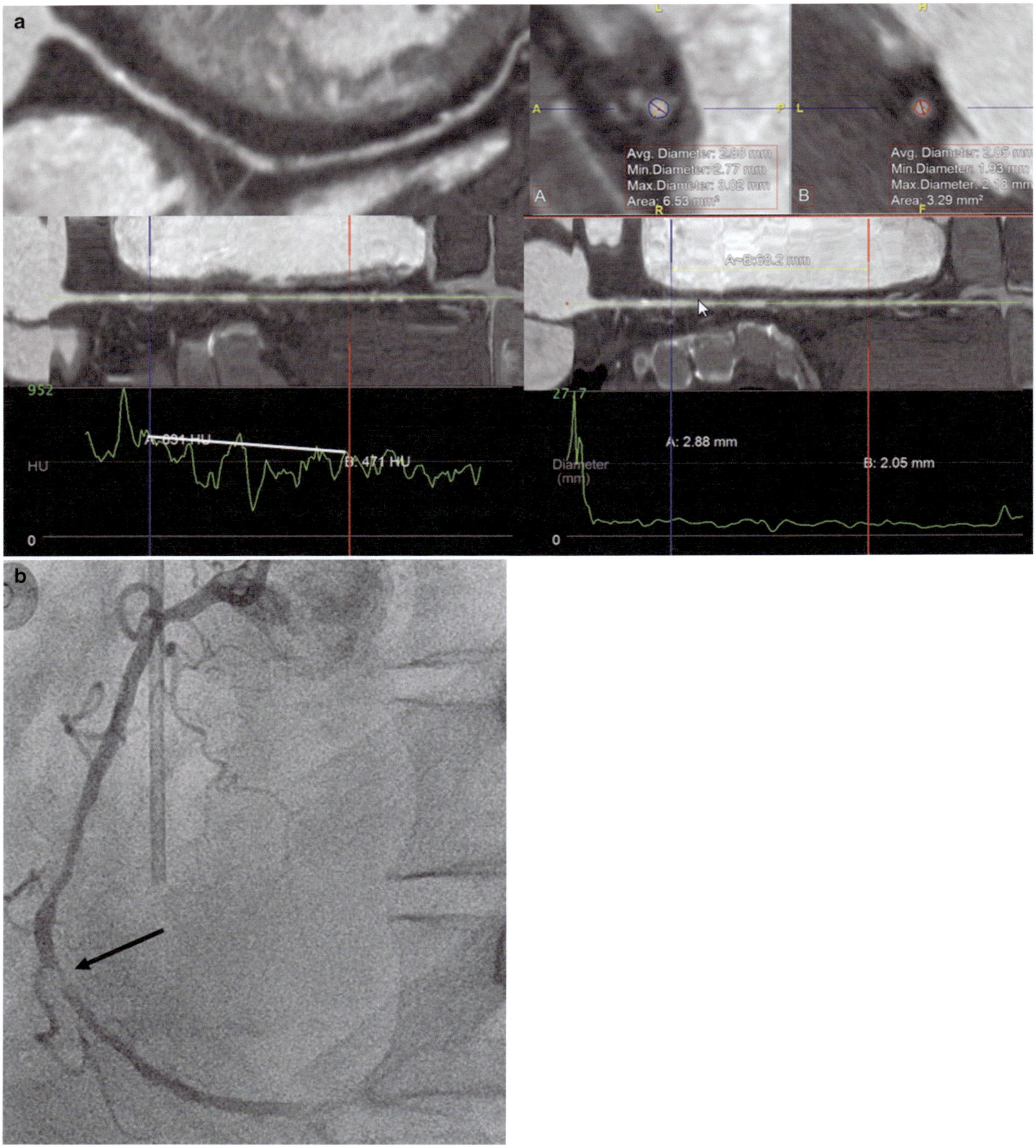

Fig. 59.7 Comparison of TAG and TDG. (**a**) TAG was −23.5 HU/cm (−3.7%/cm), and TDG was −0.12/cm (−4.3%/cm). (**b**) Invasive coronary angiography shows severe stenosis (arrow) in the mid-RCA

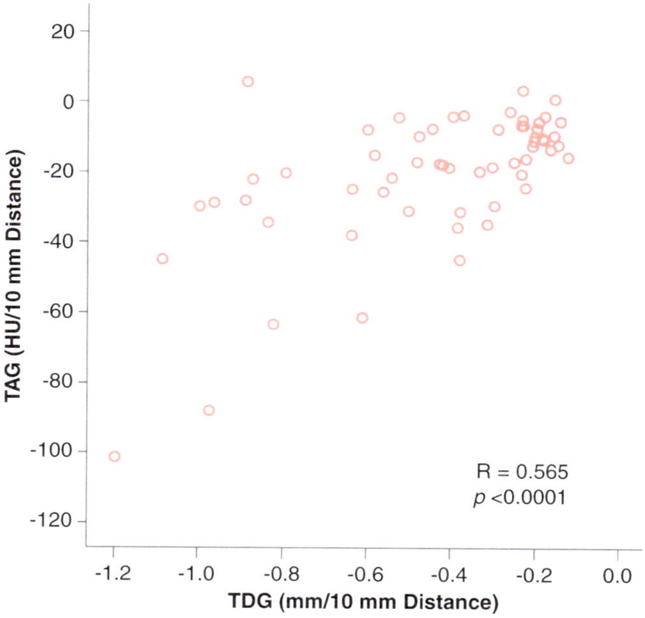

Fig. 59.8 Correlation between TAG and TDG. Significant correlation was found in patients with significant stenosis. (From Park et al. [14], with permission)

Experimental Studies: Effects of Cardiac Output and Vessel Diameters on TAG

Funama et al. investigated TAG values at different scan acquisition points along the time-density curve (TDC) after contrast material injection using a flow phantom and a 320-row CT scanner [15]. At a cardiac output of 2.0 and 4.0 L/min with 0% stenosis, TAG exhibited smaller variations at each time point along the TDC (−3.02 to +0.55 HU/cm at 2.0 L/min, −2.63 to +0.43 HU/cm at 4.0 L/min) compared to 70% stenosis [15]. Compared with a cardiac output of 2.0 L/min with 70% stenosis, the TAG curve for a cardiac output of 4.0 L/min gradually changed with time (−6.64 to +1.18 HU/cm at 2.0 L/min vs. −3.46 to +2.75 HU/cm at 4.0 L/min). The TAG value was affected by acquisition timing after contrast material injection and cardiac output; however, the size of the connecting tube (with and without stenosis) was identical.

In a study by Park et al. [14], a vessel phantom was constructed with 25 tubular holes in a 5-cm-thick polyethylene disk. The diameter of each hole was 5.0, 4.5, 4.0, 3.5, 3.0, and 2.9–1.0 mm with 0.1 mm intervals, simulating vessels of different diameters. The phantom was immersed in two different mixtures of an iodine contrast agent and saline, approximating attenuations of 800 and 600 HU at 100 kVp, with all tubular holes completely filled with contrast mixture. CT scans were performed with the phantom immersed in the 600 HU contrast mixture using 80, 100, and 120 kVp. Then, the phantom was immersed in the 800 HU contrast mixture and scanned using 100 kVp. Even though all holes were filled with the same contrast mixture, intraluminal attenuation was observed to gradually decline along with decreasing vessel diameter. The reduction of intraluminal attenuation was much greater as the diameters became smaller. The same findings were observed regardless of the acquisition's tube voltage or the concentration of contrast mixture.

In an animal study conducted by the same investigator, a dynamic CT scan was performed in 3 canines using a 320-row CT system (Fig. 59.3) [14]. Small distal coronary arteries exhibited only 55–78% of the maximum enhancement of proximal segments, regardless of which coronary artery was being evaluated. The animal study revealed that the length of the coronary artery was an important factor in calculating TAG. For example, normal vessels that were short with rapid changes in diameter exhibited higher TAG values.

Clinical Evidences of TAG

The diagnostic estimates and AUCs of ROC analyses for TAG, CCTA, and the combination of CCTA and TAG in the literature are presented in Table 59.1.

In a study by Choi et al. that used invasive coronary angiography as the reference standard, TAG decreased as stenosis severity increased from −2.37 ± 4.67 HU/cm for a diameter stenosis between 0% and 49% to −13.46 ± 9.59 HU/cm for a diameter stenosis of 100% ($p < 0.0001$) (Fig. 59.9) [12]. The accuracy in determining stenosis severity classification by CCTA, as compared with ICA, improved significantly when TAG was considered (*c*-statistic 0.932 ± 0.012 vs. 0.951 ± 0.010, $p = 0.001$; global chi-square 254.381 vs. 265.899, $p = 0.001$). The improved diagnostic accuracy was mainly driven by increased specificity (89.7% [95% CI, 83.0–94.4] vs. 93.7% [95% CI, 87.9–97.2]). Additionally, the accuracy of stenosis severity classification of calcified stenoses by CCTA significantly increased when TAG was taken into account (*c*-statistic, $p < 0.0001$; global chi-square, $p = 0.001$). The addition of TAG resulted in a reclassification of stenosis severity in a significant number of vessels with calcified lesions (net reclassification improvement [NRI] 0.095, net proportion of patients reclassified 3.15%; $p = 0.046$). TAG also improved the accuracy for determining stenosis severity caused by noncalcified plaques (*c*-statistic, $p = 0.048$; global chi-square, $p = 0.012$). However, the addition of TAG did not result in significant stenosis severity reclassification in vessels with noncalcified lesions (NRI −0.006; $p = 0.56$) or the entire cohort (NRI 0.036; $p = 0.06$).

According to Wong et al., median TAG_{320} in FFR-significant vessels was significantly lower when compared with nonsignificant vessels (−19 [−26 to −13] vs. −10 [−16 to −5] HU/cm, $p < 0.001$) [23].

Table 59.1 Diagnostic estimates of TAG, CCTA, and combination of TAG and CCTA according to studies

Authors (reference)	Number of patients	Number of vessels analyzed	CT scanner	TAG cutoff (HU/cm)	Reference standard (threshold value)	Sensitivity (%)	Specificity (%)	Positive predictive value (%)	Negative predictive value (%)	Diagnostic accuracy (%)	AUC
Choi et al. [12]	126	370	64-slice	−1.8	CAG	92.6 84.0 *59*	69.1 89.7 *94*	85.3 94.0 *83*	82.9 74.3 *82*		0.860[a] 0.932[a] *0.951*[a]
Zheng et al. [24]	107	309	128-slice DS	−11.33	CAG	73.4 94.7 *94.0*	92.1 77.7 *93.8*	89.3 83.9 *90.2*	79.6 92.3 *96.3*		0.827 0.924 *0.983*
Choi et al. [26]	63	97	64-slice DS or 64-slice SS	−6.54	FFR (0.80)	47.5 92.5 *90*	91.2 52.6 *63.2*	79.2 57.8 *63.2*	71.2 90.9 *90.0*	73.2 69.0 *74.2*	0.696[a] 0.726[a] *0.809*[a]
Yoon et al. [6]	62	82	64-slice DS or 64-slice SS	−6.54	FFR (0.80)	37.5 71.9[b]	88.0 68.0[b]	66.7 59.0[b]	68.8 79.1[b]		0.63 0.73[b]
Wang et al. [28]	32	32	64-slice DS or 128-slice DS	−15.1	FFR (0.80)	37 100	58 54	23 42	73 100		0.67
Nakanishi et al. [27]	103	146	64-slice or higher	−6.54	FFR (0.80)	63.5 84.6	28.7 39.4	33.0 43.6	58.7 82.2	41.1 55.5	0.54 0.62 *0.64*
Hell et al. [22]	59	72	128-slice DS	−6.5	FFR (0.8)	57	61	28	31		0.56 0.61
Stuijfzand et al. [25]	85	253	256-slice	−7.51	FFR (0.80)	69 95 *95*	44 75 *76*	83 98 *98*	27 54 *54*		NA 0.85 *0.87*
Wong et al. [23]	75	97	320-slice	−15.1	FFR (0.80)	71 89 *73*	77 65 *97*	63 57 *92*	83 92 *87*		NA 0.77[a] *0.84*[a]
Ko et al. [13]	51	82	320-slice	−15.37	FFR (0.80)	58.3 79.2 *45.8*	86.2 58.6 *98.3*	63.6 44.2 *91.7*	83.3 87.2 *81.4*		0.72 0.69 *0.72*
Ko et al. [29]	27	51	320-slice	−15.1 (rest)	FFR (0.80)	76.5 76.5 *58.8*	85.3 55.9 *94.1*	72.2 46.4 *83.3*	87.9 82.6 *82.1*	82.4 62.7 *82.4*	0.78 0.66 *0.76*
Ko et al. [29]	27	35	320-slice	−10 (stress)	FFR (0.80)	75 *50*	61 *78*	50 *55*	82 *75*	65.7 *68.6*	0.75 *0.64*

Numbers in the second lines represent diagnostic values with CCTA for diameter stenosis >50%. Numbers in italic represent diagnostic values with combination of CCTA and TAG. All results were analyzed on a per-vessel basis

Abbreviations: *AUC* area under curve, *CAG* invasive coronary angiography, *CCTA* coronary CT angiography, *DS* dual source, *HU* Hounsfield unit, *FFR* fractional flow reserve, *NA* not assessed, *SS* single source, *TAG* transluminal attenuation gradient

[a]C-statistic

[b]CCTA stenosis >70%

In a study by Zheng et al., the impact of plaque composition, Agatston scores, and lesion length ratio on TAG was analyzed in 107 patients [24]. TAG decreased progressively as ICA-determined stenosis severity increased, from −6.10 ± 6.97 HU/cm for stenosis <50% to −20.45 ± 13.69 HU/cm for stenosis of 70–99% ($p = 0.002$). This tendency was similar in calcified vessels. In calcified lesions, TAG decreased progressively as Agatston scores increased, from −13.93 ± 14.84 HU/cm for scores <100 to −28.64 ± 18.26 HU/cm for scores >300 ($p = 0.000$). Notably, there was no significant difference in TAG between scores <100 and scores between 100 and 300 (−13.93 ± 14.84 vs. −17.25 ± 13.91, $p = 0.198$). TAG improved the diagnostic accuracy of CCTA (c-statistic =0.982 vs. 0.942, $p = 0.0001$)

in calcified lesions. In calcified vessels, CCTA showed moderate sensitivity [70%; 95% CI =57–82%] and low specificity (66%; 95% CI =54–76%), while TAG showed moderate sensitivity (72%; 95% CI =64–79%) and high specificity (91%; 95% CI =86–95%). The addition of TAG to CCTA markedly improved the diagnostic performance of CCTA for calcified lesions and resulted in increased sensitivity (84%; 95% CI = 72–92%) and specificity (89%; 95% CI =77–96%) (Fig. 59.10). Adding TAG to CCTA resulted in a reclassification of stenosis severity in a large number of vessels with calcified lesions (NRI 0.093, net proportion of patients reclassified 5.31%; $p = 0.022$); however, the addition of TAG to CCTA did not result in significant stenosis severity reclassification among all vessels (NRI 0.009; $p = 0.09$). TAG also decreased as lesion length ratio (LLR) increased, from −10.90 ± 10.19 HU/cm for LLR <1/3 to −32.61 ± 16.64 HU/cm for LLR between 1/2 and 2/3 ($p = 0.000$). Interestingly, the TAG for LLR >2/3 was −14.51 ± 10.58 HU/cm, which was not lower than the cohort with LLR between 1/2 and 2/3.

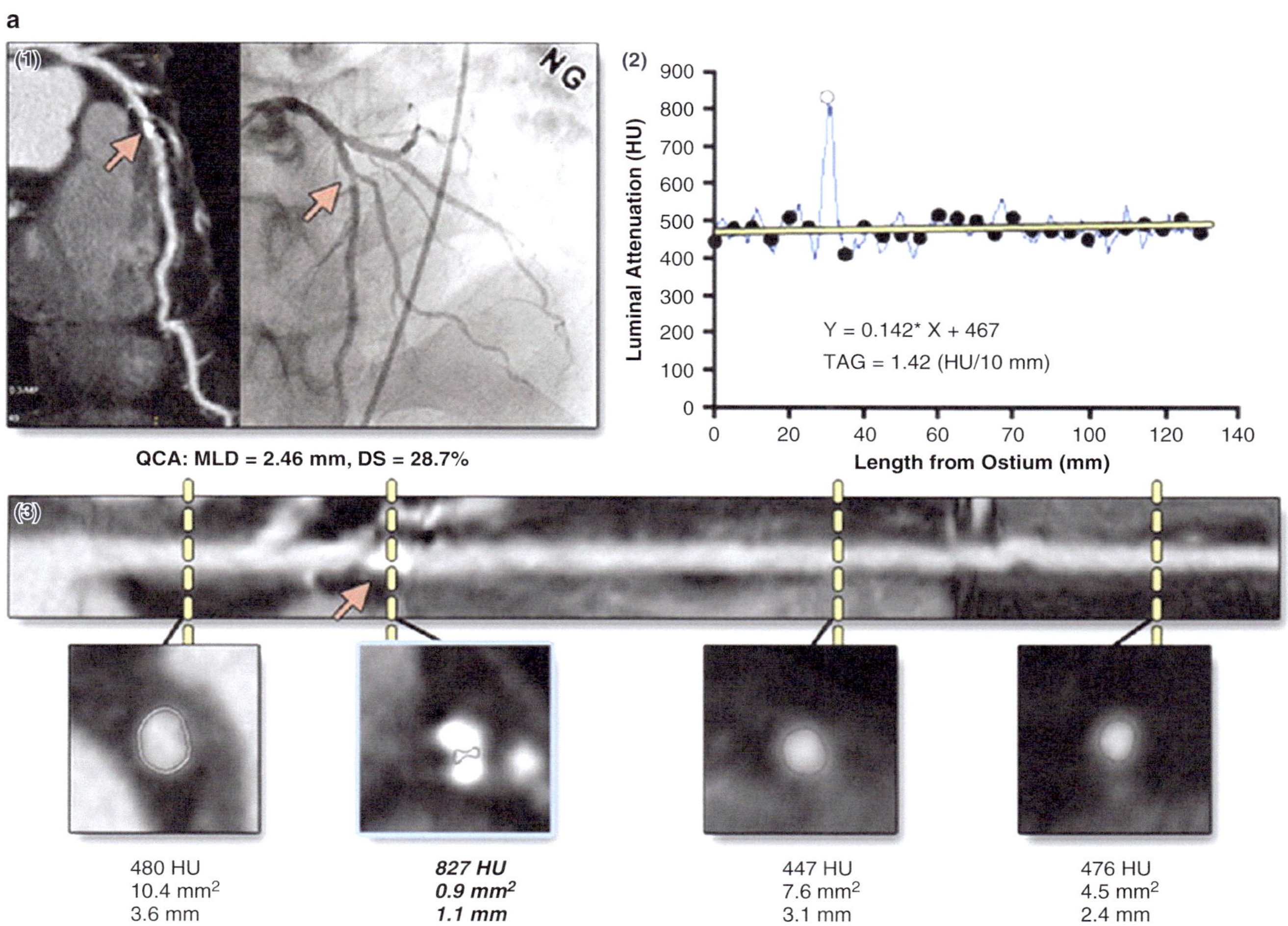

Fig. 59.9 Transluminal attenuation gradient measurement. (**a**) Calcified lesion in the mid-left anterior descending (LAD) artery that was indeterminate by CCTA, but diameter stenosis (DS) was 28.7% by quantitative coronary angiography (1). Red arrows indicate the most severe stenotic sites. Gray dots represent intervals that were excluded because of significant calcification or significant (DS 50%) stenosis (2). Cross-sectional views with gray border and sloped legend in italics represent excluded intervals. The intraluminal attenuation in the distal LAD artery does not decrease, demonstrating no significant obstruction. (**b**) CCTA demonstrates calcified lesions in the proximal LAD artery and moderate stenosis in the mid-LAD artery, confirmed by invasive coronary angiography (1). The linear correlation coefficient of black dots, TAG, is negatively sloped (−11.95 HU/cm) (2). Decrease of intraluminal attenuation in the distal vessel is shown (3). (From Choi et al. [12], with permission)

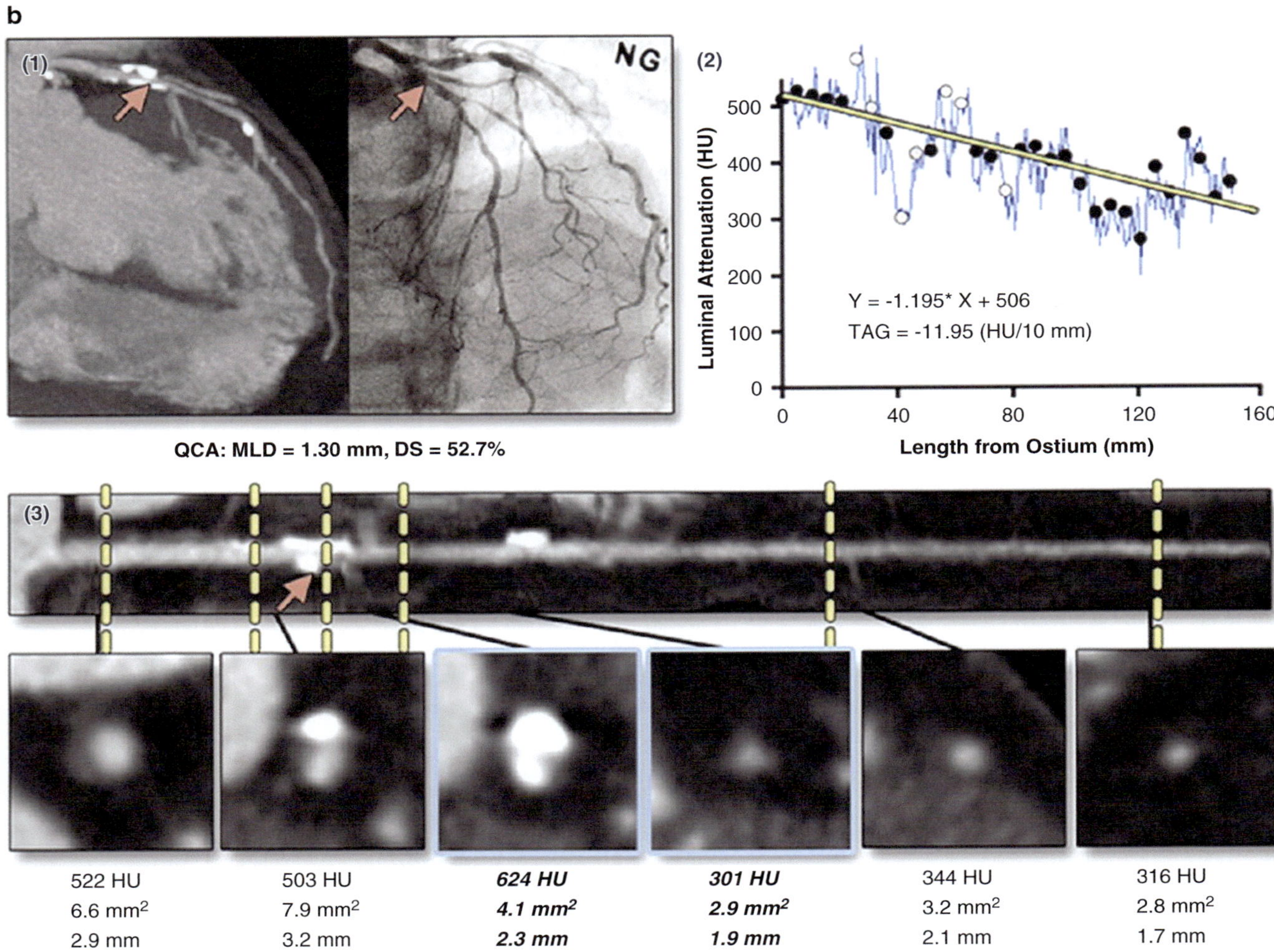

Fig. 59.9 (continued)

Comparison of TAG and CCO

In a study by Stuijfzand et al., TAG did not provide incremental diagnostic value over 256-slice coronary CTA alone for assessing the hemodynamic significance of a coronary stenosis. Step-and-shoot 256-slice CCTA was used to evaluate TAG, TAG-CCO (relating coronary density to corresponding descending aortic opacification), and TAG-ExC (excluding calcified coronary segments) analyses in 85 patients [25]. TAG and TAG-ExC did not discriminate between vessels with or without hemodynamically significant lesions with FFR values >0.8 or ≤0.8 (−13.5 ± 17.1 HU/cm vs. −11.6 ± 13.3 HU/cm, $p = 0.36$; and −13.1 ± 15.9 HU/cm vs. −11.4 ± 11.7 HU/cm, $p = 0.77$, respectively). TAG-CCO was significantly lower in vessels with a hemodynamically significant lesion (−0.050 ± 0.051/cm vs. −0.036 ± 0.034/cm, $p = 0.03$), and TAG-ExC resulted in a slight improvement of NRI (0.021, $p < 0.05$). However, TAG-CCO was no longer significantly lower when subgroup analysis was performed for vessels with a diameter stenosis ≥50% on CCTA ($n = 104$, $p = 0.07$).

Choi et al. compared TAG and CCO of CCTA with invasively measured FFR in 63 patients [26]. The overall diagnostic performance of TAG and CCO was similar and moderate on a per-vessel basis (c-statistic = 0.696 vs. 0.637, $p = 0.29$). The sensitivity, specificity, and positive and negative predictive values of TAG using a cutoff ≤−6.54 HU/cm for FFR < 0.80 were 47.5, 91.2, 79.2, and 71.2%. Using CCO and a cutoff >0.063 provided sensitivity, specificity, and positive and negative predictive values of 65.0, 61.4, 54.2, and 71.4%, respectively. TAG demonstrated incremental value to the diagnostic performance of CCTA alone; however, the added value was not observed for CCO (c-statistic = 0.726 vs. 0.809, $p = 0.025$; c-statistic = 0.726 vs. 0.784, $p = 0.09$). In NRI analysis, the addition of TAG to CCTA did not result in significant reclassification (NRI = 1.0%, $p = 0.41$), while the addition of CCO to CCTA resulted in negative reclassification (NRI = −9.3%, $p = 0.036$).

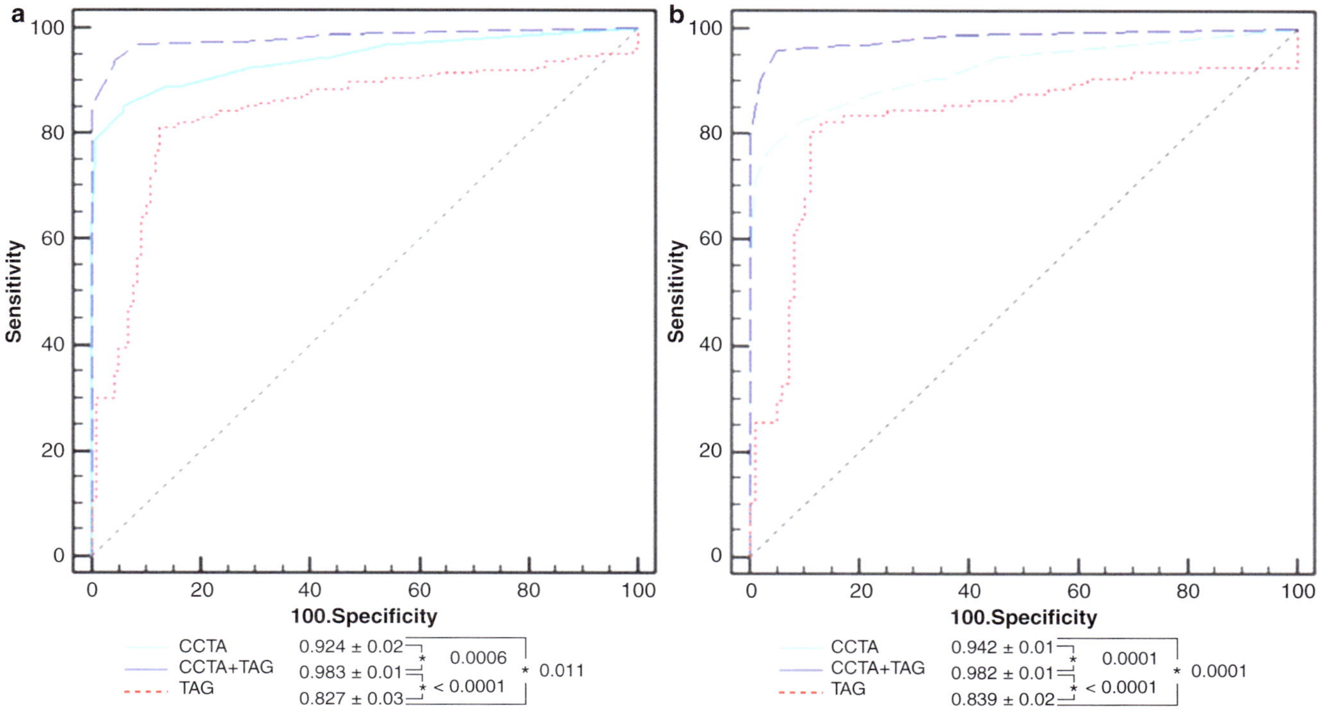

Fig. 59.10 Predicted probability of TAG in addition to CCTA stenosis severity. (**a**) Predicted probability of TAG in addition to CCTA stenosis severity in total relevant vessels on a reference of results from CAG. (**b**) Predicted probability of TAG in calcified vessels in addition to CCTA stenosis severity on a reference of results from CAG. Area under the ROC curve is shown as mean ± SD. TAG transluminal attenuation gradient, CAG coronary angiography, CCTA coronary computed tomography angiography. (From Zheng et al. [24], with permission)

Comparison of CT-FFR and TAG

Noninvasive FFR computed from CCTA provides a better diagnostic performance for the diagnosis of lesion-specific ischemia compared to CCTA stenosis and TAG [6, 13, 27].

Ko et al. compared the diagnostic performance of 320-detector row CCTA-derived computed FFR (FFR_{CT}), TAG (TAG_{320}), and CCTA alone to diagnose hemodynamically significant stenosis as determined by invasive FFR [13]. The median TAG_{320} was significantly lower in vessels with hemodynamically significant stenoses compared to vessels without significant stenosis, −17.2 HU/cm (IQR, −20.0 to −6.40) versus −8.86 HU/cm (IQR, −13.2 to −3.83) ($p = 0.002$). By using TAG_{320}, a modest yet statistically significant correlation with invasive FFR was demonstrated (Spearman $\rho = 0.47$; $p < 0.001$). FFR_{CT} demonstrated a strong and statistically significant correlation with invasive FFR (Spearman $\rho = 0.78$; $p < 0.001$). The ROC curve analysis for TAG_{320} demonstrated an AUC of 0.72 ($p = 0.002$), which was not found to be superior to the AUC of CCTA (0.72 vs. 0.68; $p = 0.67$) (Fig. 59.11). NRI for TAG_{320} when compared with CCTA was 0.89 ± 0.24 (standard error; $p < 0.001$). There was a slight difference in AUC when CCTA with TAG was compared with CCTA alone (0.72 vs 0.69; $p = 0.59$). By using a FFR_{CT} threshold ≤0.80, FFR_{CT} demonstrated an AUC of 0.93 ($p < 0.001$), which was significantly superior to both CCTA ($p = 0.008$) and TAG_{320} ($p = 0.003$).

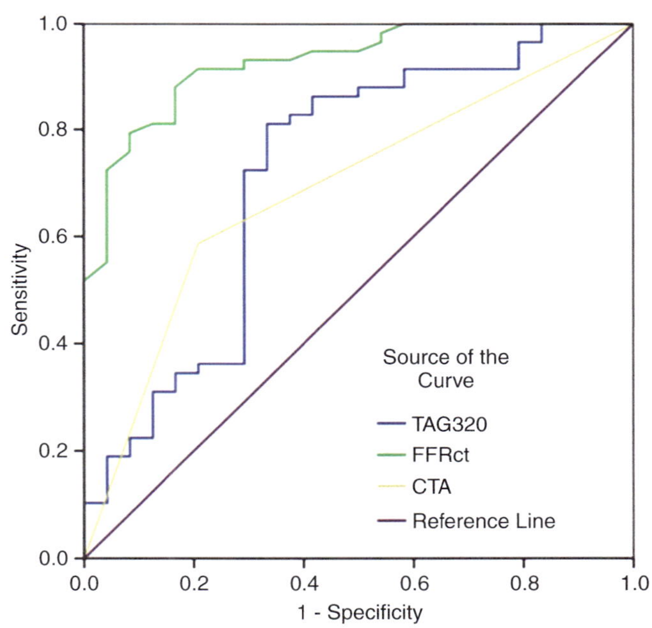

Fig. 59.11 Areas under the ROC curve (AUC) of CT angiography (*CTA*), TAG320, and FFRCT, with a reference line for comparison. (From Ko et al. [13], with permission)

Overall per-vessel accuracy, sensitivity, specificity, and positive and negative predictive values for TAG_{320} (<−15.37) were 78%, 58%, 86%, 64%, and 83%, respectively; the same values for FFR_{CT} were 83%, 92%, 79%, 65%, and 96%, respectively. NRI for FFR_{CT} compared with CCTA was 1.42 ± 0.24 ($p < 0.001$).

According to Nakanishi et al., FFR_{CT} allowed for the identification of lesion-specific ischemia with greater diagnostic accuracy than TAG, CCTA, or the combination of the two with invasive FFR used as the reference standard. In 103 patients with suspected or known CAD, the sensitivity, specificity, positive predictive value, and negative predictive value were 53.8, 45.7, 35.4, and 64.2% for TAG; 84.6, 39.4, 43.6, and 82.2% for CCTA; and 82.7, 74.5, 64.2, and 88.6% for FFR_{CT}, respectively [27]. On a per-patient basis, the AUC by ROC curve analysis for FFR_{CT} (0.77) demonstrated greater performance for predicting hemodynamically significant ischemia compared to the AUC of obstructive stenosis on CCTA (0.55, $p < 0.0001$ vs. FFR_{CT}) and TAG + CCTA. AUCs for TAG analyses with varying thresholds were as follows: ≤−11/cm (0.52, $p = 0.0001$ vs. FFR_{CT}), ≤−6.54/cm (0.56, $p = 0.0006$ vs. FFR_{CT}), and ≤−15.1/cm (0.54, $p < 0.0001$ vs. FFR_{CT}) (Fig. 59.12). Compared to CCTA alone (AUC, 0.62), the combination of TAG and

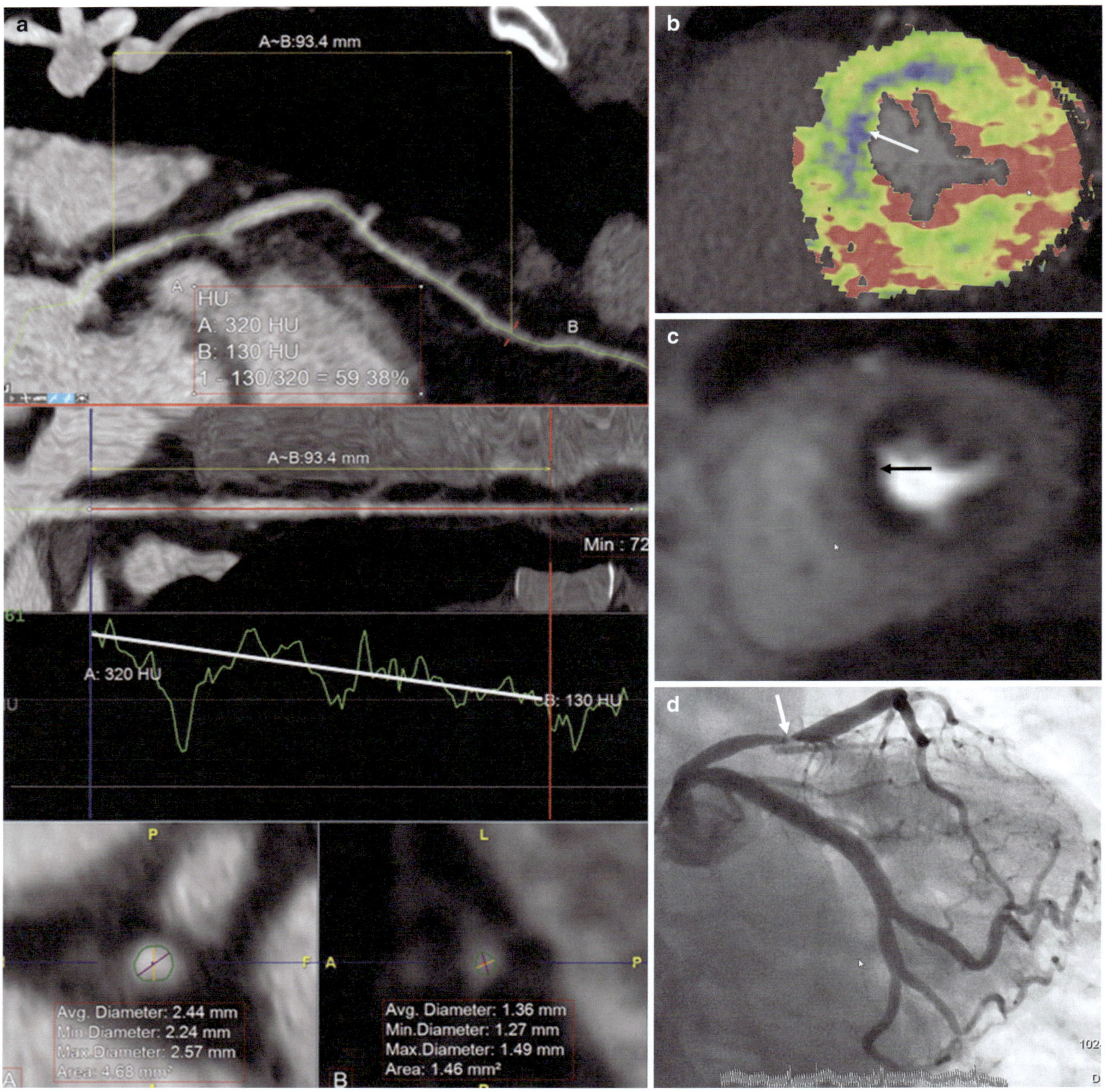

Fig. 59.12 Integration of CCTA, TAG, and stress CT perfusion imaging. (**a**) TAG measures −20.3 HU/cm. (**b**) Adenosine-stress CT perfusion imaging shows a perfusion defect (arrow) in the anteroseptal wall. (**c**) Adenosine-stress MRI confirms the presence of myocardial ischemia as a perfusion defect (arrow). (**d**) Invasive coronary angiography shows severe stenosis in the proximal LAD branch with FFR = 0.48

CCTA did not significantly improve the diagnostic value (AUC, 0.63 for ≤−11/cm, $p = 0.76$; AUC, 0.64 for ≤−6.54/cm, $p = 0.43$; AUC, 0.64 for ≤−15.1/cm, $p = 0.36$).

According to Wang et al., TAG with an AUC of 0.67 ($p = 0.152$) was unable to discriminate between vessels with or without hemodynamically significant lesions [28]. The authors calculated lesion length/minimal luminal diameter^4 (LL/MLD^4), TAG, CCO, and CT-FFR in 32 patients. A Poiseuille-based index (LL/MLD^4) was calculated as the LL divided by the 4th power of the minimal luminal diameter (MLD^4). A ratio of LL/MLD^4 > 3.86 was used to define a hemodynamically significant coronary stenosis. Compared to invasive FFR, the per-vessel sensitivity and specificity of CCTA, CT-FFR, LL/MLD^4, CCO, and TAG (≤−15.1 HU/cm) for detecting hemodynamically significant lesions were 100% and 54%, 100% and 91%, 85% and 92%, 66% and 88%, and 37% and 58%, respectively. ROC analysis resulted in an AUC of 0.91 for CT-FFR ($p = 0.0005$), 0.88 for LL/MLD^4 ($p < 0.0001$), and 0.85 for CCO ($p < 0.0001$). CT-FFR, LL/MLD^4, and CCO provided enhanced diagnostic performance over CCTA analysis alone for the discrimination of hemodynamically significant coronary stenosis.

According to Yoon et al. [6], the TAG was significantly lower in vessels with ischemia (−5.8 ± 8.0 HU/cm) compared to vessels without ischemia (−2.3 ± 4.8 HU/cm, $p = 0.029$). ROC curve analysis for TAG showed an AUC of 0.63 ($p = 0.037$) with an optimal cutoff value of ≤−6.54 HU/cm. The sensitivity, specificity, PPV, NPV, positive likelihood ratio, and negative likelihood ratio of TAG ≤−6.54 HU/cm were 37.5% (21.7–56.3%), 88.0% (75.0–95.3%), 66.7% (41.2–85.6%), 68.8% (55.8–79.4%), 3.13 (1.30–7.49), and 0.71 (0.54–0.93), respectively (Fig. 59.12). The ROC curve analysis for FFR_{CT} demonstrated an AUC of 0.94 ($p < 0.001$) with an optimal cutoff value of ≤0.77. The sensitivity, specificity, PPV, NPV, positive likelihood ratio, and negative likelihood ratio of FFR_{CT} ≤ 0.77 were 81.3% (63.0–92.1%), 94.0% (82.5–98.4%), 89.7% (71.5–97.3%), 88.7% (76.3–95.3%), 13.54 (4.46–41.08), and 0.20 (0.10–0.41), respectively. In all vessels, the AUC for FFR_{CT} (0.94) was significantly greater than CCTA (0.73, $p < 0.001$) and TAG (0.63, $p < 0.001$). In a subgroup with noncalcified or partially calcified plaque ($n = 58$), the AUC for FFR_{CT} (0.94) was greater compared to TAG (0.63, $p < 0.001$) and CCTA (0.70, $p < 0.001$). In a subgroup with calcified plaque ($n = 24$), the AUC for FFR_{CT} (0.92) was not significantly different from the AUC for TAG (0.75, $p = 0.168$) and CCTA (0.80, $p = 0.195$).

Comparison of TAG with CT Perfusion

Wong et al. compared the diagnostic accuracy of combined CT perfusion (CTP) + CCTA, TAG by 320-detector row CT (TAG_{320}, cutoff value of −15.1 HU/cm) + CCTA, and CTP + TAG_{320} + CCTA (CT-integrated protocol [MDCT-IP]) assessment in predicting significant FFR (Fig. 59.12) [23]. The MDCT-IP approach resulted in a marked increase in sensitivity and a mild decrease in specificity compared with CCTA + CTP and CCTA + TAG_{320}. Functionally significant coronary stenosis was defined as FFR ≤ 0.8. The cohort included 75 patients (age 64.1 ± 10.8 years, 52 men) and 44 (35%) FFR-significant vessels. In 127 vessels, CCTA predicted FFR-significant stenosis with 89% sensitivity and 65% specificity compared with MDCT-IP, which showed 88% sensitivity and 83% specificity. Using the generalized estimating equation, the predictive values of CTP + CCTA ($p = 0.003$) and TAG_{320} + CCTA ($p = 0.002$) were comparable. The c-statistics for the combined assessment of CTP + CCTA (0.845) and TAG_{320} + CCTA (0.844) were also comparable ($p = 0.98$). The c-statistic for MDCT-IP was 0.905. The diagnostic accuracy of MDCT-IP (AUC = 0.91) was superior to both TAG_{320} + CCTA and CTP + CCTA ($p = 0.01$). There was an incremental value of adding CTP and TAG_{320} to CCTA assessment (MDCT-IP) for the detection of significant FFR for NRI (1.46, $p < 0.0001$) and the integrated discrimination improvement index (IDI) (0.26, $p < 0.0001$). In addition, MDCT-IP also had incremental value over TAG_{320} + CCTA assessment for NRI (0.93, $p < 0.0001$) and IDI (0.12, $p < 0.0001$). MDCT-IP also had incremental value over CTP + CCTA assessment for NRI (1.45, $p < 0.0001$) and IDI (0.10, $p < 0.0001$).

Rest and Stress TAG

Ko et al. compared TAG values (TAG_{320}) during rest and vasodilator stress conditions on a 320-slice scanner [29]. Stress TAG_{320} was not interpretable in 16 vessels (31.4%). ROC analysis showed a comparable AUC for rest/stress TAG_{320} (0.78 and 0.75), which was higher than CCTA alone (0.68) and rest/stress contrast opacification (CO) difference (0.76 and 0.67). There was incremental predictive value when rest TAG_{320} was added to CCTA assessment based on the IDI (0.33, $p < 0.0001$) and NRI (1.24, $p < 0.0001$). There was incremental predictive value when stress TAG_{320} was added to CCTA assessment based on NRI (0.72, $p = 0.04$). The mean rest CO difference using a threshold of 55 HU predicted FFR ≤ 0.80 with a sensitivity, specificity, PPV, and NPV of 82%, 44%, 42%, and 83%, respectively. The corresponding values for mean stress CO difference using a threshold of 62 HU were 75%, 65%, 53%, and 83%. The ROC AUC for mean rest/stress CO difference was 0.76 (95% CI 0.60–0.93) and 0.67 (95% CI 0.48–0.86), respectively, which were not significantly different ($p = 0.37$).

Reverse Attenuation Sign and TAG in Patients with Chronic Total Occlusion, Stent, and Myocardial Bridging

The reverse attenuation gradient (RAG) sign is defined as a reverse intraluminal opacification gradient of vessels distal to occlusive lesions (Fig. 59.13). Therefore, the RAG sign represents the retrograde collateral flow distal to an occlusive

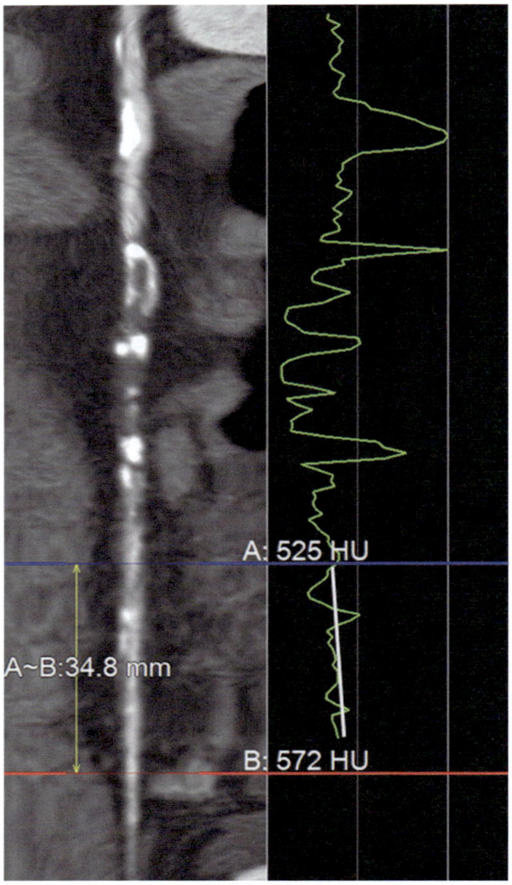

Fig. 59.13 Reverse attenuation sign and TAG in a patient with chronic total occlusion of RCA. The degree of attenuation in the more distal segment is higher than that of the more proximal segment and TAG in this segment distal to occlusion measures 13.4 HU/cm

lesion. This sign seems to be useful for the detection of chronic total occlusion (CTO) and helps differentiate CTO from subtotal occlusion (STO). In a study by Li et al., the CTO group had the RAG sign significantly more frequently than the STO group (65% [32/49] vs. 7% [3/45]; $p < 0.001$) [30]. Similarly, a significant difference in measurements of the attenuation gradient (5.1 HU/cm ± 13.4 vs. –13.4 HU/cm ± 8.7; $p < 0.001$) and lesion length (23.6 mm ± 22.7 vs. 6 mm ± 3; $p < 0.001$) was noted between the groups. All segments with RAG at CCTA were shown by means of ICA to be supplied by retrograde collateral vessels. When a combination of all those parameters was used for the diagnosis of CTO, sensitivity and specificity were 90% (44/49) and 93% (42/45), respectively.

According to Li et al. [31], RAG sign was present in 59.3% (35/59) of all stent occlusions. Superior diagnostic performance was confirmed by ROC analysis with an AUC of 0.898 when a combination of the traditional diagnosing criterion and RAG sign was employed.

According to Choi et al., coronary arteries with CTO showed longer occlusion length (cutoff ≥15 mm), higher distal TAG (cutoff ≥ −0.9 HU/cm), more frequent side branches, blunted stump, cross-sectional calcification ≥50%, and collateral vessels compared with coronaries with STO ($p < 0.001$, all) [32]. The combination of these findings could distinguish CTO from STO (c-statistics = 0.88 [95% confidence interval 0.94–0.90], sensitivity 83%, specificity 77%, positive predictive value 55%, negative predictive value 93%; $p < 0.001$). TAG from the ostium to the distal vessel (TAG_{all}) [CTO −11.0 (−19.3 to −4.5) HU/cm vs. STO −12.9 (−21.6 to −6.9) HU/cm; $p = 0.006$] and TAG distal to the occlusion (TAG_{distal}) [CTO −0.1 (−3.2 to −2.2) HU/cm vs. STO −3.0 (−4.7 to −1.1) HU/cm; $p < 0.001$] were higher in CTO versus STO. However, according to Zheng et al., the TAG (−17.96 ± 20.36 HU/cm) for CTO was not significantly lower than TAG for stenosis between 70% and 99% (−20.45 ± 13.69 HU/cm) [24].

The degree of invasive coronary angiography-assessed systolic compression of myocardial bridging (MB) significantly correlates with TAG, but not MB depth or length [33]. In a study by Li et al., TAG was lowest (−17.4 ± 6.7 HU/cm) in patients with significant dynamic compression (systolic compression ≥50%) and highest in patients without MB compression (−9.5 ± 4.3 HU/cm, $p < 0.001$). Linear correlation revealed a moderate relationship between the percentage of systolic compression and TAG (Pearson correlation, $r = -0.52$; $p < 0.001$), but no significant relationship between the percentage of systolic compression and MB depth or length. ROC curve analysis determined the optimal cutoff value of TAG as −14.8HU/cm (area under curve = 0.813; 95% confidence interval = 0.764–0.855; $p < 0.001$), which yielded high diagnostic accuracy (82.1%, 248/302).

Summary and Conclusions

TAG depends on vessel diameter, vessel-specific branching patterns, luminal stenosis, scan timing, and cardiac output. The range of thresholds of TAG to predict lesion-specific ischemia has varied widely, ranging from −1.8 HU/cm (64-slice CT) to −15.1 HU/cm (320-slice CT). TAG in FFR-significant vessels may be significantly lower when compared with nonsignificant vessels, and TAG may improve diagnostic accuracy of CCTA in calcified lesions. TAG and RAG sign may be useful in the diagnosis of CTO and stent evaluation; however, TAG assessment is susceptible to the influence of calcification and artifact throughout the entire coronary artery course. Notably, the diagnostic utility of TAG remains uncertain in branched vessel disease. In vessels without significant calcification or artifact, the combination of TAG and CCTA may provide comparable diagnostic accuracy for functional assessment of coronary artery stenosis. Regarding the current literature, the clinical value of TAG and TAG-CCO is controversial and still requires validation; however, TAG-CCO may overcome the temporal difference in coronary attenuations among imaging slabs on multi-beat CT acquisitions. There is a significant correlation between TAG and TDG. CT-FFR provides superior diagnostic performance for the diagnosis of lesion-specific ischemia compared to CCTA stenosis and TAG in noncalcified lesions.

References

1. Dweck MR, Williams MC, Moss AJ, Newby DE, Fayad ZA. Computed tomography and cardiac magnetic resonance in ischemic heart disease. J Am Coll Cardiol. 2016;68:2201–16.
2. Kim YJ, Yong HS, Kim SM, Kim JA, Yang DH, Hong YJ. Korean guidelines for the appropriate use of cardiac CT. Korean J Radiol. 2015;16:251–85.
3. Min JH, Kim SM, Lee S, Choi JH, Chang SA, Choe YH. Diagnostic performance of algorithm for computer-assisted detection of significant coronary artery disease in patients with acute chest pain: comparison with invasive coronary angiography. AJR Am J Roentgenol. 2014;202:730–7.
4. Rief M, Kranz A, Hartmann L, Roehle R, Laule M, Dewey M. Computer-aided CT coronary artery stenosis detection: comparison with human reading and quantitative coronary angiography. Int J Cardiovasc Imaging. 2014;30:1621–7.
5. Koo HJ, Yang DH, Kim YH, Kang JW, Kang SJ, Kweon J, et al. CT-based myocardial ischemia evaluation: quantitative angiography, transluminal attenuation gradient, myocardial perfusion, and CT-derived fractional flow reserve. Int J Cardiovasc Imaging. 2016;32(Suppl 1):1–19.
6. Yoon YE, Choi JH, Kim JH, Park KW, Doh JH, Kim YJ, et al. Noninvasive diagnosis of ischemia-causing coronary stenosis using CT angiography: diagnostic value of transluminal attenuation gradient and fractional flow reserve computed from coronary CT angiography compared to invasively measured fractional flow reserve. JACC Cardiovasc Imaging. 2012;5:1088–96.
7. Yoon YE, Lim TH. Current roles and future applications of cardiac CT: risk stratification of coronary artery disease. Korean J Radiol. 2014;15:4–11.
8. Zhu X, Zhu Y, Xu H, Tang L, Xu Y. The influence of body mass index and gender on coronary arterial attenuation with fixed iodine load per body weight at dual-source CT coronary angiography. Acta Radiol. 2012;53:637–42.
9. Ofili EO, Kern MJ, Labovitz AJ, St Vrain JA, Segal J, Aguirre FV, et al. Analysis of coronary blood flow velocity dynamics in angiographically normal and stenosed arteries before and after endolumen enlargement by angioplasty. J Am Coll Cardiol. 1993;21:308–16.
10. Youn HJ, Foster E. Demonstration of coronary artery flow using transthoracic Doppler echocardiography. J Am Soc Echocardiogr. 2004;17:178–85.
11. Steigner ML, Mitsouras D, Whitmore AG, Otero HJ, Wang C, Buckley O, et al. Iodinated contrast opacification gradients in normal coronary arteries imaged with prospectively ECG-gated single heart beat 320-detector row computed tomography. Circ Cardiovasc Imaging. 2010;3:179–86.
12. Choi JH, Min JK, Labounty TM, Lin FY, Mendoza DD, Shin DH, et al. Intracoronary transluminal attenuation gradient in coronary CT angiography for determining coronary artery stenosis. JACC Cardiovasc Imaging. 2011;4:1149–57.
13. Ko BS, Wong DT, Norgaard BL, Leong DP, Cameron JD, Gaur S, et al. Diagnostic performance of transluminal attenuation gradient and noninvasive fractional flow reserve derived from 320-detector row CT angiography to diagnose hemodynamically significant coronary stenosis: an NXT substudy. Radiology. 2016;279:75–83.
14. Park EA, Lee W, Park SJ, Kim YK, Hwang HY. Influence of coronary artery diameter on intracoronary transluminal attenuation gradient during CT angiography. JACC Cardiovasc Imaging. 2016;9:1074–83.
15. Funama Y, Utsunomiya D, Oda S, Shimonobo T, Nakaura T, Mukunoki T, et al. Transluminal attenuation-gradient coronary CT angiography on a 320-MDCT volume scanner: effect of scan timing, coronary artery stenosis, and cardiac output using a contrast medium flow phantom. Phys Med. 2016;32(11):1415–21.
16. Krug KB, Bovenschulte H, Geissler HJ, Flesch M, Schneider T, Brackrogge D, et al. In-vivo measurements of coronary blood flow using 16-slice multidetector spiral computed tomography (MDCT) in a porcine model. Rofo. 2009;181:220–9.
17. Chow BJ, Kass M, Gagne O, Chen L, Yam Y, Dick A, et al. Can differences in corrected coronary opacification measured with computed tomography predict resting coronary artery flow? J Am Coll Cardiol. 2011;57:1280–8.
18. Chatzizisis YS, George E, Cai T, Fulwadhva UP, Kumamaru KK, Schultz K, et al. Accuracy and reproducibility of automated, standardized coronary transluminal attenuation gradient measurements. Int J Cardiovasc Imaging. 2014;30:1181–9.
19. Lackner K, Bovenschulte H, Stutzer H, Just T, Al-Hassani H, Krug B. In vitro measurements of flow using multislice computed tomography (MSCT). Int J Cardiovasc Imaging. 2011;27:795–804.
20. Bovenschulte H, Krug B, Schneider T, Schwabe H, Kabbasch C, Bangard C, et al. CT coronary angiography: coronary CT-flow quantification supplements morphological stenosis analysis. Eur J Radiol. 2013;82:608–16.
21. Lardo AC, Rahsepar AA, Seo JH, Eslami P, Korley F, Kishi S, et al. Estimating coronary blood flow using CT transluminal attenuation flow encoding: formulation, preclinical validation, and clinical feasibility. J Cardiovasc Comput Tomogr. 2015;9:559–566. e551.
22. Hell MM, Dey D, Marwan M, Achenbach S, Schmid J, Schuhbaeck A. Non-invasive prediction of hemodynamically significant coronary artery stenoses by contrast density difference in coronary CT angiography. Eur J Radiol. 2015;84:1502–8.
23. Wong DT, Ko BS, Cameron JD, Leong DP, Leung MC, Malaiapan Y, et al. Comparison of diagnostic accuracy of combined assessment using adenosine stress computed tomography perfusion + computed tomography angiography with transluminal attenuation gradient + computed tomography angiography against invasive fractional flow reserve. J Am Coll Cardiol. 2014;63:1904–12.
24. Zheng M, Wei M, Wen D, Zhao H, Liu Y, Li J, et al. Transluminal attenuation gradient in coronary computed tomography angiography for determining stenosis severity of calcified coronary artery: a primary study with dual-source CT. Eur Radiol. 2015;25:1219–28.
25. Stuijfzand WJ, Danad I, Raijmakers PG, Marcu CB, Heymans MW, van Kuijk CC, et al. Additional value of transluminal attenuation gradient in CT angiography to predict hemodynamic significance of coronary artery stenosis. JACC Cardiovasc Imaging. 2014;7:374–86.
26. Choi JH, Koo BK, Yoon YE, Min JK, Song YB, Hahn JY, et al. Diagnostic performance of intracoronary gradient-based methods by coronary computed tomography angiography for the evaluation of physiologically significant coronary artery stenoses: a validation study with fractional flow reserve. Eur Heart J Cardiovasc Imaging. 2012;13:1001–7.
27. Nakanishi R, Matsumoto S, Alani A, Li D, Kitslaar PH, Broersen A, et al. Diagnostic performance of transluminal attenuation gradient and fractional flow reserve by coronary computed tomographic

angiography (FFR(CT)) compared to invasive FFR: a sub-group analysis from the DISCOVER-FLOW and DeFACTO studies. Int J Cardiovasc Imaging. 2015;31:1251–9.

28. Wang R, Renker M, Schoepf UJ, Wichmann JL, Fuller SR, Rier JD, et al. Diagnostic value of quantitative stenosis predictors with coronary CT angiography compared to invasive fractional flow reserve. Eur J Radiol. 2015;84:1509–15.
29. Ko BS, Seneviratne S, Cameron JD, Gutman S, Crossett M, Munnur K, et al. Rest and stress transluminal attenuation gradient and contrast opacification difference for detection of hemodynamically significant stenoses in patients with suspected coronary artery disease. Int J Cardiovasc Imaging. 2016;32:1131–41.
30. Li M, Zhang J, Pan J, Lu Z. Obstructive coronary artery disease: reverse attenuation gradient sign at CT indicates distal retrograde flow--a useful sign for differentiating chronic total occlusion from subtotal occlusion. Radiology. 2013;266:766–72.
31. Li M, Zhang J, Zhang Q, Pan J, Lu Z, Wei M. Coronary stent occlusion: reverse attenuation gradient sign observed at computed tomography angiography improves diagnostic performance. Eur Radiol. 2015;25:568–74.
32. Choi JH, Kim EK, Kim SM, Kim H, Song YB, Hahn JY, et al. Noninvasive discrimination of coronary chronic total occlusion and subtotal occlusion by coronary computed tomography angiography. JACC Cardiovasc Interv. 2015;8:1143–53.
33. Li Y, Yu M, Zhang J, Li M, Lu Z, Wei M. Non-invasive imaging of myocardial bridge by coronary computed tomography angiography: the value of transluminal attenuation gradient to predict significant dynamic compression. Eur Radiol. 2017;27(5):1971–9.

60 CT Angiography-Derived Fractional Flow Reserve

Adriaan Coenen, Frank Gijsen, and Koen Nieman

Coronary CT angiography allows for noninvasive evaluation of the coronary anatomy and angiographic assessment of coronary artery disease. Limitations are the tendency to overestimate stenosis severity in comparison to invasive angiography and its inability to assess the hemodynamic severity of stenosis. Invasive fractional flow reserve (FFR) is widely regarded as the clinical reference for the hemodynamic evaluation and therapeutic management of coronary artery disease. Computational fluid dynamics (CFD) is a field of mathematics and fluid mechanics concerned with the simulation of fluid motion. CFD is applied in various industries, to model the interaction between flow and structures. In addition to various industries, CFD has been used to investigate blood flow in the human body and in the context of various pathophysiologies. With the spatial resolution provided by contemporary computed tomography, it has become possible to use computational fluid dynamics to simulate the spatial distribution of flow and pressure in the coronary arteries from anatomical information. CT angiography-derived fractional flow reserve (CT-FFR) is a new technique that allows for assessment of the hemodynamic significance of epicardial coronary artery disease from standard CT angiographic images.

Invasive FFR

Invasive measurement of the FFR has become the clinical reference to determine the hemodynamic significance of epicardial coronary artery disease. While the name suggests measurement of flow, FFR is in fact the pressure ratio over a stenotic lesion during hyperemia. The FFR procedure consists of placement of a wire that allows for the measurement of pressure across the lesion of interest. A vasodilator, often adenosine, is administrated directly into the coronary artery or intravenously to temporarily create a hyperemic state. Adenosine causes maximum vasodilation of the microvasculature and increases flow through the coronary arteries by a factor of 4–5. Blood pressure is measured simultaneously in the coronary artery and in the aorta through the guiding catheter. The FFR is a lesion-specific index calculated as the fraction between the pressure in the coronary artery and the aorta. In case of multiple lesions, a pullback pressure curve can be performed to assess the area of most severe hemodynamic obstruction. Several landmark trials have established the clinical value of FFR in the management of coronary artery disease. The DEFER trial demonstrated that in patients with an intermediate-grade stenosis and normal FFR value (>0.75), intervention can be deferred with comparable short- and long-term outcome. The landmark FAME trial randomized patients between revascularization guided by angiography and FFR and showed that the latter was associated with a lower adverse event rate (death, myocardial infarction, and revascularization). The use of FFR to assess hemodynamic severity of stable coronary artery disease is supported by European and American guidelines, particularly when the presence of myocardial ischemia has not been established by noninvasive tests [1, 2].

Principles

CFD is focused on the simulation of the flow of fluids. Computational fluid dynamics is applied in various areas of engineering and industrial design, for instance, the behavior of a flying aircraft or the blood flow interaction of mechanical heart valves or ventricular assist devices. For the purpose of CT-FFR, CFD is applied to the anatomy from a CTA scan to simulate coronary blood flow. This simulation allows for

A. Coenen
Departments of Radiology and Cardiology, Erasmus University Medical Center, Rotterdam, The Netherlands

F. Gijsen
Department of Biomedical Engineering, Erasmus University Medical Center, Rotterdam, The Netherlands

K. Nieman (✉)
Stanford University, School of Medicine, Cardiovascular Institute, Stanford, CA, USA
e-mail: knieman@stanford.edu

U. J. Schoepf (ed.), *CT of the Heart*, Contemporary Medical Imaging, https://doi.org/10.1007/978-1-60327-237-7_60

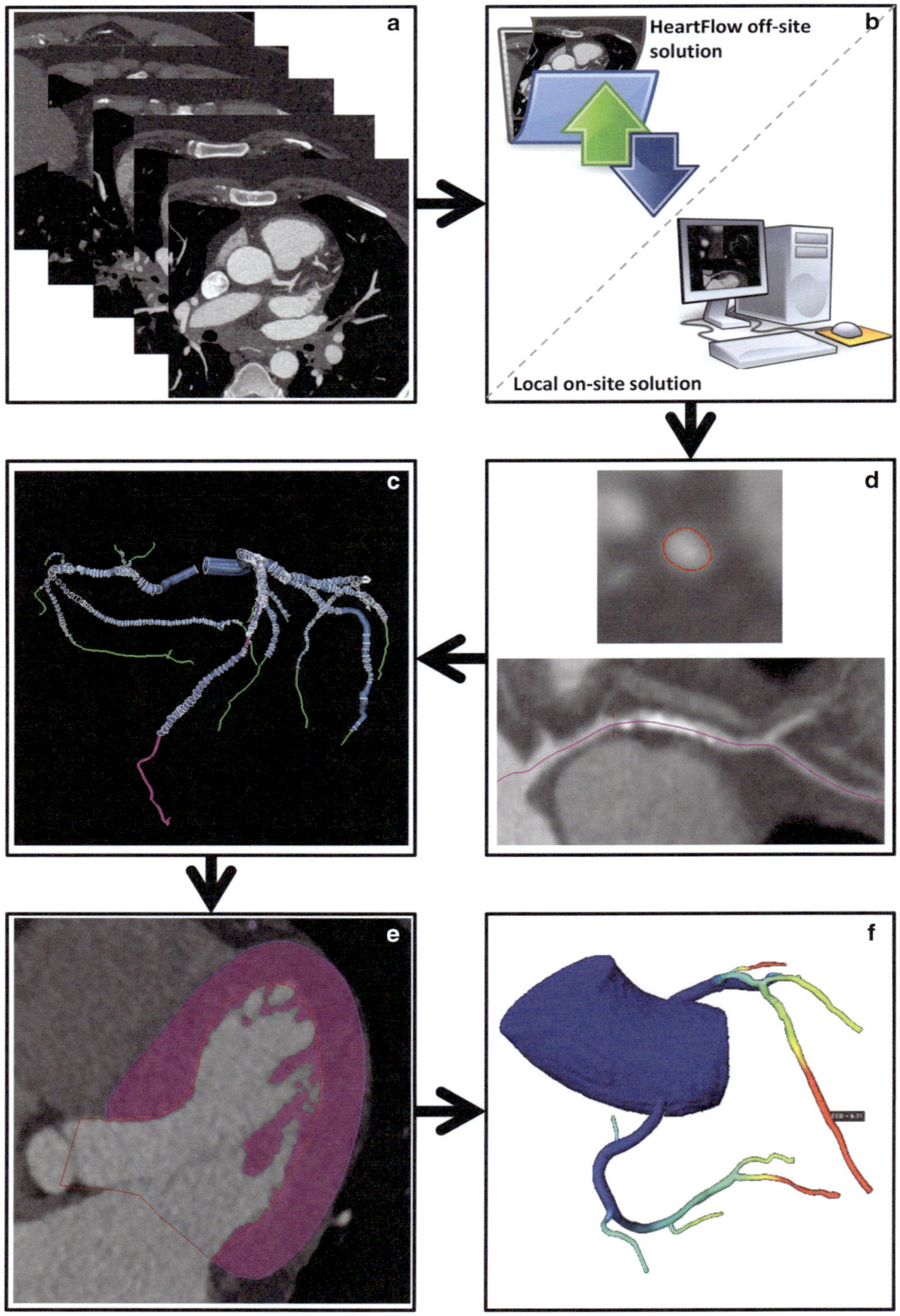

Fig. 60.1 Overview of the CT-FFR procedure. The CTA images are transferred to the central HeartFlow facilities or loaded onto a local CT-FFR application (panel **a** and **b**). From the CTA images, the coronary artery lumen contours are segmented (panel **c** and **d**). The left ventricular myocardium is segmented from the CTA (panel **e**). The resting total coronary blood flow is estimated based on the left ventricular myocardium volume (panel **e**). The microvascular resistance is reduced and a hyperemic state is simulated. The Navier-Stokes equations are solved either for a full 3D model in the HeartFlow solution or in a simplified model for the locally operated applications. The CT-FFR outcome is presented as a color-coded map (panel **f**)

computation of the flow, velocity, and pressure. Information needed to simulate flow are (1) 3D geometrical contours of the lumen of the artery; (2) the inflow and boundary conditions, for instance, pressure; and (3) characteristics of the fluid, for instance, blood viscosity. Several CT-FFR algorithms have been described in the public domain, all of which apply CFD in a slightly different manner. However, to compute the fractional flow reserve from a CT angiogram, most algorithms share a number of fundamental steps (Fig. 60.1) [3, 4].

Obtaining the Anatomical Structure

From the CT angiogram, the lumen of the entire coronary artery tree, to the extent the spatial resolution of the scan allows, needs to be segmented. While efforts are made to automate the coronary segmentation process, a substantial degree of manual correction is often still required. In the case of the algorithm by HeartFlow Inc., the segmentation, as well as other steps, is performed at the central facilities after transferring the CT data. The HeartFlow algorithm applies a subvoxel resolution technique to improve segmentation of the coronary arteries [5, 6]. Other algorithms require local operators and expertise to perform and/or correct the coronary segmentation, which can be a time-consuming process.

Estimation of the Global and Local Resting Flow

First, the total coronary flow is estimated from the total myocardial mass. Allometric scaling laws describe the relationship between the size of an organ and the required blood supply. The main work to determine the relationship between the resting coronary blood flow and the size of the heart was done by Choy et al. [7]. From the CTA the left ventricular myocardium can be segmented automatically, and based on this mass, the total resting coronary blood flow can be estimated [5, 8]. The total coronary blood flow is then distributed over the 3D coronary model. The pattern of distribution is determined by the diameter size of the coronary branches based on the principle that form (diameter) will follow function (flow demand).

Computation of the Coronary Blood Flow and Pressure

Simulated flow is governed by the Navier-Stokes equations, and computation of the coronary blood flow requires solving these equations throughout the 3D model. The Navier-Stokes equations describe the application of Newton's second law (force is determined by mass and acceleration) to fluid motion, combined with the conservation of mass. First the 3D model needs to be discretized, i.e., the model is divided into small volumetric elements. The size of the elements may be varied, using larger elements around constant flow patterns for improved efficiency, and smaller elements where flow alterations are expected. For each element in this volumetric mesh, or finite-element model, the Navier-Stokes equations need to be solved, as the outcome from one element is transferred to the adjacent elements. To do this for the 3D coronary mesh, an enormous number of computations need to be performed. To reduce the computational time, parallel supercomputers are being used [3]. While the HeartFlow algorithm is a full 3D computational flow simulation throughout the coronary artery tree, other applications incorporate simplifications to allow for on-site CT-FFR simulations on more or less regular workstations. These locally performed CT-FFR applications with simplified models reduce the computational intensity based on the principal that for computation of a pressure drop, it is not necessary to compute the entire flow field at each point in the coronary artery [8–10]. This approach does have limitations as, for example, shear stress computations are no longer possible.

Simulation of Hyperemia and CT-FFR Computation

The CTA was acquired in a resting state, while the FFR is normally measured during hyperemia. Wilson et al. investigated the effect of adenosine on the coronary circulation and demonstrated that adenosine reduces the microvascular resistance by a factor of 0.21–0.24 [11]. To simulate a state of hyperemia, the microvascular resistance of the coronary arteries is virtually reduced, mimicking the vasodilatory effect of adenosine. By performing the CFD simulation and computing the coronary blood flow and pressure during virtual hyperemia, an FFR value can be calculated by dividing the intracoronary pressure by the aortic pressure. Pressure and FFR values are calculated throughout the coronary artery tree and often displayed onto a three-dimensional coronary model using color coding.

CT-FFR Applications

Performance of CFD onto coronary CT images including the aortic root was developed by Charles Taylor and colleagues at Stanford University and later commercialized by HeartFlow Inc. (Redwood City, CA) [12]. HeartFlow offers CT-FFR as a remotely performed, full-service solution. The client transfers the CT images and clinical information to HeartFlow, where the complete workflow is performed. After the CFD computation is completed, currently within 24 h, the CT-FFR results are available by log-in into a secure HeartFlow environment (Figs. 60.2 and 60.3). Several alternative approaches to CT-FFR are under development. A CT-FFR solution was developed by Siemens (cFFR, Forchheim, Germany), which can be performed locally on a regular workstation (Fig. 60.4) [8]. Also Toshiba Medical Systems (Odawara, Japan) developed a CT-FFR algorithm that can be processed on a regular computer, which was recently evaluated in a clinical study [13]. Finally, Philips

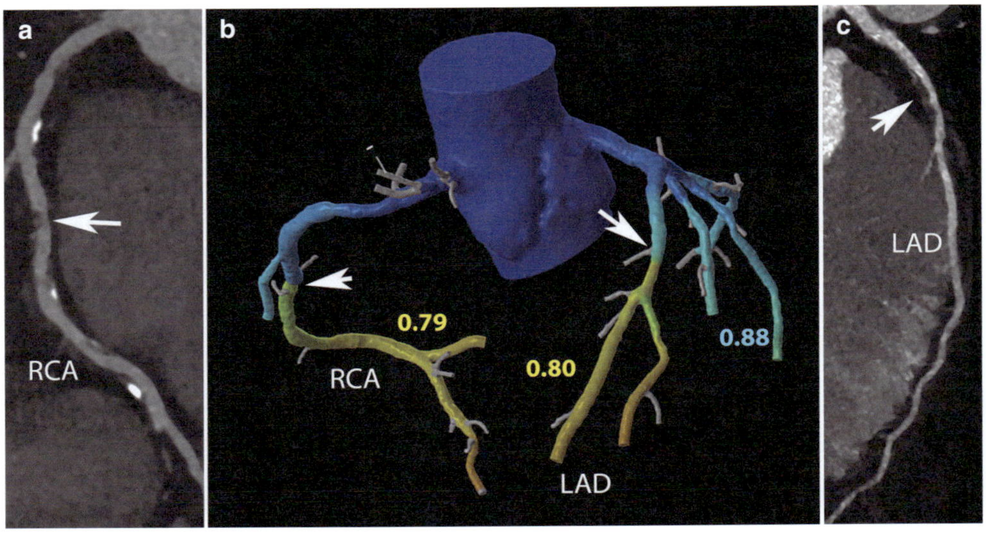

Fig. 60.2 Patient with extensive atherosclerosis and moderate stenosis (arrows) of the right (RCA, panel **a**) and left anterior descending coronary artery (LAD, panel **c**) by coronary CT angiography. CT-FFR (HeartFlow) shows a decrease in FFR toward the 0.80 threshold in both the LAD and RCA (panel **b**). In the absence of severe angina complaints, the patient was treated medically for the time being

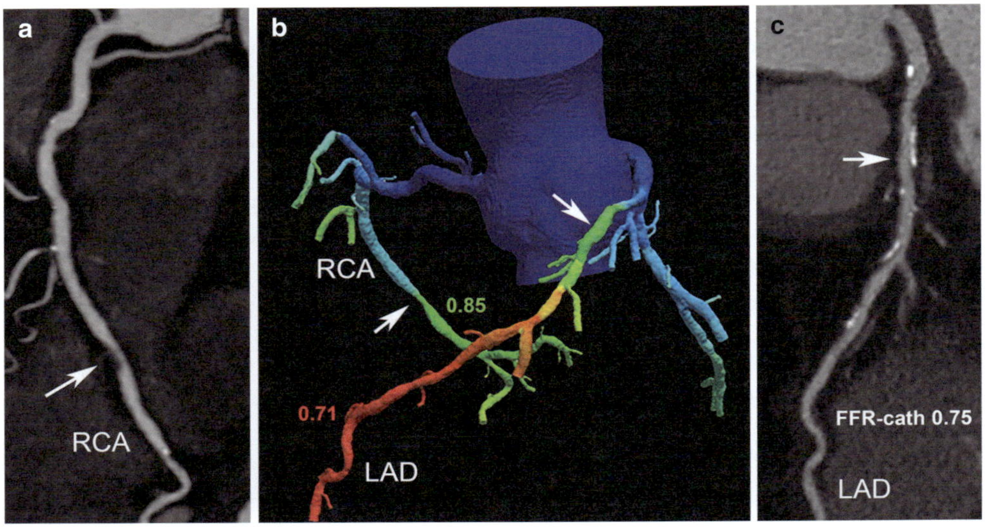

Fig. 60.3 Coronary CT angiography performed in a patient who underwent percutaneous coronary intervention of the left anterior descending coronary artery (LAD) with implantation of a bioresorbable scaffold (arrow, panel **b** and **c**) 5 years before (panel **b** and **c**). Although there is no single lesion causing more than 50% stenosis, diffuse atherosclerotic disease did result in an FFR of 0.71 by CT-FFR (panel **b**) and 0.75 by invasive FFR (panel **c**). A moderate stenosis (arrow) in the right coronary artery (RCA) did not cause a significant drop in CT-FFR (panel **a** and **b**)

Healthcare recently presented a workstation-based FFR model as well [14]. None of these on-site performed CT-FFR solutions have been commercially released yet.

Recently, a new approach for FFR computation, where machine-learning is used to predict the hemodynamic impact based on angiographic anatomy instead of performing individual CFD computation, was introduced. The machine-learning approach greatly reduces the computational intensity and allows for CT-FFR computations in mere seconds [15]. Clinical validation of a machine-learning-based application is currently being undertaken.

Validation of CT-Based Fractional Flow Reserve

The HeartFlow Application

The CT-FFR solution by HeartFlow has been extensively evaluated (Table 60.1) [12, 16, 17]. The most recent NXT trial demonstrated in a cohort of 251 patients that CT-FFR correlates well with invasive FFR, with a per-patient and per-vessel sensitivity of 86% and 84%, specificity of 79% and 86%, positive predictive value of 65% and 61%, negative predictive value of 93% and 95%, and accuracy of 81% and 86%, respectively. Restricted to lesions with an intermediate stenosis severity (30–70%), where CT-FFR is most likely to

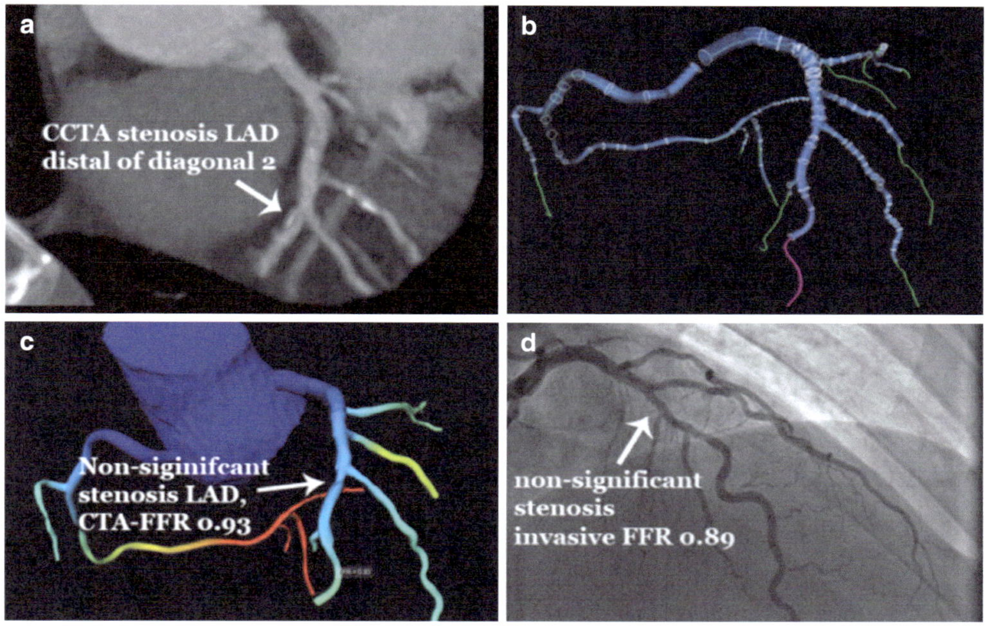

Fig. 60.4 Case example using the Siemens cFFR application. A 40-year-old man presented with exercise-related chest pain. In panel (**a**) multiplanar reformation of the CT angiogram shows moderate stenosis of the distal LAD just distal to the second diagonal branch. Panel (**b**) shows the 3D coronary model segmented from the CTA. The CT-FFR value was 0.93 indicating that the stenosis in the LAD is not flow limiting (panel **c**). Panel (**d**) displays the invasive coronary angiogram. Invasive FFR measurements confirmed the absence of a flow-limiting stenosis (FFR 0.89)

Table 60.1 Per-vessel performance of CT angiography-derived FFR versus invasive FFR

	Design	CT	Patient (vessel)	FFR ≤0.80	*R*	Sensitivity (CTA)	Specificity (CTA)	Accuracy (CTA)	AUC (CTA)
HeartFlow									
Discover-flow [12]	Multicenter prospective	64CT+	103 (159)	36%	0.72	88% (91%)	82% (40%)	84% (59%)	0.90 (0.75)
DEFACTO [16]	Multicenter prospective	64CT+	252 (407)	37%	0.63	80%	61%	69%	0.81 (0.68)
NXT [17]	Multicenter prospective	64CT+	251 (484)	21%	0.82	86% (83%)	84% (60%)	86% (65%)	0.93 (0.79)
Kawaji [45]	Single-center prospective	320CT	43 (70)	40%	NA	93%	52%	69%	0.87
Siemens									
Renker [20]	Single-center retrospective	DSCT	53 (67)	30%	0.66	85% (90%)	85% (34%)	–	0.92 (0.72)
Coenen [21]	Single-center retrospective	DSCT	106 (189)	42%	0.59	88% (81%)	65% (31%)	75% (56%)	0.83 (0.64)
Kruk [22]	Single-center retrospective	DSCT	90 (96)	43%	0.67	76% (100%)	72% (2%)	74% (44%)	0.84 (0.66)
Yang [25]	Single-center retrospective	DSCT	72 (138)	39%	0.67	87% (94%)	77% (66%)	81% (78%)	0.89 (0.85)
De Geer [24]	Single-center retrospective	DSCT	21 (23)	29%	0.77	83%	76%	78%	
Kurata [23]	Single-center retrospective	DSCT	21 (29)	48%	0.74	100%	87%	93%	
Toshiba									
Ko [13]	Single-center prospective	320CT	30 (58)	48%	0.57	78% (79%)	87% (74%)	84% (78%)	0.88 (0.77)

Diagnostic performance reported on a per-vessel basis using invasive fractional flow reserve as the reference. Number of analyzed patients and vessels with direct CT-FFR versus invasive FFR comparison. Sensitivity, specificity, and accuracy are on a per-vessel basis

FFR fractional flow reserve, *R* coefficient of correlation between CT-FFR and invasive FFR. Sensitivity, specificity, accuracy for CT-based FFR (and for CT angiography). *AUC* area under the receiver operator curve (and for CTA), *DSCT* first- and second-generation dual-source CT

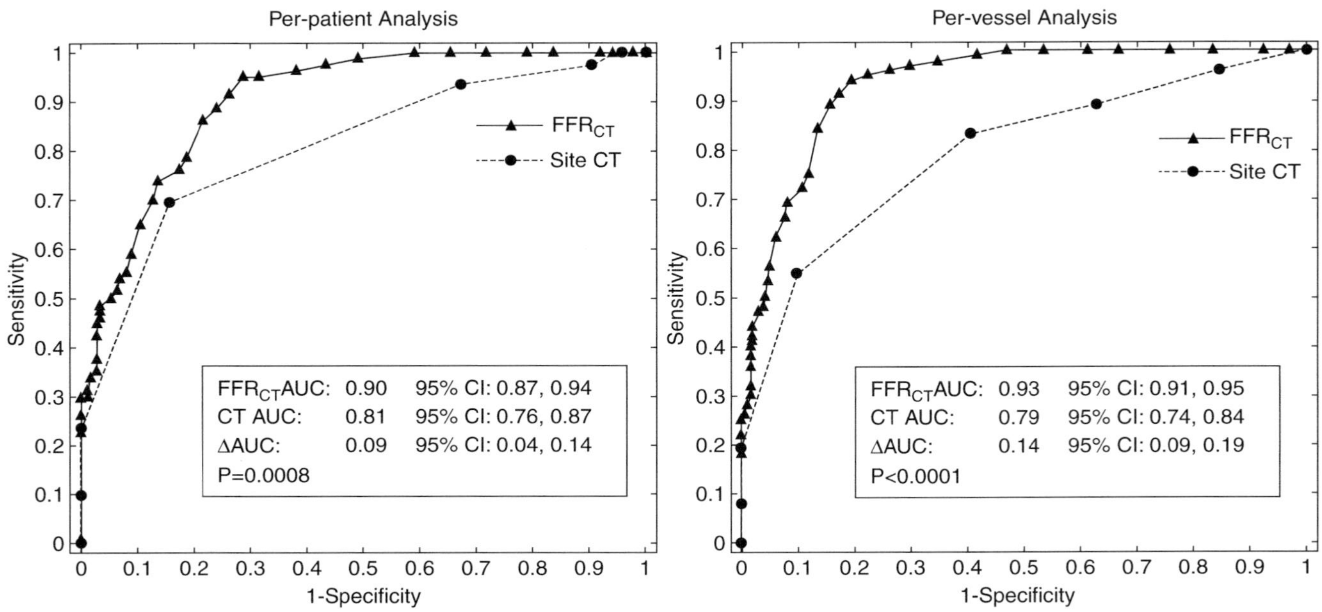

Fig. 60.5 Receiver operator curves from the NXT trial based on 251 patients, 484 vessels. In panel (**a**) the per-patient performance and in panel (**b**) the per-vessel performance. CT-FFR resulted in a significantly larger area under the curve (AUC) compared with CTA, both on a per-patient and on a per-vessel basis. (From Norgaard et al. [17], with permission)

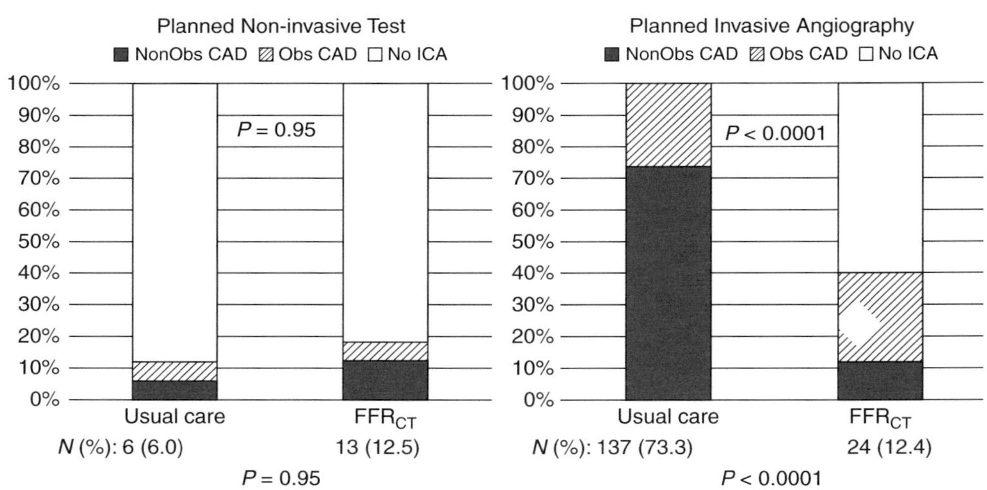

Fig. 60.6 Results from the platform trial, which evaluated the performance and diagnostic yield of invasive angiography, in patients either referred for noninvasive testing or invasive coronary angiography, in two consecutive cohorts of which the second underwent coronary CT angiography and CT-FFR in a proportion. Particularly in patients referred for invasive angiography, the use of CTA and CT-FFR reduced the number of performed catheterizations and increased the proportion of positive invasive angiograms. (From Douglas et al. [18], with permission)

be implemented, sensitivity (80%) and specificity (85%) remained good. The diagnostic performance of CT-FFR was superior to CTA alone (Table 60.1, Fig. 60.5) and allowed for correct reclassification of 68% of patients with false-positive CTA diagnoses [17]. The platform trial, which assessed the impact of CT-FFR on clinical management in consecutive cohorts, demonstrated that in patients referred for invasive angiography, the use of CTA with CT-FFR reduced the proportion of normal invasive angiograms and led to significant cost savings (Fig. 60.6) [18, 19]. The HeartFlow application has been approved and is available for clinical use in many parts of the world.

Workstation-Based CT-FFR Applications

The first generation of CT-FFR developed by Siemens was evaluated in a number of single-center studies [20–25]. These cohorts were mostly retrospective cohorts of patients with a clinical indication for invasive FFR, which may have increased the proportion of diffuse and/or intermediate severity angiographic disease (Fig. 60.7). Sensitivities in the range of 76–88% and specificities in the range of 65–85% were reported for CT-FFR, compared to relatively poor performances for CTA, in particularly specificity, in these challenging populations. Outside the borderline CT-FFR range of 0.75–0.85, the accuracy of CT-FFR can reach 95%, which allows for confident exclusion or confirmation of hemodynamic coronary disease without further need for testing [22]. The most recent CT-FFR solution by Siemens, which applies a morphological analysis to predict hemodynamical significance based on machine-learning, is under investigation in the multicenter machine study. The first, overall promising results using the CT-FFR application by Toshiba in a relatively small, but prospective cohort were recently reported [13]. Other techniques that use simplified models based on geometry data that can be extracted from CT are currently under development [26].

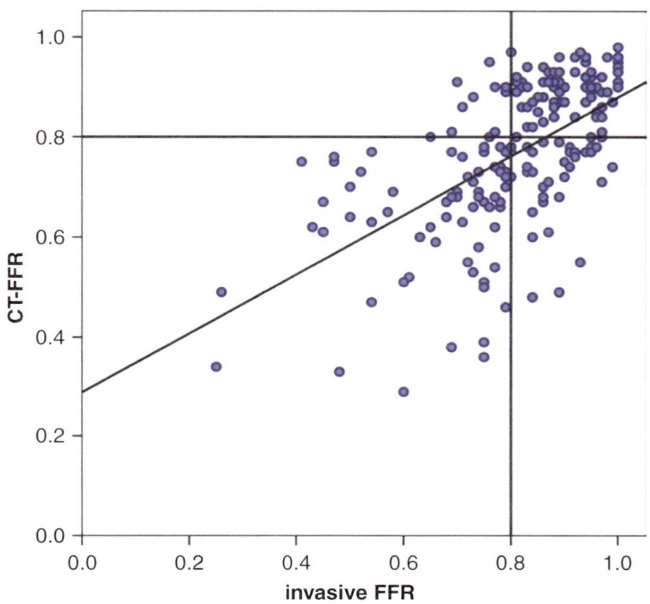

Fig. 60.7 Technical validation of an on-site performed CT-FFR application in a patient's cohort with clinically indicated coronary CT angiography and invasive FFR measurements showed promising diagnostic performance. The correlation coefficient between CT-FFR and invasive FFR was 0.59. CT-FFR improved the specificity of coronary CT angiography from 31% to 65%. (From Coenen et al. [21], with permission)

CT-FFR Compared to Other Techniques

In a substudy of the NXT trial, CT-FFR demonstrated superior diagnostic performance in comparison to the transluminal attenuation gradient along the coronary artery on CT angiography [10]. CT-FFR by Siemens was shown to perform similarly well as static CT myocardial perfusion imaging, while integration of CT-FFR with dynamic CT perfusion imaging provided incremental value over each technique separately (Fig. 60.8) [25, 27]. Although in meta-analyses CT-FFR performs well in comparison to other stress imaging techniques, no direct comparisons have been performed. No comparisons between the respective CT-FFR applications have been published either.

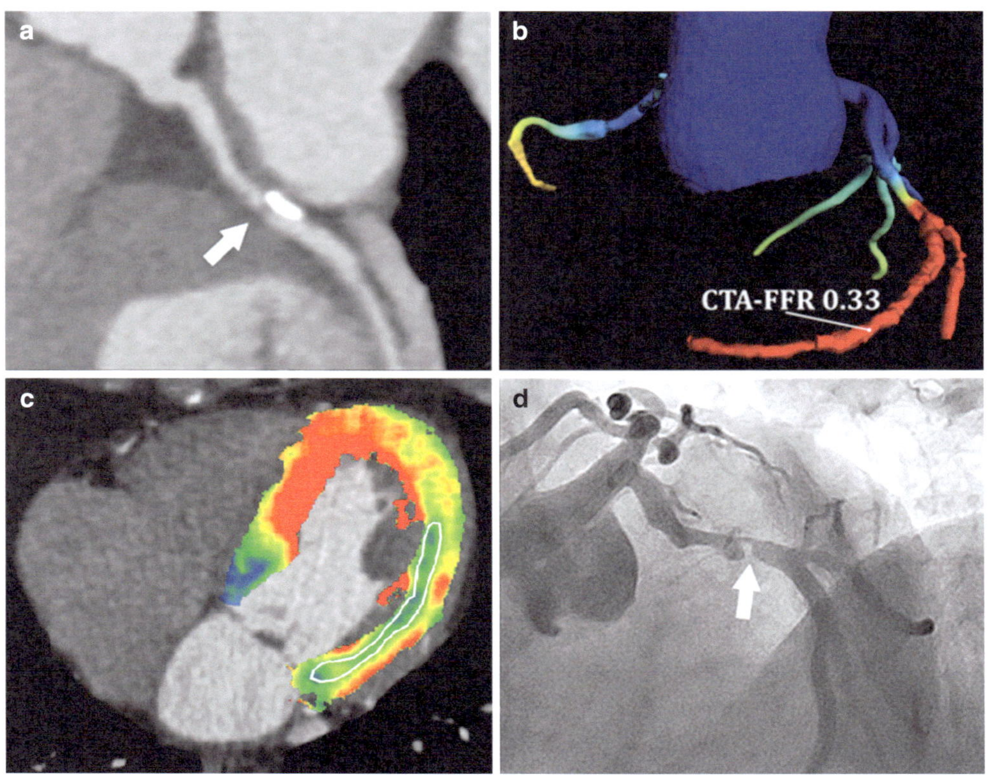

Fig. 60.8 Case example of a 61-year-old man presenting with stable chest pain. CTA demonstrated a partially calcified, severely stenosed lesion in the LCX (panel **a**). The CT-FFR simulation demonstrated a significant pressure drop (CT-FFR 0.33) over the lesion (panel **b**). CT-MPI, image fused with the CT angiogram, shows a perfusion defect in the basal lateral wall (panel **c**). The corresponding invasive angiography confirmed the short, severe stenosis, with an invasively measured FFR of 0.48 (panel **d**)

Challenges and Limitations

While the CT-FFR approach represents an attractive means to derive functional information without the need for additional testing after CT angiography, there are also challenges. Generally, the algorithms rely on artifact-free imaging for reconstruction of the coronary artery models. Adherence to CT imaging recommendations for optimal image quality is explicitly recommended. In particular vessel discontinuity between slabs as a result of arrhythmia or other displacements affects the performance of CT-FFR negatively. Although calcifications obscure the coronary lumen and compromise delineation of the coronary lumen, a substantial negative effect of calcifications on diagnostic performance could not be demonstrated [8, 28]. The diagnostic performance of CT-FFR in STEMI patients with multivessel disease was only modest [29], suggesting that the role of CT-FFR in STEMI patients is limited. CT-FFR has not been validated in patients with bypass graft, stents, prior myocardial infarction, congenital heart disease, or other out-of-the-ordinary cardiac morphologies. Momentarily, CT-FFR cannot be used to assess dynamic coronary compression (myocardial bridging, intra-arterial course of coronary anomaly), microvascular disease, or functional coronary artery disease (spasm).

The HeartFlow approach is most extensively validated and currently the only commercially available CT-FFR application. Datasets are transferred to and processed by the HeartFlow company. Off-site processing has the advantage that no local expertise or time investment, beyond the acquisition of high-quality CT data, is required. Drawbacks include the need to transfer patient data and the substantial costs. Return times are currently around 24 h, but expected to shorten in the future. On-site CT-FFR approaches, as developed by Siemens and Toshiba, leave the local investigator in control of the post-processing but demand substantial effort. User operation requires training and manual processing times are still substantial. Segmentation of the coronary arteries is particularly time-consuming, but may become more acceptable with the development of more automatic segmentation tools. Although none of the locally performed CT-FFR applications have been commercially released, costs are expected to be less than the HeartFlow application.

Further Development

Revascularization Planning

In addition to the present coronary status, simulations can also be performed on altered coronary models. By restoring dimensions of a stenotic vessel and simulation of the implantation of a coronary stent, the potential hemodynamic benefit of percutaneous intervention can be predicted [30]. Simulated stenting and treatment optimization would be especially of interest in patients with serial stenosis or complex bifurcation lesions where selection of the stenosis most benefiting from revascularization is not straightforward. Surgical revascularization can be simulated in a similar fashion, although the accuracy would be limited by uncertainty about the status and dimensions of available grafting material.

Predicting Events

Coronary endothelial cells respond to blood flow-induced shear stress; low shear stress regions are prone to plaque development. The mechanism behind atherosclerotic plaque development and shear stress levels is multifactorial and currently still being investigated. The initial response of the arterial wall to plaque development is outward or positive remodeling, also called the Glagov effect [31]. However, if plaque progression continues, also the coronary lumen will become affected. This reduction of the coronary lumen will result in an increase in local velocity and shear stress. While the exact pathophysiology is still under debate [32], increased shear stress is associated with increased plaque vulnerability [33, 34]. These findings are corroborated by clinical studies that associate the location of plaque rupture with high wall shear stress [34–37]. Most clinical computation of wall shear stress is based on intracoronary imaging, which can be supplemented by cardiac CT for vessel orientation in 3D space. Although coronary CT angiography does not provide the same spatial resolution as intravascular ultrasound or optical coherence tomography, preliminary data suggest that shear stress can be computed based on CT alone [38, 39]. In the EMERALD study, hemodynamic forces calculated with CFD from CT scans performed prior up to 2 years before myocardial infarction differentiated the ultimate culprit lesions from stable plaque. This suggests that the hemodynamic force onto coronary plaques can possibly predict future events [40].

Intracardiac Blood Flow Simulation

CFD can be used to investigate contractile cardiac function [41]. The high spatial resolution of the CT allows for precise anatomical differentiation of the lumen in all cardiac phases. CFD computations could be used to visualize the simulated cardiac function and blood flow through the main cardiac cavities and vessels. Better understanding of intracardiac flow patterns could provide valuable insights, for example, in ventricular dyssynchrony [42]. Lantz et al. presented a framework for CFD simulation of the global cardiac function from time-resolved CT angiography and computed blood flow in the pulmonary veins, atriums, left ventricle, aortic valve, aortic sinus, coronary arteries, and part of the ascending aorta. Because of the high spatial resolution of CT, even flow patterns around the papillary muscles can be visualized [43]. CFD simulations of diseased cardiac valves could improve our understanding of hemodynamic impact [44]. CFD simulation can also be used to assess the hemodynamic performance of prosthetic valves. However, large studies evaluating the clinical application of CFD computations of the cardiac and valvular function by CT are currently lacking.

References

1. Authors/Task Force members, Windecker S, Kolh P, Alfonso F, Collet JP, Cremer J, et al. 2014 ESC/EACTS guidelines on myocardial revascularization: the task force on myocardial revascularization of the European Society of Cardiology (ESC) and the European Association for Cardio-Thoracic Surgery (EACTS) developed with the special contribution of the European Association of Percutaneous Cardiovascular Interventions (EAPCI). Eur Heart J. 2014;35(37):2541–619.
2. Levine GN, Bates ER, Blankenship JC, Bailey SR, Bittl JA, Cercek B, et al. 2011 ACCF/AHA/SCAI guideline for percutaneous coronary intervention: a report of the American College of Cardiology Foundation/American Heart Association task force on practice guidelines and the Society for Cardiovascular Angiography and Interventions. Circulation. 2011;124(23):e574–651.
3. Taylor CA, Fonte TA, Min JK. Computational fluid dynamics applied to cardiac computed tomography for noninvasive quantification of fractional flow reserve: scientific basis. J Am Coll Cardiol. 2013;61(22):2233–41.
4. Morris PD, Narracott A, von Tengg-Kobligk H, Silva Soto DA, Hsiao S, Lungu A, et al. Computational fluid dynamics modelling in cardiovascular medicine. Heart. 2016;102(1):18–28.
5. Min JK, Taylor CA, Achenbach S, Koo BK, Leipsic J, Norgaard BL, et al. Noninvasive fractional flow reserve derived from coronary CT angiography: clinical data and scientific principles. JACC Cardiovasc Imaging. 2015;8(10):1209–22.
6. Schaap M, van Walsum T, Neefjes L, Metz C, Capuano E, de Bruijne M, et al. Robust shape regression for supervised vessel segmentation and its application to coronary segmentation in CTA. IEEE Trans Med Imaging. 2011;30(11):1974–86.
7. Choy JS, Kassab GS. Scaling of myocardial mass to flow and morphometry of coronary arteries. J Appl Physiol. 2008;104(5):1281–6.
8. Coenen A, Lubbers MM, Kurata A, Kono A, Dedic A, Chelu RG, et al. Coronary CT angiography derived fractional flow reserve: methodology and evaluation of a point of care algorithm. J Cardiovasc Comput Tomogr. 2016;10(2):105–13.
9. Itu L, Sharma P, Mihalef V, Kamen A, Suciu C, Lomaniciu D, editors. A patient-specific reduced-order model for coronary circulation. 2012 9th IEEE international symposium on biomedical imaging (ISBI); 2012. 2–5 May 2012.
10. Ko BS, Wong DT, Norgaard BL, Leong DP, Cameron JD, Gaur S, et al. Diagnostic performance of transluminal attenuation gradient and noninvasive fractional flow reserve derived from 320-detector row CT angiography to diagnose hemodynamically significant coronary stenosis: an NXT substudy. Radiology. 2016;279(1):75–83.
11. Wilson RF, Wyche K, Christensen BV, Zimmer S, Laxson DD. Effects of adenosine on human coronary arterial circulation. Circulation. 1990;82(5):1595–606.
12. Koo BK, Erglis A, Doh JH, Daniels DV, Jegere S, Kim HS, et al. Diagnosis of ischemia-causing coronary stenoses by noninvasive fractional flow reserve computed from coronary computed tomographic angiograms. Results from the prospective multicenter DISCOVER-FLOW (Diagnosis of Ischemia-Causing Stenoses Obtained Via Noninvasive Fractional Flow Reserve) study. J Am Coll Cardiol. 2011;58(19):1989–97.
13. Ko BS, Cameron JD, Munnur RK, Wong DT, Fujisawa Y, Sakaguchi T, et al. Noninvasive CT-derived FFR based on structural and fluid analysis: a comparison with invasive FFR for detection of functionally significant stenosis. JACC Cardiovasc Imaging. 2017;10(6):663–73.
14. Nickisch H, Lamash Y, Prevrhal S, Freiman M, Vembar M, Goshen L, et al. Learning patient-specific lumped models for interactive coronary blood flow simulations. In: Navab N, Hornegger J, Wells WM, Frangi AF, editors. Medical image computing and computer-assisted intervention – MICCAI 2015: 18th international conference, Munich, Germany, October 5–9, 2015, proceedings, part II. Cham: Springer International Publishing; 2015. p. 433–41.
15. Itu L, Rapaka S, Passerini T, Georgescu B, Schwemmer C, Schoebinger M, et al. A machine-learning approach for computation of fractional flow reserve from coronary computed tomography. J Appl Physiol. 2016;121(1):42–52.
16. Min JK, Leipsic J, Pencina MJ, Berman DS, Koo BK, van Mieghem C, et al. Diagnostic accuracy of fractional flow reserve from anatomic CT angiography. JAMA. 2012;308(12):1237–45.
17. Norgaard BL, Leipsic J, Gaur S, Seneviratne S, Ko BS, Ito H, et al. Diagnostic performance of noninvasive fractional flow reserve derived from coronary computed tomography angiography in suspected coronary artery disease the NXT trial (analysis of coronary blood flow using CT angiography: next steps). J Am Coll Cardiol. 2014;63(12):1145–55.
18. Douglas PS, Pontone G, Hlatky MA, Patel MR, Norgaard BL, Byrne RA, et al. Clinical outcomes of fractional flow reserve by computed tomographic angiography-guided diagnostic strategies vs. usual care in patients with suspected coronary artery disease: the prospective longitudinal trial of FFR(CT): outcome and resource impacts study. Eur Heart J. 2015;36(47):3359–67.
19. Douglas PS, De Bruyne B, Pontone G, Patel MR, Norgaard BL, Byrne RA, et al. 1-year outcomes of FFRCT-guided care in patients with suspected coronary disease: the PLATFORM study. J Am Coll Cardiol. 2016;68(5):435–45.
20. Renker M, Schoepf UJ, Wang R, Meinel FG, Rier JD, Bayer RR, et al. Comparison of diagnostic value of a novel noninvasive coronary computed tomography angiography method versus standard coronary angiography for assessing fractional flow reserve. Am J Cardiol. 2014;114(9):1303–8.
21. Coenen A, Lubbers MM, Kurata A, Kono A, Dedic A, Chelu RG, et al. Fractional flow reserve computed from noninvasive CT angiography data: diagnostic performance of an on-site clinician-operated computational fluid dynamics algorithm. Radiology. 2015;274(3):674–83.
22. Kruk M, Wardziak L, Demkow M, Pleban W, Pregowski J, Dzielinska Z, et al. Workstation-based calculation of CTA-based FFR for intermediate stenosis. JACC Cardiovasc Imaging. 2016;9(6):690–9.
23. Kurata A, Coenen A, Lubbers MM, Nieman K, Kido T, Kido T, et al. The effect of blood pressure on non-invasive fractional flow reserve derived from coronary computed tomography angiography. Eur Radiol. 2017;27(4):1416–23.
24. De Geer J, Sandstedt M, Bjorkholm A, Alfredsson J, Janzon M, Engvall J, et al. Software-based on-site estimation of fractional flow reserve using standard coronary CT angiography data. Acta Radiol. 2016;57(10):1186–92.
25. Yang DH, Kim YH, Roh JH, Kang JW, Ahn JM, Kweon J, et al. Diagnostic performance of on-site CT-derived fractional flow

reserve versus CT perfusion. Eur Heart J Cardiovasc Imaging. 2017;18(4):432–40.
26. Schrauwen JT, Koeze DJ, Wentzel JJ, van de Vosse FN, van der Steen AF, Gijsen FJ. Fast and accurate pressure-drop prediction in straightened atherosclerotic coronary arteries. Ann Biomed Eng. 2015;43(1):59–67.
27. Coenen A, Rossi A, Lubbers MM, Kurata A, Kono AK, Chelu RG, Segreto S, Dijkshoorn ML, Wragg A, van Geuns RM, Pugliese F, Nieman K. Integrating CT myocardial perfusion and CT-FFR in the work-up of coronary artery disease. JACC Cardiovasc Imaging. 2017;10(7):760–70.
28. Norgaard BL, Gaur S, Leipsic J, Ito H, Miyoshi T, Park SJ, et al. Influence of coronary calcification on the diagnostic performance of CT angiography derived FFR in coronary artery disease a substudy of the NXT trial. JACC Cardiovasc Imaging. 2015;8(9):1045–55.
29. Gaur S, Taylor CA, Jensen JM, Botker HE, Christiansen EH, Kaltoft AK, et al. FFR derived from coronary CT angiography in nonculprit lesions of patients with recent STEMI. JACC Cardiovasc Imaging. 2017;10(4):424–33.
30. Kim KH, Doh JH, Koo BK, Min JK, Erglis A, Yang HM, et al. A novel noninvasive technology for treatment planning using virtual coronary stenting and computed tomography-derived computed fractional flow reserve. JACC Cardiovasc Interv. 2014;7(1):72–8.
31. Glagov S, Weisenberg E, Zarins CK, Stankunavicius R, Kolettis GJ. Compensatory enlargement of human atherosclerotic coronary arteries. N Engl J Med. 1987;316(22):1371–5.
32. Wentzel JJ, Chatzizisis YS, Gijsen FJ, Giannoglou GD, Feldman CL, Stone PH. Endothelial shear stress in the evolution of coronary atherosclerotic plaque and vascular remodelling: current understanding and remaining questions. Cardiovasc Res. 2012;96(2):234–43.
33. Gijsen FJ, Wentzel JJ, Thury A, Mastik F, Schaar JA, Schuurbiers JC, et al. Strain distribution over plaques in human coronary arteries relates to shear stress. Am J Physiol Heart Circ Physiol. 2008;295(4):H1608–14.
34. Samady H, Eshtehardi P, McDaniel MC, Suo J, Dhawan SS, Maynard C, et al. Coronary artery wall shear stress is associated with progression and transformation of atherosclerotic plaque and arterial remodeling in patients with coronary artery disease. Circulation. 2011;124(7):779–88.
35. Gijsen F, van der Giessen A, van der Steen A, Wentzel J. Shear stress and advanced atherosclerosis in human coronary arteries. J Biomech. 2013;46(2):240–7.
36. Cicha I, Worner A, Urschel K, Beronov K, Goppelt-Struebe M, Verhoeven E, et al. Carotid plaque vulnerability: a positive feedback between hemodynamic and biochemical mechanisms. Stroke. 2011;42(12):3502–10.
37. Fujii K, Kobayashi Y, Mintz GS, Takebayashi H, Dangas G, Moussa I, et al. Intravascular ultrasound assessment of ulcerated ruptured plaques: a comparison of culprit and nonculprit lesions of patients with acute coronary syndromes and lesions in patients without acute coronary syndromes. Circulation. 2003;108(20):2473–8.
38. Zhang JM, Luo T, Tan SY, Lomarda AM, Wong AS, Keng FY, et al. Hemodynamic analysis of patient-specific coronary artery tree. Int J Numer Method Biomed Eng. 2015;31(4):e02708.
39. van der Giessen AG, Groen HC, Doriot PA, de Feyter PJ, van der Steen AF, van de Vosse FN, et al. The influence of boundary conditions on wall shear stress distribution in patients specific coronary trees. J Biomech. 2011;44(6):1089–95.
40. Koo BK. Haemodynamic force analysis improves non-invasive prediction of risk of ACS: the results of first-in-man EMERALD study (exploring the mechanism of the plaque rupture in acute coronary syndrome using coronary CT angiography and computational fluid dynamics). Imaging and functional assessment presented at: EuroPCR; May 16–19, 2016; Paris. 2016.
41. Chan BT, Lim E, Chee KH, Abu Osman NA. Review on CFD simulation in heart with dilated cardiomyopathy and myocardial infarction. Comput Biol Med. 2013;43(4):377–85.
42. Aguado-Sierra J, Krishnamurthy A, Villongco C, Chuang J, Howard E, Gonzales MJ, et al. Patient-specific modeling of dyssynchronous heart failure: a case study. Prog Biophys Mol Biol. 2011;107(1):147–55.
43. Lantz J, Henriksson L, Persson A, Karlsson M, Ebbers T. Patient-specific simulation of cardiac blood flow from high-resolution computed tomography. J Biomech Eng. 2016;138(12):121004.
44. Astorino M, Hamers J, Shadden SC, Gerbeau JF. A robust and efficient valve model based on resistive immersed surfaces. Int J Numer Method Biomed Eng. 2012;28(9):937–59.
45. Kawaji T, Shiomi H, Morishita H, Morimoto T, Taylor CA, Kanao S, et al. Feasibility and diagnostic performance of fractional flow reserve measurement derived from coronary computed tomography angiography in real clinical practice. Int J Cardiovasc Imaging. 2017;33(2):271–81.

CT Myocardial Perfusion Imaging: Arterial First-Pass Imaging

61

Florian Schwarz, Amadeus Altenburger, Michael Gebhard, and Christian Thilo

Coronary computed tomography angiography (CCTA) is well established for its high reliability in the exclusion of coronary artery disease (CAD) based on abundant high-class evidence demonstrating excellent negative likelihood ratios both in emergency and elective settings [1–4].

On the other hand, when coronary stenoses are detected, an estimation of their hemodynamic relevance remains difficult, and typically, CCTA-based estimations of hemodynamic relevance correlate only moderately with perfusion-based modalities [5].

The recognition of the hemodynamic relevance of stenoses, however, is of high importance as it has considerable prognostic implications and directly influences treatment decisions [6, 7]: nonobstructive CAD is associated with better outcomes when treated with best medical therapy, while patients with flow-limiting stenoses usually benefit from angioplasty and stent implantation or coronary artery bypass surgery.

In particular, the detection of intermediate-degree coronary stenoses in CCTA frequently results in the recommendation for additional tests for the visualization of potential myocardial ischemia with the treatment consequences determined only after this perfusion information is obtained.

Physiological Background

The contractile function of the heart depends on aerobic metabolism and thus oxygen supply via the coronary arteries. Due to the high oxygen extraction fraction of the heart even under rest conditions, any excess oxygen demand of the heart during increased activity can only be satisfied by an increase in coronary blood flow. For this purpose, coronary arteries have a substantial capacity for autoregulation of blood flow. This autoregulation has long been recognized as the reason why coronary stenoses under rest conditions become flow-limiting (and thus create myocardial ischemia) only when reaching at least 85% diameter stenosis [8]. At lower degrees of stenosis, autoregulation will counteract any potentially hemodynamic effect under rest conditions.

On the other hand, when coronary blood flow increases due to increased cardiac oxygen demand or due to the administration of vasodilatory drugs (i.e., pharmacological stress by application of dipyridamole, adenosine, or regadenoson), the autoregulatory capacity will be "overwhelmed" at lower degrees of coronary stenosis with segmental myocardial ischemia detectable at intermediate stenoses in the 50% range [8, 9]. Therefore, the administration of pharmacological stress agents will significantly improve sensitivity for stenosis detection. Most traditional imaging modalities based on the direct visualization of myocardial ischemia include acquisitions of myocardial perfusion under stress as well as under rest to detect reversible and nonreversible perfusion defects.

General Technical Considerations

It has long been hypothesized that the visualization and quantification of segmental myocardial contrast uptake in principle would be feasible with CT – initial experiments in myocardial infarcts date back to the late 1970s [10–12] with more specific reports on the quantification of myocardial perfusion for the electron-beam CT platform [8, 13–17].

Approaches for the analysis of perfusion in CT are based on the visualization of the first pass of iodinated contrast material after i.v. administration, similarly as in dynamic contrast-enhanced MRI.

Clinically available iodinated contrast materials are nonionic small molecules which distribute freely in the

F. Schwarz (✉) · A. Altenburger · M. Gebhard
Department of Diagnostic and Interventional Radiology and Neuroradiology, Klinikum Augsburg, Augsburg, Germany
e-mail: Florian.Schwarz@klinikum-augsburg.de

C. Thilo
Department of Cardiology, Klinikum Augsburg, Herzzentrum Augsburg-Schwaben, Augsburg, Germany

U. J. Schoepf (ed.), *CT of the Heart*, Contemporary Medical Imaging, https://doi.org/10.1007/978-1-60327-237-7_61

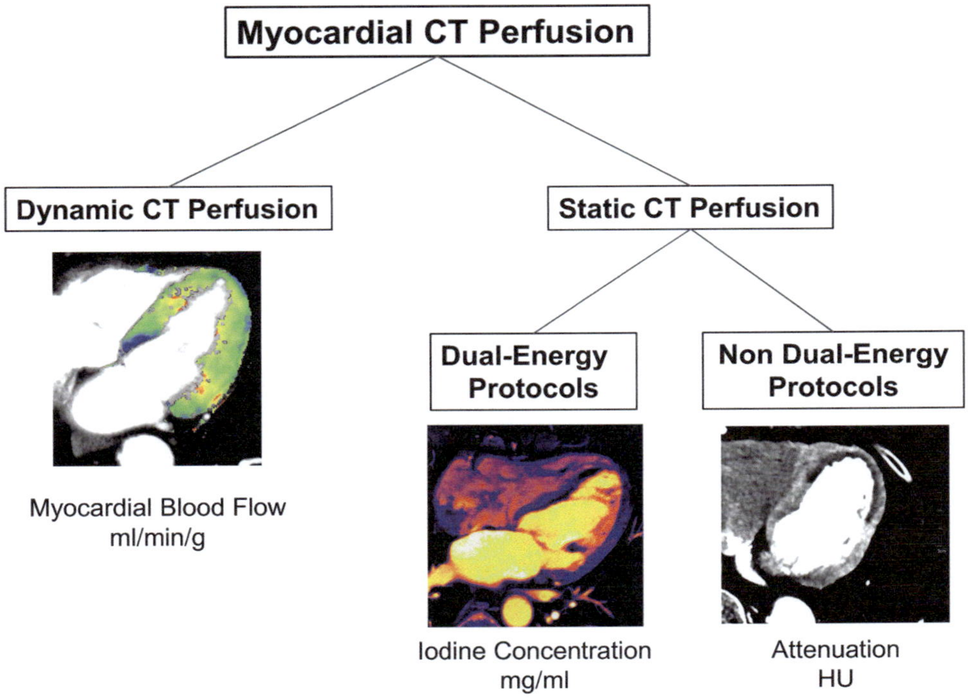

Fig. 61.1 Overview of the different scan protocols which have been applied to the visualization of myocardial perfusion in CT along with exemplary images and the major derivable parameter as the basis for perfusion evaluation: Dynamic CT perfusion allows for a true quantification of myocardial blood flow. Static CT perfusion approaches implementing a dual-energy acquisition technique still allow for a precise absolute quantification of iodine content within the myocardium which might serve as a surrogate marker for myocardial blood flow. Static CT perfusion approaches finally must rely on attenuation differences which due to the linear relationship with iodine concentration allow for an assessment of relative differences in myocardial iodine uptake

intravascular and with little delay in the extracellular space but do not enter cells to any relevant extent. It has been reported that the administration of iodinated contrast agents has an influence on coronary blood flow, inducing an initial reduction of blood flow followed by a hyperemic response [18]. This, however, seems to play a considerably smaller role for low-osmolarity nonionic contrast agents [19]. Importantly, there is significant diffusion of the contrast agents into the interstitial space. The first-pass extraction of iodinated contrast is around 1/3 with maximal vasodilation and even higher at lower flow rates [20].

Since for a given tube voltage attenuation behaves virtually linear to iodine concentration [21], hypoperfused areas of the myocardium can be appreciated by hypoattenuation of ischemic myocardial segments in comparison with normal myocardium.

Despite the mentioned early attempts, a widespread clinical application of myocardial CT perfusion imaging has remained elusive until very recently. Only with the introduction of the recent scanner generations, the visualization of myocardial perfusion has become feasible, and the prospect of coronary CT as a true "one-stop" shop modality has spurred considerable scientific interest and research activity in this direction [22].

In general, technical solutions for the visualization of myocardial perfusion in CT can be grouped into one of two major approaches: dynamic or static CT perfusion imaging (Fig. 61.1).

Dynamic CT Perfusion

"Dynamic CT perfusion" imaging refers to approaches in which repeated ECG-synchronized acquisitions of the left ventricular myocardium are performed during the first pass of iodinated contrast material, similar to the scan sequences underlying first-pass myocardial perfusion in MRI [23]. Thereby the left ventricular myocardium is repeatedly sampled during the first pass of contrast material. After motion correction, the multiphasic dataset can be used to generate time-attenuation curves for each voxel of the LV myocardium on which the typical perfusion models can be applied yielding quantitative perfusion parameters such as myocardial blood flow [24].

The technical prerequisite for these approaches either is a detector width covering the entire extension of the heart along the z-axis or – in the case of narrow detectors – a shuttle-mode acquisition. For a full discussion of the underlying technical prerequisites as well as the specific advantages of these approaches, the reader is referred to Chap. 63 for more details.

Static CT Perfusion

"Static CT perfusion" imaging on the other hand encompasses approaches which are based on a single scan of the myocardium during contrast inflow. This group has also been referred to as "arterial first-pass imaging" or "single-shot acquisition."

The rationale of this approach is to acquire the image at a timepoint at which the hemodynamic effect of flow-limiting stenosis is most apparent, i.e., in which due to the flow-limiting nature of the stenosis, contrast material will not have washed into myocardial segments distal to stenoses, while myocardial segments not affected by coronary stenoses will already show normal myocardial enhancement.

In principle, all CT acquisition techniques are feasible for static CT perfusion imaging (i.e., retrospective ECG gating, prospective ECG triggering, and prospective ECG acquisition with high-pitch factor). A closer look at the time-attenuation curves of ischemic vs. normal myocardial segments (Fig. 61.2) fosters an understanding of the concept of static vs. dynamic perfusion evaluation. In comparison with normal myocardial segments, the enhancement in ischemic myocardium starts later, has a shallower upslope, and is overall significantly less pronounced. While dynamic acquisitions permit an extensive sampling of time-attenuation curves from which all mentioned curve features can be derived, the static acquisition technique must rely on the differences in maximal attenuations (in HU), while other curve parameters will remain unaddressed.

Consequentially, with the acquisition of only a singular timepoint, the correct acquisition timing in relation to the contrast material bolus will be critical – much more so than for dynamic approaches where a wide temporal window is recorded beginning prior to the arrival of the contrast bolus in the myocardium. The optimal time of image acquisition will be when the difference in attenuations between normal and ischemic myocardium is most pronounced.

In comparison with dynamic approaches, static CT perfusion approaches are associated with considerably lower effective doses, as low as 0.9 ± 0.1 mSv for static stress CT perfusion acquisitions [25]. Furthermore, only in static CT perfusion, the acquisition of the coronary CTA dataset can be combined with myocardial perfusion under rest conditions, while in dynamic perfusion this acquisition must be performed as a distinct scan.

A technical variety of static CT perfusion is the use of a dual-energy acquisition technique (Fig. 61.1). Dual-energy acquisition protocols promise to combine the higher contrast resolution of a low-kV dataset with the lower noise of a high-kV dataset and thus facilitate the visualization of perfusion heterogeneities within the myocardium, i.e., ischemic segments [26–28]. It has been confirmed that the detection of ischemia is improved by use of a dual-energy acquisition technique [29]. Furthermore, the attenuation characteristics at distinct photon energy spectra can be used to calculate the

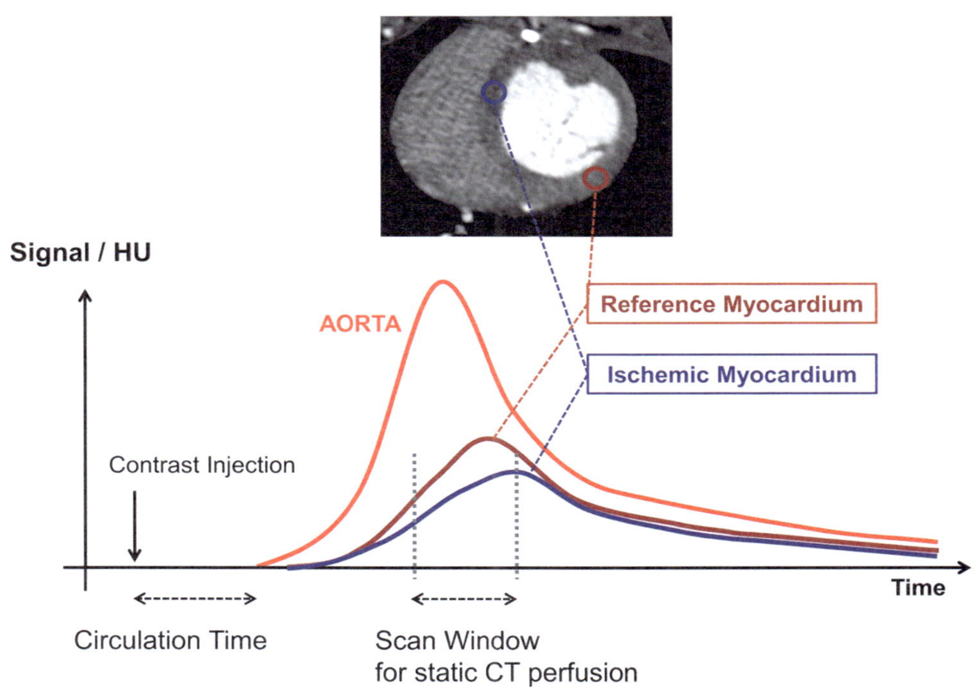

Fig. 61.2 Time-attenuation curves (TAC) of ischemic vs. reference myocardium during first pass of intravenously administered contrast material. TAC in ischemic segments begins to rise later, runs shallower, and has a later peak. This creates a window of approx. 8 s for the visualization of ischemic segments using static CT perfusion protocols

absolute concentration of iodine in each voxel [30]. It is conceivable that the absolute iodine concentrations in the myocardium during first pass of contrast material might show some correlation with MBF values thus permitting quantitative statements about myocardial perfusion. Again, a full discussion of the physical background of the various technical implementations by different vendors and the available clinical evidence is beyond the scope of this chapter, and the reader is referred to Chap. 62.

Scan Protocol Considerations in Static CT Perfusion Imaging

To facilitate a distinction between ischemic myocardium and scar tissue, it has traditionally been considered a prerequisite to acquire perfusion scans under rest as well as under stress conditions and thereby determine whether perfusion defects are "reversible" (which proves ischemia) or fixed (which favors scar tissue, i.e., an old myocardial infarct).

In static CT perfusion imaging, careful planning of the scan delay allows the same dataset to be used for the CT coronary angiogram as well as the visualization of myocardial perfusion under rest conditions (Fig. 61.3). As we will see in the following paragraphs, the myocardial contrast wash-in kinetics are such that this holds true even when scan protocols are used that acquire data during several heartbeats, i.e., prospective triggering or retrospective gating.

The dataset used for the analysis of myocardial stress perfusion, however, does currently not lend itself to the visualization of the coronary arteries themselves since the administration of vasodilatory drugs to trigger an increase in coronary blood flow usually results in a compensatory increase in heart rate of approximately 20 bpms even when beta-blockers had been administered previously [31].

Sequence of Stress and Rest Acquisitions

According to the order of the acquisition of rest and stress CT perfusion (with acquisitions at rest being simultaneously used for the visualization of the coronary arteries), a stress-rest approach (stress perfusion first) and a rest-stress (rest perfusion first) approach can be distinguished which both have specific advantages and disadvantages.

The main advantage of the stress-rest approach is that the visualization of hypoattenuated ischemic myocardial segments during stress perfusion is not compromised by any prior administration of contrast material, a phenomenon also referred to as contrast material contamination of the myocardium. Because of the small molecule nature of iodinated contrast material, there is extravasation into the extracellular space, a phenomenon utilized for late enhancement in scar tissue. When performing two perfusion acquisitions in sequence, there will be residual extracellular contrast material both within the myocardium and within scar tissue. This residual contrast material can be problematic as it will further mitigate the already small attenuation difference between normal and ischemic myocardium in the second scan potentially resulting in lower sensitivity for ischemia detection. This phenomenon is to be expected for at least 15 min after contrast administration. Since the stress perfusion scan should self-evidently have highest diagnostic accuracy for the detection (and thus also exclusion) of myocardial perfusion defects, a stress-first approach would seem advantageous.

Similarly, a stress-first approach guarantees that the administration of both a beta-blocker and of sublingual nitrates – encouraged prior to the CCTA/rest perfusion acquisition – will not interfere with the perfusion situation during stress perfusion. Particularly for beta-blockers, there is some evidence from the nuclear medicine myocardial perfusion literature that their application can hide or reduce the size and/or severity of myocardial perfusion deficits with potentially negative effects on the sensitivity of myocardial perfusion imaging [32]. However, in the CORE320 study in which an aggressive beta-blocker regime was applied at the beginning of a rest-stress CT perfusion protocol, no negative effect of metoprolol on the diagnostic accuracy of CT perfusion was observed, and CT perfusion still had higher diagnostic accuracy than SPECT myocardial perfusion imaging for the detection of significant CAD.

A rest-stress approach (i.e., rest perfusion/CCTA first) has the main advantage that it more closely follows the logical diagnostic pathway for CAD and reduces unnecessary stress perfusion acquisitions: in all patients in whom the CCTA component already excludes obstructive CAD, a stress perfusion scan can be omitted, thus resulting in considerable reduction of total effective dose. If the CCTA component shows obstructive CAD, the stress perfusion can then be performed with a specific diagnostic objective.

Furthermore, a rest-stress approach results in lower heart rates during the CTA acquisition, which is desirable for highest possible image quality of the CTA scan: George et al. showed that in the wake of a recent adenosine-stress perfusion acquisition, heart rates during CTA will be 7 bpms higher than at baseline, suggesting that adenosine (or contrast administration) triggers effects that persist despite the very short biological half-life of adenosine [33]. These effects can be expected to be even more pronounced when regadenoson is used due to its longer half-life.

This conundrum of the optimal order of scans will most likely be resolved by integrating the pretest probability for obstructive CAD, as first pointed out by Techasith et al. [34] and readily taken up by other authors [35]: in patients with an intermediate to high likelihood of obstructive CAD, the

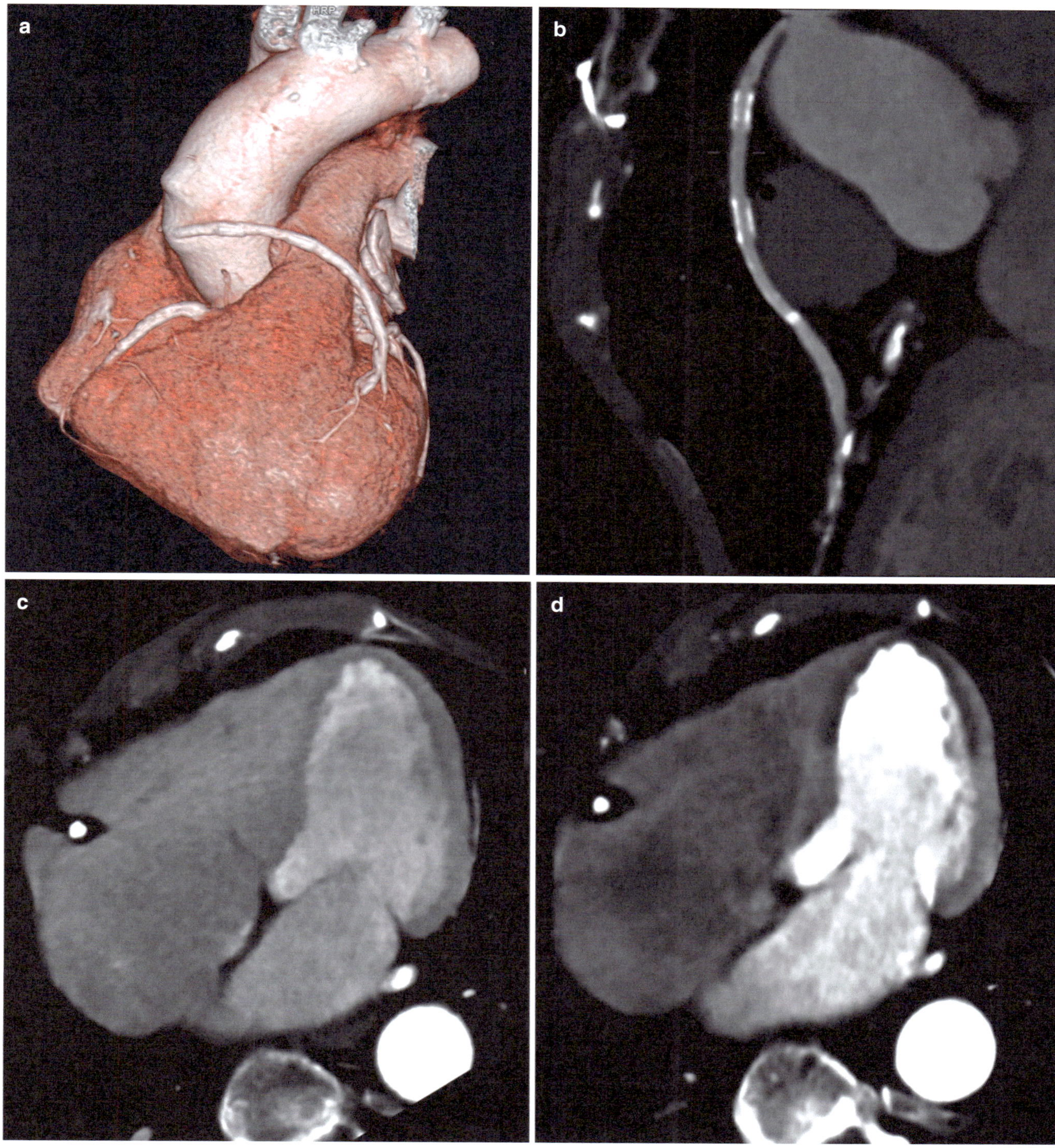

Fig. 61.3 A 59-year-old patient with recurrence of stable angina 8 years after coronary artery bypass surgery. (**a**) Volume-rendering technique (VRT) reconstruction demonstrates ACVB to LAD. (**b**) Curved planar reformation (CPR) of the venous bypass demonstrates normal vessel patency without any obvious high-grade stenoses – however, the exact status of the distal anastomosis remained uncertain. (**c**) Four-chamber view of rest perfusion shows very mild subendocardial hypoattenuation in the apex. (**d**) Four-chamber view of stress perfusion acquired 3 min after starting a continuous infusion of adenosine with an increase in heart rate from 75 to 90 bpm demonstrates severe subendocardial hypoattenuation, consistent with a reversible perfusion defect in the left ventricular anterior wall and apical region

stress-rest approach (i.e., stress perfusion first) seems more advantageous as the proportion of unnecessary stress perfusion scans will be small – defined as cases in which the stress perfusion acquisition will retrospectively prove unnecessary since CCTA excludes obstructive CAD. On the other hand, in patients with low pretest probability for obstructive CAD, the rest-stress approach clearly seems to be favorable since in most of these patients, the stress perfusion will be omissible.

Optimal Scan Delay for Static CT Myocardial Perfusion

Bischoff et al. [36], Tanabe et al. [37], and Pelgrim et al. [38] have investigated the optimal time window for image acquisition in relation to the contrast bolus by a detailed analysis of the time-attenuation curves derived from dynamic stress CT perfusion datasets acquired in the context of recent clinical studies. All three groups report a time window of approximately 8–9 s, in which the difference in contrast enhancement between ischemic and normal myocardial segments is optimal. Furthermore, the presented data support the feasibility of a bolus-triggering technique within the ascending aorta and a delay of approx. 7 s after reaching a threshold of 150 HU.

Importantly, this relatively long time window of 8–9 s implies the presence of an attenuation difference between ischemic and normal segments over several heartbeats. This demonstrates that even when selecting scan protocols that acquire data over two or three heartbeats, the evaluation of myocardial perfusion should be feasible.

It should be noted that in all three studies, the maximum difference in attenuation was approximately 20–25 HU on a background of approximately 100 HU, highlighting the relatively low contrast resolution or signal intensity that static CT perfusion techniques are associated with.

Optimal RR Phase for the Evaluation of Static CT Myocardial Perfusion

Ghoshhajra et al. analyzed the conspicuity of perfusion defects on systolic vs. diastolic reconstructions of retrospectively acquired static CT stress perfusion datasets and reported similar diagnostic accuracies of 61% for both cardiac phases with considerable higher sensitivity in end-diastolic acquisitions and higher specificity in systolic acquisitions [39].

Using the data from the CORE320 study, Steveson et al. analyzed the influence of heart rate on image quality and optimal reconstruction phase for the evaluation of stress perfusion within the confines of the diastolic acquisitions of CORE320 [31]. In this cohort undergoing a rest-stress static CT perfusion protocol prospectively triggered to 75%–95% of the RR interval, 80% of patients had excellent or good image quality and only 3% of participants poor image quality. Poor image quality was observed most frequently in heart rates ≥80 bpm (overall, 3%; in the subgroup with HR ≥80 bpm, 6%). The optimal diastolic phase for the assessment of myocardial perfusion was earlier in diastole for lower heart rates and later in diastole for higher heart rates (optimal phase: from 77% in patients with heart rates of <65 bpm to 90% in patients with ≥80 bpm) [31].

Reconstruction and Postprocessing

There is some evidence suggesting that the optimal postprocessing tool differs between diastolic and systolic acquisitions: comparing the effects of diastolic and systolic reconstructions and various postprocessing modes (MPRs, MinIPs, MIPs) on ischemia conspicuity, Ghoshhajra et al. reported highest sensitivities in diastolic datasets using 8 mm MPRs, while for systolic reconstructions, 3 mm MinIPs showed highest specificity and accuracy [39].

One of the technical challenges associated with static CT perfusion imaging has traditionally been the higher susceptibility to beam-hardening artifacts created by the high attenuation within the left ventricle and particularly within the descending aorta which lies directly adjacent to a segment of the free wall of the left ventricle. It has been shown that by using dedicated beam-hardening correction reconstruction algorithms, these artifacts can be reduced significantly [40, 41].

Depending on the acquisition protocols of rest and stress CT perfusion, the phases with least cardiac motion of the myocardium should be selected, with sharpest epi- and endocardial borders and least contour doubling [42].

Image Analysis

The images reconstructed from the perfusion datasets should be evaluated in the three traditional cardiac axes, short axis, horizontal long axis, and vertical long axis, allowing for an assessment of each myocardial segment in at least two planes. In general, a narrow window width and level (300/150) should be applied [42]. These window settings maximize the differences between normal and ischemic myocardium and help to identify fat and vessels and calcifications outside of this window width. For each patient, identical window settings should be applied for the analysis of rest and stress CT perfusion images.

Unlike in research and clinical study environments, the routine clinical application of myocardial CT perfusion will certainly employ a combined interpretation of functional and anatomic datasets.

Coronary CTA is extensively validated as the most sensitive noninvasive test for CAD, and due to its wide distribution, most imaging centers are well experienced in its performance and interpretation. In general, findings should be reported according to established guidelines [43].

Once a potentially significant stenosis is identified on CCTA, the role of myocardial CT perfusion is (1) to unambiguously prove or exclude its functional significance, (2) to differentiate between reversible and fixed perfusion defects, and (3) to provide a quantitative parameter for the overall myocardial burden of ischemia [42].

Qualitative analysis of static CT perfusion is performed by visual comparison of the images acquired during stress and rest conditions. Typically, standard cardiac long-axis and short-axis planes are reconstructed as thick multiplanar reconstructions with 5–8 mm slice thickness for optimal signal-to-noise ratio. These are then interpreted for the presence and extent of perfusion defects [42].

Several software tools are available to support the reader in the analysis of myocardial perfusion. Some software tools derive secondary parameters from the myocardial tissue attenuation values, such as the transmural perfusion ratio (TPR) – this is a semiquantitative index parameter for each segment which relates subendocardial attenuation of a particular segment with the mean epicardial attenuation of the entire heart. TPR has been initially validated for stress MRI [44] but has been implemented to aid CT perfusion analysis [33, 45] and can best be visualized by bull's eye plots.

TPR is not reliable in the presence of prior infarcts or significant artifacts in several myocardial segments since both phenomena distort mean epicardial attenuation as the denominator for the calculation of TPR. Therefore, the radiologic interpretation should not rely on this parameter alone but always be regarded as complementary to an initial visual assessment of the perfusion images.

Typical Artifacts

All CT perfusion scans should be evaluated for the presence and extent of artifacts which should be included in the written report. Common artifacts which can result in false-positive or false-negative evaluation of myocardial perfusion are due to motion, beam-hardening, reconstruction, or partial dataset misalignment artifacts.

Motion

Both the heartbeat and breathing are potential sources of motion artifacts. Both can be detected by analysis of reconstructions with a large field of view on which they are typically revealed by signs of contour doubling or haziness of anatomic edges. These artifacts can mimic or mask perfusion deficits when they appear as focal hypo- and/or hyperdensities.

Therefore, if the scan protocol selected for stress and rest perfusion permits distinct reconstructions across the RR interval, perfusion defects should be confirmed by their presence at several timepoints of the RR interval.

The only effective strategy against breathing artifacts remains their prevention by investing time in detailed instructions to and training with the patient prior to performing the CT scan.

Beam Hardening

This artifact occurs in parts of the myocardium lying adjacent to large hyperdense structures, in which low-energy photons are preferentially absorbed, resulting in a relative increase in high-energy photons in the remaining photon beam (i.e., beam hardening). Therefore, the x-ray photon beam will have slightly different spectral properties during the sampling of these adjacent myocardial segments, which will cause differences in attenuation values attributed to the respective myocardial segments. This artifact is most apparent in the basal inferior wall due to the contrast-filled descending aorta and the anterior wall of the left ventricle which can be affected by the LV cavity or overlying ribs. Severe beam-hardening artifacts affecting the interventricular septum but also the midventricular and apical lateral wall of the left ventricle can also be observed in the presence of prominent pacemaker electrodes in the right ventricle (Fig. 61.4).

Special reconstruction algorithms have been developed to take beam hardening into account [40, 41]. In general, beam-hardening artifacts appear in the plane of the x-ray beam and can thus be identified by analyzing the distribution using multiplanar reformations on the dataset during image interpretation. Usually, beam hardening creates transmural hypoattenuation and occurs directly adjacent to highly attenuating structures.

Reconstruction Artifacts

The most relevant reconstruction artifact is the cone-beam artifact which results from the fan configuration of the x-ray beam along the z-axis. This becomes most relevant for modern wide-range detectors, in particular for the 320-detector CT with cone angles of up to 15.2° [46]. Cone-beam artifacts typically present as low- and high-attenuation bands but usually extend beyond the range of the myocardium into adjacent mediastinal and lung structures.

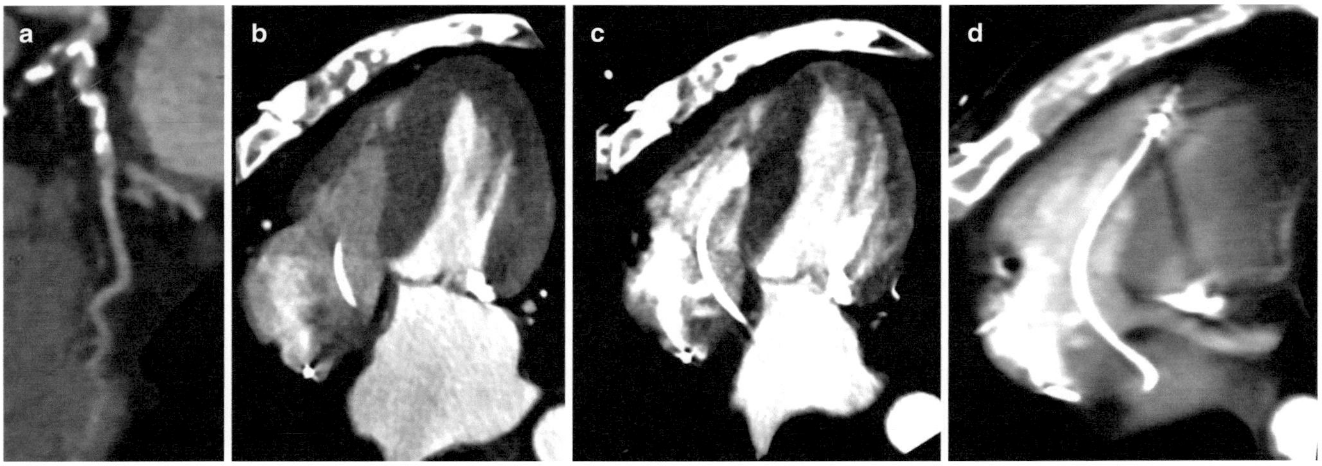

Fig. 61.4 A 62-year-old patient with a history of atypical chest pain underwent coronary CTA (**a**, **b**) followed by adenosine-stress CT perfusion (**c**, **d**). Coronary CTA demonstrated severe calcifications of the LAD (**a**) whose hemodynamic significance remained uncertain. (**b**) demonstrates four-chamber view of myocardial perfusion at rest. (**c**) shows an adenosine-stress myocardial perfusion dataset in the same orientation, revealing subendocardial hypoattenuation in the anterolateral myocardial segments, consistent with a reversible perfusion defect. The hypoattenuation of the interventricular septum in the stress image is due to an artifact by the very prominent pacemaker electrode in the right ventricular apex – notice the hypodense bands originating at the tip of the electrode (**d**)

Partial Dataset Misalignment Artifacts

As in coronary CTA, misalignment artifacts can occur when the final image is composed of image stacks acquired during different heartbeats, such as in step-and-shoot image acquisition protocols. More than when evaluating the coronary arteries, however, the differences in the exact acquisition timepoint between adjacent image stacks can be problematic, since they are acquired during different timepoints of the contrast bolus and thus make comparisons of myocardial enhancement problematic.

Image Interpretation

Rest Image Interpretation and the Assessment of Prior Infarcts

It is important to identify prior infarcts on rest perfusion images to be able to discern them from areas of ischemia during stress perfusion (Fig. 61.5). Typically, prior myocardial infarcts are characterized by the presence of subendocardial or transmural hypoattenuation during rest perfusion due to the high proportion of scar tissue, by relative myocardial thinning and the myocardial inclusion of fat in chronic infarcts. Older large infarcts often exhibit calcifications, aneurysmal dilatation, or mural thrombus formation.

Stress Image Interpretation and the Assessment of Ischemia

Stress CT perfusion images carefully need to be assessed for the presence of stress-induced subendocardial or transmural areas of hypoattenuation not present at rest, changes which are highly suggestive for (reversible) myocardial ischemia. Furthermore, in large infarcts apparent on the rest images, a relative enhancement may be appreciated on the stress images if a rest-stress protocol is applied.

Defect Severity and Ischemic Burden

Similarly to the method established in the nuclear medicine SPECT literature, the extent of segmental myocardial ischemia can be expressed in a semiquantitative manner for each myocardial segment [47], assigning a semiquantitative value expressing the severity of ischemia (0 = normal myocardial perfusion; 1 = mild perfusion deficit, i.e., <1/3 transmurality; 2 = moderate, i.e., <50% transmurality; 3 = severe, i.e., >50% transmurality).

The ischemic burden of the left ventricle can be qualitatively assessed by describing the myocardial segments involved. Semiquantitative measures for global ischemic burden can be generated by calculating the sum of all segmental ischemia values: the summed rest score (SRS),

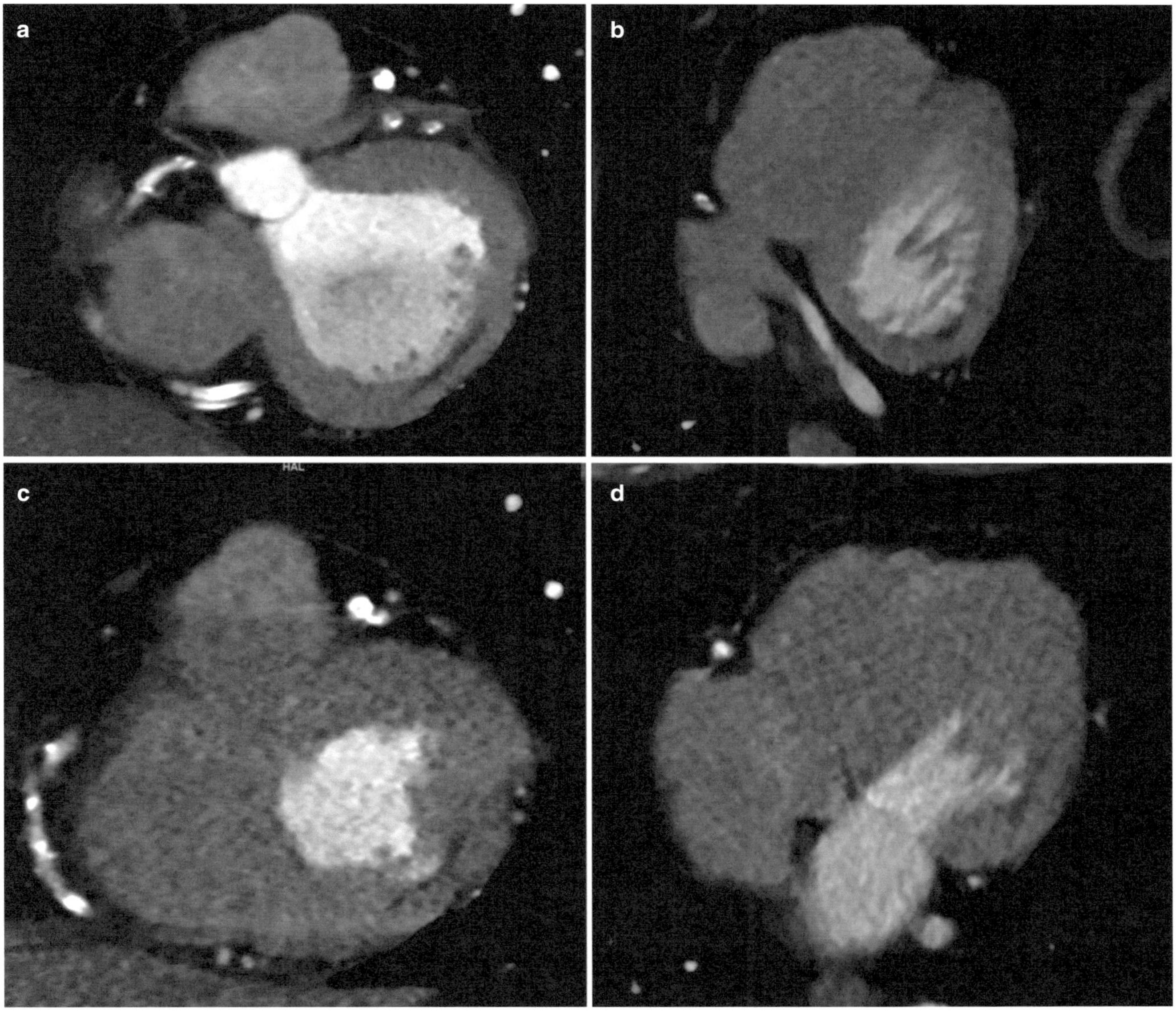

Fig. 61.5 A 55-year-old patient with a long-standing history of diabetes and stable angina who underwent retrospectively ECG-gated coronary CTA (**a–d**, **a–b**, diastolic reconstruction; **c–d**, systolic reconstruction) followed by static adenosine-stress perfusion (**e**, **f**). Subendocardial hypoattenuation in the basal inferolateral myocardial segment can be appreciated in diastolic and systolic reconstructions even under rest. Under adenosine stress, the hypoattenuated area is considerably larger (**e**, **f**), consistent with a partially reversible perfusion defect and highly suggestive of on older non-transmural infarct with significant adjacent ischemia

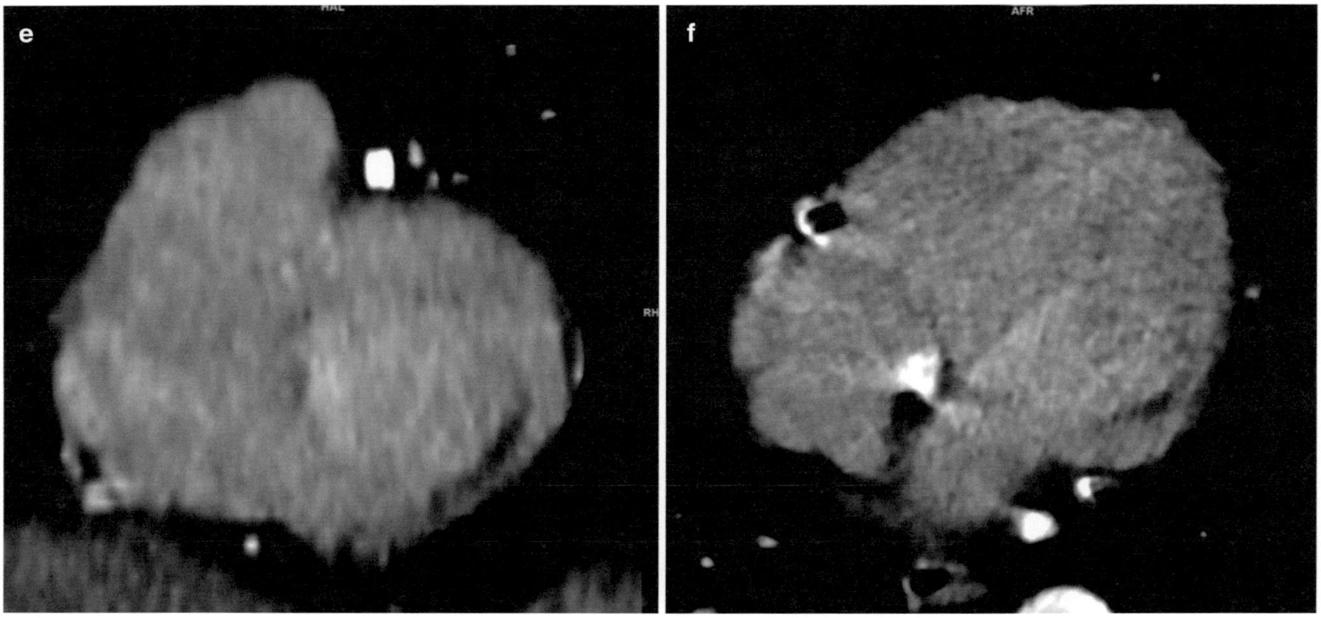

Fig. 61.5 (continued)

summed stress score (SSS), and the summed difference score (SDS). The SRS and the SSS are calculated by adding the ischemia scores for all segments at rest or stress, respectively, and the SDS is the difference between both. The diagnostic and prognostic validity of this method still needs to be confirmed for CT perfusion.

Correlation of Coronary Anatomy with Myocardial Perfusion Information

Ultimately, myocardial perfusion information will have to be matched to coronary anatomy both in respect to the individual vessel anatomy and stenoses identified on CCTA. By aligning anatomic with functional information, subtle changes in myocardial perfusion will likely be detected with higher sensitivity and perfusion defects without attributable coronary stenosis easier identified as false-positive findings.

Evidence from Clinical Studies

By now substantial clinical evidence has been accumulated demonstrating good diagnostic accuracy of static CT perfusion for the detection of segmental myocardial ischemia, both from single-center and multicenter studies.

Single-Center Studies

Various single-center studies with often small sample sizes and heterogeneous reference standards have analyzed diagnostic accuracy and/or potentially incremental value of static CT perfusion in diverse clinical scenarios.

Bettencourt et al. have investigated 90 symptomatic patients with suspected CAD who underwent static adenosine-stress CT perfusion followed by CCTA and ICA and report a significant increase in diagnostic accuracy for the detection of stenoses ≥50% and ≥70% by the addition of perfusion information [48]. Particularly for the detection of higher-grade CAD, the AUC increased from 0.8 for isolated CCTA to 0.93 for the integrated approach.

Wong et al. analyzed 75 symptomatic patients who underwent CCTA/rest CT perfusion, static adenosine-stress CT perfusion, and ICA/FFR assessment within 2 months at a single institution [49]. The authors compared the diagnostic performance for the prediction of FFR-relevant coronary artery stenosis between CCTA only, CCTA + stress CT perfusion information, CCTA + transluminal attenuation gradient information, and an integrated protocol combining all three sources of information (i.e., CCTA + stress-rest CT perfusion + transluminal attenuation gradient).

For CCTA only the authors reported sensitivities and specificities of 89% and 65% for the prediction of FFR-relevant coronary artery stenosis, while for CCTA + CT perfusion, sensitivity and specificity were 88% and 83%. Diagnostic accuracy was highest for the integrated protocol (AUC = 0.91).

Yang et al. have recently reported results from a single-center study including 75 patients with suspected CAD (ClinicalTrials.gov, NCT 01696006), in whom stress-rest static CT perfusion using adenosine was compared with ICA + FFR [50]. The authors performed retrospectively ECG-gated acquisitions for both the stress and rest CT perfusion acquisition. The per-patient sensitivity and specificity of a visual assessment of myocardial perfusion CT data for all patients were 89% and 86%, respectively. In severely calcified vessels, visual assessment of myocardial perfusion CT data in combination with CCTA provided incremental value over CCTA alone for the detection of myocardial ischemia.

Meta-analyses

Some recent meta-analyses have reported pooled data from various single-center trials on myocardial perfusion CT. Pelgrim et al. pooled data from six studies (including one multicenter study) and reported for combined coronary CT angiography and static stress CT perfusion a vessel-based sensitivity and specificity for the detection of ICA-based >50% stenoses of 84% and 93% [22]. Gonzalez et al. pooled 18 studies in which CCTA was complemented with stress CT perfusion or CT-FFR and report that CT perfusion increased the specificity of CCTA from 0.43 to 0.77 for the detection of >50% stenoses as assessed by ICA [51]. It is important to note, however, that Gonzalez et al. pooled data regardless of whether a static or dynamic CT perfusion protocol was used.

Multicenter Studies

CORE320 Study (www.clinicaltrials.gov, NCT00934037)

The CORE320 study (www.clinicaltrials.gov, NCT00934037) is the most comprehensive trial so far addressing the feasibility and accuracy of rest-stress static CT perfusion in symptomatic patients.

As a prospective, multicenter, multinational diagnostic study, it included 381 patients and was designed for the main primary objective to evaluate the diagnostic accuracy of 320-MDCT for detecting coronary artery luminal stenosis and corresponding myocardial perfusion deficits using a rest-stress static CT perfusion approach in patients with suspected CAD. The reference standard was invasive coronary angiography (ICA) and SPECT myocardial perfusion imaging [52].

The study population consisted of patients 45–85 years old who were referred for clinically indicated conventional angiography for suspected or known CAD [52]. 30% of patients had had prior percutaneous intervention, and 28% were status post coronary stent implantation. Prevalence of anatomically significant CAD as assessed by quantitative ICA was 60%.

The CT protocol comprised an unenhanced coronary artery calcium score acquisition, followed by rest CCTA (used for coronary CT angiography as well as rest perfusion) after administration of beta-blocker and sublingual nitrates, followed by adenosine-stress CT perfusion imaging with 20-min delay prior to stress perfusion acquisition. All patients underwent rest-stress SPECT myocardial perfusion imaging as well as invasive coronary angiography within 60 days.

The authors report that the addition of myocardial perfusion to CCTA significantly increased the accuracy for the detection of flow-limiting CAD as assessed by ICA-SPECT. This was demonstrated by a significant increase in the area under the curve (AUC) for the detection of ≥50% stenosis from 0.82 to 0.87 by CCTA alone vs. CCTA-CTP ($p \leq 0.001$). The highest test performance was observed in the subgroup of patients without known CAD (AUC = 0.93).

The authors conclude that the combination of CTA and perfusion correctly identifies patients with flow-limiting CAD defined as ≥50% stenosis by ICA causing perfusion defect by SPECT/MPI.

Furthermore, in head-to-head comparisons, the overall performance of stress CTP imaging in the diagnosis of anatomic coronary stenosis ≥50% (with ICA as gold standard) was higher than that of SPECT, driven in part by the higher sensitivity for left main and multivessel disease [53]. The AUC for the detection of any coronary stenosis ≥50% was 0.78 for rest-stress CT perfusion imaging and 0.69 for rest-stress SPECT imaging ($p = 0.001$). In comparison with SPECT, CT perfusion exhibited slightly lower specificity (55% vs. 67%, $p = 0.02$) but considerably higher sensitivity (88% vs. 62%, $p < 0.001$) [53, 54].

Radiation exposure of rest and stress CCTA was 3.16 (2.82–3.63) and 5.31 (3.81–6.04) mSv, respectively, with higher doses required for the stress acquisition. This was mostly due to the higher heart rates during adenosine stress (69 vs. 54 bpm). On the other hand, radiation exposure of rest-stress SPECT and of ICA were 9.75 (9.1–13) mSv and 12.0 (7.6–18.0) mSv, respectively [55].

Regadenoson Crossover Study (www.clinicaltrials.gov, NCT01334918)

Cury et al. recently published the results of a multicenter, multivendor, randomized, crossover clinical trial comparing regadenoson stress-rest static CT perfusion with regadenoson stress-rest SPECT in 110 patients with known or suspected CAD (moderate or high risk) and a clinical indication for stress-rest SPECT or CCTA [56].

The vast majority of patients underwent a retrospectively ECG-gated acquisition for stress CT perfusion after regadenoson administration followed by prospectively ECG-triggered rest CT perfusion/CCTA. Patients were randomized into either having the stress-rest SPECT on the day before or after stress-rest CT perfusion [57].

Due to the potentially higher adverse event rate of regadenoson upon initial administration (on the first day of the study), patients were randomized into either possible sequence of scans (i.e., SPECT-CT vs. CT-SPECT).

In this study, stress CT perfusion was noninferior to SPECT for detecting or excluding reversible ischemia with an agreement rate of 0.87 and sensitivity and specificity of 0.9 and 0.84, respectively [56]. Total mean radiation dose was significantly higher for stress-rest CT perfusion (17.7 ± 6.8 mSv) compared with stress-rest SPECT (11.2 ± 1.8 mSv, $p = 0.001$).

Bischoff et al. 2016

Results from a smaller multicenter study evaluating stress-rest static CT perfusion in symptomatic patients with prior revascularization in comparison with stress-rest SPECT and ICA were recently reported by Bischoff et al. [25]. Thirty-six patients who presented with new onset symptoms requiring ICA were included and underwent a stress-rest static CT perfusion protocol (with injection of the radionuclide for stress SPECT MPI during stress CT perfusion imaging) immediately followed by stress and rest SPECT acquisition and ICA within 1 week prior to or after the CT scan.

The stress CT protocol consisted of a prospectively ECG-triggered high-pitch spiral acquisition planned to scan the entire heart in the same systolic phase (commencing at 5% of the RR interval) during adenosine or after regadenoson injection. After a delay of 15–20 min, beta-blockers and sublingual nitroglycerine were administered prior to a prospectively ECG-triggered CCTA with relatively broad acquisition of systole and diastole.

The authors report that in this cohort of patients with known CAD and extensive vessel calcifications, the overall diagnostic accuracy for the detection of hemodynamically relevant coronary artery stenosis was only 31% for CCTA alone and could be increased to 78% when integrating the information obtained from stress-rest CT perfusion. Importantly, the high-pitch acquisition of the heart in systole had an effective dose of only 0.9 ± 0.1 mSv.

Clinical Studies Involving Protocol Modifications

Nakamori et al. have recently suggested that in patients with high calcium scores (>400 Agatston units) and/or prior stents, a static CT stress perfusion-only acquisition might suffice [58]. In these patients, the authors argue, the rate of nondiagnostic coronary artery segments will be not negligible for both the stress and the rest acquisition. Therefore, the addition of an acquisition at rest yields comparably little additional information. In 35 patients with high calcium scores and/or stents who underwent stress-rest static CT perfusion as well as ICA/FFR, stress CT perfusion had an AUC of 0.97 for the detection of hemodynamically significant stenoses which was not improved by the addition of the rest perfusion/CCTA [58].

Conclusion

The high pace of technological innovations in cardiac CT has extended its reach to the evaluation of ischemic cardiomyopathy, enabling pharmacological stress myocardial CT perfusion imaging. This extension promises to cover one of the traditionally weaker flanks of cardiac CT: the specificity and positive predictive value in the detection of hemodynamically significant stenoses. Furthermore, diagnostic accuracy in the assessment of stent patency and severely calcified coronary trees may be increased.

Future clinical studies will have to address the differences between static and dynamic acquisition protocols, as the former cannot provide fully quantitative data but come at considerably lower radiation doses.

Regarding further technical progress, the best is yet to come: further improvements in hardware will result in wider detectors and higher temporal and spatial resolution. Someday, photon-counting detectors with energy discrimination capabilities might make their way into clinical practice. On the software side, much is to be expected in the short term from further refinements in reconstruction algorithms such as more advanced versions of iterative reconstruction and raw data-based motion correction algorithms and in the medium term from the full implementation of neural network-/deep learning-based raw data postprocessing and data interpretation. Furthermore, the full digitalization of the interface between the image information and all other patient data in conjunction with the expected rapid implementation of artificial intelligence to a wide spectrum of clinical problems will result in considerably improved and individually tailored diagnostic and prognostic results for each and every patient.

With the already proven excellent diagnostic accuracy of stress CT perfusion for the detection of myocardial ischemia and thus the hemodynamic relevance of coronary artery stenoses in conjunction with the unsurpassed capability of characterizing coronary artery plaques among noninvasive imaging modalities, the one-stop shop in cardiac imaging that has been heralded so fervently and repeatedly now more than ever seems to be just around the corner.

References

1. Menke J, Kowalski J. Diagnostic accuracy and utility of coronary CT angiography with consideration of unevaluable results: a systematic review and multivariate Bayesian random-effects meta-analysis with intention to diagnose. Eur Radiol. 2016;26(2):451–8.
2. von Ballmoos MW, et al. Meta-analysis: diagnostic performance of low-radiation-dose coronary computed tomography angiography. Ann Intern Med. 2011;154(6):413–20.
3. Samad Z, et al. A meta-analysis and systematic review of computed tomography angiography as a diagnostic triage tool for patients with chest pain presenting to the emergency department. J Nucl Cardiol. 2012;19(2):364–76.

4. Hulten E, et al. Outcomes after coronary computed tomography angiography in the emergency department: a systematic review and meta-analysis of randomized, controlled trials. J Am Coll Cardiol. 2013;61(8):880–92.
5. Di Carli MF, et al. Relationship between CT coronary angiography and stress perfusion imaging in patients with suspected ischemic heart disease assessed by integrated PET-CT imaging. J Nuclear Cardiol. 2007;14(6):799–809.
6. Pijls NHJ, et al. Fractional flow reserve versus angiography for guiding percutaneous coronary intervention in patients with multivessel coronary artery disease: 2-year follow-up of the FAME (Fractional Flow Reserve Versus Angiography for Multivessel Evaluation) study. J Am Coll Cardiol. 2010;56(3):177–84.
7. Shaw LJ, et al. Optimal medical therapy with or without percutaneous coronary intervention to reduce ischemic burden: results from the Clinical Outcomes Utilizing Revascularization and Aggressive Drug Evaluation (COURAGE) trial nuclear substudy. Circulation. 2008;117(10):1283–91.
8. Gould KL, Lipscomb K, Hamilton GW. Physiologic basis for assessing critical coronary stenosis. Instantaneous flow response and regional distribution during coronary hyperemia as measures of coronary flow reserve. Am J Cardiol. 1974;33(1):87–94.
9. Uren NG, et al. Relation between myocardial blood flow and the severity of coronary-artery stenosis. N Engl J Med. 1994;330(25):1782–8.
10. Adams D, et al. Computed tomography of the normal and infarcted myocardium. Am J Roentgenol. 1976;126(4):786–91.
11. Powell WJ, et al. Detection of edema associated with myocardial ischemia by computerized tomography in isolated, arrested canine hearts. Circulation. 1977;55(1):99–108.
12. Siemers PT, et al. Detection, quantitation and contrast enhancement of myocardial infarction utilizing computerized axial tomography: comparison with histochemical staining and 99mTc-pyrophosphate imaging. Investig Radiol. 1978;13(2):103–9.
13. Wolfkiel CJ, et al. Measurement of myocardial blood flow by ultrafast computed tomography. Circulation. 1987;76(6):1262–73.
14. Rumberger JA, Feiring AJ, et al. Use of ultrafast computed tomography to quantitate regional myocardial perfusion: a preliminary report. J Am Coll Cardiol. 1987;9(1):59–69.
15. Rumberger JA, Stanford W, Marcus ML. Quantitation of regional myocardial perfusion by ultrafast CT: promises and pitfalls. Am J Card Imaging. 1987;1(4):336–43.
16. Gould RG. Perfusion quantitation by ultrafast computed tomography. Investig Radiol. 1992;27(Suppl 2):S18–21.
17. Bell MR, Lerman LO, Rumberger JA. Validation of minimally invasive measurement of myocardial perfusion using electron beam computed tomography and application in human volunteers. Heart. 1999;81(6):628–35.
18. Salerno M, Beller GA. Noninvasive assessment of myocardial perfusion. Circ Cardiovasc Imaging. 2009;2(5):412–24.
19. Dawson P. Cardiovascular effects of contrast agents. Am J Cardiol. 1989;64(9):2E–9E.
20. Canty JM, et al. First-pass entry of nonionic contrast agent into the myocardial extravascular space. Effects on radiographic estimates of transit time and blood volume. Circulation. 1991;84(5):2071–8.
21. Bae KT. Intravenous contrast medium administration and scan timing at CT: considerations and approaches 1. Radiology. 2010;256(1):32–61.
22. Pelgrim GJ, et al. The dream of a one-stop-shop: meta-analysis on myocardial perfusion CT. Eur J Radiol. 2015;84(12):2411–20.
23. Caruso D, et al. Dynamic CT myocardial perfusion imaging. Eur J Radiol. 2016;85(10):1893–9.
24. Cannaò PM, et al. Technical prerequisites and imaging protocols for dynamic and dual energy myocardial perfusion imaging. Eur J Radiol. 2015;84(12):2401–10.
25. Bischoff B, et al. Myocardial ischemia detection with single-phase CT perfusion in symptomatic patients using high-pitch helical image acquisition technique. Int J Cardiovasc Imaging. 2017;33(4):569–76.
26. Jin KN, et al. Myocardial perfusion imaging with dual energy CT. Eur J Radiol. 2016;85(10):1914–21.
27. De Cecco CN, et al. White paper of the Society of Computed Body Tomography and Magnetic Resonance on dual-energy CT, part 3: vascular, cardiac, pulmonary, and musculoskeletal applications. J Comput Assist Tomogr. 2017;41(1):1–7.
28. Meinel FG, et al. First–arterial-pass dual-energy CT for assessment of myocardial blood supply: do we need rest, stress, and delayed acquisition? Comparison with SPECT. Radiology. 2014;270(3):708–16.
29. Arnoldi E, et al. CT detection of myocardial blood volume deficits: dual-energy CT compared with single-energy CT spectra. J Cardiovasc Comput Tomogr. 2011;5(6):421–9.
30. Koonce JD, et al. Accuracy of dual-energy computed tomography for the measurement of iodine concentration using cardiac CT protocols: validation in a phantom model. Eur Radiol. 2014;24(2):512–8.
31. Steveson C, et al. The effect of heart rate on exposure window and best phase for stress perfusion computed tomography. J Comput Assist Tomogr. 2017;41(2):242–8.
32. Taillefer R, et al. Acute beta-blockade reduces the extent and severity of myocardial perfusion defects with dipyridamole Tc-99m sestamibi SPECT imaging. J Am Coll Cardiol. 2003;42(8):1475–83.
33. George RT, et al. Adenosine stress 64- and 256-row detector computed tomography angiography and perfusion imaging: a pilot study evaluating the transmural extent of perfusion abnormalities to predict atherosclerosis causing myocardial ischemia. Circ Cardiovasc Imaging. 2009;2(3):174–82.
34. Techasith T, Cury RC. Stress myocardial CT perfusion: an update and future perspective. JACC Cardiovasc Imaging. 2011;4(8):905–16.
35. Seitun S, et al. Stress computed tomography myocardial perfusion imaging: a new topic in cardiology. Rev Esp Cardiol (English Edition). 2016;69(2):188–200.
36. Bischoff B, et al. Optimal timing for first-pass stress CT myocardial perfusion imaging. Int J Cardiovasc Imaging. 2013;29(2):435–42.
37. Tanabe Y, et al. Optimal scan time for single-phase myocardial computed tomography perfusion to detect myocardial ischemia–derivation cohort from dynamic myocardial computed tomography perfusion. Circ J. 2016;80(12):2506–12.
38. Pelgrim GJ, et al. Optimal timing of image acquisition for arterial first pass CT myocardial perfusion imaging. Eur J Radiol. 2017;86:227–33.
39. Ghoshhajra BB, et al. A comparison of reconstruction and viewing parameters on image quality and accuracy of stress myocardial CT perfusion. J Cardiovasc Comput Tomogr. 2011;5(6):459–66.
40. Kitagawa K, et al. Characterization and correction of beam-hardening artifacts during dynamic volume CT assessment of myocardial perfusion. Radiology. 2010;256(1):111–8.
41. Bucher AM, et al. Quantitative evaluation of beam-hardening artefact correction in dual-energy CT myocardial perfusion imaging. Eur Radiol. 2016;26(9):3215–22.
42. Mehra VC, Valdiviezo C, et al. A stepwise approach to the visual interpretation of CT-based myocardial perfusion. J Cardiovasc Comput Tomogr. 2011;5(6):357–69.
43. Raff GL, et al. SCCT guidelines for the interpretation and reporting of coronary computed tomographic angiography. J Cardiovasc Comput Tomogr. 2009;3(2):122–36.
44. Keijer JT, et al. Magnetic resonance imaging of regional myocardial perfusion in patients with single-vessel coronary artery disease: quantitative comparison with (201)Thallium-SPECT and coronary angiography. J Magn Reson Imaging. 2000;11(6):607–15.

45. Mehra VC, Ambrose M, et al. CT-based myocardial perfusion imaging-practical considerations: acquisition, image analysis, interpretation, and challenges. J Cardiovasc Transl Res. 2011;4(4):437–48.
46. Kitagawa K, et al. Prospective ECG-gated 320 row detector computed tomography: implications for CT angiography and perfusion imaging. Int J Cardiovasc Imaging. 2009;25(2):201.
47. Palmas W, et al. Incremental prognostic value of exercise thallium-201 myocardial single-photon emission computed tomography late after coronary artery bypass surgery. J Am Coll Cardiol. 1995;25(2):403–9.
48. Bettencourt N, et al. Incremental value of an integrated adenosine stress-rest MDCT perfusion protocol for detection of obstructive coronary artery disease. J Cardiovasc Comput Tomogr. 2011;5(6):392–405.
49. Wong DTL, et al. Comparison of diagnostic accuracy of combined assessment using adenosine stress computed tomography perfusion + computed tomography angiography with transluminal attenuation gradient + computed tomography angiography against invasive fractional flow reserve. J Am Coll Cardiol. 2014;63(18):1904–12.
50. Yang DH, et al. Stress myocardial perfusion CT in patients suspected of having coronary artery disease: visual and quantitative analysis-validation by using fractional flow reserve. Radiology. 2015;276(3):715–23.
51. Gonzalez JA, et al. Meta-analysis of diagnostic performance of coronary computed tomography angiography, computed tomography perfusion, and computed tomography-fractional flow reserve in functional myocardial ischemia assessment versus invasive fractional flow reserve. Am J Cardiol. 2015;116(9):1469–78.
52. George RT, et al. Diagnostic performance of combined noninvasive coronary angiography and myocardial perfusion imaging using 320-MDCT: the CT angiography and perfusion methods of the CORE320 multicenter multinational diagnostic study. AJR Am J Roentgenol. 2011;197(4):829–37.
53. George RT, et al. Myocardial CT perfusion imaging and SPECT for the diagnosis of coronary artery disease: a head-to-head comparison from the CORE320 multicenter diagnostic performance study. Radiology. 2014;272(2):407–16.
54. Magalhães TA, et al. Combined coronary angiography and myocardial perfusion by computed tomography in the identification of flow-limiting stenosis – the CORE320 study: an integrated analysis of CT coronary angiography and myocardial perfusion. J Cardiovasc Comput Tomogr. 2015;9(5):438–45.
55. Rochitte CE, et al. Computed tomography angiography and perfusion to assess coronary artery stenosis causing perfusion defects by single photon emission computed tomography: the CORE320 study. Eur Heart J. 2014;35(17):1120–30.
56. Cury RC, et al. A randomized, multicenter, multivendor study of myocardial perfusion imaging with regadenoson CT perfusion vs single photon emission CT. J Cardiovasc Comput Tomogr. 2015;9(2):103–12–2.
57. Cury RC, et al. Regadenoson-stress myocardial CT perfusion and single-photon emission CT: rationale, design, and acquisition methods of a prospective, multicenter, multivendor comparison. J Cardiovasc Comput Tomogr. 2014;8(1):2–12.
58. Nakamori S, et al. Feasibility of stress-alone cardiac CT for detecting hemodynamically significant coronary stenosis in the presence of high coronary calcium score and coronary stents. Cardiovasc Imaging Asia. 2017;1(1):38–48.

Myocardial Perfusion Imaging: Dual-Energy Approaches

62

Domenico De Santis, Marwen Eid, Taylor M. Duguay, and Carlo N. De Cecco

The evaluation of patients presenting with symptoms suggestive of myocardial ischemia is one of the most common and challenging scenarios clinicians face. Despite considerable advances in treatment, more than 50% of acute myocardial infarctions (AMI) resulting in death occur in patients before undergoing cardiac catheterization. Thus, risk stratification plays a central role in averting major adverse cardiac events [1].

The current WHO rating attributes more than 25% of deaths worldwide to cardiovascular disease (CVD) [2]. Despite a decreasing trend in the last decade, CVD is the leading cause of death in the United States and worldwide. On average there is approximately one CVD-related death every 40 s, resulting in the death of over 2000 Americans each day. The estimated direct and indirect cost of CVD in 2015 was $320.1 billion and is projected to be $918 billion by 2030 [3, 4].

According to the current appropriate use criteria, coronary CT angiography (CCTA) is a robust imaging technique that provides a noninvasive, morphological assessment of the coronary arteries which can accurately depict coronary anatomy and atherosclerotic plaque burden. Thanks to its power to exclude significant coronary artery stenosis in patients with low and intermediate coronary artery disease (CAD) risk profiles [5], CCTA has become an integral part of the noninvasive diagnostic workup for the anatomic evaluation of the coronary arteries in patients with suspected CAD [5–8]. A growing body of evidence has validated CCTA as the noninvasive imaging technique with the highest sensitivity and specificity in detecting CAD, with a pooled sensitivity and specificity of 98% and 89%, respectively [6, 9]. These results compare favorably with alternative noninvasive imaging tests, where SPECT reaches sensitivities and specificities of 88% and 61%, PET of 84% and 81%, and cardiac magnetic resonance imaging (CMR) of 89% and 76%, respectively [10].

Although CCTA remains a morphological technique that can accurately depict coronary anatomy and atherosclerotic plaque burden, it is hampered by several limitations in the assessment of the hemodynamic significant coronary stenosis. The FAME and COURAGE trials [11, 12], two major studies validating the impact of functional tests in coronary revascularization, have shown that the hemodynamic relevance of coronary stenosis is not adequately predicted by purely anatomical tests. Additionally, without functional data, ICA and CCTA can only provide limited correlation with myocardial perfusion defects [13, 14]. As revascularization should be guided by information on the state of myocardial perfusion, increasing efforts aim at determining the functional relevance of lesions by CCTA. Thus, noninvasive evaluation of patients with suspected CAD has started to shift focus from morphological CAD assessment to a complex, comprehensive morphological and functional evaluation. Furthermore, patient evaluation, management, and prognostication are more reliable and effective when morphological and functional assessments are used in concert [11, 12, 14, 15].

Multiple CT techniques have the potential to provide a functional analysis. Some of these techniques are based on post-processing analysis of CCTA dataset and are focused on the direct assessment of coronary stenosis significance, such as CCTA-derived fractional flow reserve (CT-FFR) and transluminal attenuation gradient (TAG). CT-FFR relies on principles of computational fluid dynamics to calculate the ratio between the maximum coronary flow in the presence of

D. De Santis
Division of Cardiovascular Imaging, Department of Radiology and Radiological Science, Medical University of South Carolina, Charleston, SC, USA

Department of Radiological Sciences, Oncological and Pathological Sciences, University of Rome "Sapienza", Latina, Italy

T. M. Duguay (✉)
Division of Cardiovascular Imaging, Department of Radiology and Radiological Science, Medical University of South Carolina, Charleston, SC, USA
e-mail: duguay@musc.edu

M. Eid · C. N. De Cecco
Department of Radiology and Radiological Science, Medical University of South Carolina, Charleston, SC, USA

U. J. Schoepf (ed.), *CT of the Heart*, Contemporary Medical Imaging, https://doi.org/10.1007/978-1-60327-237-7_62

a coronary stenosis and the hypothetical maximum coronary flow in absence of stenosis. Despite excellent results in terms of diagnostic accuracy, the only CT-FFR software that has been granted FDA approval to date requires complex offsite analysis [16]. TAG represents the contrast attenuation gradient along the course of a coronary artery. The reliability of this technique is often hampered by extensive coronary calcifications or temporal inhomogeneity due to the acquisition window covering multiple heartbeats [17]. The correlation between coronary density and the corresponding aortic attenuation at the same axial slice, formally known as CCO (corrected coronary opacification), has been proposed as a method to achieve more robust results. However, TAG and CCO have inferior diagnostic performance when compared to other functional tests [18].

Other techniques based on CT data are focused on direct assessment of myocardial ischemia. Due to recent advancements in CT technology, in fact, in addition to its role in assessing coronary morphology and left ventricular function, CCTA has been utilized in the evaluation of a third aspect in the diagnostic algorithm of ischemic heart disease – myocardial perfusion. Computed tomography myocardial perfusion imaging (CTMPI) offers the possibility to directly detect the presence of perfusion defects in the myocardium following the administration of pharmacological stressing agent. Providing diagnostic information for each of these three cornerstones of ischemic heart disease workup, this emerging technology has the potential to become the stand-alone method for the evaluation of patients with suspected CAD using a single imaging modality and within a single imaging session [19].

CTMPI: General Overview

CT myocardial perfusion imaging (CTMPI) uses the distribution of iodinated contrast media (CM) in the myocardium as a surrogate for myocardial blood flow. Perfusion defects are thus identified as hypo-attenuating areas containing reduced amounts of CM [20]. For this purpose, two different CT techniques have been developed. *Static CTMPI* uses the static myocardial distribution of CM during the early arterial phase of the first-pass contrast enhancement to detect myocardial attenuation abnormalities [21]. In contrast, *Dynamic CTMPI* uses several consecutive acquisitions throughout the cardiac cycle to generate time attenuation curves (TAC) of myocardial perfusion. Static CTMPI can be further categorized into single-energy and dual-energy approaches.

The single-energy technique provides a *qualitative* visual assessment of a snapshot of myocardial iodine contrast attenuation at a single time point. Dual-energy CT (DECT) uses two simultaneous acquisitions of the same body region at two different kV values to generate a similar snapshot of the myocardial iodine distribution [22]. Since iodine concentration reflects myocardial perfusion, the per-voxel amount of iodine can be used to quantify the myocardial blood pool [23]. Iodine concentration is reduced in the myocardial areas with hypoperfusion and/or reduced intravascular blood volume [24]. This chapter will provide an overview of dual-energy CTPMI.

Dual-Energy CT Myocardial Perfusion Imaging

Technical Considerations

Computed tomography is based on the emission of a beam of x-rays from the x-ray tube. Two main determinants are responsible for the x-ray beam characteristics: intensity and energy. The intensity of the x-rays represents the amount of photons produced and is related to the tube current (milliamperage, mA). The energy of the x-ray beam is proportional to the difference of potential applied between the anode and the cathode of the x-ray tube and is measured in kilovolts (kV). When a certain kV value is selected, the chosen number represents the maximum kV that will be reached by the x-ray tube. Therefore, the maximum energy of the photons is determined by the peak kV; however the generated x-ray beam can be represented as a broad spectrum characterized by different photon energies (Fig. 62.1).

Dual-energy CT, also called spectral CT, by means of different technical solutions obtains two x-ray spectra. Different materials, such as iodine, calcium, and soft tissues, are characterized by different attenuation profiles at different energy levels (Fig. 62.2). Based on this tenant, dual-energy CT is able to differentiate materials with different atomic numbers, such as calcium and iodine, that look similar when scanned in single energy. Different vendor-specific CT technologies have been developed to perform DE acquisitions for the evaluation of myocardial perfusion:

- Single source – Sequential DECT (Canon Medical Systems, Otawara, Japan)
- Single source – Fast kV switching (GE Healthcare, Milwaukee, WI)
- Dual-source CT (Siemens Healthineers, Forchheim, Germany)
- Single source – Dual-layer detector (Philips Medical Systems, Cleveland, OH)
- Single source – Twin beam (Siemens Healthineers, Forchheim, Germany)

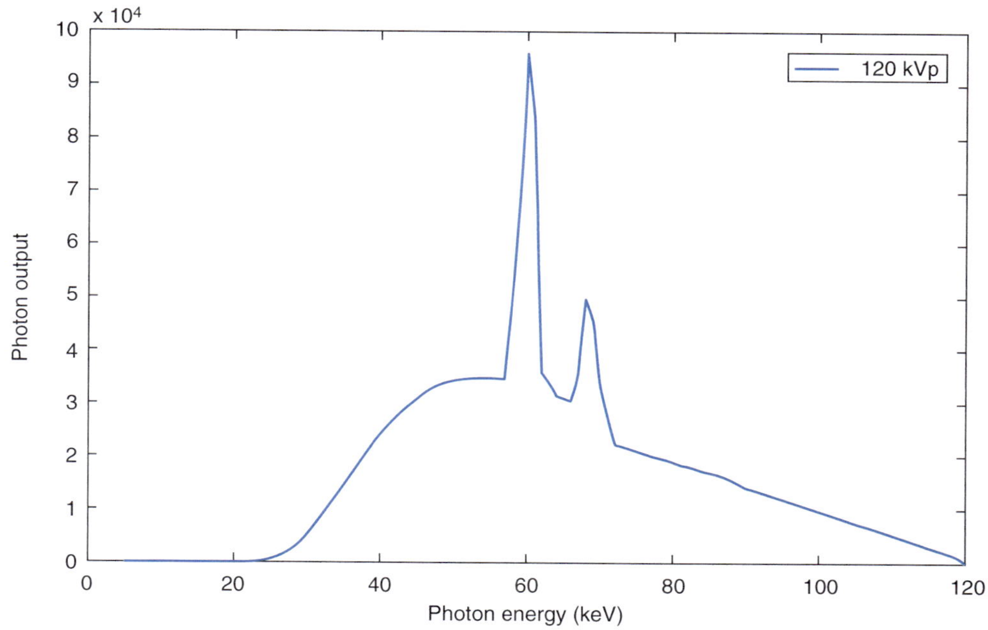

Fig. 62.1 Standard 120 kVp x-ray spectrum. The peak kV determines the maximum photon energy. However, the x-ray beam can be represented as a broad spectrum characterized by different photon energies. The spectrum is formed by the *bremsstrahlung radiation* (German word meaning "braking radiation") and two spikes representing the *characteristic radiations* of tungsten, the main material forming the anode target. The lower-energy x-rays don't contribute to the image, but they are responsible for part of the radiation dose since they are absorbed by the tissues

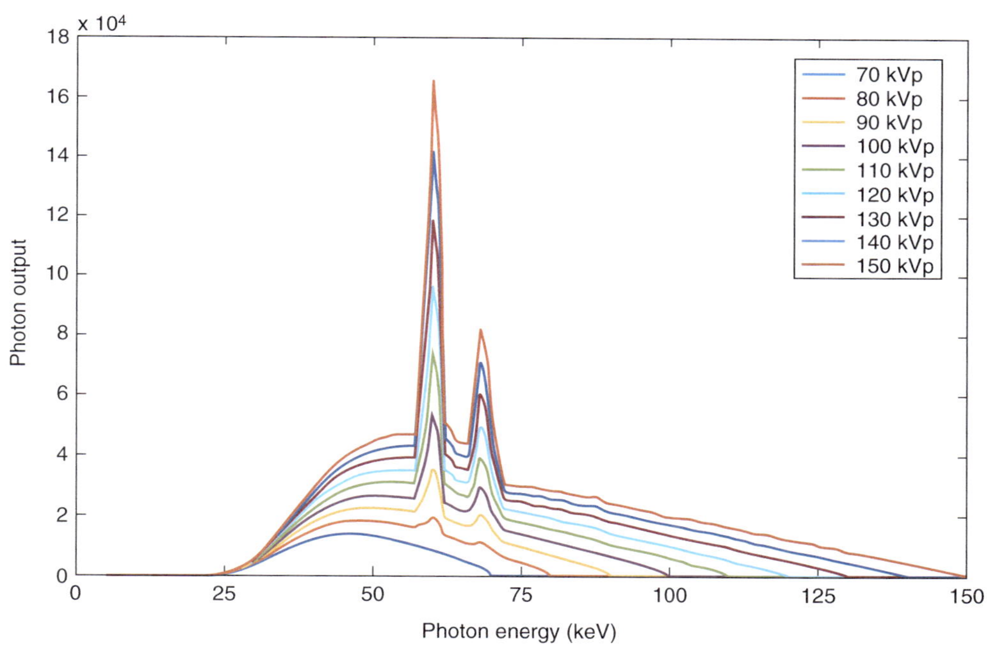

Fig. 62.2 Range of x-ray spectra that can be generated in dual-energy CT. The data of a low-energy spectrum and those derived from a high-energy spectrum are simultaneously analyzed to derive dual-energy datasets and material-specific information. The higher the kVp, the higher the number of output photons, reflecting in a *bremsstrahlung radiation* moving to the right of the graph (better x-ray quality) and higher peak for *characteristic radiations* (higher quantity of x-rays). It is worth noting that changes in kVp have no effect on the energies of the characteristic radiation and that the characteristic x-rays do not occur at kVp lower than 70 keV

The sequential DECT acquires DE data through ultrafast sequential rotations acquired in volume or helical mode. In volume mode, two single-rotation acquisitions at different kV levels are performed. In helical mode, the tube switches between the two kV levels at each rotation while the table is moving, resulting in a pitch characterized by partial overlap among the two kV levels [25] (Fig. 62.3a). The fast kV switching technique relies on a single x-ray tube able to switch between high- and low-kV settings within the same gantry rotation coupled with detectors able to register data

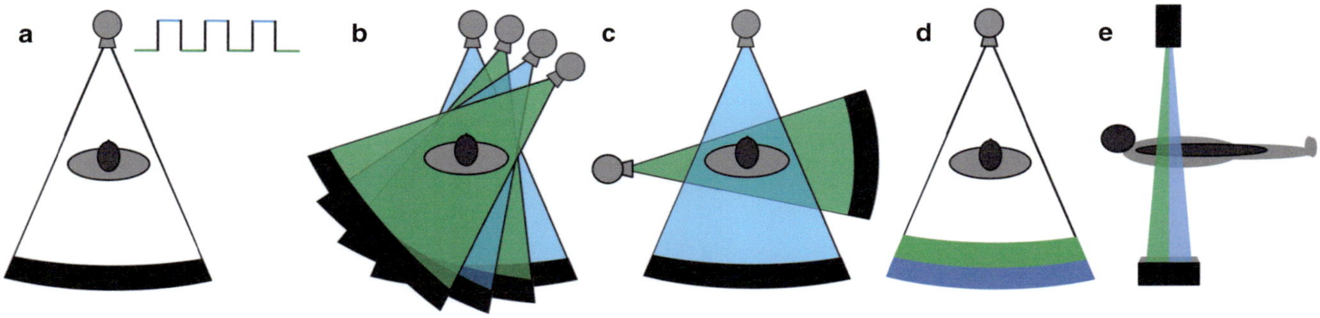

Fig. 62.3 Different DECT technologies: single source, sequential DECT (**a**); single source, fast kV switching (**b**); dual-source CT (**c**); single source, dual-layer detector (**d**); and single source, twin beam (**e**)

from both energy spectra (Fig. 62.3b) [26]. Dual-source dual-energy CT scanners have two different x-ray tubes mounted with an offset of approximately 90 degrees and are simultaneously operated at low- and high-tube voltages. Each tube is coupled with a dedicated detector layer (Fig. 62.3c). A third technical approach is represented by the dual-layer detector CT scanner (Fig. 62.3d) characterized by a single x-ray tube coupled with a detector composed of two superimposed layers. The inner layer registers data from low-energy photons, while the outer layer records information from the high-energy photons [27]. Twin beam dual energy uses a single x-ray tube emitting a polychromatic x-ray beam pre-filtered on the z-axis by means of two different materials: tin (Sn) and gold (Au). The resultant post-filtered beam is split in high (Sn)- and low-energy (Au) spectra before reaching the patient (Fig. 62.3e). The dual-source approach is the most widely adopted technique [24, 28–34]. To date, the state of the art of dual-source CT is represented by the third generation of CT scanners, which are characterized by a rotation time of 0.25 s, a temporal resolution of 66 ms, and maximal volume coverage of 737 mm/s in *flash* mode and are able to offer multiple kV setting ranging from 70 kV up to 150 kV, in 10 kV increments.

Dual-energy CT exams are composed of different datasets. Low-voltage and high-voltage spectra are combined with different blending proportion to obtain a dataset similar to the conventional 120 kVp dataset that is routinely used in clinical practice. Other unique characteristics of dual-energy CT examination include the possibility to obtain color-coded iodine maps, virtual non-contrast datasets, and virtual monoenergetic images. Iodine maps are overlaid to grayscale images, allowing both qualitative and quantitative myocardial perfusion assessment. The virtual non-contrast dataset has the ability to overcome the need for a true non-enhanced scan and, thus, to lower the radiation exposure. Eventually, virtual monoenergetic images at low photon energies, approaching the iodine K-edge, reduce the beam-hardening artifacts and enhance iodine attenuation, facilitating the identification of subtle attenuation differences within the myocardium when compared to 120 kVp dataset [35]. Figure 62.4 provides an overview on dual-energy workflow.

Acquisition Technique and Radiation Dose

As in CCTA, temporal resolution is one of the most important technical prerequisites for perfusion CT. A high temporal resolution is critical to reduce motion artifacts in consideration of the increased heart rate observed during the stress phase. However, previous challenges in temporal resolution have been overcome with second-generation (75 ms) [28] or third-generation (66 ms) [36] dual-source CT scanners. Similarly to the SE static technique, DE-CTMPI generates a snapshot of the myocardial iodine distribution at a single time point using two different kV acquisitions of the same body region; this snapshot encompasses the entire left ventricle and is acquired during the early arterial phase of first-pass contrast enhancement. A reduction in beam-hardening artifacts and direct visualization of myocardial iodine content gives DECT multiple advantages over a single-energy acquisition. For these reasons, perfusion defects and late enhancement are often more easily recognized on DECT [37]. Both prospective and retrospectively ECG-gated protocols are available for the DECT acquisition. In addition, hybrid image reconstruction enables imaging even at high heart rates [28]. Scan time and radiation dose for prospective ECG-triggered or retrospectively ECG-triggered acquisition are equivalent to those of single-energy cardiac CT acquisition [38].

Since image acquisition must be performed at the moment of peak contrast concentration in the coronary arteries to detect early differences in contrast uptake, acquisition timing is crucial to preserve diagnostic integrity. The optimal time

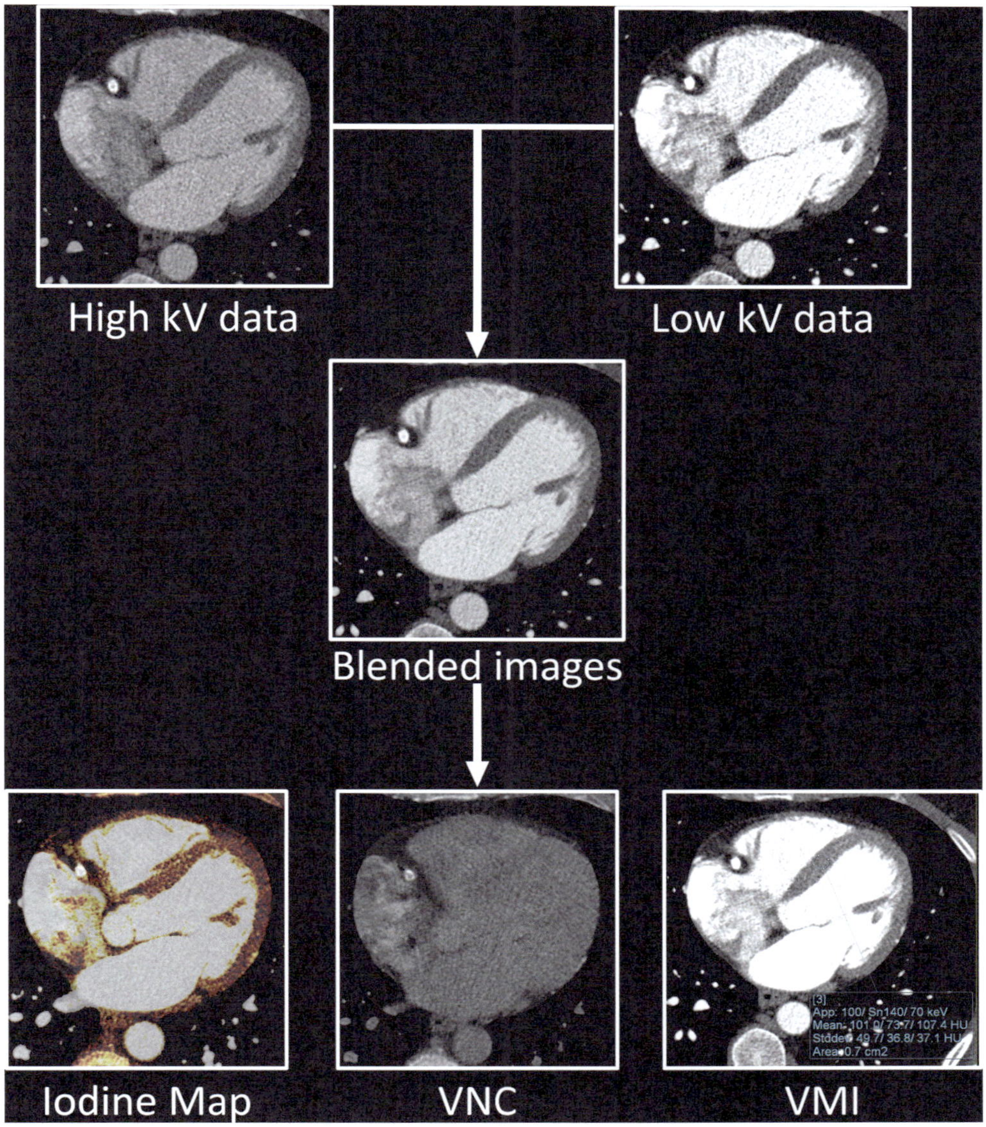

Fig. 62.4 Dual-energy CT workflow. High-kV and low-kV data are blended in order to simulate a conventional polychromatic dataset. Dual-energy CT allows to generate colored iodine maps that are superimposed on the grayscale images and lead to a qualitative and qualitative assessment of myocardial perfusion. Virtual non-contrast (VNC) images can overcome the need on the true unenhanced scan, while virtual monoenergetic images (VMI) at low keV level, approaching the k-edge of iodine, emphasize the contrast enhancement

frame for stress perfusion acquisition is between 8 s and 16 s after contrast enhancement in the aorta reaches 100 Hounsfield Units [21]. Acquisition timing may be further enhanced using bolus tracking with automatic contrast detection in the proximal ascending aorta. The right acquisition time is essential to detect the difference in early contrast uptake in myocardial tissue to ensure diagnostic accuracy. Furthermore, coronary artery assessment can be performed during the rest acquisition [37], with no additional acquisition time or radiation necessary.

If an assessment of myocardial perfusion at stress is desired, an additional acquisition during pharmacological stress can be obtained. Multiple approaches to the time order of rest and stress acquisitions have been proposed (Fig. 62.5). Starting the examination with the rest phase has the advantage that a pure CCTA study is performed before the evaluation of functional myocardial assessment [38]. On the other hand, starting the protocol with the stress phase avoids contamination of CM from the rest phase and enables maximal contrast difference between ischemic and normal myocardium [21]. However, it should be taken into account that the elevated heart rate following stress administration could impair the quality of the subsequent rest acquisition [32].

Additionally, image acquisition can be repeated after 8–10 min of CM administration in order to evaluate the delayed myocardial enhancement, where a hyperattenuating myocardial pattern is indicative of nonviable myocardium

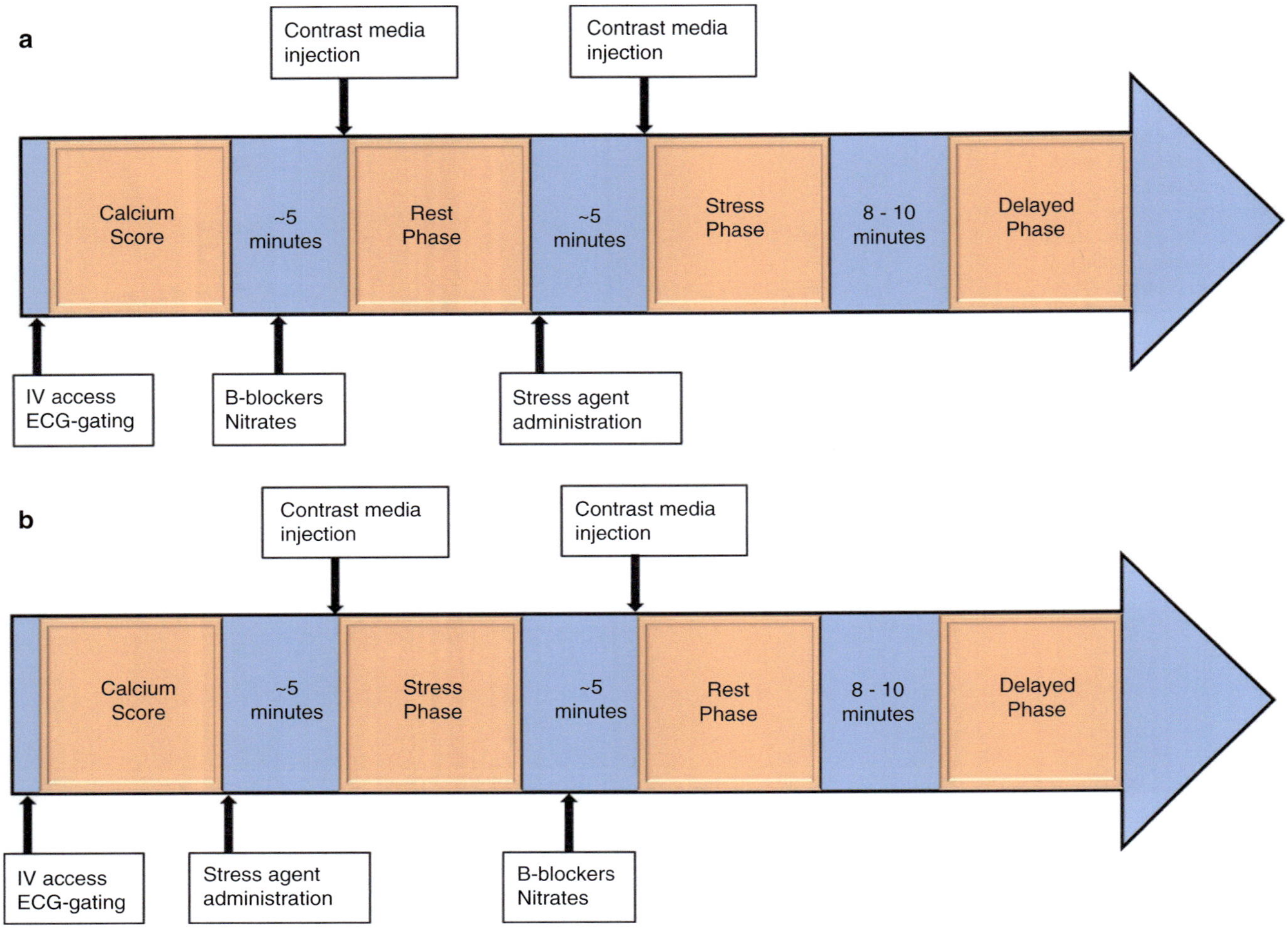

Fig. 62.5 Timeline of rest/stress (**a**) and stress/rest (**b**) DE-CTMPI protocols

(Fig. 62.6). Acquisitions utilizing this delayed enhancement, performed after invasive revascularization by percutaneous coronary intervention (PCI) procedures without additional administration of CM, have been proven to be a reliable method for evaluating transmurality and infarct size, representing an interesting alternative to CMR [39–41]. However, compared with late enhancement in CMR however, CT provides a lower signal-to-noise ratio, making the detection of infarction more challenging [23]. Additionally, Meinel et al. [42] recently demonstrated that the addition of a delayed phase acquisition for late iodine enhancement does not provide improvements in diagnostic accuracy and can thus be safely omitted in order to reduce the radiation dose.

Data sets obtained at high and low kV values in DECT can be used to create iodine concentration maps combining the lower noise of high-energy acquisitions with the higher contrast resolution of lower-energy acquisitions [33].

The radiation dose for comprehensive static CT perfusion studies (including rest and stress perfusion imaging) varies greatly depending on the specific acquisition protocol. Effective dose values between 4.2 and 16.5 mSv have been reported (Table 62.1) with an average radiation exposure of 9 mSv [43–55]. The radiation dose of CT myocardial perfusion imaging generally compares favorably with traditional nuclear imaging approaches [56–58] and is expected to decrease as new technologies are developed. Currently, the radiation dose of a comprehensive stress/rest static CTMPI protocol can be as low as 4.2 mSv [59, 60]. In terms of radiation dose, moreover, prospectively ECG-triggered or retrospectively ECG-triggered acquisitions are equivalent to those of CCTA acquisition, in which the rest and the stress acquisitions deliver a combined average dose of 12 mSv. This value may be decreased using recent technological advancements, including iterative reconstruction and low-kV acquisition [49, 61, 62].

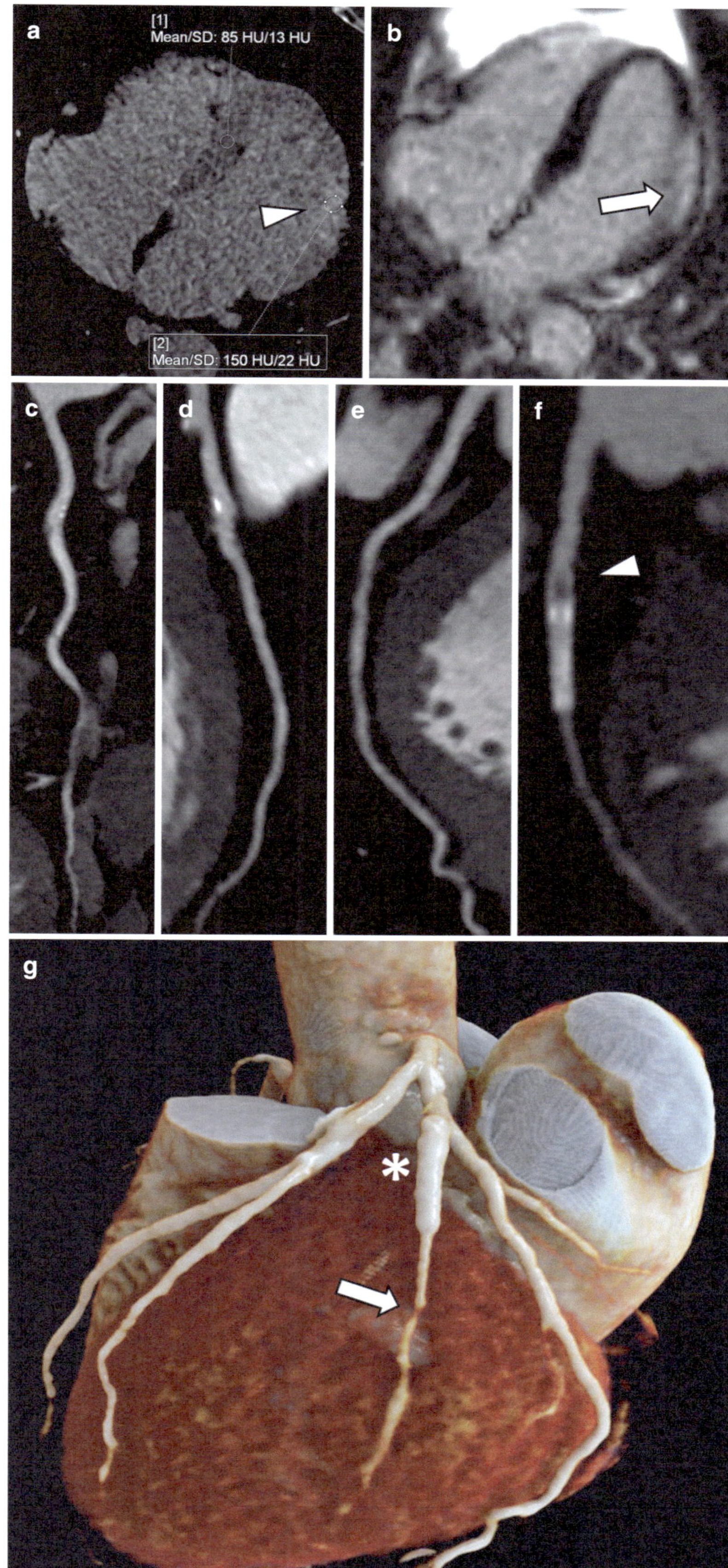

Fig. 62.6 A 63-year-old female. (**a**) CTMPI acquired 10 min administration of contrast media demonstrates a transmural area of hyperattenuating myocardial pattern in the lateral wall and is indicative of nonviable myocardium (arrowhead). The same patient underwent a CMRI (**b**) showing an extensive area of late enhancement in the corresponding myocardial wall (arrow). Curved multi-planar reformats of the coronary arteries show no significant stenosis at the RCA (**c**), LAD (**d**), and LCx (**e**). On the contrary, the first obtuse marginal branch (**f**) previously stented is affected by proximal intimal hyperplasia resulting in severe in-stent stenosis (arrowhead). (**g**) Cinematic Rendering clearly depicts the stent (asterisk) and the filiform caudal segment (arrow), poorly opacified by the contrast media

Table 62.1 Static dual-energy CT myocardial perfusion studies

Author	Patient population	CT technology	CT perfusionprotocol	AverageCT dose (mSv)	Reference technique	Level of analysis	Sensitivity (%)	Specificity (%)	PPV (%)	NPV (%)
Ruzsics (2009) [46]	36	First DSCT	Rest	14	SPECT	Segment Patient	92 97	93 67	83 93	97 80
Bauer (2010) [92]	36	First DSCT	Rest	9.7	CMR	Segment	77	97	85	96
Nagao (2010) [93]	10	First DSCT	Stress	NR	SPECT, ICA	Vessel	86	75	NR	NR
Nance (2011) [41]	12	First DSCT	Rest	NR	ICA	Segment	91	95	82	98
Ko (2011) [44]	41	First DSCT	Stress	8.6	CMR	Segment	89	78	74	91
Wang (2011) [63]	31	First DSCT	Rest	10.5	SPECT	Segment Vessel	68 81	93 92	82 89	86 85
Meyer (2012) [45]	50	Second DSCT	Rest/stress/delayed	13.4	CMR	Patient	90	71	NR	NR
Ko (2012) [69]	45	First DSCT	Rest/stress	16.5	ICA	Vessel	89	74	80	85
Weininger (2012) [70]	20	Second DSCT	Stress	12.8	SPECT CMR	Segment Segment	94 93	98 99	92 92	94 96
Delgado (2013) [71]	56	Second DSCT	Stress	8.2	CMR	Segment	76	99	89	98
Ko (2014) [59]	40	First DSCT	Rest Stress	4.2 4.6	CMR, ICA	Vessel[a] Vessel[b]	42 87	83 79	59 71	70 91
Ko (2014) [60]	100	First DSCT	Stress	4.2	CMR	Segment Vessel Patient	76 89 97	80 74 36	63 73 82	88 90 82
Kim (2014) [68]	50	Second DSCT	Stress/rest	11.4	CMR	Segment Patient	77 94	94 71	53 60	98 96
Zhao (2014) [94]	60	Second DSCT	Rest	NR	ICA	Segment	94	91	88	96
Kido (2014) [95]	21	First and second DSCT	Stress	7.7	ICA	Vessel	67	92	84	82

De Cecco (2014) [75]	29	Second DSCT	Rest Stress	5.8 6.6	ICA	Patient – morphological analysis	95[c] 95[d] 100[e] 90[f]	50[c] 50[d] 33[e] 67[f]	NR	NR
					SPECT	Patient – hemodynamic analysis	91[c] 95[d] 100[e] 86[f]	38[c] 75[d] 38[e] 75[f]		
Delgado (2016) [72]	36	Second DSCT	Stress	5.4	CMR	Segment	72.6[g] 72.6[h]	95.7[g] 94.7[h]	73.6[g] 68.8[h]	95.5[g] 95.5[h]
						Vessel	87.5[g] 91.6[h]	86.2[g] 85.9[h]	72.4[g] 73.5[h]	94.5[g] 96[h]
						Patient	100[g] 100[h]	90[g] 91[h]	92[g] 32[h]	100[g] 100[h]

Abbreviations: *PPV* positive predictive value, *NPV* negative predictive value, *CMR* cardiovascular magnetic resonance, *DSCT* dual-source computed tomography, *ICA* invasive coronary angiography, *SPECT* single-photon emission computed tomography, *NR* not reported

[a]Combined CT angiography and rest CT perfusion
[b]Combined CT angiography and stress CT perfusion
[c]Rest
[d]Stress
[e]Combined – either positive
[f]Combined – both positive
[g]Reader 1
[h]Reader 2

Pharmacological Stress Agents

Diseased coronary arteries have a limited compensatory dilation, since they are already operating within a dilatory reserve capacity to compensate for reduced perfusion. On the contrary, healthy coronary vessels maintain a dilating capacity when oxygen demand is increased [25–27]. Hypo-attenuated myocardium during pharmacological stress is classified by comparison with images in rest conditions. Areas with constant hypo-attenuation during both phases correspond to irreversible ischemia. Reversible ischemia can be suspected if hypo-attenuation is present only in stress phase or if the hypo-attenuated area increases significantly [1].

Since the reversible myocardial perfusion defects (MPD) occur prior to fixed MPD, sensitivity for the detection of reversible perfusion defects significantly improves under pharmacological stress [26]. The various agents available to induce pharmacological stress include dobutamine, dipyridamole, adenosine, and regadenoson [28]. Due to safety considerations, the two most commonly utilized agents in CT perfusion are adenosine and regadenoson.

The first adenosine stress myocardial perfusion CT study was conducted with an electron-beam CT scanner in an experimental dog model in 1987 [29]. Adenosine is a nonselective adenosine receptor agonist. Its action is a direct vasodilation of the coronary arteries and has an extremely short half-life of a few seconds. It is administered in continuous infusion with a dose of 140 μg/kg/min for at least 2 min to induce a heart rate increase of 10–20 beats above the resting heart rate. Regadenoson is a selective A_{2A} receptor agonist. It is advantageous as it can be administered in a single bolus, making stress CT studies more time efficient [28]. Regadenoson stress, moreover, causes fewer systemic side effects, which is beneficial for patients with asthma or chronic obstructive pulmonary disease [30, 31]. On the other hand, to take into account the longer-lasting effects of regadenoson, sufficient time needs to be allowed before rest acquisition (15–20 min). Alternatively, theophylline can be administered as a countermeasure [32]. The use of regadenoson showed greater efficiency over dipyridamole and adenosine in a stress/rest protocol [28]. This was attributed mostly to the administration of the substance, because regadenoson is available as a pre-drawn single-dose syringe. Typical side effects of both agents are headache, flushing, and dyspnea. Both drugs may cause moderate to severe complications [33, 34]. Ventricular tachycardia and transient asymptomatic atrial-ventricular block occur in 0.14% of patients. Recent case reports indicate that adenosine and regadenoson may cause acute myocardial infarction and death [34–36].

Dipyridamole and dobutamine can also be used as stress agents. Dipyridamole acts as an indirect vasodilator, increasing the endogenous level of adenosine by blocking cellular uptake. It is also administered through continuous infusion with a dose 140 μg/kg/min for 4–6 min. Since its half-life is longer than adenosine, aminophylline, an adenosine receptor antagonist, is required to reverse its effects.

Dobutamine is a synthetic catecholamine characterized by strong β1-receptor and mild α1- and β2-receptor agonist activity. When used in low doses, marked inotropic effects are encountered, mediated by both α1- and β1-receptor stimulation. These effects are used for treatment of heart failure and the identification of dysfunctional, but viable, cardiac muscle. When used in high doses, the heart rate is progressively increased (mediated by β1-receptor stimulation). Despite a clear increase in cardiac output, systemic blood pressure usually only increases minimally due to a decrease in systemic vascular resistance because the peripheral vasoconstrictive effects (mediated by α1-receptor stimulation) are overwhelmed by the vasodilative effects (mediated by β2-receptor stimulation) [37]. As a result of the hemodynamic changes, there is an increase in oxygen demand resulting in a secondary dilation of the coronary arteries and, thus, an increase in blood flow. Additionally, dobutamine may also have a (minor) direct vasodilative effect on coronary vessels. Table 62.2 provides a comprehensive overview of the pharmacological stress agent aforementioned.

Data Analysis

For the evaluation of SE static CTMPI, myocardial perfusion defects are assessed by visual evaluation of contrast enhancement in the left ventricle. According to the literature [46, 63], a visual evaluation can be affected by bias, as interpretation of defects in the myocardial blood pool is often highly user-dependent when compared to the absolute quantitative assessment obtained with dynamic perfusion imaging.

In the case of DECT, independent from the technology used, an iodine distribution map can be generated analyzing the differences in attenuation of iodine between both energy spectra and by merging the low and high kV datasets [64, 65]. Dedicated software typically generates the color-coded iodine distribution map overlay on top of a virtual non-contrasted image. The iodine concentrations are normalized to the myocardial areas with normal perfusion [24]. As myocardial iodine concentration has a direct relationship with myocardial perfusion, the myocardial blood pool can be quantified based on the per-voxel amount of iodine (Fig. 62.7) [23].

Table 62.2 Overview of pharmacological agents used in stress myocardial perfusion

	Mechanism of action	Effect	Dosage	Contraindications	Advantages	Common side effects
Adenosine	Nonselective adenosine receptor agonist	Coronary artery vasodilator	140 μg/kg/min for 3–6 min	High-grade AV block Asthma or COPD Sinus bradycardia Systemic hypotension (BP < 90 mmHg) Severe carotid stenosis	Good sensitivity and specificity	Flushing Headache Dyspnea May provoke acute ischemia
Regadenoson	A_{2A}-selective adenosine receptor agonist	Coronary artery vasodilator	Bolus of 400 μg in 10–20 s	High-grade AV block Sinus bradycardia Systemic hypotension (BP < 90 mmHg) Severe carotid stenosis	Dose independent from weight Fewer side effects in patients with asthma and COPD	Dyspnea Headache Flushing May provoke acute ischemia
Dobutamine	Stimulator of β1-adrenergic receptors	Increases heart rate, blood pressure, and myocardial contractility	High-dose protocol: IV dobutamine infusion in 3 min stages (10, 20, 30, 40 μg/kg/min) Low-dose protocol: 5–10 μg/kg/min	Concomitant therapy with β-blockers Severe hypertension (>220/120 mmHg) Congestive heart failure Unstable angina Aortic valve stenosis (peak gradient >50 mmHg) Hypertrophic cardiomyopathy Complex arrhythmias Myocarditis Pericarditis	Physiological mechanism Increased oxygen consumption in the myocardium	Tachycardia May provoke acute ischemia
Dipyridamole	Increases availability of adenosine by inhibiting adenosine deaminase	Indirect coronary artery vasodilator	140 μg/kg/min for 4 min	High-grade AV block Asthma or COPD Sinus bradycardia Systemic hypotension (BP < 90 mmHg) Severe carotid stenosis	Good sensitivity and specificity Inexpensive	Headache Hypotension Flushing Dyspnea

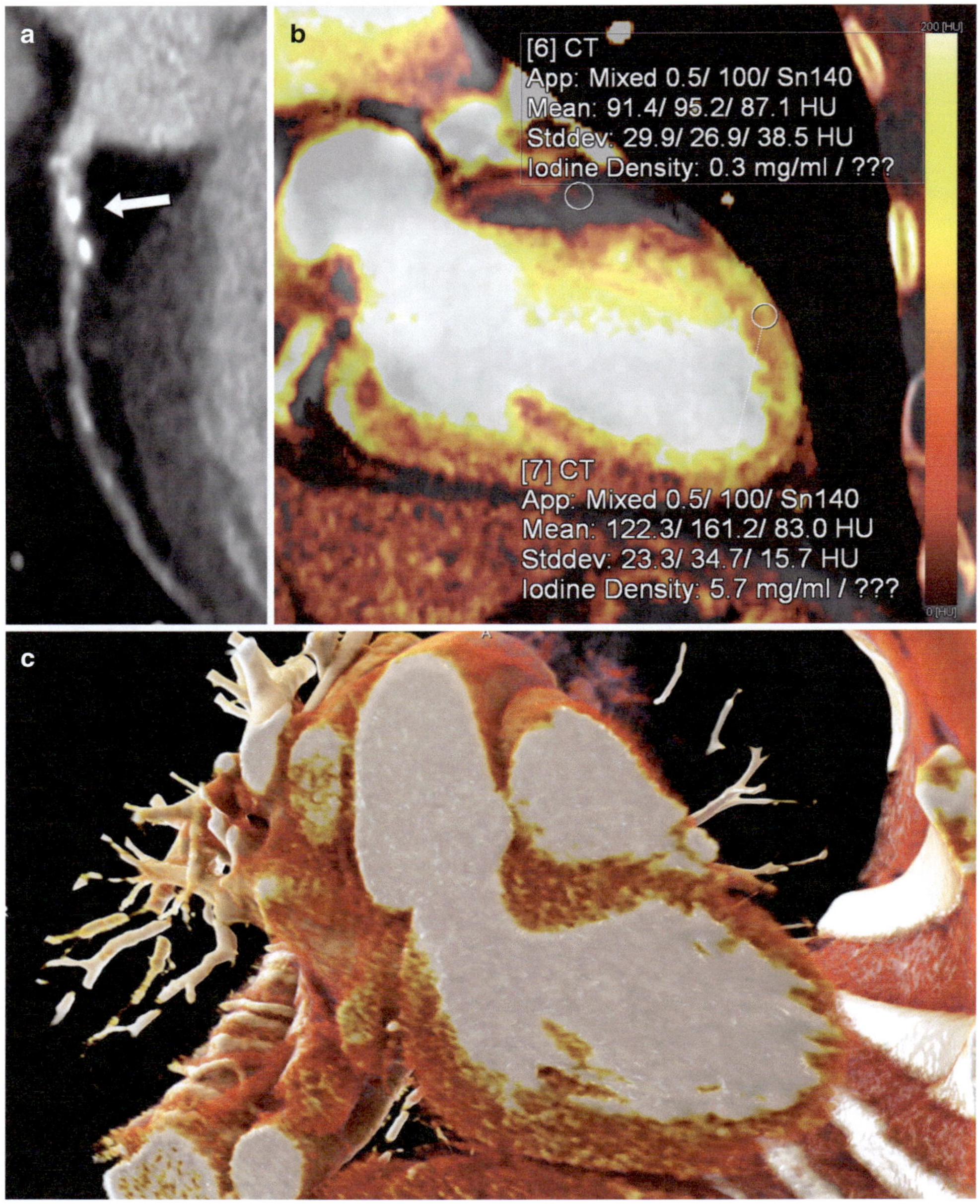

Fig. 62.7 A 57-year-old male. (**a**) Calcified eccentric plaques of the proximal LAD cause a 70% occlusion. (**b**) Stress DE-CTMPI-derived iodine map shows an area of hypoperfusion in the basal anterior myocardial segment, suggestive for myocardial infarct. Iodine map provides both qualitative and quantitative assessment of the myocardial wall. Despite the fact that the two ROIs return slightly similar attenuation values for mixed images (91.4 versus 122.3 HU), there is a substantial difference in iodine density between the hypoperfused area (0.3 mg/mL) and the remote myocardium without visual perfusion defect (5.7 mg/mL). Cinematic rendering (**c**) of the long axis plane provides extremely detailed anatomic details, albeit unable to visually demonstrate attenuation differences within the myocardial wall

A comprehensive CT myocardial perfusion examination including both rest and stress acquisitions allows to differentiate reversible from fixed MPD [23]. Reversible ischemia is suspected when hypo-attenuating myocardial areas are present only in the stress phase (Fig. 62.8), whereas a myocardial infarction is characterized by a myocardial perfusion defect persisting at rest (Fig. 62.9). Flow-limiting stenosis can cause hypo-attenuation during the rest phase as well, but the diagnostic sensitivity of the rest phase is lower compared to that of the stress acquisition, and the distinction between reversible and fixed defects is not possible (Fig. 62.10). CTMPI datasets are evaluated in the left ventricle short-axis view. The myocardium is schematically divided into 17 segments based on the American Heart Association model [66]. Although the blood supply of the left ventricle is characterized by a great variability, segments 1, 2, 7, 8, 13, 14, and 17 are traditionally assigned to the left anterior descending artery (LAD). Segments 3, 4, 10, and 15 are assigned to the

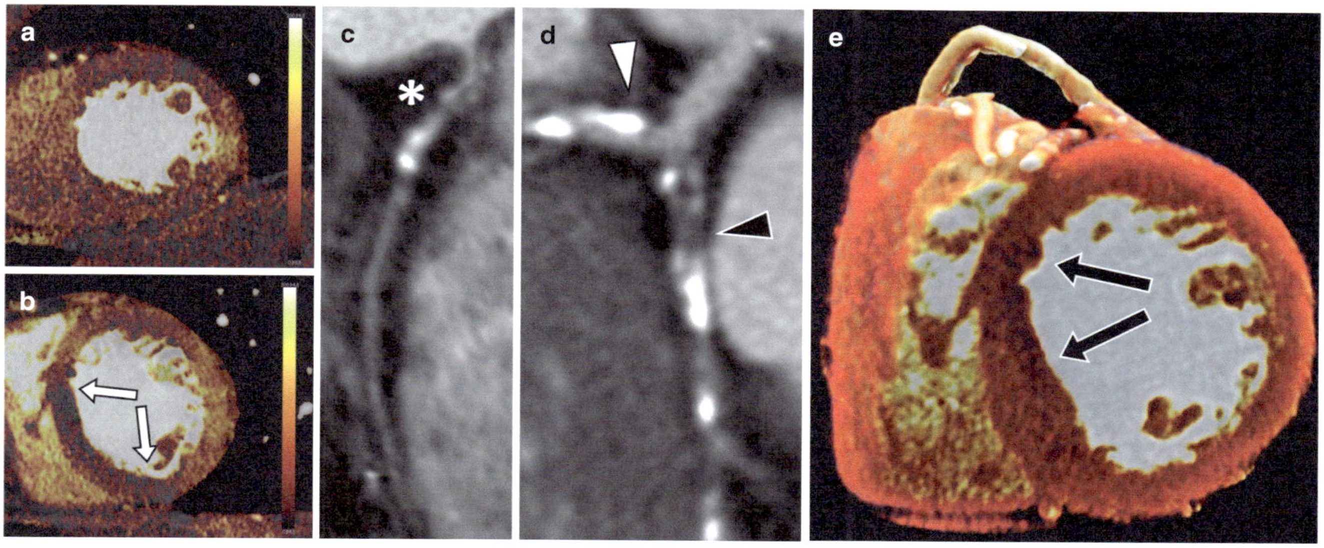

Fig. 62.8 (**a**, **b**) Short axis view of dual-energy CT myocardial perfusion of a 56-year-old male with multivessel disease and previous CABG. Rest phase (**a**) shows no perfusion defects in the ventricular wall, while the stress phase (**b**) depicts an area of hypo-attenuation in the inferior and infero-septal mid-ventricular wall (white arrows), suggestive for myocardial inducible ischemia. Curved multi-planar reformats of the coronary arteries (**c** and **d**) show a calcified and narrowed RCA (**c**, asterisk), multiple calcified plaques of the LCx (**d**, white arrowhead), and mixed plaques of the LAD (**d**, black arrowhead). Cinematic rendering (**e**) depicts the hypo-attenuation of the septal ventricular wall (black arrows)

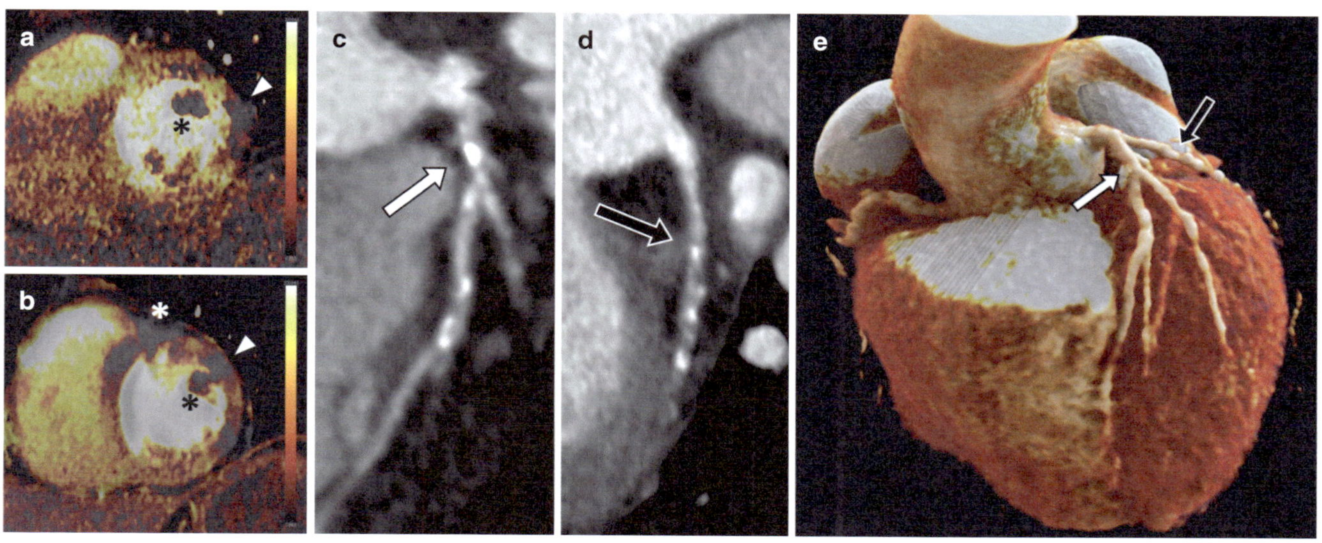

Fig. 62.9 (**a**, **b**) Short axis view of dual-energy CT myocardial perfusion of a 65-year-old male. Both rest (**a**) and stress (**b**) phases show a fixed perfusion defect in the lateral wall (arrowheads) and in the anterior papillary muscle (black asterisk). The stress phase also unveils inducible perfusion defect in the anteroseptal wall (white asterisk). Curved multi-planar reformats of the coronary arteries (**c** and **d**) show a calcified plaque of the proximal LAD (**c**, white arrow) causing approximately a 50% stenosis and a diffuse atherosclerosis of the LCx (**d**, black arrow) responsible of a 70% vessel stenosis. Cinematic rendering (**e**) depicts the diseased LAD (white arrow) and LCx (black arrow) with high-anatomical details

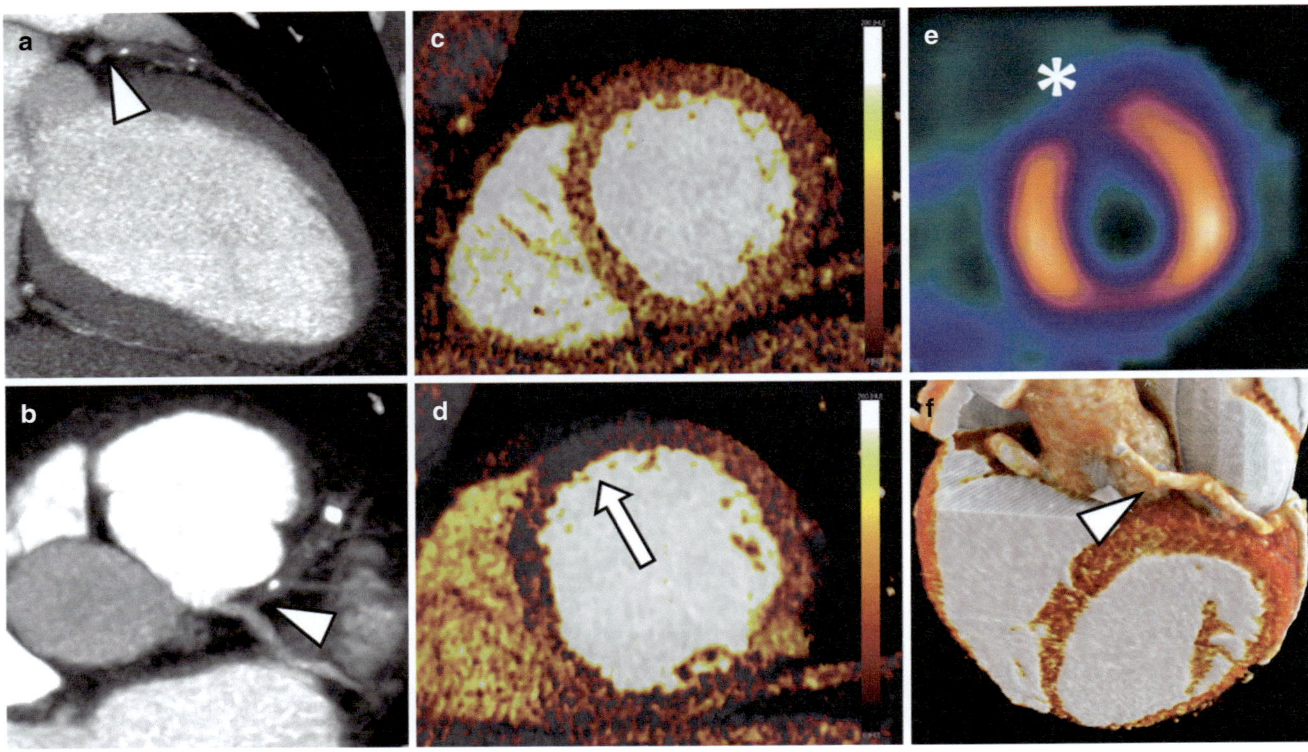

Fig. 62.10 Long-axis (**a**) and axial (**b**) maximum intensity projections of dual-energy CT myocardial perfusion of a 46-year-old male with unstable angina show an ostial occlusion of the LAD (arrowheads). DE-CTMPI at rest (**c**) does not identify any myocardial perfusion defect, while the stress phase with superimposed iodine map (**d**) unveils a basal anterior- and anteroseptal perfusion defect (arrow) suggestive for inducible ischemia. Stress myocardial SPECT (**e**) confirms the inducible ischemia (asterisk). Cinematic rendering (**f**) clearly depicts the ostial LAD occlusion (arrowhead)

Fig. 62.11 Model of 17 left ventricular segmentation proposed by the American Heart Association with corresponding feeding vessels. Segments assigned to LAD are in red, segments assigned to RCA are in green, and segments assigned to LCx are in blue

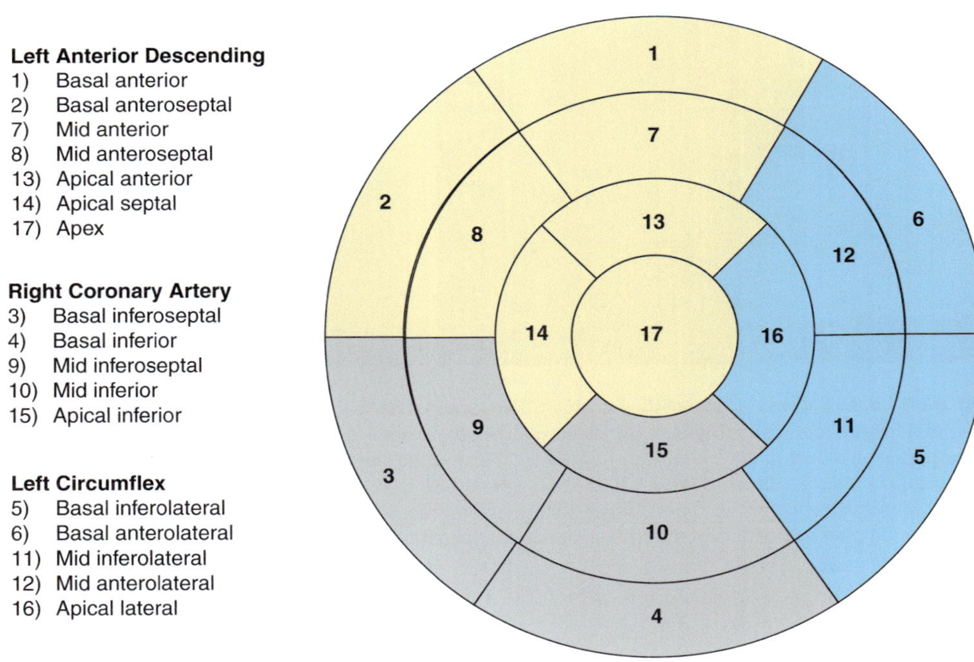

right coronary artery (RCA) when this vessel is dominant. Segments 5, 6, 11, 12, and 16 are assigned to the left circumflex coronary artery (LCx) [67]. In clinical practice, the anterior wall and the anterior septum are assigned to the LAD, the inferior wall and septum are assigned to the RCA, and the lateral wall is assigned to the LCx. The correspondence between the coronary arterial anatomy and the supplied myocardium is depicted in Fig. 62.11.

Clinical Results

Dual-energy CTMPI studies performed during rest or stress protocols showed good accuracy compared to various reference modalities (Table 62.1) [44, 46, 59, 60, 63, 68–73]. Ruzsics et al. investigated the feasibility of rest myocardial perfusion imaging using a first-generation dual-source CT system compared to SPECT in 36 patients and reported a sensitivity and specificity of 92% and 93%, respectively [46]. The incremental benefit of DE-CTMPI stress series was demonstrated in an early feasibility study by Blankstein et al. [43] where sensitivity was increased from 76% to 92% and specificity was similarly increased from 67% to 85% against the gold standard of PCI. Diagnostic accuracy was found comparable to that of SPECT. In a meta-analysis performed by Pelgrim et al., stress DE-CTMPI reported a segment-based sensitivity of 75% and a specificity of 95% in comparison to stress MRI, based on a population of 196 patients [74]. Ko et al. demonstrated the incremental diagnostic value of combined CCTA and CT perfusion compared to CCTA alone with a marked increase in sensitivity (91.8–93.5%), specificity (67.7–85.5%), positive predictive value (73.6–88.3%), and negative predictive value (87.5–91.4%) [69]. Compared to the reference standard of SPECT, Wang et al. showed increased sensitivity, specificity, and accuracy of detecting coronary stenosis >50% by addition of DE-CTMPI from 82%, 91%, and 86% with CCTA alone to 90%, 86%, and 88%, respectively [63]. A recent study reported that the combined analysis of CCTA and DE-CTMPI increases the specificity from 50% to 67% in a population at high risk for coronary artery disease (yielding a 17% higher specificity than that of either individual test) and outperforms the anatomical test of CCTA alone for detection of hemodynamically significant coronary artery stenosis [75]. A trial of 50 patients comparing DECT and SPECT for the detection of obstructive CAD against a gold standard of CMR reported higher sensitivity (90% compared to 85%) and specificity (71% vs. 58%) with DE-CTMPI than with SPECT (Fig. 62.12) [45]. The most recent studies by Ko et al. and Kim et al. demonstrated similar accuracy compared to the reference modality, cardiac CMR [59, 68]. Ko et al. additionally found fair agreement between rest and stress DECT iodine maps and described an incremental value of the stress protocol (accuracy of 83%) compared to rest protocol (accuracy of 62%) for the detection of hemodynamically significant CAD [59]. A number of studies comparing DE-CTMPI with SPECT made the interesting observation that the modalities may lead to divergent classification of perfusion defects [55, 63, 76]. Nearly one-half of perfusion defects that are reversible at SPECT are reclassified as fixed with DECT [55]. Rocha-Filho et al. [73] demonstrated considerable improvements in sensitivity (from 83% to 91%), specificity (from 71% to 91%), positive predictive value (from 66% to 86%), and negative predictive value (from 87% to 93%) by adding a stress phase to CCTA for detection of stenosis greater than 50% against a standard of invasive angiography in 35 patients with a high risk of CAD.

The first multicenter trial [56] evaluating 381 patients in comparison with combined invasive coronary angiography (ICA) and SPECT confirmed the higher diagnostic performance of combined CCTA and CTMPI. The sensitivity, specificity, positive predictive value, and negative predictive value of the combined methods in the patient-based analysis were 80%, 74%, 65%, and 86%, respectively. Also the identification of patients with hemodynamically significant CAD was significantly improved by the addition of CTMPI. The patient-based diagnostic accuracy of combined CCTA and static CTMPI in patients without prior myocardial infarction or CAD was 90% and 93%, respectively, and 87% in the whole patient population.

The DE technique demonstrated superior diagnostic performance compared to SE due to the use of iodine maps for the detection of perfusion defects with SPECT as the reference standard [42]. In the existing literature, areas with reduced myocardial iodine content at DECT perfusion studies are mainly evaluated with a qualitative approach, which can introduce bias given that myocardial blood pool defect interpretation is often highly user-dependent compared to the absolute quantitative assessment obtained with dynamic perfusion. Multiple quantitative evaluations performed in phantom and clinical studies demonstrated high accuracy for myocardial iodine quantification and the role of quantitative measurement in the differentiation between healthy and ischemic or necrotic myocardium [23, 72, 77]. A recently published experiment confirmed the accuracy of the state-of-the-art dual-source and dual-layer DE scanners in the quantification of iodine concentration, with slightly more accurate results provided by the dual-source system operating with the 150Sn/70 kVp or 150Sn/80 kVp combinations compared to the dual-layer scanner operating at 140 kVp [78].

Additionally, in a direct comparison of the different image datasets generated by DECT, iodine maps showed the highest sensitivity and specificity among all DECT datasets for the detection of myocardial perfusion defects in the DE-CTMPI [79].

In a porcine model, beam-hardening reduction through DE prospective rapid kV switching has been demonstrated [80]. In a direct comparison with SE-CTMPI, the diagnostic performance of DE-CTMPI remained unaffected by the presence of beam-hardening artifacts [81]. Moreover, a novel algorithm for beam-hardening artifact correction was proven to be effective in avoiding false-positive findings and increase the specificity of DE-CTMPI [82]. The DECIDE-Gold trial, a multicenter randomized study with the objective to determine a comprehensive assessment of the diagnostic accuracy of the DECT and DE-CTMPI in the assessment of hemodynamic significance of CAD compared to ICA, is currently ongoing [83].

In a comparison between DE and SE-CTMPI in the detection of mixed perfusion defects with SPECT as the reference

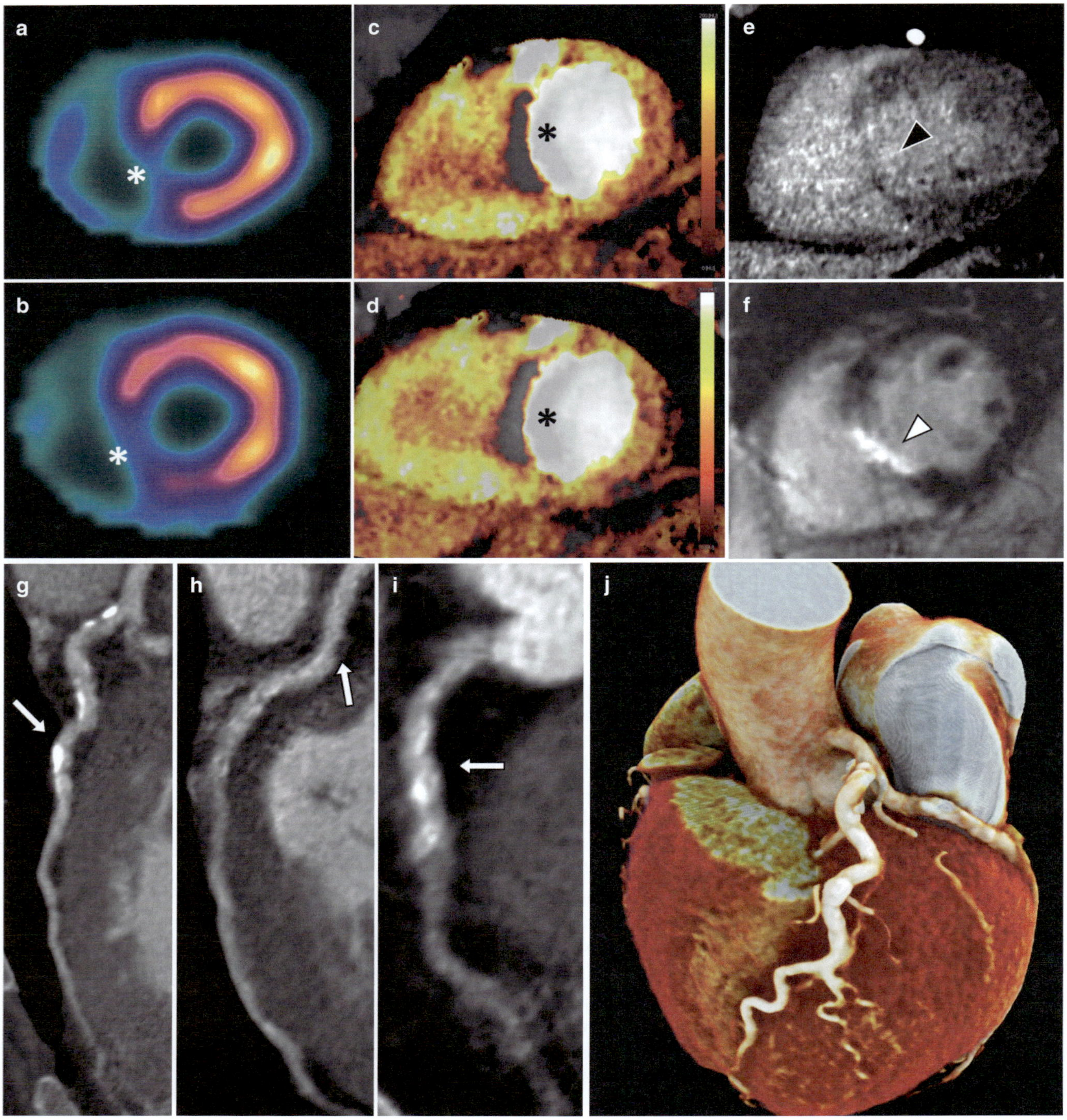

Fig. 62.12 A 68-year-old male. Myocardial SPECT at rest (**a**) and peak stress (**b**) show a fixed perfusion defect in the anteroseptal wall (white asterisks). Dual-energy CT myocardial perfusion at rest (**c**) and stress (**d**) phase with superimposed iodine maps confirms the fixed perfusion defect (black asterisks). The acquisition at the delayed phase (**e**) shows an area of late enhancement in the corresponding left ventricular segment (black arrowhead). The CTMPI is consistent with the CMR (**f**) that clearly demonstrates the transmural delayed enhancement with high contrast resolution in comparison with the healthy myocardium. All these findings are suggestive of myocardial infarct. Curved multi-planar reformats of the LAD, LCx, and RCA (**g**, **h**, and **i**, respectively) depict multiple calcified and mixed coronary plaques (arrows). Cinematic rendering (**j**) provides a detailed overview of the coronary arteries

standard, DE-CTMPI showed better results in terms of sensitivity (91% versus 55%), negative predictive value (97% versus 86%) and accuracy (93% versus 85%). However, SE-CTMPI showed a higher specificity (98% versus 94%) [42].

Limitations

The main limitation of static SE- and DE-CTMPI techniques resides in their reliance upon the acquisition timing, which can significantly influence the diagnostic accuracy. As single-shot techniques only acquire a single data set, the peak contrast attenuation could be missed [21]. Furthermore, the data collection from consecutive parts of the heart may be performed during different cardiac cycles depending on the CT system and acquisition technique, resulting in heterogeneous apicobasal attenuation. In addition, several types of artifacts may be associated with single-shot image acquisitions, such as beam-hardening, motion, and partial scan artifacts [84–86].

Cost-Effectiveness

As healthcare costs have continued to rise, the cost-effectiveness of novel techniques has been an area of increasing interest. This holds true across all fields of medicine, including CT. There have been extensive investigations comparing the cost-effectiveness of CCTA to that of SPECT. It is well established that individuals without known CAD who undergo CCTA as an initial diagnostic test, compared with those who underwent myocardial SPECT, incurred lower healthcare costs [87, 88]. Moreover, CCTA is the most cost-effective diagnostic strategy for patients with suspected acute coronary syndrome and negative troponin [89]. The state-of-the-art scanners available today in clinical practice are also cost-effective for challenging patients with CAD, such as obese patients, patients with high or irregular heartbeat, and patients who have high levels of coronary calcium or a previous stent or bypass graft [90].

To date, only a single study comparing the cost-effectiveness of DE-CTMPI versus SPECT was performed in the United States and published in 2012. Meyer et al. investigated the performance of a stress-rest DE-CTMPI protocol versus a stress-rest SPECT protocol in 50 patients with CAD, using CMR as reference standard. DE-CTMPI resulted in lower costs in comparison to routine myocardial perfusion SPECT ($2631 versus $2938, respectively; $P < 0.001$), better results in terms of quality-adjusted life-years (QALY) (14.13 versus 13.49 QALY), and, eventually, a more convenient cost profile of $3191 incremental cost-effectiveness ratio (ICER) in comparison to SPECT ($3557, $P < 0.001$). Hence, DE-CTMPI has been proven to be a cost-effective first-line imaging modality in the workup of patients with CAD [45].

Summary

A growing body of clinical evidence shows that combined CCTA and CTMPI enable the morphological and functional assessment of CAD with high accuracy in a single technique. CTMPI is most likely to be used as an add-on to CCTA to increase the specificity for hemodynamically relevant lesions, in particular in the setting of a stenosis of intermediate severity [91]. DE-CTMPI has been extensively investigated and it has shown its usefulness in various clinical settings. As such, it may play a role in the short- and long-term management of patients with CAD. This is owed to the fact that DE-CTMPI provides a comprehensive and accurate evaluation of coronary arteries and left ventricular function and ultimately enables physicians to provide the best and most advanced therapy to their patients. However, future studies are required to further evaluate the cost-effectiveness of DE-CTMPI, its place in clinical management, and its role in CAD diagnosis in comparison with dynamic CTMPI, especially in light of new emerging noninvasive functional coronary diagnostic techniques such as CT-FFR.

References

1. Bucher AM, De Cecco CN, Schoepf UJ, Wang R, Meinel FG, Binukrishnan SR, et al. Cardiac CT for myocardial ischaemia detection and characterization–comparative analysis. Br J Radiol. 2014;87:20140159.
2. World Health Organization. The top 10 causes of death. http://www.who.int/en/news-room/fact-sheets/detail/the-top-10-causes-of-death
3. Writing Group M, Mozaffarian D, Benjamin EJ, Go AS, Arnett DK, Blaha MJ, et al. Heart disease and stroke statistics-2016 update: a report from the American Heart Association. Circulation. 2016;133:e38–360.
4. American Heart Association. Heart disease and stroke statistics–at-a-glance. 2015. https://www.heart.org/idc/groups/ahamah-public/@wcm/@sop/@smd/documents/downloadable/ucm_470704.pdf
5. Taylor AJ, Cerqueira M, Hodgson JM, Mark D, Min J, O'Gara P, et al. ACCF/SCCT/ACR/AHA/ASE/ASNC/NASCI/SCAI/SCMR 2010 appropriate use criteria for cardiac computed tomography. A report of the American College of Cardiology Foundation Appropriate Use Criteria Task Force, the Society of Cardiovascular Computed Tomography, the American College of Radiology, the American Heart Association, the American Society of Echocardiography, the American Society of Nuclear Cardiology, the North American Society for Cardiovascular Imaging, the Society for Cardiovascular Angiography and Interventions, and the Society for Cardiovascular Magnetic Resonance. Circulation. 2010;122:e525–55.
6. De Cecco CN, Meinel FG, Chiaramida SA, Costello P, Bamberg F, Schoepf UJ. Coronary artery computed tomography scanning. Circulation. 2014;129:1341–5.
7. Ohnesorge BM, Hofmann LK, Flohr TG, Schoepf UJ. CT for imaging coronary artery disease: defining the paradigm for its application. Int J Cardiovasc Imaging. 2005;21:85–104.

8. Flohr TG, Schoepf UJ, Ohnesorge BM. Chasing the heart: new developments for cardiac CT. J Thorac Imaging. 2007;22:4–16.
9. von Ballmoos MW, Haring B, Juillerat P, Alkadhi H. Meta-analysis: diagnostic performance of low-radiation-dose coronary computed tomography angiography. Ann Intern Med. 2011;154:413–20.
10. Jaarsma C, Leiner T, Bekkers SC, Crijns HJ, Wildberger JE, Nagel E, et al. Diagnostic performance of noninvasive myocardial perfusion imaging using single-photon emission computed tomography, cardiac magnetic resonance, and positron emission tomography imaging for the detection of obstructive coronary artery disease: a meta-analysis. J Am Coll Cardiol. 2012;59:1719–28.
11. Pijls NH, Fearon WF, Tonino PA, Siebert U, Ikeno F, Bornschein B, et al. Fractional flow reserve versus angiography for guiding percutaneous coronary intervention in patients with multivessel coronary artery disease: 2-year follow-up of the FAME (Fractional Flow Reserve Versus Angiography for Multivessel Evaluation) study. J Am Coll Cardiol. 2010;56:177–84.
12. Shaw LJ, Berman DS, Maron DJ, Mancini GB, Hayes SW, Hartigan PM, et al. Optimal medical therapy with or without percutaneous coronary intervention to reduce ischemic burden: results from the Clinical Outcomes Utilizing Revascularization and Aggressive Drug Evaluation (COURAGE) trial nuclear substudy. Circulation. 2008;117:1283–91.
13. Kern MJ, Samady H. Current concepts of integrated coronary physiology in the catheterization laboratory. J Am Coll Cardiol. 2010;55:173–85.
14. Meijboom WB, Van Mieghem CA, van Pelt N, Weustink A, Pugliese F, Mollet NR, et al. Comprehensive assessment of coronary artery stenoses: computed tomography coronary angiography versus conventional coronary angiography and correlation with fractional flow reserve in patients with stable angina. J Am Coll Cardiol. 2008;52:636–43.
15. Sarno G, Decraemer I, Vanhoenacker PK, De Bruyne B, Hamilos M, Cuisset T, et al. On the inappropriateness of noninvasive multidetector computed tomography coronary angiography to trigger coronary revascularization: a comparison with invasive angiography. JACC Cardiovasc Interv. 2009;2:550–7.
16. Stuijfzand WJ, Danad I, Raijmakers PG, Marcu CB, Heymans MW, van Kuijk CC, et al. Additional value of transluminal attenuation gradient in CT angiography to predict hemodynamic significance of coronary artery stenosis. J Am Coll Cardiol Img. 2014;7:374–86.
17. De Cecco CN, Varga-Szemes A, Meinel FG, Renker M, Schoepf UJ. Beyond stenosis detection: computed tomography approaches for determining the functional relevance of coronary artery disease. Radiol Clin N Am. 2015;53:317–34.
18. Wang R, Renker M, Schoepf UJ, Wichmann JL, Fuller SR, Rier JD, et al. Diagnostic value of quantitative stenosis predictors with coronary CT angiography compared to invasive fractional flow reserve. Eur J Radiol. 2015;84:1509–15.
19. Varga-Szemes A, Meinel FG, De Cecco CN, Fuller SR, Bayer RR 2nd, Schoepf UJ. CT myocardial perfusion imaging. AJR Am J Roentgenol. 2015;204:487–97.
20. George RT, Silva C, Cordeiro MA, DiPaula A, Thompson DR, McCarthy WF, et al. Multidetector computed tomography myocardial perfusion imaging during adenosine stress. J Am Coll Cardiol. 2006;48:153–60.
21. Bischoff B, Bamberg F, Marcus R, Schwarz F, Becker HC, Becker A, et al. Optimal timing for first-pass stress CT myocardial perfusion imaging. Int J Cardiovasc Imaging. 2013;29:435–42.
22. Cannao PM, Schoepf UJ, Muscogiuri G, Wichmann JL, Fuller SR, Secchi F, et al. Technical prerequisites and imaging protocols for dynamic and dual energy myocardial perfusion imaging. Eur J Radiol. 2015;84:2401–10.
23. Koonce JD, Vliegenthart R, Schoepf UJ, Schmidt B, Wahlquist AE, Nietert PJ, et al. Accuracy of dual-energy computed tomography for the measurement of iodine concentration using cardiac CT protocols: validation in a phantom model. Eur Radiol. 2014;24:512–8.
24. Kang DK, Schoepf UJ, Bastarrika G, Nance JW Jr, Abro JA, Ruzsics B. Dual-energy computed tomography for integrative imaging of coronary artery disease: principles and clinical applications. Semin Ultrasound CT MR. 2010;31:276–91.
25. Siegel MJ, Kaza RK, Bolus DN, Boll DT, Rofsky NM, De Cecco CN, et al. White paper of the society of computed body tomography and magnetic resonance on dual-energy CT, part 1: technology and terminology. J Comput Assist Tomogr. 2016;40:841–5.
26. Matsumoto K, Jinzaki M, Tanami Y, Ueno A, Yamada M, Kuribayashi S. Virtual monochromatic spectral imaging with fast kilovoltage switching: improved image quality as compared with that obtained with conventional 120-kVp CT. Radiology. 2011;259:257–62.
27. Gabbai M, Leichter I, Mahgerefteh S, Sosna J. Spectral material characterization with dual-energy CT: comparison of commercial and investigative technologies in phantoms. Acta Radiol. 2015;56:960–9.
28. Nance JW Jr, Bastarrika G, Kang DK, Ruzsics B, Vogt S, Schmidt B, et al. High-temporal resolution dual-energy computed tomography of the heart using a novel hybrid image reconstruction algorithm: initial experience. J Comput Assist Tomogr. 2011;35:119–25.
29. Arnoldi E, Lee YS, Ruzsics B, Weininger M, Spears JR, Rowley CP, et al. CT detection of myocardial blood volume deficits: dual-energy CT compared with single-energy CT spectra. J Cardiovasc Comput Tomogr. 2011;5:421–9.
30. Blankstein R, Shturman LD, Rogers IS, Rocha-Filho JA, Okada DR, Sarwar A, et al. Adenosine-induced stress myocardial perfusion imaging using dual-source cardiac computed tomography. J Am Coll Cardiol. 2009;54:1072–84.
31. Ko SM, Choi JW, Song MG, Shin JK, Chee HK, Chung HW, et al. Myocardial perfusion imaging using adenosine-induced stress dual-energy computed tomography of the heart: comparison with cardiac magnetic resonance imaging and conventional coronary angiography. Eur Radiol. 2011;21:26–35.
32. Meyer M, Nance JW Jr, Schoepf UJ, Moscariello A, Weininger M, Rowe GW, et al. Cost-effectiveness of substituting dual-energy CT for SPECT in the assessment of myocardial perfusion for the workup of coronary artery disease. Eur J Radiol. 2012;81:3719–25.
33. Ruzsics B, Schwarz F, Schoepf UJ, Lee YS, Bastarrika G, Chiaramida SA, et al. Comparison of dual-energy computed tomography of the heart with single photon emission computed tomography for assessment of coronary artery stenosis and of the myocardial blood supply. Am J Cardiol. 2009;104:318–26.
34. Ruzsics B, Lee H, Powers ER, Flohr TG, Costello P, Schoepf UJ. Images in cardiovascular medicine. Myocardial ischemia diagnosed by dual-energy computed tomography: correlation with single-photon emission computed tomography. Circulation. 2008;117:1244–5.
35. Fahmi R, Eck BL, Levi J, Fares A, Dhanantwari A, Vembar M, et al. Quantitative myocardial perfusion imaging in a porcine ischemia model using a prototype spectral detector CT system. Phys Med Biol. 2016;61:2407–31.
36. Meinel FG, Canstein C, Schoepf UJ, Sedlmaier M, Schmidt B, Harris BS, et al. Image quality and radiation dose of low tube voltage 3rd generation dual-source coronary CT angiography in obese patients: a phantom study. Eur Radiol. 2014;24:1643–50.
37. Vliegenthart R, Pelgrim GJ, Ebersberger U, Rowe GW, Oudkerk M, Schoepf UJ. Dual-energy CT of the heart. AJR Am J Roentgenol. 2012;199:S54–63.
38. George RT, Arbab-Zadeh A, Miller JM, Vavere AL, Bengel FM, Lardo AC, et al. Computed tomography myocardial perfusion imaging with 320-row detector computed tomography accurately

detects myocardial ischemia in patients with obstructive coronary artery disease. Circ Cardiovasc Imaging. 2012;5:333–40.
39. Habis M, Capderou A, Sigal-Cinqualbre A, Ghostine S, Rahal S, Riou JY, et al. Comparison of delayed enhancement patterns on multislice computed tomography immediately after coronary angiography and cardiac magnetic resonance imaging in acute myocardial infarction. Heart. 2009;95:624–9.
40. Deseive S, Bauer RW, Lehmann R, Kettner M, Kaiser C, Korkusuz H, et al. Dual-energy computed tomography for the detection of late enhancement in reperfused chronic infarction: a comparison to magnetic resonance imaging and histopathology in a porcine model. Investig Radiol. 2011;46:450–6.
41. Meinel FG, De Cecco CN, Schoepf UJ, Nance JW Jr, Silverman JR, Flowers BA, et al. First-arterial-pass dual-energy CT for assessment of myocardial blood supply: do we need rest, stress, and delayed acquisition? Comparison with SPECT. Radiology. 2014;270:708–16.
42. Dole WP, Yamada N, Bishop VS, Olsson RA. Role of adenosine in coronary blood flow regulation after reductions in perfusion pressure. Circ Res. 1985;56:517–24.
43. Gould KL, Lipscomb K. Effects of coronary stenoses on coronary flow reserve and resistance. Am J Cardiol. 1974;34:48–55.
44. Sambuceti G, Marzilli M, Marraccini P, Schneider-Eicke J, Gliozheni E, Parodi O, et al. Coronary vasoconstriction during myocardial ischemia induced by rises in metabolic demand in patients with coronary artery disease. Circulation. 1997;95:2652–9.
45. Kurata A, Mochizuki T, Koyama Y, Haraikawa T, Suzuki J, Shigematsu Y, et al. Myocardial perfusion imaging using adenosine triphosphate stress multi-slice spiral computed tomography: alternative to stress myocardial perfusion scintigraphy. Circ J. 2005;69:550–7.
46. Rumberger JA, Feiring AJ, Lipton MJ, Higgins CB, Ell SR, Marcus ML. Use of ultrafast computed tomography to quantitate regional myocardial perfusion: a preliminary report. J Am Coll Cardiol. 1987;9:59–69.
47. Mahmarian JJ, Cerqueira MD, Iskandrian AE, Bateman TM, Thomas GS, Hendel RC, et al. Regadenoson induces comparable left ventricular perfusion defects as adenosine: a quantitative analysis from the ADVANCE MPI 2 trial. JACC Cardiovasc Imaging. 2009;2:959–68.
48. Salgado Garcia C, Jimenez Heffernan A, Sanchez de Mora E, Ramos Font C, Lopez Martin J, Rivera de los Santos F, et al. Comparative study of the safety of regadenoson between patients with mild/moderate chronic obstructive pulmonary disease and asthma. Eur J Nucl Med Mol Imaging. 2014;41:119–25.
49. Becker A, Becker C. CT imaging of myocardial perfusion: possibilities and perspectives. J Nucl Cardiol. 2013;20:289–96.
50. Iskandrian AE, Bateman TM, Belardinelli L, Blackburn B, Cerqueira MD, Hendel RC, et al. Adenosine versus regadenoson comparative evaluation in myocardial perfusion imaging: results of the ADVANCE phase 3 multicenter international trial. J Nucl Cardiol. 2007;14:645–58.
51. Luu JM, Filipchuk NG, Friedrich MG. Indications, safety and image quality of cardiovascular magnetic resonance: experience in >5,000 North American patients. Int J Cardiol. 2013;168:3807–11.
52. Shah S, Parra D, Rosenstein RS. Acute myocardial infarction during regadenoson myocardial perfusion imaging. Pharmacotherapy. 2013;33:e90–5.
53. Hsi DH, Marreddy R, Moshiyakhov M, Luft U. Regadenoson induced acute ST-segment elevation myocardial infarction and multivessel coronary thrombosis. J Nucl Cardiol. 2013;20:481–4.
54. Geleijnse ML, Elhendy A, Fioretti PM, Roelandt JR. Dobutamine stress myocardial perfusion imaging. J Am Coll Cardiol. 2000;36:2017–27.
55. Jin KN, De Cecco CN, Caruso D, Tesche C, Spandorfer A, Varga-Szemes A, et al. Myocardial perfusion imaging with dual energy CT. Eur J Radiol. 2016;85:1914–21.
56. Rochitte CE, George RT, Chen MY, Arbab-Zadeh A, Dewey M, Miller JM, et al. Computed tomography angiography and perfusion to assess coronary artery stenosis causing perfusion defects by single photon emission computed tomography: the CORE320 study. Eur Heart J. 2014;35:1120–30.
57. Dey D, Slomka PJ, Berman DS. Achieving very-low-dose radiation exposure in cardiac computed tomography, single-photon emission computed tomography, and positron emission tomography. Circ Cardiovasc Imaging. 2014;7:723–34.
58. Goldstein JA, Chinnaiyan KM, Abidov A, Achenbach S, Berman DS, Hayes SW, et al. The CT-STAT (Coronary Computed Tomographic Angiography for Systematic Triage of Acute Chest Pain Patients to Treatment) trial. J Am Coll Cardiol. 2011;58:1414–22.
59. Ko SM, Park JH, Hwang HK, Song MG. Direct comparison of stress- and rest-dual-energy computed tomography for detection of myocardial perfusion defect. Int J Cardiovasc Imaging. 2014;30(Suppl 1):41–53.
60. Ko SM, Song MG, Chee HK, Hwang HK, Feuchtner GM, Min JK. Diagnostic performance of dual-energy CT stress myocardial perfusion imaging: direct comparison with cardiovascular MRI. AJR Am J Roentgenol. 2014;203:W605–13.
61. Yin WH, Lu B, Hou ZH, Li N, Han L, Wu YJ, et al. Detection of coronary artery stenosis with sub-milliSievert radiation dose by prospectively ECG-triggered high-pitch spiral CT angiography and iterative reconstruction. Eur Radiol. 2013;23:2927–33.
62. Zhang LJ, Qi L, Wang J, Tang CX, Zhou CS, Ji XM, et al. Feasibility of prospectively ECG-triggered high-pitch coronary CT angiography with 30 mL iodinated contrast agent at 70 kVp: initial experience. Eur Radiol. 2014;24:1537–46.
63. Wang R, Yu W, Wang Y, He Y, Yang L, Bi T, et al. Incremental value of dual-energy CT to coronary CT angiography for the detection of significant coronary stenosis: comparison with quantitative coronary angiography and single photon emission computed tomography. Int J Cardiovasc Imaging. 2011;27:647–56.
64. Coursey CA, Nelson RC, Boll DT, Paulson EK, Ho LM, Neville AM, et al. Dual-energy multidetector CT: how does it work, what can it tell us, and when can we use it in abdominopelvic imaging? Radiographics. 2010;30:1037–55.
65. Williams MC, Newby DE. CT myocardial perfusion imaging: current status and future directions. Clin Radiol. 2016;71:739–49.
66. Cerqueira MD, Weissman NJ, Dilsizian V, Jacobs AK, Kaul S, Laskey WK, et al. Standardized myocardial segmentation and nomenclature for tomographic imaging of the heart. A statement for healthcare professionals from the Cardiac Imaging Committee of the Council on Clinical Cardiology of the American Heart Association. Circulation. 2002;105:539–42.
67. Donato P, Coelho P, Santos C, Bernardes A, Caseiro-Alves F. Correspondence between left ventricular 17 myocardial segments and coronary anatomy obtained by multi-detector computed tomography: an ex vivo contribution. Surg Radiol Anat. 2012;34:805–10.
68. Kim SM, Chang SA, Shin W, Choe YH. Dual-energy CT perfusion during pharmacologic stress for the assessment of myocardial perfusion defects using a second-generation dual-source CT: a comparison with cardiac magnetic resonance imaging. J Comput Assist Tomogr. 2014;38:44–52.
69. Ko SM, Choi JW, Hwang HK, Song MG, Shin JK, Chee HK. Diagnostic performance of combined noninvasive anatomic and functional assessment with dual-source CT and adenosine-induced stress dual-energy CT for detection of significant coronary stenosis. AJR Am J Roentgenol. 2012;198:512–20.
70. Weininger M, Schoepf UJ, Ramachandra A, Fink C, Rowe GW, Costello P, et al. Adenosine-stress dynamic real-time myocardial

perfusion CT and adenosine-stress first-pass dual-energy myocardial perfusion CT for the assessment of acute chest pain: initial results. Eur J Radiol. 2012;81:3703–10.
71. Delgado C, Vazquez M, Oca R, Vilar M, Trinidad C, Sanmartin M. Myocardial ischemia evaluation with dual-source computed tomography: comparison with magnetic resonance imaging. Rev Esp Cardiol (Engl Ed). 2013;66:864–70.
72. Delgado Sanchez-Gracian C, Oca Pernas R, Trinidad Lopez C, Santos Armentia E, Vaamonde Liste A, Vazquez Caamano M, et al. Quantitative myocardial perfusion with stress dual-energy CT: iodine concentration differences between normal and ischemic or necrotic myocardium. Initial experience. Eur Radiol. 2016;26:3199–207.
73. Rocha-Filho JA, Blankstein R, Shturman LD, Bezerra HG, Okada DR, Rogers IS, et al. Incremental value of adenosine-induced stress myocardial perfusion imaging with dual-source CT at cardiac CT angiography. Radiology. 2010;254:410–9.
74. Pelgrim GJ, Dorrius M, Xie X, den Dekker MA, Schoepf UJ, Henzler T, et al. The dream of a one-stop-shop: meta-analysis on myocardial perfusion CT. Eur J Radiol. 2015;84:2411–20.
75. De Cecco CN, Harris BS, Schoepf UJ, Silverman JR, McWhite CB, Krazinski AW, et al. Incremental value of pharmacological stress cardiac dual-energy CT over coronary CT angiography alone for the assessment of coronary artery disease in a high-risk population. AJR Am J Roentgenol. 2014;203:W70–7.
76. Vliegenthart R, Henzler T, Moscariello A, Ruzsics B, Bastarrika G, Oudkerk M, et al. CT of coronary heart disease: part 1, CT of myocardial infarction, ischemia, and viability. AJR Am J Roentgenol. 2012;198:531–47.
77. Thilo C, Hanley M, Bastarrika G, Ruzsics B, Schoepf UJ. Integrative computed tomographic imaging of cardiac structure, function, perfusion, and viability. Cardiol Rev. 2010;18:219–29.
78. Pelgrim GJ, van Hamersvelt RW, Willemink MJ, Schmidt BT, Flohr T, Schilham A, et al. Accuracy of iodine quantification using dual energy CT in latest generation dual source and dual layer CT. Eur Radiol. 2017;27(9):3904–12.
79. Li W, Zhu X, Li J, Peng C, Chen N, Qi Z, et al. Comparison of the sensitivity and specificity of 5 image sets of dual-energy computed tomography for detecting first-pass myocardial perfusion defects compared with positron emission tomography. Medicine. 2014;93:e329.
80. So A, Hsieh J, Imai Y, Narayanan S, Kramer J, Procknow K, et al. Prospectively ECG-triggered rapid kV-switching dual-energy CT for quantitative imaging of myocardial perfusion. JACC Cardiovasc Imaging. 2012;5:829–36.
81. Carrascosa PM, Cury RC, Deviggiano A, Capunay C, Campisi R, Lopez de Munain M, et al. Comparison of myocardial perfusion evaluation with single versus dual-energy CT and effect of beam-hardening artifacts. Acad Radiol. 2015;22:591–9.
82. Bucher AM, Wichmann JL, Schoepf UJ, Wolla CD, Canstein C, McQuiston AD, et al. Quantitative evaluation of beam-hardening artefact correction in dual-energy CT myocardial perfusion imaging. Eur Radiol. 2016;26:3215–22.
83. Truong QA, Knaapen P, Pontone G, Andreini D, Leipsic J, Carrascosa P, et al. Rationale and design of the dual-energy computed tomography for ischemia determination compared to "gold standard" non-invasive and invasive techniques (DECIDE-Gold): a multicenter international efficacy diagnostic study of rest-stress dual-energy computed tomography angiography with perfusion. J Nucl Cardiol. 2015;22:1031–40.
84. Nagao M, Matsuoka H, Kawakami H, Higashino H, Mochizuki T, Ohshita A, et al. Detection of myocardial ischemia using 64-slice MDCT. Circ J. 2009;73:905–11.
85. Busch JL, Alessio AM, Caldwell JH, Gupta M, Mao S, Kadakia J, et al. Myocardial hypo-enhancement on resting computed tomography angiography images accurately identifies myocardial hypoperfusion. J Cardiovasc Comput Tomogr. 2011;5:412–20.
86. Stenner P, Schmidt B, Bruder H, Allmendinger T, Haberland U, Flohr T, et al. Partial scan artifact reduction (PSAR) for the assessment of cardiac perfusion in dynamic phase-correlated CT. Med Phys. 2009;36:5683–94.
87. Min JK, Kang N, Shaw LJ, Devereux RB, Robinson M, Lin F, et al. Costs and clinical outcomes after coronary multidetector CT angiography in patients without known coronary artery disease: comparison to myocardial perfusion SPECT. Radiology. 2008;249:62–70.
88. Min JK, Shaw LJ, Berman DS, Gilmore A, Kang N. Costs and clinical outcomes in individuals without known coronary artery disease undergoing coronary computed tomographic angiography from an analysis of Medicare category III transaction codes. Am J Cardiol. 2008;102:672–8.
89. Goodacre S, Thokala P, Carroll C, Stevens JW, Leaviss J, Al Khalaf M, et al. Systematic review, meta-analysis and economic modelling of diagnostic strategies for suspected acute coronary syndrome. Health Technol Assess. 2013;17:v-vi, 1–188.
90. Westwood M, Al M, Burgers L, Redekop K, Lhachimi S, Armstrong N, et al. A systematic review and economic evaluation of new-generation computed tomography scanners for imaging in coronary artery disease and congenital heart disease: Somatom Definition Flash, Aquilion ONE, Brilliance iCT and Discovery CT750 HD. Health Technol Assess. 2013;17:1–243.
91. Boiselle PM, Choe YH, Leipsic J, Pugliese F, Schoepf UJ, Vliegenthart R. Expert opinion: how and when to perform CT myocardial perfusion imaging. J Thorac Imaging. 2015;30:167–8.
92. Bauer RW, Kerl JM, Fischer N, Burkhard T, Larson MC, Ackermann H, et al. Dual-energy CT for the assessment of chronic myocardial infarction in patients with chronic coronary artery disease: comparison with 3-T MRI. AJR Am J Roentgenol. 2010;195:639–46.
93. Nagao M, Kido T, Watanabe K, Saeki H, Okayama H, Kurata A, et al. Functional assessment of coronary artery flow using adenosine stress dual-energy CT: a preliminary study. Int J Cardiovasc Imaging. 2011;27:471–81.
94. Zhao RP, Hao ZR, Song ZJ. Diagnostic value of Flash dual-source CT coronary artery imaging combined with dual-energy myocardial perfusion imaging for coronary heart disease. Exp Ther Med. 2014;7:865–8.
95. Kido T, Watanabe K, Saeki H, Shigemi S, Matsuda T, Yamamoto M, et al. Adenosine triphosphate stress dual-source computed tomography to identify myocardial ischemia: comparison with invasive coronary angiography. Springerplus. 2014;3:75.

Dynamic Myocardial CT Perfusion Imaging

63

Marly van Assen, Gert Jan Pelgrim, and Rozemarijn Vliegenthart

Several noninvasive imaging techniques are available for the evaluation of myocardial perfusion. Nuclear techniques are positron emission tomography (PET) and single-photon emission computed tomography (SPECT). PET is the current gold standard for quantitative evaluation of myocardial perfusion, while SPECT is the most commonly used imaging method for myocardial ischemia [1]. Cardiac magnetic resonance (MRI) perfusion imaging has, however, shown better accuracy for the detection of myocardial perfusion defects [2].

In a meta-analysis involving 11,826 patients [3], myocardial perfusion evaluation with PET had a higher sensitivity for myocardial ischemia than evaluation with SPECT, 92.6% compared to 88.3%, respectively. There was no significant difference between the specificity of PET and SPECT, 81.3% compared to 76.0%. Jaarsma et al. [1] showed in a recent meta-analysis (17,901 patients) a pooled sensitivity of 84%, 88%, and 89% for PET, SPECT, and MRI, respectively, with a pooled specificity of 81%, 61%, and 76%. They concluded that both PET and MRI showed higher diagnostic accuracy than SPECT.

None of the abovementioned techniques allow simultaneous anatomical and functional evaluation of coronary artery disease (CAD). Computed tomography (CT), however, is able to evaluate both with state-of-the-art imaging techniques. Coronary CT angiography (CCTA) is often used for noninvasive evaluation of coronary anatomy, yielding a very high sensitivity and negative predictive value close to 100% [4]. Combining CT myocardial perfusion imaging (CTMPI) with CCTA allows for anatomical and functional evaluation of CAD using a single modality and examination.

Dynamic CTMPI uses multiple acquisitions to capture the first pass of contrast medium during its wash in and washout through the myocardium; this is in contrast to static CT perfusion imaging which only shows contrast distribution across the myocardium at a single point in time [5–8].

The main advantage of dynamic CTMPI is the potential of quantitative analysis of myocardial blood flow (MBF), myocardial blood volume (MBV), and other perfusion-related parameters directly from the CT images, for both the whole heart and for individual myocardial segments. Static CT does not provide a quantitative measure of perfusion but a relative map of single-time-point myocardial contrast distribution. Quantification of MBF could especially improve the detection of ischemia in patients with three-vessel disease because this approach relies on absolute values of MBF rather than on the differences between normal and ischemic myocardium. Also, subtle subclinical decreases in MBF can be detected by quantifying perfusion, while not yet visible as gross perfusion defects [9].

CTMPI was first studied in a number of animal studies. Studies in pigs and dogs showed that dynamic CTMPI was able to determine accurate MBF values, using 16- or 64-multidetector CT (MDCT) during rest and stress. CTMPI-determined semiquantitative and quantitative MBF values as well as rest/stress MBF ratios were shown to have a high correlation with microsphere-derived MBF [10–12]. In studies by Mahnken et al. [13] and Bamberg et al. [14], a dual-source CT (DSCT) system with alternating table positions ("shuttle mode") allowed for whole heart imaging in pigs, with a total coverage of 73 mm compared to 38 mm using only one table position. DSCT scanners have an improved temporal resolution due to

M. van Assen
Department of Radiology, University of Groningen, University Medical Center Groningen, Groningen, The Netherlands

Department of Radiology and Radiological Science, Division of Cardiovascular Imaging, Medical University of South Carolina Charleston, SC, USA
e-mail: vanasse@musc.edu

G. J. Pelgrim
Department of Radiology, University of Groningen, University Medical Center Groningen, Groningen, The Netherlands

R. Vliegenthart (✉)
Department of Radiology, University of Groningen, University Medical Center Groningen, Groningen, The Netherlands

Department of Radiology and Radiological Science, Division of Cardiovascular Imaging, Medical University of South Carolina Charleston, SC, USA
e-mail: r.vliegenthart@umcg.nl

U. J. Schoepf (ed.), *CT of the Heart*, Contemporary Medical Imaging, https://doi.org/10.1007/978-1-60327-237-7_63

the use of two X-ray sources, resulting in the possibility to scan a slab in less than 150 ms. Using DSCT in shuttle mode, they were able to show the hemodynamic effect of a coronary stenosis with dynamic CTMPI in stress phase and concluded that CT-determined MBF measurements could differentiate ischemic from nonischemic myocardium. However, MBF was underestimated compared to microsphere-determined MBF. Rossi et al. [15] showed that dynamic dual-source CTMPI is able to distinguish regions with reduced MBF during stress phase imaging with a good correlation with FFR measurements. They used a higher dose of adenosine as a stressor agent, 500 µg/kg/min, compared to Bamberg et al. and Mahnken et al. who used 140 µg/kg/min and 240 µg/kg/min, respectively. Contrast agent was injected directly into the pulmonary vein, whereas in the studies of Bamberg et al. and Mahnken et al., the contrast agent was injected into a peripheral vein. Rossi et al. [15] found higher MBF values than the studies of Bamberg et al. and Mahnken et al. 2.68 (2.31–2.81) ml/g/min compared to 1.10(±0.25) ml/g/min and 117.4(±18.6) ml/100 ml/min in nonischemic myocardium during stress phase, possibly caused by the differences in experimental setup. Apart from animal validation studies, in recent years a number of patient studies have been performed, evaluating the feasibility of CTMPI in a clinical setting. These studies will be discussed later in this chapter, after discussing the technical issues in CTMPI.

Technical Information

Heart Coverage

The accuracy of dynamic CTMPI logically depends on the heart coverage of the available CT systems. The first systems used for dynamic CTMPI in clinical patients were DSCT systems. Second-generation DSCT scanners allow coverage of most of the left ventricle (7.3 cm) using a shuttle mode in systolic phase. The shuttle mode consists of back-and-forth table movements alternated with sequential scanning to cover the left ventricle in two separate scans, which are later combined to reconstruct one image. Third-generation DSCT systems have wider detectors compared to second-generation scanners, enabling whole heart imaging in systolic phase with a total range of 10.2 cm. Although the shuttle mode enables the coverage of a larger portion of the heart, the movement between the two table positions lowers the temporal sampling rate, especially at high heart rates. A low temporal sampling rate results in a decrease in information on in- and outflow of contrast medium in the myocardium, the so-called first-pass perfusion, and could thereby cause inaccurate estimation of MBF values [16]. Another problem introduced by the moving table positions is the possibility of motion artifacts, decreasing the accuracy of the measurements. Single-tube multi-detector CT (MDCT) scanners with 256 or 320 detector rows cover 8 and 16 cm, respectively. Wide detector coverage enables (nearly) full left ventricle imaging with a stationary table position, allowing a higher temporal sampling rate. These CT systems offer the same or even more coverage compared to DSCT scanners without the disadvantage of table movement in shuttle mode, so far however at the disadvantage of higher radiation dose.

Cardiac Phase for Acquisition

Image acquisition is possible in systolic or diastolic phase. Motwani et al. [17, 18] studied the effect of systolic and diastolic acquisition on quantitative MRI perfusion imaging and reported higher diastolic stress MBF values compared to systolic stress MBF. However, diagnostic accuracy for myocardial ischemia was similar for systolic and diastolic acquisition. There are several important advantages for CT acquisition during the systolic phase. Firstly, the heart is contracted during systole, with maximal contraction at end systole, resulting in a smaller total heart volume, in particular a shorter basal-apical length. Thus, the range that needs to be covered for visualizing the entire heart within one scan cycle is reduced. Because of the maximal contraction, the myocardium is thicker in systole and allows for easier delineation during analysis. Secondly, although the systolic phase is shorter than the diastolic phase, the systolic phase has a constant duration (200 ms approximately) independent of heart rate and is less sensitive to arrhythmia. Thirdly, image acquisition during the systolic phase results in a lower-contrast dose in the left ventricle and, thus, reduces beam-hardening artifacts [8, 18, 19].

Radiation Dose

Cardiac imaging is a major contributor to the average population medical radiation exposure [7, 20]. Dynamic CTMPI is associated with a relatively high radiation dose since it requires multiple scan acquisitions during the first pass of contrast.

Effective radiation doses between 5 and 13 mSv, with an average dose of 9.2 mSV, have been reported for dynamic CTMPI procedures (Tables 63.1 and 63.2). Cardiac patients often undergo multiple imaging procedures in their life, increasing their cumulative radiation exposure [5, 6, 20]. One particular advantage of CT, however, is that both coronary stenosis and resulting myocardial ischemia can be evaluated with one imaging modality. In view of the significant reduction in radiation dose with newest CT systems for coronary imaging, the total radiation dose of CTA plus CTMPI does not need to exceed 10 mSv [39–41].

The effective radiation dose of CT perfusion procedures is within the range of nuclear perfusion imaging procedures. SPECT perfusion studies show radiation doses of 6.6 mSv for stress-only imaging and 11.3 mSv for both rest and stress phase imaging. PET perfusion studies need a radiation ranging from 2.4 mSv to 13.5 mSv [42].

Table 63.1 Dynamic CT myocardial perfusion patient studies using visual analysis

Study	Year	Number of patients	CT scanner	Radiation dose (mSv)	Reference	Analysis	Sens	Spec
Yang [21]	2016	72	Second-generation DSCT	7.8	ICA + FFR	Territory	79	91
Baxa [22]	2015	27	Second-generation DSCT	8.9	ICA	Territory	97	95
						Segmental	98	96
Weininger [23]	2012	10	Second-generation DSCT	12.8	MRI	Segmental	86	98
					SPECT	Segmental	84	92
Wang [24]	2012	30	Second-generation DSCT	9.5	CCTA + SPECT SPECT	Segment	100	76
Bastarrika [25]	2010	10	Second-generation DSCT	18.8	MRI	Segmental	86	98

Note: *DSCT*, dual-source *CT*; *MDCT*, multi-detector CT; *ICA*, invasive coronary angiography; *FFR*, fractional flow reserve; *MRI*, cardiac magnetic resonance; *SPECT*, single-photon emission CT

Radiation dose reduction techniques in CTMPI show promising results. Performing a scan only in stress instead of both in rest and stress phase considerably reduces the radiation dose. A rest/stress phase combination, for example, in MR and PET perfusion imaging, is normally performed to acquire information about the reversibility of a perfusion defect, which could help to differentiate ischemia from myocardial infarction; see Fig. 63.1. However, in symptomatic patients without history of myocardial infarction, the probability of a persistent perfusion defect is low. In these patients, the main reason for CT imaging is to detect hemodynamically significant CAD, where presence of coronary stenosis is combined with evaluation of ischemia in the same vascular territory. Danad et al. [43] showed that the stress MBF value has a higher diagnostic accuracy than an index parameter comparing rest and stress acquisitions acquired using PET. This implies that a single MBF measurement during stress phase could be sufficient to evaluate the significance of a coronary stenosis. Delayed enhancement scans are used to detect myocardial scarring and also to determine the difference between ischemic and infarcted myocardium in patients with history of heart disease. Delayed enhancement CT falls outside the scope of the current chapter.

Another option to reduce radiation dose is by lowering the tube voltage in patients with a normal body mass index (BMI) from 100 kVp to 80 or 70 kVp [44]. This reduces the radiation dose up to 40% compared to 100 kVp, where 100 kVp can be reserved for patients with a BMI higher than 25 kg/m [2, 44]. Kim et al. [39] showed that automatic dose-modulation techniques combined with a decreased scan duration during the first pass limit the radiation dose significantly without compromising the image quality. Of course, when decreasing scan duration, it is important that the entire upslope of the contrast at first pass is acquired. Iterative reconstruction techniques can be used to compensate the loss of image quality when using a lower-tube current [45].

Despite the developments in dose reduction techniques, CTMPI procedures still yield a relatively high radiation exposure compared to other CT examinations. Patient-tailored CTMPI protocols are essential to reduce unnecessary radiation exposure.

Temporal Sampling Rate

The temporal resolution of dynamic CTMPI needs to exceed the timescale of the fastest process observed; otherwise, the perfusion parameters may be incorrect and most likely be underestimated. The fastest process in contrast medium kinetics is typically the vascular transit time. For example, in dynamic brain perfusion imaging, the minimal temporal sampling rate is 2 s. Several articles imply that a low temporal sampling rate in cardiac imaging, for example, in shuttle mode, leads to underestimation of the MBF in dynamic CTMPI [16, 46]. Temporal sampling rates of one acquisition every second heartbeat for low heart rates, up to one acquisition per four heartbeats at high heart rates (which are common in stress situations), are reported using a DSCT system in shuttle mode [13, 16, 46]. These temporal sampling rates may be insufficient to accurately capture the first-pass contrast enhancement curve.

Patient Preparation and Scanning Protocol

There are a number of points to consider in patient preparation. Patients should not use caffeine (coffee, tea, bananas, chocolate, etc.) for preferably 24 h or more before the examination, because of the interfering effects of caffeine on the effectiveness of the stressor agent. During the CCTA, beta-blockers may be needed to lower the heart rate in order to optimize image quality. Some studies have found that the use of beta-blockers may have a negative effect on the detection of myocardial ischemia by increasing the diastolic perfusion time [47, 48]. Sublingual nitrates, also commonly used in CCTA, have been shown to decrease the ischemic area on perfusion images [47].

At this time, CTMPI is not yet clinically used apart from certain centers in Asia. The exact position of CTMPI in the work-up of CAD is still under investigation. When considering implementing CCTA with CTMPI, it is still a point of debate whether CCTA or CTMPI should be the first in the examination order. In patients with a high probability or known CAD (after stenting or bypass grafting) in whom myocardial ischemia is likely, CCTA can be performed after the stress CTMPI procedure; see Fig. 63.2. This eliminates

Table 63.2 Dynamic CT myocardial perfusion patient studies using (semi)quantitative analysis

Study	Year	Number of patients	CT scanner	Radiation dose (mSv)	Reference	Analysis	Parameter	Model used	Sens	Spec	Cutoff (ml/100 ml/min)
Tanabe [26]	2016	53	256 row MDCT	10.5	SPECT	Segment	MBF	Singular value decomposition	80	86	0.92 mL/g/min
					MRI				82	87	0.98 mL/g/min
Wichmann [27]	2016	71	Second-generation DSCT	8.2	Visual CT	Patient	MBF (3 territories)	Two-compartment model + upslope (Siemens)	100	100	88
							MBF (2 territories)		81	91	15
							MBF (1 territory)		76	87	109
							MBV (3 territories)		100	88	16
							MBV (2 territories)		75	91	136
							MBV (1 territory)		86	45	20
Wichmann [28]	2015	137	Second-generation DSCT	643.8 (mGy. Cm)	CCTA	Territory	MBF	Patlak (Siemens)	82	81	103
							MBF ratio		91	93	0.71
Bamberg [29]	2014	31	Second-generation DSCT	11.1	MRI	Territory	MBF	Patlak (Siemens)	100	75	88
						Segment			78	75	
						Patient			100	75	
Ebersberger [30]	2014	37	Second-generation DSCT	9.6	SPECT	Segment	MBF	Patlak (Siemens)	86	96	Individual thresholds
							MBV		81	96	
Kono [31]	2014	42	Second-generation DSCT	9.4	ICA + FFR	Territory	MBF	Patlak (Siemens)	89	48	103
							MBF ratio		98	70	0.85
Rossi [32]	2013	80	Second-generation DSCT	9.4	ICA	Territory	MBF	Patlak (Siemens)	88	90	78
						Patient			90	88	
Huber [33]	2013	32	256 row MDCT	9.5	ICA + FFR	Territory	MBF	Linear fit+upslope method	76	100	1.64 ml/g/min
							Upslope	–	83	88	
Greif [34]	2013	65	Second-generation DSCT	9.7	ICA + FFR	Territory	MBF	Patlak (Siemens)	95	74	75
						Patient			97	66	
So [35]	2012	26	64-MDCT	9.7	SPECT		MPR	Distributed parameter model	95	35	2.5 ml/g/min
							MVR		97	24	1.4
Bamberg [36]	2011	33	Second-generation DSCT	10	ICA + FFR	Territory	MBF	Patlak (Siemens)	93	87	75
						Segment			91	98	
						Patient			95	64	
Ho [37]	2010	35	Second-generation DSCT	9.2	ICA	Segment	MBF	Patlak (Siemens)	83	78	–
Kido [38]	2008	14	16- MDCT	–	QCA	Territory	MBF	Patlak plot analysis	73	81	1.5 ml/g/min
					SPECT				88	79	

Note: *DSCT*, dual-source CT; *MDCT*, multi-detector CT; *CCTA*, coronary CT angiography; *ICA*, invasive coronary angiography; *FFR*, fractional flow reserve; *QCA*, quantitative coronary angiography; *MRI*, cardiac magnetic resonance; *SPECT*, single-photon emission CT; *MBF*, myocardial blood flow; *MBV*, myocardial blood volume; *MPR*, myocardial perfusion reserve; *MVR*, myocardial volume reserve the influence of beta-blockers and nitroglycerin on the stress CTMPI acquisition. In view of the relatively high radiation dose of CTMPI, in less-than-high probability patients it would be preferable to start with CCTA, in order to avoid unnecessary radiation dose in the case of no stenosis. This, however, would require direct reading of CCTA, which may not be logistically feasible. An advantage could be that beta-blockers given for CCTA may, if CTMPI follows, result in lower maximum heart rate during stress, which can lead to higher temporal sampling rate.

Compared to normal CCTA equipment, an additional infusion pump may be needed for the administration of the stressor agent and an additional intravenous catheter unless contrast medium and stressor are administered into the same arm such as in the case of regadenoson. Patients should be observed continuously during the CTMPI procedure with a 12-lead ECG and a blood-pressure monitor.

An optional, delayed acquisition (10–15 min after last contrast bolus) can be considered in order to differentiate between ischemic and infarcted myocardium in patients with known CAD. With a delayed enhancement (DE) scan, infarcted myocardium can be identified owing to the delayed in- and outflow of contrast of infarcted myocardium. This results in increased HU values in DE imaging. For this DE scan, administration of contrast medium beyond that administered during the stress or rest phase is not needed. However, DE scan acquisition might not be needed for the differentiation between ischemia and infarction. Bamberg et al. [29] showed that myocardial blood volume (MBV) is decreased in infarcted myocardium compared to ischemic myocardium, while MBF is reduced in both conditions. Also, actual MBF cutoff values may allow distinguishing between ischemia and infarction, as MBF in infarcted segments was found to be lower than in merely ischemic segments according to a study comparing CTMPI to MRI and SPECT [26].

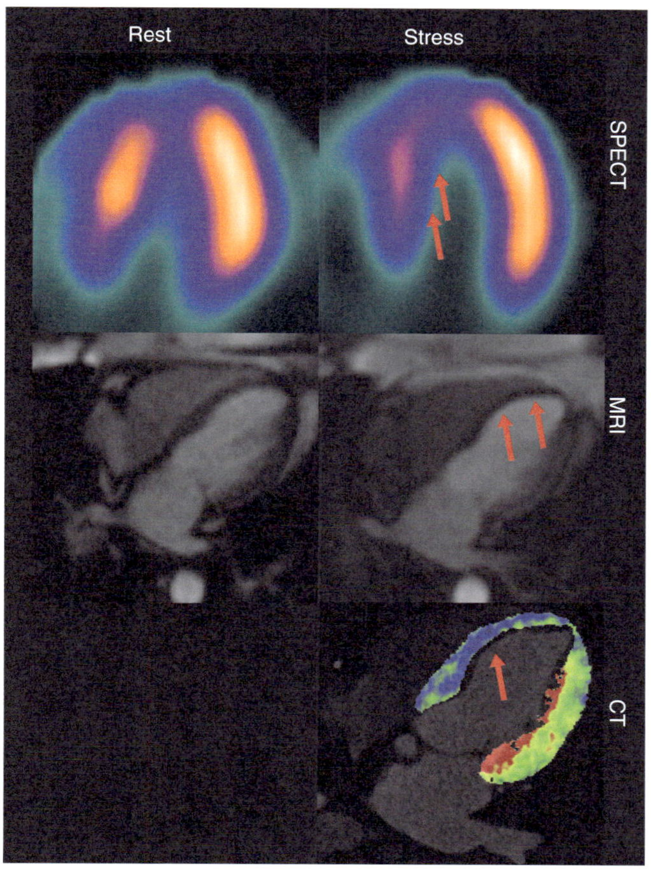

Fig. 63.1 Rest and stress perfusion images made by SPECT and MRI. For dynamic CTMPI stress imaging only could be sufficient

Image Analysis

Analysis of dynamic CTMPI images is based on the distribution of contrast medium throughout the myocardium. The distribution of iodine contrast medium can be described in two time-intensity curves. The tissue attenuation curve (TAC) describes the concentration of contrast medium in the myocardium over time, and the arterial input function (AIF) describes the concentration of contrast medium in the supplying artery (assessed at aorta or left ventricle).

Assessment of myocardial perfusion can be performed visually, semiquantitatively, or quantitatively. It should be

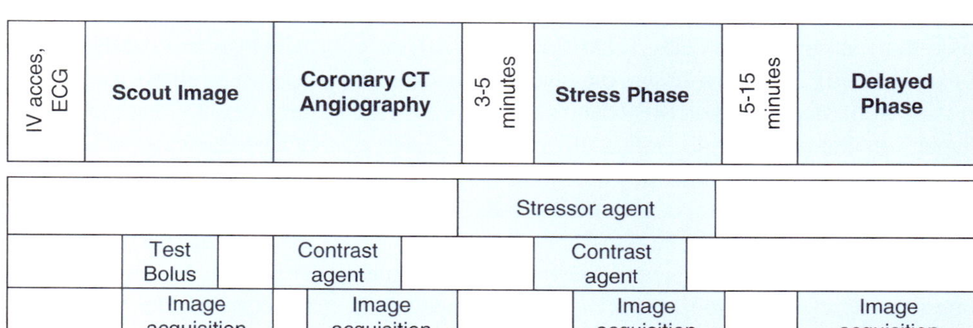

Fig. 63.2 Schematic representation of complete cardiac evaluation protocol, including anatomical (CCTA) and functional (dynamic CTMPI) evaluation. A third, optional scan is the delayed enhancement scan for the detection of infarcted myocardium

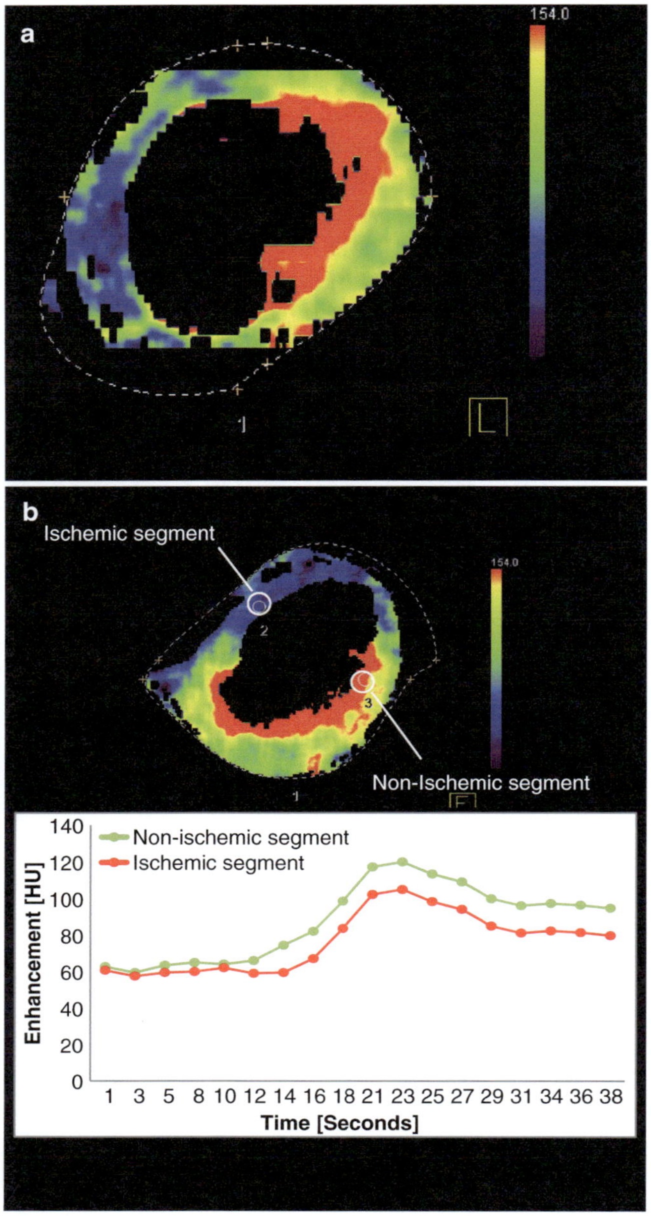

Fig. 63.3 (**a**) Color-coded perfusion map of myocardial blood flow. (**b**) The color-coded map is based on quantitative data. Regions of interest (white circles) represent a tissue attenuation curve (TAC) specific for that area

noted that, in contrast to static CTMPI, visual analysis of dynamic CTMPI is often based on quantitative data, by creating color maps based on MBF data; see Fig. 63.3. In this chapter qualitative analysis refers to visual analysis of CTMPI data without the use of any quantitative measure and may include the visual assessment of color-coded maps.

Myocardial perfusion can be assessed on a segment, territory, or patient basis. For segmental analysis, the 16-segment American Heart Association model is recommended [49]. This segmentation uses three imaging slices at basal, mid-cavity, and apical level. The basal and mid-cavity slices are each divided into six equal segments, whereas the apical slice is divided into four equal segments. The apex (segment 17) is often not taken into account for perfusion analysis because the limited scan width of most scanners does not allow the apex to be imaged [49]. Segmental CT perfusion analysis can be compared to other perfusion modalities such as MRI, PET, or SPECT. Perfusion analysis of vessel territories is based on a three-vessel division, namely, the left descending artery (LAD), the right coronary artery (RCA), and the circumflex artery (LCx) territory. Perfusion parameters are calculated per segment, after which multiple segments are averaged to represent a territory. Segments 1, 2, 7, 8, 13, and 14 are assigned to the LAD territory; segments 3, 4, 9, 10, and 15 are assigned to RCA territory; and segments 5, 6, 11, 12, and 16 are generally assigned to the LCx territory, depending on coronary dominance [49]. Anatomic variations in supplying arteries, however, may pose a problem. Territory analysis can be additionally compared with methods which analyze CAD severity on vessel level such as ICA and FFR methods. With nuclear modalities and MRI, it is also possible to analyze perfusion on a territory level.

For clinical purposes it is important to know whether a patient has myocardial ischemia and is in need of an intervention. Therefore, per-patient analysis is important for clinical diagnostics, while segment- and territory-based analyses are mostly used to validate the technique.

Qualitative, Visual Analysis

Qualitative analysis of dynamic CTMPI data can be done by visually inspecting the enhancement of myocardial tissue during the first pass of iodine contrast on dynamic series. Myocardium with reduced perfusion is hypo-attenuated and enhances later compared to normally perfused myocardium on CTMPI scans. Hypo-attenuation can in principle indicate both ischemic and infarcted myocardium. Visual analysis of dynamic CTMPI images is often done by analysis of color-coded maps; see Fig. 63.4. It is important to realize that these color-coded maps are actually based on quantitative information of myocardial perfusion. In contrast to SPECT, which primarily allows evaluation of relative perfusion of myocardial areas within a patient, the color map based on dynamic CTMPI represents actual MBF values, which allows assessment of globally reduced perfusion in three-vessel disease [50]. Below we describe the quantification of the underlying perfusion parameters.

Semiquantitative Analysis

Semiquantitative parameters can be derived from the TAC curves. The upslope method, in which the upslope of the TAC

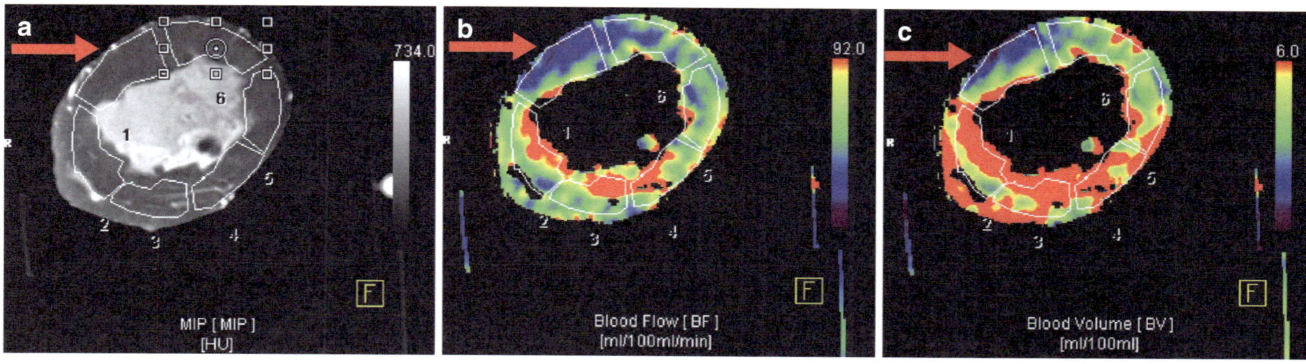

Fig. 63.4 (**a**) Mid ventricular slice of a dynamic CTMPI of a porcine heart with corresponding color-coded map representing (**b**) myocardial blood flow (MBF) in ml/100/ml/min and (**c**) myocardial blood volume (MBV) in ml/100 constructed with Volume Perfusion CT (VPCT) myocardium software (MMWP VA41A, Siemens). The AHA segmentation is projected onto the CT images. The red arrows point two the perfusion defects present in both hearts corresponding to both a decrease in MBF as in MBV

curve is taken as an indirect measure of perfusion, is a popular method to analyze CTMPI data. The upslope is calculated by making a linear fit of the upslope of the TAC curve. The main advantage of using the upslope is the possibility of shortening the scan time and thereby reducing the radiation dose since only knowledge of the wash in of contrast medium is required. For the upslope method, timing of the scan window is highly important. When the entire upslope of the curve is not included, the upslope method becomes inaccurate.

With the upslope method, MBF can be estimated with the following equation:

$$\mathrm{MBF} = \frac{\mathrm{Maxupslope}(\mathrm{TAC})}{\mathrm{Maximum}(\mathrm{AIF})} \qquad (63.1)$$

where the maximum upslope of the TAC (Maxupslope(TAC)) is divided by the maximum value of the AIF curve (Maximum(AIF)); see Fig. 63.5.

The upslope method accurately estimates MBF if the maximum slope of the TAC curve is within the mean tissue transit time, the time that a certain blood volume spends in the myocardium. In stress phase the mean tissue transit time is decreased, more so in normal myocardium than in ischemic myocardium. This decrease can cause an underestimation of MBF [51]. Another issue arising with the use of the upslope method is the inaccuracy of the AIF and TAC in the case of low temporal sampling rates. When temporal sampling rate is too low, the AIF and TAC consist of only a few measurement points during upslope, and important characteristics of both AIF and TAC can be missed.

Other semiquantitative parameters are peak enhancement, time to peak, and area under the curve, all derived from the TAC. From these semiquantitative parameters, the upslope is the most commonly used in MRI studies on semiquantitative analysis of myocardial perfusion [52–54].

Quantitative Analysis

There are several methods to perform true quantitative analysis of perfusion data, based on the AIF and TAC; see Fig. 63.6. Of these methods, the model-dependent deconvolution method is most frequently used in recent literature on cardiac and brain MRI perfusion analysis [51, 55]. Considering that the contrast media currently used in MRI (gadolinium) and CT (iodine) behave according to the same kinetic principles, the same approach can be used [51, 55, 56].

Quantitative CT perfusion analysis using model-dependent convolution can be divided in two phases. First, the signal-time curves (AIF and TAC) should be transformed into iodine concentration-time curves [10, 51]. In comparison with MRI, this is relatively easy for CT data since the change in HU values is linearly related to the iodine concentration [10].

Thus, the iodine concentration is proportional to the signal enhancement:

$$c(t) = k * \left(\mathrm{HU}(t) - \mathrm{HU}_0\right) \qquad (63.2)$$

In this formula, $c(t)$ is the iodine concentration over time, and HU_0 is the baseline HU value (i.e., before iodine injection). *K* is an unknown scale constant that is automatically corrected for during the second phase, assuming that *k* is tissue independent [51].

Second, a model-dependent deconvolution approach can be used to describe the perfusion process in the myocardium. This convolution theory-based approach is similar to deconvolution methods and models used in cardiac MRI studies [51, 57]. The iodine concentration in the myocardium over time is related to the iodine concentration in the supplying artery, convoluted (⊗) by an impulse response

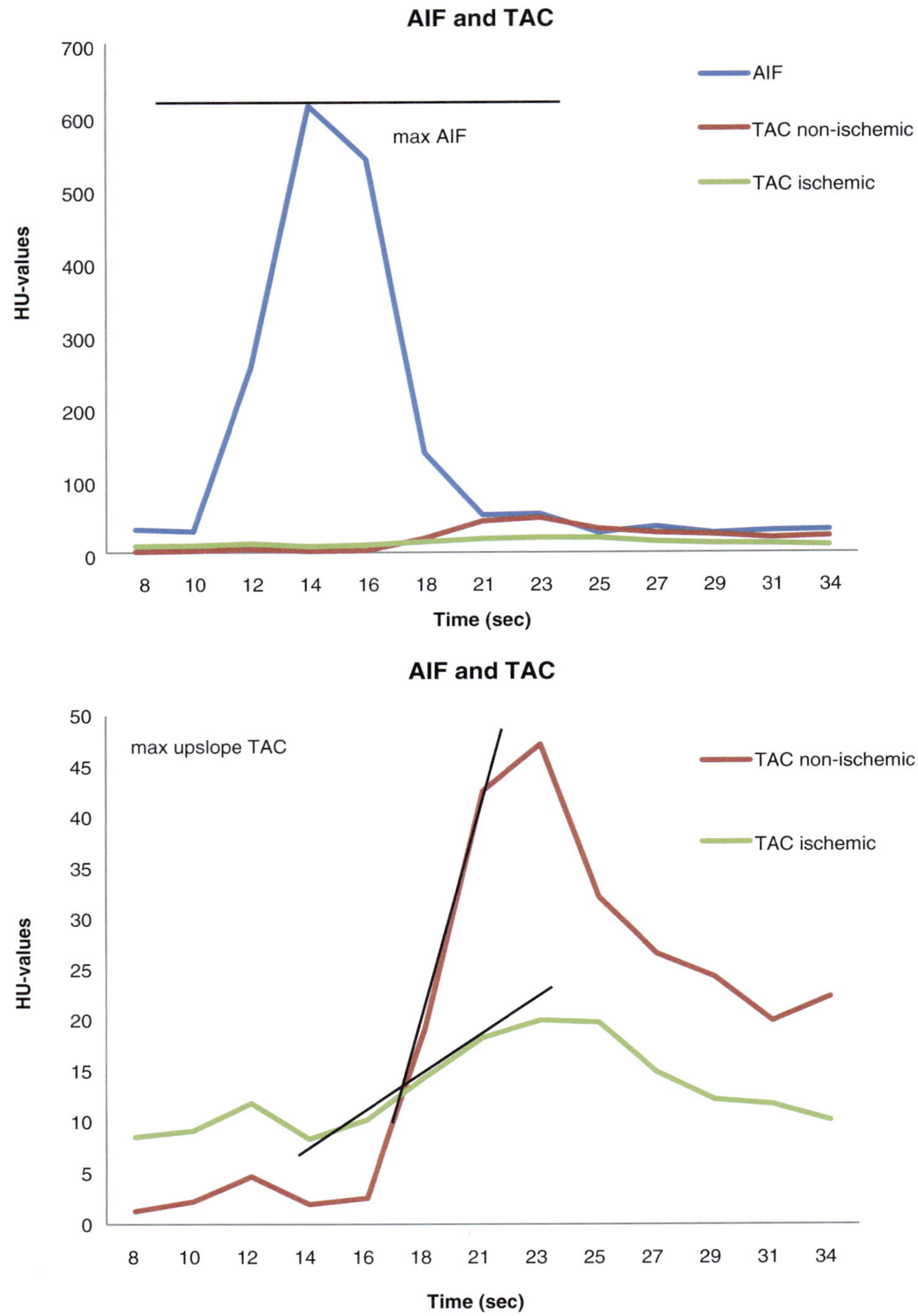

Fig. 63.5 The left figure shows the arterial input function (AIF) and the tissue attenuation curves (TAC) of a nonischemic segment and an ischemic segment. The ischemic segment shows a decreased inflow of contrast compared to the nonischemic segments. On the right is an extended graph showing the TAC in more detail. The maximum AIF value and maximum upslope of the TAC curve, used to calculate the myocardial blood flow, are indicated by black lines

function (IRF). This relation is described by the following equation [55, 56, 58]:

$$\mathrm{TAC}(t) = \mathrm{MBF} * \mathrm{AIF}(t) \otimes \mathrm{IRF}(t) \qquad (63.3)$$

where TAC(t) is the tissue attenuation curve over time (seconds) in HU values, MBF is the myocardial blood flow, AIF(t) is the arterial input function over time in HU values, and IRF(t) is the impulse response function over time.

If IRF(t) is known, the TAC can be obtained as a summation of adjusted IRFs; see Fig. 63.7. In dynamic CTMPI AIF and TAC are known parameters, measured from the CT images, whereas IRF(t) is the unknown parameter. The reversed process to reconstruct the IRF(t) is called deconvolution. The main issue with a deconvolution approach is that in contrast with convolution, deconvolution cannot give a unique solution because there are multiple IRF(t) estimations possible that would result in the same TAC(t)

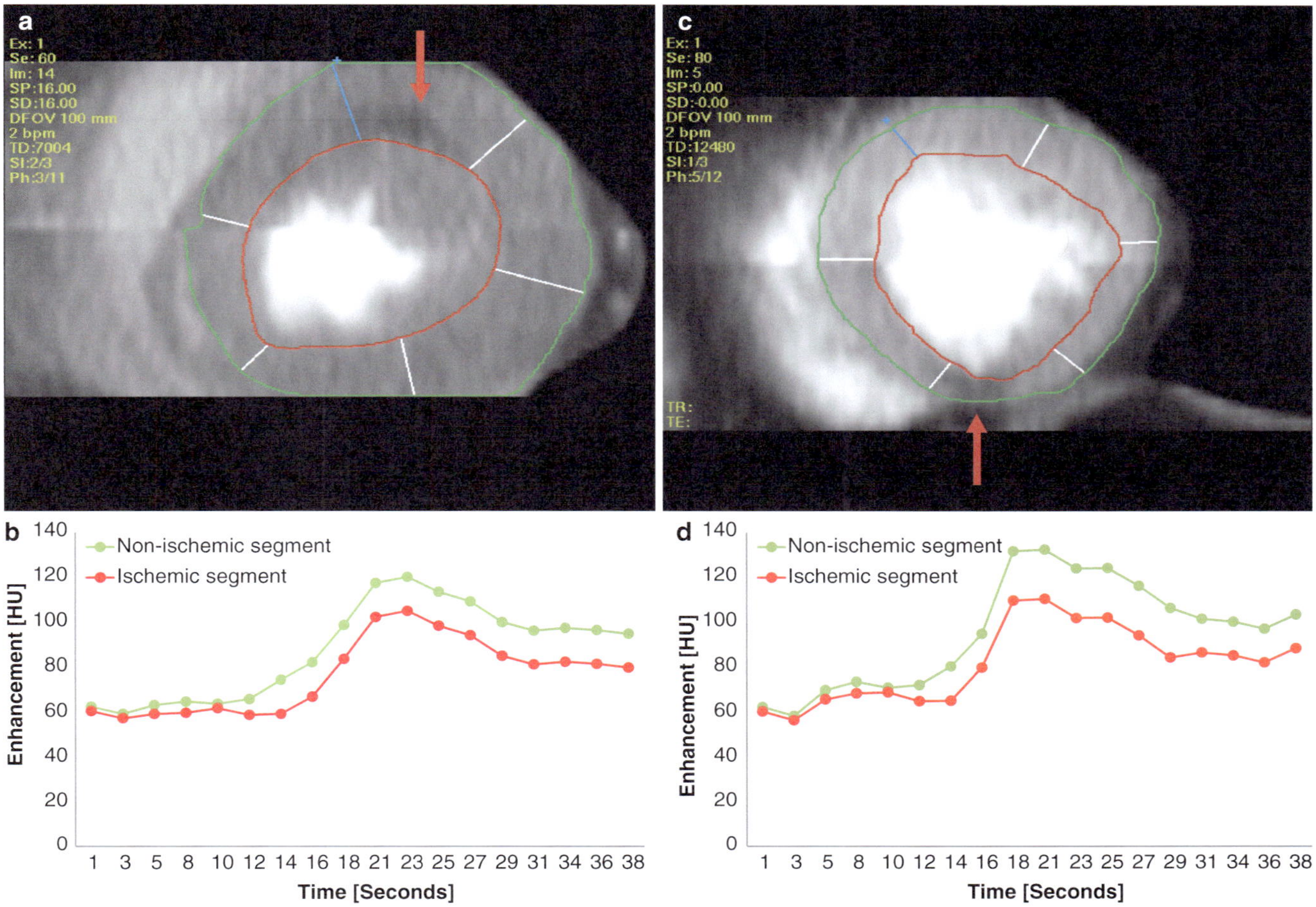

Fig. 63.6 (**a–c**) both show a midventricular slice of a dynamic CTMPI scan with a segmental overlay. A perfusion defect is visible in both scans (red arrows). (**b–d**) give the corresponding tissue attenuation curve (TAC) of a nonischemic segment without the perfusion defect (green) and of the ischemic segment with a perfusion defect (red) during multiple time points, where the TAC of the ischemic segments in both scans shows a decreased enhancement

or even a better approximation of the TAC(t). This problem is solved in model-dependent deconvolution by determining a generic model to represent the IRF(t) and setting predefined boundaries for the estimated parameters describing this model [55].

In the model-dependent deconvolution method, a tracer-kinetic model is assumed to represent IRF(t), after which the model parameters can be optimized to best fit Eq. (63.3) to the measured TAC data [51, 55, 56]. From the fitted model of the estimated IRF(t), the MBF value can be derived using Eq. 63.3, with known TAC(t), AIF(t), and IRF(t).

Convolution and deconvolution techniques are difficult because noise in either the AIF or TAC data can influence the model optimization and result in an unstable solution for IRF(t) and unreliable MBF values [58]. Noise in CTMPI data can be caused, for example, by inaccurate HU values, measured during different cardiac phases. Reducing noise is therefore an important issue in dynamic CTMPI.

Tracer-Kinetic Models

A wide variety of tracer-kinetic models can be used to represent IRF(t). Each of these models has its merits and limitations; the optimal model for CTMPI analysis has yet to be determined.

The microcirculation of the myocardium is depicted in Fig. 63.8a. Iodine is considered an extravasating contrast medium. The contrast medium distributes across the intravascular space and the extracellular extravascular space, both defined by volume and transit time parameters. High-order perfusion models try to describe the complexity of these dynamics. The two-compartment model and the distributed parameter model, both using four free parameters, are examples of high-order perfusion models.

When only limited data are available or the quality of the data is low, it becomes difficult to accurately assess all parameters in high-order models. Simplified models with fewer free parameters are useful in these situations, for example, the extended Toft model (three free parameters). These tracer-kinetic models fix

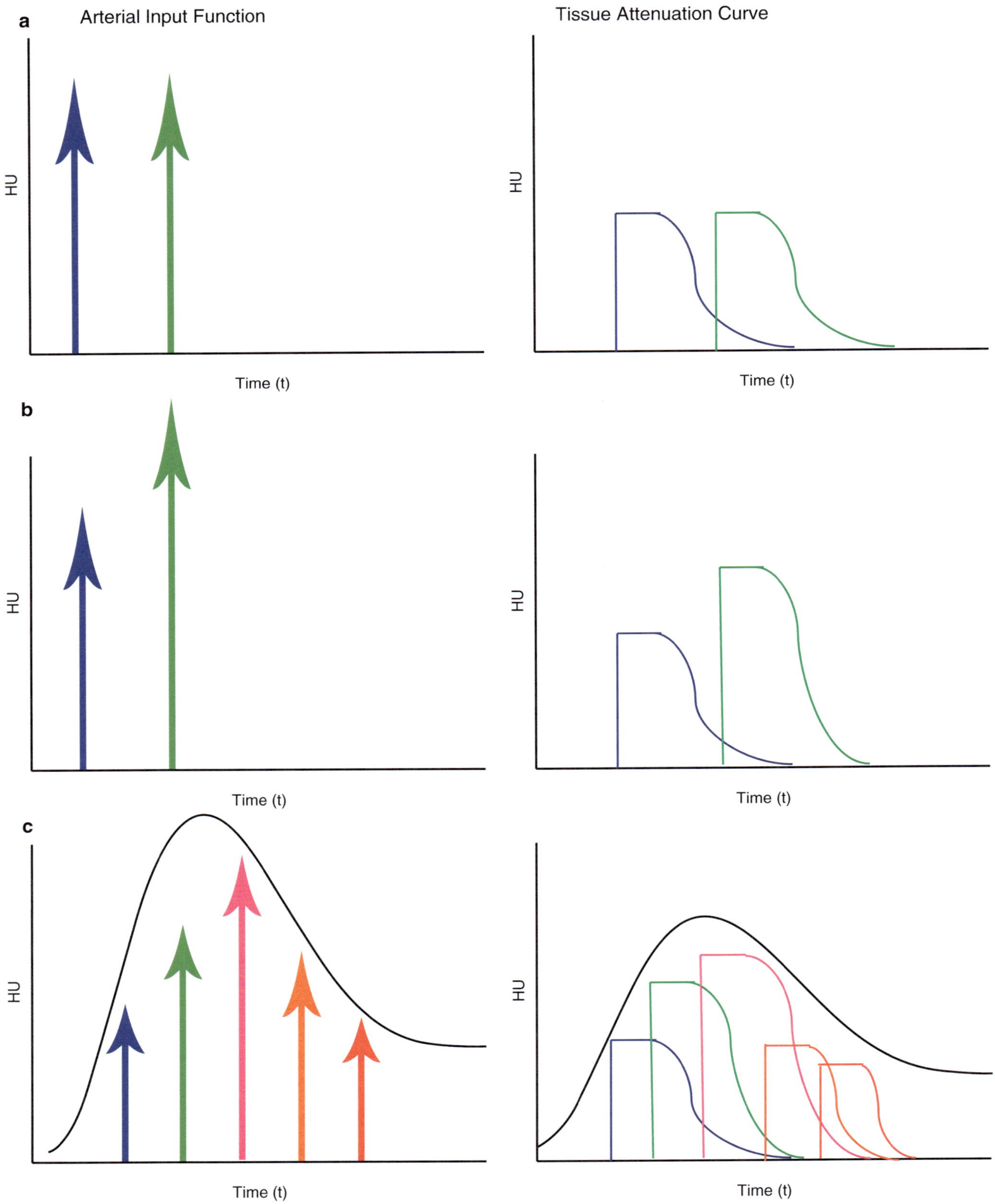

Fig. 63.7 (**a**) When two identical bolus injections of the same concentration (left) are given, then the IRF (right) will be the same for each injection. For each bolus, the IRF shows an abrupt increase in HU values (if the injection is given directly to arterial input); it then stabilizes for a period of time while the bolus passes through the tissue and finally shows a gradual return back to baseline level. The plateau represents the mean transit time. (**b**) When the bolus injections have different properties, for example, different concentrations (left), the corresponding IRFs (right) will be different. (**c**) Contrast medium inflow represented as a series of bolus injections of different concentrations (left) and corresponding IRFs (right). The tissue attenuation curve (TAC) is the sum of all IRFs corresponding to the bolus injections attenuated by the effects of blood flow

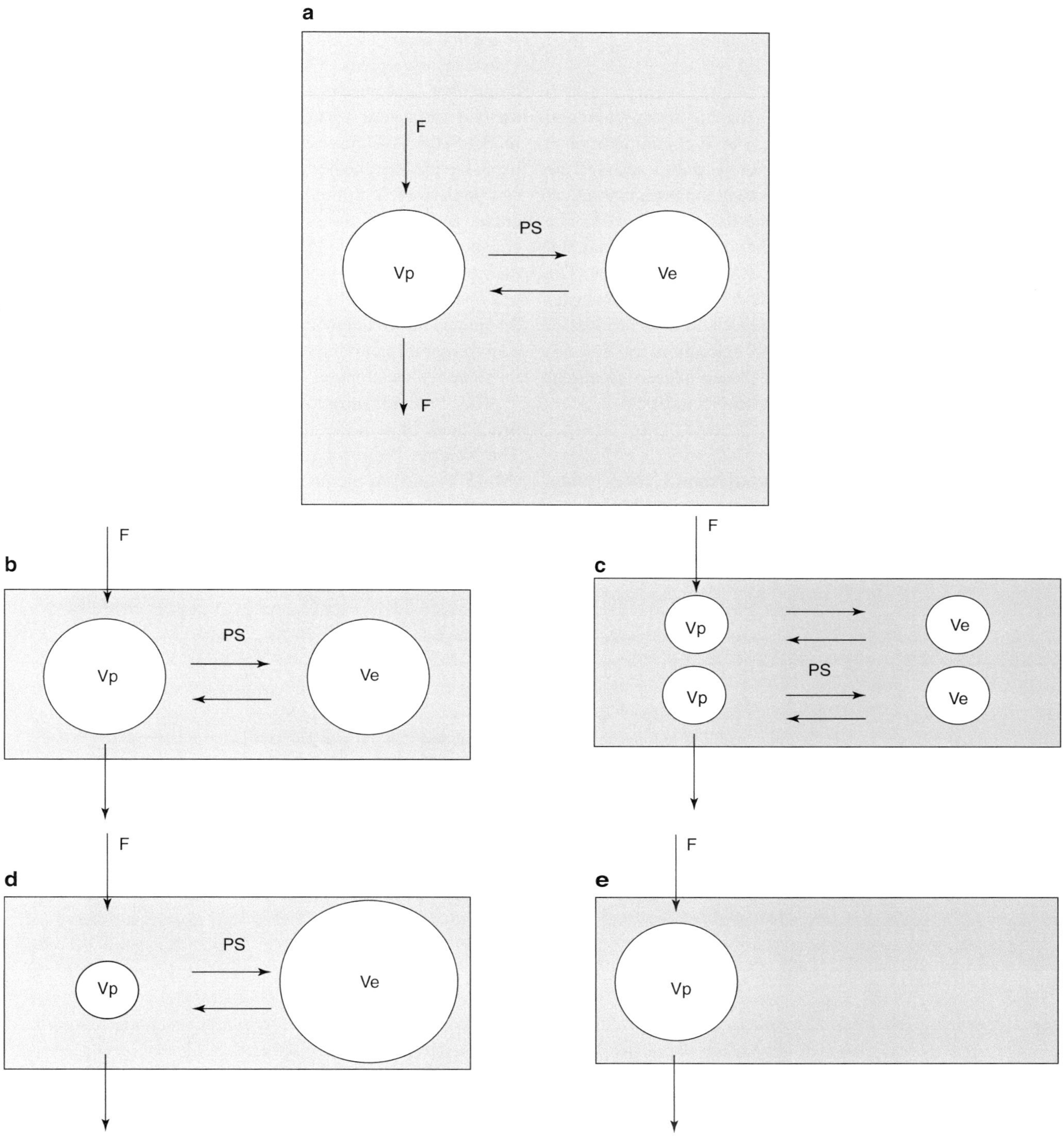

Fig. 63.8 Schematic representation of tracer-kinetic models. (**a**) Schematic representation of the myocardial microcirculation. The **b**lood plasma flows to the vascular space (Vp) driving the myocardial blood flow (F). The Vp compartment exchanges molecules via a flow (PS) with the extracellular extravascular space (Ve). (**b**) Schematics of the two-compartment model. The Vp space can only exchange contrast medium with the Ve space. (**c**) Schematics of the distributed parameter model. The Vp and Ve spaces are represented by multiple small compartments. The contrast medium can only exchange between neighboring compartments. (**d**) Schematics of the extended Toft model, where infinite flow (F) is assumed. (**e**) Schematics of the Fermi model. This mathematical model has only nonphysiological parameters and only the flow (F) can be derived

one (or more) parameters at a constant value resulting in an accurate parameter estimation with less free parameters.

Two-Compartment Model

The two-compartment model describes the intravascular and the extracellular extravascular space as two compartments; see Fig. 63.8b. This model does not take into account the transit times; therefore, the IRF of a two-compartment model does not have a stable plateau as the IRFs in Fig. 63.7. The transit time parameters represent the time a specific amount of blood volume is present in the tissue or capillaries. The peak value of the IRF corresponds to the volume transfer coefficient K_{trans}. This parameter is defined as a product of myocardial blood flow (MBF) and extraction fraction (E) and represents the inflow into the extravascular extracellular space and thereby the delivery of nutrients to tissue.

Patlak Method

This method is used in the majority of dynamic CTMPI patient studies (see Table 63.2) and is a hybrid method based on a two-compartment model combined with the upslope method. In the first phase, the TAC curve is reconstructed from the individual measurements of iodine concentration in the myocardium over time, using a convolution approach. The Patlak method uses a least square fit method to fit a two-compartment model to the TAC curve. Subsequently the MBF is calculated using the upslope method; see Eq. 63.1. The maximal upslope can be derived from the IRF(t) function, describing the TAC curve. Because of the convolution approach to estimate an equation (IRF) describing the TAC, this method is ideal for CT data with low temporal sampling rates where the use of only an upslope method results in inaccurate MBF values because of the limited information on TAC and AIF curves. An example of a low temporal sampling scan mode is the ECG-triggered shuttle mode with a temporal sampling rate of 2–3 s [51].

This method substantially simplifies the mathematical procedures of a model-dependent deconvolution approach. The Volume Perfusion CT (VPCT) myocardium software (MMWP VA41A, Siemens) adopted this method to calculate the MBF in dynamic CTMPI data (Fig. 63.9). Although this

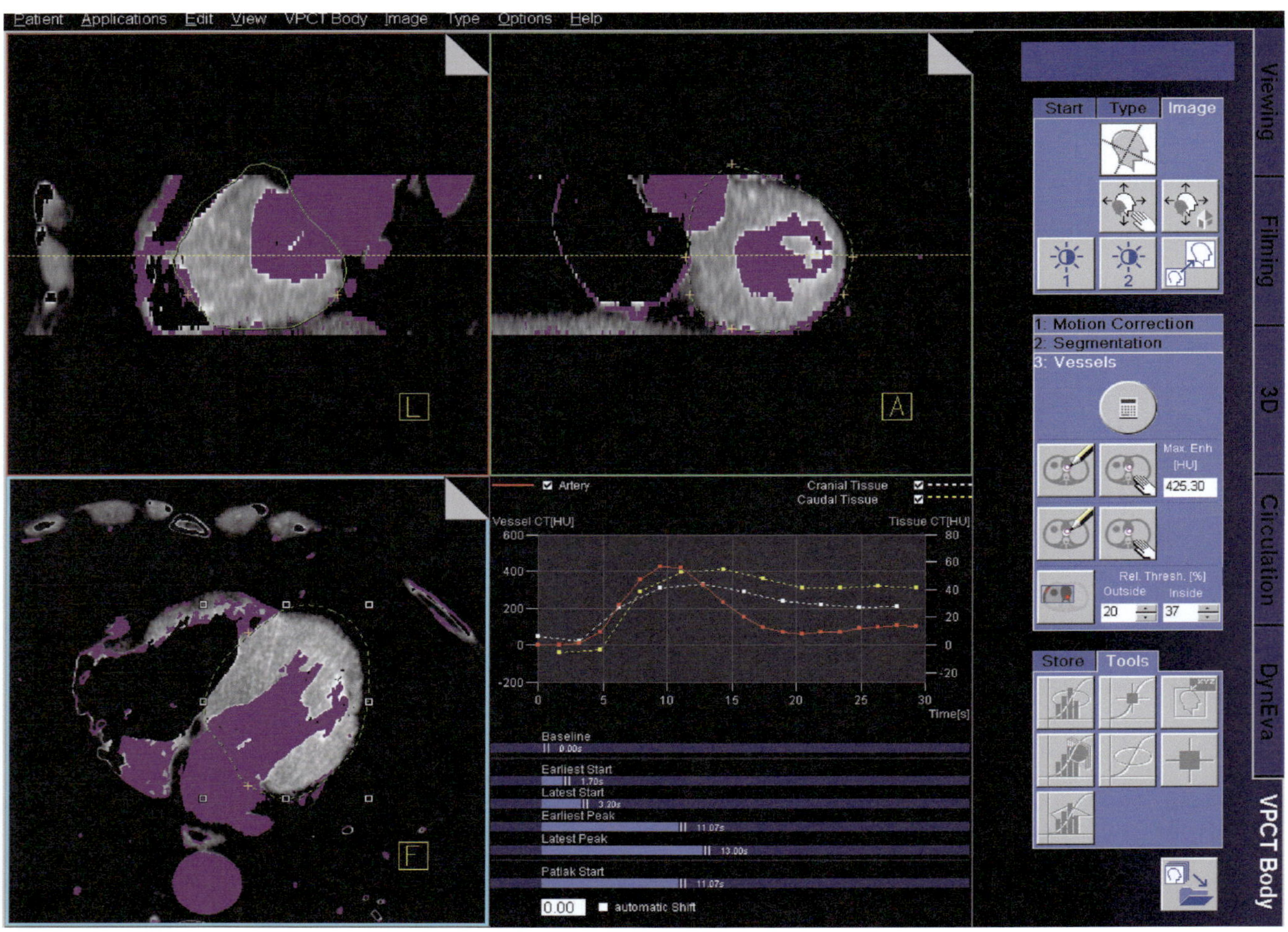

Fig. 63.9 An overview of the Volume Perfusion CT (VPCT) myocardium software (MMWP VA41A, Siemens). Multiple windows allow to visualize different CT axis, show the signal intensity curves for the drawn regions of interest and give corresponding quantitative results

method gives a good estimation and is able to distinguish ischemic myocardium from normal myocardium, MBF is substantially underestimated [16].

More accurate MBF values could be obtained by using Eq. 63.3 to calculate the MBF directly instead of using a hybrid approach with the upslope method (Eq. 63.1). However, this comes at the cost of higher computational complexity.

Distributed Parameter Model

The distributed parameter model is one of the more complex models, taking into account all aspects of contrast medium kinetics. Contrast medium is assumed to exchange between spaces. This model estimates volume, flow, and transit time parameters, providing a full description of the perfusion process [51]. In comparison with other models, the distributed parameter represents both the extracellular extravascular and the vascular space as a series of compartments, Fig. 63.8c. Each extracellular extravascular space compartment interacts only with the nearest vascular space compartment and vice versa. The use of the distributed parameter model is limited by the temporal sampling rate of the CT system. If the temporal sampling rate is too low, accurate estimation of the mean transit times becomes impossible. With higher perfusion flow, the mean transit time decreases, requiring an even higher temporal sampling rate and a compact contrast medium bolus. Because of the complexity of the distributed parameter model, complex fitting methods are required, making the system more susceptible to errors [55]. So et al. [35] used the distributed parameter model to calculate myocardial blood flow using 64-MDCT system. The myocardial perfusion ratio, a ratio between normal and remote myocardium, had 95% sensitivity and 35% specificity to identify ischemic myocardium, with SPECT as reference method.

Extended Toft Model

The extended Toft model has one fixed parameter and three free parameters. It is a simplified variation of the two-compartment model and the distributed parameter model by assuming an infinite flow; see Fig. 63.8d. This means that the MBF cannot be measured with this model; instead the volume transfer coefficient K_{trans} is obtained. Although describing a key part of the perfusion process, this model cannot be used to measure flow and should therefore not be compared to flow-measuring models. However, in situations where the flow cannot be measured accurately due to low temporal sampling rate, the extended Toft model can provide an alternative direct proxy measure for perfusion instead of MBF [51, 55]. So far this model has not been applied in any published dynamic CTMPI study in patients.

Fermi Model

The Fermi model assumes that the contrast medium does not leave the intravascular space. The Fermi model is a mathematical model providing only a functional representation of an IRF. This model does not allow a physiological interpretation of the parameters used in the model; the parameters are simply used as shaping parameters; see Fig. 63.8e. However, the flow (MBF) can still be estimated by the above-described model-dependent deconvolution technique [51, 55]. This model is successfully used in studies on MRI analysis of myocardium perfusion [10, 59–62].

Diagnostic Accuracy

Only a limited number of patient studies (n = 18) has been published on dynamic CTMPI including a total of 805 patients. They are mostly small single-center studies with large inter-study heterogeneity in protocols, scanner type, stressor agent, reference value, analysis method, and cutoff value, making it difficult to compare results.

Visual Analysis

Five studies used visual analysis to evaluate dynamic CTMPI data, including a total of 149 patients with a median of 27 patients per study. These dynamic CTMPI publications using visual analysis are listed in Table 63.1. Sensitivity was found to range from 84% to 98% and specificity from 76% to 98%. All studies with visual analysis of dynamic CT data so far used a second-generation DSCT system.

Two studies analyzed individual segments and two studies analyzed vessel territories. Baxa et al. [22] analyzed both segments and territories. They showed 97% sensitivity and 95% specificity for territory-based analysis, and 98% sensitivity and 96% specificity for segment-based analysis, comparing visual analysis of CTMPI data with ICA. None of the studies performed with visual analysis of dynamic CTMPI data assessed diagnostic accuracy on a per-patient level.

Two visual analysis studies document interobserver agreement between dynamic CTMPI and other perfusion modalities. Weininger et al. [23] compared visual analysis of dynamic CTMPI to SPECT and MRI perfusion and obtained similar results. Interobserver agreement between CTMPI and MRI and CTMPI and SPECT was high with kappa values of 0.85 and 0.82, respectively. Wang et al. [24] compared visual analysis of dynamic CTMPI analysis to SPECT and found high interobserver agreement for detecting perfusion defects with CTMPI and SPECT with kappa values of 0.81 and 0.83, respectively.

Semiquantitative Analysis

Huber et al. [33] is the only study using a semiquantitative parameter (upslope), and they compared it with a quantitative parameter (linear fit+upslope method) using a 256 row MDCT system with ICA and FFR measurements as a reference standard. The quantitative measured MBF yielded a sensitivity and specificity of 76% and 100%, while the semi-quantitative upslope measure resulted in a reported sensitivity and specificity of 83% and 88%, respectively.

Quantitative Analysis

A total of 13 dynamic CTMPI reports with quantitative analysis are shown in Table 63.2. Included were 656 patients with a median of 37 patients per study. Respective sensitivity and specificity of MBF cutoffs for myocardial ischemia ranged from 73% to 100% and 48% to 100% for MBF. For MBV, sensitivity varied between 75% and 100% and specificity between 24% and 91%. Reference techniques include SPECT, MRI, and ICA + FFR. It should be noted that of these reference techniques only MRI is able to provide a quantitative measure of MBF and MBV values. In studies of Tanabe et al. [26], Huber et al. [33], So et al. [35], and Kido et al. [38], a MDCT system was used; in all other studies, a second-generation DSCT system in shuttle mode was used.

Segment, Territory, and Patient

Bamberg et al. [29, 36] determined the diagnostic accuracy of MBF on segment-, territory-, and patient-based analysis in two separate studies, compared to, respectively, MRI and FFR. Segment-based analysis showed sensitivity of 78% and 91%, respectively, compared to 100% and 93% on territory basis and 100% and 95% on patient basis. Rossi et al. [32] analyzed their MBF data on both per-territory and per-patient level resulting in 88–90% sensitivity and specificity, compared to ICA alone.

Cutoff Values

A wide range of cutoff values (75–103 ml/100 ml/min for MBF) has been proposed to distinguish ischemic from non-ischemic myocardial segments. Studies using DSCT combined with *VPCT* software have reported cutoff values in ml/100 ml/min, while studies using MDCT have reported cutoff values in ml/g/min. Ebersberger et al. [30] used individual cutoff values instead of a generic MBF cutoff value and reported a sensitivity of 86% and a specificity of 96% with SPECT as reference modality. The cutoff values were calculated by subtracting the standard deviation of all segments from the average value of the respective measurement. Kim et al. [63] assessed the range of CTMPI-determined MBF in 19 healthy volunteers in rest and in stress using 128-slice DSCT. Results showed considerable heterogeneity in absolute MBF values. Women had higher MBF values at rest compared to men but had lower MBF values during stress imaging. Danad et al. [64] showed in a myocardial PET perfusion study that gender, age, and weight influence MBF values and that reference MBF values vary significantly within the general population. These results indicate that using a general cutoff value for perfusion parameters may be sub-optimal.

Absolute vs. Relative MBF Values

As mentioned previously, a wide variety of absolute MBF cutoff values have been reported for discriminating ischemic from nonischemic myocardium, as well as a high heterogeneity of MBF values in the normal population. This issue could be avoided by using a relative instead of an absolute measure of MBF. A relative measure comparing normally perfused myocardium with ischemic myocardium may be more accurate for the identification of myocardial ischemia in the individual patient. However, absolute values offer advantage in the diagnosis of global ischemia when normally perfused myocardium is absent.

Wichmann et al. [28] compared absolute MBF values and relative MBF values to CCTA results in 137 patients using a second-generation DSCT. Relative MBF values yielded a higher diagnostic accuracy than absolute MBF values on a territory level, with a sensitivity and specificity of 91% and 93% compared to 82% and 81%. Kono et al. [31] reported similar results in 42 patients using a second-generation DSCT, comparing relative MBF values and absolute MBF values to combined ICA and FFR results. They reported 98% sensitivity and 70% specificity for relative MBF values compared to 89% sensitivity and 48% specificity for absolute MBF values. Both studies used a two-compartment model combined with upslope analysis to calculate MBF.

Myocardial Blood Volume

Myocardial blood volume (MBV) could be another parameter for the detection of myocardial perfusion defects. In ischemic myocardium vasodilation of the arterioles compensates for the decreased flow in the stenotic artery, thereby changing the volume of blood in the myocardium. Bamberg et al. [29] showed that MBV values are lower in infarcted myocardium compared to ischemic myocardium and could therefore help to differentiate between the two states. Three studies evaluated the diagnostic accuracy of both MBF and MBV to detect ischemic myocardium. So et al. [35] used myocardial perfusion reserve (MPR) and myocardial volume reserve (MVR) to detect ischemic areas with SPECT as reference. MPR and MVR were defined as the ratio of MBV and MBF values in stress and rest imaging. They reported sensitivity and specificity of 95% and 35% using MPR, and 97% and 24% using MVR, compared to SPECT results. Ebersberger et al. [30] determined absolute MBF and MBV values and reported a slightly lower sensitivity for MBV than for MBF (81% compared to 86%) with comparable specificity, comparing dynamic CTMPI results to SPECT. Wichmann et al. [27] also determined absolute MBF and MBV values, analyzing one-, two-, or three-vessel territories and compared quantitative analysis of the CTMPI data to visual analysis of perfusion defects of the same CTMPI data. Global MBV values showed lower specificity compared to MBF values. Bamberg et al. [36] compared MBF and MBV values to combined ICA and FFR measurements. They reported that MBF had a significantly higher discriminatory power than MBV to detect myocardial ischemia. The combination of MBF and MBV values was found to be useful in discriminating ischemic and infarcted myocardium from normal myocardium.

Comparison of Visual, Semiquantitative, and Quantitative Analysis

Huber et al. [33] showed a similar diagnostic accuracy for semiquantitative parameters compared to a quantitative measure of MBF in dynamic CTMPI, with combined ICA and FFR results as a reference. The reported sensitivity and specificity were 83% and 88% for the semiquantitative upslope parameter CTMPI, respectively, and 76% and 100% for the quantitative MBF parameter. The range of reported specificities among studies is larger for quantitative analysis, indicating that diagnostic accuracy for a quantitative approach is less robust. However, quantification of myocardial perfusion may be useful in diagnosing three-vessel disease, where there is no nonischemic myocardium present as reference and in the case of global hypoperfusion of the left ventricular myocardium. Three-vessel disease and global hypoperfusion are known to cause false-negative results in SPECT. Meinel et al. [50] investigated whether quantification of global MBF is feasible and showed that global MBF is gradually lower in patients with increasing territorial perfusion defects and is correlated to the number of obstructed vessels. Global MBF showed a moderate correlation with visual CTMPI assessment and CCTA findings [50]. A study of Vliegenthart et al. [9] investigated whether absolute global perfusion parameters as MBF and MBV could detect subclinical changes in perfusion parameters in patients with hypertension and diabetes. This offers the opportunity to use absolute MBF values for the risk stratification of CAD prior to the presence of evident myocardial ischemia. The diagnosis of microvascular disease is another process that could benefit from absolute quantification of MBF with dynamic CTMPI. Microvascular disease is characterized by a decrease in (global) perfusion without correlation to an anatomical abnormality of the coronary arteries. Dynamic CTMPI combined with CTA could possibly be used to diagnose microvascular disease and exclude CAD.

Comparison of Static and Dynamic CTMPI

In an animal study, Schwarz et al. [65] concluded that dynamic CTMPI may be more sensitive for detection of smaller perfusion defects compared to static CTMPI. However, Huber et al. [33] showed that diagnostic accuracy of the dynamic CTMPI parameter was similar to that derived from static CTMPI data using combined ICA and FFR measurements as a reference. More studies are needed to investigate in which patients dynamic CTMPI has additional value beyond visual analysis of myocardial ischemia based on myocardial blood supply imaging.

Comparison with Other Modalities

Currently there are no patient studies comparing dynamic CTMPI and other ischemia imaging modalities against the same reference standard.

Future Perspectives

The limited number of dynamic CTMPI studies in patients shows promising results with regard to the diagnostic value of dynamic CT for the detection of myocardial ischemia. However, several issues need to be addressed before clinical implementation of this technique can be considered.

The currently published patient studies are difficult to compare due to heterogeneity in imaging protocols, reference standards, and analysis techniques. An optimal and robust protocol for dynamic CTMPI is yet to be determined.

The main advantage of dynamic CTMPI compared to other perfusion imaging techniques is the possibility to truly quantify myocardial blood flow, making it possible to accurately identify perfusion defects even in the absence of normally perfused myocardium. Absolute perfusion values offer the possibility of improving CAD risk stratification, diagnosing multivessel CAD, discriminating between infarcted and ischemic myocardium, and identifying early subclinically reduced myocardial perfusion such as in microvascular disease.

Although the quantification of perfusion parameters is assumed to have multiple advantages compared to visual analysis, it is yet to be proven that more accurate MBF (or MBV) values aid in the diagnosis of myocardial ischemia and are able to improve patient outcome. Dynamic CTMPI can be analyzed visually by looking at the dynamic series and quantitatively by either looking at color-coded maps based on absolute values or by analyzing the absolute perfusion parameters directly. Until now there is no study comparing the use of color-coded maps with absolute values to identify ischemic myocardium. The question remains which of the analysis methods yields highest diagnostic accuracy and best clinical feasibility.

A disadvantage of dynamic CTMPI compared to other modalities is the radiation dose, especially when CCTA and dynamic CTMPI are combined. Patient-tailored protocols to reduce radiation dose should be developed. This could be done by patient-specific tube current and kV modulation and iterative image reconstruction. Static CTMPI is unable to quantify MBF but has a lower radiation dose than dynamic CTMPI. Whether the increased radiation dose of dynamic CTMPI weighs up to the benefits of absolute quantification, and in which patients, is yet to be determined.

Although the main benefit of dynamic CTMPI is the possibility to quantify perfusion, several issues arise with the use of this quantitative imaging method. One of the challenges with dynamic CTMPI is underestimation of MBF compared to other quantitative modalities. Studies with PET-determined MBF [66, 67] have reported stress values between 3 and 5 ml/min/g, whereas dynamic CTMPI studies [24, 32, 36]. report stress MBF values between 1.0 and 1.4 ml/min/g. Studies of Bindschadler et al. [46] and Ishida et al. [16] suggest that a limited temporal sampling rate is the main cause of the underestimation of MBF determined by dynamic CTMPI. Further research should investigate the effect of temporal sampling rate on absolute MBF values and the influence on diagnostic accuracy. A second cause for underestimation of MBF values with dynamic CTMPI could be the use of combining a tracer-kinetic model with the Patlak method to calculate MBF. Possibly this method estimates K_{trans} instead of MBF [16]. By calculating the MBF using a method purely based on deconvolution, MBF values could be more accurate compared to the most widely used hybrid method combining deconvolution and upslope calculation. Each model has its own advantages and disadvantages. Further research is needed to determine which tracer-kinetic model optimally approximates the true value of MBF in CTMPI. Currently, the effect of quantitative perfusion parameters on the diagnostic accuracy in the detection of CAD and myocardial ischemia is still unknown.

There are a few studies comparing the diagnostic accuracy of different perfusion modalities [1, 3]; however, these do not include dynamic CTMPI. The performance of (dynamic) CTMPI with regard to SPECT, PET, and MRI, potentially in combination with anatomical evaluation procedures, needs to be determined in large patient studies including patient outcomes and analysis of cost-effectiveness. Large multicenter studies could also aid in the search for the optimal perfusion cutoff values for several subpopulations in order to increase the diagnostic accuracy. It should be established if dynamic CTMPI in patients with previous coronary artery bypass graft surgery or stent placements has an added value in the diagnostic process. The SPECIFIC study may answer some of these remaining questions. The objective of the multicenter SPECIFIC study is to determine the diagnostic accuracy of CTMPI for the detection of hemodynamically relevant coronary stenosis in patients with suspected or known CAD. A subgroup of patients will also undergo perfusion MRI. The diagnostic accuracy of MRI versus dynamic CTMPI for the detection of perfusion defects will be compared to the reference standard, ICA plus FFR.

In conclusion, the few patient studies focusing on dynamic CTMPI for myocardial ischemia detection show promising results. Absolute quantification of perfusion parameters offers great potential, not only in the diagnosis of myocardial ischemia but potentially also in the detection of early signs of reduced myocardial blood flow as well as the diagnosis of microvascular disease and three-vessel disease. With the advent of new dose reduction techniques and new developments in CT systems, resulting in faster scanning times and wider detectors, clinical implementation of dynamic CTMPI becomes closer.

References

1. Jaarsma C, Leiner T, Bekkers SC, et al. Diagnostic performance of noninvasive myocardial perfusion imaging using single-photon emission computed tomography, cardiac magnetic resonance, and positron emission tomography imaging for the detection of obstructive coronary artery disease. J Am Coll Cardiol. 2012;59(19):1719–28. https://doi.org/10.1016/j.jacc.2011.12.040.
2. Schwitter J, Wacker CM, van Rossum AC, et al. MR-IMPACT: comparison of perfusion-cardiac magnetic resonance with single-photon emission computed tomography for the detection of coronary artery disease in a multicentre, multivendor, randomized trial. Eur Heart J. 2008;29(4):480–9. https://doi.org/10.1093/eurheartj/ehm617.
3. Parker MW, Iskandar A, Limone B, et al. Diagnostic accuracy of cardiac positron emission tomography versus single photon emission computed tomography for coronary artery disease: a bivariate meta-analysis. Circ Cardiovasc Imaging. 2012;5(6):700–7. https://doi.org/10.1161/CIRCIMAGING.112.978270.
4. Hulten EA, Carbonaro S, Petrillo SP, Mitchell JD, Villines TC. Prognostic value of cardiac computed tomography angiography: a systematic review and meta-analysis. J Am Coll Cardiol. 2011;57(10):1237–47. https://doi.org/10.1016/j.jacc.2010.10.011.
5. Pelgrim GJ, Dorrius M, Xie X, et al. The dream of a one-stop-shop: meta-analysis on myocardial perfusion CT. Eur J Radiol. 2015;84(12):2411–20. https://doi.org/10.1016/j.ejrad.2014.12.032.
6. Danad I, Szymonifka J, Schulman-Marcus J, Min JK. Static and dynamic assessment of myocardial perfusion by computed tomography. Eur Hear J Cardiovasc Imaging. 2016;17:836–44. https://doi.org/10.1093/ehjci/jew044.
7. Williams MC, Newby DE. CT myocardial perfusion imaging: current status and future directions. Clin Radiol. 2016;71(8):1–11. https://doi.org/10.1016/j.crad.2016.03.006.
8. Caruso D, Eid M, Schoepf UJ, et al. Dynamic CT myocardial perfusion imaging. Eur J Radiol. 2016;85:1893. https://doi.org/10.1016/j.ejrad.2016.07.017.
9. Vliegenthart R, De Cecco CN, Wichmann JL, et al. Dynamic CT myocardial perfusion imaging identifies early perfusion abnormalities in diabetes and hypertension: insights from a multicenter registry. J Cardiovasc Comput Tomogr. 2016;10(4):301–8. https://doi.org/10.1016/j.jcct.2016.05.005.

10. George RT, Jerosch-Herold M, Silva C, et al. Quantification of myocardial perfusion using dynamic 64-detector computed tomography. Investig Radiol. 2007;42(12):815–22. https://doi.org/10.1097/RLI.0b013e318124a884.
11. Christian TF, Frankish ML, Sisemoore JH, et al. Myocardial perfusion imaging with first-pass computed tomographic imaging: measurement of coronary flow reserve in an animal model of regional hyperemia. J Nucl Cardiol. 2010;17(4):625–30. https://doi.org/10.1007/s12350-010-9206-6.
12. So A, Hsieh J, Li J-Y, Hadway J, Kong H-F, Lee T-Y. Quantitative myocardial perfusion measurement using CT perfusion: a validation study in a porcine model of reperfused acute myocardial infarction. Int J Cardiovasc Imaging. 2012;28(5):1237–48. https://doi.org/10.1007/s10554-011-9927-x.
13. Mahnken AH, Klotz E, Pietsch H, et al. Quantitative whole heart stress perfusion CT imaging as noninvasive assessment of hemodynamics in coronary artery stenosis: preliminary animal experience. Investig Radiol. 2010;45(6):298–305. https://doi.org/10.1097/RLI.0b013e3181dfa3cf.
14. Bamberg F, Hinkel R, Schwarz F, Sandner TA, Baloch E, Marcus R, Becker A, Kupatt C, Wintersperger BJ, Johnson TR, Theisen DKM. Accuracy of dynamic computed tomography adenosine stress myocardial perfusion imaging in estimating myocardial blood flow at various degrees of coronary artery stenosis using a porcine animal model. Investig Radiol. 2012;47(1):71–7.
15. Rossi A, Uitterdijk A, Dijkshoorn M, et al. Quantification of myocardial blood flow by adenosine-stress CT perfusion imaging in pigs during various degrees of stenosis correlates well with coronary artery blood flow and fractional flow reserve. Eur Heart J Cardiovasc Imaging. 2013;14(4):331–8. https://doi.org/10.1093/ehjci/jes150.
16. Ishida M, Kitagawa K, Ichihara T, et al. Underestimation of myocardial blood flow by dynamic perfusion CT: explanations by two-compartment model analysis and limited temporal sampling of dynamic CT. J Cardiovasc Comput Tomogr. 2016;10:1–8. https://doi.org/10.1016/j.jcct.2016.01.008.
17. Motwani M, Fairbairn TA, Larghat A, et al. Systolic versus diastolic acquisition in myocardial perfusion MR imaging. Radiology. 2012;262(3):816–23. https://doi.org/10.1148/radiol.11111549.
18. Motwani M, Kidambi A, Sourbron S, et al. Quantitative three-dimensional cardiovascular magnetic resonance myocardial perfusion imaging in systole and diastole at 3.0 T. Heart. 2013;99:A56–7. https://doi.org/10.1186/1532-429X-16-19.
19. Rossi A, Merkus D, Klotz E, Mollet N, de Feyter PJ, Krestin GP. Stress myocardial perfusion: imaging with multidetector CT. Radiology. 2014;270(1):25–46. https://doi.org/10.1148/radiol.13112739.
20. Einstein AJ. Effects of radiation exposure from cardiac imaging: how good. J Am College Cardiol. 2012;59(6):553–65. https://doi.org/10.1016/j.jacc.2011.08.079.Effects.
21. Yang DH, Kim Y-H, Roh JH, et al. Diagnostic performance of on-site CT-derived fractional flow reserve versus CT perfusion. Eur Heart J Cardiovasc Imaging. 2016;18:432. https://doi.org/10.1093/ehjci/jew094.
22. Baxa J, Hromádka M, Šedivý J, et al. Regadenoson-stress dynamic myocardial perfusion improves diagnostic performance of CT angiography in assessment of intermediate coronary artery stenosis in asymptomatic patients. Biomed Res Int. 2015;2015:105629. https://doi.org/10.1155/2015/105629.
23. Weininger M, Schoepf UJ, Ramachandra A, et al. Adenosine-stress dynamic real-time myocardial perfusion CT and adenosine-stress first-pass dual-energy myocardial perfusion CT for the assessment of acute chest pain: initial results. Eur J Radiol. 2012;81(12):3703–10. https://doi.org/10.1016/j.ejrad.2010.11.022.
24. Wang Y, Qin L, Shi X, et al. Adenosine-stress dynamic myocardial perfusion imaging with second-generation dual-source CT: comparison with conventional catheter coronary angiography and SPECT nuclear myocardial perfusion imaging. Am J Roentgenol. 2012;198(3):521–9. https://doi.org/10.2214/AJR.11.7830.
25. Bastarrika G, Ramos-Duran L, Rosenblum MA, Kang DK, Rowe GW, Schoepf UJ. Adenosine-stress dynamic myocardial CT perfusion imaging: initial clinical experience. Investig Radiol. 2010;45(6):306–13. https://doi.org/10.1097/RLI.0b013e3181dfa2f2.
26. Tanabe Y, Kido T, Uetani T, et al. Differentiation of myocardial ischemia and infarction assessed by dynamic computed tomography perfusion imaging and comparison with cardiac magnetic resonance and single-photon emission computed tomography. Eur Radiol. 2016:1–12. http://www.embase.com/search/results?subaction=viewrecord&from=export&id=L608199060.
27. Wichmann JL, Meinel FG, Schoepf UJ, et al. Semiautomated global quantification of left ventricular myocardial perfusion at stress dynamic ct: diagnostic accuracy for detection of territorial myocardial perfusion deficits compared to visual assessment. Acad Radiol. 2016;23(4):429–37. https://doi.org/10.1016/j.acra.2015.12.005.
28. Wichmann JL, Meinel FG, Schoepf UJ, et al. Absolute versus relative myocardial blood flow by dynamic CT myocardial perfusion imaging in patients with anatomic coronary artery disease. Am J Roentgenol. 2015;205(1):W67–72. https://doi.org/10.2214/AJR.14.14087.
29. Bamberg F, Marcus RP, Becker A, et al. Dynamic myocardial CT perfusion imaging for evaluation of myocardial ischemia as determined by MR imaging. JACC Cardiovasc Imaging. 2014;7(3):267–77. https://doi.org/10.1016/j.jcmg.2013.06.008.
30. Ebersberger U, Marcus RP, Schoepf UJ, et al. Dynamic CT myocardial perfusion imaging: performance of 3D semi-automated evaluation software. Eur Radiol. 2014;24(1):191–9. https://doi.org/10.1007/s00330-013-2997-5.
31. Kono AK, Coenen A, Lubbers M, et al. Relative myocardial blood flow by dynamic computed tomographic perfusion imaging predicts hemodynamic significance of coronary stenosis better than absolute blood flow. Investig Radiol. 2014;49(12):801–7. https://doi.org/10.1097/RLI.0000000000000087.
32. Rossi A, Dharampal A, Wragg A, et al. Diagnostic performance of hyperaemic myocardial blood flow index obtained by dynamic computed tomography: does it predict functionally significant coronary lesions? Eur Heart J Cardiovasc Imaging. 2014;15(1):85–94. https://doi.org/10.1093/ehjci/jet133.
33. Huber AM, Leber V, Gramer BM, et al. Myocardium: dynamic versus single-shot CT perfusion imaging. Radiology. 2013;269(2):1–8. https://doi.org/10.1148/radiol.13121441.
34. Greif M, von Ziegler F, Bamberg F, et al. CT stress perfusion imaging for detection of haemodynamically relevant coronary stenosis as defined by FFR. Heart. 2013;99(14):1004–11. https://doi.org/10.1136/heartjnl-2013-303794.
35. So A, Wisenberg G, Islam A, et al. Non-invasive assessment of functionally relevant coronary artery stenoses with quantitative CT perfusion: preliminary clinical experiences. Eur Radiol. 2012;22(1):39–50. https://doi.org/10.1007/s00330-011-2260-x.
36. Bamberg F, Becker A, Schwarz F, et al. Detection of hemodynamically significant coronary artery stenosis : incremental diagnostic value of dynamic CT-based. Radiology. 2011;260(3):689–98. https://doi.org/10.1148/radiol.11110638/-/DC1.
37. Ho KT, Chua KC, Klotz E, Panknin C. Stress and rest dynamic myocardial perfusion imaging by evaluation of complete time-attenuation curves with dual-source CT. JACC Cardiovasc Imaging. 2010;3(8):811–20. https://doi.org/10.1016/j.jcmg.2010.05.009.
38. Kido T, Kurata A, Higashino H, Inoue Y. Quantification of regional myocardial blood flow using. Circ J. 2008;72:1086–91.
39. Kim SM, Kim YN, Choe YH. Adenosine-stress dynamic myocardial perfusion imaging using 128-slice dual-source CT: optimization of the CT protocol to reduce the radiation dose. Int J

Cardiovasc Imaging. 2013;29(4):875–84. https://doi.org/10.1007/s10554-012-0138-x.
40. Deseive S, Pugliese Md F, Meave A, et al. Image quality and radiation dose of a prospectively electrocardiography-triggered high-pitch data acquisition strategy for coronary CT angiography: the multicenter, randomized PROTECTION IV study. J Cardiovasc Comput Tomogr. 2015;9:278–85. https://doi.org/10.1016/j.jcct.2015.03.001.
41. Gordic S, Desbiolles L, Sedlmair M, et al. Optimizing radiation dose by using advanced modelled iterative reconstruction in high-pitch coronary CT angiography. Eur Radiol. 2016;26(2):459–68. https://doi.org/10.1007/s00330-015-3862-5.
42. Einstein AJ, Moser KW, Thompson RC, Cerqueira MD, Henzlova MJ. Radiation dose to patients from cardiac diagnostic imaging. Circulation. 2007;116(11):1290–305. https://doi.org/10.1161/CIRCULATIONAHA.107.688101.
43. Danad I, Raijmakers PG, Appelman YE, et al. Hybrid imaging using quantitative H215O PET and CT-based coronary angiography for the detection of coronary artery disease. J Nucl Med. 2013;54(1):55–63. https://doi.org/10.2967/jnumed.112.104687.
44. Fujita M, Kitagawa K, Ito T, et al. Dose reduction in dynamic CT stress myocardial perfusion imaging: comparison of 80-kV/370-mAs and 100-kV/300-mAs protocols. Eur Radiol. 2014;24(3):748–55. https://doi.org/10.1007/s00330-013-3063-z.
45. Gramer BM, Muenzel D, Leber V, et al. Impact of iterative reconstruction on CNR and SNR in dynamic myocardial perfusion imaging in an animal model. Eur Radiol. 2012;22(12):2654–61. https://doi.org/10.1007/s00330-012-2525-z.
46. Bindschadler M, Modgil D, Branch KR, La Riviere PJ, Alessio AM. Comparison of blood flow models and acquisitions for quantitative myocardial perfusion estimation from dynamic CT. Phys Med Biol. 2008;141(4):520–9. https://doi.org/10.1016/j.surg.2006.10.010.Use.
47. Zoghbi GJ, Dorfman TA, Iskandrian AE. The effects of medications on myocardial perfusion. J Am Coll Cardiol. 2008;52(6):401–16. https://doi.org/10.1016/j.jacc.2008.04.035.
48. Machecourt J, Longère P, Fagret D, et al. Prognostic value of thallium-201 single-photon emission computed tomographic myocardial perfusion imaging according to extent of myocardial defect. Study in 1,926 patients with foilow-up at 33 months. J Am Coll Cardiol. 1994;23(5):1096–106. https://doi.org/10.1016/0735-1097(94)90597-5.
49. Cerqueira MD, Weissman NJ, Dilsizian V, et al. Standardized myocardial segmentation and nomenclature for tomographic imaging of the heart. Circulation. 2002;105:539–42.
50. Meinel FG, Ebersberger U, Schoepf UJ, et al. Global quantification of left ventricular myocardial perfusion at dynamic CT: feasibility in a multicenter patient population. Am J Roentgenol. 2014;203(2):174–80. https://doi.org/10.2214/AJR.13.12328.
51. Ingrisch M, Sourbron S. Tracer-kinetic modeling of dynamic contrast-enhanced MRI and CT: a primer. J Pharmacokinet Pharmacodyn. 2013;40(3, SI):281–300. https://doi.org/10.1007/s10928-013-9315-3.
52. Al-Saadi N, Nagel E, Gross M, et al. Noninvasive detection of myocardial ischemia from perfusion reserve based on cardiovascular magnetic resonance. Circulation. 2000;101(12):1379–83.
53. Al-Saadi N, Nagel E, Gross M, et al. Improvement of myocardial perfusion reserve early after coronary intervention: assessment with cardiac magnetic resonance imaging. J Am Coll Cardiol. 2000;36(5):1557–64.
54. Schwitter J, Nanz D, Kneifel S, et al. Assessment of myocardial perfusion in coronary artery disease by magnetic resonance: a comparison with positron emission tomography and coronary angiography. Circulation. 2001;103(18):2230–5.
55. Pelgrim G, Handayani A, Dijkstra H, et al. Quantitative myocardial perfusion with dynamic contrast-enhanced imaging in MRI and CT : theoretical models and current implementation. Biomed Res Int. 2016;2016:1.
56. Lee TY. Functional CT: physiological models. Trends Biotechnol. 2002;20(8):3–10. https://doi.org/10.1016/S0167-7799(02)02035-8.
57. Larghat AM, Maredia N, Biglands J, et al. Reproducibility of first-pass cardiovascular magnetic resonance myocardial perfusion. J Magn Reson Imaging. 2013;37(4):865–74. https://doi.org/10.1002/jmri.23889.
58. Gamel BJ, Katholi CR, Mesel E. Pitfalls in digital computation of the impulse response of vascular beds from indicator-dilution curves. Circ Res. 1973;32(April):516–23.
59. Papanastasiou G, Williams MC, Kershaw LE, et al. Measurement of myocardial blood flow by cardiovascular magnetic resonance perfusion: comparison of distributed parameter and Fermi models with single and dual bolus. J Cardiovasc Magn Reson. 2015;17:17. https://doi.org/10.1186/s12968-015-0125-1.
60. Futamatsu H, Wilke N, Klassen C, et al. Evaluation of cardiac magnetic resonance imaging parameters to detect anatomically and hemodynamically significant coronary artery disease. Am Heart J. 2007;154(2):298–305. https://doi.org/10.1016/j.ahj.2007.04.024.
61. Maredia N, Plein S, Younger JF, et al. Detection of triple vessel coronary artery disease by visual and quantitative first pass CMR myocardial perfusion imaging in the CE-MARC study. J Cardiovasc Magn Reson. 2011;13. http://www.embase.com/search/results?subaction=viewrecord&from=export&id=L70465436:O29.
62. Sammut E, Zarinabad N, Wesolowski R, et al. Feasibility of high-resolution quantitative perfusion analysis in patients with heart failure. J Cardiovasc Magn Reson. 2015;17:13. https://doi.org/10.1186/s12968-015-0124-2.
63. Kim EY, Chung WJ, Sung YM, et al. Normal range and regional heterogeneity of myocardial perfusion in healthy human myocardium: assessment on dynamic perfusion CT using 128-slice dual-source CT. Int J Cardiovasc Imaging. 2014;30(SUPPL. 1):33–40. https://doi.org/10.1007/s10554-014-0432-x.
64. Danad I, Raijmakers PG, Appelman YE, et al. Coronary risk factors and myocardial blood flow in patients evaluated for coronary artery disease: a quantitative [15O]H2O PET/CT study. Eur J Nucl Med Mol Imaging. 2012;39(1):102–12. https://doi.org/10.1007/s00259-011-1956-0.
65. Schwarz F, Hinkel R, Baloch E, et al. Myocardial CT perfusion imaging in a large animal model: comparison of dynamic versus single-phase acquisitions. JACC Cardiovasc Imaging. 2013;6(12):1229–38. https://doi.org/10.1016/j.jcmg.2013.05.018.
66. Kajander SA, Joutsiniemi E, Saraste M, et al. Clinical value of absolute quantification of myocardial perfusion with (15)O-water in coronary artery disease. Circ Cardiovasc Imaging. 2011;4(6):678–84. https://doi.org/10.1161/CIRCIMAGING.110.960732.
67. Bol A, Melin JA, Vanoverschelde JL, et al. Direct comparison of [13N]ammonia and [15O]water estimates of perfusion with quantification of regional myocardial blood flow by microspheres. Circulation. 1993;87(2):512–25. https://doi.org/10.1161/01.CIR.87.2.512.

CT's Role for Myocardial Viability Assessment

64

Ahmed Hamdy and Kakuya Kitagawa

Why Assessing Myocardial Viability?

To Revascularize or Not to Revascularize, That Is the Question

If Shakespeare were to consider a career shift to become a cardiologist, that would be his most celebrated quote ever. The degree of left ventricular (LV) dysfunction is an undisputable determinant of long-term survival in ischemic heart disease (IHD) [1–5]. Broadly speaking, the LV dysfunction following an ischemic event can be the result of one of four possible scenarios depending on the stage and reversibility state of the ischemic myocardium: (1) the acute irreversible myocardial injury, i.e., myocardial necrosis in acute myocardial infarction (MI), (2) the chronic irreversible injury, i.e., myocardial scarring in chronic/old MI, (3) the acute reversible injury, i.e., myocardial stunning that refers to viable but acutely dysfunctional myocardium despite already restored myocardial perfusion following an acute ischemic event. The condition can take up to several weeks to resolve, but eventually, the stunned myocardium restores its contractility, and (4) chronic reversible injury, i.e., myocardial hibernation that refers to viable but chronically dysfunctional myocardium due to severe coronary artery disease (CAD) with perfusion impairment at rest. Revascularization in the latter group of patients (those with viable hibernating myocardium) is associated with substantial survival benefit, symptomatic improvement, and improved LV function [6]. For this reason, identifying viable and nonviable myocardium and hence differentiating between reversible and irreversible LV dysfunction is of utmost importance. In a meta-analysis by Allman et al. involving more than 3000 patients, the authors demonstrated a strong association between myocardial viability on noninvasive testing and improved survival after revascularization in patients with chronic CAD and LV dysfunction [7]. In the case of viable myocardium, the annual death rate in patients treated with revascularization was brought significantly down to 3% compared to 16% in those treated medically. In the case of nonviable myocardium, however, the opposite scenario was encountered where the annual death rate was 7.7% vs 6.2% in the revascularization and medical treatment groups, respectively. The results of the analysis signify the fact that revascularization for the nonviable myocardium does not – at best – improve LV function nor survival rates but carries an additional risk for the already burdened patients. In short, myocardial viability assessment – whatever the tool used for the purpose – is critical for the clinical decision-making through proper selection of patients who will benefit most from revascularization.

Why CT?

Myocardial Assessment, Achilles Heel of Cardiac CT?

So far, the main clinical application for cardiac CT is reserved for the evaluation of the coronary arteries where it dominates over other noninvasive methods and is regarded as a gatekeeper for invasive catheterization [8]. On the contrary, its role for myocardial viability assessment has always been regarded premature and vulnerable. The very first attempts to find a place for CT in myocardial evaluation date back to the late 1970s and early 1980s [9–12]. These were animal studies performed with early generations of CT scanners. Frustrated with the slow machines, frequent artifacts and low-resolution images, the modality was not further pursued as a clinical tool. Alternatively, cardiac magnetic resonance (CMR) emerged as a tissue characterizing modality that soon became a mature clinical tool for viability assessment; mainly by identifying areas of late gadolinium enhancement (LGE-MRI). Nearly 20 years later, the introduction of fast rotating, multi-slice CT (MSCT) technology made the door wide open for cardiac CT researchers to rediscover its potential in infarct imaging. This technical evolution accompanied with the fact that both iodinated and gadolinium-based extracellular contrast materials used for CT and MRI respectively share almost the same pharmacodynamics, led to renewed

A. Hamdy · K. Kitagawa (✉)
Department of Radiology, Mie University Hospital, Tsu, Japan
e-mail: kakuya@clin.medic.mie-u.ac.jp

U. J. Schoepf (ed.), *CT of the Heart*, Contemporary Medical Imaging, https://doi.org/10.1007/978-1-60327-237-7_64

interest particularly in late enhancement CT (LE-CT) for viability assessment. In their prominent study, Gerber et al. demonstrated good agreement (82%) between both LE-CT and LGE-MRI for the detection of the late-enhanced areas with an excellent agreement on localization [13]. On the histological level, Lardo et al. found that areas of LE correlated well with histopathological findings in terms of detection, localization, and transmurality assessment for both the acute and chronic infarctions [14]. These – among other studies – are only examples of how cardiac CT has evolved beyond the scope of coronary vessels assessment into a potential clinical tool for infarction imaging.

CT and Rivals, the Pros and Cons

Several rivals compete to prove superiority in myocardial viability assessment, the list of which contains single-photon emission computed tomography (SPECT), fluorine-18-labeled deoxyglucose (FDG)-positron emission tomography (PET), dobutamine echocardiography, CMR, and recently CT. Despite no consensus has been yet available, LGE-MRI is regarded as the gold standard for infarction assessment [15]. The choice of the appropriate technique depends on many factors such as the availability, experience, cost, machine, and patient's characteristics. The pros and cons as well as the underlying mechanism by which these techniques assess viability also differ as summarized in Table 64.1. Comparing LE-CT to LGE-MRI is of particular interest because both methods share the same pathophysiological principle for infarction detection and because LGE-MRI is the current gold standard for viability assessment as previously pointed out.

The reasons why CMR is dominating the field of viability assessment are its superior tissue characterization, lack of ionizing radiation, and the relatively low nephrotoxicity of its contrast agents. CMR, however, is not flawless. It requires a complex infrastructure, long scanning times, is expensive, and contraindicated in implanted electronic devices that are commonly encountered in patients with ischemic cardiomyopathy.

In the United States, centers providing cardiac CT are nearly triple the number of available cardiac MRI centers. The same rule applies to the number of cardiac CT and MRI scans performed annually. Statistically speaking, a quick analysis of the Medicare Provider Utilization and Payment Data for the year 2013 reveals that the number of cardiac CT service providers in the United States was 1147 compared to 418 providers of cardiac MRI service. The number of cardiac CT scans was 40,511 compared to 12,076 cardiac MRI scans [16]. This obvious lead in service availability should act as propelling force toward more clinical role for cardiac CT in viability assessment.

An important advantage of CT over MRI is the greatly reduced slice thickness. The widely available MSCT scanners provide slice thicknesses as thin as 0.5 mm, 10–20 times thinner than that in a typical MRI viability study. This has great clinical implications through reducing the partial volume effects that occur when the slice thickness exceeds the size of the imaged structure of interest. Another independent advantage of the reduced slice thickness is the greatly improved spatial resolution in the z axis which in turn enables the production of true 3-dimensional images and retrograde reconstruction of virtually any arbitrary slice orientation from the original stack of axial images. LGE-MRI also allows production of any arbitrary slice orientation, but this is only possible at the

Table 64.1 Summary of pathophysiological principles, pros and cons of the different viability assessment imaging modalities

Modality	Principle	Pros	Cons
Dobutamine echocardiography	Contractile reserve	Most available Validated No radiation	Operator dependency Occasional acoustic window inadequacy
SPECT	Intact cell membrane	Available Extensive validation and experience	Use of radioisotopes Low spatial resolution
Thallium-201			
Technetium-99 m-sestamibi			
FDG-PET	Glucose metabolism	High accuracy Good spatial resolution	Use of radioisotopes. Relatively limited availability
MRI		Highest accuracy; considered gold standard Best spatial resolution and contrast No radiation	Incompatible with implanted intra-cardiac devices or in claustrophobic patients.
Dobutamine cine MRI	Contractile reserve		
LGE-MRI	*AMI: Ruptured cell membranes* *Chronic MI: Expanded extracellular matrix*		
LE-CT		*Available* *Rapid scan* *Best spatial resolution* *Combines CT coronary angiography*	*Radiation* *Limited validation and experience*

time of data acquisition; a process that is heavily dependent on operator interaction and obviously time consuming. This latter, i.e., scan time, is another disappointment in LGE-MRI. A single slice would take about 20 s to be acquired compared to 10 s for the entire myocardium using the currently commercially available CT scanners.

Strategies for Infarct Detection and Myocardial Viability Assessment with CT

In the United States, 195,000 silent MIs are estimated to occur annually [17]. Updates from Framingham study showed that the 10-year mortality rate in unrecognized MI patients was 45% compared to 39% in patients with recognized MI [18]. These numbers demonstrate the importance of previous unrecognized MI detection and how this can help provide the appropriate care and consequently decrease mortality rates. CT can detect previous MI through identifying areas of lipomatous metaplasia, myocardial calcification, wall thinning, or abnormal enhancement.

Non-contrast or Non-cardiac CT

Lipomatous Metaplasia

The term describes the process of adipose tissue/fat deposition in the myocardium, occurring most commonly secondary to infarction, hence regarded as an indirect sign of nonviable myocardium. The first report for identifying areas of fat metaplasia in explanted hearts dates back to 1997 [19]. Ever since, the exact etiology and pathophysiology of the phenomenon remained largely unknown. In their study on explanted hearts, Su et al. found that fat metaplasia prevailed in 84% of the healed MI lesions [20]. They hypothesized that modern therapies in the management of IHD (e.g., angiotensin-converting-enzyme inhibitors, statins) may promote the development of adiposity within scar tissue which can explain the lack of reports before 1997. In addition, very recently, Kami et al. showed that cardiac pluripotent stem cells differentiated into adipocytes through certain transcription factors within an ischemic reperfused model [21].

The prognostic value of the deposited adipose tissue and its impact on cardiac electrophysiology have been totally unclear until very recently when researchers proved that lipomatous tissue was associated with increased propensity of ventricular tachycardia (VT) and VT circuit sites [22, 23].

From this standpoint, CT seems to be taking the lead in visualizing areas of lipomatous metaplasia. Echocardiography does not allow myocardial fat characterization, and CMR requires acquisition of T1 pulse sequences, whereas fat can be clearly visualized throughout any phase of cardiac CT including the non-contrast scan (Fig. 64.1). Ichikawa et al. found a prevalence of 62% of cardiac adiposity in MI patients compared to 3% of controls [24]. They also found a strong correlation with infarct age of more than 3 years. Ahn et al. found areas of lipomatous metaplasia in 22.4% of MI patients and was more frequently associated with a longer post-infarct period, milder coronary artery stenosis, fewer number of diseased vessels, and more severe regional wall motion abnormalities [25]. Gupta et al. compared non-contrast cardiac CT with SPECT for detection of chronic/old MI depending on lipomatous metaplasia visualization on CT. Non-contrast CT yielded high sensitivity of 92% and specificity of 72%. Based on a ROC curve, a reference Hounsfield unit (HU) of 21.7 achieved sensitivity of 97.4% and specificity of 98.7% [26].

Myocardial Scar Calcification

Previous myocardial infarction is the most common cause of extra-coronary cardiac calcification [27]. Cell necrosis and

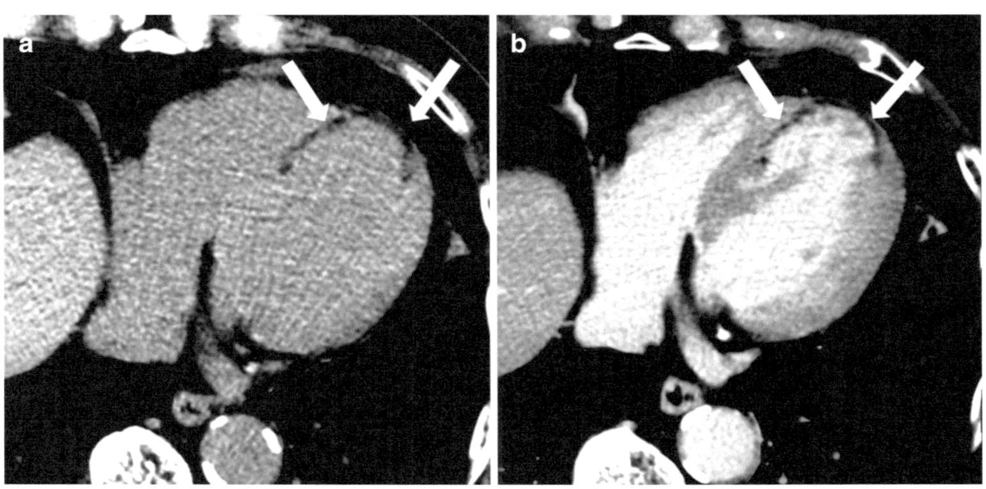

Fig. 64.1 Lipomatous metaplasia (arrows) in a patient with long-standing anteroseptal MI presenting as subendocardial fat density in both pre-contrast (**a**) and LE-CT (**b**)

membrane rupture during MI initiates the process of calcium deposition which is then accentuated by the ischemia-induced microenvironment. In 1975, calcification was reported to be present in 8% of myocardial infarctions older than 6 years using plain radiographs [28]. On echocardiography, myocardial calcifications appear as echogenic foci causing back shadowing, while at CMR they appear as low-signal foci in all pulse sequences. CT is obviously the modality of choice for calcium detection. Old MI causes associate dystrophic calcification that typically appears as thin curvilinear sheets of high-density calcium along the periphery of the infarct [29] (Fig. 64.2). It is worth noting that myocardial scar calcifications can appear on non-cardiac or non-gated cardiac CT scans; though gated scans obviously offer the best image quality. The prognostic value of myocardial calcification occurring on top of previous MI is not yet known and warrants research to resolve its relation specifically to ventricular function and electrophysiology.

Contrast-Enhanced Cardiac CT

Wall Thinning

Following MI, the inflammatory process starts removing the necrotic myocardium which ultimately leads to focal wall thinning. It is easily expected that the infarcted part of the ventricular wall becomes thinner with time. Nieman et al. confirmed that expectation, showing that patients with long-standing MI had significantly thinner myocardium that reached 5 mm or less in about 50% of cases. In acute MI, no significant differences were found when compared with controls [30]. One complication of severe myocardial thinning following transmural infarction is the development of ventricular aneurysm which is readily visualized on CT (Fig. 64.3). No studies are available on the value of wall thinning evaluated with CT for prediction of viability and subsequent functional recovery after revascularization, though CMR studies show that left ventricular wall thickness more than 5.5 mm can predict viability with a sensitivity of 92% and a specificity of 56% [31].

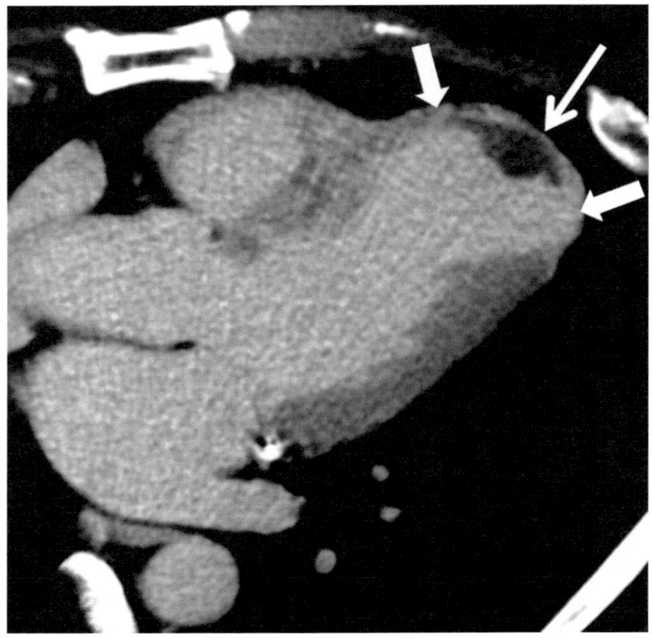

Fig. 64.3 LE-CT showing an apical LV aneurysm developing after anteroseptal MI involving the apex (block arrows). A hypodense thrombus is seen within the aneurysm (open arrow)

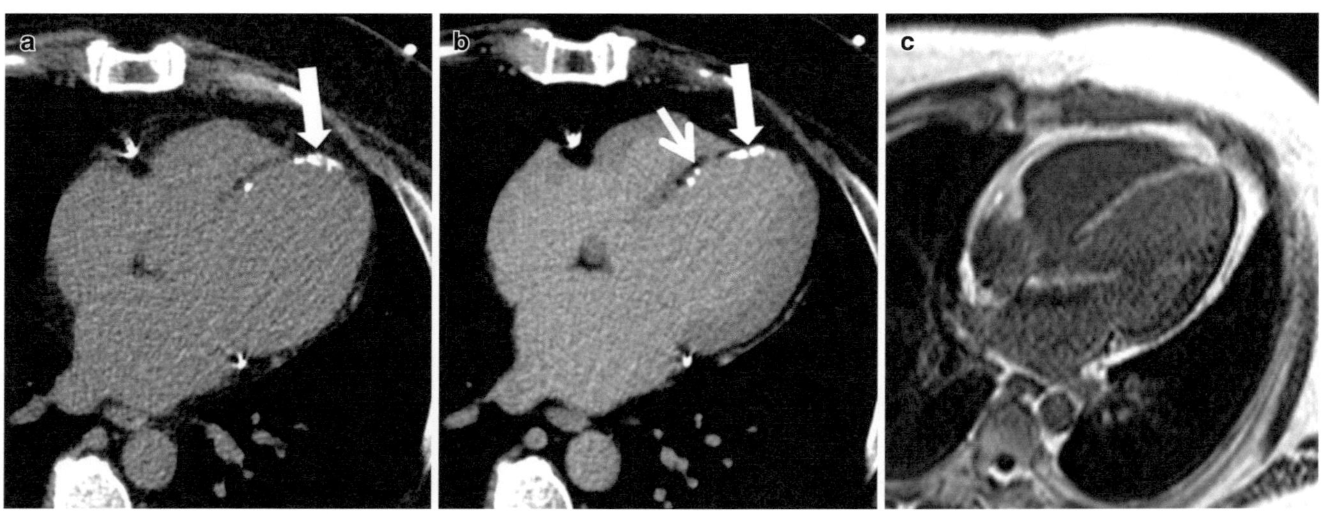

Fig. 64.2 Subendocardial curvilinear calcium density representing dystrophic calcification (block arrows) in this long-standing anteroseptal MI patient; (**a**) unenhanced CT and (**b**) LE-CT. Associated lipomatous metaplasia can also be noted (open arrow). Note that calcium is not detected with LGE-MRI (**c**)

First-Pass Arterial Phase Scan

The first-pass arterial phase CT (basically a standard coronary CT angiography study or a myocardial perfusion CT) can be used to detect infarcted myocardium. This is based on the fact that contrast enhancement of the myocardium during arterial phase CT is directly related to myocardial perfusion. Infarcted myocardium typically appears as hypoattenuated perfusion defects (Figs. 64.4 and 64.5). In one of the first studies on animal models, Hoffmann et al. found significant reductions in CT attenuation of the acute infarcts when compared to reference myocardium ($p < 0.001$). These differences in attenuation also correlated well with differences in microsphere-determined blood flow ($p < 0.01$) [32]. In a clinical study by Nikolaou et al., arterial phase cardiac CT yielded a sensitivity of 85%, specificity of 91%, and accuracy of 90% for detecting MIs [33]. The mean attenuation value for the infarcted areas was 54 ± 19 HU vs 117 ± 28 HU for non-infarcted myocardium ($p < 0.01$). These results are in concordance with the study of Francone et al. who demonstrated a sensitivity of 83% and specificity of 91% compared to a clinical reference with mean attenuation value for the infarcted areas and normal myocardium being 38.9 ± 14 HU vs 104.0 ± 16 HU, respectively ($p < 0.01$) [34]. Nieman et al. used arterial phase cardiac CT to differentiate between acute and chronic infarctions. They found significantly lower CT attenuation values in patients with long-standing MI (−13 ± 37 HU) than in those with acute MI (26 ± 26HU) and normal controls (73 ± 14 HU, $p < 0.001$) which can be attributed to lipomatous metaplasia [30].

First-pass arterial cardiac CT was also compared to other methods of viability assessment. When compared to LGE-MRI, it had a sensitivity of about 91%, specificity of 81%, and diagnostic accuracy of 86% but with tendency to underestimate infarcts sizes [35]. This underestimation was also found by Mahnken et al. who found the mean infarct size to be 24.5 ± 18.3% per slice for early-phase arterial MSCT and 31.2 ± 22.5% on MRI[36]. The frequent underestimation is probably because only a part of the infarcted tissue shows a

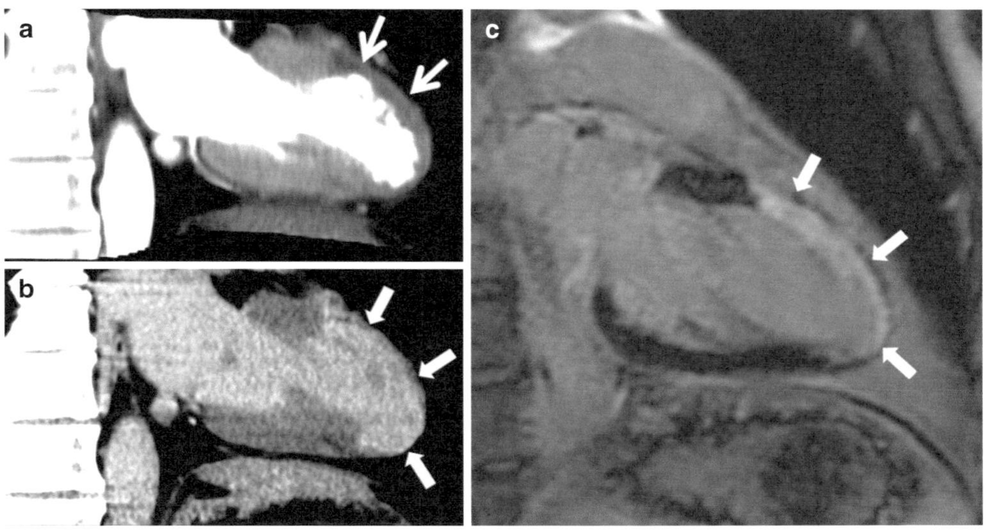

Fig. 64.4 Sagittal reformatted images of the arterial phase (**a**) showing a hypodense perfusion defect (open arrows) and LE-CT (**b**) showing an area of late enhancement at the anteroseptal wall of LV (block arrows). Note that the hypodense area appears smaller than the hyperenhanced area in LE-CT (**b**) and LGE-MRI (**c**). On the other hand, excellent correlation can be noted between LE-CT and LGE-MRI

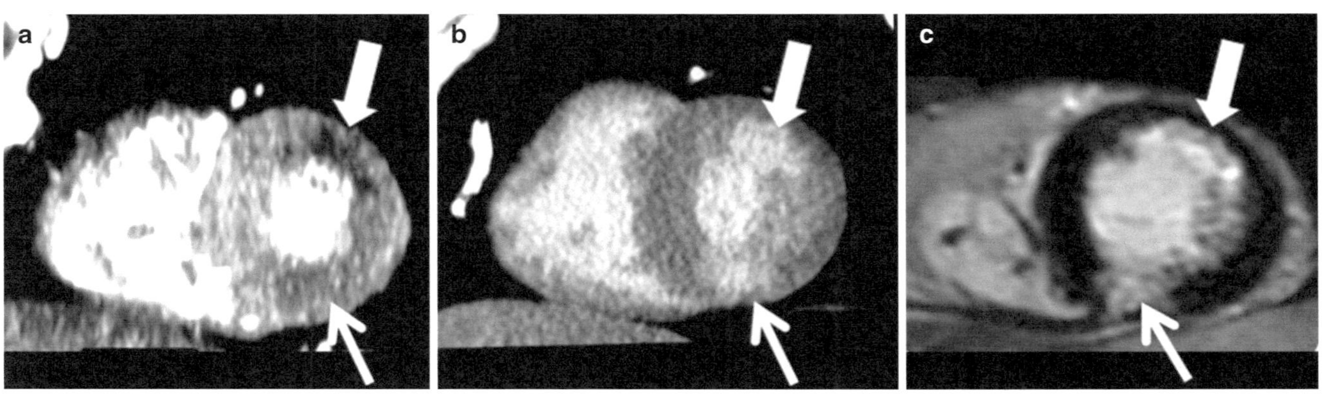

Fig. 64.5 Short-axis reformatted images of stress perfusion CT(**a**) and LE-CT (**b**), showing good correspondence to short-axis LGE-MRI (**c**) for the anterior (block arrows) and inferior (open arrows) walls MI

perfusion defect on the arterial phase, while the whole infarcted tissue becomes hyperenhanced in late phase of the study. When compared to SPECT, Hennman et al. showed an overall agreement reaching up to 96% between arterial phase CT and SPECT for detection of rest perfusion defects of old MIs [37, 38].

From a clinical prospective, the hypoattenuated areas are not exclusively seen in the infarcted myocardium. In fact, they are encountered in other conditions including lipomatous metaplasia with or without chronic MI, microvascular obstruction (MO) in reperfused acute MI, and the severely ischemic but viable myocardium in critical coronary artery stenosis. Beam hardening artifacts from dense contrast material and adjacent metalic objects as well as motion artifact can also be the source of hypoattenuation. One should be aware of these myocardial hypoattenuation-causing conditions. Combination of the hypoattenuated areas with the thinned myocardial walls, however, is in most cases an indicative of old MI of the involved segment.

Late Contrast Enhancement

LE-CT shares the same pathophysiological principle with LGE-MRI which is current clinical gold standard for infarct detection and viability assessment, owing to the proven fact that both iodinated and gadolinium-based contrast materials share almost the same pharmacodynamics [13]. In the acute phase of MI, the ruptured cell membranes allow the originally extracellular, interstitial contrast material to enter the necrotic myocytes with resultant increased volume of distribution. In old MI, the necrotic tissue is replaced with fibrotic, collagen-rich scar tissue that leads to the same result; an increased distribution volume of contrast material (Figs. 64.4 and 64.5).

Several animal studies were conducted to investigate feasibility and diagnostic accuracy of LE-CT. One of the first studies by Beucker et al. using a 16-slice MSCT demonstrated the feasibility of the technique for acute MI detection in porcine model, its ability to differentiate between reperfused and non-reperfused infarctions and good correlation with MRI and triphenyltetrazolium chloride (TTC) staining for infarct's size estimation [39]. Same results were obtained with 64-slice MSCT by Baks et al. using an acute reperfused MI model, Brodoefel et al. using both acute and subacute MI models, and Qu et al. using acute and chronic MI models [40–42]. Lardo et al. investigated LE-CT using a 32-slice MSCT in both acute canine and chronic porcine MI models. They found excellent correlation with TTC staining regarding morphology, transmurality as well as infarct volume estimation. Volumes by LE-CT compared to TTC were 21.1% ± 7.2% vs 20.4% ± 7.4% in acute infarcts (mean difference, 0.7%) and 4.15% ± 1.93% vs 4.92 ± 2.06% in chronic infarcts (mean difference, 20.76%) [14]. Mahnken et al. used LE-CT for assessment of infarction at different phases (at 0, 7, 28, and 90 days after induced MI and reperfusion). On day 0, the mean MI size was 23.7 ± 11.8% on CT and 24.5 ± 10.6% on CMR. On day 90, MI sizes decreased significantly to 16.9 ± 8.4% and 18.9 ± 8.0%, respectively ($p = 0.0019$). On TTC staining the size of MI was 16.8 ± 8.2%. Good agreement between LE-CT and LGE-MRI was found [43].

Human studies went side by side with animal studies. Head to head comparison was made in most cases with LGE-MRI. Mahnken et al. demonstrated excellent agreement of acute reperfused MI size for LE-CT and LGE-MRI (33.3% ± 23.8% compared with 31.2% ± 22.5%, respectively) [36]. The mean CT values of the normal and infarcted myocardium at the late phase were 74.5 ± 11 and 108 ± 15.9 HU, respectively. In their study on acute and chronic MI patients, Gerber et al. found good agreement (82%, $k = 0.61$, $p < 0.001$) for the identification of the hyperenhanced infarcted regions between both techniques on segmental basis and also high correlation for infarct size estimation [13]. The mean CT values of the normal and infarcted myocardium at the late phase were 97 ± 11 and 131 ± 16 HU, respectively. Choe et al. also compared LE-CT and LGE-MRI in 63 acute and chronic MI patients. LE-CT was able to detect the infarcted myocardium in all patients and correlated well with MRI for infarct's volume fraction estimation (correlation coefficient of 0.81, $p < 0.0001$). The mean CT values of the normal and infarcted myocardium at the late phase were 82.2 ± 23.2 and 115 ± 24.3 HU, respectively [44]. These studies consistently reported good agreement between LE-CT and LGE-MRI and, at the same time, low HU difference (≈30 HU) between normal and infarcted myocardium which makes contrast material reduction difficult. For example, Nieman et al. performed LE-CT with administration of smaller amount of contrast material than previous studies (75–90 mL, 320 mg of iodine per mL). In spite of good correlation between LE-CT and LGE-MRI for infarcted myocardium fraction estimation (13% ± 9 vs 15% ± 7; mean difference of −2% ± 6, $p = 0.37$) [45], late enhancement was present in only 11 of the 15 patients examined because of excessive image noise, streak artifacts, or non-detectable late enhancement. The mean CT values of the remote and infarcted myocardium at the late phase were 72 ± 10 and 93 ± 15 HU, respectively.

LE-CT was also compared to methods other than MRI. Habis et al. compared LE-CT to low-dose dobutamine echocardiography. In 36 patients with acute MI, 64-slice CT was used to acquire late CT images after invasive coronary angiography (mean delay of 24 ± 11 min) with no contrast injection, whereas echocardiography was performed 2–4 weeks later. LE-CT had a 98% sensitivity, 94% specificity, 97% accuracy, and 99% positive and 79% negative predictive values for detecting viable myocardial segments compared to echocardiography [46]. Chiou et al. compared

LE-CT to thallium SPECT and dobutamine echocardiography in patients with previous MI. By per-patient analysis, CT detected MI in 96% of the patients while SPECT detected only 87%. Among segments with late enhancement >75% segmental thickness, SPECT and echocardiography detected nonviable segments in 87.8% and 92.2%, respectively [47]. LE-CT was also compared with FDG-PET and SPECT by Lee et al. where CT had 84.2% and 89.2% agreement with SPECT and PET, respectively, for MI localization and sensitivity, specificity, and diagnostic accuracy of 73.5%, 79.4%, and 78.4% compared with combined PET and SPECT [48]. However, Dwivedi et al. found less impressive agreement with PET, reaching a modest value of 70% with qualitative analysis that increased to 77% with quantitative analysis [49].

When comparing SPECT or FDG-PET with LE-CT, one has to keep in mind that these techniques depend on different principles for viability assessment. This has significant implications when comparing their sensitivities, specificities, and diagnostic accuracies. SPECT and PET, for example, visualize the viable myocytes, while the nonviable myocytes appear as defective, invisible areas on imaging, a result of decreased cellular metabolism. This is the opposite in case of LE-CT and LGE-MRI, which visualize the nonviable myocytes rather than the viable ones, a result of the expanded extracellular matrix in the infarcted myocardium.

Extracellular Volume Fraction

Based on the abovementioned fact, it would make perfect sense to actually quantify the extracellular volume (ECV) fraction as an indirect indicator for the presence of MI. Pre- and post-contrast T1 mapping MRI is a validated method for ECV estimation. Using MRI, Sado et al. found higher ECV values in previous MI patients than in healthy subjects, Fabry disease, dilated and hypertrophic cardiomyopathies, aortic stenosis, and cardiac amyloidosis patients [50]. Publications on the value of CT for the same purpose are scarce. In a recent study by Jablonowski et al., CT was used to quantify ECV in animal models of acute MI of different forms (patchy microinfarcts induced with injection of 16 and 32 mm^3 microemboli, contiguous massive infarct induced by left anterior descending artery ligation and, combined micro- and massive infarcts) [51]. Interestingly, mean ECV values correlated with the severity of infarcts ranging from 36% ± 3 and 41% ± 3 for the 16 and 32 mm^3 microemboli-induced microinfarcts, respectively, to 55% ± 5 and 56% ± 4 for the contiguous massive and combined infarcts, respectively. Regression analysis also revealed excellent correlation between CT-derived ECV values and histological postmortem microscopy ($r^2 = 0.92$). The results not only demonstrate the potential use of ECV as a biomarker of myocardial viability but also as a discriminator between different degrees of myocardial injury and as a detector of peri-procedural complications, including dislodged microemboli and reperfusion microvascular injury.

The true power of ECV, however, lies in the detection and quantification of the diffuse interstitial type of myocardial fibrosis, extending well beyond the confines of focal replacement fibrosis usually found in infarct scars. For that purpose, CT-derived ECV values were validated against MRI as the imaging reference standard. Nacif et al. found good agreement between both methods in their study on 24 healthy and heart failure subjects. As expected, ECV values were higher in heart failure patients than in healthy individuals (33.5% ± 5.9 vs 29.3% ± 2.7, respectively; $p = 0.03$) and were inversely related to ejection fraction [52]. Bandula et al. also compared ECV values obtained by equilibrium CT and CMR and validated the results against histology in 23 patients with aortic stenosis undergoing valve replacement surgery [53]. There was a significant correlation between both CT- and MR-derived ECV and percentage of histologic fibrosis ($r = 0.71$ [$p < 0.001$] and $r = 0.84$ [$p < 0.0001$], respectively). Also, CT-derived ECV was significantly correlated to MR-derived ECV ($r = 0.73$). In cardiac amyloidosis, Triebel et al. have shown good correlation between dynamic equilibrium CT- and MR-derived ECV with good tracking of clinical markers of amyloidosis severity [54]. Recently, we demonstrated significant correlation between CT- and MR-derived ECV ($R^2 = 0.84, p < 0.001$) with a mean difference of −3.3% [55]. We also demonstrated that CT measurement of myocardial ECV in subjects without clinical CAD is feasible with high inter- and intra-observer reproducibility [56]. In this study we reported that mean ECV in males was lower compared with females (25.5 ± 2.0% vs 27.1 ± 1.8%, $p = 0.02$) and that it was positively related to age ($r = 0.46$, $p = 0.003$). There was no statistically significant difference in ECV between different left ventricular segments.

Post-percutaneous Coronary Intervention (PCI) LE-CT

Another strategy for LE-CT imaging is acquiring late-phase scan within 30 min after conventional coronary angiography or PCI. The strategy makes perfect use of the intra-arterial contrast material injected directly into coronary arteries (Fig. 64.6). While the earliest study to apply the idea used a non-gated conventional chest CT [57], subsequent studies used a dedicated ECG-gated cardiac CT scan that yielded 98% sensitivity, 94% specificity, and 97% accuracy for viability detection at a very early stage of acute MI [46].

Very recently, Jang et al. used a hybrid interventional therapeutic CT system in subacute MI swine model. Late scan images were obtained at 2, 5, 7, 10, 15, and 20 min after the end of angiography. Interestingly, the 2 min time point yielded the highest CT values for the nonviable and viable myocardium as well as maximum mean difference in CT attenuation between them. Such findings at such an

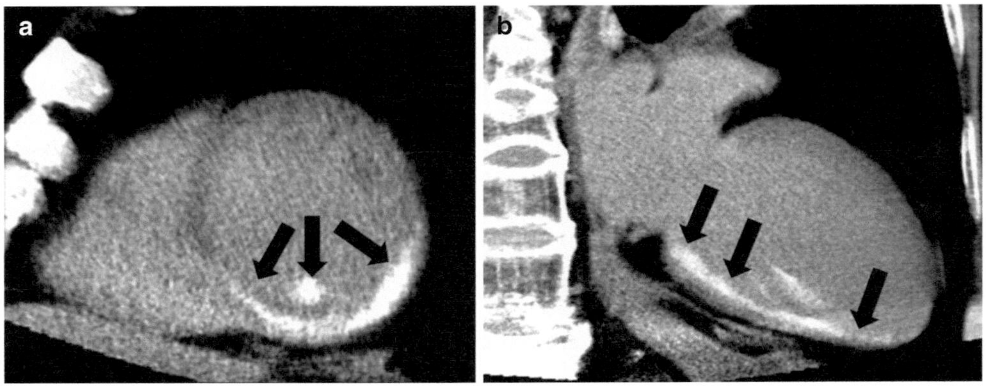

Fig. 64.6 Short-axis (**a**) and sagittal (**b**) reformatted images of cardiac CT performed immediately after primary PCI to right coronary artery in this 81-year-old man with inferior acute MI. Note the hyperenhanced infarction region (arrows)

early time point can be attributed to the intra-coronary injection of the contrast material. When correlated to TTC staining on histology, mean percentage difference of MI size at 2 min (8.5% ± 1.8%) was also the lowest [58].

Dual-Energy CT for Late Enhancement Imaging

Dual-energy imaging allows material decomposition and can theoretically provide better detection of infarcted myocardium at late phase by exploiting the increased iodine contrast enhancement of low-kV monochromatic images or through direct mapping of iodine distribution.

In a porcine model of reperfused chronic MI, Deseive et al. demonstrated a high accuracy and a good correlation of dual-energy LE-CT to LGE-MRI and histopathology [59]. In a patient study, Wichmann et al. reported a sensitivity of 89%, specificity of 98%, and accuracy of 96% for monochromatic LE-CT with LGE-MRI as the reference standard, while iodine distribution analysis provided inferior performance (52% sensitivity, 88% specificity, 81% accuracy) [60]. More recently, Truong et al. compared late enhancement by standard single-energy (at both 80 kV and 100 kV) to dual-energy LE-CT. The authors used a chronic MI porcine model and correlated results to histopathology. Interestingly, standard single-energy LE-CT (particularly at 100 kV) showed the best correlation to histopathology for scar volume and also the highest contrast-to-noise ratio while dual-energy LE-CT overestimated infarct's size the most [61]. In light of the results by Truong et al. and most of the previous studies, the theoretical assumption of superior infarction detection with dual-energy CT over single-energy CT is yet to be confirmed.

In ECV estimation, a different story is told. Lee et al. used iodine maps to estimate ECV in healthy subjects and in those with non-ischemic cardiomyopathy [62]. Interobserver agreement for ECV at CT was excellent (ICC = 0.987). In addition, Bland-Altman analysis between MRI and CT showed good agreement, with 95% limits of agreement of −1.19 and 1.79. Since pre-contrast images are not required to estimate ECV with the strategy, dose reduction and elimination of misregistration can potentially be expected compared to single-energy approach.

The Wikihow of Late Enhancement Cardiac CT

How to Do It

The perfect formula for a good LE-CT scan should be one that achieves the best diagnostic image quality with the least exposure to radiation and minimal volume of contrast material. This formula is not secret but involves many technical aspects that – so far – are not standardized among different institutes. In fact, variations of the technique among cardiac CT centers are so evident owing to differences in the used CT scanners, contrast volume, injection protocols, timing between injection and image acquisition, tube settings, and image reconstruction methods. In many cases, it is just a matter of time before cardiac CT staff build their own personal experiences and preferences. Below, we will try to explore the different techniques for late enhancement scan and present our personal experiences, tips, and tricks.

Contrast Material Volume

Despite advances in CT technology have made it possible to acquire coronary CT angiography studies using as low as 50 ml of contrast material, this is still not true for viability imaging with late-phase scan. For myocardial infarct delineation, adequate concentration gradient of the contrast material has to be achieved across vascular and expanded extracellular spaces of the infarct. Relatively high volumes of contrast material are needed to achieve this gradient. In animal studies, 700–1500 mg iodine/kg was administered. In a 75 kg human subject, this would equal an average of 250 mL of contrast material. On the other hand, human studies used quantities between 300 and 700 mg iodine/kg. Based on experimental and clinical evidence, volumes from as low as 120 mL to as high as 175 mL are commonly used.

From our personal experience, ≥600 mg iodine/kg produces sufficient late enhancement [63]. For contrast materials with iodine concentration of 370 mg/kg, this means a total of approximately 120 mL contrast agent.

Injection Protocol

Two main protocols for contrast material delivery are used; the bolus and the bolus-continuous infusion protocols. In the more commonly used bolus protocol, no further contrast material is injected after the contrast bolus of routine coronary CT angiography. The second protocol involves continuous slow infusion of 30–90 mL of contrast material after the bolus used for coronary angiography until the late-phase scan at a rate of 0.1–0.3 mL/sec. The theory behind continuous infusion technique is to maintain a persistently high intravascular concentration gradient that maintains a slow wash-in of the contrast material to extracellular spaces of the myocardial infarct. Eventually, this should result in accentuated contrast between the infarcted and healthy myocardium.

Till this moment, there is no consensus on which injection protocol to use. However, Brodoefel et al. compared both protocols in reperfused acute and subacute porcine models and reported that bolus-continuous infusion protocol yielded better image quality than did single-bolus protocol due to increased attenuation difference between viable and nonviable myocardium ($p \leq 0.003$) and between left ventricular blood pool and nonviable myocardium ($p < 0.001$) [64]. When correlated to MRI for MI size estimation, good correlation was found for both protocols although continuous infusion tended to have better correlation coefficient, reaching a maximal of 0.96 compared to 0.92 in single-bolus technique.

One matter should be taken into consideration. The continuously infused contrast agent leads to simultaneously increased LV blood pool attenuation which can mask small subendocardial infarcts. To avoid this, additional waiting time of about 5 min after infusion ends is recommended to allow for adequate washout of the contrast material from the left ventricular cavity. This increases the total time interval between coronary and late scans to an average of 15 min and makes it difficult to go below 10 min.

The single-bolus technique, on the other hand, is easier, more suitable for the clinical setting, and can save 5–10 min. In fact, the vast majority of publications on LE-CT and its diagnostic accuracy use a single-bolus protocol.

In a comprehensive protocol to be discussed later, contrast agent will be injected over the different phases of the study including coronary angiography, perfusion scan and even the test bolus. This is similar in principle to the split-dose protocol used by Goetti et al. [65].

Timing of Late Image Acquisition

This is yet another point of huge debate in cardiac CT community. Human studies reported variable time points for image acquisition ranging from 5 up to 15 min after contrast administration (Table 64.2). Jacquier et al. found no significant difference between the myocardial infarct area measured using LE-CT acquired at 5 and 10 min after injection and MRI in ST elevated MI patients [66]. In Brodoefel et al., the bolus injection protocol achieved maximal contrast between the viable and nonviable myocardium at 3 and 5 min time points, while the infusion protocol achieved that at 10 and 15 min time points [64]. This is an example of how injection protocol can affect the choice of the perfect time point for MI visualization among other factors such as the volume of the contrast agent and patient's hemodynamics. In a busy clinical facility where the luxury of a dedicated cardiac CT scanner is not available, it becomes more important to determine the earliest possible time point that allows for accurate diagnosis.

Based on our experience and yet unpublished data, 5 and 7 min after contrast agent administration equally allow for adequate wash-in of the contrast material (Fig. 64.7). Earlier time points are mostly too early for contrast accumulation in infarct scars, while later time points are accompanied with excessive washout. That said, some questions pop into one's mind. Is an early image acquisition time point totally useless? Can it act in the same way as early gadolinium enhancement in CMR to better detect MO or thrombi? Will imaging at multiple time points do better than a single one? And if so, will the benefit overweigh the increased radiation dose? These and other questions need to be raised and answered by dedicated studies.

Tube Settings, Radiation Dose, and Enhancing Image Quality

Acquiring a good image quality with a low-dose scan is a never-ending quest. A common strategy to lower radiation dose is to use a low tube voltage. Brodoefel et al. compared tube currents of 80 and 120 kV for late-phase imaging in a porcine model of reperfused acute MI [67]. The 80 kV protocol not only resulted in 65% reduction of radiation dose but also provided better contrast-to-noise ratio than did the 120 kV protocol. This, however, was not true for tube current.

Table 64.2 Examples of reported time points for LE-CTacquisition in different human studies

Study	Timing
Mahnken et al. (2005) [36]	15 min
Lardo et al. (2006) [14]	5 min
Gerber et al. (2006) [13]	10 min
Lessick et al. (2007) [81]	6 min
Nieman et al. (2008) [45]	7 min
Boussel et al. (2008) [89]	10 min
Choe et al. (2008) [44]	10 min
Kang et al. (2010) [90]	6 min
George et al. (2012) [91]	5 min
Kurobe et al. (2014) [63]	7 min
Kurita et al. (2016) [56]	7 min

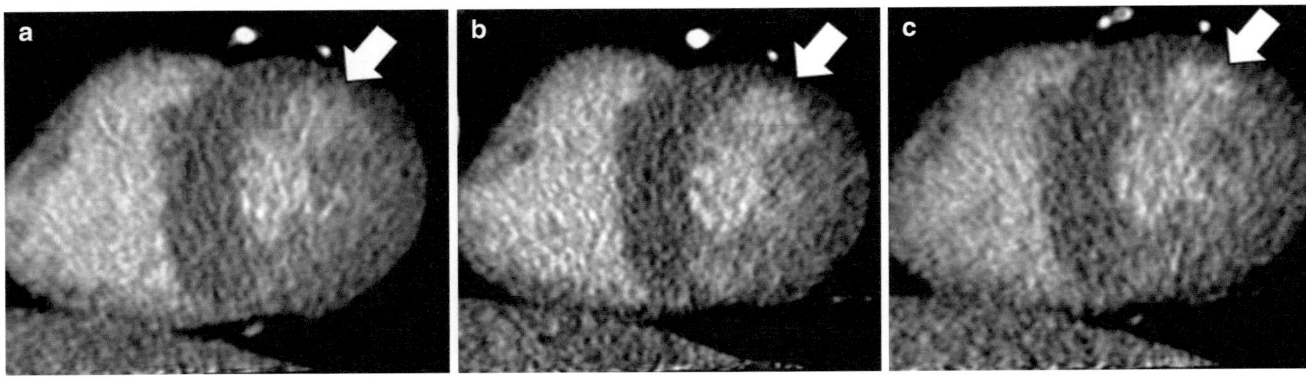

Fig. 64.7 Comparison between 3(a), 5(b), and 7(c) min time points for LE-CT acquisition in a patient with small anterior MI. Maximal contrast accumulation and best scar visualization are seen at 7 min in this patient

When the authors compared 400 mAs to the standard 800 mAs, they reported further lowering of radiation dose, the cost of which was an unacceptable degradation of image quality that interfered with accurate diagnosis. Mahnken et al. also reported highest contrast-to-noise ratio and best correlation with LGE-MRI and histology for the 80 kV protocol compared to 100 and 120 kV [68]. Reimann et al. demonstrated feasibility of low tube voltage and current protocol with doses as low as 1.19 mSv [69].

Another strategy for dose lowering is using prospective electrocardiographic (ECG) gating. Prospective triggering can significantly reduce radiation dose to as low as 1 mSv showing good agreement with both retrospective ECG gating and LGE-MRI [70, 71].

In addition, the high-pitch mode available on second and third dual-source CT scanners can lead to further reduction in radiation dose. Using a high-pitch mode, Geotti et al. achieved ultra-low radiation dose of 0.89 ± 0.07 mSv with sensitivity, specificity, and diagnostic accuracy of 90.0%, 92.9%, and 91.7%, respectively, for MI diagnosis on per-patient analysis as compared to MRI [65].

These methods might have reduced radiation exposure to unprecedented levels, but this was not the case with the persistent poor signal-to-noise ratio, inhomogeneous myocardial signal, and streaking artifacts inherit for LE-CT. As a solution, we adopted a novel image reconstruction algorithm known as targeted spatial frequency filtration (TSFF). TSFF was originally developed for cardiac dynamic perfusion CT using the cardiac shuttle mode which acquires images at two alternating table positions, to produce a hybrid algorithm of the conventional half-scan and full-scan reconstruction in dual-source CT [72]. The benefit of this algorithm is that it can achieve both high temporal resolution and diminished artifactual variations in CT number which means improved stability of myocardial signal and better image quality. We took a further step toward reducing image noise by acquiring 4 stacks of TSFF images in one breath hold and averaging them by means of non-rigid registration into one image data set [63]. Compared to conventional half-scan, TSFF with averaging resulted in significantly lower prevalence of inhomogeneous myocardial signal (65% vs 90%; $p = 0.002$), poor contrast between LV lumen and myocardium (15% vs 63%; $p < 0.001$), and streaking artifact (5% vs 63%; $p < 0.001$). When compared to the gold standard, LGE-MRI, TSFF with averaging also demonstrated better agreement, higher interobserver agreement, and reproducibility than did half-scan (Fig. 64.8). For best results, we use a combination of all the above; low tube settings of 80 kV and 370 mAs, prospective ECG gating, cardiac shuttle mode for the dual-source CT with TSFF reconstruction algorithm, and image averaging. The result is much improved image quality with relatively low-radiation dose of 1.8 mSv.

Imaging for ECV Estimation

ECV is calculated with the following equation: $ECV = (\Delta HUm/\Delta HUb) \times (1 - Hct)$, where ΔHUm is the change in attenuation of the myocardium in Hounsfield unit (HU), ΔHUb is the change in attenuation of the blood pool, and Hct is the hematocrit level. ΔHU = HUlate-HUpre, where HUlate and HUpre are attenuation values at late phase and pre-contrast CT, respectively. This means that for ECV calculation, we need to obtain a pre-contrast, post-contrast (late phase) studies and a hematocrit value.

Same scanning parameters should be applied in pre- and post-contrast scans to allow for the next step which is non-rigid registration/subtraction of both scans. This is followed by calculating change in blood pool attenuation values by the used software application and finally providing a hematocrit value to obtain an ECV map. It is worth noting that the pre-contrast study can also be used for calcium scoring [52].

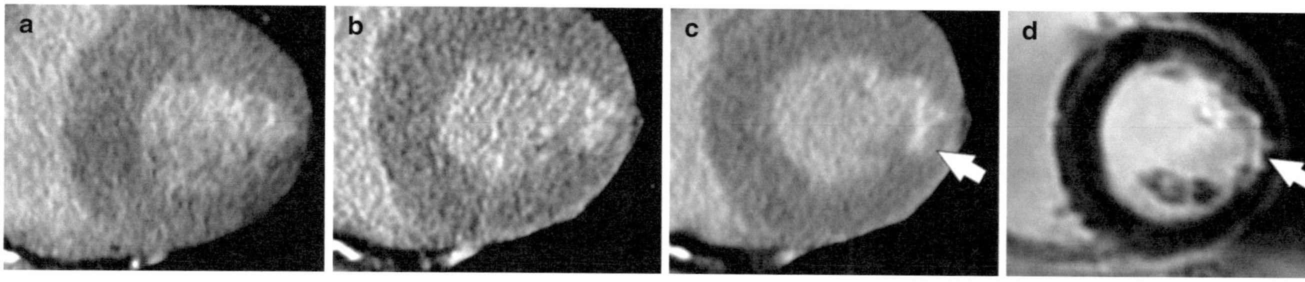

Fig. 64.8 Comparison between c conventional half-scan (**a**), TSFF (**b**) and TSFF with averaging (**c**). Best contrast-to-noise ratio and scar visualization is achieved by TSFF with averaging technique in comparison with LGE-MRI (**d**) (arrows)

How to Interpret

Image Post-processing

Before starting reading of LE-CT scan, some image setting manipulation can lead to improved MI visualization. The best combination of image settings includes: multiplanar reformation (MPR), slice thickness between 4 and 8 mm, average intensity projection (AIP), and narrow window settings; window width (WW) of 150–200 and window level (WL) $\simeq$ 100 (Fig. 64.9). MPR allows assessment in different left ventricular axes including most importantly the short and long axes. Thick slices decrease image noise and allow for better delineation of MI. AIP is preferred over maximum and minimum intensity projections (MIP and MinIP respectively) as MIP causes strong contrast accentuation which can overestimate infarct's size while MinIP causes accentuation of the inherit low-density artifacts causing grainy image and infarct's size underestimation. Finally, narrow window settings achieve higher contrast-to-noise ratio than wide window settings.

The Basics

As already known, infarcted myocardium appears as areas of delayed hyperenhancement, hence the common saying "bright is dead." As basic as it may sound, this mantra is not entirely accurate. In many conditions, the late-enhanced (bright) myocardium is not necessarily infarcted (dead) but rather reflects an expanded extracellular matrix; a condition that is encountered in many myocardial diseases including non-ischemic cardiomyopathies, amyloidosis, sarcoidosis, and many others. For this reason, differentiating ischemic from non-ischemic late enhancement is too fundamental to ignore. Late enhancement patterns on CT are identical to those on LGE-MRI. A typical infarction at late enhancement study is limited to a vascular territory and always starts at a subendocardial location because of the trans-myocardial perfusion gradients known as the wavefront phenomenon of myocardial necrosis [73]. Depending on the duration of coronary occlusion, variable degrees of transmural infarction can result. Semi-quantitative assessment of the degree of transmurality is advised in clinical setting ($\leq$25%, 26–50%, 51–75%, and $\geq$76%). The location of MI should be accurately reported according to the 17-segment model of the American Heart Association and tracked back to its culprit artery.

MO or no-reflow phenomenon is an established complication of coronary reperfusion therapy for acute MI that needs to be reported. MO can be seen at the core of acute MI as a subendocardial rim of hypodensity surrounded with the hyperenhanced infarcted tissue (Fig. 64.10). Chronic infarct-related complications such as ventricular aneurysms and thrombosis are also readily visible at LE-CT (Fig. 64.3).

Side-by-Side Assessment with Arterial Phase Scan

In general, three patterns which have different prognostic implications can be encountered when assessing LE-CT side by side with early arterial phase or perfusion CT scans. In the first, the arterial phase shows no perfusion defect, while the late phase shows a hyperenhanced lesion. In the second, the arterial phase shows a perfusion defect that disappears at late phase to be replaced with hyperenhancement. In the third pattern, an early perfusion defect persists within the core of late hyperenhancement [74]. The residual perfusion defect described in the third scenario represents mainly post-reperfusion injury in acute MI, i.e., microvascular obstruction. It may also represent a trickier condition where the residual perfusion defect is nothing but lipomatous metaplasia in long-standing MI. Clinical history, myocardial wall thinning, and fat density on pre-contrast scans allow for easy differentiation between MO and fat metaplasia. This side-by-side assessment is of utmost importance for prognosis prediction as will be discussed.

How to Predict Functional Recovery on Cardiac CT

The role of cardiac CT extends beyond its ability to detect infarction to providing vital information on possible clinical outcomes and prognosis after acute MI. Several studies assessed one or more of the most important CT-derived prognosticators including transmural extension, enhancement

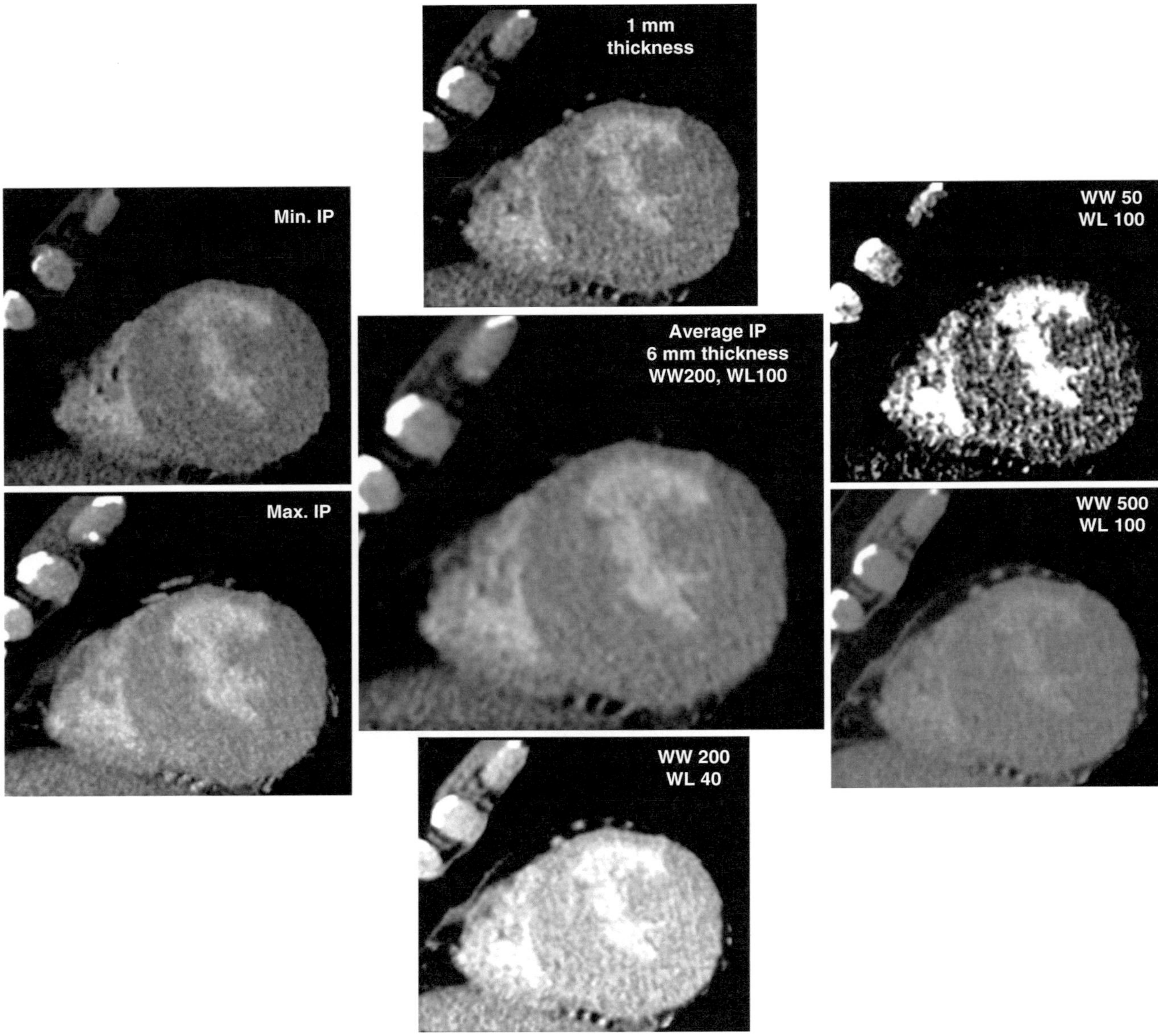

Fig. 64.9 Different post-processing image parameters. Best MI visualization is achieved with thick slices, average IP, and narrow window settings (center)

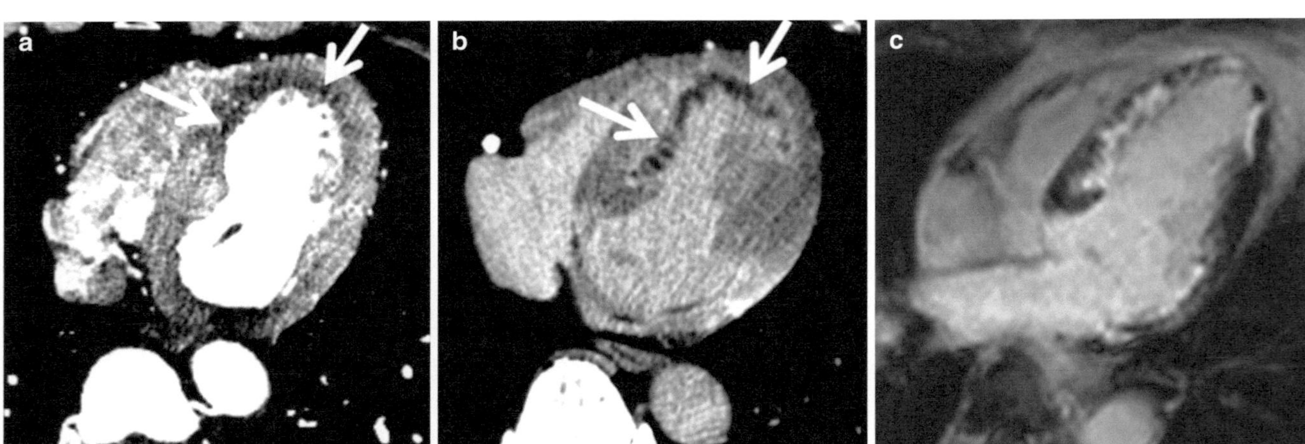

Fig. 64.10 Reperfused anteroseptal acute MI in long-axis view showing hypodense perfusion defect at arterial phase CT (**a**), that persists through LE-CT scan (**b**), representing post-reperfusion injury; MO (arrows). LGE-MRI performed 20 days later shows remnants of MO (**c**)

pattern revealed from side-by-side assessment of early arterial and late-phase scans and finally infarct's size.

Transmural Extent

Wada et al. compared transmural with subendocardial early arterial perfusion defects in reperfused anterior acute MI patients [75]. Although no functional differences were observed at the acute phase, the 6-months' scans showed poor recovery of LV function in transmural MI group and good recovery in subendocardial MI group ($p = 0.03$). These results were confirmed later on by Shapiro et al. [76]. On post-PCI LE-CT, Sato et al. demonstrated that LV remodeling ($p = 0.001$) and number of re-hospitalization for heart failure ($p = 0.0017$) were more significantly observed in transmural MI compared to subendocardial MI groups [77].

Enhancement Pattern

Koyama et al. were the first to compare functional recovery among different patterns of enhancement observed by combined assessment of early- and late-phase scans. Infarctions showing persistent hypodensity in late scan showed the greatest wall thinning and lowest ejection fraction at intermediate and long follow-up scans followed by those showing nonpersistent hypodense perfusion defects and finally those with no perfusion defect at early scan [74]. Recently, this prognosticator gained more momentum and was evaluated by using post-PCI LE-CT. In one study by Ogasawara et al., 17.5% of reperfused acute MIs showed hypodense areas at LE-CT; all of which were transmural infarctions with significantly higher infarct volumes. Both hypoenhanced lesions on late scans and larger MI sizes could predict major adverse cardiovascular events (MACE). However, the interesting part is that the incidence of MACE was significantly higher in patients with hypoenhancement at delayed scans compared to those without hypoenhancement regardless of infarct's volume ($p = 0.003$) denoting a superior prognostic performance [78]. In another study, Watabe et al. also demonstrated that heterogeneous enhancement (defined by the authors as concomitant presence of hyper- and hypoenhancement within the infarcted myocardium at LE-CT) along with infarct's relative CT density of more than 2.2 could predict MO and had a significant association with left ventricular remodeling [79].

Kim et al. assessed both transmurality and enhancement patterns as prognostic factors and concluded that transmural early perfusion defects had better correlation with follow-up myocardial dysfunction than did transmural delayed enhancement and that both had better correlation than subendocardial abnormalities. They also confirmed that persistent hypodense defects in late-phase CT were the most powerful, single-independent predictor of myocardial dysfunction [80].

Infarct Size

When assessing the impact of acute MI size as quantified from cardiac CT on functional recovery, Lessick et al. found that the presence and size of early perfusion defects and late enhancement were closely related to myocardial dysfunction on follow-up [81]. Sato et al. also showed higher risk of MACE in patients with large late enhancement size detected by post-PCI LE-CT [82]. On arterial phase CT, Kühl et al. confirmed that the degree of transmural involvement and extent of early rest perfusion defects are strongly linked to adverse outcomes in non ST-segment elevation MI patients [83].

Myocardial Viability Assessment as a Part of the Comprehensive Cardiac CT: The One-Stop Shop Around the Corner

In classic cardiology practice, most IHD patients still have to undergo multiple investigations for comprehensive assessment of function, morphology, perfusion, and viability prior to establishing a diagnosis and setting up a management plan. Finding a single comprehensive assessment modality would significantly cut expenses, save time, improve diagnosis, and make it easier for an already exhausted cardiac patient. Among the currently available cardiac imaging techniques, CMR and CT have the potential to be such comprehensive tests. Despite CMR is superior in terms of function and viability assessment, its use for coronary imaging is not as robust. On the contrary, cardiac CT's ability to visualize coronary arteries is surpassed only by invasive angiography and has proven – at the same time – to be of reliable diagnostic accuracy for function, perfusion, and viability assessment.

A typical comprehensive cardiac CT protocol comprises routine calcium scoring, coronary angiography, function or cine images, stress perfusion scan, and finally LE-CT. The protocol can be tailored to match personalized patient's care, e.g., addition of pre-contrast scan for ECV estimation. Some centers also prefer to start with perfusion study before coronary angiography or to combine rest and stress-induced LV function assessment. In a comprehensive protocol, an average of 120 ml contrast material is used throughout different phases of the study which is sufficient to perform a late phase viability scan with no need for additional administration. Recent advances in CT technology have made it possible to perform a comprehensive cardiac CT study with radiation doses of approximately 10 mSv [63, 84, 85]. Even more, ultra-low dose of 2.24 mSv was reported [86]. A comprehensive protocol not only highlights functionally significant coronary plaques but also improves both perfusion and viability assessment. As mentioned before, a perfusion defect on perfusion CT can be attributed to ischemic but viable

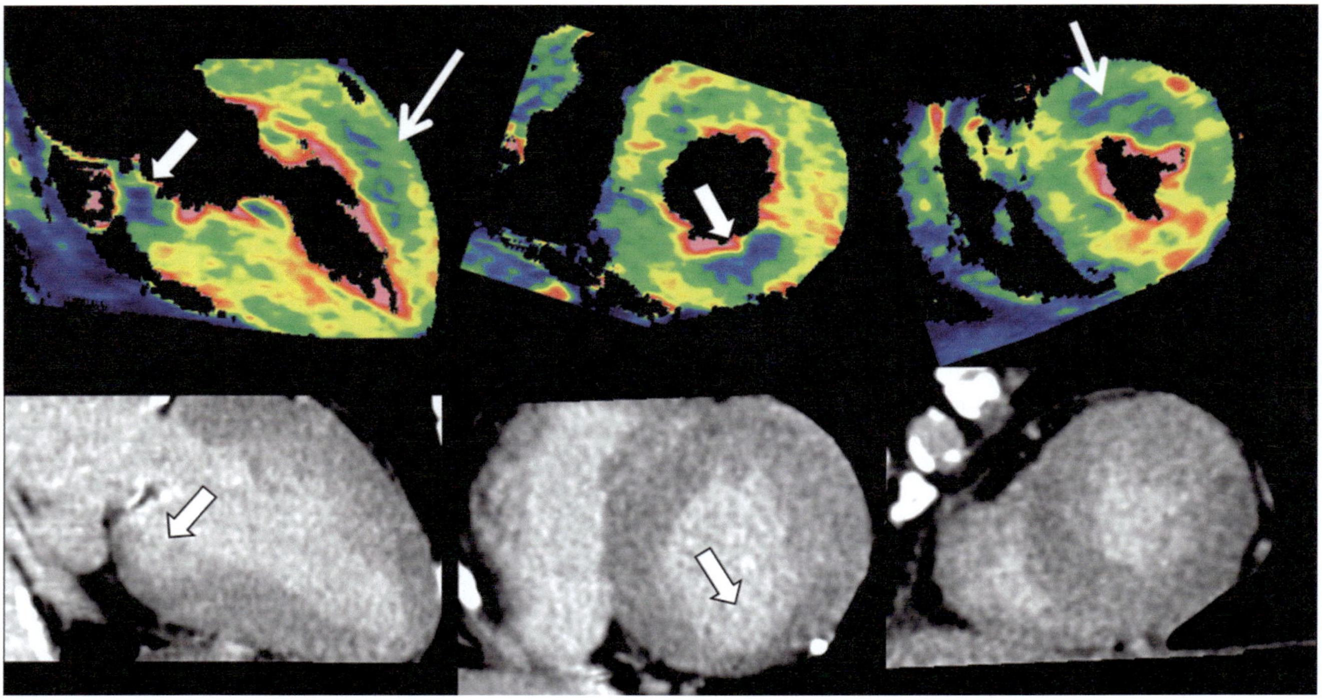

Fig. 64.11 Post-PCI, 66-years-old female with no history of previous MI. Upper row of images represents dynamic perfusion CT and shows anterior and inferior walls perfusion defects. LE-CT (lower row) could detect an irreversible ischemic defect at the inferior wall due to an old silent MI. Bock arrows represent infarctions; open arrows represent reversible ischemic defects

myocardium, MO, or previous MI. Side-by-side interpretation of perfusion and late-phase scans helps identify false-positive perfusion defects particularly in post-revascularization patients and hence increase specificity of perfusion CT (Fig. 64.11). This is important as well in patients with previous silent MI coming for initial assessment of their CAD. We demonstrated that in patients with obstructive CAD but without history of previous MI referred for comprehensive cardiac CT, up to 20% of perfusion defects on dynamic perfusion scan were attributable to silent MI as revealed from LE-CT [87]. However, Bettencourt et al. investigated whether diagnostic accuracy of a comprehensive protocol to detect significant CAD is improved by adding a late-phase viability scan and reported that LE-CT did not have such additional value [88]. These results, however, are simply explained by (1) the presence of concomitant reversible ischemic perfusion defects in the majority of patients with previous MI, (2) the presence of MI in few patients with normal coronary arteries, and (3) the lack of per-segment analysis in the study.

It is common sense to assume that diagnosis of MI becomes more reliable when assessing different phases of the comprehensive study. In an interesting research by Ghoshhajra et al., patients with intermediate-to-high probability for CAD were recruited for comprehensive cardiac CT protocol [84]. Assessment of infarctions using a combination of regional wall motion abnormalities, rest perfusion defects, and late enhancement (cine+ rest+ LE) was compared to each individual component separately using the universal definition of MI as the gold standard. The combined assessment yielded the highest diagnostic accuracy on per-patient analysis (90%) with sensitivity of 88% and specificity of 92%.

Future Directions

Cardiac CT is expected to play a greater role in viability assessment and to witness more involvement in everyday clinical practice, only when certain issues are to be addressed. The first of these is standardization of scan protocols including contrast material volume, method of its delivery, and timing of image acquisition. Much effort has been and is still being dedicated for the sake of radiation dose lowering. With next generations of state-of-the-art CT scanners and with the help of more optimized protocols, radiation doses are expected to go even lower. Much attention has also to be paid for continuous image quality improvement through developing effective image reconstruction algorithms. More validation studies and large multicenter researches have to be carried out to assess diagnostic performance and prognostic power of viability cardiac CT. ECV is also an attractive area of research in cardiac CT and holds potentials beyond viability assessment. Comprehensive cardiac CT is indeed an invaluable tool that can assess anatomy, function, perfusion, and viability in one scan and needs to be validated and tailored in a fashion that is suitable for clinical setting. Finally, dual-energy CT is expected to gain more popularity, but extensive work is still needed to reduce artifacts and improve image quality before it can be favored over conventional single-energy CT for infarct detection.

References

1. Hammermeister K, DeRouen T, Dodge H. Variables predictive of survival in patients with coronary disease. Selection by univariate and multivariate analyses from the clinical, electrocardiographic, exercise, arteriographic, and quantitative angiographic evaluations. Circulation. 1979;59(3):421–30.
2. Harris PJ, et al. Survival in medically treated coronary artery disease. Circulation. 1979;60(6):1259–69.
3. Muhlbaier LH, et al. Observational comparison of event-free survival with medical and surgical therapy in patients with coronary artery disease. 20 years of follow-up. Circulation. 1992;86(5 Suppl):II198–204.
4. Emond M, et al. Long-term survival of medically treated patients in the Coronary Artery Surgery Study (CASS) Registry. Circulation. 1994;90(6):2645–57.
5. Burns RJ, et al. The relationships of left ventricular ejection fraction, end-systolic volume index and infarct size to six-month mortality after hospital discharge following myocardial infarction treated by thrombolysis. J Am Coll Cardiol. 2002;39(1):30–6.
6. Baker DW, et al. Management of heart failure: III. The role of revascularization in the treatment of patients with moderate or severe left ventricular systolic dysfunction. JAMA. 1994;272(19):1528–34.
7. Allman KC, et al. Myocardial viability testing and impact of revascularization on prognosis in patients with coronary artery disease and left ventricular dysfunction: a meta-analysis. J Am Coll Cardiol. 2002;39(7):1151–8.
8. Shaw LJ, et al. Coronary computed tomographic angiography as a gatekeeper to invasive diagnostic and surgical procedures: results from the multicenter CONFIRM (Coronary CT angiography evaluation for clinical outcomes: an international multicenter) registry. J Am Coll Cardiol. 2012;60(20):2103–14.
9. Gray WR, et al. Computed tomography for localization and sizing of experimental acute myocardial infarcts. Circulation. 1978;58(3):497–504.
10. Higgins CB, et al. Evaluation of myocardial ischemic damage of various ages by computerized transmission tomography. Time-dependent effects of contrast material. Circulation. 1979;60(2):284–91.
11. Doherty PW, et al. Detection and quantitation of myocardial infarction in vivo using transmission computed tomography. Circulation. 1981;63(3):597–606.
12. Huber DJ, Lapray J, Hessel S. In vivo evaluation of experimental myocardial infarcts by ungated computed tomography. Am J Roentgenol. 1981;136(3):469–73.
13. Gerber BL, et al. Characterization of acute and chronic myocardial infarcts by multidetector computed tomography comparison with contrast-enhanced magnetic resonance. Circulation. 2006;113(6):823–33.
14. Lardo AC, et al. Contrast-enhanced multidetector computed tomography viability imaging after myocardial infarction characterization of myocyte death, microvascular obstruction, and chronic scar. Circulation. 2006;113(3):394–404.
15. Swoboda PP, Plein S. Established and emerging cardiovascular magnetic resonance techniques for prognostication and guiding therapy in heart failure. Expert Rev Cardiovasc Ther. 2014;12(1):45–55.
16. Medicare, C.f. and M. Services. Medicare provider utilization and payment data. Retrieved from https://www.cms.gov/Research-Statistics-Data-and-Systems/Statistics-Trends-and-Reports/Medicare-Provider-Charge-Data/Physician-and-Other-Supplier2013.html
17. Shriki JE, et al. Incidental myocardial infarct on conventional nongated CT: a review of the spectrum of findings with gated CT and cardiac MRI correlation. Am J Roentgenol. 2012;198(3):496–504.
18. Kannel WB, Abbott RD. Incidence and prognosis of unrecognized myocardial infarction: an update on the Framingham study. N Engl J Med. 1984;311(18):1144–7.
19. Baroldi G, et al. Lipomatous metaplasia in left ventricular scar. Can J Cardiol. 1997;13(1):65–71.
20. Su L, Siegel JE, Fishbein MC. Adipose tissue in myocardial infarction. Cardiovasc Pathol. 2004;13(2):98–102.
21. Kami D, et al. Cardiac mesenchymal progenitors differentiate into adipocytes via Klf4 and c-Myc. Cell Death Dis. 2016;7(4):e2190.
22. Pouliopoulos J, et al. Intramyocardial adiposity post-myocardial infarction: new implications of a substrate for ventricular tachycardia. Circulation. 2013;128(21):2296–308. https://doi.org/10.1161/CIRCULATIONAHA.113.002238
23. Sasaki T, et al. New insight into scar-related ventricular tachycardia circuits in ischemic cardiomyopathy: fat deposition after myocardial infarction on computed tomography--a pilot study. Heart Rhythm. 2015;12(7):1508–18.
24. Ichikawa Y, et al. Adipose tissue detected by multislice computed tomography in patients after myocardial infarction. JACC Cardiovasc Imaging. 2009;2(5):548–55.
25. Ahn SS, et al. CT detection of subendocardial fat in myocardial infarction. Am J Roentgenol. 2009;192(2):532–7.
26. Gupta M, et al. Non-contrast cardiac computed tomography can accurately detect chronic myocardial infarction: validation study. J Nucl Cardiol. 2011;18(1):96–103.
27. Nance JW, et al. Myocardial calcifications: pathophysiology, etiologies, differential diagnoses, and imaging findings. J Cardiovasc Comput Tomogr. 2015;9(1):58–67.
28. Freundlich I, Lind T. Calcification of the heart and great vessels. CRC Crit Rev Clin Radiol Nucl Med. 1975;6(2):171–216.
29. Gowda RM, Boxt LM. Calcifications of the heart. Radiol Clin N Am. 2004;42(3):603–17.
30. Nieman K, et al. Differentiation of recent and chronic myocardial infarction by cardiac computed tomography. Am J Cardiol. 2006;98(3):303–8.
31. Baer FM, et al. Comparison of low-dose dobutamine–gradient-echo magnetic resonance imaging and positron emission tomography with [18F] fluorodeoxyglucose in patients with chronic coronary artery disease a functional and morphological approach to the detection of residual myocardial viability. Circulation. 1995;91(4):1006–15.
32. Hoffmann U, et al. Acute myocardial infarction: contrast-enhanced multi–detector row CT in a porcine model 1. Radiology. 2004;231(3):697–701.
33. Nikolaou K, et al. Assessment of myocardial infarctions using multidetector-row computed tomography. J Comput Assist Tomogr. 2004;28(2):286–92.
34. Francone M, et al. ECG-gated multi-detector row spiral CT in the assessment of myocardial infarction: correlation with non-invasive angiographic findings. Eur Radiol. 2006;16(1):15–24.
35. Sanz J, et al. Detection of healed myocardial infarction with multidetector-row computed tomography and comparison with cardiac magnetic resonance delayed hyperenhancement. Am J Cardiol. 2006;98(2):149–55.
36. Mahnken AH, et al. Assessment of myocardial viability in reperfused acute myocardial infarction using 16-slice computed tomog-

raphy in comparison to magnetic resonance imaging. J Am Coll Cardiol. 2005;45(12):2042–7.
37. Henneman M, et al. Comprehensive cardiac assessment with multislice computed tomography: evaluation of left ventricular function and perfusion in addition to coronary anatomy in patients with previous myocardial infarction. Heart. 2006;92(12):1779–83.
38. Henneman MM, et al. Comparison of multislice computed tomography to gated single-photon emission computed tomography for imaging of healed myocardial infarcts. Am J Cardiol. 2008;101(2):144–8.
39. Buecker A, et al. A feasibility study of contrast enhancement of acute myocardial infarction in multislice computed tomography: comparison with magnetic resonance imaging and gross morphology in pigs. Investig Radiol. 2005;40(11):700–4.
40. Baks T, et al. Multislice computed tomography and magnetic resonance imaging for the assessment of reperfused acute myocardial infarction. J Am Coll Cardiol. 2006;48(1):144–52.
41. Brodoefel H, et al. Sixty-four-MSCT in the characterization of porcine acute and subacute myocardial infarction: determination of transmurality in comparison to magnetic resonance imaging and histopathology. Eur J Radiol. 2007;62(2):235–46.
42. Qu X, et al. Acute and chronic myocardial infarction in a pig model: utility of multi-slice cardiac computed tomography in assessing myocardial viability and infarct parameters. Eur J Radiol. 2012;81(4):e431–7.
43. Mahnken AH, et al. Late-phase MSCT in the different stages of myocardial infarction: animal experiments. Eur Radiol. 2007;17(9):2310–7.
44. Choe YH, et al. Comparison of MDCT and MRI in the detection and sizing of acute and chronic myocardial infarcts. Eur J Radiol. 2008;66(2):292–9.
45. Nieman K, et al. Reperfused myocardial infarction: contrast-enhanced 64-section CT in comparison to MR imaging 1. Radiology. 2008;247(1):49–56.
46. Habis M, et al. Acute myocardial infarction early viability assessment by 64-slice computed tomography immediately after coronary angiography: comparison with low-dose dobutamine echocardiography. J Am Coll Cardiol. 2007;49(11):1178–85.
47. Chiou K-R, et al. Identification and viability assessment of infarcted myocardium with late enhancement multidetector computed tomography: comparison with thallium single photon emission computed tomography and echocardiography. Am Heart J. 2008;155(4):738–45.
48. Lee IH, et al. Comparison of multidetector CT with F-18-FDG-PET and SPECT in the assessment of myocardial viability in patients with myocardial infarction: a preliminary study. Eur J Radiol. 2009;72(3):401–5.
49. Dwivedi G, et al. Scar imaging using multislice computed tomography versus metabolic imaging by F-18 FDG positron emission tomography: a pilot study. Int J Cardiol. 2013;168(2):739–45.
50. Sado DM, et al. Cardiovascular magnetic resonance measurement of myocardial extracellular volume in health and disease. Heart. 2012;98(19):1436–41. https://doi.org/10.1136/heartjnl-2012-302346
51. Jablonowski R, et al. Multidetector CT measurement of myocardial extracellular volume in acute patchy and contiguous infarction: validation with microscopic measurement. Radiology. 2014;274(2):370–8.
52. Nacif MS, et al. Interstitial myocardial fibrosis assessed as extracellular volume fraction with low-radiation-dose cardiac CT. Radiology. 2012;264(3):876–83.
53. Bandula S, et al. Measurement of myocardial extracellular volume fraction by using equilibrium contrast-enhanced CT: validation against histologic findings. Radiology. 2013;269(2):396–403.
54. Treibel TA, et al. Extracellular volume quantification by dynamic equilibrium cardiac computed tomography in cardiac amyloidosis. J Cardiovasc Comput Tomogr. 2015;9(6):585–92.
55. Kurita Y, et al. Data on correlation between CT-derived and MRI-derived myocardial extracellular volume. Data Brief. 2016;7:1045–7.
56. Kurita Y, et al. Estimation of myocardial extracellular volume fraction with cardiac CT in subjects without clinical coronary artery disease: a feasibility study. J Cardiovasc Comput Tomogr. 2016;10(3):237–41.
57. Kato M, et al. Plain computed tomography for assessment of early coronary microcirculatory damage after revascularization therapy in acute myocardial infarction. Circ J. 2006;70(11):1475–80.
58. Jang Y, et al. Viability assessment after conventional coronary angiography using a novel cardiovascular interventional therapeutic CT system: comparison with gross morphology in a subacute infarct swine model. J Cardiovasc Comput Tomogr. 2015;9(4):321–8.
59. Deseive S, et al. Dual-energy computed tomography for the detection of late enhancement in reperfused chronic infarction: a comparison to magnetic resonance imaging and histopathology in a porcine model. Investig Radiol. 2011;46(7):450–6.
60. Wichmann JL, et al. Diagnostic accuracy of late iodine–enhancement dual-energy computed tomography for the detection of chronic myocardial infarction compared with late gadolinium–enhancement 3-T magnetic resonance imaging. Investig Radiol. 2013;48(12):851–6.
61. Truong QA, et al. Myocardial scar imaging by standard single-energy and dual-energy late enhancement CT: comparison with pathology and electroanatomic map in an experimental chronic infarct porcine model. J Cardiovasc Comput Tomogr. 2015;9(4):313–20.
62. Lee H-J, et al. Myocardial extracellular volume fraction with dual-energy equilibrium contrast-enhanced cardiac CT in nonischemic cardiomyopathy: a prospective comparison with cardiac MR imaging. Radiology. 2016;280(1):49–57. https://doi.org/10.1148/radiol.2016151289
63. Kurobe Y, et al. Myocardial delayed enhancement with dual-source CT: advantages of targeted spatial frequency filtration and image averaging over half-scan reconstruction. J Cardiovasc Comput Tomogr. 2014;8(4):289–98.
64. Brodoefel H, et al. Assessment of myocardial viability in a reperfused porcine model: evaluation of different MSCT contrast protocols in acute and subacute infarct stages in comparison with MRI. J Comput Assist Tomogr. 2007;31(2):290–8.
65. Goetti R, et al. Delayed enhancement imaging of myocardial viability: low-dose high-pitch CT versus MRI. Eur Radiol. 2011;21(10):2091–9.
66. Jacquier A, et al. Multidetector computed tomography in reperfused acute myocardial infarction: assessment of infarct size and no-reflow in comparison with cardiac magnetic resonance imaging. Investig Radiol. 2008;43(11):773–81.
67. Brodoefel H, et al. Late myocardial enhancement assessed by 64-MSCT in reperfused porcine myocardial infarction: diagnostic accuracy of low-dose CT protocols in comparison with magnetic resonance imaging. Eur Radiol. 2007;17(2):475–83.
68. Mahnken AH, et al. Low tube voltage improves computed tomography imaging of delayed myocardial contrast enhancement in an experimental acute myocardial infarction model. Investig Radiol. 2007;42(2):123–9.
69. Reimann AJ, et al. Late enhancement using multidetector row computer tomography: a feasibility study with low dose 80kV protocol. Eur J Radiol. 2008;66(1):127–33.
70. Chang H-J, et al. Prospective electrocardiogram-gated delayed enhanced multidetector computed tomography accurately quantifies infarct size and reduces radiation exposure. JACC Cardiovasc Imaging. 2009;2(4):412–20.
71. Wang R, et al. Low dose prospective ECG-gated delayed enhanced dual-source computed tomography in reperfused acute myocar-

dial infarction comparison with cardiac magnetic resonance. Eur J Radiol. 2011;80(2):326–30.
72. Ramirez-Giraldo JC, et al. A strategy to decrease partial scan reconstruction artifacts in myocardial perfusion CT: phantom and in vivo evaluation. Med Phys. 2012;39(1):214–23.
73. Reimer KA, et al. The wavefront phenomenon of ischemic cell death. 1. Myocardial infarct size vs duration of coronary occlusion in dogs. Circulation. 1977;56(5):786–94.
74. Koyama Y, et al. Assessment of reperfused acute myocardial infarction with two-phase contrast-enhanced helical ct: prediction of left ventricular function and wall thickness 1. Radiology. 2005;235(3):804–11.
75. Wada H, et al. Multi-detector computed tomography for imaging of subendocardial infarction-prediction of wall motion recovery after Reperfused anterior myocardial infarction. Circ J. 2004;68(5):512–4.
76. Shapiro MD, et al. Cardiac computed tomography for prediction of myocardial viability after reperfused acute myocardial infarction. J Cardiovasc Comput Tomogr. 2010;4(4):267–73.
77. Sato A, et al. Early validation study of 64-slice multidetector computed tomography for the assessment of myocardial viability and the prediction of left ventricular remodelling after acute myocardial infarction. Eur Heart J. 2008 Feb;29(4):490–8.
78. Ogasawara S, et al. Presence of myocardial hypoenhancement on multidetector computed tomography after primary percutaneous coronary intervention in acute myocardial infarction predicts poor prognosis. Int J Cardiol. 2015;184:101–7.
79. Watabe H, et al. Enhancement patterns detected by multidetector computed tomography are associated with microvascular obstruction and left ventricular remodelling in patients with acute myocardial infarction. Eur Heart J. 2016;37(8):684–92.
80. Kim T, et al. Assessment of myocardial viability using multidetector computed tomography in patients with reperfused acute myocardial infarction. Clin Radiol. 2012;67(8):754–65.
81. Lessick J, et al. Is functional improvement after myocardial infarction predicted with myocardial enhancement patterns at multidetector CT? 1. Radiology. 2007;244(3):736–44.
82. Sato A, et al. Prognostic value of myocardial contrast delayed enhancement with 64-slice multidetector computed tomography after acute myocardial infarction. J Am Coll Cardiol. 2012;59(8):730–8.
83. Kühl JT, et al. The transmural extent and severity of myocardial hypoperfusion predicts long-term outcome in NSTEMI: an MDCT study. JACC Cardiovasc Imaging. 2015;8(6):684–94.
84. Ghoshhajra BB, et al. Infarct detection with a comprehensive cardiac CT protocol. J Cardiovasc Comput Tomogr. 2012;6(1): 14–23.
85. Williams M, et al. Cardiac and coronary CT comprehensive imaging approach in the assessment of coronary heart disease. Heart. 2011;97(15):1198–205.
86. Williams MC, et al. A low-dose comprehensive cardiac CT protocol assessing anatomy, function, perfusion, and viability. J Cardiovasc Comput Tomogr. 2013;7(1):69–72.
87. Nakamura S, et al. Frequency of perfusion abnormality on quantitative myocardial CT perfusion imaging in patients with no, nonobstructive, and obstructive coronary artery disease on coronary CT angiography. 11th annual scientific meeting abstracts, 2016. poster no. 161.
88. Bettencourt N, et al. CAD detection in patients with intermediate-high pre-test probability: low-dose CT delayed enhancement detects ischemic myocardial scar with moderate accuracy but does not improve performance of a stress-rest CT perfusion protocol. JACC Cardiovasc Imaging. 2013;6(10):1062–71.
89. Boussel L, et al. Assessment of acute myocardial infarction using MDCT after percutaneous coronary intervention: comparison with MRI. Am J Roentgenol. 2008;191(2):441–7.
90. Kang DK, et al. Dual-energy computed tomography for integrative imaging of coronary artery disease: principles and clinical applications. In: Seminars in ultrasound, CT and MRI. New York: Elsevier; 2010.
91. George RT, et al. Computed tomography myocardial perfusion imaging with 320-row detector computed tomography accurately detects myocardial ischemia in patients with obstructive coronary artery disease. Circ Cardiovasc Imaging. 2012;5(3):333–40.

Part XVI

Where We Are Going: The Road Ahead

65 Coronary CT Angiography as the Gatekeeper to the Cath Lab: Where Are We?

Christoph Artzner, Lynne M. Hurwitz, and Fabian Bamberg

Coronary disease is highly prevalent, affecting approximately 18% of men and 11% of women over the age of 65 years and 19% and 16% over the age of 75 years, respectively [1]. For patients with stable chest pain symptoms, accurately identifying patients with coronary artery disease (CAD) is a central part of cardiovascular medicine. If there is clinical concern for coronary artery disease, societal guidelines recommend determining patients' pretest probability based on history and physical examination and those categorized as intermediate risk referred for noninvasive testing (NIT) and those categorized as high risk referred for invasive coronary angiography [2–4].

Despite these guidelines and studies suggesting cost-effectiveness of selective referral to ICA [5–7], NIT prior to ICA is often not performed. Patel et al. evaluated 661,063 patients undergoing elective catheterization without history of CAD in the National Cardiovascular Data Registry's CathPCI Registry between July 2009 and December 2011. Only 64% received at least one pre-procedural NIT [8]. The most common NIT was stress SPECT MPI (78.1%), followed by stress echo (11.6%), stress ECG (9.8%), CCTA (2.1%), and stress CMR (0.8%) [8]. In this patient population, ICA demonstrated nonobstructive CAD (all stenoses <50%) in 58.4% of patients. Rates of obstructive CAD exceeded rates of nonobstructive disease only among those patients with abnormal NIT and high-risk findings (67.5% vs. 32.5%) [8]. Thus, it is not surprising that 18.3% of patients undergoing ICA had only evidence of moderate atherosclerosis (stenoses between 20% and 49%) and 40.1% of patients had minimal or no stenosis at all (all stenoses <20%).

Referral to ICA should be made carefully, since the interventional procedure is associated with risks and discomfort for patients. Major complications while rare (less than 1% of procedures) include death, myocardial infarction, cerebral infarction, or major embolization [9, 10]. Vascular access complications, reported to be as high as 6% in some series, remain the leading cause of morbidity after a cardiac catheterization procedure [11, 12]. Complications range from hematoma at femoral access, retroperitoneal hematoma, pseudoaneurysm, dissection, arteriovenous fistulae, and infections [12]. Although studies of closure devices have been developed to improve patients comfort, safety and efficacy remain unclear [12]. ICA with intra-arterial application of contrast media is also associated with higher risk for contrast-induced nephropathy [13].

While there are various NIT to assess for CAD, cardiac CT angiography (CCTA) has evolved as a robust modality to directly detect and characterize CAD and in contrast to other noninvasive studies assesses the vessels directly and not the end muscle or electrical signals. Major technical advances include substantially improved spatial (0.5 mm) and temporal resolution (66 msec) allowing optimal image quality for a broad range of patients, as well as sensitive detector technology to improve IQ for calcified lesions and additional low kV acquisitions, and iterative reconstruction approaches that have lowered radiation exposure to as low as one millisievert.

Given that great potential of a CCTA to detect and characterize CAD, in this chapter, we critically review the current scientific evidence showing whether CCTA can be effectively utilized as a gatekeeper to ICA to reduce the number of unnecessary, purely diagnostic procedures.

C. Artzner (✉)
Department of Radiology, Duke University Medical Center, Durham, NC, USA

Department of Diagnostic and Interventional Radiology, University of Tuebingen, Tubingen, Germany
e-mail: Christoph.Schabel@duke.edu

L. M. Hurwitz
Department of Radiology, Duke University Medical Center, Durham, NC, USA

F. Bamberg
Department of Diagnostic and Interventional Radiology, University of Tuebingen, Tubingen, Germany

U. J. Schoepf (ed.), *CT of the Heart*, Contemporary Medical Imaging, https://doi.org/10.1007/978-1-60327-237-7_65

Ability of CCTA to Depict and Characterize CAD

Three prospective multicenter trials and hundreds of single-center evaluations assessed the diagnostic performance of CCTA for identification of coronary stenoses. CCTA has a sensitivity from 94% to 99% with a specificity of 64–83% across a wide range of disease prevalence and stage of disease (acute and stable CP) for the detection of CAD. It has been shown that CCTA features a very favorable negative predictive value (NPV) of 97–99% to exclude obstructive anatomic stenosis (<50%) which means that a CT-based approach can effectively rule out anatomic CAD with good predictive capabilities for patients without coronary stenoses [14–18]. Interestingly, sensitivity and specificity were reported not to be affected by body size or by heart rates, whereas calcium scores >400 reduced the specificity significantly [15, 19]. However, significant false-positive rates are a result of the average to low specificity with overestimation of CAD severity by CCTA [14, 15, 20]. This has mainly been attributed to cases with poor image quality and presence of calcium.

Role of Morphologic CAD Assessment by CCTA as a Gatekeeper in Stable Angina

Based on the high diagnostic performance of CCTA to detect CAD and the high negative predictive value to exclude CAD as compared with ICA [14–18], it has been assumed that the presence of CAD can easily be excluded in a relevant portion of patients. Therefore, it was expected that ICA rates would be decreased by the utilization of CCTA. However, despite single-center observations or case reports, existing studies based on anatomic assessment of CAD are controversial. A clear trend toward gatekeeping capabilities of CCTA for ICA was not found, relating to the low specificity regarding ischemia resulting from CAD and because optimal thresholds of stenoses might not have been found yet from a functional perspective [14, 15].

In 2011 a retrospective, observational cohort study by Shreibati et al. assessed Medicare records of 282,830 without prior history of CAD who received nonemergent, noninvasive testing for CAD. Compared with stress myocardial perfusion scintigraphy (MPS), CCTA was associated with an increased likelihood of subsequent cardiac catheterization (22.9% vs. 12.1%), percutaneous coronary intervention (7.8% vs. 3.4%), and coronary artery bypass graft surgery (3.7% vs. 1.3%). CCTA was also associated with higher total healthcare spending, which was mainly attributable to CAD. At 180 days, CCTA was associated with a similar likelihood of all-cause mortality (1.05% vs. 1.28) and a slightly lower likelihood of hospitalization for acute myocardial infarction (0.19% vs. 0.43%). The data indicated that individuals who underwent CCTA in a non-acute setting were more likely to undergo subsequent invasive cardiac procedures and have higher CAD-related spending than patients who underwent stress testing [21].

It was hoped that the recently published PROMISE trial (Prospective Multicenter Imaging Study for Evaluation of Chest Pain) would elucidate CCTA regarding its gatekeeping capabilities. It was designed to compare functional testing by multiple modalities and anatomic evaluation of stenosis severity by CCTA [22]. In this study, more than 10,000 symptomatic patients underwent CCTA or to functional testing (exercise electrocardiography, nuclear stress testing, or stress echocardiography). The mean pretest likelihood of obstructive CAD was 53 ± 21% and an anticipated event rate of 9%. The study was powered for a 20% reduction to show superiority and a 10% margin for noninferiority. Over a median follow-up period of 25 months, the composite primary end point (death, myocardial infarction, hospitalization for unstable angina, or major procedural complication) occurred only in 3.3% of patients in the CTA group and 3.0% in the functional-testing group (adjusted hazard ratio, 1.04; 95% confidence interval, 0.83–1.29; $p = 0.75$). However, CTA was associated with fewer catheterizations showing no obstructive CAD than was functional testing (3.4% vs. 4.3%, $p = 0.02$), although more patients in the CTA group underwent catheterization within 90 days after randomization (12.2% vs. 8.1%). The median cumulative radiation exposure per patient was lower in the CTA group than in the functional-testing group (10.0 mSv vs. 11.3 mSv) if functional NIT involved iodizing radiation. This study concluded that initial CTA provides similar clinical outcomes over a median follow-up of 2 years [22].

Since PROMISE indicated similar clinical, economic, and safety-based outcomes for CCTA and functional testing, these results have been the subject of ongoing discussion, and optimal NIT strategy has not yet been determined [22, 23]. Criticism of the PROMISE trial is that for routinely performed CCTA, stenosis evaluation alone discards important functional data, and for perfusion analysis, myocardial perfusion scintigraphy (MPS) evaluation alone discards important anatomic information, but a combined assessment may identify a superior methodology [24].

Additionally, a recent open-label, parallel-group, multicenter trial of CCTA in patients with suspected angina due to coronary heart disease (SCOT-HEART) assessed the benefit of CCTA. The study included 4146 patients that were randomly assigned either to standard care or standard care plus CCTA. Of these participants, 47% had a baseline clinic diagnosis of coronary heart disease, and 36% had angina due to coronary heart disease. Compared to standard care, CTCA reclassified the diagnosis of coronary heart disease in 27% patients and the diagnosis of angina due to coronary heart disease in 23% patients vs. 1% and 1% ($p < 0.0001$). CCTA demonstrated increased certainty for both coronary heart disease and the diagnosis of angina due to coronary heart disease. Interestingly the frequency of coronary heart disease increased, and the diagnosis of angina due to coronary showed a decreasing trend. In this study, CTA lead to an increase of planned investigations (94 additional ICAs were indicated and 29 were cancelled) and treatments (375 initiated and 189 were cancelled) compared to standard care (8 and 1 and 95 and 14, respectively) but did not affect 6-week symptom severity or subsequent hospital admissions for chest pain [25]. In follow-up of these patients at 1.7 years, CTCA was associated with a 38% reduction in fatal and nonfatal myocardial infarction (26 vs. 42, HR 0.62, 95% CI 0.38–1.01; $p = 0.053$) [25]. The study concluded that CCTA clarifies the diagnosis, enables targeting of interventions, and might reduce the future risk of myocardial infarction [25]. Again, the topic of CCTA as a gatekeeper remains highly controversial. A newly published prospective, single-center study of 340 patients compared a CCTA-based approach and a traditional primarily ICA-based approach. The study showed a decreased need for ICA in the group of patients that received CCTA imaging initially (14% of patients received additional ICA) compared to the ICA group (100% of patients received ICA). Over a median follow-up of 3.3 years, rates of major adverse cardiovascular events were similar with 4.2% in the CCTA group and 3.7% in the coronary angiography group (adjusted hazard ratio 0.90, 95% confidence interval 0.30–2.69, $p = 0.86$). Patient comfort and time to patient discharge were found to be superior for the CCTA subgroup [26].

Role of Functional CAD Assessment by CCTA as a Gatekeeper

The anatomical assessment of coronary artery stenosis does not correlate well with functional significance of coronary stenosis. Thus, the hemodynamic significance of an angiographically intermediate stenosis remains relevant before referral for revascularization treatment [20]. The goal of CCTA like other vascular CTA exams has been for the assessment of anatomic stenosis with vessel narrowing of 50% or less considered non-flow limiting. This model for management of vascular disease is limited in that the demonstration of end-organ ischemia is not determined from a static anatomic dataset. A major criticism of the PROMISE trial was that for routinely performed CCTA, stenosis evaluation alone discards important functional data [24]. Although CCTA has demonstrated excellent sensitivity and specificity for characterization of luminal stenosis, the moderate specificity of CTA in the PROMISE trial increased the rate of invasive catheterization by almost 50% compared with functional testing, with over a quarter of these patients not having obstructive CAD on invasive angiography [27]. Given the great potential of a combined morphological and functional assessment by CT for both anatomic stenosis and functional significant of areas of stenosis, tremendous research efforts have been undertaken to develop tools and techniques to also evaluate coronary and myocardial function. Major developments include the derivation of the fractional flow reserve based on CCTA image data (FFR_{CT}) as well as the assessment of myocardial perfusion by either static or dynamic scan acquisitions (Figs. 65.1 and 65.2).

FFR_{CT} is based on computational fluid dynamics and simulated maximal coronary hyperemia. Recent advances in computational fluid dynamics enable calculation of coronary flow and pressure fields from anatomic image data and validated it to invasive FFR performed during invasive catheterization. This technology allows for calculation of FFR_{CT} feasible without additional imaging or medications or radiation [28, 29]. Multiple studies showed superiority of CTA with FFRCT vs. CCTA.

The DISCOVER-FLOW (Diagnosis of Ischemia-Causing Stenoses Obtained Via Noninvasive Fractional Flow Reserve) compared invasive FFR with FFRCT and CCTA in 103 patients. On a per-vessel basis, the accuracy (84.7 vs. 58.5%) and specificity (82.2 vs. 39.6%) and the positive predictive value (73.9 vs. 46.5%) improved substantially with similar sensitivities and negative predictive values for FFR. The area under the receiver operating characteristic curve was 0.90 for FFRCT and 0.75 for CCTA ($p = 0.001$) [30]. The DeFACTO (Determination of Fractional Flow Reserve by Anatomic Computed Tomographic Angiography) trial evaluated FFRCT against CTA for diagnostic accuracy of ischemia. The study included 252 patients with 137 patients (54.4%) showing an abnormal FFR determined by ICA. This study showed on a per-patient basis slightly lower values for diagnostic accuracy (73%), sensitivity (90%), specificity (54%), positive predictive value (67%), and negative predictive value (84%) of FFRCT plus CT. When FFR findings were compared with obstructive CAD diagnosed by CT alone, area under the receiver operating characteristic curve was in favor of FFR CT with AUC 0.81 (0.75–0.86) vs. AUC 0.68 (0.62–0.74; $p < 0.001$) [31]. Thus, these studies indicate that the inclusion of FFR_{CT} might improve gatekeeping capabilities of CCTA.

To address the clinical utility of this new method and how its use may affect patient care and clinical outcomes, the PLATFORM (Prospective Longitudinal Trial of FFR_{CT} Outcome and Resource Impacts) trial included 584 patients at 11 sites with new-onset chest pain who were prospectively assigned to receive either usual testing ($n = 287$) or CTA/FFR_{CT} ($n = 297$). The primary end point was the percentage of ICA with no significant obstructive CAD. The patient collective showed a pretest probability of obstructive CAD

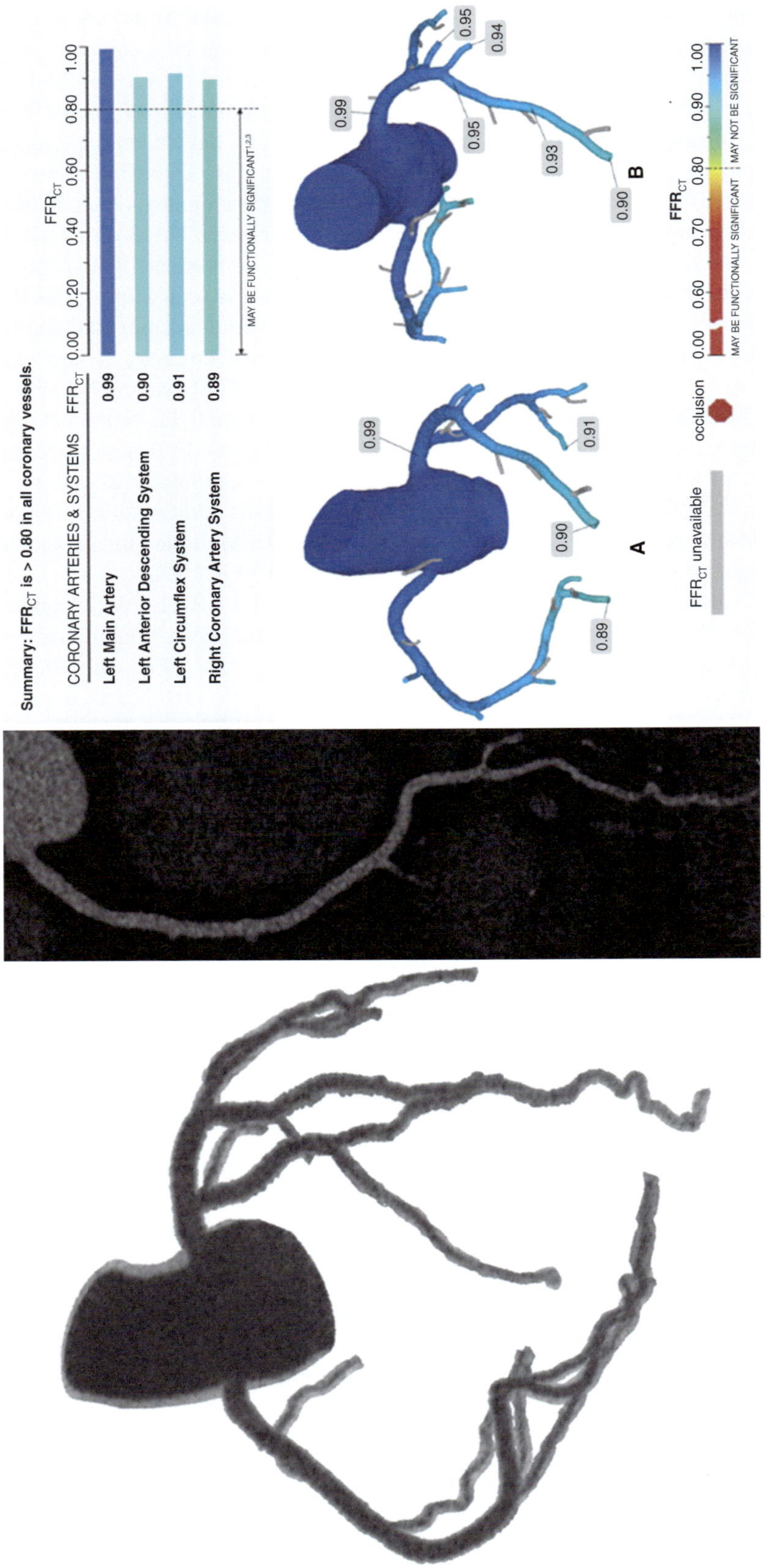

Fig. 65.1 Example of a negative CCTA demonstrating the absence of CAD. FFR_{CT} were calculated by HeartFlow, Redwood City, CA, USA

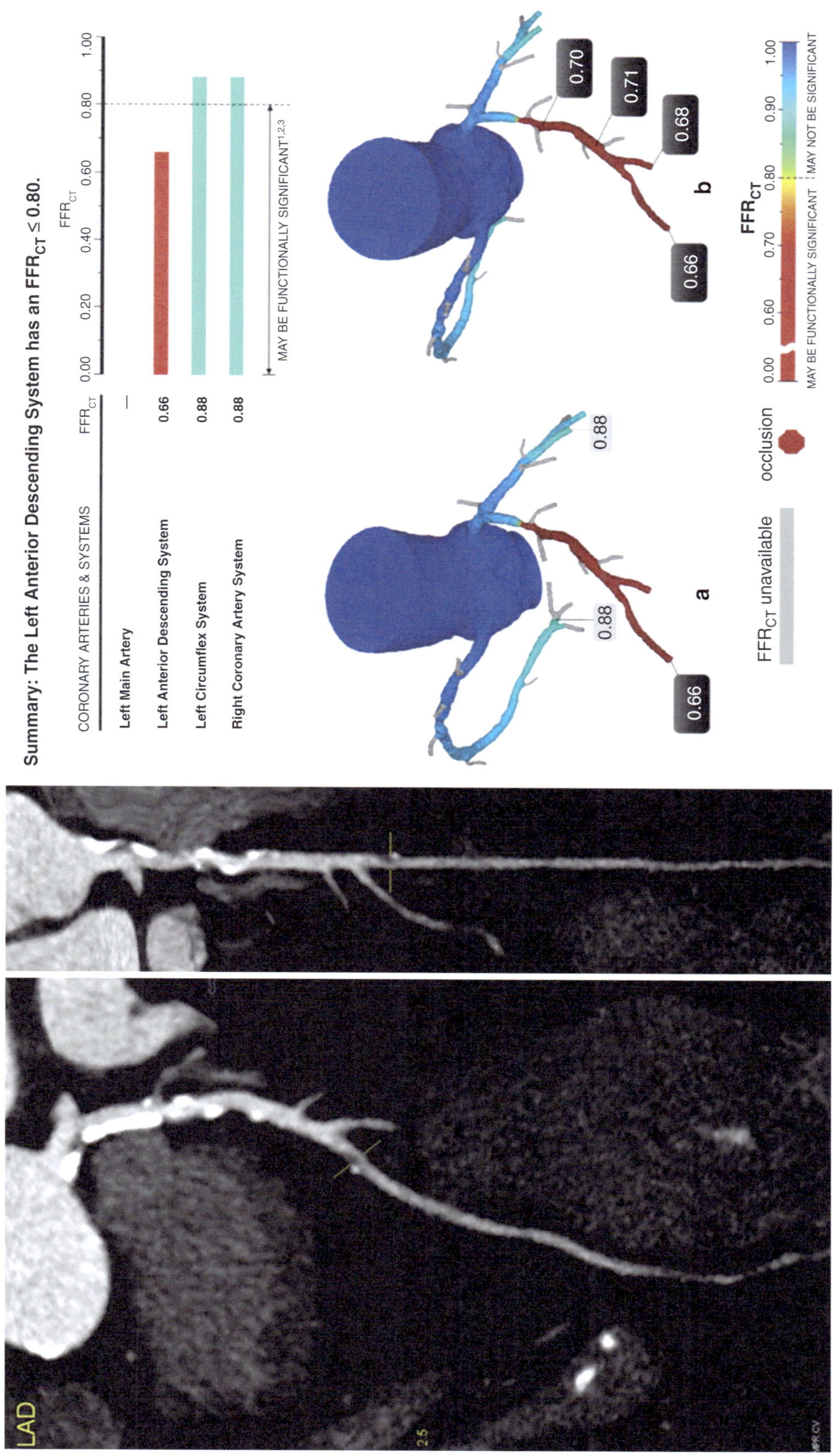

Fig. 65.2 Example of positive CCTA demonstrating stenosis in LAD. FFR_{CT} were calculated by HeartFlow, Redwood City, CA, USA

of 49 ± 17%. Indication for ICA was FFR_{CT} guided in 193 patients vs. 187 in usual care, and no obstructive CAD was found at ICA in 24 patients (12%) for CTA/FFR_{CT} and 137 patients (73%) in the usual care arm (risk difference 61%, 95% confidence interval 53–69, $p < 0.0001$). Clinical event rates within 90 days were low for usual care and CTA with FFR_{CT}. Thus, the authors concluded CTA with FFR_{CT} was a feasible and safe alternative to ICA and associated with a significantly lower rate of invasive angiography showing no obstructive CAD [27].

These findings were also supported by the NXT (Analysis of Coronary Blood Flow Using CT Angiography: Next Steps). In this prospective multicenter trial, 254 patients with suspected CAD were included and underwent clinically indicated ICA. Coronary CTA was performed before ICA. The area under the receiver operating characteristic curve for FFR_{CT} was 0.90 versus 0.81 for coronary CTA ($p = 0.0008$). Per-patient sensitivity and specificity to identify myocardial ischemia were 86% and 79% for FFRCT versus 94% and 34% for coronary CTA and 64% and 83% for ICA, respectively [32]. These results are very promising in that they indicate the combination of CCTA and FFR in patients with CAD can decrease the rates of negative ICA procedures and thus act as a decision-maker for ICA. But to date, no study addresses the gatekeeping capabilities of a comprehensive CCTA CAD assessment including FFR when compared with functional diagnostics, like MPS, which is still widely accepted as standard of care.

Subsequently, the Computed TomogRaphic Evaluation of Atherosclerotic DEtermiNants of Myocardial IsChEmia (CREDENCE) trial was initiated as a prospective multicenter cross-sectional study to further investigate the performance of CCTA as a gatekeeper for ICA and to incorporate latest CCTA data-based techniques beyond luminal stenosis severity alone for the diagnosis of lesion-specific ischemia including atherosclerotic plaque characteristics (APCs) and calculation of fractional flow reserve (FFRCT) [24]. This study is meant to mitigate the limitations and critics of the PROMISE trial. For this purpose, 618 participants underwent clinically indicated CCTA, MPS, ICA, and FFR with either MPS or CCTA/FFRCT performed as part of the study. This design was chosen because despite availability of multiple functional imaging techniques (echocardiography, cardiac magnetic resonance, MPS), MPS remained the clinical standard for functional imaging to identify ischemia by detecting stress-induced regional myocardial perfusion defects [2, 3]. Although MPS can determine the severity and extent of myocardial ischemia with high performance by single-photon emission computed tomography (SPECT) or positron emission tomography (PET) at a per-patient level [24, 33, 34]. However, its accuracy to correctly discriminate ischemia on a per-vessel basis is less robust [24, 35] and compromised in patients with multi-vessel CAD [24, 36]. Therefore, it is questionable whether MPS will be able to identify vessels that would benefit from revascularization accurately [24, 37]. On the other hand, the addition of FFR_{CT} and atherosclerotic plaque characteristics (APCs) by coronary CCTA to coronary CTA may allow for a comprehensive anatomic and functional assessment of CAD in a manner potentially promoting beneficial clinical and cost outcomes. At the current stage, recruitment into the CREDENCE trial has been completed, and results of the study are highly anticipated [24].

Future concepts to improve CCTA beyond anatomic lesion assessment include APC evaluation, which has demonstrated high agreement with invasive methods of plaque assessment and has shown to improve discrimination of ischemia causing culprit coronary lesions [24, 38]. APC evaluates lesions regarding aggregate plaque volume (APV), positive remodeling (PR), low attenuation plaque (LAP), and spotty calcification (SC) [39]. A single-center study by Park et al. including 252 patients showed an association of APV and LAP with an increased risk of ischemia in stenosis >50%, whereas PR was found to be a predictor of ischemia independently of severity of stenosis [39].

As a second major development, CT perfusion imaging has been introduced recently. This approach becomes feasible with further improvement of CT acquisition technique and therefore higher temporal resolution to visualize myocardial enhancement as the contrast medium passes through the heart [40, 41]. Based on these first feasibility studies, it remains unclear whether this technique will yield sufficient diagnostic performance and robustness to be potentially implemented into clinical workflow. First prospective studies are planned, but patient recruitment has not started.

Impact of CCTA in Patients with Acute Chest Pain on Diagnostic Cath Rates

A study of Hoffmann et al. assessed 1000 patients with presentation of acute coronary syndromes in the emergency department. ROMICAT-II was designed as a randomized, controlled, multicenter trial to compare an evaluation and management strategy facilitating CCTA as a first diagnostic test with a standard emergency department evaluation for patients with acute chest pain and suggested acute coronary syndrome. A total of 75 patients (8%) had a final diagnosis of an acute coronary syndrome. ICA was performed in 54 (11%) and 36 (7%) patients in the CCTA group and standard group, respectively ($p = 0.06$). Percutaneous interventions were performed in 24 and 14 patients ($p = 0.14$) and bypass surgery in 5 and 4 patients ($p = 0.99$) in the CCTA group and standard group, respectively. In this study, more diagnostic testing was performed in the CCTA group than in the standard evaluation group ($p < 0.001$), and CTA was demonstrated to reduce the length of the stay by 7.6 h, and less patients were admitted to an observation unit but discharged directly from the emergency department (47% vs. 12%). From a cost-effectiveness standpoint, both strategies were evaluated as equivalent. Number of diagnostic tests and radiation exposure were found to be higher in the CCTA group. No acute coronary syndromes were missed, and no significant differences in major adverse cardiovascular events were found during 28 days of follow-up [42].

A further study assessing a similar scenario was performed by Litt et al. In this study 1370 patients were included with a randomized assignment of 2:1 to a CCTA-based or a conventional strategy. Of the 908 patients in the CCTA subgroup, 767 individuals received a CCTA. ICA was performed in 37 of 908 patients in the CCTA subgroup vs. 18 of 462 patients in the traditional care group at index visit. The rate of maximal stenosis <50% was lower in the CCTA subgroup than in the traditional care group, 9 of 37 and 10 of 18 patients, respectively; and hence the rate of significant stenosis was higher in the CCTA group than in the traditional care group, 28 of 37 and 8 of 18 patients, respectively. Within 30 days after index visit, the use of invasive angiography was similar (5.1% and 4.2%; difference, 0.9%; 95% CI, −4.8 to 6.6) or in the rate of revascularization (2.7% and 1.3%; difference, 1.4%; 95% CI, −4.3 to 7.0). Nevertheless, negative findings on invasive angiography were less likely in the CCTA subgroup (29% vs. 53%; difference, −23.7% points; 95% CI, −48.8 to 3.3). There was no significant between-group difference in the likelihood of a repeat emergency department visit, hospitalization, or cardiologist office visit or rate of major cardiac events. The study showed similar results compared to Hoffmann et al. with shorter hospital stay and more direct discharges from emergency department. Overall, coronary disease was more likely to be diagnosed in patients in the CCTA group than in patients in the traditional care group (9.0% vs. 3.5%; difference, 5.6% points; 95% CI, 0–11.2), but prognostic impact was not assessed [43].

Summary and Future Outlook

Accounting for the excellent negative predictive value of CCTA for CTA, it has been a long-standing goal to utilize it as a gatekeeper for invasive coronary angiography to utilize resources more efficiently and further reduce patient's treatment burden. However, this idea is not supported by available scientific evidence in prospective, multicenter studies contradicting numerous case reports and single-center observations. This scientific evidence will be challenged by the CONSERVE (Coronary Computed Tomographic Angiography for Selective Cardiac Catheterization) trial (NCT01810198), which is directly testing the concept of CCTA as a gatekeeper to ICA [44].

For stable angina, large, randomized trials found no superior methodology comparing the standard of care and a CCTA-based strategy but found slight increase of ICA rates in the CCTA groups. For acute chest pain, both strategies showed an identical safety profile with similar proportion of purely diagnostic ICAs, but with the tendency to have less negative findings in ICA and a higher likelihood to diagnose CAD compared with traditional standard of care, which in consequence does not result in functional apparent symptoms in all subjects. It is hypothesized that these subjects without functional impairment, who receive treated accordingly to current guidelines, will have improved survival rates. Nevertheless, this assumption is not supported by available scientific evidence.

Despite the sole use of CCTA for anatomic assessment of CAD, FFR_{CT} along with anatomic assessment of CAD are showing promising results and potential for more robust decision-making potential for patient management and long-term outcomes. Prospective, multicenter studies are currently under way, and results are expected to be released soon.

References

1. Go AS, Mozaffarian D, Roger VL, Benjamin EJ, Berry JD, Blaha MJ, Dai S, Ford ES, Fox CS, Franco S, Fullerton HJ, Gillespie C, Hailpern SM, Heit JA, Howard VJ, Huffman MD, Judd SE, Kissela BM, Kittner SJ, Lackland DT, Lichtman JH, Lisabeth LD, Mackey RH, Magid DJ, Marcus GM, Marelli A, Matchar DB, McGuire DK, Mohler ER 3rd, Moy CS, Mussolino ME, Neumar RW, Nichol G, Pandey DK, Paynter NP, Reeves MJ, Sorlie PD, Stein J, Towfighi A, Turan TN, Virani SS, Wong ND, Woo D, Turner MB, American Heart Association Statistics C, Stroke Statistics S. Heart disease and stroke statistics–2014 update: a report from the American Heart Association. Circulation. 2014;129(3):e28–e292. https://doi.org/10.1161/01.cir.0000441139.02102.80.
2. Fraker TD Jr, Fihn SD, Chronic Stable Angina Writing C, American College of C, American Heart A, Gibbons RJ, Abrams J, Chatterjee K, Daley J, Deedwania PC, Douglas JS, Ferguson TB Jr, Gardin JM, O'Rourke RA, Williams SV, Smith SC Jr, Jacobs AK, Adams CD, Anderson JL, Buller CE, Creager MA, Ettinger SM, Halperin JL, Hunt SA, Krumholz HM, Kushner FG, Lytle BW, Nishimura R, Page RL, Riegel B, Tarkington LG, Yancy CW. 2007 chronic angina focused update of the ACC/AHA 2002 guidelines for the management of patients with chronic stable angina: a report of the American College of Cardiology/American Heart Association Task Force on Practice Guidelines Writing Group to develop the focused update of the 2002 guidelines for the management of patients with chronic stable angina. J Am Coll Cardiol. 2007;50(23):2264–74. https://doi.org/10.1016/j.jacc.2007.08.002.
3. Klocke FJ, Baird MG, Lorell BH, Bateman TM, Messer JV, Berman DS, O'Gara PT, Carabello BA, Russell RO Jr, Cerqueira MD, St John Sutton MG, DeMaria AN, Udelson JE, Kennedy JW, Verani MS, Williams KA, Antman EM, Smith SC Jr, Alpert JS, Gregoratos G, Anderson JL, Hiratzka LF, Faxon DP, Hunt SA, Fuster V, Jacobs AK, Gibbons RJ, Russell RO, American College of C, American Heart A, American Society for Nuclear C. ACC/AHA/ASNC guidelines for the clinical use of cardiac radionuclide imaging--executive summary: a report of the American College of

Cardiology/American Heart Association Task Force on Practice Guidelines (ACC/AHA/ASNC Committee to Revise the 1995 Guidelines for the Clinical Use of Cardiac Radionuclide Imaging). J Am Coll Cardiol. 2003;42(7):1318–33.
4. Cheitlin MD, Armstrong WF, Aurigemma GP, Beller GA, Bierman FZ, Davis JL, Douglas PS, Faxon DP, Gillam LD, Kimball TR, Kussmaul WG, Pearlman AS, Philbrick JT, Rakowski H, Thys DM, Antman EM, Smith SC Jr, Alpert JS, Gregoratos G, Anderson JL, Hiratzka LF, Faxon DP, Hunt SA, Fuster V, Jacobs AK, Gibbons RJ, Russell RO, Acc, Aha, Ase. ACC/AHA/ASE 2003 guideline update for the clinical application of echocardiography: summary article. A report of the American College of Cardiology/American Heart Association Task Force on Practice Guidelines (ACC/AHA/ASE Committee to Update the 1997 Guidelines for the Clinical Application of Echocardiography). J Am Soc Echocardiogr. 2003;16(10):1091–110. https://doi.org/10.1016/S0894-7317(03)00685-0.
5. Shaw LJ, Hachamovitch R, Berman DS, Marwick TH, Lauer MS, Heller GV, Iskandrian AE, Kesler KL, Travin MI, Lewin HC, Hendel RC, Borges-Neto S, Miller DD. The economic consequences of available diagnostic and prognostic strategies for the evaluation of stable angina patients: an observational assessment of the value of precatheterization ischemia. Economics of Noninvasive Diagnosis (END) Multicenter Study Group. J Am Coll Cardiol. 1999;33(3):661–9.
6. Nance JW Jr, Bamberg F, Schoepf UJ. Coronary computed tomography angiography in patients with chronic chest pain: systematic review of evidence base and cost-effectiveness. J Thorac Imaging. 2012;27(5):277–88. https://doi.org/10.1097/RTI.0b013e3182631c5c.
7. Toutouzas K, Synetos A, Karanasos A, Drakopoulou M, Tsiamis E, Lerakis S, Stefanadis C. Percutaneous coronary intervention in chronic stable angina. Am J Med Sci. 2010;339(6):568–72. https://doi.org/10.1097/MAJ.0b013e3181d673d7.
8. Patel MR, Dai D, Hernandez AF, Douglas PS, Messenger J, Garratt KN, Maddox TM, Peterson ED, Roe MT. Prevalence and predictors of nonobstructive coronary artery disease identified with coronary angiography in contemporary clinical practice. Am Heart J. 2014;167(6):846–52 e842. https://doi.org/10.1016/j.ahj.2014.03.001.
9. Segal AZ, Abernethy WB, Palacios IF, BeLue R, Rordorf G. Stroke as a complication of cardiac catheterization: risk factors and clinical features. Neurology. 2001;56(7):975–7.
10. Ammann P, Brunner-La Rocca HP, Angehrn W, Roelli H, Sagmeister M, Rickli H. Procedural complications following diagnostic coronary angiography are related to the operator's experience and the catheter size. Catheter Cardiovasc Interv. 2003;59(1):13–8. https://doi.org/10.1002/ccd.10489.
11. Meyerson SL, Feldman T, Desai TR, Leef J, Schwartz LB, McKinsey JF. Angiographic access site complications in the era of arterial closure devices. Vasc Endovasc Surg. 2002;36(2):137–44.
12. Patel MR, Jneid H, Derdeyn CP, Klein LW, Levine GN, Lookstein RA, White CJ, Yeghiazarians Y, Rosenfield K, American Heart Association D, Interventional Cardiac Catheterization Committee of the Council on Clinical Cardiology CoCR, Intervention CoPVDCoCS, Anesthesia, Stroke C. Arteriotomy closure devices for cardiovascular procedures: a scientific statement from the American Heart Association. Circulation. 2010;122(18):1882–93. https://doi.org/10.1161/CIR.0b013e3181f9b345.
13. Wichmann JL, Katzberg RW, Litwin SE, Zwerner PL, De Cecco CN, Vogl TJ, Costello P, Schoepf UJ. Contrast-induced nephropathy. Circulation. 2015;132(20):1931–6. https://doi.org/10.1161/CIRCULATIONAHA.115.014672.
14. Meijboom WB, Meijs MF, Schuijf JD, Cramer MJ, Mollet NR, van Mieghem CA, Nieman K, van Werkhoven JM, Pundziute G, Weustink AC, de Vos AM, Pugliese F, Rensing B, Jukema JW, Bax JJ, Prokop M, Doevendans PA, Hunink MG, Krestin GP, de Feyter PJ. Diagnostic accuracy of 64-slice computed tomography coronary angiography: a prospective, multicenter, multivendor study. J Am Coll Cardiol. 2008;52(25):2135–44. https://doi.org/10.1016/j.jacc.2008.08.058.
15. Budoff MJ, Dowe D, Jollis JG, Gitter M, Sutherland J, Halamert E, Scherer M, Bellinger R, Martin A, Benton R, Delago A, Min JK. Diagnostic performance of 64-multidetector row coronary computed tomographic angiography for evaluation of coronary artery stenosis in individuals without known coronary artery disease: results from the prospective multicenter ACCURACY (Assessment by Coronary Computed Tomographic Angiography of Individuals Undergoing Invasive Coronary Angiography) trial. J Am Coll Cardiol. 2008;52(21):1724–32. https://doi.org/10.1016/j.jacc.2008.07.031.
16. Marwan M, Hausleiter J, Abbara S, Hoffmann U, Becker C, Ovrehus K, Ropers D, Bathina R, Berman D, Anders K, Uder M, Meave A, Alexanderson E, Achenbach S. Multicenter Evaluation Of Coronary Dual-Source CT angiography in patients with intermediate Risk of Coronary Artery Stenoses (MEDIC): study design and rationale. J Cardiovasc Comput Tomogr. 2014;8(3):183–8. https://doi.org/10.1016/j.jcct.2014.04.006.
17. Hadamitzky M, Taubert S, Deseive S, Byrne RA, Martinoff S, Schomig A, Hausleiter J. Prognostic value of coronary computed tomography angiography during 5 years of follow-up in patients with suspected coronary artery disease. Eur Heart J. 2013;34(42):3277–85. https://doi.org/10.1093/eurheartj/eht293.
18. Hoffmann U, Bamberg F, Chae CU, Nichols JH, Rogers IS, Seneviratne SK, Truong QA, Cury RC, Abbara S, Shapiro MD, Moloo J, Butler J, Ferencik M, Lee H, Jang IK, Parry BA, Brown DF, Udelson JE, Achenbach S, Brady TJ, Nagurney JT. Coronary computed tomography angiography for early triage of patients with acute chest pain: the ROMICAT (Rule Out Myocardial Infarction using Computer Assisted Tomography) trial. J Am Coll Cardiol. 2009;53(18):1642–50. https://doi.org/10.1016/j.jacc.2009.01.052.
19. Mangold S, Wichmann JL, Schoepf UJ, Caruso D, Tesche C, Steinberg DH, Varga-Szemes A, Stubenrauch AC, Bayer RR 2nd, Biancalana M, Nikolaou K, De Cecco CN. Diagnostic accuracy of coronary CT angiography using 3rd-generation dual-source CT and automated tube voltage selection: clinical application in a non-obese and obese patient population. Eur Radiol. 2016. https://doi.org/10.1007/s00330-016-4601-2.
20. Meijboom WB, Van Mieghem CA, van Pelt N, Weustink A, Pugliese F, Mollet NR, Boersma E, Regar E, van Geuns RJ, de Jaegere PJ, Serruys PW, Krestin GP, de Feyter PJ. Comprehensive assessment of coronary artery stenoses: computed tomography coronary angiography versus conventional coronary angiography and correlation with fractional flow reserve in patients with stable angina. J Am Coll Cardiol. 2008;52(8):636–43. https://doi.org/10.1016/j.jacc.2008.05.024.
21. Shreibati JB, Baker LC, Hlatky MA. Association of coronary CT angiography or stress testing with subsequent utilization and spending among Medicare beneficiaries. JAMA. 2011;306(19):2128–36. https://doi.org/10.1001/jama.2011.1652.
22. Douglas PS, Hoffmann U, Patel MR, Mark DB, Al-Khalidi HR, Cavanaugh B, Cole J, Dolor RJ, Fordyce CB, Huang M, Khan MA, Kosinski AS, Krucoff MW, Malhotra V, Picard MH, Udelson JE, Velazquez EJ, Yow E, Cooper LS, Lee KL, Investigators P. Outcomes of anatomical versus functional testing for coronary artery disease. N Engl J Med. 2015;372(14):1291–300. https://doi.org/10.1056/NEJMoa1415516.
23. Mark DB, Federspiel JJ, Cowper PA, Anstrom KJ, Hoffmann U, Patel MR, Davidson-Ray L, Daniels MR, Cooper LS, Knight JD, Lee KL, Douglas PS, Investigators P. Economic outcomes with anatomical versus functional diagnostic testing for coronary

artery disease. Ann Intern Med. 2016;165(2):94–102. https://doi.org/10.7326/M15-2639.
24. Rizvi A, Hartaigh BO, Knaapen P, Leipsic J, Shaw LJ, Andreini D, Pontone G, Raman S, Khan MA, Ridner M, Nabi F, Gimelli A, Jang J, Cole J, Nakazato R, Zarins C, Han D, Lee JH, Szymonifika J, Gomez MJ, Truong QA, Chang HJ, Lin FY, Min JK. Rationale and design of the CREDENCE trial: computed tomog raphic evaluation of atherosclerotic determinants of myocardial IsChEmia. BMC Cardiovasc Disord. 2016;16(1):190. https://doi.org/10.1186/s12872-016-0360-x.
25. Investigators S-H. CT coronary angiography in patients with suspected angina due to coronary heart disease (SCOT-HEART): an open-label, parallel-group, multicentre trial. Lancet. 2015;385(9985):2383–91. https://doi.org/10.1016/S0140-6736(15)60291-4.
26. Dewey M, Rief M, Martus P, Kendziora B, Feger S, Dreger H, Priem S, Knebel F, Bohm M, Schlattmann P, Hamm B, Schonenberger E, Laule M, Zimmermann E. Evaluation of computed tomography in patients with atypical angina or chest pain clinically referred for invasive coronary angiography: randomised controlled trial. BMJ. 2016;355:i5441. https://doi.org/10.1136/bmj.i5441.
27. Douglas PS, Pontone G, Hlatky MA, Patel MR, Norgaard BL, Byrne RA, Curzen N, Purcell I, Gutberlet M, Rioufol G, Hink U, Schuchlenz HW, Feuchtner G, Gilard M, Andreini D, Jensen JM, Hadamitzky M, Chiswell K, Cyr D, Wilk A, Wang F, Rogers C, De Bruyne B, Investigators P. Clinical outcomes of fractional flow reserve by computed tomographic angiography-guided diagnostic strategies vs. usual care in patients with suspected coronary artery disease: the prospective longitudinal trial of FFR(CT): outcome and resource impacts study. Eur Heart J. 2015;36(47):3359–67. https://doi.org/10.1093/eurheartj/ehv444.
28. Taylor CA, Fonte TA, Min JK. Computational fluid dynamics applied to cardiac computed tomography for noninvasive quantification of fractional flow reserve: scientific basis. J Am Coll Cardiol. 2013;61(22):2233–41. https://doi.org/10.1016/j.jacc.2012.11.083.
29. Kim HJ, Vignon-Clementel IE, Coogan JS, Figueroa CA, Jansen KE, Taylor CA. Patient-specific modeling of blood flow and pressure in human coronary arteries. Ann Biomed Eng. 2010;38(10):3195–209. https://doi.org/10.1007/s10439-010-0083-6.
30. Koo BK, Erglis A, Doh JH, Daniels DV, Jegere S, Kim HS, Dunning A, DeFrance T, Lansky A, Leipsic J, Min JK. Diagnosis of ischemia-causing coronary stenoses by noninvasive fractional flow reserve computed from coronary computed tomographic angiograms. Results from the prospective multicenter DISCOVER-FLOW (Diagnosis of Ischemia-Causing Stenoses Obtained Via Noninvasive Fractional Flow Reserve) study. J Am Coll Cardiol. 2011;58(19):1989–97. https://doi.org/10.1016/j.jacc.2011.06.066.
31. Min JK, Leipsic J, Pencina MJ, Berman DS, Koo BK, van Mieghem C, Erglis A, Lin FY, Dunning AM, Apruzzese P, Budoff MJ, Cole JH, Jaffer FA, Leon MB, Malpeso J, Mancini GB, Park SJ, Schwartz RS, Shaw LJ, Mauri L. Diagnostic accuracy of fractional flow reserve from anatomic CT angiography. JAMA. 2012;308(12):1237–45. https://doi.org/10.1001/2012.jama.11274.
32. Norgaard BL, Leipsic J, Gaur S, Seneviratne S, Ko BS, Ito H, Jensen JM, Mauri L, De Bruyne B, Bezerra H, Osawa K, Marwan M, Naber C, Erglis A, Park SJ, Christiansen EH, Kaltoft A, Lassen JF, Botker HE, Achenbach S, Group NXTTS. Diagnostic performance of noninvasive fractional flow reserve derived from coronary computed tomography angiography in suspected coronary artery disease: the NXT trial (Analysis of Coronary Blood Flow Using CT Angiography: Next Steps). J Am Coll Cardiol. 2014;63(12):1145–55. https://doi.org/10.1016/j.jacc.2013.11.043.
33. Klocke FJ, Baird MG, Lorell BH, Bateman TM, Messer JV, Berman DS, O'Gara PT, Carabello BA, Russell RO Jr, Cerqueira MD, St John Sutton MG, DeMaria AN, Udelson JE, Kennedy JW, Verani MS, Williams KA, Antman EM, Smith SC Jr, Alpert JS, Gregoratos G, Anderson JL, Hiratzka LF, Faxon DP, Hunt SA, Fuster V, Jacobs AK, Gibbons RJ, Russell RO, American College of C, American Heart Association Task Force on Practice G, American Society for Nuclear C. ACC/AHA/ASNC guidelines for the clinical use of cardiac radionuclide imaging–executive summary: a report of the American College of Cardiology/American Heart Association Task Force on Practice Guidelines (ACC/AHA/ASNC Committee to Revise the 1995 Guidelines for the Clinical Use of Cardiac Radionuclide Imaging). Circulation. 2003;108(11):1404–18. https://doi.org/10.1161/01.CIR.0000080946.42225.4D.
34. Kim C, Kwok YS, Heagerty P, Redberg R. Pharmacologic stress testing for coronary disease diagnosis: a meta-analysis. Am Heart J. 2001;142(6):934–44. https://doi.org/10.1067/mhj.2001.119761.
35. Elhendy A, Schinkel AF, Bax JJ, van Domburg RT, Valkema R, Biagini E, Feringa HH, Poldermans D. Accuracy of stress Tc-99m tetrofosmin myocardial perfusion tomography for the diagnosis and localization of coronary artery disease in women. J Nucl Cardiol. 2006;13(5):629–34. https://doi.org/10.1016/j.nuclcard.2006.06.128.
36. Melikian N, De Bondt P, Tonino P, De Winter O, Wyffels E, Bartunek J, Heyndrickx GR, Fearon WF, Pijls NH, Wijns W, De Bruyne B. Fractional flow reserve and myocardial perfusion imaging in patients with angiographic multivessel coronary artery disease. JACC Cardiovasc Interv. 2010;3(3):307–14. https://doi.org/10.1016/j.jcin.2009.12.010.
37. Beller GA, Ragosta M. Decision making in multivessel coronary disease: the need for physiological lesion assessment. JACC Cardiovasc Interv. 2010;3(3):315–7. https://doi.org/10.1016/j.jcin.2010.01.007.
38. Voros S, Rinehart S, Qian Z, Joshi P, Vazquez G, Fischer C, Belur P, Hulten E, Villines TC. Coronary atherosclerosis imaging by coronary CT angiography: current status, correlation with intravascular interrogation and meta-analysis. JACC Cardiovasc Imaging. 2011;4(5):537–48. https://doi.org/10.1016/j.jcmg.2011.03.006.
39. Park HB, Heo R, o Hartaigh B, Cho I, Gransar H, Nakazato R, Leipsic J, Mancini GB, Koo BK, Otake H, Budoff MJ, Berman DS, Erglis A, Chang HJ, Min JK. Atherosclerotic plaque characteristics by CT angiography identify coronary lesions that cause ischemia: a direct comparison to fractional flow reserve. JACC Cardiovasc Imaging. 2015;8(1):1–10. https://doi.org/10.1016/j.jcmg.2014.11.002.
40. Bamberg F, Becker A, Schwarz F, Marcus RP, Greif M, von Ziegler F, Blankstein R, Hoffmann U, Sommer WH, Hoffmann VS, Johnson TR, Becker HC, Wintersperger BJ, Reiser MF, Nikolaou K. Detection of hemodynamically significant coronary artery stenosis: incremental diagnostic value of dynamic CT-based myocardial perfusion imaging. Radiology. 2011;260(3):689–98. https://doi.org/10.1148/radiol.11110638.
41. Rossi A, Merkus D, Klotz E, Mollet N, de Feyter PJ, Krestin GP. Stress myocardial perfusion: imaging with multidetector CT. Radiology. 2014;270(1):25–46. https://doi.org/10.1148/radiol.13112739.
42. Hoffmann U, Truong QA, Schoenfeld DA, Chou ET, Woodard PK, Nagurney JT, Pope JH, Hauser TH, White CS, Weiner SG, Kalanjian S, Mullins ME, Mikati I, Peacock WF, Zakroysky P, Hayden D, Goehler A, Lee H, Gazelle GS, Wiviott SD, Fleg JL, Udelson JE, Investigators R-I. Coronary CT angiography versus standard evaluation in acute chest pain. N Engl J Med. 2012;367(4):299–308. https://doi.org/10.1056/NEJMoa1201161.
43. Litt HI, Gatsonis C, Snyder B, Singh H, Miller CD, Entrikin DW, Leaming JM, Gavin LJ, Pacella CB, Hollander JE. CT angiography for safe discharge of patients with possible acute coronary syndromes. N Engl J Med. 2012;366(15):1393–403. https://doi.org/10.1056/NEJMoa1201163.
44. Marwick TH, Cho I, OH B, Min JK. Finding the gatekeeper to the cardiac catheterization laboratory: coronary CT angiography or stress testing? J Am Coll Cardiol. 2015;65(25):2747–56. https://doi.org/10.1016/j.jacc.2015.04.060.

3D Printing from Cardiac CT Images

66

Karin E. Dill, Leonid Chepelev, Todd Pietila, and Frank J. Rybicki

Medical 3D printing is a culmination of several steps, which broadly involve acquisition of volumetric imaging datasets (in this case, cardiac CT studies), segmentation to extract the relevant anatomy, post-processing, and fabrication of anatomical structures using dedicated printing hardware. The resultant 3D printed models enable detailed visual inspection and direct manipulation of cardiac anatomy and pathology depicted by CT in a manner that bypasses the limitations of two-dimensionality from a computer monitor. This enables intuitive model exploration, allowing for presurgical planning and practice on the 3D printed models for a personalized, patient-specific intervention strategy. While 3D printing has a rich history within medicine, recent hardware and software advances have catalyzed an exponential growth in the interest and practical implementation of this new modality in the clinical arena. Already established in numerous technology sectors, 3D printing has reached medicine and, with cardiac CT imaging advances, resulted in successes paralleling those seen in other specialties. Presently, cardiac CT imaging-derived applications of 3D printing primarily focus on clinical use of these models for patient and physician education, procedure simulation, and device design.

Elements to ensure a technically optimal cardiac CT acquisition and image segmentation are further detailed. The crucial difference between traditional segmentation and segmentation for 3D printing is highlighted. The latter relies on a new paradigm focused on translating mathematical models visualized as images on the computer screen to physical models that can be fabricated in the real world and implemented in a clinical workflow. Accurate 3D printable segmentation and computer-aided design (CAD) will be highlighted.

This chapter is divided into three parts. The first part reviews fundamentals of 3D printing, with an introductory overview designed to provide a cardiovascular imager with the foundation to understand 3D printing from cardiac CT DICOM images. The second part of this chapter uses leading commercial software (Mimics Medical and Mimics inPrint, Materialise) to illustrate the process of conversion of a DICOM dataset to a 3D printable model. The final part briefly discusses clinical applications.

Fundamentals of 3D Printing

The essential steps in creating a 3D printed model are image acquisition, anatomy segmentation, model post-processing, and model fabrication [1, 2]. Determining the clinical setting and appropriateness of such a model is a prerequisite and guides subsequent steps. The functionality and accuracy of a 3D printed model is predicated by collaborative interactions. Imagers, referring specialists, technicians, engineers, and other parties involved in model creation need to work closely to ensure appropriate execution of each step [3]. Figure 66.1 illustrates a clinical cardiovascular 3D-printing workflow.

Data Acquisition

3D printing from medical images requires volumetric data with a signal-to-noise ratio that allows segmentation of the anatomy of interest. In cardiovascular imaging, sufficient contrast opacification of the organ in question and reducing imaging artifact is required. The majority of CT studies produced for diagnostic purposes already satisfy these criteria by utilizing improved scanning and reconstruction techniques, though insufficient contrast opacification may limit

K. E. Dill
Department of Radiology, UMass Medical Center, Worcester, MA, USA

L. Chepelev · F. J. Rybicki (✉)
Department of Radiology, University of Ottawa Faculty of Medicine, Ottawa, ON, Canada

Ottawa Hospital Research Institute, Ottawa, ON, Canada
e-mail: frybicki@toh.ca

T. Pietila
Materialise USA Biomedical Engineering, Plymouth, MI, USA

U. J. Schoepf (ed.), *CT of the Heart*, Contemporary Medical Imaging, https://doi.org/10.1007/978-1-60327-237-7_66

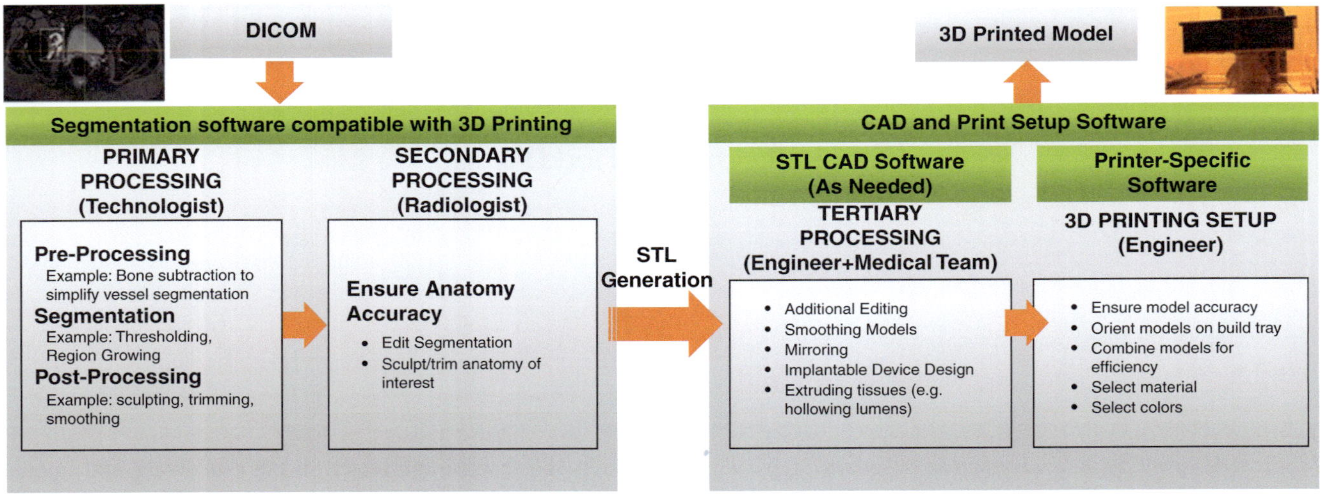

Fig. 66.1 Typical cardiac CT 3D printing workflow

segmentation accuracy. Specifically, minimized contrast doses, post-contrast saline flushes, and contrast admixture should be carefully considered in studies intended for 3D printing since enhancement of the entirety of the imaged structure with high concentration contrast media is necessary to optimize model quality. Contrast administration should be tailored to the imaged anatomy – in cases where the entirety of the heart is included in the segmentation, all cardiac chambers must be opacified, while cases focused on coronary arteries may require only limited opacification of the heart. In some situations, referring physicians may request modifications to the original model to include a broader portion of the anatomy, which necessitates complete opacification of the cardiovascular anatomy included in the field of view.

In addition to appropriate contrast administration, other factors influence model quality [4]. Spatial resolution of CT image reconstruction is a key factor in deciding the resolution of the final segmented model. Ideally, the voxels within a volumetric dataset should be isotropic with each voxel side measuring no more than 1 mm, smaller if fine vascular detail requires depiction. The disadvantage of minimizing voxel sizes is the computational and manpower cost associated with manipulating datasets containing significantly more images, some of which may not be amenable to automated segmentation. Minimizing the impact of cardiac motion, stair-step artifact, and breathing artifact will streamline model segmentation. Finally, the post-processing itself should not introduce artifact.

While the majority of relevant features of a cardiovascular 3D printed model can be obtained from coronary CT images that are now considered routine, results of CT-enabled cardiovascular anatomy segmentation may need to be fused with models obtained from multiple additional modalities, including 3D transthoracic or transoesophageal echocardiography, magnetic resonance imaging, or 3D rotational digital subtraction angiography. In such cases, the CT imaging data typically serves as an overall scaffold, allowing reconstruction of major cardiac chambers and major vessels, while echocardiography provides the data for valve segmentation and angiography (e.g., MRI or rotational angiography) provides finer detail of vascular anatomy.

Segmentation of Relevant Anatomy

Segmentation is the second step in the 3D printing workflow and involves the separation of the anatomy of interest from background anatomy. While many advances have been achieved in developing semi- and fully automated software solutions for this task, no solution has yet been able to circumvent the need for careful assessment by a human expert with deep knowledge of anatomy, disease pathophysiology, and imaging to ensure accuracy and appropriateness for a specific clinical scenario. Optimal image quality and contrast opacification improve the automated segmentation accuracy, thus allowing segmentation to focus on small adjustments to optimize quality. Where image quality is inferior, segmentation may involve bypassing all automation in favor of manual selection of the relevant anatomy on every relevant image within the CT dataset. More frequently, with higher study quality, the task of segmentation involves thresholding (i.e., selecting the upper and lower Hounsfield unit values for voxels included in the model), followed by definition of a bounding box and manual refinement of the resultant collection of voxels using various sculpting tools, as discussed using a practical example below.

Segmentation as outlined above is similar for clinical cardiac CT and by itself is not sufficient for 3D printing, since the output remains an abstract collection of cubic or cuboid voxels. The transformation to a printable model occurs where an interpolation between the vertices of the voxels is performed to define the various surfaces of a three-dimensional geometry. For example, a collection of cubic voxels may represent a sphere with a two-voxel-thick wall. Converting this collection of voxels to a printable sphere involves defining the surfaces of the outer and inner walls of this sphere and encoding this information into a file format that a 3D printer can convert directly or indirectly into a series of instructions, such as printer head movement, filament extrusion, or advancing to the next layer.

The most commonly used file format for 3D model representation is the Standard Tessellation Language (STL) file format. Although other file formats may supersede STL by enabling more powerful model definition and annotation, essentially all medical 3D printing at the time of writing uses STL files. Just as typical workstations use Digital Imaging and Communications in Medicine (DICOM) files to render patient data in the form of an image on a computer screen, 3D printers use STL files to fabricate and describe geometric shapes. An STL file allows the definition of the surface of a 3D shape by approximating it as a collection of triangles. The term tessellation refers to the process of representing an arbitrary surface as a collection of connected triangles that form a mesh overlying this surface. Typical commercial software solutions provide tools to minimize or eliminate possible printing failures. These tools are typically seamlessly integrated with the modules responsible for the conversion of voxel collections or regions of interest to a printable model represented in an STL file.

One possible source of print failure is the incorporation of geometry elements (non-manifold geometry) that can only exist as abstract geometrical constructs. Some examples of this include shapes that meet at a single point or a single line, self-intersecting surfaces, and disconnected surfaces or surfaces with holes. In each of these cases, the incorporation of these geometry elements precludes the definition of a reproducible real-world shape that occupies a specific volume. Most standard software solutions currently provide rapid and automatic built-in routines for model validation and error correction. Careful review by human experts following automated adjustments is necessary to optimize and further refine model quality [5].

Computer-Aided Design

Once the relevant cardiovascular anatomy has been segmented, converted to a three-dimensional object, and reviewed by domain experts for accuracy, further model manipulation typically takes place using computer-aided design (CAD) software. Since visualization of cardiac chambers and relevant vascular structures in cardiovascular CT imaging is achieved using intravenous contrast agents, segmentation of cardiovascular anatomy typically reflects the intraluminal contrast rather than the myocardium and vessel walls. To avoid tedious manual segmentation of vessel walls and the myocardium, CAD tools may be used to automatically construct walls surrounding intraluminal contrast. These models can then be used within the same CAD software to design patient-specific instrumentation or to adjust the size of the existent general tools and implants. Finally, manipulations of resultant models may be performed to optimize the printable model quality (wrapping or smoothing), adding or subtracting parts for better visualization of relevant pathology (trimming, coloring, extruding) and planning for model presentation by adding connectors between discrete isolated structures of interest. Operations such as Boolean additions and subtractions allow model fusion and removal of a three-dimensional, precisely defined region of space, respectively. Boolean operations are indispensable in the creation and manipulation of additional model features superimposed upon the existing models.

CAD tools capable of editing STL files to create any conceivable geometry are available for a widely ranging audience and at a wide range of price points. These include industry-standard tools such as those provided by Materialise, as well as a large array of software packages that have been approved by the FDA. Recent FDA commentary has clarified that approved software is required for the major steps of medical modeling intended for clinical use [5, 6]. While free, open-source software is available and can be applied to medical images, it should not be used for clinical care, including the generation of 3D models designed for patient education and patient consent for intervention. Commonly used techniques and approaches to patient-specific 3D printed model design and creation will be practically demonstrated in the second part of this chapter using as an example the design of a ventricular septal defect (VSD) patch.

Model Fabrication

Model fabrication is the final step of the process. The manufacturing process starts with the selection of the appropriate materials and printing technologies to address model requirements. For example, a model used for education alone can be produced with lower-cost materials. Models used for clinical practice on the other hand would have to reasonably match the flexibility and compliance of a human heart tissue, adhere to a quality assurance review, and be sufficiently accurate to avoid providing misleading information to the clinician or surgeon ultimately responsible for the intervention. The choice of a printing technology and material would therefore be guided by the application of the resultant models, in the context of additional factors, such as material and printer cost and the capabilities of the materials, ranging from available colors, sterilization capability, biocompatibility, and physical properties of the available materials.

Step-by-Step 3D Model Creation and Printing Guide

While theoretical discussion of 3D printing using cardiovascular CT images is important, equally important is exposure to the specific steps involved in the preparation of a clinically usable 3D printed model. Since the majority of time and efforts in a 3D printing laboratory will be spent on segmentation and additional image post-processing, we illustrate the key concepts, typical tasks, and the overall software workflow with a case previously reported and used for education at the 2015 annual meeting of the Radiological Society of North America [7]. In this case, the patient in question has a double outlet right ventricle (DORV) with a ventricular septal defect. Illustrated is a patient-specific customized patch using segmentation and computer-aided design software. The basic steps involved in this work will use common terminology [8] and will be illustrated using Materialise software, including inPrint and 3-matic (Materialise Inc., Leuven, Belgium).

Segmentation software converts 2D cross-sectional imaging data to high-quality 3D printable models, operating on voxel data to generate 3D models represented as meshes, typically in STL format, for printing or further manipulation. The resultant models can also be optimized for further processing in computational analysis, such as in flow dynamics for the assessment of computed fractional flow reserve. In the final step, setting up model printing will be briefly discussed in general terms, as 3D printer-specific software that enables printing STL files from any 3D CAD application is ubiquitous and relatively simple, allowing printing tray placement, job cost estimation, and job control.

Model Preparation

Model preparation should ideally be initiated at the point of study protocolling and guided by the specific setting, for example, an educational application or preoperative cardiovascular intervention. Once a DICOM file containing appropriately acquired CT image data is obtained, it is exported in a decompressed form from an institutional PACS system for further manipulation. DICOM decompression is an essential step as specific image compression approaches may not be universally compatible with segmentation software. The import of uncompressed DICOM data is a simple task in most segmentation software solutions and is accessible through a simple wizard in the inPrint software (Figs. 66.2 and 66.3).

Additional image data reformatting may be performed at the loading step, including image realignment and voxel size minimization using the existing voxel data to improve the resolution of the models resulting from subsequent segmentation steps.

Segmentation of the Heart and Great Vessels

Segmentation is the essential next step to separate the relevant cardiac anatomy. Segmentation in the context of cardiovascular CT imaging is quite similar to segmentation in the established visualization applications and involves the application of manual or semi-automated approaches to separate the anatomical structure of interest from the background anatomy.

In the most basic terms, the two key discriminators of relevant voxels are typically voxel attenuation values and the presence of the selected voxels within a specific region of space (a specific adjustable bounding box), typically in association with similar voxels (Fig. 66.4).

The segmentation of cardiac anatomy in the case of our patient begins with the identification of the intravenous contrast bolus and involves setting minimum (310 HU) and maximum (3071 HU) Hounsfield unit thresholds to select only the voxels that correspond to intravenous contrast (Fig. 66.5). This task is termed thresholding and results in the selection of voxels that include those corresponding to the intravenous contrast. Unfortunately, skeletal structures within the bounding box are also selected.

Isolating the desired ROI from the background requires the selection of a single voxel in a given ROI by simply clicking on the desired anatomy to keep, in this case intraluminal contrast, in any of the CT reconstructions (Fig. 66.6).

Since the skeletal structures are irrelevant in this setting, we shall remove them using the region growing semi-automated algorithm. This algorithm uses a seed point placed by the segmenter within the structure of interest to identify all the voxels that are contiguous with the voxel at the seed point. A typical variation of algorithm includes the ability to consider only the 6 possible voxel neighbors connected face-to-face or to include all 26 immediate neighbors of a given voxel.

The resultant intermediate model is termed a region of interest (ROI) or a mask, to reflect the fact that at this point, the model is not a 3D printable object but rather a three-dimensional collection of voxels that satisfies the three criteria set above. Further manipulations are required to ensure

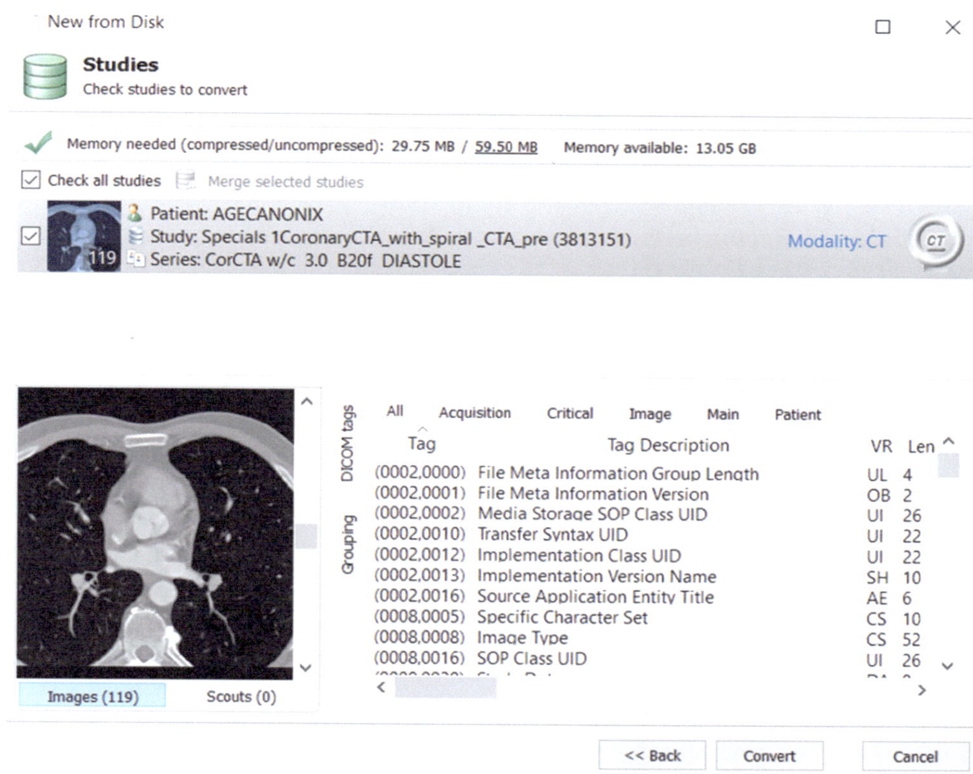

Fig. 66.2 Import wizard in the inPrint software. The specific series within a study can be selected. The associated images and DICOM annotations can be previewed to identify the optimal series

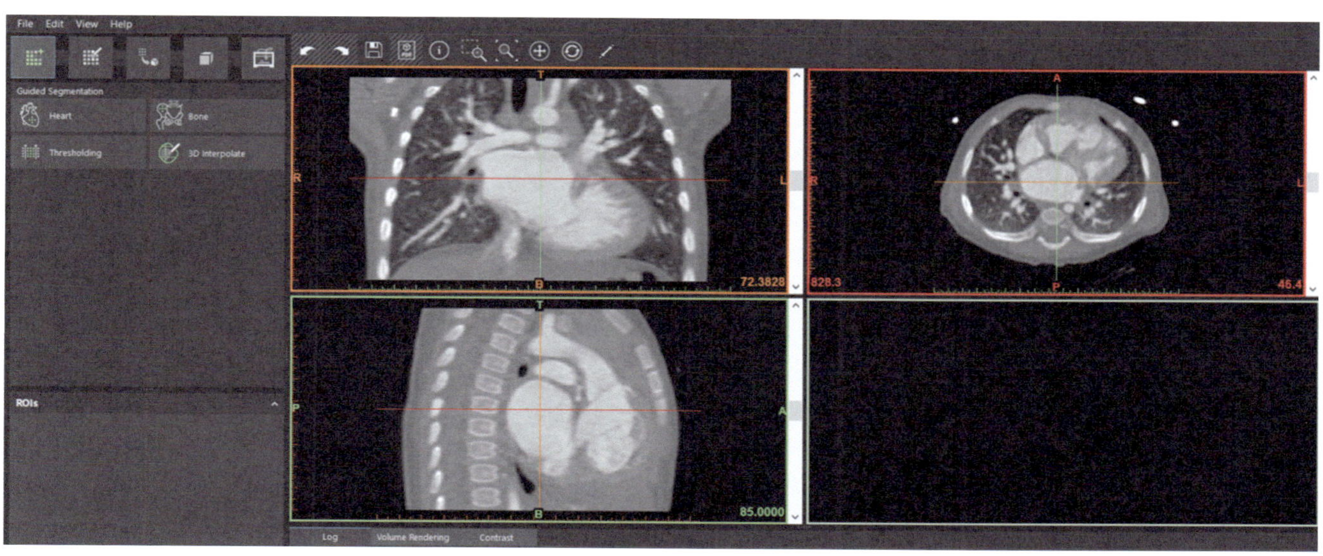

Fig. 66.3 Loaded DICOM data within the inPrint software. The segmentation and 3D object manipulation selections are in the top left corner. The available operations are shown in the left middle panel (here, guided segmentation operations including segmentation of the heart and bone). The ROIs and parts are listed on the left. The three DICOM image data reconstructions are shown on the right, with a window to render 3D models on the bottom right, currently empty

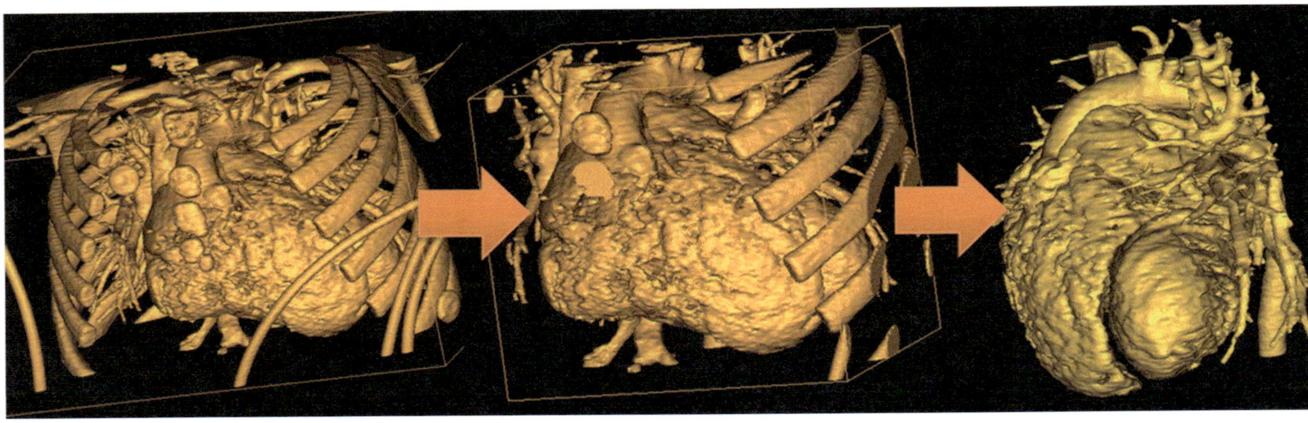

Fig. 66.4 Incremental refinement of cardiac segmentation. Thresholding in a wide bounding box (left) results in a wide region of interest, which can be narrowed by decreasing bounding box size (middle). Inclusion of adjacency criteria with a seed point in cardiac contrast segments isolated cardiovascular anatomy (right)

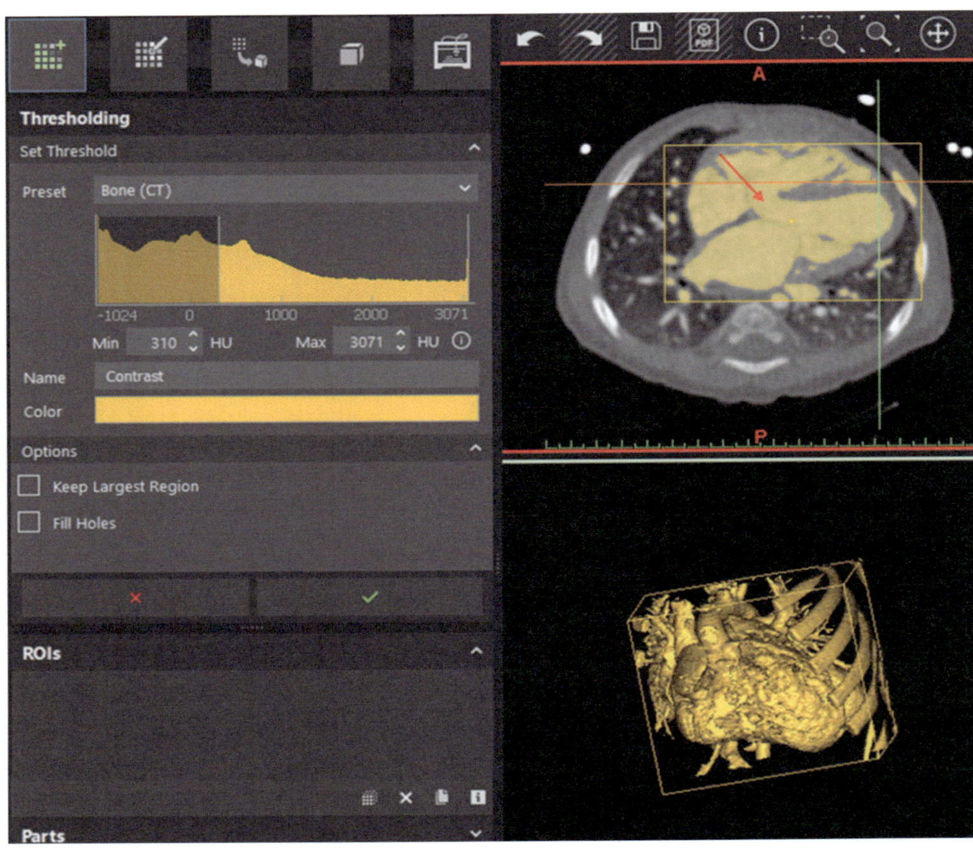

Fig. 66.5 Thresholding settings and resultant ROI. The bounding box may be adjusted by clicking and dragging the outline of the bounding box on the three reconstructions (orange box in the top right). Note the ventricular septal defect on the axial CT image (arrow)

3D printability. The quality of this ROI directly reflects the quality of the image acquisition and the adequacy of contrast administration. Optimization of image acquisition to reduce beam hardening, blooming, and motion artifact, optimize contrast dose, and minimize isotropic voxel size is therefore crucial in ensuring a relatively accurate and rapid segmentation.

In the setting of a study that has not been tailored for 3D printing, further segmentation is required, akin to direct planimetry in 3D visualization. Alternatively, unnecessary anatomic parts may be trimmed manually after the 3D object has been generated if a clear separation plane can be identified.

For this example, high-quality acquisition has resulted in facile segmentation of the relevant cardiovascular anatomy,

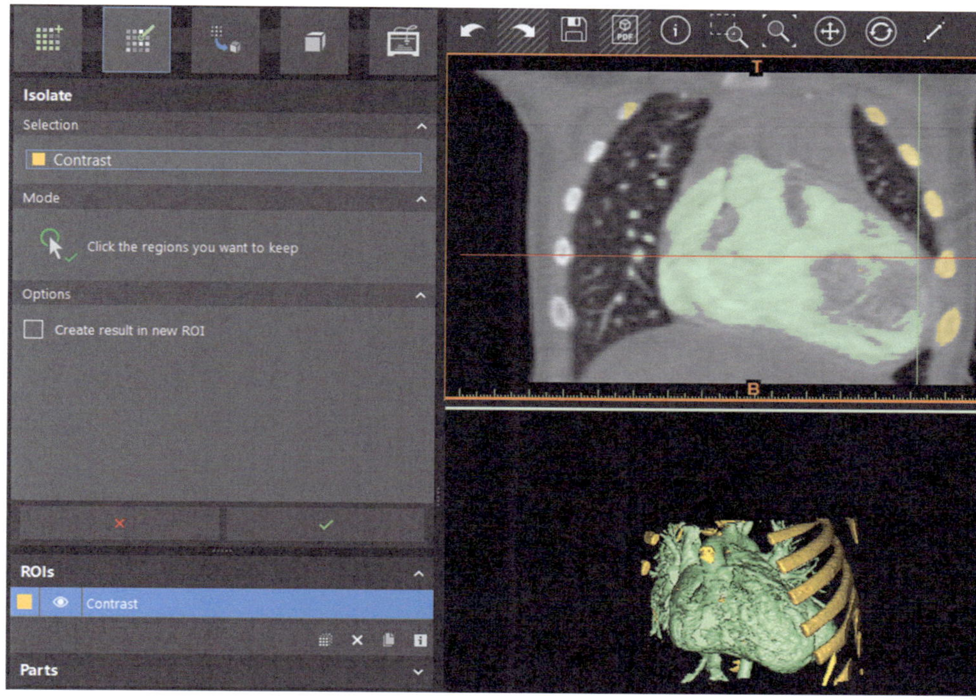

Fig. 66.6 Application of the region growing algorithm by using the Isolate tool from the Edit ROI menu (second on the left)

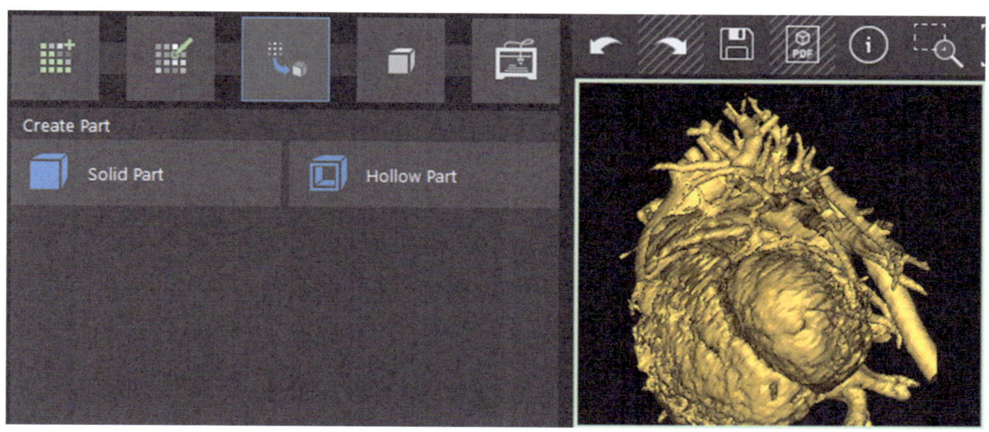

Fig. 66.7 Create Part menu (third from left in the top row), offering options of creating a solid or a hollow part. In this case, a solid part needs to be created using the contrast-containing ROI

as defined by intraluminal contrast, and the creation of an accurate ROI depicting intraluminal contrast. To enable further manipulations, an actionable 3D model needs to be generated using the ROI outline (Fig. 66.7).

The 3D models defined as a surface composed of triangles, describing a 3D object (as opposed to voxel collections in ROI), are termed "parts." When part creation is complete, the ROI list collapses, and the part list is presented in the bottom left. Furthermore, the annotations on the three CT images change to denote the outline of the created 3D object (Fig. 66.8).

Since this object contains multiple surface imperfections and abrupt edges, it may be smoothed using the Smooth tool in the Edit Part menu (Fig. 66.9). Special care needs to be taken to not smooth the printed part to an extent that erases the relevant anatomy or closes relevant cavities within the model, by selecting appropriate detail and filling parameters. While a smoothed model may be easy to manufacture, handle, and appreciate, physicians have to be cognizant of the dangers of excessive smoothing in model interpretation.

The resultant object depicts a smoothed version of intraluminal contrast and can be printed directly with or without an additional wrapping operation (typically used to further smooth model outlines, ensure printability, and fill any thin holes). In this scenario, the intraluminal contrast is used merely to identify the extent and configuration of the ventricular septal defect in order to design a patient-specific patch (Fig. 66.10).

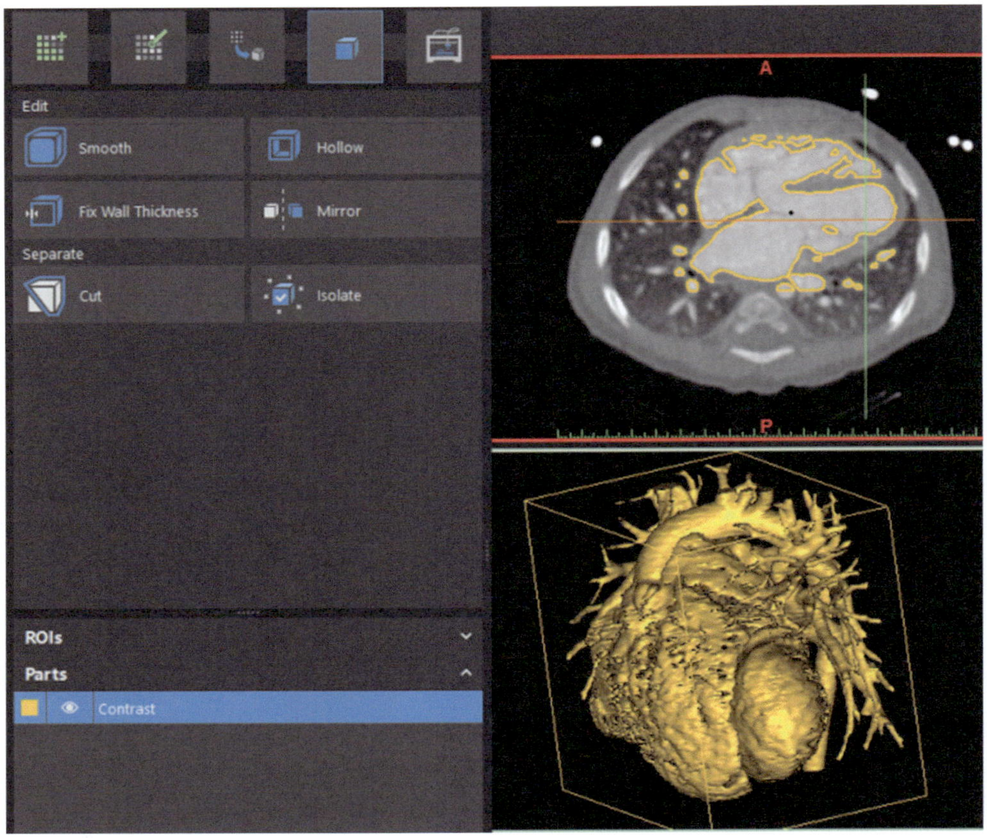

Fig. 66.8 Result of the solid part creation operation. Note the automatic switch to the edit part menu with the appearance of appropriate options on the top left panel. The parts list contains the *Contrast* part. The depiction of this part has changed on the axial image to describe its outer surface, which has been smoothed during the part creation process. The degree of smoothing can typically be controlled

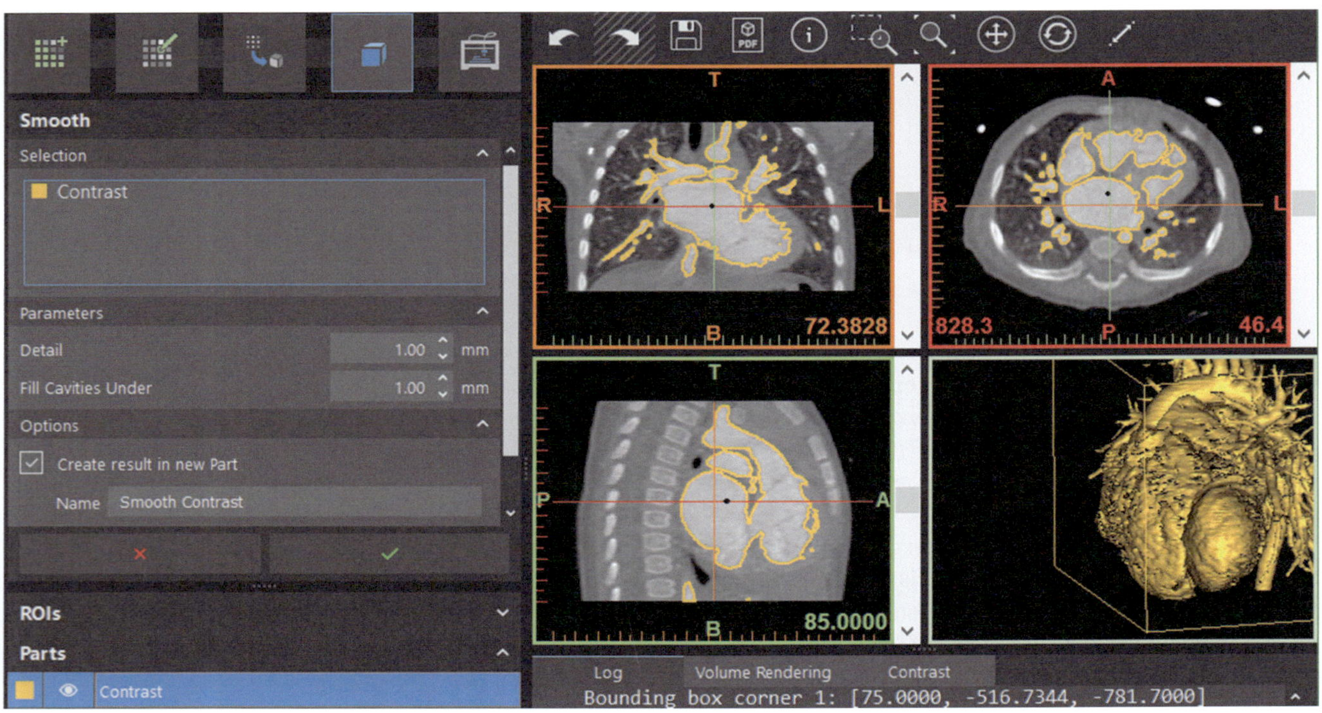

Fig. 66.9 Smoothing operation, with minimal detail of 1 mm and option to fill cavities under 1 mm. Using the Contrast object in the selection menu (top left), a new part called "Smooth Contrast" will be created

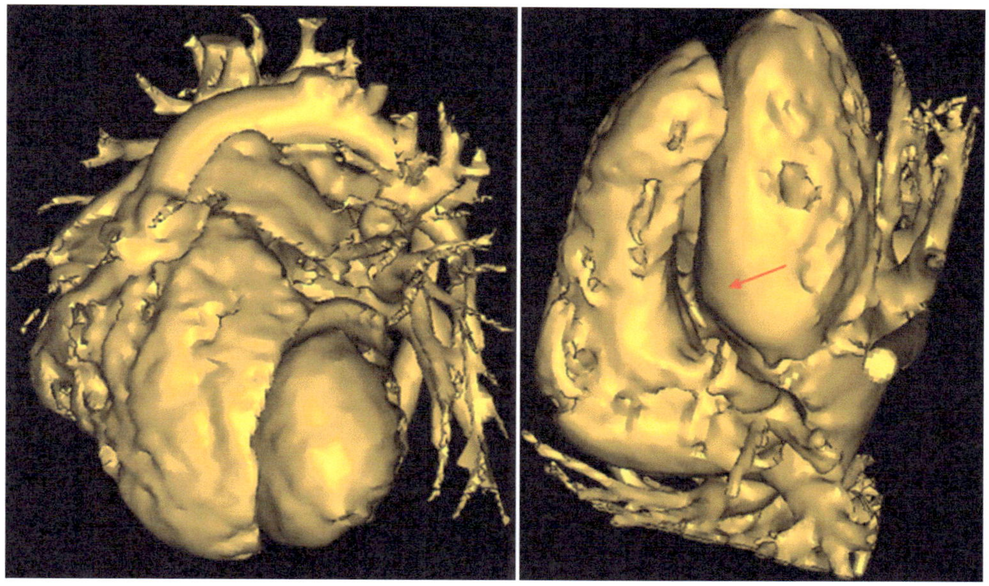

Fig. 66.10 Smoothed contrast model, from the cardiac apex (left) and from the inferior view (right) demonstrating the contrast bridge between the left and right ventricles, corresponding to the ventricular septal defect (arrow)

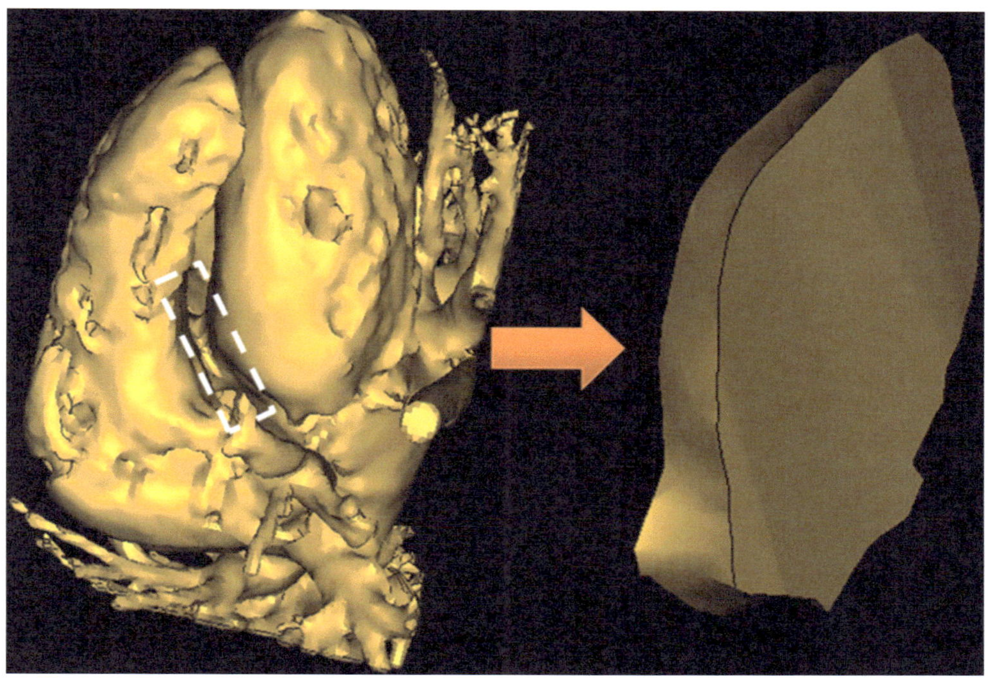

Fig. 66.11 Using the Cut tool from the Edit Part menu on the intraluminal contrast model will result in isolation of the contrast that occupies the septal defect

A reasonable approximation of a septal defect patch could be obtained by cutting out the contrast portion that corresponds to the septal defect communication using the Cut tool from the Edit Part menu (Fig. 66.11). The resultant model would provide an excellent representation of the septal defect extent and will allow implant sizing.

More extensive manipulations can be enabled by emulating the myocardial and vascular walls, however. The same model used for defect patch design may be used for further implant and tool sizing or simulating minimally invasive procedures. For these applications, the simulation of cardiac and vessel walls is indispensable. This is enabled by the application of the Hollow tool from the Edit Part menu. This tool creates a hollow model that completely envelops an existing model (intraluminal contrast), providing a reasonable simulation of the walls surrounding the intraluminal contrast (Fig. 66.12).

Since the defect patch needs to be created from the inside, an approach needs to be made to visualize the defect. This

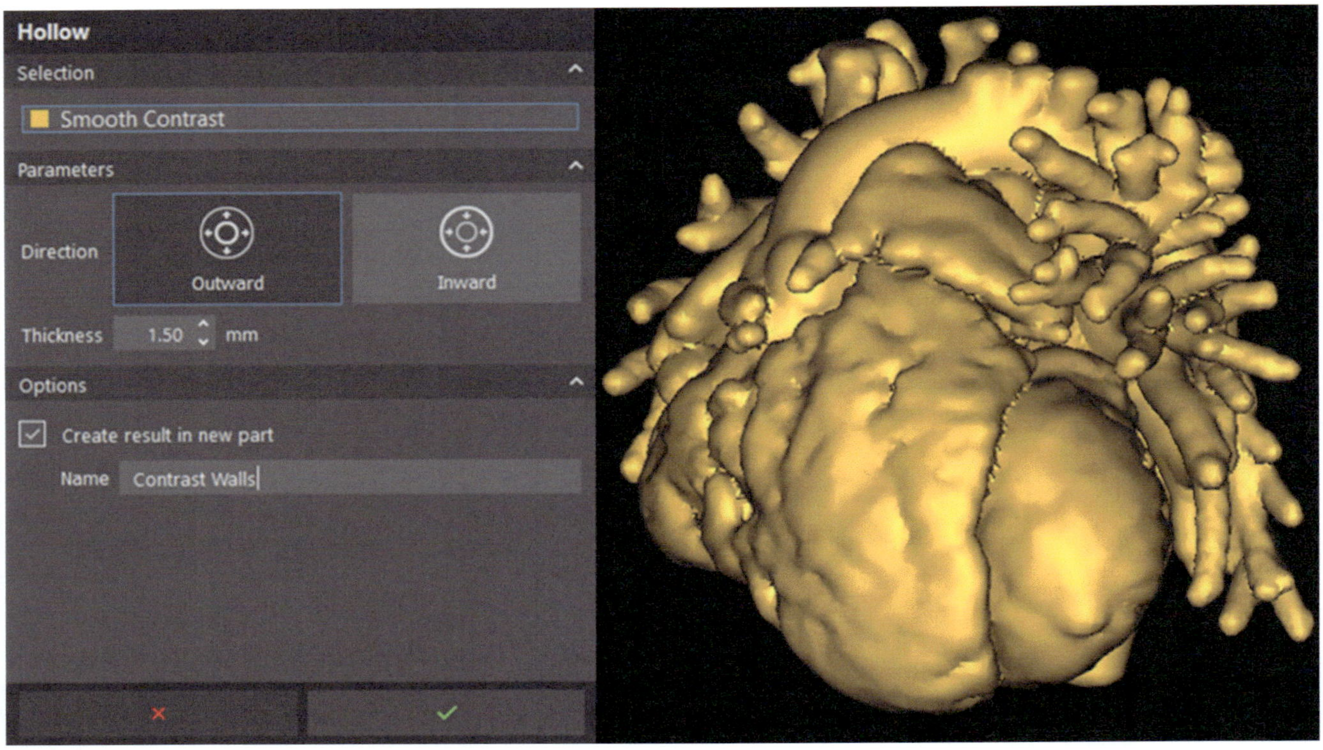

Fig. 66.12 Hollow operation menu allowing the creation of a new part called "Contrast Walls" (left) by growing existing model outward, by 1.5 mm in this case. Note that the new part is larger and smoother than the previously shown smoothed contrast model

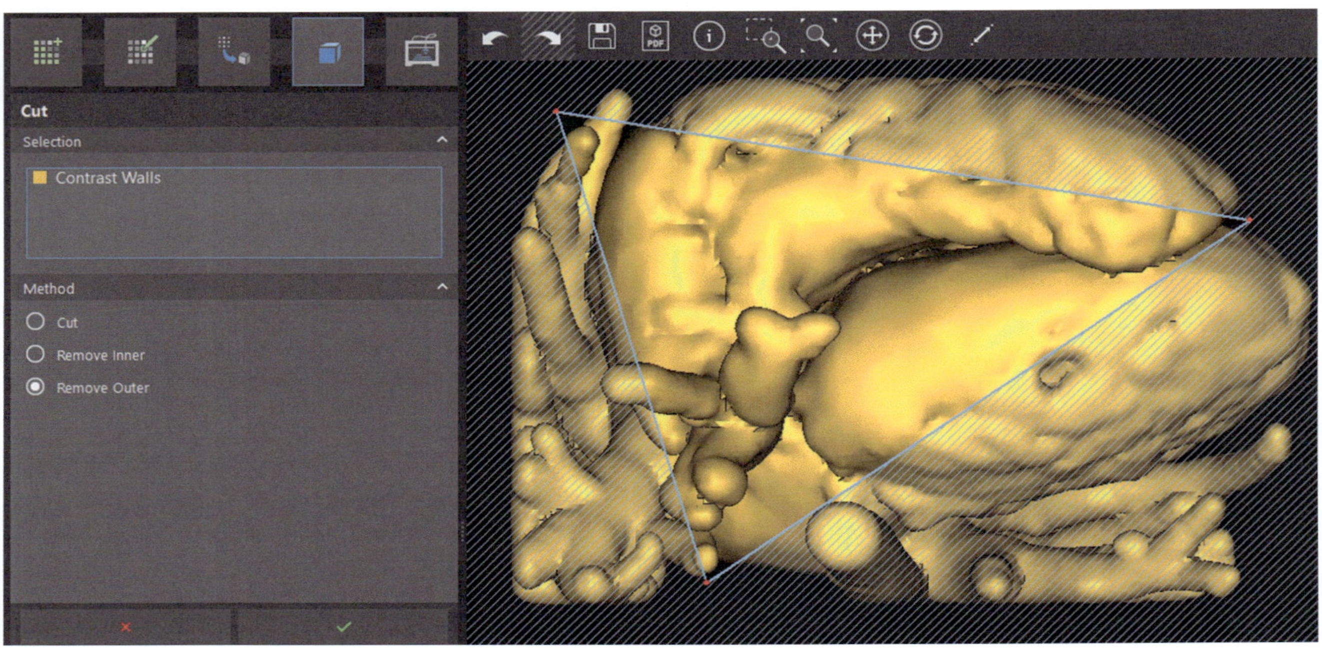

Fig. 66.13 Intermediate step in the application of the Cut tool from the Edit Part menu. Note that in the selected model, "Contrast Walls" has been visualized using the bottom view (accessible from the View menu), and points were selected at the apex and just outside both atria. By removing the outer area (dashed), the septal defect is exposed

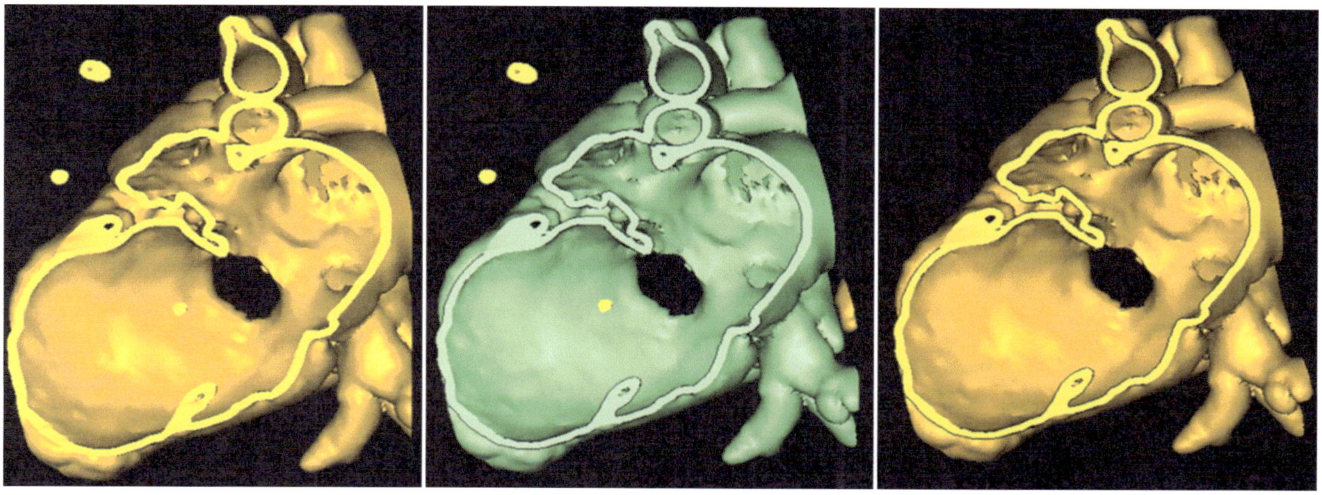

Fig. 66.14 The septal defect is visualized following the cut operation (left). Multiple floating loose model fragments are removed by using the Isolate tool from the Edit Part menu and selecting the model to keep (green, middle), resulting in a clean simulation of the ventricular septal defect

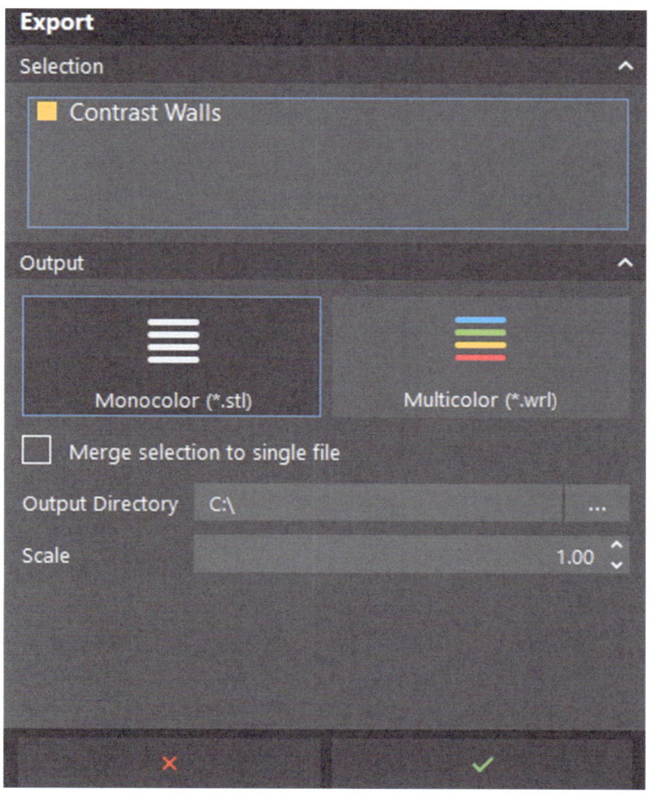

Fig. 66.15 Export model dialogue. The Contrast Walls model is being exported to the C:\ directory, in a 1:1 scale and as an STL file, presently the most widespread file format for 3D printing

can be achieved by resecting the outer cardiac walls using the Cut tool (Fig. 66.13). The resultant model lacks ventricular sidewalls, thus exposing the septal defect (Fig. 66.14).

Segmentation concludes with the creation of a model depicting the relevant anatomy. Further manipulations to create a medical device de novo are the domain of computer-aided design (CAD), which is carried out in the 3-matic software. To bring the model to the 3-matic software, the model can be exported using the Export tool from the Prepare Print menu as an STL file (Fig. 66.15).

This model can be imported into the 3-matic software using the built-in import wizard (Fig. 66.16). As the 3-matic software is loaded, you will note that the 3-matic window contains the menus and tabs on the top, the Scene Tree with all 3D objects and their components in a hierarchical distribution on the top right, the operations tab to set all relevant operation parameters at the bottom right, and process logger on the bottom.

The next step is to design the patch. This will be done in three steps. First, a curve will be drawn to create the outer outline of the septal defect patch ensuring adequate defect coverage is provided (Fig. 66.17). This curve may be partially drawn and the Close Curve algorithm may be used to approximate the ends of the curve (Fig. 66.18).

The next step in patch creation is the conversion of the newly created curve to a surface. For this, the curve is first

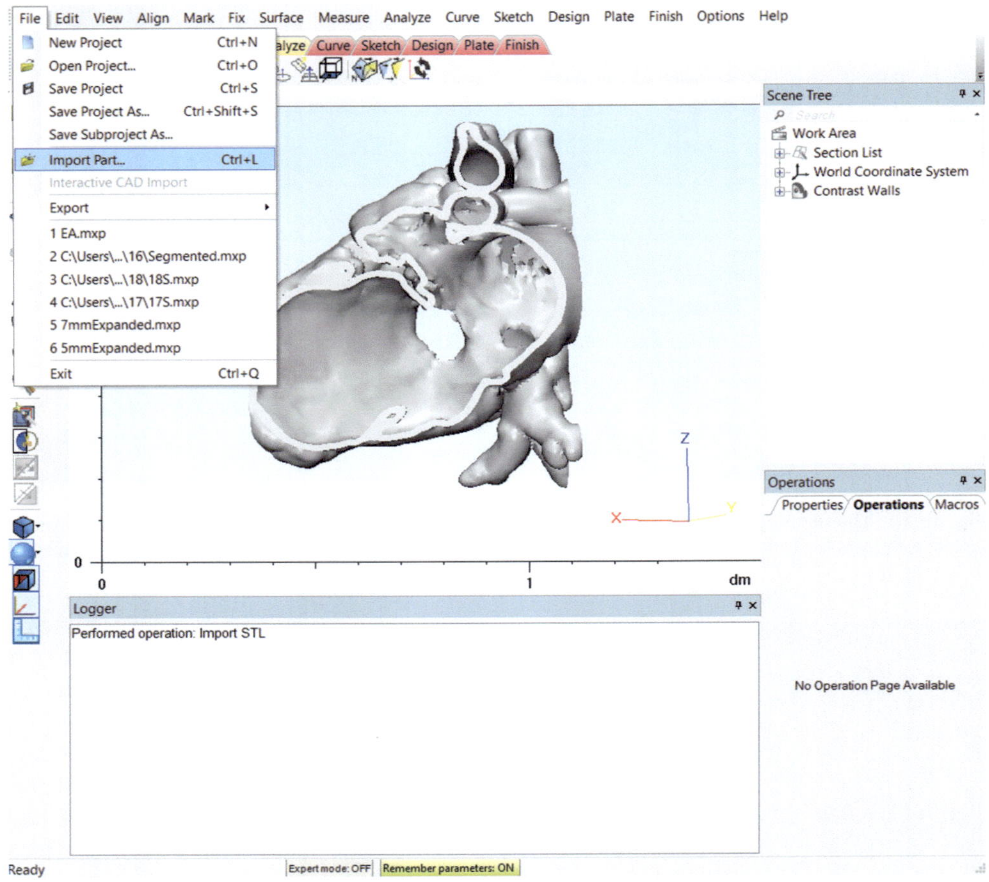

Fig. 66.16 Importing the heart simulation using the Import Part wizard

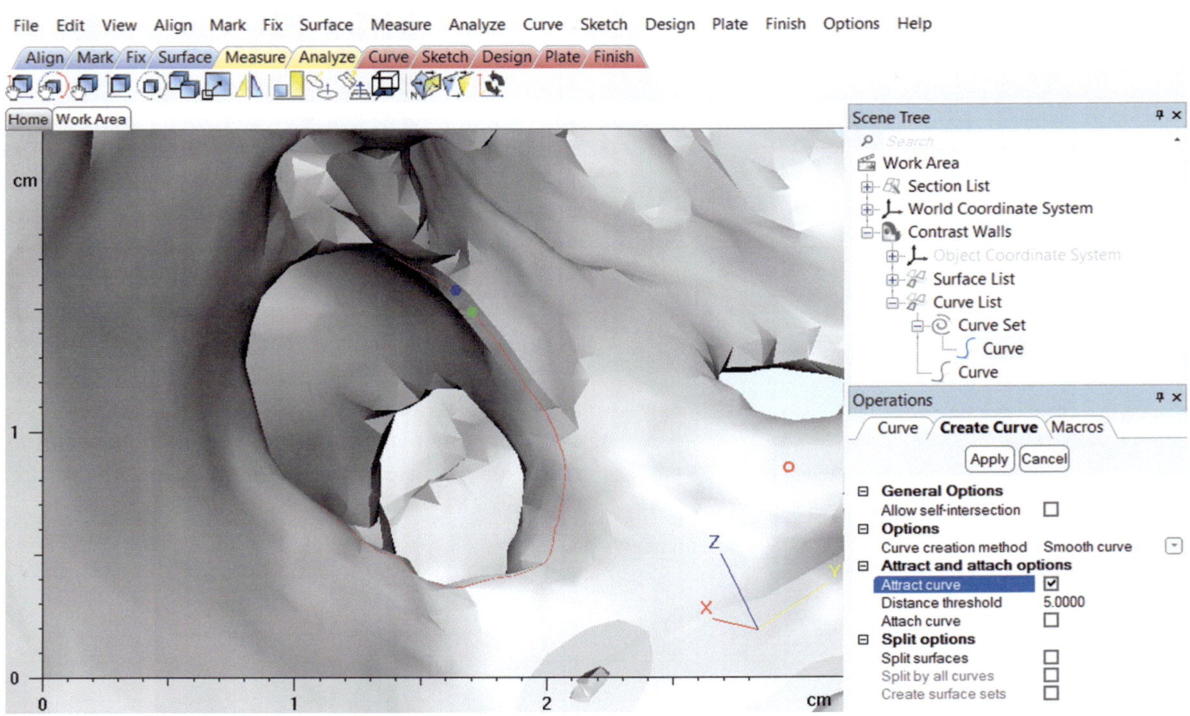

Fig. 66.17 Creating the curve describing the defect patch from the Curve > Create Curve operation. A smooth curve is created, with attract curve option selected to attract the curve to the surface on which it is drawn, avoiding free-hanging edges and creating good approximation with the simulated wall. Note that the curve is incomplete here and can be closed automatically

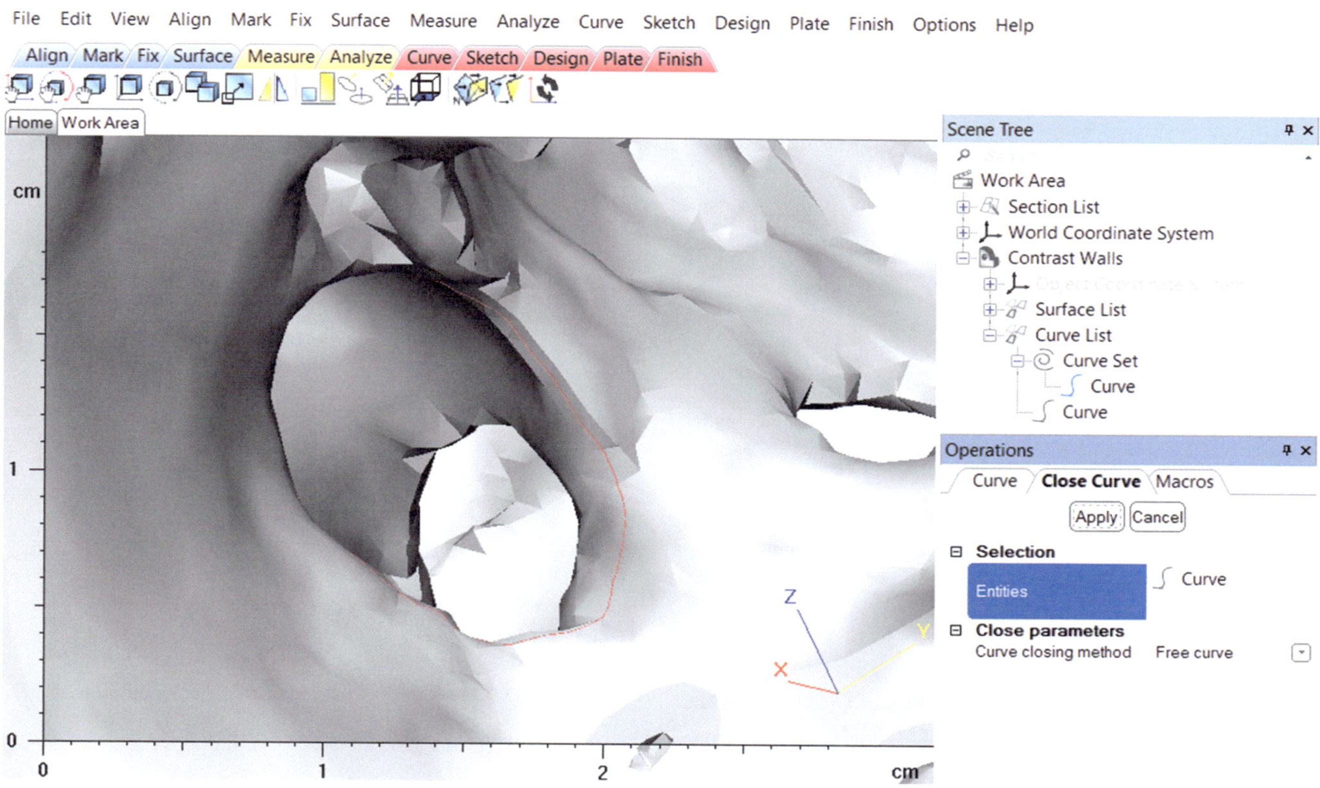

Fig. 66.18 Closing the curve using the Curve > Close Curve operation. Please note the selection of the curve named "Curve" from the Scene Tree object hierarchy at the top right. Once the Apply button is pressed, the curve closing operation is complete (left)

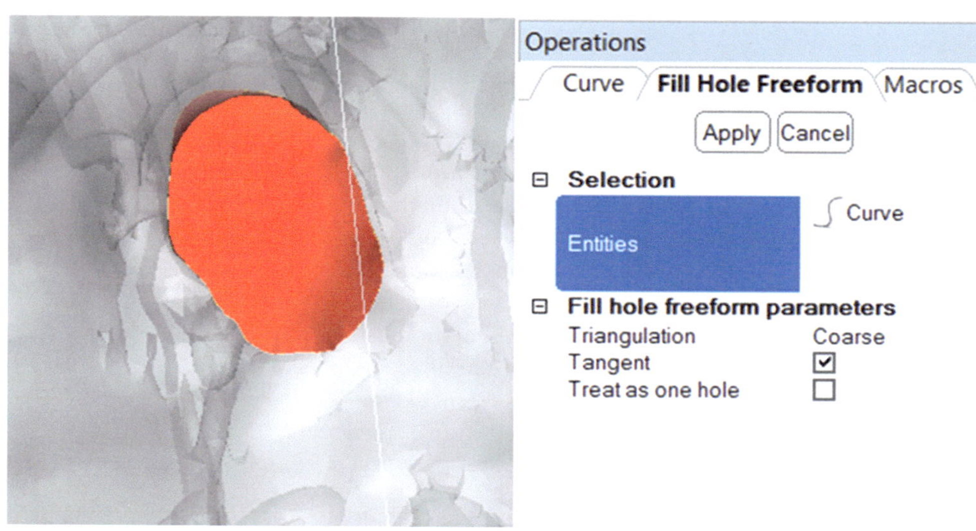

Fig. 66.19 Setup and result of the Fill Hole Freeform operation. Note that the curve from the new part which was renamed to "Patch" in the Scene Tree (not shown) is selected in the Entities list

separated into a new part (right click the curve in the Scene Tree, Separate > Move to Part > Create New), followed by the application of the Fill Hole Freeform operation to create a surface that describes a single plane of the patch (Fig. 66.19).

The final step in patch creation is the addition of thickness to the resultant abstract plane. This is achieved using the Uniform Offset operation, which creates a predefined offset based on a provided surface to generate a three-dimensional object that can be printed (Fig. 66.20).

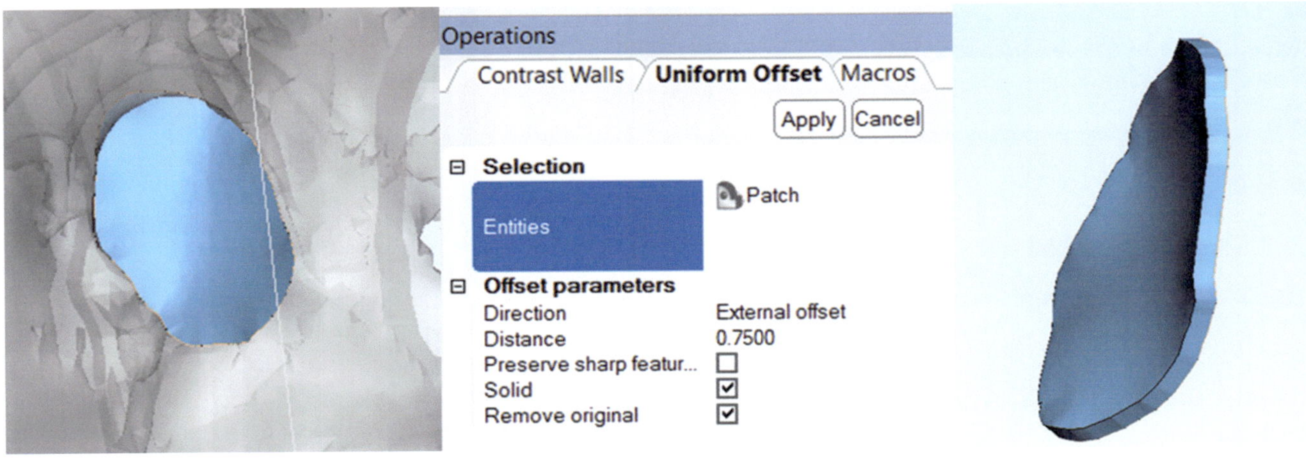

Fig. 66.20 Generating a three-dimensional patch using the Design > Offset > Uniform Offset operation, with a distance of 0.75 mm to create a 1.5 mm – thick patch as the offset applies in two directions outward from the plane used to create the patch. Please note the new Patch object is selected in the Entities list

The septal defect patch is now ready to be printed. It may be exported from 3-matic using the File > Export operation, in a process identical to that demonstrated for the cardiac wall simulation model. The resultant STL may then be printed after loading it in any of a wide range of printer-specific software solutions, arranging the object on the printer tray, selecting print materials, and finally submitting the job to the printer.

Summary

The collective term 3D visualization refers to all image post-processing commonly used in current medical imaging, including cardiac CT. These include multi-planar reformatted images, maximum intensity projections, and volume rendering. All of these currently used manipulations use DICOM images to render volumetric data on a 2D computer screen. 3D printing represents a paradigm shift in representing imaging data, using novel formats to define the surface of a 3D shape by approximating it as a collection of triangles. These files can be modified and printed using a variety of technologies for medical diagnosis, preprocedure planning, device creation, and education.

References

1. Mitsouras D, Liacouras P, Imanzadeh A, Giannopoulos A, Cai T, Kumamaru KK, George E, Wake N, Caterson EJ, Pomahac B, Ho V, Grant GT, Rybicki FJ. Medical 3D printing for the radiologist. Radiographics. 2015;35(7):1965–88.
2. Matsumoto JS, Morris JM, Foley TA, et al. Three-dimensional physical modeling: applications and experience at Mayo Clinic. Radiographics. 2015;35(7):1989–2006.
3. Giannopoulos A, Mitsouras D, Yoo S-J, Liu P, Chatzizisis Y, Rybicki FJ. Applications of 3D printing in cardiovascular diseases. Nat Rev Cardiol. 2017;13(12):701–18.
4. George E, Liacouras P, Rybicki FJ, Mitsouras D. Measuring and establishing the accuracy & reproducibility of 3D-printed medical models. Radiographics. 2017;37(5):1424–50.
5. Christensen A, Rybicki FJ. Maintaining safety and efficacy for 3D printing in medicine. 3D Print Med. 2017;3:1. https://doi.org/10.1186/s41205-016-0009-5.
6. Di Prima M, Coburn J, Hwang D, Kelly J, Khairuzzaman A, Ricles L. Additively manufactured medical products–the FDA perspective. 3D Print Med. 2016;2(1):1–6.
7. Giannopoulos AA*, Chepelev L*, Sheikh A, Wang A, Dang W, Akyuz E, Hong C, Wake N, Pietila P, Dydynski PB, Mitsouras D, Rybicki FJ. (*Both authors contributed equally.) 3D printed ventricular septal defect patch: a primer for the 2015 Radiological Society of North America (RSNA) hands-on course in 3D printing. 3D Print Med. 2015;1:3. https://doi.org/10.1186/s41205-015-0002-4.
8. Chepelev L, Giannopoulos A, Tang A, Mitsouras D, Rybicki FJ. Medical 3D printing: methods to standardize terminology and report trends. 3D Print Med. 2017;3:4. https://doi.org/10.1186/s41205-017-0012-5.

Future Technological Advances in Cardiac CT

67

Thomas G. Flohr, Thomas Allmendinger, Herbert Bruder, Chris Schwemmer, Steffen Kappler, and Bernhard Schmidt

Challenges in Cardiac CT

Imaging of the heart with computed tomography (CT) is technically demanding. It is fair to say that the technological advancement of CT during the past 15 years has been mainly driven by the ongoing refinement of cardiac CT.

Adequate visualization of the moving anatomy of the heart and the coronary arteries requires a short "exposure time" per image – technically speaking the CT scanner has to provide high temporal resolution. The coronary arteries have diameters of only few millimeters, and plaque and stenosis need to be reliably and at best quantitatively evaluated. Therefore, excellent spatial resolution is needed in addition.

Synchronization of data acquisition with the patient's electrocardiogram (ECG) is a prerequisite to image the heart in a phase-consistent way – e. g., in the diastolic rest phase or the end-systolic phase at higher heart rates. Finally, the radiation exposure to the patient has to be as low as reasonably achievable. A summary of challenges in cardiac CT and recent developments may also be found in [1].

Temporal Resolution

In ECG-controlled CT examinations of the heart, dedicated image reconstruction approaches using only the very minimum of scan data are used to minimize the "exposure time" per image and to optimize temporal resolution. The minimum amount of scan data for image reconstruction in the entire scan field of view (SFOV) is a partial scan, comprising an angular range of 180° of fan-beam data (half a gantry rotation) plus the total fan angle of the detector (~50° for a typical SFOV of 50 cm) plus a transition angle for smooth data weighting, in total 240–260° of fan-beam data. This corresponds to a temporal resolution of about 2/3 of the CT scanner's gantry rotation time. In the center of the CT gantry, where the heart is typically located, 180° of scan data (a half-scan segment) plus the transition angle are sufficient for image reconstruction. In refined image reconstruction approaches for cardiac CT, only the very minimum of scan data needed to reconstruct that pixel is used for every image pixel. Therefore, close to the isocenter, the temporal resolution is about half the gantry rotation time of the respective CT system [2].

During the past 15 years, technical developments have aimed at improving the temporal resolution of CT scanners to make cardiac CT more robust in clinical practice and applicable to a wider range of patients.

The most straightforward approach to reduce the "exposure time" per image is faster gantry rotation. Gantry rotation times dropped from 0.5 s with the first generation of four-slice CT systems (resulting in a temporal resolution of 250 ms close to the isocenter) to 0.25 s with the latest generation of multi-detector row CT (MDCT) systems (corresponding to 125 ms temporal resolution). With state-of-the-art MDCT, robust visualization of the coronary arteries can be achieved in clinical routine at moderate and reasonably regular heart rates but is still challenging in patients with high and irregular heart rates. Larger variability of the heart rate is known to negatively affect the image quality of coronary CT angiography (CTA) [3]. Therefore, the administration of beta-blockers is frequently recommended to lower and stabilize the patients' heart rates.

Even faster gantry rotation to further improve temporal resolution is technically demanding because of significant gravitational forces which are challenging in particular for the x-ray tube design. Rotation times of less than 0.2 s, needed to achieve a temporal resolution better than 100 ms, appear to be beyond today's mechanical limits. As an additional challenge, the more the gantry rotation time is decreased, the more the x-ray tube power has to be increased

T. G. Flohr · T. Allmendinger · H. Bruder · C. Schwemmer · S. Kappler
B. Schmidt (✉)
Department of Computed Tomography, Siemens Healthcare GmbH, Forchheim, Germany
e-mail: bernhard.schmidt@siemens.com

U. J. Schoepf (ed.), *CT of the Heart*, Contemporary Medical Imaging, https://doi.org/10.1007/978-1-60327-237-7_67

to maintain adequate contrast-to-noise ratio (CNR) in images with shorter exposure time. As a consequence, extrapolating from the power reserves of today's MDCT systems about 150 kW tube power would be needed for adequate CNR in the desired sub-mm images at rotation times of less than 0.2 s. Again, the required power densities in a small focal spot on the anode plate appear to be beyond today's technical limits.

An alternative approach to improve temporal resolution of mechanical CT systems is the dual-source principle. Dual-source CT (DSCT) systems are equipped with two x-ray tubes and two corresponding detectors offset by about 90° [4] (Fig. 67.1). Since 2005, three generations of DSCT systems have been commercially introduced. Enabled by simultaneous data acquisition of both measurement systems, DSCT scanners provide a temporal resolution close to a quarter of the gantry rotation time [5] – 83 ms for the first-generation DSCT, 75 ms for the second-generation DSCT, and 66 ms for the third-generation DSCT. Meanwhile, clinical studies have demonstrated the potential of DSCT for clinically robust coronary CTA examinations with little or no dependence of the diagnostic performance on the patient's heart rate [6–9]. In a meta-analysis of 33 studies published between 2006 and 2011 which compared the diagnostic accuracy of first- and second-generation DSCT coronary angiography for the detection of >50% stenosis with invasive catheter angiography as a reference standard [10], the authors found a pooled sensitivity of 98% and a pooled specificity of 88% on a per-patient basis, with no significant differences in sensitivity or specificity in the subgroup of studies with and without heart rate control. The median radiation dose, however, was smaller in the studies with heart rate control (1.6 mSv) than in the studies without heart rate control (8 mSv).

CT scanner designs with more than two x-ray tubes – detector pairs [11], combined with refined approaches to improve temporal resolution even further by decoupling of the source rotation from the detector rotation – appear to be mechanically too complex for a practical realization. An experimental CT design, referred to as "multisource interior tomography" [12], has not left the concept stage so far. Multisource interior tomography intends to enable ultrafast imaging by only irradiating a small region of interest, such as the heart, with narrow x-ray beams defined by many source – detector pairs surrounding the patient (Fig. 67.2). Images covering this region of interest can then be reconstructed using the interior tomography approach. Again, the practical realization of the proposed setup seems to be extremely challenging, and the clinical field of application of such systems would be very limited.

Yet another attempt to improve temporal resolution is the design of nonmechanical CT systems without mechanically rotating gantry ring. Already in 1984, an electron beam CT (EBCT) was introduced as a noninvasive imaging modality for the diagnosis of coronary artery disease [13, 14]. It consisted of a stationary x-ray tube and a stationary detector

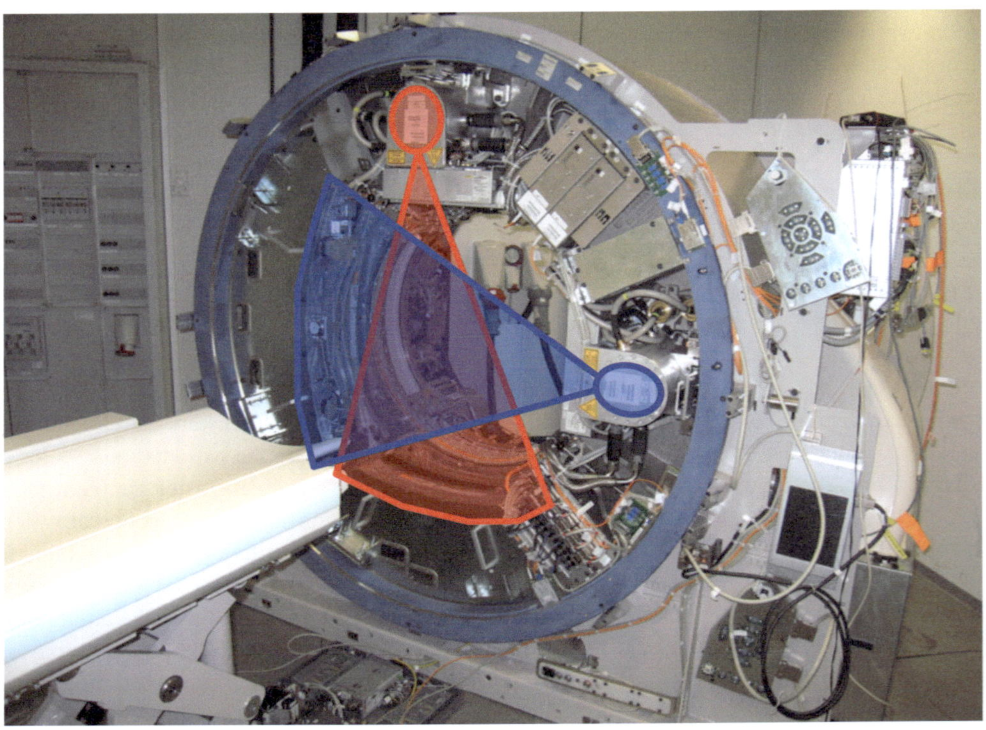

Fig. 67.1 DSCT with two independent measurement systems at an angle of 90° (first generation) or 95° (second and third generation)

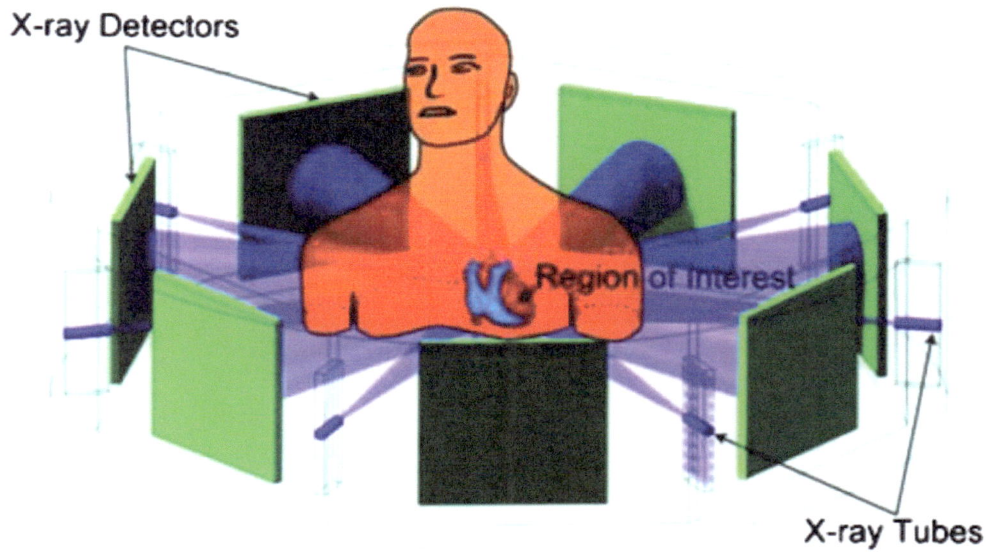

Fig. 67.2 Proposed setup for a multisource interior tomography system

ring. An electron beam was emitted from a powerful electron gun and magnetically deflected to hit a semicircular anode surrounding the patient, thus generating an x-ray source that virtually rotated around the patient. Given the absence of mechanically moving parts, a sweep is needed as little as 50 ms. However, because of inherent disadvantages such as excessive scattered radiation as a consequence of missing anti-scatter grids or lack of sufficient tube power and therefore suboptimal CNR in the images, EBCT systems never made their way into clinical routine, and the EBCT principle has been abandoned by now.

Unfortunately, no other convincing concept for a nonmechanical CT design has been proposed so far, and a clinical introduction of such systems in the near future appears unlikely.

From the very beginning of cardiac CT, approaches to reduce the exposure time per image by mechanical advancements such as faster gantry rotation times, and design changes such as dual-source CT, went hand in hand with attempts to improve temporal resolution by algorithmic approaches. Multi-segment reconstruction, the combination of small scan data segments from multiple consecutive heartbeats to build up the half-scan data segment needed for image reconstruction while reducing the data acquisition window per heart cycle, was introduced in the first years of cardiac CT but is meanwhile only rarely used in clinical practice. It can only improve image quality at higher heart rates when the heart rate is regular, and it results in increased radiation dose (see, e.g., [15], who found an average radiation dose of 4.8 mSv for a 1-beat scan and 7.8 mSv for a 2-beat scan in the CORE320 trial).

Algorithmic approaches to achieve improved "virtual" temporal resolution in the CT images beyond the mechanical limits of the respective CT system have been proposed recently [16–21]. In essence two different strategies are pursued. One attempt is based on using less scan data than theoretically needed for image reconstruction (i.e., less than a half-scan interval at the scanner's isocenter), thereby shortening the exposure time per image. Pertinent examples are TRI-PICCS [16] or TRIM [17]. The image artifacts caused by the insufficient scan data range need to be corrected for, e.g., by using a prior image based on a partial scan in an iterative image reconstruction approach and image regularization terms that enforce image smoothness (as in TRI-PICCS) or positivity (as in TRIM). The quantification of the actual temporal resolution of these algorithms is difficult. Latest results suggest small improvements [22, 23].

Another attempt is based on estimating the motion of the coronary arteries and compensating for it during image reconstruction. Pertinent algorithms incorporate a motion model into iterative reconstruction algorithms or approximate analytic reconstruction algorithms (see, e.g., [19, 24]). The unknown motion of the coronary arteries during the CT scan has to be estimated by suitable algorithms – this turns out to be a challenging problem. Most recent attempts aim at obtaining a motion model of the coronary arteries by minimizing a cost function such as the image entropy [20]. Figure 67.3 shows an example of the performance of a recently developed motion correction approach [25].

While algorithmic approaches to improve temporal resolution in cardiac CT beyond the mechanical system limits appear conceptually appealing, the proposed algorithms are still missing validation in large clinical studies. One approach ("Snapshot Freeze," GE Healthcare, Waukesha, USA) has meanwhile been evaluated in several smaller studies. In a study with 120 patients [26], improved image quality and coronary assessability were found in patients with higher heart rate and heart rate variability. In another study [27]

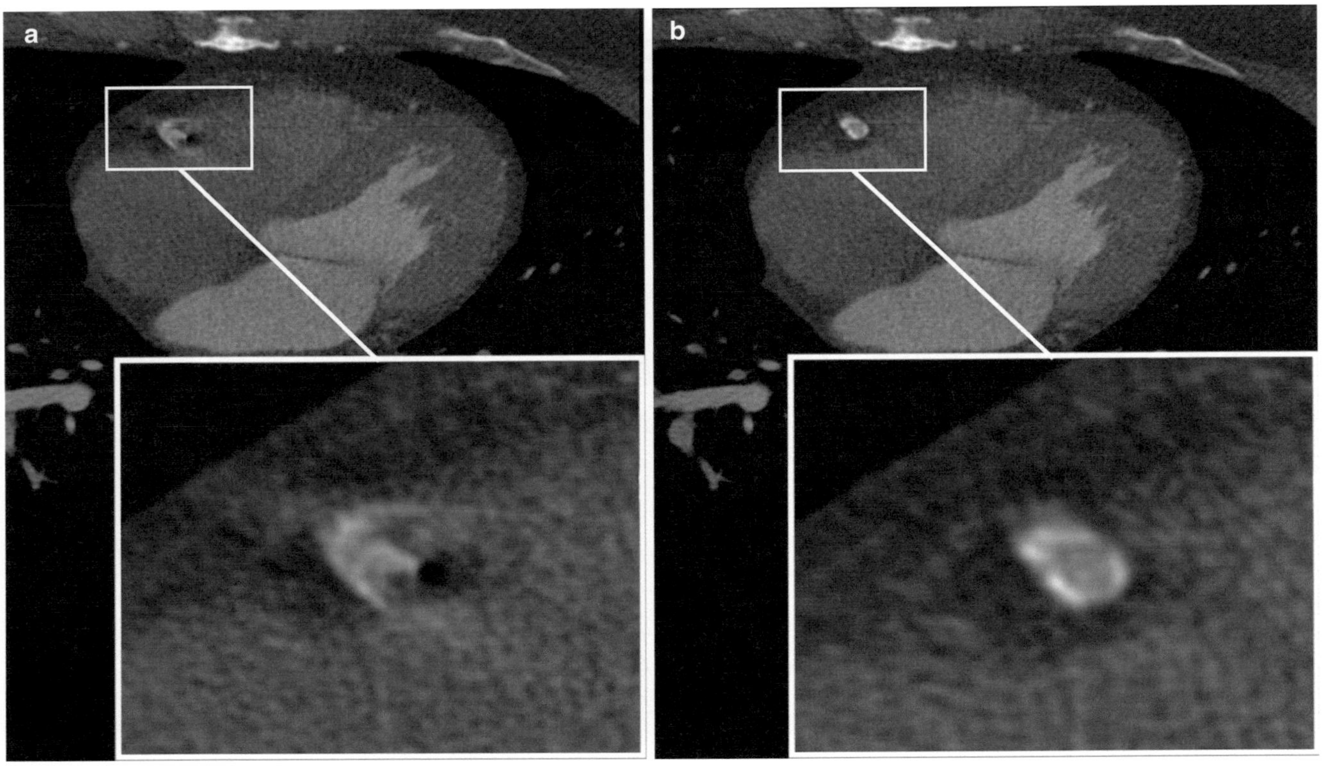

Fig. 67.3 Example for a coronary CTA image of a patient with a stent in the right coronary artery (RCA), heart rate 72 bpm, systolic reconstruction at 30% of the RR-interval, and temporal resolution 143 ms, without (**a**) and with motion correction based on a minimization of the image entropy in partial angle reconstructions (**b**). (See Ref. [25])

motion correction reduced the presence of motion artifacts and improved image quality, but did not influence the diagnostic utility – it did not reduce the percentage of nondiagnostic images. In a randomized trial with 64 patients receiving beta-blockers and 51 patients without heart rate control, motion correction improved image quality and reduced motion artifacts, but could not compensate for the absence of beta-blockers [28]. Therefore, larger studies are still needed to assess the clinical performance of current motion correction algorithms, and it is currently not possible to decide on the clinical robustness of motion correction and on its potential to reliably improve temporal resolution in cardiac CT.

Spatial Resolution

The spatial resolution of a CT system is limited by the size of the individual detector pixels and by the size of the focal spot. With typically 700–900 detector pixels per detector row covering a SFOV of usually 500 mm in diameter, the in-plane sampling distance in a modern CT system is about 0.28–0.36 mm at isocenter. By using techniques such as quarter detector offset or flying focal spot to double the in-plane sampling density, a maximum spatial resolution of about 14–18 lp/cm can be achieved. In practice, to avoid excessive image noise and streak artifacts at high-contrast structures, in-plane spatial resolution is reduced by smoothing convolution kernels. Typically, about 0.4–0.5 mm in-plane resolution, corresponding to 10–12 lp/cm, is not exceeded in coronary CTA.

Spatial resolution is not only important in the image plane but also perpendicular to it – then it is called through-plane spatial resolution. Through-plane spatial resolution is mainly determined by the slice width of the reconstructed images and by the image increment. State-of-the-art ECG-controlled scanning of the heart with 64 or more slices with 0.5 mm, 0.6 mm, or 0.625 mm collimated slice width and overlapping image reconstruction may result in 0.35–0.5 mm through-plane resolution and hence in nearly isotropic sub-millimeter resolution to visualize the coronary arteries. Figure 67.4 illustrates the progress in spatial and temporal resolution from 4-slice CT to 64-slice CT and newer CT systems.

Yet, scanning of patients with severe coronary calcifications remains a challenge because of Ca blooming: partial volume artifacts as a consequence of still insufficient spatial resolution make calcifications appear bigger as they are. This prevents reliable assessment of the coronary lumen and leads to overestimation of coronary artery stenosis. In a multicenter coronary CTA trial [29], the presence of coronary calcifica-

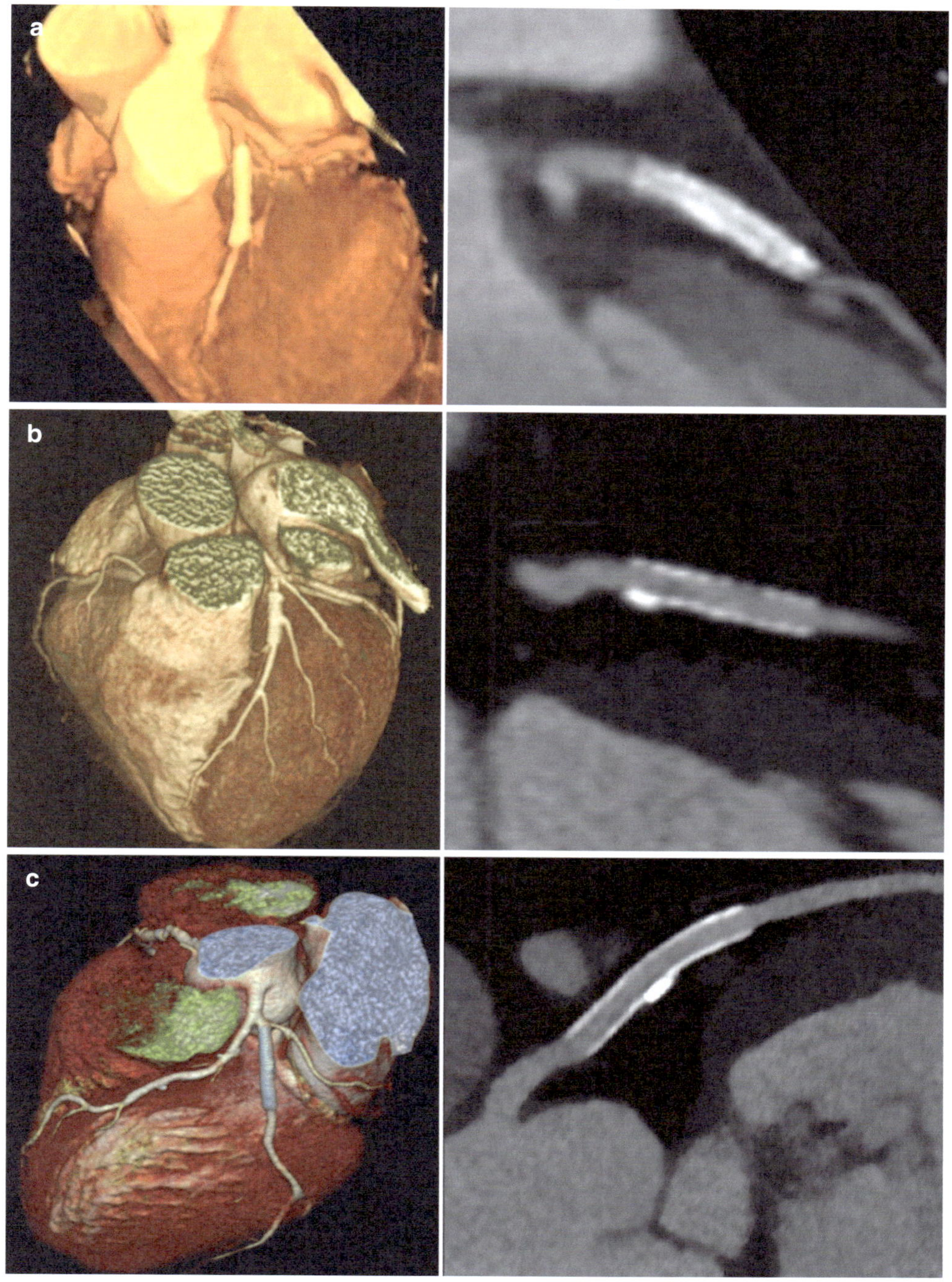

Fig. 67.4 Typical coronary CTA examinations with (**a**) a 4-slice CT scanner (temporal resolution 250 ms, spatial resolution about $0.6 \times 0.6 \times 1\ mm^3$), (**b**) a 64-slice CT scanner (temporal resolution 165 ms, spatial resolution about $0.5 \times 0.5 \times 0.4\ mm^3$), and (**c**) a second-generation dual-source CT (temporal resolution 75 ms, spatial resolution about $0.4 \times 0.4 \times 0.4\ mm^3$). The improvement of detail visualization thanks to better temporal and spatial resolution is obvious

tions with an Agatston score >1000 was the most relevant independent predictor of uninterpretable coronary segments, followed by a heart rate >80 bpm and a body mass index >40 kg/m^2. Furthermore, the limited ability of today's CT scanners to reliably and unambiguously characterize plaque composition (e.g., to distinguish lipid-rich and fibrous plaques) is mainly a result of insufficient spatial resolution. Assessments of stent patency and in-stent restenosis are related problems. Previous studies have demonstrated that image quality strongly depends on the material of the stents and on the CT equipment. Maintz et al. [30, 31] found an average lumen visibility of 50–59% for the majority of commonly used 2.5–4 mm coronary stents in a phantom experiment carried out on 64-slice CT and first-generation DSCT, with extreme values of 3.3% for a tantalum stent and 90% for a magnesium stent. In a meta-analysis of 9 studies performed with 64-slice CT [32], the authors concluded that still a relatively large proportion of coronary stents remains uninterpretable. Accordingly, only in selected patients, 64-slice CT may serve as a potential alternative noninvasive method to rule out in-stent restenosis.

Recent technical progress has resulted in improved spatial resolution in cardiac imaging to potentially overcome some of the challenges of scanning patients with coronary calcifications, plaque, and stents. The use of dedicated high-definition (HD) scan modes, aimed at improving both the angular and the in-plane sampling density, for the evaluation of 25 coronary stents resulted in significantly lower in-stent luminal attenuation. The mean measured in-stent luminal diameter was significantly larger [33]. Improved in-stent lumen assessment could be demonstrated with third-generation DSCT [34], mainly as a result of smaller detector pixels, smaller focal spot sizes, and refined iterative reconstruction approaches. Two previously evaluated stents [30, 31] presented a significantly improved in-stent lumen visibility of up to 76% and 83%, respectively, compared to visible diameters of 52% and 56.7% when using older CT equipment (Fig. 67.5).

However, significant further improvements of spatial resolution with today's CT scanner technology are unlikely. The detector pixels of today's medical MDCT systems cannot be made much smaller to further increase spatial resolution. State-of-the-art CT detectors are based on scintillating ceramic materials that convert the x-rays into visible light. Optically reflecting material has to be inserted between the individual detector pixels to prevent optical cross talk from one pixel to the next to avoid a degradation of spatial resolution. X-ray quanta that hit these separation zones between the detector pixels do not contribute to signal generation in the detector. The relative area of these "dead zones" would increase significantly for further reduced dimensions of the detector pixels, thereby reducing the radiation dose efficiency of the detector to unacceptably low values (Fig. 67.6a).

There is, however, light on the horizon. Photon-counting detectors are a promising technology for future CT systems [35, 36]. They do not require optically in-transparent layers between the individual detector pixels, which – as a consequence – can be made much smaller than the detector pixels of today's scintillation detectors (Fig. 67.6b). Small detector sizes are also needed to mitigate physical effects such as pulse pileup; see section "New CT Concepts". Therefore, CT systems with photon-counting detectors hold promise of potentially providing improved spatial resolution – at least theoretically up to a level of 0.2–0.25 mm comparable with catheter angiography. Increased spatial resolution, however, goes hand in hand with increased image noise. Consequently, to maintain adequate CNR in the images, significantly increased radiation dose is needed. This may be justified for detail examination of plaques or evaluation of in-stent patency but problematic for routine cardiac scanning. From a technical perspective, the required high power reserves to maintain adequate CNR in high-resolution images are a challenge for the x-ray tube design.

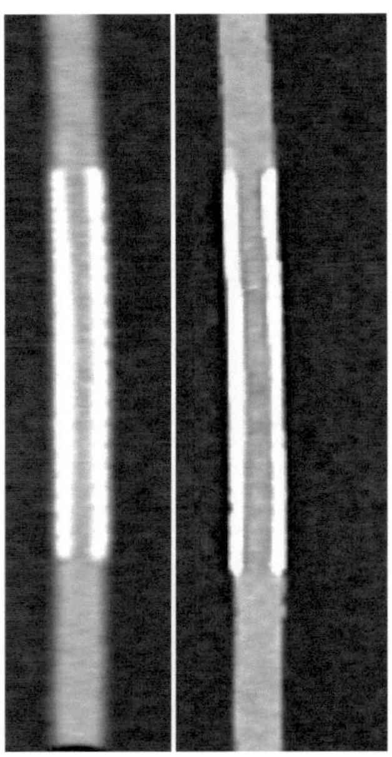

Fig. 67.5 3 mm stent in a contrast-filled tube, scanned on a 64-slice CT system (left) and on a third-generation DSCT system (right) in an ECG-triggered routine scan mode, applying the highest available spatial resolution in that scan mode. (Courtesy of T. Gassenmaier, University of Würzburg, Germany)

Radiation Dose

As a consequence of the ongoing discussion of radiation exposure by CT both in the public and in the scientific literature, the advancement of techniques to reduce radiation dose in cardiac CT examinations has been a key topic for CT manufacturers during the last years.

Radiation exposure of coronary CTA is significantly influenced by the choice of the scan technique. Prospectively ECG-triggered axial scanning has been proven to result in significantly less radiation dose to the patient than retrospectively ECG-gated spiral scanning. The pooled effective dose in a meta-analysis of 20 coronary CTA studies was 3.5 mSv with prospective triggering and 12.3 mSv with retrospective gating [37]. A further reduction in radiation exposure to values below 1 mSv was demonstrated with ECG-triggered DSCT high-pitch spiral scanning [38–41]. However, this technique is limited to patients with low to moderate regular heart rates. Another very efficient technique to lower radiation exposure is the use of low-kV protocols, i.e., scan protocols relying on 70–100 kV x-ray tube voltage instead of the "standard" 120 kV setting. Because of the increased iodine contrast at lower kV, the CNR in contrast-enhanced images

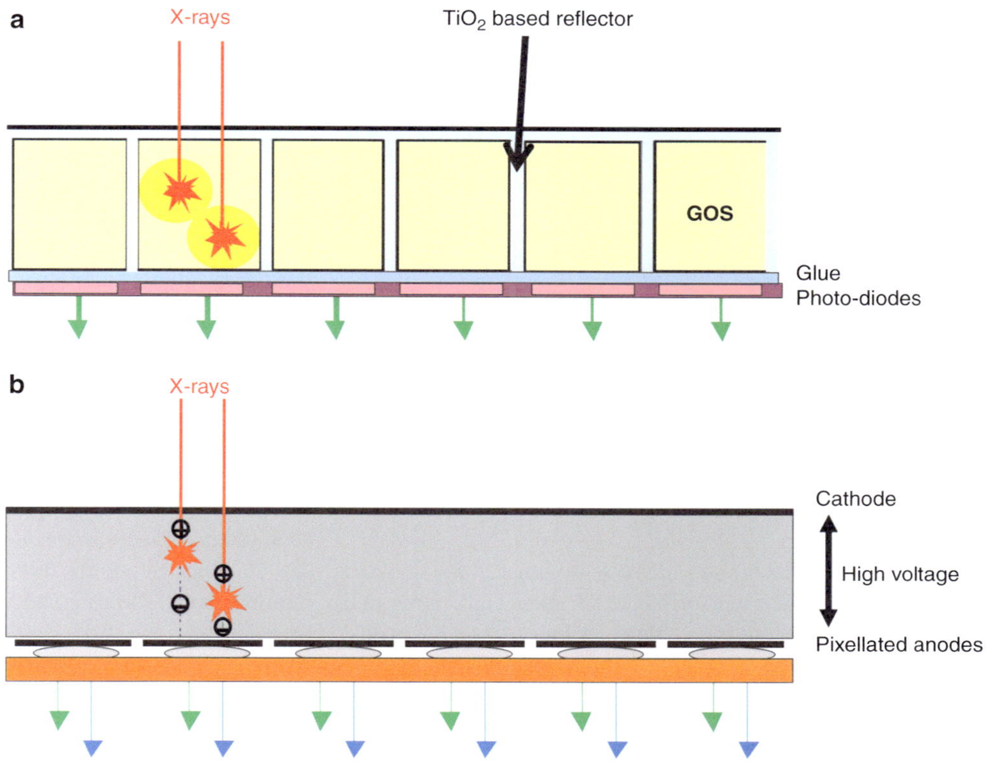

Fig. 67.6 Schematic drawing of a conventional solid-state scintillation detector (**a**) used in all commercially available medical CT systems. The x-rays are absorbed and converted into visible light which is then detected by photodiodes attached to the backside of the detector pixels. The detector pixels cannot be made much smaller than today because optically in-transparent separation layers (based on TiO_2) between them are needed to prevent optical cross talk. In novel photon-counting detectors, (**b**) the individual detector pixels are defined by a strong electric field between cathode and pixelated anodes. The absorbed x-ray quanta directly produce electron-hole pairs which induce fast current pulses. No optical separation layers between the detector pixels are necessary. Therefore, the detector pixels can be made smaller to improve spatial resolution

increases at low kV if the radiation dose is kept constant [42]. Vice versa, lower radiation dose is sufficient to maintain adequate CNR. Recent progress in x-ray tube design has led to the introduction of CT systems capable of providing high power reserves at low x-ray tube voltages of 70–100 kV. These systems have the potential to enable coronary CTA at low kV even in obese patients without compromising CNR and thus reduce radiation dose by 49–68% [43].

To further reduce radiation dose in non-contrast-enhanced CT scans of the heart, e.g., for the detection and quantification of coronary calcifications ("Ca-scoring"), spectral shaping has been proposed [44, 45]. Tin pre-filtration of the x-ray beam at 100 kV (Sn100 kV) removes unnecessary low-energy quanta and results in a mean x-ray energy similar to the 120 kV spectrum that is typically used for Ca-scoring. Although the Agatston scores were systematically lower with Sn 100 kV than with 120 kV in a study with 70 patients [45], the comparison of Agatston score categories and percentile-based cardiac risk categories showed excellent agreement. Effective radiation dose was significantly lower at Sn 100 kV than at 120 kV (0.19 mSv vs 0.82 mSv). Currently, new approaches are being investigated to enable Ca-scoring at other kV settings than 120 kV to reduce radiation dose while maintaining the Agatston score. They rely on dedicated beam-hardening corrections to correct the CT number of calcifications to their values at 120 kV.

As an add-on to the dose reduction approaches described so far, iterative image reconstruction has found its way into routine cardiac CT scanning. In an iterative reconstruction, a correction loop is introduced into the image reconstruction process [46]. While the technical realization is highly vendor-specific, all approaches aim at including the statistical properties of the acquired measurement data into the image reconstruction process in a more optimal way than traditional filtered back projection. As a result, they maintain or even improve high-contrast resolution and reduce image noise in low-contrast areas, which is the prerequisite for a potential radiation dose reduction. In particular, when combined with other dose-efficient scan techniques, such as ECG-triggered sequential scanning, ECG-triggered high-pitch scanning, and low-kV data acquisition, iterative reconstruction may enable coronary CTA at very low radiation dose levels [39, 47–49]. Figure 67.7 shows a representative clinical example for a coronary CTA acquired at very low radiation dose by combining several dose reduction technologies.

Currently, alternative image reconstruction approaches relying on machine learning and dictionary-based image representation are being evaluated [50, 51]. In a nutshell, these approaches decompose a low-dose image into small overlapping image segments and attempt to represent each of these segments by a weighted combination of image primitives

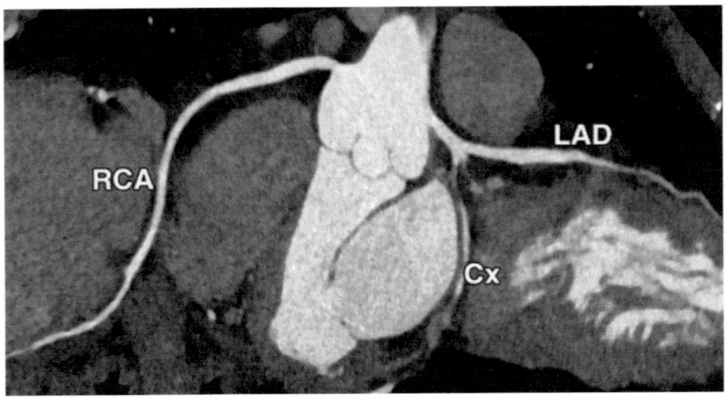

Fig. 67.7 Example of a coronary CTA examination in a patient with a heart rate of 64 bpm, acquired at very low radiation dose of 0.21 mSv by combining several dose reduction technologies: low-kV imaging at 70 kV, ECG-triggered high-pitch spiral scanning and iterative reconstruction. (Courtesy of Mannheim University, Germany)

from a high-dose dictionary, thereby de-noising the original low-dose image. The performance of such algorithms and their potential to allow for reduced radiation dose in cardiac CT examinations even below the levels of "traditional" iterative image reconstruction approaches will still have to be evaluated.

To sum up, we will probably see moderate further improvements in the already very efficient approaches to reduce radiation dose in cardiac CT, but another breakthrough cannot be expected. By adequate combination of the available dose reduction techniques, CT scans of the heart can be performed at very low radiation dose levels. This may open the potential to allow for scan protocols with somewhat higher radiation exposure in selected diagnostic situations, when, e.g., high spatial resolution or spectral information is needed to better characterize plaques in the coronary arteries.

New CT Concepts

Phase-Contrast CT

Medical CT is based on measuring and displaying the local x-ray attenuation coefficients in a slice of the patient. Phase-contrast CT is an alternative CT technique that does not measure the x-ray absorption but the phase shift of the x-rays by the measurement object. The phase-contrast CT images show the local x-ray phase shift coefficients on a gray scale. Phase-contrast imaging has recently gained considerable attention in the scientific literature as a new method with potential applications in medical imaging, in particular after its successful implementation using compact low-brilliance x-ray sources that are standard components of medical x-ray systems or CT systems [52]. For typical x-ray energies used in CT, the phase shift coefficients of relevant body materials, such as water, are three orders of magnitude larger than the attenuation coefficients. This suggests that phase-contrast CT should be much more sensitive than absorption CT and allow for significantly reduced radiation dose to the patient.

Unfortunately, this advantage can only be utilized at very high spatial resolution [53], and spectacular results demonstrating the potential of phase-contrast CT have so far been limited to small specimen scanned at very high spatial resolution; see the excised coronary artery in Fig. 67.8 [54].

At the resolution level of today's medical CT, the relative performance of phase-contrast CT is inferior to absorption CT. Increasing the resolution to a level at which the relative performance of phase-contrast CT is better than that of absorption CT would require substantially increased radiation dose to maintain adequate CNR in the images. Therefore, as of today, phase-contrast imaging is not an option for medical CT because of the predicted excessive radiation dose requirements. The root cause of the disappointing dose performance is the bad spatial coherence of today's low-brilliance x-ray sources [53]. Should new, compact x-ray tube designs with much better spatial coherence, providing high x-ray photon flux from an extremely small focal spot, become available the concept of phase-contrast CT is worth revisiting.

CT Systems with Photon-Counting Detectors

Solid-state scintillation detectors used in today's medical CT systems are a very mature technology. The two-step detection process, however, based on first converting the x-rays into visible light and then the light into an electrical current (Fig. 67.6a), has certain disadvantages. Solid-state scintillation detectors do not provide energy-resolved signals. As a consequence of the detection process, low-energy x-ray quanta that carry most of the low-contrast information of the object are down-weighted in the signal. This results in a nonoptimal CNR of the CT images in particular in contrast-enhanced CT scans. Furthermore, the spatial resolution of solid-state scintillation detectors is limited by their pixel size, which cannot be made much smaller than today.

Another type of detector that is currently being investigated directly converts the absorbed x-rays into electrical signals (Fig. 67.6b). The photon-counting detector is based on a semiconductor such as cadmium telluride (CdTe) or cadmium-zinc-telluride (CZT). A review of photon-counting detectors in medical x-ray imaging is available in [35, 36]. The absorbed x-rays directly induce short current pulses that are individually counted as soon as they exceed a threshold (Fig. 67.9). The pulse height is proportional to the x-ray energy – a photon-counting detector can therefore provide

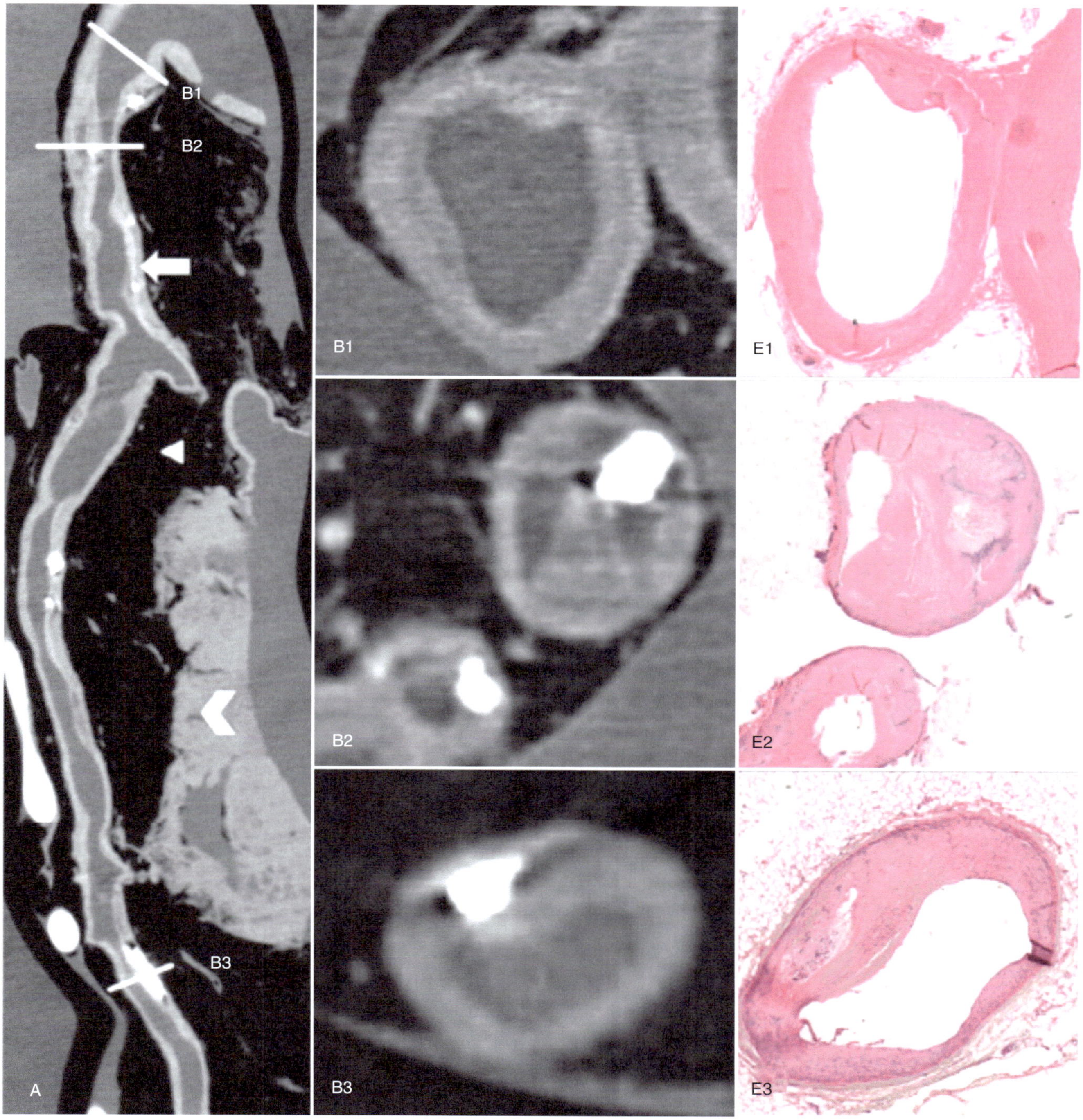

Fig. 67.8 Phase-contrast CT scan of a left anterior descending coronary artery (A and B) with corresponding histopathology (E). The vessel (arrow) is shown with surrounding epicardial fat (arrowhead) and myocardial muscle (chevron). The left main coronary artery (B1 and E1) shows mild intimal thickening. The proximal LAD (B2 and E2) shows a large eccentric plaque with fibrosis, lipid, and calcifications causing high-grade stenosis. In the distal LAD, a calcified lesion can be found (B3 and E3). (Modified from Hetterich et al. [54], with permission)

energy-resolved signals. The individual detector pixels are defined by the high electric field between common cathode and pixelated anodes (Fig. 67.6b) – in contrast to conventional scintillation detectors, no additional separation layers between the pixels are necessary. Therefore, the detector pixels can be made much smaller to improve spatial resolution.

The missing down-weighting of low-energy x-ray quanta has the potential to improve the CNR of the images, in particular in CT scans using iodinated contrast agent. In addition, different energy thresholds for energy discrimination may be introduced. The detector can then simultaneously provide CT raw data in different "energy bins" for spectrally resolved measurements, as illustrated in Figs. 67.9 and 67.10.

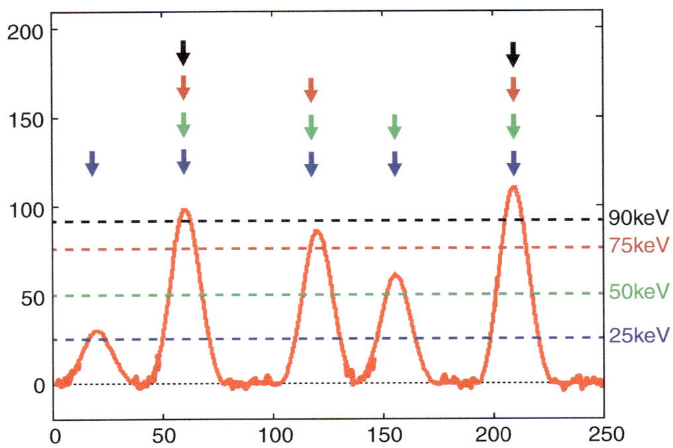

Fig. 67.9 The fast signal pulses at the anode are counted as soon as they exceed a threshold. The pulse height is proportional to the x-ray energy. By introducing more than one threshold (here, four energy thresholds are indicated), the detector provides spectral CT data. In this example, five x-ray quanta with an energy >25 keV are detected (blue arrows). Four of them are also detected in the energy band >50 keV (green arrows), but only three exceed a threshold of 75 keV (red arrows) and only two the upper threshold of 90 keV (black arrows)

By implementing two energy bins for data readout, photon-counting detectors can provide dual-energy information comparable to today's dual-energy (DE) CT approaches. Using more than two energy bins opens the potential of refined spectral analysis, e.g., K-edge imaging for material separation of three materials, with one of them having a K-edge in the accessible energy range of about 40–90 keV. In this way, different contrast agents such as iodine and gadolinium could be separated in the same scan [56, 57].

Another potential application pertinent to cardiac CT is the detection of gold- and iron-based high-density lipoprotein nanoparticle contrast agents that are claimed to attach to macrophages accumulating in atherosclerotic plaques in the coronary arteries. Spectral CT could then provide information about the macrophage content of plaques, with a high macrophage content associated with an elevated risk of plaque rupture [58]. So far, however, feasibility has only been demonstrated in small animal models, and the translation to human imaging is not straightforward, e.g., with regard to the very high amount of contrast agent that would have to be administered.

The spectral separation of a real CdTe- or CZT-based device is reduced by undesired but unavoidable physical effects, such as signal splitting at pixel borders ("charge shar-

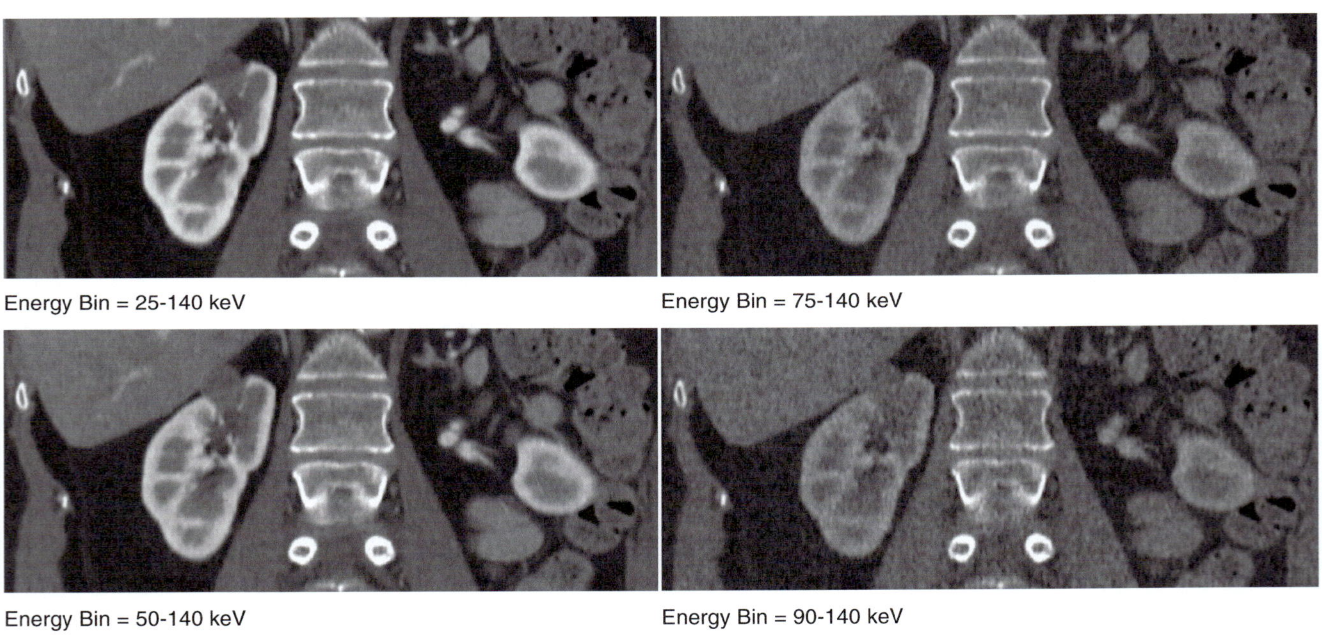

Fig. 67.10 Clinical example of a contrast-enhanced CT scan of the kidney in a 71-year-old woman, acquired on a preclinical photon-counting CT scanner at the NIH, Bethesda, USA (see also Ref. [55]). The detector provides four energy bins in a chess-pattern mode ([25–140 keV], [50–140 keV], [75–140 keV], [90–140 keV]); the corresponding images are shown (see also Fig. 67.9). As expected, iodine contrast decreases with increasing lower energy of the bin, and image noise increases because less x-ray quanta are used for image reconstruction

ing") or energy loss of the x-ray quanta due to K-escape, whereby the K-edges of the detector material lead to preferential absorption of some photon energies and the corresponding release of characteristic x-rays at lower energies within the detector itself. These mechanisms lead to a double counting of x-ray quanta at the wrong energies and therefore to a reduction of spectral separation. For a realistic detector model, the energy discrimination potential is probably equivalent to that of a dual-kV scan with optimized pre-filtration [59].

A main limitation of photon-counting detectors today is the finite pulse width of the detected x-ray pulses with a full width at half maximum (FWHM) of 10 ns and more. This leads to pulse pileup at high x-ray flux rates: overlapping low-energy pulses may be incorrectly registered as high-energy hits, and several overlapping pulses may be counted as one hit only [60]. To reduce pulse pileup, the pixels of the detector need to be small: they are divided into sub-pixels of, e.g., 0.25×0.25 mm^2 [59]. Another problem is count-rate drift at higher x-ray fluxes caused by nonhomogeneously distributed crystal defects in the sensor material. This may lead to severe ring artifacts in the images at higher flux rates.

Photon-counting detectors are a very promising new development in CT, yet the problems of pulse pileup and count-rate drift will have to be solved before these devices can be introduced into clinical CT systems. Currently, preclinical prototypes are used to evaluate the potential and limitations of photon-counting CT in clinical practice and to solve the remaining challenges for routine clinical use. A preclinical hybrid CT scanner based on a dual-source CT geometry with a conventional energy-integrating scintillation detector and a photon-counting CdTe detector was presented in 2012 [61]. Meanwhile, the performance of the hybrid CT scanner has been evaluated [62, 63]. In an IRB-approved patient study with 15 asymptomatic volunteers [55], the non-inferiority of this photon-counting device compared with standard CT has been demonstrated for abdominal imaging. Figure 67.11 illustrates the level of spatial resolution that can be achieved with the preclinical photon-counting CT scanner. Its meaningful clinical use, however, depends on the availability of sufficient radiation dose reserves and the acceptance of increased radiation dose to the patient.

In a nutshell, CT systems with photon-counting detector have the potential to provide spectral information not as an add-on but as an integral part of each scan. In combination with increased spatial resolution, new possibilities for the evaluation of coronary plaques or in-stent restenosis may be opened. The CNR in contrast-enhanced scans will be improved, leading to a potential reduction of radiation dose and/or contrast dose.

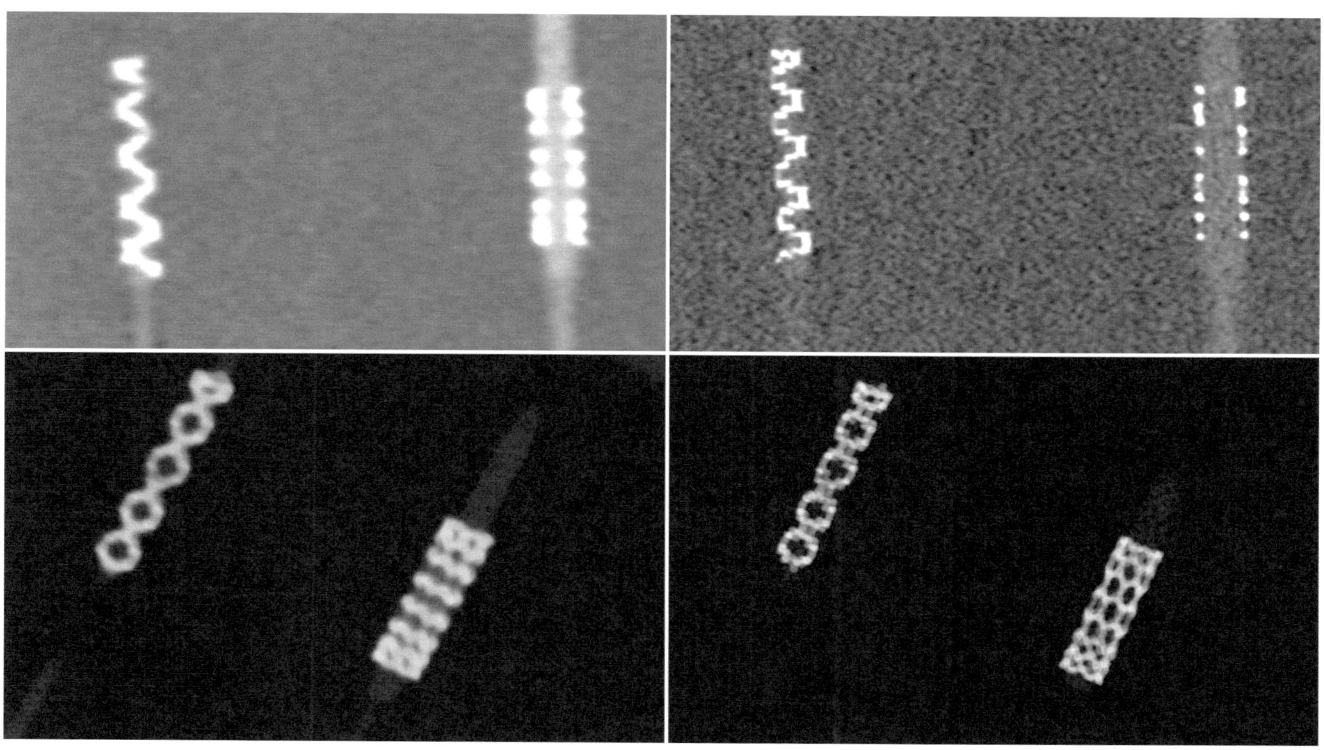

Fig. 67.11 Coronary artery phantom with stent scanned with a conventional high-end CT scanner (left) and with a preclinical photon-counting CT scanner in a high-resolution scan mode (right). Note the significantly increased spatial resolution

New Approaches Enhancing the Application Spectrum of Cardiac CT

Coronary CTA has meanwhile been established as a noninvasive alternative to invasive catheter angiography. It has demonstrated a very high negative predictive value and is primarily used to rule out coronary artery disease. However, as a consequence of still insufficient spatial resolution, it tends to overestimate the degree of coronary stenosis. Coronary CTA is a poor predictor of the hemodynamic relevance of stenosis and of myocardial ischemia [64].

During the last several years, efforts have been ongoing to improve the positive predictive value of cardiac CT for relevant coronary stenosis, with the aim of positioning CT as a singular imaging modality to assess both coronary artery morphology and the status of myocardial perfusion, at best in a single examination [65].

Reduction of Ca Blooming

Improved spatial resolution is needed for a better estimation of the actual degree of coronary stenosis, and for a reduction of Ca blooming, see section "Challenges in Cardiac CT". In addition, dual-energy-based approaches to remove calcified plaques from the coronary arteries to better reveal the true residual lumen are currently being investigated. Instead of the common material decomposition into an iodine image and a soft tissue image, a modified material decomposition into an iodine image and a calcium image is performed. With the choice of these two base materials, calcifications appear in the calcium image only and are suppressed in the iodine image, thereby revealing the actual degree of coronary stenosis. Because the two base materials iodine and calcium show much less difference in their dual-energy behavior than the typical base materials iodine and water, the resulting material images suffer from significantly increased noise which has to be reduced by refined image filtration. Figure 67.12 shows an example of the performance achieved with this technique. Clinical studies are needed to evaluate whether dual-energy-based calcium-removal has the potential to reduce the typical overestimation of the degree of coronary stenosis in coronary CTA.

First-Pass Enhancement Scanning and Dynamic Perfusion CT

Pertinent CT techniques to directly assess and visualize the local blood supply of the myocardium are first-pass enhancement scanning and dynamic perfusion CT. A review of currently available CT techniques to assess myocardial perfusion can be found in [66].

First-pass enhancement studies provide a "snapshot image" of the myocardial blood volume at a single arterial contrast phase by reusing the coronary CTA images to also evaluate the myocardium. Hypo-attenuation of the myocardium is interpreted as perfusion defect. To identify reversible ischemia, first-pass enhancement scanning has not only been performed at rest but also with the application of adenosine stress. In the recent CORE320 multicenter trial, CT first-pass rest and stress myocardial blood volume imaging showed a per-patient sensitivity and specificity for the diagnosis of CAD of 88% and 55% compared with invasive catheter angiography as the gold standard. In those patients with a >50% stenosis on coronary CTA, evaluation of CT first-pass enhancement resulted in a sensitivity, specificity, positive predictive, and negative predictive values of 80%, 74%, 65%, and 86%, respectively [67, 68].

First-pass enhancement scanning has also been performed with the use of dual-energy acquisition techniques. Dual-energy data have been used to create "iodine maps" of the myocardium as a surrogate parameter for the myocardial blood supply. DE iodine maps are potentially more sensitive for the detection of hypoperfused myocardium compared with the hypo-attenuation on single-energy CT images [69]; they allow for a potentially quantitative evaluation of the iodine content, and other sources of hypo-attenuation (e.g., fat) can be ruled out. Figure 67.13 shows a clinical example. Using first-generation dual-source CT for first-pass rest and stress DE CT scans in a group of 45 patients with known coronary artery disease, the authors found 93.2% sensitivity, 85.5% specificity, 88.3% PPV, and 91.4% NPV for the detection of significant coronary artery stenosis compared with invasive catheter angiography (ICA) as the standard of reference [70].

Because of technical limitations, problematic image quality at higher heart rates, and insufficient integration of DE cardiac CT into routine clinical workflows, this technique has so far been limited to first feasibility studies and has not yet entered clinical routine. Future CT systems which provide spectral information on a routine basis as an integral part of each standard scan, such as the photon-counting CT systems discussed in section "CT Systems with Photon-Counting Detectors", combined with excellent temporal resolution, will enable a more widespread utilization of spectral cardiac CT and an intensified analysis of its benefits and limitations on the way to routine clinical application.

The most refined CT technique to acquire information about the blood supply of the myocardium is dynamic perfusion scanning, characterized by time-resolved assessment of the in- and outflow of iodinated contrast agent in the left ventricle. The entire myocardium can be examined by either performing repeated ECG-triggered axial scans using CT systems with area detector technology (that provide 16 cm

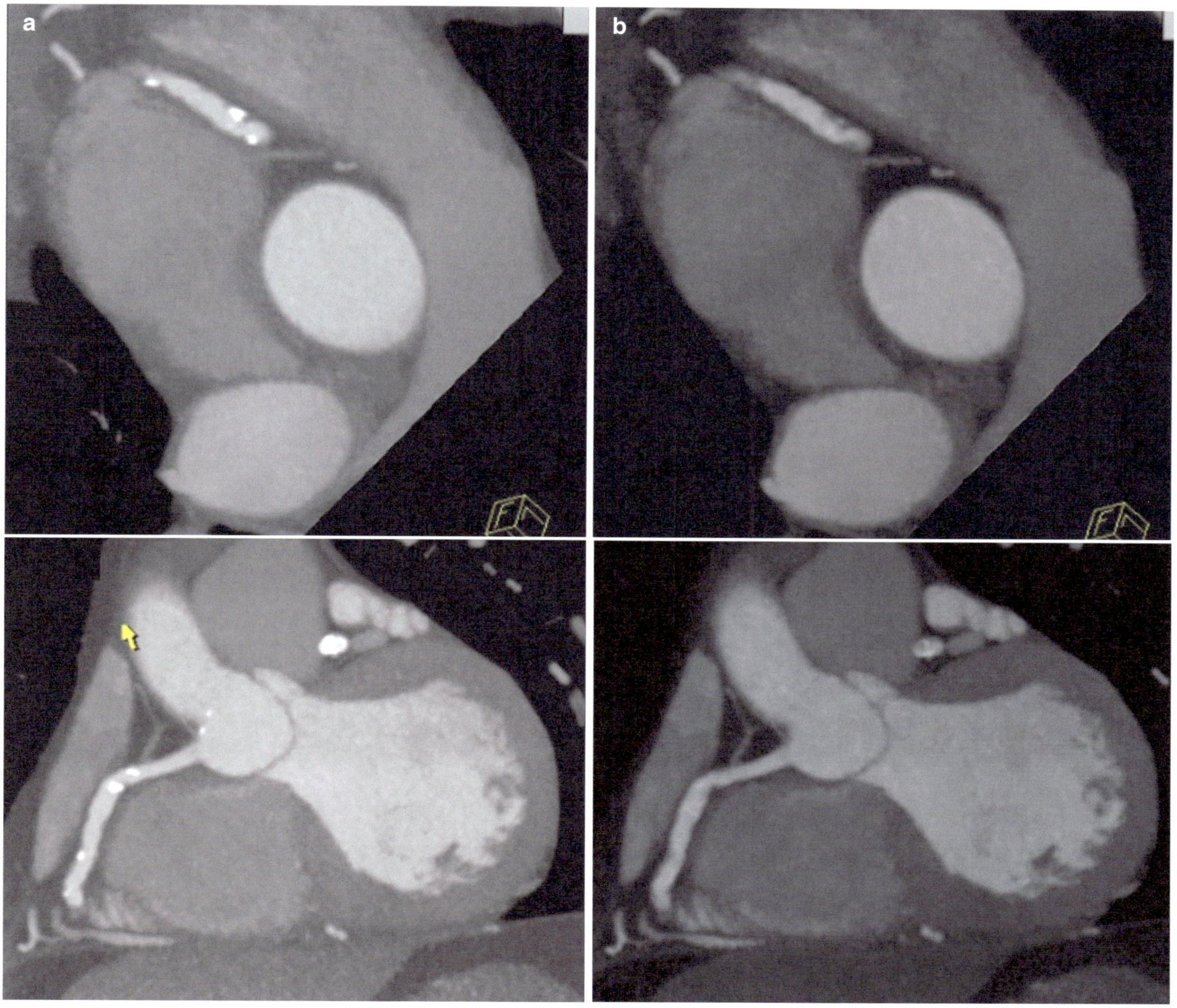

Fig. 67.12 Dual-energy coronary CTA in a patient with calcifications in the right coronary artery (RCA). Mixed images corresponding to a standard CT scan (**a**) and images with suppressed calcifications to reveal the true degree of stenosis from a dual-energy-based material decomposition using iodine and calcium as the two base materials (**b**). (Courtesy of Medical University of South Carolina, USA)

z-axis coverage at isocenter) or by performing ECG-triggered axial scans at two alternating table positions, with the table moving forward and backward between the two positions [71]. As a benefit over qualitative first-pass enhancement techniques, dynamic perfusion CT provides quantitative results for relevant perfusion parameters such as the myocardial blood flow (MBF). Dynamic perfusion CT has the potential to improve the specificity of coronary CTA for the detection of functionally significant coronary stenosis. In a recent study [72], the specificity of visual coronary CTA (69%) and quantitative coronary CTA (77%) could be improved by the subsequent use of the MBF index under stress (89%), compared with invasive FFR as the gold standard. Most important, quantitative cutoff value of the MBF index to detect functionally significant coronary lesions can be defined: 78 mL/100 mL/min [72] or – quite similar – 75 ml/100 mL/min [73].

Because of its quantitative nature, dynamic cardiac perfusion CT is particularly useful in cases where relative assessment of the functional significance of a lesion is difficult, such as in patients with multivessel disease (Fig. 67.14). In contrast to first-pass enhancement approaches, the quantitative MBF index does not rely on the assumption that the best-enhanced territory is normal and can be used as a reference [72].

The wide clinical applicability of dynamic cardiac perfusion CT will secure its future role in the comprehensive

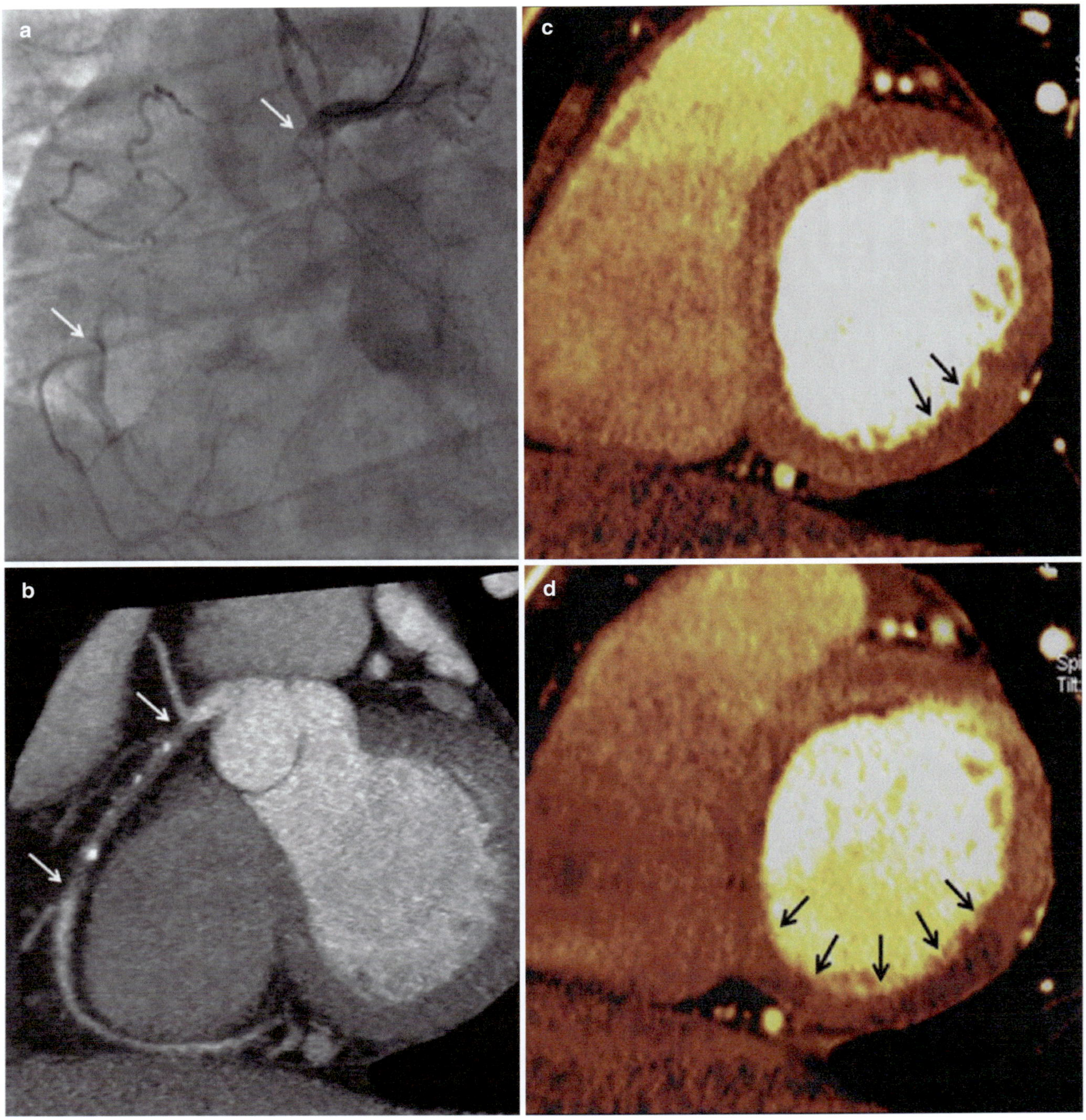

Fig. 67.13 ECG-gated dual-energy cardiac CT in a 60-year-old hypertensive man with a history of smoking, using second-generation DSCT. Both conventional catheter angiography (**a**) and CTA derived from the rest DE scan (**b**) show chronic total occlusion of the proximal RCA. The DE energy iodine maps at rest (**c**) and during stress (**d**) indicate a reversible perfusion defect (arrows). (Courtesy of Vancouver General Hospital, Vancouver, Canada)

workup of patients, despite simpler but less versatile approaches such as first-pass enhancement scanning or CT-FFR (see next section), provided the complex workflow of cardiac perfusion CT can be further simplified and streamlined, both with regard to scan data acquisition and results processing, and the radiation dose can be further reduced. Ongoing technical progress, enabling the use of 80 kV and 70 kV tube voltages for dynamic cardiac perfusion CT, holds promise to reduce radiation dose to values of 5 mSv and below [74].

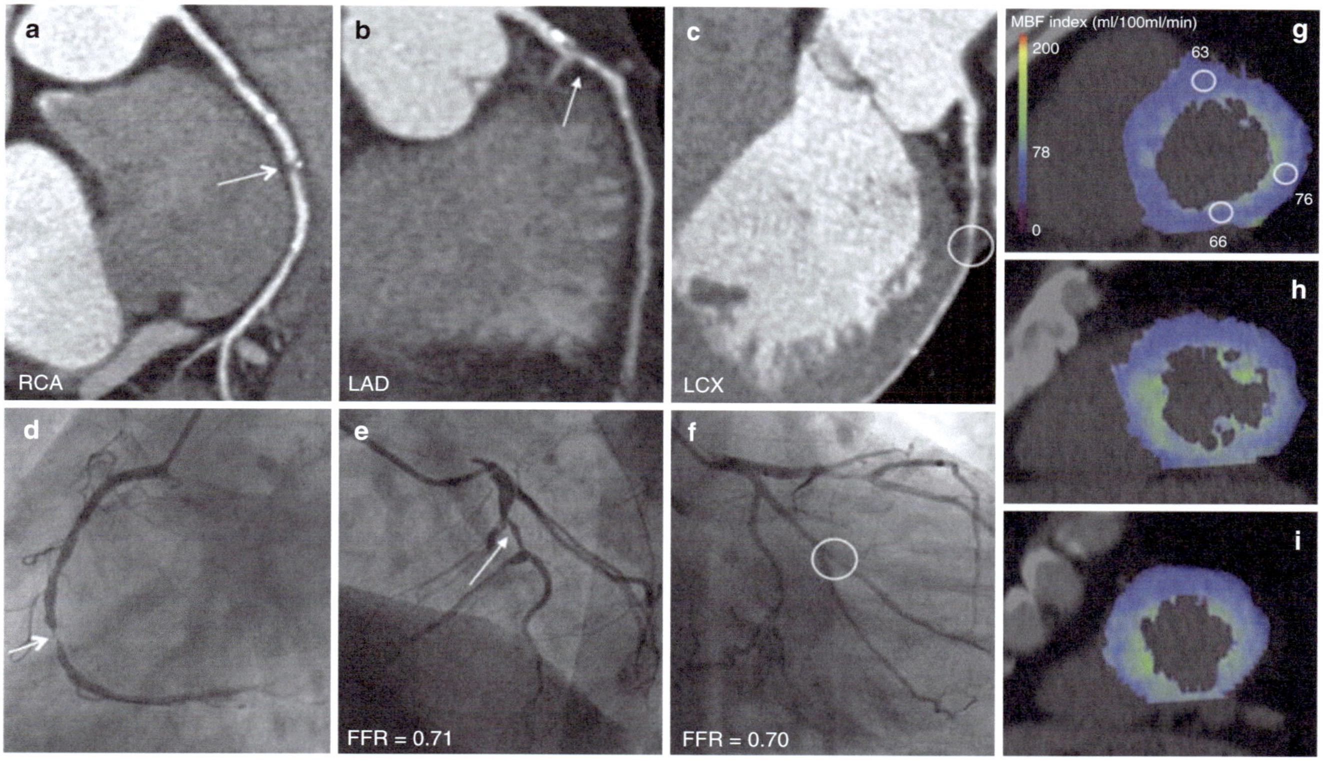

Fig. 67.14 Coronary CTA images (**a–c**) and conventional catheter angiography (**d–f**) in a patient with three-vessel disease. MBF derived from a dynamic CT perfusion scan (**g–i**) is reduced in the whole myocardium (<78 mL/100 mL/min). (From Rossi et al. [72], with permission)

Meanwhile, first attempts have been made to also derive a prognostic value from quantitative perfusion parameters. Using data of 144 patients from a multicenter trial with follow-up for 6, 12, and 18 months, Meinel et al. [75] found that global quantification of the left ventricular MBF at stress may have incremental predictive value for future major adverse cardiac events (MACE) over clinical risk factors and assessment of stenosis at coronary CTA. Patients with global MBF of <121 mL/100 mL/min were at increased risk for MACE. The number of territories with perfusion defects was strongly predictive of MACE with adjusted hazard ratios of 1.41, 3.44, and 4.76 for one, two, and three affected territories [76].

Combining several parameters derived from cardiac CT scans to improve and refine the prediction of MACE, potentially in combination with traditional risk factors and laboratory data of the patient, is a promising future research area and may significantly influence the clinical value of cardiac CT. For the analysis of larger databases, machine learning approaches will be needed.

CT Fractional Flow Reserve

Another technique to assess the hemodynamic relevance of stenosis is CT-FFR. It applies computational fluid dynamics (CFD) techniques to coronary CTA images to compute the fractional flow reserve (FFR), a measure of lesion-specific ischemia [77].

Standard coronary CTA images are used to create a patient-specific three-dimensional model of the coronary arteries. Then, by applying the principles of CFD to this model, hyperemic coronary flow and pressure can be simulated from the coronary CTA images at rest. These pressure and flow values are used to noninvasively compute the local fractional flow reserve (FFR), which is the ratio of maximal coronary blood flow through a stenotic artery to the blood flow in the hypothetical case that the artery was normal [78]. The end result is a color-coded map of computed local FFR values as an overlay to the three-dimensional model of the coronary arteries, indicating regions of low FFR <0.8 corresponding to potentially hemodynamically relevant lesions in red (Fig. 67.15).

A meta-analysis of 6 original studies comparing the performance of CT-FFR with the gold-standard invasive FFR (1354 vessels; 812 patients) in diagnosing hemodynamically relevant coronary stenosis showed a pooled per-vessel sensitivity and specificity of 0.84 [95% confidence interval (CI): 0.80–0.87] and 0.76 [95% CI: 0.73–0.79], respectively [79]. The original studies were performed with two different methods, an FDA-approved off-site approach requiring the coronary CTA images to be sent to a centralized core lab to perform coronary artery segmentation and CT-FFR computation (HeartFlow, Redwood City, California, USA) and a

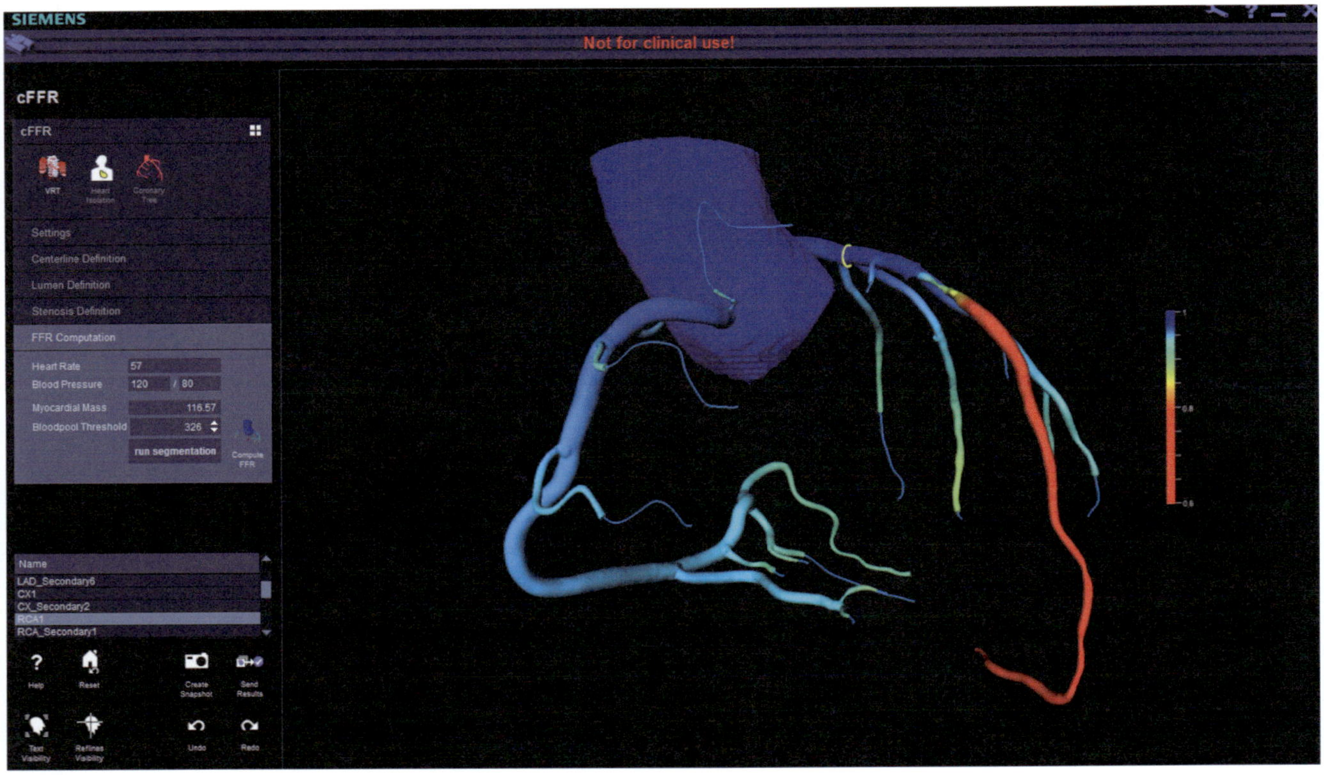

Fig. 67.15 User-interface of a prototype preclinical on-site software to compute CT-FFR

preclinical on-site approach using software installed on a local computer in the hospital (Siemens Healthcare GmbH, Forchheim, Germany). A subgroup analysis of the studies performed with the preclinical on-site approach revealed a per-vessel sensitivity and specificity of 0.87 (95% CI: 079–0.93) and 0.71 (95% CI: 0.63–0.78), respectively.

According to Panchal et al. [79], the addition of CT-FFR to coronary CTA improves the diagnostic ability of noninvasive CT to evaluate hemodynamically significant coronary lesions and might improve noninvasive clinical decision-making for patients with CAD. In the PLATFORM study [80], equivalent clinical outcomes at lower cost were demonstrated for care guided by coronary CTA and selective CT-FFR in patients with stable chest pain, compared with usual care over 1-year follow-up. As a further step, the ADVANCE Registry is planned as a multicenter, prospective registry enrolling approximately 5000 patients at 50 sites to evaluate utility, clinical outcomes, and resource utilization following CT-FFR-guided treatment in clinically stable, symptomatic patients diagnosed with CAD by coronary CTA [81].

Recently, machine learning has been used to compute CT-FFR instead of computationally expensive CFD techniques [82]. In the machine learning approach, the model is trained on a large database of synthetically generated coronary anatomies, where the target values are computed using the physics-based CFD model. The trained model predicts FFR at each point along the centerline of the coronary tree (Fig. 67.16). Correlation between machine learning and physics-based predictions is excellent [82], with a significant reduction of the average execution time by machine learning, leading to near real-time assessment of FFR.

In a study [83], on-site CT-FFR showed a comparable diagnostic accuracy as dynamic CT perfusion for identifying hemodynamically significant stenosis defined by invasive FFR. According to the authors, CT perfusion was more robust and could be successfully analyzed in all patients who had to be excluded from CT-FFR evaluation due to technical problems. CT perfusion is a complementary modality in patients with severe coronary calcifications and poor coronary CTA image quality. According to Coenen [84] diagnostic performance can be improved by combining CT-FFR and CT perfusion. A stepwise approach to improve diagnostic performance is recommended, reserving CT perfusion for patients with intermediate CT-FFR results.

According to [85], the workflow of how CT-FFR will be used in clinical practice – whether on- or off-site – remains to be determined.

In the future, machine learning is expected to go beyond providing CT-FFR numbers to predict the hemodynamic relevance of stenosis. By combining CT-FFR with other parameters, such as plaque location and composition, machine learning-based approaches may have the potential for a more exact classification of patients and prediction of future events.

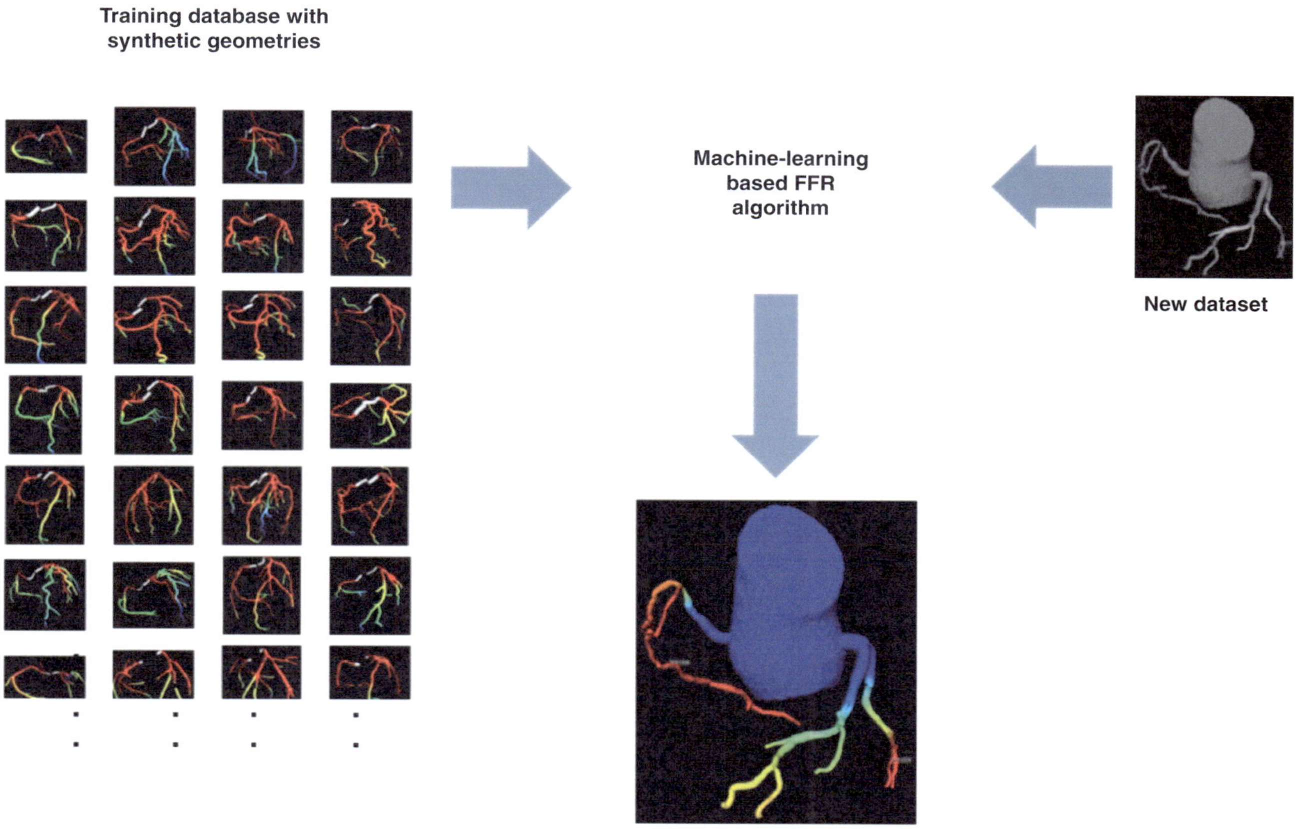

Fig. 67.16 Principle of a machine learning approach using a trained model to compute CT-FFR

Prognostic Risk Assessment

Traditional prognostic risk assessment to determine an individual's chances of developing cardiovascular disease is based on evaluating few traditional risk factors, such as age, family history of CAD, hypertension, increased cholesterol levels, or diabetes. Additional CT imaging findings, such as coronary calcifications, coronary artery stenosis, and distribution and composition of coronary plaques, add incremental improvement to the prediction of MACE (e.g., [86]).

Machine learning is a rapidly evolving field that gives computers the ability to make data-driven predictions or decisions, through building a model from test inputs. Machine learning can identify patterns in large datasets with a multitude of variables – hence it is consequent to apply it to large databases collecting CT imaging data, traditional risk factors, clinical parameters, and follow-up data of patients. Instead of evaluating just few selected clinical or imaging parameters as in traditional approaches, machine learning can combine and rank a large number of features to potentially improve and refine the prediction of MACE.

In a first feasibility study [87], the authors included 10,030 patients with suspected coronary artery disease and 5-year follow-up from the CONFIRM International Multicenter Registry. Machine learning evaluating 25 clinical and 44 coronary CTA parameters was found to predict the 5-year all-cause mortality significantly better than existing clinical or coronary CTA metrics alone.

Future clinical studies will be needed to further evaluate the potential of machine learning for prognostic risk assessment and to refine the prognosis – it is very likely, however, that machine learning-based approaches will play a rapidly increasing role in cardiac CT on its way to a comprehensive clinical imaging modality.

References

1. Flohr TG, De Cecco CN, Schmidt B, Wang R, Schoepf UJ, Meinel FG. Computed tomographic assessment of coronary artery disease: state-of-the-art imaging techniques. Radiol Clin N Am. 2015;53(2):271–85.
2. Flohr T, Ohnesorge B. Heart rate adaptive optimization of spatial and temporal resolution for ECG-gated multi-slice spiral CT of the heart. JCAT. 2001;25(6):907–23.
3. Leschka S, Wildermuth S, Boehm T, Desbiolles L, Husmann L, Plass A, Koepfli P, Schepis T, Marincek B, Kaufmann PA, Alkadhi H. Noninvasive coronary angiography with 64-section CT: effect of average heart rate and heart rate variability on image quality. Radiology. 2006;241(2):378–85.

4. Flohr TG, McCollough CH, Bruder H, Petersilka M, Gruber K, Süß C, Grasruck M, Stierstorfer K, Krauss B, Raupach R, Primak AN, Küttner A, Achenbach S, Becker C, Kopp A, Ohnesorge BM. First performance evaluation of a dual-source CT (DSCT) system. Eur Radiol. 2006;16(2):256–68.
5. McCollough CH, Schmidt B, Yu L, Primak A, Ulzheimer S, Bruder H, Flohr TG. Measurement of temporal resolution in dual source CT. Med Phys. 2008;35(2):764–8.
6. Matt D, Scheffel H, Leschka S, Flohr TG, Marincek B, Kaufmann PA, Alkadhi H. Dual-source CT coronary angiography: image quality, mean heart rate, and heart rate variability. AJR Am J Roentgenol. 2007;189(3):567–73.
7. Ropers U, Ropers D, Pflederer T, Anders K, Kuettner A, Stilianakis NI, Komatsu S, Kalender W, Bautz W, Daniel WG, Achenbach S. Influence of heart rate on the diagnostic accuracy of dual-source computed tomography coronary angiography. J Am Coll Cardiol. 2007;50(25):2393–8.
8. Scheffel H, Alkadhi H, Plass A, Vachenauer R, Desbiolles L, Gaemperli O, Schepis T, Frauenfelder T, Schertler T, Husmann L, Grunenfelder J, Genoni M, Kaufmann PA, Marincek B, Leschka S. Accuracy of dual-source CT coronary angiography: first experience in a high pre-test probability population without heart rate control. Eur Radiol. 2006;16(12):2739–47.
9. Weustink AC, Neefjes LA, Kyrzopoulos S, van Straten M, Neoh Eu R, Meijboom WB, van Mieghem CA, Capuano E, Dijkshoorn ML, Cademartiri F, Boersma E, de Feyter PJ, Krestin GP, Mollet NR. Impact of heart rate frequency and variability on radiation exposure, image quality, and diagnostic performance in dual-source spiral CT coronary angiography. Radiology. 2009;253(3):672–80.
10. Li M, Zhang GM, Zhao JS, Jiang ZW, Peng ZH, Jin ZT, Sun G. Diagnostic performance of dual-source CT coronary angiography with and without heart rate control: systematic review and meta-analysis. Clin Radiol. 2014;69(2):163–71.
11. Besson GM. New CT system architectures for high temporal resolution with applications to improved geometric dose efficiency and cardiac imaging. Med Phys. 2015;42(5):2668–78.
12. Wang G, Yu H, Ye Y. A scheme for multisource interior tomography. Med Phys. 2009;36(8):3575–81.
13. Agatston AS, Janowitz WR, Hildner FJ, Zusmer NR, Viamonte M, Detrano R. Quantification of coronary artery calcium using ultrafast computed tomography. JACC. 1990;15:827–32.
14. Budoff M, Georgiou D, Brody A, et al. Ultrafast computed tomography as a diagnostic modality in the detection of coronary artery disease: a multicenter study. Circulation. 1996;93:898–904.
15. Yoneyama K, Vavere AL, Cerci R, Ahmed R, Arai AE, Niinuma H, Rybicki FJ, Rochitte CE, Clouse ME, George RT, Lima JA, Arbab-Zadeh A. Influence of image acquisition settings on radiation dose and image quality in coronary angiography by 320-detector volume computed tomography: the CORE320 pilot experience. Heart Int. 2012;7(2):e11.
16. Tang J, Hsieh J, Chen GH. Temporal resolution improvement in cardiac CT using PICCS (TRI-PICCS): performance studies. Med Phys. 2010;37(8):4377–88.
17. Schöndube H, Allmendinger T, Stierstorfer K, Bruder H, Flohr T. Evaluation of a novel CT image reconstruction algorithm with enhanced temporal resolution, in medical imaging 2011: physics of medical imaging, vol. 7961. Lake Buena Vista/Florida: SPIE; 2011. p. 79611N.
18. Bhagalia R, Pack JD, Miller JV, Iatrou M. Nonrigid registration-based coronary artery motion correction for cardiac computed tomography. Med Phys. 2012;39(7):4245–54.
19. Tang Q, Cammin J, Srivastava S, Taguchi K. A fully four-dimensional, iterative motion estimation and compensation method for cardiac CT. Med Phys. 2012;39(7):4291–305.
20. Rohkohl C, Bruder H, Stierstorfer K, Flohr T. Improving best-phase image quality in cardiac CT by motion correction with MAM optimization. Med Phys. 2013;40(3):031901.
21. Fuchs TA, Stehli J, Dougoud S, Fiechter M, Sah BR, Buechel RR, Bull S, Gaemperli O, Kaufmann PA. Impact of a new motion-correction algorithm on image quality of low-dose coronary CT angiography in patients with insufficient heart rate control. Acad Radiol. 2014;21(3):312–7.
22. Maass C, Hofmann C, Kachelriess M. TRI-PICCS in single source and dual source CT, in IEEE NSS-MIC (nuclear science symposium- medical imaging conference). Knoxville: NSS/MIC; 2010. p. 2805–10.
23. Apfaltrer P, Schoendube H, Schoepf UJ, Allmendinger T, Tricarico F, Schindler A, Vogt S, Sunnegårdh J, Stierstorfer K, Henzler T, Fink C, Bruder H, Flohr TG, Ebersberger U. Enhanced temporal resolution at cardiac CT with a novel CT image reconstruction algorithm: initial patient experience. Eur J Radiol. 2013;82(2):270–4.
24. Isola AA, Ziegler A, Koehler T, Niessen WJ, Grass M. Motion-compensated iterative cone-beam CT image reconstruction with adapted blobs as basis functions. Phys Med Biol. 2008;53(23):6777–97.
25. Hahn J, Bruder H, Allmendinger T, Stierstorfer K, Flohr T, et al. Reduction of motion artifacts in cardiac CT based on partial angle reconstructions from short scan data. Proceedings SPIE 9783, medical imaging 2016: physics of medical imaging, 97831A (March 25, 2016).
26. Andreini D, Pontone G, Mushtaq S, Bertella E, Conte E, Segurini C, Baggiano A, Bartorelli AL, Annoni A, Formenti A, Petullà M, Beltrama V, Fiorentini C, Pepi M. Low-dose CT coronary angiography with a novel IntraCycle motion-correction algorithm in patients with high heart rate or heart rate variability. Eur Heart J Cardiovasc Imaging. 2015;16(10):1093–100.
27. Sheta HM, Egstrup K, Husic M, Heinsen LJ, Lambrechtsen J. Impact of a motion correction algorithm on quality and diagnostic utility in unselected patients undergoing coronary CT angiography. Clin Imaging. 2016;40(2):217–21.
28. Sheta HM, Egstrup K, Husic M, Heinsen LJ, Nieman K, Lambrechtsen J. Impact of a motion correction algorithm on image quality in patients undergoing CT angiography: a randomized controlled trial. Clin Imaging. 2017;42:1–6.
29. Vanhecke TE, Madder RD, Weber JE, Bielak LF, Peyser PA, Chinnaiyan KM. Development and validation of a predictive screening tool for uninterpretable coronary CT angiography results. Circ Cardiovasc Imaging. 2011;4(5):490–7.
30. Maintz D, Seifarth H, Raupach R, Flohr T, Rink M, Sommer T, Ozgün M, Heindel W, Fischbach R. 64-slice multidetector coronary CT angiography: in vitro evaluation of 68 different stents. Eur Radiol. 2006;16(4):818–26.
31. Maintz D, Burg MC, Seifarth H, Bunck AC, Ozgün M, Fischbach R, Jürgens KU, Heindel W. Update on multidetector coronary CT angiography of coronary stents: in vitro evaluation of 29 different stent types with dual-source CT. Eur Radiol. 2009;19(1):42–9.
32. Carrabba N, Schuijf JD, de Graaf FR, et al. Diagnostic accuracy of 64-slice computed tomography coronary angiography for the detection of in-stent restenosis: a meta-analysis. J Nucl Cardiol. 2010;17(3):470–8.
33. Fuchs TA, Stehli J, Fiechter M, Dougoud S, Sah BR, Gebhard C, Bull S, Gaemperli O, Kaufmann PA. First in vivo head-to-head comparison of high-definition versus standard-definition stent imaging with 64-slice computed tomography. Int J Cardiovasc Imaging. 2013;29(6):1409–16.
34. Gassenmaier T, Petri N, Allmendinger T, et al. Next generation coronary CT angiography: in vitro evaluation of 27 coronary stents. Eur Radiol. 2014;24(11):2953–61.

35. Taguchi K, Iwanczyk JS. Vision 20/20: single photon counting x-ray detectors in medical imaging. Med Phys. 2013;40(10):100901. https://doi.org/10.1118/1.4820371. Review.
36. Taguchi K. Energy-sensitive photon counting detector-based X-ray computed tomography. Radiol Phys Technol. 2017;10(1):8–22.
37. Menke J, Unterberg-Buchwald C, Staab W, Sohns JM, Seif Amir Hosseini A, Schwarz A. Head-to-head comparison of prospectively triggered vs retrospectively gated coronary computed tomography angiography: meta-analysis of diagnostic accuracy, image quality, and radiation dose. Am Heart J. 2013;165(2):154–63.
38. Neefjes LA, Dharampal AS, Rossi A, Nieman K, Weustink AC, Dijkshoorn ML, Ten Kate GJ, Dedic A, Papadopoulou SL, van Straten M, Cademartiri F, Krestin GP, de Feyter PJ, Mollet NR. Image quality and radiation exposure using different low-dose scan protocols in dual-source CT coronary angiography: randomized study. Radiology. 2011;261(3):779–86.
39. Yin WH, Lu B, Hou ZH, Li N, Han L, Wu YJ, Niu HX, Silverman JR, Nicola De Cecco C, Schoepf UJ. Detection of coronary artery stenosis with sub-milliSievert radiation dose by prospectively ECG-triggered high-pitch spiral CT angiography and iterative reconstruction. Eur Radiol. 2013;23(11):2927–33.
40. Morsbach F, Gordic S, Desbiolles L, Husarik D, Frauenfelder T, Schmidt B, Allmendinger T, Wildermuth S, Alkadhi H, Leschka S. Performance of turbo high-pitch dual-source CT for coronary CT angiography: first ex vivo and patient experience. Eur Radiol. 2014;24(8):1889–95.
41. Chinnaiyan KM, Bilolikar AN, Walsh E, Wood D, DePetris A, Gentry R, Boura J, Abbara S, Al-Mallah M, Bis K, Boswell G, Gallagher M, Arunakul IO, Halliburton S, Jacobs J, Lesser J, Schoepf UJ, Valeti US, Raff GL. CT dose reduction using prospectively triggered or fast-pitch spiral technique employed in cardiothoracic imaging (the CT dose study). J Cardiovasc Comput Tomogr. 2014;8(3):205–14.
42. McCollough CH, Primak AN, Braun N, Kofler J, Yu L, Christner J. Strategies for reducing radiation dose in CT. Radiol Clin N Am. 2009;47(1):27–40.
43. Meinel FG, Canstein C, Schoepf UJ, Sedlmaier M, Schmidt B, Harris BS, Flohr TG, De Cecco CN. Image quality and radiation dose of low tube voltage 3rd generation dual-source coronary CT angiography in obese patients: a phantom study. Eur Radiol. 2014;24(7):1643–50.
44. Vonder M, Pelgrim GJ, Huijsse SE, Meyer M, Greuter MJ, Henzler T, Flohr TG, Oudkerk M, Vliegenthart R. Feasibility of spectral shaping for detection and quantification of coronary calcifications in ultra-low dose CT. Eur Radiol. 2017;27(5):2047–54.
45. Tesche C, De Cecco CN, Vliegenthart R, Albrecht MH, Varga-Szemes A, Duguay TM, Ebersberger U, Bayer RR 2nd, Canstein C, Schmidt B, Allmendinger T, Litwin SE, Morris PB, Flohr TG, Hoffmann E, Schoepf UJ. Accuracy and radiation dose reduction using low-voltage computed tomography coronary artery calcium scoring with tin filtration. Am J Cardiol. 2017;119(4):675–80.
46. Thibault JB, Sauer KD, Bouman CA, Hsieh J. A three-dimensional statistical approach to improved image quality for multislice helical CT. Med Phys. 2007;34(11):4526–44.
47. Stehli J, Fuchs TA, Bull S, Clerc OF, Possner M, Buechel RR, Gaemperli O, Kaufmann PA. Accuracy of coronary CT angiography using a submillisievert fraction of radiation exposure: comparison with invasive coronary angiography. J Am Coll Cardiol. 2014;64(8):772–80.
48. Layritz C, Schmid J, Achenbach S, Ulzheimer S, Wuest W, May M, Ropers D, Klinghammer L, Daniel WG, Pflederer T, Lell M. Accuracy of prospectively ECG-triggered very low-dose coronary dual-source CT angiography using iterative reconstruction for the detection of coronary artery stenosis: comparison with invasive catheterization. Eur Heart J Cardiovasc Imaging. 2014;15(11):1238–45.
49. Schuhbaeck A, Achenbach S, Layritz C, Eisentopf J, Hecker F, Pflederer T, Gauss S, Rixe J, Kalender W, Daniel WG, Lell M, Ropers D. Image quality of ultra-low radiation exposure coronary CT angiography with an effective dose <0.1 mSv using high-pitch spiral acquisition and raw data-based iterative reconstruction. Eur Radiol. 2013;23(3):597–606.
50. Elad M, Aharon M. Image denoising via sparse and redundant representations over learned dictionaries. IEEE Trans Image Process. 2006;15(12):3736–45.
51. Ghadrdan S, Alirezaie J, Dillenseger JL, Babyn P. Low-dose computed tomography image denoising based on joint wavelet and sparse representation. Conf Proc IEEE Eng Med Biol Soc. 2014;2014:3325–8.
52. Pfeiffer F, Weitkamp T, Bunk O, David C. Phase retrieval and differential phase-contrast imaging with low-brilliance X-ray sources. Nat Phys. 2006;2:258–61.
53. Raupach R, Flohr T. Performance evaluation of x-ray differential phase contrast computed tomography (PCT) with respect to medical imaging. Med Phys. 2012;39(8):4761–74.
54. Hetterich H, Willner M, Habbel C, Herzen J, Hoffmann VS, Fill S, Hipp A, Marschner M, Schüller U, Auweter S, Massberg S, Reiser MF, Pfeiffer F, Saam T, Bamberg F. X-ray phase-contrast computed tomography of human coronary arteries. Investig Radiol. 2015;50(10):686–94.
55. Pourmorteza A, Symons R, Sandfort V, Mallek M, Fuld MK, Henderson G, Jones EC, Malayeri AA, Folio LR, Bluemke DA. Abdominal imaging with contrast-enhanced photon-counting CT: first human experience. Radiology. 2016;279(1):239–45.
56. Roessl E, et al. K-edge imaging in x-ray computed tomography using multi-bin photon counting detectors. Phys Med Biol. 2007;52:4679–96.
57. Schlomka JP, Roessl E, Dorscheid R, Dill S, Martens G, Istel T, Bäumer C, Herrmann C, Steadman R, Zeitler G, Livne A, Proksa R. Multienergy photon-counting K-edge imaging: potential for improved luminal depiction in vascular imaging. Radiology. 2008;249(3):1010–6.
58. Cormode DP, Roessl E, Thran A, Skajaa T, Gordon RE, Schlomka JP, Fuster V, Fisher EA, Mulder WJ, Proksa R, Fayad ZA. Atherosclerotic plaque composition: analysis with multicolor CT and targeted gold nanoparticles. Radiology. 2010;256(3):774–82.
59. Kappler S, Niederlöhner D, Stierstorfer K, Flohr T. Contrast-enhancement, image noise and dual-energy simulations for quantum-counting clinical CT. Proc SPIE Med Imaging Conf. 2010;7622:76223H.
60. Barber WC, et al. Characterization of a novel photon counting detector for clinical CT: count rate, energy resolution, and noise performance. Proc SPIE Med Imaging Conf. 2009;7258:725824.
61. Kappler S, et al. First results from a hybrid prototype CT scanner for exploring benefits of quantum-counting in clinical CT. Proc SPIE Med Imaging Conf. 2012;8313:83130X.
62. Yu Z, Leng S, Jorgensen SM, Li Z, Gutjahr R, Chen B, Halaweish AF, Kappler S, Yu L, Ritman EL, McCollough CH. Evaluation of conventional imaging performance in a research whole-body CT system with a photon-counting detector array. Phys Med Biol. 2016;61(4):1572–95.
63. Gutjahr R, Halaweish AF, Yu Z, Leng S, Yu L, Li Z, Jorgensen SM, Ritman EL, Kappler S, McCollough CH. Human imaging with photon counting-based computed tomography at clinical dose levels: contrast-to-noise ratio and cadaver studies. Investig Radiol. 2016;51(7):421–9.
64. Stolzmann P, Donati OF, Scheffel H, Azemaj N, Baumueller S, Plass A, Kozerke S, Leschka S, Grünenfelder J, Boesiger P, Marincek B, Alkadhi H. Low-dose CT coronary angiography for the prediction of myocardial ischaemia. Eur Radiol. 2010;20(1):56–64.

65. Bastarrika G, Lee YS, Huda W, Ruzsics B, Costello P, Schoepf UJ. CT of coronary artery disease. Radiology. 2009;253(2):317–38.
66. Bucher AM, De Cecco CN, Schoepf UJ, Wang R, Meinel FG, Binukrishnan SR, Spearman JV, Vogl TJ, Ruzsics B. Cardiac CT for myocardial ischaemia detection and characterization-comparative analysis. Br J Radiol. 2014;24:20140159.
67. George RT, Arbab-Zadeh A, Miller JM, Vavere AL, Bengel FM, Lardo AC, Lima JA. Computed tomography myocardial perfusion imaging with 320-row detector computed tomography accurately detects myocardial ischemia in patients with obstructive coronary artery disease. Circ Cardiovasc Imaging. 2012;5(3):333–40.
68. George RT, Mehra VC, Chen MY, Kitagawa K, Arbab-Zadeh A, Miller JM, Matheson MB, Vavere AL, Kofoed KF, Rochitte CE, Dewey M, Yaw TS, Niinuma H, Brenner W, Cox C, Clouse ME, Lima JA, Di Carli M. Myocardial CT perfusion imaging and SPECT for the diagnosis of coronary artery disease: a head-to-head comparison from the CORE320 multicenter diagnostic performance study. Radiology. 2014;272(2):407–16.
69. Ruzsics B, Schwarz F, Schoepf UJ, et al. Comparison of dual-energy computed tomography of the heart with single photon emission computed tomography for assessment of coronary artery stenosis and of the myocardial blood supply. Am J Cardiol. 2009;104(3):318–26.
70. Ko SM, Choi JW, Song MG, et al. Myocardial perfusion imaging using adenosine-induced stress dual-energy computed tomography of the heart: comparison with cardiac magnetic resonance imaging and conventional coronary angiography. Eur Radiol. 2011;21:26–35.
71. Mahnken AH, Klotz E, Pietsch H, Schmidt B, Allmendinger T, Haberland U, Kalender WA, Flohr T. Quantitative whole heart stress perfusion CT imaging as noninvasive assessment of hemodynamics in coronary artery stenosis: preliminary animal experience. Investig Radiol. 2010;45(6):298–305.
72. Rossi A, Dharampal A, Wragg A, Davies LC, van Geuns RJ, Anagnostopoulos C, Klotz E, Kitslaar P, Broersen A, Mathur A, Nieman K, Hunink MG, de Feyter PJ, Petersen SE, Pugliese F. Diagnostic performance of hyperaemic myocardial blood flow index obtained by dynamic computed tomography: does it predict functionally significant coronary lesions? Eur Heart J Cardiovasc Imaging. 2014;15(1):85–94.
73. Bamberg F, Becker A, Schwarz F, Marcus RP, Greif M, von Ziegler F, Blankstein R, Hoffmann U, Sommer WH, Hoffmann VS, Johnson TR, Becker HC, Wintersperger BJ, Reiser MF, Nikolaou K. Detection of hemodynamically significant coronary artery stenosis: incremental diagnostic value of dynamic CT-based myocardial perfusion imaging. Radiology. 2011;260(3):689–98.
74. Kim SM, Cho YK, Choe YH. Adenosine-stress dynamic myocardial perfusion imaging using 128-slice dual-source CT in patients with normal body mass indices: effect of tube voltage, tube current, and iodine concentration on image quality and radiation dose. Int J Cardiovasc Imaging. 2014;30(Suppl 2):95–103.
75. Meinel FG, Wichmann JL, Schoepf UJ, Pugliese F, Ebersberger U, Lo GG, Choe YH, Wang Y, Tesche C, Segreto S, Kunz WG, Thierfelder KM, Bamberg F, De Cecco CN. Global quantification of left ventricular myocardial perfusion at dynamic CT imaging: prognostic value. J Cardiovasc Comput Tomogr. 2017;11(1):16–24.
76. Meinel FG, Pugliese F, Schoepf UJ, Ebersberger U, Wichmann JL, Lo GG, Choe YH, Wang Y, Segreto S, Bamberg F, De Cecco CN. Prognostic value of stress dynamic myocardial perfusion CT in a multicenter population with known or suspected coronary artery disease. AJR Am J Roentgenol. 2017;8:W1–9.
77. Min JK, Berman DS, Budoff MJ, Jaffer FA, Leipsic J, Leon MB, Mancini GB, Mauri L, Schwartz RS, Shaw LJ. Rationale and design of the DeFACTO (determination of fractional flow reserve by anatomic computed tomographic AngiOgraphy) study. J Cardiovasc Comput Tomogr. 2011;5(5):301–9.
78. Taylor CA, Fonte TA, Min JK. Computational fluid dynamics applied to cardiac computed tomography for noninvasive quantification of fractional flow reserve: scientific basis. J Am Coll Cardiol. 2013;61(22):2233–41.
79. Panchal HB, Veeranki SP, Bhatheja S, Barry N, Mahmud E, Budoff M, Lavine SJ, Mamudu HM, Paul TK. Fractional flow reserve using computed tomography for assessing coronary artery disease: a meta-analysis. J Cardiovasc Med (Hagerstown). 2016;17(9):694–700.
80. Douglas PS, De Bruyne B, Pontone G, Patel MR, Norgaard BL, Byrne RA, Curzen N, Purcell I, Gutberlet M, Rioufol G, Hink U, Schuchlenz HW, Feuchtner G, Gilard M, Andreini D, Jensen JM, Hadamitzky M, Chiswell K, Cyr D, Wilk A, Wang F, Rogers C, Hlatky MA, PLATFORM Investigators. 1-year outcomes of FFRCT-guided care in patients with suspected coronary disease: The PLATFORM Study. J Am Coll Cardiol. 2016;68(5):435–45.
81. Chinnaiyan KM, Akasaka T, Amano T, Bax JJ, Blanke P, De Bruyne B, Kawasaki T, Leipsic J, Matsuo H, Morino Y, Nieman K, Norgaard BL, Patel MR, Pontone G, Rabbat M, Rogers C, Sand NP, Raff G. Rationale, design and goals of the heart flow assessing diagnostic value of non-invasive FFRCT in coronary care (ADVANCE) registry. J Cardiovasc Comput Tomogr. 2017;11(1):62–7.
82. Itu L, Rapaka S, Passerini T, Georgescu B, Schwemmer C, Schoebinger M, Flohr T, Sharma P, Comaniciu D. A machine-learning approach for computation of fractional flow reserve from coronary computed tomography. J Appl Physiol (1985). 2016;121(1):42–52.
83. Yang DH, Kim YH, Roh JH, Kang JW, Ahn JM, Kweon J, Lee JB, Choi SH, Shin ES, Park DW, Kang SJ, Lee SW, Lee CW, Park SW, Park SJ, Lim TH. Diagnostic performance of on-site CT-derived fractional flow reserve versus CT perfusion. Eur Heart J Cardiovasc Imaging. 2017;18:432–40.
84. Coenen A, Rossi A, Lubbers MM, Kurata A, Kono AK, Chelu RG, Segreto S, Dijkshoorn ML, Wragg A, van Geuns RM, Pugliese F, Nieman K. Integrating CT myocardial perfusion and CT-FFR in the work-up of coronary artery disease. JACC Cardiovasc Imaging. 2017. pii: S1936-878X(16)30975-5. https://doi.org/10.1016/j.jcmg.2016.09.028.
85. Nakazato R, Park HB, Berman DS, Gransar H, Koo BK, Erglis A, Lin FY, Dunning AM, Budoff MJ, Malpeso J, Leipsic J, Min JK. Noninvasive fractional flow reserve derived from computed tomography angiography for coronary lesions of intermediate stenosis severity: results from the DeFACTO study. Circ Cardiovasc Imaging. 2013;6(6):881–9.
86. Chow BJ, Small G, Yam Y, Chen L, Achenbach S, Al-Mallah M, Berman DS, Budoff MJ, Cademartiri F, Callister TQ, Chang H-J, Cheng V, Chinnaiyan K, Delago A, Dunning A, Hadamitzky M, Hausleiter J, Kaufmann P, Lin F, Maffei E, Raff GL, Shaw LJ, Villines TC, Min JK. Incremental prognostic value of cardiac CT in CAD using CONFIRM (COroNary computed tomography angiography evaluation for clinical outcomes: an international multicenter registry). Circ Cardiovasc Imaging. 2011;4:463–72.
87. Motwani M, Dey D, Berman DS, et al. Machine learning for prediction of all-cause mortality in patients with suspected coronary artery disease: a 5-year multicentre prospective registry analysis. Eur Heart J. 2017;38(7):500–7.

Machine Learning and Artificial Intelligence in Cardiovascular Imaging

68

Marwen Eid, James V. Spearman, Marly van Assen, Domenico De Santis, Pooyan Sahbaee, Scott P. Landreth, Brian Jacobs, and Carlo N. De Cecco

Introduction

Artificial intelligence (AI) has captured the minds of science fiction writers and the general public for quite some time. As advancements have been made in computer science and engineering research, much improved computational power and the creation of newer, more efficient algorithms such as machine learning (ML) and deep learning (DL) have enabled the feasibility of big data analysis. AI has moved from the realm of science fiction to applications used in everyday life, such as Tesla's self-driving cars, Facebook's facial recognition, Amazon's product recommendations, mobile check deposits, language translation software, and more.

As AI continues to improve, ML algorithms can now master tasks that were previously thought to be too complex for machines and are now even capable of detecting patterns that are beyond human perception [1]. This has led to a renewed and increased interest in ML as a useful tool in medical practice, particularly in the field of medical imaging [1]. Indeed, now more than ever, medicine has become a big data science, with the introduction of electronic medical records (EMR) leading to a substantial amount of patient information being recorded. This available information will only increase in the future through the use of bidirectional patient portals. Moreover, in the era of evidence-based medicine, thousands of new evidence and data are being published daily. Going through such large volumes of data to determine what is clinically relevant and actionable can be overwhelming, resulting in important information being missed by physicians. However, AI machines can now consistently perform repetitive tasks at maximum capacity, sometimes producing results faster and more efficiently than humans. Medicine is thereby a perfect testing ground for the application of ML, as these systems can augment the ability of physicians to identify key information required for patient management while presenting it in an understandable manner. In particular, because radiology directly involves extracting data consisting of specific features seen on images and interpreting them through the knowledge base acquired by the radiologist, the medical imaging field serves as an attractive arena for the incorporation of ML systems.

As advanced AI and ML systems transition from fiction to reality and steadily approach their implementation into medical and radiology practices, understanding the general methods, capabilities, and limitations of machine learning is of fundamental importance to physicians and radiologists for the effective use of these systems. This chapter will introduce some of the basic concepts of machine learning techniques, provide a basic framework for their use, and highlight current and future applications in medicine and radiology with a special focus on cardiovascular imaging.

Machine Learning and Artificial Intelligence

Basics and Learning Process

ML is the science of how computers learn from data [2, 3]; it encompasses a wide range of statistical analysis algorithms that iteratively improve with exposure to data, meaning that the performance of the system improves with time and expe-

M. Eid (✉) · J. V. Spearman · M. van Assen · S. P. Landreth
B. Jacobs
Department of Radiology and Radiological Science, Medical University of South Carolina, Charleston, SC, USA

D. De Santis
Department of Radiological Sciences, Oncological and Pathological Sciences, University of Rome "Sapienza", Latina, Italy

Division of Cardiovascular Imaging, Department of Radiology and Radiological Science, Medical University of South Carolina, Charleston, SC, USA

P. Sahbaee
Siemens Medical Solutions USA, Inc., Malvern, PA, USA

C. N. De Cecco
Department of Radiology and Radiological Science, Medical University of South Carolina, Charleston, SC, USA

Department of Radiology and Imaging Sciences, Emory University, Atlanta, GA, USA

U. J. Schoepf (ed.), *CT of the Heart*, Contemporary Medical Imaging, https://doi.org/10.1007/978-1-60327-237-7_68

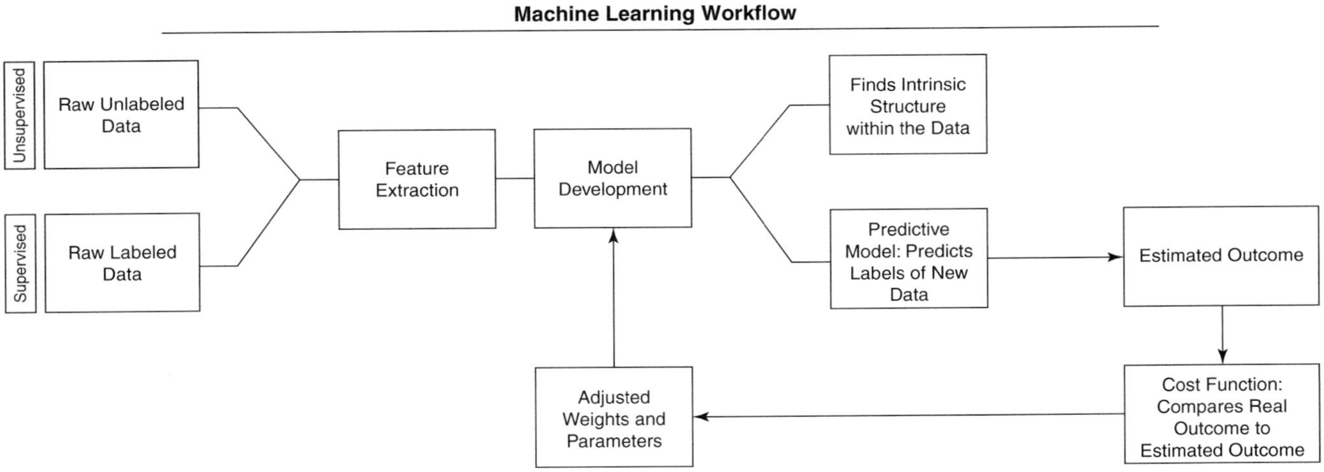

Fig. 68.1 Typical workflow of machine learning algorithms. In supervised learning, the algorithm is given labeled data, i.e., the true answer, based on which it will learn to classify this data. The estimated outcome is then compared with the true outcome, and the weights and parameters are adjusted accordingly until optimal performance is reached. On the other hand, in unsupervised learning, the algorithm is given unlabeled data, i.e., it does not know the ground truth. The objective is for the algorithm to find intrinsic meaning in the data and classify them into groups of similar characteristics

rience [4]. Thus, ML systems aim to develop mathematical models that interpret the provided data in a meaningful way in order to later predict the label of new data; in other words, to create a model for autonomous predictions (Fig. 68.1). Because ML can extract meaningful patterns from large amounts of data, which is a component of human intelligence, it is considered to be a branch of AI.

All ML algorithms require a set of input data and desired outputs [5]. Input data such as images and specific report text are fed to the neural network, which is the name given to computer systems that simulate the way in which human brains think and solve problems. This data is transmitted through a collection of nodes. The node or artificial neuron multiplies each of these inputs by a weight. Then it adds the multiplications and passes the sum to an activation function. Notice that input nodes do not have activation functions. The weights indeed reflect importance of that node or feature relative to the task at hand, such that more important features receive higher weights than less important or irrelevant features [6]. Nodes can be grouped into a hidden layer. When input data is given to the algorithm, the hidden layers act as feature detectors that play important roles in decoding the inputs and transforming them into what the output layer expects. This is referred to as the forward propagation phase. After the outcome is computed, the difference error between the calculated outcome and the given true outcome is calculated and propagated in a backward direction to estimate the contribution of each node to the total error. This is known as the back propagation phase. Based on that information, the algorithm adjusts the weights. Through a series of forward and back propagation, minimizing the error, the algorithm iteratively learns how to best approximate the desired outcome and create the best possible model for future predictions [1, 5].

Practically, there are two ways for ML systems to learn, known as supervised and unsupervised learning [7] (Fig. 68.2). In supervised learning, the input data is labeled with the correct answer. These labels can be as specific or as general as needed. The system is then given a series of validation sets, also called training sets, which will be used to train the algorithm and improve its performance until it reaches a point of no further improvement. At this point, the machine is given a test dataset in order to test the model's performance. For example, in coronary artery calcium detection, a ML algorithm undergoing supervised learning would be given a dataset of coronary arteries images with calcified plaques labeled as calcium. Once the algorithm has reached its optimal performance, it would be given an unlabeled dataset of coronary arteries with the aim of autonomously detecting calcium deposits. Most machine learning algorithms applicable to radiology use supervised learning (Figs. 68.3 and 68.4). On the other hand, in unsupervised learning, the machine is exposed to unlabeled data. The objective is for the algorithm to generate its own labels, detect patterns, and organize the data in a consequential fashion. These new labels can then be used in a supervised learning system to generate a useful prediction model; this is called semi-supervised learning.

In a classic three-layer neural network (input, hidden, and output), inputs are analyzed by a single hidden layer in order to produce an output. With advancements in processing and computational power, the combination of multiple hidden layers has now become feasible, creating deep learning (DL)

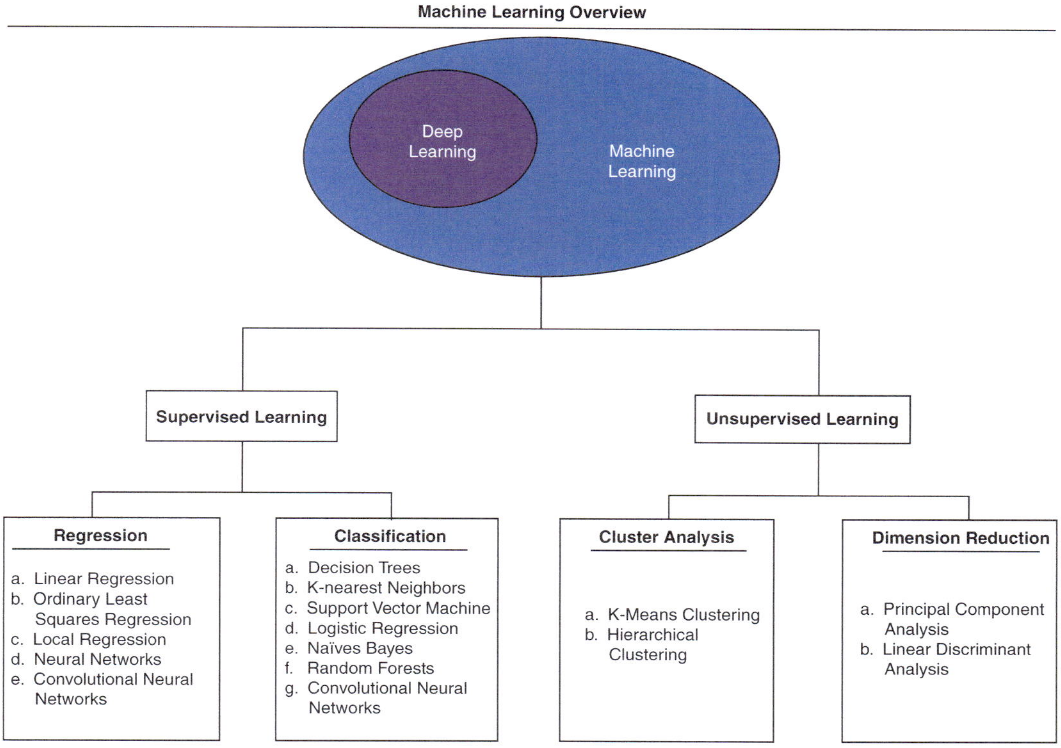

Fig. 68.2 Overview of machine learning algorithms. Machine learning algorithms can be divided into two most commonly used learning methods: supervised and unsupervised learning. The choice of the optimal algorithm greatly depends on the problem to be solved. Neural networks and convolutional neural networks deliver good performance with image feature detection and are commonly used in medical imaging. Decision tress, k-nearest neighbors, support vector machines, naive Bayes, and random forest are also common algorithms employed in medicine and radiology

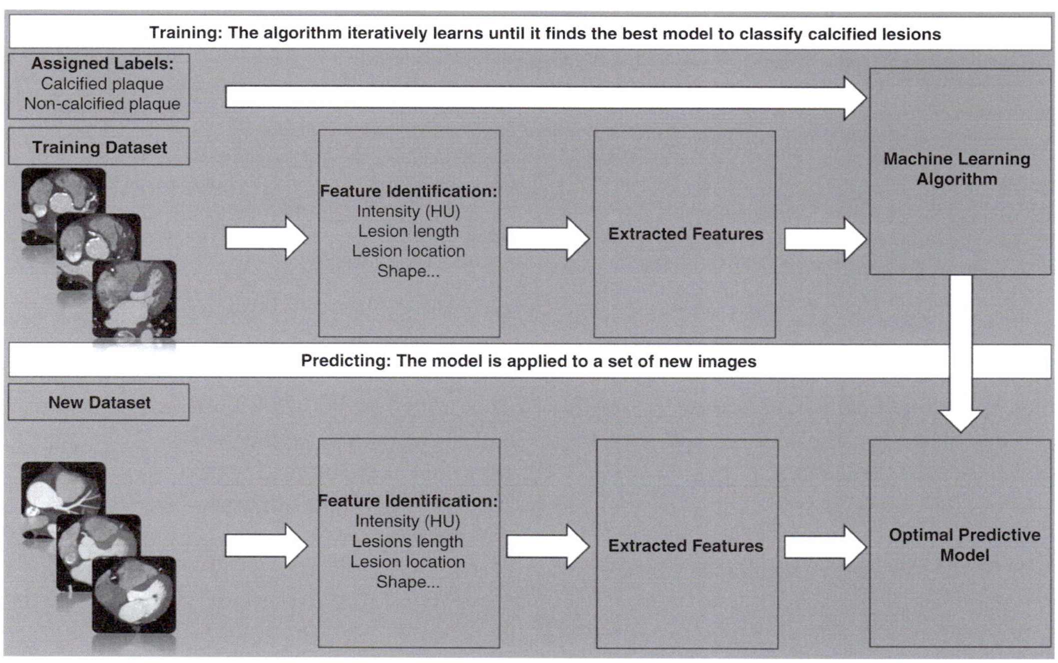

Fig. 68.3 Example of a machine learning algorithm development and training. In the training phase, the algorithm is taught to detect specific image features, based on the labeled data of the training set, which will be used to subsequently correctly classify future data. The weights for each feature are adjusted as the training progresses until the optimal predictive model is reached. In the predicting phase, the algorithm will use the features it learned and their corresponding weights to assign labels, calcified and noncalcified plaque in this example, to never before seen data

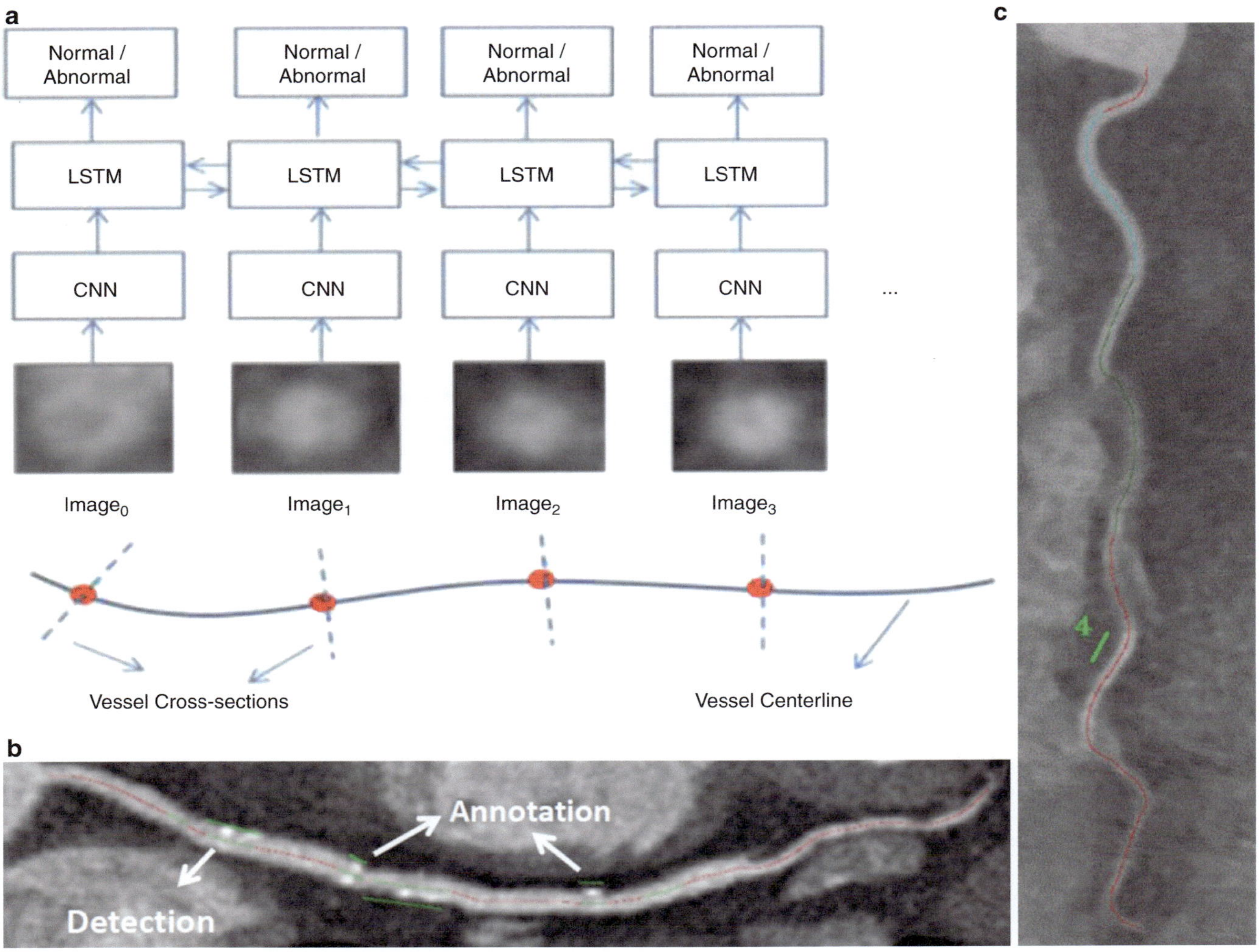

Fig. 68.4 Illustration of a machine learning algorithm for the detection of coronary artery calcium. (**a**) Scheme of a recurrent neural network with long short term memory used at our institution for the automatic detection of coronary artery calcium. (**b**) Curved multiplanar reconstruction of the left anterior descending artery where the arrows and annotation represent coronary artery calcium as manually noted by a reader and the centerline represents the automatic segmentation by the algorithm where the green portion shows automatically detected calcium and the red portion the artery segments with no detected calcium. As can be seen, the algorithm performs as accurately as the reader. (**c**) Case example of a false positive where the algorithm detects calcium in the mid and proximal parts of the right coronary artery as shown by the green centerline when in fact no calcium is present. Image courtesy of Siemens Healthineers

neural networks (Fig. 68.5). DL networks allow one to approach and solve more complex and advanced problems. In deep learning, a convolutional neural network (CNN) is a class of deep neural networks, most commonly applied to analyzing visual imagery such as medical images.

Limitations of Machine Learning Algorithms

Computer science literature is full of debate regarding the selection of algorithms and how much testing is necessary before optimal efficiency is achieved [8, 9], largely because the accuracy of the algorithm is a function of dataset size and time (i.e., computational power). Dataset size, particularly in imaging applications, has the potential to outpace computational power. For example, a coronary CT angiography study from a high-definition scanner can consume approximately half a gigabyte of storage space. A patient of interest to a study might have up to 3 or 4 of these scans and another gigabyte of medical records data, yielding 3 gigabytes of data per patient as a conservative estimate. A recent study by Motwani et al. analyzed 10,000 patients [10] which, using the previous example, would account for approximately 30 terabytes of data. The practical limitations of computational resources require the pairing of data, as was done in this study, to generate in the near term a less comprehensive dataset based on values derived from CT images or portions of medical records. In that same regard, the availability of

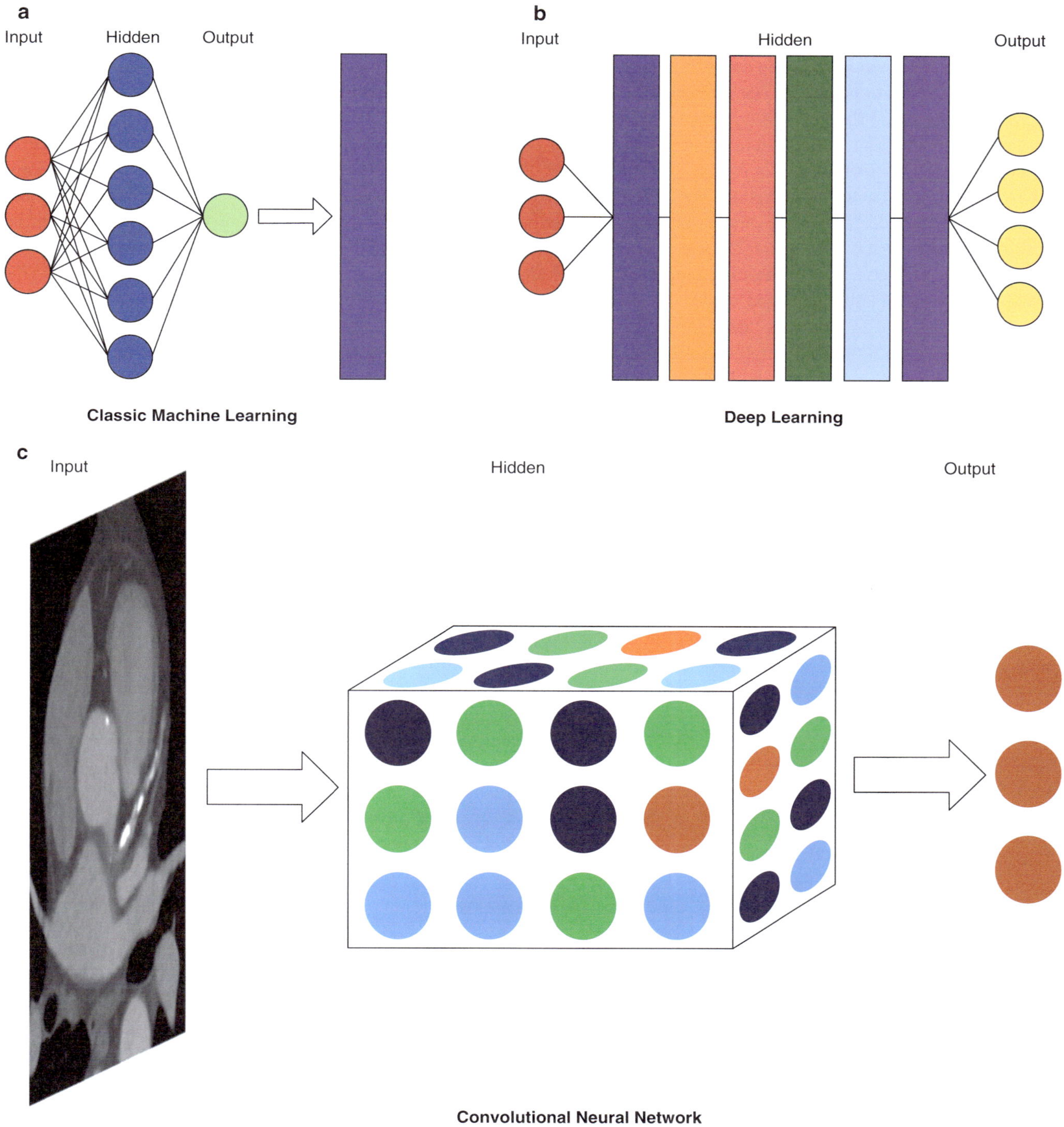

Fig. 68.5 Concepts of machine learning algorithms commonly used in medical imaging analysis. (**a**) Classic three-layer machine learning scheme where the first layer represents the input, the second layer is composed of the hidden nodes containing the weights and parameters, and the third layer is the calculated output. (**b**) With deep learning, all three layers of the classic scheme become one hidden layer. A number of hidden layers can be combined allowing much more complex problem solving. (**c**) Convolutional neural networks are a particular form of deep learning which perform particularly well with image analysis. They apply mathematical transformations on individual pixels, evaluate the outcome, and eventually identify specific portions of the image. When a number of these convolutions are combined, they can recognize more complex structures within the image

labeled data for algorithm training can also be an obstacle to ML implementation. Truly, the legal procedures to acquire medical data are complex, and even completely anonymized data must gain institutional review board approval prior to its distribution. Because ML algorithms continually improve as they learn from new data, these systems typically require tremendous amounts of data to be fully optimized for a specific task [11]. A potential solution to this problem is the creation of publically available "banks" of data, containing massive amounts of images that have been validated and annotated by experts readily available for ML training purposes [12–17]. Lastly, even with available data, the quality of the training data must be optimal to reach the algorithm's best performance. This is a well-known principle coined "garbage in, garbage out" by computer scientists, in which poor-quality input will always yield poor-quality output.

ML systems are able to make highly accurate predications or diagnoses analyzing complex relationships. However, an important pitfall of these systems when considering their application in clinical work or medical research is overfitting (Fig. 68.6). Overfitting is when a statistical model tends to describe random errors or noise rather than the true underlying relationship between the data of a training set. This typically occurs when the model is more complex than it needs to be to reach optimal efficiency. For example, having too many parameters relative to the number of observations or using too few training examples during learning can cause the algorithm to adjust to very specific but random features of the data that have no causative relationship to the ground truth. The result is a model that is too specific to the examples it was shown, rendering overly optimistic results for its accuracy while underperforming when exposed to unfamiliar real-world data.

Applications of Machine Learning in Medicine

The clinical practice of medicine is one of the fields that can largely benefit from machine learning systems. Through these algorithms, hundreds of thousands of variables such as patient information, demographics, lab values, and radiology and pathology images can be analyzed alongside medical literature and applied to patient care for risk stratification as well as to determine appropriate patient management and prognosis.

Clinical Decision Support Tool

As most clinical work is conducted in accordance with an evidence-based medicine approach, it is important for clinicians to keep abreast of novel published medical evidence. However, the sheer number of new peer-reviewed journal publications is increasing at an exponential rate, making it overwhelming for physicians to stay current with new evidence while treating patients. ML systems can be of great assistance in this regard with the ability to constantly analyze literature for new evidence which, combined with patient information, can recommend an appropriate course of treatment. IBM's AI software, Watson, is currently being investigated for such use, specifically for applications in oncology. Watson's particular advantage is its capacity for natural language processing. This refers to the ability of a computer to understand human language as it is spoken or written as opposed to requiring a highly precise programming language or very clear but brief voice commands. In a study by Seidman et al., the ability of Watson to recommend multidisciplinary

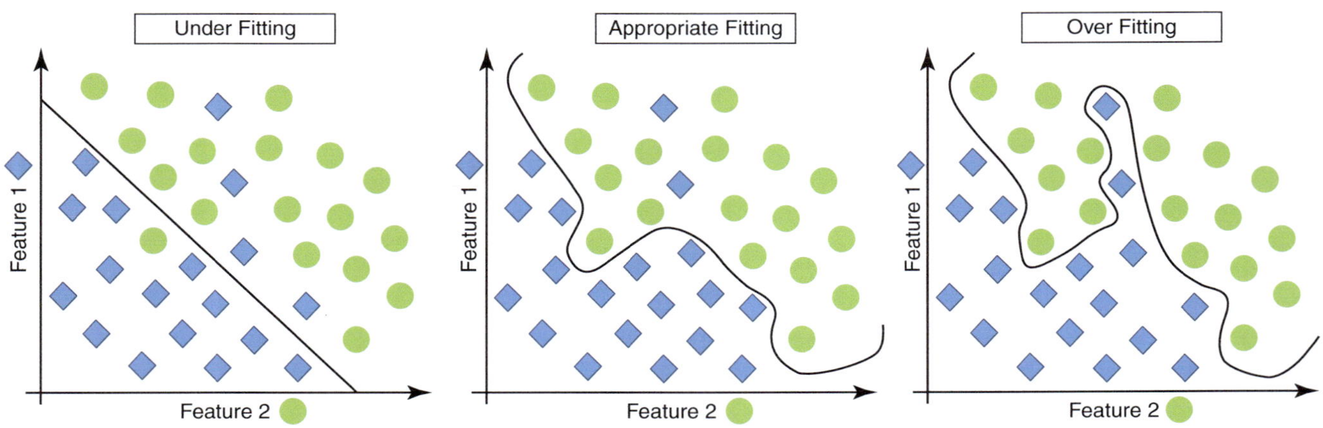

Fig. 68.6 Illustration of under- and overfitting. Underfitting occurs when the algorithm is too simple to capture the underlying trend in the data. Specifically, the algorithm shows low variance but high bias. An appropriate fit is seen when the algorithm performs well and in a balanced way on both training and test sets without being to flexible or inflexible in fitting the data. Overfitting on the other hand captures the underlying trend in the data too well and is generally too good to be true, and the model shows low bias but high variance. This tends to happen when the algorithm is excessively complex and is capturing noise as part of the data. Validation and cross-validation with test sets is crucial to prevent overfitting

patient management in early stage breast cancer was investigated [18]. The software was able to correctly recommend radiotherapy in 98% of cases, genetic counseling in 94%, and fertility preservation in 91%.

In a time when healthcare systems are facing physician shortages and increasing quantities and complexities of patient data are being recorded with the introduction of electronic health records, the increased workload for healthcare providers can result in oversight of important information. Given that correct diagnosis and appropriate patient management are the physician's most important tasks, ML systems can be implemented in situations where they can serve as highly efficient assistants by analyzing thousands of data in the form of clinical notes, lab results, radiology images, electrocardiogram tracings, and even genomic sequences. With all of this information, ML systems can then infer clinical causations that may eventually be presented to the physician in real time to assist with clinical decision-making. This application could be particularly helpful in acute care settings where physicians must make lifesaving decisions in a timely manner. One such setting in which ML systems are being evaluated is the intensive care unit (ICU). Patients admitted to the ICU typically present with acute illness and are at a higher risk of mortality. As large amounts of patient data are routinely recorded in the ICU, it seems an attractive setting to input data into ML models, infer causalities, and predict outcomes, with final predictions being presented to physicians in a clinically actionable manner [19]. In a retrospective study by Gultepe et al., the authors used ML algorithms in septic patients in the ICU to predict rising lactate levels, a sign of organ failure, as well as mortality with routinely measured data [20]. Results demonstrated the ability to predict rising lactate levels by using vital signs and white blood cell counts as inputs, achieving a discriminatory power of 0.98 by area under the curve (AUC). Moreover, their ML system was able to predict mortality with a discriminatory power and accuracy of 0.73. These results highlight the potential of using ML algorithms for early detection of sepsis and multiple organ failure, prompting a timely intervention and possible reduction of mortality.

In a more recent study by Gulshan et al., a DL algorithm was used to screen for referable diabetic retinopathy and macular edema from acquired retinal images. Using the algorithm on two different datasets, they were able to reach an AUC of 0.991 and 0.990, sensitivities of 97.5% and 96.1%, and specificities of 93.4% and 93.9% [21]. This study demonstrated the potential of integrating ML systems to enhance routine clinical workflow where simple validated tests can be analyzed to infer a diagnosis. This can be particularly helpful when a disease is very prevalent and a validated screening method requiring time and resources can be delegated to ML systems, thus allowing clinicians to focus on more important and urgent tasks.

Machine learning systems learn in an analogous way to a resident in training, from observation. The more they see, the better they get. However, one superior aspect of ML systems is that information is never forgotten. This is particularly important for rare diseases; which ML systems may potentially identify more efficiently than trained physicians to allow for timelier interventions. In this regard, Liu et al. investigated the accuracy of a ML algorithm in detecting congenital cataracts from ocular images, compared with detection by expert ophthalmologists [22]. The algorithm achieved an accuracy of 99% and suggested the correct treatment plan in 97% of cases. When applied to three sets of 100 ocular images, each containing one case of congenital cataract, the algorithm successfully identified and provided accurate treatment recommendations while making fewer mistakes than the three expert ophthalmologists. Early detection of disease often translates into improved patient prognosis and is an area of medicine where ML can be of great of use. Investigators have used DL methods to detect skin cancer, which can be lifesaving if diagnosed early. The ability of the DL algorithm to detect skin cancer was compared with 21 expert dermatologists [23]. The algorithm's performance was comparable to the dermatologists, demonstrating the ability of ML to accurately diagnose skin lesions. These two studies show the potential added value of ML applications in particularly rural areas, where access to expert clinicians is not readily available and early diagnosis of rare or fatal diseases is more likely to be missed.

Predicting Prognosis and Outcome

Predicting prognosis and outcome is a central component of clinical practice as it is directly related to choosing an appropriate management plan. Most scoring systems used are based on a limited number of clinical, laboratory, or imaging findings. ML systems have the ability to consider larger quantities and complexities of variables, potentially generating more accurate prediction models based on novel or unknown predictors. As a result, the evaluation of ML algorithms for the prediction of prognosis and outcomes in different clinical settings compared with routine scoring systems is of great importance.

One particular field of interest for this application is oncology, where diagnosis and prognosis are often derived from histopathological analysis. In a study by Beck et al., the authors investigated the ability of a ML system named "C-Path" to perform a semiquantitative analysis of breast histopathology slides and to infer patient survival rates [24]. The algorithm was able to detect 6642 morphological features used to construct a prognostic model. The features recognized by "C-Path" were independent from prognostic factors used in clinical routine and were significantly associated with patient survival (*P-value* < 0.001). Of the 11 most important features associated with patient survival, 3 were related to the stroma and proved to be the strongest predictors of survival. Interestingly, most morphological features used for prognosis in clinical practice are derived from the epithelium.

In a similar, yet more recent study by Yu et al., a ML algorithm was used to predict non-small cell lung cancer prognosis using a fully automated analysis of histopathologic features [25]. Based on 2186 histopathology slides, the algorithm was able to detect more than 9000 features to predict patient prognosis. The top 80 features were first used to accurately differentiate cancerous tissue from normal tissue, achieving an AUC of 0.85. These features were also able to differentiate between adenocarcinoma and squamous cell carcinoma with an AUC of 0.85. For both adenocarcinoma and squamous cell carcinoma, the features detected by the algorithm significantly correlated with patient survival. In contrast, the tumor grade, a marker often used clinically, was not significantly correlated with patient survival. These two studies exemplify the ability of ML systems to predict survival models based on a much greater number of features with more complexities than previously unknown by clinicians. This ability of ML has the potential to lead to a substantial change in patient management.

Machine Learning: The Road to Precision Medicine?

An exciting aspect of using ML in medicine is the possibility of precision medicine, defined by the national institute of health as "disease treatment and prevention that takes into account individual variability in genes, environment, and lifestyle for each person" [26]. Indeed, while medicine to date has been based on a population-wide diagnostic and treatment model, it is possible that in many cases the "standard of care" treatment may not be the optimal management plan. Integrating specific patient data from demographics, clinical reports, lab values, imaging results, and genomic sequences to be analyzed by the machine can be combined with decision support tools such as IBM's Watson. Decision support tools are constantly updated with the most recent literature with the potential to provide improved, patient-tailored recommendations for risk assessment, outcome prediction, and subsequent treatment and management.

An important area where such use is being extensively researched is oncology, particularly in genomic and molecular medicine. In these areas of study, the input of clinical data and patient genomic and molecular profiles into ML systems such as Watson is helping to provide a diagnosis as well as patient-tailored treatment options [27–31]. In a study by McDonald et al., a support vector machine-based algorithm to predict treatment response in patients with ovarian cancer based on individual genomic profiles was evaluated [29]. Gene expression data was found to provide accurate results by correctly predicting treatment responsiveness with 80–100% accuracy.

Since unsupervised learning allows the algorithm to detect meaningful patterns from unlabeled data, it can be an additional method suitable for precision medicine. Indeed, through unsupervised learning, thousands of patient data regarding specific diseases with particularly heterogeneous clinical presentations can be analyzed by ML algorithms to deduce more accurate risk stratification based on individual patient phenotypes. In a recent study by Shah et al., the clinical and radiological data of 397 patients diagnosed with heart failure with preserved ejection fraction were analyzed by a ML algorithm [32]. The algorithm was able to divide the patients into three clinically distinct subgroups based on clinical characteristics, cardiac structure and function, invasive hemodynamic parameters, and outcome. This study showed the potential of ML systems in creating accurate, clinically similar subcategories of patients with rather heterogeneous diseases, allowing for improved risk stratification and ultimately defining therapeutically homogeneous subclasses.

Applications of Machine Learning in Radiology

ML software has had substantial success in image feature detection and pattern recognition in daily life applications. With radiology being, at least in part, a science of detecting clinically relevant features and patterns from acquired images, it naturally serves as a prime candidate for ML applications. At their earlier stages, these systems were hampered by low computational power, limiting the amount of data that could be processed. However currently, with increased computational power, graphics processing unit-based computing, and the development of DL, the application of ML to radiology has become feasible and is gaining interest from physicians as well as computer scientists. As radiology has become a central part of patient management, with new imaging technologies constantly creating new possibilities for solving clinical problems, radiologists often find themselves dealing with an abundant amount of studies to review. Much of the time spent during the assessment of these studies is dedicated to more trivial tasks such as image segmentation, searching for lung nodules, microcalcifications in breast tissue, or looking for small bone fractures in cases that are often negative. A clinical practice where these tasks can be delegated to a ML algorithm would result in a much more enhanced workflow, allowing the radiologist to focus on more important tasks such as looking at truly emergent or complex cases and making a prompt diagnosis. The fairly recent and rapid improvements to ML have allowed these systems to handle much more complex tasks, constantly learning and improving their performance more efficiently. As a result, completion of basic tasks using ML systems has become feasible, and more applications for their use, such as computer-aided diagnosis and image segmentation, are continuously being evaluated [33].

Image segmentation is an important step in reaching an accurate diagnosis for both radiologists and ML systems if they are to reach a point of automated image analysis in the future. However, it is a time-consuming process prone to inter- and intraindividual variability. As imaging technologies improve, more detailed anatomy is being captured, and the need to perform time-consuming tasks such as segmentation will only increase. While automating this process can be beneficial by means of enhancing a radiologist's workflow, it remains a challenge for ML systems due to the high variation in human anatomy, thus requiring a tremendous amount of data to reach optimal accuracy. However, with recent advancements in ML technology and particularly the development of DL, novel algorithms are outperforming previous versions and are now capable of faster, more accurate, and even fully automated image segmentation. Recent studies are demonstrating this capability with applications for brain segmentation on MRI [34–36], rib cage, airway, pulmonary lobes and nodules from chest CT [37–39], tumor and organs-at-risk segmentation from CT images in radiation oncology [40, 41], third lumbar vertebra detection from CT [42], and fully automated abdominal analysis from CT [43].

A much anticipated application of ML in radiology is computer-aided diagnosis (CADx). While computers have been helping radiologists for decades, it is expected that increased computational power and more sophisticated algorithms such as DL will render them faster, more efficient, and more accurate in completing this task [44]. Indeed, computer systems are now much better at detecting more complex radiological findings and diagnosing a wider array of conditions. An exciting example is IBM's Watson. In acquiring Merge Healthcare in 2015 to the tune of $1 billion, IBM was able to provide Watson with over 30 billion images to learn from. Presented at the Radiological Society of North America conference in 2016, in an important step for precision medicine and CADx in radiology, Watson showcased its potential to analyze patient history and clinical data in addition to radiological images to reach a diagnosis in a number of conditions including aortic dissection, pulmonary embolism, and breast lesions. Moreover, several studies have already shown the ability of ML systems in detecting abnormalities with an accuracy comparable if not superior to that of expert radiologists for different conditions such as colonic polyps on CT colonography [45], sclerotic bone metastases and enlarged lymph nodes on body CT [44], cerebral microbleeds from MRI [46], interstitial lung disease [47], pulmonary nodules detection [48, 49] and classification [50], pulmonary embolism [51], classification of chest radiographs [52], prostate cancer [53], and breast cancer [54–57].

Machine Learning in Cardiovascular Imaging

Radiology should be at the forefront of medical specialties embracing ML applications, and cardiac imaging has proven to be one of the first specialties quickly adapting to that change. The field has seen a wide range of ML uses such as image segmentation, feature detection, CADx, risk, and prognosis prediction in a variety of modalities such as CT, MRI, nuclear imaging, and echocardiography [58–62].

Computer-Aided Diagnosis

Machine-based evaluation of cardiac datasets involving human-specified parameters is well established in clinical practice. However, new forms of analysis are emerging that allow the machine to evaluate what parameters should be measured based on a known endpoint. Early attempts at such systems struggled with the volume of data and the number of potential variables creating processing times that prohibited large, high-quality evaluation. Despite these early shortcomings, advances in both processing power and model sophistication are reaching a point where systems can be trained using information from tens of thousands of patients with hundreds of thousands of data points being evaluated. This type of analysis requires both sophisticated ML algorithms and specialized statistics to elucidate new parameters for clinical evaluation. While many of these methods are still in the nascent phase of research, some are now emerging as a part of clinical workflows.

Computational support of cardiac imaging utilizing basic algorithms is not a new concept. Quantifying image density for gross measurement of cardiac calcium scores is common place and provides meaningful clinical guidance in many diagnostic scenarios. Likewise, pattern recognition for the identification and lengthwise evaluation of coronary arteries reduces the complexity of coronary artery stenosis. Similar pattern recognition systems are being used for CT-FFR, automated cardiac volume measurements, and wall motion characterization [63]. These algorithms are early forms of ML-based clinical support applications, as the data they generate are fed into human algorithms used to predict clinical risk. These applications are categorized as diagnostic support tools.

Diagnostic support tools may rely on ML for their development, but differ fundamentally from true ML systems in that they are not adaptive. In other words, once the pattern recognition is established, it is fixed and cannot be retrained. ML systems can potentially be able to adapt to unpredicted patterns that generate errors in pattern recognition applications.

As mentioned earlier, accurate image segmentation is a crucial part of image diagnosis and a critical step in reaching a fully automated analysis of radiological studies. As opposed to the current CADx software which follow a rigid set of rules, ML systems could potentially learn as they are exposed to more data and are thus prone to adapt to the variation in individual anatomies. This inherently results in a more accurate segmentation process across the board.

In a study by Avendi et al., the authors evaluated the performance of a ML algorithm using convolutional neural networks in segmenting the left ventricle from magnetic resonance imaging datasets for the evaluation of cardiac function [64]. Their proposed algorithm performed better than previous methods by reaching good contours in 96.69% of cases and correlation coefficients of 0.98, 0.99, and 0.98 for end-diastolic volume, end-systolic volume, and ejection fraction, respectively, when compared with manual evaluation.

Myocardial perfusion imaging (MPI) is another field of cardiac imaging where ML is quickly gaining ground in terms of its application. MPI plays an important role in the diagnosis of coronary artery disease (CAD) as it provides important information regarding myocardial perfusion, which is directly related to the significance of coronary artery stenoses as well as ventricular function information. Although perfusion quantification with MPI is becoming increasingly automated [65, 66], diagnosis remains visually based by physicians who often need to supervise the segmentation process, as errors in segmentation may lead to false positives [67]. In a study performed by Betancur et al., a support vector machine-based ML algorithm was used for a more precise automated definition of the mitral valve plane during left ventricle segmentation in single-photon emission computed tomography (SPECT) [68]. The algorithm was tested on 392 patients who had undergone same-day SPECT and coronary computed tomography angiography (CCTA) after a tenfold cross-validation process and was compared with the results of two expert readers. Results determined that their ML algorithm performed just as well as the two expert readers regarding both mitral valve placement and diagnostic accuracy for perfusion defects, with no significant difference observed in correlation or AUC between the algorithm and the expert readers.

Reaching a point where machines can make a full diagnosis and radiology workflows can be fully automated remains a challenge, particularly in cardiac and chest imaging. Potential roadblocks include variation in patient anatomy as well as the high presence of motion artifacts, which make it more challenging for automated systems to accurately detect pathology. However, the accuracy of ML systems is rapidly improving. Previous studies have evaluated computer algorithms for the detection of obstructive CAD from CCTA [69–73]. While these studies all reported high sensitivity values, the corresponding specificity values were relatively low. In a recent study by Kang et al., a ML algorithm was evaluated for the detection of both obstructive and nonobstructive CAD compared with three expert readers [74]. The proposed algorithm achieved higher sensitivity, specificity, accuracy, and AUC values (93%, 95%, 94%, and 0.937, respectively) compared with previous methods which reached a sensitivity and specificity of 93% and 81%, respectively [69, 70, 73]. The ability to autonomously diagnose both obstructive and nonobstructive CAD with high accuracy, as demonstrated in this study, brings the concept of automated diagnosis in cardiac imaging one step closer to a reality.

The determination of calcium burden in the coronary arteries through coronary artery calcium scoring (CACS) is another important aspect of the diagnosis of CAD, risk stratification for adverse events, and the subsequent direction of appropriate patient management [75, 76]. CACS is usually performed following a noncontrast cardiac scan with a semiautomatic calculation of the Agatston score, which often requires manual intervention by a radiologist. In a study by Wolterink et al., a convolutional neural network-based ML algorithm was used to automatically derive calcium scores from contrast-enhanced CCTA [77]. The study included 250 patients who had undergone both CCTA and CACS scans. A two-step system was used in which the primary algorithm would first identify voxels that are likely to be calcium, followed by a secondary algorithm that definitively classifies the remaining voxels as either calcium or calcium like. Using this technique for calcium detection, a sensitivity of 71% was achieved with an average of 0.48 false positives per scan, providing a correlation of 0.944 with expert readers for calcium scores. This study shows the possibility of using ML to accurately compute CACS from CCTA, potentially precluding the need for a dedicated CACS scan. Furthermore, application of such a ML algorithm may reduce, if not eliminate, the need for manual intervention by a radiologist.

ML for diagnostic support has also been studied on cardiac echocardiography. In their study, Sengupta et al. used an associative memory classifier-based ML algorithm to differentiate constrictive pericarditis from restrictive cardiomyopathy on echocardiographic images [78]. An AUC of 0.892 was achieved using 15 variables from speckle-tracking echocardiography chosen by the algorithm. The addition of four echocardiographic features (early diastolic mitral valve velocity, ratio of early diastolic mitral flow velocity to early diastolic mitral valve annular velocity, posterior and septal wall thickness) improved the AUC to 0.962. In comparison, the AUC of the clinically used markers of early diastolic mitral valve annular velocity and left ventricular longitudinal strain were 0.821 and 0.637, respectively.

Prognosis and Outcome Prediction

As new technologies and imaging techniques are being introduced, radiology is increasingly relevant in appropriate patient management, not only for diagnostic purposes but also for the prediction of outcomes via incorporation of the many radiological features of diseases into prediction scores. However, those scores tend to rely on a limited number of factors, potentially omitting many unknown predictors from consideration. As big data analysis has become feasible through the recent advancements in ML, using these systems to predict outcomes from radiological data has gained significant interest, particularly in the field of cardiac imaging given the high morbidity and mortality rates associated with cardiovascular disease.

Indeed, coronary artery disease (CAD) is one of the most important causes of mortality and morbidity worldwide [79]. CCTA has been established as the modality of choice for the detection and characterization of atherosclerotic plaques, and several studies have shown the ability to predict future adverse events based on CCTA findings [80–83]. Thus, it is of great interest to evaluate the application of ML in predicting outcomes. In a recent prospective study including 10,030 patients by Motwani et al., the authors investigated the ability of a ML algorithm to predict 5-year all-cause mortality based on 44 CCTA features and 25 clinical features, compared with established clinical and CCTA metrics [10]. The algorithm was found to be significantly superior to routinely used scores, achieving an AUC of 0.79 vs 0.61 for the Framingham risk score, 0.64 for the segment stenosis score, 0.64 for the segment involvement score, and 0.62 for the Duke index with all P-values reported <0.001.

Dawes et al. also used a supervised ML algorithm on cardiac MRI-derived three-dimensional wall function of the right ventricle to predict outcomes in patients with pulmonary hypertension [84]. The algorithm identified certain wall contraction patterns associated with lower survival at 1 year. Particularly, loss of effective contraction in the septum and free wall as well as reduced basal longitudinal motion accurately predicted poor outcomes. When these features were added to routine hemodynamic, clinical, and functional markers, survival prediction significantly improved with an AUC of 0.73 vs 0.60 ($P < 0.001$) and was able to more accurately stratify patients between high- and low-risk groups based on median survival time (13.8 vs 10.7 years; $P < 0.001$).

In another study by Kotu et al., ML algorithms were used to extract image-based features from cardiac MRI for the classification of post-myocardial infarction patients into high and low arrhythmic risk groups [85]. The k-nearest neighbor and support vector machine-based algorithm evaluated the combination of 17 different factors for risk stratification. A combination of scar location and heterogeneity achieved an accuracy of 94.44% and an AUC of 0.965 in differentiating between high- and low-risk patients. This technique outperformed the current reference standard based on scar size and left ventricular function, which reached an accuracy and an AUC of 90.7% and 0.941, respectively.

In a study by Arsanjani et al., ML analysis was used to integrate clinical and quantitative MPI data in order to predict revascularization in patients with suspected CAD, compared with two expert readers and standalone measures of perfusion [86]. The algorithm analyzed data from 713 patients, selected 33 features, and was tested through tenfold cross-validation. Given both stress and rest perfusion data, the sensitivity of the algorithm for predicting early revascularization was comparable to readers and standalone measures of perfusion (73.6%, 73.9%, and 75.5%, respectively, $P > 0.05$). However, its specificity was found to be superior to both readers and standalone measures of perfusion (74.7 vs 67.2, 66, and 68.3, respectively), resulting in the highest AUC for ML (0.81 vs 0.81, 0.72, and 0.77, respectively). Thus, ML was found to be comparable, if not superior, to expert readers in predicting early revascularization from MPI data. This could result in a significant change in patient management, particularly in reducing unnecessary revascularization procedures via improved patient risk stratification. These studies not only suggest the ability of ML systems to predict risk and outcome in a manner comparable, if not superior to routinely used scores, but also the possibility of discovering new valid and potentially more accurate predictors that were previously unknown to clinicians and radiologists alike.

Adapting to Machine Learning

Although medicine has been slower than other fields in pursuing ML applications, early studies show very promising results. As computational power and ML algorithms improve at an exponential speed, it is only a matter of time before AI becomes a central part of medicine. Thus, it would seem wise for medical practices to start planning for such a future, with pathology and radiology being at the forefront of this change [87]. While some experts fear or even predict pathologists and radiologists to be completely replaced by ML applications, this is a premature statement due to the many remaining challenges in adapting to ML.

In order for ML systems to be optimally efficient in analyzing big data and integrated into clinical routine, they must be seamlessly interfaced with electronic medical records and other established systems. For example, in the field of radiology, ML systems must be integrated into image interpretation systems to avoid impeding clinical workflow. This is crucial for implementation, as it would not be feasible to manually enter hundreds of data points for each patient into the ML system to generate a recommendation or risk score.

Furthermore, regarding the enhancement of clinical workflows, further multicenter large-scale clinical trials are needed to validate the accuracy and efficiency of ML systems reported in previous studies. Particularly, results shown in single-center trials must be validated in studies spanning over a larger range of patient demographics, image qualities, and disease patterns and prevalence, as these often vary in different populations. The argument for further validation through multicenter trials centers on the idea that ML algorithms will have to adapt to such variations to reach maximal accuracy in real-world scenarios. This then raises the important question: how is accuracy determined? Indeed, diagnostic accuracy is modeled on the reference standard used in clinical practice. However, reference standards are not available in many situations, and even when it is, opinions vary between experts regarding diagnosis and treatment management. Consequently, it will be important to determine the appropriate reference standard to evaluate the accuracy of ML systems. Furthermore, ML systems will need to learn every "normal" in different clinical scenarios. For example, the brain of a 70-year-old patient might look completely different from that of a younger person without necessarily having clinical implications.

Another important challenge arises when considering both ethical and legal concerns. Electronic health records are slowly becoming the standard in clinical practices, which raises concerns for patient security and privacy. Despite this software being advertised as secure and impenetrable, information stored on servers is always at risk of breaches. In fact, recently targeted medical institutions all around the world were compromised, with valuable patient information being held for ransom [88]. Adding more technological components such as ML systems to the medical field will only increase the complexity of this problem. Thus, finding an effective way of securing ML systems will be central to their integration into clinical workflows. Moreover, in a future where machines could potentially diagnose and even recommend treatment options, the questions of general patient reception and legal responsibility for system errors remain ambiguous. Would it be the treating physician who is responsible for mistakes, the medical institution, the system's company, or the software's developer? What happens if a physician chooses to follow his experience-based clinical judgment rather than a ML system recommendation, resulting in an adverse event? These are just on the surface of potential obstacles that must be addressed before ML can find its way into routine clinical practice.

Since ML will be able to integrate much more data than humanly possible, it has the potential to lead to new correlations that were previously unknown to clinicians. However, these new findings require interpretation with a critical eye in order to avoid overdiagnosing, overtreating, and potentially harming patients. In a recent study by Moss et al., a ML algorithm was used to analyze patient ECG tracings in the ICU [89]. The algorithm was able to detect atrial fibrillation, which was classified as clinical when already documented and subclinical when undocumented by the clinicians. However, upon further analysis, subclinical arrhythmia was not found to be related to clinical outcomes or worsened prognosis. Although ML was better suited to detect subclinical atrial fibrillation, this had no clinical significance and could lead to overtreatment, possibly harming patients. As a result, ML data should be interpreted in light of clinical judgment.

Finally, a potential obstacle for the implementation of ML systems in medical practice is physician resistance. As ML systems exponentially improve and eventually overcome current shortcomings, physicians, particularly radiologists, fear that such systems could eventually replace them. Indeed, as these systems perfect themselves overtime and are immune to fatigue, a future where medical institutions favor machine analysis over human analysis is imaginable. In a recent article, Chockley et al. coined the term "ultimate threat to radiology" while describing ML, expressing the very real possibility of the end of radiology as a specialty within the next 10 years. Chockley particularly emphasized the public's skepticism about driverless cars not more than a decade ago, and how far that technology has reached today [90]. However, if the extinction of radiology as a specialty were to occur, it is still quite far from becoming reality. In fact, a capable radiologist is trained to detect 2613 findings and account for more than 20,000 medical conditions across all imaging domains and modalities. As it takes substantial effort in terms of time and data needed to create an algorithm accurate in the detection of a very specific finding on a single modality, it begs the question: If ever possible, how long it will take to create algorithms that can accurately detect all findings across all modalities so as to completely replace radiologists? In the coming years, it is likely that ML will at least displace some of the more routine work done by radiologists that can easily and safely be delegated to machines [91]. As Jha et al. stated, a higher education is not essential for recognizing patterns and specific signs on an image [87]. However, they argue that radiologists will still be needed as "information specialists" to interpret and highlight the important information provided by the machine while considering the patient's clinical setting. Furthermore, radiologists will remain desirable for the foreseeable future to help guide the treating team toward a diagnosis and further patient management.

Summary

The recent advancements in computational power and the development of novel, more sophisticated ML algorithms have made big data analysis in medicine feasible. Thus, ML is seeing an increasingly important role in clinical practice with a variety of applications such as clinical decision support, precision medicine, risk stratification, and prognosis prediction. As these systems become particularly apt at recognizing patterns from images, cardiovascular imaging is seeing an increased role of ML in clinical practice for image segmentation, CADx, and mortality prediction. The more likely applications in the coming years will be to enhance clinical workflow through highly accurate tools to better detect disease, assess risk, and stratify patients. Thus, ML should be viewed as an opportunity in a positive light, as optimized systems will utilize all patient data to improve quality, efficiency, and outcomes, leading to optimized patient and patient-specific care.

References

1. Erickson BJ, Korfiatis P, Akkus Z, Kline TL. Machine learning for medical imaging. Radiographics. 2017;37(2):505–15. https://doi.org/10.1148/rg.2017160130.
2. Friedman J, Hastie T, Tibshirani R. The elements of statistical learning: Springer series in statistics. Berlin: Springer; 2001.
3. Abu-Mostafa YS, Magdon-Ismail M, Lin H-T. Learning from data. New York: AMLBook; 2012.
4. Jordan M, Mitchell T. Machine learning: trends, perspectives, and prospects. Science. 2015;349(6245):255–60.
5. Kohli M, Prevedello LM, Filice RW, Geis JR. Implementing machine learning in radiology practice and research. AJR Am J Roentgenol. 2017;208(4):754–60.
6. Martinez TR, Zeng X. Feature weighting using neural networks. In: Proceedings of the IEEE International Joint Conference on Neural Networks IJCNN'04; 2004. p. 1327–30.
7. Alpaydin E. Introduction to machine learning. Cambridge: The MIT Press; 2014.
8. Langley P. Machine learning as an experimental science. Mach Learn. 1988;3(1):5–8.
9. Özöğür-Akyüz S, Ünay D, Smola A. Guest editorial: model selection and optimization in machine learning. Mach Learn. 2011;85(1):1.
10. Motwani M, Dey D, Berman DS, Germano G, Achenbach S, Al-Mallah MH, et al. Machine learning for prediction of all-cause mortality in patients with suspected coronary artery disease: a 5-year multicentre prospective registry analysis. Eur Heart J. 2017;38(7):500–7.
11. Greenspan H, van Ginneken B, Summers RM. Guest editorial deep learning in medical imaging: Overview and future promise of an exciting new technique. IEEE Trans Med Imaging. 2016;35(5):1153–9.
12. Petersen SE, Matthews PM, Bamberg F, Bluemke DA, Francis JM, Friedrich MG, et al. Imaging in population science: cardiovascular magnetic resonance in 100,000 participants of UK Biobank-rationale, challenges and approaches. J Cardiovasc Magn Reson. 2013;15(1):46.
13. Fonseca CG, Backhaus M, Bluemke DA, Britten RD, Do Chung J, Cowan BR, et al. The Cardiac Atlas Project—an imaging database for computational modeling and statistical atlases of the heart. Bioinformatics. 2011;27(16):2288–95.
14. del Toro OAJ, Goksel O, Menze B, Müller H, Langs G, Weber M-A, et al. VISCERAL–VISual Concept Extraction challenge in RAdioLogy: ISBI 2014 challenge organization. Proceedings of the VISCERAL Challenge at ISBI. 2014;1194:6–15.
15. Kirişli H, Schaap M, Metz C, Dharampal A, Meijboom WB, Papadopoulou S-L, et al. Standardized evaluation framework for evaluating coronary artery stenosis detection, stenosis quantification and lumen segmentation algorithms in computed tomography angiography. Med Image Anal. 2013;17(8):859–76.
16. Grand Challenges in Biomedical Imaging. 2016. Available from: https://grand-challenge.org/All_Challenges/.
17. Data Science Bowl. 2016. Available from: https://www.kaggle.com/c/second-annual-data-science-bowl.
18. Seidman AD, Pilewskie ML, Robson ME, Kelvin JF, Zauderer MG, Epstein AS, et al. Integration of multi-modality treatment planning for early stage breast cancer (BC) into Watson for Oncology, a Decision Support System: Seeing the forest and the trees. J Clin Oncol. 2015;33(15_suppl):e12042–e.
19. Johnson AE, Ghassemi MM, Nemati S, Niehaus KE, Clifton DA, Clifford GD. Machine learning and decision support in critical care. Proc IEEE. 2016;104(2):444–66.
20. Gultepe E, Green JP, Nguyen H, Adams J, Albertson T, Tagkopoulos I. From vital signs to clinical outcomes for patients with sepsis: a machine learning basis for a clinical decision support system. J Am Med Inform Assoc. 2014;21(2):315–25.
21. Gulshan V, Peng L, Coram M, Stumpe MC, Wu D, Narayanaswamy A, et al. Development and validation of a deep learning algorithm for detection of diabetic retinopathy in retinal fundus photographs. JAMA. 2016;316(22):2402–10.
22. Long E, Lin H, Liu Z, Wu X, Wang L, Jiang J, et al. An artificial intelligence platform for the multihospital collaborative management of congenital cataracts. Nat Biomed Eng. 2017;1:0024.
23. Esteva A, Kuprel B, Novoa RA, Ko J, Swetter SM, Blau HM, et al. Dermatologist-level classification of skin cancer with deep neural networks. Nature. 2017;542(7639):115–8.
24. Beck AH, Sangoi AR, Leung S, Marinelli RJ, Nielsen TO, van de Vijver MJ, et al. Systematic analysis of breast cancer morphology uncovers stromal features associated with survival. Sci Transl Med. 2011;3(108):108ra13.
25. Yu KH, Zhang C, Berry GJ, Altman RB, Re C, Rubin DL, et al. Predicting non-small cell lung cancer prognosis by fully automated microscopic pathology image features. Nat Commun. 2016;7:12474.
26. Precision Medicine Initiative. 2016. Available from: https://www.nih.gov/news-events/news-releases/nih-awards-55-million-build-million-person-precision-medicine-study https://www.nimhd.nih.gov/programs/collab/pmi/ https://syndication.nih.gov/multimedia/pmi/infographics/pmi-infographic.pdf.
27. Artificial Intelligence Used To Detect Rare Leukemia Type In Japan. 2016. Available from: http://www.ndtv.com/health/artificial-intelligence-used-to-detect-rare-leukemia-type-in-japan-1440789.
28. Sharpless N. As seen on 60 minutes: Watson accelerates precision oncology. 2016. Available from: https://www.ibm.com/blogs/think/2016/10/sharpless/.
29. McDonald JF, Mezencev R, Long TQ, Benigno B, Bonta I, Priore GD. Accurate prediction of optimal cancer drug therapies from molecular profiles by a machine-learning algorithm. J Clin Oncol. 2015;33(15_suppl):e22182–e.
30. Ramarajan N, Badwe RA, Perry P, Srivastava G, Nair NS, Gupta S. A machine learning approach to enable evidence based oncology practice: ranking grade and applicability of RCTs to individual patients. J Clin Oncol. 2016;34(15_suppl):e18165–e.
31. Sidaway P. Immunotherapy: genomic and immunological features predict a response. Nat Rev Clin Oncol. 2017;14(5):263.
32. Shah SJ, Katz DH, Selvaraj S, Burke MA, Yancy CW, Gheorghiade M, et al. Phenomapping for novel classification of heart failure with preserved ejection fraction. Circulation. 2015;131(3):269–79. https://doi.org/10.1161/CIRCULATIONAHA.114.010637.
33. Wang S, Summers RM. Machine learning and radiology. Med Image Anal. 2012;16(5):933–51.
34. Akkus Z, Galimzianova A, Hoogi A, Rubin DL, Erickson BJ. Deep learning for brain MRI segmentation: state of the art and future directions. J Digit Imaging. 2017;30:449.

35. Kamnitsas K, Ledig C, Newcombe VFJ, Simpson JP, Kane AD, Menon DK, et al. Efficient multi-scale 3D CNN with fully connected CRF for accurate brain lesion segmentation. Med Image Anal. 2017;36:61–78.
36. Havaei M, Davy A, Warde-Farley D, Biard A, Courville A, Bengio Y, et al. Brain tumor segmentation with deep neural networks. Med Image Anal. 2017;35:18–31.
37. van Ginneken B. Fifty years of computer analysis in chest imaging: rule-based, machine learning, deep learning. Radiol Phys Technol. 2017;10(1):23–32.
38. Doel T, Gavaghan DJ, Grau V. Review of automatic pulmonary lobe segmentation methods from CT. Comput Med Imaging Graph. 2015;40:13–29.
39. Mansoor A, Bagci U, Foster B, Xu Z, Papadakis GZ, Folio LR, et al. Segmentation and image analysis of abnormal lungs at CT: current approaches, challenges, and future trends. Radiographics. 2015;35(4):1056–76.
40. Ikushima K, Arimura H, Jin Z, Yabu-Uchi H, Kuwazuru J, Shioyama Y, et al. Computer-assisted framework for machine-learning-based delineation of GTV regions on datasets of planning CT and PET/CT images. J Radiat Res. 2017;58(1):123–34.
41. Ibragimov B, Xing L. Segmentation of organs-at-risks in head and neck CT images using convolutional neural networks. Med Phys. 2017;44(2):547–57.
42. Belharbi S, Chatelain C, Herault R, Adam S, Thureau S, Chastan M, et al. Spotting L3 slice in CT scans using deep convolutional network and transfer learning. Comput Biol Med. 2017;87:95–103.
43. Summers RM. Progress in fully automated abdominal CT interpretation. AJR Am J Roentgenol. 2016;207(1):67–79.
44. Roth HR, Lu L, Liu J, Yao J, Seff A, Cherry K, et al. Improving computer-aided detection using convolutional neural networks and random view aggregation. IEEE Trans Med Imaging. 2016;35(5):1170–81.
45. Näppi JJ, Hironaka T, Regge D, Yoshida H, editors. Deep transfer learning of virtual endoluminal views for the detection of polyps in CT colonography. San Diego: Proc SPIE; 2016.
46. Qi D, Hao C, Lequan Y, Lei Z, Jing Q, Defeng W, et al. Automatic detection of cerebral microbleeds from MR images via 3D convolutional neural networks. IEEE Trans Med Imaging. 2016;35(5):1182–95.
47. Anthimopoulos M, Christodoulidis S, Ebner L, Christe A, Mougiakakou S. Lung pattern classification for interstitial lung diseases using a deep convolutional neural network. IEEE Trans Med Imaging. 2016;35(5):1207–16.
48. Bergtholdt M, Wiemker R, Klinder T, editors. Pulmonary nodule detection using a cascaded SVM classifier. SPIE Medical Imaging; 2016. International Society for Optics and Photonics.
49. Setio AA, Ciompi F, Litjens G, Gerke P, Jacobs C, van Riel SJ, et al. Pulmonary nodule detection in CT images: false positive reduction using multi-view convolutional networks. IEEE Trans Med Imaging. 2016;35(5):1160–9.
50. Ciompi F, Chung K, Van Riel SJ, Setio AAA, Gerke PK, Jacobs C, et al. Towards automatic pulmonary nodule management in lung cancer screening with deep learning. Sci Rep. 2017;7:46479.
51. Rucco M, Sousa-Rodrigues D, Merelli E, Johnson JH, Falsetti L, Nitti C, et al. Neural hypernetwork approach for pulmonary embolism diagnosis. BMC Res Notes. 2015;8:617.
52. Rajkomar A, Lingam S, Taylor AG, Blum M, Mongan J. High-throughput classification of radiographs using deep convolutional neural networks. J Digit Imaging. 2017;30(1):95–101.
53. Rampun A, Tiddeman B, Zwiggelaar R, Malcolm P. Computer aided diagnosis of prostate cancer: a texton based approach. Med Phys. 2016;43(10):5412.
54. Dhungel N, Carneiro G, Bradley AP. A deep learning approach for the analysis of masses in mammograms with minimal user intervention. Med Image Anal. 2017;37:114–28.
55. Kooi T, Litjens G, van Ginneken B, Gubern-Mérida A, Sánchez CI, Mann R, et al. Large scale deep learning for computer aided detection of mammographic lesions. Med Image Anal. 2017;35:303–12.
56. Lassen B, van Rikxoort EM, Schmidt M, Kerkstra S, van Ginneken B, Kuhnigk J-M. Automatic segmentation of the pulmonary lobes from chest CT scans based on fissures, vessels, and bronchi. IEEE Trans Med Imaging. 2013;32(2):210–22.
57. Wang J, Yang X, Cai H, Tan W, Jin C, Li L. Discrimination of breast cancer with microcalcifications on mammography by deep learning. Sci Rep. 2016;6:27327.
58. Dilsizian SE, Siegel EL. Artificial intelligence in medicine and cardiac imaging: harnessing big data and advanced computing to provide personalized medical diagnosis and treatment. Curr Cardiol Rep. 2013;16(1):441.
59. Krittanawong C, Zhang H, Wang Z, Aydar M, Kitai T. Artificial intelligence in precision cardiovascular medicine. J Am Coll Cardiol. 2017;69(21):2657–64.
60. Slomka PJ, Dey D, Sitek A, Motwani M, Berman DS, Germano G. Cardiac imaging: working towards fully-automated machine analysis & interpretation. Expert Rev Med Devices. 2017;14(3):197–212.
61. Douglas PS, Cerqueira MD, Berman DS, Chinnaiyan K, Cohen MS, Lundbye JB, et al. The future of cardiac imaging: report of a think tank convened by the American College of Cardiology. JACC Cardiovasc Imaging. 2016;9(10):1211–23.
62. Nagueh SF. Unleashing the potential of machine-based learning for the diagnosis of cardiac diseases. Am Heart Assoc; 2016; 9(6).
63. Tesche C, De Cecco CN, Albrecht MH, Duguay TM, Bayer RR 2nd, Litwin SE, et al. Coronary CT angiography-derived fractional flow reserve. Radiology. 2017;285(1):17–33.
64. Avendi MR, Kheradvar A, Jafarkhani H. A combined deep-learning and deformable-model approach to fully automatic segmentation of the left ventricle in cardiac MRI. Med Image Anal. 2016;30:108–19.
65. Germano G, Kavanagh PB, Slomka PJ, Van Kriekinge SD, Pollard G, Berman DS. Quantitation in gated perfusion SPECT imaging: the Cedars-Sinai approach. J Nucl Cardiol. 2007;14(4):433–54.
66. Garcia EV, Faber TL, Cooke CD, Folks RD, Chen J, Santana C. The increasing role of quantification in clinical nuclear cardiology: the Emory approach. J Nucl Cardiol. 2007;14(4):420–32.
67. Arsanjani R, Xu Y, Hayes SW, Fish M, Lemley M, Gerlach J, et al. Comparison of fully automated computer analysis and visual scoring for detection of coronary artery disease from myocardial perfusion SPECT in a large population. J Nucl Med. 2013;54(2):221–8.
68. Betancur J, Rubeaux M, Fuchs T, Otaki Y, Arnson Y, Slipczuk L, et al. Automatic valve plane localization in myocardial perfusion SPECT/CT by machine learning: anatomical and clinical validation. J Nucl Med. 2017;58(6):961–7.
69. Arnoldi E, Gebregziabher M, Schoepf UJ, Goldenberg R, Ramos-Duran L, Zwerner PL, et al. Automated computer-aided stenosis detection at coronary CT angiography: initial experience. Eur Radiol. 2010;20(5):1160–7.
70. Halpern EJ, Halpern DJ. Diagnosis of coronary stenosis with CT angiography: comparison of automated computer diagnosis with expert readings. Acad Radiol. 2011;18(3):324–33.
71. Goldenberg R, Eilot D, Begelman G, Walach E, Ben-Ishai E, Peled N. Computer-aided simple triage (CAST) for coronary CT angiography (CCTA). Int J Comput Assist Radiol Surg. 2012;7(6):819–27.
72. Kang K-W, Chang H-J, Shim H, Kim Y-J, Choi B-W, Yang W-I, et al. Feasibility of an automatic computer-assisted algorithm for the detection of significant coronary artery disease in patients presenting with acute chest pain. Eur J Radiol. 2012;81(4):e640–e6.
73. Kang D, Slomka P, Nakazato R, Cheng VY, Min JK, Li D, et al., editors. Automatic detection of significant and subtle arterial lesions from coronary CT angiography. SPIE Medical Imaging; 2012. International Society for Optics and Photonics.

74. Kang D, Dey D, Slomka PJ, Arsanjani R, Nakazato R, Ko H, et al. Structured learning algorithm for detection of nonobstructive and obstructive coronary plaque lesions from computed tomography angiography. J Med Imaging (Bellingham, Wash). 2015;2(1):014003.
75. Agatston AS, Janowitz WR, Hildner FJ, Zusmer NR, Viamonte M Jr, Detrano R. Quantification of coronary artery calcium using ultrafast computed tomography. J Am Coll Cardiol. 1990;15(4):827–32.
76. Kondos GT, Hoff JA, Sevrukov A, Daviglus ML, Garside DB, Devries SS, et al. Electron-beam tomography coronary artery calcium and cardiac events: a 37-month follow-up of 5635 initially asymptomatic low- to intermediate-risk adults. Circulation. 2003;107(20):2571–6.
77. Wolterink JM, Leiner T, de Vos BD, van Hamersvelt RW, Viergever MA, Išgum I. Automatic coronary artery calcium scoring in cardiac CT angiography using paired convolutional neural networks. Med Image Anal. 2016;34:123–36.
78. Sengupta PP, Huang YM, Bansal M, Ashrafi A, Fisher M, Shameer K, et al. Cognitive machine-learning algorithm for cardiac imaging: a pilot study for differentiating constrictive pericarditis from restrictive cardiomyopathy. Circ Cardiovasc Imaging. 2016;9(6):e004330.
79. Mahmood SS, Levy D, Vasan RS, Wang TJ. The Framingham Heart Study and the epidemiology of cardiovascular disease: a historical perspective. Lancet. 2014;383(9921):999–1008.
80. Budoff MJ, Dowe D, Jollis JG, Gitter M, Sutherland J, Halamert E, et al. Diagnostic performance of 64-multidetector row coronary computed tomographic angiography for evaluation of coronary artery stenosis in individuals without known coronary artery disease: results from the prospective multicenter ACCURACY (Assessment by Coronary Computed Tomographic Angiography of Individuals Undergoing Invasive Coronary Angiography) trial. J Am Coll Cardiol. 2008;52(21):1724–32.
81. Chow BJ, Small G, Yam Y, Chen L, Achenbach S, Al-Mallah M, et al. Incremental prognostic value of cardiac computed tomography in coronary artery disease using CONFIRMClinical perspective. Circ Cardiovasc Imaging. 2011;4(5):463–72.
82. Hadamitzky M, Freißmuth B, Meyer T, Hein F, Kastrati A, Martinoff S, et al. Prognostic value of coronary computed tomographic angiography for prediction of cardiac events in patients with suspected coronary artery disease. JACC Cardiovasc Imaging. 2009;2(4):404–11.
83. Hadamitzky M, Taubert S, Deseive S, Byrne RA, Martinoff S, Schomig A, et al. Prognostic value of coronary computed tomography angiography during 5 years of follow-up in patients with suspected coronary artery disease. Eur Heart J. 2013;34(42):3277–85.
84. Dawes TJ, de Marvao A, Shi W, Fletcher T, Watson GM, Wharton J, et al. Machine learning of three-dimensional right ventricular motion enables outcome prediction in pulmonary hypertension: a cardiac MR imaging study. Radiology. 2017;283(2):381–90.
85. Kotu LP, Engan K, Borhani R, Katsaggelos AK, Orn S, Woie L, et al. Cardiac magnetic resonance image-based classification of the risk of arrhythmias in post-myocardial infarction patients. Artif Intell Med. 2015;64(3):205–15.
86. Arsanjani R, Dey D, Khachatryan T, Shalev A, Hayes SW, Fish M, et al. Prediction of revascularization after myocardial perfusion SPECT by machine learning in a large population. J Nucl Cardiol. 2015;22(5):877–84.
87. Jha S, Topol EJ. Adapting to artificial intelligence: radiologists and pathologists as information specialists. JAMA. 2016;316(22):2353–4.
88. Chinthapalli K. The hackers holding hospitals to ransom. BMJ. 2017;357:j 2214.
89. Moss TJ, Calland JF, Enfield KB, Gomez-Manjarres DC, Ruminski C, DiMarco JP, et al. New-onset atrial fibrillation in the critically ill. Crit Care Med. 2017;45(5):790.
90. Chockley K, Emanuel E. The end of radiology? three threats to the future practice of radiology. J Am Coll Radiol. 2016;13(12):1415–20.
91. Obermeyer Z, Emanuel EJ. Predicting the future – big data, machine learning, and clinical medicine. N Engl J Med. 2016;375(13):1216–9.

Correction to: CT of the Heart

Correction to: U. J. Schoepf (ed.), CT of the Heart, Contemporary Medical Imaging, https://doi.org/10.1007/978-1-60327-237-7

This book was inadvertently published with the below error:

- The name of Dr. Pooyan Sahbaee had been missed out in the list of contributors; hence, we have now included his name in the contributors section of the front matter.

The updated online version of this book can be found at https://doi.org/10.1007/978-1-60327-237-7

U. J. Schoepf (ed.), *CT of the Heart*, Contemporary Medical Imaging, https://doi.org/10.1007/978-1-60327-237-7_69

Index

U. J. Schoepf (ed.), *CT of the Heart*, Contemporary Medical Imaging, https://doi.org/10.1007/978-1-60327-237-7

D

G

H

U

V

MIX
Papier aus verantwortungsvollen Quellen
Paper from responsible sources
FSC® C105338

If you have any concerns about our products,
you can contact us on
ProductSafety@springernature.com

In case Publisher is established outside the EU,
the EU authorized representative is:
Springer Nature Customer Service Center GmbH
Europaplatz 3, 69115 Heidelberg, Germany

Printed by Libri Plureos GmbH
in Hamburg, Germany